Wilson and Gisvold's
Textbook of

ORGANIC MEDICINAL AND PHARMACEUTICAL CHEMISTRY

T W E L F T H E D I T I O N

Edited by

John M. Beale, Jr., PhD
Associate Professor of Medicinal Chemistry
Division of Basic and Pharmaceutical Sciences
St. Louis College of Pharmacy
Saint Louis, Missouri

●

John H. Block, PhD, RPh
Professor Emeritus, Medicinal Chemistry
Department of Pharmaceutical Sciences
College of Pharmacy
Oregon State University
Corvallis, Oregon

● Wolters Kluwer | Lippincott Williams & Wilkins
Health

Philadelphia · Baltimore · New York · London
Buenos Aires · Hong Kong · Sydney · Tokyo

Editor: David B. Troy
Product Manager: Meredith L. Brittain
Vendor Manager: Kevin Johnson
Designer: Holly McLaughlin
Compositor: Absolute Service, Inc./Maryland Composition

12th Edition

Copyright © 2011 by Lippincott Williams & Wilkins, a Wolters Kluwer business.

First Edition, 1949	Fifth Edition, 1966	Ninth Edition, 1991
Second Edition, 1954	Sixth Edition, 1971	Tenth Edition, 1998
Third Edition, 1956	Seventh Edition, 1977	Eleventh Edition, 2004
Fourth Edition, 1962	Eighth Edition, 1982	

351 West Camden Street   530 Walnut Street
Baltimore, MD 21201   Philadelphia, PA 19106

Printed in The People's Republic of China

9 8 7 6 5 4 3 2 1

Library of Congress Cataloging-in-Publication Data

Wilson and Gisvold's textbook of organic medicinal and pharmaceutical chemistry. — 12th ed. / edited by John M. Beale, Jr., John H. Block.
    p. ; cm.
Includes bibliographical references and index.
ISBN 978-0-7817-7929-6
1. Pharmaceutical chemistry. 2. Chemistry, Organic. I. Wilson, Charles Owens, 1911- II. Beale, John Marlowe. III. Block, John H. IV. Title: Textbook of organic medicinal and pharmaceutical chemistry.
[DNLM: 1. Chemistry, Pharmaceutical. 2. Chemistry, Organic. QV 744 W754 2011]
RS403.T43 2011
615'.19—dc22

2009043714

DISCLAIMER

Care has been taken to confirm the accuracy of the information present and to describe generally accepted practices. However, the authors, editors, and publisher are not responsible for errors or omissions or for any consequences from application of the information in this book and make no warranty, expressed or implied, with respect to the currency, completeness, or accuracy of the contents of the publication. Application of this information in a particular situation remains the professional responsibility of the practitioner; the clinical treatments described and recommended may not be considered absolute and universal recommendations.

The authors, editors, and publisher have exerted every effort to ensure that drug selection and dosage set forth in this text are in accordance with the current recommendations and practice at the time of publication. However, in view of ongoing research, changes in government regulations, and the constant flow of information relating to drug therapy and drug reactions, the reader is urged to check the package insert for each drug for any change in indications and dosage and for added warnings and precautions. This is particularly important when the recommended agent is a new or infrequently employed drug.

Some drugs and medical devices presented in this publication have Food and Drug Administration (FDA) clearance for limited use in restricted research settings. It is the responsibility of the healthcare provider to ascertain the FDA status of each drug or device planned for use in their clinical practice.

To purchase additional copies of this book, call our customer service department at **(800) 638-3030** or fax orders to **(301) 223-2320**. International customers should call **(301) 223-2300**.

Visit Lippincott Williams & Wilkins on the Internet: http://www.lww.com. Lippincott Williams & Wilkins customer service representatives are available from 8:30 am to 6:00 pm, EST.

The 12th Edition of Wilson and Gisvold's Textbook of Organic Medicinal and Pharmaceutical Chemistry *is dedicated to the memory of Robert F. Doerge.*

Robert F. Doerge
1915–2006

Robert Doerge—pharmacist, medicinal chemist, and educator—experienced the Depression and served in the Civilian Conservation Corp in Sheridan, AR. Dr. Doerge received his B.S. in pharmacy in 1943 and his PhD in pharmaceutical chemistry, both from the University of Minnesota in 1949. The latter was under the direction of Dr. Charles O. Wilson, who, with Dr. Ole Gisvold, started this well-respected medicinal chemistry textbook. Dr. Doerge began his professional career as an assistant professor in the University of Texas-Austin School of Pharmacy before becoming a research chemist with the former Smith Kline and French Laboratories in Philadelphia. Beginning in 1960, he returned to academia as professor and chair of the pharmaceutical chemistry department in Oregon State University's College of Pharmacy. Prior to his retirement as professor emeritus in 1981, he was the assistant dean.

Dr. Doerge's initial publications were on the topic of synthesis of anticonvulsants. At Smith Kline and French, his work included publications on vitamin stability, and at Oregon State University, his papers focused on the heterocyclic phenylindolizines. Dr. Doerge was a volunteer abstractor for *Chemical Abstracts*. As an educator, Dr. Doerge was an author of chapters in *Wilson and Gisvold's Textbook of Organic Medicinal and Pharmaceutical Chemistry*, coeditor of the 6th and 7th editions, and editor of the 8th edition. His skill and dedication in the classroom were recognized by the students and university with several teaching awards.

We certainly miss this fine gentleman who put the students first and advanced the teaching of medicinal chemistry as a chapter author, coeditor, and editor of the Wilson and Gisvold textbook series.

John H. Block

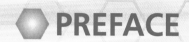

PREFACE

For 6 decades, *Wilson and Gisvold's Textbook of Organic Medicinal and Pharmaceutical Chemistry* has been a standard in the literature of medicinal chemistry. Generations of students and faculty have depended on this textbook not only for undergraduate courses in medicinal chemistry but also as a supplement for graduate studies. Moreover, students in other health sciences have found certain chapters useful. The current editors and authors worked on the 12th edition with the objective of continuing the tradition of a modern textbook for undergraduate students and also for graduate students who need a general review of medicinal chemistry. Because the chapters include a blend of chemical and pharmacological principles necessary for understanding structure–activity relationships and molecular mechanisms of drug action, the book should be useful in supporting courses in medicinal chemistry and in complementing pharmacology courses.

ABOUT THE 12TH EDITION

The 12th edition follows in the footsteps of the 11th edition by reflecting the dynamic changes occurring in medicinal chemistry. With increased knowledge of the disease process and the identification of the key steps in the biochemical process, the chapters have been updated, expanded, and reorganized. At the same time, to streamline the presentation of the content, some topics were combined into existing chapters. For example, Chapter 2, "Drug Design Strategies," incorporates material from 11th edition Chapters 2, 3, and 28, and Chapter 3, "Metabolic Changes of Drugs and Related Organic Compounds," includes the content from 11th edition Chapter 5, "Prodrugs and Drug Latentiation." In addition, with the newer drugs that have entered the pharmaceutical armamentarium since publication of the 11th edition, coverage of the following topics has been expanded in the 12th edition: Central Dopaminergic Signaling Agents (Chapter 13), Anticonvulsants (Chapter 14), Hormone-Related Disorders: Nonsteroidal Therapies (Chapter 20), Agents Treating Bone Disorders (Chapter 21), and Anesthetics (Chapter 22).

New features of the 12th edition include a chapter overview at the beginning of each chapter to introduce material to be covered in the chapter and review questions at the end of each chapter to reinforce concepts learned in the chapter (answers to these questions are available to students on the book's companion Web site; see next section).

ADDITIONAL RESOURCES

Wilson and Gisvold's Textbook of Organic Medicinal and Pharmaceutical Chemistry, 12th Edition, includes additional resources for both instructors and students that are available on the book's companion Web site at http://www.thePoint.lww.com/Beale12e.

Instructors

Approved adopting instructors will be given access to the following additional resources:

• Image bank of all the figures and tables in the book

Students

Students who have purchased *Wilson and Gisvold's Textbook of Organic Medicinal and Pharmaceutical Chemistry*, 12th Edition, have access to the following additional resources:

• The answers to the review questions found in the book

In addition, purchasers of the text can access the searchable Full Text On-line by going to the *Wilson and Gisvold's Textbook of Organic Medicinal and Pharmaceutical Chemistry*, 12th Edition, Web site at http://www.thePoint.lww.com/Beale12e. See the inside front cover of this text for more details, including the passcode you will need to gain access to the Web site.

⬡ ACKNOWLEDGMENTS

The editors welcome the new contributors to the 12th edition: Jeffrey J. Christoff, A. Michael Crider, Carolyn J. Friel, Ronald A. Hill, Shengquan Liu, Matthias C. Lu, Marcello J. Nieto, and Kenneth A. Witt. The editors extend thanks to all of the authors who have cooperated in the preparation of the current edition. Collectively, the authors represent many years of teaching and research experience in medicinal chemistry. Their chapters include summaries of current research trends that lead the reader to the original literature. Documentation and references continue to be an important feature of the book.

We continue to be indebted to Professors Charles O. Wilson and Ole Gisvold, the originators of the book and editors of five editions, Professor Robert Doerge, who joined Professors Wilson and Gisvold for the 6th and 7th editions and single-handedly edited the 8th edition, and Professors Jaime Delgado and William Remers, who edited the 9th and 10th editions. They and the authors have contributed significantly to the education of countless pharmacists, medicinal chemists, and other pharmaceutical scientists.

John M. Beale, Jr.
John H. Block

1st	1949	Wilson and Gisvold (*Organic Chemistry in Pharmacy*)	6th	1971	Wilson, Gisvold, and Doerge
			7th	1977	Wilson, Gisvold, and Doerge
2nd	1954	Wilson and Gisvold	8th	1982	Doerge
3rd	1956	Wilson	9th	1991	Delgado and Remers
4th	1962	Wilson and Gisvold	10th	1998	Delgado and Remers
5th	1966	Wilson	11th	2004	Block and Beale

CONTRIBUTORS

John M. Beale, Jr., PhD
Associate Professor of Medicinal
 Chemistry
Division of Basic and Pharmaceutical
 Sciences
St. Louis College of Pharmacy
Saint Louis, Missouri

John H. Block, PhD, RPh
Professor Emeritus, Medicinal
 Chemistry
Department of Pharmaceutical
 Sciences
College of Pharmacy
Oregon State University
Corvallis, Oregon

**Jeffrey J. Christoff,
 PhD, RPh**
Professor
Department of Pharmaceutical
 and Biomedical Sciences
College of Pharmacy, Ohio Northern
 University
Ada, Ohio

C. Randall Clark, PhD
Professor
Department of Pharmaceutical
 Sciences
Auburn University School of
 Pharmacy
Auburn, Alabama

A. Michael Crider, PhD
Chair and Professor
Department of Pharmaceutical
 Sciences
Southern Illinois University
 Edwardsville
Edwardsville, Illinois

Horace G. Cutler, PhD
Senior Research Professor
College of Pharmacy and Health
 Sciences
Mercer University
Atlanta, Georgia

Stephen J. Cutler
Chair and Professor
Department of Medicinal Chemistry
University of Mississippi
Oxford, Mississippi

**Michael J. Deimling,
 RPh, PhD**
Department of Pharmaceutical
 Sciences
School of Pharmacy
Georgia Campus—Philadelphia
 College of Osteopathic Medicine
Suwanee, Georgia

Jack DeRuiter, MS, PhD
Professor
Department of Pharmaceutical
 Sciences
Auburn University School of
 Pharmacy
Auburn, Alabama

**Carolyn J. Friel,
 RPh, PhD**
Associate Professor of Medicinal
 Chemistry
Department of Pharmaceutical
 Sciences
Massachusetts College of Pharmacy
 and Health Sciences—Worcester
Worcester, Massachusetts

Ronald A. Hill, PhD
Associate Professor
Department of Basic Pharmaceutical
 Sciences
The University of Louisiana at
 Monroe
Monroe, Louisiana

**Thomas J. Holmes, Jr.,
 PhD**
Professor
Department of Pharmaceutical
 Sciences
Campbell University College of
 Pharmacy and the Health Sciences
Buies Creek, New Carolina

**M. O. Faruk Khan,
 BPharm, MPharm, PhD**
Assistant Professor of Medicinal
 Chemistry
Department of Pharmaceutical
 Sciences
Southwestern Oklahoma State
 University College of Pharmacy
Weatherford, Oklahoma

Matthias C. Lu, PhD
Professor and Assistant Head for
 Curricular Affairs
Department of Medicinal Chemistry
 and Pharmacognosy
College of Pharmacy, University of
 Illinois at Chicago
Chicago, Illinois

Shengquan Liu, PhD
Assistant Professor
Department of Medicinal Chemistry
Touro University—California
Vallejo, California

Marcello J. Nieto, PhD
Assistant Professor
Department of Pharmaceutical
 Sciences
Southern Illinois University
Edwardsville, Illinois

**Gustavo R. Ortega,
 RPh, PhD**
Professor Emeritus
Department of Pharmaceutical
 Sciences
Southwestern Oklahoma State
 University College of Pharmacy
Weatherford, Oklahoma

Philip J. Proteau, PhD
Associate Professor of Medicinal
 Chemistry
Department of Pharmaceutical
 Sciences
Oregon State University College of
 Pharmacy
Corvallis, Oregon

Forrest T. Smith, PhD
Associate Professor
Department of Pharmaceutical
 Sciences
Auburn University School of
 Pharmacy
Auburn, Alabama

Kenneth A. Witt, PhD
Assistant Professor
Department of Pharmaceutical
 Sciences
Southern Illinois University
 Edwardsville
Edwardsville, Illinois

CONTENTS

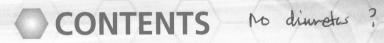 *no diuretics ?*

CHAPTER 1

Introduction

JOHN M. BEALE, JR. AND JOHN H. BLOCK

The discipline of medicinal chemistry is devoted to the discovery and development of new agents for treating diseases. Most of this activity is directed to new natural or synthetic organic compounds. Paralleling the development of medicinal agents has come a better understanding of the chemistry of the receptor. The latter has been greatly facilitated by low-cost computers running software that calculates molecular properties and structure and pictures it using high-resolution graphics. Development of organic compounds has grown beyond traditional synthetic methods. It now includes the exciting field of biotechnology using the cell's biochemistry to synthesize new compounds. Techniques ranging from recombinant DNA and site-directed mutagenesis to fusion of cell lines have greatly broadened the possibilities for new entities that treat disease. The pharmacist now dispenses modified human insulins that provide more convenient dosing schedules, cell-stimulating factors that have changed the dosing regimens for chemotherapy, humanized monoclonal antibodies that target specific tissues, and fused receptors that intercept immune cell–generated cytokines.

This 12th edition of *Wilson and Gisvold's Textbook of Organic Medicinal and Pharmaceutical Chemistry* continues the philosophy of presenting the scientific basis of medicinal chemistry originally established by Professors Charles Wilson and Ole Gisvold, describing the many aspects of organic medicinals: how they are discovered, how they act, and how they developed into clinical agents. The process of establishing a new pharmaceutical is exceedingly complex and involves the talents of people from various disciplines, including chemistry, biochemistry, molecular biology, physiology, pharmacology, pharmaceutics, and medicine. Medicinal chemistry, itself, is concerned mainly with the organic, analytical, and biochemical aspects of this process, but the chemist must interact productively with those in other disciplines. Thus, medicinal chemistry occupies a strategic position at the interface of chemistry and biology. All of the principles discussed in this book are based on fundamental organic chemistry, physical chemistry, and biochemistry. To provide an understanding of the principles of medicinal chemistry, it is necessary to consider the physicochemical properties used to develop new pharmacologically active compounds and their mechanisms of action, the drug's metabolism, including possible biological activities of the metabolites, the importance of stereochemistry in drug design, and the methods used to determine what "space" a drug occupies.

The earliest drug discoveries were made by random sampling of higher plants. Some of this sampling, although based on anecdotal evidence, led to the use of such crude plant drugs as opium, belladonna, and ephedrine that have been important for centuries. With the accidental discovery of penicillin came the screening of microorganisms and the large number of antibiotics from bacterial and fungal sources. Many of these antibiotics provided the prototypical structure that the medicinal chemist modified to obtain antibacterial drugs with better therapeutic profiles. With the changes in federal legislation reducing the efficacy requirement for "nutriceutical," the public increasingly is using so-called nontraditional or alternative medicinals that are sold over the counter, many outside of traditional pharmacy distribution channels. It is important for the pharmacist and the public to understand the rigor that is required for prescription-only and Food and Drug Administration (FDA)-approved nonprescription products to be approved relative to the nontraditional products. It is also important for all people in the healthcare field and the public to realize that whether these nontraditional products are effective as claimed or not, many of the alternate medicines contain pharmacologically active agents that can potentiate or interfere with physician-prescribed therapy.

Hundreds of thousands of new organic chemicals are prepared annually throughout the world, and many of them are entered into pharmacological screens to determine whether they have useful biological activity. This process of random screening has been considered inefficient, but it has resulted in the identification of new lead compounds whose structures have been optimized to produce clinical agents. Sometimes, a lead develops by careful observation of the pharmacological behavior of an existing drug. The discovery that amantadine protects and treats early influenza A came from a general screen for antiviral agents. The use of amantadine in long-term care facilities showed that it also could be used to treat parkinsonian disorders. More recently, automated high-throughput screening systems utilizing cell culture systems with linked enzyme assays and receptor molecules derived from gene cloning have greatly increased the efficiency of random screening. It is now practical to screen enormous libraries of peptides and nucleic acids obtained from combinatorial chemistry procedures.

Rational design, the opposite approach to high-volume screening, is also flourishing. Statistical methods based on the correlation of physicochemical properties with biological potency are used to explain and optimize biological activity. Significant advances in x-ray crystallography and nuclear magnetic resonance have made it possible to obtain detailed representations of enzymes and other drug receptors. The techniques of molecular graphics and computational chemistry have provided novel chemical structures that have led to new drugs with potent medicinal activities. Development of human immunodeficiency virus (HIV) protease inhibitors and angiotensin-converting enzyme (ACE) inhibitors came from an understanding of the geometry and chemical character of the respective enzyme's active site. Even if the receptor structure is not known in detail, rational approaches based on the physicochemical properties of lead compounds can provide new drugs. For example, the development of cimetidine involved a careful study of the changes in antagonism of H_2-histamine receptors induced by varying the physical properties of structures based on histamine.

As you proceed through the chapters, think of what problem the medicinal chemist is trying to solve. Why were certain structures selected? What modifications were made to produce more focused activity or reduce adverse reactions or produce better pharmaceutical properties? Was the prototypical molecule discovered from random screens, or did the medicinal chemist have a structural concept of the receptor or an understanding of the disease process that must be interrupted?

CHAPTER 2

Drug Design Strategies

JOHN H. BLOCK

CHAPTER OVERVIEW

Modern drug design as compared with the classical approach—*let's make a change on an existing compound or synthesize a new structure and see what happens*—continues to evolve rapidly as an approach to solving a drug design problem. The combination of increasing power and decreasing cost of desktop computing has had a major impact on solving drug design problems. Although drug design increasingly is based on modern computational chemical techniques, it also uses sophisticated knowledge of disease mechanisms and receptor properties. A good understanding of how the drug is transported into the body, distributed throughout the body compartments, metabolically altered by the liver and other organs, and excreted from the patient is required, along with the structural characteristics of the receptor. Acid–base chemistry is used to aid in formulation and biodistribution. Structural attributes and substituent patterns responsible for optimum pharmacological activity can often be predicted by statistical techniques such as regression analysis. Computerized conformational analysis permits the medicinal chemist to predict the drug's three-dimensional (3D) shape that is *seen* by the receptor. With the isolation and structural determination of specific receptors and the availability of computer software that can estimate the 3D shape of the receptor, it is possible to design molecules that will show an optimum fit to the receptor.

⬡ DRUG DISTRIBUTION

A drug is a chemical molecule. Following introduction into the body, a drug must pass through many barriers, survive alternate sites of attachment and storage, and avoid significant metabolic destruction before it reaches the site of action, usually a receptor on or in a cell (Fig. 2.1). At the receptor, the following equilibrium (Rx. 2.1) usually holds:

$$\text{Drug} + \text{Receptor} \rightleftharpoons \text{Drug-Receptor Complex}$$
$$\downarrow$$
$$\text{Pharmacologic Response}$$

$$(\text{Rx. 2.1})$$

The ideal drug molecule will show favorable binding characteristics to the receptor, and the equilibrium will lie to the right. At the same time, the drug will be expected to dissociate from the receptor and reenter the systemic circulation to be excreted. Major exceptions include the alkylating agents used in cancer chemotherapy (see Chapter 10), a few inhibitors of the enzyme acetylcholinesterase (see Chapter 17), suicide inhibitors of monoamine oxidase (see Chapter 16), and the aromatase inhibitors 4-hydroxyandrostenedione and exemestane (see Chapter 25). These pharmacological agents form covalent bonds with the receptor, usually an enzyme's active site. In these cases, the cell must destroy the receptor or enzyme, or, in the case of the alkylating agents, the cell would be replaced, ideally with a normal cell. In other words, the usual use of drugs in medical treatment calls for the drug's effect to last for a finite period of time. Then, if it is to be repeated, the drug will be administered again. If the patient does not tolerate the drug well, it is even more important that the agent dissociate from the receptor and be excreted from the body.

Oral Administration

An examination of the *obstacle course* (Fig. 2.1) faced by the drug will give a better understanding of what is involved in developing a commercially feasible product. Assume that the drug is administered orally. The drug must go into solution to pass through the gastrointestinal mucosa. Even drugs administered as true solutions may not remain in solution as they enter the acidic stomach and then pass into the alkaline intestinal tract. (This is explained further in the discussion on acid–base chemistry.) The ability of the drug to dissolve is governed by several factors, including its chemical structure, variation in particle size and particle surface area, nature of the crystal form, type of tablet coating, and type of tablet matrix. By varying the dosage form and physical characteristics of the drug, it is possible to have a drug dissolve quickly or slowly, with the latter being the situation for many of the sustained-action products. An example is orally administered sodium phenytoin, with which variation of both the crystal form and tablet adjuvants can significantly alter the bioavailability of this drug widely used in the treatment of epilepsy.

Chemical modification is also used to a limited extent to facilitate a drug reaching its desired target (see Chapter 3). An example is olsalazine, used in the treatment of ulcerative colitis. This drug is a dimer of the pharmacologically active mesalamine (5-aminosalicylic acid). The latter is not effective orally because it is metabolized to inactive forms before reaching the colon. The dimeric form passes

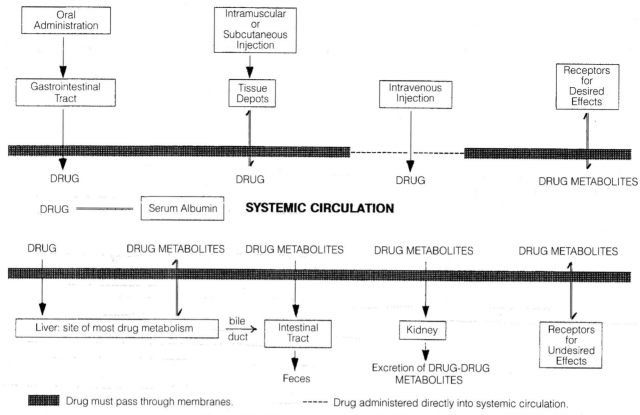

Figure 2.1 ● Summary of drug distribution.

through a significant portion of the intestinal tract before being cleaved by the intestinal bacteria to two equivalents of mesalamine.

Olsalazine

Mesalamine

As illustrated by olsalazine, any compound passing through the gastrointestinal tract will encounter a large number and variety of digestive and bacterial enzymes, which, in theory, can degrade the drug molecule. In practice, a new drug entity under investigation will likely be dropped from further consideration if it cannot survive in the intestinal tract or its oral bioavailability is low, necessitating parenteral dosage forms only. An exception would be a drug for which there is no effective alternative or which is more effective than existing products and can be administered by an alternate route, including parenteral, buccal, or transdermal.

In contrast, these same digestive enzymes can be used to advantage. Chloramphenicol is water soluble enough

(2.5 mg/mL) to come in contact with the taste receptors on the tongue, producing an unpalatable bitterness. To mask this intense bitter taste, the palmitic acid moiety is added as an ester of chloramphenicol's primary alcohol. This reduces the parent drug's water solubility (1.05 mg/mL), enough so that it can be formulated as a suspension that passes over the bitter taste receptors on the tongue. Once in the intestinal tract, the ester linkage is hydrolyzed by the digestive esterases to the active antibiotic chloramphenicol and the very common dietary fatty acid palmitic acid.

Chloramphenicol: R = H
Chloramphenicol Palmitate: R = CO(CH_2)_{14}CH_3

Olsalazine and chloramphenicol palmitate are examples of *prodrugs*. Most prodrugs are compounds that are inactive in their native form but are easily metabolized to the active agent. Olsalazine and chloramphenicol palmitate are examples of prodrugs that are cleaved to smaller compounds, one of which is the active drug. Others are metabolic precursors to the active form. An example of this type of prodrug is menadione, a simple naphthoquinone that is converted in the liver to phytonadione (vitamin K_{2(20)}).

Menadione

↓

Phytonadione (Vitamin $K_{2(20)}$)

Occasionally, the prodrug approach is used to enhance the absorption of a drug that is poorly absorbed from the gastrointestinal tract. Enalapril is the ethyl ester of enaprilic acid, an active inhibitor of angiotensin-converting enzyme (ACE). The ester prodrug is much more readily absorbed orally than the pharmacologically active carboxylic acid.

Enalapril: R = C_2H_5
Enaprilic Acid: R = H

Unless the drug is intended to act locally in the gastrointestinal tract, it will have to pass through the gastrointestinal mucosal barrier into venous circulation to reach the site of the receptor. The drug's route involves distribution or partitioning between the aqueous environment of the gastrointestinal tract, the lipid bilayer cell membrane of the mucosal cells, possibly the aqueous interior of the mucosal cells, the lipid bilayer membranes on the venous side of the gastrointestinal tract, and the aqueous environment of venous circulation. Some very lipid-soluble drugs may follow the route of dietary lipids by becoming part of the mixed micelles, incorporating into the chylomicrons in the mucosal cells into the lymph ducts, servicing the intestines, and finally entering venous circulation via the thoracic duct.

The drug's passage through the mucosal cells can be passive or active. As is discussed later in this chapter, the lipid membranes are very complex with a highly ordered structure. Part of this membrane is a series of channels or tunnels that form, disappear, and reform. There are receptors that move compounds into the cell by a process called *pinocytosis*. Drugs that resemble a normal metabolic precursor or intermediate may be actively transported into the cell by the same system that transports the endogenous compound. On the other hand, most drug

molecules are too large to enter the cell by an active transport mechanism through the passages. The latter, many times, pass into the patient's circulatory system by passive diffusion.

Parenteral Administration

Many times, there will be therapeutic advantages in bypassing the intestinal barrier by using parenteral (injectable) dosage forms. This is common in patients who, because of illness, cannot tolerate or are incapable of accepting drugs orally. Some drugs are so rapidly and completely metabolized to inactive products in the liver (first-pass effect) that oral administration is precluded. But that does not mean that the drug administered by injection is not confronted by obstacles (Fig. 2.1). Intravenous administration places the drug directly into the circulatory system, where it will be rapidly distributed throughout the body, including tissue depots and the liver, where most biotransformations occur (see later in this chapter), in addition to the receptors. Subcutaneous and intramuscular injections slow distribution of the drug, because it must diffuse from the site of injection into systemic circulation.

It is possible to inject the drug directly into specific organs or areas of the body. Intraspinal and intracerebral routes will place the drug directly into the spinal fluid or brain, respectively. This bypasses a specialized epithelial tissue, the blood-brain barrier, which protects the brain from exposure to a large number of metabolites and chemicals. The blood-brain barrier is composed of membranes of tightly joined epithelial cells lining the cerebral capillaries. The net result is that the brain is not exposed to the same variety of compounds that other organs are. Local anesthetics are examples of administration of a drug directly onto the desired nerve. A spinal block is a form of anesthesia performed by injecting a local anesthetic directly into the spinal cord at a specific location to block transmission along specific neurons.

Most of the injections a patient will experience in a lifetime will be subcutaneous or intramuscular. These parenteral routes produce a depot in the tissues (Fig. 2.1), from which the drug must reach the blood or lymph. Once in systemic circulation, the drug will undergo the same distributive phenomena as orally and intravenously administered agents before reaching the target receptor. In general, the same factors that control the drug's passage through the gastrointestinal mucosa will also determine the rate of movement out of the tissue depot.

The prodrug approach described previously can also be used to alter the solubility characteristics, which, in turn, can increase the flexibility in formulating dosage forms. The solubility of methylprednisolone can be altered from essentially water-insoluble methylprednisolone acetate to slightly water-insoluble methylprednisolone to water-soluble methylprednisolone sodium succinate. The water-soluble sodium hemisuccinate salt is used in oral, intravenous, and intramuscular dosage forms. Methylprednisolone itself is normally found in tablets. The acetate ester is found in topical ointments and sterile aqueous suspensions for intramuscular injection. Both the succinate and acetate esters are hydrolyzed to the active methylprednisolone by the patient's own systemic hydrolytic enzymes (esterases).

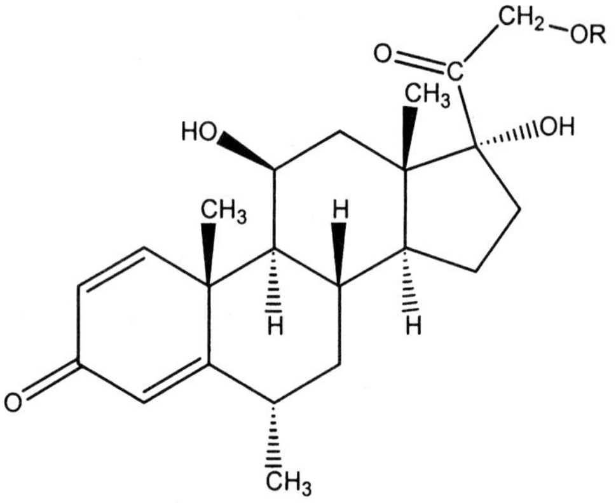

Methylprednisolone: R = H

Methylprednisolone Acetate: R = C(=O)CH₃

Methylprednisolone Sodium Succinate: R = C(=O)CH₂CH₂COO⁻ Na⁺

Another example of how prodrug design can significantly alter biodistribution and biological half-life is illustrated by two drugs based on the retinoic acid structure used systemically to treat psoriasis, a nonmalignant hyperplasia. Etretinate has a 120-day *terminal* half-life after 6 months of therapy. In contrast, the active metabolite, acitretin, has a 33- to 96-hour *terminal* half-life. Both drugs are potentially teratogenic. Women of childbearing age must sign statements that they are aware of the risks and usually are administered a pregnancy test before a prescription is issued. Acitretin, with its shorter half-life, is recommended for a woman who would like to become pregnant, because it can clear her body within a reasonable time frame. When effective, etretinate can keep a patient clear of psoriasis lesions for several months.

Protein Binding

Once the drug enters the systemic circulation (Fig. 2.1), it can undergo several events. It may stay in solution, but many drugs will be bound to the serum proteins, usually albumin (Rx. 2.2). Thus, a new equilibrium must be considered. Depending on the equilibrium constant, the drug can remain in systemic circulation bound to albumin for a considerable period and not be available to the sites of biotransformation, the pharmacological receptors, and excretion.

Drug + Albumin $\rightleftharpoons$ Drug-Albumin Complex   (Rx. 2.2)

Protein binding can have a profound effect on the drug's effective solubility, biodistribution, half-life in the body, and interaction with other drugs. A drug with such poor water solubility that therapeutic concentrations of the unbound (active) drug normally cannot be maintained still can be a very effective agent. The albumin–drug complex acts as a reservoir by providing large enough concentrations of free drug to cause a pharmacological response at the receptor.

Protein binding may also limit access to certain body compartments. The placenta is able to block passage of proteins from maternal to fetal circulation. Thus, drugs that normally would be expected to cross the placental barrier and possibly harm the fetus are retained in the maternal circulation, bound to the mother's serum proteins.

Protein binding also can prolong the drug's duration of action. The drug–protein complex is too large to pass through the renal glomerular membranes, preventing rapid excretion of the drug. Protein binding limits the amount of drug available for biotransformation (see later in this chapter and Chapter 3) and for interaction with specific receptor sites. For

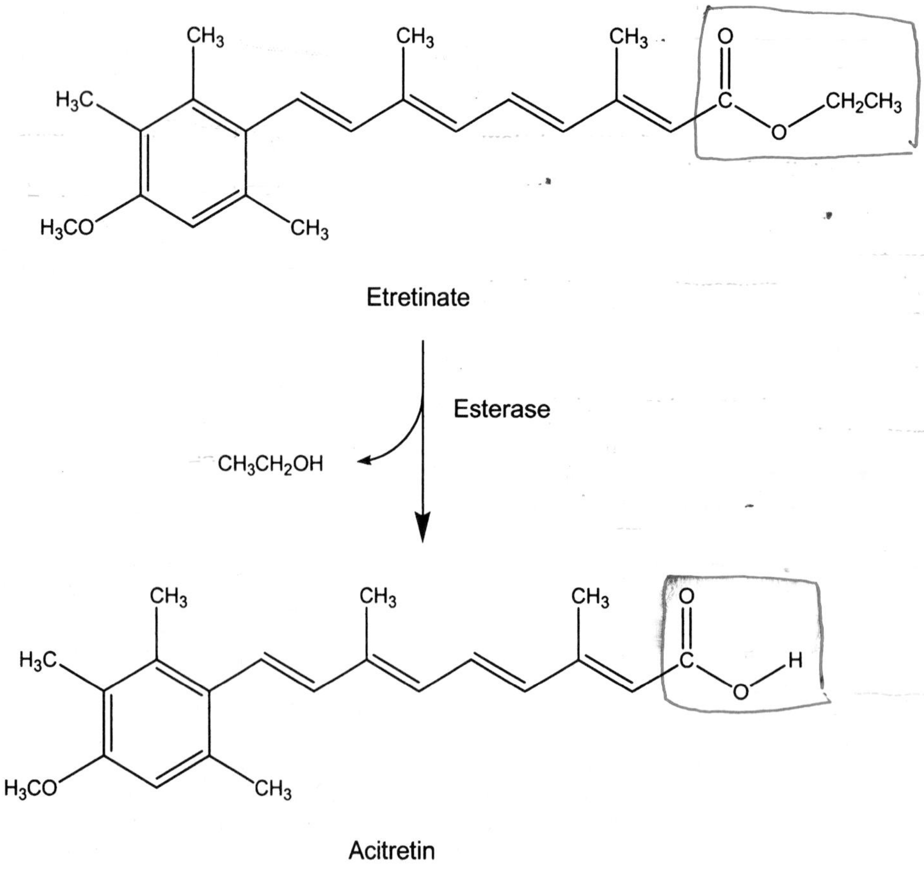

Etretinate

Esterase

CH₃CH₂OH

Acitretin

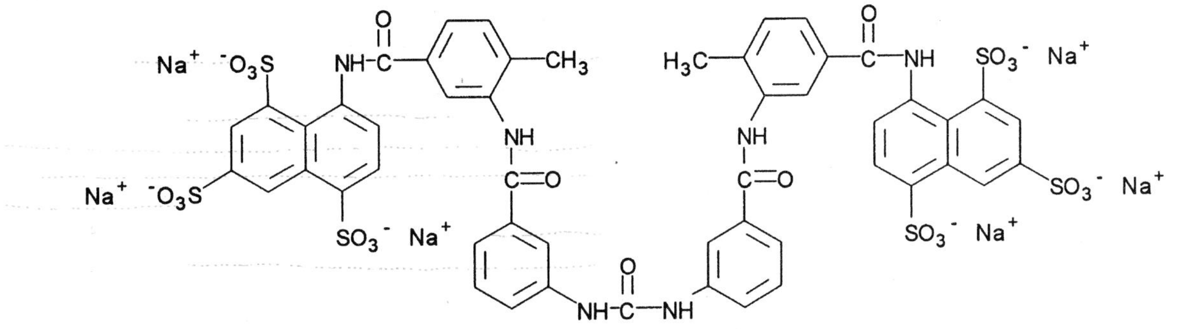

Suramin Sodium

example, the large, polar trypanocide suramin remains in the body in the protein-bound form for as long as 3 months ($t_{1/2}$ = 50 days). The maintenance dose for this drug is based on weekly administration. At first, this might seem to be an advantage to the patient. It can be, but it also means that, should the patient have serious adverse reactions, a significant length of time will be required before the concentration of drug falls below toxic levels.

The drug–protein binding phenomenon can lead to some clinically significant drug–drug interactions that result when one drug displaces another from the binding site on albumin. A large number of drugs can displace the anticoagulant warfarin from its albumin-binding sites. This increases the effective concentration of warfarin at the receptor, leading to an increased prothrombin time (increased time for clot formation) and potential hemorrhage.

Tissue Depots

The drug can also be stored in tissue depots. Neutral fat constitutes some 20% to 50% of body weight and constitutes a depot of considerable importance. The more lipophilic the drug, the more likely it will concentrate in these pharmacologically inert depots. The ultra–short-acting, lipophilic barbiturate thiopental's concentration rapidly decreases below its effective concentration following administration. It *disappears* into tissue protein, redistributes into body fat, and then slowly diffuses back out of the tissue depots but in concentrations too low for a pharmacological response. Thus, only the initially administered thiopental is present in high enough concentrations to combine with its receptors. The remaining thiopental diffuses out of the tissue depots into systemic circulation in concentrations too small to be effective (Fig. 2.1), is metabolized in the liver, and is excreted.

In general, structural changes in the barbiturate series (see Chapter 12) that favor partitioning into the lipid tissue stores decrease duration of action but increase central nervous system (CNS) depression. Conversely, the barbiturates with the slowest onset of action and longest duration of action contain the more polar side chains. This latter group of barbiturates both enters and leaves the CNS more slowly than the more lipophilic thiopental.

Drug Metabolism

All substances in the circulatory system, including drugs, metabolites, and nutrients, will pass through the liver. Most molecules absorbed from the gastrointestinal tract enter the portal vein and are initially transported to the liver. A significant proportion of a drug will partition or be transported into the hepatocyte, where it may be metabolized by hepatic enzymes to inactive chemicals during the initial trip through the liver, by what is known as the first-pass effect (see Chapter 3).

Lidocaine is a classic example of the significance of the first-pass effect. Over 60% of this local anesthetic antiarrhythmic agent is metabolized during its initial passage through the liver, resulting in it being impractical to administer orally. When used for cardiac arrhythmias, it is administered intravenously. This rapid metabolism of lidocaine is used to advantage when stabilizing a patient with cardiac arrhythmias. Should too much lidocaine be administered intravenously, toxic responses will tend to decrease because of rapid biotransformation to inactive metabolites. An understanding of the metabolic labile site on lidocaine led to the development of the primary amine analog tocainide. In contrast to lidocaine's half-life of less than 2 hours, tocainide's half-life is approximately 15 hours, with 40% of the drug excreted unchanged. The development of orally active antiarrhythmic agents is discussed in more detail in Chapter 19.

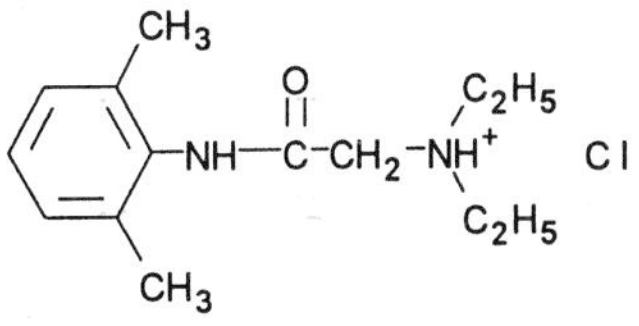

Lidocaine

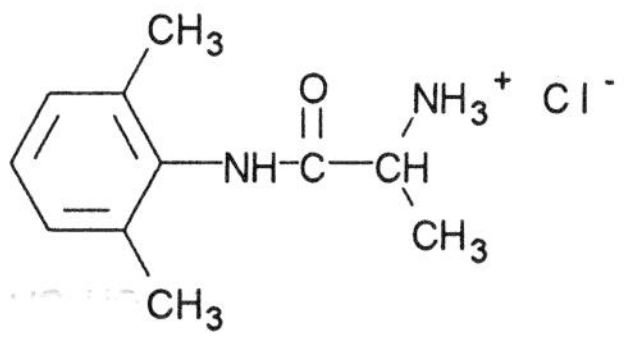

Tocainide

A study of the metabolic fate of a drug is required for all new drug products. Often it is found that the metabolites are also active. Sometimes the metabolite is the pharmacologically active molecule. These drug metabolites can provide leads for additional investigations of potentially new products. Examples of an inactive parent drug that is converted to an active metabolite include the nonsteroidal antiinflammatory agent sulindac being reduced to the active sulfide metabolite, the immunosuppressant azathioprine being cleaved to the purine antimetabolite 6-mercaptopurine, and purine and pyrimidine antimetabolites and antiviral agents being conjugated to their nucleotide form (acyclovir phosphorylated to acyclovir triphosphate). Often both the parent drug and its metabolite are active, which has led to additional commercial products, instead of just one being marketed. About 75% to 80% of phenacetin (now withdrawn from the U.S. market) is converted to acetaminophen. In the tricyclic antidepressant series (see Chapter 12), imipramine and amitriptyline are *N*-demethylated to desipramine and nortriptyline, respectively. All four compounds have been marketed in the United States. Drug metabolism is discussed more fully in Chapter 3.

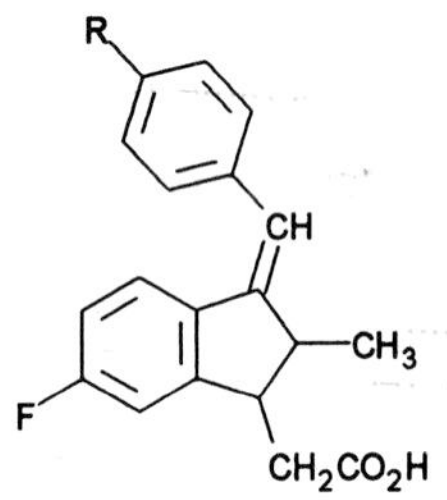

Sulindac: R = CH₃S(=O)
Active Sulfide Metabolite: R = CH₃S

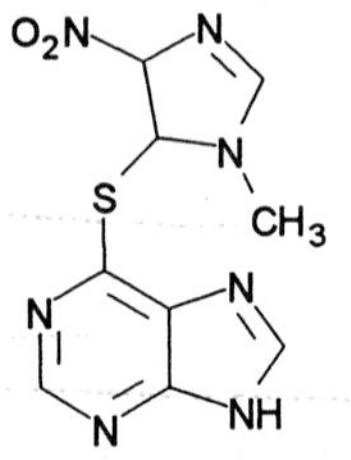

Azathioprine 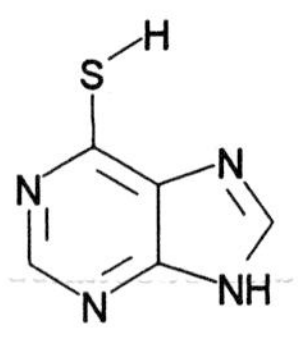   6-Mercaptopurine

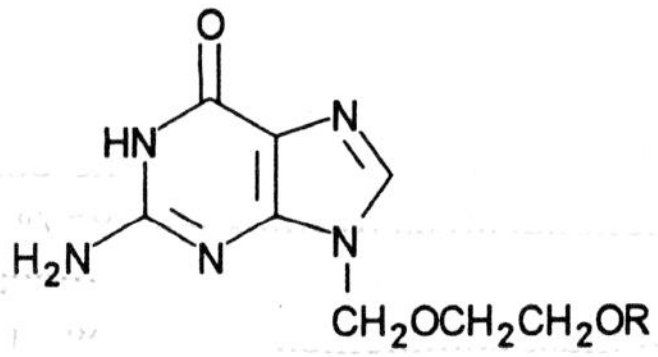

Acyclovir: R = H
Acyclovir triphosphate: R = O-P-O-P-O-P

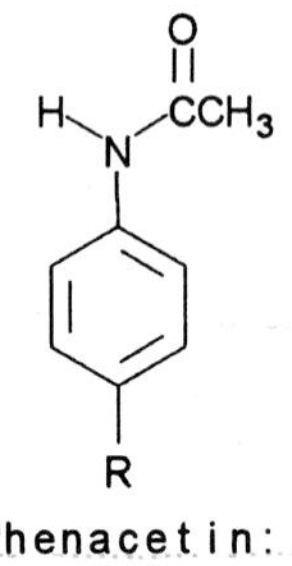

Phenacetin: R = OC₂H₅
Acetaminophen: R = OH

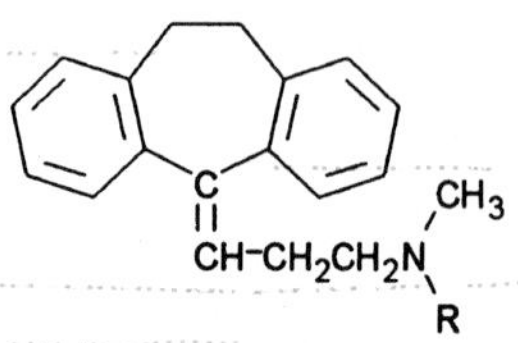

Amitriptyline: R = CH₃
Nortriptyline: R = H

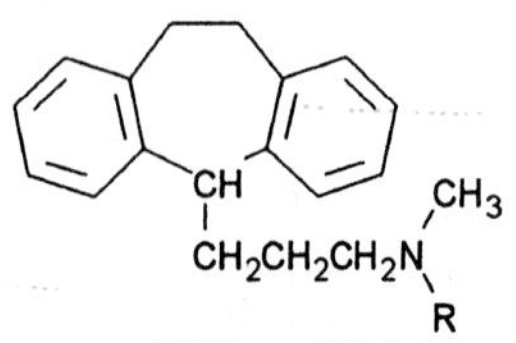

Imipramine: R = CH₃
Desipramine: R = H

Although a drug's metabolism can be a source of frustration for the medicinal chemist, pharmacist, and physician and lead to inconvenience and compliance problems with the patient, it is fortunate that the body has the ability to metabolize foreign molecules (xenobiotics). Otherwise, many of these substances could remain in the body for years. This has been the complaint against certain lipophilic chemical pollutants, including the once very popular insecticide dichlorodiphenyltrichloroethane (DDT). After entering the body, these chemicals reside in body tissues, slowly diffusing out of the depots and potentially harming the individual on a chronic basis for several years. They can also reside in tissues of commercial food animals that have been slaughtered before the drug has *washed out* of the body.

Excretion

The main route of excretion of a drug and its metabolites is through the kidney. For some drugs, enterohepatic circulation (Fig. 2.1), in which the drug reenters the intestinal tract from the liver through the bile duct, can be an important part of the agent's distribution in the body and route of excretion. Either the drug or drug metabolite can reenter systemic circulation by passing once again through the intestinal mucosa. A portion of either also may be excreted in the feces. Nursing mothers must be concerned, because drugs and their metabolites can be excreted in human milk and be ingested by the nursing infant.

One should keep a sense of perspective when learning about drug metabolism. As explained in Chapter 3, drug metabolism can be conceptualized as occurring in two stages or phases. Intermediate metabolites that are pharmacologically active usually are produced by phase I reactions. The products from the phase I chemistry are converted into inactive, usually water-soluble end products by phase II reactions. The latter, commonly called *conjugation* reactions, can be thought of as synthetic reactions that involve addition of water-soluble substituents. In human drug metabolism, the main conjugation reactions add glucuronic acid, sulfate, or glutathione. Obviously, drugs that are bound to serum protein or show favorable partitioning into tissue depots are going to be metabolized and excreted more slowly for the reasons discussed previously.

This does not mean that drugs that remain in the body for longer periods of time can be administered in lower doses or be taken fewer times per day by the patient. Several variables determine dosing regimens, of which the affinity of the drug for the receptor is crucial. Reexamine Reaction 2.1 and Figure 2.1. If the equilibrium does not favor formation of the drug–receptor complex, higher and usually more frequent doses must be administered. Further, if partitioning into tissue stores or metabolic degradation and/or excretion is favored, it will take more of the drug and usually more frequent administration to maintain therapeutic concentrations at the receptor.

The Receptor

With the possible exception of general anesthetics (see Chapter 22), the working model for a pharmacological response consists of a drug binding to a specific receptor. Many drug receptors are the same as those used by endogenously produced ligands. Cholinergic agents interact with the same receptors as the neurotransmitter acetylcholine.

Synthetic corticosteroids bind to the same receptors as cortisone and hydrocortisone. Often, receptors for the same ligand are found in various tissues throughout the body. The nonsteroidal anti-inflammatory agents (see Chapter 26) inhibit the prostaglandin-forming enzyme cyclooxygenase, which is found in nearly every tissue. This class of drugs has a long list of side effects with many patient complaints. Note in Figure 2.1 that, depending on which receptors contain bound drug, there may be desired or undesired effects. This is because various receptors with similar structural requirements are found in several organs and tissues. Thus, the nonsteroidal anti-inflammatory drugs combine with the desired cyclooxygenase receptors at the site of the inflammation and the undesired cyclooxygenase receptors in the gastrointestinal mucosa, causing severe discomfort and sometimes ulceration. One of the *second-generation* antihistamines, fexofenadine, is claimed to cause less sedation because it does not readily penetrate the blood-brain barrier. The rationale is that less of this antihistamine is available for the receptors in the CNS, which are responsible for the sedation response characteristic of antihistamines. In contrast, some antihistamines are used for their CNS depressant activity because a significant proportion of the administered dose is crossing the blood-brain barrier relative to binding to the histamine H_1 receptors in the periphery.

Although it is normal to think of side effects as undesirable, they sometimes can be beneficial and lead to new products. The successful development of oral hypoglycemic agents used in the treatment of diabetes began when it was found that certain sulfonamides had a hypoglycemic effect. Nevertheless, a real problem in drug therapy is patient compliance in taking the drug as directed. Drugs that cause serious problems and discomfort tend to be avoided by patients.

At this point, let us assume that the drug has entered the systemic circulation (Fig. 2.1), passed through the lipid barriers, and is now going to make contact with the receptor. As illustrated in Reaction 2.1, this is an equilibrium process. A good ability to fit the receptor favors binding and the desired pharmacological response. In contrast, a poor fit favors the reverse reaction. With only a small amount of drug bound to the receptor, there will be a much smaller pharmacological effect. If the amount of drug bound to the receptor is too small, there may be no discernible response. Many variables contribute to a drug's binding to the receptor. These include the structural class, the 3D shape of the molecule, and the types of chemical bonding involved in the binding of the drug to the receptor.

Most drugs that belong to the same pharmacological class have certain structural features in common. The barbiturates act on specific CNS receptors, causing depressant effects; hydantoins act on CNS receptors, producing an anticonvulsant response; benzodiazepines combine with the γ-aminobutyric acid (GABA) receptors, with resulting anxiolytic activity; steroids can be divided into such classes as corticosteroids, anabolic steroids, progestogens, and estrogens, each acting on specific receptors; nonsteroidal anti-inflammatory agents inhibit enzymes required for the prostaglandin cascade; penicillins and cephalosporins inhibit enzymes required to construct the bacterial cell wall; and tetracyclines act on bacterial ribosomes.

With the isolation and characterization of receptors becoming a common occurrence, it is hard to realize that the concept of receptors began as a postulate. It had been realized

early that molecules with certain structural features would elucidate a specific biological response. Very slight changes in structure could cause significant changes in biological activity. These structural variations could increase or decrease activity or change an agonist into an antagonist. This early and fundamentally correct interpretation called for the drug (ligand) to fit onto some surface (the receptor) that had fairly strict structural requirements for proper binding of the drug. The initial receptor model was based on a rigid lock-and-key concept, with the drug (key) fitting into a receptor (lock). It has been used to explain why certain structural attributes produce a predictable pharmacological action. This model still is useful, although one must realize that both the drug and the receptor can have considerable flexibility. Molecular graphics, using programs that calculate the preferred conformations of drug and receptor, show that the receptor can undergo an adjustment in 3D structure when the drug makes contact. Using space-age language, the drug *docks* with the receptor.

More complex receptors now are being isolated, characterized, and cloned. The first receptors to be isolated and characterized were the reactive and regulatory sites on enzymes. Acetylcholinesterase, dihydrofolate reductase, angiotensin, and human immunodeficiency virus (HIV) protease-converting enzyme are examples of enzymes whose active sites (the receptors) have been modeled. Most drug receptors probably are receptors for natural ligands used to regulate cellular biochemistry and function and to communicate between cells. Receptors include a relatively small region of a macromolecule, which may be an isolatable enzyme, a structural and functional component of a cell membrane, or a specific intracellular substance such as a protein or nucleic acid. Specific regions of these macromolecules are visualized as being oriented in space in a manner that permits their functional groups to interact with the complementary functional groups of the drug. This interaction initiates changes in structure and function of the macromolecule, which lead ultimately to the observable biological response. The concept of spatially oriented functional areas forming a receptor leads directly to specific structural requirements for functional groups of a drug, which must complement the receptor.

It now is possible to isolate membrane-bound receptors, although it still is difficult to elucidate their structural chemistry, because once separated from the cell membranes, these receptors may lose their native shape. This is because the membrane is required to hold the receptor in its correct tertiary structure. One method of receptor isolation is affinity chromatography. In this technique, a ligand, often an altered drug molecule known to combine with the receptor, is attached to a chromatographic support phase. A solution containing the desired receptor is passed over this column. The receptor will combine with the ligand. It is common to add a chemically reactive grouping to the drug, resulting in the receptor and drug covalently binding with each other. The drug–receptor complex is washed from the column and then characterized further.

A more recent technique uses recombinant DNA. The gene for the receptor is located and cloned. It is transferred into a bacterium, yeast, or animal, which then produces the receptor in large enough quantities to permit further study. Sometimes it is possible to determine the DNA sequence of the cloned gene. By using the genetic code for amino acids, the amino acid sequence of the protein component of the receptor can be determined, and the receptor then modeled, producing an estimated 3D shape. The model for the receptor becomes the template for designing new ligands. Genome mapping has greatly increased the information on receptors. Besides the human genome, the genetic composition of viruses, bacteria, fungi, and parasites has increased the possible sites for drugs to act. The new field of proteomics studies the proteins produced by structural genes.

The earlier discussion in this chapter emphasizes that the cell membrane is a highly organized, dynamic structure that interacts with small molecules in specific ways; its focus is on the lipid bilayer component of this complex structure. The receptor components of the membranes appear to be mainly protein. They constitute a highly organized, intertwined region of the cell membrane. The same type of molecular specificity seen in such proteins as enzymes and antibodies is also a property of drug receptors. The nature of the amide link in proteins provides a unique opportunity for the formation of multiple internal hydrogen bonds, as well as internal formation of hydrophobic, van der Waals, and ionic bonds by side chain groups, leading to such organized structures as the α-helix, which contains about four amino acid residues for each turn of the helix. An organized protein structure would hold the amino acid side chains at relatively fixed positions in space and available for specific interactions with a small molecule.

Proteins can potentially adopt many different conformations in space without breaking their covalent amide linkages. They may shift from highly coiled structures to partially disorganized structures, with parts of the molecule existing in *random chain* or *folded sheet* structures, contingent on the environment. In the monolayer of a cell membrane, the interaction of a small foreign molecule with an organized protein may lead to a significant change in the structural and physical properties of the membrane. Such changes could well be the initiating events in the tissue or organ response to a drug, such as the ion-translocation effects produced by interaction of acetylcholine and the cholinergic receptor.

The large body of information now available on relationships between chemical structure and biological activity strongly supports the concept of flexible receptors. The fit of drugs onto or into macromolecules is rarely an all-or-none

process as pictured by the earlier lock-and-key concept of a receptor. Rather, the binding or partial insertion of groups of moderate size onto or into a macromolecular pouch appears to be a continuous process, at least over a limited range, as indicated by the frequently occurring regular increase and decrease in biological activity as one ascends a homologous series of drugs. A range of productive associations between drug and receptor may be pictured, which leads to agonist responses, such as those produced by cholinergic and adrenergic drugs. Similarly, strong associations may lead to unproductive changes in the configuration of the macromolecule, leading to an antagonistic or blocking response, such as that produced by anticholinergic agents and HIV protease inhibitors. Although the fundamental structural unit of the drug receptor is generally considered to be protein, it may be supplemented by its associations with other units, such as mucopolysaccharides and nucleic acids.

Humans (and mammals in general) are very complex organisms that have developed specialized organ systems. It is not surprising that receptors are not distributed equally throughout the body. It now is realized that, depending on the organ in which it is located, the same receptor class may behave differently. This can be advantageous by focusing drug therapy on a specific organ system, but it can also cause adverse drug responses because the drug is exerting two different responses based on the location of the receptors. An example is the selective estrogen receptor modulators (SERMs). They cannot be classified simply as agonists or antagonists. Rather, they can be considered variable agonists and antagonists. Their selectivity is very complex because it depends on the organ in which the receptor is located.

This complexity can be illustrated with tamoxifen and raloxifene (Fig. 2.2). Tamoxifen is used for estrogen-sensitive breast cancer and for reducing bone loss from osteoporosis. Unfortunately, prolonged treatment increases the risk of endometrial cancer because of the response from the uterine estrogen receptors. Thus, tamoxifen is an estrogen antagonist in the mammary gland and an agonist in the uterus and bone. In contrast, raloxifene does not appear to have much agonist property in the uterus but, like tamoxifen, is an antagonist in the breast and agonist in the bone.

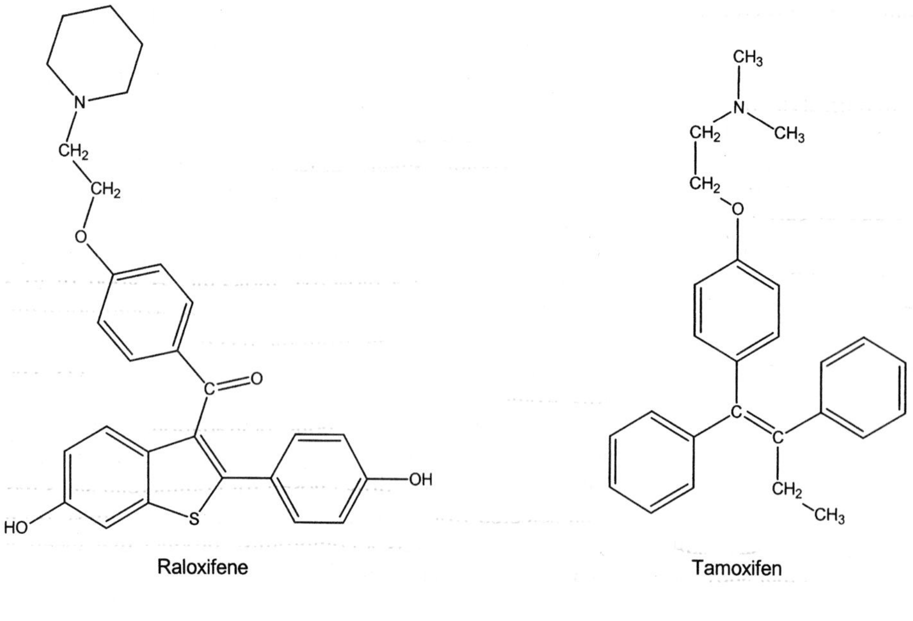

Raloxifene   Tamoxifen   **Figure 2.2** ● Selective SERMs.

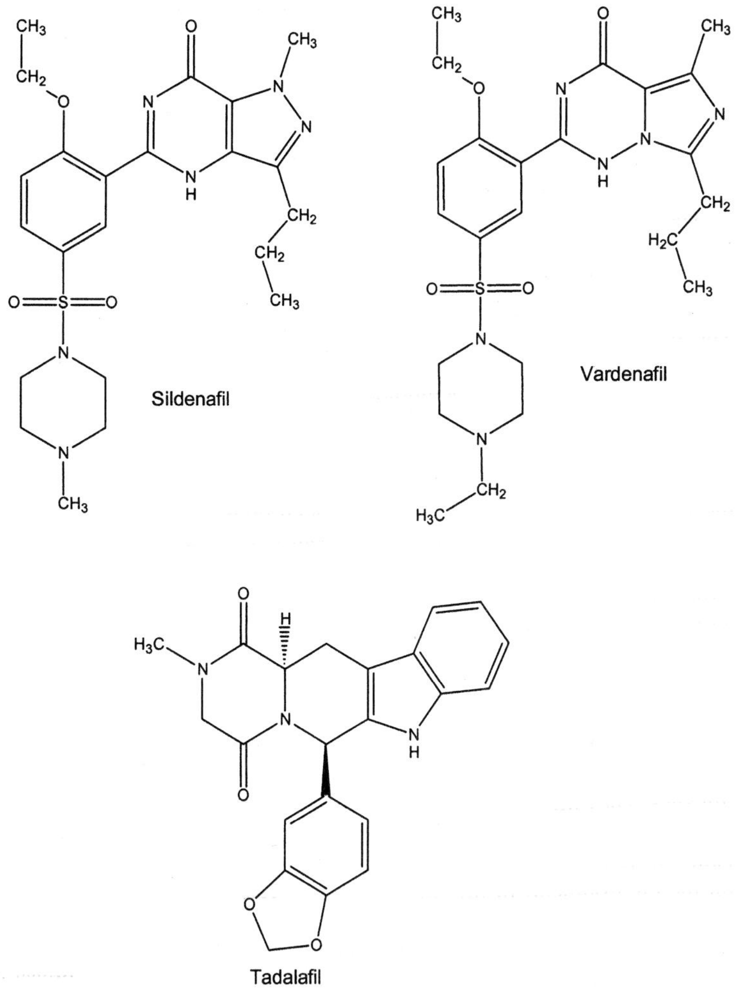

Figure 2.3 ● Examples of phosphodiesterase type 5 inhibitors.

There are a wide variety of phosphodiesterases through-out the body. These enzymes hydrolyze the cyclic phosphate esters of adenosine monophosphate (cAMP) and guanosine monophosphate (cGMP). Although the substrates for this family of enzymes are cAMP and cGMP, there are differences in the active sites. Figure 2.3 illustrates three drugs used to treat erectile dysfunction (sildenafil, tadalafil, and vardenafil). These three take advantage of the differences in active site structural requirements between phosphodiesterase type 5 and the other phosphodiesterases. They have an important role in maintaining a desired lifestyle: treatment of erectile dysfunction caused by various medical conditions. The drugs approved for this indication were discovered by accident. The goal was to develop a newer treatment of angina. The approach was to develop phosphodiesterase inhibitors that would prolong the activity of cGMP. The end result was drugs that were not effective inhibitors of the phosphodiesterase that would treat angina, but were effective inhibitors of the one found in the corpus cavernosum. The vasodilation in this organ results in penile erection.

Summary

One of the goals is to design drugs that will interact with receptors at specific tissues. There are several ways to do this, including (a) altering the molecule, which, in turn, can change the biodistribution; (b) searching for structures that show in-creased specificity for the target receptor that will produce the desired pharmacological response while decreasing the affinity for undesired receptors that produce adverse responses; and (c) the still experimental approach of attaching the drug to a monoclonal antibody (see Chapter 5) that will bind to a specific tissue antigenic for the antibody. Biodistribution can be altered by changing the drug's solubility, enhancing its ability to resist being metabolized (usually in the liver), altering the formulation or physical characteristics of the drug, and changing the route of administration. If a drug molecule can be designed so that its binding to the desired receptor is enhanced relative to the undesired receptor and biodistribution remains favorable, smaller doses of the drug can be administered. This, in turn, reduces the amount of drug available for binding to those receptors responsible for its adverse effects.

The medicinal chemist is confronted with several challenges in designing a bioactive molecule. A good fit to a specific receptor is desirable, but the drug would normally be expected to dissociate from the receptor eventually. The specificity for the receptor would minimize side effects. The drug would be expected to clear the body within a reasonable time. Its rate of metabolic degradation should allow reasonable dosing schedules and, ideally, oral administration. Many times, the drug chosen for commercial sales has been selected from hundreds of compounds that have been screened. It usually is a compromise product that meets a medical need while demonstrating good patient acceptance.

⬡ ACID–BASE PROPERTIES

Most drugs used today can be classified as acids or bases. As is noted shortly, a large number of drugs can behave as either acids or bases as they begin their journey into the patient in different dosage forms and end up in systemic circulation. A drug's acid–base properties can greatly influence its biodistribution and partitioning characteristics.

Over the years, at least four major definitions of acids and bases have been developed. The model commonly used in pharmacy and biochemistry was developed independently by Lowry and Brønsted. In their definition, an *acid* is defined as a proton donor and a *base* is defined as a proton acceptor. Notice that for a base, *there is no mention of the hydroxide ion*. In the Brønsted-Lowry model, the acid plus base reaction can be expressed as:

$$\text{Acid} + \text{Base} \rightleftharpoons \text{Conjuate Acid} + \text{Conjugate Base}$$

(Rx. 2.3)

Acid/Base–Conjugate Acid/Conjugate Base Pairs

Representative pairings of acids with their conjugate bases and bases with their conjugate acids are shown in Table 2.1. Careful study of this table shows water functioning as a proton acceptor (base) in reactions *a, c, e, g, i, k,* and *m* and a proton donor (base) in reactions *b, d, f, h, j, l,* and *n.* Hence, water is known as an *amphoteric* substance. Water can be either a weak base accepting a proton to form the strongly acidic hydrated proton or hydronium ion H_3O^+ (reactions *a, c, e, g, i, k,* and *m*), or a weak acid donating a proton to form the strongly basic (proton accepting) hydroxide anion OH^- (reactions *b, d, f, h, j, l,* and *n*).

Also note the shift between un-ionized and ionized forms in Table 2.1. Examples of un-ionized acids donating their protons forming ionized conjugate bases are acetic acid-acetate (reaction *g*), phenobarbital-phenobarbiturate (reaction *i*), and saccharin-saccharate (reaction *k*). In contrast, examples of ionized acids yielding un-ionized conjugate bases are ammonium chloride-ammonia (reaction *e*) and ephedrine hydrochloride (reaction *m*). A similar shift between un-ionized and ionized forms is seen with bases and their conjugate acids. Examples of un-ionized bases yielding their ionized conjugate acids include ammonia and ammonium (reaction *f*) and ephedrine and protonated ephedrine (reaction *n*). Whereas examples of ionized bases yielding un-ionized conjugate acids are acetate forming acetic acid (reaction *h*), phenobarbiturate yielding phenobarbital (reaction *j*), and saccharate yielding saccharin (reaction *l*). Complicated as it may seem at first, conjugate acids and conjugate bases are nothing more than the products of an acid–base reaction. In other words, they appear to the right of the reaction arrows.

Representative examples of pharmaceutically important acidic drugs are listed in Table 2.1. Each acid, or proton donor, yields a *conjugate base.* The latter is the product after the proton is lost from the acid. Conjugate bases range from the chloride ion (reaction *a*), which does not accept a proton in aqueous media, to ephedrine (reaction *h*), which is an excellent proton acceptor.

Acid Strength

While any acid–base reaction can be written as an equilibrium reaction, an attempt has been made in Table 2.1 to indicate which sequences are unidirectional or show only a small reversal. For hydrochloric acid (reaction *a*), the conjugate base, Cl^-, is such a weak base that it essentially does not function as a proton acceptor. In a similar manner, water is such a weak conjugate acid that there is little reverse reaction involving water donating a proton to the hydroxide anion of sodium hydroxide (reaction *b*).

Two logical questions to ask at this point are how one predicts in which direction an acid–base reaction lies and to what extent the reaction goes to completion. The common physical chemical measurement that contains this information is known as the pK_a. The pK_a is the negative logarithm of the modified equilibrium constant, K_a (Eq. 2.1), for an acid–base reaction written so that water is the base or proton acceptor (reactions *a, c, e, g, i, k, m,* Table 2.1).

$$K_a = \frac{[\text{conj. acid}][\text{conj. base}]}{\text{acid}} \quad \text{(Eq. 2.1)}$$

Equation 2.1 is based on Rx. 2.3. The square brackets indicate molar concentrations. Because the molar concentration of water (the base in these acid–base reactions) is considered constant in the dilute solutions used in pharmacy and medicine, it is incorporated into the K_a. Rewriting Equation 2.1 by taking the negative logarithm of the K_a, results in the familiar Henderson-Hasselbalch equation (Eq. 2.2).

$$pH = pK_a + \log \frac{[\text{conj. base}]}{[\text{acid}]} \quad \text{(Eq. 2.2)}$$

Warning! It is *important* to recognize that a pK_a for a base is in reality the pK_a of the conjugate acid (acid donor or protonated form, BH^+) of the base. The pK_a is listed in the Appendix as 9.6 for ephedrine and as 9.3 for ammonia. In reality, this is the pK_a of the protonated form, such as ephedrine hydrochloride (reaction *m* in Table 2.1) and ammonium chloride (reaction *e* in Table 2.1), respectively. This is confusing to students, pharmacists, clinicians, and experienced scientists. It is crucial that the chemistry of the drug be understood when interpreting a pK_a value. When reading tables of pK_a values, such as those found in the Appendix, one must realize that the listed value is for the proton donor form of the molecule, no matter what form is indicated by the name. See Table 2.2 for several worked examples of how the pK_a is used to calculate pHs of solutions, required ratios of [conjugate base]/[acid], and percent ionization (discussed later) at specific pHs.

Just how strong or weak are the acids whose reactions in water are illustrated in Table 2.1? Remember that the K_as or pK_a's are modified equilibrium constants that indicate the extent to which the acid (proton donor) reacts with water to form conjugate acid and conjugate base. The equilibrium for a strong acid (low pK_a) in water lies to the right, favoring the formation of products (conjugate acid and conjugate base). The equilibrium for a weak acid (high pK_a) in water lies to the left, meaning that the conjugate acid is a better proton donor than the parent acid is or that the conjugate base is a good proton acceptor.

Refer back to Equation 2.1 and, using the K_a values in Table 2.3, substitute the K_a term for each of the acids. For

TABLE 2.1 **Examples of Acid–Base Reactions (with the Exception of Hydrochloric Acid, Whose Conjugate Base [Cl⁻] Has No Basic Properties in Water, and Sodium Hydroxide, which Generates Hydroxide, the Reaction of the Conjugate Base in Water Is Shown for Each Acid)**

Acid	+	Base	⇌	Conjugate Acid	+	Conjugate Base
Hydrochloric acid						
(a) HCl	+	H_2O	⟶	H_3O^+	+	Cl^-
Sodium hydroxide						
(b) H_2O	+	$NaOH$	⟶	H_2O	+	$OH^-(Na^+)^a$
Sodium dihydrogen phosphate and its conjugate base, sodium monohydrogen phosphate						
(c) $H_2PO_4^-(Na^+)^a$	+	H_2O	⇌	H_3O^+	+	$HPO_4^{2-}(Na^+)^a$
(d) H_2O	+	$HPO_4^{2-}(2Na^+)^a$	⇌	$H_2PO_4^-(Na^+)^a$	+	$OH^-(Na^+)^a$
Ammonium chloride and its conjugate base, ammonia						
(e) $NH_4^+(Cl^-)^a$	+	H_2O	⇌	$H_3O^+(Cl^-)^a$	+	NH_3
(f) H_2O	+	NH_3	⇌	NH_4^+	+	OH^-
Acetic acid and its conjugate base, sodium acetate						
(g) CH_3COOH	+	H_2O	⇌	H_3O^+	+	CH_3COO^-
(h) H_2O	+	$CH_3COO^-(Na^+)^a$	⇌	CH_3COOH	+	$OH^-(Na^+)^a$

Indomethacin and its conjugate base, indomethacin sodium, show the identical acid–base chemistry as acetic acid and sodium acetate, respectively.

Phenobarbital and its conjugate base, phenobarbital sodium

| (i) | + | H_2O | ⇌ | H_3O^+ | + | |
| (j) H_2O | + | | ⇌ | | + | $OH^-(Na^+)^a$ |

Saccharin and its conjugate base, saccharin sodium

| (k) | + | H_2O | ⇌ | H_3O^+ | + | |
| (l) H_2O | + | | ⇌ | | + | $OH^-(Na^+)^a$ |

Ephedrine HCl and its conjugate base, ephedrine

| (m) | + | H_2O | ⇌ | $H_3O^+(Cl^-)^a$ | + | |
| (n) H_2O | + | | ⇌ | | + | OH^- |

^{a}The chloride anion and sodium cation are present only to maintain charge balance. These anions play no other acid–base role.

TABLE 2.2 Examples of Calculations Requiring the pK$_a$

1. What is the ratio of ephedrine to ephedrine HCl (pK$_a$ 9.6) in the intestinal tract at pH 8.0? Use Equation 2.2.

$$8.0 = 9.6 + \log\frac{[\text{ephedrine}]}{[\text{ephedrine HCl}]} = -1.6$$

$$\frac{[\text{ephedrine}]}{[\text{ephedrine HCl}]} = 0.025$$

The number whose log is −1.6 is 0.025, meaning that there are 25 parts ephedrine for every 1,000 parts ephedrine HCl in the intestinal tract whose environment is pH 8.0.

2. What is the pH of a buffer containing 0.1-M acetic acid (pK$_a$ 4.8) and 0.08-M sodium acetate? Use Equation 2.2.

$$pH = 4.8 + \log\frac{0.08}{0.1} = 4.7$$

3. What is the pH of a 0.1-M acetic acid solution? Use the following equation for calculating the pH of a solution containing either an HA or BH$^+$ acid.

$$pH = \frac{pK_a - \log[\text{acid}]}{2} = 2.9$$

4. What is the pH of a 0.08-M sodium acetate solution? Remember, even though this is the conjugate base of acetic acid, the pK$_a$ is still used. The pK$_w$ term in the following equation corrects for the fact that a proton acceptor (acetate anion) is present in the solution. The equation for calculating the pH of a solution containing either an A$^-$ or B base is

$$pH = \frac{pK_w + pK_a + \log[\text{base}]}{2} = 8.9$$

5. What is the pH of an ammonium acetate solution? The pK$_a$ of the ammonium (NH$_4^+$) cation is 9.3. Always bear in mind that the pK$_a$ refers to the ability of the proton donor form to release the proton into water to form H$_3$O$^+$. Since this is the salt of a weak acid (NH$_4^+$) and the conjugate base of a weak acid (acetate anion), the following equation is used. Note that molar concentration is not a variable in this calculation.

$$pH = \frac{pK_{a_1} + pK_{a_2}}{2} = 7.1$$

6. What is the percentage ionization of ephedrine HCl (pK$_a$ 9.6) in an intestinal tract buffered at pH 8.0 (see example 1)? Use Equation 2.4 because this is a BH$^+$ acid.

$$\% \text{ ionization} = \frac{100}{1 + 10^{(8.0-9.6)}} = 97.6\%$$

Only 2.4% of ephedrine is present as the un-ionized conjugate base.

7. What is the percentage ionization of indomethacin (pK$_a$ 4.5) in an intestinal tract buffered at pH 8.0? Use Equation 2.3 because this is an HA acid.

$$\% \text{ ionization} = \frac{100}{1 + 10^{(4.5-8.0)}} = 99.97\%$$

For all practical purposes, indomethacin is present only as the anionic conjugate base in that region of the intestine buffered at pH 8.0.

TABLE 2.3 Representative K_a and pK$_a$ Values from the Reactions Listed in Table 2.1 (See the Appendix)

Hydrochloric acid	1.26×10^6	−6.1
Dihydrogen phosphate	6.31×10^{-8}	7.2
Ammonia (ammonium)	5.01×10^{-10}	9.3
Acetic acid	1.58×10^{-5}	4.8
Phenobarbital	3.16×10^{-8}	7.5
Saccharin	2.51×10^{-2}	1.6
Indomethacin	3.16×10^{-5}	4.5
Ephedrine (as the HCl salt)	2.51×10^{-10}	9.6

hydrochloric acid, a K_a of 1.26×10^6 means that the product of the molar concentrations of the conjugate acid, [H$_3$O$^+$], and the conjugate base, [Cl$^-$], is huge relative to the denominator term, [HCl]. In other words, there essentially is no unreacted HCl left in an aqueous solution of hydrochloric acid. At the other extreme is ephedrine HCl with a pK$_a$ of 9.6 or a K_a of 2.51×10^{-10}. Here, the denominator representing the concentration of ephedrine HCl greatly predominates over that of the products, which, in this example, is ephedrine (conjugate base) and H$_3$O$^+$ (conjugate acid). In other words, the protonated form of ephedrine is a very poor proton donor. It holds onto the proton. Free ephedrine (the conjugate base in this reaction) is an excellent proton acceptor.

A general rule for determining whether a chemical is strong or weak acid or base is

- pK$_a$ <2: strong acid; conjugate base has no meaningful basic properties in water
- pK$_a$ 4 to 6: weak acid; weak conjugate base
- pK$_a$ 8 to 10: very weak acid; conjugate base getting stronger
- pK$_a$ >12: essentially no acidic properties in water; strong conjugate base

This delineation is only approximate. Other properties also become important when considering cautions in handling acids and bases. Phenol has a pK$_a$ of 9.9, slightly less than that of ephedrine HCl. Why is phenol considered corrosive to the skin, whereas ephedrine HCl or free ephedrine is considered innocuous when applied to the skin? Phenol has the ability to partition through the normally protective lipid layers of the skin. Because of this property, this extremely weak acid has carried the name carbolic acid. Thus, the pK$_a$ simply tells a person the acid properties of the protonated form of the chemical. It does not represent anything else concerning other potential toxicities.

Percent Ionization

Using the drug's pK$_a$, the formulation or compounding pharmacist can adjust the pH to ensure maximum water solubility (ionic form of the drug) or maximum solubility in nonpolar media (un-ionic form). This is where understanding the drug's acid–base chemistry becomes important. Note Reactions 2.4 and 2.5:

Acid	Base	Conj. Acid	Conj. Base	
HA$_{(\text{un-ionized})}$ +	H$_2$O	$\rightleftharpoons$ H$_3$O$^+$ +	A$^-_{(\text{ionized})}$	(Rx. 2.4)

Acid	Base	Conj. Acid	Conj. Base	
BH$^+_{(\text{ionized})}$ +	H$_2$O	$\rightleftharpoons$ H$_3$O$^+$ +	B$_{(\text{un-ionized})}$	(Rx. 2.5)

Acids can be divided into two types, HA and BH$^+$, on the basis of the ionic form of the acid (or conjugate base). HA acids go from un-ionized acids to ionized conjugate bases (Rx. 2.4). In contrast, BH$^+$ acids go from ionized (polar) acids to un-ionized (nonpolar) conjugate bases (Rx. 2.5). In general, pharmaceutically important HA acids include the inorganic acids (e.g., HCl, H$_2$SO$_4$), enols (e.g., barbiturates, hydantoins), carboxylic acids (e.g., low–molecular-weight organic acids, arylacetic acids, *N*-aryl anthranilic acids, salicylic acids), and amides and imides (e.g., sulfonamides and saccharin, respectively). The chemistry is simpler for the pharmaceutically important BH$^+$ acids: They are all protonated amines. A polyfunctional drug can have several pK$_a$'s (e.g., amoxicillin). The latter's ionic state is based on amoxicillin's ionic state at physiological pH 7.4.

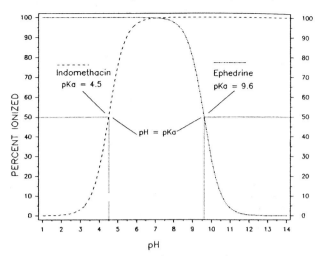

Figure 2.4 ● Percent ionized versus pH for indomethacin (pK$_a$ 4.5) and ephedrine (pK$_a$ 9.6).

pK$_{a3}$ = 9.6

pK$_{a2}$ = 7.4

pK$_{a1}$ = 2.4

Amoxicillin

The percent ionization of a drug is calculated by using Equation 2.3 for HA acids and Equation 2.4 for BH$^+$ acids.

$$\% \text{ ionization} = \frac{100}{1 + 10^{(\text{pK}_a - \text{pH})}} \qquad \text{(Eq. 2.3)}$$

$$\% \text{ ionization} = \frac{100}{1 + 10^{(\text{pH} - \text{pK}_a)}} \qquad \text{(Eq. 2.4)}$$

A plot of percent ionization versus pH illustrates how the degree of ionization can be shifted significantly with small changes in pH. The curves for an HA acid (indomethacin) and BH$^+$ (protonated ephedrine, Table 2.1, reaction *m*) are shown in Figure 2.4. First, note that when pH = pK$_a$, the compound is 50% ionized (or 50% un-ionized). In other words, when the pK$_a$ is equal to the pH, the molar concentration of the acid equals the molar concentration of its conjugate base. In the Henderson-Hasselbalch equation, pK$_a$ = pH when log [conjugate base]/[acid] = 1. An increase of 1 pH unit from the pK$_a$ (increase in alkalinity) causes an HA acid (indomethacin) to become 90.9% in the

ionized conjugate base form but results in a BH$^+$ acid (ephedrine HCl) decreasing its percent ionization to only 9.1%. An increase of 2 pH units essentially shifts an HA acid to complete ionization (99%) and a BH$^+$ acid to the nonionic conjugate base form (0.99%).

Just the opposite is seen when the medium is made more acidic relative to the drug's pK$_a$ value. Increasing the hydrogen ion concentration (decreasing the pH) will shift the equilibrium to the left, thereby increasing the concentration of the acid and decreasing the concentration of conjugate base. In the case of indomethacin, a decrease of 1 pH unit below the pK$_a$ will increase the concentration of un-ionized (protonated) indomethacin to 9.1%. Similarly, a decrease of 2 pH units results in only 0.99% of the indomethacin being present in the ionized conjugate base form. The opposite is seen for the BH$^+$ acids. The percentage of ephedrine present as the ionized (protonated) acid is 90.9% at 1 pH unit below the pK$_a$ and is 99.0% at 2 pH units below the pK$_a$. These results are summarized in Table 2.4.

With this knowledge in mind, return to the drawing of amoxicillin. At physiological pH, the carboxylic acid (HA acid; pK$_{a1}$ 2.4) will be in the ionized carboxylate form, the primary amine (BH$^+$ acid; pK$_{a2}$ 7.4) will be 50% protonated and 50% in the free amine form, and the phenol (HA acid; pK$_{a3}$ 9.6) will be in the un-ionized protonated form. Knowledge of percent ionization makes it easier to explain and predict why the use of some preparations can cause

Acid   Base   Conj. Acid   Conj. Base

+ H$_2$O ⇌ H$_3$O$^+$ +

Indomethacin

TABLE 2.4 Percentage Ionization Relative to the pK_a

	Ionization (%)	
	HA Acids	**BH Acids**
pK_a − 2 pH units	0.99	99.0
pK_a − 1 pH unit	9.1	90.9
pK_a = pH	50.0	50.0
pK_a + 1 pH unit	90.9	9.1
pK_a + 2 pH units	99.0	0.99

problems and discomfort as a result of pH extremes. Phenytoin (HA acid; pK_a 8.3) injection must be adjusted to pH 12 with sodium hydroxide to ensure complete ionization and maximize water solubility. In theory, a pH of 10.3 will result in 99.0% of the drug being an anionic water-soluble conjugate base. To lower the concentration of phenytoin in the insoluble acid form even further and maintain excess alkalinity, the pH is raised to 12 to obtain 99.98% of the drug in the ionized form. Even then, a cosolvent system of 40% propylene glycol, 10% ethyl alcohol, and 50% water for injection is used to ensure complete solution. This highly alkaline solution is irritating to the patient and generally cannot be administered as an admixture with other intravenous fluids that are buffered more closely at physiological pH 7.4. This decrease in pH would result in the parent unionized phenytoin precipitating out of solution.

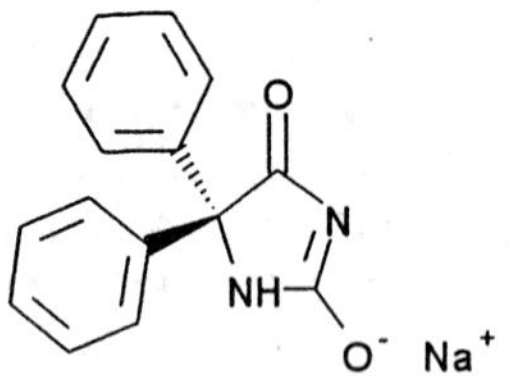

Phenytoin Sodium

Tropicamide is an anticholinergic drug administered as eye drops for its mydriatic response during eye examinations. With a pK_a of 5.2, the drug has to be buffered near pH 4 to obtain more than 90% ionization. The acidic eye drops can sting. Some optometrists and ophthalmologists use local anesthetic eye drops to minimize the patient's discomfort. The only atom with a meaningful pK_a is the pyridine nitrogen. The amide nitrogen has no acid–base properties in aqueous media.

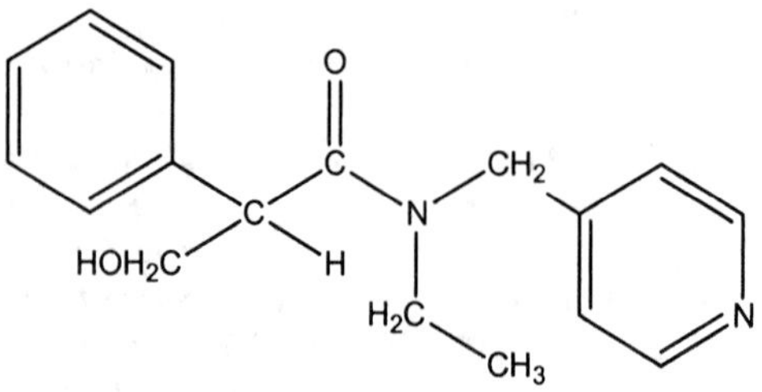

Tropicamide

Adjustments in pH to maintain water solubility can sometimes lead to chemical stability problems. An example is indomethacin (HA acid; pK_a 4.5), which is unstable in alkaline media. Therefore, the preferred oral liquid dosage form is a suspension buffered at pH 4 to 5. Because this is

near the drug's pK_a, only 50% will be in the water-soluble form. There is a medical indication requiring intravenous administration of indomethacin to premature infants. The intravenous dosage form is the lyophilized (freeze-dried) sodium salt, which is reconstituted just prior to use.

Drug Distribution and pK_a

The pK_a can have a pronounced effect on the pharmacokinetics of the drug. As discussed previously, drugs are transported in the aqueous environment of the blood. Those drugs in an ionized form will tend to distribute throughout the body more rapidly than will un-ionized (nonpolar) molecules. With few exceptions, the drug must leave the polar environment of the plasma to reach the site of action. In general, drugs pass through the nonpolar membranes of capillary walls, cell membranes, and the blood-brain barrier in the un-ionized (nonpolar) form. For HA acids, it is the parent acid that will readily cross these membranes (Fig. 2.5). The situation is just the opposite for the BH^+ acids. The unionized conjugate base (free amine) is the species most readily crossing the nonpolar membranes (Fig. 2.6).

Consider the changing pH environment experienced by the drug molecule orally administered. The drug first encounters the acidic stomach, where the pH can range from 2 to 6 depending on the presence of food. HA acids with pK_a's of 4 to 5 will tend to be nonionic and be absorbed partially through the gastric mucosa. (The main reason most acidic drugs are absorbed from the intestinal tract rather than the stomach is that the microvilli of the intestinal mucosa provide a large surface area relative to that found in the gastric mucosa of the stomach.) In contrast, amines (pK_a 9–10) will be protonated (BH^+ acids) in the acidic stomach and usually will not be absorbed until reaching the mildly alkaline intestinal tract (pH 8). Even here, only a portion of the amine-containing drugs will be in their nonpolar conjugate base form (Fig. 2.4). Remember that the reactions shown in Figures 2.3 and 2.4 are equilibrium reactions with K_a values. Therefore, whenever the nonpolar form of either an HA acid (as the acid) or a B base (the conjugate base of the BH^+ acid) passes the lipid barrier, the ratio of conjugate base to acid (percent ionization) will be maintained. Based on Equations 2.3 and 2.4, this ratio depends on the pK_a (a constant) and the pH of the medium.

For example, once in systemic circulation, the plasma pH of 7.4 will be one of the determinants of whether the drug will tend to remain in the aqueous environment of the blood or partition across lipid membranes into hepatic tissue to be metabolized, into the kidney for excretion, into tissue depots, or to the receptor tissue. A useful exercise is to calculate either the [conjugate base]/[acid] ratio using the Henderson-Hasselbalch equation (Eq. 2.2) or percent

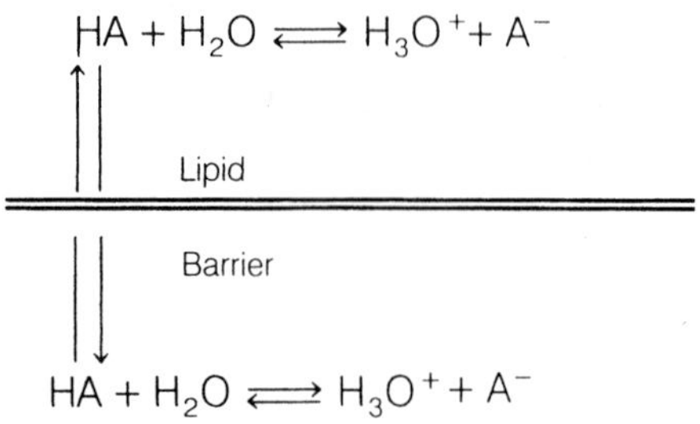

$$HA + H_2O \rightleftharpoons H_3O^+ + A^-$$

Lipid

Barrier

$$HA + H_2O \rightleftharpoons H_3O^+ + A^-$$

Figure 2.5 ● Passage of HA acids through lipid barriers.

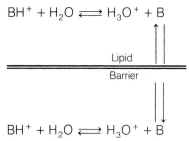

$$BH^+ + H_2O \rightleftharpoons H_3O^+ + B$$

Lipid
Barrier

$$BH^+ + H_2O \rightleftharpoons H_3O^+ + B$$

Figure 2.6 ● **Passage of BH^+ acids through lipid barriers.**

ionization for ephedrine (pK_a 9.6; Eq. 2.4) and indomethacin (pK_a 4.5; Eq. 2.3) at pH 3.5 (stomach), pH 8.0 (intestine), and pH 7.4 (plasma) (see examples 1, 6, and 7 in Table 2.2). Of course, the effect of protein binding, discussed previously, can greatly alter any prediction of biodistribution based solely on pK_a.

⬡ COMPUTER-AIDED DRUG DESIGN: EARLY METHODS

Initially, the design of new drugs was based on starting with a prototypical molecule, usually a natural product and making structural modifications. Examples include steroidal hormones based on naturally occurring cortisone, testosterone, progesterone and estrogen; adrenergic drugs based on epinephrine; local anesthetics based on cocaine; opiate analgesics based on morphine; antibiotics based on penicillin, cephalosporin and tetracycline. Examples of prototypical molecules that were not natural in origin include the antipsychotic phenothiazines, bisphosphonates for osteoporosis, benzodiazepines indicated for various CNS treatments. Although prototypical molecules have produced significant advancements in treating diseases, this approach to drug development is limited to the initial discovery of the prototypical molecule. Today, it is more common to take a *holistic* approach that, where possible, involves understanding the etiology of the disease and the structure of the receptor where the ligand (drug) will bind. Increasing computer power coupled with applicable software, both at reasonable cost, has lead to more focused approaches for the development of new drugs. Computational methodologies include mathematical equations correlating structure with biological activity, searching chemical databases for leads and rapid docking of ligand to the receptor. The latter requires 3D structure information of the receptor. Originally crystallized enzymes were the common receptors, and their spatial arrangements determined by x-ray crystallography. Today's software can calculate possible 3D structures of protein starting with the amino acid sequence.

Statistical Prediction of Pharmacological Activity

Just as mathematical modeling is used to explain and model many chemical processes, it has been the goal of medicinal chemists to quantify the effect of a structural change on a defined pharmacological response. This would meet three goals in drug design: (a) to predict biological activity in untested compounds, (b) to define the structural requirements required for a good fit between the drug molecule and the receptor, and

(c) to design a test set of compounds to maximize the amount of information concerning structural requirements for activity from a minimum number of compounds tested. This aspect of medicinal chemistry is commonly referred to as quantitative structure–activity relationships (QSAR).

The goals of QSAR studies were first proposed about 1865 to 1870 by Crum-Brown and Fraser, who showed that the gradual chemical modification in the molecular structure of a series of poisons produced some important differences in their action.[1] They postulated that the physiological action, ϕ, of a molecule is a function of its chemical constitution, C. This can be expressed in Equation 2.5:

$$\phi = f(C) \qquad \text{(Eq. 2.5)}$$

Equation 2.5 states that a defined change in chemical structure results in a predictable change in physiological action. The problem now becomes one of numerically defining chemical structure. It still is a fertile area of research. What has been found is that biological response can be predicted from physical chemical properties such as vapor pressure, water solubility, electronic parameters, steric descriptors, and partition coefficients (Eq. 2.6). Today, the partition coefficient has become the single most important physical chemical measurement for QSAR studies. Note that Equation 2.6 is the equation for a straight line ($Y = mx + b$).

$$\log BR = a(\text{physical chemical property}) + c \qquad \text{(Eq. 2.6)}$$

where

BR = a defined pharmacological response usually expressed in millimoles such as the inhibitory constant K_i, the effective dose in 50% of the subjects (ED_{50}), the lethal dose in 50% of the subjects (LD_{50}), or the minimum inhibitory concentration (MIC). It is common to express the biological response as a reciprocal, $1/BR$ or $1/C$

a = the regression coefficient or slope of the straight line

c = the intercept term on the y axis (when the physical chemical property equals zero)

To understand the concepts in the next few paragraphs, it is necessary to know how to interpret defined pharmacological concepts such as the ED_{50}, which is the amount of the drug needed to obtain the defined pharmacological response in 50% of the test subjects. Let us assume that drug A's ED_{50} is 1 mmol and drug B's ED_{50} is 2 mmol. Drug A is twice as potent as drug B. In other words, the smaller the ED_{50} (or ED_{90}, LD_{50}, MIC, etc.), the more potent is the substance being tested.

The logarithmic value of the dependent variable (concentration necessary to obtain a defined biological response) is used to linearize the data. As shown later in this chapter, QSARs are not always linear. Nevertheless, using logarithms is an acceptable statistical technique (taking reciprocals obtained from a Michaelis-Menton study produces the linear Lineweaver-Burke plots found in any biochemistry textbook).

Now, why is the biological response usually expressed as a reciprocal? Sometimes, one obtains a statistically more valid relationship. More importantly, expressing the biological response as a reciprocal usually produces a positive slope (Fig. 2.7). Let us examine the following published example (Table 2.5). The BR is the LD_{100} (lethal dose in 100% of the subjects). The mechanism of death is general depression of the CNS.

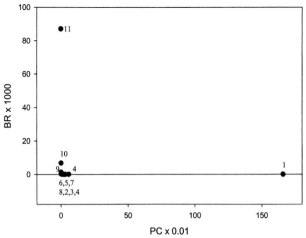

Figure 2.7 ● Plot of (BR × 1,000) versus (PC × 0.01).

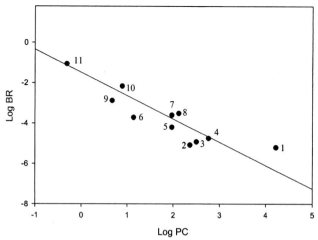

Figure 2.8 ● Plot of log BR versus log PC.

The most lethal compound in this assay was chlorpromazine, with a BR (LD$_{100}$) of only 0.00000631 mmol; and the least active was ethanol, with a BR of 0.087096 mmol. In other words, it takes about 13,800 times as many millimoles of ethanol than of chlorpromazine to kill 100% of the test subjects in this particular assay.

Plotting BR versus PC (partition coefficient) produces the nonlinear scatter shown in Figure 2.7. Note that compounds 1 and 11 lie at a considerable distance from the remaining nine compounds. In addition to the 13,800 times difference in activity, there is a 33,900 times difference in the octanol/water partition coefficient. An attempt at obtaining a linear regression equation produces the meaningless Equation. 2.7 whose equation is:

$$BR = -0.0000 \ PC + 0.0117 \qquad (Eq. \ 2.7)$$

It is meaningless statistically. The slope is 0, meaning that the partition coefficient has no effect on biological activity, and yet from the plot and Table 2.5, it is obvious that the higher the octanol/water partition coefficient, the more toxic the compound. The correlation coefficient (r^2) is 0.05, meaning that there is no significant statistical relationship between activity and partition coefficient.

Now, let us see if the data can be linearized by using the logarithms of the biological activity and partition coefficient. Notice the logarithmic terms. The difference between the LD$_{100}$ of chlorpromazine and ethanol is only 4.14

logarithmic units. Similarly, the difference between chlorpromazine's partition coefficient and that of ethanol is 4.53 logarithmic units. Figure 2.8 shows the plot and regression line for log BR versus log PC. It is an inverse relationship (Eq. 2.8) between physicochemical property and biological response. Otherwise, the regression equation is excellent with a correlation coefficient of 0.9191.

$$\log BR = -1.1517 \log PC - 1.4888 \qquad (Eq. \ 2.8)$$

Although there is no statistical advantage to using the log of the reciprocal of the biological response, the positive relationship is consistent with common observation that the biological activity increases as the partition coefficient (or other physicochemical parameter) increases. In interpreting plots such as that in Figure 2.9, remember that biological activity is increasing as the amount of compound required to obtain the defined biological response is decreasing. The equation for the line in Figure 2.9 is identical to Equation 2.8, except for the change to positive slope and sign of the intercept. The correlation coefficient also remains the same at 0.9191.

$$\log 1/BR = 1.517 \log PC + 1.4888 \qquad (Eq. \ 2.9)$$

Partition Coefficient

The most common physicochemical descriptor is the molecule's partition coefficient in an octanol/water system. As

---

TABLE 2.5 Data Used for a Quantitative Structure–Activity Relationship Study

Compound	Log 1/BR	1/BR	BR	BR × 1,000	Log BR	Log PC	PC × 0.01
1. Chlorpromazine	5.20	158,489.32	0.000006	0.006310	−5.2000	4.22	165.95869
2. Propoxyphene	5.08	120,226.44	0.000008	0.008318	−5.0800	2.36	2.2908677
3. Amitriptyline	4.92	83,176.38	0.000012	0.012023	−4.9200	2.50	3.1622777
4. Dothiepin	4.75	56,234.13	0.000018	0.017783	−4.7500	2.76	5.7543994
5. Secobarbital	4.19	15,488.17	0.000065	0.064565	−4.1900	1.97	0.9332543
6. Phenobarbital	3.71	5,128.61	0.000195	0.194984	−3.7100	.1.14	0.1380384
7. Chloroform	3.60	3,981.07	0.000251	0.251189	−3.6000	1.97	0.9332543
8. Chlormethiazole	3.51	3,235.94	0.000309	0.309030	−3.5100	2.12	1.3182567
9. Paraldehyde	2.88	758.58	0.001318	1.318257	−2.8800	0.67	0.0467735
10. Ether	2.17	147.91	0.006761	6.760830	−2.1700	0.89	0.0776247
11. Ethanol	1.06	11.48	0.087096	87.096359	−1.0600	−0.31	0.0048978

Source: Hansch, C., Björkroth, J. P., and Leo, A.: J. Pharm. Sci. 76:663, 1987.
BR is defined as the LD$_{100}$, and PC is the octanol/water partition coefficient.

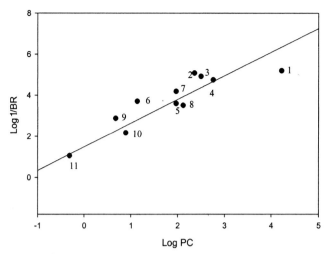

Figure 2.9 ● Plot of log 1/BR versus log PC.

percentage will be in their anionic forms. An assumption is made that the ionic form is water-soluble and will remain in the water phase of an octanol/water system. This *reality* has led to the use of log D, which is defined as the equilibrium ratio of both the ionized and un-ionized species of the molecule in an octanol/water system (Eq. 2.12). The percent ionization of ionized HA acids and BH protonated amines and acids can be estimated from Equations 2.3 and 2.4 and the log D from Equations 2.13 and 2.14, respectively.

$$\log D = \log\left(\frac{[\text{solute}]_{\text{oct}}}{[\text{solute}]_{\text{aq}}^{\text{ionized}} + [\text{solute}]_{\text{aq}}^{\text{nonionized}}}\right) \quad \text{(Eq. 2.12)}$$

$$\log D_{\text{acids}} = \log P = \log\left[\frac{1}{(1 + 10^{(\text{pH}-\text{pK}_a')})}\right] \quad \text{(Eq. 2.13)}$$

$$\log D_{\text{bases}} = \log P = \log\left[\frac{1}{(1 + 10^{(\text{pK}_a-\text{pH})})}\right] \quad \text{(Eq. 2.14)}$$

Because much of the time the drug's movement across membranes is a partitioning process, the partition coefficient has become the most common physicochemical property. The question that now must be asked is what immiscible nonpolar solvent system best mimics the water/lipid membrane barriers found in the body? It is now realized that the *n*-octanol/water system is an excellent estimator of drug partitioning in biological systems. One could argue that it was fortuitous that *n*-octanol was available in reasonable purity for the early partition coefficient determinations. To appreciate why this is so, one must understand the chemical nature of the lipid membranes.

These membranes are not exclusively anhydrous fatty or oily structures. As a first approximation, they can be considered bilayers composed of lipids consisting of a polar cap and large hydrophobic tail. Phosphoglycerides are major components of lipid bilayers (Fig. 2.10). Other groups of bifunctional lipids include the sphingomyelins, galactocerebrosides, and plasmalogens. The hydrophobic portion is composed largely of unsaturated fatty acids, mostly with *cis* double bonds. In addition, there are considerable amounts of cholesterol esters, protein, and charged mucopolysaccharides in the lipid membranes. The final result is that these membranes are highly organized structures composed of channels for transport of important molecules such as metabolites, chemical regulators (hormones), amino acids, glucose, and fatty acids into the cell and removal of waste products and biochemically produced products out of the

emphasized previously, the drug will go through a series of partitioning steps: (a) leaving the aqueous extracellular fluids, (b) passing through lipid membranes, and (c) entering other aqueous environments before reaching the receptor (Fig. 2.1). In this sense, a drug is undergoing the same partitioning phenomenon that happens to any chemical in a separatory funnel containing water and a nonpolar solvent such as hexane, chloroform, or ether. The partition coefficient (P) is the ratio of the molar concentration of chemical in the nonaqueous phase (usually 1-octanol) versus that in the aqueous phase (Eq. 2.10). For reasons already discussed, it is more common to use the logarithmic expression (Eq. 2.11). The difference between the separatory funnel model and what actually occurs in the body is that the partitioning in the funnel will reach an equilibrium at which the rate of chemical leaving the aqueous phase and entering the organic phase will equal the rate of the chemical moving from the organic phase to the aqueous phase. This is not the physiological situation. Refer to Figure 2.1 and note that dynamic changes are occurring to the drug, such as it being metabolized, bound to serum albumin, excreted from the body, and bound to receptors. The environment for the drug is not static. Upon administration, the drug will be *pushed* through the membranes because of the high concentration of drug in the extracellular fluids relative to the concentration in the intracellular compartments. In an attempt to maintain equilibrium ratios, the flow of the drug will be from systemic circulation through the membranes onto the receptors. As the drug is metabolized and excreted from the body, it will be *pulled* back across the membranes, and the concentration of drug at the receptors will decrease.

$$P = \frac{[\text{chemical}]_{\text{oct}}}{[\text{chemical}]_{\text{aq}}} \quad \text{(Eq. 2.10)}$$

$$\log P = \log\left(\frac{[\text{solute}]_{\text{oct}}}{[\text{solute}]_{\text{aq}}}\right) \quad \text{(Eq. 2.11)}$$

Equations 2.10 and 2.11 assume that the drug is in the nonpolar state. A large percentage of drugs are amines whose pK_a is such that at physiological pH 7.4, a significant percentage of the drug will be in its protonated, ionized form. A similar statement can be made for the HA acids (carboxyl, sulfonamide, imide) in that at physiological pH, a significant

Hydrophobic Tail

Lecithin: R = $OCH_2CH_2N^+(CH_3)_3$

Cephalin: R = $OCH_2CH_2NH_3^+$

Figure 2.10 ● General structure of a bifunctional phospholipid. Many of the fatty acid esters will be *cis* unsaturated.

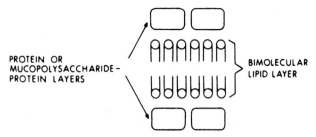

Figure 2.11 ● Schematic representation of the cell membrane.

PROTEIN OR MUCOPOLYSACCHARIDE-PROTEIN LAYERS

BIMOLECULAR LIPID LAYER

cell. The cellular membranes are dynamic, with the channels forming and disappearing depending on the cell's and body's needs (Fig. 2.11). So complex is this system that it is not uncommon to have situations where there is poor correlation between the partition coefficient of a series of molecules and the biological response.[2]

In addition, the membranes on the surface of nucleated cells have specific antigenic markers, major histocompatibility complex (MHC), by which the immune system monitors the cell's status. There are receptors on the cell surface where hormones such as epinephrine and insulin bind, setting off a series of biochemical events within the cell. Some of these receptors are used by viruses to gain entrance into the cells, where the virus reproduces. As newer instrumental techniques are developed, and genetic cloning permits isolation of the genetic material responsible for forming and regulating the structures on the cell surface, the image of a passive lipid membrane has disappeared to be replaced by a very complex, highly organized, dynamically functioning structure.

For purposes of the partitioning phenomenon, picture the cellular membranes as two layers of lipids (Fig. 2.9). The two outer layers, one facing the interior and the other facing the exterior of the cell, consist of the polar ends of the bifunctional lipids. Keep in mind that these surfaces are exposed to an aqueous polar environment. The polar ends of the charged phospholipids and other bifunctional lipids are solvated by the water molecules. There are also considerable amounts of charged proteins and mucopolysaccharides present on the surface. In contrast, the interior of the membrane is populated by the hydrophobic aliphatic chains from the fatty acid esters.

With this representation in mind, a partial explanation can be presented as to why the *n*-octanol/water partitioning system seems to mimic the lipid membranes/water systems found in the body. It turns out that *n*-octanol is not as nonpolar as initially might be predicted. Water-saturated octanol contains 2.3 M water because the small water molecule easily clusters around octanol's hydroxy moiety. *n*-Octanol–saturated water contains little of the organic phase because of the large hydrophobic 8-carbon chain of octanol. The water in the *n*-octanol phase apparently approximates the polar properties of the lipid bilayer, whereas the lack of octanol in the water phase mimics the physiological aqueous compartments, which are relatively free of nonpolar components. In contrast, partitioning systems such as hexane/water and chloroform/water contain so little water in the organic phase that they are poor models for the lipid bilayer/water system found in the body. At the same time, remember that the *n*-octanol/water system is only an approximation of the actual environment found in the interface between the cellular membranes and the extracellular/intracellular fluids.

Experimental determination of octanol/water partition coefficients is tedious and time consuming. Today, most are calculated. The accuracy of these calculations is only as good as the assumptions made by the writers of the software. These include atomic fragment values, correction factors, spatial properties, effects of resonance and induction, internal secondary bonding forces, etc. There are over 30 different software packages for calculating a molecules partition coefficient, and their accuracy varies widely.[3,4]

Other Physicochemical and Descriptor Parameters

There is a series of other descriptors that measure the contribution by substituents to the molecule's total physicochemical properties. These include Hammett's ϕ constant; Taft's steric parameter, E_s; Charton's steric parameter, v; Verloop's multidimensional steric parameters, L, B_1, B_5; and molar refractivity, MR, number of hydrogen bond donors and acceptors, pK_a, polar surface area, number of rotatable bonds, connectivity indices, and the list goes into the thousands. Although directories of these have been published, it is common to calculate them. Table 2.6 lists a very small set and illustrates several items that must be kept in mind when selecting substituents to be evaluated in terms of the type of factors that influence a biological response. For electronic parameters such as ϕ, the location on an aromatic ring is important because of resonance versus inductive effects. Notice the twofold differences seen between ϕ_{meta} and ϕ_{para} for the three aliphatic substituents and iodo, and severalfold difference for methoxy, amino, fluoro, and phenolic hydroxyl.

Selection of substituents from a certain chemical class may not really test the influence of a parameter on biological activity. There is little numerical difference among the ϕ_{meta} or ϕ_{para} values for the four aliphatic groups or the four halogens. It is not uncommon to go to the tables and find missing parameters such as the E_s values for acetyl and *N*-acyl.

TABLE 2.6 **Sampling of Physicochemical Parameters Used in Quantitative Structure–Activity Relationships Investigations**

Substituent Group	π	σ_{meta}	σ_{para}	E_s	MR
—H	0.00	0.00	0.00	0.00	1.03
—CH$_3$	0.56	−0.07	−0.17	−1.24	5.65
—CH$_2$CH$_3$	1.02	−0.07	−0.15	−1.31	10.30
—CH$_2$CH$_2$CH$_3$	1.55	−0.07	−0.13	−1.60	14.96
—C(CH$_3$)$_2$	1.53	−0.07	−0.15	−1.71	14.96
—OCH$_3$	−0.02	0.12	−0.27	−0.55	7.87
—NH$_2$	−1.23	−0.16	−0.66	−0.61	5.42
—F	0.14	0.34	0.06	−0.46	0.92
—Cl	0.71	0.37	0.23	−0.97	6.03
—Br	0.86	0.39	0.23	−1.16	8.88
—I	1.12	0.35	0.18	−1.40	13.94
—CF$_3$	0.88	0.43	0.54	−2.40	5.02
—OH	−0.67	0.12	−0.37	−0.55	2.85
—COCH$_3$	−0.55	0.38	0.50		11.18
—NHCOCH$_3$	−0.97	0.21	0.00		14.93
—NO$_2$	−0.8	0.71	0.78	−2.52	7.36
—CN	−0.57	0.56	0.66	−0.51	6.33

Reprinted with permission from Hansch, C., and Leo, A. J.: Substituent Constants for Correlation Analysis in Chemistry and Biology. New York, John Wiley & Sons, 1979.

Nevertheless, medicinal chemists can use information from extensive tables of physicochemical parameters to minimize the number of substituents required to find out if the biological response is sensitive to electronic, steric, and/or partitioning effects.[5] This is done by selecting substituents in each of the numerical ranges for the different parameters. In Table 2.6, there are three ranges of B values (-1.23 to -0.55, -0.28 to 0.56, and 0.71 to 1.55); three ranges of MR values (0.92–2.85, 5.02–8.88, and 10.30–14.96); and two main clusters of ϕ values, one for the aliphatic substituents and the other for the halogens. In the ideal situation, substituents are selected from each of the clusters to determine the dependence of the biological response over the largest possible variable space. Depending on the biological responses obtained from testing the new compounds, it is possible to determine if lipophilicity (partitioning), steric bulk (molar refraction), or electron-withdrawing/donating properties are important determinants of the desired biological response.

With this background in mind, two examples of QSAR equations taken from the medicinal chemistry literature are presented. A study of a group of griseofulvin analogs showed a linear relationship (Eq. 2.15) between the biological response and both lipophilicity (log P) and electronic character (σ).[6] It was suggested that the antibiotic activity may depend on the enone system facilitating the addition of griseofulvin to a nucleophilic group such as the SH moiety in a fungal enzyme.

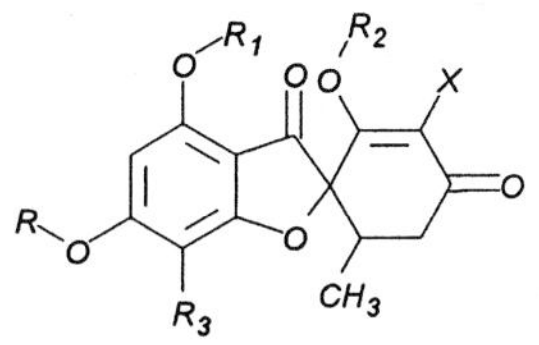

Griseofulvin: $R = R_1 = R_2 = OCH_3$; $R_3 = Cl$; $X = H$

$$\log BR = (0.56)\log P + (2.19)\sigma_x - 1.32 \quad \text{(Eq. 2.15)}$$

A parabolic relationship (Eq. 2.16) was reported for a series of substituted acetylated salicylates (substituted aspirins) tested for anti-inflammatory activity.[7] A nonlinear relationship exists between the biological response and lipophilicity, and a significant detrimental steric effect

is seen with substituents at position 4. The two sterimol parameters used in this equation were L, defined as the length of the substituent along the axis of the bond between the first atom of the substituent and the parent molecule, and B_2, defined as a width parameter. Steric effects were not considered statistically significant at position 3, as shown by the sterimol parameters for substituents at position 3 not being part of Equation 2.16. The optimal partition coefficient (log P_o) for the substituted aspirins in this assay was 2.6. At the same time, increasing bulk, as measured by the sterimol parameters, decreases activity.

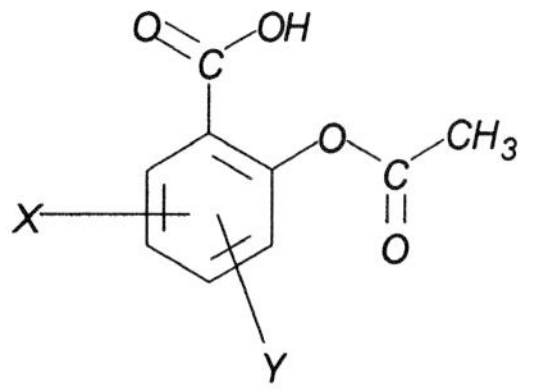

Aspirin: $X = Y = H$

$$\log 1/ED_{50} = 1.03 \log P - 0.20(\log P)^2$$
$$-0.05 L_{(4)} - 0.24 B_{2(4)} + 2.29 \quad \text{(Eq. 2.16)}$$

At this point, it is appropriate to ask the question, "are all the determinations of partition coefficients and compilation of physical chemical parameters useful only when a statistically valid QSAR model is obtained?" The answer is a firm *no*. One of the most useful spinoffs from the field of QSAR has been the application of experimental design to the selection of new compounds to be synthesized and tested. Let us assume that a new series of drug molecules is to be synthesized based on the following structure. The goal is to test the effect of the 16-substituents in Table 2.6 at each of the three positions on our new series. The number of possible analogs is equal to 16^3, or 4,096, compounds, assuming that all three positions will always be substituted with one of the substituents from Table 2.7. If hydrogen is included when a position is not substituted, there are 17^3, or 4,913, different combinations. The problem is to select a small number of substituents that represent the different ranges or clusters of values for lipophilicity, electronic influence, and bulk. An initial design set could include the methyl and propyl from the

TABLE 2.7 Connectivity Table for Hydrogen-Suppressed Phenylalanine

Atom	O-1	C-2	O-3	C-4	N-5	C-6	C-7	C-8	C-9	C-10	C-11	C-12
O-1		X										
C-2	X		X	X								
O-3		X										
C-4		X			X	X						
N-5				X								
C-6				X			X					
C-7						X		X				X
C-8							X		X			
C-9								X		X		
C-10									X		X	
C-11										X		X
C-12						X					X	

aliphatic cluster, fluorine and chlorine from the halogen cluster, *N*-acetyl and phenol from the substituents showing hydrophilicity, and a range of electronic and bulk values. Including hydrogen, there will be 7^3, or 343, different combinations. Obviously, that is too many for an initial evaluation. Instead, certain rules have been devised to maximize the information obtained from a minimum number of compounds. These include the following:

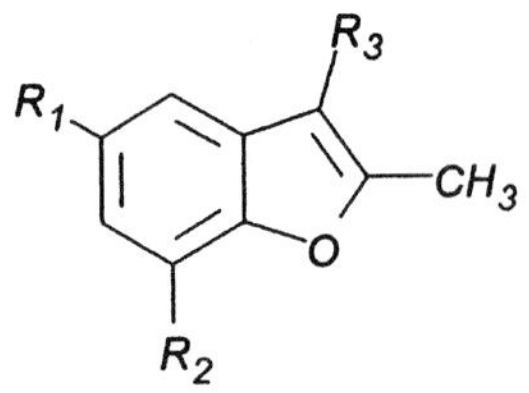

1. Each substituent must occur more than once at each position on which it is found.
2. The number of times that each substituent at a particular position appears should be approximately equal.
3. No two substituents should be present in a constant combination.
4. When combinations of substituents are a necessity, they should not occur more frequently than any other combination.

Following these guidelines, the initial test set can be reduced to 24 to 26 compounds. Depending on the precision of the biological tests, it will be possible to see if the data will fit a QSAR model. Even an approximate model usually will indicate the types of substituents to test further and what positions on the molecules are sensitive to substitution and, if sensitive, to what degree variation in lipophilic, electronic, or bulk character is important. Just to ensure that the model is valid, it is a good idea to synthesize a couple of compounds that the model predicts would be inactive. As each group of new compounds is tested, the QSAR model is refined until the investigators have a pretty good idea what substituent patterns are important for the desired activity. These same techniques used to develop potent compounds with desired activity also can be used to evaluate the influence of substituent patterns on undesired toxic effects and pharmacokinetic properties.

Topological Descriptors

An alternate method of describing molecular structure is based on graph theory, in which the bonds connecting the atoms is considered a path that is traversed from one atom to another. Consider Figure 2.12 containing D-phenylalanine

and its hydrogen-suppressed graph representation. The numbering is arbitrary and not based on International Union of Pure and Applied Chemistry (IUPAC) or *Chemical Abstracts* nomenclature rules. A connectivity table, Table 2.7, is constructed.

Table 2.7 is a two-dimensional connectivity table for the hydrogen-suppressed phenylalanine molecule. No 3D representation is implied. Further, this type of connectivity table will be the same for molecules with asymmetric atoms (D vs. L) or for those that can exist in more than one conformation (i.e., *chair* vs. *boat* conformation, *anti* vs. *gauche* vs. *eclipsed*).

Graph theory is not limited to the paths followed by chemical bonds. In its purest form, the atoms in the phenyl ring of phenylalanine would have paths connecting atom 7 with atoms 9, 10, 11, and 12; atom 8 with atoms 10, 11, and 12; atom 9 with atoms 11 and 12; and atom 10 with atom 12. Also, the graph itself might differentiate neither single, double, and triple bonds nor the type of atom (C, O, and N in the phenylalanine example). Connectivity tables can be coded to indicate the type of bond.

The most common application of graph theory used by medicinal chemistry is called *molecular connectivity*. It limits the paths to the molecule's actual chemical bonds. Table 2.8 shows several possible paths for phenylalanine, including linear paths and clusters or branching. Numerical values for each path or path-cluster are based on the number of nonhydrogen bonds to each atom. Let us examine oxygen atom 1. There is only one nonhydrogen bond, and it connects oxygen atom 1 to carbon atom 2. The formula is the reciprocal square root of the number of bonds. For oxygen 1, the connectivity value is 1. For carbonyl oxygen 2, it is $2^{-1/2}$, or 0.707. Note that there is no difference between oxygen 1 and nitrogen 5. Both have only one nonhydrogen bond and a connectivity value of 1. Similarly, there is no difference in values for a carbonyl oxygen and a methylene carbon, each having two nonhydrogen bonds. The final connectivity values for a path are the reciprocal square roots of the products of each path. For the second-order path 2C-4C-6C, the reciprocal square root $(3 \times 3 \times 2)^{-1/2}$ is 4.243. The values for each path order are calculated and summed.

As noted previously, the method as described so far cannot distinguish between atoms that have the same number of nonhydrogen bonds. A method to distinguish heteroatoms from each other and carbon atoms is based on the difference between the number of valence electrons and possible hydrogen atoms (which are suppressed in the graph). The *valence* connectivity term for an alcoholic oxygen would be 6 valence electrons minus 1 hydrogen, or 5. The *valence* connectivity term for a primary amine

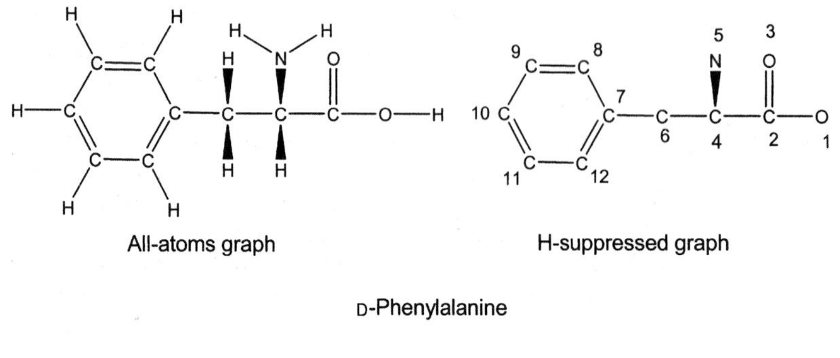

All-atoms graph   H-suppressed graph

D-Phenylalanine

Figure 2.12 ● Hydrogen-suppressed graphic representation of phenylalanine.

TABLE 2.8 Examples of Paths Found in the Phenylalanine Molecule

1st Order Path	2nd Order Path	3rd Order Path	4th Order Path	5th Order Path	Path-Cluster
1O-2C	1O-2C-3O	1O-2C-4C-6C	1O-2C-4C-6C-7C	1O-2C-4C-6C-7C-8C	1O-2C-3O-4C
2C-3O	1O-2C-4C	3O-2C-4C-5N	3O-2C-4C-6C-7C	1O-2C-4O-6C-7C-12C	2C-4C-5N-6C
2C-4C	3O-2C-4C	3O-2C-4C-6C	2C-4C-6C-7C-8C	2C-4C-6C-7C-8C-9C	6C-7C-8C-12C
4C-5N	2C-4C-5N	1O-2C-4C-5N	2C-4C-6C-7C-12C	2C-4C-6C-7C-12C-11C	
4C-6C	2C-4C-6C	2C-4C-6C-7C	4C-6C-7C-8C-9C	3O-2C-4C-6C-7C-8C	
6C-7C	5N-4C-6C	5N-4C-6C-7C	4C-6C-7C-12C-11C	3O-2C-4C-6C-7C-12C	
7C-8C	4C-6C-7C	4C-6C-7C-8C	5N-4C-6C-7C-8C	4C-6C-7C-8C-9C-10C	
8C-9C	6C-7C-8C	4C-6C-7C-12C	5N-4C-6C-7C-12C	4C-6C-7C-12C-11C-10C	
7C-12C	6C-7C-12C	6C-7C-8C-9C	6C-7C-8C-9C-10C	5N-4C-6C-7C-8C-9C	
9C-10C	7C-8C-9C	6C-7C-12C-11C	6C-7C-12C-11C-10C	5N-4C-6C-7C-12C-11C	
10C-11C	7C-12C-11C	7C-8C-9C-10C	7C-8C-9C-10C-11C	6C-7C-8C-9C-10C-11C	
11C-12C	8C-9C-10C	7C-12C-11C-10C	7C-12C-11C-10C-9C	6C-7C-12C-11C-10C	
	9C-10C-11C	8C-9C-10C-11C	8C-9C-10C-11C-12C	7C-8C-9C-10C-11C-12C	
	10C-11C-12C	9C-10C-11C-12C		7C-12C-11C-10C-9C-8C	

nitrogen would be 5 valence electrons minus 2 hydrogens, or 3. There are various additional modifications that are done to further differentiate atoms and define their environments within the molecule.

Excellent regression equations using topological indices have been obtained. A problem is interpreting what they mean. Is it lipophilicity, steric bulk, or electronic terms that define activity? The topological indices can be correlated with all of these common physicochemical descriptors. Another problem is that it is difficult to use the equation to decide what molecular modifications can be made to enhance activity further, again because of ambiguities in physicochemical interpretation. Should the medicinal chemist increase or decrease lipophilicity at a particular location on the molecule? Should specific substituents be increased or decreased? On the other hand, topological indices can be very valuable in classification schemes that are described later in this chapter. They do describe the structure in terms of rings, branching, flexibility, etc.

Classification Methods

Besides regression analysis, there are other statistical techniques used in drug design. These fit under the classification of multivariate statistics and include discriminant analysis, principal component analysis, and pattern recognition. The latter can consist of a mixture of statistical and nonstatistical methodologies. The goal usually is to try to ascertain what physicochemical parameters and structural attributes contribute to a class or type of biological activity. Then, the chemicals are classified into groupings such as carcinogenic/noncarcinogenic, sweet/bitter, active/inactive, and depressant/stimulant.

The term *multivariate* is used because of the wide variety and number of independent or descriptor variables that may be used. The same physicochemical parameters seen in QSAR analyses are used, but in addition, the software in the computer programs *breaks* the molecule down into substructures. These structural fragments also become variables. Examples of the typical substructures used include carbonyls, enones, conjugation, rings of different sizes and types, N-substitution patterns, and aliphatic substitution patterns such as 1,3- or 1,2-disubstituted. The end result is that for even a moderate-size molecule typical of most drugs, there can be 50 to 100 variables.

The technique is to develop a large set of chemicals well characterized in terms of the biological activity that is going to be predicted. This is known as the *training set*. Ideally, it should contain hundreds, if not thousands, of compounds, divided into active and inactive types. In reality, sets smaller than 100 are studied. Most of these investigations are retrospective ones in which the investigator locates large data sets from several sources. This means that the biological testing likely followed different protocols. That is why classification techniques tend to avoid using continuous variables such as ED_{50}, LD_{50}, and MIC. Instead, arbitrary end points such as active or inactive, stimulant or depressant, sweet or sour, are used.

Once the training set is established, the multivariate technique is carried out. The algorithms are designed to group the underlying commonalities and select the variables that have the greatest influence on biological activity. The predictive ability is then tested with a test set of compounds that have been put through the same biological tests used for the training set. For the classification model to be valid, the investigator must select data sets whose results are not intuitively obvious and could not be classified by a trained medicinal chemist. Properly done, classification methods can identify structural and physicochemical descriptors that can be powerful predictors and determinants of biological activity.

There are several examples of successful applications of this technique.[8] One study consisted of a diverse group of 140 tranquilizers and 79 sedatives subjected to a two-way classification study (tranquilizers vs. sedatives). The ring types included phenothiazines, indoles, benzodiazepines, barbiturates, diphenylmethanes, and various heterocyclics. Sixty-nine descriptors were used initially to characterize the molecules. Eleven of these descriptors were crucial to the classification, 54 had intermediate use and depended on the composition of the training set, and 4 were of little use. The overall range of prediction accuracy was 88% to 92%. The results with the 54 descriptors indicate an important limitation when large numbers of descriptors are used. The inclusion or exclusion of descriptors and parameters can depend on the composition of the training set. The training set must be representative of the population of chemicals that are going to be evaluated. Repeating the study on different randomly selected training sets is important.

Classification techniques lend themselves to studies lacking quantitative data. An interesting classification problem involved olfactory stimulants, in which the goal was to select chemicals that had a musk odor. A group of 300 unique compounds was selected from a group of odorants that included 60 musk odorants plus 49 camphor, 44 floral, 32 ethereal, 41 mint, 51 pungent, and 23 putrid odorants. Initially, 68 descriptors were evaluated. Depending on the approach, the number of descriptors was reduced to 11 to 16, consisting mostly of bond types. Using this small number, the 60 musk odorants could be selected from the remaining 240 compounds, with an accuracy of 95% to 97%.

The use of classification techniques in medicinal chemistry has matured over years of general use. The types of descriptors have expanded to spatial measurements in 3D space similar to those used in 3D-QSAR (see discussion that follows). Increasingly, databases of existing compounds are scanned for molecules that possess what appear to be the desired parameters. If the scan is successful, compounds that are predicted to be active provide the starting point for synthesizing new compounds for testing. One can see parallels between the search of chemical databases and screening plant, animal, and microbial sources for new compounds. Although the statistical and pattern recognition methodologies have been in use for a very long time, there still needs to be considerable research into their proper use, and further testing of their predictive power is needed. The goal of scanning databases of already synthesized compounds to select compounds for pharmacological evaluation will require considerable additional development of the various multivariate techniques.

This chapter is limited to fairly simple computational techniques using readily available, low-cost software. The QSAR approach, including classification methods has at its disposal literally thousands of different descriptors, each with its advocates, and many computational approaches starting with the previously discussed linear regression to neural networks, decision trees and support vector machines. Thus, it is fair to ask if drug discoveries have been made with these computational techniques. The answer is in the ambiguous *yes-and-no* category depending on who is asked. There is general agreement

that QSAR provided the foundation to better understand the relationship between *chemical space* and *pharmacological space*. Consider these two pairs of active molecules. For classification purposes, acetylcholine and nicotine are nicotinic agonists, and dopamine and pergolide are dopaminergic agonists. Using the various measures of similarity and their descriptors, fingerprints, and fragments, these two pairs come up as dissimilar. It is true that the pharmacological profiles of acetylcholine—nicotine and dopamine—pergolide vary so much that nicotine is not used as a nicotinic agonist and pergolide is falling into disuse.[9,10] Without being trite, computational drug design techniques are not going to replace the medicinal chemist who has an open, inquiring mind.

Has QSAR Been Successful?

The answer to this question depends on what are the expectations.[11] In their original development, it was hoped that QSAR equations would lead to commercially successful drugs. This has not occurred. Over the years, methodologies to develop these equations have changed. In the early development of QSAR equations, all of the compounds in a data set were used followed by random holding out of compounds to see if the equation changed. If there are enough compounds, it is now more common to begin with a *training set* and evaluate its validity with a *test set*. This has led to recommendations on the most reliable statistical measurements of validity.[12–14]

Paralleling the evolution in the use of different statistical measures of validity, deriving these equations has lead to the development of a wide variety of descriptors ranging from descriptive, physicochemical and topological. What can be frustrating is that the quality of predictions is dependent on the descriptor set.[15] It must be remembered that most of descriptors are only as good as the algorithms used to calculate them. Further, it can be difficult to interpret exactly what the descriptors are measuring in chemical space. QSAR equations must explain physical reality if predictions for future compounds are to be made.[16]

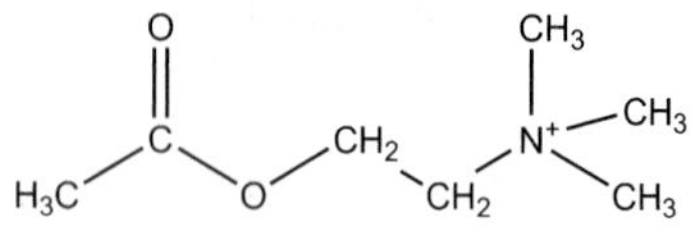

Acetylcholine

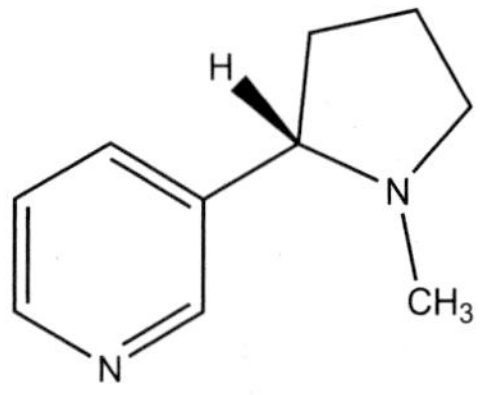

Nicotine

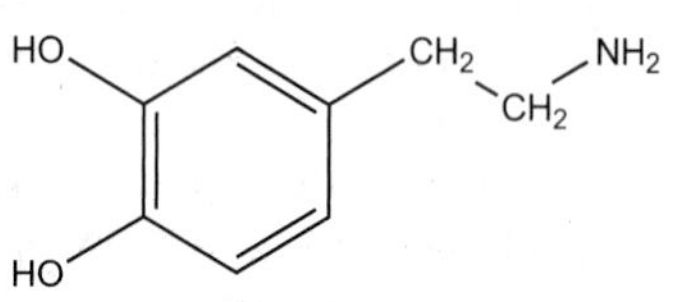

Dopamine

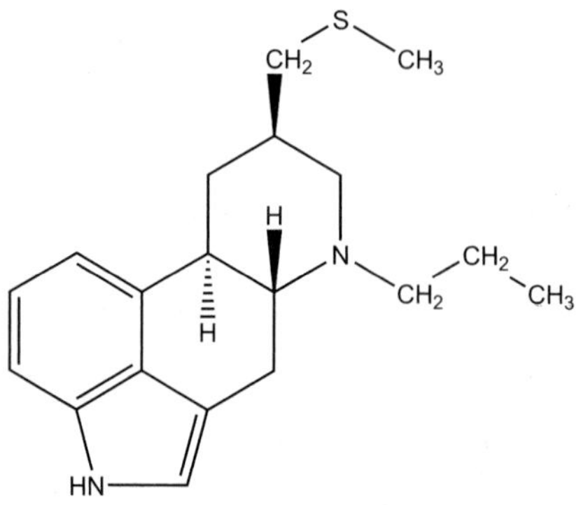

Pergolide

◉ COMPUTER-AIDED DRUG DESIGN: NEWER METHODS

Because powerful computing power, high-resolution computer graphics, and applicable software has reached the desktop, computational drug design methods are widely used in both industrial and academic environments. Through the use of computer graphics, structures of organic molecules can be entered into a computer and manipulated in many ways. Computational chemistry methods are used to calculate molecular properties and generate pharmacophore hypotheses. Once a pharmacophore hypothesis has been developed, structural databases (commercial, corporate, and/or public) of 3D structures can be searched rapidly for *hits* (i.e., existing compounds that are available with the required functional groups and permissible spatial orientations as defined by the search query). It has become popular to carry out *in silico* (computer as opposed to biological) screening of drug–receptor candidate interactions, known as *virtual* high-throughput screening (*v*HTS), for future development. The realistic goal of *v*HTS is to identify potential lead compounds. The drug–receptor fit and predicted physicochemical properties are used to *score* and *rank* compounds according to penalty functions and information filters (molecular weight, number of hydrogen bonds, hydrophobicity, etc.). Although medicinal chemists have always been aware of *a*bsorption, *d*istribution, *m*etabolism, *e*limination, and *t*oxicity (ADMET or ADME/Tox), in recent years, a much more focused approach addresses these issues in the early design stages. Increased efforts to develop computer-based absorption, distribution, metabolism, and elimination (ADME) models are being pursued aggressively. Many of the *predictive* ADME models use QSAR methods described earlier in this chapter. In general, understanding what chemical space descriptors are critical for druglike molecules helps provide insight into the design of chemical libraries for biological evaluation.

Today's computers and software give the medicinal chemist the ability to *design* the molecule on the basis of an estimated fit onto a receptor or have similar spatial characteristics found in the prototypical lead compound. Of course, this assumes that the molecular structure of the receptor is known in enough detail for a reasonable estimation of its 3D shape. When a good understanding of the geometry of the active site is known, databases containing the 3D coordinates of the chemicals in the database can be searched rapidly by computer programs that select candidates likely to fit in the active site. As shown later, there have been some dramatic successes with use of this approach, but first one must have an understanding of ligand (drug)–receptor interactions and conformational analysis.

Forces Involved with Drug–Receptor Interactions

Keep in mind that a biological response is produced by the interaction of a drug with a functional or organized group of molecules. This interaction would be expected to take place by using the same bonding forces as are involved when simple molecules interact. These, together with typical examples, are collected in Table 2.9.

TABLE 2.9 Types of Chemical Bonds

Bond Type	Bond Strength (kcal/mol)	Example
Covalent	40–140	$CH_3—OH$
Reinforced ionic	10	
Ionic	5	$R_4N^{\oplus} \cdots {}^{\ominus}I$
Hydrogen	1–7	
Ion–dipole	1–7	$R_4N^{\oplus} \cdots :NR_3$
Dipole–dipole	1–7	
van der Waals	0.5–1	
Hydrophobic	1	See text

Source: Albert, A.: Selective Toxicity. New York, John Wiley & Sons, 1986, p. 183.

Most drugs do not possess functional groups of a type that would lead to ready formation of strong and essentially irreversible covalent bonds between drug and biological receptors. In most cases, it is desirable to have the drug leave the receptor site when the concentration decreases in the extracellular fluids. Therefore, most useful drugs are held to their receptors by ionic or weaker bonds. When relatively long-lasting or irreversible effects are desired (e.g., antibacterial, anticancer), drugs that form covalent bonds with the receptor are effective and useful. The alkylating agents, such as the nitrogen mustards used in cancer chemotherapy, furnish an example of drugs that act by formation of covalent bonds (see Chapter 10).

Covalent bond formation between drug and receptor is the basis of Baker's concept of *active-site-directed irreversible inhibition.*[17] Considerable experimental evidence on the nature of enzyme inhibitors supports this concept. Compounds studied possess appropriate structural features for reversible and highly selective association with an enzyme. If, in addition, the compounds carry reactive groups capable of forming covalent bonds, the substrate may be irreversibly bound to the drug–receptor complex by covalent bond formation with reactive groups adjacent to the active site. The diuretic drug ethacrynic acid (see Chapter 19) is an α,β-unsaturated ketone, thought to act by covalent bond formation with sulfhydryl groups of ion transport systems in the renal tubules. Another example of a drug that covalently binds to the receptor is selegiline (see Chapter 13), an inhibitor of monoamine oxidase-B. Other examples of covalent bond formation between drug and biological receptor site include the reaction of arsenicals and mercurials with cysteine sulfhydryl groups, the acylation of bacterial cell wall constituents by penicillin, and the phosphorylation of the serine hydroxyl moiety at the active site of cholinesterase by organic phosphates.

Ethacrynic Acid

Selegiline

Keep in mind that it is desirable to have most drug effects reversible. For this to occur, relatively weak forces must be involved in the drug–receptor complex yet be strong enough that other binding sites will not competitively deplete the site of action. Compounds with high structural specificity may orient several weakly binding groups so that the summation of their interactions with specifically oriented complementary groups on the receptor provides total bond strength sufficient for a stable combination. Consequently, most drugs acting by virtue of their structural specificity will bind to the receptor site by hydrogen bonds, ionic bonds, ion–dipole and dipole–dipole interactions, and van der Waals and hydrophobic forces.

Considering the wide variety of functional groups found on a drug molecule and receptor, there will be a variety of secondary bonding forces. Ionization at physiological pH would normally occur with the carboxyl, sulfonamido, and aliphatic amino groups, as well as the quaternary ammonium group at any pH. These sources of potential ionic bonds are frequently found in active drugs. Differences in electronegativity between carbon and other atoms, such as oxygen and nitrogen, lead to an asymmetric distribution of electrons (dipoles) that are also capable of forming weak bonds with regions of high or low electron density, such as ions or other dipoles. Carbonyl, ester, amide, ether, nitrile, and related groups that contain such dipolar functions are frequently found in equivalent locations in structurally specific drugs.

The relative importance of the *hydrogen bond* in the formation of a drug–receptor complex is difficult to assess. Many drugs possess groups such as carbonyl, hydroxyl, amino, and imino, with the structural capabilities of acting as acceptors or donors in the formation of hydrogen bonds. However, such groups would usually be solvated by water, as would the corresponding groups on a biological receptor. Relatively little net change in free energy would be expected in exchanging a hydrogen bond with a water molecule for one between drug and receptor. However, in a drug–receptor combination, several forces could be involved, including the hydrogen bond, which would contribute to the stability of the interaction. Where multiple hydrogen bonds may be formed, the total effect may be sizable, such as that demonstrated by the stability of the protein α-helix and by the stabilizing influence of hydrogen bonds between specific base pairs in the double-helical structure of DNA.

Van der Waals forces are attractive forces created by the polarizability of molecules and are exerted when any two uncharged atoms approach each other very closely. Their strength is inversely proportional to the seventh power of the distance. Although individually weak, the summation of their forces provides a significant bonding factor in higher–molecular-weight compounds. For example, it is not possible to distill normal alkanes with more than 80 carbon atoms, because the energy of 80 kcal/mol required to separate the molecules is approximately equal to the energy required to break a carbon–carbon covalent bond. Flat structures, such as aromatic rings, permit close approach of atoms. The aromatic ring is frequently found in active drugs, and a reasonable explanation for its requirement for many types of biological activity may be derived from the contributions of this flat surface to van der Waals binding to a correspondingly flat receptor area.

The *hydrophobic bond* is a concept used to explain attractive interactions between nonpolar regions of the receptor and the drug. Explanations such as the *isopropyl moiety of the drug fits into a hydrophobic cleft on the receptor composed of the hydrocarbon side chains of the amino acids valine, isoleucine, and leucine* are commonly used to explain why a nonpolar substituent at a particular position on the drug molecule is important for activity. Over the years, the concept of hydrophobic bonds has developed. There has been considerable controversy over whether the bond actually exists. Thermodynamic arguments on the gain in entropy (decrease in ordered state) when hydrophobic groups cause a partial collapse of the ordered water structure on the surface of the receptor have been proposed to validate a hydrophobic bonding model. There are two problems with this concept. First, the term *hydrophobic* implies repulsion. The term for attraction is *hydrophilicity*. Second, and perhaps more important, there is no truly water-free region on the receptor. This is true even in the areas populated by the nonpolar amino acid side chains. An alternate approach is to consider only the concept of hydrophilicity and lipophilicity. The predominating water molecules solvate polar moieties, effectively squeezing the nonpolar residues toward each other.

STERIC FEATURES OF DRUGS

Regardless of the ultimate mechanism by which the drug and the receptor interact, the drug must approach the receptor and fit closely to its surface. Steric factors determined by the stereochemistry of the receptor site surface and that of the drug molecules are, therefore, of primary importance in determining the nature and the efficiency of the drug–receptor interaction. With the possible exception of the general anesthetics, such drugs must possess a high structural specificity to initiate a response at a particular receptor.

Some structural features contribute a high structural rigidity to the molecule. For example, aromatic rings are planar, and the atoms attached directly to these rings are held in the plane of the aromatic ring. Hence, the quaternary

Neostigmine

nitrogen and carbamate oxygen attached directly to the benzene ring in the cholinesterase inhibitor neostigmine are restricted to the plane of the ring, and consequently, the spatial arrangement of at least these atoms is established.

The relative positions of atoms attached directly to multiple bonds are also fixed. For the double bond, *cis*- and *trans*-isomers result. For example, diethylstilbestrol exists in two fixed stereoisomeric forms: *trans*-diethylstilbestrol is estrogenic, whereas the *cis*-isomer is only 7% as active. In *trans*-diethylstilbestrol, resonance interactions and minimal steric interference tend to hold the two aromatic rings and connecting ethylene carbon atoms in the same plane.

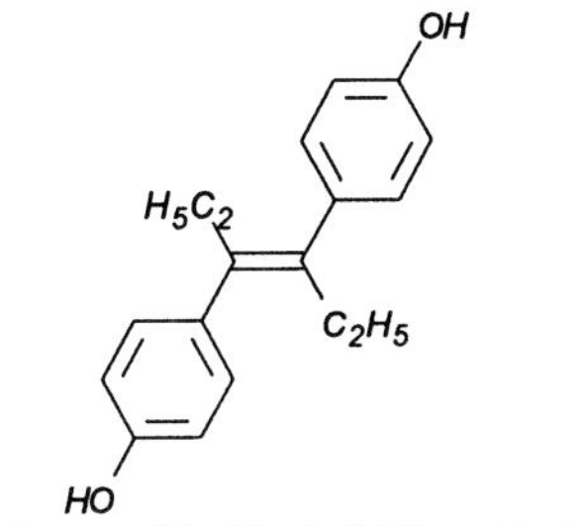

Geometric isomers, such as the *cis*- and the *trans*-isomers, hold structural features at different relative positions in space. These isomers also have significantly different physical and chemical properties. Therefore, their distributions in the biological medium are different, as are their capabilities for interacting with a biological receptor in a structurally specific manner. The *United States Pharmacopeia* recognizes that there are drugs with vinyl groups whose commercial form contains both their *E*- and *Z*-isomers. Figure 2.13 provides four examples of these mixtures.

More subtle differences exist for *conformational* isomers. Like geometric isomers, these exist as different arrangements in space for the atoms or groups in a single classic structure. Rotation about bonds allows interconversion of conformational isomers. However, an energy barrier between isomers is often high enough for their independent existence and reaction. Differences in reactivity of functional groups or interaction with biological receptors may be caused by differences in steric requirements of the receptors. In certain semirigid ring systems, conformational isomers show significant differences in biological activities. Methods for calculating these energy barriers are described next.

Open chains of atoms, which form an important part of many drug molecules, are not equally free to assume all possible conformations; some are sterically preferred. Energy barriers to free rotation of the chains are present because of interactions of nonbonded atoms. For example, the atoms tend to position themselves in space so that they occupy staggered positions, with no two atoms directly facing each other (eclipsed). Nonbonded interactions in polymethylene

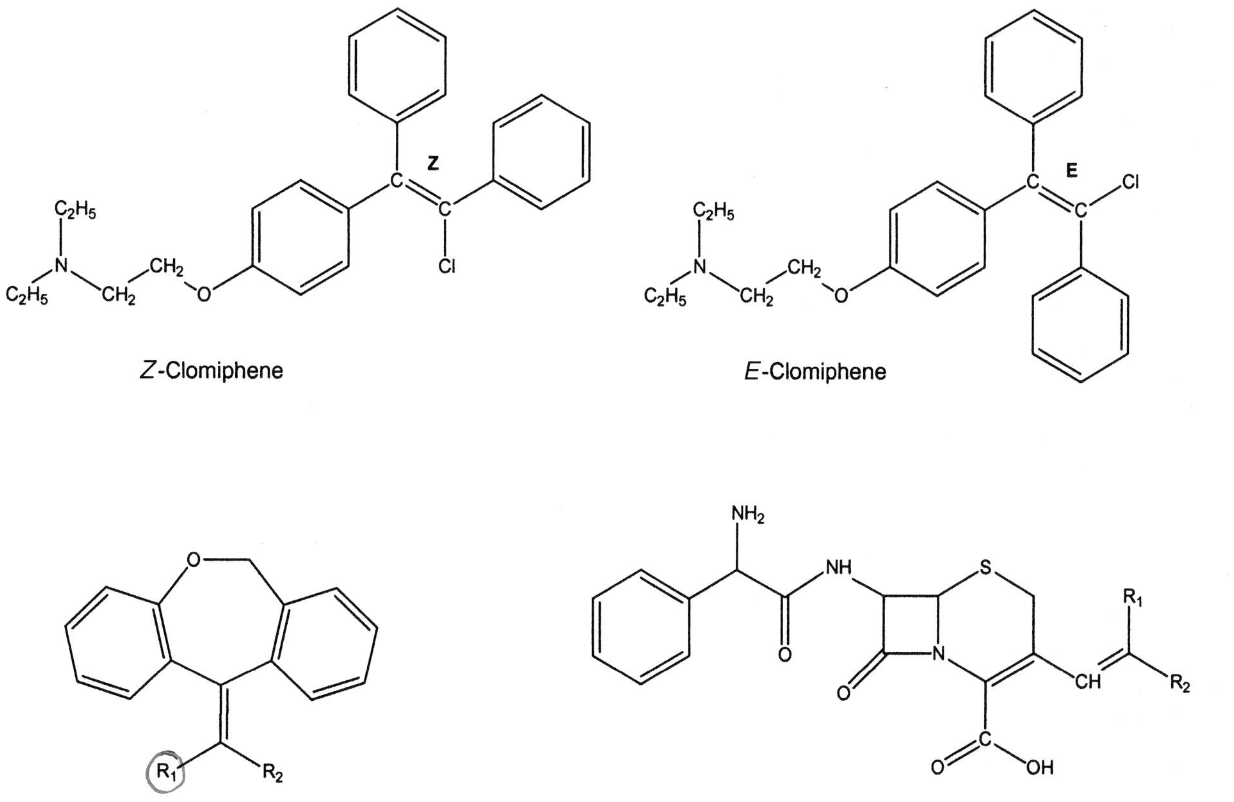

trans-Diethylstilbestrol

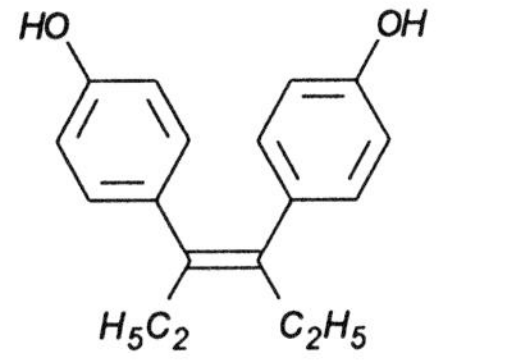

cis-Diethylstilbestrol

Z-Clomiphene

E-Clomiphene

Z-Doxepin: R_1 = $CH_2CH_2N(CH_3)_2$; R_2 = H
E-Doxepin: R_1 = H; R_2 = $CH_2CH_2N(CH_3)_2$

Z-Cefprozil: R_1 = H; R_2 = CH_3
E-Cefprozil: R_1 = CH_3; R_2 = H

Figure 2.13 ● Examples of *E*- and *Z*-isomers.

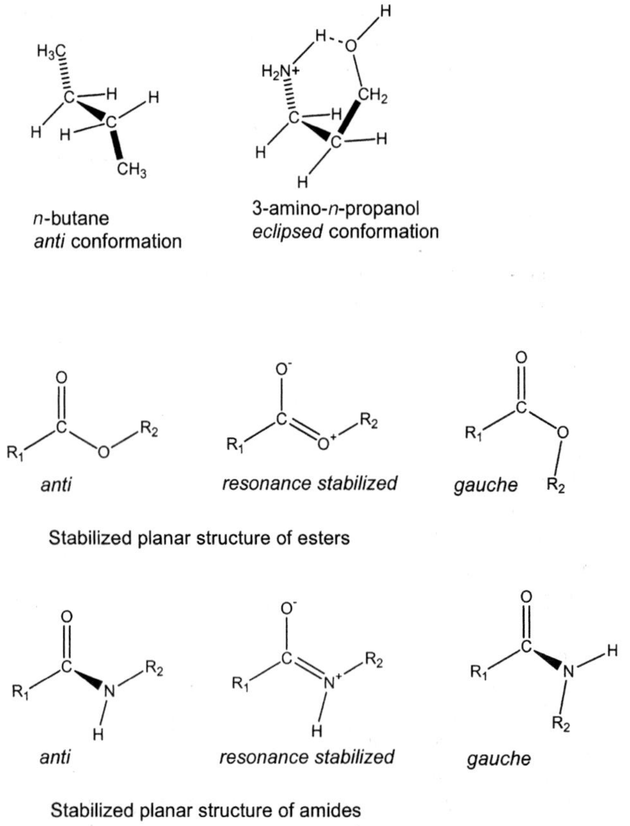

n-butane
anti conformation

3-amino-n-propanol
eclipsed conformation

anti   *resonance stabilized*   *gauche*

Stabilized planar structure of esters

anti   *resonance stabilized*   *gauche*

Stabilized planar structure of amides

Figure 2.14 ● Effect of noncarbon atoms on a molecule's configuration.

chains tend to favor the most extended *anti* conformations, although some of the partially extended *gauche* conformations also exist. Intramolecular bonding between substituent groups can make what might first appear to be an unfavorable conformation favorable.

The introduction of atoms other than carbon into a chain strongly influences the conformation of the chain (Fig. 2.14). Because of resonance contributions of forms in which a double bond occupies the central bonds of esters and amides, a planar configuration is favored in which minimal steric interference of bulky substituents occurs. Hence, an ester may exist mainly in the *anti*, rather than the *gauche*, form. For the same reason, the amide linkage is essentially planar, with the more bulky substituents occupying the *anti* position. Therefore, ester and amide linkages in a chain tend to hold bulky groups in a plane and to separate them as far as possible. As components of the side chains of drugs, ester and amide groups favor fully extended chains and also add polar character to that segment of the chain.

In some cases, *dipole–dipole interactions* appear to influence structure in solution. Methadone may exist partially in a cyclic form in solution because of dipolar attractive forces between the basic nitrogen and carbonyl group or because of hydrogen bonding between the hydrogen on the nitrogen and the carbonyl oxygen (Fig. 2.15). In either conformation, methadone may resemble the conformationally more rigid potent analgesics including morphine, meperidine, and their analogs (see Chapter 24), and it may be this form that interacts with the analgesic receptor. Once the interaction between the drug and its receptor begins, a flexible drug molecule may assume a different conformation than that predicted from solution chemistry.

An intramolecular *hydrogen bond* usually formed between donor hydroxy and amino groups and acceptor oxygen and nitrogen atoms, might be expected to add stability to a particular conformation of a drug in solution. However, in aqueous solution, donor and acceptor groups tend to be bonded to water, and little gain in free energy would be achieved by the formation of an intramolecular hydrogen bond, particularly if unfavorable steric factors involving nonbonded interactions were introduced in the

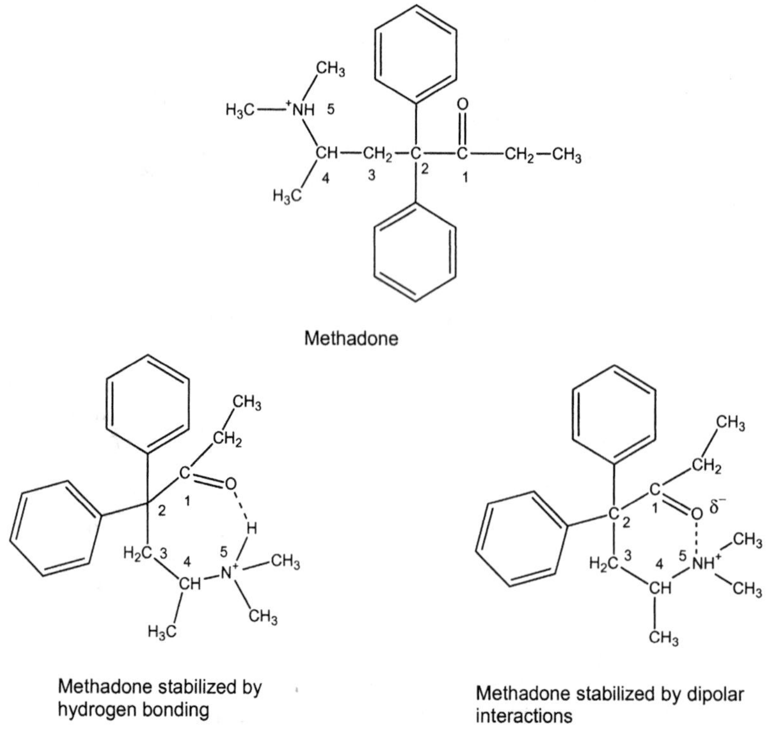

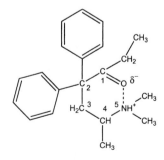

Methadone

Methadone stabilized by hydrogen bonding

Methadone stabilized by dipolar interactions

Figure 2.15 ● Stabilization of conformations by secondary bonding forces.

process. Therefore, internal hydrogen bonds likely play only a secondary role to steric factors in determining the conformational distribution of flexible drug molecules.

Hydrogen-bonding donor groups

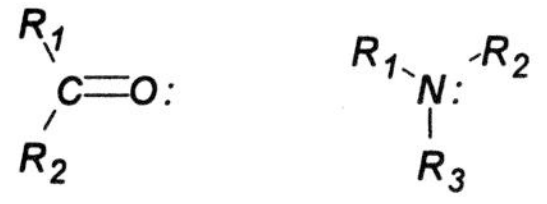

Hydrogen-bonding acceptor groups

Conformational Flexibility and Multiple Modes of Action

It has been proposed that the conformational flexibility of most open-chain neurohormones, such as acetylcholine, epinephrine, serotonin, histamine, and related physiologically active biomolecules, permits multiple biological effects to be produced by each molecule, by virtue of their ability to interact in a different and unique conformation with different biological receptors. Thus, it has been suggested that acetylcholine may interact with the muscarinic receptor of postganglionic parasympathetic nerves and with acetylcholinesterase in the fully extended conforma-

tion and, in a different, more folded structure, with the nicotinic receptors at ganglia and at neuromuscular junctions (Fig. 2.16).

Conformationally rigid acetylcholine-like molecules have been used to study the relationships between these various possible conformations of acetylcholine and their biological effects (Fig. 2.16). (+)-*trans*-2-Acetoxycyclopropyl trimethylammonium iodide, in which the quaternary nitrogen atom and acetoxyl groups are held apart in a conformation approximating that of the extended conformation of acetylcholine, was about five times more active than acetylcholine in its muscarinic effect on dog blood pressure and was as active as acetylcholine in its muscarinic effect on the guinea pig ileum.[18] The (+)-*trans*-isomer was hydrolyzed by acetylcholinesterase at a rate equal to the rate of hydrolysis of acetylcholine. It was inactive as a nicotinic agonist. In contrast, the (−)-*trans*-isomer and the mixed (±)-*cis*-isomers were, respectively, 1/500 and 1/10,000 as active as acetylcholine in muscarinic tests on guinea pig ileum and were inactive as nicotinic agonists. Similarly, the *trans* diaxial relationship between the quaternary nitrogen and acetoxyl group led to maximal muscarinic response and rate of hydrolysis by true acetylcholinesterase in a series of isomeric 3-trimethylammonium-2-acetoxydecalins.[19] These results could be interpreted as either that acetylcholine was acting in a *trans* conformation at the muscarinic receptor and not acting in a *cisoid* conformation at the nicotinic receptor or that the nicotinic response is highly sensitive to steric effects of substituents being used to orient the

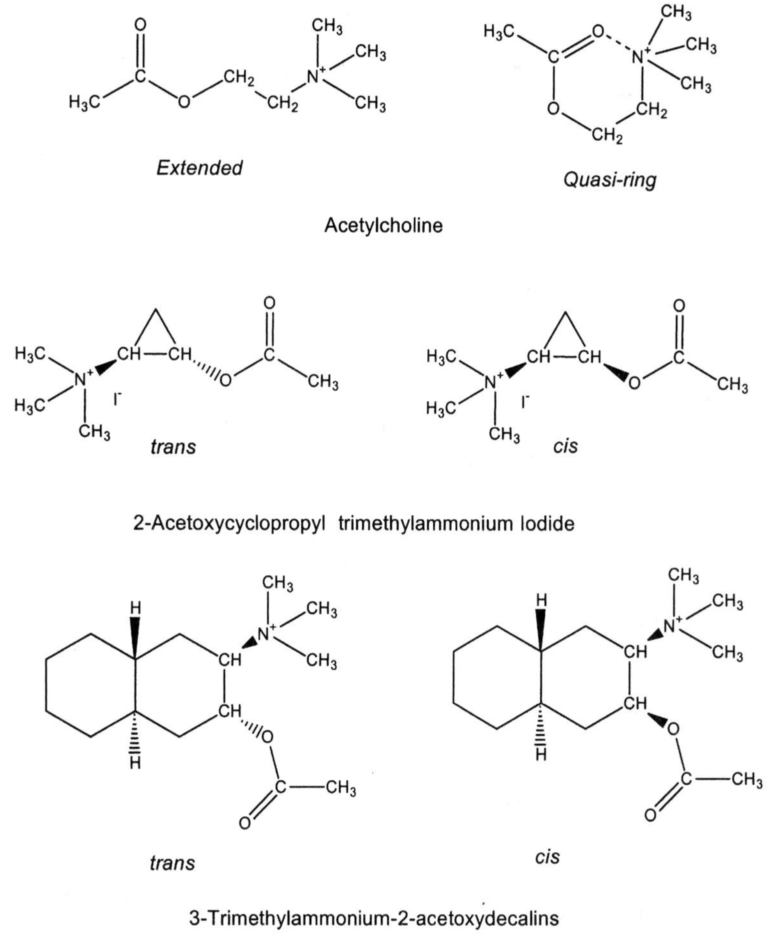

Extended

Quasi-ring

Acetylcholine

trans

cis

2-Acetoxycyclopropyl trimethylammonium Iodide

trans

cis

3-Trimethylammonium-2-acetoxydecalins

Figure 2.16 ● Acetylcholine conformations (only one each of the two possible *trans*- and *cis*-isomers is represented).

molecule. This approach in studying the cholinergic receptor is covered in more detail in Chapter 17.

Optical Isomerism and Biological Activity

The widespread occurrence of differences in biological activities for *optical activities* has been of particular importance in the development of theories on the nature of drug–receptor interactions. Most commercial drugs are asymmetric, meaning that they cannot be divided into symmetrical halves. Although D- and L-isomers have the same physical properties, a large number of drugs are *diastereomeric*, meaning that they have two or more asymmetric centers. Diastereomers have different physical properties. Examples are the diastereomers ephedrine and pseudoephedrine. The former has a melting point of 79° and is soluble in water, whereas pseudoephedrine's melting

point is 118°, and it is only sparingly soluble in water. Keep in mind that receptors will be asymmetric because they are mostly protein, meaning that they are constructed from L-amino acids. A ligand fitting the hypothetical receptor shown in Figure 2.18 will have to have a positively charged moiety in the upper left corner and a hydrophobic region in the upper right. Therefore, one would predict that optical isomers will also have different biological properties. Well-known examples of this phenomenon include (−)-hyoscyamine, which exhibits 15 to 20 times more mydriatic activity than (+)-hyoscyamine, and (−)-ephedrine, which shows three times more pressor activity than (+)-ephedrine, five times more pressor activity than (+)-pseudoephedrine, and 36 times more pressor activity than (−)-pseudoephedrine. All of ascorbic acid's antiscorbutic properties reside in the (+) isomer. A postulated fit to epinephrine's receptor can explain why (−)-epinephrine exhibits 12 to 15 times more vasoconstrictor activity than (+)-epinephrine. This is the classical three-point attachment model. For epinephrine, the benzene ring, benzylic hydroxyl, and protonated amine must have the stereochemistry seen with the (−) isomer to match up with the hydrophobic or aromatic region, anionic site, and a hydrogen-bonding center on the receptor. The (+) isomer (the mirror image) will not align properly on the receptor.

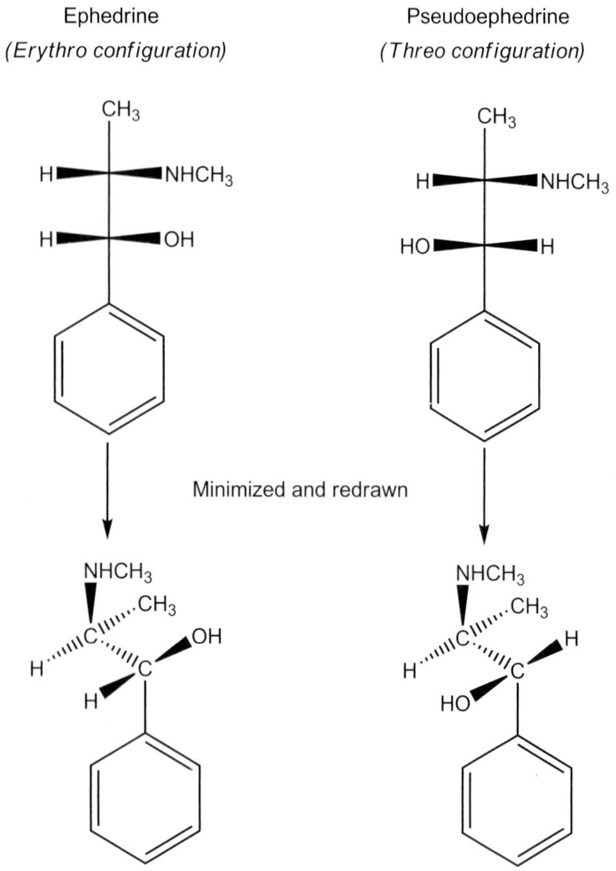

Frequently, the generic name indicates a specific stereoisomer. Examples include levodopa, dextroamphetamine, dextromethorphan, levamisole, dexmethylphenidate, levobupivacaine, dexlansoprazole, and levothyroxine. Sometimes, the difference in pharmacological activity between stereoisomers is dramatic. The dextrorotatory isomers in the morphine series are cough suppressants with less risk of substance abuse, whereas the levorotatory isomers (Fig. 2.19) contain the analgesic activity and significant risk of substance abuse. Although the direction of optical rotation is opposite to that of the morphine series, dextropropoxyphene contains the analgesic activity, and the *levo*-isomer contains antitussive activity. More recently drugs originally marketed as racemic mixtures are reintroduced using the active isomer. The generic name of the latter does not readily indicate that the *new* product is a specific stereoisomer of a product already in use. Examples include racemic citalopram and its S-enantiomer escitalopram; racemic omeprazole and its S-enantiomer esomeprazole; and racemic modafinil and its R-enantiomer armodafinil.

Figure 2.17 contains examples of drugs with asymmetric carbons. Some were originally approved as racemic mixtures, and later a specific isomer was marketed with claims of having fewer adverse reactions in patients. An example of the latter is the local anesthetic levobupivacaine, which is the *S*-isomer of bupivacaine. Both the *R*- and *S*-isomers have good local anesthetic activity, but the *R*-isomer may cause depression of the myocardium leading to decreased cardiac output, heart block hypotension, bradycardia, and ventricular arrhythmias. In contrast, the *S*-isomer shows less cardiotoxic responses but still good local anesthetic activity. Escitalopram is the *S*-isomer of the antidepressant citalopram. There is some evidence that the *R*-isomer, which contains little of the desired selective serotonin reuptake inhibition, contributes more to the adverse reactions than does the *S*-isomer.

As dramatic as the previous examples of stereoselectivity may be, sometimes it may not be cost-effective to resolve

Ephedrine
(Erythro configuration)

Pseudoephedrine
(Threo configuration)

Minimized and redrawn

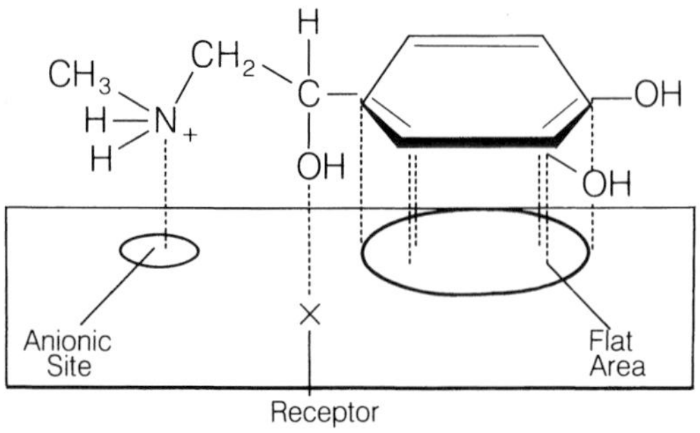

(−)-Epinephrine — more active

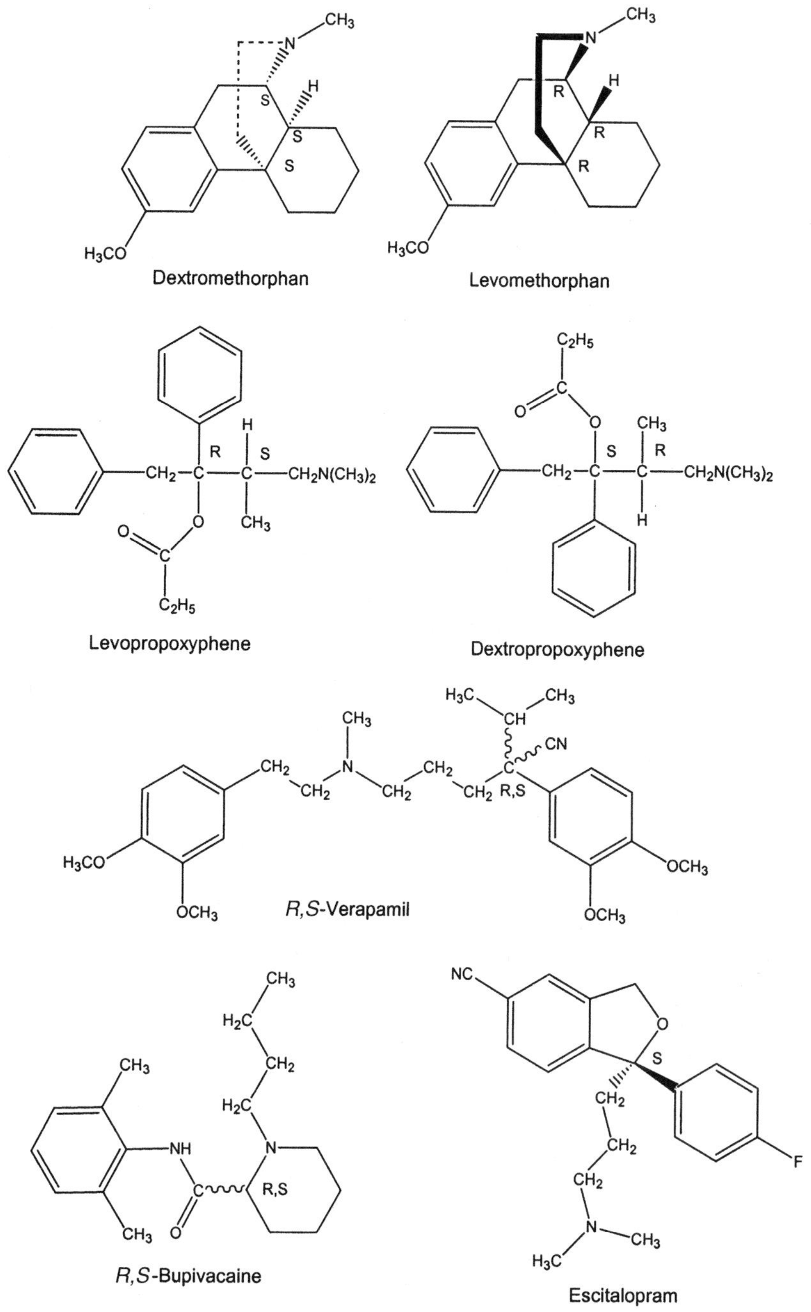

Figure 2.17 ● Examples of drug stereoisomers.

the drug into its stereoisomers. An example is the calcium channel antagonist verapamil, which illustrates why it is difficult to conclude that one isomer is superior to the other. *S*-Verapamil is a more active pharmacological stereoisomer than *R*-verapamil, but the former is more rapidly metabolized by the first-pass effect. First-pass refers to orally administered drugs that are extensively metabolized as they pass through the liver (see Chapter 3). *S*- and *R*-warfarin are metabolized by two different cytochrome P450 isozymes. Drugs that either inhibit or induce these enzymes can significantly affect warfarin's anticoagulation activity.

Because of biotransformations after the drug is administered, it sometimes makes little difference whether a racemic mixture or one isomer is administered. The popular nonsteroidal anti-inflammatory drug (NSAID) ibuprofen is sold as the racemic mixture. The S-enantiomer contains the anti-inflammatory activity by inhibiting cyclooxygenase. The *R*-isomer does have centrally acting analgesic activity, but it is converted to the *S* form in vivo (Fig. 2.18).

In addition to the fact that most receptors are asymmetric, there are other reasons why stereoisomers show different biological responses. Active transport mechanisms involve asymmetric carrier molecules, which means that there will be preferential binding of one stereoisomer over others. When differences in physical properties exist, the distribution of isomers between body fluids and tissues where the receptors are located will differ. The enzymes responsible for drug metabolism are asymmetric, which means that biological half-lives will differ among possible stereoisomers of the same molecule. The latter may be a very important variable because the metabolite may actually be the active molecule.

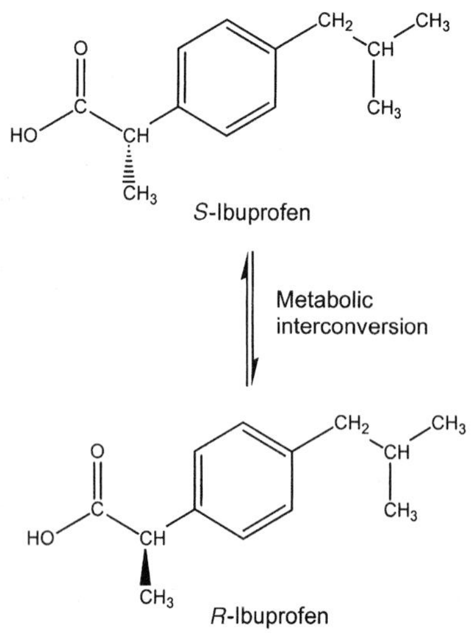

Figure 2.18 ● Metabolic interconversion of *R*- and *S*-ibuprofen.

Calculated Conformations

It should now be obvious that medicinal chemists must obtain an accurate understanding of the active conformation of the drug molecule. Originally, molecular models were constructed from kits containing various atoms of different valence and oxidation states. Thus, there would be carbons suitable for carbon–carbon single, double, and triple bonds; carbon–oxygen bonds for alcohols or ethers and the carbonyl moiety; carbon–nitrogen bonds for amines, amides, imines, and nitrites; and carbons for three-, four-, five-, and larger-member rings. More complete sets include various heteroatoms including nitrogen, oxygen, and sulfur in various oxidation states. These kits might be ball and stick, stick or wire only, or space filling. The latter contained attempts at realistically visualizing the effect of a larger atom such as sulfur relative to the smaller oxygen. The diameters of the atoms in these kits are proportional to the van der Waals radii, usually corrected for overlap effects. In contrast, the wire models usually depict accurate intra-atomic distances between atoms. A skilled chemist using these kits usually can obtain a reasonably accurate 3D representation. This is particularly true if it is a moderately simple molecule with considerable rigidity. An extreme example is a steroid with the relatively inflexible fused-ring system. In contrast, molecules with chains consisting of several atoms can assume many shapes. Yet, there will be a *best* shape or conformation that can be expected to fit onto the receptor. The number of conformers can be estimated from Equation 2.17. Calculating the *global minimum*, the lowest-energy conformation, can be a difficult computational problem. Assume that there are three carbon–carbon freely rotatable single bonds that are rotated in 10-degree increments. Equation 2.17 states that there are 46,656 different conformations.

$$\text{Number of conformers} = \left(\frac{360}{\text{angle increment}}\right)^{\text{No. rotatable bonds}}$$

(Eq. 2.17)

There are three common quantitative ways to obtain estimations of preferred molecular shapes required for a good fit at the receptor. The first, which is the oldest and considered the most accurate, is x-ray crystallography. When properly done, resolution down to a few angstrom units can be obtained. This permits an accurate mathematical description of the molecule, providing atomic coordinates in 3D space that can be drawn by using a chemical graphics program. A serious limitation of this technique is the requirement for a carefully grown crystal. Some chemicals will not form crystals. Others form crystals with mixed symmetries. Nevertheless, with the newer computational techniques, including high-speed computers, large databases of x-ray crystallographic data are now available. These databases can be searched for structures, including substructures, similar to the molecule of interest. Depending on how close is the match, it is possible to obtain a pretty good idea of the low-energy conformation of the drug molecule. This is a common procedure for proteins and nucleic acids after obtaining the amino acid and nucleotide sequences, respectively. Obtaining these sequences is now largely an automated process.

There also is the *debate* that asks if the conformation found in the crystal represents the conformation *seen* by the receptor. For rigid molecules, it probably is. The question is very difficult to answer for flexible molecules. A common technique is to determine the crystal structure of a protein accurately and then *soak* the crystal in a nonaqueous solution of the drug. This allows the drug molecules to diffuse into the active site. The resulting crystal is reanalyzed using different techniques, and the bound conformation of the drug can be determined rapidly without redoing the entire protein. Often, the structure of a bound drug can be determined in a day or less.

Because of the drawbacks to x-ray crystallography, two purely computational methods that require only a knowledge of the molecular structure are used. The two approaches are known as *quantum mechanics* and *molecular mechanics*. Both are based on assumptions that (a) a molecule's 3D geometry is a function of the forces acting on the molecule and (b) these forces can be expressed by a set of equations that pertain to all molecules. For the most part, both computational techniques assume that the molecule is in an isolated system. Solvation effects from water, which are common to any biological system, tend to be ignored, although this is changing with increased computational power. Calculations now can include limited numbers of water molecules, where the number depends on the amount of available computer time. Interestingly, many crystals grown for x-ray analysis can contain water in the crystal lattice. High-resolution nuclear magnetic resonance (NMR) provides another means of obtaining the structures of macromolecules and drugs in solution.

There are fundamental differences between the quantum and molecular mechanics approaches, and they illustrate the dilemma that can confront the medicinal chemist. Quantum mechanics is derived from basic theoretical principles at the atomic level. The model itself is exact, but the equations used in the technique are only approximate. The molecular properties are derived from the electronic structure of the molecule. The assumption is made that the distribution of electrons within a molecule can be described by a linear sum of functions that represent an atomic orbital. (For carbon, this would be s, p_x, p_y, etc.) Quantum mechanics is computation intensive, with the calculation time for obtaining an approximate solution increasing by approximately N^4 times, where N is the number of such functions. Until the advent of the high-speed supercomputers, quantum mechanics in its *pure* form was restricted to small molecules. In other words, it was not practical to conduct a quantum mechanical analysis of a drug molecule.

To make this technique more practical, simplifying techniques have been developed. Whereas the computing time is decreased, the accuracy of the outcome is also lessened. In general, use of calculations of the quantum mechanics type in medicinal chemistry is a method that is *still waiting to happen*. It is being used by laboratories with access to large-scale computing, but there is considerable debate about its utility, because so many simplifying approximations must be made for larger molecules.

To overcome the limitation of quantum mechanics, there has been motivation to develop alternative approaches to calculation conformations of flexible molecules. The reason is that manipulation of computer models is much superior to the use of traditional physical models. Mathematical models using quantum mechanics or the more common force field methods (see later) better account for the inherent flexibility of molecules than do hard sphere physical models. In addition, it is easy to superimpose one or more molecular models on a computer and to color each structure separately for ease of viewing. Medicinal chemists use the superimposed structures to identify the necessary structural features and the 3D orientation (pharmacophore) responsible for the observed biological activity. The display of the multiple conformations available to a single molecule can provide valuable information about the conformational space available to druglike molecules. Rather than measuring bond distances with a ruler, as was done years ago with handheld models, it is relatively easy to query a computer-generated molecular display. Because the coordinates for each atom are stored in computer memory, rapid data retrieval is achieved. Moreover, the shape and size of a molecular system can be visualized and quantified, unlike the situation with handheld models, when only visual inspections are possible. Exactly how much energy does it cost to rotate torsion angles from one position to the next? Understanding drug volumes and molecular shapes is critically important when defining the complementary (negative volume image) receptor sites needed to accommodate the drug molecule.

High-resolution computer graphics that accompany the conformation calculations have revolutionized the way drug design is carried out. Once a molecular structure has been entered into a molecular modeling software program, the structure can be viewed from any desired perspective. The dihedral angles can be rotated to generate new conformations, and functional groups can be eliminated or modified almost effortlessly. As indicated previously, the molecular features (bond lengths, bond angles, nonbonded distances, etc.) can be calculated readily from the stored 3D coordinates.

Because of ease of calculations relative to quantum mechanics, medicinal chemists are embracing molecular mechanics. Force field calculations rest on the fundamental concept that a ball-and-spring model may be used to approximate a molecule.[20,21] That is, the stable relative positions of the atoms in a molecule are a function of through-bond and through-space interactions, which may be described by relatively simple mathematical relationships. The complexity of the mathematical equations used to describe the ball-and-spring model is a function of the nature, size, and shape of the structures. Moreover, the fundamental equations used in force fields are much less complicated than those found in quantum mechanics. For example, small strained organic molecules require greater detail than less strained systems such as peptides and proteins. Furthermore, it is assumed that the total energy of the molecule is a summation of the individual energy components, as outlined in Equation 2.18. In other words, the total energy (E_{total}) is divided into energy components, which are attributed to bond stretching ($E_{stretching}$), angle bending ($E_{bending}$), nonbonded interactions ($E_{nonbonded}$), torsion interactions ($E_{torsion}$), and coupled energy terms ($E_{cross-terms}$). The cross-terms combine two interrelated motions (bend–stretch, stretch–stretch, torsion–stretch, etc.). The division of the total energy into terms associated with distortions from equilibrium values is the way most chemists and biological scientists tend to think about molecules.

$$E_{total} = \Sigma_{bonds}E_{stretching} + \Sigma_{angles}E_{bending}$$
$$+ \Sigma_{nonbonded}(E_{VDW} + E_{electrostatics})$$
$$+ \Sigma_{dihedrals}E_{torsion} + \Sigma E_{cross-terms} \quad \text{(Eq. 2.18)}$$

Each atom is defined (parameterized) in terms of these energy terms. What this means is that the validity of molecular mechanics depends on the accuracy of the parameterization process. Historically, saturated hydrocarbons have proved easy to parameterize, followed by selective heteroatoms such as ether oxygens and amines. Unsaturated systems, including aromaticity, caused problems because of the delocalization of the electrons, but this seems to have been solved. Charged atoms such as the carboxylate anion and protonated amine can prove to be a real problem, particularly if the charge is delocalized. Nevertheless, molecular mechanics is being used increasingly by medicinal chemists to gain a better understanding of the preferred conformation of drug molecules and the macromolecules that compose a receptor. The computer programs are readily available and run on relatively inexpensive, but powerful, desktop computers.

The only way to test the validity of the outcome from either quantum or molecular mechanics calculations is to compare the calculated structure or property with actual experimental data. Obviously, crystallographic data provide a reliable measure of the accuracy of at least one of the low-energy conformers. Because that is not always feasible, other physical chemical measurements are used for comparison. These include comparing calculated vibrational energies, heats of formation, dipole moments, and relative conformational energies with measured values. When results are inconsistent, the parameter values are adjusted. This readjustment of the parameters is analogous to the fragment approach for calculating octanol/water partition coefficients. The values for the fragments and the accompanying correction factors are determined by comparing calculated partition coefficients with a large population of experimentally determined partition coefficients.

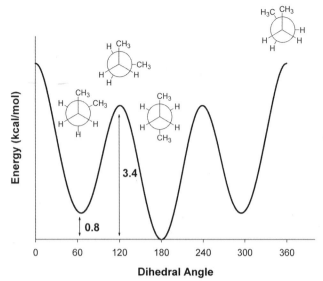

Figure 2.19 ● Potential energy for butane. The energy (kcal/mol) is plotted on the *y*-axis versus the torsion angle C_{sp3}-C_{sp3}-C_{sp3}-C_{sp3}, which is plotted on the *x*-axis. There are three minima. The two *gauche* conformers are higher in energy that the *anti* conformer by approximately 0.9 kcal/mol.

A simplified energy diagram for the hydrocarbon butane is shown in Figure 2.19. It illustrates that the energy rises and falls during rotation around the central C_{sp3}–C_{sp3} bond as a function of the relative positions of the methyl groups. The peaks on the curve correspond to energy maxima, whereas the valleys correspond to energy minima. For butane, there are two different types of minima: one is for the *anti* butane conformation and the other two correspond to the *gauche* butane conformations. The *anti* conformation is the global minimum, meaning it has the absolute lowest energy of the three possible low-energy conformations. The differences in the conformational energies cannot be attributed to steric interactions alone. Structures with more than one rotatable bond have multiple minima available. Knowing the permissible conformations available to druglike molecules is important for design purposes.

A more typical energy diagram is shown in Figure 2.20. Notice that some of the minima are nearly equivalent, and it is easy to move from one minimum to another. From energy diagrams alone, it is difficult to answer the question, which of the ligand's low or moderately low conformations fits onto the receptor? This question can be answered partially by assuming that lower-energy conformations are more highly populated and thus more likely to interact with the receptor. Nevertheless, specific interactions such as hydrogen bond formation and dipole–dipole interactions can affect the energy levels of different conformations. Therefore, the bound conformation of a drug is seldom its lowest-energy conformation.

Because looking solely at the molecule can lead to ambiguous conclusions regarding the conformation when docking at the receptor, this has lead to calculating conformations of the macromolecule that is the receptor and visualizing the results. A capability that today's graphics software is representing molecular structures in many

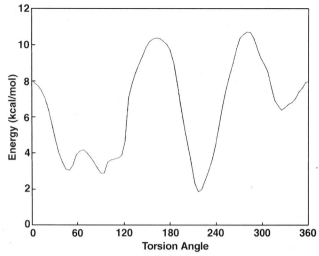

Figure 2.20 ● Diagram showing the energy maxima and minima as two substituted carbons connected by a single bond are rotated 360 degrees relative to each other.

different ways, depending on the properties one decides to highlight. Dorzolamide is a good example of a drug that involved computer-aided drug design (CADD) methods in its development.[22] Figure 2.21 shows a standard representation of dorzolamide from a molecular modeling software package. The atoms can be color coded in various ways according to the different properties that one might want to highlight. As noted previously, however, it is important to know the size and shape of the molecule. Various representations are possible. A convenient visualization technique is to have the atoms and bonds displayed simultaneously with the van der Waals surface represented by an even distribution of dots. These dot surfaces are convenient, in that the atomic connectivity is shown along with the appropriate size and shape of the molecular surface. As computer graphics technology has improved, it has become possible to represent the surface as a translucent volume, shown in Figure 2.22, in which the

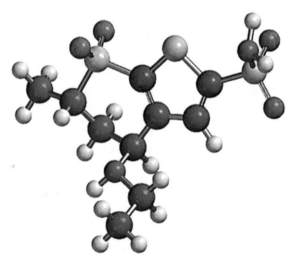

Figure 2.21 ● A computer-generated representation of dorzolamide. The structure has been energy minimized using Spartan '08.

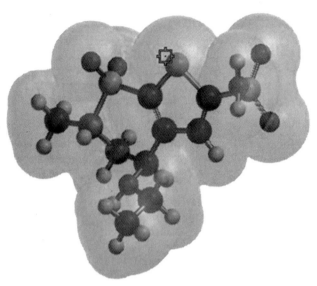

Figure 2.22 ● The ball-and-stick minimized model is displayed with superimposed translucent van der Waals surface showing both atomic connectivity of the molecular structure and its 3D shape and size.

molecular structure appears to be embedded in a clear gelatin material.

Dorzolamide

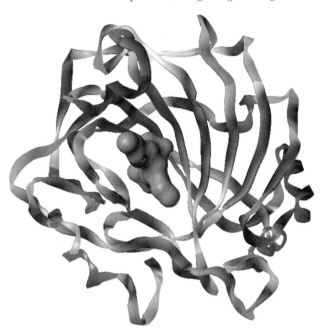

Figure 2.23 ● A computer-generated representation of a thienothipyran-2-sulfonamide bound to the active site of carbonic anhydrase. Note that the ribbon has been traced through the protein backbone. Proteins are commonly displayed this way.

Finally, computer graphics images of drug–receptor interactions, whether taken from x-ray crystal data or in silico generated, provide insight into the binding interactions, as shown in Figure 2.23. A full display of all the atomic centers in a protein structure gives too much detail. Most commonly, as shown in Figure 2.23, a ribbon structure traces the backbone of the protein main chain.[23] The Richardson approach is another commonly used display to highlight secondary structural features, in which cylinders denote α-helices, arrows denote β-sheets, and tubes are used for coils and turns.[24]

Because drug molecules make contact with solvents and receptor sites through surface contacts, it is paramount to have accurate methods to represent molecular surfaces correctly. Algorithms have been developed for such purposes, and they continue to be improved. The most straightforward way to represent a molecular shape is by the so-called van der Waals surface (Fig. 2.22), in which each constituent atom contributes its exposed surface to the overall molecular surface. Each atom is assigned a volume corresponding to its van der Waals radius, and only the union of atomic spheres contributes. These van der Waals surfaces have

small crevices and pockets that cannot make contact with solvent molecules. Another surface, known as the solvent accessible or Connolly surface, can be generated.[25] The algorithm takes the van der Waals surface and rolls a sphere, having the volume of a water molecule with a radius of 1.4 Å, across it. Wherever the sphere makes contact with the original surface, a new surface is created. This expanded surface is a more realistic representation of what water molecules contact. Another similar solvent-accessible surface is known as the Lee and Richards surface.[26] This surface is constructed in an analogous way, with a sphere rolled over the van der Waals surface, but the boundary is taken as a line connecting the center of mass of the sphere from point to point. Also, it is possible to calculate the solvent excluded surface. The polar and nonpolar surface areas can be used as QSAR descriptors, and many computer models for solvation use solvent-accessible surface areas (SASA). Commonly, the electrostatic density may be displayed on the surface of a molecular structure, providing an easily recognized color coded grid that may be used to infer the complementary binding functional groups of the putative receptor.

A goal of docking programs is to screen large dataset to locate compounds that appear to have the atomic structure and conformation to dock readily at the receptor. Although there are several software programs available, their ability to differentiate between known ligands and decoys has not reached a level that this approach to searching databases has become standard. In other words, the programs will selected valid ligands and show them docking accordingly with the receptor, but they also docked the decoys and also usually do a poor job of predicting ligand binding affinity.[27,28] So challenging is this problem that a database of docking decoys has been created.[29]

Three-Dimensional Quantitative Structure–Activity Relationships

With molecular modeling becoming more common, the QSAR paradigm that traditionally used physicochemical descriptors on a two-dimensional molecule can be adapted to 3D space. Essentially, the method requires knowledge of the 3D shape of the molecule. Accurate modeling of the molecule is crucial. A reference (possibly the prototype molecule) or shape is selected against which all other molecules are compared. The original method called for overlapping the test molecules with the reference molecule and minimizing the differences in overlap. Then, distances were calculated between arbitrary locations on the molecule. These distances were used as variables in QSAR regression equations. Although overlapping rigid ring systems such as tetracyclines, steroids, and penicillins are relatively easy, flexible molecules can prove challenging. Examine the following hypothetical molecule. Depending on the size of the various R groups and the type of atom represented by X, a family of compounds represented by this molecule could have various conformations. Even when the conformations might be known with reasonable certainty, the reference points crucial for activity must be identified. Is the overlap involving the tetrahedral carbon important for activity? Or should the five-membered ring provide the reference points? And which way should it be rotated? Assuming that R_b is an important part of the pharmacophore, should the five-membered ring be rotated so that R_b is pointed down or up? These are not trivial questions, and successful 3D-QSAR studies have depended on just how the investigator positions the molecules relative to each other. There are several instances in which apparently very similar structures have been shown to bind to a given receptor in different orientations.

There are various algorithms for measuring the degree of conformational and shape similarities, including molecular shape analysis (MSA),[30] distance geometry,[31] and molecular similarity matrices.[32,33] Many of the algorithms use graph theory, in which the bonds that connect the atoms of a molecule can be thought of as paths between specific points on the molecule. Molecular connectivity is a commonly used application of graph theory.[34–36]

Besides comparing how well a family of molecules overlaps with a reference molecule, there are sophisticated software packages that determine the physicochemical parameters located at specific distances from the surface of the molecule. An example of this approach is comparative molecular field analysis (CoMFA).[37,38] The hypothetical molecule is placed in a grid (Fig. 2.24) and its surface sampled at a specified distance. The parameter types include steric, Lennard-Jones potentials and other quantum chemical parameters, electrostatic and steric parameters, and partition coefficients. The result is thousands of independent variables. Standard regression analysis requires that the dimensionality be reduced and rigorous tests of validity be used. Partial least squares (PLS) has been the most common statistical method used. Elegant as the CoMFA algorithm is for explaining ligand–receptor interactions for a set of molecules, the method alone does not readily point the

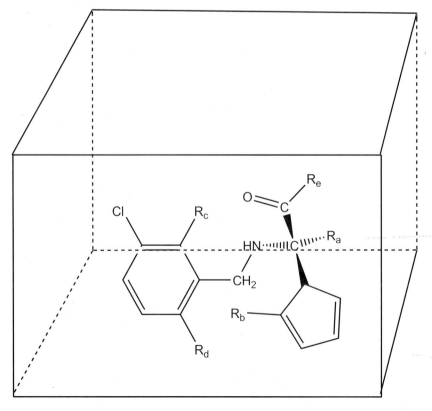

Figure 2.24 • Molecule situated in a CoMFA grid.

investigator toward the next molecule that should be synthesized. To get around the problem of strict alignment of one particular conformation with another, there are methods that sample several possible conformations of a set of possible ligands. This is called 4D-QSAR.[39]

The CoMFA methodology is used in similarity analyses comparing molecular conformers' ability to bind to a receptor. This is called comparative molecular similarity indices analysis or CoMSIA.[40] It is similar to CoMFA in that the molecules are aligned in a grid, but differs in the type of indices or descriptors with Gaussian functions producing descriptors that describe binding to the receptor being the most useful.

Database Searching and Mining

As pointed out previously, receptors can be isolated and cloned. This means that it is possible to determine their structures. Most are proteins and that means having to determine their amino acid sequence. This can be done either by degrading the protein or by obtaining the nucleotide sequence of the structural gene coding for the receptor and using the triplet genetic code to determine the amino acid sequence. The parts of the receptor that bind the drug (ligand) can be determined by site-directed mutagenesis. This alters the nucleotide sequence at specific points on the gene and, therefore, changes specific amino acids. Also, keep in mind that many enzymes become receptors when the goal is to alter their activity. Examples of the latter include acetylcholinesterase, monoamine oxidase, HIV protease, rennin, ACE, and tetrahydrofolate reductase.

The starting point is a database of chemical structures. They may belong to large pharmaceutical or agrochemical firms that literally have synthesized the compounds in the database and have them *sitting on the shelf.* Alternatively, the database may be constructed so that several different chemical classes and substituent patterns are represented. (See discussion of isosterism in the next section.) The first step is to convert the traditional or historical two-dimensional molecules into 3D structures whose intramolecular distances are known. Keeping in mind the problems of finding the "correct" conformation for flexible molecule, false hits and misses might result from the search. Next, the dimensions of the active site must be determined. Ideally, the receptor has been crystallized, and from the coordinates, the intramolecular distances between what are assumed to be key locations are obtained. If the receptor cannot be crystallized, there are methods for estimating the 3D shape based on searching crystallographic databases and matching amino acid sequences of proteins whose tertiary structure has been determined.

Fortunately, the crystal structures of literally thousands of proteins have been determined, and their structures have been stored in the Brookhaven Protein Databank. It is now known that proteins with similar functions have similar amino acid sequences in various regions of the protein. These sequences tend to show the same shapes in terms of α-helix, parallel and antiparallel β-pleated forms, turns in the chain, etc. Using this information plus molecular mechanics parameters, the shape of the protein and the dimensions of the active site can be estimated. Figure 2.25 contains the significant components of a hypothetical active site. Notice that four amino acid residues at positions

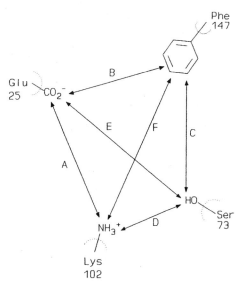

Figure 2.25 ● Diagram of a hypothetical receptor site, showing distances between functional groups.

25, 73, 102, and 147 have been identified as important either for binding the ligand to the site or for the receptor's intrinsic activity. Keep in mind that Figure 2.25 is a two-dimensional representation of a 3D image. Therefore, the distances between amino acid residues must take into account the fact that each residue is above or below the planes of the other three residues. For an artificial ligand to "dock," or fit into the site, six distances must be considered: (a) Lys–Glu, (b) Glu–Phe, (c) Phe–Ser, (d) Ser–Lys, (e) Glu–Phe, and (f) Lys–Phe. In reality, not all six distances may be important. In selecting potential ligands, candidates might include a positively charged residue (protonated amine), aromatic ring, hydrogen bond donor or acceptor (hydroxy, phenol, amine, nitro), and hydrogen bond acceptor or a negatively charged residue (carboxylate) that will interact with the aspartate, phenylalanine, serine, and lysine residues, respectively. A template is constructed containing the appropriate residues at the proper distances with correct geometries, and the chemical database is searched for molecules that fit the template. A degree of fit or match is obtained for each "hit." Their biological responses are obtained, and the model for the receptor is further refined. New, better-defined ligands may be synthesized.

In addition to the interatomic distances, the chemical databases will contain important physicochemical values including partition coefficients, electronic terms, molar refractivity, pK$_a$'s, solubilities, and steric values. Arrangements of atoms may be coded by molecular connectivity or other topological descriptors. The result is a "flood of data" that requires interpretation, large amounts of data storage, and rapid means of analysis. Compounds usually must fit within defined limits that estimate ADME.

Chemical databases can contain hundreds of thousands of molecules that could be suitable ligands for a receptor. But, no matter how good the fit is to the receptor, the candidate molecule is of no use if the absorption is poor or if the drug is excreted too slowly from the body. An analysis of 2,245 drugs has led to a set of "rules" called the *Lipinski*

Rule of Five.[41,42] A candidate molecule is more likely to have poor absorption or permeability if:

1. The molecular weight exceeds 500.
2. The calculated octanol/water partition coefficient exceeds 5.
3. There are more than 5 H-bond donors expressed as the sum of O–H and N–H groups.
4. There are more than 10 H-bond acceptors expressed as the sum of N and O atoms.

Because of *misses* when searching or mining databases, there have been two suggested changes. The first of these is to take into account the fact that many compounds will be significantly ionized at physiological pH and, therefore, use the distribution coefficient log D with an upper limit of 5.5 rather than a log P of 5.[43] Similar results have been found when evaluating herbicides and pesticides.[44] A second suggested modification of the Rule of Five gives specific ranges for log P, molar refractivity, molecular weight and number of atoms (Table 2.10).[45]

The rapid evaluation of large numbers of molecules is sometimes called *high-throughput screening* (Fig. 2.26). The screening can be in vitro, often measuring how well the tested molecules bind to cloned receptors or enzyme active sites. Robotic devices are available for this testing. Based on the results, the search for viable structures is narrowed, and new compounds are synthesized. The criteria for activity will be based on structure and physicochemical values. QSAR, including 3D-QSAR, models can be developed to aid in designing new active ligands.

Alternatively, the search may be virtual. Again starting with the same type of database and the dimensions of the active site, the ability of the compounds in the database to fit or bind is estimated. The virtual receptor will include both its

TABLE 2.10 Suggested Modifications to the Lipinski Rule of Five

	Druglike Range	Preferred Range	Mean
Log P	−0.4–5.6	1.3–4.1	2.3
Molar Refractivity	40–130	70–110	97
Molecular Weight	160–480	230–390	360
No. of Atom	20–70	30–55	48

Source: Ghose, A. K., Viswanadhan, V. N., and Wendoloski, J. J.: J. Comb. Chem. 1:55, 1999.

dimensions and physicochemical characteristic. Keeping in mind that the receptor is a protein, there will be hydrogen bond acceptors and donors (serine, threonine, tyrosine), positively and negatively charged side chains (lysine, histidine, glutamic acid, aspartic acid), nonpolar or hydrophobic side chains (leucine, isoleucine, valine, alanine), and induced dipoles (phenylalanine, tyrosine). The type of groups that will be attracted or repulsed by the type of amino acid side chain is coded into the chemical database. The virtual screening will lead to development of a refined model for good binding, and the search is repeated. When the model is considered valid, it must be tested by actual screening in biological test systems and by synthesizing new compounds to test its validity.

Another approach to searching a database of compounds is the use of the chemical fragments described earlier. There is ongoing debate regarding what type of fragments will result in the most *hits*. Nevertheless, there now are fragment libraries constructed around the range of the fragments' physicochemical properties, solubilities, molecular diversity, and drug likeness based on their presence in existing compounds.[46]

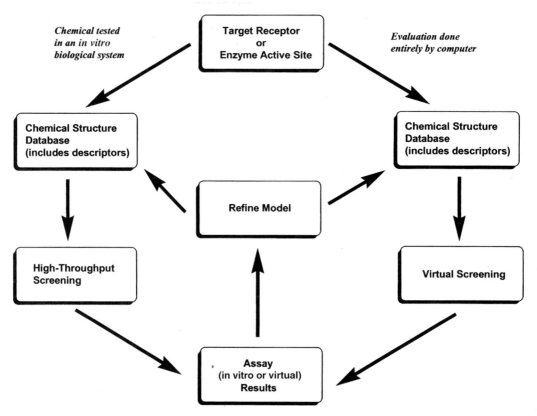

Figure 2.26 ● High-throughput screening.

Isosterism

In the process of designing new pharmacologically active compounds or searching databases, it is important to not restrict the definition of the structures to specific atoms. An important concept is *isosterism*, a term that has been used widely to describe the selection of structural components—the steric, electronic, and solubility characteristics that make them interchangeable in drugs of the same pharmacological class. The concept of isosterism has evolved and changed significantly in the years since its introduction by Langmuir in 1919.[47] Langmuir, while seeking a correlation that would explain similarities in physical properties for nonisomeric molecules, defined *isosteres* as compounds or groups of atoms having the same number and arrangement of electrons. Isosteres that were isoelectric (i.e., with the same total charge as well as the same number of electrons) would possess similar physical properties. For example, the molecules N_2 and CO both possess 14 total electrons and no charge and show similar physical properties. Related examples described by Langmuir were CO_2, N_2O, N_3^-, and NCO^- (Table 2.11).

With increased understanding of the structures of molecules, less emphasis has been placed on the number of electrons involved, because variations in hybridization during bond formation may lead to considerable differences in the angles, lengths, and polarities of bonds formed by atoms with the same number of peripheral electrons. Even the same atom may vary widely in its structural and electronic characteristics when it forms part of a different functional group. Thus, nitrogen is part of a planar structure in the nitro group but forms the apex of a pyramidal structure in ammonia and amines.

Groups of atoms that impart similar physical or chemical properties to a molecule because of similarities in size, electronegativity, or stereochemistry are now frequently referred to by the general term of *isostere*. The early recognition that benzene and thiophene were alike in many of their properties (Fig. 2.27) led to the term *ring equivalents* for the vinylene group (—CH=CH—) and divalent sulfur (—S—). This concept has led to replacement of the sulfur atom in the phenothiazine ring system of tranquilizing agents with the vinylene

TABLE 2.11 Commonly Used Alicyclic Chemical Isosteres

A. Univalent atoms and groups				
(1) —CH₃	—NH₂	—OH	—F	—Cl
(2) —Cl	—SH			
(3) —Br	—*i*—Pr			
B. Bivalent atoms and groups				
(1) —CH₂—	—NH—	—O—	—S—	
(2) —COCH₂R	—CONHR			
(3) —CO₂R	—COSR			
C. Trivalent atoms and groups				
(1) —CH=	—N=			

Source: Silverman, R. B.: The Organic Chemistry of Drug Design and Drug Action. New York, Academic Press, 1992.

group to produce the dibenzodiazepine class of antidepressant drugs. The vinylene group in an aromatic ring system may be replaced by other atoms isosteric to sulfur, such as oxygen (furan) or NH (pyrrole); however, in such cases, aromatic character is significantly decreased (Fig. 2.27).

Examples of isosteric pairs that possess similar steric and electronic configurations are the carboxylate (COO⁻) and sulfonamide (SO₂NR⁻) ions; ketone (C=O) and sulfone (O=S=O); chloride (Cl⁻) and trifluoromethyl (CF₃); hydrogen (—H) and fluorine (—F); hydroxy (—OH) and amine (—NH₂); hydroxy (—OH) and thiol (—SH). Divalent ether (—O—), sulfide (—S—), amine (—NH—), and methylene (—CH₂—) groups, although dissimilar electronically, are sufficiently alike in their steric nature to be frequently interchangeable in designing new drugs.[48]

Compounds may be altered by isosteric replacements of atoms or groups, to develop analogs with select biological effects or to act as antagonists to normal metabolites. Each series of compounds showing a specific biological effect must be considered separately, because there are no general rules that predict whether biological activity will be increased or decreased. Some examples of this type follow.

When a group is present in a part of a molecule in which it may be involved in an essential interaction or may influence

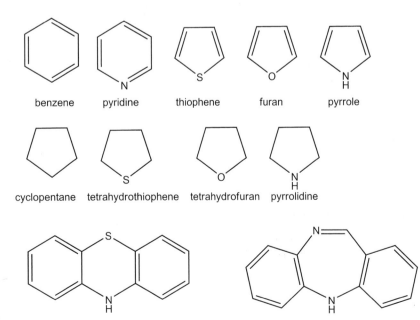

Figure 2.27 ● Examples of isosteric ring systems.

benzene   pyridine   thiophene   furan   pyrrole

cyclopentane   tetrahydrothiophene   tetrahydrofuran   pyrrolidine

phenothiazine   dibenzodiazepine

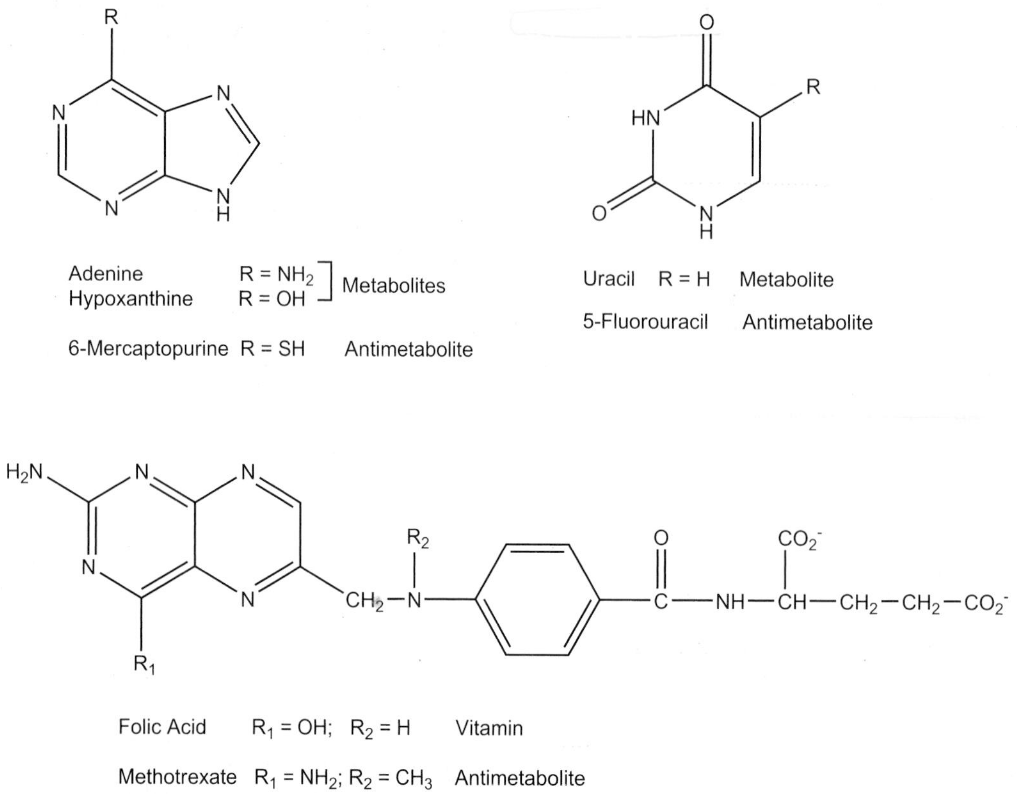

Adenine   R = NH₂

Hypoxanthine   R = OH   Metabolites

6-Mercaptopurine   R = SH   Antimetabolite

Uracil   R = H   Metabolite

5-Fluorouracil   Antimetabolite

Folic Acid R_1 = OH; R_2 = H   Vitamin

Methotrexate R_1 = NH₂; R_2 = CH₃   Antimetabolite

Figure 2.28 • Examples of how isosterism produces drugs that inhibit the activity of the native metabolite.

the reactions of neighboring groups, isosteric replacement sometimes produces analogs that act as antagonists. The 6-NH_2 and 6-OH groups appear to play essential roles in the hydrogen-bonding interactions of base pairs during nucleic acid replication in cells (Fig. 2.28). Adenine, hypoxanthine and the antineoplastic 6-mercaptopurine illustrate how substitution of the significantly weaker hydrogen-bonding isosteric sulfhydryl groups results in a partial blockage of this interaction and a decrease in the rate of cellular synthesis. Similarly, replacement of the hydroxyl group of pteroylglutamic acid (folic acid) by the isosteric amino group and addition of the methyl group to the *p*-aminobenzoate leads to the widely used methotrexate, a folate antimetabolite. Replacement of the hydrogen at the 5-position of uracil with the isosteric fluorine producing 5-fluorouracil blocks the methylation step leading to thymine.

As a better understanding of the nature of the interactions between drug-metabolizing enzymes and biological receptors develops, selection of isosteric groups with particular electronic, solubility, and steric properties should permit the rational preparation of drugs that act more selectively. At the same time, results obtained by the systematic application of the principles of isosteric replacement are aiding in the understanding of the nature of these receptors.

Are There Drugs Developed Using the Newer Computer-Aided Drug Design Methods?

The same question asked in the discussion of QSAR must be asked regarding the newer CADD methods. Are their commercial products that were discovered using these techniques?

Here, the answer is *yes*. The example of dorzolamide is one. Others include the ACE-inhibitor captopril and HIV protease inhibitors nelfinavir and amprenavir. In reality, modern CADD is used in combination with structure-based drug design and QSAR. These methods permit the medicinal chemist to focus more quickly on the structural components that enhance activity and provide receptor specificity.[49,50]

SELECTED WEB PAGES

The field of drug design, particularly those aspects that are computer intensive, is increasingly being featured on Web pages. Faculty and students might find it instructive to search the Web at regular intervals. Many university chemistry departments have organized Web pages that provide excellent linkages. Listed are a small number of representative sites that feature drug design linkages. Some have excellent illustrations. These listings should not be considered any type of endorsement by the author, editors, or publisher. Indeed, some of these sites may disappear.

http://www.nih.gov/
(Search terms: QSAR; molecular modeling)
http://www.cooper.edu/engineering/chemechem/monte.html
http://www.clunet.edu/BioDev/omm/gallery.htm
http://www.netsci.org/Science/Compchem/feature19.html
http://www.pomona.edu/
(Search terms: QSAR; medicinal chemistry)
http://www.umass.edu/microbio/rasmol/index2.htm
http://www.webmo.net/
http://www.molinspiration.com/cgi-bin/properties
http://www.pharma-algorithms.com/webboxes/

1. Name at least two ways that a drug's pharmacological half-life may be shortened following administration.

2. Define conjugate acid and conjugate base.

3. Estimate the percent ionization of acetic acid (pK_a 4.8) at pH 3.8 and at pH 5.8.

4. Would you expect selegiline to be more water soluble or insoluble at physiological pH. (Look up selegiline's pK_a in the Appendix.)

5. What does each of the following acronyms represent? QSAR, CADD, CoMFA, CoMSIA, Log P, Log D, HTS

6. Rank order the following bond types from weakest to strongest: van der Waals, covalent, hydrogen, ionic, dipole–dipole.

7. What is Lipinski Rule of Five? Give one application where it can be applied.

REFERENCES

1. Crum Brown, A., and Fraser, T.: R. Soc. Edinburgh 25:151, 1868–1869.
2. Grime, J. M. A., Edwards, M. A., Rudd, N. C., et al.: Proc. Nat. Acad. Sci. 105:14277, 2008.
3. Benfenati, E., Gini, G., Piclin, N., et al.: Chemosphere 53:1155, 2003.
4. Mannhold, R., Poda, G. I., Ostermann, C. E., et al.: J. Pharm. Sci. 98:861, 2009.
5. Hansch, C., Leo, A., and Hoekman, D.: Exploring QSAR: Hydrophobic, Electronic, and Steric Constants. Washington, DC, American Chemical Society, 1995.
6. Hansch, C., and Lien, E. J.: J. Med. Chem. 14:653, 1971.
7. Dearden, J. C., and George, E.: J. Pharm. Pharmacol. 31:S45P, 1979.
8. Stuper, A. J., Brügger, W. E., and Jurs, P. C.: Computer Assisted Studies of Chemical Structure and Biological Function. New York, John Wiley & Sons, 1979.
9. Martin, Y. C., Kofron, J. L., and Traphagen, L. M.: J. Med. Chem. 45:4350, 2002.
10. Maggiora, G. M.: J. Chem. Inf. Model. 46:1535, 2006.
11. Doweyko, A. M.: J. Computer-Aided Molec. Design 22:81, 2008.
12. Eriksson, L. E., Jaworska, J., Worth, A. P., et al.: Environmental Health Perspectives 111:1361, 2003.
13. Konovalov, D. A., Llewellyn, L. E., Heyden, Y. V., et al.: J. Chem. Inf. Model. 48:2081, 2008.
14. Roy, P. P., Paul, S., Mitra, I., et al.: Molecules 14:1660, 2009.
15. Gedeck, P., Rohde, B., and Bartels, C.: J. Chem. Inf. Model. 46:1924, 2006.
16. Johnson, S. R.: J. Chem. Inf. Model. 48:25, 2008.
17. Baker, B. R.: J. Pharm. Sci. 53:347, 1964.
18. Chiou, C. Y., Long, J. P., Cannon, J. G., et al.: J. Pharmacol. Exp. Ther. 166:243, 1969.
19. Smissman, E., Nelson, W., Day, J., et al.: J. Med. Chem. 9:458, 1966.
20. Burkert, U., and Allinger, N. L.: Molecular Mechanics. ACS Monograph 177. Washington, DC, American Chemical Society, 1982.
21. Rappe, A. K., and Casewit, C.: Molecular Mechanics Across Chemistry. Sausalito, CA, University Science Books, 1992.
22. Greer, J., Erickson, J. W., Baldwin, J. J., et al.: J. Med. Chem. 37:1035, 1994.
23. Carson, M., and Bugg, C. E.: J. Mol. Graphics 4:121, 1986.
24. Richardson, J. S., and Richardson, D. C.: Trends Biochem. Sci. 14:304, 1989.
25. Connolly, M. L.: Science 221:709, 1983.
26. Lee, B., and Richards, F. M.: J. Mol. Biol. 55:379, 1971.
27. Warren, G. L., Andrews, C. W., Capelli, A., et al.: J. Med. Chem. 49:5912, 2006.
28. Leach, A. R., Shoichet, B. K., and Peishoff, C. E.: J. Med. Chem.: 49: 5851, 2006.
29. Huang, H., Shoichet, B. K., and Irwin, J. J.: J. Med. Chem.: 49:6789, 2006.
30. Hopfinger, A. J., and Burke, B. J.: Molecular shape analysis: a formalism to quantitatively establish spatial molecular similarity. In Johnson, M. A., and Maggiora, G. M. (eds.). Concepts and Applications of Molecular Similarity. New York, John Wiley & Sons, 1990.
31. Srivastava, S., Richardson, W. W., Bradely, M. P., et al.: Three dimensional receptor modeling using distance geometry and Voronoi polyhydra. In Kubinyi, H. (ed.). 3D QSAR in Drug Design: Theory, Methods and Applications. Leiden, The Netherlands, ESCOM, 1993.
32. Good, A. C., Peterson, S. J., and Richards, W. G.: J. Med. Chem. 36:2929, 1993.
33. Good, A. C., and Richards, W. G.: Drug Inf. J. 30:371, 1996.
34. Kier, L. B., and Hall, L. H.: Molecular Connectivity in Chemistry and Drug Research. New York, Academic Press, 1976.
35. Kier, L. B., and Hall, L. H.: Molecular Connectivity in Structure Activity Analysis. New York, Research Studies Press (Wiley), 1986.
36. Bonchev, D.: Information Theoretic Indices for Characterization of Chemical Structures. New York, Research Studies Press (Wiley), 1983.
37. Cramer III, R. D., Patterson, D. E., and Bunce, J. D.: J. Am. Chem. Soc. 110:5959, 1988.
38. Marshall, G. R., and Cramer III, R. D.: Trends Pharmacol. Sci. 9:285, 1988.
39. Krasowski, M. D., Hong, X., Hopfinger, A. J., et al.: J. Med. Chem. 45:3210, 2002.
40. Kleve, G.: 3D QSAR in Drug Design. In Kubinyi, H., Folkers, G., and Martin, Y. C. (eds.). Three-Dimensional Quantitative Structure-Activity Relationships, vol. 3. New York, Springer, 1998.
41. Lipinski, C. A.: J. Pharmacol. Toxicol. Methods 44:235, 2000.
42. Lipinski, C. A., Lombardo, F., Dominy, B. W., et al.: Adv. Drug Deliv. Rev. 46:3, 2001.
43. Bhal, S. K., Kassam, K., Peirson, I. G., et al.: Mol. Pharm. 4:556, 2007.
44. Kah, M., and Brown, C. D.: Chemosphere 72:1401, 2008.
45. Ghose, A. K., Viswanadhan, V. N., and Wendoloski, J. J.: J. Comb. Chem. 1:55, 1999.
46. Congreve, M., Chessari, G., Tisi, D., et al.: J. Med. Chem. 51:3661, 2008.
47. Langmuir, I.: J. Am. Chem. Soc. 41:1543, 1919.
48. Patani, G. A., and LaVoie, E. J.: Chem Rev. 96:3147, 1996.
49. Kubinyi, H.: Success Stories of Computer-Aided Design. In Ekins, S. (ed.). Computer Applications in Pharmaceutical Research and Development. New York, Wiley-Interscience, 2006, p. 377.
50. Boyd, D. B.: In Lipkowitz, K. B. and Cundari, T. R., (eds.). Reviews in Computational Chemistry. 23:401, 2007.

SELECTED READING

Abraham, D. (ed.): Burger's Medicinal Chemistry and Drug Discovery, 6th ed. New York, Wiley-Interscience, 2003.
Albert, A.: Selective Toxicity, 7th ed. New York, Chapman & Hall, 1985.
Cramer, C. J.: Essentials of Computational Chemistry: Theories and Models. New York, Wiley, 2002.
Dean, P. M. (ed.): Molecular Similarity in Drug Design. New York, Chapman & Hall, 1995.
Devillers, J., and Balaban, A. T., (eds.): Topological Indices and Related Descriptors in QSAR and QSPR. Amsterdam, Gordon and Breach, 1999.
Franke, R.: Theoretical drug design methods. In Nauta, W. T., and Rekker, R. F. (eds.). Pharmacochemistry Library, vol. 7. New York, Elsevier, 1984.

Güner, O. F. (ed.): Pharmacophore Perception, Development, and Use in Drug Design. La Jolla, CA, International University Line, 2000.

Hansch, C., and Leo, A.: Exploring QSAR, vol. 1. Fundamentals and Applications in Chemistry and Biology. Washington, DC, American Chemical Society, 1995.

Hehre, W. J.: A Guide to Molecular Mechanics and Quantum Chemical Calculations. Irvine, CA, Wavefunction, 2003.

Höltje, H.-D., Sippl, W., Rognan, D., and Folkers, G.: Molecular Modeling: Basic Principles and Applications. 2nd ed. New York, Wiley-VCH, 2003.

Keverling Buisman, J. A.: Biological activity and chemical structure. In Nauta, W. T., Rekker, R. F. (eds.). Pharmacochemistry Library, vol. 2. New York, Elsevier, 1977.

Kier, L. B., and Hall, L. H.: Molecular Connectivity in Structure-Activity Analysis. New York, John Wiley & Sons, 1986.

Kier, L. B., and Hall, L. H.: Molecular Structure Description, the Electrotopological State. New York, Academic Press, 1999.

Leach, A. R.: Molecular Modeling Principles and Applications. Essex, England, Longman, 1996.

Leo, A., Hansch, C., and Hoekman, D.: Exploring QSAR, vol. 2. Hydrophobic, Electronic, and Steric Constants. Washington, DC, American Chemical Society, 1995.

Martin, Y. C.: Quantitative drug design. In Grunewald, G. (ed.). Medicinal Research, vol. 8. New York, Dekker, 1978.

Mutschler, E., and Windterfeldt, E. (eds.): Trends in Medicinal Chemistry. Berlin, VCH Publishers, 1987.

Olson, E. C., and Christoffersen, R. E.: Computer-assisted drug design. In Comstock, M. J. (ed.). ACS Symposium Series, vol. 112. Washington, DC, American Chemical Society, 1979.

Rappé, A. K., and Casewit, C. J.: Molecular Mechanics Across Chemistry. Sausalito, CA, 1997.

Silverman, R. B.: The Organic Chemistry of Drug Design and Drug Action. New York, Academic Press, 1992.

Smith, H. J.: Smith and Williams' Introduction to the Principles of Drug Design and Action, 4th ed. New York, CRC Taylor & Francis, 2006.

Todeschini, R., and Consonni, V.: Handbook of Molecular Descriptors. In Mannhold, R., Kubinyi, H., and Timmerman, H. (eds.). New York, Wiley-VCH, 2000.

Topliss, J. G.: Quantitative Structure-Activity Relationships of Drugs. Medicinal Chemistry, A Series of Monographs, vol. 19. New York, Academic Press, 1983.

Wermuth, C. G. (ed): The Practice of Medicinal Chemistry, 2nd ed. New York, Academic Press, 2003.

Witten, I. H., and Frank, E.: Data Mining: Practical Machine Learning Tools and Techniques, 2nd ed. New York, Elsevier Morgan Kaufmann, 2005.

Young, D.: Computational Chemistry: A Practical Guide for Applying Techniques to Real World Problems. New York, Wiley-Interscience, 2001.

CHAPTER 3

Metabolic Changes of Drugs and Related Organic Compounds

STEPHEN J. CUTLER AND JOHN H. BLOCK

CHAPTER OVERVIEW

Metabolic Changes of Drugs and Related Organic Compounds describes the human metabolic processes of various functional groups found in therapeutic agents. The importance of a chapter on metabolism lies in the fact that drug interactions are based on these processes. For pharmacists to be good practitioners, it is necessary for them to understand why certain drugs are contraindicated with other drugs. This chapter attempts to describe the various phases of drug metabolism, the sites where these biotransformations will occur, the role of specific enzymes, metabolism of specific functional groups, and several examples of the metabolism of currently used therapeutic agents.

Metabolism plays a central role in the elimination of drugs and other foreign compounds (*xenobiotics*) from the body. A solid understanding of drug metabolic pathways is an essential tool for pharmacists in their role of selecting and monitoring appropriate drug therapy for their patients. Most organic compounds entering the body are relatively lipid soluble (*lipophilic*). To be absorbed, they must traverse the lipoprotein membranes of the lumen walls of the gastrointestinal (GI) tract. Then, once in the bloodstream, these molecules can diffuse passively through other membranes and be distributed effectively to reach various target organs to exert their pharmacological actions. Because of reabsorption in the renal tubules, lipophilic compounds are not excreted to any substantial extent in the urine. Xenobiotics then meet their metabolic fate through various enzyme systems that change the parent compound to render it more water soluble (*hydrophilic*). Once the metabolite is sufficiently water soluble, it may be excreted from the body. The previous statements show that a working knowledge of the ADME (absorption, distribution, metabolism, and excretion) principles is vital for successful determination of drug regimens.

If lipophilic drugs, or xenobiotics, were not metabolized to polar, readily excretable water-soluble products, they would remain indefinitely in the body, eliciting their biological effects. Thus, the formation of water-soluble metabolites not only enhances drug elimination, but also leads to compounds that are generally pharmacologically inactive and relatively nontoxic. Consequently, drug metabolism reactions have traditionally been regarded as *detoxication* (or *detoxification*) processes.[1] Unfortunately, it is incorrect to assume that drug metabolism reactions are always detoxifying. Many drugs are biotransformed to pharmacologically active metabolites. These metabolites may have significant activity that contributes substantially to the pharmacological or toxicological effect(s) ascribed to the parent drug. Occasionally, the parent compound is inactive when administered and must be metabolically converted to a biologically active drug (metabolite).[2,3] These types of compounds are referred to as *prodrugs*. In addition, it is becoming increasingly clear that not all metabolites are nontoxic. Indeed, many adverse effects (e.g., tissue necrosis, carcinogenicity, teratogenicity) of drugs and environmental contaminants can be attributed directly to the formation of chemically reactive metabolites that are highly detrimental to the body.[4–6] This concept is more important when the patient has a disease state that inhibits or expedites xenobiotic metabolism. Also, more and more drug metabolites are being found in our sewage systems. These compounds may be nontoxic to humans but harmful to other animals or the environment.

GENERAL PATHWAYS OF DRUG METABOLISM

Drug metabolism reactions have been divided into two categories: phase I (*functionalization*) and phase II (*conjugation*) reactions.[1,7] Phase I, or functionalization reactions, include oxidative, reductive, and hydrolytic biotransformations (Table 3.1).[8] The purpose of these reactions is to introduce a functional polar group(s) (e.g., OH, COOH, NH₂, SH) into the xenobiotic molecule to produce a more water-soluble compound. This can be achieved by direct introduction of the functional group (e.g., aromatic and aliphatic hydroxylation) or by modifying or "unmasking" existing functionalities (e.g., reduction of ketones and aldehydes to alcohols; oxidation of alcohols to acids; hydrolysis of ester and amides to yield COOH, NH₂, and OH groups; reduction of azo and nitro compounds to give NH₂ moieties; oxidative N-, O-, and S-dealkylation to give NH₂, OH, and SH groups). Although phase I reactions may not produce sufficiently hydrophilic or inactive metabolites, they generally tend to provide a functional group or "handle" on the molecule that can undergo subsequent phase II reactions.

The purpose of phase II reactions is to attach small, polar, and ionizable endogenous compounds such as glucuronic acid, sulfate, glycine, and other amino acids to the functional handles of phase I metabolites or parent compounds that already have suitable existing functional groups to form water-soluble conjugated products. Conjugated metabolites are readily excreted in the urine

TABLE 3.1 General Summary of Phase I and Phase II Metabolic Pathways

Phase I or Functionalization Reactions

Oxidative Reactions
Oxidation of aromatic moieties
Oxidation of olefins
Oxidation at benzylic, allylic carbon atoms, and carbon atoms α to carbonyl and imines
Oxidation at aliphatic and alicyclic carbon atoms
Oxidation involving carbon–heteroatom systems:
  Carbon–nitrogen systems (aliphatic and aromatic amines; includes *N*-dealkylation, oxidative deamination, *N*-oxide formation, *N*-hydroxylation)
  Carbon–oxygen systems (*O*-dealkylation)
  Carbon–sulfur systems (*S*-dealkylation, *S*-oxidation, and desulfuration)
Oxidation of alcohols and aldehydes
Other miscellaneous oxidative reactions

Reductive Reactions
Reduction of aldehydes and ketones
Reduction of nitro and azo compounds
Miscellaneous reductive reactions

Hydrolytic Reactions
Hydrolysis of esters and amides
Hydration of epoxides and arene oxides by epoxide hydrase

Phase II or Conjugation Reactions

Glucuronic acid conjugation
Sulfate conjugation
Conjugation with glycine, glutamine, and other amino acids
Glutathione or mercapturic acid conjugation
Acetylation
Methylation

ment one another in detoxifying, and facilitating the elimination of, drugs and xenobiotics.

To illustrate, consider the principal psychoactive constituent of marijuana, Δ^9-tetrahydrocannabinol (Δ^9-THC, also known as Δ^1-THC, depending on the numbering system being used). This lipophilic molecule (octanol/water partition coefficient $\sim$6,000)[9] undergoes allylic hydroxylation to give 11-hydroxy-Δ^9-THC in humans.[10,11] More polar than its parent compound, the 11-hydroxy metabolite is further oxidized to the corresponding carboxylic acid derivative Δ^9-THC-11-oic acid, which is ionized (pK$_a$ COOH $\sim$5) at physiological pH. Subsequent conjugation of this metabolite (either at the COOH or phenolic OH) with glucuronic acid leads to water-soluble products that are readily eliminated in the urine.[12]

In the series of biotransformations, the parent Δ^9-THC molecule is made increasingly polar, ionizable, and hydrophilic. The attachment of the glucuronyl moiety (with its ionized carboxylate group and three polar hydroxyl groups; see structure) to the Δ^9-THC metabolites notably favors partitioning of the conjugated metabolites into an aqueous medium. This is an important point in using urinalysis to identify illegal drugs.

The purpose of this chapter is to provide students with a broad overview of drug metabolism. Various phase I and phase II biotransformation pathways (see Table 3.1) are outlined, and representative drug examples for each pathway are presented. Drug metabolism examples in humans are emphasized, although discussion of metabolism in other mammalian systems is necessary. The central role of the cytochrome P450 (CYP) monooxygenase system in oxidative drug biotransformation is elaborated. Discussion of other enzyme systems involved in phase I and phase II reactions is presented in their respective sections. In addition to stereochemical factors that may affect drug metabolism, biological factors such as age, sex, heredity, disease state, and species variation are considered. The effects of enzyme induction and inhibition on drug metabolism and a section on pharmacologically active metabolites are included.

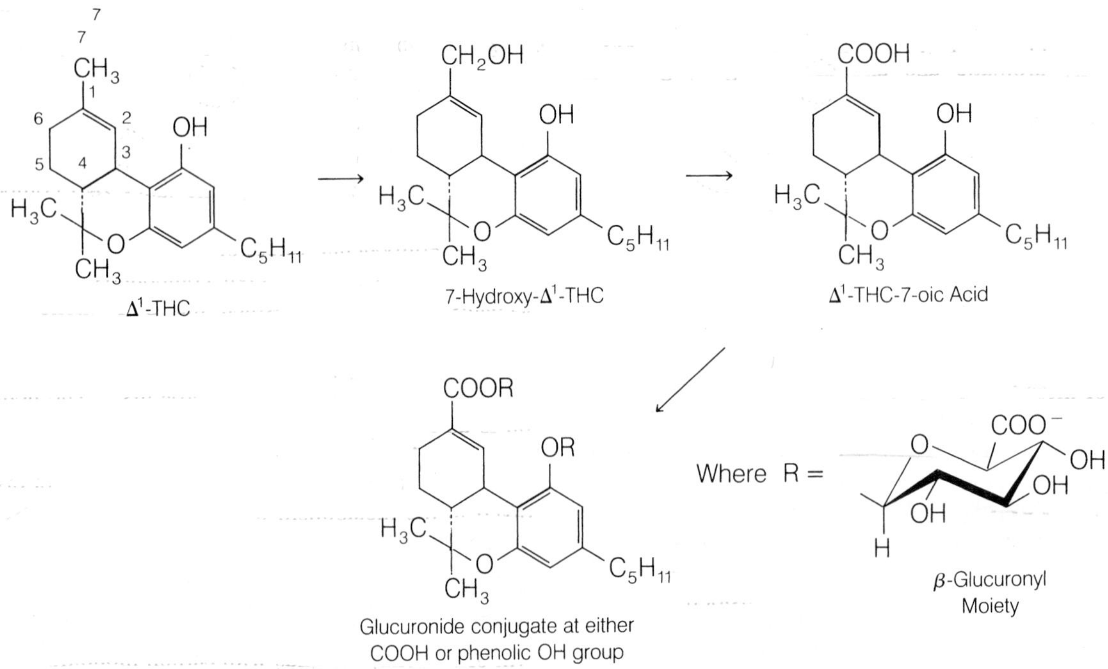

and are generally devoid of pharmacological activity and toxicity in humans. Other phase II pathways, such as methylation and acetylation, terminate or attenuate biological activity, whereas glutathione (GSH) conjugation protects the body against chemically reactive compounds or metabolites. Thus, phase I and phase II reactions complement

Δ^1-THC

7-Hydroxy-Δ^1-THC

Δ^1-THC-7-oic Acid

Where R =

β-Glucuronyl Moiety

Glucuronide conjugate at either COOH or phenolic OH group

⬡ SITES OF DRUG BIOTRANSFORMATION

Although biotransformation reactions may occur in many tissues, the liver is, by far, the most important organ in drug metabolism and detoxification of endogenous and exogenous compounds.[13] Another important site, especially for orally administered drugs, is the intestinal mucosa. The latter contains the CYP3A4 isozyme (see discussion on cytochrome nomenclature) and P-glycoprotein that can capture the drug and secrete it back into the intestinal tract. In contrast, the liver, a well-perfused organ, is particularly rich in almost all of the drug-metabolizing enzymes discussed in this chapter. Orally administered drugs that are absorbed into the bloodstream through the GI tract must pass through the liver before being further distributed into body compartments. Therefore, they are susceptible to hepatic metabolism known as the *first-pass effect* before reaching the systemic circulation. Depending on the drug, this metabolism can sometimes be quite significant and results in decreased oral bioavailability. For example, in humans, several drugs are metabolized extensively by the first-pass effect.[14] The following list includes some of those drugs:

Isoproterenol *	Morphine	Propoxyphene
Lidocaine	Nitroglycerin	Propranolol *
Meperidine	Pentazocine	Salicylamide

Some drugs (e.g., lidocaine) are removed so effectively by first-pass metabolism that they are ineffective when given orally.[15] Nitroglycerin is administered buccally to bypass the liver.

Because most drugs are administered orally, the intestine appears to play an important role in the extrahepatic metabolism of xenobiotics. For example, in humans, orally administered isoproterenol undergoes considerable sulfate conjugation in the intestinal wall.[16] Several other drugs (e.g., levodopa, chlorpromazine, and diethylstilbestrol)[17] are also reportedly metabolized in the GI tract. Esterases and lipases present in the intestine may be particularly[18] important in carrying out hydrolysis of many ester prodrugs (see "Hydrolytic Reactions"). Bacterial flora present in the intestine and colon appear to play an important role in the reduction of many aromatic azo and nitro drugs (e.g., sulfasalazine).[19,20] Intestinal β-glucuronidase enzymes can hydrolyze glucuronide conjugates excreted in the bile, thereby liberating the free drug or its metabolite for possible reabsorption (enterohepatic circulation or recycling).[21]

Although other tissues, such as kidney, lungs, adrenal glands, placenta, brain, and skin, have some drug-metabolizing capability, the biotransformations that they carry out are often more substrate selective and more limited to particular types of reaction (e.g., oxidation, glucuronidation).[22] In many instances, the full metabolic capabilities of these tissues have not been explored fully.

⬡ ROLE OF CYTOCHROME P450 MONOOXYGENASES IN OXIDATIVE BIOTRANSFORMATIONS

Of the various phase I reactions that are considered in this chapter, oxidative biotransformation processes are, by far, the most common and important in drug metabolism. The

TABLE 3.2 **Cytochrome P450 Enzymes Nomenclature**

CYP-Arabic Number-Capital Letter-Arabic Number
1. CYP: Cytochrome P450 enzymes
2. Arabic number: Family (CYP1, CYP2, CYP3, etc.)
   Must have more than 40% identical amino acid sequence
3. Capital letter: Subfamily (CYP1A, CYP2C, CYP3A, etc.)
   Must have more than 55% identical amino acid sequence
4. Arabic number: Individual enzyme in a subfamily (CYP1A2, CYP2C9, CYP2D6, CYP2E1, CYP3A4, etc.)
   Identity of amino acid sequences can exceed 90%

general stoichiometry that describes the oxidation of many xenobiotics (R-H) to their corresponding oxidized metabolites (R-OH) is given by the following equation:[23]

$$RH + NADPH + O_2 + H^+ \rightarrow ROH + NADP^+ + H_2O$$

The enzyme systems carrying out this biotransformation are referred to as *mixed-function oxidases* or *monooxygenases*.[24,25] There is a large family that carry out the same basic chemical reactions. Their nomenclature is based on amino acid homology and is summarized in Table 3.2. There are four components to the name. CYP refers to the cytochrome system. This is followed by the Arabic number that specifies the cytochrome family (CYP1, CYP2, CYP3, etc.). Next is a capital letter that represents the subfamily (CYP1A, CYP1B, CYP2A, CYP2B, CYP3A, CYP3B, etc.). Finally, the cytochrome name ends with another Arabic number that specifies the specific enzyme responsible for a particular reaction (CYP1A2, CYP2C9, CYP2C19, CYP3A4, etc.).

The reaction requires both molecular oxygen and the reducing agent NADPH (reduced form of nicotinamide adenosine dinucleotide phosphate). During this oxidative process, one atom of molecular oxygen (O_2) is introduced into the substrate R-H to form R-OH and the other oxygen atom is incorporated into water. The mixed-function oxidase system[26] is actually made up of several components, the most important being the superfamily of CYP enzymes (currently at 57 genes [http://drnelson.utmem.edu/CytochromeP450.html]), which are responsible for transferring an *oxygen atom* to the substrate R-H. Other important components of this system include the NADPH-dependent CYP reductase and the NADH-linked cytochrome b₅. The latter two components, along with the cofactors NADPH and NADH, supply the reducing equivalents (electrons) needed in the overall metabolic oxidation of foreign compounds. The proposed mechanistic scheme by which the CYP monooxygenase system catalyzes the conversion of molecular oxygen to an "activated oxygen" species is elaborated below.

The CYP enzymes are heme proteins.[27] The heme portion is an iron-containing porphyrin called *protoporphyrin IX*, and the protein portion is called the *apoprotein*. CYP is found in high concentrations in the liver, the major organ involved in the metabolism of xenobiotics. The presence of this enzyme in many other tissues (e.g., lung, kidney, intestine, skin, placenta, adrenal cortex) shows that these tissues have drug-oxidizing capability too. The name *cytochrome P450* is derived from the fact that the reduced (Fe^{2+}) form of this enzyme binds with carbon monoxide to form a complex that has a distinguishing spectroscopic absorption maximum at 450 nm.[28]

One important feature of the hepatic CYP mixed-function oxidase system is its ability to metabolize an almost unlimited number of diverse substrates by various oxidative transformations.[29] This versatility is believed to be a result of the substrate nonspecificity of CYP as well as the presence of multiple forms of the enzyme.[30] Some of these P450 enzymes are selectively inducible by various chemicals (e.g., phenobarbital, benzo[α]pyrene, 3-methylcholanthrene).[31] One of these inducible forms of the enzyme (cytochrome P448)[32] is of particular interest and is discussed later in this section.

The CYP monooxygenases are located in the endoplasmic reticulum, a highly organized and complex network of intracellular membranes that is particularly abundant in tissues such as the liver.[33] When these tissues are disrupted by homogenization, the endoplasmic reticulum loses its structure and is converted into small vesicular bodies known as *microsomes.* Mitochondria house many of the cytochrome enzymes that are responsible for the biosynthesis of steroidal hormones and metabolism of certain vitamins.

Microsomes isolated from hepatic tissue appear to retain all of the mixed-function oxidase capabilities of intact hepatocytes; because of this, microsomal preparations (with the necessary cofactors, e.g., NADPH, Mg^{2+}) are used frequently for in vitro drug metabolism studies. Because of its membrane-bound nature, the CYP monooxygenase system appears to be housed in a lipoidal environment. This may explain, in part, why lipophilic xenobiotics are generally good substrates for the monooxygenase system.[34]

The catalytic role that the CYP monooxygenase system plays in the oxidation of xenobiotics is summarized in the cycle shown in Figure 3.1.[35–37] The initial step of this catalytic reaction cycle starts with the binding of the substrate to the oxidized (Fe^{3+}) resting state of CYP to form a P450-substrate complex. The next step involves the transfer of one electron from NADPH-dependent CYP reductase to the P450-substrate complex. This one-electron transfer reduces Fe^{3+} to Fe^{2+}. It is this reduced (Fe^{2+}) P450-substrate complex that is capable of binding dioxygen (O_2). The dioxygen–P450-substrate complex that is formed then undergoes another one-electron reduction (by CYP reductase-NADPH and/or cytochrome b_5 reductase-NADH) to yield what is believed to be a peroxide dianion–P450 (Fe^{3+})-substrate complex. Water (containing one of the oxygen atoms from the original dioxygen molecule) is released from the latter intermediate to form an activated oxygen–P450-substrate complex (Fig. 3.2). The activated oxygen $[FeO]^{3+}$ in this complex is highly electron deficient and a potent oxidizing agent. The activated oxygen is transferred to the substrate (R-H), and the oxidized substrate product (R-OH) is released from the enzyme complex to regenerate the oxidized form of CYP.

The key sequence of events appears to center around the alteration of a dioxygen–P450-substrate complex to an activated oxygen–P450-substrate complex, which can then effect the critical transfer of oxygen from P450 to the substrate.[37,38] In view of the potent oxidizing nature of the activated oxygen being transferred, it is not surprising CYP

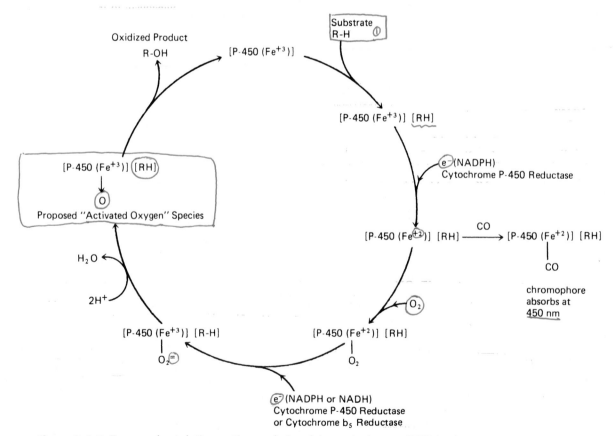

Figure 3.1 ● Proposed catalytic reaction cycle involving cytochrome P450 in the oxidation of xenobiotics.

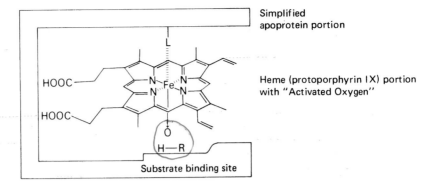

Figure 3.2 ● Simplified depiction of the proposed activated oxygen–cytochrome P450-substrate complex. Note the simplified apoprotein portion and the heme (protoporphyrin IX) portion or cytochrome P450 and the proximity of the substrate R-H undergoing oxidation.

can oxidize numerous substrates. The mechanistic details of oxygen activation and transfer in CYP-catalyzed reactions continue to be an active area of research in drug metabolism.[34] The many types of oxidative reaction carried out by CYP are enumerated in the sections below. Many of these oxidative pathways are summarized schematically in Figure 3.3 (see also Table 3.1).[37]

The versatility of CYP in carrying out various oxidation reactions on a multitude of substrates may be attributed to the multiple forms of the enzyme. Consequently, students must realize that the biotransformation of a parent xenobiotic to several oxidized metabolites is carried out not just by one form of P450 but, more likely, by several different forms. Extensive studies indicate that the apoprotein portions of various CYPs differ from one another in their tertiary structure (because of differences in amino acid sequence or the makeup of the polypeptide chain).[27,30,39–41] Because the apoprotein portion is important in substrate binding and catalytic transfer of activated

oxygen, these structural differences may account for some substrates being preferentially or more efficiently oxidized by one particular form of CYP. Finally, because of the enormous number of uncommon reactions that are catalyzed by P450, the reader is directed to other articles of interest.[42]

⬡ OXIDATIVE REACTIONS

Oxidation of Aromatic Moieties

Aromatic hydroxylation refers to the mixed-function oxidation of aromatic compounds (*arenes*) to their corresponding phenolic metabolites (*arenols*).[43] Almost all aromatic hydroxylation reactions are believed to proceed initially through an epoxide intermediate called an "arene oxide," which rearranges rapidly and spontaneously to the arenol product in most instances. The importance of arene oxides in the formation of arenols and in other metabolic and toxicologic

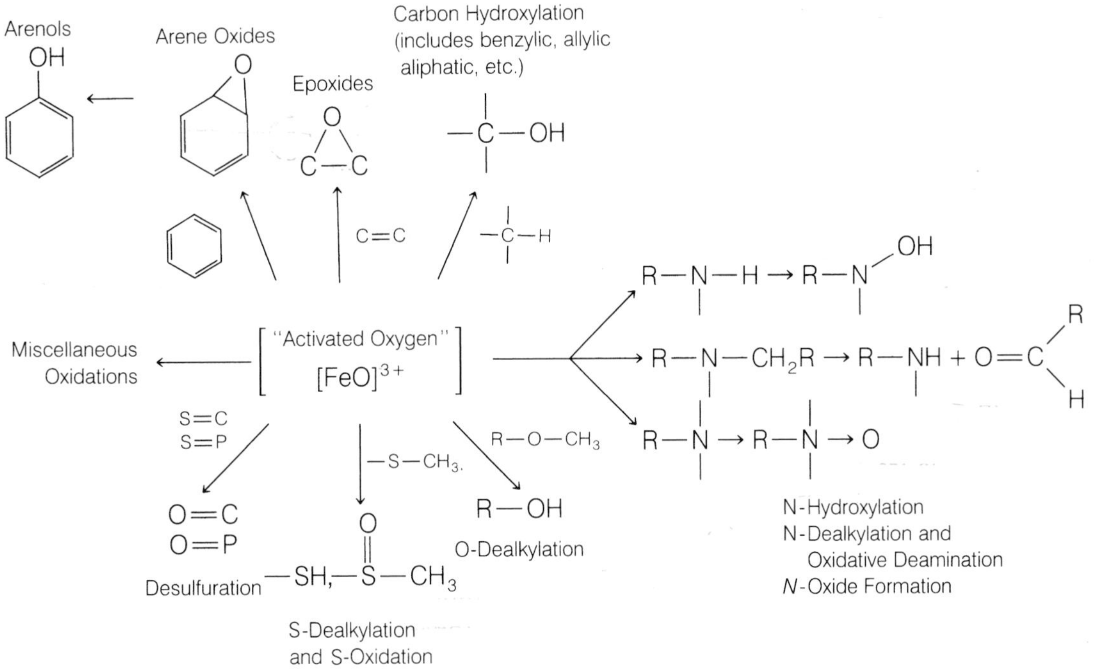

Figure 3.3 ● Schematic summary of cytochrome P450-catalyzed oxidation reactions. (Adapted from Ullrich, V.: Top. Curr. Chem. 83:68, 1979.)

reactions is discussed below.[44,45] Our attention now focuses on the aromatic hydroxylation of several drugs and xenobiotics.

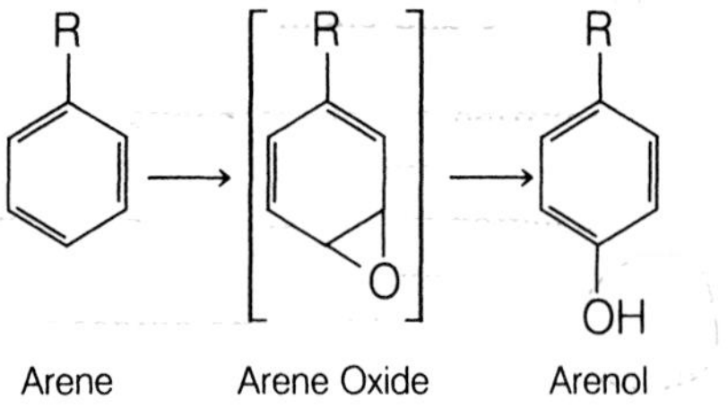

Arene   Arene Oxide   Arenol

Most foreign compounds containing aromatic moieties are susceptible to aromatic oxidation. In humans, aromatic hydroxylation is a major route of metabolism for many drugs containing phenyl groups. Important therapeutic agents such as propranolol,[46,47] phenobarbital,[48] phenytoin,[49,50] phenylbutazone,[51,52] atorvastatin,[53] 17α-ethinylestradiol,[54,55] and $(S)(-)$-warfarin,[56] among others, undergo extensive aromatic oxidation (Fig. 3.4 shows structure and site of hydroxylation). In most of the drugs just mentioned, hydroxylation occurs at the *para* position.[57] Most phenolic metabolites formed from aromatic oxidation undergo further conversion to polar and water-soluble glucuronide or sulfate conjugates, which are readily excreted in the urine. For example, the major urinary metabolite of phenytoin found in humans is the *O*-glucuronide conjugate of *p*-hydroxyphenytoin.[49,50] Interestingly, the *para*-hydroxylated metabolite of phenylbutazone, oxyphenbutazone, is pharmacologically active and has been marketed itself as an anti-inflammatory agent (Tandearil, Oxalid).[51,52] Of the two enantiomeric forms of the oral anticoagulant warfarin (Coumadin), only the more active $S(-)$ enantiomer has been shown to undergo substantial aromatic hydroxylation to 7-hydroxywarfarin in humans.[56] In contrast, the $(R)(+)$ enantiomer is metabolized by keto reduction[56] (see "Stereochemical Aspects of Drug Metabolism").

Often, the substituents attached to the aromatic ring may influence the ease of hydroxylation.[57] As a general rule, microsomal aromatic hydroxylation reactions appear to proceed most readily in activated (electron-rich) rings, whereas deactivated aromatic rings (e.g., those containing electron-withdrawing groups Cl, $-N^+R_3$, COOH, SO_2NHR) are generally slow or resistant to hydroxylation. The deactivating groups (Cl, $-N^+H=C$) present in the antihypertensive clonidine (Catapres) may explain why this drug undergoes little aromatic hydroxylation in humans.[58,59] The uricosuric agent probenecid (Benemid), with its electron-withdrawing carboxy and sulfamido groups, has not been reported to undergo any aromatic hydroxylation.[60]

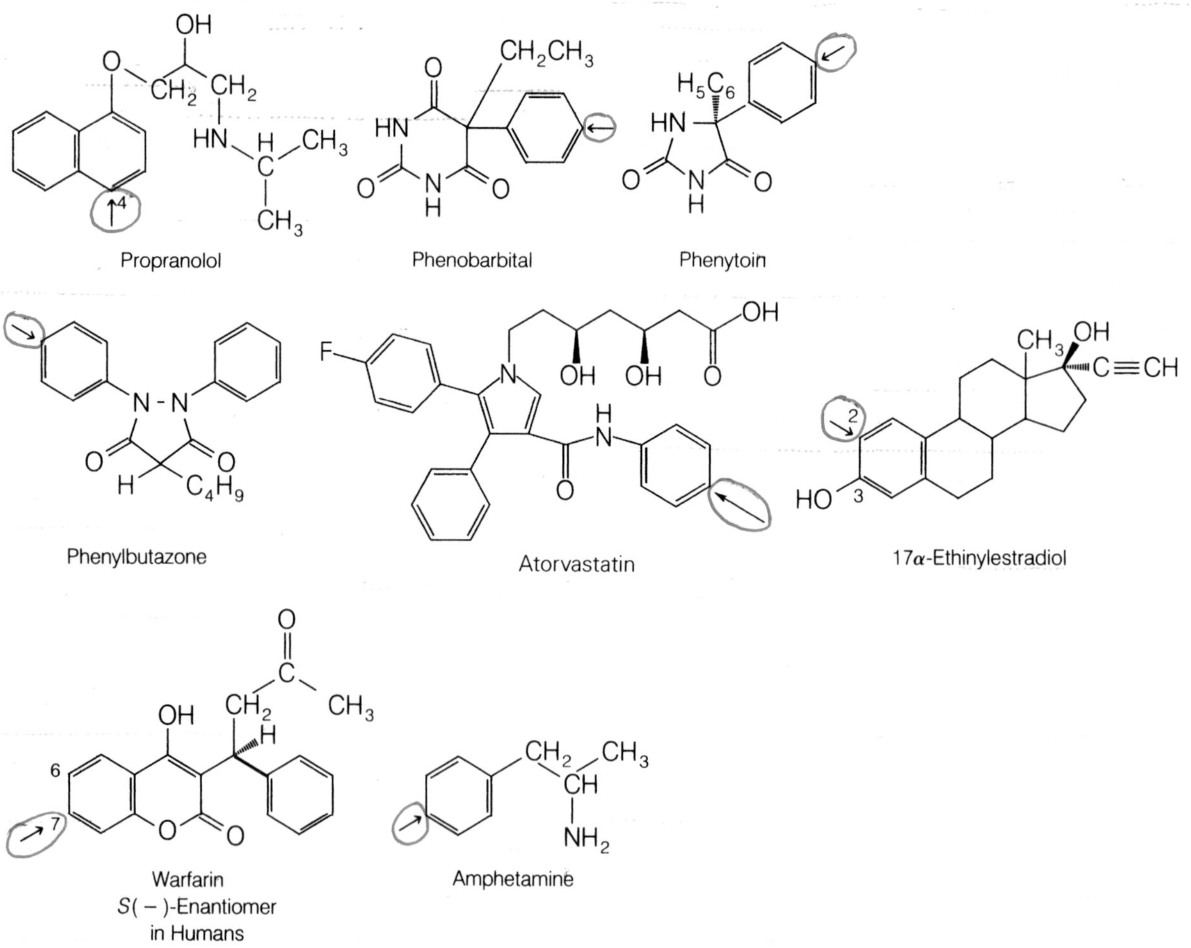

Figure 3.4 ● Examples of drugs and xenobiotics that undergo aromatic hydroxylation in humans. *Arrow* indicates site of aromatic hydroxylation.

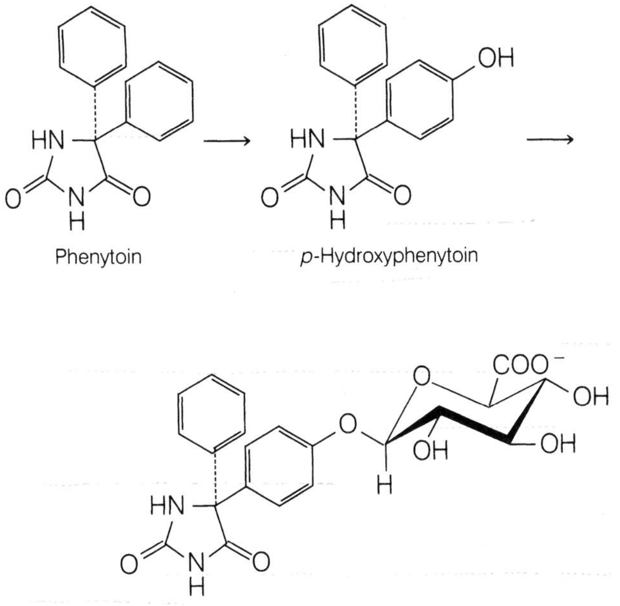

Phenytoin

p-Hydroxyphenytoin

O-Glucuronide Conjugate

In compounds with two aromatic rings, hydroxylation occurs preferentially in the more electron-rich ring. For example, aromatic hydroxylation of diazepam (Valium) occurs primarily in the more activated ring to yield 4′-hydroxydiazepam.[61] A similar situation is seen in the 7-hydroxylation of the antipsychotic agent chlorpromazine (Thorazine)[62] and in the *para*-hydroxylation of *p*-chlorobiphenyl to *p*-chloro-*p*′-hydroxybiphenyl.[63]

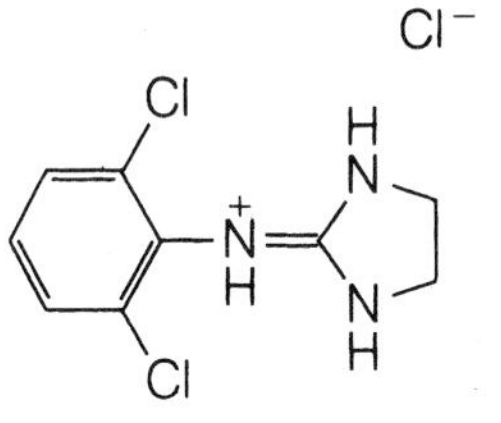

Clonidine Hydrochloride

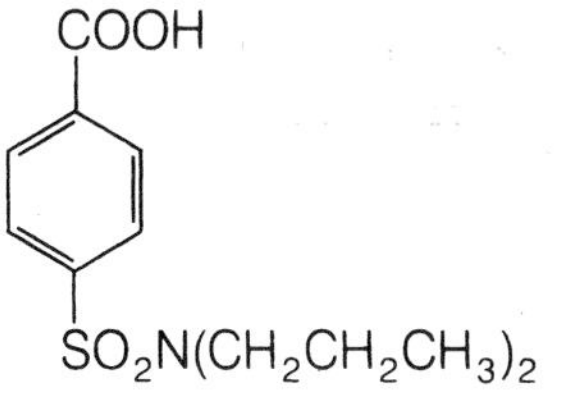

Probenecid

Recent environmental pollutants, such as polychlorinated biphenyls (PCBs) and 2,3,7,8-tetrachlorodibenzo-*p*-dioxin (TCDD), have attracted considerable public concern over their toxicity and health hazards. These compounds appear to be resistant to aromatic oxidation because of the numerous electronegative chlorine atoms in their aromatic rings. The metabolic stability coupled to the lipophilicity of these environmental contaminants probably explains their long persistence in the body once absorbed.[64–66]

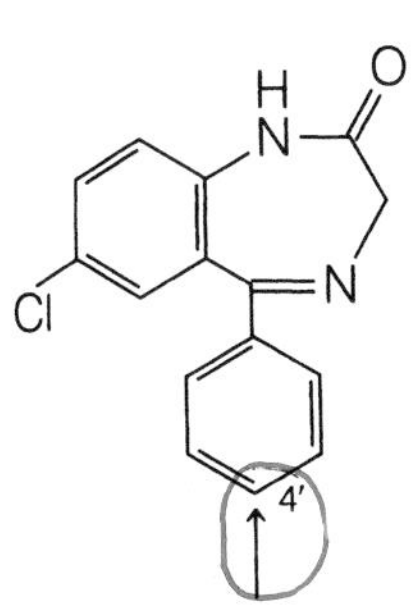

Diazepam

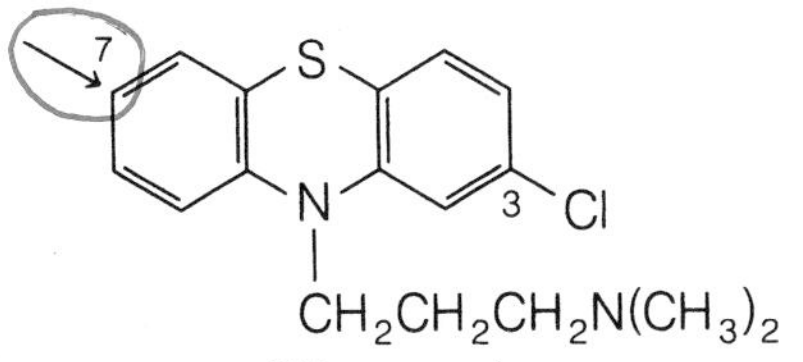

Chlorpromazine

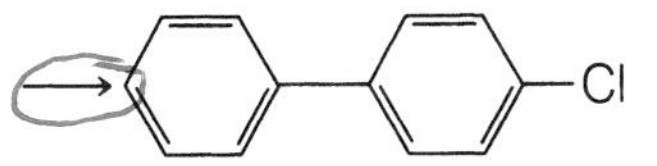

p-Chlorobiphenyl

Arene oxide intermediates are formed when a double bond in aromatic moieties is epoxidized. Arene oxides are of significant toxicologic concern because these intermediates are electrophilic and chemically reactive (because of the strained three-membered epoxide ring). Arene oxides are mainly detoxified by spontaneous rearrangement to arenols, but enzymatic hydration to *trans*-dihydrodiols and enzymatic conjugation with GSH also play very important roles (Fig. 3.5).[43,44] If not effectively detoxified by the first three pathways in Figure 3.5, arene oxides will bind covalently with nucleophilic groups present on proteins, deoxyribonucleic acid (DNA), and ribonucleic acid (RNA), thereby leading to serious cellular damage.[5,43] This, in part, helps explain why benzene can be so toxic to mammalian systems.

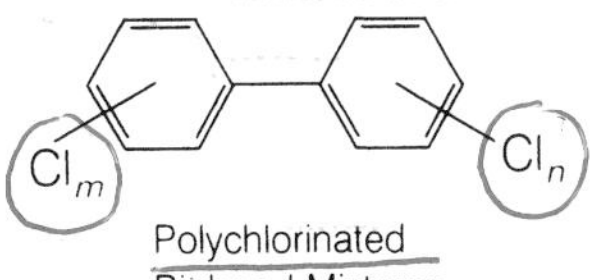

Polychlorinated
Biphenyl Mixtures

2.3.7.8-Tetrachlorodibenzo-*p*-dioxin
(TCDD)

The number of chlorine atoms (*m*.*n*) present in two aromatic rings varies considerably

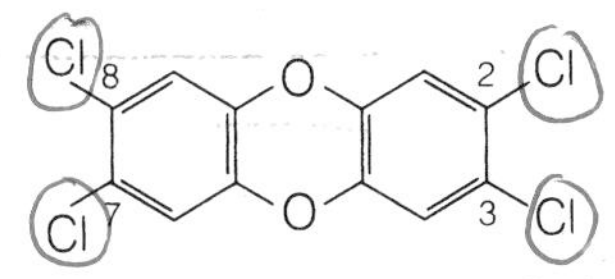

Quantitatively, the most important detoxification reaction for arene oxides is the spontaneous rearrangement to corresponding arenols. Often, this rearrangement is accompanied by a novel intramolecular hydride (deuteride) migration called the "NIH shift."[67] It was named after the National Institutes of Health (NIH) laboratory in Bethesda, Maryland, where this process was discovered. The general features of the NIH shift are illustrated with the mixed-function aromatic oxidation of 4-deuterioanisole to 3-deuterio-4-hydroxyanisole in Figure 3.6.[68]

After its metabolic formation, the arene oxide ring opens in the direction that generates the most resonance-stabilized carbocation (positive charge on C-3 carbon is resonance stabilized by the OCH$_3$ group). The zwitterionic species (positive charge on the C-3 carbon atom and negative charge on the oxygen atom) then undergoes a 1,2-deuteride shift (NIH shift) to form the dienone. Final transformation of the dienone to 3-deuterio-4-hydroxyanisole occurs with the preferential loss of a proton because of the weaker bond energy of the C–H bond (compared with the C–D bond). Thus, the deuterium is retained in the molecule by undergoing this intramolecular NIH shift. The experimental observation of an NIH shift for aromatic hydroxylation of a drug or xenobiotic is taken as indirect evidence for the involvement of an arene oxide.

In addition to the NIH shift, the zwitterionic species may undergo direct loss of D$^+$ to generate 4-hydroxyanisole, in which there is no retention of deuterium (Fig. 3.6). The alternative pathway (direct loss of D$^+$) may be more favorable than the NIH shift in some aromatic oxidation reactions. Therefore, depending on the substituent group on the arene, some aromatic hydroxylation reactions do not display any NIH shift.

Two extremely important enzymatic reactions also aid in neutralizing the reactivity of arene oxides. The first of these involves the hydration (i.e., nucleophilic attack of water on the

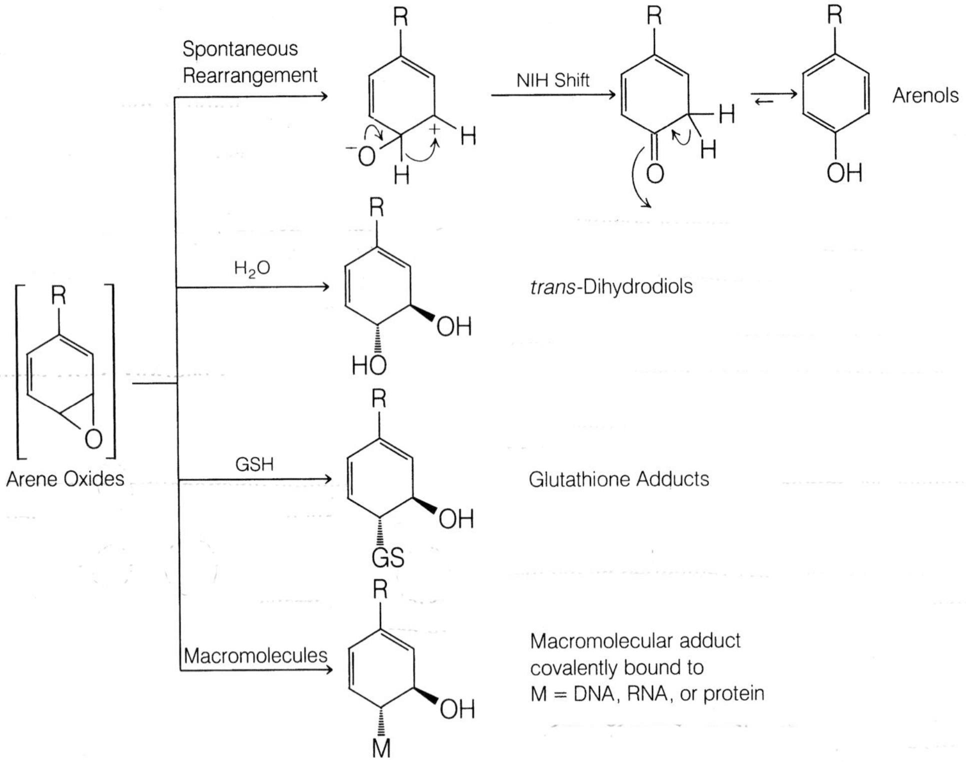

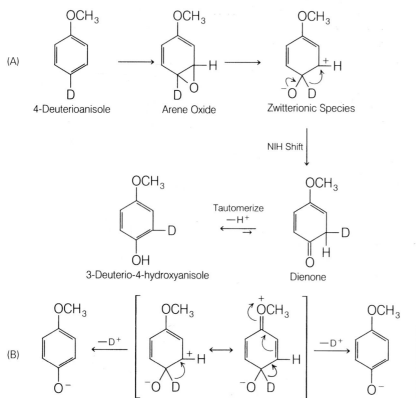

Figure 3.5 ● Possible reaction pathways for arene oxides. (Data are from Daly, J. W., et al.: *Experientia* 28:1129, 1972; Jerina, D. M., and Daly, J. W.: *Science* 185:573, 1974; and Kaminsky, L. S.: In Anders, M. W. [ed.]. Bioactivation of Foreign Compounds. New York, Academic Press, 1985, p. 157.)

Figure 3.6 ● **A.** General features of the NIH shift or 1,2-hydride (deuteride) shift in the mixed-function oxidation of 4-deuterio-4-hydroxyanisole. **B.** Direct loss of D$^+$ from zwitterionic species, leading to no retention of deuterium in 4-hydroxyanisole.

epoxide) of arene oxides to yield inactive *trans*-dihydrodiol metabolites (Fig. 3.5). This reaction is catalyzed by microsomal enzymes called *epoxide hydrases*.[69,70] Often, epoxide hydrase inhibitors, such as cyclohexene oxide and 1,1,1-trichloropropene-2,3-oxide, have been used to demonstrate the detoxification role of these enzymes. Addition of these inhibitors is accompanied frequently by increased toxicity of the arene oxide being tested, because formation of nontoxic dihydrodiols is blocked. For example, the mutagenicity of benzo[α]pyrene-4,5-oxide, as measured by the Ames *Salmonella typhimurium* test system, is potentiated when cyclohexene oxide is added.[71] Dihydrodiol metabolites have been reported in the metabolism of several aromatic hydrocarbons (e.g., naphthalene, benzo[α]pyrene, and other related polycyclic aromatic hydrocarbons).[43] A few drugs (e.g., phenytoin,[72] phenobarbital,[73] glutethimide[74]) also yield dihydrodiol products as minor metabolites in humans. Dihydrodiol products are susceptible to conjugation with glucuronic acid, as well as enzymatic dehydrogenation to the corresponding catechol metabolite, as exemplified by the metabolism of phenytoin.[72]

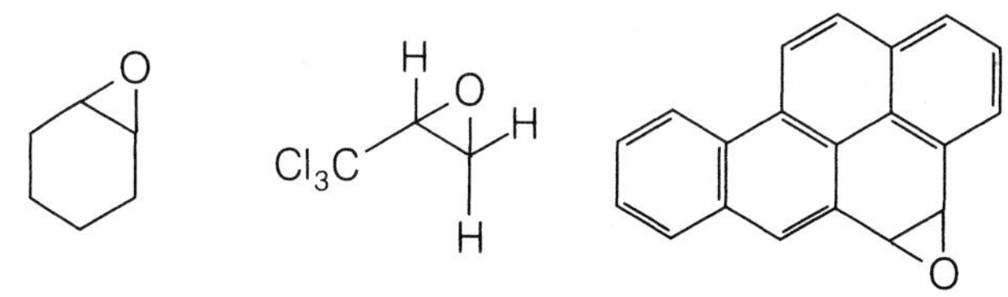

A second enzymatic reaction involves nucleophilic ring opening of the arene oxide by the sulfhydryl (SH) group present in GSH to yield the corresponding *trans*-1,2-dihydro-1-*S*-glutathionyl-2-hydroxy adduct, or GSH adduct (Fig. 3.5).[44] The reaction is catalyzed by various GSH *S*-transferases.[75] Because GSH is found in practically all mammalian tissues, it plays an important role in the detoxification not only of arene oxides but also of other various chemically reactive and potentially toxic intermediates. Initially, GSH adducts formed from arene oxides are modified in a series of reactions to yield "premercapturic acid" or mercapturic acid metabolites.[76] Because it is classified as a phase II pathway, GSH conjugation is covered in greater detail later in this chapter.

Because of their electrophilic and reactive nature, arene oxides also may undergo spontaneous reactions with nucleophilic functionalities present on biomacromolecules.[44,45] Such reactions lead to modified protein, DNA, and RNA structures and often cause dramatic alterations in how these macromolecules function. Much of the cytotoxicity and irreversible lesions caused by arene oxides are presumed to result from their covalent binding to cellular components. Several well-established examples of reactive arene oxides that cause serious toxicity are presented below.

Administration of bromobenzene to rats causes severe liver necrosis.[77] Extensive in vivo and in vitro studies indicate that the liver damage results from the interaction of a chemically reactive metabolite, 4-bromobenzene oxide, with hepatocytes.[78] Extensive covalent binding to hepatic

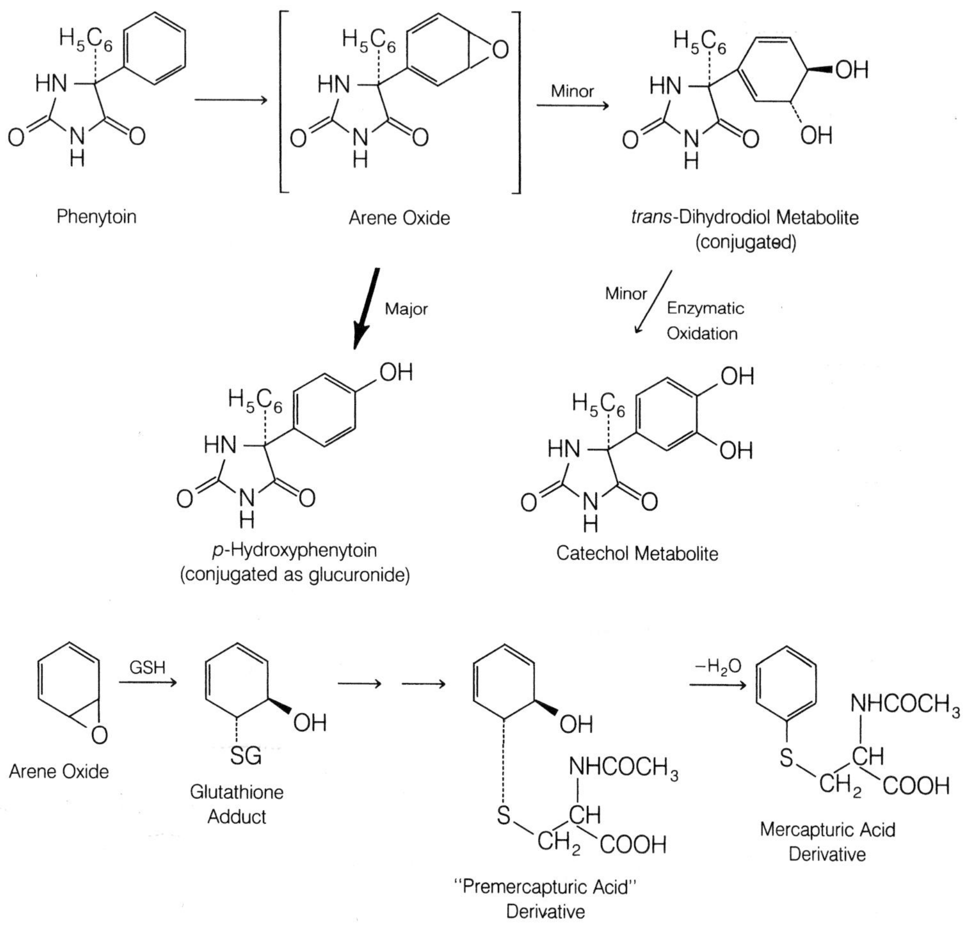

Cyclohexane oxide

1,1,1-Trichloropropene 2,3-oxide

Benzo[*a*]pyrene 4,5-oxide

Phenytoin

Arene Oxide

trans-Dihydrodiol Metabolite (conjugated)

Major

Minor / Enzymatic Oxidation

p-Hydroxyphenytoin (conjugated as glucuronide)

Catechol Metabolite

Arene Oxide

Glutathione Adduct

"Premercapturic Acid" Derivative

Mercapturic Acid Derivative

tissue was confirmed by use of radiolabeled bromobenzene. The severity of necrosis correlated well with the amount of covalent binding to hepatic tissue. Use of diethyl maleate or large doses of bromobenzene in rats showed that the depletion of hepatic GSH led to more severe liver necrosis.

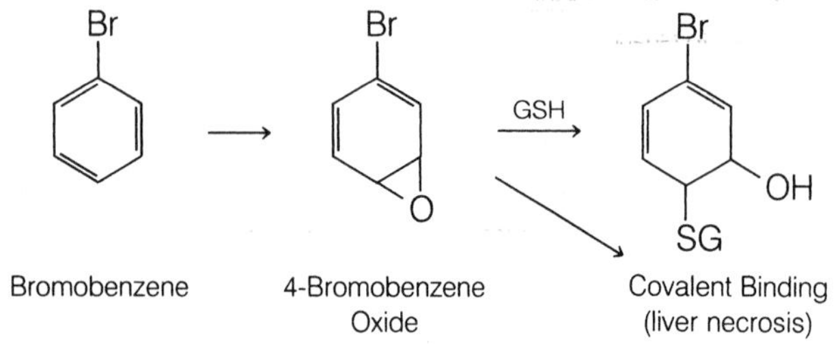

Polycyclic aromatic hydrocarbons are ubiquitous environmental contaminants that are formed from auto emission, refuse burning, industrial processes, cigarette smoke, and other combustion processes. Benzo[α]pyrene, a potent carcinogenic agent, is perhaps the most extensively studied of the polycyclic aromatic hydrocarbons.[79] Inspection of its structure reveals that aromatic hydroxylation of benzo[α]pyrene can occur at several positions. The identification of several dihydrodiol metabolites is viewed as indirect evidence for the formation and involvement of arene oxides in the metabolism of benzo[α]pyrene. Although certain arene oxides of benzo[α]pyrene (e.g., 4,5-oxide, 7,8-oxide, 9,10-oxide) appear to display some mutagenic and tumorigenic activity, it does not appear that they represent the ultimate reactive species responsible for benzo[α]pyrene's carcinogenicity. In recent years, extensive studies have led to the characterization of a specific sequence of metabolic reactions (Fig. 3.7) that generate a highly reactive intermediate that covalently binds to DNA. Metabolic activation of benzo[α]pyrene to the ultimate carcinogenic species involves an initial epoxidation reaction to form the 7,8-oxide, which is then converted by epoxide hydrase to (−)-7(R),8(R)-dihydroxy-7,8-dihydrobenzo[α]pyrene.[80] The two-step enzymatic formation of this *trans*-dihydrodiol is stereospecific. Subsequent epoxidation at the 9,10-double bond of the latter metabolite generates predominantly (+)-7(R),8(S)-dihydroxy-9(R),10(R)-oxy-7,8,9,10-tetrahydrobenzo[α]pyrene or (+)7,8-diol-9,10-epoxide. It is this key electrophilic diol epoxide metabolite that readily reacts with DNA to form many covalently bound adducts.[81–83] Careful degradation studies have shown that the principal adduct involves attack of the C-2 amino group of deoxyguanosine at C-10 of the diol epoxide. Clearly, these reactions are responsible for genetic code alterations that ultimately lead to the malignant transformations. Covalent binding of the diol epoxide metabolite to deoxyadenosine and to deoxycytidine also has been established.[84]

Another carcinogenic polycyclic aromatic hydrocarbon, 7,12-dimethylbenz[α]anthracene, also forms covalent adducts with nucleic acids (RNA).[85] The ultimate carcinogenic reactive species apparently is the 5,6-oxide that results from epoxidation of the 5,6-double bond in this aromatic hydrocarbon. The arene oxide intermediate binds covalently to guanosine residues of RNA to yield the two adducts.

Oxidation of Olefins

The metabolic oxidation of olefinic carbon–carbon double bonds leads to the corresponding epoxide (or oxirane). Epoxides derived from olefins generally tend to be somewhat more stable than the arene oxides formed from aromatic compounds. A few epoxides are stable enough to be directly measurable in biological fluids (e.g., plasma, urine). Like their arene oxide counterparts, epoxides are susceptible to enzymatic hydration by epoxide hydrase to form *trans*-1,2-dihydrodiols (also called *1,2-diols* or *1,2-dihydroxy*

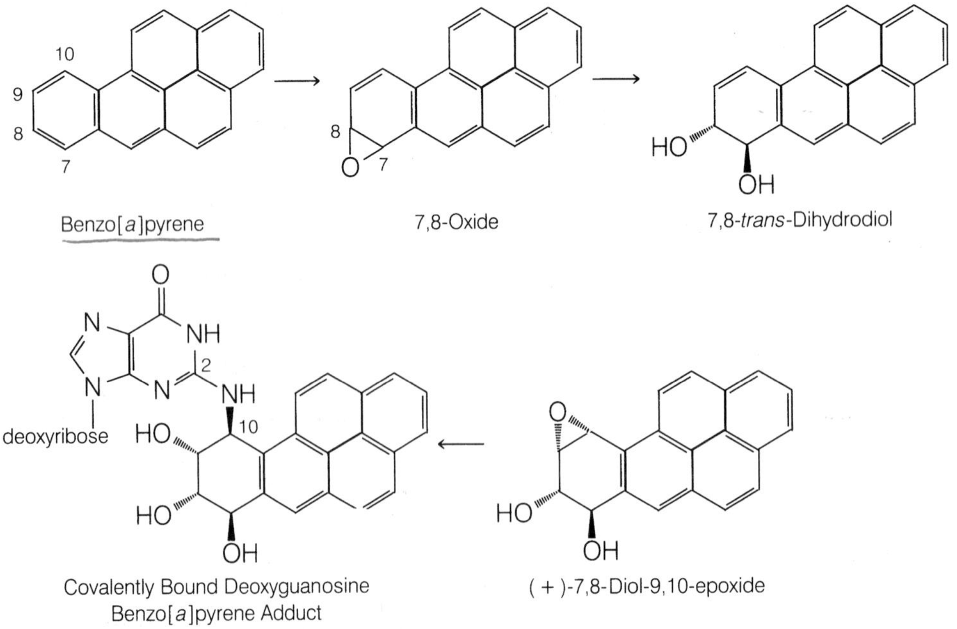

Figure 3.7 ● Metabolic sequence leading to the formation of the ultimate carcinogenic species of benzo[α]pyrene: (+)-7R, 8S-dihydroxy-9R, 10-oxy-7,8,9,10-tetrahydrobenzo[α]pyrene or (+)-7,8-diol-9,10-epoxide.

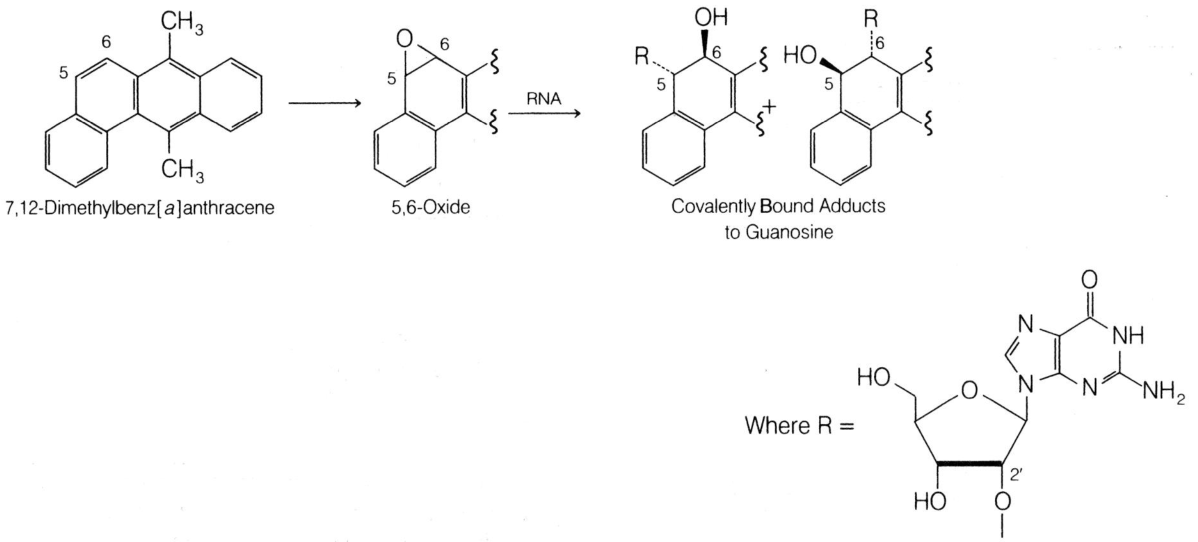

7,12-Dimethylbenz[*a*]anthracene

5,6-Oxide

Covalently Bound Adducts
to Guanosine

Where R =

compounds).[69,70] In addition, several epoxides undergo GSH conjugation.[86]

A well-known example of olefinic epoxidation is the metabolism, in humans, of the anticonvulsant drug carbamazepine (Tegretol) to carbamazepine-10,11-epoxide.[87] The epoxide is reasonably stable and can be measured quantitatively in the plasma of patients receiving the parent drug. The epoxide metabolite may have marked anticonvulsant activity and, therefore, may contribute substantially to the therapeutic effect of the parent drug.[88] Subsequent hydration of the epoxide produces 10,11-dihydroxycarbamazepine, an important urinary metabolite (10%–30%) in humans.[87]

Epoxidation of the olefinic 10,11-double bond in the antipsychotic agent protriptyline (Vivactil)[89] and in the H$_1$-histamine antagonist cyproheptadine (Periactin)[90]

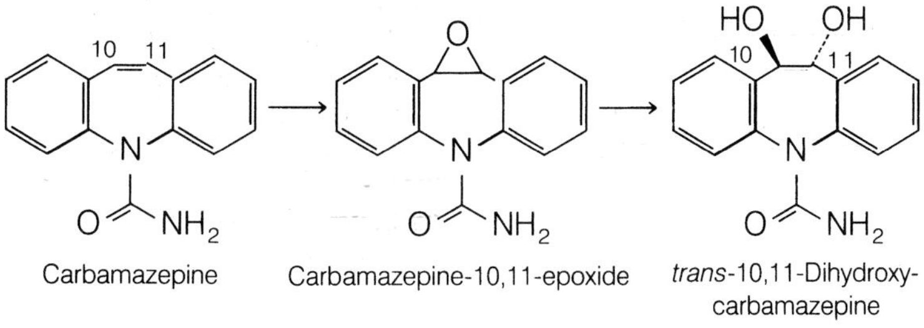

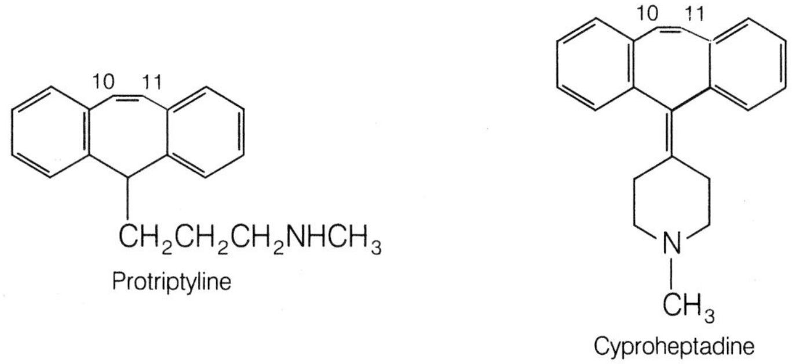

Carbamazepine

Carbamazepine-10,11-epoxide

trans-10,11-Dihydroxy-carbamazepine

Protriptyline

Cyproheptadine

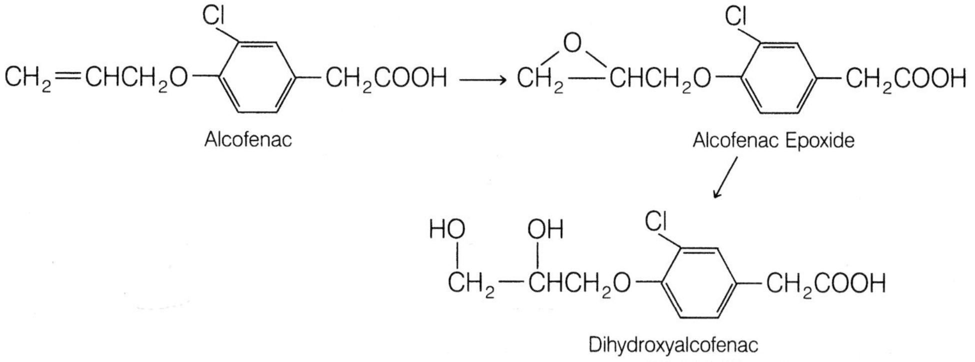

Alcofenac

Alcofenac Epoxide

Dihydroxyalcofenac

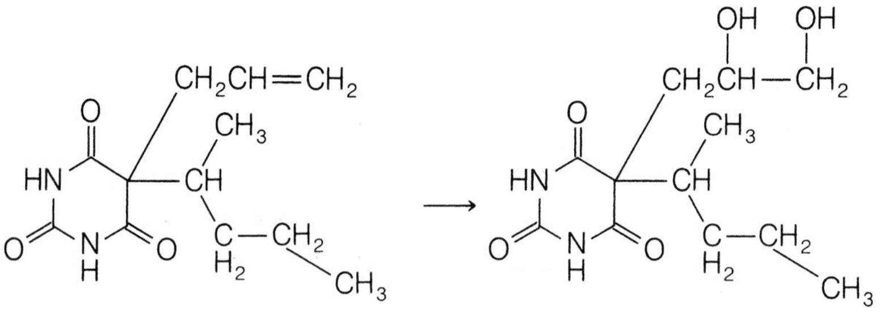

Secobarbital

Secodiol
5-(2,3-Dihydroxypropyl)-5-
(1-methylbutyl)-barbituric Acid

also occurs. Frequently, the epoxides formed from the biotransformation of an olefinic compound are minor products, because of their further conversion to the corresponding 1,2-diols. For instance, dihydroxyalcofenac is a major human urinary metabolite of the once clinically useful anti-inflammatory agent alclofenac.[91] The epoxide metabolite from which it is derived, however, is present in minute amounts. The presence of the dihydroxy metabolite (secodiol) of secobarbital, but not the epoxide product, has been reported in humans.[92]

Indirect evidence for the formation of epoxides comes also from the isolation of GSH or mercapturic acid metabolites. After administration of styrene to rats, two urinary metabolites were identified as the isomeric mercapturic acid derivatives resulting from nucleophilic attack of GSH on the intermediate epoxide.[93] In addition, styrene oxide covalently binds to rat liver microsomal proteins and nucleic acids.[94] These results indicate that styrene oxide is relatively reactive toward nucleophiles (e.g., GSH and nucleophilic groups on protein and nucleic acids).

There are, apparently, diverse metabolically generated epoxides that display similar chemical reactivity toward nucleophilic functionalities. Accordingly, the toxicity of some olefinic compounds may result from their metabolic conversion to chemically reactive epoxides.[95] One example that clearly links metabolic epoxidation as a biotoxification pathway involves aflatoxin B_1. This naturally occurring carcinogenic agent contains an olefinic (C2–C3) double bond adjacent to a cyclic ether oxygen. The hepatocarcinogenicity of aflatoxin B_1 has been clearly linked to its metabolic oxidation to the corresponding 2,3-oxide, which is extremely reactive.[96,97] Extensive in vitro and in vivo metabolic studies indicate that this 2,3-oxide binds covalently to DNA, RNA, and proteins. A major DNA adduct has been isolated and characterized as 2,3-dihydro-2-(N^7-guanyl)-3-hydroxyaflatoxin B_1.[98,99]

Other olefinic compounds, such as vinyl chloride,[100] stilbene,[101] and the carcinogenic estrogenic agent diethylstilbestrol (DES),[102,103] undergo metabolic epoxidation. The corresponding epoxide metabolites may be the reactive

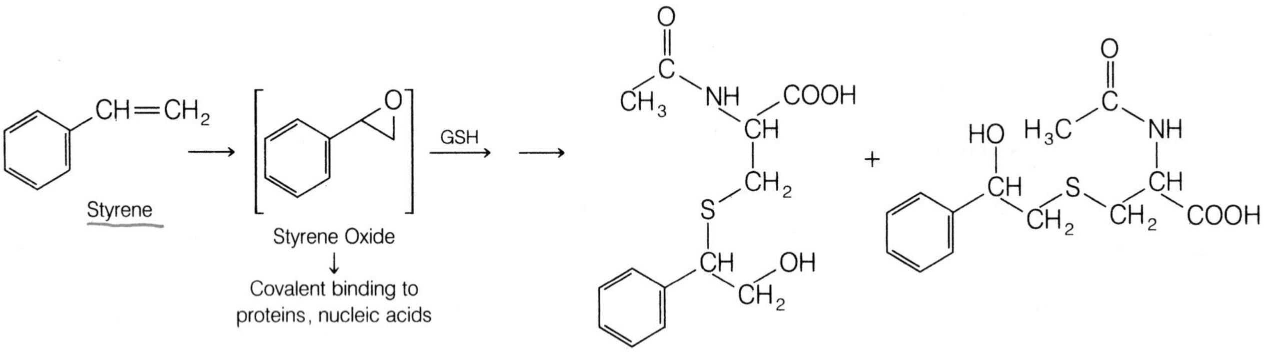

Styrene

Styrene Oxide

↓
Covalent binding to
proteins, nucleic acids

Mercapturic Acid
Derivative (major)

Mercapturic Acid
Derivative (minor)

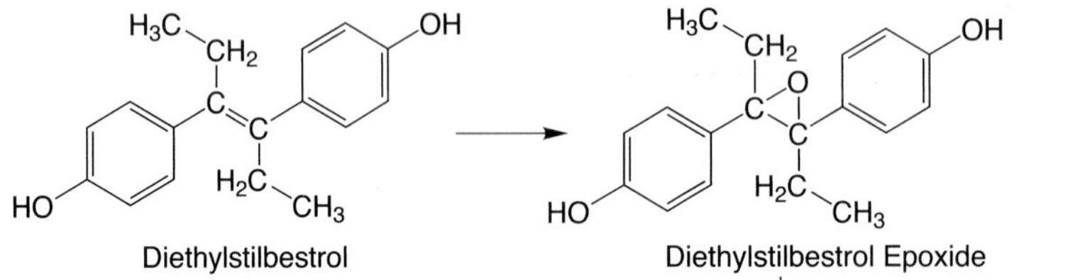

Diethylstilbestrol

Diethylstilbestrol Epoxide

↓
Possible covalent binding to
proteins and/or nucleic acids

species responsible for the cellular toxicity seen with these compounds.

An interesting group of olefin-containing compounds causes the destruction of CYP.[104,105] Compounds belonging to this group include allylisopropylacetamide,[106,107] secobarbital,[108,109] and the volatile anesthetic agent fluroxene.[110] It is believed that the olefinic moiety present in these compounds is activated metabolically by CYP to form a very reactive intermediate that covalently binds to the heme portion of CYP.[111–113] The abnormal heme derivatives, or "green pigments," that result from this covalent interaction have been characterized as N-alkylated protoporphyrins in which the N-alkyl moiety is derived directly from the olefin administered.[104,105,111–113] Long-term administration of the above-mentioned three agents is expected to lead to inhibition of oxidative drug metabolism, potential drug interactions, and prolonged pharmacological effects.

Oxidation at Benzylic Carbon Atoms

Carbon atoms attached to aromatic rings (benzylic position) are susceptible to oxidation, thereby forming the corresponding alcohol (or carbinol) metabolite.[114,115] Primary alcohol metabolites are often oxidized further to aldehydes and carboxylic acids ($CH_2OH \rightarrow CHO \rightarrow COOH$), and secondary alcohols are converted to ketones by soluble alcohol and aldehyde dehydrogenases.[116] Alternatively, the alcohol may be conjugated directly with glucuronic acid.[117] The benzylic carbon atom present in the oral hypoglycemic agent tolbutamide (Orinase) is oxidized extensively to the corresponding alcohol and carboxylic acid. Both metabolites have been isolated from human urine.[118] Similarly, the "benzylic" methyl group in the anti-inflammatory agent tolmetin (Tolectin) undergoes oxidation to yield the dicarboxylic acid product as the major metabolite in humans.[119,120] The selective cyclooxygenase 2 (COX-2) anti-inflammatory agent celecoxib undergoes benzylic oxidation at its C-5 methyl group to give hydroxycelecoxib as a major metabolite.[121] Significant benzylic hydroxy-

lation occurs in the metabolism of the β-adrenergic blocker metoprolol (Lopressor) to yield α-hydroxymetoprolol.[122,123] Additional examples of drugs and xenobiotics undergoing benzylic oxidation are shown in Figure 3.8.

Oxidation at Allylic Carbon Atoms

Microsomal hydroxylation at allylic carbon atoms is commonly observed in drug metabolism. An illustrative example of allylic oxidation is given by the psychoactive component of marijuana, Δ^1-tetrahydrocannabinol Δ^1-THC. This molecule contains three allylic carbon centers (C-7, C-6, and C-3). Allylic hydroxylation occurs extensively at C-7 to yield 7-hydroxy-Δ^1-THC as the major plasma metabolite in humans.[10,11] Pharmacological studies show that this 7-hydroxy metabolite is as active as, or even more active than, Δ^1-THC per se and may contribute significantly to the overall central nervous system (CNS) psychotomimetic effects of the parent compound.[124,125] Hydroxylation also occurs to a minor extent at the allylic C-6 position to give both the epimeric 6α- and 6β-hydroxy metabolites.[10,11] Metabolism does not occur at C-3, presumably because of steric hindrance.

The antiarrhythmic agent quinidine is metabolized by allylic hydroxylation to 3-hydroxyquinidine, the principal plasma metabolite found in humans.[126,127] This metabolite shows significant antiarrhythmic activity in animals and possibly in humans.[128]

Other examples of allylic oxidation include the sedative–hypnotic hexobarbital (Sombulex) and the analgesic pentazocine (Talwin). The 3'-hydroxylated metabolite formed from hexobarbital is susceptible to glucuronide conjugation as well as further oxidation to the 3'-oxo compound.[129,130] Hexobarbital is a chiral barbiturate derivative that exists in two enantiomeric forms. Studies in humans indicate that the pharmacologically less active (R)(−) enantiomer is metabolized more rapidly than its (S)(+)-isomer.[131] Pentazocine undergoes allylic hydroxylation at the two

(text continues on page 58)

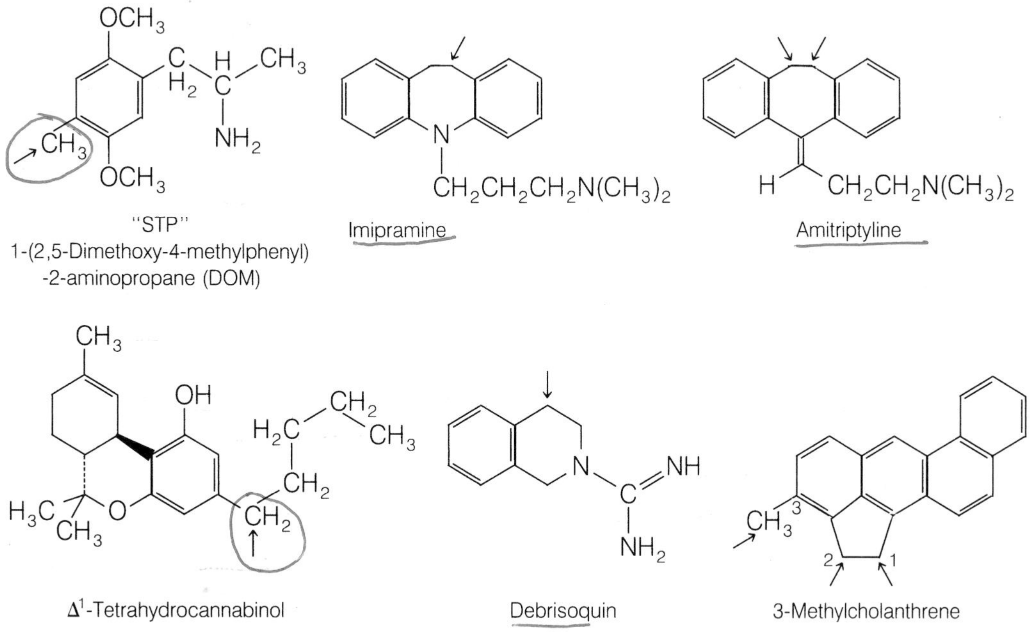

Figure 3.8 ● Examples of drugs and xenobiotics undergoing benzylic hydroxylation. *Arrow* indicates site of hydroxylation.

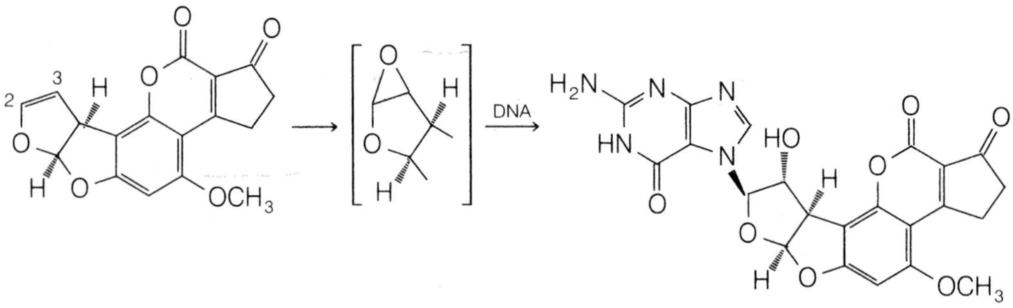

Aflatoxin B$_1$ → 2,3-Expoxide → 2,3-Dihydro-2-(N^7-guanyl)-3-hydroxyaflatoxin B$_1$

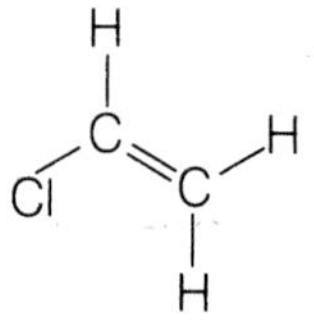

Vinyl Chloride

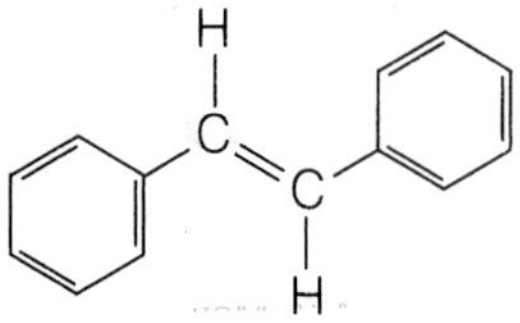

Stilbene

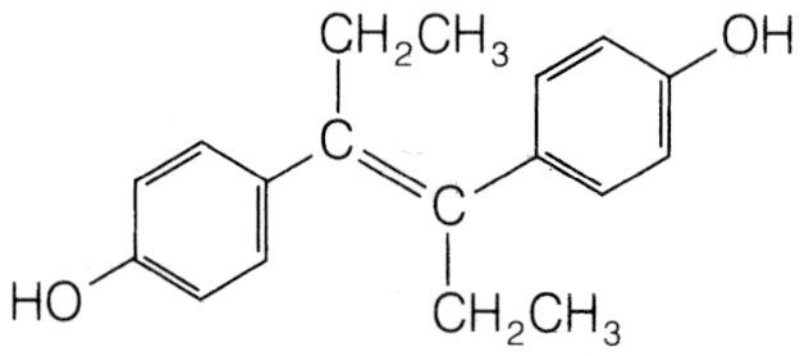

Diethylstilbestrol (DES)

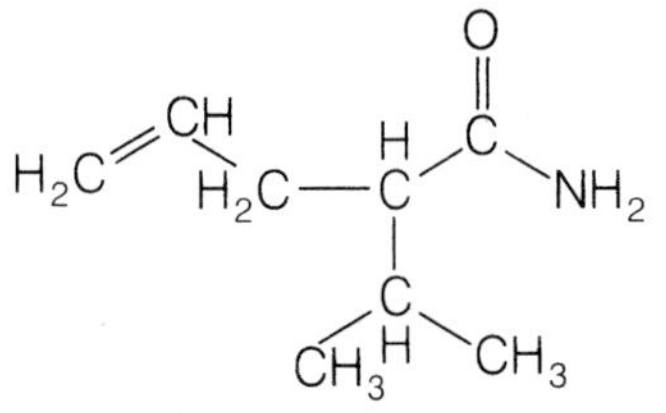

Allylisopropylacetamide

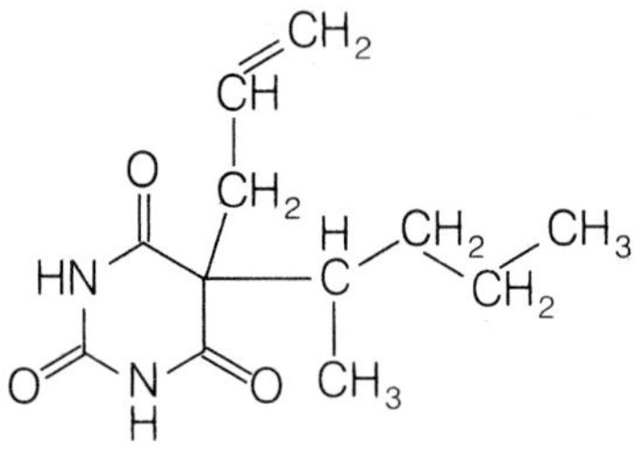

Secobarbital

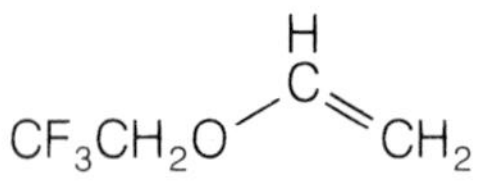

Fluroxene

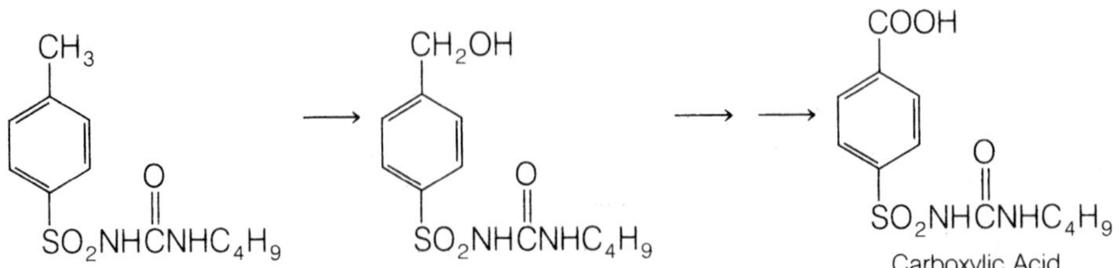

$CF_3CH_2O-CH=CH_2$

Tolbutamide → Alcohol Metabolite → Carboxylic Acid Metabolite

$SO_2NHCNHC_4H_9$

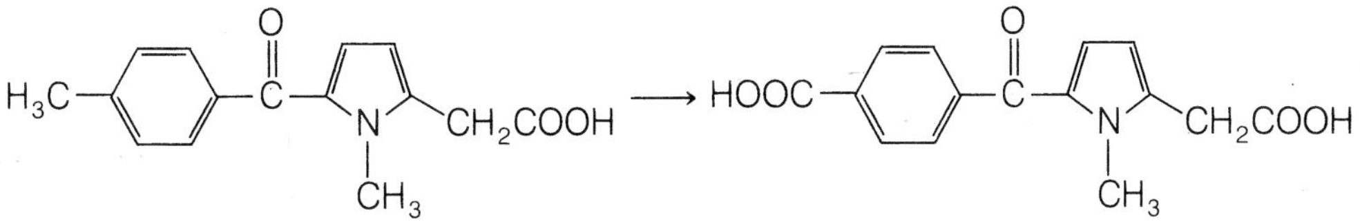

Tolmetin → Dicarboxylic Acid Metabolite

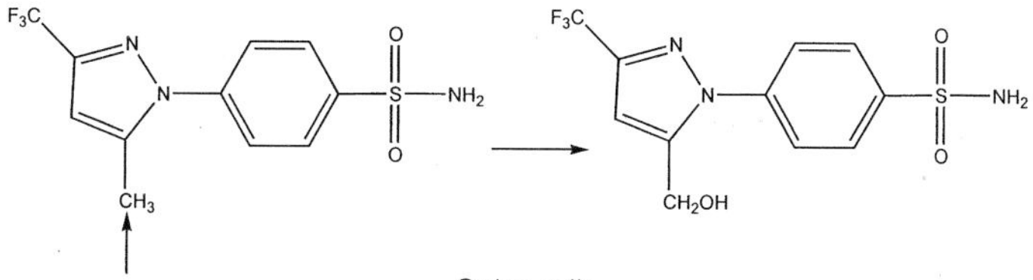

Celecoxib
4-(5-Methyl-3-trifluoromethyl-pyrazol-1-yl)-benzenesulfonamide

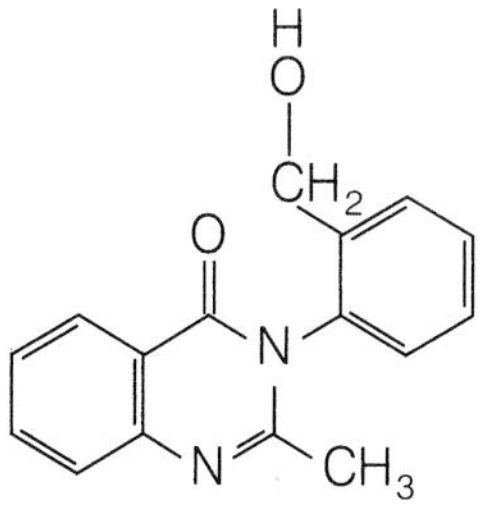

2'-Hydroxymethylmethaqualone

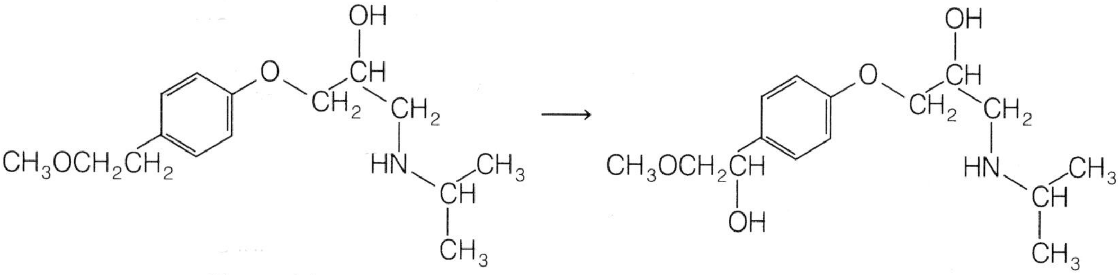

Metroprolol

α-Hydroxymetroprolol

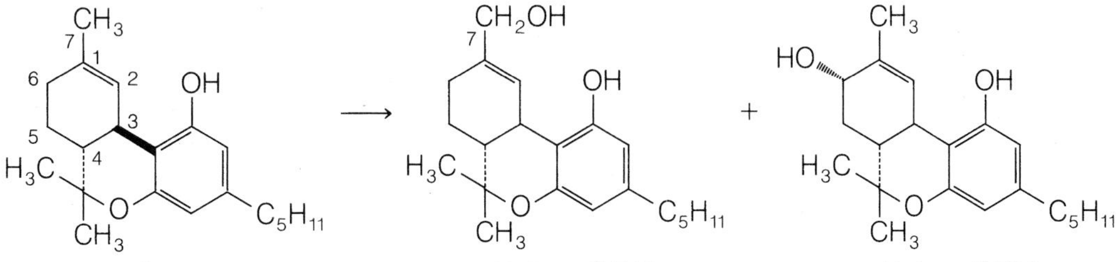

Δ^1-THC

7-Hydroxy-Δ^1-THC

6α-Hydroxy-Δ^1-THC

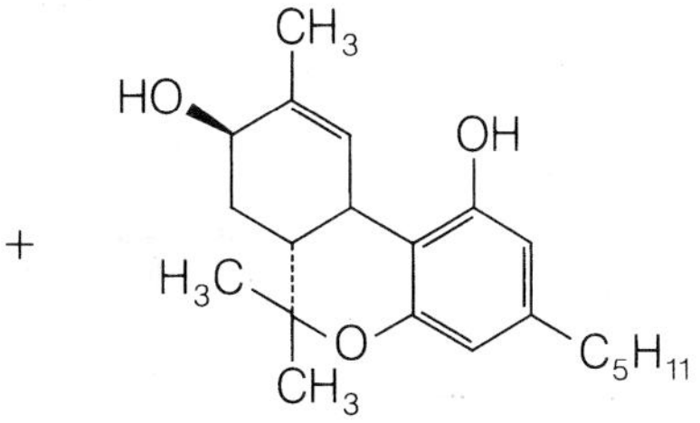

6β-Hydroxy-Δ^1-THC

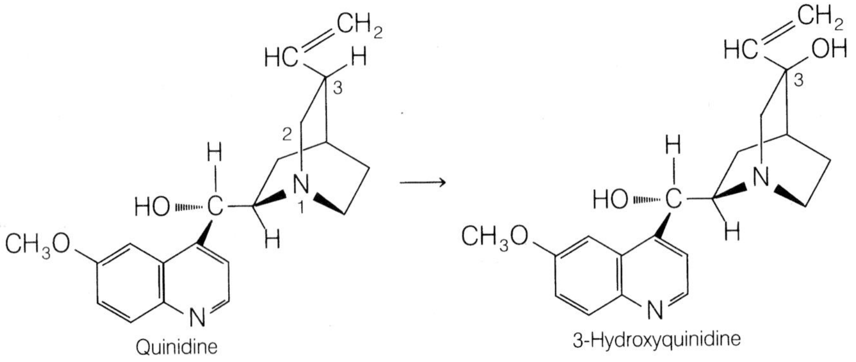

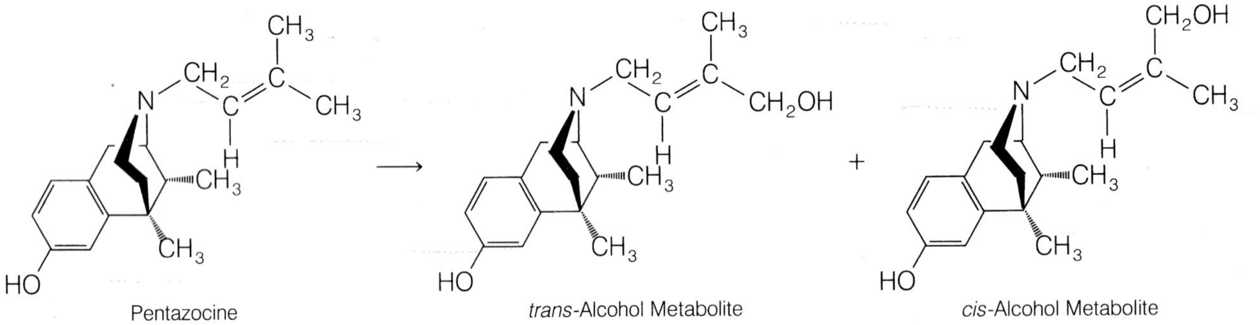

Quinidine → 3-Hydroxyquinidine

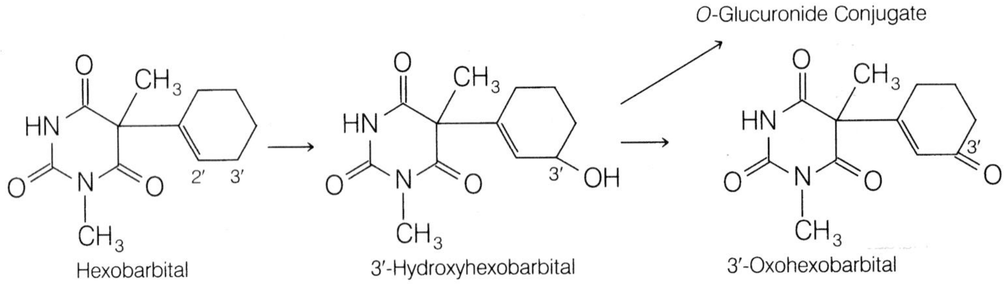

O-Glucuronide Conjugate

Hexobarbital → 3'-Hydroxyhexobarbital → 3'-Oxohexobarbital

Pentazocine → *trans*-Alcohol Metabolite + *cis*-Alcohol Metabolite

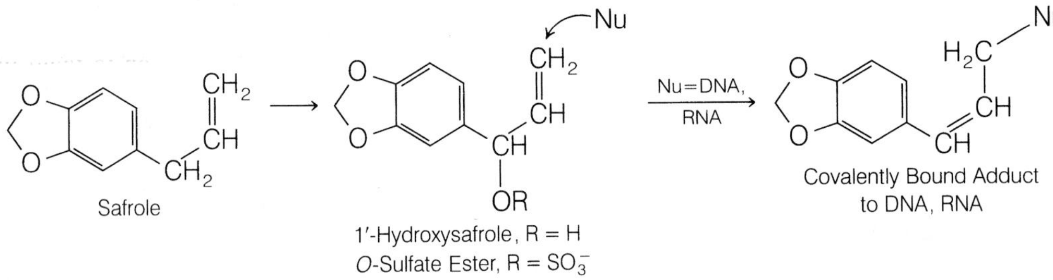

Safrole → 1'-Hydroxysafrole, R = H / O-Sulfate Ester, R = SO$_3^-$ → Covalently Bound Adduct to DNA, RNA

Nu=DNA, RNA

terminal methyl groups of its *N*-butenyl side chain to yield either the *cis* or *trans* alcohol metabolites shown in the diagrams. In humans, more of the *trans* alcohol is formed.[132,133]

For the hepatocarcinogenic agent safrole, allylic hydroxylation is involved in a bioactivation pathway leading to the formation of chemically reactive metabolites.[134] This process involves initial hydroxylation at the C-1' carbon of safrole, which is both allylic and benzylic. The hydroxylated metabolite then undergoes further conjugation to form a sulfate ester. This chemically reactive ester intermediate presumably undergoes nucleophilic displacement reactions with DNA or RNA in vitro to form covalently bound adducts.[135] As shown in the scheme, nucleophilic attack by DNA, RNA, or other nucleophiles is facilitated by a good leaving group (e.g., SO$_4^{2-}$) at the C-1 position. The leaving group tendency of the alcohol OH group itself is not

enough to facilitate displacement reactions. Importantly, allylic hydroxylation generally does not lead to the generation of reactive intermediates. Its involvement in the biotoxification of safrole appears to be an exception.

Oxidation at Carbon Atoms α to Carbonyls and Imines

The mixed-function oxidase system also oxidizes carbon atoms adjacent (i.e., α) to carbonyl and imino (C=N) functionalities. An important class of drugs undergoing this type of oxidation is the benzodiazepines. For example, diazepam (Valium), flurazepam (Dalmane), and nimetazepam are oxidized to their corresponding 3-hydroxy metabolites.[136–138] The C-3 carbon atom undergoing hydroxylation is α to both a lactam carbonyl and an imino functionality.

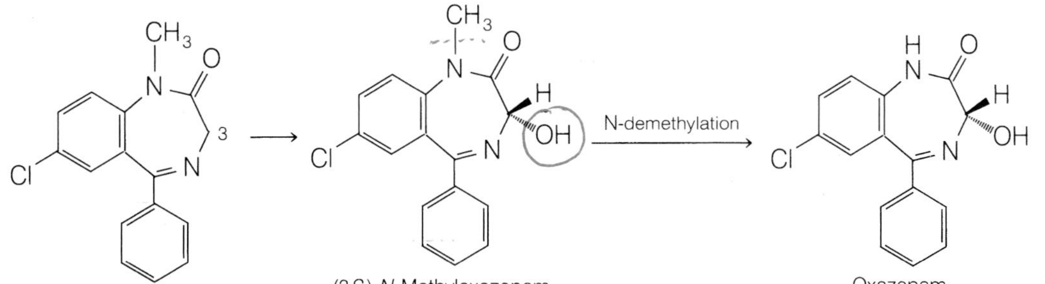

Diazepam → (3*S*) *N*-Methyloxazepam or 3-Hydroxydiazepam → N-demethylation → Oxazepam

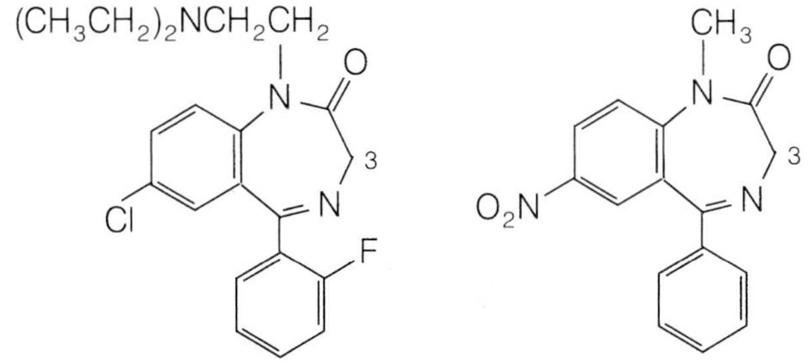

Flurazepam

Nimetazepam

For diazepam, the hydroxylation reaction proceeds with remarkable stereoselectivity to form primarily (90%) 3-hydroxydiazepam (also called *N*-methyloxazepam), with the (*S*) absolute configuration at C-3.[139] Further *N*-demethylation of the latter metabolite gives rise to the pharmacologically active 3(*S*)(+)-oxazepam.

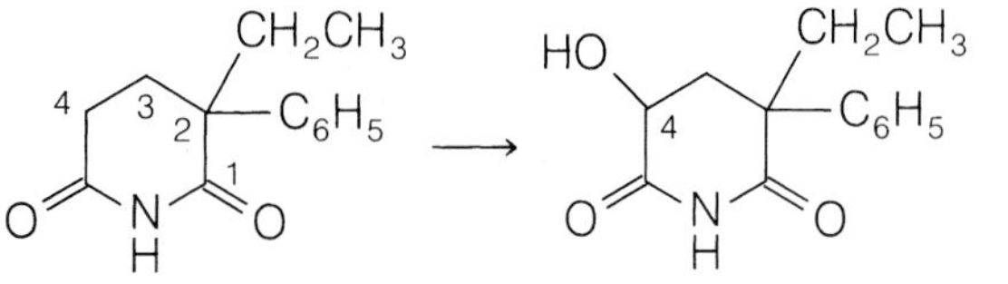

Glutethimide → 4-Hydroxyglutethimide

ω Oxidation

ω − 1 Oxidation

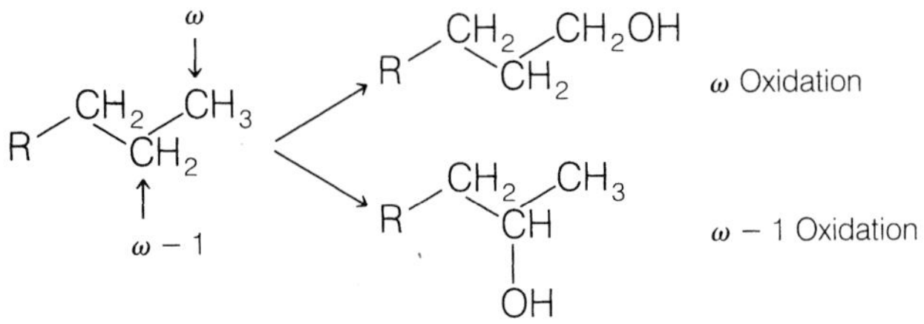

Hydroxylation of the carbon atom α to carbonyl functionalities generally occurs only to a limited extent in drug metabolism. An illustrative example involves the hydroxylation of the sedative–hypnotic glutethimide (Doriden) to 4-hydroxyglutethimide.[140,141]

Oxidation at Aliphatic and Alicyclic Carbon Atoms

Alkyl or aliphatic carbon centers are subject to mixed-function oxidation. Metabolic oxidation at the terminal methyl group often is referred to as *ω-oxidation*, and oxidation of the penultimate carbon atom (i.e., next-to-the-last carbon) is called *ω–1 oxidation*.[114,115] The initial alcohol metabolites formed from these enzymatic ω and ω–1 oxidations are susceptible to further oxidation to yield aldehyde, ketones, or carboxylic acids. Alternatively, the alcohol metabolites may undergo glucuronide conjugation.

Aliphatic ω and ω–1 hydroxylations commonly take place in drug molecules with straight or branched alkyl chains. Thus, the antiepileptic agent valproic acid (Depakene) undergoes both ω and ω–1 oxidation to the 5-hydroxy and 4-hydroxy metabolites, respectively.[142,143] Further oxidation of the 5-hydroxy metabolite yields 2-*n*-propylglutaric acid.

Numerous barbiturates and oral hypoglycemic sulfonylureas also have aliphatic side chains that are susceptible to oxidation. Note that the sedative–hypnotic amobarbital (Amytal) undergoes extensive ω–1 oxidation to the corresponding 3′-hydroxylated metabolite.[144] Other barbiturates, such as pentobarbital,[145,146] thiamylal,[147] and secobarbital,[92] reportedly are metabolized by way of ω and ω–1 oxidation. The *n*-propyl side chain attached to the oral hypoglycemic agent chlorpropamide (Diabinese) undergoes extensive ω–1 hydroxylation to yield the secondary alcohol 2′-hydroxychlorpropamide as a major urinary metabolite in humans.[148]

Omega and ω–1 oxidation of the isobutyl moiety present in the anti-inflammatory agent ibuprofen (Motrin) yields the corresponding carboxylic acid and tertiary alcohol metabolites.[149] Additional examples of drugs reported to undergo aliphatic hydroxylation include meprobamate,[150] glutethimide,[140,141] ethosuximide,[151] and phenylbutazone.[152]

The cyclohexyl group is commonly found in many medicinal agents, and is also susceptible to mixed-function oxidation (alicyclic hydroxylation).[114,115] Enzymatic introduction of a hydroxyl group into a monosubstituted cyclohexane ring generally occurs at C-3 or C-4 and can lead to *cis* and *trans* conformational stereoisomers, as shown in the diagrammed scheme.

An example of this hydroxylation pathway is seen in the metabolism of the oral hypoglycemic agent acetohexamide (Dymelor). In humans, the *trans*-4-hydroxycyclohexyl product is reportedly a major metabolite.[153] Small amounts of the other possible stereoisomers (namely, the *cis*-4-, *cis*-3-, and *trans*-3-hydroxycyclohexyl derivatives) also have been detected. Another related oral hypoglycemic agent, glipizide, is oxidized in humans to the *trans*-4- and *cis*-3-hydroxylcyclohexyl metabolites in about a 6:1 ratio.[154]

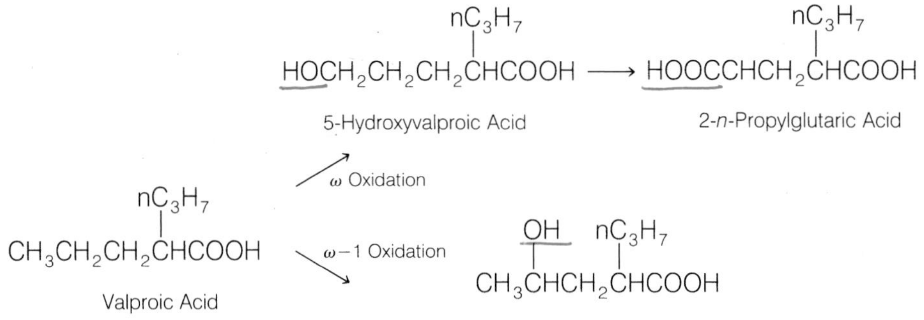

$$\underline{HOCH_2CH_2CH_2}\overset{\overset{\displaystyle nC_3H_7}{|}}{C}HCOOH \longrightarrow \underline{HOOCCHCH_2}\overset{\overset{\displaystyle nC_3H_7}{|}}{C}HCOOH$$

5-Hydroxyvalproic Acid   2-*n*-Propylglutaric Acid

$$CH_3CH_2CH_2\overset{\overset{\displaystyle nC_3H_7}{|}}{C}HCOOH$$

Valproic Acid

ω Oxidation

ω−1 Oxidation

$$CH_3\overset{\overset{\displaystyle OH}{|}}{C}H CH_2\overset{\overset{\displaystyle nC_3H_7}{|}}{C}HCOOH$$

4-Hydroxyvalproic Acid

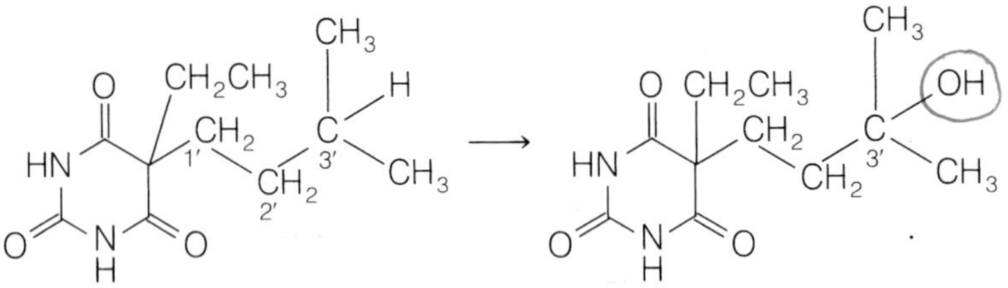

Amobarbital   3'-Hydroxyamobarbital

Two human urinary metabolites of phencyclidine (PCP) have been identified as the 4-hydroxypiperidyl and 4-hydroxycyclohexyl derivatives of the parent compound.[155,156] Thus, from these results, it appears that "alicyclic" hydroxylation of the six-membered piperidyl moiety may parallel closely the hydroxylation pattern of the cyclohexyl moiety. The stereochemistry of the hydroxylated centers in the two metabolites has not been clearly established. Biotransformation of the antihypertensive agent minoxidil (Loniten) yields the 4'-hydroxypiperidyl metabolite. In dogs, this product is a major urinary metabolite (29%–47%), whereas in humans it is detected in small amounts (~3%).[157,158]

Oxidation Involving Carbon–Heteroatom Systems

Nitrogen and oxygen functionalities are commonly found in most drugs and foreign compounds; sulfur functionalities occur only occasionally. Metabolic oxidation of carbon–nitrogen, carbon–oxygen, and carbon–sulfur systems principally involves two basic types of biotransformation processes:

1. Hydroxylation of the α-carbon atom attached directly to the heteroatom (*N*, *O*, *S*). The resulting intermediate is often unstable and decomposes with the cleavage of the carbon–heteroatom bond:

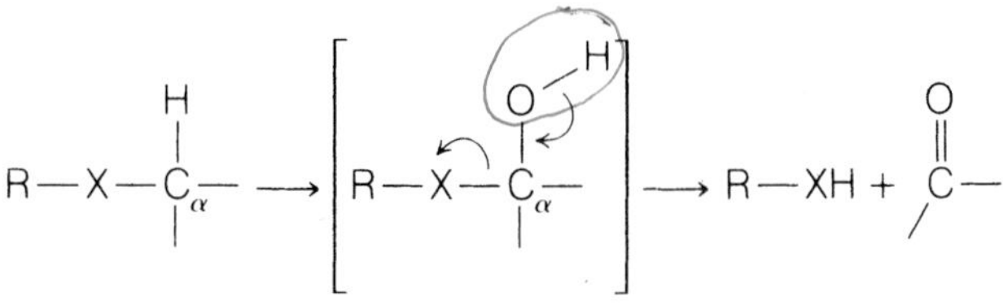

$$R-X-\overset{|}{\underset{|}{C}}_\alpha - \longrightarrow \left[R-X-\overset{\overset{\displaystyle O-H}{|}}{\underset{|}{C}}_\alpha - \right] \longrightarrow R-XH + \overset{\displaystyle O}{\underset{\displaystyle \diagup}{C}}-$$

Where X = N,O,S   Usually Unstable

Oxidative *N*-, *O*-, and *S*-dealkylation as well as oxidative deamination reactions fall under this mechanistic pathway.

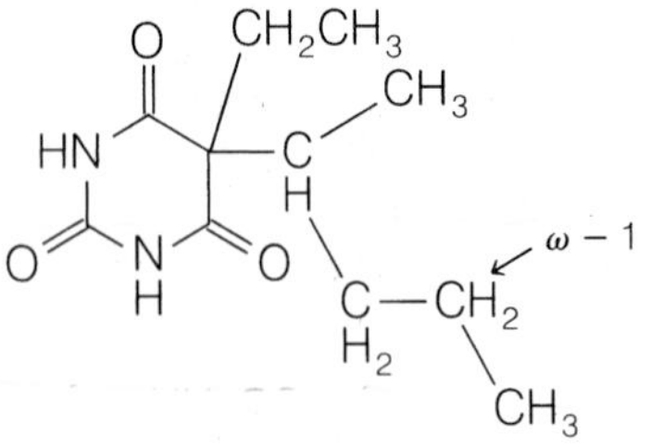

Pentobarbital 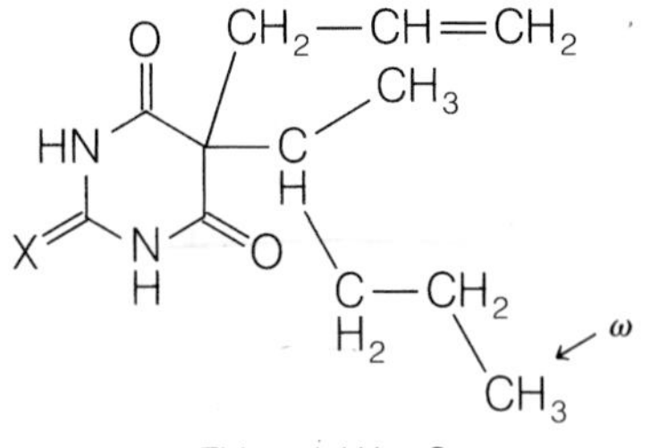   Thiamylal X = S
                                       Secobarbital X = O

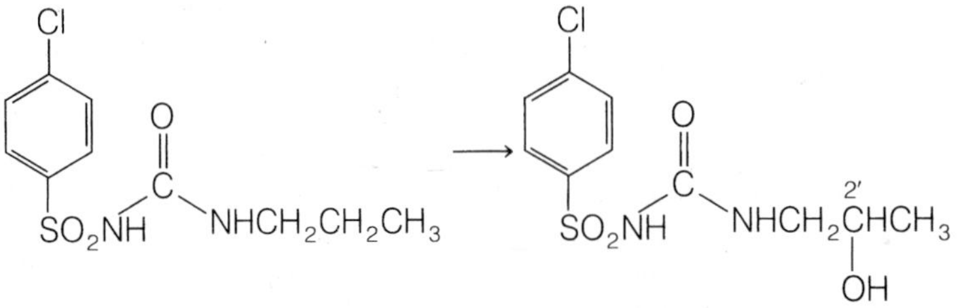

Chlorpropamide   2'-Hydroxychlorpropamide

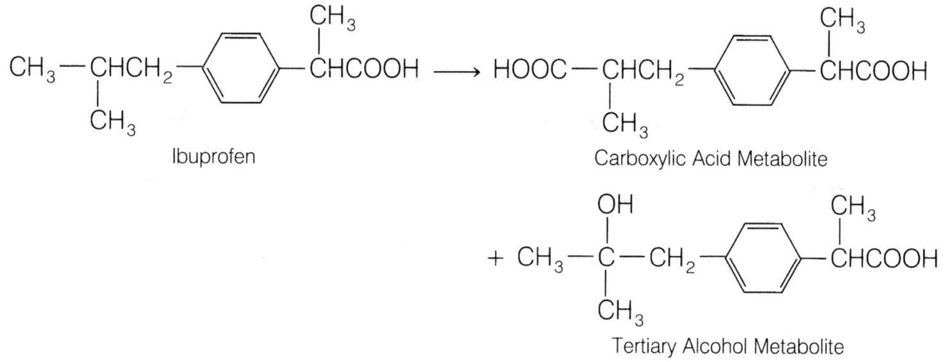

Ibuprofen → Carboxylic Acid Metabolite

+ Tertiary Alcohol Metabolite

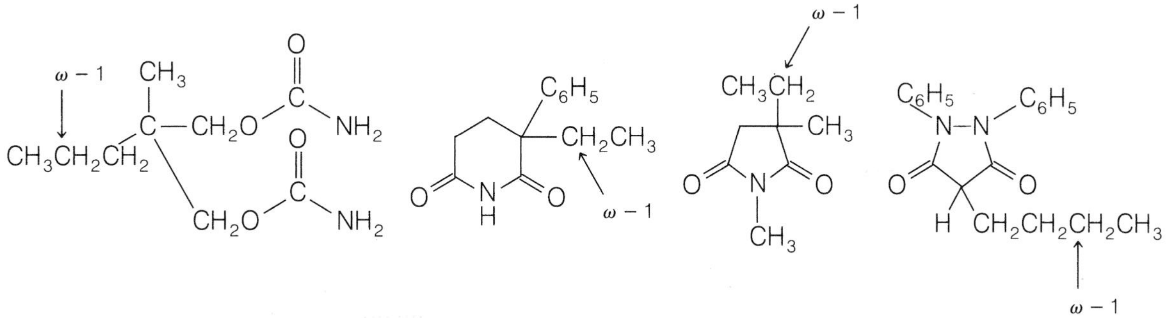

Meprobamate Glutethimide Ethosuximide Phenylbutazone

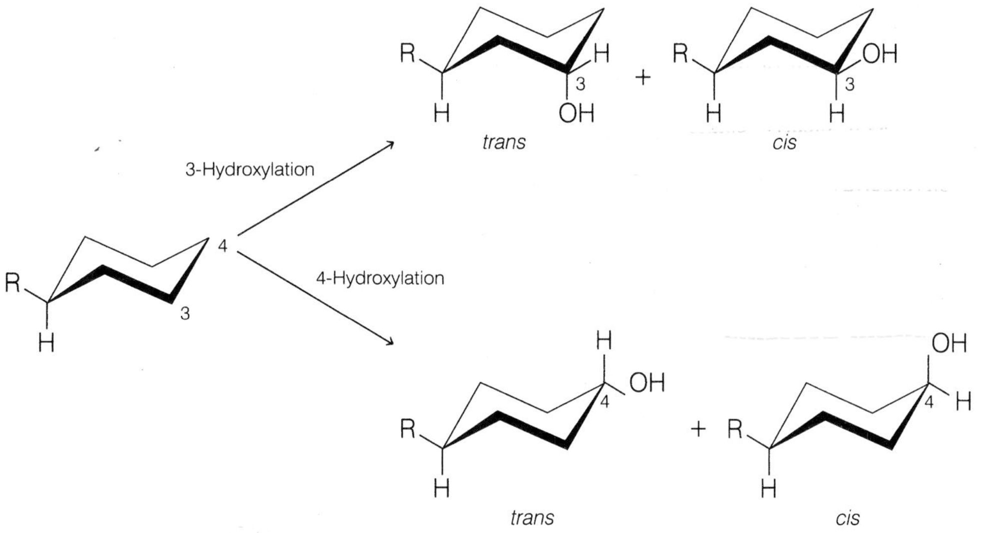

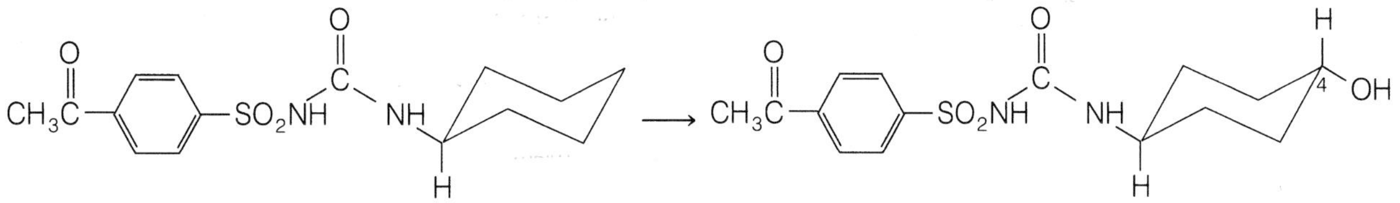

3-Hydroxylation

trans + *cis*

4-Hydroxylation

trans + *cis*

Acetohexamide → *trans*-4-Hydroxyacetohexamide

2. Hydroxylation or oxidation of the heteroatom (*N, S* only, e.g., *N*-hydroxylation, *N*-oxide formation, sulfoxide, and sulfone formation).

Several structural features frequently determine which pathway will predominate, especially in carbon–nitrogen systems. Metabolism of some nitrogen-containing compounds is complicated by the fact that carbon- or nitrogen-hydroxylated products may undergo secondary reactions to form other, more complex metabolic products (e.g., oxime, nitrone, nitroso, imino). Other oxidative processes that do not fall under these two basic categories are discussed individually in the appropriate carbon–heteroatom section. The metabolism of carbon–nitrogen systems will be discussed first, followed by the metabolism of carbon–oxygen and carbon–sulfur systems.

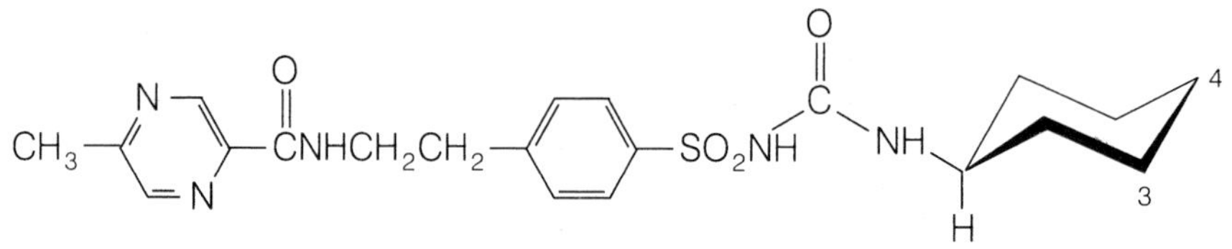

Glipizide

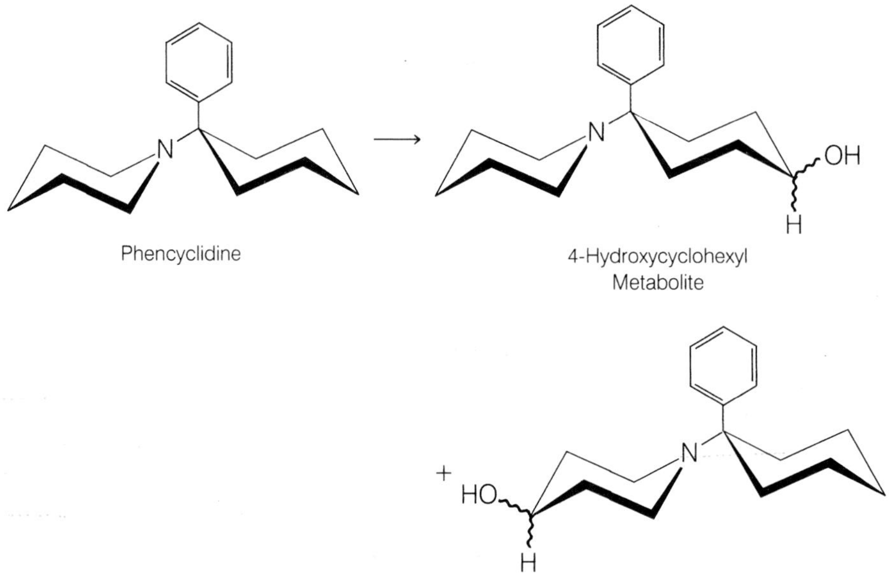

Phencyclidine → 4-Hydroxycyclohexyl Metabolite

4-Hydroxypiperidyl Metabolite

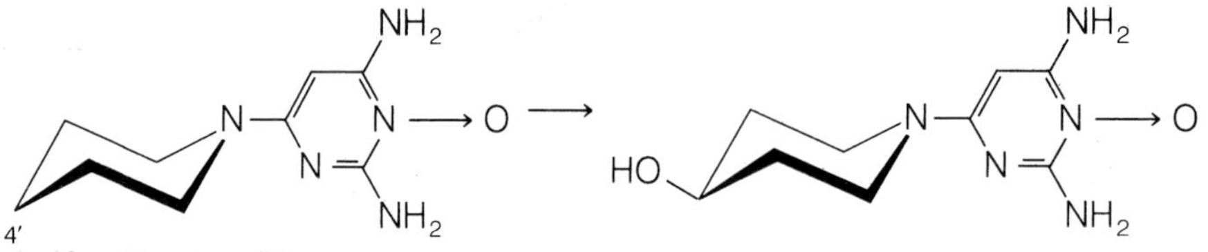

Minoxidil → 4'-Hydroxyminoxidil

OXIDATION INVOLVING CARBON–NITROGEN SYSTEMS

Metabolism of nitrogen functionalities (e.g., amines, amides) is important because such functional groups are found in many natural products (e.g., morphine, cocaine, nicotine) and in numerous important drugs (e.g., phenothiazines, antihistamines, tricyclic antidepressants, β-adrenergic agents, sympathomimetic phenylethylamines, benzodiazepines).[159] The following discussion divides nitrogen-containing compounds into three basic classes:

1. Aliphatic (primary, secondary, and tertiary) and alicyclic (secondary and tertiary) amines
2. Aromatic and heterocyclic nitrogen compounds
3. Amides

The susceptibility of each class of these nitrogen compounds to either α-carbon hydroxylation or N-oxidation and the metabolic products that are formed are discussed.

The hepatic enzymes responsible for carrying out α-carbon hydroxylation reactions are the CYP mixed-function oxidases. The N-hydroxylation or N-oxidation reactions, however, appear to be catalyzed not only by CYP but also by a second class of hepatic mixed-function oxidases called amine oxidases (sometimes called N-oxidases).[160] These enzymes are NADPH-dependent flavoproteins and do not contain CYP.[161,162] They require NADPH and molecular oxygen to carry out N-oxidation.

N-Dealkylation

Tertiary Aliphatic and Alicyclic Amines. The oxidative removal of alkyl groups (particularly methyl groups) from tertiary aliphatic and alicyclic amines is carried out by hepatic CYP mixed-function oxidase enzymes. This reaction is commonly referred to as *oxidative N-dealkylation*.[163] The initial step involves α-carbon hydroxylation to form a carbinolamine intermediate, which is unstable and undergoes spontaneous heterolytic cleavage of the C–N bond to give a secondary amine and a carbonyl moiety (aldehyde or ketone).[164,165] In general, small alkyl groups, such as methyl, ethyl, and isopropyl, are removed rapidly.[163] N-dealkylation of the *t*-butyl group is not possible by the carbinolamine pathway because α-carbon hydroxylation cannot occur. The first alkyl group from a tertiary amine is removed more rapidly than the second alkyl group. In some instances, bisdealkylation of the tertiary aliphatic amine to the corresponding primary aliphatic amine occurs very slowly.[163] For example, the tertiary amine imipramine

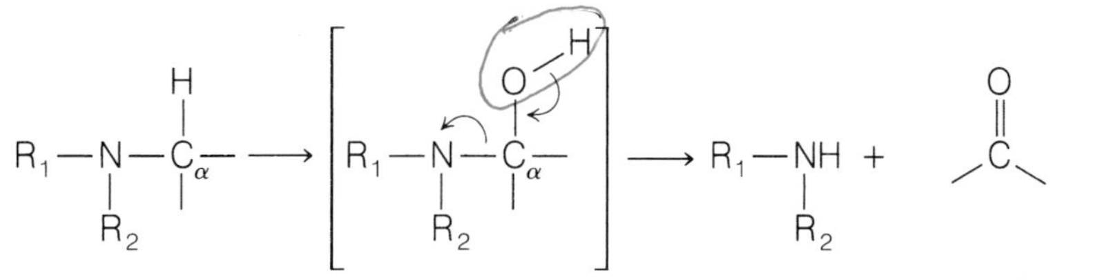

Good to use

Tertiary Amine → Carbinolamine → Secondary Amine + Carbonyl Moiety (aldehyde or ketone)

(Tofranil) is monodemethylated to desmethylimipramine (desipramine).[166,167] This major plasma metabolite is pharmacologically active in humans and contributes substantially to the antidepressant activity of the parent drug.[168] Very little of the bisdemethylated metabolite of imipramine is detected. In contrast, the local anesthetic and antiarrhythmic agent lidocaine is metabolized extensively by N-deethylation to both monoethylglycylxylidine and glycyl-2,6-xylidine in humans.[169,170]

Numerous other tertiary aliphatic amine drugs are metabolized principally by oxidative N-dealkylation. Some of these include the antiarrhythmic disopyramide (Norpace),[171,172] the antiestrogenic agent tamoxifen (Nolvadex),[173] diphenhydramine (Benadryl),[174,175] chlorpromazine (Thorazine),[176,177] and (+)-α-propoxyphene (Darvon).[178] When the tertiary amine contains several different substituents capable of undergoing dealkylation, the smaller alkyl group is removed preferentially and more rapidly. For example, in benzphetamine (Didrex), the methyl group is removed much more rapidly than the benzyl moiety.[179]

An interesting cyclization reaction occurs with methadone on N-demethylation. The demethylated metabolite normethadone undergoes spontaneous cyclization to form the enamine metabolite 2-ethylidene-1,5-dimethyl-3,3-diphenyl-pyrrolidine (EDDP).[180] Subsequent N-demethylation of EDDP and isomerization of the double bond leads to 2-ethyl-5-methyl-3,3-diphenyl-1-pyrroline (EMDP).

Many times, bisdealkylation of a tertiary amine leads to the corresponding primary aliphatic amine metabolite, which is susceptible to further oxidation. For example, the

bisdesmethyl metabolite of the H_1-histamine antagonist brompheniramine (Dimetane) undergoes oxidative deamination and further oxidation to the corresponding propionic acid metabolite.[181] Oxidative deamination is discussed in greater detail when we examine the metabolic reactions of secondary and primary amines.

Like their aliphatic counterparts, alicyclic tertiary amines are susceptible to oxidative N-dealkylation reactions. For example, the analgesic meperidine (Demerol) is metabolized principally by this pathway to yield normeperidine as a major plasma metabolite in humans.[182] Morphine, N-ethylnormorphine, and dextromethorphan also undergo some N-dealkylation.[183]

Direct N-dealkylation of t-butyl groups, as discussed below, is not possible by the α-carbon hydroxylation pathway. In vitro studies indicate, however, that N-t-butylnorchlorocyclizine is, indeed, metabolized to significant amounts of norchlorocyclizine, whereby the t-butyl group is lost.[184] Careful studies showed that the t-butyl group is removed by initial hydroxylation of one of the methyl groups of the t-butyl moiety to the carbinol or alcohol product.[185] Further oxidation generates the corresponding carboxylic acid that, on decarboxylation, forms the N-isopropyl derivative. The N-isopropyl intermediate is dealkylated by the normal α-carbon hydroxylation (i.e., carbinolamine) pathway to give norchlorocyclizine and acetone. Whether this is a general method for the loss of t-butyl groups from amines is still unclear. Indirect N-dealkylation of t-butyl groups is not observed significantly. The N-t-butyl group present in many β-adrenergic antagonists, such as terbutaline and

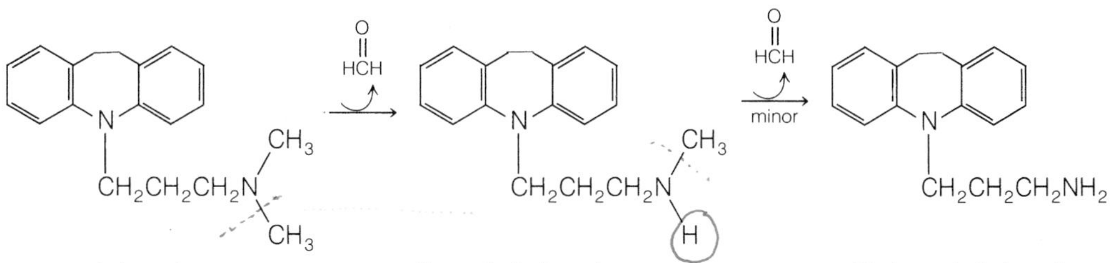

Imipramine → Desmethylimipramine (desipramine) → Bisdesmethylimipramine

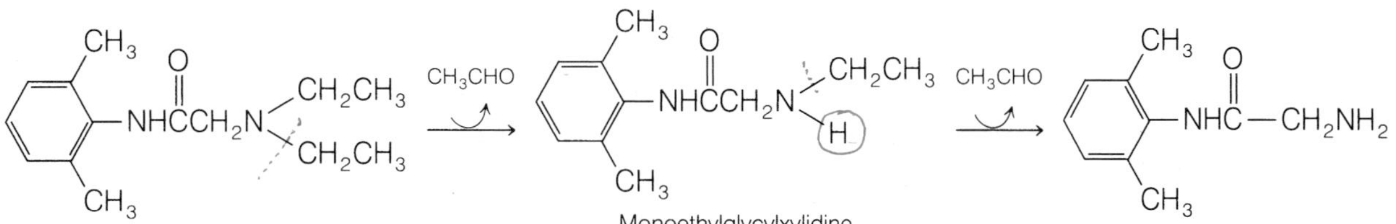

Lidocaine → Monoethylglycylxylidine (MEGX) → Glycyl-2,6-xylidine

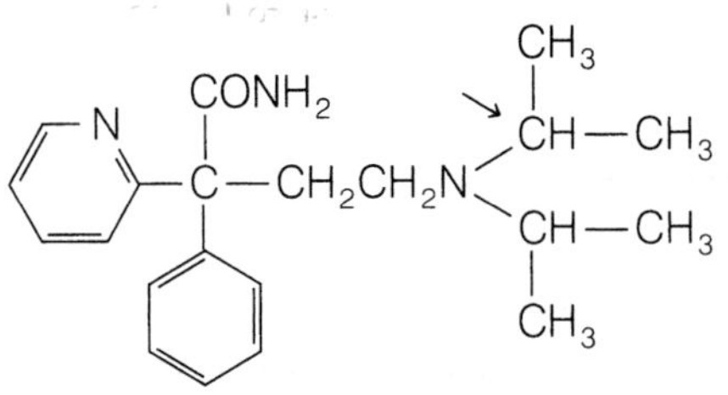

Disopyramide

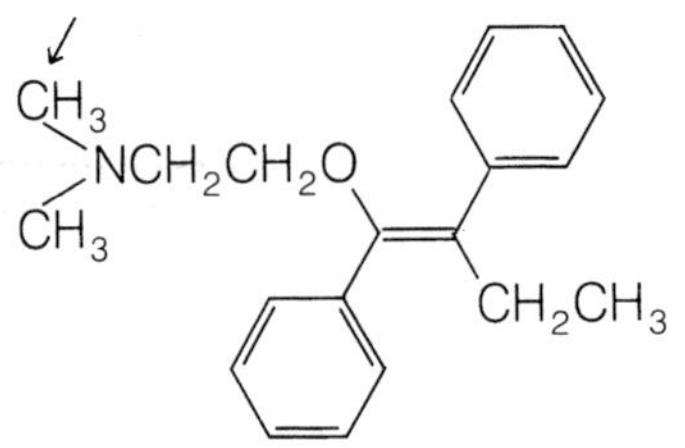

Tamoxifen

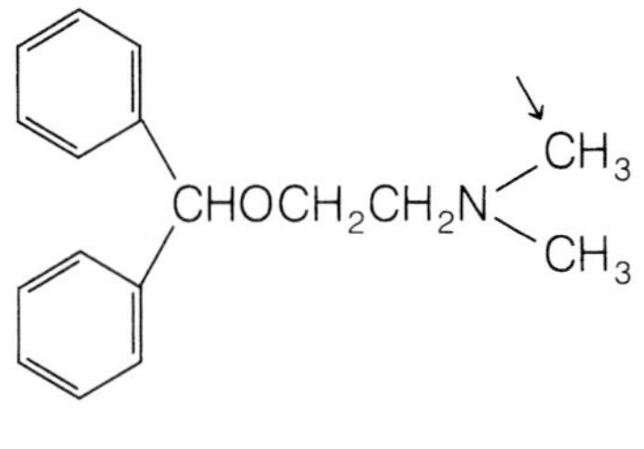

Diphenhydramine

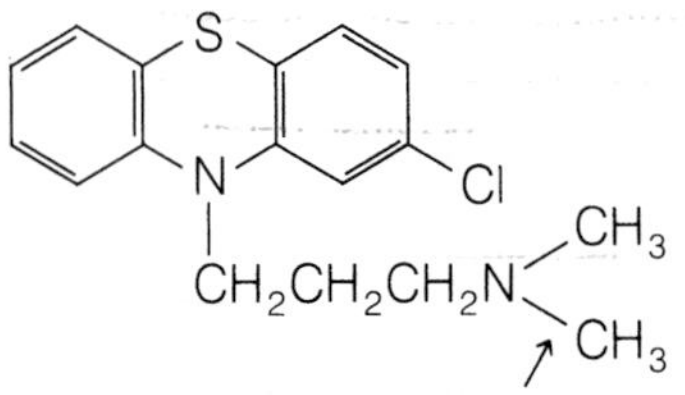

Chlorpromazine

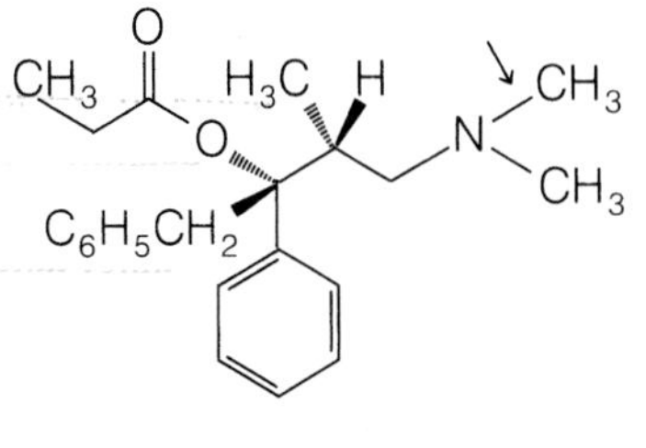

(+)-α-Propoxyphene

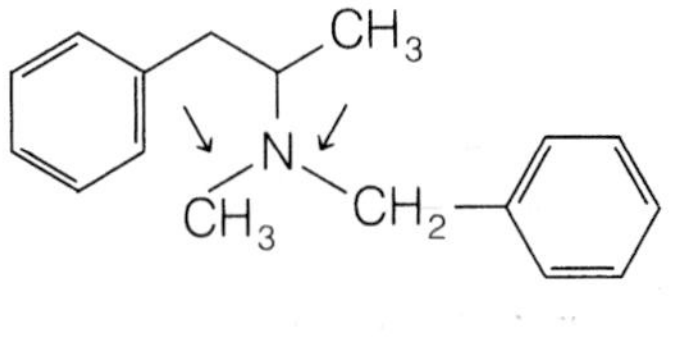

Benzphetamine
(N-demethylation
and N-debenzylation)

salbutamol, remains intact and does not appear to undergo any significant metabolism.[186]

Alicyclic tertiary amines often generate lactam metabolites by α-carbon hydroxylation reactions. For example, the tobacco alkaloid nicotine is hydroxylated initially at the ring carbon atom α to the nitrogen to yield a carbinolamine intermediate. Furthermore, enzymatic oxidation of this cyclic carbinolamine generates the lactam metabolite cotinine.[187,188]

Formation of lactam metabolites also has been reported to occur to a minor extent for the antihistamine cyprohep-

tadine (Periactin)[189,190] and the antiemetic diphenidol (Vontrol).[191]

N-oxidation of tertiary amines occurs with several drugs.[192] The true extent of *N*-oxide formation often is complicated by the susceptibility of *N*-oxides to undergo in vivo reduction back to the parent tertiary amine. Tertiary amines such as H_1-histamine antagonists (e.g., orphenadrine, tripelennamine), phenothiazines (e.g., chlorpromazine), tricyclic antidepressants (e.g., imipramine), and narcotic analgesics (e.g., morphine, codeine, and meperidine) reportedly form

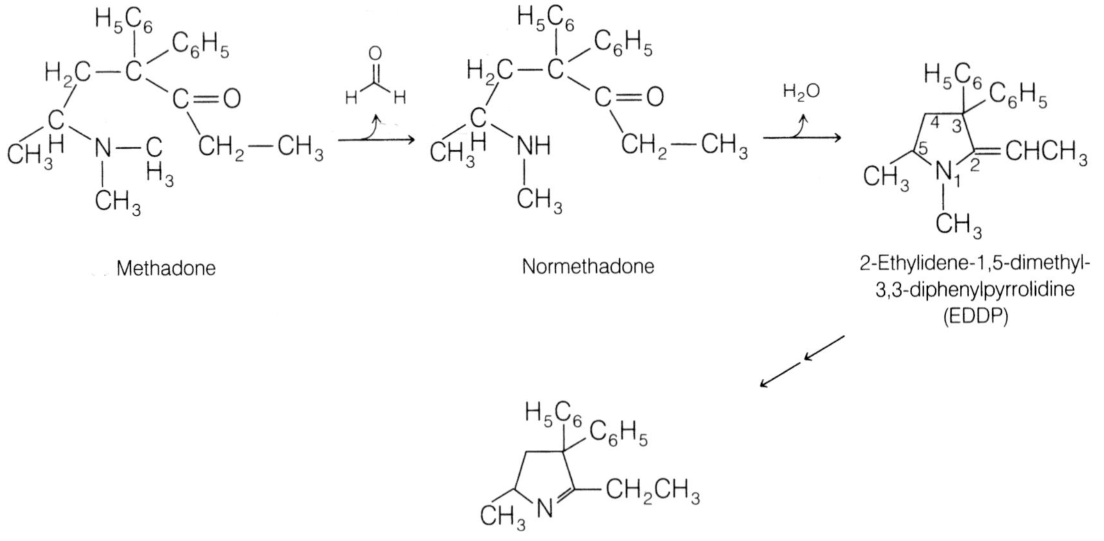

Methadone

Normethadone

2-Ethylidene-1,5-dimethyl-
3,3-diphenylpyrrolidine
(EDDP)

2-Ethyl-5-methyl-
3,3-diphenyl-1-pyrroline
(EMDP)

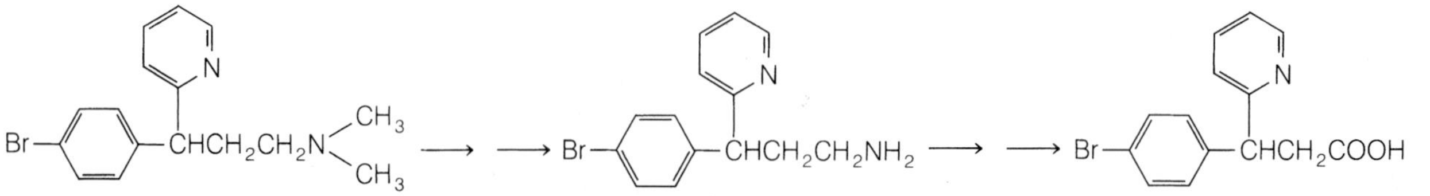

Brompheniramine

Bisdesmethyl Metabolite

3-(*p*-Bromophenyl)-3-pyridyl-
propionic acid

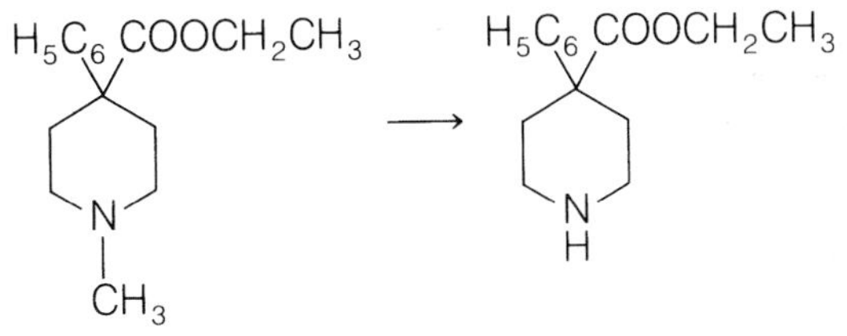

Meperidine → Normeperidine

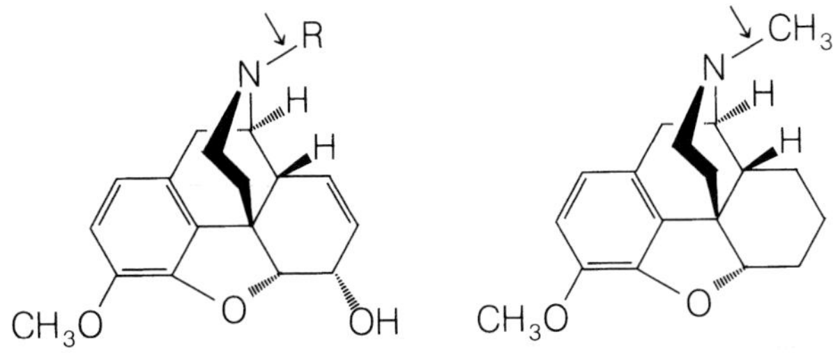

Morphine   R = CH₃
N-Ethylnormorphine R = CH₂CH₃

Dextromethorphan

N-oxide products. In some instances, N-oxides possess pharmacological activity.[193] A comparison of imipramine N-oxide with imipramine indicates that the N-oxide itself possesses antidepressant and cardiovascular activity similar to that of the parent drug.[194,195]

Secondary and Primary Amines. Secondary amines (either parent compounds or metabolites) are susceptible to oxidative N-dealkylation, oxidative deamination, and N-oxidation reactions.[163,196] As in tertiary amines, N-dealkylation of secondary amines proceeds by the carbinolamine pathway. Dealkylation of secondary amines gives rise to the corresponding primary amine metabolite. For example, the α-adrenergic blockers propranolol[46,47] and

oxprenolol[197] undergo N-deisopropylation to the corresponding primary amines. N-dealkylation appears to be a significant biotransformation pathway for the secondary amine drugs methamphetamine[198,199] and ketamine,[200,201] yielding amphetamine and norketamine, respectively.

The primary amine metabolites formed from oxidative dealkylation are susceptible to *oxidative deamination*. This process is similar to N-dealkylation, in that it involves an initial α-carbon hydroxylation reaction to form a carbinolamine intermediate, which then undergoes subsequent carbon–nitrogen cleavage to the carbonyl metabolite and ammonia. If α-carbon hydroxylation cannot occur, then oxidative deamination is not possible. For example, deamination does not occur for norketamine because α-carbon hydroxylation cannot take place.[200,201] With methamphetamine, oxidative deamination of primary amine metabolite amphetamine produces phenylacetone.[198,199]

In general, dealkylation of secondary amines is believed to occur before oxidative deamination. Some evidence indicates, however, that this may not always be true. Direct deamination of the secondary amine also has occurred. For example, in addition to undergoing deamination through its desisopropyl primary amine metabolite, propranolol can undergo a direct oxidative deamination reaction (also by α-carbon hydroxylation) to yield the aldehyde metabolite and isopropylamine (Fig. 3.9).[202] How much direct oxidative deamination contributes to the metabolism of secondary amines remains unclear.

Some secondary alicyclic amines, like their tertiary amine analogs, are metabolized to their corresponding lactam derivatives. For example, the anorectic agent phenmetrazine (Preludin) is metabolized principally to the lactam product 3-oxophenmetrazine.[203] In humans, this lactam metabolite is a major urinary product. Methylphenidate (Ritalin) also reportedly yields a lactam metabolite, 6-oxori-

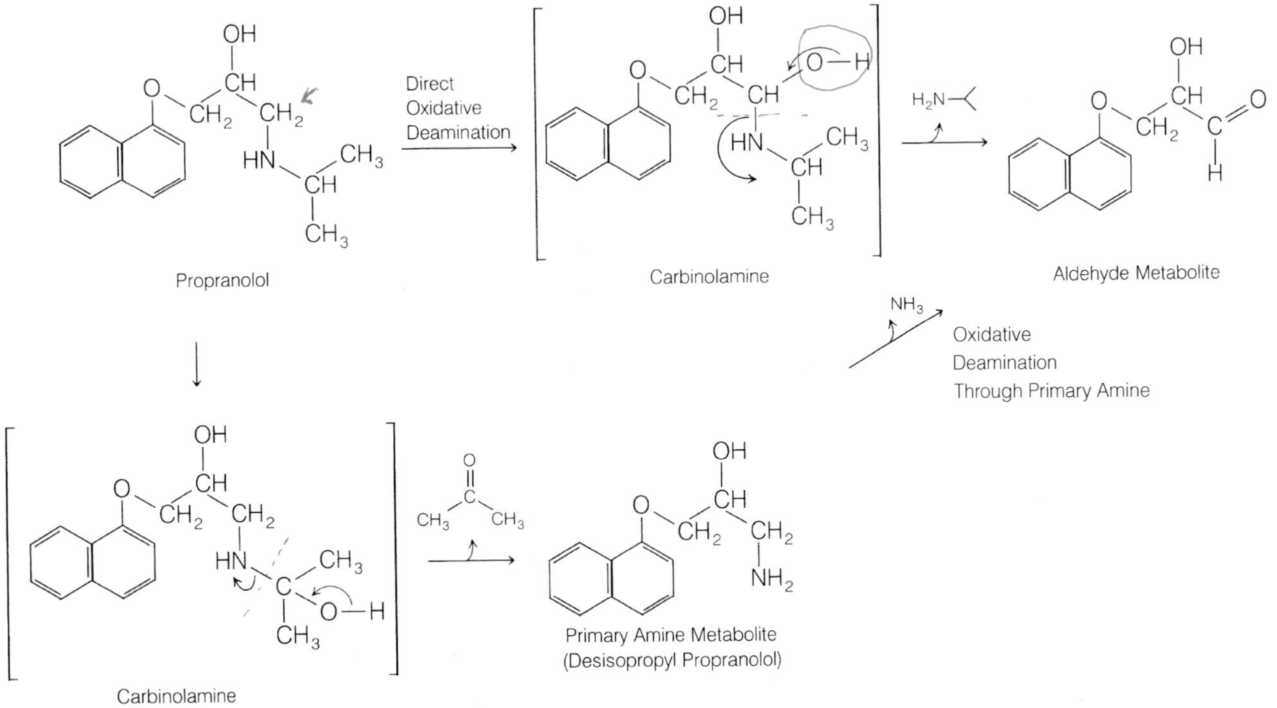

Figure 3.9 ● Metabolism of propranolol to its aldehyde metabolite by direct deamination of the parent compound and by deamination of its primary amine metabolite, desisopropyl propranolol.

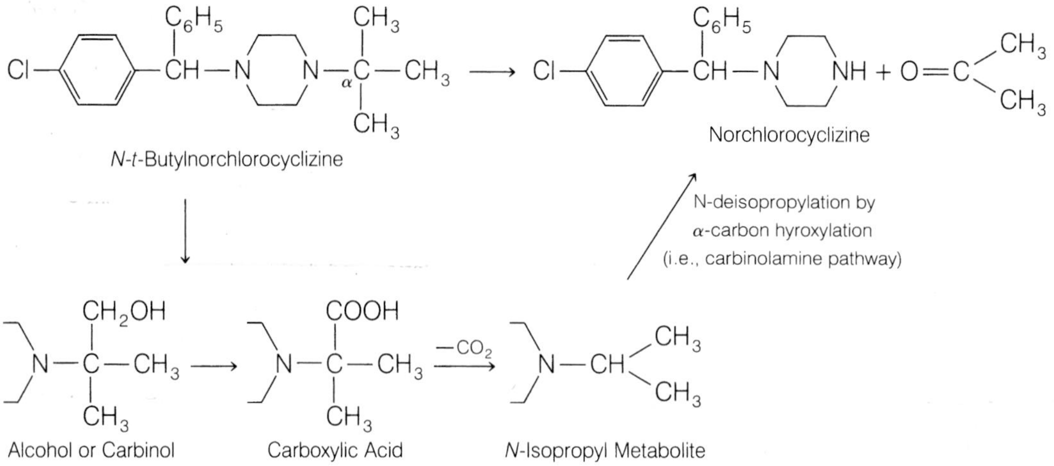

N-t-Butylnorchlorocyclizine → Norchlorocyclizine + O=C(CH₃)₂

N-deisopropylation by α-carbon hyroxylation (i.e., carbinolamine pathway)

Alcohol or Carbinol → Carboxylic Acid —CO₂→ *N*-Isopropyl Metabolite

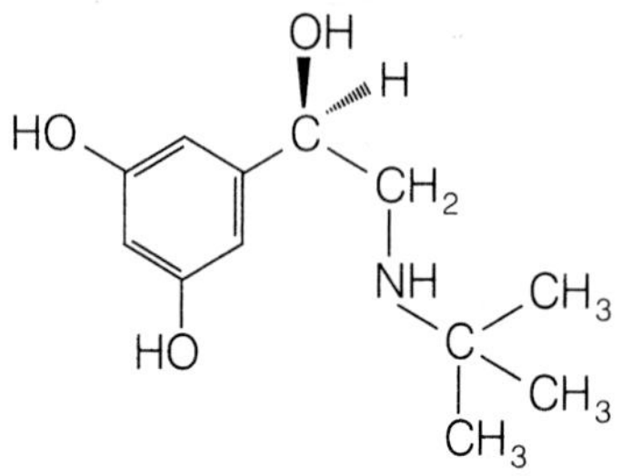

Terbutaline

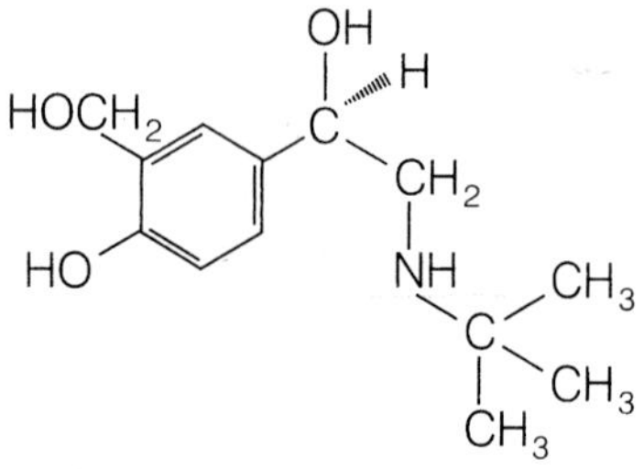

Salbutamol

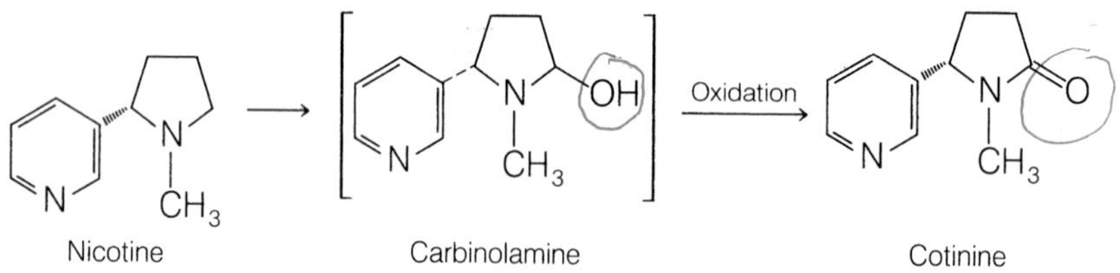

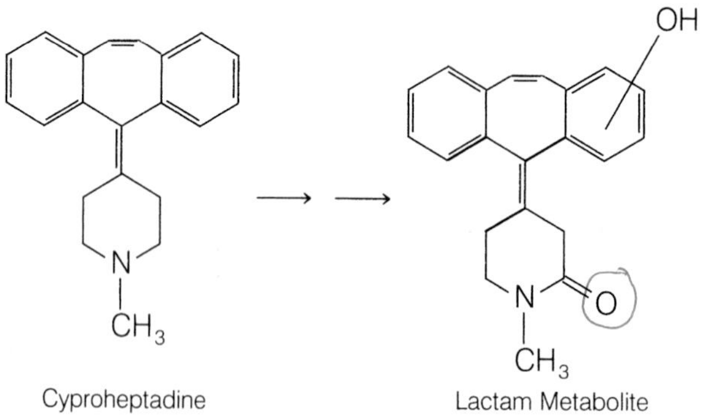

Nicotine → Carbinolamine —Oxidation→ Cotinine

Cyproheptadine → Lactam Metabolite

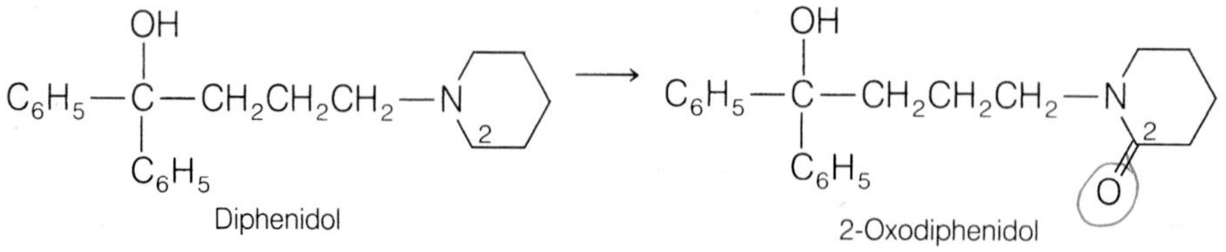

Diphenidol → 2-Oxodiphenidol

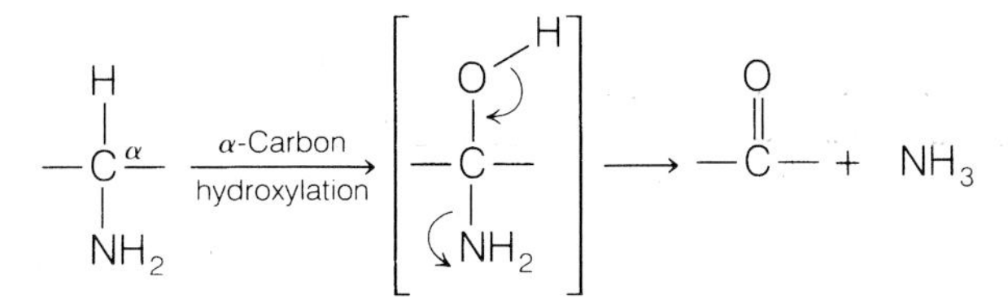

Primary Amine   Carbinolamine   Carbonyl   Ammonia

talinic acid, by oxidation of its hydrolyzed metabolite, ritalinic acid, in humans.[204]

Metabolic *N*-oxidation of secondary aliphatic and alicyclic amines leads to several *N*-oxygenated products.[196] *N*-hydroxylation of secondary amines generates the corresponding *N*-hydroxylamine metabolites. Often, these

hydroxylamine products are susceptible to further oxidation (either spontaneous or enzymatic) to the corresponding nitrone derivatives. *N*-benzylamphetamine undergoes metabolism to both the corresponding *N*-hydroxylamine and the nitrone metabolites.[205] In humans, the nitrone metabolite of phenmetrazine (Preludin), found in the urine, is believed to be formed by further oxidation of the *N*-hydroxylamine intermediate *N*-hydroxyphenmetrazine.[203] Importantly, much less *N*-oxidation occurs for secondary amines than oxidative dealkylation and deamination.

Primary aliphatic amines (whether parent drugs or metabolites) are biotransformed by oxidative deamination (through the carbinolamine pathway) or by *N*-oxidation. In general, oxidative deamination of most exogenous primary amines is

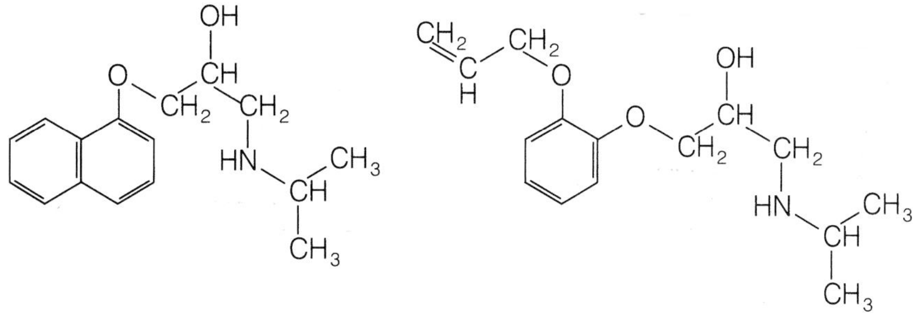

Propranolol

Oxprenolol

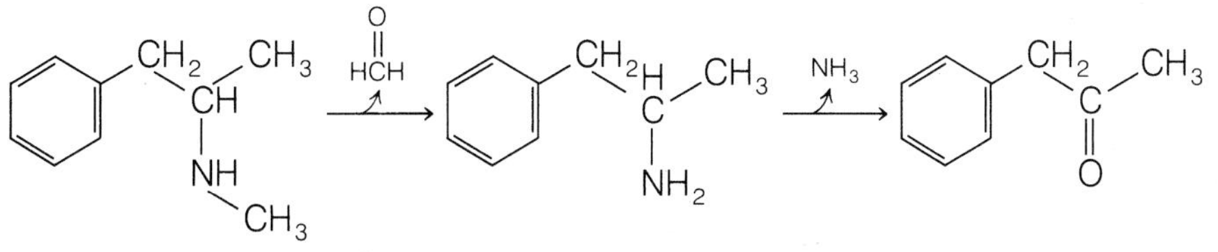

Methamphetamine

Amphetamine

Phenylacetone

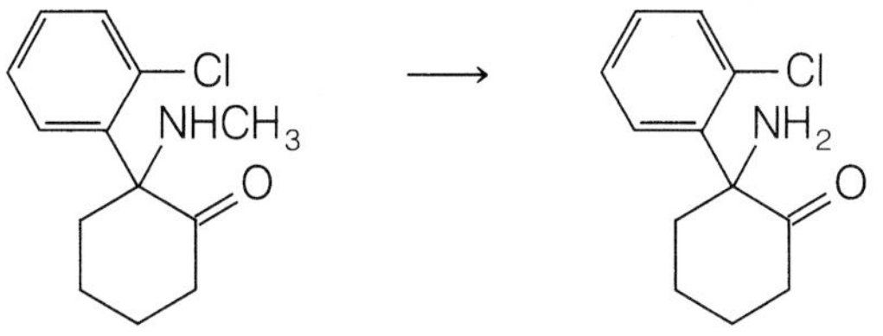

Ketamine

Norketamine

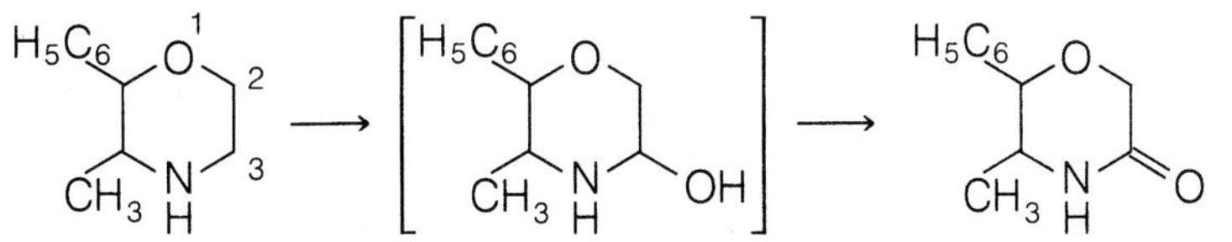

Phenmetrazine

Carbinolamine Intermediate

3-Oxophenmetrazine

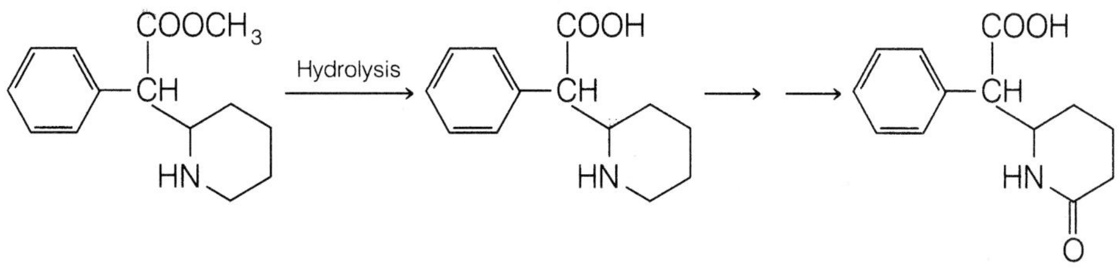

Methylphenidate

Ritalinic Acid

6-Oxoritalinic Acid

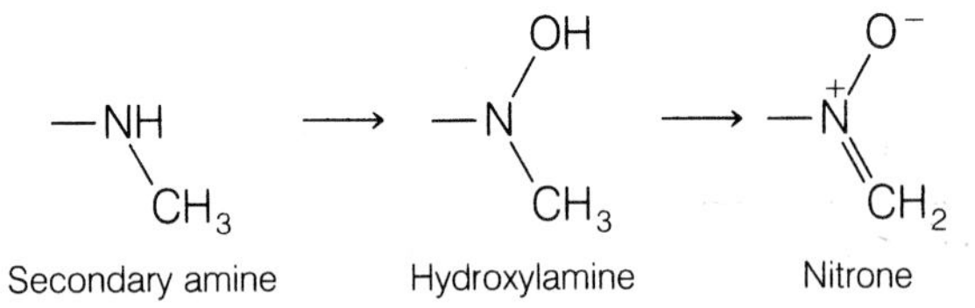

Secondary amine → Hydroxylamine → Nitrone

carried out by the mixed-function oxidases discussed previously. Endogenous primary amines (e.g., dopamine, norepinephrine, tryptamine, and serotonin) and xenobiotics based on the structures of these endogenous neurotransmitters are metabolized, however, via oxidative deamination by a specialized family of enzymes called *monoamine oxidases* (MAOs).[206]

MAO is a flavin (FAD)-dependent enzyme found in two isozyme forms, MAO-A and MAO-B, and widely distributed in both the CNS and peripheral organs. In contrast, CYP exists in a wide variety of isozyme forms and is an NADP-dependent system. Also the greatest variety of CYP isozymes, at least the ones associated with the metabolism of xenobiotics, are found mostly in the liver and intestinal mucosa. MAO-A and MAO-B are coded by two genes, both on the X-chromosome and have about 70% amino acid sequence homology. Another difference between the CYP and MAO

families is cellular location. CYP enzymes are found on the endoplasmic reticulum of the cell's cytosol, whereas the MAO enzymes are on the outer mitochondrial membrane. In addition to the xenobiotics illustrated in the reaction schemes, other drugs metabolized by the MAO system include phenylephrine, propranolol, timolol and other β-adrenergic agonists and antagonists, and various phenylethylamines.[206]

Structural features, especially the α-substituents of the primary amine, often determine whether carbon or nitrogen oxidation will occur. For example, compare amphetamine with its α-methyl homologue phentermine. In amphetamine, α-carbon hydroxylation can occur to form the carbinolamine intermediate, which is converted to the oxidatively deaminated product phenylacetone.[67] With phentermine, α-carbon hydroxylation is not possible and precludes oxidative deamination for this drug. Consequently, phentermine would be expected to undergo N-oxidation readily. In humans, p-hydroxylation and N-oxidation are the main pathways for biotransformation of phentermine.[207]

Indeed, *N*-hydroxyphentermine is an important (5%) urinary metabolite in humans.[207] As discussed below, *N*-hydroxylamine metabolites are susceptible to further oxidation to yield other *N*-oxygenated products.

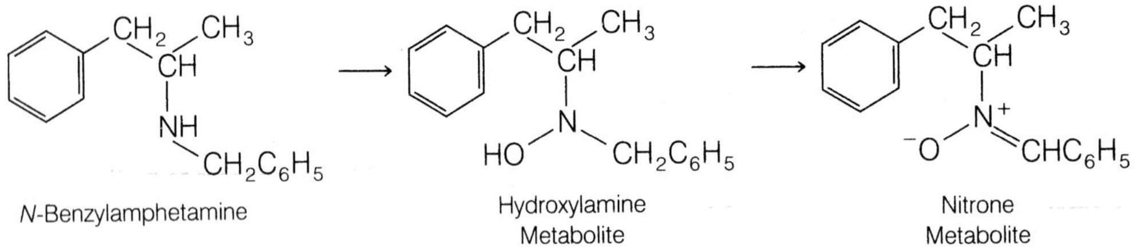

N-Benzylamphetamine → Hydroxylamine Metabolite → Nitrone Metabolite

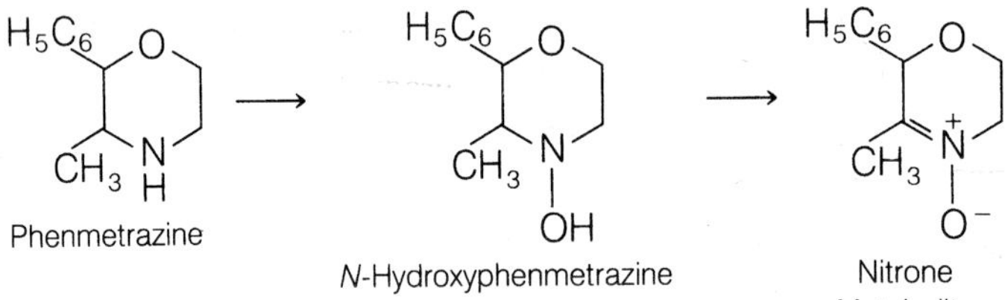

Phenmetrazine → *N*-Hydroxyphenmetrazine → Nitrone Metabolite

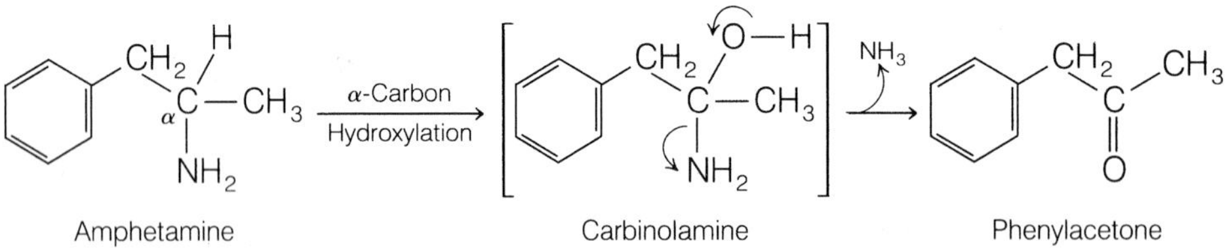

Amphetamine → [Carbinolamine] → Phenylacetone

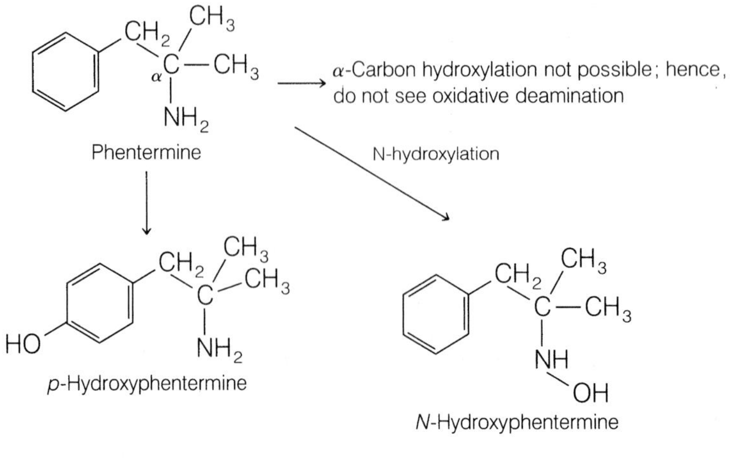

Phentermine — α-Carbon hydroxylation not possible; hence, do not see oxidative deamination

N-hydroxylation

p-Hydroxyphentermine

N-Hydroxyphentermine

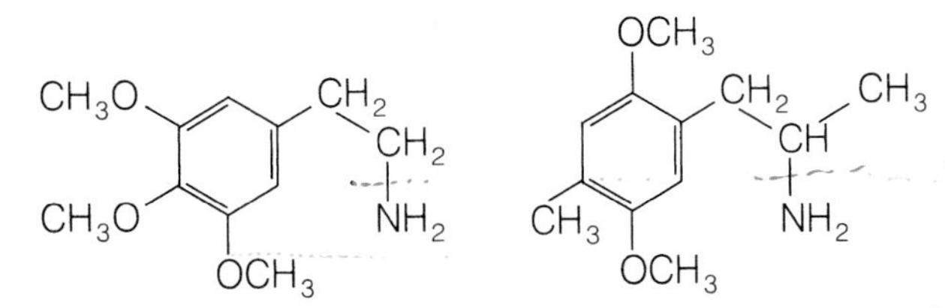

Mescaline

1-(2,5-Dimethoxy-4-methylphenyl)-
2-aminopropane
DOM or "STP"

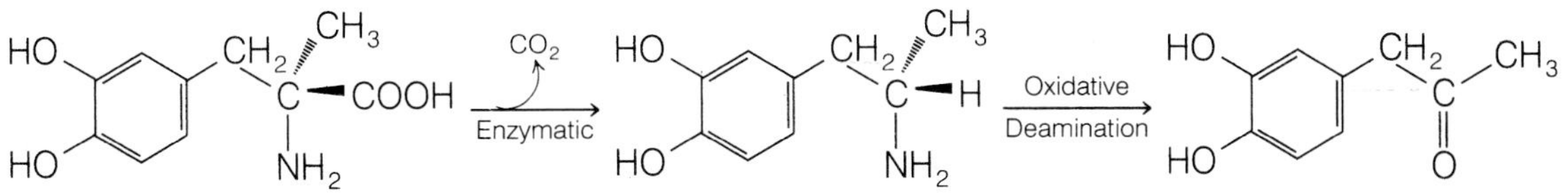

$S(-)$-α-Methyldopa $S(+)$-α-Methyldopamine   3,4-Dihydroxyphenylacetone

Xenobiotics, such as the hallucinogenic agents mescaline[208,209] and 1-(2,5-dimethoxy-4-methylphenyl)-2-aminopropane (DOM or "STP"),[210,211] are oxidatively deaminated. Primary amine metabolites arising from *N*-dealkylation or decarboxylation reactions also undergo deamination. The example of the bisdesmethyl primary amine metabolite derived from bromopheniramine is discussed previously in this chapter (see section on tertiary aliphatic and alicyclic amines).[181] In addition, many tertiary aliphatic amines (e.g., antihistamines) and secondary aliphatic amines (e.g., propranolol) are dealkylated to their corresponding primary amine metabolites, which are amenable to oxidative deamination. $(S)(+)$-α-Methyldopamine resulting from decarboxylation of the antihypertensive agent $(S)(-)$-α-methyldopa (Aldomet) is deaminated to the corresponding ketone metabolite 3,4-dihydroxyphenylacetone.[212] In humans, this ketone is a major urinary metabolite.

The *N*-hydroxylation reaction is not restricted to α-substituted primary amines such as phentermine. Amphetamine has been observed to undergo some *N*-hydroxylation in vitro to *N*-hydroxyamphetamine.[213,214] *N*-Hydroxyamphetamine is, however, susceptible to further conversion to the imine or oxidation to the oxime intermediate. Note that the oxime intermediate arising from this *N*-oxidation pathway can undergo hydrolytic cleavage to yield phenylacetone, the same product obtained by the α-carbon hydroxylation (carbinolamine)

pathway.[215,216] Thus, amphetamine may be converted to phenylacetone through either the α-carbon hydroxylation or the *N*-oxidation pathway. The debate concerning the relative importance of the two pathways is ongoing.[217–219] The consensus, however, is that both metabolic pathways (carbon and nitrogen oxidation) are probably operative. Whether α-carbon or nitrogen oxidation predominates in the metabolism of amphetamine appears to be species dependent.

In primary aliphatic amines, such as phentermine,[207] chlorphentermine (*p*-chlorphentermine),[219] and amantadine,[220] *N*-oxidation appears to be the major biotransformation pathway because α-carbon hydroxylation cannot occur. In humans, chlorphentermine is *N*-hydroxylated extensively. About 30% of a dose of chlorphentermine is found in the urine (48 hours) as *N*-hydroxychlorphentermine (free and conjugated) and an additional 18% as other products of *N*-oxidation (presumably the nitroso and nitro metabolites).[219] In general, *N*-hydroxylamines are chemically unstable and susceptible to spontaneous or enzymatic oxidation to the nitroso and nitro derivatives. For example, the *N*-hydroxylamine metabolite of phentermine undergoes further oxidation to the nitroso and nitro products.[207] The antiviral and antiparkinsonian agent amantadine (Symmetrel) reportedly undergoes *N*-oxidation to yield the corresponding *N*-hydroxy and nitroso metabolites in vitro.[220]

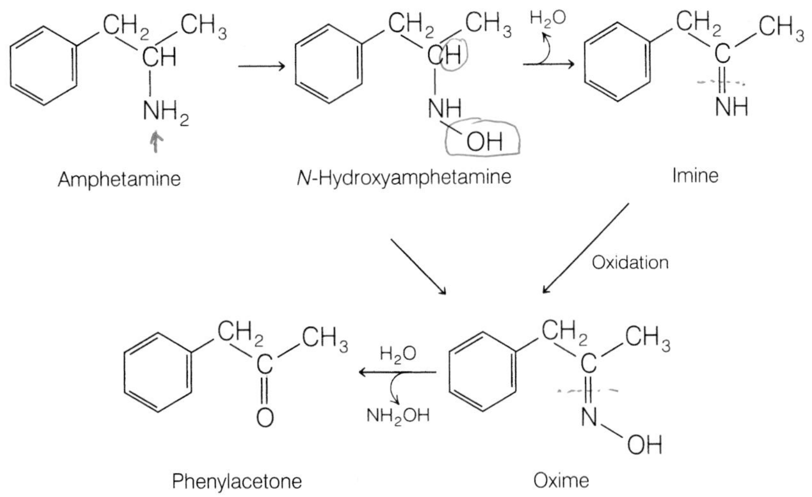

Amphetamine   *N*-Hydroxyamphetamine   Imine

Oxidation

Phenylacetone   Oxime

Aromatic Amines and Heterocyclic Nitrogen Compounds. The biotransformation of aromatic amines parallels the carbon and nitrogen oxidation reactions seen for aliphatic amines.[221–223] For tertiary aromatic amines, such as *N,N*-dimethylaniline, oxidative *N*-dealkylation as well as *N*-oxide formation take place.[224] Secondary aromatic amines may undergo *N*-dealkylation or *N*-hydroxylation to give the corresponding *N*-hydroxylamines. Further oxidation of the *N*-hydroxylamine leads to nitrone products, which in turn may be hydrolyzed to primary hydroxylamines.[225] Tertiary and secondary aromatic amines are encountered rarely in medicinal agents. In contrast, primary aromatic amines are found in many drugs and are often generated from enzymatic reduction of aromatic nitro compounds, reductive cleavage of azo compounds, and hydrolysis of aromatic amides.

N-oxidation of primary aromatic amines generates the *N*-hydroxylamine metabolite. One such case is aniline, which is metabolized to the corresponding *N*-hydroxy product.[223] Oxidation of the hydroxylamine derivative to the nitroso derivative also can occur. When one considers primary aromatic amine drugs or metabolites, *N*-oxidation constitutes only a minor pathway in comparison with other biotransformation pathways, such as *N*-acetylation and aromatic hydroxylation, in humans. Some *N*-oxygenated metabolites have been reported, however. For example, the antileprotic agent dapsone and its *N*-acetylated metabolite are metabolized significantly to their corresponding *N*-hydroxylamine derivatives.[226] The *N*-hydroxy metabolites are further conjugated with glucuronic acid.

Methemoglobinemia toxicity is caused by several aromatic amines, including aniline and dapsone, and is a result of the bioconversion of the aromatic amine to its *N*-hydroxy derivative. Apparently, the *N*-hydroxylamine oxidizes the Fe^{2+} form of hemoglobin to its Fe^{3+} form. This oxidized (Fe^{3+}) state of hemoglobin (called *methemoglobin* or *ferrihemoglobin*) can no longer transport oxygen, which leads to serious hypoxia or anemia, a unique type of chemical suffocation.[227]

Diverse aromatic amines (especially azoamino dyes) are known to be carcinogenic. *N*-oxidation plays an important role in bioactivating these aromatic amines to potentially reactive electrophilic species that covalently bind to cellular protein, DNA, or RNA. A well-studied example is the carcinogenic agent *N*-methyl-4-aminoazobenzene.[228,229] *N*-oxidation of this compound leads to the corresponding hydroxylamine, which undergoes sulfate conjugation. Because of the good leaving-group ability of the sulfate (SO_4^{2-}) anion, this conjugate can ionize spontaneously to form a highly reactive, resonance-stabilized nitrenium species. Covalent adducts between this species and DNA, RNA, and proteins have been characterized.[230,231] The sulfate ester is believed to be the ultimate carcinogenic species. Thus, the example indicates that certain aromatic amines can be bioactivated to reactive intermediates by *N*-hydroxylation and *O*-sulfate conjugation. Whether primary hydroxylamines can be bioactivated similarly is unclear. In addition, it is not known if this biotoxification pathway plays any substantial role in the toxicity of aromatic amine drugs.

N-oxidation of the nitrogen atoms present in aromatic heterocyclic moieties of many drugs occurs to a minor extent. Clearly, in humans, *N*-oxidation of the folic acid antagonist trimethoprim (Proloprim, Trimpex) has yielded approximately equal amounts of the isomeric 1-*N*-oxide and 3-*N*-oxide as minor metabolites.[232] The pyridinyl nitrogen atom present in nicotinine (the major metabolite of nicotine) undergoes oxidation to yield the corresponding *N*-oxide metabolite.[233] Another therapeutic agent that has been observed to undergo formation of an *N*-oxide metabolite is metronidazole.[234]

Amides. Amide functionalities are susceptible to oxidative carbon–nitrogen bond cleavage (via α-carbon hydroxylation) and *N*-hydroxylation reactions. Oxidative dealkylation of many *N*-substituted amide drugs and xenobiotics has been reported. Mechanistically, oxidative dealkylation proceeds via an initially formed carbinolamide, which is unstable and fragments to form the *N*-dealkylated product. For example, diazepam undergoes extensive *N*-demethylation to the pharmacologically active metabolite desmethyldiazepam.[235]

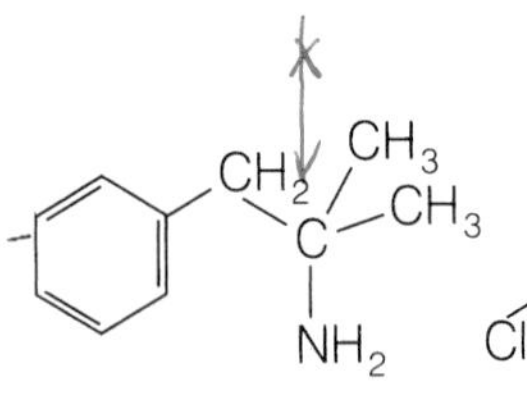

Phentermine 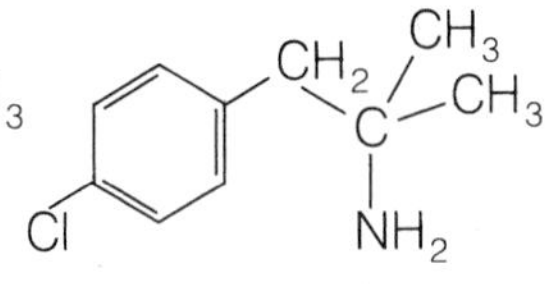   Chlorphentermine 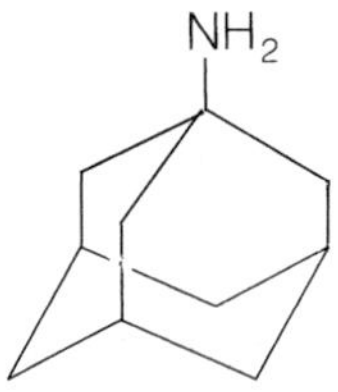   Amantadine

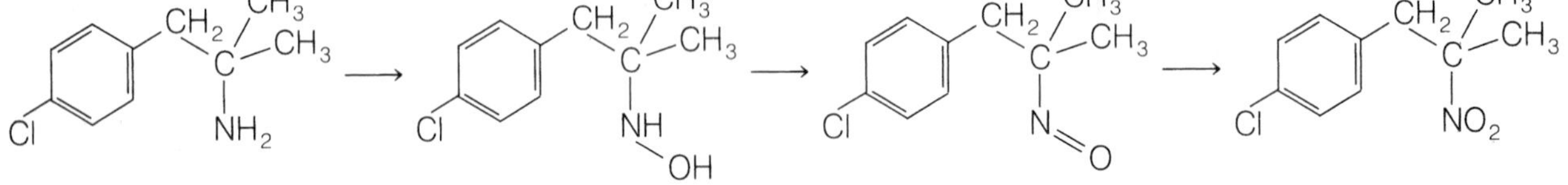

Chlorphentermine   *N*-Hydroxychlorphentermine   Nitroso Metabolite   Nitro Metabolite

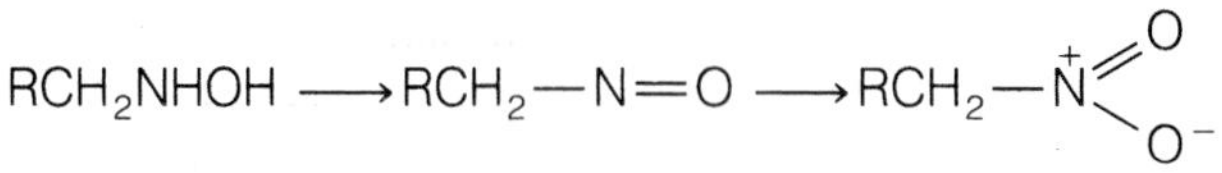

$$RCH_2NHOH \longrightarrow RCH_2-N=O \longrightarrow RCH_2-\overset{+}{N}\underset{O^-}{\overset{O}{\diagup}}$$

Hydroxylamine   Nitroso   Nitro

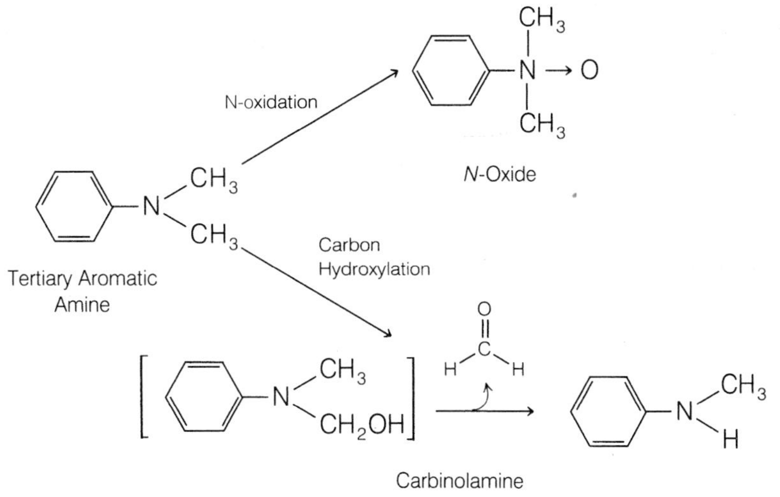

Tertiary Aromatic Amine

N-oxidation → *N*-Oxide

Carbon Hydroxylation → Carbinolamine

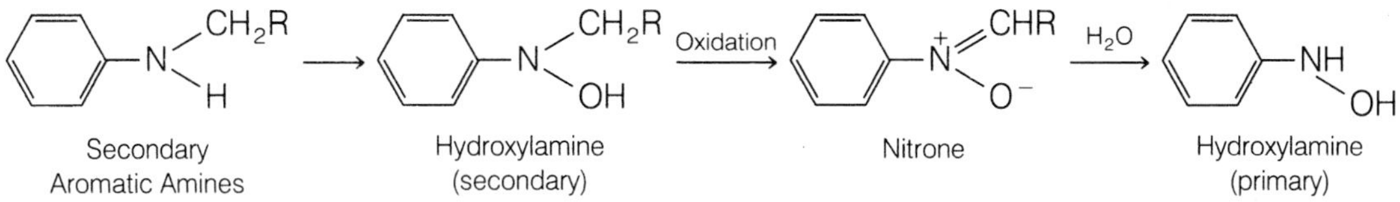

Secondary Aromatic Amines → Hydroxylamine (secondary) → Oxidation → Nitrone → H₂O → Hydroxylamine (primary)

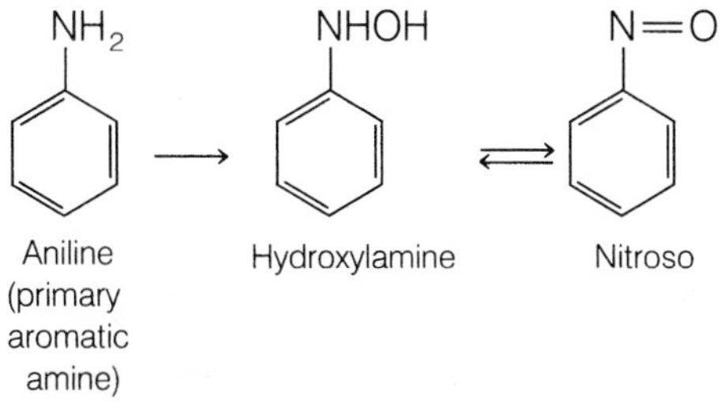

Aniline (primary aromatic amine) → Hydroxylamine ⇌ Nitroso

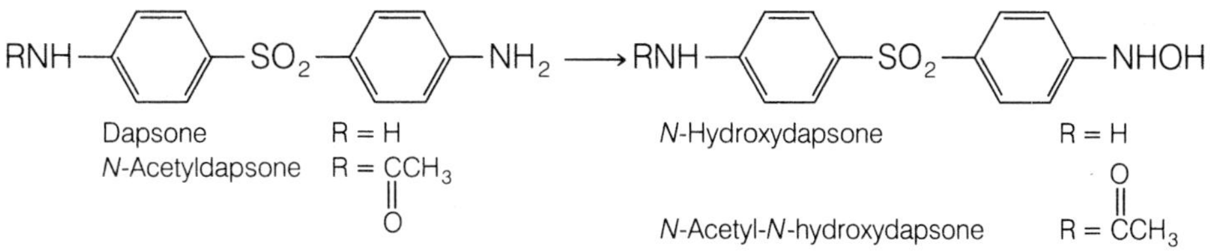

Dapsone   R = H
N-Acetyldapsone   R = CCH₃
                        ‖
                        O

N-Hydroxydapsone   R = H

N-Acetyl-*N*-hydroxydapsone   R = CCH₃
                                    ‖
                                    O

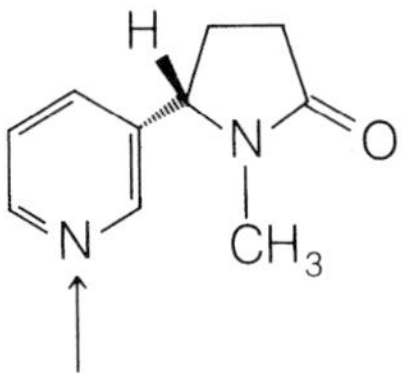

Cotinine

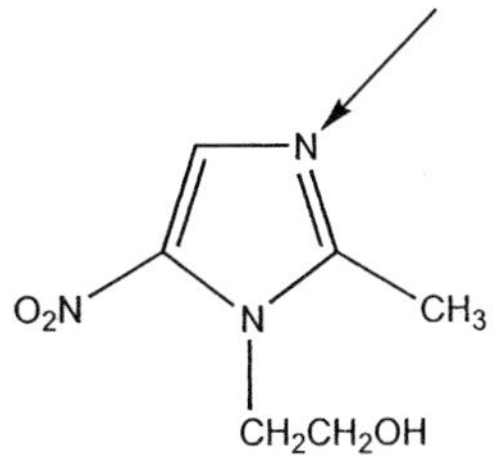

Metronidazole
2-(2-Methyl-5-nitro-imidazol-1-yl)-ethanol

Various other *N*-alkyl substituents present in benzodiazepines (e.g., flurazepam)[136–138] and in barbiturates (e.g., hexobarbital and mephobarbital)[128] are similarly oxidatively *N*-dealkylated. Alkyl groups attached to the amide moiety of some sulfonylureas, such as the oral hypoglycemic chlorpropamide,[236] also are subject to dealkylation to a minor extent.

In the cyclic amides or lactams, hydroxylation of the alicyclic carbon α to the nitrogen atom also leads to carbinolamides. An example of this pathway is the conversion of cotinine to 5-hydroxycotinine. Interestingly, the latter carbinolamide intermediate is in tautomeric equilibrium with the ring-opened metabolite γ-(3-pyridyl)-γ-oxo-*N*-methylbutyramide.[237]

Metabolism of the important cancer chemotherapeutic agent cyclophosphamide (Cytoxan) follows a hydroxylation pathway similar to that just described for cyclic amides. This

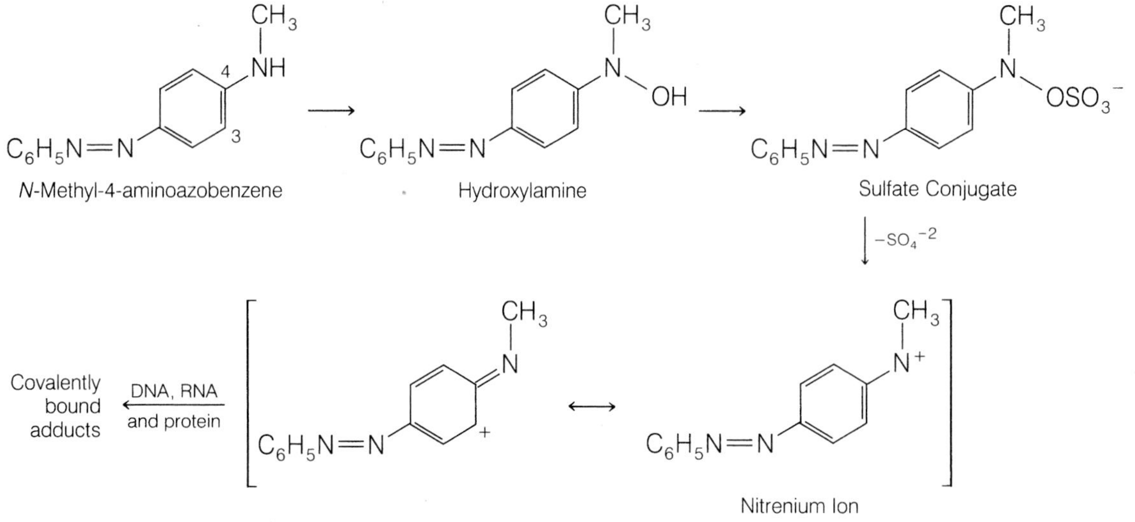

N-Methyl-4-aminoazobenzene → Hydroxylamine → Sulfate Conjugate

Covalently bound adducts ← DNA, RNA and protein — Nitrenium Ion

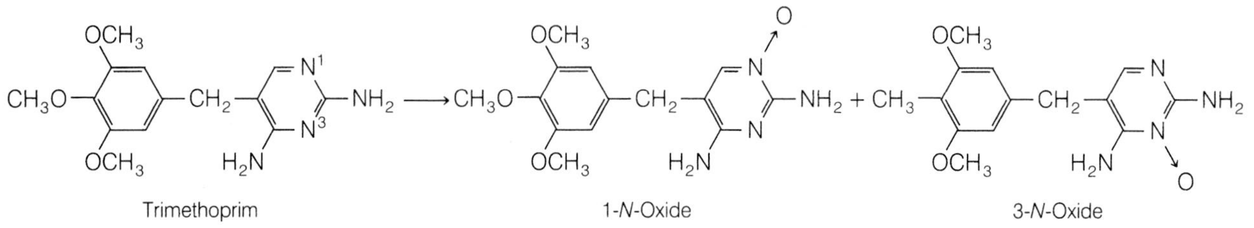

Trimethoprim → 1-N-Oxide + 3-N-Oxide

drug is a cyclic phosphoramide derivative and, for the most part, is the phosphorous counterpart of a cyclic amide. Because cyclophosphamide itself is pharmacologically inactive,[238] metabolic bioactivation is required for the drug to mediate its antitumorigenic or cytotoxic effects. The key biotransformation pathway leading to the active metabolite involves an initial carbon hydroxylation reaction at C-4 to form the carbinolamide 4-hydroxycyclophosphamide.[239,240]

4-Hydroxycyclophosphamide is in equilibrium with the ring-opened dealkylated metabolite aldophosphamide. Although it has potent cytotoxic properties, aldophosphamide undergoes a further elimination reaction (reverse Michael reaction) to generate acrolein and the phosphoramide mustard *N,N*-bis(2-chloro-ethyl)phosphorodiamidic acid. The latter is the principal species responsible for cyclophosphamide's antitumorigenic properties and

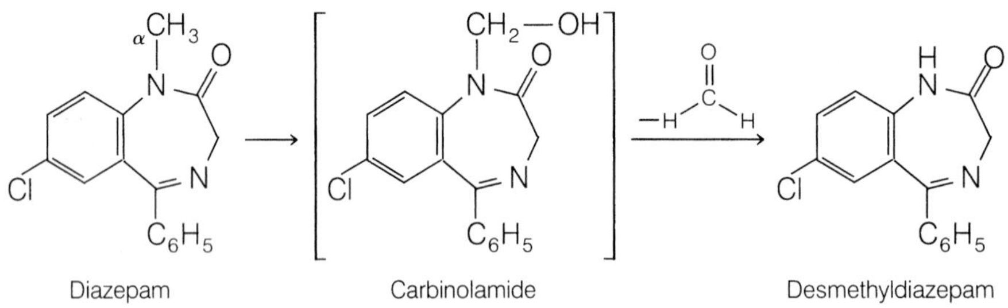

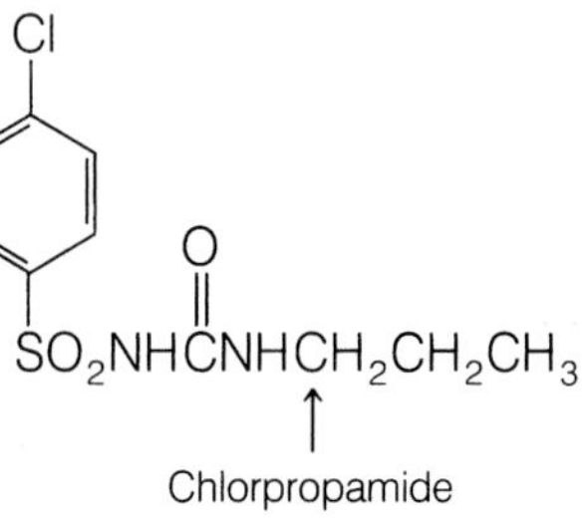

Diazepam → Carbinolamide → Desmethyldiazepam

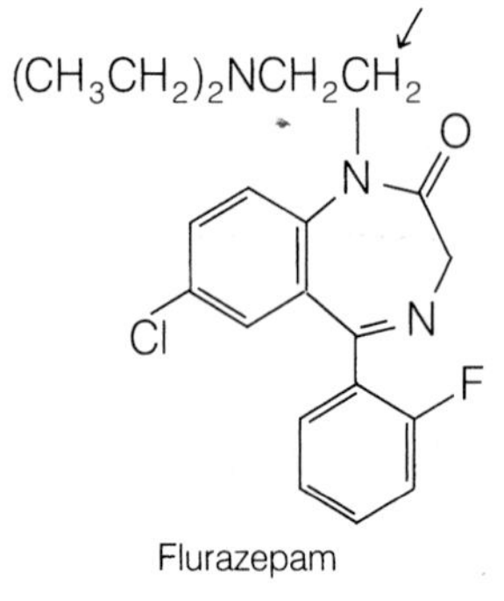

Flurazepam

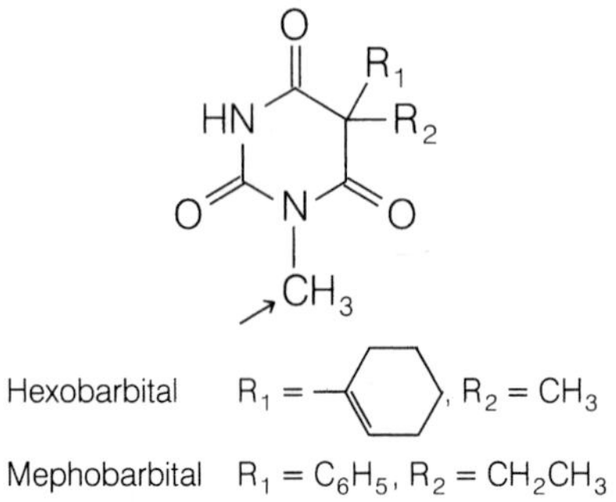

Hexobarbital $R_1 = $ cyclohexenyl, $R_2 = CH_3$

Mephobarbital $R_1 = C_6H_5$, $R_2 = CH_2CH_3$

Chlorpropamide

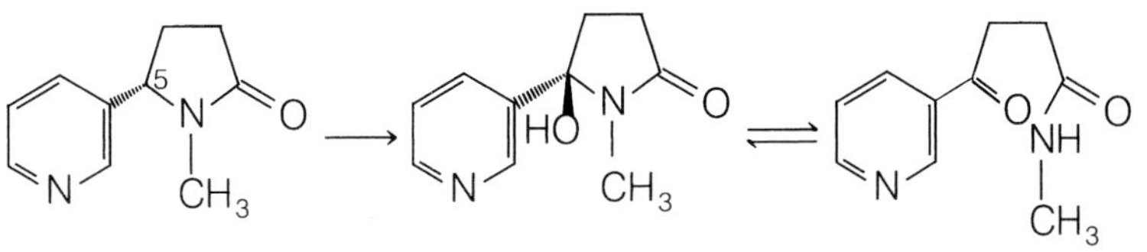

Cotinine   5-Hydroxycotinine   γ-(3-Pyridyl)-γ-oxo-*N*-methylbutyramide

chemotherapeutic effect. Enzymatic oxidation of 4-hydroxy-cyclophosphamide and aldophosphamide leads to the relatively nontoxic metabolites 4-ketocyclophosphamide and carboxycyclophosphamide, respectively.

N-hydroxylation of aromatic amides, which occurs to a minor extent, is of some toxicological interest, because this biotransformation pathway may lead to the formation of chemically reactive intermediates. Several examples of cytotoxicity or carcinogenicity associated with metabolic *N*-hydroxylation of the parent aromatic amide have been reported. For example, the well-known hepatocarcinogenic 2-acetylaminofluorene (AAF) undergoes an *N*-hydroxylation reaction catalyzed by CYP to form the corresponding *N*-hydroxy metabolite (also called a *hydroxamic acid*).[241] Further conjugation of this hydroxamic acid produces the corresponding *O*-sulfate ester, which ionizes to generate the electrophilic nitrenium species. Covalent binding of this reactive intermediate to DNA is known to occur and is likely to be the initial event that ultimately leads to malignant tumor formation.[242] Sulfate conjugation plays an important role in this biotoxification pathway (see "Sulfate Conjugation," for further discussion).

Acetaminophen is a relatively safe and nontoxic analgesic agent if used at therapeutic doses. Its metabolism illustrates the fact that a xenobiotic commonly produces more than one metabolite. Its metabolism also illustrates the effect of age, because infants and young children carry out sulfation rather than glucuronidation (see discussion at the end of this chapter). New pharmacists must realize that at one time acetanilide and phenacetin were more widely used than acetaminophen, even though both are considered more toxic because they pro-

duce aniline derivatives. Besides producing toxic aniline and *p*-phenetidin, these two analgesics also produce acetaminophen. When large doses of the latter drug are ingested, extensive liver necrosis is produced in humans and animals.[243,244] Considerable evidence argues that this hepatotoxicity depends on the formation of a metabolically generated reactive intermediate.[245] Until recently,[246,247] the accepted bioactivation pathway was believed to involve an initial *N*-hydroxylation reaction to form *N*-hydroxyacetaminophen.[248]

Spontaneous dehydration of this *N*-hydroxyamide produces *N*-acetylimidoquinone, the proposed reactive metabolite. Usually, the GSH present in the liver combines with this reactive metabolite to form the corresponding GSH conjugate. If GSH levels are sufficiently depleted by large doses of acetaminophen, covalent binding of the reactive intermediate occurs with macromolecules present in the liver, thereby leading to cellular necrosis. Studies indicate, however, that the reactive *N*-acetylimidoquinone intermediate is not formed from *N*-hydroxyacetaminophen.[245–247] It probably arises through some other oxidative process. Therefore, the mechanistic formation of the reactive metabolite of acetaminophen remains unclear.

OXIDATION INVOLVING CARBON–OXYGEN SYSTEMS

Oxidative *O*-dealkylation of carbon–oxygen systems (principally ethers) is catalyzed by microsomal mixed function oxidases.[163] Mechanistically, the biotransformation involves an initial α-carbon hydroxylation to form either a hemiacetal or a hemiketal, which undergoes spontaneous carbon–oxygen

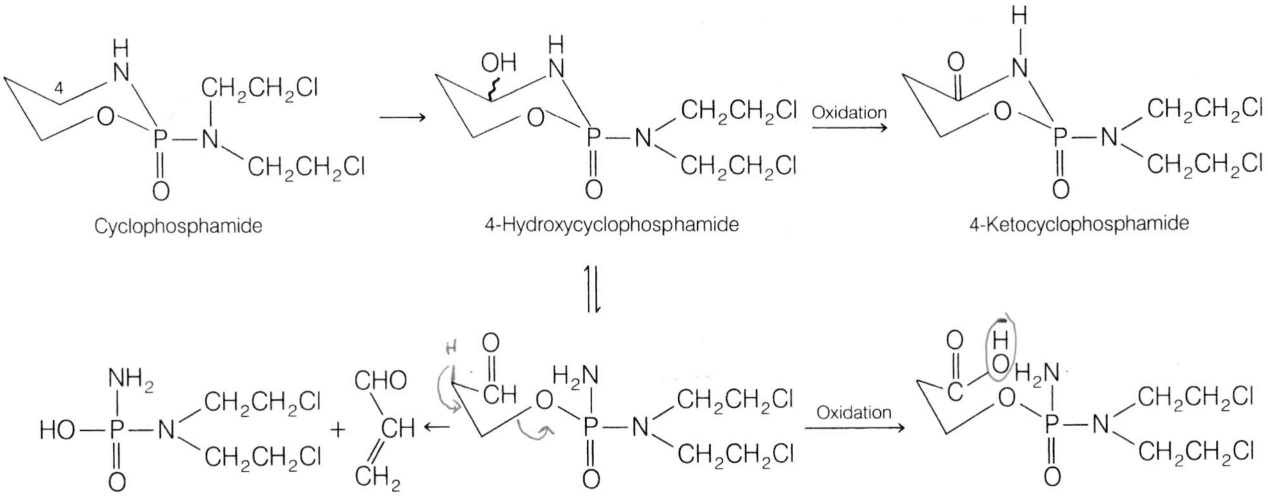

Cyclophosphamide   4-Hydroxycyclophosphamide   4-Ketocyclophosphamide

Phosphoramide Mustard, *N,N*-bis(2-Chloroethyl)-phosphorodiamidic Acid   Acrolein   Aldophosphamide   Carboxyphosphamide

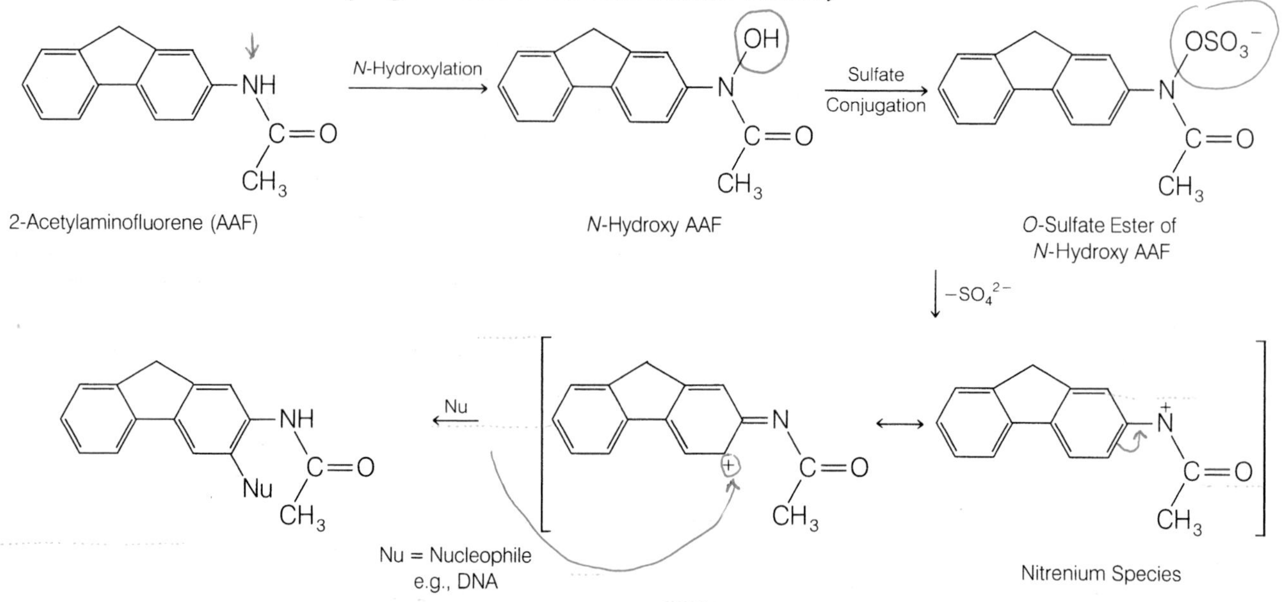

2-Acetylaminofluorene (AAF)

N-Hydroxylation

N-Hydroxy AAF

Sulfate Conjugation

O-Sulfate Ester of *N*-Hydroxy AAF

$-SO_4^{2-}$

Nu

Nu = Nucleophile e.g., DNA

Nitrenium Species

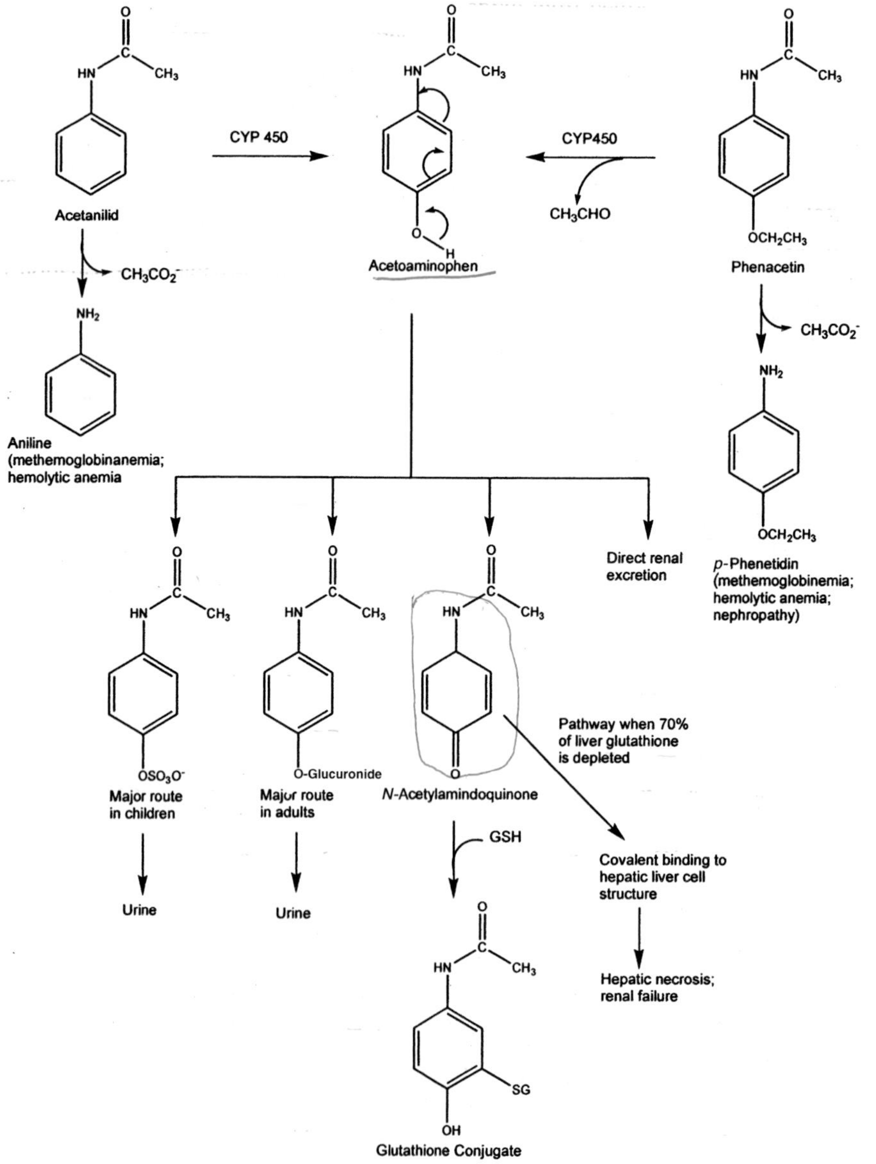

CYP 450

Acetanilid

CYP450

CH_3CHO

Acetoaminophen

Phenacetin

$CH_3CO_2^-$

Aniline (methemoglobinanemia; hemolytic anemia

$CH_3CO_2^-$

p-Phenetidin (methemoglobinemia; hemolytic anemia; nephropathy)

Direct renal excretion

OSO_3O^-
Major route in children

O-Glucuronide
Major route in adults

N-Acetylamindoquinone

Pathway when 70% of liver glutathione is depleted

Urine

Urine

GSH

Covalent binding to hepatic liver cell structure

Hepatic necrosis; renal failure

Glutathione Conjugate

bond cleavage to yield the dealkylated oxygen species (phenol or alcohol) and a carbon moiety (aldehyde or ketone). Small alkyl groups (e.g., methyl or ethyl) attached to oxygen are *O*-dealkylated rapidly. For example, morphine is the metabolic product of *O*-demethylation of codeine.[249] The antipyretic and analgesic activities of phenacetin (see drawing of acetaminophen metabolism) in humans appear to be a consequence of *O*-deethylation to the active metabolite acetaminophen.[250] Several other drugs containing ether groups, such as indomethacin (Indocin),[251,252] prazosin (Minipress),[253,254] and metoprolol (Lopressor),[122,123] have reportedly undergone significant *O*-demethylation to their corresponding phenolic or alcoholic metabolites, which are further conjugated. In many drugs that have several nonequivalent methoxy groups, one particular methoxy group often appears to be *O*-demethylated selectively or preferentially. For example, the 3,4,5-trimethoxyphenyl moiety in both mescaline[255] and trimethoprim[232] undergoes *O*-demethylation to yield predominantly the corresponding 3-*O*-demethylated metabolites. 4-*O*-demethylation also occurs to a minor extent for both drugs. The phenolic and alcoholic metabolites formed from oxidative *O*-demethylation are susceptible to conjugation, particularly glucuronidation.

OXIDATION INVOLVING CARBON–SULFUR SYSTEMS

Carbon–sulfur functional groups are susceptible to metabolic *S*-dealkylation, desulfuration, and *S*-oxidation reactions. The first two processes involve oxidative

carbon–sulfur bond cleavage. *S*-dealkylation is analogous to *O*- and *N*-dealkylation mechanistically (i.e., it involves α-carbon hydroxylation) and has been observed for various sulfur xenobiotics.[163,256] For example, 6-(methylthio)purine is demethylated oxidatively in rats to 6-mercaptopurine.[257,258] *S*-demethylation of methitural[259] and *S*-debenzylation of 2-benzylthio-5-trifluoromethylbenzoic acid also have been reported. In contrast to *O*- and *N*-dealkylation, examples of drugs undergoing *S*-dealkylation in humans are limited because of the small number of sulfur-containing medicinals and the competing metabolic *S*-oxidation processes (see diagram).

Oxidative conversion of carbon–sulfur double bonds (C=S) (thiono) to the corresponding carbon–oxygen double bond (C=O) is called *desulfuration*. A well-known drug example of this metabolic process is the biotransformation of thiopental to its corresponding oxygen analog pentobarbital.[260,261] An analogous desulfuration reaction also occurs with the P=S moiety present in several organophosphate insecticides, such as parathion.[262,263] Desulfuration of parathion leads to the formation of paraoxon, which is the active metabolite responsible for the anticholinesterase activity of the parent drug. The mechanistic details of desulfuration are poorly understood, but it appears to involve microsomal oxidation of the C=S or P=S double bond.[264]

Organosulfur xenobiotics commonly undergo *S*-oxidation to yield sulfoxide derivatives. Several phenothiazine derivatives are metabolized by this pathway. For example, both sulfur atoms present in thioridazine (Mellaril)[265,266] are susceptible to *S*-oxidation. Oxidation of the 2-methylthio

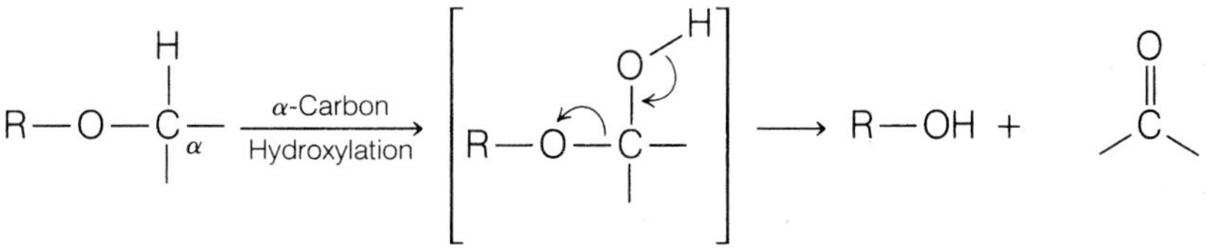

Ether → Hemiacetal or Hemiketal → Phenol or Alcohol + Carbonyl Moiety (aldehyde or ketone)

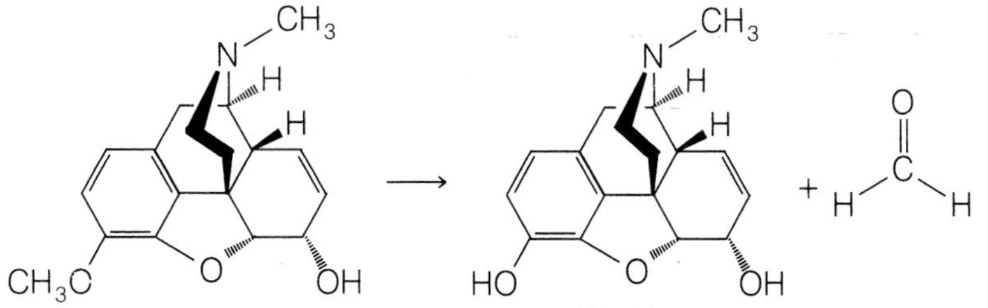

Codeine → Morphine

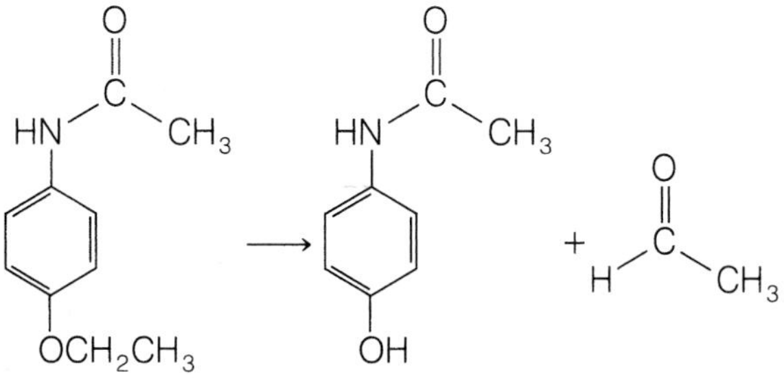

Phenacetin → Acetaminophen

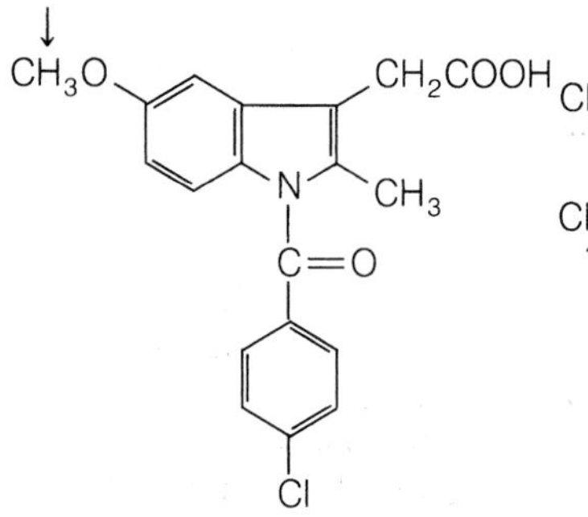

Indomethacin

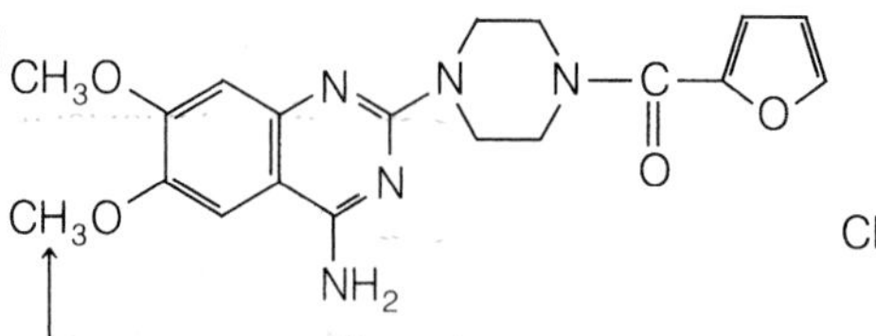

Prazosin

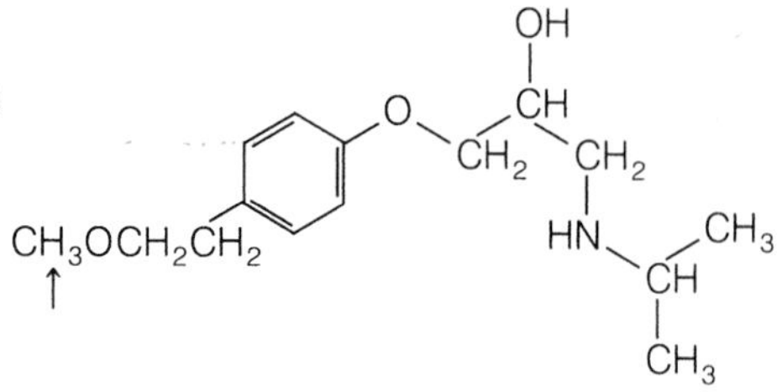

Metoprolol

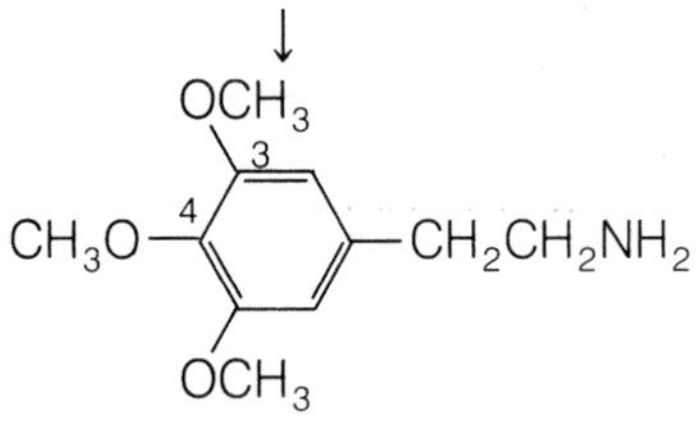

Mescaline

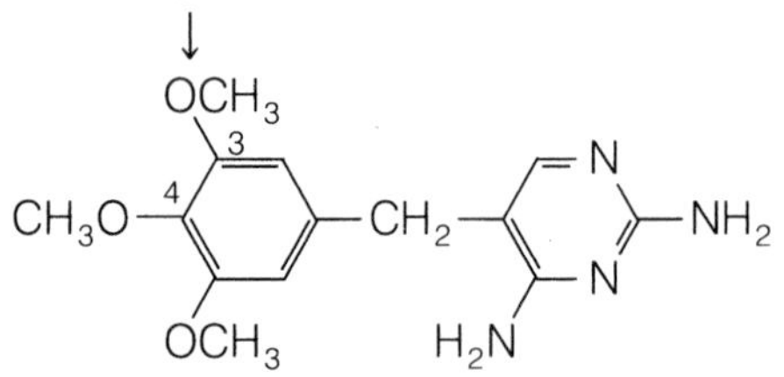

Trimethoprim

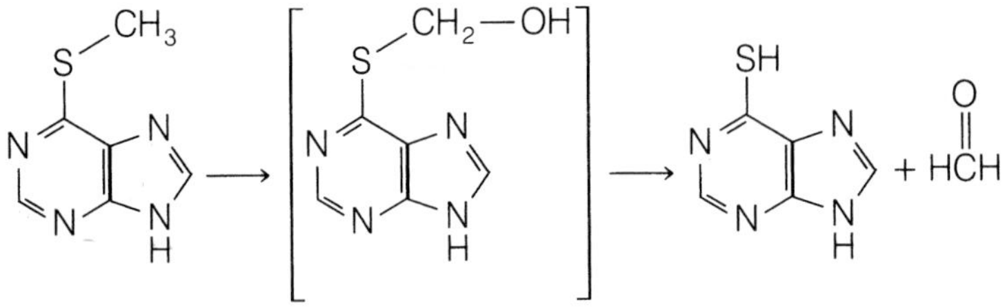

6-(Methylthio)-purine

6-Mercaptopurine

group yields the active sulfoxide metabolite mesoridazine. Interestingly, mesoridazine is twice as potent an antipsychotic agent as thioridazine in humans and has been introduced into clinical use as Serentil.[267]

S-oxidation constitutes an important pathway in the metabolism of the H$_2$-histamine antagonists cimetidine (Tagamet)[268] and metiamide.[269] The corresponding sulfoxide derivatives are the major human urinary metabolites.

Sulfoxide drugs and metabolites may be further oxidized to sulfones (-SO$_2$-). The sulfoxide group present in the immunosuppressive agent oxisuran is metabolized to a sulfone moiety.[270] In humans, dimethylsulfoxide (DMSO) is found primarily in the urine as the oxidized product dimethylsulfone. Sulfoxide metabolites, such as those of thioridazine, reportedly undergo further oxidation to their sulfone -SO$_2$- derivatives.[265,266]

Oxidation of Alcohols and Aldehydes

Many oxidative processes (e.g., benzylic, allylic, alicyclic, or aliphatic hydroxylation) generate alcohol or carbinol metabolites as intermediate products. If not conjugated, these alcohol products are further oxidized to aldehydes (if primary alcohols) or to ketones (if secondary alcohols). Aldehyde metabolites resulting from oxidation of primary alcohols or from oxidative deamination of primary aliphatic amines often undergo facile oxidation to generate polar carboxylic acid derivatives.[116] As a general rule, primary alcoholic groups and aldehyde functionalities are quite vulnerable to oxidation. Several drug examples in which primary alcohol metabolites and aldehyde metabolites are oxidized to carboxylic acid products are cited in previous sections.

Although secondary alcohols are susceptible to oxidation, this reaction is not often important because the reverse reaction, namely, reduction of the ketone back to the secondary alcohol, occurs quite readily. In addition, the secondary alcohol group, being polar and functionalized, is more likely to be conjugated than the ketone moiety.

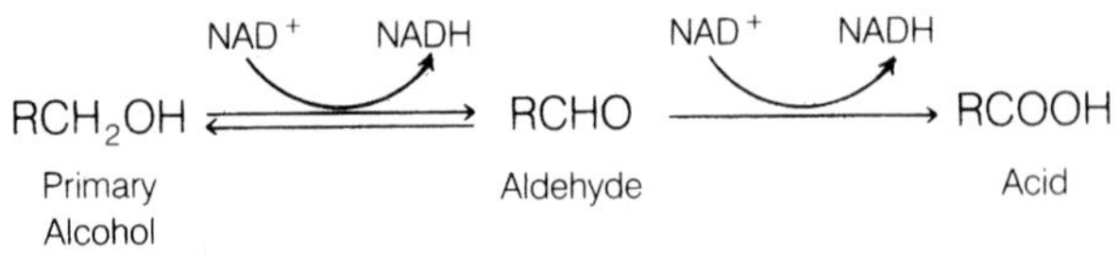

The bioconversion of alcohols to aldehydes and ketones is catalyzed by soluble alcohol dehydrogenases present in the liver and other tissues. NAD$^+$ is required as a coenzyme, although NADP$^+$ also may serve as a coenzyme. The reaction catalyzed by alcohol dehydrogenase is reversible but often proceeds to the right because the aldehyde formed

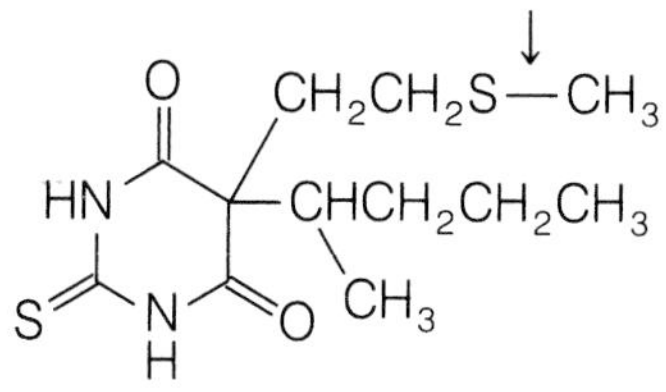

Methitural

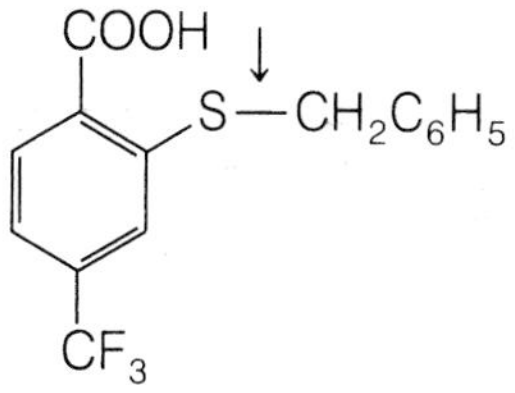

2-Benzylthio-5-
trifluoromethylbenzoic Acid

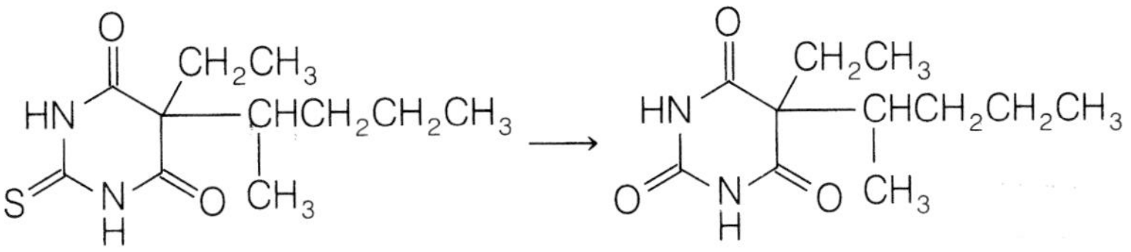

Thiopental

Pentobarbital

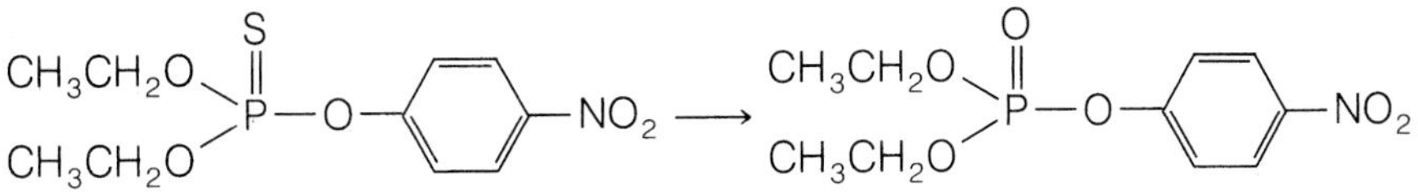

Parathion

Paraoxon

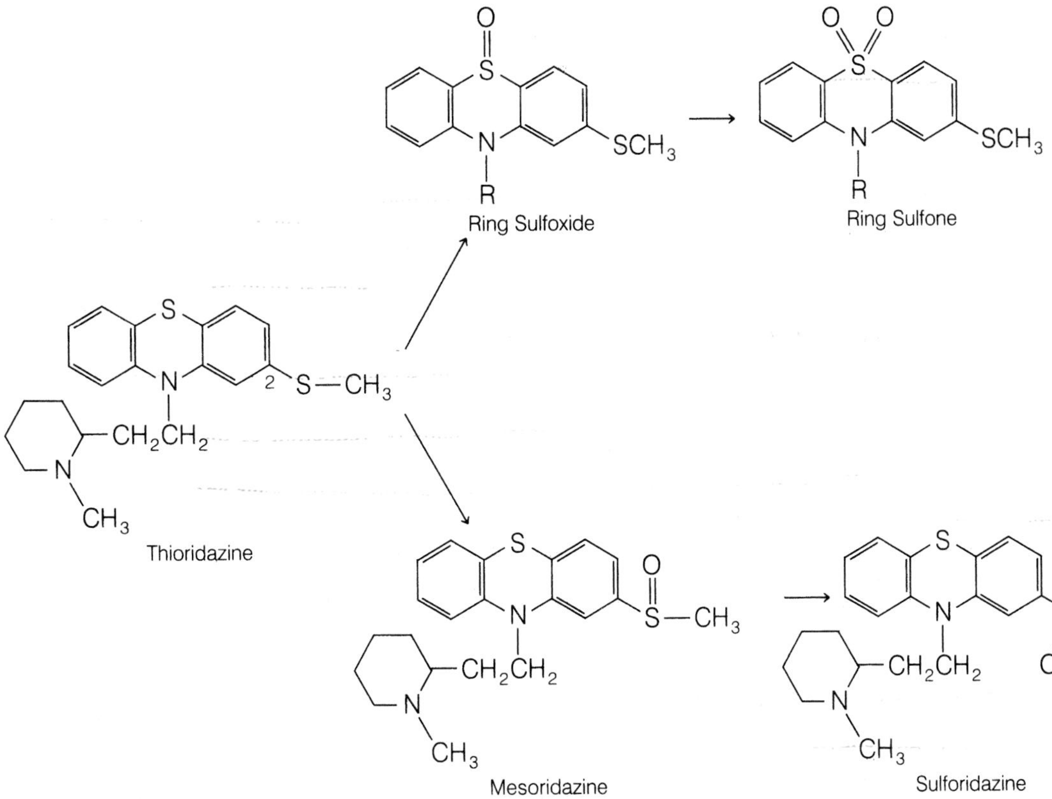

Ring Sulfoxide

Ring Sulfone

Thioridazine

Mesoridazine

Sulforidazine

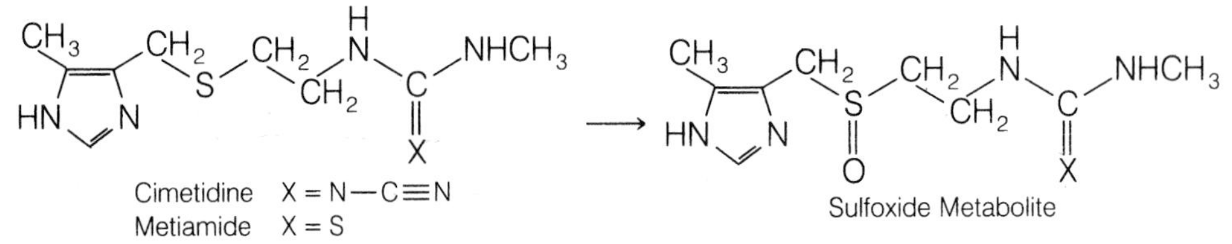

Cimetidine   X = N — C ≡ N
Metiamide   X = S

Sulfoxide Metabolite

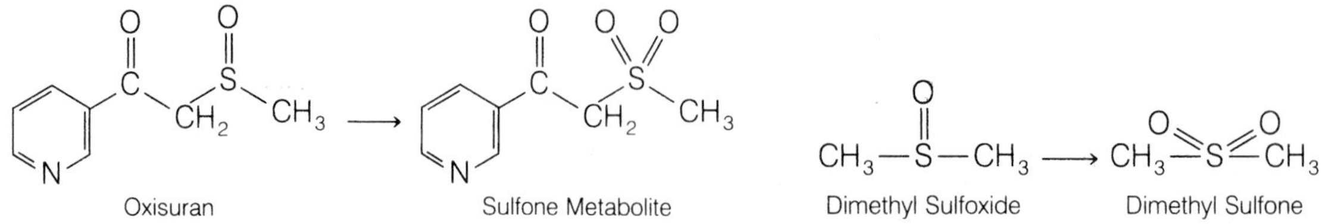

Oxisuran

Sulfone Metabolite

Dimethyl Sulfoxide

Dimethyl Sulfone

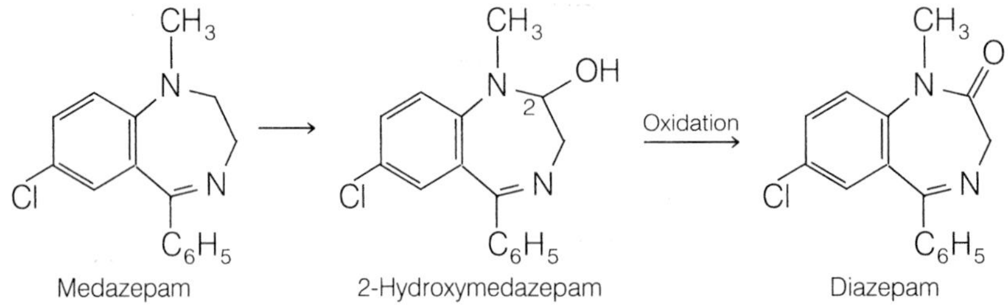

Medazepam

2-Hydroxymedazepam

Oxidation

Diazepam

is further oxidized to the acid. Several aldehyde dehydrogenases, including aldehyde oxidase and xanthine oxidase, carry out the oxidation of aldehydes to their corresponding acids.[116,271–273]

Metabolism of cyclic amines to their lactam metabolites has been observed for various drugs (e.g., nicotine, phenmetrazine, and methylphenidate). It appears that soluble or microsomal dehydrogenase and oxidases are involved in oxidizing the carbinol group of the intermediate carbinolamine to a carbonyl moiety.[273] For example, in the metabolism of medazepam to diazepam, the intermediate carbinolamine (2-hydroxymedazepam) undergoes oxidation of its 2-hydroxy group to a carbonyl moiety. A microsomal dehydrogenase carries out this oxidation.[274]

Other Oxidative Biotransformation Pathways

In addition to the many oxidative biotransformations discussed previously in this chapter, oxidative aromatization or dehydrogenation and oxidative dehalogenation reactions also occur. Metabolic aromatization has been reported for norgestrel. Aromatization or dehydrogenation of the A ring present in this steroid leads to the corresponding phenolic product 17α-ethinyl-18-homoestradiol as a minor metabolite in women.[275] In mice, the terpene ring of Δ^1-THC or $\Delta^{1,6}$-THC undergoes aromatization to give cannabinol.[276,277]

Many halogen-containing drugs and xenobiotics are metabolized by oxidative dehalogenation. For example, the volatile anesthetic agent halothane is metabolized principally to trifluoroacetic acid in humans.[278,279] It has been postulated that this metabolite arises from CYP-mediated hydroxylation of halothane to form an initial carbinol intermediate that spontaneously eliminates hydrogen bromide (dehalogenation) to yield trifluoroacetyl

chloride. The latter acyl chloride is chemically reactive and reacts rapidly with water to form trifluoroacetic acid. Alternatively, it can acylate tissue nucleophiles. Indeed, in vitro studies indicate that halothane is metabolized to a reactive intermediate (presumably trifluoroacetyl chloride), which covalently binds to liver microsomal proteins.[280,281] Chloroform also appears to be metabolized oxidatively by a similar dehalogenation pathway to yield the chemically reactive species phosgene. Phosgene may be responsible for the hepatotoxicity and nephrotoxicity associated with chloroform.[282]

A final example of oxidative dehalogenation concerns the antibiotic chloramphenicol. In vitro studies have shown that the dichloroacetamide portion of the molecule undergoes oxidative dechlorination to yield a chemically reactive oxamyl chloride intermediate that can react with water to form the corresponding oxamic acid metabolite or can acylate microsomal proteins.[283,284] Thus, it appears that in several instances, oxidative dehalogenation can lead to the formation of toxic and reactive acyl halide intermediates.

⬡ REDUCTIVE REACTIONS

Reductive processes play an important role in the metabolism of many compounds containing carbonyl, nitro, and azo groups. Bioreduction of carbonyl compounds generates alcohol derivatives,[116,285] whereas nitro and azo reductions lead to amino derivatives.[286] The hydroxyl and amino moieties of the metabolites are much more susceptible to conjugation than the functional groups of the parent compounds. Hence, reductive processes, as such, facilitate drug elimination.

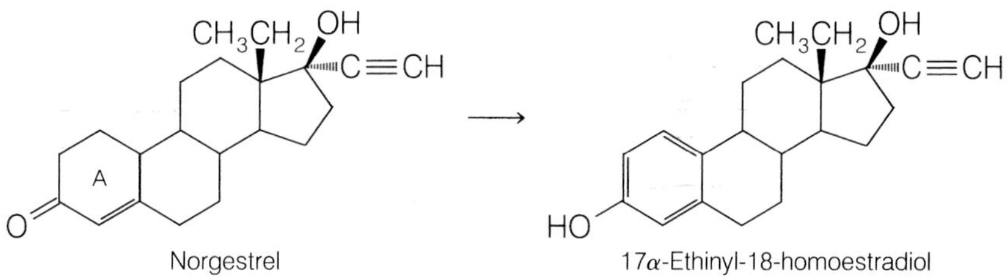

Norgestrel → 17α-Ethinyl-18-homoestradiol

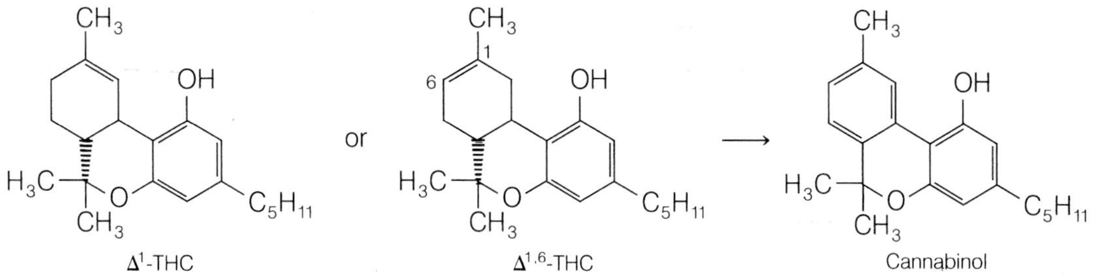

Δ¹-THC   or   Δ¹,⁶-THC   →   Cannabinol

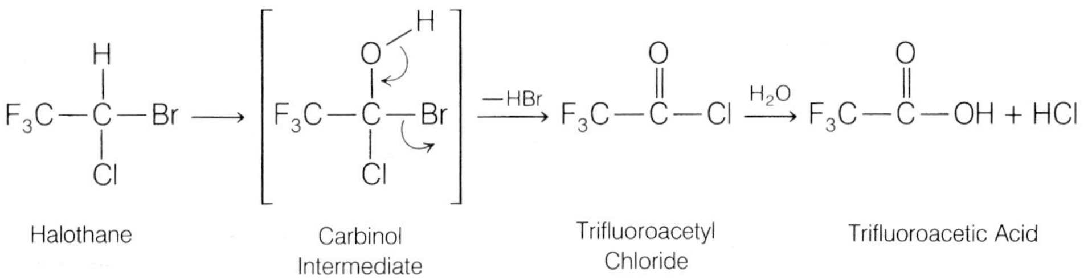

Halothane → Carbinol Intermediate → Trifluoroacetyl Chloride → Trifluoroacetic Acid

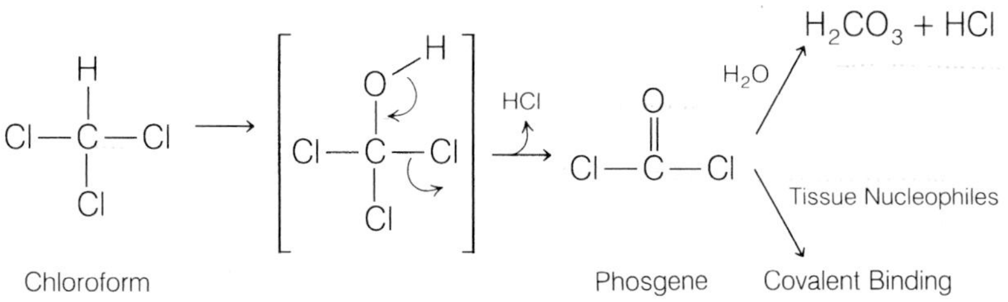

Chloroform → Phosgene → H_2CO_3 + HCl / Tissue Nucleophiles → Covalent Binding

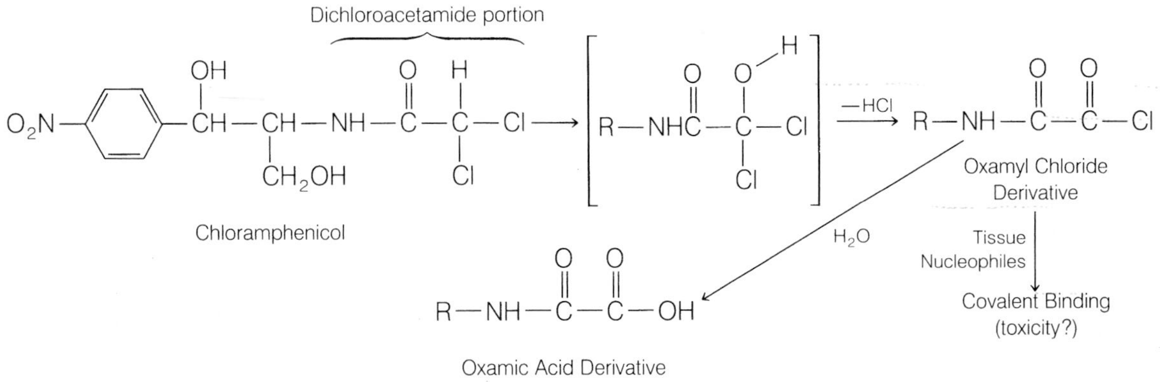

Dichloroacetamide portion

Chloramphenicol → Oxamyl Chloride Derivative → Oxamic Acid Derivative / Tissue Nucleophiles → Covalent Binding (toxicity?)

Reductive pathways that are encountered less frequently in drug metabolism include reduction of *N*-oxides to their corresponding tertiary amines and reduction of sulfoxides to sulfides. Reductive cleavage of disulfide linkages and reduction of carbon–carbon double bonds also occur, but constitute only minor pathways in drug metabolism.

Reduction of Aldehyde and Ketone Carbonyls

The carbonyl moiety, particularly the ketone group, is encountered frequently in many drugs. In addition, metabolites containing ketone and aldehyde functionalities often arise from oxidative deamination of xenobiotics (e.g., propranolol, chlorpheniramine, amphetamine). Because of their ease of oxidation, aldehydes are metabolized mainly to carboxylic acids. Occasionally, aldehydes are reduced to primary alcohols. Ketones, however, are generally resistant to oxidation and are reduced mainly to secondary alcohols. Alcohol metabolites arising from reduction of carbonyl compounds generally undergo further conjugation (e.g., glucuronidation).

Aldehyde → Primary Alcohols

Ketone → Secondary Alcohols
(stereoisomeric products possible)

Diverse soluble enzymes, called *aldo-keto reductases*, carry out bioreduction of aldehydes and ketones.[116,287] They are found in the liver and other tissues (e.g., kidney). As a general class, these soluble enzymes have similar physiochemical properties and broad substrate specificities and require NADPH as a cofactor. Oxidoreductase enzymes that carry out both oxidation and reduction reactions also can reduce aldehydes and ketones.[287] For example, the important liver alcohol dehydrogenase is an NAD⁺-dependent–oxidoreductase that oxidizes ethanol and other aliphatic alcohols to aldehydes and ketones. In the presence of NADH or NADPH, however, the same enzyme system can reduce carbonyl derivatives to their corresponding alcohols.[116]

Few aldehydes undergo bioreduction because of the relative ease of oxidation of aldehydes to carboxylic acids. However, one frequently cited example of a parent aldehyde drug undergoing extensive enzymatic reduction is the sedative–hypnotic chloral hydrate. Bioreduction of this hydrated aldehyde yields trichloroethanol as the major metabolite in humans.[288] Interestingly, this alcohol metabolite is pharmacologically active. Further glucuronidation of the alcohol leads to an inactive conjugated product that is readily excreted in the urine.

Chloral Hydrate   Chloral   Trichloroethanol

Aldehyde metabolites resulting from oxidative deamination of drugs also undergo reduction to a minor extent. For example, in humans the β-adrenergic blocker propranolol is converted to an intermediate aldehyde by *N*-dealkylation and oxidative deamination. Although the aldehyde is oxidized primarily to the corresponding carboxylic acid (naphthoxylactic acid), a small fraction is also reduced to the alcohol derivative (propranolol glycol).[289]

Two major polar urinary metabolites of the histamine H₁-antagonist chlorpheniramine have been identified in dogs as the alcohol and carboxylic acid products (conjugated) derived, respectively, by reduction and oxidation of an aldehyde metabolite. The aldehyde precursor arises from bis-*N*-demethylation and oxidative deamination of chlorpheniramine.[290]

Bioreduction of ketones often leads to the creation of an asymmetric center and, thereby, two possible stereoisomeric alcohols.[116,291] For example, reduction of acetophenone by a soluble rabbit kidney reductase leads to the enantiomeric alcohols (*S*)(−)- and (*R*)(+)-methylphenylcarbinol, with the (*S*)(−)-isomer predominating (3:1 ratio).[292] The preferential formation of one stereoisomer over the other is termed *product stereoselectivity* in drug metabolism.[291] Mechanistically, ketone reduction involves a "hydride" transfer from the reduced nicotinamide moiety of the cofactor NADPH or NADH to the carbonyl carbon atom of the ketone. It is generally agreed that this step proceeds with considerable *stereoselectivity*.[116,291] Consequently, it is not surprising to find many reports of xenobiotic ketones that are reduced preferentially to a predominant stereoisomer. Often, ketone reduction yields alcohol metabolites that are pharmacologically active.

Although many ketone-containing drugs undergo significant reduction, only a few selected examples are presented in detail here. The xenobiotics that are not discussed in the text have been structurally tabulated in Figure 3.10. The keto group undergoing reduction is designated with an arrow.

Ketones lacking asymmetric centers in their molecules, such as acetophenone or the oral hypoglycemic acetohexamide, usually give rise to predominantly one enantiomer on reduction. In humans, acetohexamide is metabolized rapidly in the liver to give principally (*S*)(−)-hydroxyhexamide.[293,294] This metabolite is as active a hypoglycemic agent as its parent compound and is eliminated through the kidneys.[295] Acetohexamide usually is not recommended in diabetic patients with renal failure, because of the possible accumulation of its active metabolite, hydroxyhexamide.

When chiral ketones are reduced, they yield two possible diastereomeric or epimeric alcohols. For example, the (*R*)(+) enantiomer of the oral anticoagulant warfarin undergoes extensive reduction of its side chain keto group to generate the (*R*,*S*)(+) alcohol as the major plasma metabolite in humans.[56,296] Small amounts of the (*R*,*R*)(+) diastereomer are also formed. In contrast, the (*S*)(−) enantiomer undergoes little ketone reduction and is primarily 7-hydroxylated (i.e., aromatic hydroxylation) in humans.

Reduction of the 6-keto functionality in the narcotic antagonist naltrexone can lead to either the epimeric 6α- or 6β-hydroxy metabolites, depending on the animal species.[297,298] In humans and rabbits, bioreduction of naltrexone is highly stereoselective and generates only 6β-naltrexol, whereas in chickens, reduction yields only 6α-

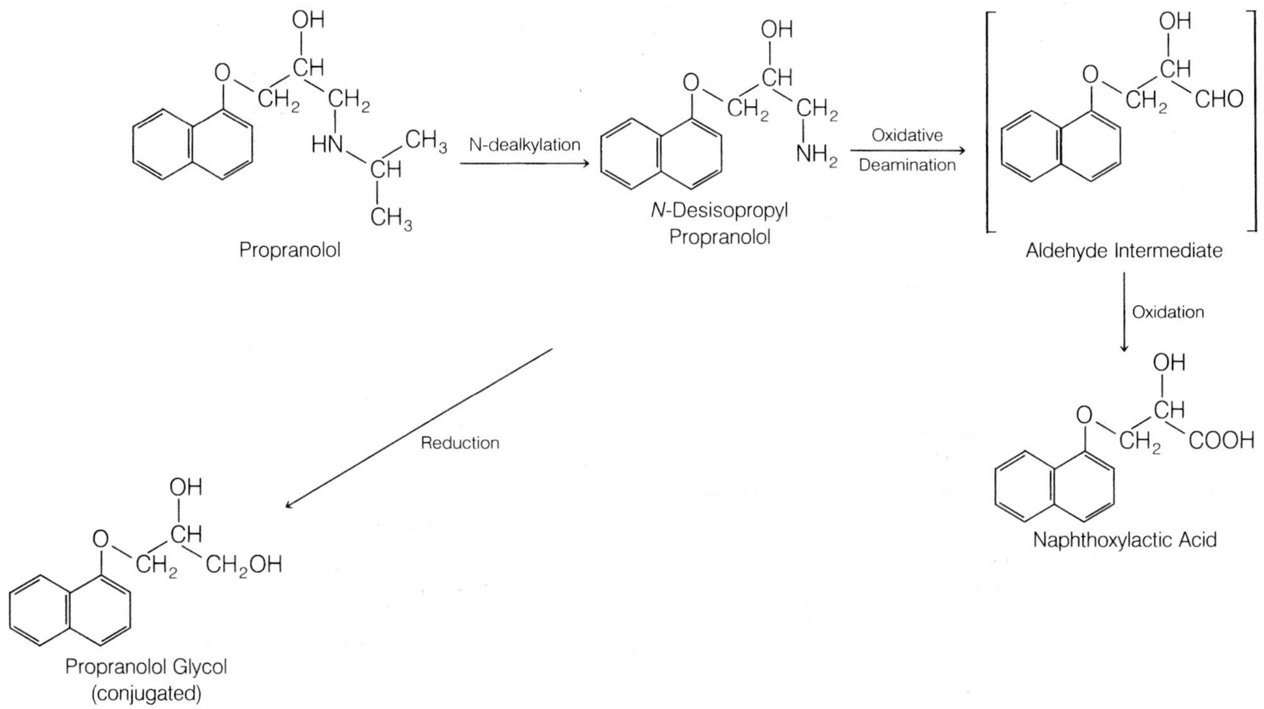

Propranolol → N-dealkylation → *N*-Desisopropyl Propranolol → Oxidative Deamination → Aldehyde Intermediate → Oxidation → Naphthoxylactic Acid

Reduction → Propranolol Glycol (conjugated)

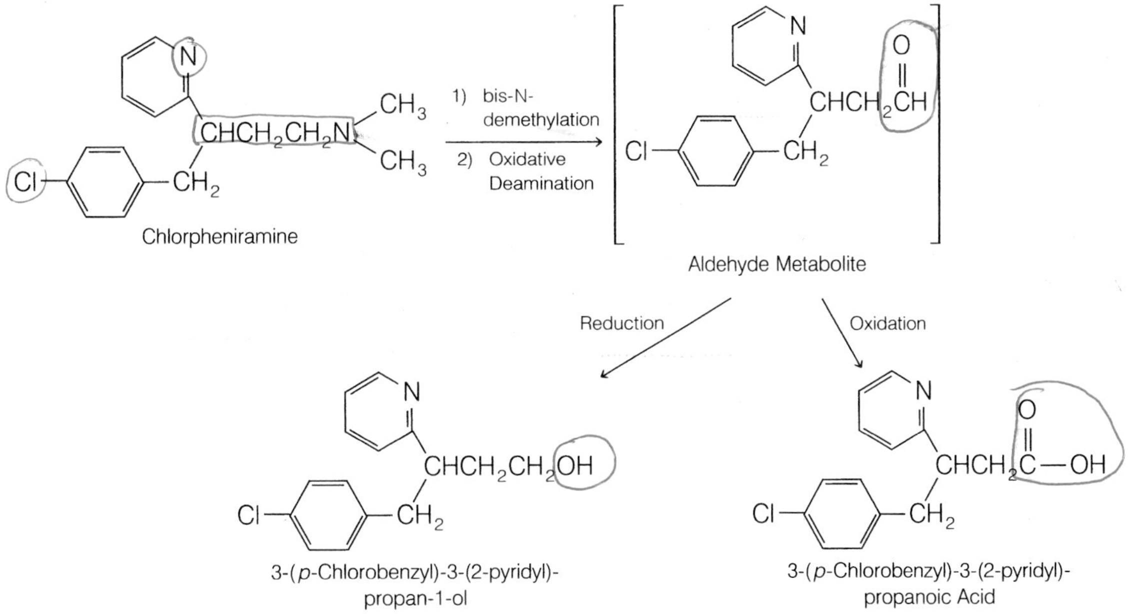

Chlorpheniramine → 1) bis-N-demethylation 2) Oxidative Deamination → Aldehyde Metabolite

Reduction → 3-(*p*-Chlorobenzyl)-3-(2-pyridyl)-propan-1-ol

Oxidation → 3-(*p*-Chlorobenzyl)-3-(2-pyridyl)-propanoic Acid

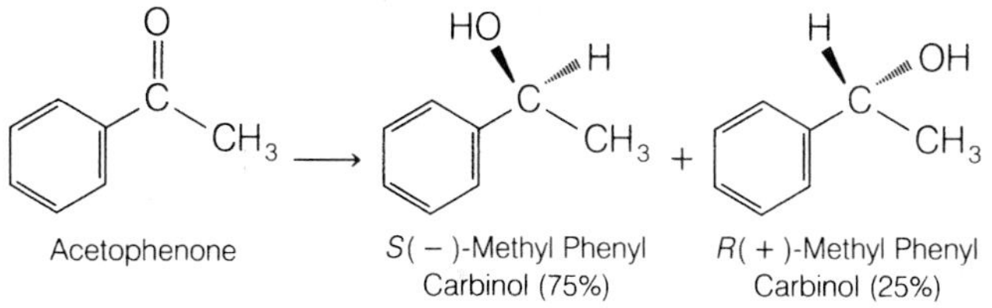

Acetophenone → $S(-)$-Methyl Phenyl Carbinol (75%) + $R(+)$-Methyl Phenyl Carbinol (25%)

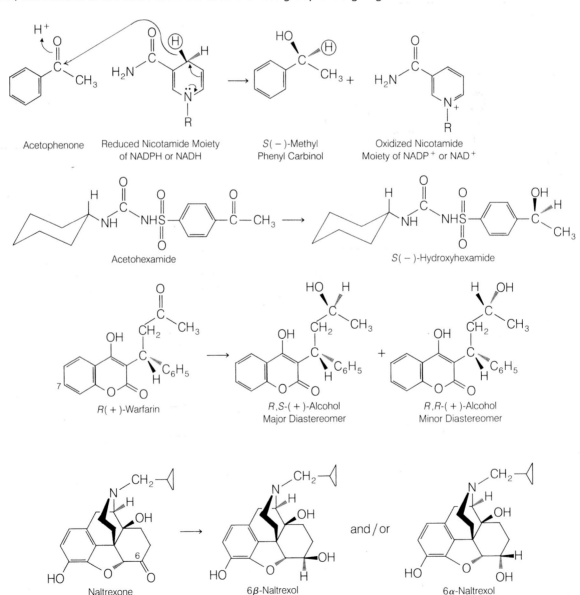

Figure 3.10 ● Additional examples of xenobiotics that undergo extensive ketone reduction, not covered in the text. *Arrow* indicates the keto group undergoing reduction.

naltrexol.[297–299] In monkeys and guinea pigs, however, both epimeric alcohols are formed (predominantly 6β-naltrexol).[300,301] Apparently, in the latter two species, reduction of naltrexone to the epimeric 6α- and 6β-alcohols is carried out by two distinctly different reductases found in the liver.[299–301]

Reduction of oxisuran appears not to be an important pathway by which the parent drug mediates its immunosuppressive effects. Studies indicate that oxisuran has its greatest immunosuppressive effects in those species that form alcohols as their major metabolic products (e.g., human, rat).[302–306] In species in which reduction is a minor pathway (e.g., dog), oxisuran shows little immunosuppressive activity.[304–306] These findings indicate that the oxisuran alcohols (oxisuranols) are pharmacologically active and contribute substantially to the overall immunosuppressive effect of the parent drug. The sulfoxide group in oxisuran is chiral, by virtue of the lone pair of electrons on sulfur. Therefore, reduction of oxisuran leads to diastereomeric alcohols.

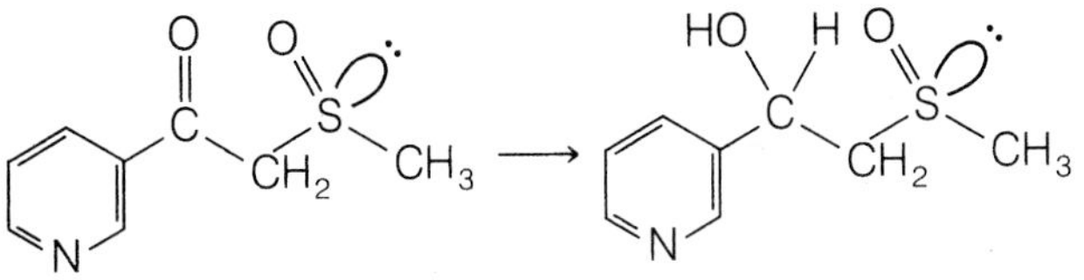

Oxisuran

Oxisuranols
(diastereomeric mixture)

Reduction of α,β-unsaturated ketones results in reduction not only of the ketone group but of the carbon–carbon double bond as well. Steroidal drugs often fall into this class, including norethindrone, a synthetic progestin found in many oral contraceptive drug combinations. In women, the major plasma and urinary metabolite of norethindrone is the 3β,5β-tetrahydro derivative.[307]

Ketones resulting from metabolic oxidative deamination processes are also susceptible to reduction. For instance, rabbit liver microsomal preparations metabolize amphetamine to phenylacetone, which is reduced subsequently to 1-phenyl-2-propanol.[308] In humans, a minor urinary metabolite of (−)-ephedrine has been identified as the diol derivative formed from keto reduction of the oxidatively deaminated product 1-hydroxy-1-phenylpropan-2-one.[309]

Reduction of Nitro and Azo Compounds

The reduction of aromatic nitro and azo xenobiotics leads to aromatic primary amine metabolites.[286] Aromatic nitro compounds are reduced initially to the nitroso and hydroxylamine intermediates, as shown in the following metabolic sequence:

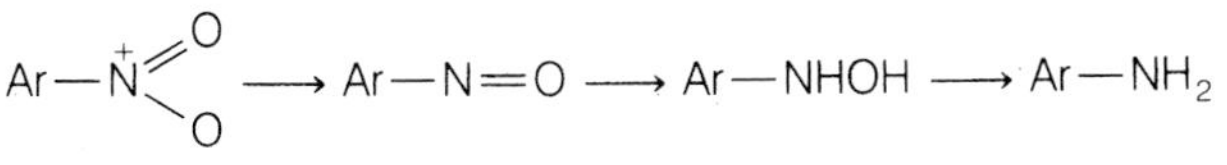

$$Ar-\overset{+}{N}\overset{O}{\underset{O}{\diagup}} \longrightarrow Ar-N=O \longrightarrow Ar-NHOH \longrightarrow Ar-NH_2$$

Nitro   Nitroso   Hydroxylamine   Amine

Azo reduction, however, is believed to proceed via a hydrazo intermediate (-NH-NH-) that subsequently is cleaved reductively to yield the corresponding aromatic amines:

$$Ar-N=N-Ar' \longrightarrow Ar-NH-NH-Ar' \longrightarrow$$

Azo   Hydrazo

$$Ar-NH_2 + H_2N-Ar'$$

Amines

Bioreduction of nitro compounds is carried out by NADPH-dependent microsomal and soluble nitro reductases present in the liver. A multicomponent hepatic microsomal

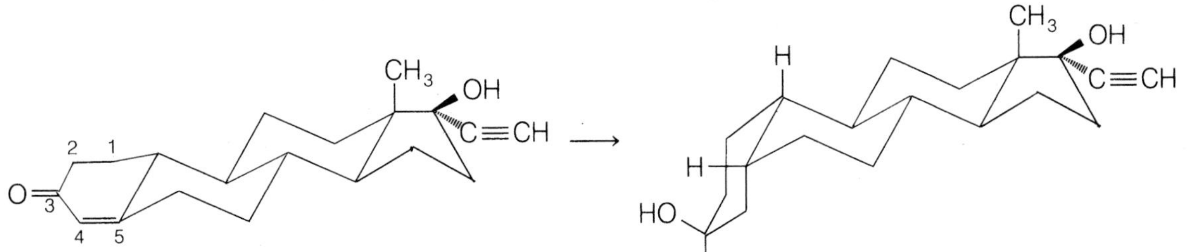

Norethindrone

3β,5β-Tetrahydronorethindrone

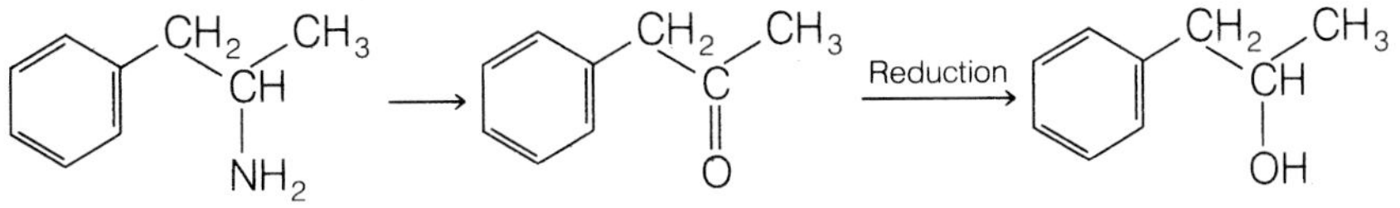

Amphetamine

Phenylacetone

1-Phenyl-2-propanol

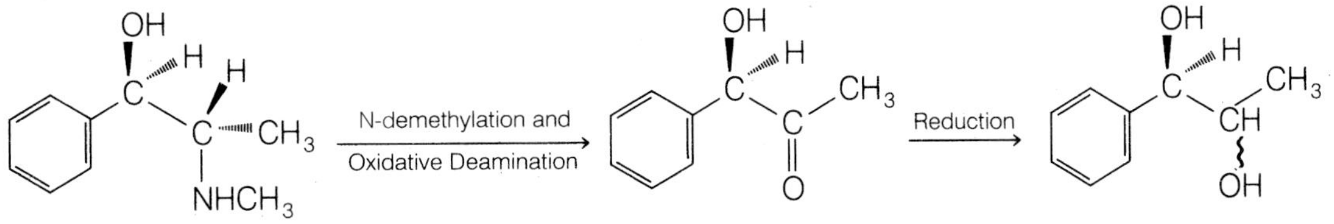

(−)-Ephedrine

1-Hydroxy-1-phenyl-propan-2-one

1-Phenyl-1,2-propanediol
(as glucuronide conjugate)

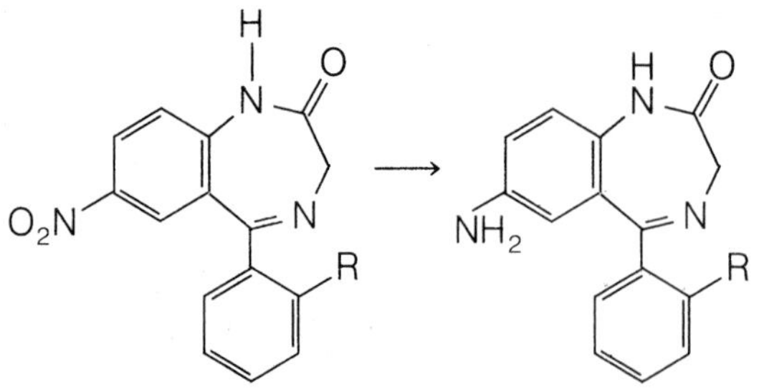

Clonazepam, R = Cl
Nitrazepam, R = H

7-Amino Metabolite

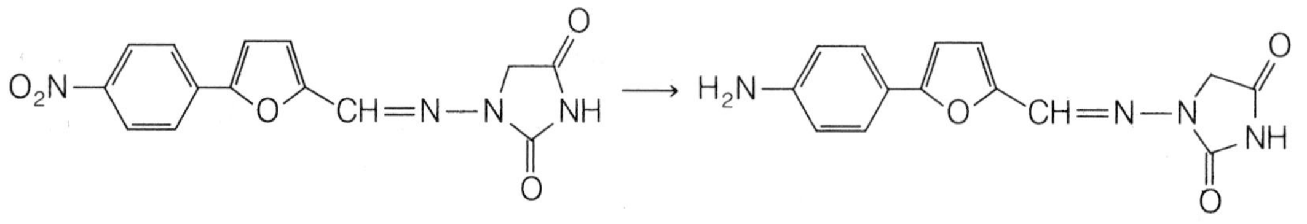

Dantrolene

Aminodantrolene

reductase system requiring NADPH appears to be responsible for azo reduction.[310–312] In addition, bacterial reductases present in the intestine can reduce nitro and azo compounds, especially those that are absorbed poorly or excreted mainly in the bile.[313,314]

Various aromatic nitro drugs undergo enzymatic reduction to the corresponding aromatic amines. For example, the 7-nitro benzodiazepine derivatives clonazepam and nitrazepam are metabolized extensively to their respective 7-amino metabolites in humans.[315,316] The skeletal muscle relaxant dantrolene (Dantrium) also reportedly undergoes reduction to aminodantrolene in humans.[317,318]

For some nitro xenobiotics, bioreduction appears to be a minor metabolic pathway in vivo, because of competing oxidative and conjugative reactions. Under artificial anaerobic in vitro incubation conditions, however, these same nitro xenobiotics are enzymatically reduced rapidly. For example, most of the urinary metabolites of metronidazole found in humans are either oxidation or conjugation products. Reduced metabolites of metronidazole have not been detected.[319] When incubated anaerobically with guinea pig liver preparations, however, metronidazole undergoes considerable nitro reduction.[320]

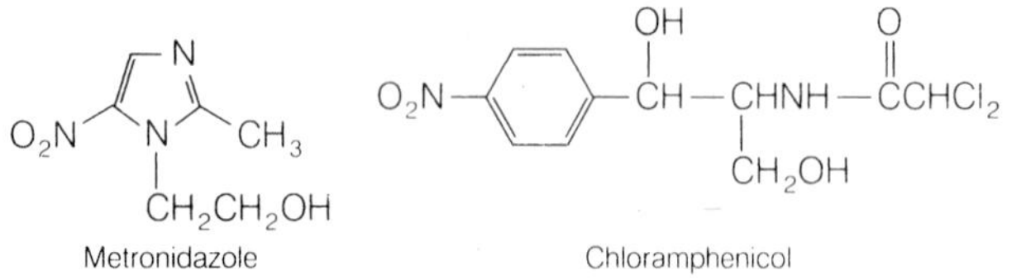

Metronidazole

Chloramphenicol

Bacterial reductase present in the intestine also tends to complicate in vivo interpretations of nitro reduction. For example, in rats, the antibiotic chloramphenicol is not reduced in vivo by the liver but is excreted in the bile and, subsequently, reduced by intestinal flora to form the amino metabolite.[321,322]

The enzymatic reduction of azo compounds is best exemplified by the conversion of sulfamidochrysoidine (Prontosil) to the active sulfanilamide metabolite in the liver.[323] This reaction has historical significance, for it led to the discovery of sulfanilamide as an antibiotic and eventually to the development of many of the therapeutic sulfonamide drugs. Bacterial reductases present in the intestine play a significant role in reducing azo xenobiotics, particularly those that are absorbed poorly.[313,314] Accordingly, the two azo dyes tartrazine[324,325] and amaranth[326] have poor oral absorption because of the many polar and ionized zsulfonic acid groups present in their structures.

Therefore, these two azo compounds are metabolized primarily by bacterial reductases present in the intestine. The importance of intestinal reduction is further revealed in the metabolism of sulfasalazine (formerly salicylazosulfapyridine, Azulfidine), a drug used in the treatment of ulcerative colitis. The drug is absorbed poorly and undergoes reductive cleavage of the azo linkage to yield sulfapyridine and 5-aminosalicylic acid.[327,328] The reaction occurs primarily in the colon and is carried out principally by intestinal bacteria. Studies in germfree rats, lacking intestinal flora, have demonstrated that sulfasalazine is not reduced to any appreciable extent.[329]

Miscellaneous Reductions

Several minor reductive reactions also occur. Reduction of N-oxides to the corresponding tertiary amine occurs to some extent. This reductive pathway is of interest because several tertiary amines are oxidized to form polar and water-soluble N-oxide metabolites. If reduction of N-oxide metabolites occurs to a significant extent, drug elimination of the parent tertiary amine is impeded. N-Oxide reduction often is assessed by administering the pure synthetic N-oxide in vitro or in vivo and then attempting to detect the formation of the tertiary amine. For example, imipramine N-oxide undergoes reduction in rat liver preparations.[330]

Reduction of sulfur-containing functional groups, such as the disulfide and sulfoxide moieties, also constitutes a minor reductive pathway. Reductive cleavage of the disulfide bond in disulfiram (Antabuse) yields N,N-diethyldithiocarbamic acid (free or glucuronidated) as a major metabolite in humans.[331,332] Although sulfoxide functionalities are oxidized mainly to sulfones (-SO_2-), they sometimes undergo reduction to sulfides. The

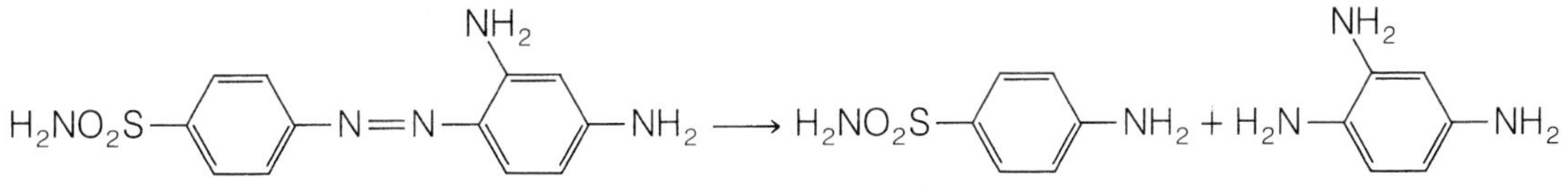

Sulfamidochrysoidine
(Prontosil) → Sulfanilamide + 1,2,4-Triaminobenzene

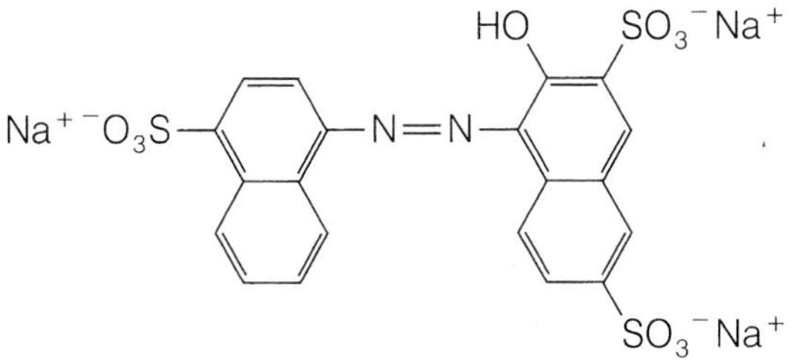

Tartrazine

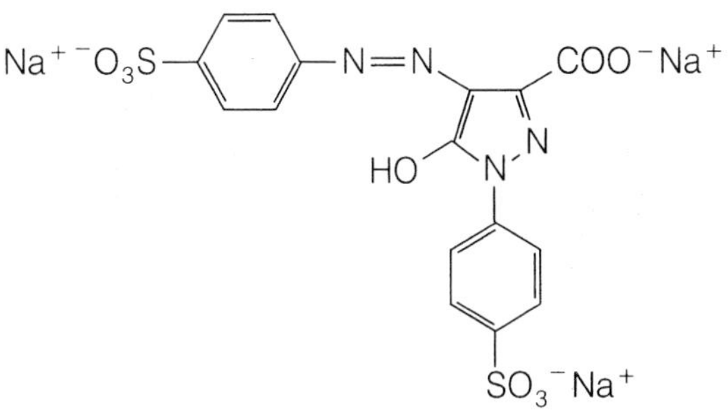

Amaranth

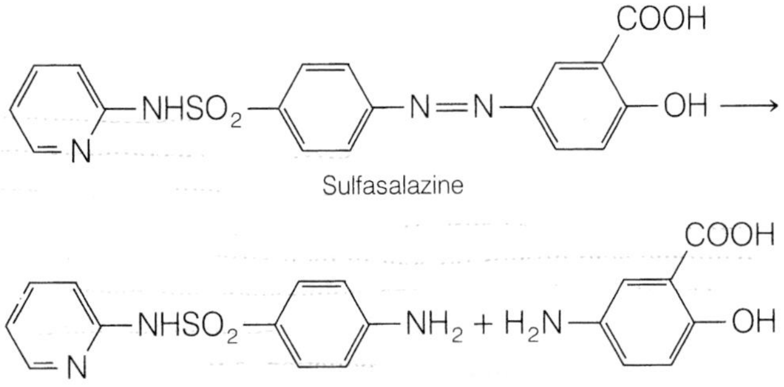

Sulfasalazine →

Sulfapyridine + 5-Aminosalicylic Acid

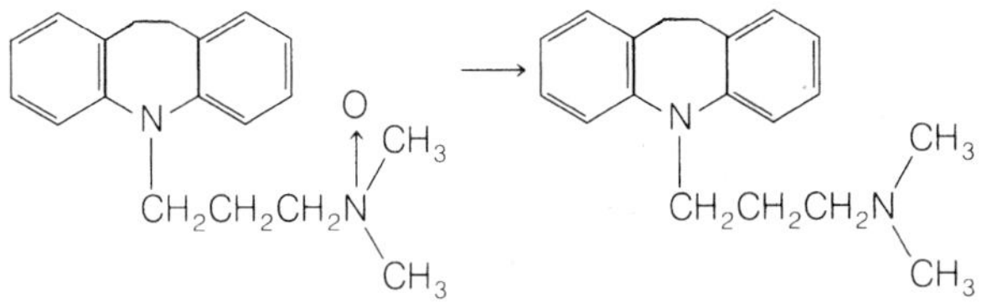

Imipramine *N*-Oxide → Imipramine

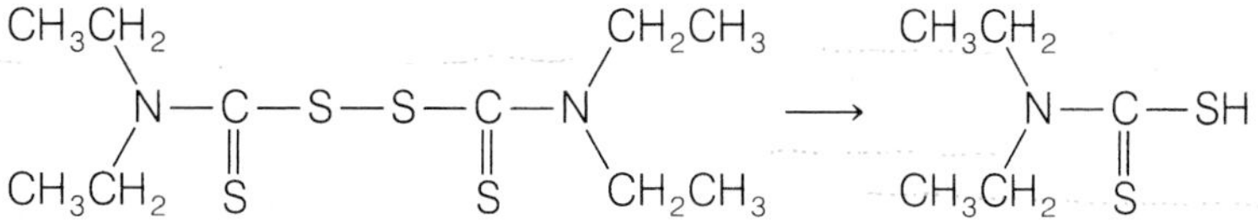

Disulfiram → *N,N*-Diethylthiocarbamic Acid

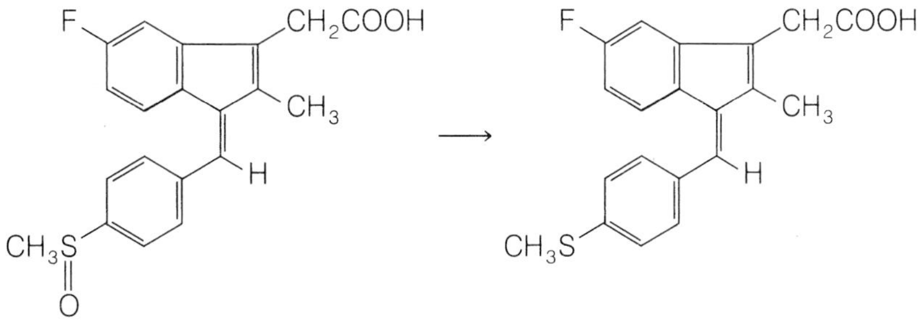

Sulindac → Sulindac Sulfide Metabolite

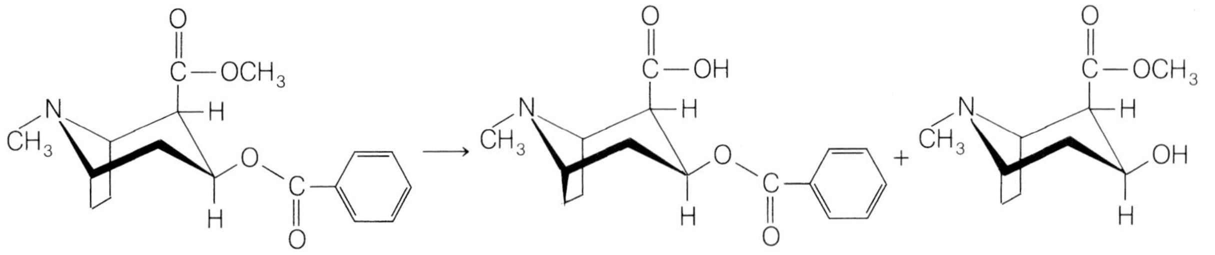

Cocaine → Benzoylecgonine + Methylecgonine

importance of this reductive pathway is seen in the metabolism of the anti-inflammatory agent sulindac (Clinoril). Studies in humans show that sulindac undergoes reduction to an active sulfide that is responsible for the overall anti-inflammatory effect of the parent drug.[333,334] Sulindac or its sulfone metabolite exhibits little anti-inflammatory activity. Another example of sulfide formation involves the reduction of DMSO to dimethyl sulfide. In humans, DMSO is metabolized to a minor extent by this pathway. The characteristic unpleasant odor of dimethyl sulfide is evident on the breath of patients who use this agent.[335]

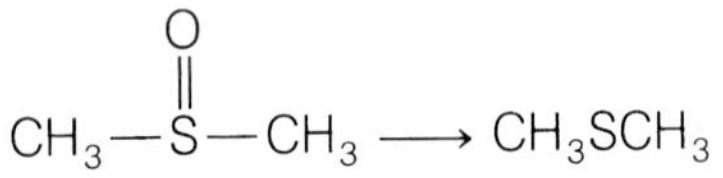

Dimethyl Sulfoxide → Dimethyl Sulfide

⬡ HYDROLYTIC REACTIONS

Hydrolysis of Esters and Amides

The metabolism of ester and amide linkages in many drugs is catalyzed by hydrolytic enzymes present in various tissues and in plasma. The metabolic products formed (carboxylic acids, alcohols, phenols, and amines) generally are polar and functionally more susceptible to conjugation and excretion than the parent ester or amide drugs. The enzymes carrying out ester hydrolysis include several nonspecific esterases found in the liver, kidney, and intestine as well as the pseudocholinesterases present in plasma.[336,337] Amide hydrolysis appears to be mediated by liver microsomal amidases, esterases, and deacylases.[337]

Hydrolysis is a major biotransformation pathway for drugs containing an ester functionality. This is because of the relative ease of hydrolyzing the ester linkage. A classic example of ester hydrolysis is the metabolic conversion of aspirin (acetylsalicylic acid) to salicylic acid.[338] Of the two ester moieties present in cocaine, it appears that, in general, the methyl group is hydrolyzed preferentially to yield benzoylecgonine as the major human urinary metabolite.[339] The hydrolysis of cocaine to methyl ecgonine, however, also occurs in plasma and, to a minor extent, blood.[340,341] Methylphenidate (Ritalin) is biotransformed rapidly by hydrolysis to yield ritalinic acid as the major urinary metabolite in humans.[342] Often, ester hydrolysis of the parent drug leads to pharmacologically active metabolites. For example, hydrolysis of diphenoxylate in humans leads to diphenoxylic acid (difenoxin), which is, apparently, 5 times more potent an antidiarrheal agent than the parent ester.[343] The rapid metabolism of clofibrate

(Atromid-S) yields *p*-chlorophenoxyisobutyric acid (CPIB) as the major plasma metabolite in humans.[344] Studies in rats indicate that the free acid CPIB is responsible for clofibrate's hypolipidemic effect.[345]

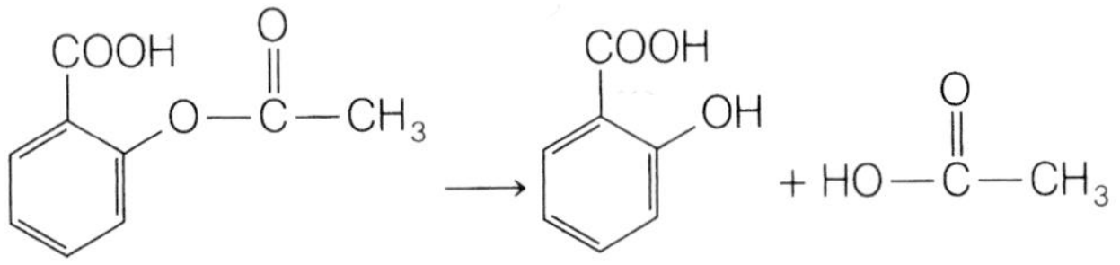

Aspirin (Acetylsalicylic acid) → Salicylic Acid + Acetic Acid

Many parent drugs have been chemically modified or derivatized to generate so-called prodrugs to overcome some undesirable property (e.g., bitter taste, poor absorption, poor solubility, irritation at site of injection). The rationale behind the prodrug concept was to develop an agent that, once inside the biological system, would be biotransformed to the active parent drug.[18] The presence of esterases in many tissues and plasma makes ester derivatives logical prodrug candidates, because hydrolysis would cause the ester prodrug to revert to the parent compound. Accordingly, antibiotics such as chloramphenicol and clindamycin have been derivatized as their palmitate esters to minimize their bitter taste and to improve their palatability in pediatric liquid suspensions.[346,347] After oral administration, intestinal esterases and lipases hydrolyze the palmitate esters to the free antibiotics. To improve the poor oral absorption of carbenicillin, a lipophilic indanyl ester has been formulated (Geocillin).[348] Once orally absorbed, the ester is hydrolyzed rapidly to the parent drug. A final example involves derivatization of prednisolone to its C-21 hemisuccinate sodium salt. This water-soluble derivative is extremely useful for parenteral administration and is metabolized to the parent steroid drug by plasma and tissue esterases.[349]

Amides are hydrolyzed slowly in comparison to esters.[337] Consequently, hydrolysis of the amide bond of procainamide is relatively slow compared with hydrolysis of the ester linkage in procaine.[336,350] Drugs in which amide cleavage has been reported to occur, to some extent, include lidocaine,[351] carbamazepine,[87] indomethacin,[251,252] and prazosin (Minipress).[253,254] Amide linkages present in barbiturates (e.g., hexobarbital)[352,353] as well as in hydantoins (e.g., 5-phenylhydantoin)[354,355] and succinimides (phensuximide)[354,355] are also susceptible to hydrolysis.

Miscellaneous Hydrolytic Reactions

Hydrolysis of recombinant human peptide drugs and hormones at the N- or C-terminal amino acids by carboxypeptidase and aminopeptidase and proteases in blood and other

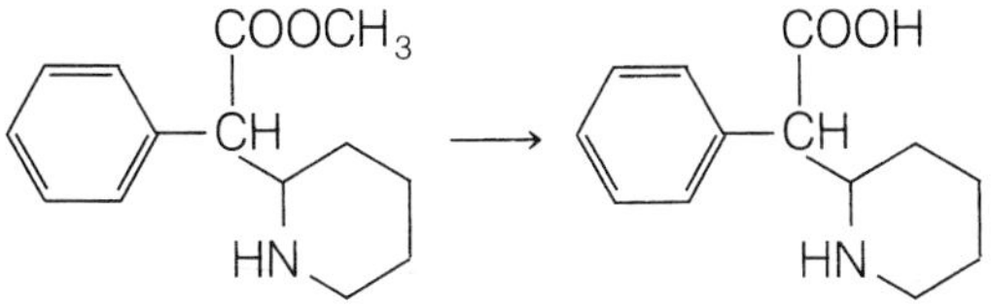

Methylphenidate → Ritalinic Acid

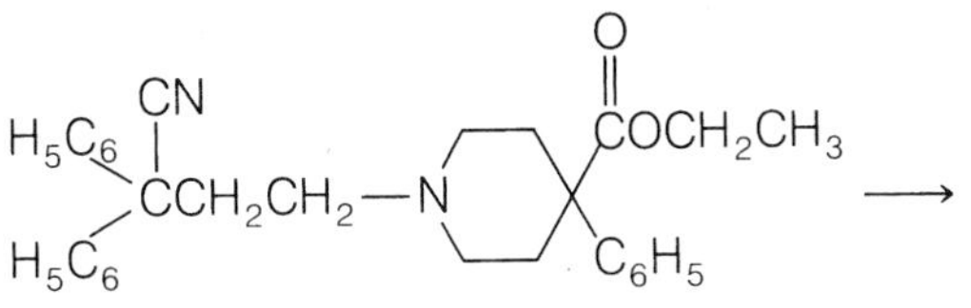

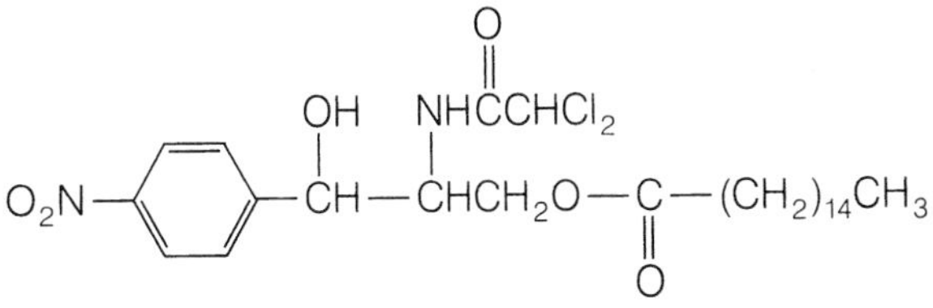

Chloramphenicol Palmitate

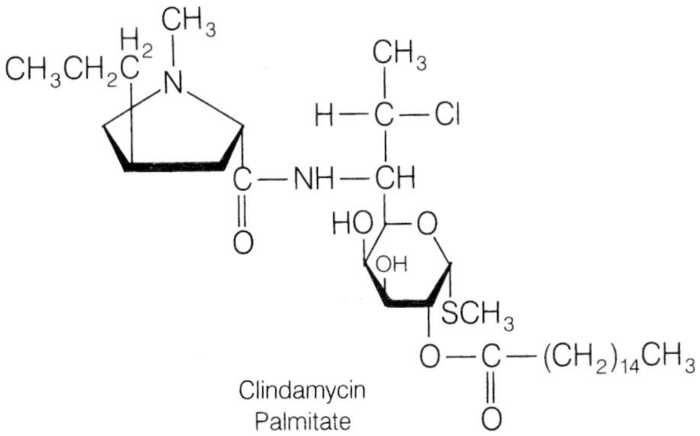

Diphenoxylate →

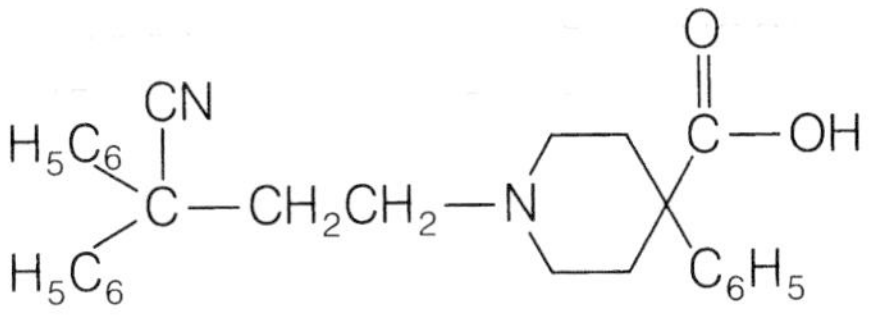

Diphenoxylic Acid (Difenoxin)

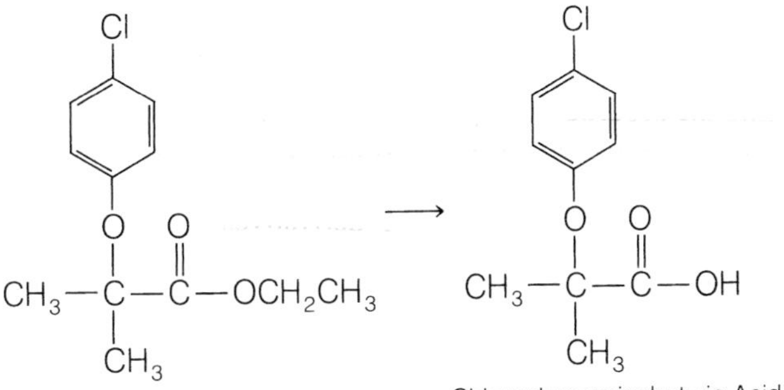

Clindamycin Palmitate

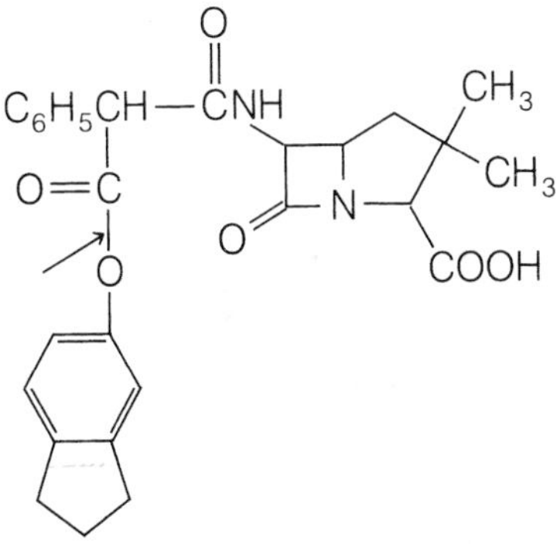

Clofibrate → p-Chlorophenoxyisobutyric Acid

Carbenicillin Indanyl Ester

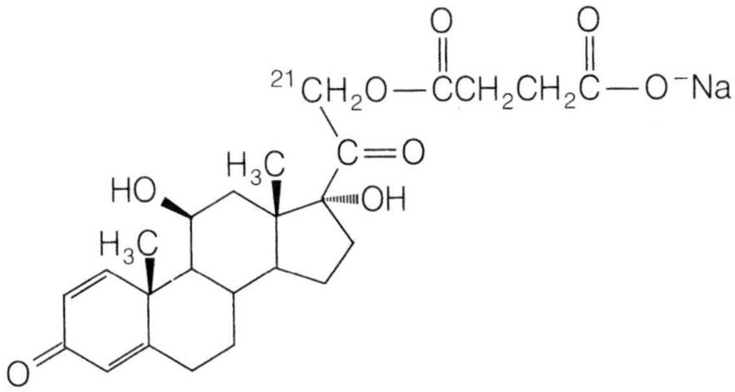

tissues is a well-recognized hydrolytic reaction.[356,357] Examples of peptides or protein hormones undergoing hydrolysis include human <u>insulin</u>, growth hormone (GH), prolactin, parathyroid hormone (PTH), and atrial natriuretic factor (ANF).[358]

In addition to hydrolysis of amides and esters, hydrolytic cleavage of other moieties occurs to a minor extent in drug metabolism,[8] including the <u>hydrolysis of phosphate esters</u> (e.g., diethylstilbestrol diphosphate), <u>sulfonylureas</u>, cardiac glycosides, carbamate esters, and organophosphate compounds. Glucuronide and sulfate conjugates also can undergo hydrolytic cleavage by <u>β-glucuronidase and sulfatase</u> enzymes. These hydrolytic reactions are discussed in the following section. Finally, the hydration or hydrolytic cleavage of epoxides and arene oxides by epoxide hydrase is considered a hydrolytic reaction.

Miscellaneous Bioactivation of Prodrugs

Throughout this chapter, the metabolism of produgs to an active form is presented. However, in the cases presented earlier, there was a chemical functional group that was subject to phase I metabolism to release the active drug molecule.

Prednisolone Hemisuccinate Sodium Salt

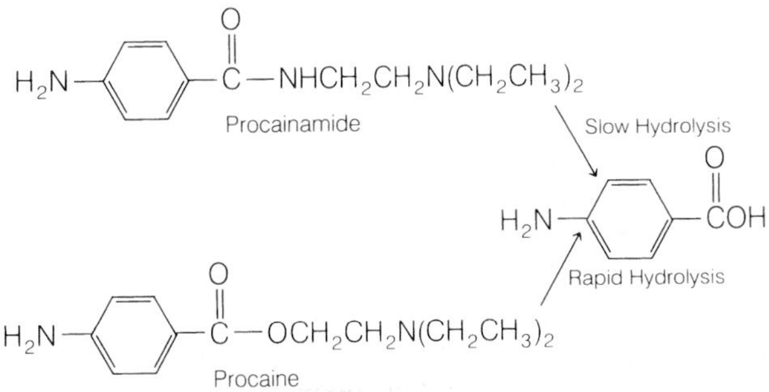

Procainamide

Procaine

Slow Hydrolysis

Rapid Hydrolysis

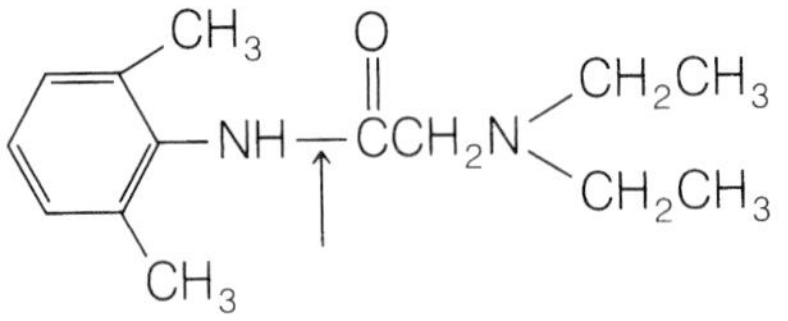

Lidocaine

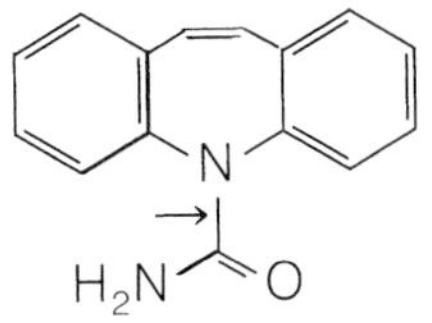

Carbamazepine

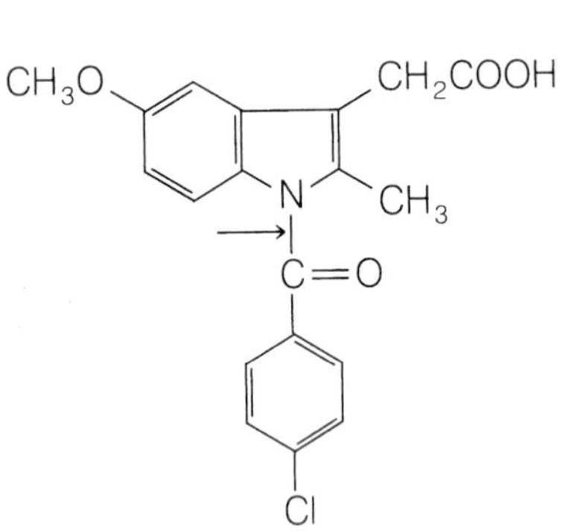

Indomethacin

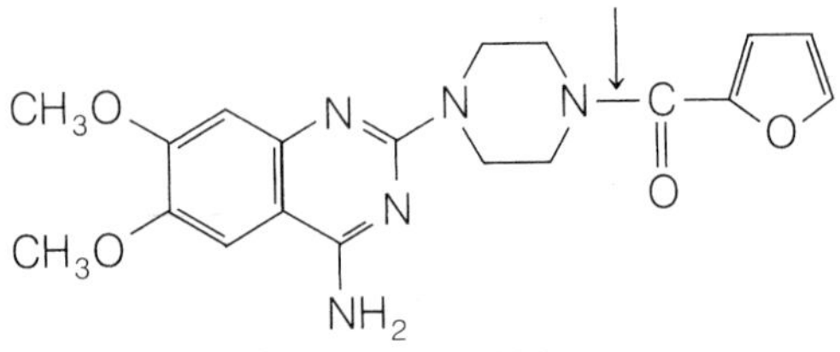

Prazosin

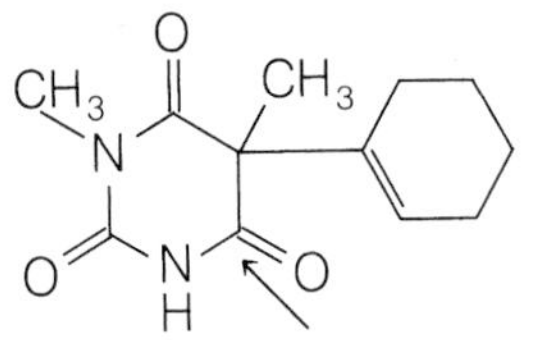

Hexobarbital 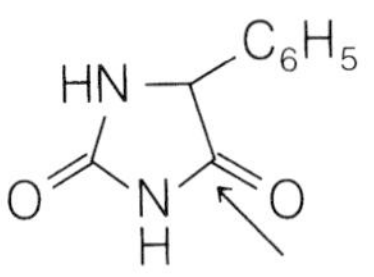   5-Phenylhydantoin 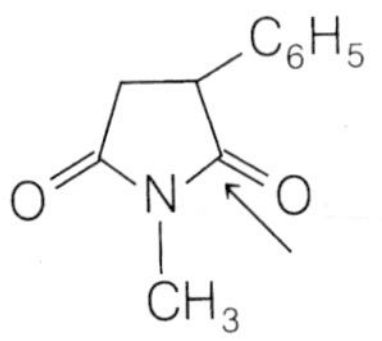   Phensuximide

The metabolic reactions included oxidative activation, reductive activation, hydrolytic activation, etc. One reaction that is of particular interest involves chemical activation as seen with the proton pump inhibitors, which are clinically used to treat gastric ulceration. When administered to a patient, the drug is dosed orally, allowing for systemic distribution. When the proton pump inhibitor arrives at an acidic region of the body, such as the parietal cells of the stomach, chemical activation occurs. The highly acidic environment in and around the parietal cell allows for protonation of nitrogen on the benzimidazole ring, followed by attachment of the pyridine nitrogen. Ring opening of the intermediate then yields the sulfenic acid that subsequently cyclizes with the loss of water. This intermediate is highly susceptible to nucleophilic attack by the SH moieties of the cysteine residues associated with proteins, including the proton pump of the parietal cells. This pump is responsible for exchange of K+ with H+ from parietal cell into gastric lumen, and through this inhibition, there is regulation of the acidic environment of stomach.

PHASE II OR CONJUGATION REACTIONS

Phase I or functionalization reactions do not always produce hydrophilic or pharmacologically inactive metabolites. Various phase II or conjugation reactions, however, can convert these metabolites to more polar and water-soluble products. Many conjugative enzymes accomplish this objective by attaching small, polar, and ionizable endogenous molecules, such as glucuronic acid, sulfate, glycine, and glutamine, to the phase I metabolite or parent xenobiotic. The resulting conjugated products are relatively water soluble and readily excretable. In addition, they generally are biologically inactive and nontoxic. Other phase II reactions, such as methylation and acetylation, do not generally increase water solubility but mainly serve to terminate or attenuate pharmacological activity. The role of GSH is to combine with chemically reactive compounds to prevent damage to important biomacromolecules, such as DNA, RNA, and proteins. Thus, phase II reactions can be regarded as truly detoxifying pathways in drug metabolism, with a few exceptions.

A distinguishing feature of most phase II reactions is that the conjugating group (glucuronic acid, sulfate, methyl, and acetyl) is activated initially in the form of a coenzyme before transfer or attachment of the group to the accepting substrate by the appropriate transferase enzyme. In other cases, such as glycine and glutamine conjugation, the substrate is activated initially. Many endogenous compounds, such as bilirubin, steroids, catecholamines, and histamine, also undergo conjugation reactions and use the same coenzymes, although they appear to be mediated by more specific transferase enzymes. The phase II conjugative pathways

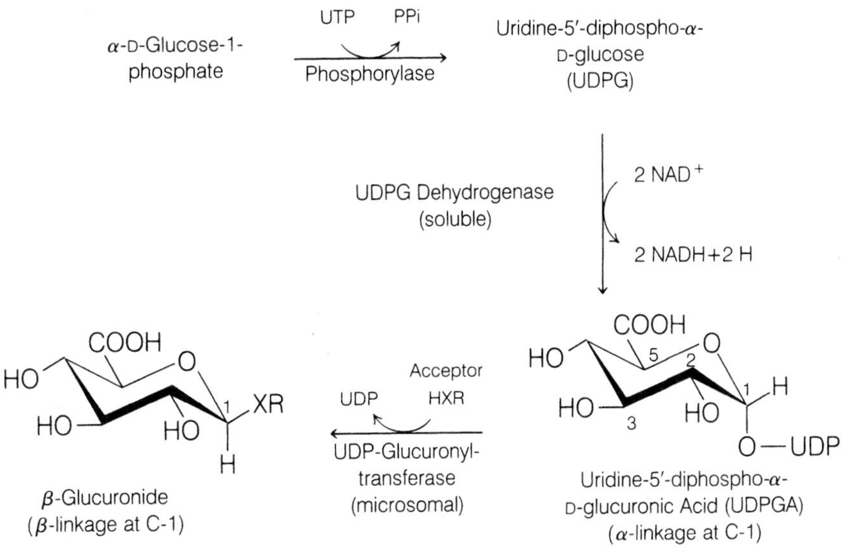

Figure 3.11 ● Formation of UDPGA and β-glucuronide conjugates.

Glucuronic Acid Conjugation

discussed include those previously listed in this chapter. Although other conjugative pathways exist (e.g., conjugation with glycosides, phosphate, and other amino acids and conversion of cyanide to thiocyanate), they are of minor importance in drug metabolism and are not covered in this chapter.

Glucuronidation is the most common conjugative pathway in drug metabolism for several reasons: (a) a readily available supply of D-glucuronic acid (derived from D-glucose), (b) numerous functional groups that can combine enzymatically with glucuronic acid, and (c) the glucuronyl moiety (with its ionized carboxylate [pK$_a$ 3.2] and polar hydroxyl groups), which, when attached to xenobiotic substrates, greatly increases the water solubility of the conjugated product.[117,359-361] Formation of β-glucuronides involves two steps: synthesis of an activated coenzyme, uridine-5'-diphospho-α-D-glucuronic acid (UDPGA), and subsequent transfer of the glucuronyl group from UDPGA to an appropriate substrate.[117,360,361] The transfer step is catalyzed by microsomal enzymes called *UDP-glucuronyltransferases*. They are found primarily in the liver but also occur in many other tissues, including kidney, intestine, skin, lung, and brain.[360,361] The sequence of events involved in glucuronidation is summarized in Figure 3.11.[117,360,361] The synthesis of the coenzyme UDPGA uses α-D-glucose-1-phosphate as its initial precursor. Note that all glucuronide conjugates have the β-configuration or β-linkage at C-1 (hence, the term *β-glucuronides*). In contrast, the coenzyme UDPGA has an α-linkage. In the enzymatic transfer step, it appears that nucleophilic displacement of the α-linked UDP moiety from UDPGA by the substrate RXH proceeds with complete inversion of configuration at C-1 to give the β-glucuronide. Glucuronidation of one functional group usually suffices to effect excretion of the conjugated metabolite; diglucuronide conjugates do not usually occur.

The diversity of functional groups undergoing glucuronidation is illustrated in Table 3.3 and Figure 3.12.

Metabolic products are classified as oxygen–, nitrogen–, sulfur–, or carbon–glucuronide, according to the heteroatom attached to the C-1 atom of the glucuronyl group. Two important functionalities, the hydroxy and carboxy, form *O*-glucuronides. Phenolic and alcoholic hydroxyls are the most common functional groups undergoing glucuronidation in drug metabolism. As we have seen, phenolic and alcoholic hydroxyl groups are present in many parent compounds and arise through various phase I metabolic pathways. Morphine,[362,363] acetaminophen,[364] and *p*-hydroxyphenytoin (the major metabolite of phenytoin)[49,50] are a few examples of phenolic compounds that undergo considerable glucuronidation. Alcoholic

TABLE 3.3 Types of Compounds Forming Oxygen, Nitrogen, Sulfur, and Carbon Glucuronides[a]

Oxygen Glucuronides

Hydroxyl compounds
Phenols: morphine, acetaminophen, *p*-hydroxyphenytoin
Alcohols: tricholoroethanol, chloramphenicol, propranolol
Enols: 4-hydroxycoumarin
N-Hydroxyamines: *N*-hydroxydapsone
N-Hydroxyamides: *N*-hydroxy-2-acetylaminofluorene

Carboxyl compounds
Aryl acids: benzoic acid, salicylic acid
Arylalkyl acids: naproxen, fenoprofen

Nitrogen Glucuronides

Arylamines: 7-amino-5-nitroindazole
Alkylamines: desipramine
Amides: meprobamate
Sulfonamides: sulfisoxazole
Tertiary amines: cyproheptadine, tripelennamine

Sulfur Glucuronides

Sulfhydryl groups: methimazole, propylthiouracil, diethylthiocarbamic acid

Carbon Glucuronides

3,5-Pyrazolidinedione: phenylbutazone, sulfinpyrazone

[a]For structures and site of β-glucuronide attachment, see Figure 4.12.

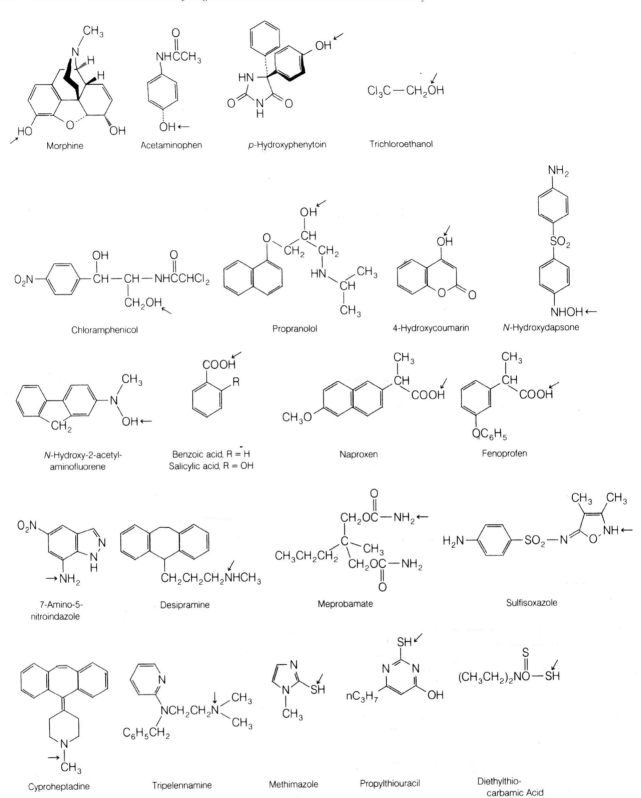

Figure 3.12 ● Structure of compounds that undergo glucuronidation. *Arrows* indicate sites of β-glucuronide attachment.

hydroxyls, such as those present in trichloroethanol (major metabolite of chloral hydrate),[288] chloramphenicol,[365] and propranolol,[366,367] are also commonly glucuronidated. Less frequent is glucuronidation of other hydroxyl groups, such as enols,[368] *N*-hydroxylamines,[226] and *N*-hydroxylamides.[241] For examples, refer to the list of glucuronides in Table 3.3.

The carboxy group is also subject to conjugation with glucuronic acid. For example, arylaliphatic acids, such as the anti-inflammatory agents naproxen[369] and fenoprofen,[370,371] are excreted primarily as their *O*-glucuronide derivatives in humans. Carboxylic acid metabolites such as those arising from chlorpheniramine[290] and propranolol[289] (see "Reduction of Aldehyde and Ketone Carbonyls,") form *O*-glucuronide conjugates. Aryl acids (e.g., benzoic acid,[372] salicylic acid[373,374]) also undergo conjugation with glucuronic acid, but conjugation with glycine appears to be a more important pathway for these compounds.

Occasionally, *N*-glucuronides are formed with aromatic amines, aliphatic amines, amides, and sulfonamides. Representative examples are found in the list of glucuronides in Table 3.3. Glucuronidation of aromatic and aliphatic amines is generally a minor pathway in comparison with *N*-acetylation or oxidative processes (e.g., oxidative deamination). Tertiary amines, such as the antihistaminic agents cyproheptadine (Periactin)[375] and tripelennamine,[376] form interesting quaternary ammonium glucuronide metabolites.

Because the thiol group (SH) does not commonly occur in xenobiotics, *S*-glucuronide products have been reported for only a few drugs. For instance, the thiol groups present in methimazole (Tapazole),[377] propylthiouracil,[378,379] and *N*,*N*-diethyldithiocarbamic acid (major reduced metabolite of disulfiram, Antabuse)[380] undergo conjugation with glucuronic acid.

The formation of glucuronides attached directly to a carbon atom is relatively novel in drug metabolism. Studies in humans have shown that conjugation of phenylbutazone (Butazolidin)[381,382] and sulfinpyrazone (Anturane)[383] yield the corresponding *C*-glucuronide metabolites:

C-Glucuronide Metabolite

Phenylbutazone, R = CH₂CH₂CH₂CH₃
Sulfinpyrazone, R = CH₂CH₂SC₆H₅
                              ‖
                              O

Besides xenobiotics, several endogenous substrates, notably bilirubin[384] and steroids,[385] are eliminated as gluc-uronide conjugates, which are excreted primarily in the urine. As the relative molecular mass of the conjugate exceeds 300 Da, however, biliary excretion may become an important route of elimination.[386] Glucuronides that are excreted in the bile are susceptible to hydrolysis by β-glucuronidase enzymes present in the intestine. The hydrolyzed product may be reabsorbed in the intestine, thus leading to enterohepatic recycling.[22] β-Glucuronidases are also present in many other tissues, including the liver, the endocrine system, and the reproductive organs. Although the function of these hydrolytic enzymes in drug metabolism is unclear, it appears that, in terms of hormonal and endocrine regulation, β-glucuronidases may liberate active hormones (e.g., steroids) from their inactive glucuronide conjugates.[22]

In neonates and children, glucuronidating processes are often not developed fully. In such subjects, drugs and endogenous compounds (e.g., bilirubin) that are metabolized normally by glucuronidation may accumulate and cause serious toxicity. For example, neonatal hyperbilirubinemia may be attributable to the inability of newborns to conjugate bilirubin with glucuronic acid.[387] Similarly, the inability of infants to glucuronidate chloramphenicol has been suggested to be responsible for the *gray baby syndrome*, which results from accumulation of toxic levels of the free antibiotic.[388]

Sulfate Conjugation

Conjugation of xenobiotics with sulfate occurs primarily with phenols and, occasionally, with alcohols, aromatic amines, and *N*-hydroxy compounds.[389–391] In contrast to glucuronic acid, the amount of available sulfate is rather limited. The body uses a significant portion of the sulfate pool to conjugate numerous endogenous compounds such as steroids, heparin, chondroitin, catecholamines, and thyroxine. The sulfate conjugation process involves activation of inorganic sulfate to the coenzyme 3′-phosphoadenosine-5′-phosphosulfate (PAPS). Subsequent transfer of the sulfate group from PAPS to the accepting substrate is catalyzed by various soluble sulfotransferases present in the liver and other tissues (e.g., kidney, intestine).[392] The sequence of events involved in sulfoconjugation is depicted in Figure 3.13. Sulfate conjugation generally leads to water-soluble and inactive metabolites. It appears, however, that the *O*-sulfate conjugates of some *N*-hydroxy compounds give rise to chemically reactive intermediates that are toxic.[241]

Phenols compose the main group of substrates undergoing sulfate conjugation. Thus, drugs containing phenolic moieties are often susceptible to sulfate formation. For example, the antihypertensive agent α-methyldopa (Aldomet) is metabolized extensively to its 3-*O*-sulfate ester in humans.[393,394] The β-adrenergic bronchodilators salbutamol (albuterol)[395] and terbutaline (Brethine, Bricanyl)[396] also undergo sulfate conjugation as their

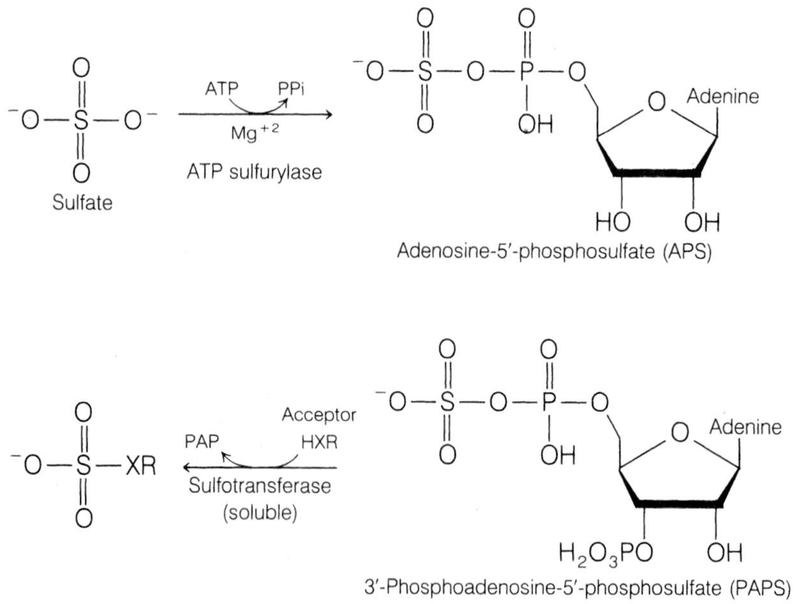

Figure 3.13 ● Formation of PAPS and sulfate conjugates.

principal route of metabolism in humans. For many phenols, however, sulfoconjugation may represent only a minor pathway. Glucuronidation of phenols is frequently a competing reaction and may predominate as the conjugative route for some phenolic drugs. In adults, the major urinary metabolite of the analgesic acetaminophen is the *O*-glucuronide conjugate, with the concomitant *O*-sulfate conjugate being formed in small amounts.[364] Interestingly, infants and young children (ages 3–9 years) exhibit a different urinary excretion pattern: the *O*-sulfate conjugate is the main urinary product.[397,398] The explanation for this reversal stems from the fact that neonates and young children have a decreased glucuronidating capacity because of undeveloped glucuronyltransferases or low levels of these enzymes. Sulfate conjugation, however, is well developed and becomes the main route of acetaminophen conjugation in this pediatric group.

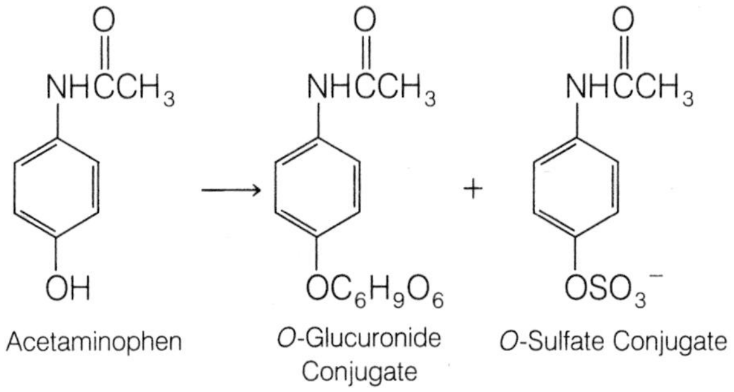

Other functionalities, such as alcohols (e.g., aliphatic C_1 to C_5 alcohols, diethylene glycol)[399,400] and aromatic amines (e.g., aniline, 2-naphthylamine),[401,402] can also form sulfate conjugates. These reactions, however, have only minor importance in drug metabolism. The sulfate conjugation of

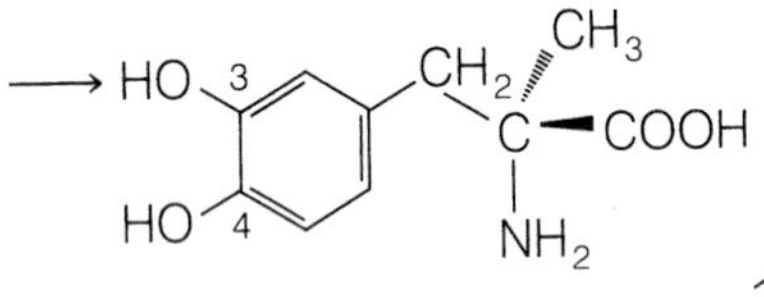

α-Methyldopa

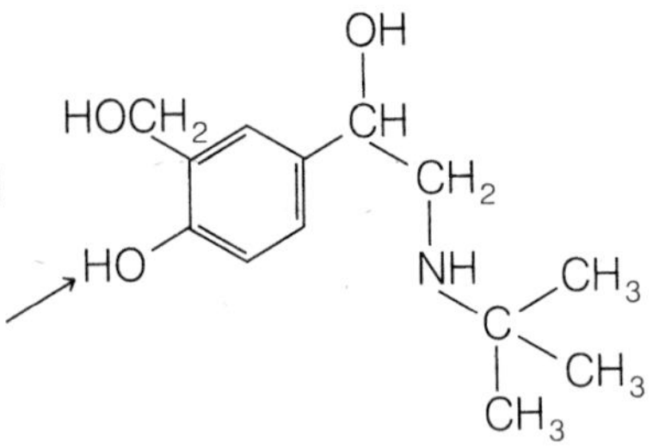

Salbutamol
(Albuterol)

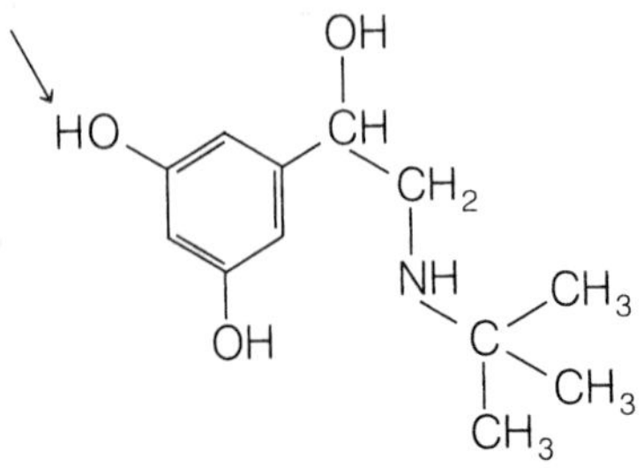

Terbutaline

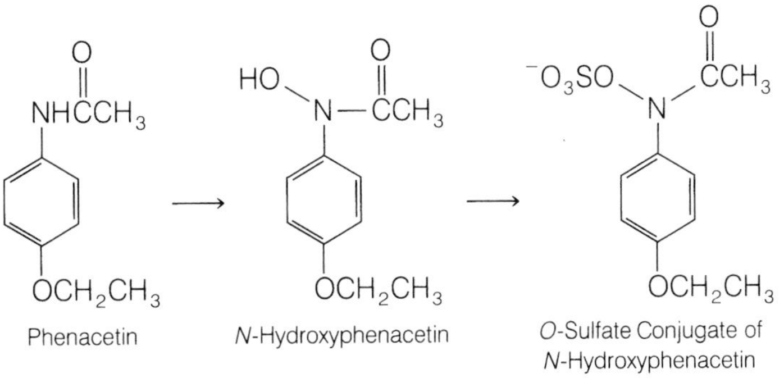

N-hydroxylamines and *N*-hydroxylamides takes place as well, occasionally. *O*-Sulfate ester conjugates of *N*-hydroxy compounds are of considerable toxicological concern because they can lead to reactive intermediates that are responsible for cellular toxicity. The carcinogenic agents *N*-methyl-4-aminoazobenzene and 2-AAF are believed to mediate their toxicity through *N*-hydroxylation to the corresponding *N*-hydroxy compounds (see earlier section on *N*-hydroxylation of amines and amides). Sulfoconjugation of the *N*-hydroxy metabolites yields *O*-sulfate esters, which presumably are the ultimate carcinogenic species. Loss of SO_4^{2-} from the foregoing sulfate conjugates generates electrophilic nitrenium species, which may react with nucleophilic groups (e.g., NH_2, OH, SH) present in proteins, DNA, and RNA to form covalent linkages that lead to structural and functional alteration of these crucial biomacromolecules.[403] The consequences of this are cellular toxicity (tissue necrosis) or alteration of the genetic code, eventually leading to cancer. Some evidence supporting the role of sulfate conjugation in the metabolic activation of *N*-hydroxy compounds to reactive intermediates comes from the observation that the degree of hepatotoxicity and hepatocarcinogenicity of *N*-hydroxy-2-acetylaminofluorene depends markedly on the level of sulfotransferase activity in the liver.[404,405]

The discontinued analgesic phenacetin is metabolized to *N*-hydroxyphenacetin and subsequently conjugated with sulfate.[406] The *O*-sulfate conjugate of *N*-hydroxyphenacetin binds covalently to microsomal proteins.[407]

This pathway may represent one route leading to reactive intermediates that are responsible for the hepatotoxicity and nephrotoxicity associated with phenacetin. Other pathways (e.g., arene oxides) leading to reactive electrophilic intermediates are also possible.[6]

Conjugation with Glycine, Glutamine, and Other Amino Acids

The amino acids glycine and glutamine are used by mammalian systems to conjugate carboxylic acids, particularly aromatic acids and arylalkyl acids.[408,409] Glycine conjugation is common to most mammals, whereas glutamine conjugation appears to be confined mainly to humans and other primates. The quantity of amino acid conjugates formed from xenobiotics is minute because of the limited availability of amino acids in the body and competition with glucuronidation for carboxylic acid substrates. In contrast with glucuronic acid and sulfate, glycine and glutamine are not converted to activated coenzymes. Instead, the carboxylic acid substrate is activated with adenosine triphosphate (ATP) and coenzyme A (CoA) to form an acyl-CoA complex. The latter intermediate, in turn, acylates glycine or glutamine under the influence of specific glycine or glutamine *N*-acyltransferase enzymes. The activation and acylation steps take place in the mitochondria of liver and kidney cells. The sequence of metabolic events associated with glycine and glutamine conjugation of phenylacetic acid is summarized in Figure 3.14. Amino acid conju-

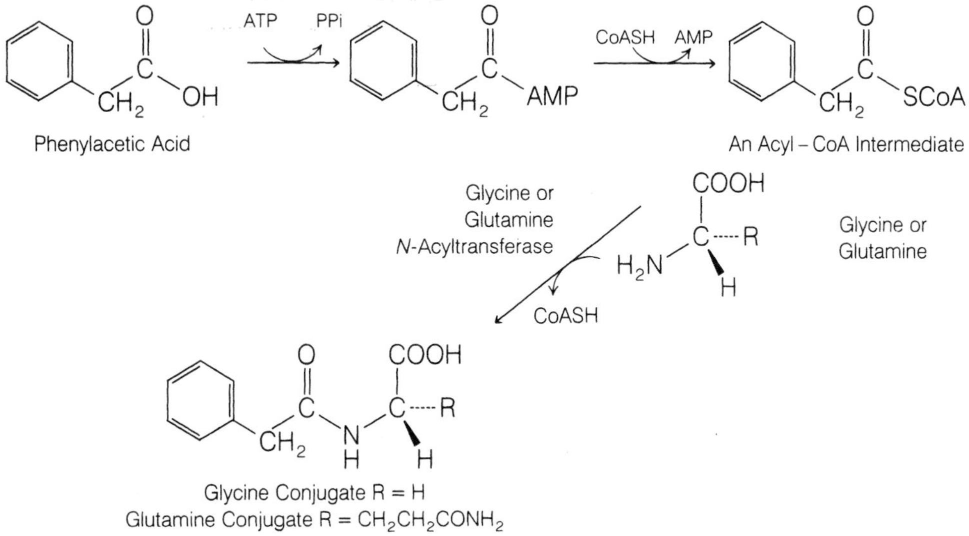

Glycine Conjugate R = H
Glutamine Conjugate R = $CH_2CH_2CONH_2$

Figure 3.14 ● Formation of glycine and glutamine conjugates of phenylacetic acid.

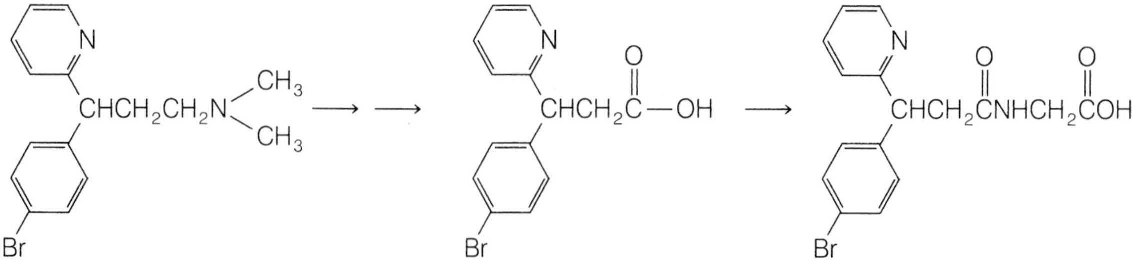

Bromcpheniramine → 3-(*p*-Bromophenyl)-3-(2-pyridyl)-propionic Acid → Glycine Conjugate

gates, being polar and water soluble, are excreted mainly renally and, sometimes, in the bile.

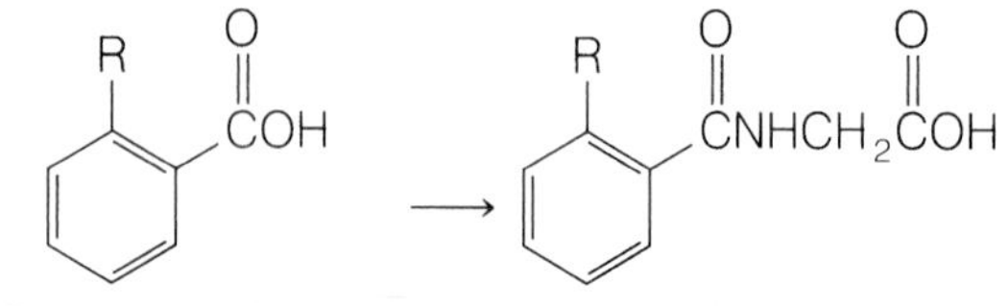

Benzoic Acid, R = H   Hippuric Acid, R = H
Salicylic Acid, R = OH   Salicyluric Acid, R = OH

Aromatic acids and arylalkyl acids are the major substrates undergoing glycine conjugation. The conversion of benzoic acid to its glycine conjugate, hippuric acid, is a well-known metabolic reaction in many mammalian systems.[410] The extensive metabolism of salicylic acid (75% of dose) to salicyluric acid in humans is another illustrative example.[411,412] Carboxylic acid metabolites resulting from oxidation or hydrolysis of many drugs are also susceptible to glycine conjugation. For example, the H_1-histamine antagonist brompheniramine is oxidized to a propionic acid metabolite that is conjugated with glycine in both human and dog.[181] Similarly, *p*-fluorophenylacetic acid, derived from the metabolism of the antipsychotic agent haloperidol (Haldol), is found as the glycine conjugate in the urine of rats.[413] Phenylacetic acid and isonicotinic acid, resulting from the hydrolysis of, respectively, the anticonvulsant phenacemide (Phenurone)[414] and the antituberculosis agent isoniazid,[415] also are conjugated with glycine to some extent.

Glutamine conjugation occurs mainly with arylacetic acids, including endogenous phenylacetic[416] and 3-indolylacetic acid.[417] A few glutamine conjugates of drug metabolites have been reported. For example, in humans, the 3,4-dihydroxy-5-methoxyphenylacetic acid metabolite of mescaline is found as a conjugate of glutamine.[418] Diphenylmethoxyacetic acid, a metabolite of the antihistamine diphenhydramine (Benadryl), is biotransformed further to the corresponding glutamine derivative in the rhesus monkey.[419]

Several other amino acids are involved in the conjugation of carboxylic acids, but these reactions occur only occasionally and appear to be highly substrate and species dependent.[409,420] Ornithine (in birds), aspartic acid and serine (in rats), alanine (in mouse and hamster), taurine ($H_2NCH_2CH_2SO_3H$) (in mammals and pigeons), and histidine (in African bats) are among these amino acids.[420]

GSH or Mercapturic Acid Conjugates

GSH conjugation is an important pathway for detoxifying chemically reactive electrophilic compounds.[421–428] It is now generally accepted that reactive electrophilic species manifest their toxicity (e.g., tissue necrosis, carcinogenicity, mutagenicity, teratogenicity) by combining covalently with nucleophilic groups present in vital cellular proteins and nucleic acids.[4,429] Many serious drug toxicities may be explained also in terms of covalent interaction of metabolically generated electrophilic intermediates with cellular nucleophiles.[5,6] GSH protects vital cellular constituents against chemically reactive species by virtue of its nucleophilic SH group. The SH group reacts with electron-deficient compounds to form *S*-substituted GSH adducts (Fig. 3.15).[421–428]

GSH is a tripeptide (γ-glutamyl-cysteinylglycine) found in most tissues. Xenobiotics conjugated with GSH usually are not excreted as such, but undergo further biotransformation to give *S*-substituted *N*-acetylcysteine products called mercapturic acids.[76,86,424–428] This process involves enzymatic cleavage of two amino acids (namely, glutamic acid and glycine) from the initially formed GSH adduct and subsequent *N*-acetylation of the remaining *S*-substituted cysteine residue. The formation of GSH conjugates and their conversion to mercapturic acid derivatives are outlined in Figure 3.15.

Conjugation of a wide spectrum of substrates with GSH is catalyzed by a family of cytoplasmic enzymes known as GSH *S*-transferases.[75] These enzymes are found in most tissues, particularly the liver and kidney. Degradation of GSH conjugates to mercapturic acids is carried out principally by renal and hepatic microsomal enzymes (Fig. 3.15).[76] Unlike other conjugative phase II reactions, GSH conjugation does not require the initial formation of an activated coenzyme or substrate. The inherent reactivity of the nucleophilic GSH toward an electrophilic substrate usually provides sufficient driving force. The substrates susceptible to GSH conjugation are quite varied and encompass many chemically different classes of compounds. A major prerequisite is that the substrate be sufficiently electrophilic. Compounds that react with GSH do so by two general mechanisms: (a) nucleophilic displacement at an electron-deficient carbon or heteroatom or (b) nucleophilic addition to an electron-deficient double bond.[421–423]

Many aliphatic and arylalkyl halides (Cl, Br, I), sulfates (OSO_3^-), sulfonates (OSO_2R), nitrates (NO_2), and organophosphates ($O-P[OR]_2$) possess electron-deficient carbon atoms that react with GSH (by aliphatic nucleophilic displacement) to form GSH conjugates, as shown:

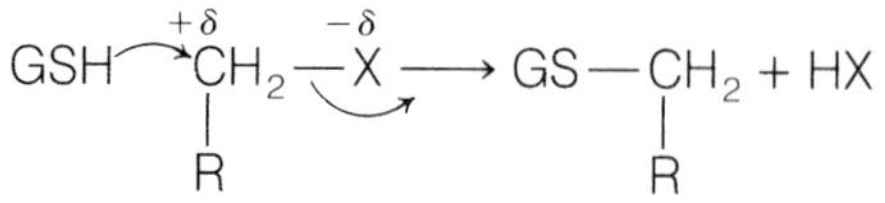

R = Alkyl, Aryl, Benzylic, Allylic
X = Br, Cl, I, OSO_3^-, OSO_2R, $OPO(OR)_2$

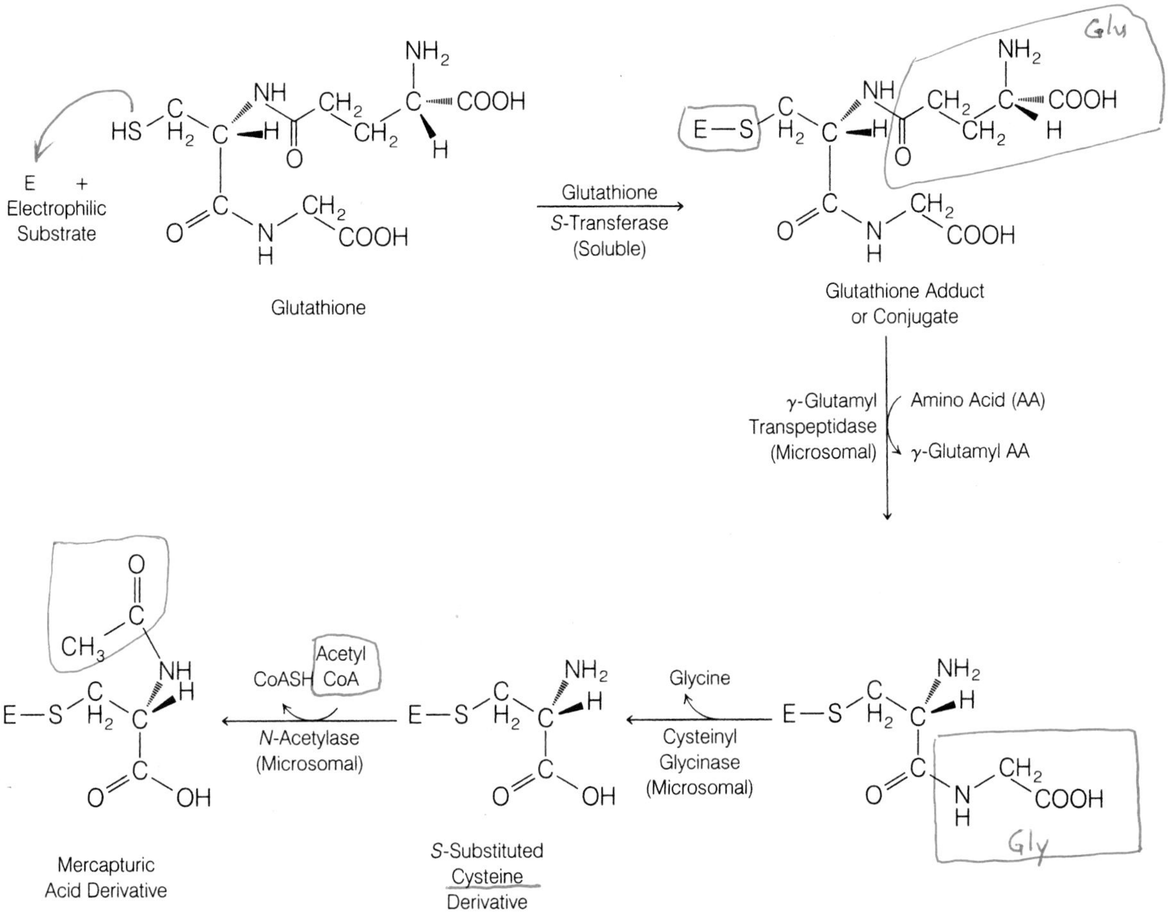

Figure 3.15 ● Formation of GSH conjugates of electrophilic xenobiotics or metabolites (*E*) and their conversion to mercapturic acids.

The carbon center is rendered electrophilic as a result of the electron-withdrawing group (e.g., halide, sulfate, phosphate) attached to it. Nucleophilic displacement often is facilitated when the carbon atom is benzylic or allylic or when X is a good leaving group (e.g., halide, sulfate). Many industrial chemicals, such as benzyl chloride ($C_6H_5CH_2Cl$), allyl chloride (CH_2=$CHCH_2Cl$), and methyl iodide, are known to be toxic and carcinogenic. The reactivity of these three halides toward GSH conjugation in mammalian systems is demonstrated by the formation of the corresponding mercapturic acid derivatives.[424–428] Organophosphate insecticides, such as methyl parathion, are detoxified by two different GSH pathways.[430,431] Pathway "a" involves aliphatic nucleophilic substitution and yields *S*-methylglu-

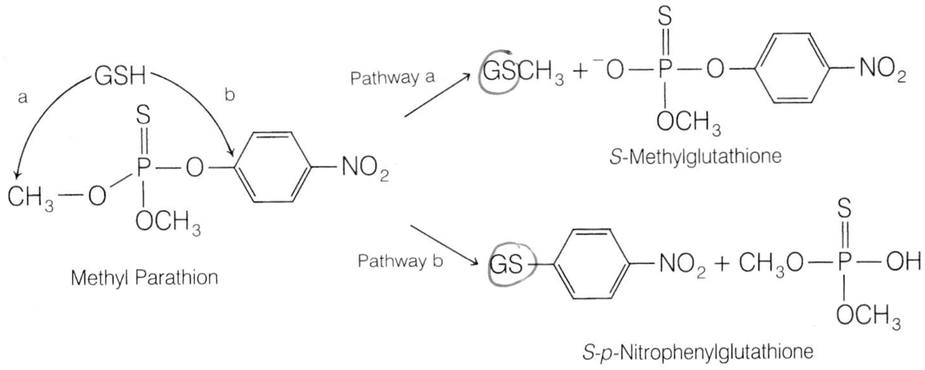

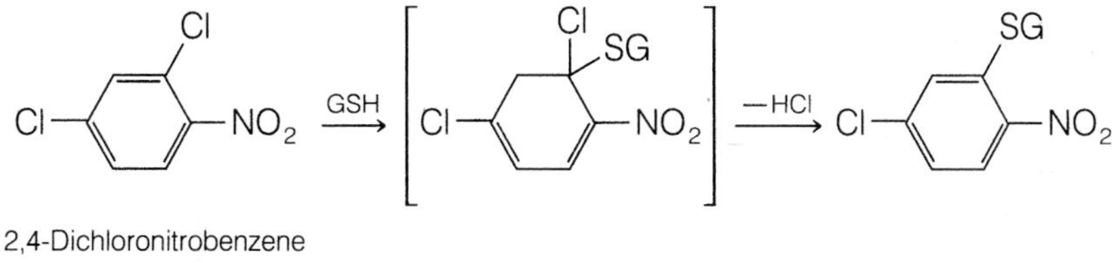

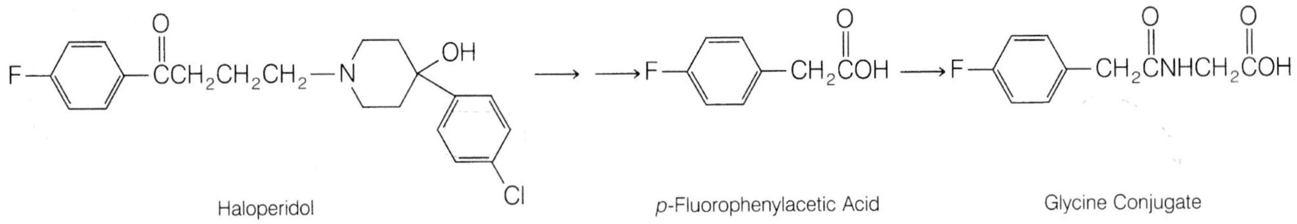

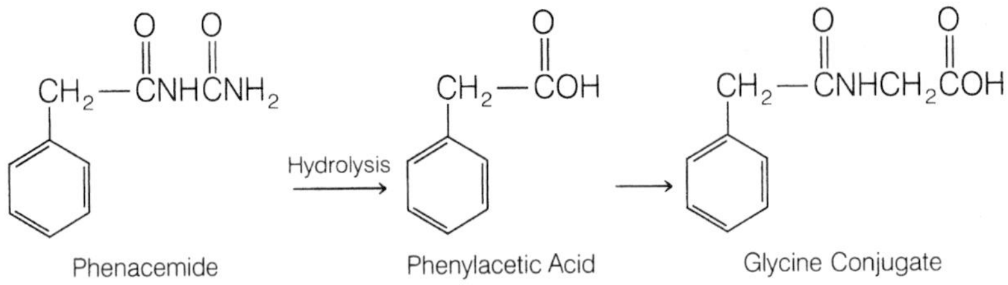

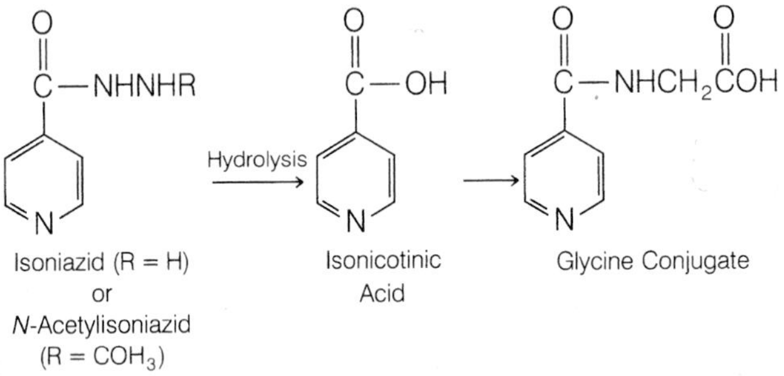

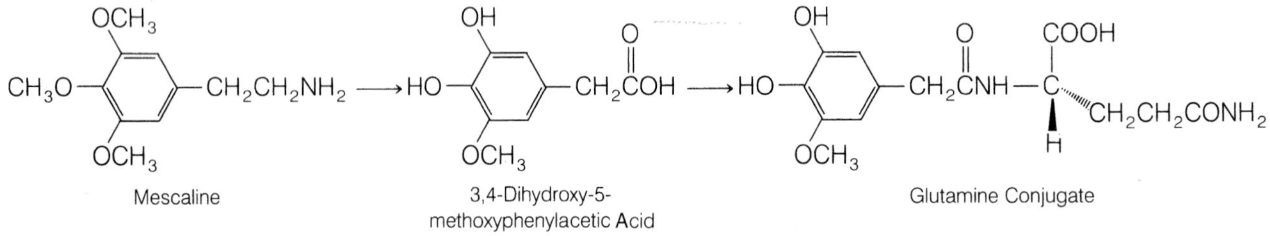

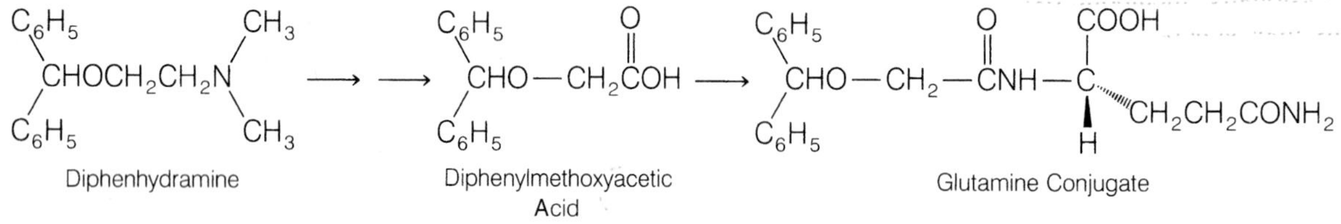

Haloperidol → p-Fluorophenylacetic Acid → Glycine Conjugate

Phenacemide → (Hydrolysis) → Phenylacetic Acid → Glycine Conjugate

Isoniazid (R = H) or N-Acetylisoniazid (R = COH$_3$) → (Hydrolysis) → Isonicotinic Acid → Glycine Conjugate

Mescaline → 3,4-Dihydroxy-5-methoxyphenylacetic Acid → Glutamine Conjugate

Diphenhydramine → Diphenylmethoxyacetic Acid → Glutamine Conjugate

tathione. Pathway "b" involves aromatic nucleophilic substitution and produces S-p-nitrophenylglutathione. Aromatic or heteroaromatic nucleophilic substitution reactions with GSH occur only when the ring is rendered sufficiently electrondeficient by the presence of one or more strongly electron-withdrawing substituents (e.g., NO$_2$, Cl). For example, 2,4-dichloronitrobenzene is susceptible to nucleophilic substitution by GSH, whereas chlorobenzene is not.[432]

The metabolism of the immunosuppressive drug azathioprine (Imuran) to 1-methyl-4-nitro-5-(S-glutathionyl)imidazole and 6-mercaptopurine is an example of heteroaromatic nucleophilic substitution involving GSH.[433–435] Interestingly, 6-mercaptopurine formed in this reaction appears to be responsible for azathioprine's immunosuppressive activity.[436]

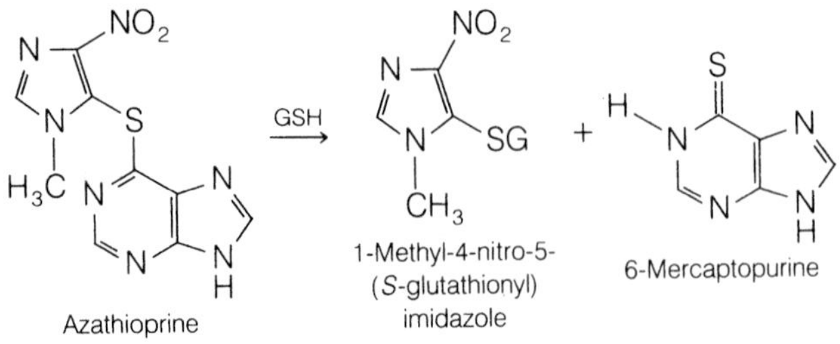

Azathioprine → (GSH) → 1-Methyl-4-nitro-5-(S-glutathionyl)imidazole + 6-Mercaptopurine

Arene oxides and aliphatic epoxides (or oxiranes) represent a very important class of substrates that are conjugated and detoxified by GSH.[437] The three-membered oxygen-containing ring in these compounds is highly strained and, therefore, reactive toward ring cleavage by nucleophiles (e.g., GSH, H$_2$O, or nucleophilic groups present on cellular macromolecules). As discussed previously, arene oxides and epoxides are intermediary products formed from CYP oxidation of aromatic compounds (arenes) and olefins, respectively. If reactive arene oxides (e.g., benzo[α]pyrene-4,5-oxide, 4-bromobenzene oxide) and aliphatic epoxides (e.g., styrene oxide) are not "neutralized" or detoxified by GSH *S*-transferase, epoxide hydrase, or other pathways, they ultimately covalently bind to cellular macromolecules and cause serious cytotoxicity and carcinogenicity. The isolation of GSH or mercapturic acid adducts from benzo[α]pyrene, bromobenzene, and styrene clearly demonstrates the importance of GSH in reacting with the reactive epoxide metabolites generated from these compounds.

GSH conjugation involving substitution at heteroatoms, such as oxygen, is seen often with organic nitrates. For example, nitroglycerin (Nitrostat) and isosorbide dinitrate (Isordil) are metabolized by a pathway involving an initial GSH conjugation reaction. The GSH conjugate products, however, are not metabolized to mercapturic acids but instead are converted enzymatically to the corresponding alcohol derivatives and glutathione disulfide (GSSG).[438]

The nucleophilic addition of GSH to electron-deficient carbon–carbon double bonds occurs mainly in compounds with α,β-unsaturated double bonds. In most instances, the double bond is rendered electron deficient by resonance or conjugation with a carbonyl group (ketone or aldehyde), ester, nitrile, or other. Such α,β-unsaturated systems undergo so-called Michael addition reactions with GSH to yield the corresponding GSH adduct.[421–428] For example, in rats and dogs, the diuretic agent ethacrynic acid (Edecrin) reacts with GSH to form the corresponding GSH or mercapturic acid derivatives.[439] Not all α,β-unsaturated compounds are conjugated with GSH. Many steroidal agents with α,β-unsaturated carbonyl moieties, such as prednisone and digitoxigenin, have evinced no significant conjugation with GSH. Steric factors, decreased reactivity of the double bond, and other factors (e.g., susceptibility to metabolic reduction of the ketone or the C=C double bond) may account for these observations.

Occasionally, metabolic oxidative biotransformation reactions may generate chemically reactive α,β-unsaturated systems that react with GSH. For example, metabolic oxidation of acetaminophen presumably generates the chemically reactive intermediate *N*-acetylimidoquinone. Michael addition of GSH to the imidoquinone leads to the corresponding mercapturic acid derivative in both animals and humans.[245,248] 2-Hydroxyestrogens, such as 2-hydroxy-17β-estradiol, undergo conjugation with GSH to yield the two isomeric mercapturic acid or GSH derivatives. Although the exact mechanism is unclear, it appears that 2-hydroxyestrogen is oxidized to a chemically reactive orthoquinone or semiquinone intermediate that reacts with GSH at either the electrophilic C-1 or C-4 position.[440,441]

In most instances, GSH conjugation is regarded as a detoxifying pathway that protects cellular macromolecules such as protein and DNA against harmful electrophiles. In a few cases, GSH conjugation has been implicated in causing toxicity. Often, this is because the GSH conjugates are themselves electrophilic (e.g., vicinal dihaloethanes) or give rise to metabolic intermediates (e.g., cysteine metabolites of haloalkenes) that are electrophilic.[424–428] 1,2-Dichloroethane, for example, reacts with GSH to produce *S*-(2-chloroethyl)glutathione; the nucleophilic sulfur group in this conjugate can internally dis-

place the chlorine group to give rise to an electrophilic three-membered ring episulfonium ion. The covalent interaction of the episulfonium intermediate with the guanosine moiety of DNA may contribute to the mutagenic and carcinogenic effects observed for 1,2-dichloroethane.[425–427] The metabolic conversion of GSH conjugates to reactive cysteine metabolites is responsible for the nephrotoxicity associated with some halogenated alkanes and alkenes.[428] The activation pathway appears to involve γ-glutamyl transpeptidase and cysteine conjugate β-lyase, two enzymes that apparently target the conjugates to the kidney.

Acetylation

Acetylation constitutes an important metabolic route for drugs containing primary amino groups.[408,442,443] This encompasses primary aromatic amines ($ArNH_2$), sulfonamides ($H_2NC_6H_4SO_2NHR$), hydrazines (—$NHNH_2$), hydrazides (—$CONHNH_2$), and primary aliphatic amines. The amide derivatives formed from acetylation of these amino functionalities are generally inactive and nontoxic. Because water solubility is not enhanced greatly by *N*-acetylation, it appears that the primary function of acetylation is to terminate pharmacological activity and detoxification. A few reports indicate, however, that acetylated metabolites may be as active as (e.g., *N*-acetylprocainamide),[444,445] or more toxic than (e.g., *N*-acetylisoniazid),[446,447] their corresponding parent compounds.

The acetyl group used in *N*-acetylation of xenobiotics is supplied by acetyl-CoA.[408] Transfer of the acetyl group from this cofactor to the accepting amino substrate is carried out by soluble *N*-acetyltransferases present in hepatic reticuloendothelial cells. Other extrahepatic tissues, such as the lung, spleen, gastric mucosa, red blood cells, and lymphocytes, also show acetylation capability. *N*-Acetyltransferase enzymes display broad substrate specificity and catalyze the acetylation of several drugs and xenobiotics (Fig. 3.16).[442,443] Aromatic compounds with a primary amino group, such as aniline,[408] *p*-aminobenzoic acid,[448,449] *p*-aminosalicylic acid,[418] procainamide (Pronestyl),[444,445,448,449] and dapsone (Avlosulfon),[450] are especially susceptible to *N*-acetylation. Aromatic amine metabolites resulting from the reduction of aryl nitro compounds also are *N*-acetylated. For example, the anticonvulsant clonazepam (Klonopin) undergoes nitro reduction to its 7-amino metabolite, which in turn is *N*-acetylated.[315] Another related benzodiazepam analog, nitrazepam, follows a similar pathway.[316]

The metabolism of several sulfonamides, such as sulfanilamide,[451] sulfamethoxazole (Gantanol),[452] sulfisoxazole (Gantrisin),[452] sulfapyridine[453] (major metabolite from azo reduction of sulfasalazine, Azulfidine), and sulfamethazine,[408] occurs mainly by acetylation at the N-4 position. With sulfanilamide, acetylation also takes place at the sulfamido N-1 position.[451] *N*-Acetylated metabolites of sulfonamides tend to be less water soluble than their parent compounds and have the potential of crystallizing out in renal tubules (*crystalluria*), thereby causing kidney damage. The frequency of crystalluria and renal toxicity is especially high with older sulfonamide derivatives, such as sulfathiazole.[1,420] Newer sulfonamides, such as sulfisoxazole and sulfamethoxazole, however, are metabolized to relatively water-soluble acetylated derivatives, which are less likely to precipitate out.

(text continues on page 101)

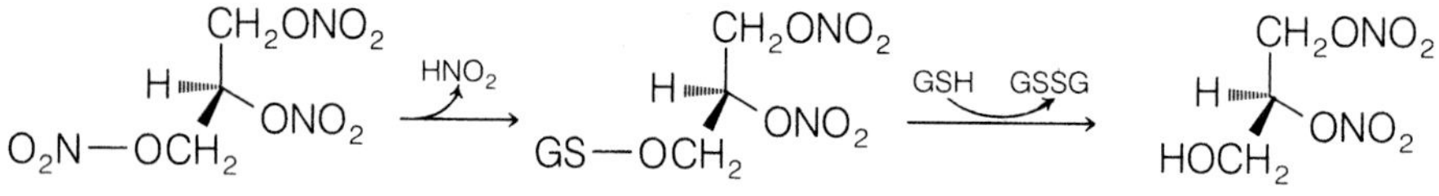

HSG
Nitroglycerin

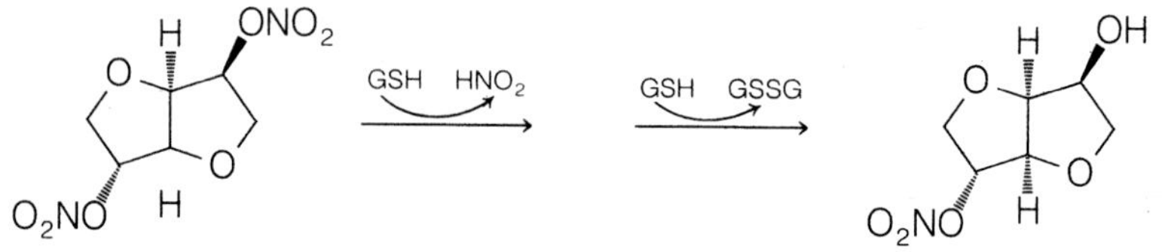

Isosorbide

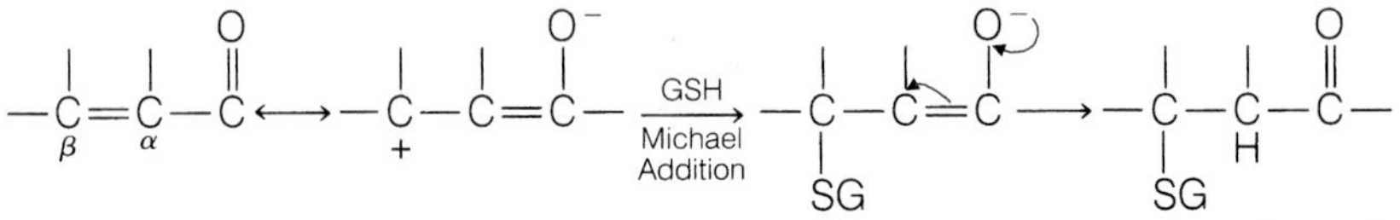

α-β-Unsaturated
System

Glutathione
Adduct

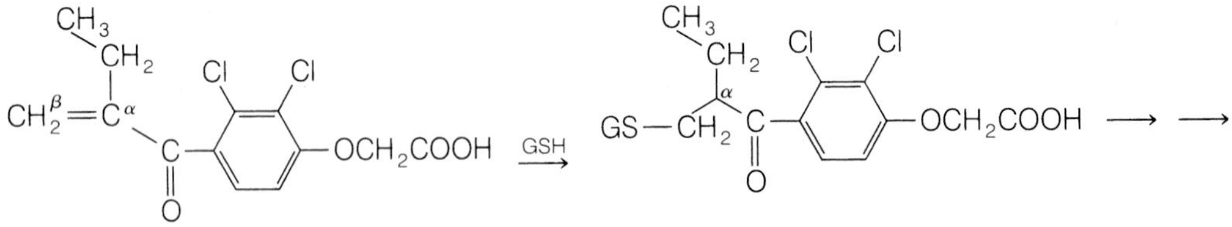

Ethacrynic Acid
(note α,β-unsaturated
ketone moiety)

Glutathione adduct
of Ethacrynic Acid

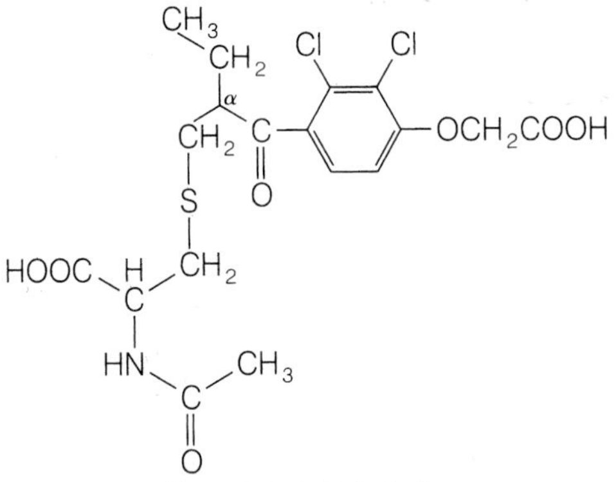

Mercapturic Acid Derivative

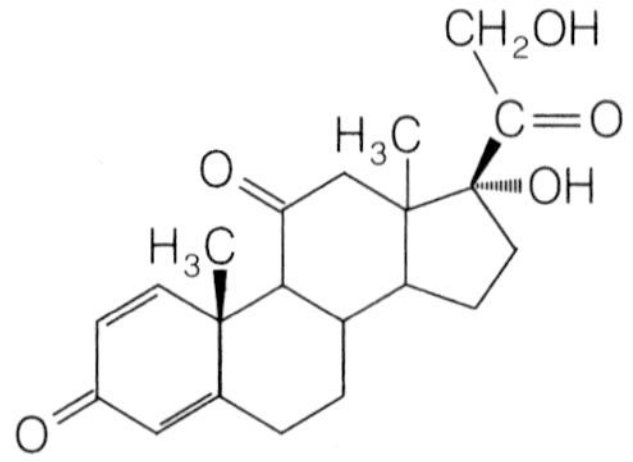

Prednisone

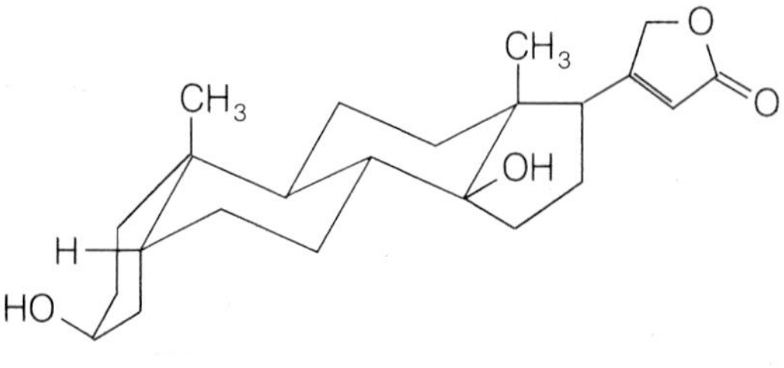

Digitoxigenin

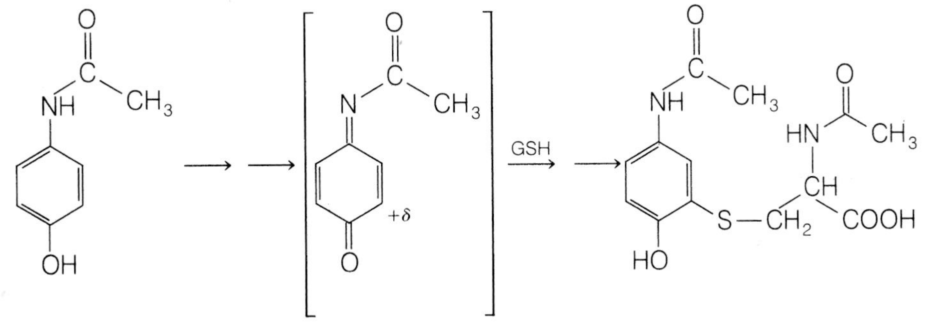

Acetaminophen → *N*-Acetylimidoquinone → Mercapturic Acid Derivative

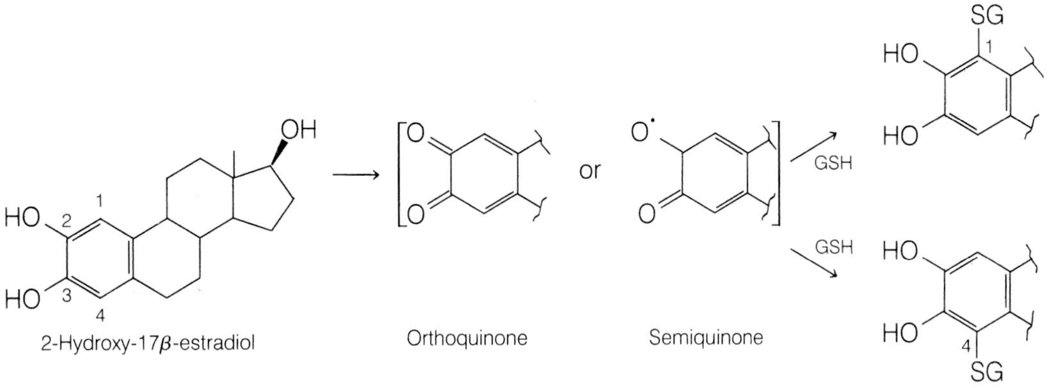

2-Hydroxy-17β-estradiol → Orthoquinone or Semiquinone → (GSH products)

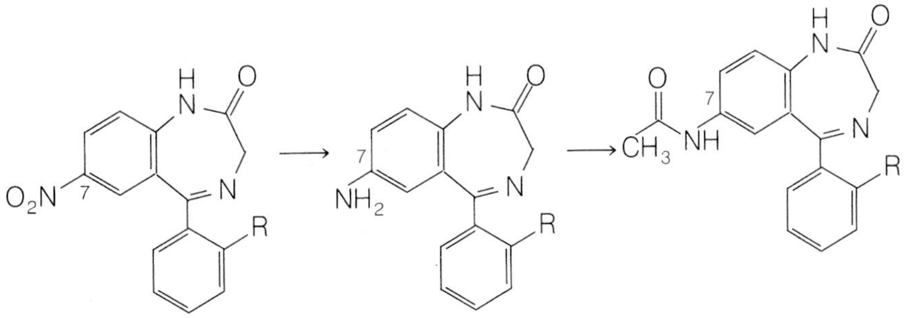

Clonazepam, R = Cl
Nitrazepam, R = H

7-Amino Metabolite

7-Acetamido Metabolite
or
N-Acetylated Metabolite

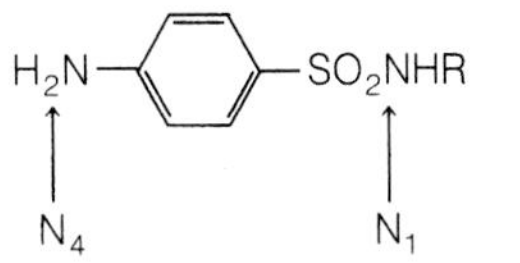

H_2N—〈 〉—SO_2NHR

N_4 N_1
Sulfonamide Nomenclature

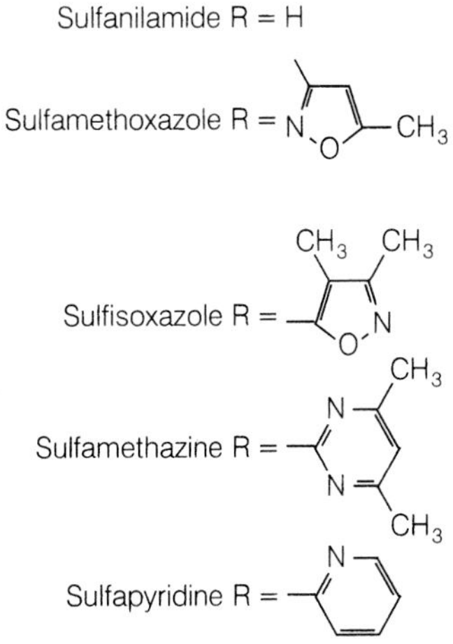

Sulfanilamide R = H

Sulfamethoxazole R =

Sulfisoxazole R =

Sulfamethazine R =

Sulfapyridine R =

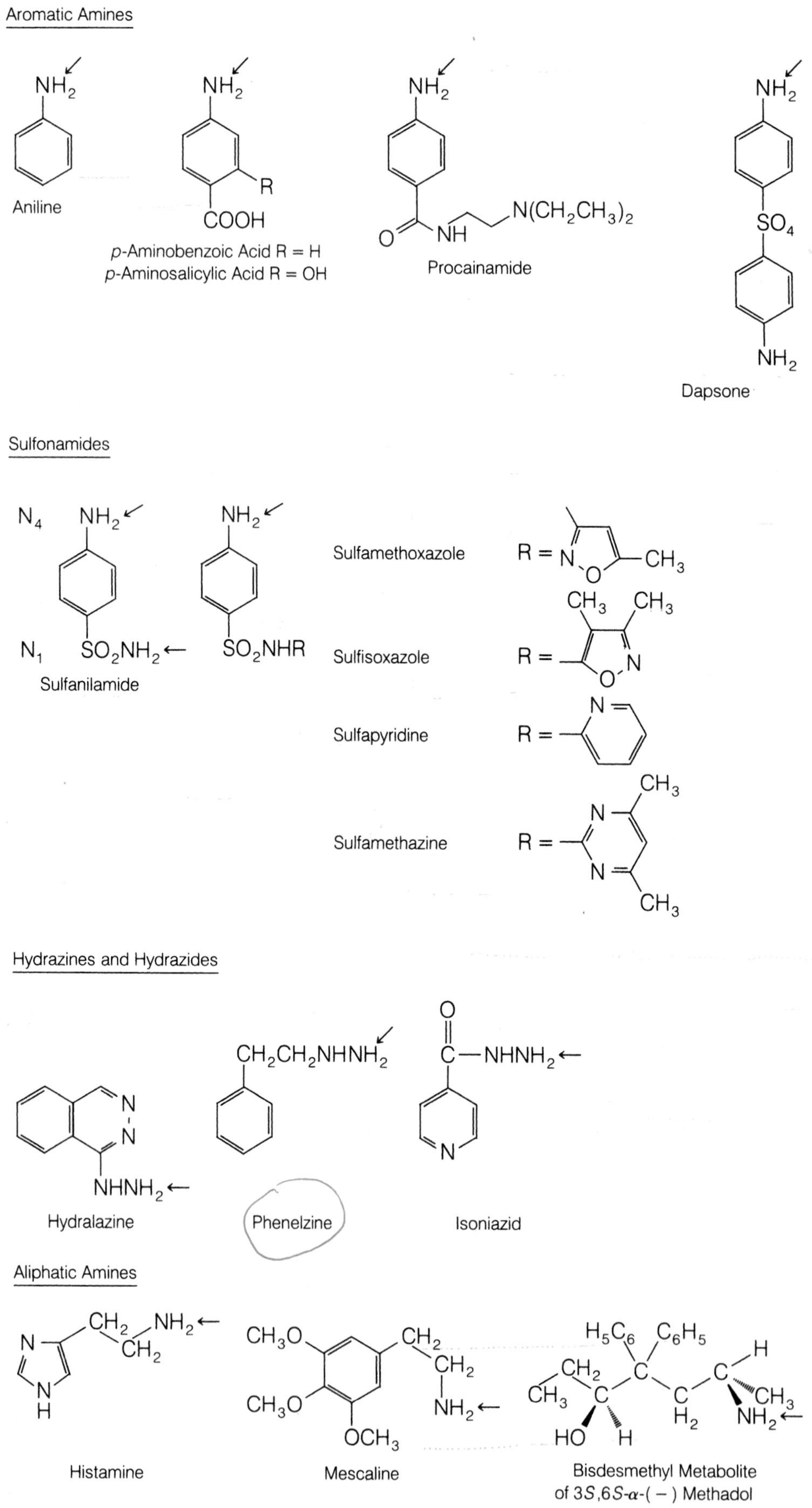

Aromatic Amines

Aniline

p-Aminobenzoic Acid R = H
p-Aminosalicylic Acid R = OH

Procainamide

Dapsone

Sulfonamides

Sulfanilamide

Sulfamethoxazole
Sulfisoxazole
Sulfapyridine
Sulfamethazine

Hydrazines and Hydrazides

Hydralazine

Phenelzine

Isoniazid

Aliphatic Amines

Histamine

Mescaline

Bisdesmethyl Metabolite
of 3S,6S-α-(−) Methadol

Figure 3.16 ● Examples of different types of compound undergoing *N*-acetylation. *Arrows* indicate sites of *N*-acetylation.

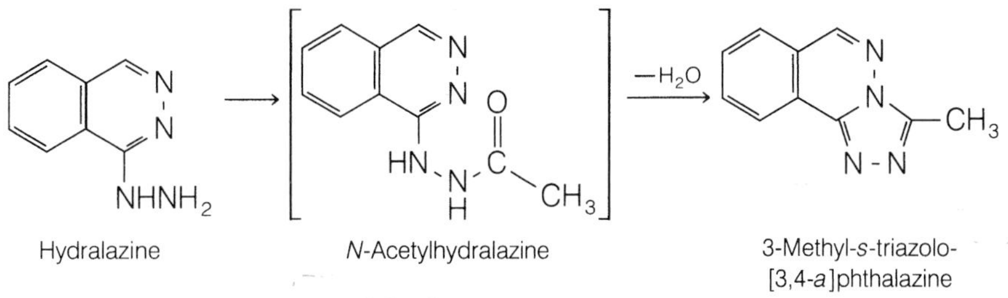

Hydralazine → N-Acetylhydralazine → 3-Methyl-s-triazolo-[3,4-a]phthalazine

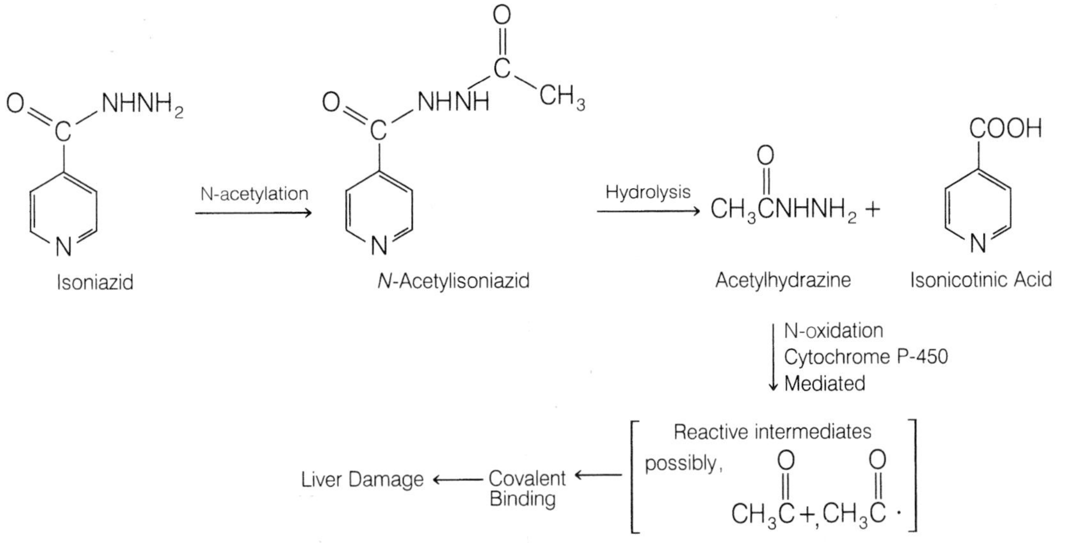

Isoniazid → N-Acetylisoniazid → Acetylhydrazine + Isonicotinic Acid

N-oxidation Cytochrome P-450 Mediated

Liver Damage ← Covalent Binding ← Reactive intermediates possibly, $CH_3C+, CH_3C\cdot$

The biotransformation of hydrazine and hydrazide derivatives also proceeds by acetylation. The antihypertensive hydralazine (Apresoline)[454,455] and the MAO inhibitor phenelzine (Nardil)[456] are two representative hydrazine compounds that are metabolized by this pathway. The initially formed N-acetyl derivative of hydralazine is unstable and cyclizes intramolecularly to form 3-methyl-s-triazolo[3,4-α]phthalazine as the major isolable hydralazine metabolite in humans.[454,455] The antituberculosis drug isoniazid or isonicotinic acid hydrazide (INH) is metabolized extensively to N-acetylisoniazid.[446,447]

The acetylation of some primary aliphatic amines such as histamine,[457] mescaline,[208,209] and the bis-N-demethylated metabolite of α(−)-methadol[458–460] also has been reported. In comparison with oxidative deamination processes, N-acetylation is only a minor pathway in the metabolism of this class of compounds.

The acetylation pattern of several drugs (e.g., isoniazid, hydralazine, procainamide) in the human population displays a bimodal character in which the drug is conjugated either rapidly or slowly with acetyl-CoA.[461,462] This phenomenon is termed *acetylation polymorphism*. Individuals are classified as having either slow or rapid acetylator phenotypes. This variation in acetylating ability is genetic and is caused mainly by differences in N-acetyltransferase activity. The proportion of rapid and slow acetylators varies widely among different ethnic groups throughout the world. Oddly, a high proportion of Eskimos and Asians are rapid acetylators, whereas Egyptians and some Western European groups are mainly slow acetylators.[462] Other populations are intermediate between these two

extremes. Because of the bimodal distribution of the human population into rapid and slow acetylators, there appears to be significant individual variation in therapeutic and toxicological responses to drugs displaying acetylation polymorphism.[408,461,462] Slow acetylators seem more likely to develop adverse reactions, whereas rapid acetylators are more likely to show an inadequate therapeutic response to standard drug doses.

The antituberculosis drug isoniazid illustrates many of these points. The plasma half-life of isoniazid in rapid acetylators ranges from 45 to 80 minutes; in slow acetylators, the half-life is about 140 to 200 minutes.[463] Thus, for a given fixed-dosing regimen, slow acetylators tend to accumulate higher plasma concentrations of isoniazid than do rapid acetylators. Higher concentrations of isoniazid may explain the greater therapeutic response (i.e., higher cure rate) among slow acetylators, but they probably also account for the greater incidence of adverse effects (e.g., peripheral neuritis and drug-induced systemic lupus erythematosus syndrome) observed among slow acetylators.[462] Slow acetylators of isoniazid apparently are also more susceptible to certain drug interactions involving drug metabolism. For example, phenytoin toxicity associated with concomitant use with isoniazid appears to be more prevalent in slow acetylators than in rapid acetylators.[464] Isoniazid inhibits the metabolism of phenytoin, thereby leading to an accumulation of high and toxic plasma levels of phenytoin.

Interestingly, patients who are rapid acetylators appear to be more likely to develop isoniazid-associated hepatitis.[446,447] This liver toxicity presumably arises from initial hydrolysis of the N-acetylated metabolite N-acetylisoniazid to acetylhydrazine. The latter metabolite is further converted (by CYP enzyme systems) to chemically reactive acylating intermediates that covalently bind to hepatic tissue, causing necrosis. Pathological and biochemical studies in experimental animals appear to support this hypothesis. Therefore, rapid acetylators run a greater risk of incurring liver injury by virtue of producing more acetylhydrazine.

The tendency of drugs such as hydralazine and procainamide to cause lupus erythematosus syndrome and to elicit formation of antinuclear antibodies (ANAs) appears related to acetylator phenotype, with greater prevalence in slow acetylators.[465,466] Rapid acetylation may prevent the immunological triggering of ANA formation and the lupus syndrome. Interestingly, the *N*-acetylated metabolite of procainamide is as active an antiarrhythmic agent as the parent drug[444,445] and has a half-life twice as long in humans.[467] These findings indicate that *N*-acetylprocainamide may be a promising alternative to procainamide as an antiarrhythmic agent with less lupus-inducing potential.

Methylation

Methylation reactions play an important role in the biosynthesis of many endogenous compounds (e.g., epinephrine and melatonin) and in the inactivation of numerous physiologically active biogenic amines (e.g., norepinephrine, dopamine, serotonin, and histamine).[468] Methylation, however, constitutes only a minor pathway for conjugating drugs and xenobiotics. Methylation generally does not lead to polar or water-soluble metabolites, except when it creates a quaternary ammonium derivative. Most methylated products tend to be pharmacologically inactive, although there are a few exceptions.

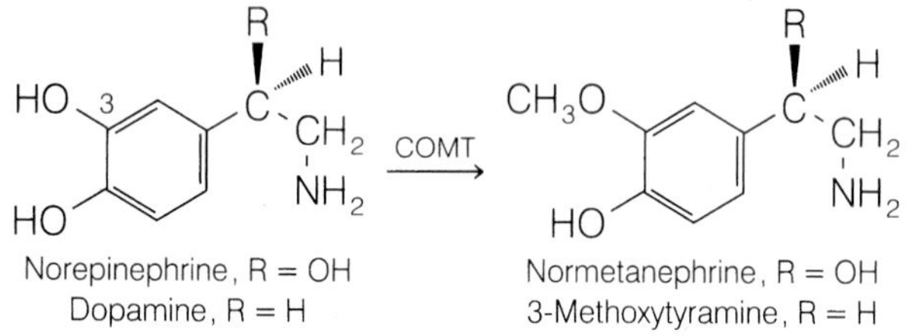

Norepinephrine, R = OH
Dopamine, R = H

Normetanephrine, R = OH
3-Methoxytyramine, R = H

The coenzyme involved in methylation reactions is *S*-adenosylmethionine (SAM). The transfer of the activated

methyl group from this coenzyme to the acceptor substrate is catalyzed by various cytoplasmic and microsomal methyltransferases (Fig. 3.17).[468,469] Methyltransferases of particular importance in the metabolism of foreign compounds include catechol-*O*-methyltransferase (COMT), phenol-*O*-methyltransferase, and nonspecific *N*-methyltransferases and *S*-methyltransferases.[358] One of these enzymes, COMT, should be familiar because it carries out *O*-methylation of such important neurotransmitters as norepinephrine and dopamine and thus terminates their activity. Besides being present in the central and peripheral nerves, COMT is distributed widely in other mammalian tissues, particularly the liver and kidney. The other methyltransferases mentioned are located primarily in the liver, kidney, or lungs. Transferases that specifically methylate histamine, serotonin, and epinephrine are not usually involved in the metabolism of xenobiotics.[468]

Foreign compounds that undergo methylation include catechols, phenols, amines, and *N*-heterocyclic and thiol compounds. Catechol and catecholamine-like drugs are metabolized by COMT to inactive monomethylated catechol products. Examples of drugs that undergo significant *O*-methylation by COMT in humans include the antihypertensive (*S*)(−)α-methyldopa (Aldomet),[470,471] the antiparkinsonism agent (*S*)(−)-dopa (Levodopa),[472] isoproterenol (Isuprel),[473] and dobutamine (Dobutrex).[474] The student should note the marked structural similarities between these drugs and the endogenous catecholamines such as norepinephrine and dopamine. In the foregoing four drugs, COMT selectively *O*-methylates only the phenolic OH at C-3. Bismethylation does not occur. Catechol metabolites arising from aromatic hydroxylation of phenols (e.g., 2-hydroxylation of 17α-ethinylestradiol)[54,55] and from the arene oxide dihydrodiol–catechol pathway (see section on oxidation of aromatic moieties, e.g., the catechol metabolite of phenytoin)[475] also undergo *O*-methylation. Substrates undergoing *O*-methylation by COMT must contain an aromatic 1,2-dihydroxy group (i.e., catechol group). Resorcinol (1,3-dihydroxybenzene) or *p*-hydroquinone (1,4-dihydroxybenzene) derivatives are not substrates for COMT. This explains why isoproterenol undergoes extensive *O*-methylation[473] but terbutaline (which contains a resorcinol moiety) does not.[396]

Occasionally, phenols have been reported to undergo *O*-methylation but only to a minor extent.[468] One interesting

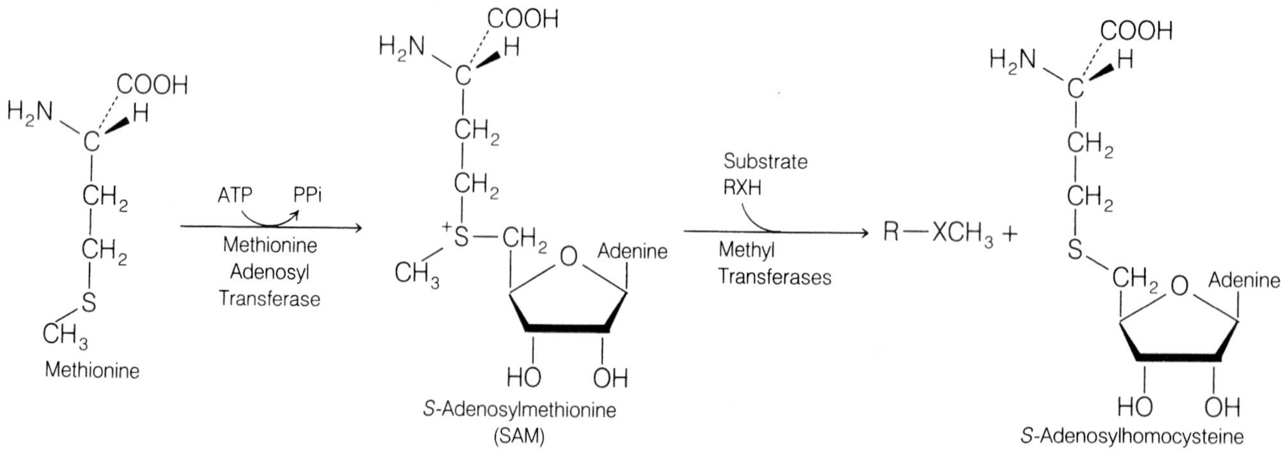

Figure 3.17 • Conjugation of exogenous and endogenous substrates (*RXH*) by methylation.

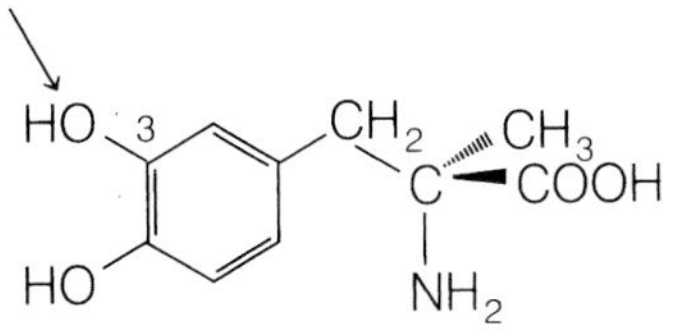

S(−)-α-Methyldopa

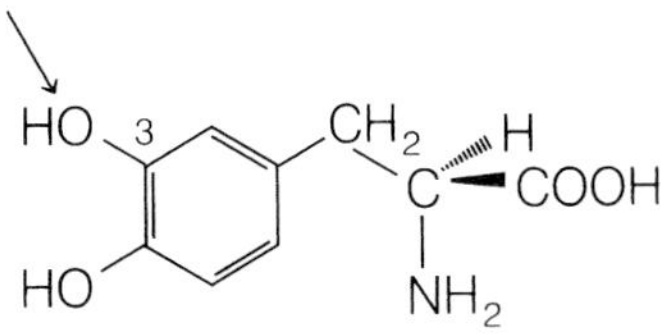

S(−)-Dopa

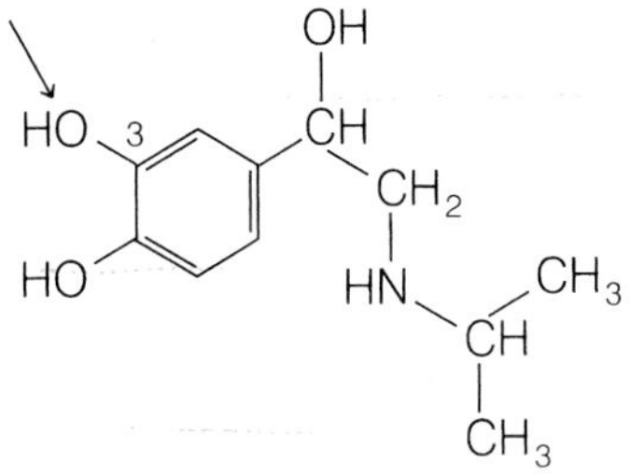

Isoproterenol

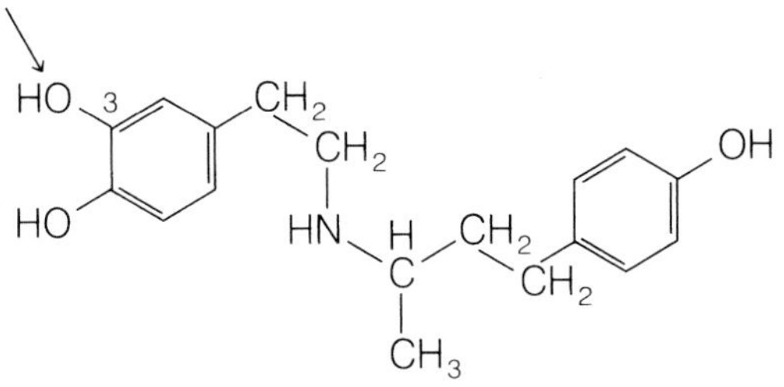

Dobutamine

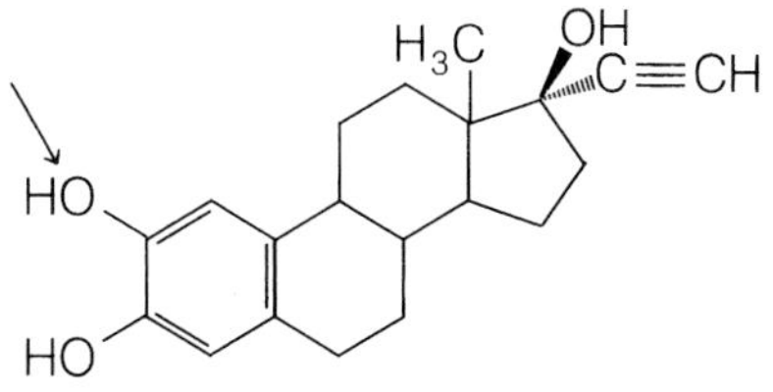

2-Hydroxy-17α-ethinylestradiol

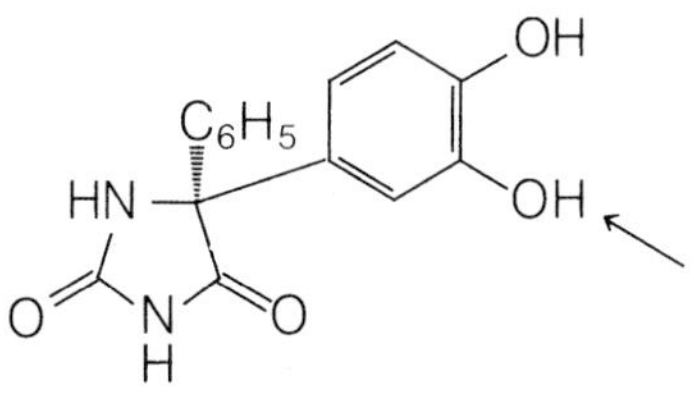

Catechol Metabolite
of Phenytoin

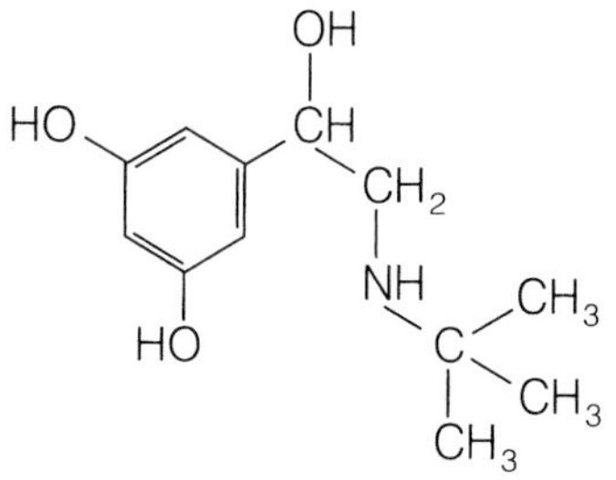

Terbutaline
(not a substrate for COMT)

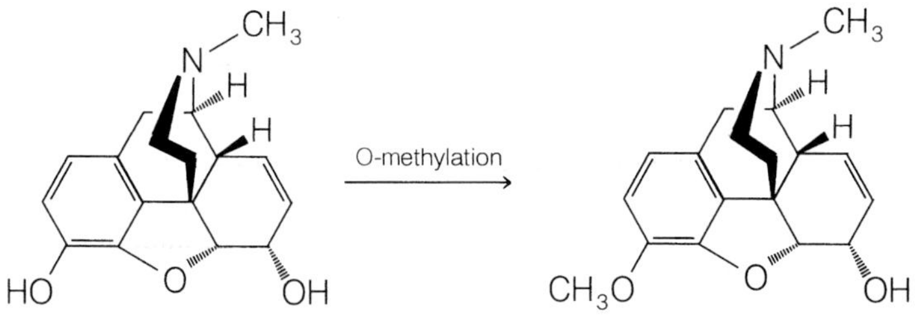

Morphine

O-methylation

Codeine

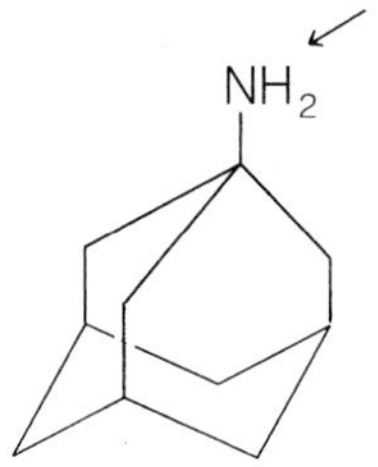

Amantadine

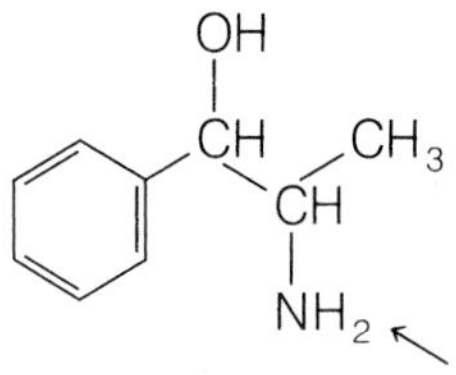

Norephedrine

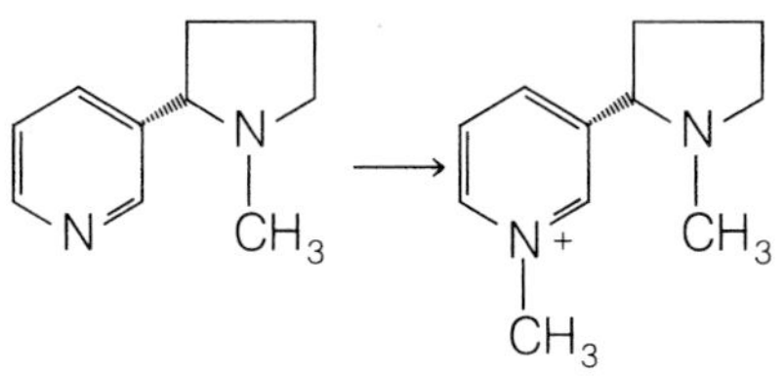

Nicotine

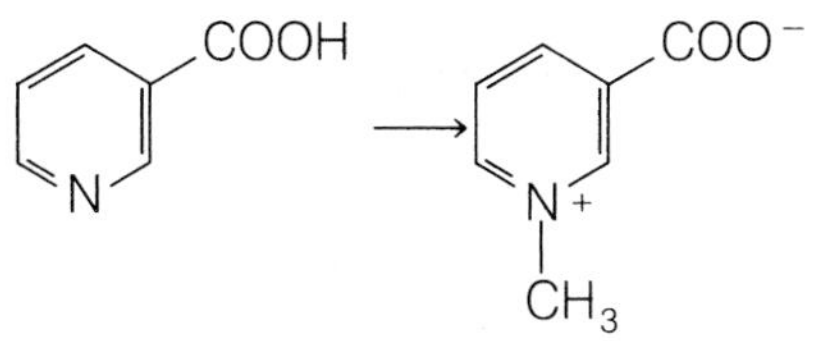

Nicotinic Acid

Trigonelline

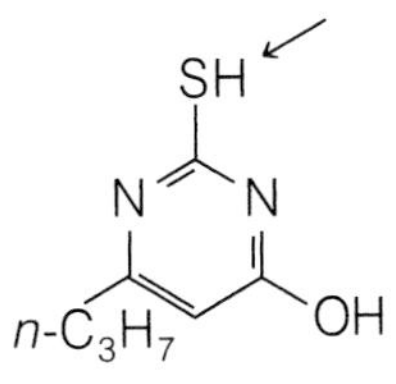

Propylthiouracil

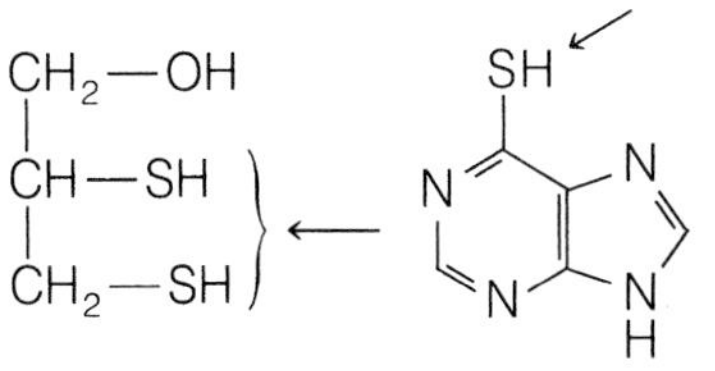

2,3-Dimercapto-1-
propanol (BAL)

6-Mercaptopurine

example involves the conversion of morphine to its *O*-methylated derivative, codeine, in humans. This metabolite is formed in significant amounts in tolerant subjects and may account for up to 10% of the morphine dose.[476]

Although *N*-methylation of endogenous amines (e.g., histamine, norepinephrine) occurs commonly, biotransformation of nitrogen-containing xenobiotics to *N*-methylated metabolites occurs to only a limited extent. Some examples reported include the *N*-methylation of the antiviral and antiparkinsonism agent amantadine (Symmetrel) in dogs[477] and the in vitro *N*-methylation of norephedrine in rabbit lung preparations.[468] *N*-methylation of nitrogen atoms present in heterocyclic compounds (e.g., pyridine derivatives) also takes place. For example, the pyridinyl nitrogens of nicotine[187,188] and nicotinic acid[478] are *N*-methylated to yield quaternary ammonium products.

Thiol-containing drugs, such as propylthiouracil,[479] 2,3-dimercapto-1-propanol (BAL),[480] and 6-mercaptopurine,[481,482] also have been reported to undergo *S*-methylation.

FACTORS AFFECTING DRUG METABOLISM

Drugs and xenobiotics often are metabolized by several different phase I and phase II pathways to give several metabolites. The relative amount of any particular metabolite is determined by the concentration and activity of the enzyme(s) responsible for the biotransformation. The rate of metabolism of a drug is particularly important for its pharmacological action as well as its toxicity. For example, if the rate of metabolism of a drug is decreased, this generally increases the intensity and duration of the drug action. In addition, decreased metabolic elimination may lead to accumulation of toxic levels of the drug. Conversely, an increased rate of metabolism decreases the intensity and duration of action as well as the drug's efficacy. Many factors may affect drug metabolism, and they are discussed in the following sections. These include age, species and strain, genetic or hereditary factors, sex, enzyme induction, and enzyme inhibition.[32,483–486]

Age Differences

Age-related differences in drug metabolism are generally quite apparent in the newborn.[487,488] In most fetal and newborn animals, undeveloped or deficient oxidative and conjugative enzymes are chiefly responsible for the reduced metabolic capability seen. In general, the ability to carry out metabolic reactions increases rapidly after birth and approaches adult levels in about 1 to 2 months. An illustration of the influence of age on drug metabolism is seen in the duration of action (sleep time) of hexobarbital in newborn and adult mice.[489] When given a dose of 10 mg/kg of body weight, the newborn mouse sleeps more than 6 hours. In contrast, the adult mouse sleeps for fewer than 5 minutes when given the same dose.

In humans, oxidative and conjugative (e.g., glucuronidation) capabilities of newborns are also low compared with those of adults. For example, the oxidative (CYP) metabolism of tolbutamide appears to be markedly lower in newborns.[490] Compared with the half-life of 8 hours in adults, the plasma half-life of tolbutamide in infants is more than 40 hours. As discussed previously, infants possess poor glucuronidating ability because of a deficiency in glucuronyltransferase activity. The inability of infants to conjugate chloramphenicol with glucuronic acid appears to be responsible for the accumulation of toxic levels of this antibiotic, resulting in the so-called gray baby syndrome.[388] Similarly, neonatal hyperbilirubinemia (or kernicterus) results from the inability of newborn babies to glucuronidate bilirubin.[387]

The effect of old age on drug metabolism has not been as well studied. There is some evidence in animals and humans that drug metabolism diminishes with old age.[491,492] Much of the evidence, however, is based on prolonged plasma half-lives of drugs that are metabolized totally or mainly by hepatic microsomal enzymes (e.g., antipyrine, phenobarbital, acetaminophen). In evaluating the effect of age on drug metabolism, one must differentiate between "normal" loss of enzymatic activity with aging and the effect of a diseased liver from hepatitis, cirrhosis, etc., plus decreased renal function, because much of the water-soluble conjugation products are excreted in the liver.

Species and Strain Differences

The metabolism of many drugs and foreign compounds is often species dependent. Different animal species may biotransform a particular xenobiotic by similar or markedly different metabolic pathways. Even within the same species, individual variations (strain differences) may result in significant differences in a specific metabolic pathway.[493,494] This is a problem when a new drug is under development. A new drug application requires the developer to account for the product as it moves from the site of administration to final elimination from the body. It is difficult enough to find appropriate animal models for a disease. It is even harder to find animal models that mimic human drug metabolism.

Species variation has been observed in many oxidative biotransformation reactions. For example, metabolism of amphetamine occurs by two main pathways: oxidative deamination or aromatic hydroxylation. In human, rabbit, and guinea pig, oxidative deamination appears to be the predominant pathway; in the rat, aromatic hydroxylation appears to be the more important route.[495] Phenytoin is another drug that shows marked species differences in metabolism. In the human, phenytoin undergoes aromatic oxidation to yield primarily $(S)(-)$-*p*-hydroxyphenytoin; in the dog, oxidation occurs to give mainly $(R)(+)$-*m*-hydroxyphenytoin.[496] There is a dramatic difference not only in the position (i.e., *meta* or *para*) of aromatic hydroxylation but also in which of the two phenyl rings (at C-5 of phenytoin) undergoes aromatic oxidation.

Species differences in many conjugation reactions also have been observed. Often, these differences are caused by the presence or absence of transferase enzymes involved in the conjugative process. For example, cats lack glucuronyltransferase enzymes and, therefore, tend to conjugate phenolic xenobiotics by sulfation instead.[497] In pigs, the situation is reversed: pigs are not able to conjugate phenols with sulfate (because of lack of sulfotransferase enzymes) but appear to have good glucuronidation capability.[497] The conjugation of aromatic acids with amino acids (e.g., glycine, glutamine) depends on the animal species as well as on the substrate. For example, glycine conjugation is a common conjugation pathway for benzoic acid in many animals. In certain birds (e.g., duck, goose, turkey), however, glycine is replaced by the amino acid ornithine.[498] Phenylacetic acid is a substrate for both glycine and glutamine conjugation in humans and other primates. However, nonprimates, such as rabbit and rat, excrete phenylacetic acid only as the glycine conjugate.[499] The metabolism of the urinary antiseptic, phenazopyridine (Pyridium) depends strongly on the animal. The diazo linkage remains intact in over half of the metabolites in humans, whereas 40% of the metabolites in the guinea pig result from its cleavage. The metabolic product pattern in human or guinea pig does not correlate with that of either rat or mouse (Fig. 3.18).[500]

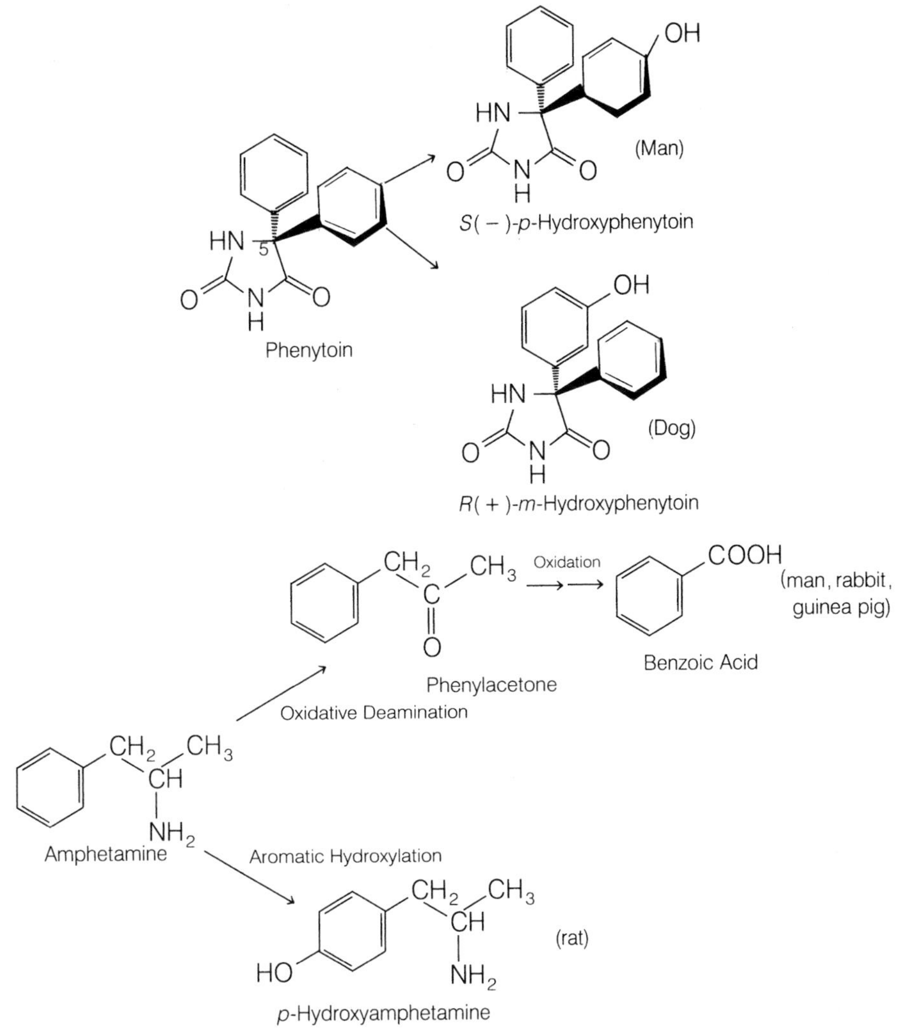

Strain differences in drug metabolism exist, particularly in inbred mice and rabbits. These differences apparently are caused by genetic variations in the amount of metabolizing enzyme present among the different strains. For example, in vitro studies indicate that cottontail rabbit liver microsomes metabolize hexobarbital about 10 times faster than New Zealand rabbit liver microsomes.[501] Interindividual differences in drug metabolism in humans are considered in the section that follows.

Hereditary or Genetic Factors

Marked individual differences in the metabolism of several drugs exist in humans.[463] Many of these genetic or heredi-

tary factors are responsible for the large differences seen in the rate of metabolism of these drugs. The frequently cited example of the biotransformation of the antituberculosis agent isoniazid is discussed previously under acylation. Genetic factors also appear to influence the rate of oxidation of drugs such as phenytoin, phenylbutazone, dicumarol, and nortriptyline.[502,503] The rate of oxidation of these drugs varies widely among different individuals; however, these differences do not appear to be distributed bimodally, as in acetylation. In general, individuals who tend to oxidize one drug rapidly are also likely to oxidize other drugs rapidly. Numerous studies in twins (identical and fraternal) and in families indicate that oxidation of these drugs is under genetic control.[503]

Many patients state that they do not respond to codeine and codeine analogs. It now is realized that their CYP2D6 isozyme does not readily *O*-demethylate codeine to form morphine. This genetic polymorphism is seen in about 8% of Caucasians, 4% of African Americans, and less than 1% of Asians.[504] Genetic polymorphism with CYP isozymes is well documented as evidenced by the many examples in this chapter. There is limited evidence of polymorphism involving MAO-A and MAO-B. The chemical imbalances seen with some mental diseases may be the cause.[206]

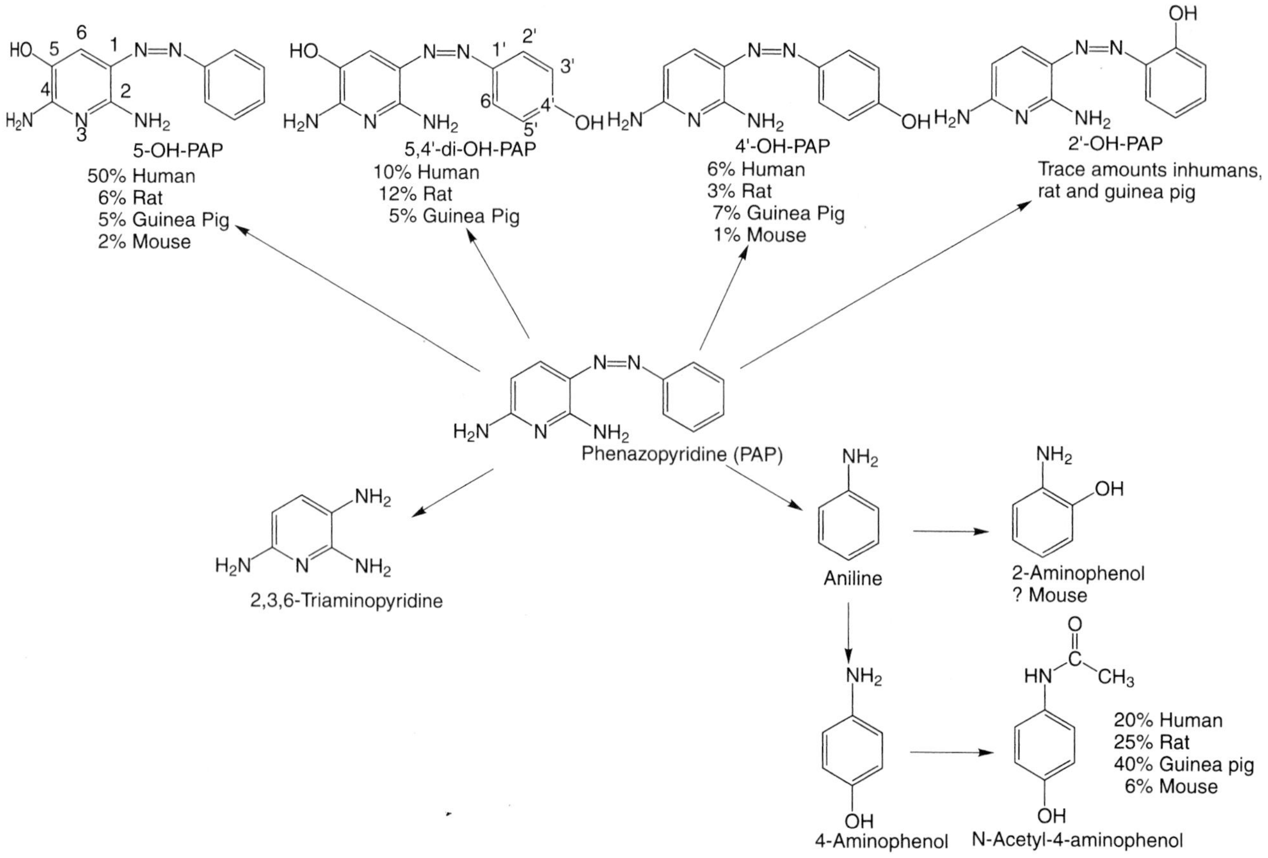

Figure 3.18 • Phenazopyridine metabolism in humans, guinea pigs, rats, and mice.

Sex Differences

The rate of metabolism of xenobiotics also varies according to gender in some animal species. A marked difference is observed between female and male rats. Adult male rats metabolize several foreign compounds at a much faster rate than female rats (e.g., *N*-demethylation of aminopyrine, hexobarbital oxidation, glucuronidation of *o*-aminophenol). Apparently, this sex difference also depends on the substrate, because some xenobiotics are metabolized at the same rate in both female and male rats. Differences in microsomal oxidation are under the control of sex hormones, particularly androgens; the anabolic action of androgens seems to increase metabolism.[505]

Sex differences in drug metabolism appear to be species dependent. Rabbits and mice, for example, do not show a significant sex difference in drug metabolism.[505] In humans, there have been a few reports of sex differences in metabolism. For instance, nicotine and aspirin seem to be metabolized differently in women and men.[506,507] On the other hand, gender differences can become significant in terms of drug–drug interactions based on the drug's metabolism. For women, the focus is on drugs used for contraception. Note in Table 3.4 that the antibiotic rifampin, a CYP3A4 inducer, can shorten the half-life of oral contraceptives.

Enzyme Induction

The activity of hepatic microsomal enzymes, such as the CYP mixed-function oxidase system, can be increased markedly by exposure to diverse drugs, pesticides, polycyclic aromatic hydrocarbons, and environmental xenobiotics. The process by which the activity of these drug-metabolizing enzymes is increased is termed *enzyme induction*.[508–511] The increased activity is apparently caused by an increased amount of newly synthesized enzyme. Enzyme induction often increases the rate of drug metabolism and decreases the duration of drug action. (See Table 3.4 for a list of clinically significant drug–drug interactions based on one drug inducing the metabolism of a second drug.)

Inducing agents may increase the rate of their own metabolism as well as those of other unrelated drugs or foreign compounds (Table 3.4).[32] Concomitant administration of two or more drugs often may lead to serious drug interactions as a result of enzyme induction. For instance, a clinically critical drug interaction occurs with phenobarbital and warfarin.[512] Induction of microsomal enzymes by phenobarbital increases the metabolism of warfarin and, consequently, markedly decreases the anticoagulant effect. Therefore, if a patient is receiving warfarin anticoagulant therapy and begins taking phenobarbital, careful attention must be paid to readjustment of the warfarin dose. Dosage readjustment is also needed if a patient receiving both warfarin and phenobarbital therapy suddenly stops taking the barbiturate. The ineffectiveness of oral contraceptives in women on concurrent phenobarbital or rifampin therapy has been attributed to the enhanced metabolism of estrogens (e.g., 17α-ethinylestradiol) caused by phenobarbital[513] and rifampin[514] induction.

TABLE 3.4 Clinically Significant Cytochrome P450-Based Drug–Drug Interactions

Agent	Substrates	Inhibitors	Inducers	Agent	Substrates	Inhibitors	Inducers
CYP 1A2	Amitriptyline	Cimetidine	Carbamazepine		Imipramine		
	Clomipramine	Ciprofloxacin	Phenobarbital		Meperidine		
	Clozapine	Clarithromycin	Phenytoin		Methadone		
	Desipramine	Enoxacin	Primidone		Mexiletine		
	Fluvoxamine	Erythromycin	Rifampin		Nortriptyline		
	Haloperidol	Fluvoxamine	Ritonavir		Oxycodone		
	Imipramine	Isoniazid	Smoking		Propafenone		
	Ropinirole	Nalidixic acid	St. John's wort		Propoxyphene		
	Tacrine	Norfloxacin			Thioridazine		
	Theophylline	Troleandomycin			Tramadol		
	(R)-Warfarin	Zileuton			Trazodone		
CYP 2C9	Diazepam	Amiodarone	Carbamazepine		Alfentanil	Amiodarone	Carbamazepine
	Phenytoin	Chloramphenicol	Phenobarbital	CYP 3A4	Alprazolam	Cimetidine	Efavirenz
	(S)-Warfarin	Cimetidine	Phenytoin		Amlodipine	Ciprofloxacin	Ethosuximide
		Fluconazole	Primidone		Atorvastatin	Clarithromycin	Garlic supplements
		Fluoxetine	Rifampin		Busulfan	Cyclosporine	Modafinil
		Fluvoxamine	Rifapentine		Carbamazepine	Delavirdine	Nevirapine
		Isoniazid			Cisapride	Diltiazem	Oxcarbazepine
		Metronidazole			Clarithromycin	Efavirenz	Phenobarbital
		Voriconazole			Cyclosporine	Erythromycin	Phenytoin
		Zafirlukast			Dihydroergotamine	Fluconazole	Primidone
CYP 2C19	Phenytoin	Fluoxetine	Carbamazepine		Disopyramide	Fluoxetine	Rifabutin
	Thioridazine	Fluvoxamine	Phenobarbital		Doxorubicin	Fluvoxamine	Rifampin
		Modafinil	Phenytoin		Dronabinol	Grapefruit	Rifapentine
		Omeprazole			Ergotamine	Indinavir	St. John's wort
		Topiramate			Erythromycin	Isoniazid	
CYP 2D6	Amitriptyline	Amiodarone	St. John's wort		Estrogens, oral contraceptives	Itraconazole	
	Atomoxetine	Cimetidine			Ethinyl estradiol	Ketoconazole	
	Codeine	Fluoxetine			Ethosuximide	Metronidazole	
	Desipramine	Paroxetine			Etoposide	Miconazole	
	Dextromethorphan	Quinidine			Felodipine	Nefazodone	
	Donepezil	Ritonavir			Fentanyl	Nelfinavir	
	Doxepin	Sertraline			Indinavir	Nifedipine	
	Fentanyl				Isradipine	Norfloxacin	
	Flecainide				Itraconazole	Quinine	
	Haloperidol					Ritonavir	
	Hydrocodone						

Abstracted from Levien, T. L., and Baker, D. E.: Pharmacist's Letter, December 2002, Detail-Document #150400. (Pharmacist's Letter used as sources: Hansten, P. D., and Horn, J. R.: Drug Interactions Analysis and Management. Vancouver, WA, Applied Therapeutics, 2002; and Tatro, D. S. [ed.]: Drug Interaction Facts. St. Louis, Facts & Comparisons, 2002.)

Inducers of microsomal enzymes also may enhance the metabolism of endogenous compounds, such as steroidal hormones and bilirubin. For instance, phenobarbital can increase the metabolism of cortisol, testosterone, vitamin D, and bilirubin in humans.[508,509] The enhanced metabolism of vitamin D_3 induced by phenobarbital and phenytoin appears to be responsible for the osteomalacia seen in patients on long-term therapy with these two anticonvulsant drugs.[515] Interestingly, phenobarbital induces glucuronyltransferase enzymes, thereby enhancing the conjugation of bilirubin with glucuronic acid. Phenobarbital has been used occasionally to treat hyperbilirubinemia in neonates.[516]

In addition to drugs, other chemicals, such as polycyclic aromatic hydrocarbons (e.g., benzo[α]pyrene, 3-methyl-cholanthrene) and environmental pollutants (e.g., pesticides, PCBs, TCDD), may induce certain oxidative pathways and, thereby, alter drug response.[508,509,511] Cigarette smoke contains minute amounts of polycyclic aromatic hydrocarbons, such as benzo[α]pyrene, which are potent inducers of microsomal CYP enzymes. This induction increases the oxidation of some drugs in smokers. For example, theophylline is metabolized more rapidly in smokers than in nonsmokers. This difference is reflected in the marked difference in the plasma half-life of theophylline between smokers ($t_{1/2}$ 4.1 hours) and nonsmokers ($t_{1/2}$ 7.2 hours).[517] Other drugs, such as phenacetin, pentazocine, and propoxyphene, also reportedly undergo more rapid metabolism in smokers than in nonsmokers.[518–520]

Occupational and accidental exposure to chlorinated pesticides and insecticides can also stimulate drug metabolism. For instance, the half-life of antipyrine in workers occupationally exposed to the insecticides lindane and dichlorodiphenyltrichloroethane (DDT) is reportedly significantly shorter (7.7 vs. 11.7 hours) than in control subjects.[521] A case was reported in which a worker exposed to chlorinated insecticides failed to respond (i.e., decreased anticoagulant effect) to a therapeutic dose of warfarin.[522]

As discussed previously in this chapter, multiple forms (isozymes) of CYP have been demonstrated.[31,40–42] Many chemicals selectively induce one or more distinct forms of CYP[31] (see Table 3.4.) Enzyme induction also may affect toxicity of some drugs by enhancing the metabolic formation of chemically reactive metabolites. Particularly important is the induction of CYP enzymes involved in the oxidation of drugs to reactive intermediates. For example, the oxidation of acetaminophen to a reactive imidoquinone metabolite appears to be carried out by a phenobarbital-inducible form of CYP in rats and mice. Numerous studies in these two animals indicate that phenobarbital pretreatment increases in vivo hepatotoxicity and covalent binding as well as increases formation of reactive metabolite in microsomal incubation mixtures.[243–245,248] Induction of cytochrome P448 is of toxicological concern because this particular enzyme is involved in the metabolism of polycyclic aromatic hydrocarbons to reactive and carcinogenic intermediates.[80,523] Consequently, the metabolic bioactivation of benzo[α]pyrene to its ultimate carcinogenic diol epoxide intermediate is carried out by cytochrome P448 (see section on aromatic oxidation for the bioactivation pathway of benzo[α]pyrene to its diol epoxide).[523] Thus, it is becoming increasingly apparent that enzyme induction may enhance the toxicity of some xenobiotics by increasing the rate of formation of reactive metabolites.

Enzyme Inhibition

Several drugs, other xenobiotics including grapefruit, and possibly other foods can inhibit drug metabolism (Table 3.5).[32,483–486] With decreased metabolism, a drug often accumulates, leading to prolonged drug action and serious adverse effects. Enzyme inhibition can occur by diverse mechanisms, including substrate competition, interference with protein synthesis, inactivation of drug-metabolizing enzymes, and hepatotoxicity leading to impairment of enzyme activity. Some drug interactions resulting from enzyme inhibition have been reported in humans.[524,525] For example, phenylbutazone (limited to veterinary use) stereoselectively inhibits the metabolism of the more potent (S)(−) enantiomer of warfarin. This inhibition may explain the excessive hypoprothrombinemia (increased anticoagulant effect) and many instances of hemorrhaging seen in patients on both warfarin and phenylbutazone therapy.[56] The metabolism of phenytoin is inhibited by drugs such as chloramphenicol, disulfiram, and isoniazid.[512] Interestingly, phenytoin toxicity as a result of enzyme inhibition by isoniazid appears to occur primarily in slow acetylators.[464] Several drugs, such as dicumarol, chloramphenicol, and phenylbutazone,[512] inhibit the biotransformation of tolbutamide, which may lead to a hypoglycemic response.

The grapefruit–drug interaction is complex. It may be caused by the bioflavonoids or the furanocoumarins. Grapefruit's main bioflavonoid, naringin, is a weak CYP inhibitor, but the product of the intestinal flora, naringenin, does inhibit CYP3A4. The literature is very confusing because many of the studies were done in vitro, and they cannot always be substantiated under in vivo conditions. In addition, components in grapefruit also activate P-glycoprotein, which would activate the efflux pump in the gastric mucosa and thus interfere with oral absorption of the certain drugs. The combination of CYP enzyme inhibition and P-glycoprotein activation can lead to inconclusive results.[526] The general recommendation when a drug interaction is suspected is that the patient avoid grapefruit and its juice.

Miscellaneous Factors Affecting Drug Metabolism[32,483–486]

Other factors also may influence drug metabolism. Dietary factors, such as the protein-to-carbohydrate ratio, affect the metabolism of a few drugs. Indoles present in vegetables such as Brussels sprouts, cabbage, and cauliflower, and polycyclic aromatic hydrocarbons present in charcoal-broiled beef induce enzymes and stimulate the metabolism of some drugs. Vitamins, minerals, starvation, and malnutrition also apparently influence drug metabolism. Finally, physiological factors, such as the pathological state of the liver (e.g., hepatic cancer, cirrhosis, hepatitis), pregnancy, hormonal disturbances (e.g., thyroxine, steroids), and circadian rhythm, may markedly affect drug metabolism.

Stereochemical Aspects of Drug Metabolism

Many drugs (e.g., warfarin, propranolol, hexobarbital, glutethimide, cyclophosphamide, ketamine, and ibuprofen) often are administered as racemic mixtures in humans. The two enantiomers present in a racemic mixture may differ in pharmacological activity. Usually, one enantiomer tends to be much more active than the other. For example, the (S)(−)

TABLE 3.5 Potential Drug–Grapefruit Interactions Based on Grapefruit Inhibition of CYP 3A4

Drug	Result
Amiodarone	Increased bioavailability
Diazepam	Increased AUC
Carbamazepine	Increased AUC, peak and trough plasma concentrations
Cisapride	Increased AUC
Cyclosporine, tacrolimus	Increased AUC and serum concentrations
Atorvastatin, simvastatin	Increased absorption and plasma concentrations
Saquinavir	Increased absorption and plasma concentrations

Abstracted from Kehoe, W. A.: Pharmacist's Letter, 18, September 2002, Detail Document #180905.
AUC, area under the curve.

enantiomer of warfarin is 5 times more potent as an oral anticoagulant than the $(R)(+)$ enantiomer.[527] In some instances, the two enantiomers may have totally different pharmacological activities. For example, $(+)$-α-propoxyphene (Darvon) is an analgesic, whereas $(-)$-α-propoxyphene (Novrad) is an antitussive.[528] Such differences in activity between stereoisomers should not be surprising, because Chapter 2 explains that stereochemical factors generally have a dramatic influence on how the drug molecule interacts with the target receptors to elicit its pharmacological response. By the same token, the preferential interaction of one stereoisomer with drug-metabolizing enzymes may lead one to anticipate differences in metabolism for the two enantiomers of a racemic mixture. Indeed, individual enantiomers of a racemic drug often are metabolized at different rates. For instance, studies in humans indicate that the less active $(+)$ enantiomer of propranolol undergoes more rapid metabolism than the corresponding $(-)$ enantiomer.[529] Allylic hydroxylation of hexobarbital occurs more rapidly with the $R(-)$ enantiomer in humans.[530] The term *substrate stereoselectivity* is used frequently to denote a preference for one stereoisomer as a substrate for a metabolizing enzyme or metabolic process.[291]

Individual enantiomers of a racemic mixture also may be metabolized by different pathways. For instance, in dogs, the $(+)$ enantiomer of the sedative–hypnotic glutethimide (Doriden) is hydroxylated primarily α to the carbonyl to yield 4-hydroxyglutethimide, whereas the $(-)$ enantiomer undergoes aliphatic $\omega-1$ hydroxylation of its C-2 ethyl

group.[140,141] Dramatic differences in the metabolic profile of two enantiomers of warfarin also have been noted. In humans, the more active $(S)(-)$-isomer is 7-hydroxylated (aromatic hydroxylation), whereas the $(R)(+)$-isomer undergoes keto reduction to yield primarily the (R,S) warfarin alcohol as the major plasma metabolite.[56,296] Although numerous other examples of substrate stereoselectivity or enantioselectivity in drug metabolism exist, the examples presented should suffice to emphasize the point.[291,531]

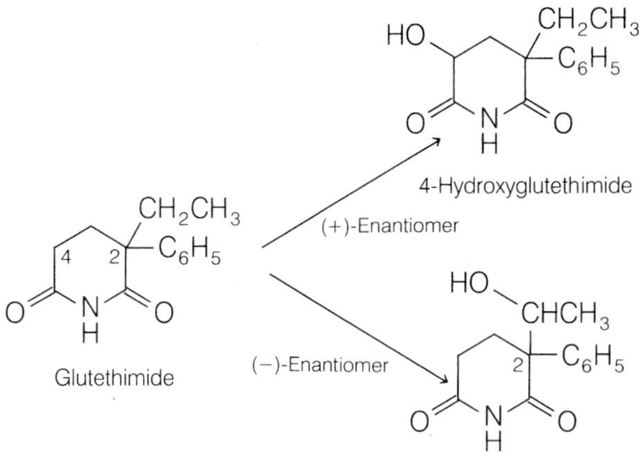

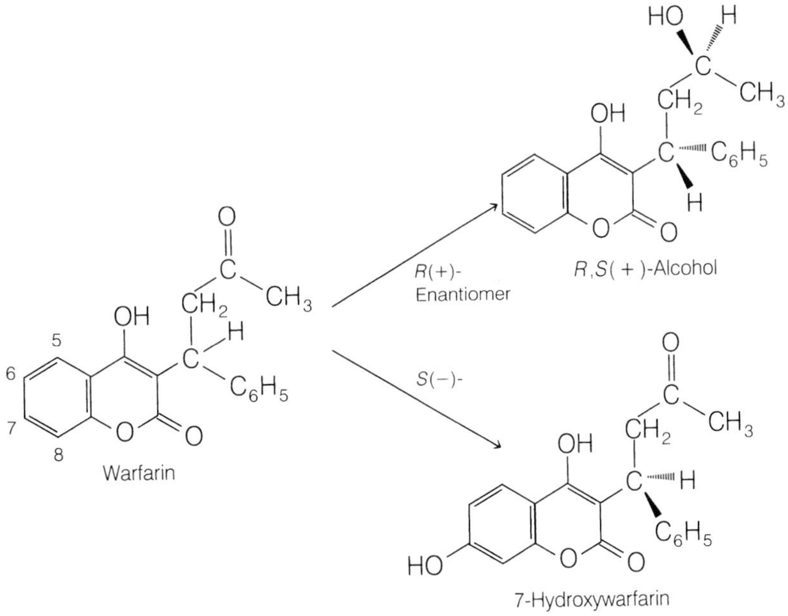

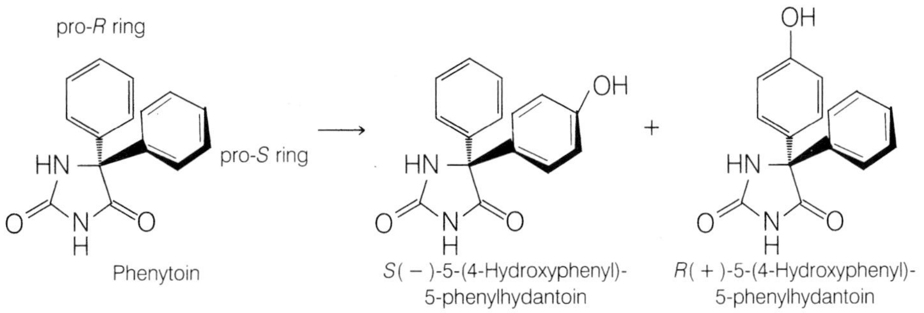

Drug biotransformation processes often lead to the creation of a new asymmetric center in the metabolite (i.e., stereoisomeric or enantiomeric products). The preferential metabolic formation of a stereoisomeric product is called *product stereoselectivity*.[291] Thus, bioreduction of ketone xenobiotics, as a general rule, produces predominantly one stereoisomeric alcohol (see "Reduction of Ketone Carbonyls").[116,291] The preferential formation of $(S)(-)$-hydroxyhexamide from the hypoglycemic agent acetohexamide[293,294] and the exclusive generation of 6β-naltrexol from naltrexone[297,298] (see "Reduction of Ketone Carbonyls" for structure) are two examples of highly stereoselective bioreduction processes in humans.

Oxidative biotransformations display product stereoselectivity, too. For example, phenytoin contains two phenyl rings in its structure, both of which a priori should be susceptible to aromatic hydroxylation. In humans, however, p-hydroxylation occurs preferentially ($\sim90\%$) at the pro-(S)-phenyl ring to give primarily $(S)(-)$-5-(4-hydroxyphenyl)-5-phenylhydantoin. Although the other phenyl ring also is p-hydroxylated, it occurs only to a minor extent (10%).[496] Microsomal hydroxylation of the C-3 carbon of diazepam and desmethyldiazepam (using mouse liver preparations) has been reported to proceed with remarkable stereoselectivity to yield optically active metabolites with the 3(S) absolute configuration.[139] Interestingly, these two metabolites are pharmacologically active and one of them, oxazepam, is marketed as a drug (Serax). The allylic hydroxylation of the N-butenyl side group of the analgesic pentazocine (Talwin) leads to two possible alcohols (*cis* and *trans* alcohols). In human, mouse, and monkey, pentazocine is metabolized predominantly to the *trans* alcohol metabolite, whereas the rat primarily tends to form the *cis* alcohol.[129,130] The product stereoselectivity observed in this biotransformation involves *cis* and *trans* geometric stereoisomers.

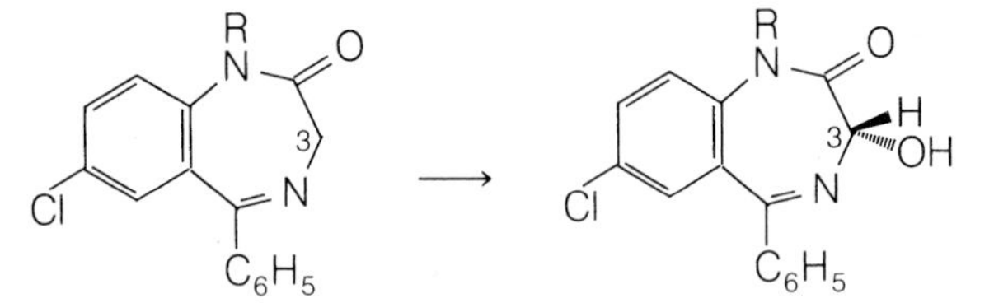

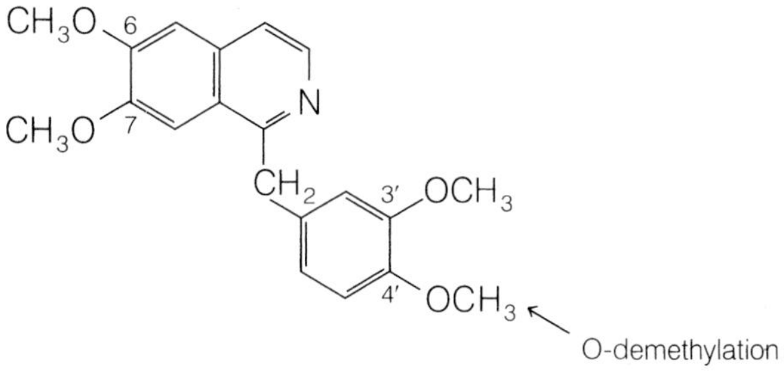

Papaverine

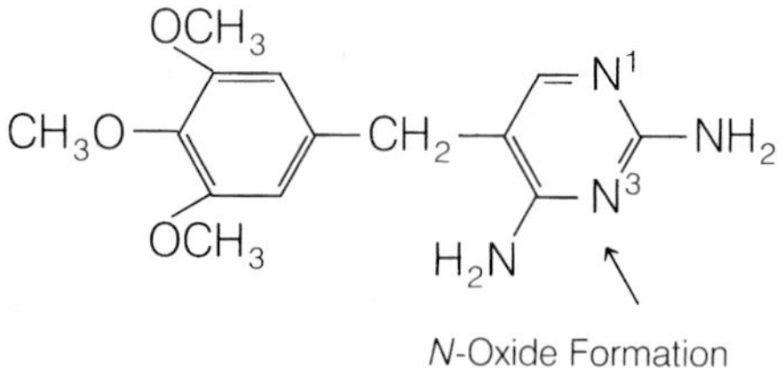

Trimethoprim

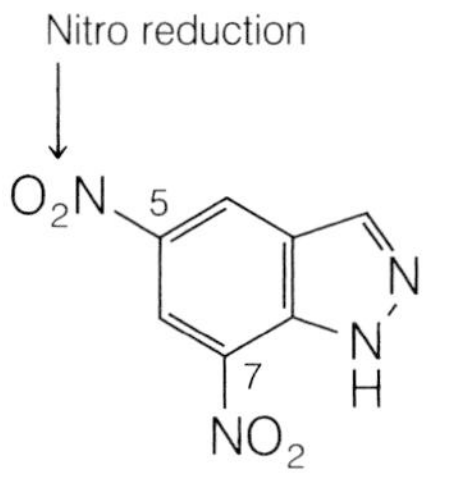

5,7-Dinitroindazole

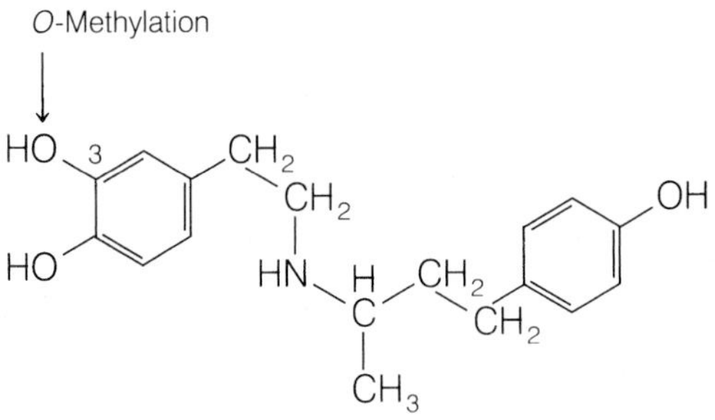

Diazepam, R = CH₃
Desmethyldiazepam, R = H

(3S) N-Methyloxazepam, R = CH₃
S(+)-Oxazepam, R = H

Dobutamine

The term *regioselectivity*[532] has been introduced in drug metabolism to denote the selective metabolism of two or more similar functional groups (e.g., OCH_3, OH, NO_2) or two or more similar atoms that are positioned in different regions of a molecule. For example, of the four methoxy groups present in papaverine, the 4-OCH_3 group is regioselectively O-demethylated in several species

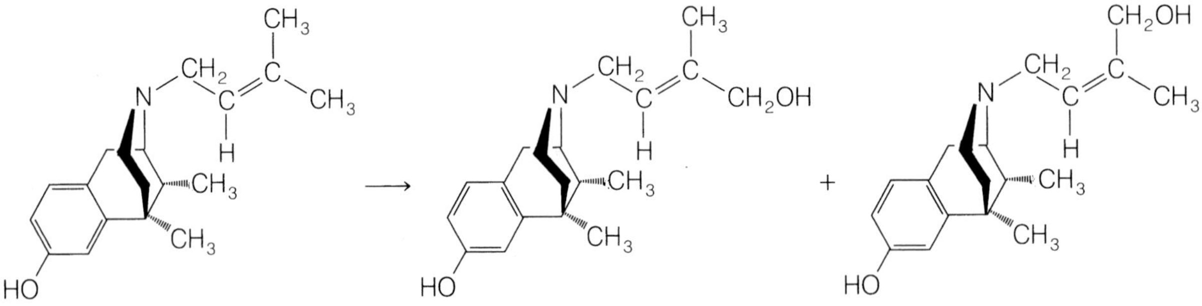

Pentazocine

trans-Alcohol

cis-Alcohol

(e.g., rat, guinea pig, rabbit, and dog).[533] Trimethoprim (Trimex, Proloprim) has two heterocyclic sp^2 nitrogen atoms (N^1 and N^3) in its structure. In dogs, it appears that oxidation occurs regioselectively at N^3 to give the corresponding 3-N-oxide.[232] Nitroreduction of the 7-nitro group in 5,7-dinitroindazole to yield the 7-amino derivative in the mouse and rat occurs with high regioselectivity.[534] Substrates amenable to *O*-methylation by COMT appear to proceed with remarkable regioselectivity, as typified by the cardiotonic agent dobutamine (Dobutrex). *O*-methylation occurs exclusively with the phenolic hydroxy group at C-3.[474]

Pharmacologically Active Metabolites

The traditional notion that drug metabolites are inactive and insignificant in drug therapy has changed dramatically in recent years. Increasing evidence indicates that many drugs are biotransformed to pharmacologically active metabolites that contribute to the therapeutic as well as toxic effects of the parent compound. Metabolites shown to have significant therapeutic activity in humans are listed in Table 3.4.[2,535] The parent drug from which the metabolite is derived and the biotransformation process involved also are given.

How significantly an active metabolite contributes to the therapeutic or toxic effects ascribed to the parent drug depend on its relative activity and quantitative importance (e.g., plasma concentration). In addition, whether the metabolite accumulates after repeated administration (e.g., desmethyldiazepam in geriatric patients) or in patients with renal failure is determinant.

From a clinical standpoint, active metabolites are especially important in patients with decreased renal function. If renal excretion is the major pathway for elimination of the active metabolite, then accumulation is likely to occur in patients with renal failure. Especially with drugs such as procainamide, clofibrate, and digitoxin, caution should be exercised in treating patients with renal failure.[2,413]

Many of the toxic effects seen for these drugs have been attributed to high-plasma levels of their active metabolites. For example, the combination of severe muscle weakness and tenderness (myopathy) seen with clofibrate in renal failure patients is believed to be caused by high levels of the active metabolite chlorophenoxyisobutyric acid.[536,537] Cardiovascular toxicity owing to digitoxin and procainamide in anephric subjects has been attributed to high plasma levels of digoxin and N-acetylprocainamide, respectively. In such situations, appropriate reduction in dosage and careful monitoring of plasma levels of the parent drug and its active metabolite often are recommended.

The pharmacological activity of some metabolites has led many manufacturers to synthesize these metabolites and to market them as separate drug entities (Table 3.6). For example, oxyphenbutazone (Tandearil, Oxalid) is the *p*-hydroxylated metabolite of the anti-inflammatory agent phenylbutazone (Butazolidin, Azolid), nortriptyline (Aventyl) is the N-demethylated metabolite of the tricyclic antidepressant amitriptyline (Elavil), oxazepam (Serax) is the N-demethylated and 3-hydroxylated metabolite of diazepam (Valium), and mesoridazine (Serentil) is the sulfoxide metabolite of the antipsychotic agent thioridazine (Mellaril).

Antivirals that are used in treating herpes simplex virus, varicella-zoster virus, and/or human cytomegalovirus must be bioactivated.[538] These include acyclovir, valacyclovir, penciclovir, famciclovir, and ganciclovir, which must be phosphorylated on the pentoselike side chain to the triphosphate derivative to be effective in inhibiting the enzyme DNA polymerase. The antiviral cidovir is dispensed as a monophosphate and only needs to be diphosphylated for conversion to the active triphosphate metabolite. The nucleoside antivirals that are used in treating acquired immunodeficiency syndrome/human immunodeficiency virus (AIDS/HIV) must also undergo a similar metabolic conversion to the triphosphate metabolite.[539] The triphosphate derivative acts as a competitive inhibitor of the enzyme, reverse transcriptase, which normally uses the triphosphorylated form of

TABLE 3.6 Pharmacologically Active Metabolites in Humans

Parent Drug	Metabolite	Biotransformation Process
Acetohexamide	Hydroxyhexamide	Ketone reduction
Acetylmethadol	Noracetylmethadol	*N*-Demethylation
Amitriptyline	Nortriptyline	*N*-Demethylation
Azathioprine	6-Mercaptopurine	Glutathione conjugation
Carbamazepine	Carbamazepine-9,10-epoxide	Epoxidation
Chloral hydrate	Trichloroethanol	Aldehyde reduction
Chlorpromazine	7-Hydroxychlorpromazine	Aromatic hydroxylation
Clofibrate	Chlorophenoxyisobutyric acid	Ester hydrolysis
Cortisone	Hydrocortisone	Ketone reduction
Diazepam	Desmethyldiazepam and oxazepam	*N*-Demethylation and 3-hydroxylation
Digitoxin	Digoxin	Alicyclic hydroxylation
Diphenoxylate	Diphenoxylic acid	Ester hydrolysis
Imipramine	Desipramine	*N*-Demethylation
Mephobarbital	Phenobarbital	*N*-Demethylation
Metoprolol	α-Hydroxymethylmetoprolol	Benzylic hydroxylation
Phenacetin	Acetaminophen	*O*-Deethylation
Phenylbutazone	Oxybutazone	Aromatic hydroxylation
Prednisone	Prednisolone	Ketone reduction
Primidone	Phenobarbital	Hydroxylation and oxidation to ketone
Procainamide	*N*-Acetylprocainamide	*N*-Acetylation
Propranolol	4-Hydroxypropranolol	Aromatic hydroxylation
Quinidine	3-Hydroxyquinidine	Allylic hydroxylation
Sulindac	Sulfide metabolite of sulindac	Sulfoxide reduction
Thioridazine	Mesoridazine	*S*-oxidation
Warfarin	Warfarin alcohols	Ketone reduction

nucleic acids. Examples include zidovudine, stavudine, zalcitabine, lamivudine, and didanosine.

One of the more recent uses of drug metabolism in the development of a novel agent includes the example of oseltamivir, a neuraminidase inhibitor used in treating influenza. Ro-64-0802, the lead drug, showed promise against both influenza A and B viruses in vitro but was not very effective when used in vivo. To improve the oral bioavailability, the ethyl ester, oseltamivir, was developed as a prodrug. Administration of the more lipophilic oseltamivir allowed good penetration of the active metabolite in various tissues, especially in the lower respiratory tract. The metabolism proceeds via a simple ester hydrolysis to yield the active free carboxylic acid.[540]

◆ R E V I E W   Q U E S T I O N S ◆

1. What would be the logical primary metabolite of a phase I reaction for the following drug molecule?

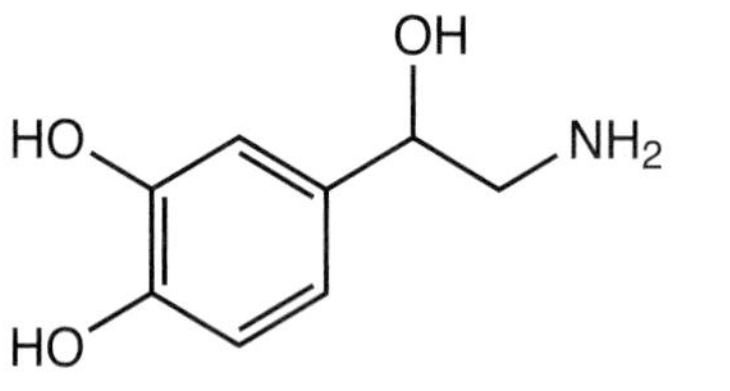

norepinephrine

a.

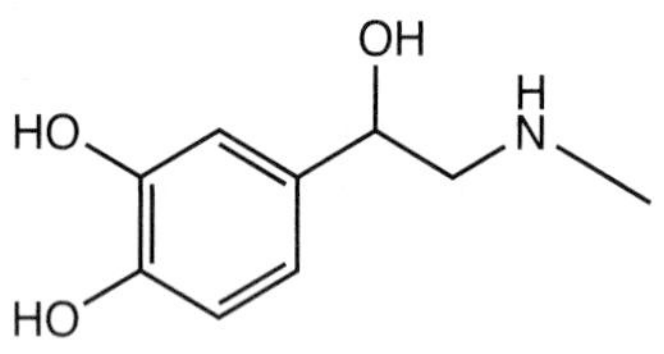

b.

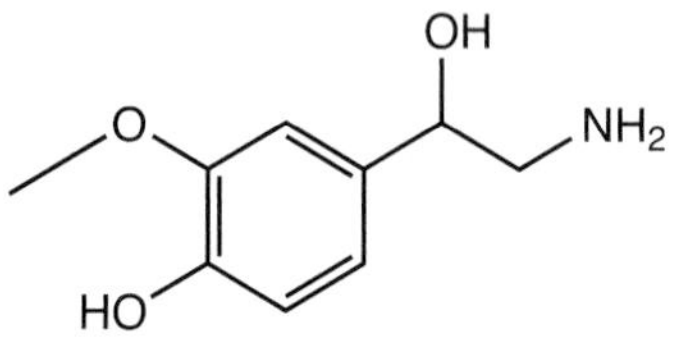

c.

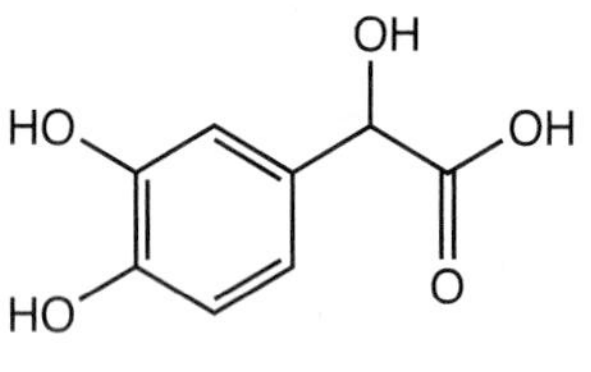

d.

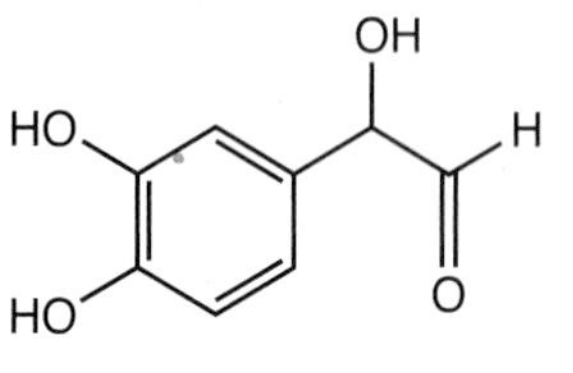

e.

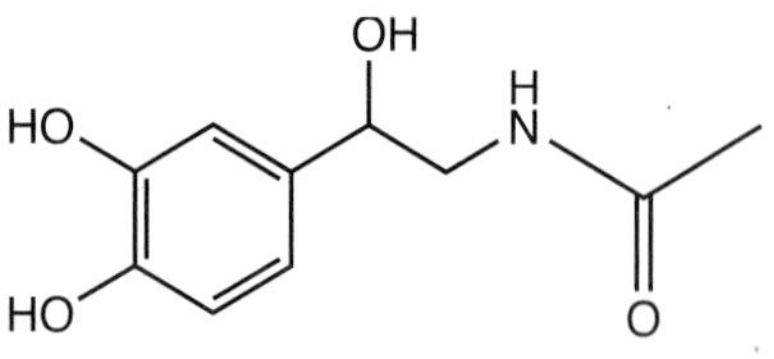

2. Using the agent represented, identify which of the following metabolic pathways might occur.

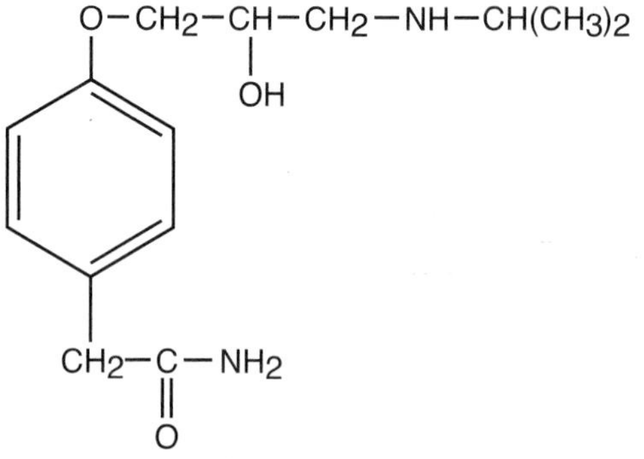

Atenolol (Tenormin)

a. hydrolysis by amidase enzymes
b. oxidative *N*-dealkylation
c. oxidative *O*-dealkylation
d. All of the above are possible.
e. Only a and b are correct.

3. Using the structure for Esmolol (Brevibloc), an antiarrhythmic beta-blocking agent, identify which of the following is/are true:

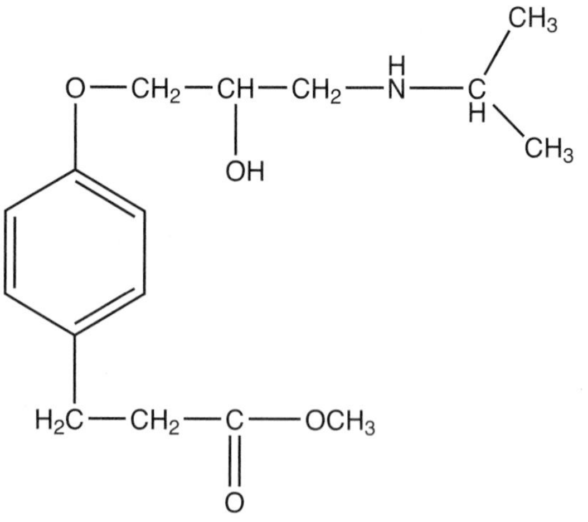

a. The agent has a very short $t_{1/2}$ because of its susceptibility of hydrolysis by esterases.
b. The agent is compatible with sodium bicarbonate.
c. The agent should not be "pushed" in an iv line that is supplying a drug to a patient that is buffered with bicarbonate.
d. All of the above are true.
e. Only a and c are true.

4. Explain your answer(s) for question number 3.

5. A patient you are monitoring has been on Telmisartan (Cozaar), an angiotensin receptor blocker for the management of their hypertension. The drug must be metabolized by CYP2C9 or CYP3A4 from a 5-methanol to a 5-carboxylic acid to exhibit its effects. After 2 years of successful therapy, their blood pressure suddenly increases. Why might this occur and what would you suggest as a substitute?

REFERENCES

1. Williams, R. T.: Detoxication Mechanisms, 2nd ed. New York, John Wiley & Sons, 1959.
2. Drayer, D. E.: Clin. Pharmacokinet. 1:426, 1976.
3. Drayer, D. E.: Drugs 24:519, 1982.
4. Jollow, D. J., et al.: Biological Reactive Intermediates. New York, Plenum Press, 1977.
5. Gillette, J. R., et al.: Annu. Rev. Pharmacol. 14:271, 1974.
6. Nelson, S. D., et al.: In Jerina, D. M. (ed.). Drug Metabolism Concepts. Washington, DC, American Chemical Society, 1977, p. 155.
7. Testa, B., and Jenner, P.: Drug Metab. Rev. 7:325, 1978.
8. Low, L. K., and Castagnoli, N., Jr.: In Wolff, M. E. (ed.). Burger's Medicinal Chemistry, Part 1, 4th ed. New York, Wiley-Interscience, 1980, p. 107.
9. Gill, E. W., et al.: Biochem. Pharmacol. 22:175, 1973.
10. Wall, M. E., et al.: J. Am. Chem. Soc. 94:8579, 1972.
11. Lemberger, L.: Drug Metab. Dispos. 1:641, 1973.
12. Green, D. E., et al.: In Vinson, J. A. (ed.). Cannabinoid Analysis in Physiological Fluids. Washington, DC, American Chemical Society, 1979, p. 93.
13. Williams, R. T.: In Brodie, B. B., and Gillette, J. R. (eds.). Concepts in Biochemical Pharmacology, Part 2. Berlin, Springer-Verlag, 1971, p. 226.
14. Rowland, M.: In Melmon, K. L., and Morelli, H. F. (eds.). Clinical Pharmacology: Basic Principles in Therapeutics, 2nd ed. New York, Macmillan, 1978, p. 25.
15. Benowitz, N. L., and Meister, W.: Clin. Pharmacokinet. 3:177, 1978.
16. Connolly, M. E., et al.: Br. J. Pharmacol. 46:458, 1972.
17. Gibaldi, M., and Perrier, D.: Drug Metab. Rev. 3:185, 1974.
18. Sinkula, A. A., and Yalkowsky, S. H.: J. Pharm. Sci. 64:181, 1975.
19. Scheline, R. R.: Pharmacol. Rev. 25:451, 1973.
20. Peppercorn, M. A., and Goldman, P.: J. Pharmacol. Exp. Ther. 181:555, 1972.
21. Levy, G. A., and Conchie, J.: In Dutton, G. J. (ed.). Glucuronic Acid, Free and Combined. New York, Academic Press, 1966, p. 301.
22. Testa, B., and Jenner, P.: Drug Metabolism: Chemical and Biochemical Aspects. New York, Marcel Dekker, 1976, p. 419.
23. Powis, G., and Jansson, I.: Pharmacol. Ther. 7:297, 1979.
24. Mason, H. S.: Annu. Rev. Biochem. 34:595, 1965.
25. Hayaishi, O.: In Hayaishi, O. (ed.). Oxygenases. New York, Academic Press, 1962, p. 1.
26. Mannering, G. J.: In LaDu, B. N., et al. (eds.). Fundamentals of Drug Metabolism and Disposition. Baltimore, Williams & Wilkins, 1971, p. 206.
27. Sato, R., and Omura, T. (eds.): Cytochrome P-450. New York, Academic Press, 1978.
28. Omura, T., and Sato, R.: J. Biol. Chem. 239:2370, 1964.
29. Gillette, J. R.: Adv. Pharmacol. 4:219, 1966.
30. Nelson, D. R., Koymans, L., Kamataki, T., et al.: Pharmacogenetics 6:1, 1996.
31. Schuetz, E. G.: Curr. Drug Metab. 2:139, 2001.
32. Claude, A.: In Gillette, J. R., et al. (eds.). Microsomes and Drug Oxidations. New York, Academic Press, 1969, p. 3.
33. Hansch, D.: Drug Metab. Rev. 1:1, 1972.
34. Ortiz de Montellano, P. R.: Cytochrome P-450. New York, Plenum Press, 1986, p. 217.
35. Estabrook, R. W., and Werringloer, J.: In Jerina, D. M. (ed.). Drug Metabolism Concepts. Washington, DC, American Chemical Society, 1977, p. 1.
36. Trager, W. F.: In Jenner, P., and Testa, B. (eds.). Concepts in Drug Metabolism, Part A. New York, Marcel Dekker, 1980, p. 177.
37. Ullrich, V.: Top. Curr. Chem. 83:68, 1979.
38. White, R. E., and Coon, M. J.: Annu. Rev. Biochem. 49:315, 1980.
39. Guengerich, F. P. (ed.): Mammalian Cytochromes P-450, vols. 1 and 2. Boca Raton, FL, CRC Press, 1987.
40. Schenkman, J. B., and Kupfer, D. (eds.): Hepatic Cytochrome P-450 Monooxygenase System. New York, Pergamon Press, 1982.
41. Ioannides, C. (ed.): Cytochromes P450: Metabolic and Toxicological Aspects. Boca Raton, FL, CRC Press, 1996.
42. Guengerich, F. P.: Curr. Drug Metab. 2:93, 2001.
43. Daly, J. W., et al.: Experientia 28:1129, 1972.
44. Jerina, D. M., and Daly, J. W.: Science 185:573, 1974.
45. Kaminsky, L. S.: In Anders, M. W. (ed.). Bioactivation of Foreign Compounds. New York, Academic Press, 1985, p. 157.
46. Walle, T., and Gaffney, T. E.: J. Pharmacol. Exp. Ther. 182:83, 1972.
47. Bond, P.: Nature 213:721, 1967.
48. Whyte, M. P., and Dekaban, A. S.: Drug Metab. Dispos. 5:63, 1977.
49. Witkin, K. M., et al.: Ther. Drug Monit. 1:11, 1979.
50. Richens, A.: Clin. Pharmacokinet. 4:153, 1979.
51. Burns, J. J., et al.: J. Pharmacol. Exp. Ther. 113:481, 1955.
52. Yü, T. F., et al.: J. Pharmacol. Exp. Ther. 123:63, 1958.
53. Black A. E., Hayes R. N., Roth B. D., et al.: Drug Metab. Dispos. 27(8):916, 1999.
54. Williams, M. C., et al.: Steroids 25:229, 1975.
55. Ranney, R. E.: J. Toxicol. Environ. Health 3:139, 1977.
56. Lewis, R. J., et al.: J. Clin. Invest. 53:1697, 1974.
57. Daly, J.: In Brodie, B. B., and Gillette, J. R. (eds.). Concepts in Biochemical Pharmacology, Part 2. Berlin, Springer-Verlag, 1971, p. 285.
58. Lowenthal, D. T.: J. Cardiovasc. Pharmacol. 2(Suppl. 1):S29, 1980.
59. Davies, D. S., et al.: Adv. Pharmacol. Ther. 7:215, 1979.
60. Dayton, P. G., et al.: Drug Metab. Dispos. 1:742, 1973.
61. Schreiber, E. E.: Annu. Rev. Pharmacol. 10:77, 1970.
62. Hollister, L. E., et al.: Res. Commun. Chem. Pathol. Pharmacol. 2:330, 1971.
63. Safe, S., et al.: J. Agric. Food Chem. 23:851, 1975.
64. Allen, J. R., et al.: Food Cosmet. Toxicol. 13:501, 1975.
65. Vinopal, J. H., et al.: Arch. Environ. Contamin. Toxicol. 1:122, 1973.
66. Hathway, D. E. (Sr. Reporter): Foreign Compound Metabolism in Mammals, vol. 4. London, Chemical Society, 1977, p. 234.
67. Guroff, G., et al.: Science 157:1524, 1967.
68. Daly, J., et al.: Arch. Biochem. Biophys. 128:517, 1968.
69. Oesch, F.: Prog. Drug Metab. 3:253, 1978.
70. Lu, A. A. H., and Miwa, G. T.: Annu. Rev. Pharmacol. Toxicol. 20:513, 1980.
71. Ames, B. N., et al.: Science 176:47, 1972.
72. Maguire, J. H., et al.: Ther. Drug Monit. 1:359, 1979.
73. Harvey, D. G., et al.: Res. Commun. Chem. Pathol. Pharmacol. 3:557, 1972.
74. Stillwell, W. G.: Res. Commun. Chem. Pathol. Pharmacol. 12:25, 1975.
75. Jakoby, W. B., et al.: In Arias, I. M., and Jakoby, W. B. (eds.). Glutathione, Metabolism and Function. New York, Raven Press, 1976, p. 189.
76. Boyland, E.: In Brodie, B. B., and Gillette, J. R. (eds.). Concepts in Biochemical Pharmacology, Part 2. Berlin, Springer-Verlag, 1971, p. 584.
77. Brodie, B. B., et al.: Proc. Natl. Acad. Sci. U. S. A. 68:160, 1971.
78. Jollow, D. J., et al.: Pharmacology 11:151, 1974.
79. Gelboin, H. V., et al.: In Jollow, D. J., et al. (eds.). Biological Reactive Intermediates. New York, Plenum Press, 1977, p. 98.
80. Thakker, D. R., et al.: Chem. Biol. Interact. 16:281, 1977.
81. Weinstein, I. B., et al.: Science 193:592, 1976.
82. Jeffrey A. M., et al.: J. Am. Chem. Soc. 98:5714, 1976.
83. Koreeda, M., et al.: J. Am. Chem. Soc. 98:6720, 1976.
84. Straub, K. M., et al.: Proc. Natl. Acad. Sci. U. S. A. 74:5285, 1977.
85. Kasai, H., et al.: J. Am. Chem. Soc. 99:8500, 1977.
86. Chausseaud, L. F.: Drug Metab. Rev. 2:185, 1973.
87. Pynnönen, S.: Ther. Drug Monit. 1:409, 1979.
88. Eadie, M. J., and Tyrer, J. H.: Anticonvulsant Therapy, 2nd ed. Edinburgh, Churchill-Livingstone, 1980, p. 142.
89. Hucker, H. B., et al.: Drug Metab. Dispos. 3:80, 1975.
90. Hintze, K. L., et al.: Drug Metab. Dispos. 3:1, 1975.

91. Slack, J. A., and Ford-Hutchinson, A. W.: Drug Metab. Dispos. 8:84, 1980.
92. Waddell, W. J.: J. Pharmacol. Exp. Ther. 149:23, 1965.
93. Seutter-Berlage, F., et al.: Xenobiotica 8:413, 1978.
94. Marniemi, J., et al.: In Ullrich, V., et al. (eds.). Microsomes and Drug Oxidations. Oxford, Pergamon Press, 1977, p. 698.
95. Garner, R. C.: Prog. Drug Metab. 1:77, 1976.
96. Swenson, D. H., et al.: Biochem. Biophys. Res. Commun. 60:1036, 1974.
97. Swenson, D. H., et al.: Biochem. Biophys. Res. Commun. 53:1260, 1973.
98. Essigman, J. M., et al.: Proc. Natl. Acad. Sci. U. S. A. 74:1870, 1977.
99. Croy, R. G., et al.: Proc. Natl. Acad. Sci. U. S. A. 75:1745, 1978.
100. Henschler, D., and Bonser, G.: Adv. Pharmacol. Ther. 9:123, 1979.
101. Watabe, T., and Akamatsu, K.: Biochem. Pharmacol. 24:442, 1975.
102. Metzler, M.: J. Toxicol. Environ. Health 1(Suppl.):21, 1976.
103. Neuman, H. G., and Metzler, M.: Adv. Pharmacol. Ther. 9:113, 1979.
104. Ortiz de Montellano, P. R., and Correia, M. A.: Annu. Rev. Pharmacol. Toxicol. 23:481, 1983.
105. Ortiz de Montellano, P. R.: In Anders, M. W. (ed.). Bioactivation of Foreign Compounds. New York, Academic Press, 1985, p. 121.
106. DeMatteis, F.: Biochem. J. 124:767, 1971.
107. Levin, W., et al.: Arch. Biochem. Biophys. 148:262, 1972.
108. Levin, W., et al.: Science 176:1341, 1972.
109. Levin, W., et al.: Drug Metab. Dispos. 1:275, 1973.
110. Ivanetich, K. M., et al.: In Ullrich, V., et al. (eds.). Microsomes and Drug Oxidations. Oxford, Pergamon Press, 1977, p. 76.
111. Ortiz de Montellano, P. R., et al.: Biochem. Biophys. Res. Commun. 83:132, 1978.
112. Ortiz de Montellano, P. R., et al.: Arch. Biochem. Biophys. 197:524, 1979.
113. Ortiz de Montellano, P. R., et al.: Biochemistry 21:1331, 1982.
114. Beckett, A. H., and Rowland, M.: J. Pharm. Pharmacol. 17:628, 1965.
115. Dring, L. G., et al.: Biochem. J. 116:425, 1970.
116. McMahon, R. E.: In Brodie, B. B., and Gillette, J. R. (eds.). Concepts in Biochemical Pharmacology, Part 2. Berlin, Springer-Verlag, 1971, p. 500.
117. Dutton, G.: In Brodie, B. B., and Gillette, J. R. (eds.). Concepts in Biochemical Pharmacology, Part 2. Berlin, Springer-Verlag, 1971, p. 378.
118. Thomas, R. C., and Ikeda, G. J.: J. Med. Chem. 9:507, 1966.
119. Selley, M. L., et al.: Clin. Pharmacol. Ther. 17:599, 1975.
120. Sumner, D. D., et al.: Drug Metab. Dispos. 3:283, 1975.
121. Tang C., Shou M., Mei Q., et al.: J. Pharmacol. Exp. Ther. 293(2):453, 2000.
122. Borg, K. O., et al.: Acta Pharmacol. Toxicol. 36(Suppl. 5):125, 1975.
123. Hoffmann, K. J.: Clin. Pharmacokinet. 5:181, 1980.
124. Lemberger, L., et al.: Science 173:72, 1971.
125. Lemberger, L., et al.: Science 177:62, 1972.
126. Carroll, F. I., et al.: J. Med. Chem. 17:985, 1974.
127. Drayer, D. E., et al.: Clin. Pharmacol. Ther. 27:72, 1980.
128. Drayer, D. E., et al.: Clin. Pharmacol. Ther. 24:31, 1978.
129. Bush, M. T., and Weller, W. L.: Drug Metab. Rev. 1:249, 1972.
130. Thompson, R. M., et al.: Drug Metab. Dispos. 1:489, 1973.
131. Breimer, D. D., and Van Rossum, J. M.: J. Pharm. Pharmacol. 25:762, 1973.
132. Pittman, K. A., et al.: Biochem. Pharmacol. 18:1673, 1969.
133. Pittman, K. A., et al.: Biochem. Pharmacol. 19:1833, 1970.
134. Miller, J. A., and Miller, E. C.: In Jollow, D. J., et al. (eds.). Biological Reactive Intermediates. New York, Plenum Press, 1977, p. 14.
135. Wislocki, P. G., et al.: Cancer Res. 36:1686, 1976.
136. Garattini, S., et al.: In Usdin, E., and Forrest, I. (eds.). Psychotherapeutic Drugs, Part 2. New York, Marcel Dekker, 1977, p. 1039.
137. Greenblatt, D. J., et al.: Clin. Pharmacol. Ther. 17:1, 1975.
138. Yanagi, Y., et al.: Xenobiotica 5:245, 1975.
139. Corbella, A., et al.: J. Chem. Soc. Chem. Commun. 721, 1973.
140. Keberle, H., et al.: Arch. Int. Pharmacodyn. 142:117, 1963.
141. Keberle, H., et al.: Experientia 18:105, 1962.
142. Ferrandes, B., and Eymark, P.: Epilepsia, 18:169, 1977.
143. Kuhara, T., and Matsumoto, J.: Biomed. Mass Spectrom. 1:291, 1974.
144. Maynert, E. W.: J. Pharmacol. Exp. Ther. 150:117, 1965.
145. Palmer, K. H.: J. Pharmacol. Exp. Ther. 175:38, 1970.
146. Holtzmann, J. L., and Thompson, J. A.: Drug Metab. Dispos. 3:113, 1975.
147. Carroll, F. J., et al.: Drug Metab. Dispos. 5:343, 1977.
148. Thomas, R. C., and Judy, R. W.: J. Med. Chem. 15:964, 1972.
149. Adams, S. S., and Buckler, J. W.: Clin. Rheum. Dis. 5:359, 1979.
150. Ludwig, B. J., et al.: J. Med. Pharm. Chem. 3:53, 1961.
151. Horning, M. G., et al.: Drug Metab. Dispos. 1:569, 1973.
152. Dieterle, W., et al.: Arzneimittelforschung 26:572, 1976.
153. McMahon, R. E., et al.: J. Pharmacol. Exp. Ther. 149:272, 1965.
154. Fuccella, L. M., et al.: J. Clin. Pharmacol. 13:68, 1973.
155. Lin, D. C. K., et al.: Biomed. Mass Spectrom. 2:206, 1975.
156. Wong, L. K., and Biemann, K.: Clin. Toxicol. 9:583, 1976.
157. Thomas, R. C., et al.: J. Pharm. Sci. 64:1360, 1366, 1975.
158. Gottlieb, T. B., et al.: Clin. Pharmacol. Ther. 13:436, 1972.
159. Gorrod, J. W. (ed.): Biological Oxidation of Nitrogen. Amsterdam, Elsevier-North Holland, 1978.
160. Gorrod, J. W.: Chem. Biol. Interact. 7:289, 1973.
161. Ziegler, D. M., et al.: Drug Metab. Dispos. 1:314, 1973.
162. Ziegler, D. M., et al.: Arch. Biochem. Biophys. 150:116, 1972.
163. Gram, T. E.: In Brodie, B. B., and Gillette, J. R. (eds.). Concepts in Biochemical Pharmacology, Part 2. Berlin, Springer-Verlag, 1971, p. 334.
164. Brodie, B. B., et al.: Annu. Rev. Biochem. 27:427, 1958.
165. McMahon, R. E.: J. Pharm. Sci. 55:457, 1966.
166. Crammer, J. L., and Scott, B.: Psychopharmacologia 8:461, 1966.
167. Nagy, A., and Johansson, R.: Arch. Pharm. (Weinheim) 290:145, 1975.
168. Gram, L. F., et al.: Psychopharmacologia 54:255, 1977.
169. Collinsworth, K. A., et al.: Circulation 50:1217, 1974.
170. Narang, P. K., et al.: Clin. Pharmacol. Ther. 24:654, 1978.
171. Hutsell, T. C., and Kraychy, S. J.: J. Chromatogr. 106:151, 1975.
172. Heel, R. C., et al.: Drugs 15:331, 1978.
173. Adam, H. K., et al.: Biochem. Pharmacol. 27:145, 1979.
174. Chang, T. K., et al.: Res. Commun. Chem. Pathol. Pharmacol. 9:391, 1974.
175. Glazko, A. J., et al.: Clin. Pharmacol. Ther. 16:1066, 1974.
176. Hammar, C. G., et al.: Anal. Biochem. 25:532, 1968.
177. Beckett, A. H., et al.: J. Pharm. Pharmacol. 25:188, 1973.
178. Due, S. L., et al.: Biomed. Mass Spectrom. 3:217, 1976.
179. Beckett, A. H., et al.: J. Pharm. Pharmacol. 23:812, 1971.
180. Pohland, A., et al.: J. Med. Chem. 14:194, 1971.
181. Bruce, R. B., et al.: J. Med. Chem. 11:1031, 1968.
182. Szeto, H. H., and Inturri, C. E.: J. Chromatogr. 125:503, 1976.
183. Misra, A. L.: In Adler, M. L., et al. (eds.). Factors Affecting the Action of Narcotics. New York, Raven Press, 1978, p. 297.
184. Kamm, J. J., et al.: J. Pharmacol. Exp. Ther. 182:507, 1972.
185. Kamm, J. J., et al.: J. Pharmacol. Exp. Ther. 184:729, 1973.
186. Goldberg, M. E. (ed.): Pharmacological and Biochemical Properties of Drug Substances, vol. 1. Washington, DC, American Pharmaceutical Association, 1977, pp. 257, 311.
187. Gorrod, J. W., and Jenner, P.: Essays Toxicol. 6:35, 1975.
188. Beckett, A. H., and Triggs, E. J.: Nature 211:1415, 1966.
189. Hucker, H. B., et al.: Drug Metab. Dispos. 2:406, 1974.
190. Wold, J. S., and Fischer, L. J.: J. Pharmacol. Exp. Ther. 183:188, 1972.
191. Kaiser, C., et al.: J. Med. Chem. 15:1146, 1972.
192. Bickel, M. H.: Pharmacol. Rev. 21:325, 1969.
193. Jenner, P.: In Gorrod, J. W. (ed.). Biological Oxidation of Nitrogen. Amsterdam, Elsevier-North Holland, 1978, p. 383.
194. Faurbye, A., et al.: Am. J. Psychiatry 120:277, 1963.
195. Theobald, W., et al.: Med. Pharmacol. Exp. 15:187, 1966.
196. Coutts, R., and Beckett, A. H.: Drug Metab. Rev. 6:51, 1977.
197. Leinweber, F. J., et al.: J. Pharm. Sci. 66:1570, 1977.
198. Beckett, A. H., and Rowland, M.: J. Pharm. Pharmacol. 17:109S, 1965.
199. Caldwell, J., et al.: Biochem. J. 129:11, 1972.
200. Wieber, J., et al.: Anesthesiology 24:260, 1975.
201. Chang, T., and Glazko, A. J.: Anesthesiology 21:401, 1972.
202. Tindell, G. L., et al.: Life Sci. 11:1029, 1972.
203. Franklin, R. B., et al.: Drug Metab. Dispos. 5:223, 1977.
204. Barlett, M. F., and Egger, H. P.: Fed. Proc. 31:537, 1972.
205. Beckett, A. H., and Gibson, G. G.: Xenobiotica 8:73, 1978.
206. Benedetti, M. S.: Fundam. Clin. Pharmacol. 15:75, 2001.
207. Beckett, A. H., and Brookes, L. G.: J. Pharm. Pharmacol. 23:288, 1971.

208. Charalampous, K. D., et al.: J. Pharmacol. Exp. Ther. 145:242, 1964.
209. Charalampous, K. D., et al.: Psychopharmacologia 9:48, 1966.
210. Ho, B. T., et al.: J. Med. Chem. 14:158, 1971.
211. Matin, S., et al.: J. Med. Chem. 17:877, 1974.
212. Au, W. Y. W., et al.: Biochem. J. 129:110, 1972.
213. Parli, C. J., et al.: Biochem. Biophys. Res. Commun. 43:1204, 1971.
214. Lindeke, B., et al.: Acta Pharm. Suecica 10:493, 1973.
215. Hucker, H. B.: Drug Metab. Dispos. 1:332, 1973.
216. Parli, C. H., et al.: Drug Metab. Dispos. 3:337, 1973.
217. Wright, J., et al.: Xenobiotica 7:257, 1977.
218. Gal, J., et al.: Res. Commun. Chem. Pathol. Pharmacol. 15:525, 1976.
219. Beckett, A. H., and Bélanger, P. M.: J. Pharm. Pharmacol. 26:205, 1974.
220. Bélanger, P. M., and Grech-Bélanger, O.: Can. J. Pharm. Sci. 12:99, 1977.
221. Weisburger, J. H., and Weisburger, E. K.: Pharmacol. Rev. 25:1, 1973.
222. Miller, E. C., and Miller, J. A.: Pharmacol. Rev. 18:805, 1966.
223. Weisburger, J. H., and Weisburger, E. K.: In Brodie, B. B., and Gillette, J. R. (eds.). Concepts in Biochemical Pharmacology, Part 2. Berlin, Springer-Verlag, 1971, p. 312.
224. Uehleke, H.: Xenobiotica 1:327, 1971.
225. Beckett, A. H., and Bélanger, P. M.: Biochem. Pharmacol. 25:211, 1976.
226. Israili, Z. H., et al.: J. Pharmacol. Exp. Ther. 187:138, 1973.
227. Kiese, M.: Pharmacol. Rev. 18:1091, 1966.
228. Lin, J. K., et al.: Cancer Res. 35:844, 1975.
229. Poirer, L. A., et al.: Cancer Res. 27:1600, 1967.
230. Lin, J. K., et al.: Biochemistry 7:1889, 1968.
231. Lin, J. K., et al.: Biochemistry 8:1573, 1969.
232. Schwartz, D. E., et al.: Arzneimittelforschung 20:1867, 1970.
233. Dagne, E., and Castagnoli, N., Jr.: J. Med. Chem. 15:840, 1972.
234. Essien E. E., Ogonor, J. I., Coker H. A., et al.: J. Pharm. Pharmacol. 39(10):843, 1987.
235. Garrattini, S., et al.: Drug Metab. Rev. 1:291, 1972.
236. Brotherton, P. M., et al.: Clin. Pharmacol. Ther. 10:505, 1969.
237. Langone, J. J., et al.: Biochemistry 12:5025, 1973.
238. Grochow, L. B., and Colvin, M.: Clin. Pharmacokinet. 4:380, 1979.
239. Colvin, M., et al.: Cancer Res. 33:915, 1973.
240. Connors, T. A., et al.: Biochem. Pharmacol. 23:115, 1974.
241. Irving, C. C.: In Fishman, W. H. (ed.). Metabolic Conjugation and Metabolic Hydrolysis, vol. 1. New York, Academic Press, 1970, p. 53.
242. Miller, J., and Miller, E. C.: In Jollow, D. J., et al. (eds.). Biological Reactive Intermediates. New York, Plenum Press, 1970, p. 6.
243. Jollow, D. J., et al.: J. Pharmacol. Exp. Ther. 187:195, 1973.
244. Prescott, L. F., et al.: Lancet 1:519, 1971.
245. Hinson, J. A.: Rev. Biochem. Toxicol. 2:103, 1980.
246. Hinson, J. A., et al.: Life Sci. 24:2133, 1979.
247. Nelson, S. D., et al.: Biochem. Pharmacol. 29:1617, 1980.
248. Potter, W. Z., et al.: J. Pharmacol. Exp. Ther. 187:203, 1973.
249. Adler, T. K., et al.: J. Pharmacol. Exp. Ther. 114:251, 1955.
250. Brodie, B. B., and Axelrod, J.: J. Pharmacol. Exp. Ther. 97:58, 1949.
251. Duggan, D. E., et al.: J. Pharmacol. Exp. Ther. 181:563, 1972.
252. Kwan, K. C., et al.: J. Pharmacokinet. Biopharm. 4:255, 1976.
253. Brogden, R. N., et al.: Drugs 14:163, 1977.
254. Taylor, J. A., et al.: Xenobiotica 7:357, 1977.
255. Daly, J., et al.: Ann. N. Y. Acad. Sci. 96:37, 1962.
256. Mazel, P., et al.: J. Pharmacol. Exp. Ther. 143:1, 1964.
257. Sarcione, E. J., and Stutzman, L.: Cancer Res. 20:387, 1960.
258. Elion, G. B., et al.: Proc. Am. Assoc. Cancer Res. 3:316, 1962.
259. Taylor, J. A.: Xenobiotica 3:151, 1973.
260. Brodie, B. B., et al.: J. Pharmacol. Exp. Ther. 98:85, 1950.
261. Spector, E., and Shideman, F. E.: Biochem. Pharmacol. 2:182, 1959.
262. Neal, R. A.: Arch. Intern. Med. 128:118, 1971.
263. Neal, R. A.: Biochem. J. 103:183, 1967.
264. Neal, R. A.: Rev. Biochem. Toxicol. 2:131, 1980.
265. Gruenke, L., et al.: Res. Commun. Chem. Pathol. Pharmacol. 10:221, 1975.
266. Zehnder, K., et al.: Biochem. Pharmacol. 11:535, 1962.
267. Aguilar, S. J.: Dis. Nerv. Syst. 36:484, 1975.
268. Taylor, D. C., et al.: Drug Metab. Dispos. 6:21, 1978.
269. Taylor, D. C.: In Wood, C. J., and Simkins, M. A. (eds.). International Symposium on Histamine H$_2$-Receptor Antagonists. Welwyn Garden City, UK, Smith, Kline & French, 1973, p. 45.
270. Crew, M. C., et al.: Xenobiotica 2:431, 1972.
271. Hucker, H. B., et al.: J. Pharmacol. Exp. Ther. 154:176, 1966.
272. Hucker, H. B., et al.: J. Pharmacol. Exp. Ther. 155:309, 1967.
273. Hathway, D. E. (Sr. Reporter): Foreign Compound Metabolism in Mammals, vol. 3. London, Chemical Society, 1975, p. 512.
274. Schwartz, M. A., and Kolis, S. J.: Drug Metab. Dispos. 1:322, 1973.
275. Sisenwine, S. F., et al.: Drug Metab. Dispos. 3:180, 1975.
276. McCallum, N. K.: Experientia 31:957, 1975.
277. McCallum, N. K.: Experientia 31:520, 1975.
278. Cohen, E. N., and Van Dyke, R. A.: Metabolism of Volatile Anesthetics. Reading, MA, Addison-Wesley, 1977.
279. Cohen, E. N., et al.: Anesthesiology 43:392, 1975.
280. Van Dyke, R. A., et al.: Drug Metab. Dispos. 3:51, 1975
281. Van Dyke, R. A., et al.: Drug Metab. Dispos. 4:40, 1976.
282. Pohl, L.: Rev. Biochem. Toxicol. 1:79, 1979.
283. Pohl, L., et al.: Biochem. Pharmacol. 27:335, 1978.
284. Pohl, L., et al.: Biochem. Pharmacol. 27:491, 1978.
285. Parke, D. V.: The Biochemistry of Foreign Compounds. Oxford, Pergamon Press, 1968, p. 218.
286. Gillette, J. R.: In Brodie, B. B., and Gillette, J. R. (eds.). Concepts in Biochemical Pharmacology, Part 2. Berlin, Springer-Verlag, 1971, p. 349.
287. Bachur, N. R.: Science 193:595, 1976.
288. Sellers, E. M., et al.: Clin. Pharmacol. Ther. 13:37, 1972.
289. Pritchard, J. F., et al.: J. Chromatogr. 162:47, 1979.
290. Osterloh, J. D., et al.: Drug Metab. Dispos. 8:12, 1980.
291. Jenner, P., and Testa, B.: Drug Metab. Rev. 2:117, 1973.
292. Culp, H. W., and McMahon, R. E.: J. Biol. Chem. 243:848, 1968.
293. McMahon, R. E., et al.: J. Pharmacol. Exp. Ther. 149:272, 1965.
294. Galloway, J. A., et al.: Diabetes 16:118, 1967.
295. Yü, T. F., et al.: Metabolism 17:309, 1968.
296. Chan, K. K., et al.: J. Med. Chem. 15:1265, 1972.
297. Pollock, S. H., and Blum, K.: In Blum, K., et al. (eds.). Alcohol and Opiates. New York, Academic Press, 1977, p. 359.
298. Chatterjie, N., et al.: Drug Metab. Dispos. 2:401, 1974.
299. Dayton, H., and Inturrisi, C. E.: Drug Metab. Dispos. 4:474, 1974.
300. Roerig, S., et al.: Drug Metab. Dispos. 4:53, 1976.
301. Malsperis, L., et al.: Res. Commun. Chem. Pathol. Pharmacol. 14:393, 1976.
302. Bachur, N. R., and Felsted, R. L.: Drug Metab. Dispos. 4:239, 1976.
303. Crew, M. C., et al.: Clin. Pharmacol. Ther. 14:1013, 1973.
304. DiCarlo, F. J., et al.: Xenobiotica 2:159, 1972.
305. Crew, M. C., et al.: Xenobiotica 2:431, 1972.
306. DiCarlo, F. J., et al.: J. Reticuloendothel. Soc. 14:387, 1973.
307. Gerhards, E., et al.: Acta Endocrinol. 68:219, 1971.
308. Wright, J., et al.: Xenobiotica 7:257, 1977.
309. Kawai, K., and Baba, S.: Chem. Pharm. Bull. (Tokyo) 24:2728, 1976.
310. Gillette, J. R., et al.: Mol. Pharmacol. 4:541, 1968.
311. Fouts, J. R., and Brodie, B. B.: J. Pharmacol. Exp. Ther. 119:197, 1957.
312. Hernandez, P. H., et al.: Biochem. Pharmacol. 16:1877, 1967.
313. Scheline, R. R.: Pharmacol. Rev. 25:451, 1973.
314. Walker, R.: Food Cosmet. Toxicol. 8:659, 1970.
315. Min, B. H., and Garland, W. A.: J. Chromatogr. 139:121, 1977.
316. Rieder, J., and Wendt, G.: In Garattini, S., et al. (eds.). The Benzodiazepines. New York, Raven Press, 1973, p. 99.
317. Conklin, J. D., et al.: J. Pharm. Sci. 62:1024, 1973.
318. Cox, P. L., et al.: J. Pharm. Sci. 58:987, 1969.
319. Stambaugh, J. E., et al.: J. Pharmacol. Exp. Ther. 161:373, 1968.
320. Mitchard, M.: Xenobiotica 1:469, 1971.
321. Glazko, A. J., et al.: J. Pharmacol. Exp. Ther. 96:445, 1949.
322. Smith, G. N., and Worrel, G. S.: Arch. Biochem. Biophys. 24:216, 1949.
323. Tréfouël, J., et al.: C. R. Seances Soc. Biol. Paris 190:756, 1935.
324. Jones, R., et al.: Food Cosmet. Toxicol. 2:447, 1966.
325. Jones, R., et al.: Food Cosmet. Toxicol. 4:419, 1966.
326. Ikeda, M., and Uesugi, T.: Biochem. Pharmacol. 22:2743, 1973.
327. Peppercorn, M. A., and Goldman, P.: J. Pharmacol. Exp. Ther. 181:555, 1972.
328. Das, E. M.: Scand. J. Gastroenterol. 9:137, 1974.
329. Schröder, H., and Gustafsson, B. E.: Xenobiotica 3:225, 1973.
330. Bickel, M. H., and Gigon, P. L.: Xenobiotica 1:631, 1971.
331. Eldjarn, L.: Scand. J. Clin. Lab. Invest. 2:202, 1950.
332. Staub, H.: Helv. Physiol. Acta 13:141, 1955.
333. Duggan, D. E., et al.: Clin. Pharmacol. Ther. 21:326, 1977.
334. Duggan, D. E., et al.: J. Pharmacol. Exp. Ther. 20:8, 1977.

335. Kolb, H. K., et al.: Arzneimittelforschung 15:1292, 1965.
336. LaDu, B. N., and Snady, H.: In Brodie, B. B., and Gillette, J. R. (eds.). Concepts in Biochemical Pharmacology, Part 2. Berlin, Springer-Verlag, 1971, p. 477.
337. Junge, W., and Krisch, K.: CRC Crit. Rev. Toxicol. 3:371, 1975.
338. Davison, C.: Ann. N. Y. Acad. Sci. 179:249, 1971.
339. Kogan, M. J., et al.: Anal. Chem. 49:1965, 1977.
340. Inaba, T., et al.: Clin. Pharmacol. Ther. 23:547, 1978.
341. Stewart, D. J., et al.: Life Sci. 1557, 1977.
342. Wells, R., et al.: Clin. Chem. 20:440, 1974.
343. Rubens, R., et al.: Arzneimittelforschung 22:256, 1972.
344. Gugler, L., and Jensen, C.: J. Chromatogr. 117:175, 1976.
345. Houin, G., et al.: Eur. J. Clin. Pharmacol. 8:433, 1975.
346. Sinkula, A. A., et al.: J. Pharm. Sci. 62:1106, 1973.
347. Martin, A. R.: In Wilson, C. O., et al. (eds.). Textbook of Organic Medicinal and Pharmaceutical Chemistry, 7th ed. Philadelphia, J. B. Lippincott, 1977, p. 304.
348. Knirsch, A. K., et al.: J. Infect. Dis. 127:S105, 1973.
349. Stella, V.: In Higuchi, T., and Stella, V. (eds.): Prodrugs as Novel Drug Delivery Systems. Washington, DC, American Chemical Society, 1975, p. 1.
350. Mark, L. C., et al.: J. Pharmacol. Exp. Ther. 102:5, 1951.
351. Nelson, S. D., et al.: J. Pharm. Sci. 66:1180, 1977.
352. Tsukamoto, H., et al.: Chem. Pharm. Bull. (Tokyo) 3:459, 1955.
353. Tsukamoto, H., et al.: Chem. Pharm. Bull. (Tokyo) 3:397, 1955.
354. Dudley, K. H., et al.: Drug Metab. Dispos. 6:133, 1978.
355. Dudley, K. H., et al.: Drug Metab. Dispos. 2:103, 1974.
356. Humphrey, M. J., and Ringrose, P. S.: Drug Metab. Rev. 17:283, 1986.
357. Kompella, U. B., and Lee, V. H. L.: Adv. Parenteral Sci. 4:391, 1992.
358. Moore, J. A., and Wroblewski, V. J.: In Ferraiolo, B. L., et al. (eds.). Protein Pharmacokinetics and Metabolism. New York, Plenum Press, 1992, p. 93.
359. Dutton, G. J., et al.: In Parke, D. V., and Smith, R. L. (eds.). Drug Metabolism: From Microbe to Man. London, Taylor & Francis, 1977, p. 71.
360. Dutton, G. J.: In Dutton, G. J. (ed.). Glucuronic Acid, Free and Combined. New York, Academic Press, 1966, p. 186.
361. Dutton, G. D., et al.: Prog. Drug Metab. 1:2, 1977.
362. Brunk, S. F., and Delle, M.: Clin. Pharmacol. Exp. Ther. 16:51, 1974.
363. Berkowitz, B. A., et al.: Clin. Pharmacol. Exp. Ther. 17:629, 1975.
364. Andrews, R. S., et al.: J. Int. Med. Res. 4(Suppl. 4):34, 1976.
365. Thies, R. L., and Fischer, L. J.: Clin. Chem. 24:778, 1978.
366. Walle, T., et al.: Fed. Proc. 35:665, 1976.
367. Walle, T., et al.: Clin. Pharmacol. Ther. 26:167, 1979.
368. Roseman, S., et al.: J. Am. Chem. Soc. 76:1650, 1954.
369. Segre, E. J.: J. Clin. Pharmacol. 15:316, 1975.
370. Rubin, A., et al.: J. Pharm. Sci. 61:739, 1972.
371. Rubin, A., et al.: J. Pharmacol. Exp. Ther. 183:449, 1972.
372. Bridges, J. W., et al.: Biochem. J. 118:47, 1970.
373. Gibson, T., et al.: Br. J. Clin. Pharmacol. 2:233, 1975.
374. Tsuichiya, T., and Levy, G.: J. Pharm. Sci. 61:800, 1972.
375. Porter, C. C., et al.: Drug Metab. Dispos. 3:189, 1975.
376. Chaundhuri, N. K., et al.: Drug Metab. Dispos. 4:372, 1976.
377. Sitar, D. S., and Thornhill, D. P.: J. Pharmacol. Exp. Ther. 184:432, 1973.
378. Lindsay, R. H., et al.: Pharmacologist 18:113, 1976.
379. Sitar, D. S., and Thornhill, D. P.: J. Pharmacol. Exp. Ther. 183:440, 1972.
380. Dutton, G. J., and Illing, H. P. A.: Biochem. J. 129:539, 1972.
381. Dieterle, W., et al.: Arzneimittelforschung 26:572, 1976.
382. Richter, J. W., et al.: Helv. Chim. Acta 58:2512, 1975.
383. Dieterle, W., et al.: Eur. J. Clin. Pharmacol. 9:135, 1975.
384. Schmid, R., and Lester, R.: In Dutton, G. J. (ed.). Glucuronic Acid, Free and Combined. New York, Academic Press, 1966, p. 493.
385. Hadd, H. E., and Blickenstaff, R. T.: Conjugates of Steroid Hormones. New York, Academic Press, 1969.
386. Smith, R. L.: The Excretory Function of Bile: The Elimination of Drugs and Toxic Substance in Bile. London, Chapman & Hall, 1973.
387. Stern, L., et al.: Am. J. Dis. Child. 120:26, 1970.
388. Weiss, C. F., et al.: N. Engl. J. Med. 262:787, 1960.
389. Dodgson, K. S.: In Parke, D. V., and Smith, R. L. (eds.). Drug Metabolism: From Microbe to Man. London, Taylor & Francis, 1977, p. 91.
390. Roy, A. B.: In Brodie, B. B., and Gillette, J. R. (eds.). Concepts in Biochemical Pharmacology, Part 2. Berlin, Springer-Verlag, 1971, p. 536.
391. Williams, R. T.: In Bernfeld, P. (ed.). Biogenesis of Natural Products, 2nd ed. Oxford, Pergamon Press, 1967, p. 611.
392. Roy, A. B.: Adv. Enzymol. 22:205, 1960.
393. Kwan, K. C., et al.: J. Pharmacol. Exp. Ther. 198:264, 1976.
394. Stenback, O., et al.: Eur. J. Clin. Pharmacol. 12:117, 1977.
395. Lin, C., et al.: Drug Metab. Dispos. 5:234, 1977.
396. Nilsson, H. T., et al.: Xenobiotica 2:363, 1972.
397. Miller, R. P., et al.: Clin. Pharmacol. Ther. 19:284, 1976.
398. Levy, G., et al.: Pediatrics 55:818, 1975.
399. James, S. P., and Waring, R. H.: Xenobiotica 1:572, 1971.
400. Bostrum, H., and Vestermark, A.: Acta Physiol. Scand. 48:88, 1960.
401. Boyland, E., et al.: Biochem. J. 65:417, 1957.
402. Roy, A. B.: Biochem. J. 74:49, 1960.
403. Irving, C. C.: In Gorrod, J. W. (ed.). Biological Oxidation of Nitrogen. Amsterdam, Elsevier-North Holland, 1978, p. 325.
404. Irving, C. C.: Cancer Res. 35:2959, 1975.
405. Jackson, C. D., and Irving, C. C.: Cancer Res. 32:1590, 1972.
406. Hinson, J. A., and Mitchell, J. R.: Drug Metab. Dispos. 4:430, 1975.
407. Mulder, G. J., et al.: Biochem. Pharmacol. 26:189, 1977.
408. Weber, W.: In Brodie, B. B., and Gillette, J. R. (eds.). Concepts in Biochemical Pharmacology, Part 2. Berlin, Springer-Verlag, 1971, p. 564.
409. Williams, R. T., and Millburn, P.: In Blaschko, H. K. F. (ed.). MTP International Review of Science, Biochemistry Series One, vol. 12, Physiological and Pharmacological Biochemistry. Baltimore, University Park Press, 1975, p. 211.
410. Bridges, J. W., et al.: Biochem. J. 118:47, 1970.
411. Wan, S. H., and Riegelman, S.: J. Pharm. Sci. 61:1284, 1972.
412. Von Lehmann, B., et al.: J. Pharm. Sci. 62:1483, 1973.
413. Braun, G. A., et al.: Eur. J. Pharmacol. 1:58, 1967.
414. Tatsumi, K, et al.: Biochem. Pharmacol. 16:1941, 1967.
415. Weber, W. W., and Hein, D. W.: Clin. Pharmacokinet. 4:401, 1979.
416. James, M. O., et al.: Proc. R. Soc. Lond. B. Biol. Sci. 182:25, 1972.
417. Smith, R. L., and Caldwell, J.: In Parke, D. V., and Smith, R. L. (eds.). Drug Metabolism: From Microbe to Man. London, Taylor & Francis, 1977, p. 331.
418. Williams, R. T.: Clin. Pharmacol. Ther. 4:234, 1963.
419. Drach, J. C., et al.: Proc. Soc. Exp. Biol. Med. 135:849, 1970.
420. Caldwell, J.: In Jenner, P., and Testa, B. (eds.). Concepts in Drug Metabolism, Part A. New York, Marcel Dekker, 1980, p. 211.
421. Jerina, D. M., and Bend, J. R.: In Jollow, D. J., et al. (eds.). Biological Reactive Intermediates. New York, Plenum Press, 1977, p. 207.
422. Chasseaud, L. F.: In Arias, I. M., and Jakoby, W. B. (eds.). Glutathione: Metabolism and Function. New York, Raven Press, 1976, p. 77.
423. Ketterer, B.: Mutat. Res. 202:343, 1988.
424. Mantle, T. J., Pickett, C. B., and Hayes, J. D. (eds.): Glutathione S-Transferases and Carcinogenesis. London, Taylor & Francis, 1987.
425. Foureman, G. L., and Reed, D. J.: Biochemistry 26:2028, 1987.
426. Rannung, U., et al.: Chem. Biol. Interact. 20:1, 1978.
427. Olson, W. A., et al.: J. Natl. Cancer Inst. 51:1993, 1973.
428. Monks, T. J., and Lau, S. S.: Toxicology 52:1, 1988.
429. Weisburger, E. K.: Annu. Rev. Pharmacol. Toxicol. 18:395, 1978.
430. Hollingworth, R. M., et al.: Life Sci. 13:191, 1973.
431. Benke, G. M., and Murphy, S. D.: Toxicol. Appl. Pharmacol. 31:254, 1975.
432. Bray, H. G., et al.: Biochem. J. 67:607, 1957.
433. Chalmers, A. H.: Biochem. Pharmacol. 23:1891, 1974.
434. de Miranda, P., et al.: J. Pharmacol. Exp. Ther. 187:588, 1973.
435. de Miranda, P., et al.: J. Pharmacol. Exp. Ther. 195:50, 1975.
436. Elion, G. B.: Fed. Proc. 26:898, 1967.
437. Jerina, D. M.: In Arias, I. M., and Jakoby, W. B. (eds.). Glutathione: Metabolism and Function. New York, Raven Press, 1976, p. 267.
438. Needleman, P.: In Needleman, P. (ed.). Organic Nitrates. Berlin, Springer-Verlag, 1975, p. 57.
439. Klaasen, C. D., and Fitzgerald, T. J.: J. Pharmacol. Exp. Ther. 191:548, 1974.
440. Kuss, E., et al.: Hoppe Seyler Z. Physiol. Chem. 352:817, 1971.
441. Nelson, S. D., et al.: Biochem. Biophys. Res. Commun. 70:1157, 1976.
442. Weber, W.: In Fishman, W. H. (ed.). Metabolic Conjugation and Metabolic Hydrolysis, vol. 3. New York, Academic Press, 1973, p. 250.

443. Williams, R. T.: Fed. Proc. 26:1029, 1967.
444. Elson, J., et al.: Clin. Pharmacol. Ther. 17:134, 1975.
445. Drayer, D. E., et al.: Proc. Soc. Exp. Biol. Med. 146:358, 1974.
446. Mitchell, J. R., et al.: Ann. Intern. Med. 84:181, 1976.
447. Nelson, S. D., et al.: Science 193:193, 1976.
448. Giardina, E. G., et al.: Clin. Pharmacol. Ther. 19:339, 1976.
449. Giardina, E. G., et al.: Clin. Pharmacol. Ther. 17:722, 1975.
450. Peters, J. H., and Levy, L.: Ann. N. Y. Acad. Sci. 179:660, 1971.
451. Reimerdes, E., and Thumim, J. H.: Arzneimittelforschung 20:1171, 1970.
452. Vree, T. B., et al.: In Merkus, F. W. H. M. (ed.). The Serum Concentration of Drugs. Amsterdam, Excerpta Medica, 1980, p. 205.
453. Garrett, E. R.: Int. J. Clin. Pharmacol. 16:155, 1978.
454. Reidenberg, M. W., et al.: Clin. Pharmacol. Ther. 14:970, 1973.
455. Israili, Z. H., et al.: Drug Metab. Rev. 6:283, 1977.
456. Evans, D. A. P., et al.: Clin. Pharmacol. Ther. 6:430, 1965.
457. Tabor, H., et al.: J. Biol. Chem. 204:127, 1953.
458. Sullivan, H. R., and Due, S. L.: J. Med. Chem. 16:909, 1973.
459. Sullivan, H. R., et al.: J. Am. Chem. Soc. 94:4050, 1972.
460. Sullivan, H. R., et al.: Life Sci. 11:1093, 1972.
461. Drayer, D. E., and Reidenberg, M. M.: Clin. Pharmacol. Ther. 22:251, 1977.
462. Lunde, P. K. M., et al.: Clin. Pharmacokinet. 2:182, 1977.
463. Kalow, W.: Pharmacogenetics: Heredity and the Response to Drugs. Philadelphia, W. B. Saunders, 1962.
464. Kutt, H., et al.: Am. Rev. Respir. Dis. 101:377, 1970.
465. Alarcon-Segovia, D.: Drugs 12:69, 1976.
466. Reidenberg, M. M., and Martin, J. H.: Drug Metab. Dispos. 2:71, 1974.
467. Strong, J. M., et al.: J. Pharmacokinet. Biopharm. 3:233, 1975.
468. Axelrod, J.: In Brodie, B. B., and Gillette, J. R. (eds.). Concepts in Biochemical Pharmacology, Part 2. Berlin, Springer-Verlag, 1971, p. 609.
469. Mudd, S. H.: In Fishman, W. H. (ed.). Metabolic Conjugation and Metabolic Hydrolysis, vol. 3. New York, Academic Press, p. 297.
470. Young, J. A., and Edwards, K. D. G.: Med. Res. 1:53, 1962.
471. Young, J. A., and Edwards, K. D. G.: J. Pharmacol. Exp. Ther. 145:102, 1964.
472. Shindo, H., et al.: Chem. Pharm. Bull. (Tokyo) 21:826, 1973.
473. Morgan, C. D., et al.: Biochem. J. 114:8P, 1969.
474. Weber, R., and Tuttle, R. R.: In Goldberg, M. E. (ed.). Pharmacological and Biochemical Properties of Drug Substances, vol. 1. Washington, DC, American Pharmaceutical Association, 1977, p. 109.
475. Glazko, A. J.: Drug Metab. Dispos. 1:711, 1973.
476. Börner, U., and Abbott, S.: Experientia 29:180, 1973.
477. Bleidner, W. E., et al.: J. Pharmacol. Exp. Ther. 150:484, 1965.
478. Komori, Y., and Sendju, Y.: J. Biochem. 6:163, 1926.
479. Lindsay, R. H., et al.: Biochem. Pharmacol. 24:463, 1975.
480. Bremer, J., and Greenberg, D. M.: Biochim. Biophys. Acta 46:217, 1961.
481. Allan, P. W., et al.: Biochim. Biophys. Acta 114:647, 1966.
482. Elion, G. B.: Fed. Proc. 26:898, 1967.
483. Testa, B., and Jenner, P.: Drug Metabolism: Chemical and Biochemical Aspects. New York, Marcel Dekker, 1976, pp. 329–418.
484. Testa, B., and Jenner, P.: Drug Metab. Rev. 12:1, 1981.
485. Murray, M., and Reidy, G. F.: Pharmacol. Ther. 42:85, 1990.
486. Murray, M.: Clin. Pharmacokinet. 23:132, 1992.
487. Ward, R. M., et al.: In Avery, G. S. (ed.). Drug Treatment, 2nd ed. Sydney, ADIS Press, 1980, p. 76.
488. Morselli, P. L.: Drug Disposition During Development. New York, Spectrum, 1977.
489. Jondorf, W. R., et al.: Biochem. Pharmacol. 1:352, 1958.
490. Nitowsky, H. M., et al.: J. Pediatr. 69:1139, 1966.
491. Crooks, J., et al.: Clin. Pharmacokinet. 1:280, 1976.
492. Crooks, J., and Stevenson, I. H. (eds.): Drugs and the Elderly. London, Macmillan, 1979.
493. Williams, R. T.: Ann. N. Y. Acad. Sci. 179:141, 1971.
494. Williams, R. T.: In LaDu, B. N., et al. (eds.). Fundamentals of Drug Metabolism and Disposition. Baltimore, Williams & Wilkins, 1971, p. 187.
495. Williams, R. T., et al.: In Snyder, S. H., and Usdin, E. (eds.). Frontiers in Catecholamine Research. New York, Pergamon Press, 1973 p. 927.
496. Butler, T. C., et al.: J. Pharmacol. Exp. Ther. 199:82, 1976.
497. Williams, R. T.: Biochem. Soc. Trans. 2:359, 1974.
498. Bridges, J. W., et al.: Biochem. J. 118:47, 1970.
499. Williams, R. T.: Fed. Proc. 26:1029, 1967.
500. Thomas, B. H., et al.: J. Pharm. Sci., 79:321, 1990.
501. Cram, R. L., et al.: Proc. Soc. Exp. Biol. Med. 118:872, 1965.
502. Kutt, H., et al.: Neurology 14:542, 1962.
503. Vesell, E. S.: Prog. Med. Genet. 9:291, 1973.
504. Pelkonen, O., et al.: In Pacifici, G. M., and Pelkonen, O. (eds.). Interindividual Variability in Human Drug Metabolism. New York, Taylor & Francis, 2001, p. 269.
505. Kato, R.: Drug Metab. Rev. 3:1, 1974.
506. Beckett, A. H., et al.: J. Pharm. Pharmacol. 23:62S, 1971.
507. Menguy, R., et al.: Nature 239:102, 1972.
508. Conney, A. H.: Pharmacol. Rev. 19:317, 1967.
509. Snyder, R., and Remmer, H.: Pharmacol. Ther. 7:203, 1979.
510. Parke, D. V.: In Parke, D. V. (ed.). Enzyme Induction. London, Plenum Press, 1975, p. 207.
511. Estabrook, R. W., and Lindenlaub, E. (eds.): The Induction of Drug Metabolism. Stuttgart, Schattauer Verlag, 1979.
512. Hansten, P. D.: Drug Interactions, 4th ed. Philadelphia, Lea & Febiger, 1979, p. 38.
513. Laenger, H., and Detering, K.: Lancet 600, 1974.
514. Skolnick, J. L., et al.: JAMA 236:1382, 1976.
515. Dent, C. E., et al.: Br. Med. J. 4:69, 1970.
516. Yeung, C. Y., and Field, C. E.: Lancet 135, 1969.
517. Jenne, J., et al.: Life Sci. 17:195, 1975.
518. Pantuck, E. J., et al.: Science 175:1248, 1972.
519. Pantuck, E. J., et al.: Clin. Pharmacol. Ther. 14:259, 1973.
520. Vaughan, D. P., et al.: Br. J. Clin. Pharmacol. 3:279, 1976.
521. Kolmodin, B., et al.: Clin. Pharmacol. Ther. 10:638, 1969.
522. Jeffrey, W. H., et al.: JAMA 236:2881, 1976.
523. Gelboin, H. V., and Ts'o, P. O. P. (eds.): Polycyclic Hydrocarbons and Cancer: Environment, Chemistry, Molecular and Cell Biology. New York, Academic Press, 1978.
524. Vesell, E. S., and Passananti, G. T.: Drug Metab. Dispos. 1:402, 1973.
525. Anders, M. W.: Annu. Rev. Pharmacol. 11:37, 1971.
526. Kehoe, W. A.: Pharmacist's Letter, 18:#180905, September 2002.
527. Hewick, D., and McEwen, J.: J. Pharm. Pharmacol. 25:458, 1973.
528. Casy, A. F.: In Burger, A. (ed.). Medicinal Chemistry, Part 1, 3rd ed. New York, Wiley-Interscience, 1970, p. 81.
529. George, C. F., et al.: Eur. J. Clin. Pharmacol. 4:74, 1972.
530. Breimer, D. D., and Van Rossum, J. M.: J. Pharm. Pharmacol. 25:762, 1973.
531. Low, L. K., and Castagnoli, N., Jr.: Annu. Rep. Med. Chem. 13:304, 1978.
532. Testa, B., and Jenner, P.: J. Pharm. Pharmacol. 28:731, 1976.
533. Belpaire, F. M., et al.: Xenobiotica 5:413, 1975.
534. Woolhouse, N. M., et al.: Xenobiotica 3:511, 1973.
535. Drayer, D. E.: US Pharm. (Hosp. Ed.) 5:H15, 1980.
536. Pierides, A. M., et al.: Lancet 2:1279, 1975.
537. Gabriel, R., and Pearce, J. M. S.: Lancet 2:906, 1976.
538. Gallois-Montbrun, S., Schneider, B., Chen, Y., et al.: J. Biol. Chem. 277(42):39953, 2002.
539. Stein, D. S., and Moore, K. H.: Pharmacotherapy 21(1), 11, 2001.
540. Sweeny, D. J., Lynch, G., Bidgood, et al.: Drug Metab. Dispos. 28(7):737, 2000.

SELECTED READING

Aitio, A. (ed.): Conjugation Reactions in Drug Biotransformation. Amsterdam, Elsevier, 1978.
Anders, M. W. (ed.): Bioactivation of Foreign Compounds. New York, Academic Press, 1985.
Baselt, R. C., and Cravey, R. H.: Disposition of Toxic Drugs and Chemicals in Man. Foster City, CA, Chemical Toxicology Institute, 1995.
Benford, D. J., Bridges, J. W., and Gibson, G. G. (eds.): Drug Metabolism—From Molecules to Man. London, Taylor & Francis, 1987.
Brodie, B. B., and Gillette, J. R. (eds.): Concepts in Biochemical Pharmacology, Part 2. Berlin, Springer-Verlag, 1971.
Caldwell, J.: Conjugation reactions in foreign compound metabolism. Drug Metab. Rev. 13:745, 1982.
Caldwell, J., and Jakoby, W. B. (eds.): Biological Basis of Detoxification. New York, Academic Press, 1983.
Caldwell, J., and Paulson, G. D. (eds.): Foreign Compound Metabolism. London, Taylor & Francis, 1984.
Creasey, W. A.: Drug Disposition in Humans. New York, Oxford University Press, 1979.

DeMatteis, F., and Lock, E. A. (eds.): Selectivity and Molecular Mechanisms of Toxicity. London, Macmillan, 1987.

Dipple, A., Micheijda, C. J., and Weisburger, E. K.: Metabolism of chemical carcinogens. Pharmacol. Ther. 27:265, 1985.

Drayer, D. E.: Pharmacologically active metabolites of drugs and other foreign compounds. Drugs 24:519, 1982.

Dutton, G. J.: Glucuronidation of Drugs and Other Compounds. Boca Raton, FL, CRC Press, 1980.

Estabrook, R. W., and Lindenlaub, E. (eds.): Induction of Drug Metabolism. Stuttgart, Schattauer Verlag, 1979.

Ferraiolo, B. L., Mohler, M. A., and Gloff, C. A. (eds.): Protein Pharmacokinetics and Metabolism. New York, Plenum Press, 1992.

Gibson, G. G., and Skett, P.: Introduction to Drug Metabolism. London, Chapman & Hall, 1986.

Gorrod, J. W. (ed.): Drug Toxicity. London, Taylor & Francis, 1979.

Gorrod, J. W., and Damani, L. A. (eds.): Biological Oxidation of Nitrogen in Organic Molecules. Chichester, UK, Ellis Horwood, 1985.

Gorrod, J. W., Oelschlager, H., and Caldwell, J. (eds.): Metabolism of Xenobiotics. London, Taylor & Francis, 1988.

Gram, T. E. (ed.): Extrahepatic Metabolism of Drugs and Other Foreign Compounds. New York, SP Medical and Scientific, 1980.

Guengerich, F. P.: Analysis and characterization of drug metabolizing enzymes. In Hayes, A. W. (ed.). Principles and Methods of Toxicology, 3rd ed. New York, Raven Press, 1994.

Guengerich, F. P. (ed.): Mammalian Cytochromes P-450, vols. 1 and 2. Boca Raton, FL, CRC Press, 1987.

Hathway, D. E.: Mechanisms of Chemical Carcinogenesis. London, Butterworths, 1986.

Hodgson, E., and Levi, P. E. (eds.): A Textbook of Modern Toxicology. New York, Elsevier, 1987.

Humphrey, M. I., and Ringrose, P. S.: Peptides and related drugs: a review of their absorption, metabolism and excretion. Drug Metab. Rev. 17:283, 1986.

Jakoby, W. B. (ed.): Detoxification and drug metabolism. Methods Enzymol. 77: 1981.

Jakoby, W. B. (ed.): Enzymatic Basis of Detoxification, vols. 1 and 2. New York, Academic Press, 1980.

Jakoby, W. B., Bend, J. R., and Caldwell, J. (eds.): Metabolic Basis of Detoxification: Metabolism of Functional Groups. New York, Academic Press, 1982.

Jeffrery, E. H.: Human Drug Metabolism. From Molecular Biology to Man. Boca Raton, FL, CRC Press, 1993.

Jenner, P., and Testa, B.: The influence of stereochemical factors on drug disposition. Drug Metab. Rev. 2:117, 1973.

Jenner, P., and Testa, B. (eds.): Concepts in Drug Metabolism, Parts A and B. New York, Marcel Dekker, 1980, 1981.

Jerina, D. M. (ed.): Drug Metabolism Concepts. Washington, DC, American Chemical Society, 1977.

Jollow, D. J., et al. (eds.): Biological Reactive Intermediates: Formation, Toxicity and Inactivation. New York, Plenum Press, 1977.

Kauffman, F. C. (ed.): Conjugation–Deconjugation Reactions in Drug Metabolism and Toxicity. Berlin, Springer-Verlag, 1994.

Klaasen, C. D. (ed.): Casarett & Doull's Toxicology, 5th ed. New York, McGraw-Hill, 1996.

La Du, B. N., Mandel, H. G., and Way, E. L. (eds.): Fundamentals of Drug Metabolism and Drug Disposition. Baltimore, Williams & Wilkins, 1971.

Low, L. K., and Castagnoli, N.: Drug biotransformations. In Wolff, M. E. (ed.). Burger's Medicinal Chemistry, Part 1, 4th ed. New York, Wiley-Interscience, 1980, p. 107.

Mitchell, J. R., and Horning, M. G. (eds.): Drug Metabolism and Drug Toxicity. New York, Raven Press, 1984.

Monks, T. J., and Lau, S. S.: Reactive intermediates and their toxicological significance. Toxicology 52:1, 1988.

Mulder, G. J. (ed.): Sulfate Metabolism and Sulfate Conjugation. London, Taylor & Francis, 1985.

Nelson, S. D.: Chemical and biological factors influencing drug biotransformation. In Wolff, M. E. (ed.). Burger's Medicinal Chemistry, Part 1, 4th ed. New York, Wiley-Interscience, 1980, p. 227.

Nelson, S. D.: Metabolic activation and drug toxicity. J. Med. Chem. 25:753, 1982.

Ortiz de Montellano, P. R. (ed.): Cytochrome P-450: Structure, Mechanism, and Biochemistry. New York, Plenum Press, 1986.

Pacifici, G. M., and Pelkonen O. (eds.): Interindividual Variability in Human Drug Metabolism, New York, Taylor & Francis, 2001.

Parke, D. V.: The Biochemistry of Foreign Compounds. New York, Pergamon Press, 1968.

Parke, D. V., and Smith, R. L. (eds.): Drug Metabolism: From Microbe to Man. London, Taylor & Francis, 1977.

Paulson, G. D., et al. (eds.): Xenobiotic Conjugation Chemistry. Washington, DC, American Chemical Society, 1986.

Reid, E., and Leppard, J. P. (eds.): Drug Metabolite Isolation and Detection. New York, Plenum Press, 1983.

Sato, R., and Omura, T. (eds.): Cytochrome P-450. New York, Academic Press, 1978.

Schenkman, J. B., and Greim, H. (eds.): Cytochrome P450. Berlin, Springer-Verlag, 1993.

Schenkman, J. B., and Kupfer, D. (eds.): Hepatic Cytochrome P-450 Monooxygenase System. New York, Pergamon Press, 1982.

Siest, G. (ed.): Drug Metabolism: Molecular Approaches and Pharmacological Implications. New York, Academic Press, 1985.

Singer, B., and Grunberger, D.: Molecular Biology of Mutagens and Carcinogens. New York, Plenum Press, 1983.

Snyder, R., et al. (eds.): Biological Reactive Intermediates II, Parts A and B. New York, Plenum Press, 1982.

Snyder, R., et al. (eds.): Biological Reactive Intermediates III: Animal Models and Human Disease, Parts A and B. New York, Plenum Press, 1986.

Tagashira, Y., and Omura, T. (eds.): P-450 and Chemical Carcinogenesis. New York, Plenum Press, 1985.

Testa, B., and Caldwell, J. (eds.): The Metabolism of Drugs and Other Xenobiotics. London, Academic Press, 1995.

Testa, B., and Jenner, P.: Drug Metabolism: Chemical and Biochemical Aspects. New York, Marcel Dekker, 1976.

Timbrell, J. A.: Principles of Biochemical Toxicology. London, Taylor & Francis, 1982.

Williams, R. T.: Detoxification Mechanisms, 2nd ed. New York, Wiley, 1959.

Biotechnology and Drug Discovery

JOHN M. BEALE, JR.

CHAPTER OVERVIEW

Developments in biotechnology in recent times have been quite dramatic. The years between 1999 and 2001 witnessed a tremendous increase in the number of biotechnology-related pharmaceutical products in development, and a number of important new drugs progressed through trials and into the clinic. A good reflection of the impact of biotechnology is the GenBank database. GenBank is an electronic repository of gene sequence information, specifically the nucleotide sequences of complementary DNA (cDNA), representing the messenger RNA (mRNA), and genomic clones that have been isolated and sequenced by scientists worldwide.[1,2] The growth of the GenBank database has been rapid, and it has been increasing steadily since about 1992.[3] Figures 4.1 and 4.2 graphically depict these growth rates.

In October 2008, the Pharmaceutical Research and Manufacturers Association (PhRMA) reported that 633 biotechnology-derived medicines were in testing at various stages and that nearly 100 diseases are being targeted by research conducted by 144 companies and the National Cancer Institute. Of these—all of which are in human trials or awaiting Food and Drug Administration (FDA) approval—244 are new drugs for cancer, 162 are new drugs for infectious diseases, 59 are new drugs for autoimmune diseases, 18 are new drugs for neurological disorders, and 34 are new drugs for human immunodeficiency virus (HIV) and acquired immunodeficiency syndrome (AIDS) and related conditions.[4] PhRMA also reported nearly 200 new medicines targeted for pediatric use.[5] Approved drugs derived from biotechnology also treat or help prevent myocardial infarction, stroke, multiple sclerosis (MS), leukemia, hepatitis, rheumatoid arthritis, breast cancer, diabetes, congestive heart failure, lymphoma, renal cancer, cystic fibrosis (CF), and other diseases. The number of biotechnology products under development for a wide variety of diseases are illustrated in Figure 4.3.

The Human Genome Project, an international effort to obtain complete genetic maps, including nucleotide sequences, of each of the 24 human chromosomes, has spawned much new knowledge and technology. It is awesome to consider that in the mere 30 years since 1972, the science has reached the stage of attempting genetic cures for some diseases, such as CF and immune deficiency disorders.

BIOTECHNOLOGY AND PHARMACEUTICAL CARE

As it affects medicine and pharmaceutical care, biotechnology has forever altered the drug discovery process and the thinking about patient care. Extensive screening programs once drove drug discovery on natural or synthetic compounds. Now, the recombinant DNA (rDNA)-driven drug discovery process is beginning to yield new avenues for the preparation of some old drugs. For example, insulin, once prepared by isolation from pancreatic tissue of bovine or porcine species, can now be prepared in a pure form identical with human insulin. Likewise, human growth hormone (hGH), once isolated from the pituitary glands of the deceased, can now be prepared in pure form. Recombinant systems, such as these, provide high-yielding, reproducible batches of the drug and uniform dosing for patients.

LITERATURE OF BIOTECHNOLOGY

Many good literature sources on biotechnology exist for the pharmacist and medicinal chemist. These cover topics such as management issues in biotechnology,[6–14] implementation of instruction on biotechnology in education,[15–22] costs of biotechnology drugs,[23–26] implementation in a practice setting,[27–42] regulatory issues,[43–46] product evaluation and formulation,[47,48] patient compliance,[49,50] and finding information.[51–53] Additionally, there are a number of general texts,[54–60] review articles,[61–65] and a general resource reference catalogue.[66] Any good biochemistry textbook is also a useful resource.

BIOTECHNOLOGY AND NEW DRUG DEVELOPMENT

The tools of biotechnology are also being brought to bear in the search for new biological targets for presently available drugs as well as for the discovery of new biological molecules with therapeutic utility. Molecular cloning of novel receptors can provide access to tremendous tools for the testing of drugs (e.g., the adrenergic receptors), whereas cloning of a novel growth factor might potentially provide a new therapeutic agent. Biotechnology is also being used to screen compounds for biological activity. By using cloned and

Base Pairs by Year

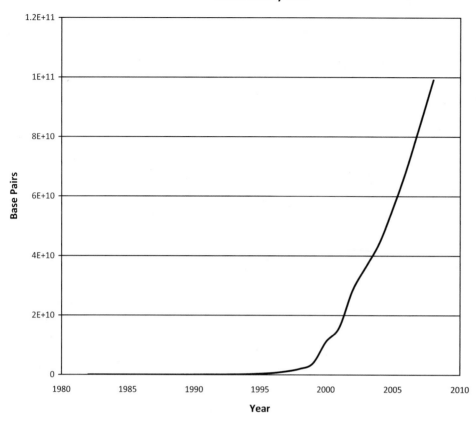

Figure 4.1 ● Yearly growth of GenBank in base pairs.

Sequences by Year

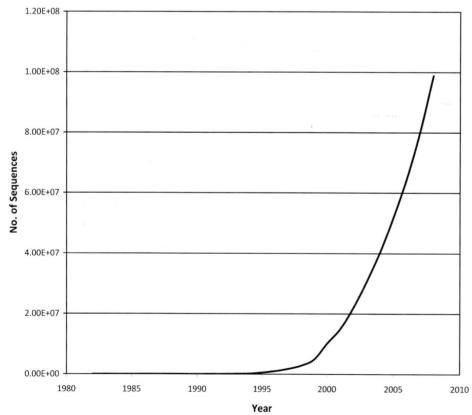

Figure 4.2 ● Yearly growth of GenBank in terms of gene sequences.

Biotechnology Drug Development by Disease State (2008-09)

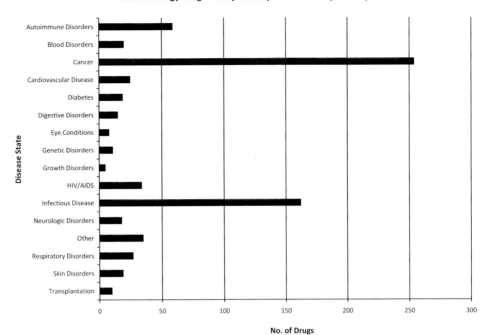

Figure 4.3 ● Yearly approvals of biotechnology-derived drugs and vaccines.

expressed genes, it is possible to generate receptor proteins to facilitate high-throughput screening of drugs in vitro or in cell culture systems rather than in animals or tissues. Biotechnology is being investigated in completely novel approaches to the battle against human disease, including the use of antisense oligonucleotides and gene replacement therapies for the treatment of diseases such as CF and the use of monoclonal antibodies (MAbs) for the treatment of cancer.

Biotechnology encompasses many subdisciplines, including genomics, proteomics, gene therapy, made-to-order molecules, computer-assisted drug design, and pharmacogenomics. A goal of biotechnology in the early 21st century is to eliminate the "one-drug-fits-all" paradigm for pharmaceutical care.[58]

The drugs that are elaborated by biotechnological methods are proteins and, hence, require special handling. There are some basic requirements of pharmaceutical care for the pharmacist working with biotechnologically derived products[41]:

- An understanding of how the handling and stability of biopharmaceuticals differs from other drugs that pharmacists dispense
- Knowledge of preparation of the product for patient use, including reconstitution or compounding if required
- Patient education on the disease, benefits of the prescribed biopharmaceutical, potential side effects or drug interactions to be aware of, and the techniques of self-administration
- Patient counseling on reimbursement issues involving an expensive product
- Monitoring of the patient for compliance

The pharmacist must maintain an adequate knowledge of agents produced through the methods of biotechnology and remain "in the loop" for new developments. The language of biotechnology encompasses organic chemistry, biochemistry, physiology, pharmacology, medicinal chemistry, immunology, molecular biology, and microbiology. A pharmacist has studied in all of these areas and is uniquely poised to use these skills to provide pharmaceutical care with biotechnological agents when needed.

The key techniques that unlocked the door to the biotechnology arena are those of rDNA, also known as *genetic engineering*. rDNA techniques allow scientists to manipulate genetic programming, create new genomes, and extract genetic material (genes) from one organism and insert it into another to produce proteins.

THE BIOTECHNOLOGY OF RECOMBINANT DNA

Since its inception in the mid-1970s, recombinant DNA (rDNA)[67–74] (genetic engineering) technology has driven much of the fundamental research and practical development of novel drug molecules and proteins. rDNA technology provides the ability to isolate genetic material from any source and insert it into cells (plant, fungal, bacterial, animal) and even live animals and plants, where it is expressed as part of the receiving organism's genome. Before discussing techniques of genetic engineering, a review of some of the basics of cellular nucleic acid and protein chemistry is relevant.[75–77]

Most of the components that contribute to cellular homeostasis are proteins—so much so that more than half of the dry weight of a cell is protein. Histones, cellular enzymes, membrane transport systems, and immunoglobulins are just a few examples of the proteins that carry out the biological functions of a living human cell. Proteins are hydrated three-dimensional structures, but at their most basic level, they are composed of linear sequences of amino acids that fold to create the spatial characteristics of the protein. These linear sequences are called the *primary structure* of the protein, and they are encoded from DNA through RNA. The information flow sequence DNA → RNA → protein has, for many years, been called the biological "Central Dogma."[78,79] The specific sequence of amino acids is encoded in genes. Genes are discrete segments of linear DNA that compose the chromosomes in the nucleus of a cell. The Human Genome Project has revealed that there are between 30,000 and 35,000 functional genes in a human, encompassing about 3,400,000,000 base pairs (bp).[80]

As depicted in Figure 4.4, in the nucleus of the cell, double-stranded DNA undergoes a process of transcription (catalyzed by RNA polymerase) to yield a single-stranded molecule of pre-mRNA. Endonucleases then excise nonfunctional RNA sequences called *introns*, from the pre-mRNA, to yield functional mRNA. In the cytoplasm, mRNA complexes with the ribosomes and the codons are read and translated into proteins. The process of protein synthesis in *Escherichia coli* begins with the activation of amino acids as aminoacyl-transfer RNA (tRNA) derivatives. All 20 of the amino acids undergo this activation, an adenosine triphosphate (ATP)-dependent step catalyzed by aminoacyltRNA synthetase. Initiation involves the mRNA template, *N*-formylmethionyl tRNA, the initiation codon (AUG), initiation factors, and the ribosomal subunits. Elongation occurs (using several elongation factors) with the aminoacyltRNAs being selected by recognition of their specific codons and forming new peptide bonds with neighboring amino acids. When biosynthesis of the specific protein is finished, a termination codon in the mRNA is recognized, and release factors disengage the protein from the elongation complex. Finally, the protein is folded and posttranslational processing occurs.[81,82] Processes that might be used in this step include removal of initiating residues and signaling sequences, proteolysis, modification of terminal residues, and attachment of phosphate, methyl, carboxyl, sulfate, carbohydrate, or prosthetic groups that help the protein achieve its final three-dimensional shape. Specialized

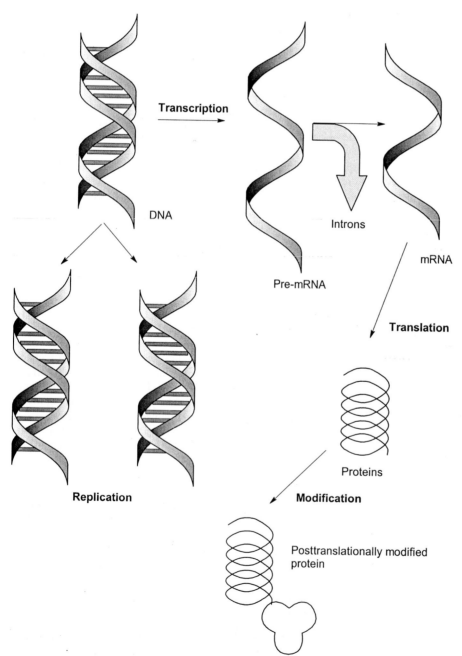

Figure 4.4 • Path from DNA to protein.

chaperone proteins can also direct the three-dimensional formation. Posttranslational modifications occur in mammalian cells in the endoplasmic reticulum or the Golgi apparatus before the protein is transported out of the cell. Most posttranslational modifications occur only in higher organisms, not in bacteria. The three-base genetic codon system is well known and has been conserved among all organisms. This allows rDNA procedures to work and facilitates the development of a model for the amino acid sequence of a protein by correlation with the codon sequence of the genome.

Recombinant DNA Technology

The fundamental techniques involved in working with rDNA include isolating or copying a gene; inserting the precise gene into a transmissible vector that can be transcribed, amplified, and propagated by a host cell's biochemical machinery; transferring it to that host cell; and facilitating the transcription into mRNA and translation into proteins. Cloned DNA can also be removed or altered by using an appropriate restriction endonuclease. Because genes encode the language of proteins, in theory, it is possible to create any protein if one can obtain a copy of the corresponding gene. rDNA methods require the following[83]:

- An efficient method for cleaving and rejoining phosphodiester bonds on fragments of DNA (genes) derived from an array of different sources
- Suitable vectors or carriers capable of replicating both themselves and the foreign DNA linked to them
- A means of introducing the rDNA into a bacterial, yeast, plant, or mammalian cell
- Procedures for screening and selecting a clone of cells that has acquired the rDNA molecule from a large population of cells

There are two primary methods for cloning DNA[84] using genomic and cDNA libraries as the primary sources of DNA fragments, which, respectively, represent either the chromosomal DNA of a particular organism or the cDNA prepared from mRNA present in a given cell, tissue, or organ. In the first method, a library of DNA fragments is created from a cell's genome, which represents all of the genes present. The library is then screened against special DNA probes. Lysing the genomic contents to generate fragments of different sizes and compositions, some of which should contain the genetic sequences that encode the specific activity that one is seeking, creates the library. With knowledge of the protein sequence that the gene specifies, DNA probes can be synthesized that should hybridize with corresponding fragments in the library. By labeling the probes with fluorescent or radioactive tags, probe molecules that hybridize and form double-helical DNA can be identified and isolated electrophoretically. The DNA from the library can then be amplified by a technique such as the polymerase chain reaction (PCR), inserted into a vector, and transferred into a host cell. A comparison of these methods is given in Table 4.1.

The second major method for cloning DNA represents only genes that are being expressed[84] at a given time and involves first the isolation of the mRNA that encodes the amino acid sequence of the protein of interest. Treating the mRNA with the viral enzyme reverse transcriptase in the presence of nucleoside triphosphates (NTPs) causes a strand of DNA to be synthesized complementary to the mRNA matrix, affording

TABLE 4.1 Characteristics of Genomic versus cDNA Libraries

Characteristic	Genomic	cDNA
Source of genetic material	Genomic DNA	Cell or tissue mRNA
Complexity (independent recombinants)	>100,000	5,000–20,000
Size range of recombinants (bp[a])	1,000–50,000	30–10,000
Presence of introns	Yes	No
Presence of regulatory elements	Yes	Maybe
Suitable for heterologous expression	Maybe	Yes

[a]bp, base pairs.

an RNA–DNA hybrid. The RNA strand is broken down in alkaline conditions, yielding a single-stranded molecule of DNA. The DNA polymerase reaction affords a complementary or copy strand of DNA (cDNA), which on fusion of a promotor sequence can be attached to a transport vector. Figure 4.5 depicts these reactions.

If the amino acid sequence of a protein (and, hence, the codon sequence) is known, automated synthesis of DNA through chemical or enzymatic means represents a third way that genes can be engineered. This method is useful only for relatively small proteins. In principle, for the preparation of a genomic library, the cellular origin of the DNA is not an issue, whereas the cellular origin of mRNA is central to the preparation of a cDNA library. Therefore, genomic libraries vary from species to species but not from tissue to tissue within that species. cDNA varies with tissue and the developmental stages of cells, tissues, or species. Another important distinction is that the fragment of DNA from eukaryotic chromosomes will contain exons (protein-coding segments) and introns (noncoding segments between exons), whereas in cDNA, the introns are spliced out.

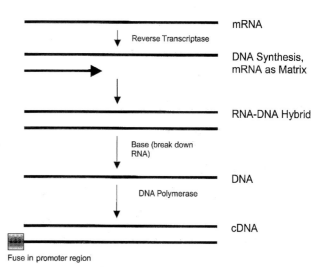

Figure 4.5 ● Method for preparation of cDNA from an mRNA transcript.

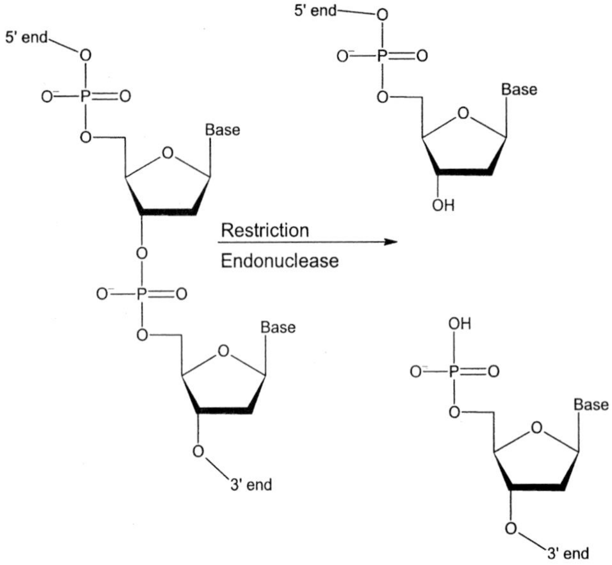

Figure 4.6 ● Mechanism of a restriction endonuclease reaction.

Restriction Endonucleases[84,85]

The restriction endonuclease (or restriction enzyme) is probably best described as a set of "molecular scissors" in nature. Restriction endonucleases are bacterial enzymes that, as the name implies, cleave internal phosphodiester bonds of a DNA molecule. The cleavage site on a segment of DNA lies within a specific nucleotide sequence of about 6 to 8 bp. More than 500 restriction endonucleases have been discovered, and these react with more than 100 different cleavage sites. The chemical reaction of the restriction endonuclease releases the 3' end of one base as an alcohol and the 5' end as a monophosphate. The general reaction is shown in Figure 4.6.

The recognition sites for restriction endonucleases are specific palindromic sequences of DNA[85] not more than 8 bp long. A number of these palindromes are listed in Table 4.2. A *palindrome* is a sequence of letters that reads the same way forward and backward, for instance: "A man, a plan, a canal: Panama!," "DNA-land," "Did Hannah see bees? Hannah did." Restriction endonucleases cleave DNA at palindromic sites to yield several types of cuts:

5' CCTAG↓

5' CCTAGG 3' → 5' CCTAG 3'

3' GGATCC 5' → 3' GATCC 5'

3' G↑

These cuts yields an overhanging C/C "sticky" end that is relatively easy to ligate with complementary ends of other DNA molecules. A cut from an endonuclease like *Hae*III:

5' CC↓GG 3' → 5' CC GG 3'

3' GG↑CC 5' → 3' GG CC 5'

requires more complicated methods to ligate into vector DNA. Palindromic cleavage sites for some selected restriction enzymes are given in Table 4.2. The *arrow* shows the cleavage site. The restriction endonucleases are a robust group of enzymes that form a toolbox for investigators working in the field of genetic engineering. About the only caveat to their use is an obvious one: They must be chosen not to make their cut inside the gene of interest.

DNA Ligases[86]

When the gene of interest has been excised from its flanking DNA by the appropriate restriction endonucleases and the vector DNA has been opened (using the same restriction endonuclease to break phosphodiester bonds), the two different DNA molecules are brought together by annealing. In the first step of this process, heating unwinds the double-stranded DNA of the vector. The insert or passenger DNA is added to the heated mixture, and subsequent cooling facilitates pairing of complementary strands. Then, phosphodiester bonds are regenerated, linking the two DNA molecules, vector and insert. A total of four such bonds must be reformed, two on each strand at the 5' and 3' sites. This process is termed *ligation*, and the enzymes that catalyze the reaction are named *DNA ligases*. Typically, ATP or another energy source is required to drive the ligation reaction, and linker fragments of DNA are used to facilitate coupling. There are several different types of ligation reactions that are used, depending on the type of restriction endonuclease product that was formed. The sticky-ended DNA, using complementary vector and insert ends that easily base pair at the cuts, is probably the easiest to accomplish, although methods exist to ligate the blunt-ended varieties, using DNA ligase.

The Vector[84]

There are several methods available for introducing DNA into host cells. DNA molecules that can maintain themselves by replication are called *replicons*. Vectors are subsets of replicons. In genetic engineering, the vector (carrier) is the most widely used method for the insertion of foreign, or passenger, genetic material into a cell. *Vectors* are genetic elements such as plasmids or viruses that can be propagated and that have been engineered so that they can accept fragments of foreign DNA. Depending on the vector, they may have many other features, including multiple cloning sites

TABLE 4.2 Palindromic Cleavage Sites

AluI	*AsuII*	*BalI*	*BamH1*	*BglII*	*ClaI*	*EcoRI*
AG↓CT	TT↓CGAA	TGG↓CCA	G↓GATCC	A↓GATCT	AT↓CGAT	G↓AATTC
EcoRV	*HaeIII*	*HhaI*	*HindII*	*HindIII*	*HpaII*	*KpnI*
GAT↓ATC	GG↓CC	GCG↓C	GTPy↓PuAC	A↓AGCTT	C↓CGG	GGTAC↓C
MboI	*PstI*	*PvuI*	*SalI*	*SmaI*	*XmaI*	*NotI*
↓GATC	CTGCA↓G	CGAT↓CG	G↓TCGAC	CCC↓GGG	C↓CCGGG	GC↓GGCCGC

(a region containing multiple restriction enzyme sites into which an insert can be installed or removed), selection markers, and transcriptional promoters. The passenger DNA must integrate into the host cell's DNA or be carried into the cell as part of a biologically active molecule that can replicate independently. If this result is not achieved, the inserted gene will not be successfully transcribed. The most commonly used biological agent for transporting genes into bacterial and yeast cells is the plasmid, such as the *E. coli* bacterial plasmid pBR322. A plasmid is a small, double-stranded, closed circular extrachromosomal DNA molecule. This plasmid contains 4,361 bp and can transport relatively small amounts of DNA. Plasmids occur in many species of bacteria and yeasts. Sometimes, plasmids carry their own genes (e.g., the highly transmissible genes for antibiotic resistance in some bacterial species). An important feature of a plasmid is that it has an origin of replication (*ori*) site that allows it to multiply independently of a host cell's DNA. Although there can be more than one copy of a plasmid in a cell, the copy number is controlled by the plasmid itself.

Another type of cloning vector is the bacteriophage (Fig. 4.7). Bacteriophage λ (lambda) possesses a genome of approximately 4.9×10^5 bp and can package large amounts of genetic material without affecting the infectivity of the phage. A large DNA library can be created, packaged in bacteriophage λ, and, when the virus infects, inserted into cells. Hybridization is then detected by screening with DNA probes.[87] In addition, there are special vectors called *phagemids*, vaccinia and adenovirus for cloning into mammalian cells, and yeast artificial chromosomes (YACs) that facilitate cloning in yeasts.[88] Differences among these vectors concern the size of the insert that they will accept, the methods used in the selection of the clones, and the procedures for propagation.

Once the passenger DNA has been created and the plasmid vector cut (both with the same restriction enzyme), the insert is ligated into the plasmid along with a promoter (a short DNA sequence that enhances the transcription of the adjacent gene). Often, a gene imparting antibiotic resistance linked to the desired gene is inserted as a selection tool. The idea behind this is that if the gene is inserted in the proper location, the bacterial cell will grow on a medium containing the antibiotic. Bacteria that do not contain the resistance gene and, hence, lack the required gene will not grow. This makes the task of screening for integration of the desired gene easier. After the molecule is ligated, the vector is finally an rDNA molecule that can be inserted into a host cell.

Host cells can be bacteria (e.g., *E. coli*), eukaryotic yeast (*Saccharomyces cerevisiae*), or mammalian cell lines, including Chinese hamster ovary (CHO), African green monkey kidney (VERO), and baby hamster kidney (BHK). It is easy to grow high concentrations of bacteria and yeast cells in fermenters to yield high protein concentrations. Mammalian cell culture systems typically give poorer protein yields, but sometimes this is acceptable, especially when the product demands the key posttranslational modifications that do not occur in bacteria. Host cells containing the vector are grown in small-scale cultures and screened for the desired gene.[89] When the clone providing the best protein yield is located, the organism is grown under carefully controlled conditions and used to inoculate pilot-scale fermentations. Parameters such as production medium composition, pH, aeration, agitation, and temperature are investigated at this stage to optimize the fermentation. The host cells divide, and the plasmids in them replicate, producing the desired "new" protein. The fermentation is scaled up into larger bioreactors for large-scale isolation of the recombinant protein. Obviously, the cultures secrete

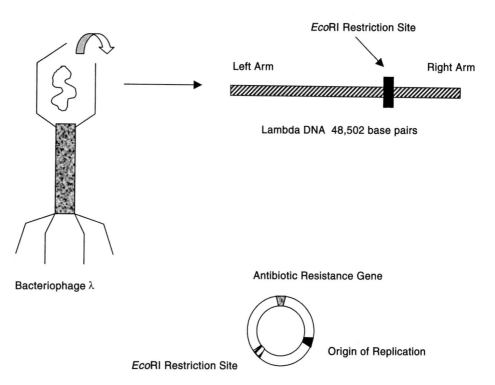

Figure 4.7 ● Types of cloning vectors: a bacteriophage and a plasmid.

Bacteriophage λ

*Eco*RI Restriction Site

Left Arm

Right Arm

Lambda DNA 48,502 base pairs

Antibiotic Resistance Gene

Origin of Replication

*Eco*RI Restriction Site

E. coli plasmid pBR322   4,361 base pairs

their own natural proteins along with the cloned protein. Purification steps are required before the recombinant protein is suitable for testing as a new, genetically engineered pharmaceutical agent. Once the host cell line expressing the recombinant gene is isolated, it is essential to maintain selection pressure on it so that it does not spontaneously lose the plasmid. Typically, this pressure is applied by maintaining the cells on medium containing an antibiotic to which they bear a resistance gene.

SOME TYPES OF CLONING

A listing of some types of cloning is given in Table 4.3.

Functional Expression Cloning[90]

Functional expression cloning focuses on obtaining a specific cDNA of known function. There are many variations on this approach, but they all rely on the ability to search for and isolate cDNAs based on some functional activity that can be measured (e.g., the electrophysiological measurement of ion conductances following expression of cDNAs in frog oocytes). By incrementally subdividing the cDNAs into pools and following the activity, it is possible to obtain a single cDNA clone that encodes the functionality. The advantage of functional expression cloning is that it does not rely on knowledge of the primary amino acid sequence. This is a definite advantage when attempting to clone proteins of low abundance.

Positional Cloning[90]

Positional cloning can be used to localize fragments of DNA representing genes prior to isolating the DNA. An example of the use of positional cloning is the cloning of the gene responsible for CF. By studying the patterns of inheritance of the disease and then comparing these with known chromosomal markers (linkage analysis), it was possible, without knowing the function of the gene, to locate the gene on human chromosome 7. Then, by using a technique known as *chromosome walking*, the gene was localized to a DNA sequence that encodes a protein now known as the cystic fibrosis transmembrane conductance regulator (CFTR). This protein, previously unknown, was shown to be defective in CF patients and could account for many of the symptoms of the disease. Like functional cloning, positional cloning has the advantage that specific knowledge of the protein is not required. It is also directly relevant to the understanding of human disease, and it can provide important new biological targets for drug development and the treatment of disease.

Homology-Based Cloning

Another cloning strategy involves the use of previously cloned genes to guide identification and cloning of evolutionarily related genes. This approach, referred to as *homology-based cloning*, takes advantage of the fact that nucleotide sequences encoding important functional domains of proteins tend to be conserved during the process of evolution. Thus, nucleotide sequences encoding regions involved with ligand binding or enzymatic activity can be used as probes that will hybridize to complementary nucleotide sequences that may be present on other genes that bind similar ligands or have similar enzymatic activity. This approach can be combined with PCR[91,92] to amplify the DNA sequences. The use of homology-based cloning has the advantages that it can be used to identify families of related genes, does not rely on the purification or functional activity of a given protein, and can provide novel targets for drug discovery. Its usefulness is offset by the possibility that the isolated fragment may not encode a complete or functional protein or that, in spite of knowledge of the shared sequence, the actual function of the clone may be difficult to identify.

TABLE 4.3 **Cloning Strategies**

Strategy	Advantages	Disadvantages	Example
Positional	Provides information underlying the genetic basis of known diseases	3.3×10^9 bp, difficult to use with diseases caused by multiple interacting alleles	Cystic fibrosis gene product
Protein purification	Yields genetic information encoding proteins of known structure and function	Protein purification, especially for low-abundance proteins, is exacting; availability of appropriate libraries, incomplete coding sequences	β_2-Adrenergic receptor
Antibody based	Yields genetic information encoding proteins of known structure and function	Involves protein purification, unrecognized cross-reactivity, incomplete coding sequences	Vitamin D receptor
Functional expression	Yields genetic information encoding a functionally active protein; does not require protein purification	Function must be compatible with existing library-screening technology	Substance K receptor
Homology based	Identification of related genes or gene families; relatively simple	Depends on preexisting gene sequence; can yield incomplete genes or genes of unknown function	Muscarinic receptor
Expressed sequence tagging	High throughput; identification of novel cDNAs	Incomplete coding sequences or genes of unknown function	
Total genomic sequencing	Knowledge of total genome; identification of all potential gene products	3.3×10^9 bp, labor intensive; genes of unknown function	*Haemophilus influenzae*

Source: PhRMA: Biotechnology Drug Development by Disease State, 2008–2009.

EXPRESSION OF CLONED DNA

Once cloned, there are many different possibilities for the expression and manipulation of DNA sequences. Because it concerns the use of cloned genes in the process of drug discovery and development, there are many obvious ways in which the expression of DNA sequences can be applied. One of the most obvious is in replacement of older technologies that involve the purification of proteins for human use from either animal sources or human byproducts, such as blood. An example of this is factor VIII, a clotting cascade protein used for the treatment of the genetically linked bleeding disorder hemophilia. Until recently, the only source of purified factor VIII was human blood, and tragically, before the impact of AIDS was fully appreciated, stocks of factor VIII had become contaminated with HIV-1, resulting in the infection of as many as 75% of the patients receiving this product. The gene encoding factor VIII has since been cloned, and recombinant factor VIII is now available as a product purified from cultured mammalian cells. Other recombinant clotting factors, including factors VIIa and IX, are under development and, together with recombinant factor VIII, will eliminate the risk of exposure to human pathogens.

Other examples in which the expression of cloned human genes offers alternatives to previously existing products include human insulin, which is now a viable replacement for purified bovine and porcine insulin for the treatment of diabetes, and hGH, which is used for the treatment of growth hormone deficiency in children (dwarfism). Unlike insulin, growth hormones from other animal species are ineffective in humans; thus, until human recombinant growth hormone became available, the only source of hGH was the pituitary glands of cadavers. This obviously limited the supply of hGH and, like factor VIII, exposed patients to potential contamination by human pathogens. Recombinant hGH (rhGH) can now be produced by expression in bacterial cells.

The expression of cloned genes can be integrated into rational drug design by providing detailed information about the structure and function of the sites of drug action. With the cloning of a gene comes knowledge of the primary amino acid sequence of an encoded receptor protein. This information can be used to model its secondary structure and in an initial attempt to define the protein's functional domains, such as its ligand-binding site. Such a model can then serve as a basis for the design of experiments that can be used to test the model and facilitate further refinement. Of particular use are mutagenesis experiments that use rDNA techniques to change a primary amino acid sequence so that the consequences can be studied. In addition, expression of a cloned target protein can be used to generate samples for various biophysical determinations, such as x-ray crystallography. This technique, which can provide detailed information about the three-dimensional molecular structure of a protein, frequently requires large amounts of protein, which, in some cases, is only available with the use of recombinant expression systems.

Like the many strategies used to clone genes, there are many strategies for their expression, involving the use of either bacterial or eukaryotic cells and specialized vectors compatible with expression in host cells. Since these cells do not normally express the protein of interest, this methodology is often referred to as *heterologous expression*. It is also possible to prepare cRNA from rDNA, which can then be used for either in vitro expression or injection directly into cells. In the former situation, purified ribosomes are used in the test tube to convert cRNA into protein; for the latter situation, the endogenous cellular ribosomes make the protein. A relatively new development for the expression of cloned genes is the use of animals that have the cloned gene stably integrated into their genome. Such transgenic animals can potentially make very large amounts of recombinant protein, which can be harvested from the milk, blood, and ascites fluid.

The choice of a particular expression system depends on several factors. Protein yield, requirements for biological activity, and compatibility of the expressed protein with the host organism are a few. An example of the compatibility issue is that bacteria do not process proteins in exactly the same way as do mammalian cells, so that the expression of human proteins in bacteria will not always yield an active product or any product at all. Cases like these may require expression in mammalian cell cultures. The choice of an expression system also reflects the available vectors and corresponding host organisms. A basic requirement for the heterologous expression of a cloned gene is the presence of a promoter that can function in the host organism and a mechanism for introducing the cloned gene into the organism. The promoter is the specific site at which DNA polymerase binds to initiate transcription and is usually specific for the host organism. As in gene cloning, the vectors are either plasmids or viruses that have been engineered to accept rDNA and that contain promoters that direct the expression of the rDNA. The techniques for introducing the vector into the organism vary widely and depend on whether one is interested in transient expression of the cloned gene or in stable expression. In the latter case, integration into the host genome is usually required; transient expression simply requires getting the vector into the host cell.

MANIPULATION OF DNA SEQUENCE INFORMATION

Perhaps the greatest impact of rDNA technology lies in its ability to alter a DNA sequence and create entirely new molecules that, if reintroduced into the genome, can be inherited and propagated in perpetuity. The ability to alter a DNA sequence, literally in a test tube, at the discretion of an individual, corporation, or nation, brings with it important questions about ownership, ethics, and social responsibility. There is no question, however, that potential benefits to the treatment of human disease are great.

There are three principal reasons for using rDNA technology to alter DNA sequences. The first is simply to clone the DNA to facilitate subsequent manipulation. The second is to intentionally introduce mutations so that the site-specific effect on protein structure and function can be studied.[93,94] The third reason is to add or remove sequences to obtain some desired attribute in the recombinant protein. For example, recent studies with factor VIII show that the protein contains a small region of amino acids that are the major determinant for the generation of anti–factor VIII antibodies in a human immune system. This autoimmune response of the patient inhibits the activity of factor VIII, which is obviously a serious therapeutic complication for patients who are using factor VIII for the treatment of hemophilia. By altering the DNA sequence encoding, this determinant, however, the amino acid sequence can be changed both to reduce the antigenicity of the factor VIII molecule and to make it transparent to any existing anti–factor VIII antibodies (i.e., changing the epitope eliminates the existing antibody recognition sites).

It is possible to combine elements of two proteins into one new recombinant protein. The resulting protein, referred to as a *chimeric* or *fusion protein*, may then have some of the functional properties of both of the original proteins. This is illustrated in Figure 4.8 for two receptors labeled *A* and *B*. Each receptor has functional domains that are responsible for ligand binding, integration into the plasma membrane, and activation of intracellular signaling pathways. Using rDNA techniques, one can exchange these functional domains to create chimeric receptors that, for example, contain the ligand-binding domain of receptor B but the transmembrane and intracellular signaling domains of receptor A. The application of the fusion protein strategy is discussed further in connection with the hGH receptor (under "Novel Drug-Screening Strategies") and with denileukin diftitox.

Another reason for combining elements of two proteins into one recombinant protein is to facilitate its expression and purification. For example, recombinant glutathione S-transferase (GST), cloned from the parasitic worm *Schistosoma japonicum*, is strongly expressed in *E. coli* and has a binding site for glutathione. Heterologous sequences encoding the functional domains from other proteins can be fused, in frame, to the carboxy terminus of GST, and the resulting fusion protein is often expressed at the same levels as GST itself. In addition, the resulting fusion protein retains the ability to bind glutathione, which means that affinity chromatography, using glutathione that has been covalently bonded to agarose, can be used for a single-step purification of the fusion protein. The functional activity of the heterologous domains that have been fused to GST can then be studied either as part of the fusion protein or separately following treatment of the fusion protein with specific proteases that cleave at the junction between GST and the heterologous domain. Purified fusion proteins can also be used to generate antibodies to the heterologous domains and for other biochemical studies. Sometimes, fusion proteins are made to provide a recombinant protein that can be easily identified. An example of this is a technique called *epitope tagging*, in which well-characterized antibody recognition sites are fused with recombinant proteins. The resulting recombinant protein can then be identified by immunofluorescence or can be purified with antibodies that recognize the epitope.

NEW BIOLOGICAL TARGETS FOR DRUG DEVELOPMENT

One of the outcomes of the progress that has been made in the identification and cloning of genes is that many proteins encoded by these genes represent entirely new targets for drug development. In some cases, the genes themselves may represent the ultimate target for the treatment of a disease in the form of gene therapy. The cloning of the CF gene is an example of both a new drug target and a gene that could potentially be used to treat the disease. The protein encoded by this gene, CFTR, is a previously unknown integral membrane protein that functions as a channel for chloride ions. Mutations in *CFTR* underlie the pathophysiology of CF, and in principle, replacement or coexpression of the defective gene with the healthy, nonmutated gene would cure the disease. It is also possible, however, that by understanding the structure and function of the healthy CFTR, drugs could be designed to interact with the mutated CFTR and improve its function.

An important outgrowth of the study of new drug targets is the recognition that many traditional targets, such as enzymes and receptors, are considerably more heterogeneous than previously thought. Thus, instead of one enzyme or receptor, there may be several closely related subtypes, or isoforms, each with the potential of representing a separate drug target. This can be illustrated with the enzyme cyclooxygenase (COX), which is pivotal to the formation of prostaglandins and which is the target of aspirin and the nonsteroidal anti-inflammatory drugs (NSAIDs). Until recently, COX was considered to be a single enzyme, but pharmacological and gene cloning studies have revealed that there are at least three enzyme forms, named COX-1, COX-2, and COX-3. Interestingly, they are differentially regulated. COX-1 is expressed constitutively in many tissues, whereas the expression of COX-2 is induced by inflammatory processes. Thus, the development of COX-2 selective agents can yield NSAIDs with the same efficacy as existing (nonselective) agents but with fewer side effects, such as those on the gastric mucosa.

The elucidation of the family of adrenergic receptors is another example in which molecular cloning studies have revealed previously unknown heterogeneity, with the consequence of providing new targets for drug development. The adrenergic receptors mediate the physiological effects of the catecholamines epinephrine and norepinephrine. They are also the targets for many drugs used in the treatment of such conditions as congestive heart failure, asthma, hypertension,

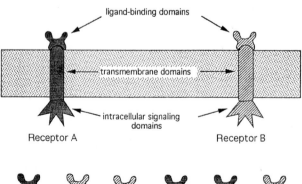

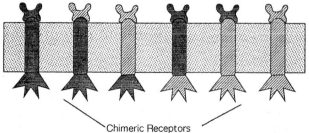

Figure 4.8 ● Chimeric receptors.

TABLE 4.4 Selected Examples of Receptor Subtype Heterogeneity

Receptor Superfamily	Original Subtypes	Present Subtypes
G-protein–coupled		
Adrenergic	β_1, β_2, α_1, α_2	β_1, β_2, β_3, α_{1A}, α_{1B}, α_{1D}, α_2A, α_2B, α_2C
Dopamine	D_1, D_2	D_1, $D_2{}^a$, D_3, D_4, D_5
Prostaglandin E_2	EP_1, EP_2, EP_3	EP_1, EP_2, $EP_3{}^a$, EP_4
Receptor tyrosine kinase neurotrophins	Nerve growth factor receptor	$TrkA^a$, TrkB, $TrkC^a$
DNA binding		
Estrogen	Estrogen receptor	ERR1, ERR2
Thyroid hormone	Thyroid hormone receptor	TRα, TRβ
Retinoic acid	Retinoic acid receptor	RARα, RARβ
Ligand-activated channels		
Glycine	Glycine and/or strychnine receptor	α_1, α_2, α_3 (multisubunit)^b
$GABA_A$	GABA and/or benzodiazepine receptor	α_1, α_2, α_3, α_4, α_5, α_6 (multisubunit)^b

^{a}Alternative mRNA splicing creates additional receptor heterogeneity.

^{b}Only the heterogeneity of the ligand-binding subunit is listed; a multisubunit structure combined with the heterogeneity of the other subunits creates a very large number of potential subtypes.

glaucoma, and benign prostatic hypertrophy. Prior to the molecular cloning and purification of adrenergic receptors, the pharmacological classification of this family of receptors consisted of four subtypes: α_1, α_2, β_1, and β_2. The initial cloning of the α-adrenergic receptor in 1986 and subsequent gene cloning studies revealed at least nine subtypes: β_1, β_2, β_3, α_{1A}, α_{1B}, α_{1D}, α_{2A}, α_{2B}, and α_{2C} (Chapter 16).

The evidence that there are nine subtypes of adrenergic receptors is very important in terms of understanding the physiology of the adrenergic receptors and of developing drugs that can selectively interact with these subtypes. For example, in the case of the α_2-agonist *p*-aminoclonidine, an agent used to lower intraocular pressure (IOP) in the treatment of glaucoma, it may now be possible to explain some of the drug's pharmacological side effects (e.g., bradycardia and sedation) by invoking interactions with the additional α_2-adrenergic receptor subtypes. Of considerable interest is the possibility that these pharmacological effects (i.e., lowering of IOP, bradycardia, and sedation) are each mediated by one of the three different α_2-receptor subtypes. If this is true, it might be possible to develop a subtype-selective α_2-agonist that lowers IOP but does not cause bradycardia or sedation. Likewise, it might even be possible to take advantage of the pharmacology and develop α_2-adrenergic agents that selectively lower heart rate or produce sedation.

The discovery of subtypes of receptors and enzymes by molecular cloning studies seems to be the rule rather than the exception and is offering a plethora of potential new drug targets (Table 4.4). To note just a few: 5 dopamine receptor subtypes have been cloned, replacing 2 defined pharmacologically (Chapter 13); 7 serotonin receptor subtypes have been cloned, replacing 3; 4 genes encoding receptors for prostaglandin E_2 have been isolated, including 12 additional alternative mRNA splice variants; and 3 receptors for nerve growth factor have been cloned, replacing 1.

⬡ NOVEL DRUG-SCREENING STRATEGIES

The combination of the heterologous expression of cloned DNA, the molecular cloning of new biological targets, and the ability to manipulate gene sequences has created powerful new tools that can be applied to the process of drug discovery and development. In its most straightforward application, the ability to simply express newly identified receptor protein targets offers a novel means of obtaining information that may be difficult, or even impossible, to obtain from more complex native biological systems. There is a reason for this. A newly identified protein can be expressed in isolation. Even for closely related enzyme or receptor subtypes, heterologous expression of the individual subtype can potentially provide data that are specific for the subtype being expressed, whereas the data from native biological systems will reflect the summation of the individual subtypes that may be present.

The potential advantage of heterologous expression is illustrated in Figure 4.9 for the interaction of a drug with multiple binding sites. In *panel A*, which can represent the data

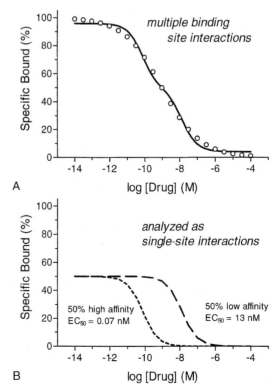

Figure 4.9 ● Convoluted data from binding to multiple receptor subtypes versus classic mass action.

obtained from a native biological system, the data are complex, and the curve reflects interactions of the drug with two populations of receptors: one with high affinity, representing 50% of the total receptor population, and one with low affinity, representing the remaining 50%. The individual contributions of these two populations of receptors are indicated in *panel B*, which could also reflect the data obtained if rDNA encoding these two receptors were expressed individually in a heterologous expression system. Although in some cases, the data, as in *panel A*, can be analyzed with success, frequently they cannot, especially if more than two subtypes are present or if any one subtype makes up less than 10% of the total receptor population or if the affinities of the drug for the two receptor populations differ by less than 10-fold.

Another important reason for integrating heterologous expression into drug-screening strategies is that data can usually be obtained for the human target protein rather than an animal substitute. This does not mean that organ preparations or animal models will be totally replaced. For the purposes of the identification of lead compounds and the optimization of selectivity, affinity, etc., however, the use of recombinant expression systems provides some obvious advantages.

By combining heterologous expression with novel functional assays, it is possible to increase both specificity and throughput (the number of compounds that can be screened per unit time). For example, reporter genes have been developed that respond to various intracellular second messengers, such as the activation of guanine nucleotide–binding proteins (G proteins), and levels of cyclic adenosine monophosphate (cAMP), or calcium. One approach to the development of novel functional assays involves the use of promoter regions in DNA that control the transcription of genes. This approach is exemplified by the *c*AMP *r*esponse *e*lement (CRE). This is a specifically defined sequence of DNA that is a binding site for the *c*AMP *r*esponse *e*lement-*b*inding (CREB) protein. In the unstimulated condition, the binding of CREB to the CRE prevents the transcription and expression of genes that follow it (Fig. 4.10). When CREB

is phosphorylated by cAMP-dependent protein kinase A (PKA), however, its conformation changes, permitting the transcription and expression of the downstream gene. Thus, increases in intracellular cAMP, such as those caused by receptors that activate adenylyl cyclase (e.g., β-adrenergic, vasopressin, etc.), will stimulate the activity of PKA, which, in turn, results in the phosphorylation of CREB and the activation of gene transcription.

In nature, there are a limited number of genes whose activity is regulated by a CRE. Biologically, however, the expression of almost any gene can be regulated in a cAMP-dependent fashion if it is placed downstream of a CRE, using rDNA techniques. If the products of the expression of the downstream gene can be easily detected, they can serve as reporters for any receptor or enzyme that can modulate the formation of cAMP in the cell. The genes encoding chloramphenicol acetyl transferase (CAT), luciferase, and β-galactosidase are three examples of potential "reporter genes," whose products can be easily detected. Sensitive enzymatic assays have been developed for all of these enzymes; thus, any changes in their transcription will be quickly reflected by changes in enzyme activity. By coexpressing the reporter gene along with the genes encoding receptors and enzymes that modulate cAMP formation, it is possible to obtain very sensitive functional measures of the activation of the coexpressed enzyme or receptor.

Another example of the use of a reporter gene for high-throughput drug screening is the *r*eceptor *s*election and *a*mplification *t*echnology (r-SAT) assay. This assay takes advantage of the fact that the activation of several different classes of receptors can cause cellular proliferation. If genes for such receptors are linked with a reporter gene, such as β-galactosidase, the activity of the reporter will be increased as the number of cells increase as a consequence of receptor activation. Initially, a limitation of this assay was that it only worked with receptors that normally coupled to cellular proliferation; by making a mutation in one of the second-messenger proteins involved with the proliferative response, however, it was possible to get additional

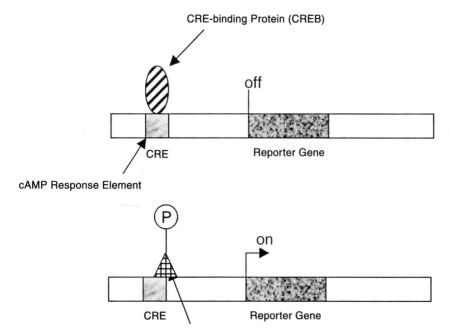

Figure 4.10 ● Activation of transcription by a cAMP response element (CRE). CREB is phosphorylated by cAMP-dependent protein kinase.

receptors to work in this assay. This second-messenger protein, G_q, was cloned, and a recombinant chimera was made that included part of another second messenger known as G_i. In native cells, receptors that activate G_i are not known for their stimulation of cell proliferation, but when such receptors are coexpressed in the r-SAT assay with the chimeric G_q, their activity can be measured.

A similar strategy involving chimeric proteins has been used for receptors whose second-messenger signaling pathways are not clearly understood. For example, the development of potential therapeutic agents acting on the hGH receptor has been difficult because of a lack of a good signaling assay. The functional activity of other receptors that are structurally and functionally related to the growth hormone receptor can be measured, however, in a cell proliferation assay. One such receptor that has been cloned is the murine receptor for granulocyte colony-stimulating factor (G-CSF). By making a recombinant chimeric receptor containing the ligand-binding domain of the hGH receptor with the second-messenger–coupling domain of the murein G-CSF receptor, it was possible to stimulate cellular proliferation with hGH.

In addition to providing a useful pharmacological screen for hGH analogs, the construction of this chimeric receptor provides considerable insight into the mechanism of agonist-induced growth hormone receptor activation. The growth hormone–binding domain is clearly localized to the extracellular amino terminus of the receptor, whereas the transmembrane and intracellular domains are implicated in the signal transduction process. It was also determined that successful signal transduction required receptor dimerization by the agonist (i.e., simultaneous interaction of two receptor molecules with one molecule of growth hormone). Based on this information, a mechanism-based strategy was used for the design of potential antagonists. Thus, hGH analogs were prepared, were incapable of producing receptor dimerization, and were found to be potent antagonists.

⬡ PROCESSING OF THE RECOMBINANT PROTEIN

Processing the fermentation contents to isolate a recombinant protein is often a difficult operation, requiring as much art as science. In the fermentation broth are whole bacterial cells, lysed cells, cellular fragments, nucleotides, normal bacterial proteins, the recombinant protein, and particulate medium components. If a Gram-negative bacterium such as *E. coli* has been used, lipopolysaccharide endotoxins (pyrogens) may be present. When animal cell cultures are used, it is commonly assumed that virus particles may be present. Viruses can also be introduced by the culture nutrients, generated by an infected cell line, or introduced by animal serum. Purification of an rDNA protein while maintaining the factors that keep it in its active three-dimensional conformation from this mixture may be difficult, because each step must be designed to ensure that the protein remains intact and pharmacologically active. Assays must be designed that allow the activity of the protein to be assessed at each purification step. Consequently, the structure and activity of the recombinant protein must be considered at all stages of purification, and assays must be conducted to measure the amount of purified, intact protein.

A general scheme for purification of an rDNA protein is as follows[95]:

- *Particulate removal.* Particulates may be removed by centrifugation, filtration, ultrafiltration, and tangential flow filtration. Virus particles may be inactivated by heating if the rDNA peptide can tolerate the procedure.
- *Concentration.* The volume of the mixture is reduced, which increases the concentration of the contents. Often, concentration is achievable by the filtration step, especially if ultrafiltration is used.
- *Initial purification.* The initial purification of the mixture is sometimes accomplished by precipitation of the proteins, using a slow, stepwise increase of the ionic strength of the solution (salting out). Ammonium sulfate is a typical salt that can be used in cold, aqueous solutions. Water-miscible organic solvents such as trichloroacetic acid and polyethylene glycol (PEG) change the dielectric constant of the solution and also effect precipitation of proteins.
- *Intermediate purification.* In this stage, the proteins may be dialyzed against water to remove salts that were used in the precipitation step. Ion exchange chromatography is used to effect a somewhat crude separation of the proteins based on their behavior in a pH or salt gradient on the resin. Another step that may be taken is size exclusion (gel filtration) chromatography. Gels of appropriate molecular weight cutoffs can yield a somewhat low-resolution separation of proteins of a desired molecular weight. If a native bacterial protein that has been carried this far is nearly the same molecular weight as the rDNA protein, no separation will occur.
- *Final purification.* Final purification usually involves the use of high-resolution chromatography, typically high-performance liquid chromatography. An abundance of commercial stationary phases allows various types of adsorption chromatography (normal and reversed phase), ion exchange chromatography, immunoaffinity chromatography, hydrophobic interaction chromatography, and size exclusion chromatography. The protein fractions are simply collected when they elute from the column and are concentrated and assayed for activity.
- *Sterilization and formulation.* This step can be accomplished by ultrafiltration to remove pyrogens or by heating if the protein can withstand this. Formulation might involve reconstitution into stable solutions for administration or determining the optimum conditions for stability when submitting for clinical trials.

Complicating factors include (a) proteins unfolding into an inactive conformation during processing (it may not be possible to refold the protein correctly) and (b) proteases that are commonly produced by bacterial, yeast, and mammalian cells, which may partially degrade the protein.

⬡ PHARMACEUTICS OF RECOMBINANT DNA-PRODUCED AGENTS

rDNA methods have facilitated the production of very pure, therapeutically useful proteins. The physicochemical and pharmaceutical properties of these agents are those of proteins, which means that pharmacists must understand the chemistry (and the chemistry of instability) of proteins to store, handle, dispense, reconstitute, and administer these protein drugs. Instabilities among proteins may be physical or chemical. In the former case, the protein might stick to glass vessels or flocculate, altering the dose that the patient will receive. In the latter case, chemical reactions taking place on the protein may alter the type or stereochemistry of the amino acids, change the position of disulfide bonds, cleave the peptide chains themselves, and alter the charge distribution of the protein. Any of these can cause unfolding (denaturation) of the protein and loss of activity, rendering the molecule useless as a drug. Chemical instability can be a problem during the purification stages of a protein, when the molecule might be subjected to acids or bases, but instability could occur at the point of administration when, for example, a lyophilized protein is reconstituted. The pharmacist must understand a few concepts of the chemical and physical instability of proteins to predict and handle potential problems.

Chemical Instability of Proteins[67]

See Figure 4.11.

- *Hydrolysis*. Hydrolytic reactions of the peptide bonds can break the polymer chain. Aspartate residues hydrolyze 100 times faster in dilute acids than do other amino acids under the same conditions. As a general rule of peptide hydrolysis, Asp-Pro > Asp-X or X-Asp bonds. This property of Asp is probably a result of an autocatalytic function of the Asp side chain carboxyl group. Asn, Asp, Gln, and Glu hydrolyze exceptionally easily if they occur next to Gly, Ser, Ala, and Pro. Within these groupings, Asn and Gln accelerate hydrolysis more at low pH, whereas Asp and Glu hydrolyze most readily at high pH, when the side chain carboxyl groups are ionized.
- *Deamidation*. Gln and Asn undergo hydrolytic reactions that deamidate their side chains. These reactions convert neutral amino acid residues into charged ones. Gln is converted to Glu and Asn to Asp. The amino acid type is changed, but the chain is not cleaved. This process is, effectively, primary sequence isomerization, and it may influence biological activity. The deamidation reaction of Asn residues is accelerated under neutral or alkaline pH conditions. A five-membered cyclic imide intermediate formed by intramolecular attack of the nitrogen atom on the carbonyl carbon of the Asn side chain is the accelerant. The cyclic imide spontaneously hydrolyzes to give a mixture of residues—the aspartyl peptide and an isoform.
- *Racemization*. Base-catalyzed racemization reactions can occur in any of the amino acids except glycine, which is achiral. Racemizations yield proteins with mixtures of L- and D-amino acid configurations. The reaction occurs following the abstraction of the α-hydrogen from the amino acid to form a carbanion. As should be expected, the stability of the carbanion controls the rate of the reaction. Asp, which undergoes racemization via a cyclic imide intermediate, racemizes 105 times faster than free Asn. By comparison, other amino acids in a protein racemize about 2 to 4 times faster than their free counterparts.
- *β-Elimination*. Proteins containing Cys, Ser, Thr, Phe, and Lys undergo facile β-elimination in alkaline conditions that facilitate formation of an α-carbanion.
- *Oxidation*. Oxidation can occur at the sulfur-containing amino acids Met and Cys and at the aromatic amino acids His, Trp, and Tyr. These reactions can occur during protein

processing as well as in storage. Methionine (CH_3—S—R) is oxidizable at low pH by hydrogen peroxide or molecular oxygen to yield a sulfoxide (R—SO—CH_3) and a sulfone (R—SO_2—CH_3). The thiol group of Cys (R—SH) can undergo successive oxidation to the corresponding sulfenic acid (R—SOH), disulfide (R—S—S—R), sulfinic acid (R—SO_2H), and sulfonic acid (R—SO_3H). Several factors, including pH, influence these reactions. Free —SH groups can be converted into disulfide bonds (—S—S—) and vice versa. In the phenomenon of disulfide exchange, disulfide bonds break and reform in different positions, causing incorrect folding of the protein. Major changes in the three-dimensional structure of the peptide can abolish activity. Oxidation of the aromatic rings of His, Trp, and Tyr residues is believed to occur with various oxidizing enzymes.

Physical Instability of Proteins[96]

Chemical alterations are not the only source of protein instability. A protein is a large, globular polymer that exists in some specific forms of secondary, tertiary, and quaternary structure. A protein is not a fixed, rigid structure. The molecule is in dynamic motion, and the structure samples an array of three-dimensional space. During this motion, noncovalent intramolecular bonds can break, reform, and break again, but the overall shape remains centered around an energy minimum that represents the most likely (and pharmacologically active) conformer of the molecule. Any major change in the conformation can abolish the activity of the protein. Small drug molecules do not demonstrate this problem. A globular protein normally folds so that the hydrophobic groups are directed to the inside and the hydrophilic groups are directed to the outside. This arrangement facilitates the water solubility of the protein. If the normal protein unfolds, it can refold to yield changes in hydrogen bonding, charge, and hydrophobic effects. The protein loses its globular structure, and the hydrophobic groups can be repositioned to the outside. The unfolded protein can subsequently undergo further physical interactions. The loss of the globular structure of a protein is referred to as *denaturation*.

Denaturation is, by far, the most widely studied aspect of protein instability. In the process, the three-dimensional folding of the native molecule is disrupted at the tertiary and, possibly, the secondary structure level. When a protein denatures, physical structure rather than chemical composition changes. The normally globular protein unfolds, exposing hydrophobic residues and abolishing the native three-dimensional structure. Factors that affect the denaturation of proteins are temperature, pH, ionic strength of the medium, inclusion of organic solutes (urea, guanidine salts, acetamide, and formamide), and the presence of organic solvents such as alcohols or acetone. Denaturation can be reversible or irreversible. If the denatured protein can regain its native form when the denaturant is removed by dialysis, reversible denaturation will occur. Denatured proteins are generally insoluble in water, lack biological activity, and become susceptible to enzymatic hydrolysis. The air–water interface presents a hydrophobic surface that can facilitate protein denaturation. Interfaces like these are commonly encountered in drug delivery devices and intravenous (IV) bags.

Surface adsorption of proteins is characterized by adhesion of the protein to surfaces, such as the walls of the containers

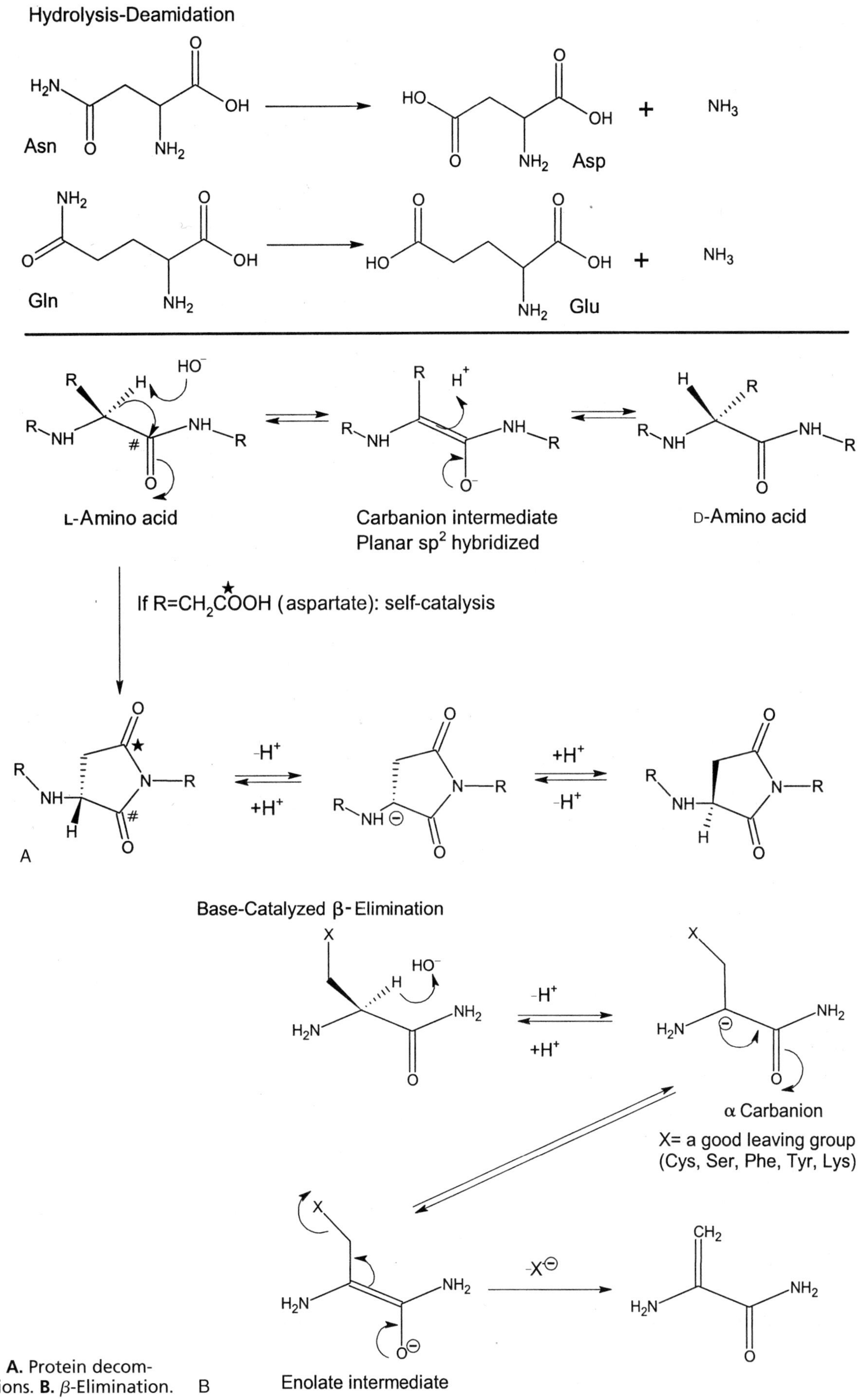

Hydrolysis-Deamidation

If R=CH₂C*OOH (aspartate): self-catalysis

Base-Catalyzed β-Elimination

X= a good leaving group
(Cys, Ser, Phe, Tyr, Lys)

Figure 4.11 ● **A.** Protein decomposition reactions. **B.** β-Elimination.

of the dosage form and drug delivery devices, ampuls, and IV tubing. Proteins can adhere to glass, plastics, rubber, polyethylene, and polyvinylchloride. This phenomenon is referred to as *flocculation*. The internal surfaces of IV delivery pumps and IV delivery bags pose particular problems of this kind. Flocculated proteins cannot be dosed properly.

Aggregation results when protein molecules, in aqueous solution, self-associate to form dimers, trimers, tetramers, hexamers, and large macromolecular aggregates. Self-association depends on the pH of the medium as well as solvent composition, ionic strength, and dielectric properties. Moderate amounts of denaturants (below the concentration that would cause denaturation) may also cause protein aggregation. Partially unfolded intermediates have a tendency to aggregate. Concentrated protein solutions, such as an immunoglobulin for injection, may aggregate with storage time on the shelf. The presence of particulates in the preparation is the pharmacist's clue that the antibody solution is defective.

Precipitation usually occurs along with denaturation. Detailed investigations have been conducted with insulin, which forms a finely divided precipitate on the walls of an infusion device or its dosage form container. It is believed that insulin undergoes denaturation at the air–water interface, facilitating the precipitation process. The concentration of zinc ion, pH, and the presence of adjuvants such as protamine also affect the precipitation reaction of insulin.

Immunogenicity of Biotechnologically Produced Drugs[97,98]

Proteins, by their very nature, are antigens. A human protein, innocuous at its typical physiological concentration, may exhibit completely different immunogenic properties when administered in the higher concentration that would be used as a drug. Unless a biotechnology-derived protein is engineered to be 100% complementary to the human form, it will differ among several major epitopes. The protein may have modifications of its amino acid sequence (substitutions of one amino acid for another). There may be additions or deletions of amino acids, N-terminal methionyl groups, incorrect or abnormal folding patterns, or oxidation of a sulfur-containing side chain of a methionine or a cysteine. Additionally, when a protein has been produced by using a bacterial vector, a finite amount of immunoreactive material may pass into the final product. All of these listed items contribute to the antigenicity of a biotechnologically produced protein. When it is administered to a human patient, the host's immune system will react to the protein just as it would to a microbial attack and neutralize it. This is why research has been undertaken to create 100% human protein drugs, such as insulin, which patients will need to take for a long time. In addition, some of the most promising biotechnology products, the MAbs, are produced in mice by use of *humanized* genes to avoid human reaction to the mouse antibody.

⬡ DELIVERY AND PHARMACOKINETICS OF BIOTECHNOLOGY PRODUCTS[99]

As with any drug class, the medicinal chemist and pharmacist must be concerned with the absorption, distribution, metabolism, and excretion (ADME) parameters of protein drugs. Biotechnology-produced drugs add complexities that are not encountered with "traditional" low–molecular-weight drug molecules. ADME parameters are necessary to compute pharmacokinetic and pharmacodynamic parameters for a given protein. As for any drug, these parameters are essential in calculating the optimum dose for a given response, determining how often to administer the drug to obtain a steady state, and adjusting the dose to obtain the best possible residence time at the receptor (pharmacodynamic parameters).

Delivery of drugs with the molecular weights and properties of proteins into the human body is a complex task. The oral route cannot be used with a protein because the acidity of the stomach will catalyze its hydrolysis unless the drug is enteric coated. Peptide bonds are chemically labile, and proteolytic enzymes that are present throughout the body can attack and destroy protein drugs. Hydrolysis and peptidase decomposition also occur during membrane transport through the vascular endothelium, at the site of administration, and at sites of reaction in the liver, blood, kidneys, and most tissues and fluids of the body. It is possible to circumvent these enzymes by saturating them with high concentrations of drug or by coadministering peptidase inhibitors. Oxidative metabolism of aromatic rings and sulfur oxidation can also occur. Proteins typically decompose into small fragments that are readily hydrolyzed, and the individual amino acids are assimilated into new peptides. A potentially serious hindrance to a pharmacokinetic profile is the tendency of proteins administered as drugs to bind to plasma proteins, such as serum albumin. If this happens, they enter a new biodistribution compartment from which they may slowly exit. Presently, the routes of administration that are available for protein drugs are largely subcutaneous (SC) and intramuscular (IM). Much ongoing research is targeted at making peptide drugs more bioavailable. An example of this is conjugation of interleukin-2 (IL-2) with PEG. These so-called pegylated proteins tend to have a slower elimination clearance and a longer $t_{1/2}$ than IL-2 alone. Another strategy being used is the installation of a prosthetic sugar moiety onto the peptide. The sugar moiety will adjust the partition coefficient of the drug, probably making it more water soluble.

⬤ RECOMBINANT DRUG PRODUCTS

Hormones

HUMAN INSULIN, RECOMBINANT[100–102]

Human insulin was the first pharmacologically active biological macromolecule to be produced through genetic engineering. The FDA approved the drug in 1982 for the treatment of type 1 (insulin-dependent) diabetes (see Chapter 27). The insulin protein is a two-chain polypeptide containing 51 amino acid residues. Chain A is composed of 21 amino acids, and chain B contains 30. The human insulin molecule has three disulfide linkages, $CysA_7$ to $CysB_7$, $CysA_{20}$ to $CysB_{19}$, and an intrachain linkage, $CysA_6$ to $CysA_{11}$. Insulin is secreted by the β-cells of the pancreatic islets of Langerhans, initially as a single peptide chain called *proinsulin*. Enzymatic cleavage of the propeptide releases the insulin.

Historically, insulin was isolated from bovine or porcine sources. Using these agents was not without difficulty. Both porcine and bovine insulin differ in amino acid sequence, with Ala replacing Thr at the C-terminus of the human B chain (B_{30}). Bovine insulin also differs in sequence from human insulin, with Ala substituting for Thr at A_8 and Val substituting for isoleucine at A_{10}. These differences, small though they may seem, result in immunological reactions in some patients. Adjustments to the formulation of bovine and porcine insulin led to products that differed in time of onset, time to peak reduction in glucose, and duration of action. These parameters were varied by addition of protamine and zinc (which yielded a particulate insulin with a longer duration of action), and adjustment of the pH to neutrality, which stabilized the preparation. Insulins were characterized as regular (short-duration Iletin, 4–12 hours), semilente (ultra-short duration), lente (intermediate [1–3 hours to peak, 24 hours duration]), and ultralente (extended duration). An additional form of insulin was NPH (neutral protamine Hagedorn), which had an intermediate time of onset and time to peak (1–3 hours) and a long duration of action (16–24 hours).

Producing a recombinant insulin that is chemically and physically indistinguishable from the human pancreatic hormone was a major accomplishment. The problem with immunoreactivity has been eliminated, the pyrogen content of the rDNA product is nil, the insulin is not contaminated with other peptides, and the hormone can be biosynthesized in larger quantities. Human insulin (rDNA) is available as Humulin, Novolin, and several analogs that differ in their pharmacokinetic profiles. Humulin is produced by using recombinant *E. coli*; Novolin is prepared by using recombinant *S. cerevisiae*, a yeast. There have been modifications in the production procedure since the initial successful biosynthesis. Prior to 1986, Humulin was produced by creating two different vectors, one for the A chain and one for the B chain, and inserting them into *E. coli*. The A chain and the B chain would be secreted into the medium, and the two were joined chemically to form rDNA insulin. Today, the entire proinsulin gene is used to create a recombinant organism, and the connecting peptide in proinsulin is cleaved by two enzymes (an endopeptidase and a carboxypeptidase B), yielding insulin (for details see Chapter 27).

Insulin rDNA is available in several[103] forms. Insulin lispro (Humalog) has a more rapid (15–30 minutes) onset and a shorter duration (3–6.5 hours) of action than regular human insulin (onset 30–60 minutes, duration 6–10 hours). It is effective when administered 15 minutes before a meal, unlike regular insulin, which must be injected 30 minutes before a meal. In lispro, the B-chain amino acids B_{28}Pro and B_{29}Lys are exchanged. Insulin aspart (NovoLog), onset 15 to 30 minutes, duration 3 to 6.5 hours, with a single amino acid substitution of Asp for Pro at B_{28}, is effective when administered 5 to 10 minutes before a meal. The ultra–long-acting agent insulin glargine has the Asp at A_{21} replaced by Gly and has two Arg residues added at the C-terminus of the B chain. Insulin glargine, administered subcutaneously, has a duration of action of 24 to 48 hours. The alteration in basicity of this agent causes it to precipitate at neutral pH, creating a depot effect.

Insulin rDNA has been very successful. The only problem has arisen in patients who have been using porcine or bovine insulin for a long time. Some patients who are switched to rDNA human insulin report difficulty in "feeling their glucose level," and these patients require extra counseling in the use of the recombinant hormone.

GLUCAGON[104]

The hormone glucagon (GlucaGen) is biosynthesized in the pancreas as a high–molecular-weight protein from which the active macromolecule is released by proteolytic cleavage. Glucagon is a single chain of 29 amino acids and generally opposes the actions of insulin. Bovine and porcine glucagons, which possess structures identical with human glucagon, have been in use for years. The rDNA form has been approved by the FDA for use in severe hypoglycemia and as a radiological diagnostic aid. Glucagon relaxes smooth muscles in the gastrointestinal (GI) tract, decreasing GI motility and improving the quality of radiological examinations. In the treatment of severe hypoglycemia in insulin-dependent diabetics, GlucaGen causes the liver to convert glycogen to glucose. Left untreated, severe hypoglycemia (low–blood-sugar reactions) can cause prolonged loss of consciousness and may be fatal. The rDNA drug has the benefit that there is no chance of acquiring bovine spongiform encephalopathy from glucagon therapy. This condition, also known as *mad cow disease*, is caused by a prion that was suspected to infect animal pancreas tissue.

HUMAN GROWTH HORMONE, RECOMBINANT[105,106]

hGH is a protein that is essential for normal growth and development in humans. hGH affects many aspects of human development and metabolism including longitudinal growth, regulation (increase) of protein synthesis and lipolysis, and regulation (decrease) of glucose metabolism. hGH has been used as a drug since the 1950s, and it has been extremely successful in the treatment of classic growth hormone deficiency, chronic renal insufficiency, Turner syndrome, failure to lactate in women, and Prader-Willi syndrome. In its long history, the hormone has been remarkably successful and free of side effects.

The primary form of hGH in the circulation is a 22-kDa, nonglycosylated protein produced in the anterior pituitary and composed of 191 amino acid residues linked by disulfide bridges in two peptide loops. The structure of hGH is globular, with four antiparallel α-helical regions. Endogenous hGH is composed of about 85% of the 22-kDa monomer, 5% to 10% of a 20-kDa monomer, and 5% of a mixture of disulfide-linked dimers, oligomers, and other modified forms. From the late 1950s, hGH was isolated from pituitary extracts of cadavers. A prion associated with the preparation was suspected to cause Creutzfeldt-Jakob disease, a fatal degenerative neurological disorder.

The first use of rhGH was reported in 1982. rhGH preparations were first produced in *E. coli*. These preparations contained a terminal methionine and 192 amino acids. Natural sequence rhGH has since been produced in mammalian (mouse) cell culture.

Somatrem, the first recombinant preparation, introduced in 1985, contains the natural 191-amino acid primary sequence plus one methionyl residue on the N-terminal end. The somatropin products all contain the 191-amino acid sequence and are identical with the hGH produced by the pituitary gland. The three-dimensional crystal structure shows that the protein is oblate, with most of its nonpolar amino acid side chains projecting toward the interior of the molecule. This rhGH is pharmacologically identical with natural hGH.

Most current formulations of rhGH are supplied in lyophilized form and must be reconstituted prior to injection. Typically, 5 to 10 mg of protein are supplied in a powdered glycine and/or mannitol phosphate buffer. The preparation is reconstituted with sterile water for injection, and the stability of the product is quite good. If stored at 2°C to 8°C, rhGH will remain stable for 2 years.

rhGH undergoes rapid, predictable metabolism in vivo in the kidney and the liver. Chemically, the metabolites are those expected for any peptide: deamidation of Asn and Gln and oxidation of Met, Trp, His, and Tyr.

FOLLICLE-STIMULATING HORMONE[107,108]

The gonadotropin follicle-stimulating hormones (FSH), follitropin alfa (Gonal-F) and follitropin beta (Follistim), are produced in the anterior lobe of the pituitary gland. FSH can function in two ways. On the one hand, it causes increased spermatogenesis in men. On the other hand, in concert with estrogen and luteinizing hormone (LH), it stimulates follicular growth and development in women. Consequently, FSH may be useful in the treatment of infertility.

FSH is a member of a superfamily of proteins, all structurally related, which includes LH, chorionic gonadotropin, and thyroid-stimulating hormone (TSH). It is a heterodimer, the α subunit contains 92 amino acids, and the β subunit contains 111 amino acids. The protein is rather heavily glycosylated and has a molecular mass of approximately 35 kDa. The traditional source for isolation of FSH was postmenopausal urine, which provided a preparation that was less than 5% pure and was significantly contaminated by LH. The recombinant human FSH (rhFSH) is produced in a mammalian cell line, the CHO.

Follitropin α and follitropin β are the same protein, but they differ with respect to the way they are formulated. Both preparations are lyophilized. The α form is formulated with sucrose (as a bulk modifying agent and a lyoprotectant) and the components of phosphate buffer. The β form contains sucrose, with sodium citrate as a stabilizer and polysorbate 20 as a lyoprotectant and a dispersant. The products are reconstituted immediately before administration. The shelf life of both preparations is 2 years when they are stored in the supplied containers at less than 30°C (not frozen) and protected from light.

THYROTROPIN ALPHA[109,110]

Human TSH, thyrotropin alpha (Thyrogen), is a heterodimeric protein of molecular mass ~28,000 to 30,000 Da. The α subunit is composed of 92 amino acids, and the β subunit, 112. The specificity of the protein is controlled by the β subunit. TSH binds to TSH receptors on normal thyroid epithelial cells or on well-differentiated cancerous thyroid tissue to stimulate iodine uptake into the gland, organification of iodine, and secretion of thyroglobulin, T_3, and T_4. The drug is used as a tool for radioiodine imaging in the diagnosis of thyroid cancer.

Cytokines

HEMATOPOIETIC GROWTH FACTORS

Among all of the events taking place in the immune system, the bone marrow, and the bloodstream, the process of hematopoiesis is probably the most complicated. All of the cells in the blood and the immune system can trace their lineage back to a common, parental hematopoietic stem cell in the bone marrow. This cell is referred to as *pluripotent* because under the proper stimulation, it can differentiate into any other cell. The processes of maturation, proliferation, and differentiation are under the strict control of several cytokines (Table 4.5) that regulate a host of cellular events. Two distinct blood cell lineages exist: the lymphoid lineage that gives rise to B and T lymphocytes, and the myeloid lineage that produces granulocytes (macrophages, neutrophils, eosinophils, basophils, and mast cells), as well as platelets and erythrocytes. As many as 20 of the hematopoiesis-associated cytokines have been cloned and expressed. Some of these are listed in Table 4.5.

The cascade is shown in Figure 4.12. A further feature of the pluripotent stem cell deserves mention. Each stem cell divides into two daughter cells, one an active hematopoietic

---

TABLE 4.5 Examples of Important Cytokines

Cytokine	Biological Function
Interleukin-1	Maturation and proliferation of B cells; activation of NK cells, inflammation, fever
Interleukin-2	Stimulates growth and differentiation of T-cell response; used to treat cancer or transplant patients
Interleukin-3	Differentiation and proliferation of myeloid stem cells
Interleukin-4	Switches B cells from IgG to IgE
Interleukin-5	Activates eosinophils
Interleukins 6 and 7	Controls differentiation of T lymphocytes
Interleukin-8	Neutrophil chemotaxis
Interleukin-9	Potentiates IgM, IgG, and IgE; stimulates mast cells
Interleukin-10	Inhibits Th1 cytokine production IFN-γ, TNFβ, IL-2
Interleukin-11	Acute-phase protein production
Interleukin-12	Controls the ratio of T_H1–T_H2
Interleukin-18	Induces production of IFN-γ, increases NK cell activity
Erythropoietin	Stimulates red cell production
Granulocyte–macrophage colony-stimulating factor	Acts with IL-3 to control myeloid branch
Granulocyte colony-stimulating factor	Neutrophil production
Macrophage colony-stimulating factor	Macrophage production
Stem cell factor	Controls activity through myeloid branch

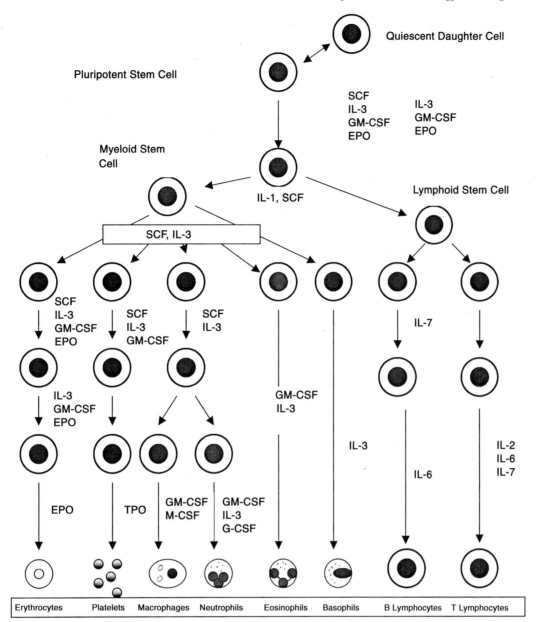

Figure 4.12 ● Cytokine-mediated cascade leading to different blood cell types. (EPO, erythropoietin; G-CSF, granulocyte colony-stimulating factor; GM-CSF, granulocyte–macrophage colony-stimulating factor; IL-X, interleukins; M-CSF, macrophage colony-stimulating factor; SCF, stem cell factor; TPO, thrombopoietin.)

progenitor and one quiescent. The active precursor matures to give hematopoietic progenitors and then circulating blood cells. The quiescent stem cells rejoin the stem cell pool. Hence, the number of parental cells is always the same. This process is termed *self-renewal.*

PRODUCTS

Erythropoietin Alfa[111–113]

Erythropoietin alfa, recombinant Epoetin Alfa, Epogen, Procrit, is a glycoprotein that stimulates red blood cell production. It is produced in the kidney, and it activates the proliferation and differentiation of specially committed erythroid progenitors in the bone marrow. Epoetin alfa (Epogen) is a 165-amino acid glycoprotein that is manufactured in mammalian cells by rDNA technology. The protein is heav-

ily glycosylated and has a molecular mass of approximately 30,400 Da. Erythropoietin is composed of four antiparallel α-helices. The rDNA protein has the same amino acid sequence as natural erythropoietin.

Epoetin is indicated to treat anemia of chronic renal failure patients, anemia in zidovudine-treated HIV-infected patients, and in cancer patients taking chemotherapy. The results in these cases have been dramatic; most patients respond with a clinically significant increase in hematocrit.

Filgrastim[114,115]

Filgrastim, G-CSF, Neupogen, stimulates the proliferation of granulocytes (especially neutrophils) by mobilizing hematopoietic stem cells in the bone marrow. Endogenous G-CSF is a glycoprotein produced by monocytes, fibroblasts, and endothelial cells. G-CSF is a protein of 174 amino acids, with a molecular mass of approximately 18,800 Da. The native protein is glycosylated.

Filgrastim selectively stimulates proliferation and differentiation of neutrophil precursors in the bone marrow. This leads to the release of mature neutrophils into the circulation from the bone marrow. Filgrastim also affects mature neutrophils by enhancing phagocytic activity, priming the cellular metabolic pathways associated with the respiratory burst, enhancing antibody-dependent killing, and increasing the expression of some functions associated with cell surface antigens.

In patients receiving chemotherapy with drugs such as cyclophosphamide, doxorubicin, and etoposide, the incidence of neutropenia accompanied by fever is rather high. Administration of G-CSF reduces the time of neutrophil recovery and duration of fever in adults with acute myelogenous leukemia. The number of infections, days that antibiotics are required, and duration of hospitalization are also reduced.

Filgrastim[116] is identical with G-CSF in its amino acid sequence, except that it contains an N-terminal methionine that is necessary for expression of the vector in *E. coli*. The protein is not glycosylated. Filgrastim is supplied in a 0.01 M sodium acetate buffer containing 5% sorbitol and 0.004% polysorbate 80. It should be stored at 2°C to 8°C without freezing. Under these conditions, the shelf life is 24 months. Avoid shaking when reconstituting; although the foaming will not harm the product, it may alter the amount of drug that is drawn into a syringe.

Sargramostim[117,118]

Sargramostim, granulocyte–macrophage colony-stimulating factor (GM-CSF), Leukine, is a glycoprotein of 127 amino acids, consisting of three molecular subunits of 19,500, 16,800, and 15,500 Da. The endogenous form of GM-CSF is produced by T lymphocytes, endothelial fibroblasts, and macrophages. Recombinant GM-CSF, produced in *S. cerevisiae*, differs from native human GM-CSF only by substitution of a leucine for an arginine at position 23. This substitution facilitates expression of the gene in the yeast. The site of glycosylation in the recombinant molecule may possibly differ from that of the native protein.

Sargramostim binds to specific receptors on target cells and induces proliferation, activation, and maturation. Administration to patients causes a dose-related increase in the peripheral white blood cell count. Unlike G-CSF, GM-CSF is a multilineage hematopoietic growth factor that induces partially committed progenitor cells to proliferate and differentiate along the granulocyte and the macrophage pathways. It also enhances the function of mature granulocytes and macrophages/monocytes. GM-CSF increases the chemotactic, antifungal, and antiparasitic activities of granulocytes and monocytes. It also increases the cytotoxicity of monocytes toward neoplastic cell lines and activates polymorphonuclear leukocytes to inhibit the growth of tumor cells.

Sargramostim is used to reconstitute the myeloid tissue after autologous bone marrow transplant and following chemotherapy in acute myelogenous leukemia. The preparation decreases the incidence of infection, decreases the number of days that antibiotics are required, and decreases the duration of hospital stays.

Sargramostim is supplied as a solution or powder (for solution). Both forms should be stored at 2°C to 8°C without freezing. The liquid and powder have expiration dates of 24 months. The reconstituted powder and the aqueous solution should not be shaken.

Becaplermin[119]

Becaplermin, Regranex Gel, an endogenous polypeptide that is released from cells that are involved in the healing process, is a recombinant human platelet–derived growth factor (rhPDGF-BB). The "BB" signifies that becaplermin is the homodimer of the B chain. Becaplermin is produced by a recombinant strain of *S. cerevisiae* containing the gene for the B chain of PDGF. The protein has a molecular mass of approximately 25 kDa and is a homodimer composed of two identical polypeptide chains that are linked by disulfide bonds. It is a growth factor that activates cell proliferation, differentiation, and function, and it is released from cells involved in the healing process.

Becaplermin is formulated as a gel recommended for topical use in the treatment of ulcerations of the skin secondary to diabetes.

Interferons

The interferons are a family of small proteins or glycoproteins of molecular masses ranging from 15,000 to 25,000 Da and 145 to 166 amino acids long. Eukaryotic cells secrete interferons in response to viral infection. Their mechanism of action is bimodal. The immediate effect is the recruitment of natural killer (NK) cells to kill the host cell harboring the virus (Fig. 4.13). Interferons then induce a state of viral resistance in cells in the immediate vicinity, preventing spread of the virus. Additionally, interferons induce a cascade of antiviral proteins from the target cell, one of which is 2′,5′-oligoadenylate synthetase. This enzyme catalyzes the conversion of ATP into 2′,5′-oligoadenylate, which activates ribonuclease R, hydrolyzing viral RNA. Interferons can be defined as cytokines that mediate antiviral, antiproliferative, and immunomodulatory activities.

Three classes of interferon (IFN) have been characterized: α (alpha), β (beta), and γ (gamma) (see Table 4.6). α-Interferons are glycoproteins derived from human leukocytes. β-Interferons are glycoproteins derived from fibroblasts and macrophages. They share a receptor with α-interferons. γ-Interferons are glycoproteins derived from human T lymphocytes and NK cells. These interferons are acid labile and used to be called "type 2 interferon." The receptor for IFN-γ is smaller than that for IFN-α and IFN-β, 90 to 95 kDa versus 95 to 110 kDa, respectively. The three classes are not homogeneous, and each may contain several different molecular species. For example, at least 18 genetically and molecularly distinct human α-interferons have

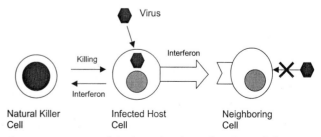

Figure 4.13 • Antiviral mechanism of action of the interferons.

TABLE 4.6 Interferons Used Therapeutically

Interferon Type	Endogenous Source	Available Drug Products
Alpha	Leukocytes	Interferon alfa-2a Interferon alfa-2b Interferon alfa-2c
Beta	Fibroblasts, macrophages	Beta-1a Beta-1b
Gamma	T Lymphocytes, natural killer cells	Gamma-1b

been identified, each differing in the amino acid substitution at positions 23 and 34. Interferons alfa-2a, alfa-2b, and alfa-2c have been purified and are either in clinical use or in development. A listing of commercially available α-interferons is given in Table 4.7.

As a class, the interferons possess some common side effects. These are flulike symptoms, headache, fever, muscle aches, back pain, chills, nausea and vomiting, and diarrhea. At the injection site, pain, edema, hemorrhage, and inflammation are common. Dizziness is also commonly reported.

For the pharmacist, when predicting drug interactions with the interferons, cytochrome P450 metabolism should always be a key consideration. Most of the interferons inhibit cytochrome P450, causing drugs that are metabolized by this route to reach higher-than-normal and, possibly, toxic concentrations in the blood and tissues.

PRODUCTS: α-INTERFERONS

Interferon Alfa-2a (Recombinant)[120]
Interferon alfa-2a (recombinant), Roferon A, is expressed in an *E. coli* system and purified by using high-affinity mouse MAb chromatography. The protein consists of 165 amino acids with a molecular mass of approximately 19,000 Da and contains lysine at position 23 and histidine at position 34.

Interferon alfa-2a is used in the treatment of hairy cell leukemia and AIDS-related Kaposi sarcoma in selected patients older than 18 years of age. It is also used to treat chronic hepatitis C, and in patients with this disease, interferon alfa-2a can normalize serum alanine aminotransferase (ALT) levels, improve liver histology, and decrease viral load. The drug has a direct antiproliferative activity against tumor cells. Modulation of the host immune response probably plays a role in the antitumor activity of interferon alfa-2a.

The interferon is supplied as a solution or as a powder for solution. The solution contains 0.72% NaCl. The powder contains 0.9% NaCl, 0.17% human serum albumin, and 0.33% phenol. The interferon vials, if properly stored at 2°C to 8°C without freezing, expire in 30 months. Prefilled syringes expire in 24 months. The solutions should not be shaken because the albumin will cause frothing.

Pegylated Interferon Alfa-2a[121]
Pegylated interferon alfa-2a, Pegasys, is a covalent conjugate of recombinant interferon alfa-2a (approximate molecular mass, 20 kDa) with a singly branched bis-monomethoxy PEG chain (approximate molecular mass, 40 kDa). The PEG moiety is linked at a single site to the interferon alfa moiety by a stable amide bond to lysine. Peginterferon alfa-2a has an approximate molecular mass of 60 kDa. Pegasys provides sustained therapeutic serum levels for up to a full week (168 hours). The drug is approved for the treatment of adults with chronic hepatitis C who have compensated liver disease and who have not been previously treated with interferon alfa. Efficacy has also been demonstrated in patients with compensated cirrhosis.

Interferon Alfa-2b (Recombinant)[122]
Interferon alfa-2b, Intron A, a water-soluble protein of 165 amino acids and an approximate molecular mass of 19,200 Da, is expressed from a recombinant strain of *E. coli*. This interferon molecule possesses an arginine at position 23 and a histidine at position 34.

Interferon alfa-2b is a broad-spectrum agent. It is indicated for hairy cell leukemia, condyloma acuminata (genital or

TABLE 4.7 Summary of the α-Interferons

	Interferon Alfa-2a	Interferon Alfa-2b	Interferon Alfa-n1	Interferon Alfa-n3	Interferon Alfacon-1
Trade name Dosage form Solvent	Roferon A Solution, powder Sodium chloride, excipients	Intron A Solution, powder Buffered saline	Wellferon Solution Buffered saline	Alferon N Solution Buffered saline	Infergen Solution Phosphate-buffered saline
Indications	Hairy cell leukemia, AIDS-related Kaposi sarcoma, chronic hepatitis C	Hairy cell leukemia, AIDS-related Kaposi sarcoma, condylomata acuminata, chronic hepatitis B, chronic hepatitis C	Chronic hepatitis C	Condylomata acuminata	Chronic hepatitis C
Routes[a]	SC, IM, IV, infusion or intralesional	SC, IM, IV, infusion or intralesional	SC or IM	Intralesional	SC
Source	*Escherichia coli*		Human lymphoblastoid cell line	Human leukocytes	*E. coli*

[a]SC, subcutaneously; IM, intramuscularly; IV, intravenously.

venereal warts), AIDS-related Kaposi sarcoma, and chronic hepatitis B and C infections.

Intron A can be administered by the SC, IM, or IV routes, by infusion or by intralesional routes. The dose is 1 to 35 million IU/day, depending on the application. The drug is supplied as a solution or as a powder for solution, and both forms contain albumin, glycine, and sodium phosphate buffer. Hence, they should not be shaken. Vials of solution should be stored at 2°C to 8°C without freezing. The powder is stable for 18 months at room temperature or 7 days at 45°C.

Interferon Alfa-n1[123]

Interferon alfa-n1, Wellferon, is a mixture of α-interferons isolated from a human lymphoblastoid cell line after induction with mouse parainfluenza virus type 1 (Sendai strain). Each of the subtypes of IFN-α in this product consists of 165 or 166 amino acids with an average molecular mass of 26,000 Da. The product is a mixture of each of the nine predominant subtypes of IFN-α.

Interferon alfa-n1 is indicated to treat chronic hepatitis C in patients 18 years of age or older who have no decompensated liver disease. The exact mechanism of action for interferon alfa-n1 in the treatment of this disease has not been elucidated.

This drug may be administered SC or IM, with a usual dose of 3 million IU 3 times per week. Interferon alfa-n1 is supplied as a solution containing tromethamine and buffered saline with human albumin as a stabilizer. Hence, the solution should not be shaken. The solution should be stored at 2°C to 8°C without freezing, and should be discarded if freezing occurs. Properly stored solution expires in 24 months.

Interferon Alfa-n3[124]

Interferon alfa-n3, Alferon N, is an α-interferon expressed from human leukocytes that are antigen-stimulated with avian Sendai virus. The Sendai virus is propagated in chicken eggs. The protein consists of at least 14 molecular subtypes. The average chain length is 166 amino acids, and the molecular mass range is 16,000 to 27,000 Da. The polydisperse interferon alfa-n3 is extremely pure, because it is processed by affinity chromatography over a bed of mouse MAbs specifically raised for the protein.

Interferon alfa-n3 is indicated for intralesional treatment of refractory or recurrent condyloma acuminata (genital warts) in patients 18 years of age or older. These warts are associated with human papillomavirus (HPV). Interferon alfa-n3 is especially useful in patients who have not responded well to other modalities (podophyllin resin, surgery, laser, or cryotherapy). Interferon alfa-n3 is also being investigated for the treatment of non-Hodgkin lymphoma, herpes simplex virus, rhinovirus, vaccinia, and varicella zoster. A usual dose in condyloma acuminata is 250,000 IU/wart, injected with a 30-gauge needle around the base of the lesion.

Interferon alfa-n3 is contraindicated in persons sensitive to mouse immunoglobulin G (IgG), egg protein, and neomycin.

Interferon alfa-n3 is supplied as a solution with the protein in phosphate-buffered saline with phenol as a preservative. The solution should be stored at 2°C to 8°C without freezing. Properly stored solution expires at 18 months.

Interferon Alfacon-1 (Recombinant)

Interferon alfacon-1 (recombinant), Infergen,[125] is a "consensus" interferon that shares structural elements of IFN-α and several subtypes. The range of activity is about the same as the other alpha species, but the specific activity is greater.

The 166-amino acid sequence of alfacon-1 is synthetic. It was developed by comparing several natural IFN-α subtypes and assigning the *most common* amino acid to each variable position. Additionally, four amino acid changes were made to facilitate synthesis. The DNA sequence is also constructed by chemical synthesis. Interferon alfacon-1 differs from interferon alfa-n2 at 20/166 amino acids, yielding 88% homology. The protein has a molecular mass of approximately 19,400 Da.

Interferon alfacon-1 is used in the treatment of chronic hepatitis C virus (HCV) infection in patients 18 years of age or older with compensated liver disease and who have anti-HCV serum antibodies or HCV RNA.

The drug is administered by the SC route in a dose of 9 μg 3 times per week. Interferon alfacon-1 is supplied as a solution in phosphate-buffered saline. It should be stored at 2°C to 8°C without freezing. Avoid shaking the solution.

PRODUCTS: β-INTERFERONS

A listing of two commercially available IFN-βs is given in Table 4.8.

Interferon Beta-1a (Recombinant)[126]

Interferon beta-1a (recombinant), Avonex, is a glycoprotein with 166 amino acids. It has a molecular mass of approximately 22,000 Da. The site of glycosylation is at the asparagine residue at position 80. Interferon beta-1a possesses a cysteine residue at position 17, as does the native molecule. Natural IFN-β and interferon beta-1a are glycosylated, with each containing a single carbohydrate moiety. The overall complex has 89% protein and 11% carbohydrate by weight. Recombinant interferon beta-1a is expressed in CHO cells containing the recombinant gene for human IFN-β and is equivalent to the human form secreted by fibroblasts.

Interferon beta-1a is indicated for the treatment of relapsing forms of MS. Patients treated with interferon beta-1a demonstrate a slower progression to disability and a less noticeable breakdown of the blood-brain barrier as observed in gadolinium-enhanced magnetic resonance imaging (MRI).

TABLE 4.8 β-Interferons

	Interferon Beta-1a (Avonex)	Interferon Beta-1b (Betaseron)
Recombinant system	CHO cells	*Escherichia coli*
Type	Asn$_{80}$ complex carbohydrate	Not glycosylated
Concentration	30 μg or 6 million IU/mL	250 μg or 8 million IU/mL
Supplied form	Powder for reconstitution	Powder for reconstitution
Diluent	Sterile water–no preservatives	NaCl 0.54% without preservatives
Storage	2°C–8°C; do not freeze	2°C–8°C; do not freeze
Dosage	30 μg once a week	250 μg every other day
Route	Intramuscular	Subcutaneous
Notable side effects	Injection site reactions, 3%; no necrosis	Injection site reactions, 85%; necrosis, 5%

Although the exact mechanism of action of interferon beta-1a in MS has not been elucidated, it is known that the drug exerts its biological effects by binding to specific receptors on the surface of human cells. This binding initiates a cascade of intracellular events that lead to the expression of interferon-induced gene products. These include $2',5'$-oligoadenylate synthetase and β_2 microglobulin. These products have been measured in the serum and in cellular fractions of blood collected from patients treated with interferon beta-1a. The functionally specific interferon-induced proteins have not been defined for MS.

Adverse effects include flulike syndrome at the start of therapy that decreases in severity as treatment progresses. Interferon beta-1a is a potential abortifacient and an inhibitor of cytochrome P450.

The dosage form is a powder for solution that is reconstituted in sterile water. Excipients are human albumin, sodium chloride, and phosphate buffer. The solution can be stored at $2°C$ to $8°C$ and should be discarded if it freezes. The lyophilized powder expires in 15 months. After reconstitution, the solution should be used within 6 hours. The solution should not be shaken because of the albumin content.

Interferon Beta-1b (Recombinant)[127]

Interferon beta-1b, Betaseron, is a protein that is expressed in a recombinant *E. coli*. It is equivalent in type to the interferon that is expressed by human fibroblasts. Interferon beta-1b possesses 165 amino acids and has an approximate molecular mass of 18.5 kDa. The native form has 166 amino acids and weighs 23 kDa. Interferon beta-1b contains a serine residue at position 17 rather than the cysteine in native IFN-β and does not contain the complex carbohydrate side chains found in the natural molecule. In addition to its antiviral activity, interferon beta-1b possesses immunomodulating activity.

Interferon beta-1b is administered SC to decrease the frequency of clinical exacerbation in ambulatory patients with relapsing–remitting multiple sclerosis (RRMS). RRMS is characterized by unpredictable attacks resulting in neurological deficits, separated by variable periods of remission.

Although it is not possible to delineate the mechanisms by which interferon beta-1b exerts its activity in MS, it is known that the interferon binds to specific receptors on cell surfaces and induces the expression of several interferon-induced gene products, such as $2',5'$-oligoadenylate synthetase and protein kinase. Additionally, interferon beta-1b blocks the synthesis of INF-γ, which is believed to be involved in MS attacks.

Interferon beta-1b is supplied as powder for solution with albumin and/or dextrose as excipients. It should be stored at $2°C$ to $8°C$ without freezing. After reconstitution, the solution can be stored in the refrigerator for 3 hours. The solution should not be shaken.

A major difference between interferon beta-1a and beta-1b is that beta-1b causes more hemorrhage and necrosis at the injection site than does interferon beta-1a.

PRODUCTS: γ-INTERFERON

Interferon Gamma-1b (Recombinant)[128]

Interferon gamma-1b, Actimmune, is a recombinant protein expressed in *E. coli*. IFN-γ is the cytokine that is secreted by human T lymphocytes and NK cells. It is a single-chain glycoprotein composed of 140 amino acids. The crystal structure of the protein reveals several helical segments arranged to approximate a toric shape.

Interferon gamma-1b is indicated for reducing the frequency and severity of serious infections associated with chronic granulomatous disease, an inherited disorder characterized by deficient phagocyte oxidase activity. In this disease, macrophages try to respond to invading organisms but lack the key oxidative enzymes to dispose of them. To compensate, additional macrophages are recruited into the infected region and form a granulomatous structure around the site. IFN-γ can stimulate the oxidative burst in macrophages and may reverse the situation.

Interferon gamma-1b is supplied as a solution in sterile water for injection. The solution must be stored at $2°C$ to $8°C$, without freezing. The product cannot tolerate more than 12 hours at room temperature.

THE INTERLEUKINS

Aldesleukin[129]

Aldesleukin, T-cell growth factor, thymocyte-stimulating factor, Proleukin, is recombinant IL-2 expressed in an engineered strain of *E. coli* containing an analog of the human IL-2 gene. The recombinant product is a highly purified protein of 133 amino acids with an approximate molecular mass of 15,300 Da. Unlike native IL-2, aldesleukin is not glycosylated, has no N-terminal alanine, and has serine substituted for Cys at site 125. Aldesleukin exists in solution as biologically active, noncovalently bound microaggregates with an average size of 27 IL-2 molecules. This contrasts with traditional solution aggregates of proteins, which often form irreversibly bound structures that are biologically inactive.

Aldesleukin enhances lymphocyte mitogenesis and stimulates long-term growth of human IL-2-dependent cell lines. IL-2 also enhances the cytotoxicity of lymphocytes. Induction of NK cell and lymphocyte-activated killer (LAK) cell activity occurs, as does induction of production. In mouse and human tumor cell lines, aldesleukin activates cellular immunity in patients with profound lymphocytosis, eosinophilia, and thrombocytopenia. Aldesleukin also activates the production of cytokines, including tumor necrosis factor (TNF), IL-1, and IFN-γ. In vivo experiments in mouse tumor models have shown inhibition of tumor growth. The mechanism of the antitumor effect of aldesleukin is unknown.

Aldesleukin is indicated for the treatment of metastatic renal cell carcinoma in adults. It is also indicated for the treatment of metastatic melanoma in adults. Research is under way on the use of aldesleukin for the treatment of various cancers (including head and neck cancers), treatment of acute myelogenous leukemia, and adjunct therapy in the treatment of Kaposi sarcoma. Renal and hepatic function is typically impaired during therapy with aldesleukin, so interaction with other drugs that undergo elimination by these organs is possible.

Aldesleukin is supplied as a powder for solution. After reconstitution, the solution should not be shaken. The preparation is solubilized with sodium dodecyl sulfate (SDS) in a phosphate buffer. Aldesleukin should be stored as nonreconstituted powder at $2°C$ to $8°C$ and never frozen. Reconstituted vials can be frozen and thawed once in 7 days without loss of activity. It expires over a period of 18 months.

Denileukin Diftitox (Recombinant)[130]

Denileukin diftitox, recombinant, Ontak, is an example of a drug that acts like a Trojan horse. One part of the molecule is involved in recognition and binds selectively with the diseased cell, and a highly toxic second part of the molecule effects a kill. Denileukin diftitox is a fusion protein expressed by a recombinant strain of *E. coli*. It is an rDNA-derived cytotoxic protein composed of the amino acid sequences for diphtheria toxin fragments A and B (Met_1-Thr_{387})-His, followed by the sequences for IL-2 (Ala_1-Thr_{133}). The fusion protein has a molecular mass of 58,000 Da. We can think of this large protein as a molecule of diphtheria toxin in which the receptor-binding domain has been replaced by IL-2 sequences, thereby changing its binding specificity. Cells that express the high-affinity (α, β, γ) IL-2 receptor bind the protein tightly. The IL-2 component is used as a director to bring the cytotoxic species in contact with tumor cells. The diphtheria toxin inhibits cellular protein synthesis and the cells die. Malignant cells in certain leukemias and lymphomas, including cutaneous T-cell lymphoma, express the high-affinity IL-2 receptor on their cell surfaces. It is these cells that denileukin diftitox targets.

Denileukin diftitox is indicated for the treatment of persistent or recurrent cutaneous T-cell lymphoma whose malignant cells express the CD25 component of the IL-2 receptor.

Denileukin diftitox is supplied as a frozen solution in water for injection. It should be stored at $-10°C$ or colder. It is suggested that the vials be thawed in a refrigerator at $2°C$ to $8°C$ for less than 24 hours or at room temperature for 1 to 2 hours. Prepared solutions should be used within 6 hours. The drug is administered by IV infusion from a bag or through a syringe pump.

Oprelvekin (Recombinant)[131,132]

Oprelvekin, Neumega, is recombinant human IL-11 that is expressed in a recombinant strain of *E. coli* as a thioredoxin and/or rhIL-11 fusion protein. The fusion protein is cleaved and purified to obtain the rhIL-11 protein. The protein is 177 amino acids in length and has a mass of approximately 19,000 Da. Oprelvekin differs from the natural 178-amino acid IL-11 by lacking an N-terminal proline. This alteration has not resulted in differences in bioactivity either in vitro or in vivo.

IL-11 is a thrombopoietic growth factor. It directly stimulates the proliferation of hematopoietic stem cells as well as megakaryocyte progenitor cells. This process induces megakaryocyte maturation and increased production of platelets. The primary hematopoietic activity of oprelvekin is stimulation of megakaryocytopoiesis and thrombopoiesis. Primary osteoblasts and mature osteoclasts express mRNAs for both IL-11 and its receptor, IL-11R alpha. Hence, both bone-forming and bone-resorbing cells are possible targets for IL-11.

Oprelvekin is indicated for the prevention of severe thrombocytopenia. It reduces the need for platelet transfusions after myelosuppressive chemotherapy in patients with nonmyeloid malignancies who are at high risk for severe thrombocytopenia. Efficacy has been demonstrated in persons who have experienced severe thrombocytopenia following a previous chemotherapy cycle.

Oprelvekin causes many adverse reactions. Among these are edema, neutropenic fever, headache, nausea and/or vomiting, dyspnea, and tachycardia. Patients must be monitored closely.

Oprelvekin is supplied as a lyophilized powder for reconstitution. Excipients include glycine and phosphate buffer components. The powder has a shelf life of 24 months. It should be stored at $2°C$ to $8°C$. If it is frozen, thaw it before reconstitution.

Tumor Necrosis Factor (Recombinant)[133–135]

The TNFs (Etanercept, Enbrel) are members of a family of cytokines that are produced primarily in the innate immune system by activated mononuclear phagocytes. Along with IL-1, TNF is typically the first cytokine to be produced upon infection, and its reactions can be both positive and negative. On the one hand, TNF can cause cytotoxicity and inflammation, and on the other hand, it serves as a signal to the adaptive immune response. The TNFs are all endogenous pyrogens, and they cause chills, fever, and flulike symptoms. There are two forms of TNF: TNFα (cachectin) and TNFβ (lymphotoxin). Both bind to the same receptor and cause similar effects.

Etanercept is a dimeric fusion protein consisting of the extracellular ligand-binding portion of the human 75-kDa (p75) TNF receptor (TNFR) linked to the Fc portion of human isotype IgG_1. The Fc component of etanercept contains the CH_2 domain, the CH_3 domain, and the hinge region, but not the CH_1 domain of IgG_1. These regions are responsible for the biological effects of immunoglobulins. Etanercept is produced in recombinant CHO cultures. It consists of a peptide chain of 934 amino acids and has a molecular mass of approximately 150 kDa. It binds specifically to TNF and blocks its interaction with cell surface TNFRs. Each etanercept molecule binds specifically to two TNF molecules in the synovial fluid of rheumatoid arthritis patients. It is equally efficacious at blocking TNFα and TNFβ. The drug is indicated for reducing signs and symptoms and inhibiting the progression of structural damage in patients with moderately to severely active rheumatoid arthritis. Etanercept is also indicated for reducing signs and symptoms of moderately to severely active polyarticular-course juvenile rheumatoid arthritis in patients 4 years of age and older who have had an inadequate response to one or more disease-modifying antirheumatic drugs (DMARDS). Etanercept is also indicated for reducing signs and symptoms of active arthritis in patients with psoriatic arthritis.

◉ ENZYMES

Blood-Clotting Factors

The blood clotting system of the human body is typically in a carefully balanced homeostatic state. If damage occurs to a blood vessel wall, a clot will form to wall off the damage so that the process of regeneration can begin. Normally this process is highly localized to the damaged region, so that the hemostatic response does not cause thrombi to migrate to distant sites or persist longer than it is needed. Lysis of blood clots occurs through the conversion of plasminogen to plasmin, which causes fibrinolysis, converting insoluble fibrin to soluble fibrinopeptides. The plasminogen–plasmin conversion is catalyzed by several blood and tissue activators, among them urokinase, kallikrein, plasminogen activators, and some undefined inhibitors. More specifically, the conversion of plasminogen to plasmin is catalyzed by two extremely specific serine proteases: a urokinase plasminogen activator (uPA) and a tissue plasminogen activator (tPA). This section focuses on tPA.

Human tPA is a serine protease that is synthesized in the vascular endothelial cells. It is a single-chain peptide composed of 527 amino acids and has a molecular mass of approximately 64,000 Da. About 7% of the mass of the molecule consists of carbohydrate. The molecule contains 35 Cys residues. These are fully paired, giving the tPA molecule 17 disulfide bonds. There are four N-linked glycosylation sites recognized by consensus sequences Asn-X-Ser/Thr at residues 117, 184, 218, and 448. It is suspected that Thr_{61} bears an *O*-fucose residue. There are two forms of tPA that differ by the presence or absence of a carbohydrate group at Asp_{184}. Type I tPA is glycosylated at Asn_{117}, Asn_{184}, and Asn_{448}, whereas type II tPA lacks a glycosyl group at Asn_{184}. Asn_{218} is typically unsubstituted in both forms. Asn_{117} contains a high-mannose oligosaccharide, whereas Asn substituents 184 and 448 are complex carbohydrate substituted. During the process of fibrinolysis the single-chain protein is cleaved between Arg_{275} and Ile_{276} by plasmin to yield two-chain tPA. Two-chain tPA consists of a heavy chain (the A chain, derived from the N-terminus) and a light chain (B chain), linked by a single disulfide bond between Cys_{264} and Cys_{395}. The A chain bears some unique structural features: the finger region (residues 6–36), the growth factor region (approximate residues 44–80), and two kringle domains. These domains are disulfide-closed loops, mostly β sheet in structure. The finger and kringle 2 are responsible for tPA binding to fibrin and for the activation of plasminogen. The function of kringle 1 is not known. The B chain contains the serine protease domain that contains the His-Asp-Ser unit that cleaves plasminogen.

TISSUE PLASMINOGEN ACTIVATOR, RECOMBINANT[136,137]

Recombinant tPA (rtPA), alteplase (Activase), is identical with endogenous tPA. rtPA lacks a glycosyl residue at Asn_{184}. At one time, rtPA was produced in two-chain form in CHO cultures. Now, large-scale cultures of recombinant human melanoma cells in fermenters are used to produce a product that is about 80% single-chain rtPA.

Alteplase is used to improve ventricular function following an acute myocardial infarction, including reducing the incidence of congestive heart failure and decreasing mortality. The drug is also used to treat acute ischemic stroke after computed tomography (CT) or other diagnostic imaging has ruled out intracranial hemorrhage. rtPA is also used in cases of acute pulmonary thromboembolism and is being investigated for unstable angina pectoris.

Alteplase is supplied as powder for injection, and in reconstituted form (normal saline or 5% dextrose in water) is intended for IV infusion only. The solution expires in 8 hours at room temperature and must be prepared just before use.

RETEPLASE

Reteplase (Retavase) is a deletion mutant variant of tPA that is produced in recombinant *E. coli*. The deletions are in domains responsible for half-life, fibrin affinity, and thrombolytic potency. It consists of the kringle-2 domain

TABLE 4.9 Comparison of the Pharmacokinetic Parameters of Alteplase and Reteplase

Pharmacokinetic Parameter	Alteplase	Reteplase
Effective $t_{1/2}$ (minutes)	5	13–16
Volume of distribution (L)	8.1	6
Plasma clearance (mL/min)	360–620	250–450

and protease domain of tPA but lacks the kringle-1 domain and the growth factor domain. It is considered a third-generation thrombolytic agent and has a mechanism of action similar to that of alteplase. Reteplase acts directly by catalyzing the cleavage of plasminogen and initiating thrombolysis. It has high thrombolytic potency. A comparison of alteplase and reteplase is given in Table 4.9.

TENECTEPLASE[137]

Tenecteplase is a tPA produced by recombinant CHO cells. The molecule is a 527-amino acid glycoprotein developed by introducing the following modifications to the cDNA construct: Thr_{103} to Asp, Asp_{117} to Gln, both within the kringle-1 domain, and a tetra-alanine substitution at amino acids 296 to 299 in the protease domain. The drug is a sterile, lyophilized powder recommended for single IV bolus administration after reconstitution with sterile water. Tenecteplase should be administered immediately after reconstitution.

FACTOR VIII[138]

Antihemophilic factor VIII (recombinant), Recombinate, Kogenate, Bioclate, Helixate, is a plasma protein that functions in the normal blood-clotting cascade by increasing the V_{max} for the activation of clotting factor X by factor IXa in the presence of calcium ions and negatively charged phospholipids. Factor VIII is used in the treatment of hemophilia A. Hemophilia A is a congenital disorder characterized by bleeding. The introduction of factor VIII as a drug has improved the quality of life and the life expectancy of individuals with this disorder. Unfortunately, it has been necessary to rely on an unsure source (human plasma) for the factor. Exposure of patients to alloantigens and viruses has been a concern. Factor VIII derived from a recombinant source will potentially eliminate many of these problems and provide an essentially unlimited supply of the drug.

Factor VIII is biosynthesized as a single-chain polypeptide of 2,332 amino acids. The protein is very heavily glycosylated. Shortly after biosynthesis, peptide cleavage occurs and plasma factor VIII circulates as an 80-kDa light chain associated with a series of heavy chains of approximately 210 kDa in a metal ion-stabilized complex. Factor VIII possesses 25 potential N-linked glycosylation sites and 22 Cys residues. The 210-kDa heavy chain is further cleaved by proteases to yield a series of proteins of molecular mass 90 to 188 kDa. The 90- to 188-kDa protein molecules form a metal ion-stabilized complex with the light chain.

Recombinant factor VIII is produced in two recombinant systems: in batch culture of transfected CHO cells or in continuous culture of BHK cells. There are four types of recombinant factor VIII available. All four are produced by inserting a cDNA construct encoding the entire peptide sequence into the

CHO cell or BHK cell line. The CHO cell product contains a Galα[1→3]Gal unit, whereas the BHK enzyme does not. Recombinant factor VIII is polydisperse, containing multiple peptide homologues including an 80-kDa protein and various modifications of an approximately 90-kDa subunit protein. The product contains no blood products and is free of microbes and pyrogens.

Recombinant factor VIII is indicated for the treatment of classical hemophilia (hemophilia A) and for the prevention and treatment of hemorrhagic episodes and perioperative management of patients with hemophilia A. The drug is also indicated for the treatment of hemophilia A in persons who possess inhibitors to factor VIII.

Recombinant factor VIII is supplied in sterile, single-dose vials. The product is stabilized with human albumin and lyophilized. The product must be stored at 2°C to 8°C, without freezing. In some instances, the powder may be stored at room temperature for up to 3 months without loss of biological activity. Shaking of the reconstituted product should be avoided because of the presence of the albumin. The drug must be administered by IV bolus or drip infusion within 3 hours of reconstitution.

Because trace amounts of mouse or hamster protein may copurify with recombinant factor VIII, one should be cautious when administering the drug to individuals with known hypersensitivity to plasma-derived antihemophilic factor or with hypersensitivity to biological preparations with trace amounts of mouse or hamster proteins.

CLOTTING FACTOR IX (RECOMBINANT)[139,140]

When a person is deficient in clotting factor IX (Christmas factor), hemophilia B results. Hemophilia B affects primarily males and accounts for about 15% of all cases of hemophilia. Treatment involves replacement of factor IX so that the blood will clot. Recombinant coagulation factor IX (BeneFIX) is a highly purified protein produced in recombinant CHO cells, free of blood products. The product is a glycoprotein of molecular mass approximately 55,000 Da. It consists of 415 amino acids in a single chain. The primary amino acid sequence of BeneFIX is identical with the Ala$_{148}$ allelic form of plasma-derived factor IX, and it has structural and functional characteristics similar to those of the endogenous protein. The recombinant protein is purified by chromatography, followed by membrane filtration. SDS-polyacrylamide gel electrophoresis shows that the product exists primarily as a single component.

Clotting factor IX, recombinant, is indicated for the control and prevention of hemorrhagic episodes in persons with hemophilia B (Christmas disease), including the control and prevention of bleeding in surgical procedures.

BeneFIX is supplied as a sterile lyophilized powder. It should be stored at 2°C to 8°C. The product will tolerate storage at room temperature not above 25°C for 6 months. The drug becomes unstable, following reconstitution, and must be used within 3 hours.

DROTRECOGIN ALFA[141]

About 750,000 people are diagnosed with sepsis in the United States each year, and of these, an estimated 30% will die from it, despite treatment with IV antibiotics and supportive care. Patients with severe sepsis often experience failures of various systems in the body, including the circulatory system, the kidneys, and clotting. Drotrecogin alfa (activated), drotrecogin alfa (activated; Xigris), is a recombinant form of human activated protein C. Activated protein C exerts an antithrombotic effect by inhibiting factors Va and VIIIa. In vitro data indicate that activated protein C has indirect profibrinolytic activity through its ability to inhibit plasminogen activator inhibitor-1 (PAI-1) and to limit generation of activated thrombin-activatable fibrinolysis inhibitor. Additionally, in vitro data indicate that activated protein C may exert an anti-inflammatory effect by inhibiting TNF production by monocytes, by blocking leukocyte adhesion to selectins, and by limiting the thrombin-induced inflammatory responses within the microvascular epithelium.

Vials of drotrecogin alfa should be stored at 2°C to 8°C without freezing. The reconstituted solution is stable for 14 hours at 25°C.

Anticoagulant

LEPIRUDIN, RECOMBINANT[142]

Leeches *(Hirudo medicinalis)* have been used medicinally for centuries to treat injuries in which blood engorges the tissues. The logic behind this is solid: leeches produce an agent known as *hirudin* that is a potent, specific thrombin inhibitor. Leeches have been used to prevent thrombosis in the microvasculature of reattached digits. Lepirudin (Refludan) is an rDNA-derived protein produced in yeast. It has a molecular mass of approximately 7,000 Da. Lepirudin differs from the natural polypeptide, in that it has an N-terminal leucine instead of isoleucine and is missing a sulfate function at Tyr$_{63}$.

Other Enzymes

RECOMBINANT HUMAN DEOXYRIBONUCLEASE I (DNASE)[143]

DNAse is a human endonuclease, normally present in saliva, urine, pancreatic secretions, and blood. The enzyme catalyzes the hydrolysis of extracellular DNA into oligonucleotides. Aerosolized recombinant human deoxyribonuclease I (rhDNAse), dornase alfa, Pulmozyme, has been formulated into an inhalation agent for the treatment of pulmonary disease in patients with CF.

Among the clinical manifestations of CF are obstruction of the airways by viscous, dehydrated mucus. Pulmonary function is diminished, and microbes can become entrapped in the viscid matrix. A cycle of pulmonary obstruction and infection leads to progressive lung destruction and eventual death before the age of 30 for most CF patients. The immune system responds by sending in neutrophils, and these accumulate and eventually degenerate, releasing large amounts of DNA. The high levels of extracellular DNA released and the mucous glycoproteins are responsible for the degenerating lung function. The DNA-rich secretions also bind to aminoglycoside antibiotics typically used to treat the infections. In vitro studies showed that the viscosity of the secretions could be reduced by application of DNAse I.

Before DNAse was purified and sequenced from human sources, a partial DNA sequence from bovine DNAse (263 amino acids) was used to create a library that could be used to screen a human pancreatic DNA library. This facilitated the development of the human recombinant protein. The endogenous human and recombinant protein sequences are identical.

rhDNAse was cloned, sequenced, and expressed to examine the potential of DNAse I as a drug for use in CF. It has been shown that cleavage of high–molecular-weight DNA into smaller fragments by treatment with aerosolized rhDNAse improves the clearance of mucus from the lungs and reduces the exacerbations of respiratory symptoms requiring parenteral antibiotics.

rhDNAse I is a monomeric glycoprotein consisting of 260 amino acids produced in CHO cell culture. The molecule possesses four Cys residues and two sites that probably contain N-linked glycosides. The molecular mass of the molecule is about 29 kDa. DNAse I is an endonuclease that cleaves double-stranded DNA (and to some extent, single-stranded DNA) into 5′-phosphate-terminated polynucleotides. Activity depends on the presence of calcium and magnesium ions.

Pulmozyme is approved for use in the treatment of CF patients, in conjunction with standard therapies, to reduce the frequency of respiratory infections requiring parenteral antibiotics and to improve pulmonary function. The dose is delivered at a level of 2.5 mg daily with a nebulizer. Pulmozyme is not a replacement for antibiotics, bronchodilators, and daily physical therapy.

CEREZYME

Type 1 Gaucher disease is a hereditary condition occurring in about 1:40,000 individuals. It is characterized by a functional deficiency in β-glucocerebrosidase enzyme activity and the resulting accumulation of lipid glucocerebroside in tissue macrophages, which become engorged and are termed *Gaucher cells*. Gaucher cells typically accumulate in the liver, spleen, and bone marrow and, occasionally, in lung, kidney, and intestine. Secondary hematological sequelae include severe anemia and thrombocytopenia in addition to characteristic progressive hepatosplenomegaly. Skeletal complications are common and are frequently the most debilitating and disabling feature of Gaucher disease. Possible skeletal complications are osteonecrosis, osteopenia with secondary pathological fractures, remodeling failure, osteosclerosis, and bone crises.

Cerezyme (Imiglucerase)[144] is a recombinant, macrophage-targeted variant of human β-glucocerebrosidase, purified from CHO cells. It catalyzes the hydrolysis of the glycolipid glucocerebroside to glucose and ceramide following the normal degradation pathway for membrane lipids.

Cerezyme is supplied as a lyophilized powder for reconstitution. The powder should be stored at 2°C to 8°C until used. The reconstituted product for IV infusion is stable for 12 hours at room temperature.

⬡ VACCINES

Vaccines and immunizing biologicals are covered thoroughly in Chapter 5 of this text, so no lengthy discussion is given here. Vaccine production is a natural application of rDNA technology, aimed at achieving highly pure and efficacious products. Currently, there are four rDNA vaccines approved for human use. A number of others are in clinical trials for some rather exotic uses. It would appear that biotechnological approaches to vaccines will bring about some very useful drugs.

Products

RECOMBIVAX AND ENGERIX-B[145]

Recombivax and Engerix-B are interchangeable for immunization against hepatitis B virus (HBV, serum hepatitis). Both contain a 226-amino acid polypeptide composing 22-nm diameter particles that possess the antigenic epitopes of the HBV surface coat (S) protein. The products from two manufacturers are expressed from recombinant *S. cerevisiae*. It is recommended that patients receive 3 doses, with the second dose 1 month after the first and the third dose 6 months after the first. The route and site of injection are IM in deltoid muscle or, for infants and young children, in the anterolateral thigh. The vaccines achieve 94% to 98% immunogenicity among adults 20 to 39 years of age, 1 to 2 months after the third dose. Adults older than 40 years of age reach 89% immunogenicity. Infants, young children, and adolescents achieve 96% to 99% immunogenicity.

The vaccine is supplied as a suspension adsorbed to aluminum hydroxide. The shelf life is 36 months. The vaccine should be stored at 2°C to 8°C and should be discarded if frozen. Freezing destroys potency.

LYMErix[146]

Lyme disease is caused by the spirochete *Borrelia burgdorferi*. The microorganism is transmitted primarily by ticks and is endemic in heavily wooded areas and forests. The disease produces arthritis-like symptoms. A vaccine against Lyme disease was created by developing a recombinant *E. coli* that contains the gene for the bacterial outer surface protein. This protein (OspA) is a single polypeptide chain of 257 amino acids with covalently bound lipids at the N-terminus. The vaccine is formulated as a suspension with aluminum hydroxide as an adsorption adjuvant. In testing, subjects between 15 and 70 years immunized with 3 doses of LYMErix at 0, 1, and 12 months demonstrated a 78% decrease in the likelihood of infection.

LYMErix has a shelf life of 24 months. It should be stored at 2°C to 8°C and must be discarded if frozen. If necessary, the vaccine can tolerate 4 days at room temperature.

COMVAX

Comvax is a combination of *Haemophilus influenzae* type b conjugate and hepatitis B (recombinant). It was recently approved by the Advisory Committee on Immunization Practices (ACIP). Each 0.5-mL dose contains 7.5 μg of *H. influenzae* type b polyribosylribitol phosphate (PRP), 125 μg of *Neisseria meningitidis* outer membrane protein complex (OMPC), and 5 μg of hepatitis B surface antigen (HBsAg) on an aluminum hydroxide adjuvant. The Committee on Infectious Diseases, the American Academy of Pediatrics, and the Advisory Academy of Family Physicians recommend that all infants receive the vaccine. Three doses should be administered at ages 2, 4, and 12 to 15 months. The vaccine should not be administered to infants younger than 6 weeks because of potential suppression of the immune response to PRP-OMPC with subsequent doses of Comvax TM. The series should be completed by 12 to 15 months.

TABLE 4.10 **Vaccines Developed Using Biotechnology**

Vaccine	Type	Use
MAGE-12: 170–178	Vaccine	Breast, colorectal, lung cancers; melanoma; sarcoma
MART-1 melanoma vaccine	Vaccine	Metastatic melanoma
Mylovenge	Vaccine	Multiple myeloma
Myeloma-derived idiotypic Ag vaccine	Vaccine	Multiple myeloma
Melacine melanoma theraccine, therapeutic vaccine	Therapeutic vaccine	Stage IV malignant melanoma
NBI-6024	Peptide therapeutic vaccine	Type 1 diabetes
Antigastrin therapeutic vaccine	Vaccine	Gastroesophageal reflux disease
Helivax *Helicobacter pylori* vaccine	Cellular vaccine	*H. pylori* infection
Hepatitis E vaccine	Recombinant subunit vaccine	Hepatitis E prophylaxis
StreptAvax	Vaccine	Group A streptococci, including necrotizing fasciitis, strep throat, and rheumatic fever
Hepatitis B vaccine	Recombinant vaccine	Hepatitis B prophylaxis

Vaccines in Development

Quite a number of biotechnology-generated vaccines are in development (Table 4.10).

Some of them are in the category of "therapeutic vaccines." These vaccines are designed to bind to cellular receptors, endogenous molecules, and so on, producing specific pharmacological effects. For example, if a cell has a particular receptor that binds a ligand to activate the cell, binding an antibody raised by a specific vaccine to the receptor will prevent activation. If a tumor has a requirement for such a receptor–ligand binding, using a vaccine to develop antibody to the receptor or the ligand should prevent or slow cellular proliferation.

 ## PREPARATION OF ANTIBODIES[147–149]

Hybridoma (Monoclonal Antibody) Techniques

In a humoral immune response, B-lymphocyte–derived plasma cells produce antibodies with variations in chemical structure. Biologically, these variations extend the utility of the secreted antibody. These variations are caused by affinity maturation, the tendency for the affinity of antibody for antigen to increase with each challenge, and mutation at the time of somatic recombination. These phenomena produce antibodies with slightly different specificities. Because the clones of antibody-producing cells provide more than one structural type of antibody, they are called *polyclonal antibodies*. Another type of antibody consists of highly homogeneous populations of hybrid proteins produced by one clone of specially prepared B lymphocytes. These antibodies, lacking structural variations, are highly "focused" on their antigenic counterparts' determinants or epitopes, and are called *monoclonal*.

A problem with creating MAbs is that one cannot simply prepare an antibody-producing B lymphocyte and propagate it. Such cells live only briefly in the laboratory environment. Instead, antibody-producing cells are fused with an immortal (tumor) cell line to create *hybridomas*—long-lived, antibody-secreting cells. The trick is to select the monoclonal cells that produce the desired antibody. The hybridoma technique has opened the door to new therapeutic antibodies, imaging agents, radiological diagnostic test kits, targeted radionuclide delivery agents, and home test kits.

In the hybridoma method (Fig. 4.14), a mouse or other small animal is sensitized with an antigen. When a high enough titer of antibody against the selected antigen has been attained, the animal is sacrificed and its spleen cells are collected. The spleen cells contain a large number of B lymphocytes, and it is certain that some will be able to produce antigen-specific antibodies. Because the spleen cells are normal B lymphocytes, they have a very short lifetime in cell cultures. Therefore, a method must be used to extend their lifetime.

To produce MAbs, B cells are fused with immortal myeloma cells in the presence of fusogens such as PEG. This procedure produces genetically half-normal and half-myeloma cells. Because the myeloma cells are immortal, the longevity problem is solved. The selection process depends on two different myeloma cell lines: one lacking the enzyme hypoxanthine-guanine phosphoribosyl transferase (HGPRT), a key enzyme in the nucleotide salvage pathways, and the other lacking the *Tk* gene, a key gene in the pyrimidine biosynthetic pathways. The spleen B cells are HGPRT and *Tk* (+), whereas the myeloma cells are HGPRT and *Tk* (−). This myeloma cell line cannot survive in a medium containing aminopterin, a thymidylate synthetase inhibitor, because it cannot synthesize pyrimidines. The HGPRT (−) cell line cannot use the purine salvage pathways to make nucleotides, forcing it to use thymidylate synthetase. With thymidylate synthetase inhibited, the cell dies. After fusion, cells are maintained on a medium containing hypoxanthine, aminopterin, and thymidine (HAT). Only cells that are "correctly" fused between one spleen cell (HGPRT [+]) and one myeloma cell (immortal), that is, a hybridoma, can survive in HAT medium. Fused myeloma cells (myeloma–myeloma) lack the correct genes and cannot survive. Fused spleen cells (spleen–spleen) cannot grow in culture. Thus, only the fused hybridoma (myeloma–spleen) survives. Hypoxanthine and thymidine furnish precursors for the growth of HGPRT (+) cells. Aminopterin suppresses cells that failed to fuse. Hybridomas can be isolated in a 96-well plate and transferred into larger cultures for proliferation. The culture medium will eventually contain a high concentration of MAb against the original antigen. This antibody can be purified to homogeneity.

MAbs, being proteins, tend to be highly immunogenic in humans. This is especially true of the MAbs produced in mouse culture. Humans begin to develop antibodies to

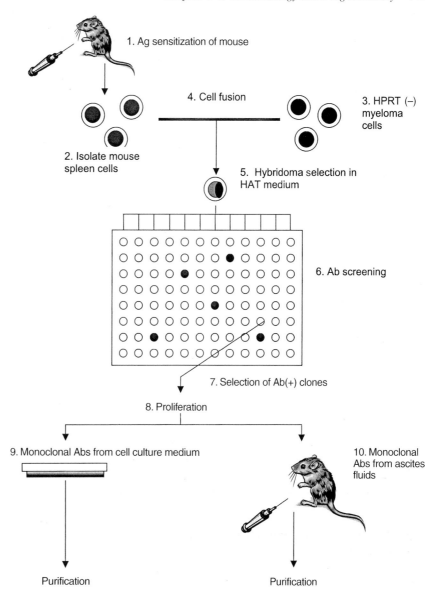

1. Ag sensitization of mouse

4. Cell fusion

3. HPRT (−) myeloma cells

2. Isolate mouse spleen cells

5. Hybridoma selection in HAT medium

6. Ab screening

7. Selection of Ab(+) clones

8. Proliferation

9. Monoclonal Abs from cell culture medium

10. Monoclonal Abs from ascites fluids

Purification

Purification

Figure 4.14 ● General method for the preparation of monoclonal antibodies, using hybridomas and HAT medium. (Ab, antibody; Ag, antigen.)

mouse MAbs after a single dose. This is natural. The human host is mounting an antibody response to a foreign antigen. The human antimouse antibody (known as *HAMA*) response has tended to limit the use of monoclonals in human therapy.

In developing a method for making MAbs useful in humans, it is necessary to remove the mouse immunogenic characteristics from the MAb. The antigen-recognition region (Fab) of the MAb must retain its ability to bind to the antigen, however. If this feature is altered, the antibody will likely be useless. Within the light and heavy chains of the Fab portions of antibody molecules are regions that are called *complementarity-determining regions* or CDRs. Each chain possesses three of these. One of the CDRs, CDR3, is located at the juncture of the variable and common domains. CDR3 is also referred to as the *hypervariable region* because most of the variability of the antibody molecule is concentrated there. These must be intact for specific antigen–antibody binding. Immune responses against murine MAb are directed against not only the variable regions, but also the constant regions. Hence, to decrease the

immunogenicity of an MAb one must create antibodies that have been "humanized." In MAb production, usually the V_H and V_L domains of a human antibody are replaced by the corresponding regions from the mouse antibody, leaving the specificity intact, but using human constant regions that should not be immunogenic. Antibodies like these are called *chimeric*, and they are less immunogenic and have a longer half-life in human patients. Examples of chimeric MAbs are abciximab, rituximab, infliximab, and basiliximab.

Methods are available for the development of MAbs with 95% to 100% human sequence. By using transgenic mice, all of the essential human antibody genes can be expressed.

Monoclonal Antibody Drugs

RITUXIMAB[150,151]

Rituximab (Rituxan, Chimeric) is an MAb directed against the CD20 antigen expressed on the surfaces of normal and malignant B lymphocytes. The MAb is produced in mammalian (CHO) suspension culture and is a chimeric (murine/human) MAb of the $IgG_1 \kappa$ type. The protein is composed of murine light and heavy chain variable regions and human constant regions. Rituximab is indicated for the treatment of patients with relapsed or refractory, low-grade or follicular, CD20(+) B-cell non-Hodgkin lymphoma. Rituximab binds specifically to antigen CD20 (human B-lymphocyte–restricted differentiation antigen, a hydrophobic transmembrane protein expressed on pre-B and mature B lymphocytes). CD20 is a protein of 35 to 37 kDa, and it may play a role in B cell activation and regulation and may be a calcium ion channel. The antigen is also expressed on more than 90% of non-Hodgkin lymphoma B cells but is not found on hematopoietic stem cells, pro-B cells, normal plasma cells, or other normal tissues. CD20 regulates the early steps in the activation process for cell cycle initiation and differentiation.

GEMTUZUMAB OZOGAMICIN[152,153]

Gemtuzumab ozogamicin (Mylotarg, fusion molecule) is an MAb derived from the CD33 antigen, a sialic acid-dependent adhesion protein expressed on the surface of leukemia blasts and immature normal cells of myelomonocytic origin but not on normal hematopoietic stem cells. CD33 binds sialic acid and appears to regulate signaling in myeloid cells. The antibody is recombinant, humanized IgG$_4$ κ, linked with the cytotoxic antitumor antibiotic ozogamicin (from the calicheamicin family). More than 98.3% of the amino acids of gemtuzumab are of human origin. The constant region of the MAb contains human sequences, whereas the CDRs derive from a murine antibody that binds CD33. The antibody is linked to N-acetyl-γ-calicheamicin via a bifunctional linker.

Gemtuzumab ozogamicin is indicated for the treatment of patients with CD33-positive acute myeloid leukemia in first relapse among adults 60 years of age or older who are not considered candidates for cytotoxic chemotherapy.

Gemtuzumab ozogamicin binds to the CD33 antigen expressed by hematopoietic cells. This antigen is expressed on the surface of leukemic blasts in more than 80% of patients with acute myeloid leukemia. CD33 is also expressed on normal and leukemic myeloid colony-forming cells, including leukemic clonogenic precursors, but it is not expressed on pluripotent hematopoietic stem cells or nonhematopoietic cells. Binding of the anti-CD33 antibody results in a complex that is internalized. On internalization the calicheamicin derivative is released inside the lysosomes of the myeloid cells. The released calicheamicin derivative binds to the minor groove of DNA and causes double-strand breaks and cell death.

ALEMTUZUMAB[154,155]

Alemtuzumab (Campath) is humanized MAb (Campath-1H) that is directed against the 21- to 28-kDa cell surface glycoprotein CD52. CD52 is expressed on the surface of normal and malignant B and T lymphocytes, NK cells, monocytes, macrophages, and tissues of the male reproductive system. The Campath-1H antibody is an IgG$_1$ κ form with humanized variable and constant regions and CDRs from a rat MAb, Campath-1G.

Alemtuzumab is indicated for the treatment of B-cell chronic lymphocytic leukemia in patients who have been treated with alkylating agents and who have failed on this therapy. Alemtuzumab binds to CD52, a nonmodulating

antigen that is present on the surface of essentially all B and T lymphocytes; most monocytes, macrophages, and NK cells, and a subpopulation of granulocytes. The proposed mechanism of action is antibody-dependent lysis of leukemic cells following cell surface binding.

BASILIXIMAB[156–158]

Basiliximab (Simulect, Chimeric) is an MAb produced by a mouse monoclonal cell line that has been engineered to produce the basiliximab IgG$_1$ κ antibody glycoprotein. The product is chimeric (murine/human). Basiliximab is indicated for prophylaxis of acute organ rejection in patients receiving renal transplantation when used as part of a regimen of immunosuppressants and corticosteroids. Basiliximab is also indicated in pediatric renal transplantation.

Basiliximab specifically binds to the IL-2 receptor α-chain (the CD25 antigen, part of the three-component IL-2 receptor site). These sites are expressed on the surfaces of activated T lymphocytes. Once bound, it blocks the IL-2α receptor with extremely high affinity. This specific, high-affinity binding to IL-2α competitively inhibits IL-2-mediated activation of lymphocytes, a critical event in the cellular immune response in allograft rejection.

DACLIZUMAB[159,160]

Molecularly, daclizumab (Zenapax, Chimeric) is an IgG$_1$ MAb that binds specifically to the α subunit of the IL-2 receptor (the complete, high-affinity activated IL-2 receptor consists of interacting α, β, and γ subunits). IL-2 receptors are expressed on the surfaces of activated lymphocytes, where they mediate lymphocyte clonal expansion and differentiation. Daclizumab is a chimeric protein (90% human and 10% mouse) IgG$_1$. The MAb targets only recently activated T cells that have interacted with antigen and have developed from their naive form into their activated form. It is at this time that the IL-2 receptors are expressed. The human amino acid sequences of daclizumab derive from constant domains of human IgG, and the variable domains are derived from the fused Eu myeloma antibody. The murine sequences derive from CDRs of a mouse anti-IL2α antibody.

The indications for daclizumab are prophylaxis of acute organ rejection in patients receiving renal transplants, as part of an immunosuppressant regimen including cyclosporine and corticosteroids. The mechanism of action is the same as that of basiliximab.

MUROMONAB-CD3[161–163]

Muromonab-CD3 (murine, Orthoclone-OKT3) is an unmodified mouse immunoglobulin, an IgG$_{2a}$, monoclonal. It binds a glycoprotein on the surface of mature T lymphocytes. Mature T cells have, as part of the signal transduction machinery of the T-cell receptor complex, a set of three glycoproteins that are collectively called CD3. Together with the protein zeta, the CD3 molecules become phosphorylated when the T-cell receptor is bound to a peptide fragment and the major histocompatibility complex. The phosphorylated CD3 and zeta molecules transmit information into the cell, ultimately producing transcription factors that enter the nucleus and direct the T-cell activity. By binding to CD3, muromonab-CD3 prevents signal transduction into T cells.

Muromonab-CD3 blocks the function of T cells that are involved in acute renal rejection. Hence, it is indicated for the treatment of acute allograft rejection in heart and liver transplant recipients resistant to standard steroid therapies.

ABCIXIMAB[164,165]

Abciximab (ReoPro, chimeric) is an MAb engineered from the glycoprotein IIb/IIIa receptor of human platelets. The preparation is fragmented, containing only the Fab portion of the antibody molecule. This MAb is a chimeric human–mouse immunoglobulin. The Fab fragments may contain mouse variable heavy- and light-chain regions and human constant heavy- and light-chain regions.

Abciximab is indicated as an adjunct to percutaneous transluminal coronary angioplasty or atherectomy for the prevention of acute cardiac ischemic complications in patients at high risk for abrupt closure of a treated coronary vessel. Abciximab appears to decrease the incidence of myocardial infarction.

Abciximab binds to the intact GPIIb/GPIIIa receptor, which is a member of the integrin family of adhesion receptors and the major platelet-specific receptors involved in aggregation. The antibody prevents platelet aggregation by preventing the binding of fibrinogen, the von Willebrand factor, and other adhesion molecules on activated platelets. The inhibition of binding to the surface receptors may be a result of steric hindrance or conformational effects preventing large molecules from approaching the receptor.

TRASTUZUMAB[166,167]

Trastuzumab (Herceptin, humanized) is an MAb engineered from the human epidermal growth factor receptor type 2 (HER2) protein. This MAb is a human–murine immunoglobulin. It contains human structural domains (framework) and the CDR of a murine antibody (4D5) that binds specifically to HER2. IgG_1 κ is the type structure, and the antibody is monoclonal. The protein inhibits the proliferation of human tumor cells that overexpress HER2.

Trastuzumab is indicated for use as a single agent for the treatment of patients with metastatic breast cancer whose tumors overexpress the HER2 protein and who have not received chemotherapy for their metastatic disease.

The HER2 proto-oncogene encodes a transmembrane receptor protein of 185 kDa that is structurally related to the epidermal growth factor receptor HER2. Overexpression of this protein is observed in 25% to 30% of primary breast cancers. Trastuzumab binds with high affinity to the extracellular domain of HER2. It inhibits the proliferation of human tumor cells that overexpress HER2. Trastuzumab also mediates the process of antibody-mediated cellular cytotoxicity (ADCC). This process, leading to cell death, is preferentially exerted on HER2-overexpressing cancer cells over those that do not overexpress HER2.

INFLIXIMAB[168,169]

The MAb infliximab (Remicade, chimeric) is produced from cells that have been sensitized with human $TNF\alpha$. The MAb is a chimeric human–mouse immunoglobulin. The constant regions are of human peptide sequence and the variable regions are murine. The MAb is of type IgG_1 κ.

Infliximab is indicated for the treatment of moderately to severely active Crohn disease to decrease signs and symptoms in patients who had an inadequate response to conventional treatments. Infliximab binds specifically to $TNF\alpha$. It neutralizes the biological activity of $TNF\alpha$ by binding with high affinity to soluble and transmembrane forms of the TNF. Infliximab destroys $TNF\alpha$-producing cells. An additional mechanism by which infliximab could work is as follows: by inhibiting $TNF\alpha$, pathways leading to IL-1 and IL-6 are inhibited. These interleukins are inflammatory cytokines. Inhibiting their production blocks some of the inflammation common to Crohn disease.

Monoclonal Antibody Radionuclide Test Kits

ARCITUMOMAB[170]

Arcitumomab (CEA-Scan) is a murine monoclonal Fab′ fragment of IMMU-4, an MAb generated in murine ascites fluid. Both IMMU-4 and arcitumomab react with carcinoembryonic antigen (CEA), a tumor-associated antigen whose expression is increased in various carcinomas, especially those of the GI tract. The preparation is a protein, murine Ig Fab fragment from IgG_1, for chemical labeling with Tc-99m.

Arcitumomab/Tc-99m is for use with standard diagnostic evaluations for detecting the presence, location, and extent of recurrent or metastatic colorectal carcinoma involving the liver, extrahepatic abdomen, and pelvis, with a histologically confirmed diagnosis. IMMU-4 (and the Fab′ fragments of arcitumomab) bind to carcinoembryonic antigen (CEA), whose expression is increased in carcinoma. Arcitumomab/Tc-99m is injected, and the radionuclide scan is read 2 to 5 hours later.

NOFETUMOMAB MERPENTAN[171]

Nofetumomab merpentan (Verluma Kit) is the Fab fragment derived from the murine MAb NR-LU-10. The product is a protein, IgG_{2b}, monoclonal that has been fragmented from NR-LU-10. Nofetumomab possesses only the Fab portion. NR-LU-10 and nofetumomab are directed against a 40-kDa protein antigen that is expressed in various cancers and some normal tissues.

Nofetumomab is indicated for the detection and evaluation of extensive-stage disease in patients with biopsy-confirmed, previously untreated small cell lung cancer by bone scan, CT scan (head, chest, abdomen), or chest x-ray.

Nofetumomab merpentan possesses a linker and a chelator that binds the technetium to the peptide. This is a phenthioate ligand, 2,3,5,6-tetrafluorophenyl-4,5-bis-*S*-[1-ethoxyethyl]-thioacetoamidopentanoate, hence the name *merpentan*.

SATUMOMAB PENDETIDE[172]

Satumomab pendetide (OncoScint, murine) is a kit for In-111. Satumomab is prepared from a murine antibody raised to a membrane-enriched extract of human breast carcinoma hepatic metastasis. It is a protein, IgG_1 κ antibody, and monoclonal. The MAb recognizes tumor-associated glycoprotein (TAG) 72, a mucinlike molecule with a mass greater than 100,000 Da.

Satumomab is indicated as a diagnostic aid in determining the extent and location of extrahepatic malignant disease in patients with known colorectal and ovarian cancer. This agent is used after standard diagnostic tests are completed and when additional information is needed. The cancer must be recurrent or previously diagnosed by other methods.

Satumomab localizes to TAG 72. The antibody is chemically modified so that it links to radioactive indium-111, which is mixed with the antibody just prior to injection. Imaging techniques will reveal the localization of the satumomab as "hot spots." To link the indium-111 to the satumomab protein, a linker-chelator is used. This is glycyl-tyrosyl-(N,ε-diethylenetriaminepentaacetic acid)-lysine hydrochloride.

IMCIROMAB PENTETATE[173]

Imciromab pentetate (murine; Myoscint Kit for the preparation of indium-111 imciromab pentetate) is a murine immunoglobulin fragment raised to the heavy chain of human myosin. The drug is a protein of the IgG$_2$ κ class. It is monoclonal, consisting of the Fab-binding fragments only, and it is bound to the linker-chelator diethylenetriamine pentaacetic acid for labeling with indium-111. Imciromab binds to the heavy chain of human myosin, the intracellular protein found in cardiac and skeletal muscle cells.

Imciromab pentetate is indicated for detecting the presence and location of myocardial injury in patients after a suspected myocardial infarction. In normal myocardium, intracellular proteins such as myosin are isolated from the extravascular space by the cell membrane and are inaccessible to antibody binding. After myocyte injury, the cell membrane loses integrity and becomes permeable to macromolecules, which allows Imciromab-In-111 to enter the cells, where it binds to intracellular myosin. The drug localizes in infarcted tissues, where radionuclide scanning can visualize it.

CAPROMAB PENDETIDE[174]

Capromab (ProstaScint Kit for the preparation of In-111 capromab pendetide, murine) is an MAb (murine IgG$_1$ κ) that derives from an initial sensitization with a glycoprotein expressed by prostate epithelium known as *prostate surface membrane antigen* (PSMA). The MAb recognizes PSMA specifically and thus is specific for prostate adenocarcinomas. The drug is used in newly diagnosed patients with proven prostate cancer who are at high risk for pelvic lymph metastasis. PSMA has been found in many primary and metastatic prostate cancer lesions. The cytoplasmic domain marker 7E11-C5.3 reacts with more than 95% of adenocarcinomas evaluated.

To join the indium-111 to the antibody, a linker-chelator is used. This moiety is glycyltyrosyl-(N-ethylenetriaminepentaacetic acid)-lysine HCl.

A Therapeutic Radionuclide Monoclonal Antibody[175]

IBRITUMOMAB TIUXETAN

Ibritumomab (Zevalin kits to prepare In-111 Zevalin and Y-90 Zevalin, murine) is an MAb derived from an initial sensitization with CD20 antigen, expressed on the surface of normal and malignant B cells. The antibody is a murine IgG$_1$ κ subtype, directed against CD20 antigen. It is produced in a CHO cell line. Ibritumomab is indicated for use as a multistage regimen to treat patients with relapsed or refractory low-grade, follicular, or transformed B-cell non-Hodgkin lymphoma, including patients with rituximab-refractory follicular non-Hodgkin lymphoma.

Ibritumomab tiuxetan binds specifically to CD20 antigen (human B-lymphocyte–restricted differentiation antigen). CD20 is expressed on pre-B and mature B lymphocytes and on more than 90% of B-cell non-Hodgkin lymphoma. When the CDR of ibritumomab tiutuxan binds to the CD20 antigen, apoptosis is initiated. The tiutuxan chelate binds indium-111 and yttrium-90 tightly. Beta emission induces cellular damage by forming free radicals in the target cells and neighboring cells. Tiutuxan is [N-[2-bis(carboxymethyl)amino]-3-(p-isothiocyanatophenyl)propyl]-[N-[2-bis(carboxymethyl)amino]2-(methyl)-ethyl]glycine.

In-Home Test Kits[176]

There are various MAb-based in-home test kits that are designed to detect pregnancy and ovulation. For example, a pregnancy test kit targets the antigen human chorionic gonadotropin and displays a certain sign if the test is positive. The other type of test kit predicts ovulation by targeting LH in the urine. Just before ovulation, LH surges. The test kit is designed to detect and signal the time of ovulation. These test kits, based on the complex techniques of MAbs, are designed to be as simple and error-free as possible for patients.

GENOMICS

Genomics[177] is a term that means "a study of genes and their functions." Currently, genomics is probably the central driving force for new drug discovery and for novel treatments for disease. Gene therapy is a concept that is often discussed. The human genome project, which was largely completed in the year 2000, provided over 4 billion bp of data that have been deposited in public databases. Sequencing the genome itself was an enormous task, but the correlation of genomic data with disease states, sites of microbial attachment, and drug receptor sites is still in its infancy. Once these problems are solved, genomic data will be used to diagnose and treat disease and to develop new drugs specifically for disease states (and possibly specific for a patient). Studying the genetics of biochemical pathways will provide an entry into enzyme-based therapies. There will undoubtedly be a host of new targets for drug therapy. Because deciphering the information that the genomic sequence provides is a complex undertaking, these benefits are probably going to occur years in the future.

Unraveling the Genomic Code to Determine Structure–Function Relationships: Bioinformatics

When considering the topic of bioinformatics, one must recognize that this is a broad term, covering many different research areas. The roots of bioinformatics lie in the decades-old field of computational biology. Advances in computer technology that yielded faster computations fueled the expansion of this field into many different scientific areas, as did the development of new mathematical algorithms that allowed highly sophisticated problems to be solved quickly. For instance, with the computer technology available in 2003, it is relatively straightforward to determine a three-dimensional structure of a protein by x-ray crystallography, by nuclear magnetic resonance–distance geometry–molecular dynamics approaches, or to compare a large set of genes structurally. Out of bioinformatics have grown some new scientific disciplines: functional genomics, structural genomics, and evolutionary genomics. The term *bioinformatics* is routinely applied to experiments in genomics that rely on sophisticated computations.

One reason why computational methods are so critical is that biological macromolecules must be simulated in a three-dimensional environment for realistic comparisons and visualizations to be made. A typical molecule is represented in a computer by a set of three Cartesian coordinates per atom that specify the position of each atom in space. There are sets of three-atom and dihedral angles to specify interatomic connectivity, and designations for the start and end points of chains, where needed. Fortunately, it is a relatively simple matter to build or download molecules from databases. Although the Cartesian coordinate system provides the relative positions of the atoms in space, the computer offers the opportunity to let the molecule evolve in the fourth dimension, time. This is where energy minimization routines and molecular dynamics simulations are used.

Functional Genomics

Functional genomics seeks to make an *inference* about the function of a gene (Fig. 4.15). Given a novel gene sequence to be tested, the functional genomics method starts by comparing the new gene with genetic sequences in a database. In some cases, the name of the gene, a function, or a close analogy to previously identified genes can be made. The test gene is then used as a template to construct, in a computer, a three-dimensional model of the protein. The three-dimensional model is refined by searching databases for possible folded structures of the protein product. Lastly, the likely folded structure of the protein from the new gene is *inferred* by comparison with folding patterns of proteins of known structure and function.

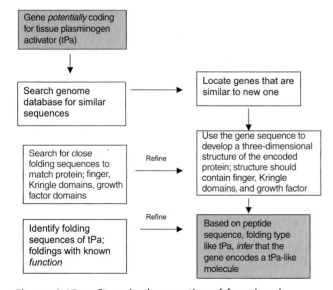

Figure 4.15 ● Steps in the practice of functional genomics.

The aforementioned method is not without difficulty. There is a lot of genetic overlap between organisms of different types. Usually, as a first step, the genomic sequences of prokaryotes and *Archaebacteria* are subtracted out, but there can still be overlap with organisms such as yeasts. In addition, the human genome possesses introns and exons, and the genetic components that encode one protein may lie on parts of one chromosome that are separated by a large number of nucleotides, or the gene may even be distributed over more than one chromosome.

DNA Microarrays[178,179]

Each cell in the human body contains a full set of chromosomes and an identical complement of genes. At any given time in a given cell, only a fraction of these genes may be expressed. It is the expressed genes that give each cell its uniqueness. We use the term *gene expression* to describe the transcription of the information contained in the DNA code into mRNA molecules that are translated into the proteins that perform the major functions of the cell. The amount and type of mRNA that is produced by a cell provides information on which genes are being expressed and how the cell responds dynamically to changing conditions (e.g., disease). Gene expression can act as an "on/off" switch to control which genes are expressed, and a level regulator, somewhat like a volume control, that increases or decreases the level of expression as necessary. Thus, genes can be on or off, and low or high.

Historically, scientists wishing to study gene expression could analyze mRNA from cell lines, but the complexity of the task meant that only a few genes could be studied at once. The advent of DNA microarray technology allows scientists to analyze expression of thousands of genes in a single experiment, quickly and efficiently. DNA microarray technology facilitates the identification and classification of DNA sequence information and takes steps toward assigning functions to the new genes. The fundamental precept of microarray technology is that any mRNA molecule can hybridize to the DNA template from which it originated.

In a typical microarray experiment, an array is constructed of many DNA samples. Automation that was developed for the silicon chip industry helps in this procedure, spotting thousands of different DNA samples on glass plates, silicon chips, or nylon wafers. mRNA isolated from probe cells is treated with a mixture of fluorescent-tagged (usually red, green, and yellow) nucleotides in the presence of reverse transcriptase. This process generates fluorescent-tagged cDNA. The fluors will emit light when excited with a laser. The labeled nucleic acids are considered *mobile probes* that, when incubated with the stationary DNA, hybridize or bind to the complementary molecules (sequences that can base pair with each other). After hybridization, bound cDNA is detected by use of a laser scanner. Data on the presence or absence of fluorescence, the color, and the intensity at the various points in the array are acquired in a computer for analysis.

As an example, we can consider two cells: cell type 1, a healthy cell, and cell type 2, a diseased cell. Both cell types contain an identical set of four genes: A, B, C, and D. mRNA is isolated from each cell type and used to create fluorescent-tagged cDNA. In this case, red and green are used. Labeled samples are mixed and incubated with a microarray that contains the immobilized genes A, B, C, and D.

The tagged molecules bind to the sites on the array corresponding to the genes being expressed in each cell. A robotic scanner, also a product of silicon chip technology, excites the fluorescent labels, and images are stored in a computer. The computer can compute the red-to-green fluorescence ratio, subtract out background noise, and so on. The computer creates a table of the intensity of red-to-green fluorescence for every point in the matrix. Perhaps both cells express the same levels of gene A, cell 1 expresses more of gene B, cell 2 (the diseased cell) expresses more of gene C, and neither cell expresses gene D. This is a simplistic explanation; experiments have been reported in which as many as 30,000 spots have been placed in the microarray.

DNA microarrays can detect changes in gene expression levels, expression patterns (e.g., the cell cycle), genomic gains and losses (e.g., lost or broken parts of chromosomes in cancer cells), and mutations in DNA (single-nucleotide polymorphism [SNPs]). SNPs are also of interest because they may provide clues about how different people respond to a single drug in different ways.

Proteomics[180,181]

The word *proteome* describes *prot*ein expressed by a gen*ome*. Proteomics is a scientific endeavor that attempts to study the sum total of all of the proteins in a cell from the point of view of their individual functions and how the interaction of specific proteins with other cellular components affects the function of these proteins. Not surprisingly, this is a very complex task. There are many more proteins than there are genes, and in biochemical pathways, a protein rarely acts by itself. At present, we know that the expression of multiple genes is involved for any given disease process. "Simply" knowing the gene sequence rarely unmasks the function of the encoded protein or its relevance to a disease. Consequently, the science of proteomics is not developed to the point at which drug discovery can be driven by gene sequence information. There have been, however, some significant technology-driven approaches to the field. High-throughput high-resolution mass spectroscopy allows the amino acid sequences of proteins to be determined very quickly. The technique of two-dimensional gel electrophoresis has likewise advanced the science of proteomics. Proteomics will, undoubtedly, eventually provide targets for drug discovery and the detection of disease states.

Pharmacogenomics[182]

When pharmaceutical companies develop new drugs for any given disease state, they are limited by a lack of knowledge about how individual patients will respond to the agent. No simple algorithms exist that facilitate prediction of whether a patient will respond negatively (an adverse drug reaction), positively (the desired outcome), or not at all. Consequently, drugs are developed for an "average" patient. The manufacturer relies on clinical studies to expose potential adverse reactions and publishes them in statistical format to guide the physician. Nevertheless, when a physician prescribes a drug to a patient he or she has no way of knowing the outcome. Statistics show clearly that a single drug does not provide a positive outcome in all patients. This "one-drug-does-not-fit-all" concept has its basis in the genetics of a patient, and the science of studying these phenomena is called *pharmacogenomics*.

A patient's response to a drug, positive or negative, is a highly complex trait that may be influenced by the activities of many different genes. ADME, as well as the receptor-binding relationship, are all under the control of proteins, lipids, and carbohydrates, which are in turn under the control of the patient's genes. When the fact that a person's genes display small variations in their DNA base content was recognized, genetic prediction of response to drugs or infectious microbes became possible. Pharmacogenomics is the science that looks at the inherited variations in genes that dictate drug response and tries to define the ways in which these variations can be used to predict if a patient will have a positive response to a drug, an adverse one, or none at all.

Cataloging the genetic variations is an important phase of present research activity. Scientists look for SNPs in a person's gene sequences. SNPs are viewed as markers for slight genomic variation. Unfortunately, traditional gene sequencing is slow and expensive, preventing for now the general use of SNPs as diagnostic tools. DNA microarrays may make it possible to identify SNPs quickly in a patient's cells. SNP screening may help to determine a response to a drug before it is prescribed. Obviously, this would be a tremendous tool for the physician.

⬡ ANTISENSE TECHNOLOGY

During the process of transcription, double-stranded DNA is separated into two strands by polymerases. These strands are named the *sense* (coding or [+] strand) and the *antisense* (template or [−] strand). The antisense DNA strand serves as the template for mRNA synthesis in the cell. Hence, the code for ribosomal protein synthesis is normally transmitted through the antisense strand. Sometimes, the sense DNA strand will code for a molecule of RNA. In this case, the resulting RNA molecule is called *antisense RNA*. Antisense RNA sequences were first reported to be naturally occurring molecules in which endogenous strands formed complementarily to cellular mRNA, resulting in the repression of gene expression. Hence, they may be natural control molecules. Rationally designed antisense oligonucleotide interactions occur when the base pairs of a synthetic, specifically designed antisense molecule align precisely with a series of bases in a target mRNA molecule.

Antisense oligonucleotides may inhibit gene expression transiently by masking the ribosome-binding site on mRNA, blocking translation and thus preventing protein synthesis, or permanently by cross-linkage between the oligonucleotide and the mRNA. Most importantly, ribonuclease H (RNase H) can recognize the DNA–RNA duplex (antisense DNA binding to mRNA), or an RNA–RNA duplex (antisense RNA interacting with mRNA), disrupting the base pairing interactions and digesting the RNA portion of the double helix. Inhibition of gene expression occurs because the digested mRNA is no longer competent for translation and resulting protein synthesis.

Antisense technology is beginning to be used to develop drugs that might be able to control disease by blocking the genetic code, interfering with damaged or malfunctioning genes. Among the possible therapeutic antisense agents under investigation are agents for chronic myelogenous leukemia, HIV infection and AIDS, cytomegalovirus retinitis in AIDS patients, and some inflammatory diseases.

⬡ GENE THERAPY

Gene therapy arguably represents the ultimate application of rDNA technology to the treatment of disease. There are two ways to envision gene therapy: (a) the replacement of a defective gene with a normal gene or (b) the addition of a gene whose product can help fight a disease such as a viral infection or cancer. In the former case, replacement of a defective gene, an actual cure can be effected instead of just treating the symptoms. For example, in CF, a defective gene has been clearly identified as the cause of the disease. It is possible that replacement of the defective gene with a corrected one could produce a cure. Similar possibilities exist for other inherited genetic disorders such as insulin-dependent diabetes, growth hormone deficiency, hemophilia, and sickle cell anemia.

The ability to transfer genes into other organisms has other important applications, including the heterologous production of recombinant proteins (discussed previously) and the development of animal models for the study of human diseases. Another area of exploration is the introduction of recombinant genes as biological response modifiers, for example, in preventing rejection following organ transplantation. If genes encoding host major histocompatibility complexes could be introduced into transplanted cells, the transplanted tissue might be recognized as "self." It might also be possible to introduce genes for substances such as transforming growth factor-β that would decrease local cell-mediated immune responses. An opposite strategy might be considered for the treatment of cancer, whereby transplanted cells could be used to target cancer cells, increasing local cell-mediated immune responses.

The transfer of genes from one organism to another is termed *transgenics*, and an animal that has received such a transgene is referred to as a *transgenic animal*. If the transgene is incorporated into the *germ cells* (eggs and sperm), it will be inherited and passed on to successive generations. If the transgene is incorporated into other cells of the body (*somatic cells*), it will be expressed only as long as the newly created transgenic cells are alive. Hence, if a terminally differentiated, postmitotic cell receives a transgene it will not undergo further cell division, whereas if a transgene is created in an undifferentiated stem cell, the product will continuously be expressed in new cells.

⬡ AFTERWORD

Clearly, biotechnology has become an integral part of pharmaceutical care. Pharmacists need to become comfortable with biotechnology and its language to deliver this kind of care to their patients. This chapter has tried to present an overview of the major biotechnological arenas present in the year 2009. The field is advancing rapidly, and every pharmacist must stay current with the literature on biotechnology.

● R E V I E W   Q U E S T I O N S ●

1. Describe the pharmaceutics-related problems with biotechnologically produced drugs.

2. Why cannot biotechnologically produced drugs be administered orally?

3. What is GenBank? Why is it important scientifically?

4. Describe pharmacogenomics. Describe proteomics. How do these two differ?

5. What are chimeric receptors?

REFERENCES

1. NCBI, NLM, NIH: Bethesda, MD 20894. e-mail info@ncbi.nlm.nih.gov.
2. Benson, D. A.: Nucl. Acids Res. 30(1):17–20, 2002.
3. GenBank, NCBI: https://www.ncbi.nlm.nih.gov/GenBank/genbankstats.html.
4. Pharmaceutical Research and Manufacturers Association: New Medicines in Biotechnology Survey. Washington, DC, Pharmaceutical Research and Manufacturers Association, 2002.
5. Pharmaceutical Research and Manufacturers Association: New Medicines in Development for Pediatrics Survey. Washington, DC, Pharmaceutical Research and Manufacturers Association, 2002.
6. Akinwande, K., et al.: Hosp. Formul. 28(9):773–780, 1993.
7. Mahoney, C. D.: Hosp. Formul. 27(Suppl. 2):2–3, 1992.
8. Wordell, C. J.: Hosp. Pharm. 27(6):521–528, 1992.
9. Seltzer, J. L., et al.: Hosp. Formul. 27(4):379–392, 1992.
10. Schneider, P. J.: Pharm. Pract. Manage. Q. 18(2):32–36, 1998.
11. Huber, S. L.: Am. J. Hosp. Pharm. 50(7 Suppl. 3):531–533, 1993.
12. Bleeker, G. C.: Am. J. Hosp. Pharm. 50(7 Suppl. 3):527–530, 1993.
13. Herfindal, E. T.: Am. J. Hosp. Pharm. 46(12):2516–2520, 1989.
14. Dasher, T.: Am. Pharm. NS35(2):9–10, 1995.
15. Vizirianakis, I. S.: Eur. J. Pharm. Sci. 15(3):243–250, 2002.
16. Baumgartner, R. P.: Hosp. Pharm. 26(11):939–946, 1991.
17. Rospond, R. M., and Do, T. T.: Hosp. Pharm. 26(9):823–827, 1991.
18. Brodie, D. C., and Smith, W. E.: Am. J. Hosp. Pharm. 42(1):81–95, 1985.
19. Slavkin, H. C.: Technol. Health Care 4(3):249–253, 1996.
20. Stewart, C. F., and Fleming, R. A.: Am. J. Hosp. Pharm. 46(11 Suppl. 2):54–58, 1989.
21. Tami, J., and Evens, R. P.: Pharmacotherapy 16(4):527–536, 1996.
22. Koeller, J. M.: Am. J. Hosp. Pharm. 46(Suppl. 2):511–515, 1989.
23. Wagner, M.: Mod. Healthcare 22(2):24–29, 1992.
24. Dana, W. J., and Farthing, K.: Pharm. Pract. Manage. Q. 18(2):23–31, 1988.
25. Santell, J. P.: Am. J. Health Syst. Pharm. 53(2):139–155, 1996.
26. Reid, B.: Nat. Biotechnol. 20(4):322, 2002.
27. Piascik, P.: Pharm. Pract. Manage. Q. 18(2):1–12, 1998.
28. Piascik, P.: Am. Pharm. NS35(6):9–10, 1995.
29. Roth, R.: Am. Pharm. NS34(4):31–33, 1994.
30. Taylor, K. S.: Hosp. Health Netw. 67(17):36–38, 1993.
31. Wade, D. A., and Levy, R. A.: Am. Pharm. NS32(9):33–37, 1992.
32. Lumisdon, K.: Hospitals 65(23):32–35, 1991.
33. Crane, V. S., Gilliland, M., and Trussell, R. G.: Top. Hosp. Pharm. Manage. 10(4):23–30, 1991.
34. Zilz, D. A.: Am. J. Hosp. Pharm. 47(8):1759–1765, 1990.
35. Zarus, S. A.: Curr. Concepts Hosp. Pharm. Manage. 11(4):12–19, 1989.
36. Schneider, P. J.: Pharm. Pract. Manage. Q. 18(2):32–36, 1998.
37. Manuel, S. M.: Am. Pharm. NS34(11):14–15, 1994.

38. Gillouzo, A.: Cell Mol. Biol. 47(8):1307–1308, 2001.
39. Sindelar, R. D.: Drug Top. 137:66–78, 1993.
40. McKinnon, B.: Drug Benefit Trends 9(12):30–34, 1997.
41. Wolf, B. A.: Ther. Drug Monit. 18(4):402–404, 1996.
42. Vermeij, P., and Blok, D.: Pharm. World Sci. 18(3):87–93, 1996.
43. Lambert, K.: Curr. Opin. Biotechnol. 8(3):347–349, 1997.
44. Beatrice, M.: Curr. Opin. Biotechnol. 8(3):370–378, 1997.
45. Romac, D. R., et al.: Formulary 30(9):520–531, 1995.
46. McGarity, T. O.: Issues Sci. Technol. 1(3):40–56, 1985.
47. Columbo P., et al.: Eur. J. Drug Metab. Pharmacokinet. 21(2):87–91, 1996.
48. Berthold, W., and Walter, J.: Biologicals 22(2):135–150, 1994.
49. Roth, R., and Constantine, L. M.: Am. Pharm. NS35(7):19–21, 1995.
50. Santell, J. P.: Am. J. Hosp. Pharm. 51(2):177–187, 1994.
51. Piascek, P.: Am. Pharm. NS33(4):18–19, 1993.
52. Piascek, M. M.: Am. J. Hosp. Pharm. 48(10 Suppl. 11):14–18, 1992.
53. Piascek, P., and Alexander, S.: Am. Pharm. NS35(11):8–9, 1995.
54. Glick, B. R., and Pasternak, J. J. (eds.): Molecular Biotechnology: Principles and Applications of Recombinant DNA, 2nd ed. Washington, DC, ASM Press, 1998.
55. Franks, F. (ed.): Protein Biotechnology. Totowa, NJ, Humana Press, 1993.
56. Bains, W.: Biotechnology from A to Z, 2nd ed. Oxford, England, Oxford University Press, 1998.
57. Alberts, B., Bray, D., Lewis, J., et al. (eds.): Molecular Biology of the Cell, 3rd ed. New York, NY, Garland Publishing, 1994.
58. Wolfe, S. L.: An Introduction to Cell and Molecular Biology. Belmont, CA, Wadsworth Publishing, 1995.
59. Williams, D. A., and Lemke, T. L. (eds.): Foye's Principles of Medicinal Chemistry, 5th ed. New York, Lippincott Williams & Wilkins, 2001, pp. 981–1015.
60. Sindelar, R. D.: Drug Top. Suppl:3–13, 2001.
61. Fields, S.: Am. Pharm. NS33:4:28–29, 1993.
62. Roth, R.: Am. Pharm. NS34(4):31–34, 1997.
63. Allen, L. V.: Am. Pharm. NS34:31–33, 1994.
64. Evens, R., Louie, S. G., Sindelar, R., et al.: Biotech. Rx: Biotechnology in Pharmacy Practice: Science, Clinical Applications, and Pharmaceutical Care—Opportunities in Therapy Management. Washington, DC, American Pharmaceutical Association, 1997.
65. Zito, S. W. (ed.): Pharmaceutical Biotechnology: A Programmed Text. Lancaster, PA, Technomic Publishing, 1992.
66. Biotechnology Resource Catalog. Philadelphia, Philadelphia College of Pharmacy and Science, 1993.
67. Watson, J. D., Hopkins, N. H., Roberts, J. W., et al.: Molecular Biology of the Gene, 4th ed. Menlo Park, CA, Benjamin Cummings, 1987.
68. Davis, L. G., Dibner, M. D., and Battey, J. F.: Basic Methods in Molecular Biology. New York, Elsevier, 1986.
69. Wu–Pong, S., and Rojanaskul, Y. (eds.): Biopharmaceutical Drug Design and Development. Totowa, NJ, Humana Press, 1999.
70. Ausubel, F. M., Brent, R., et al.: Current Protocols in Molecular Biology. New York, Greene, Wiley-Interscience, 1988.
71. Davis, L. G.: Background to Recombinant DNA Technology. In Pezzuto, J. M., Johnson, M. E., and Manasse, H. R. (eds.). Biotechnology and Pharmacy. New York, Chapman & Hall, 1993, pp. 1–38.
72. Watson, J. D., et al.: Recombinant DNA, 2nd ed. New York, Scientific American Books, 1992, pp. 13–32.
73. Greene, J. J., and Rao, V. B. (eds.): Recombinant DNA: Principles and Methodologies. New York, Marcel Dekker, 1998.
74. Kreuzer, H., and Massey, A.: Recombinant DNA and Biotechnology. Washington, DC, ASM Press, 1996.
75. Nelson, D. L., and Cox, M. M. (eds.): Lehninger: Principles of Biochemistry. New York, Worth Publishers, 2000, pp. 905–1119.
76. Devlin, T. M. (ed.): Textbook of Biochemistry with Clinical Correlations, 3rd ed. New York, John Wiley & Sons, 1992, pp. 607–766.
77. Horton, H. R., Moran, L. A., Ochs, R. S., et al. (eds.): Principles of Biochemistry, 2nd ed. Upper Saddle River, NJ, Prentice-Hall, 1996, pp. 561–692.
78. Crick, F. H. C.: Symp. Soc. Exp. Biol. 12:128–163, 1958.
79. Watson, J. D.: Molecular Biology of the Gene. New York, W. A. Benjamin, 1970.
80. Jordan, E.: Am. J. Hum. Genet. 51:1–6, 1992.
81. Voet, D., and Voet, J. G.: Biochemistry, 2nd ed. New York, John Wiley & Sons, 1995, pp. 944–945.
82. Johnson, M. E., and Kahn, M.: In Pezzuto, J. M., Johnson, M. E., and Manasse, H. R. (eds.). Biotechnology and Pharmacy. New York, 1993, pp. 369–371.
83. Paolella, P.: Introduction to Molecular Biology. Boston, WCB McGraw-Hill, 1988, p. 176.
84. Davis, L. G.: In Pezzuto, J. M., Johnson, M. E., and Manasse, H. R. (eds.). New York, Biotechnology and Pharmacy, 1993, pp. 10–11.
85. Rojanaskul, Y., and Dokka, S.: In Wu-Pong, S., and Rojanaskul, Y. (eds.). Biopharmaceutical Drug Design and Development. Totowa, NJ, Humana Press, 1999, pp. 39–40.
86. Paolella, P.: Introduction to Molecular Biology. Boston, WCB McGraw-Hill, 1988, pp. 177–178.
87. Rojanaskul, Y., and Dokka, S.: In Wu–Pong, S., and Rojanaskul, Y. (eds.). Biopharmaceutical Drug Design and Development. Totowa, NJ, Humana Press, 1999, pp. 38–39.
88. Green, E. D., and Olson, M. V.: Proc. Natl. Acad. Sci. U. S. A. 87:1213–1217, 1990.
89. Kadir, F.: Production of Biotech Compounds—Cultivation and Downstream Processing. In Crommelin, D. J. A., and Sindelar, R. D. (eds.). Pharmaceutical Biotechnology: An Introduction for Pharmacists and Pharmaceutical Scientists. Amsterdam, The Netherlands: Harwood Academic Publishers, 1997, pp. 53–70.
90. Riordan, J. R., et al.: Science 245:1066–1073, 1989.
91. Rommens, J. M., et al.: Science 245:1059–1065, 1989.
92. Heldebrand, G. E., et al.: In Pezzuto, J. M., Johnson, M. E., and Manasse, H. R. (eds.). Biotechnology and Pharmacy. New York, 1993, pp. 198–199.
93. Rojanaskul, Y., and Dokka, S.: In Wu-Pong, S., and Rojanaskul, Y. (eds.). Biopharmaceutical Drug Design and Development. Totowa, NJ, Humana Press, 1999, pp. 43–45.
94. Katz, E. D., and Dong, M. W.: BioTechniques 8:628–632, 1990.
95. Kadir, F.: Production of Biotech Compounds—Cultivation and Downstream Processing. In Crommelin, D. J. A., and Sindelar, R. D. (eds.). Pharmaceutical Biotechnology: An Introduction for Pharmacists and Pharmaceutical Scientists. Amsterdam, The Netherlands, Harwood Academic Publishers, 1997, pp. 61–65.
96. Burgess, D. J.: In Pezzuto, J. M., Johnson, M. E., and Manasse, H. R. (eds.). Biotechnology and Pharmacy. New York, 1993, pp. 118–122.
97. Dillman, R. O.: Antibody Immunoconj. Radiopharm. 1990:1–15.
98. Wettendorff, M., et al.: Proc. Natl. Acad. Sci. U. S. A. 86:3787–3791, 1989.
99. Burgess, D. J.: In Pezzuto, J. M., Johnson, M. E., and Manasse, H. R. (eds.). Biotechnology and Pharmacy. New York, 1993, pp. 124–143.
100. Facts and Comparisons. St. Louis, MO, Facts and Comparisons, 2000, pp. 287–290.
101. American Hospital Formulary Service Drug Information, 1989. Bethesda, MD, ASHP, 1989, pp. 2714–2728.
102. Beals, J. M., and Kovach, P. M.: In Crommelin, D. J. A., and Sindelar, R. D. (eds.). Pharmaceutical Biotechnology: An Introduction for Pharmacists and Pharmaceutical Scientists. Amsterdam, The Netherlands, Harwood Academic Publishers, 1997, p. 220.
103. Riley, T. N., and DeRuiter, J.: U. S. Pharm. 25(10):56–64, 2000.
104. Facts and Comparisons. St. Louis, MO, Facts and Comparisons, 2000, pp. 313–314.
105. Facts and Comparisons. St. Louis, MO, Facts and Comparisons, 2000, pp. 344–346.
106. Marian, M.: In Crommelin, D. J. A., and Sindelar, R. D. (eds.). Pharmaceutical Biotechnology: An Introduction for Pharmacists and Pharmaceutical Scientists. Amsterdam, The Netherlands, Harwood Academic Publishers, 1997, pp. 241–253.
107. Facts and Comparisons. St. Louis, MO, Facts and Comparisons, 2000, pp. 247–250.
108. Sam, T., and DeBoer, W.: Follicle Stimulating Hormone. In Crommelin, D. J. A., and Sindelar, R. D. (eds.). Pharmaceutical Biotechnology: An Introduction for Pharmacists and Pharmaceutical Scientists. Amsterdam, The Netherlands, Harwood Academic Publishers, 1997, pp. 315–320.
109. Buckland, P. R., et al.: Biochem. J. 235:879–882, 1986.
110. Pharmaceutical Research and Manufacturers Association: Biotechnology Medicines in Development. PhRMA 2002 Annual Survey. Washington, DC, Pharmaceutical Research and Manufacturers Association, 2002.
111. Graber, S. E., and Krantz, S. B.: Annu. Rev. Med. 29:51–66, 1978.
112. Egric, J. C., Strickland, T. W., Lane J., et al.: Immunobiology 72:213–224, 1986.

113. Eschenbach, J. W., et al.: Ann. Intern. Med. 111:992–1000, 1989.
114. Zsebo, K. M., Cohen, A. M., et al.: Immunobiology 72:175–184, 1986.
115. Souza, L. M., Boone, T. C., et al.: Science 232:61–65, 1986.
116. Heil, G., Hoelzer, D., et al.: Blood 90:4710–4718, 1997.
117. Metcalf, D.: Blood 67(2):257–267, 1986.
118. Vadhan-Raj, S., Keating, M., et al.: N. Engl. J. Med. 317:1545–1552, 1987.
119. Facts and Comparisons. St. Louis, MO, Facts and Comparisons, 2000, pp. 192–194.
120. Grabenstein, J. D. (ed.): Immunofacts: Vaccines and Immunologic Drugs. St. Louis, MO, Facts and Comparisons, 2002, pp. 695–704.
121. Pegasys. Roche Pharmaceuticals Company Stat/Gram. Nutley, NJ, Hoffman-LaRoche, 2003.
122. Grabenstein, J. D. (ed.): Immunofacts: Vaccines and Immunologic Drugs, St. Louis, MO, Facts and Comparisons, 2002, pp. 705–717.
123. Grabenstein, J. D. (ed.): Immunofacts: Vaccines and Immunologic Drugs, St. Louis, MO, Facts and Comparisons, 2002, pp. 737–740 and references therein.
124. Grabenstein, J. D. (ed.): Immunofacts: Vaccines and Immunologic Drugs, St. Louis, MO, Facts and Comparisons, 2002, pp. 741–745 and references therein.
125. Grabenstein, J. D. (ed.): Immunofacts: Vaccines and Immunologic Drugs, St. Louis, MO, Facts and Comparisons, 2002, pp. 746–752 and references therein.
126. Grabenstein, J. D. (ed.): Immunofacts: Vaccines and Immunologic Drugs, St. Louis, MO, Facts and Comparisons, 2002, pp. 756–764 and references therein.
127. Grabenstein, J. D. (ed.): Immunofacts: Vaccines and Immunologic Drugs, St. Louis, MO, Facts and Comparisons, 2002, pp. 765–770 and references therein.
128. Grabenstein, J. D. (ed.): Immunofacts: Vaccines and Immunologic Drugs, St. Louis, MO, Facts and Comparisons, 2002, pp. 771–775 and references therein.
129. Grabenstein, J. D. (ed.): Immunofacts: Vaccines and Immunologic Drugs, St. Louis, MO, Facts and Comparisons, 2002, pp. 776–787 and references therein.
130. Grabenstein, J. D. (ed.): Immunofacts: Vaccines and Immunologic Drugs, St. Louis, MO, Facts and Comparisons, 2002, pp. 788–794 and references therein.
131. Grabenstein, J. D. (ed.): Immunofacts: Vaccines and Immunologic Drugs, St. Louis, MO, Facts and Comparisons, 2002, pp. 795–802 and references therein.
132. Murray, K. M., and Dahl, S. L.: Ann. Pharmacother. 31(11):1335–1338, 1997.
133. Weinblatt, M., et al.: Arthritis Rheum. 40(Suppl):S126, 1997.
134. Moreland, L. W., et al.: N. Engl. J. Med. 337:141–147, 1997.
135. Verstraate, M., Lijnen, H., and Cullen, D.: Drugs 50(1):29–42, 1995.
136. Facts and Comparisons. St. Louis, MO, Facts and Comparisons, 2000, pp. 183–189.
137. Cannon, C. P., Gibson, C. M., et al.: Circulation 98:2805–2814, 1998.
138. Facts and Comparisons. St. Louis, MO, Facts and Comparisons, 2000, p. 193.
139. Shapiro, A. D., Ragni, M. V., Lusher, J. M., et al.: Thromb. Haemost. 75(1):30–35, 1996.
140. Facts and Comparisons. St. Louis, MO, Facts and Comparisons, 2000, p. 195.
141. Bernard, G. R., et al.: N. Engl. J. Med. 344:699–709, 2001.
142. Fabrizio, M.: J. Extra. Corpor. Technol. 331:117–125, 2001.
143. Facts and Comparisons. St. Louis, MO, Facts and Comparisons, 2000, pp. 679–680.
144. Facts and Comparisons. St. Louis, MO, Facts and Comparisons, 2000, pp. 355.
145. Facts and Comparisons. St. Louis, MO, Facts and Comparisons, 2000, pp. 1529–1531.
146. Facts and Comparisons. St. Louis, MO, Facts and Comparisons, 2000, pp. 1505–1508.
147. Reichmann, L., et al.: Nature 332:323–327, 1983.
148. Cobbold, S. P., and Waldmann, H.: Nature 334:460–462, 1984.
149. Adair, J. R., et al.: In Crommelin, D. J. A., and Sindelar, R. D. (eds.). Pharmaceutical Biotechnology: An Introduction for Pharmacists and Pharmaceutical Scientists. Amsterdam, The Netherlands, Harwood Academic Publishers, 1997, pp. 279–287.
150. Coiffier, B., et al.: N. Engl. J. Med. 346(4):280–282, 2002.
151. Maloney, D. G., et al.: Blood 90:2188–2195, 1997.
152. Grabenstein, J. D. (ed.): Immunofacts: Vaccines and Immunologic Drugs. St. Louis, MO, Facts and Comparisons, 2002, pp. 406–413 and references therein.
153. Voliotis, D., et al.: Ann. Oncol. 11(4):95–100, 2000.
154. Grabenstein, J. D. (ed.): Immunofacts: Vaccines and Immunologic Drugs. St. Louis, MO, Facts and Comparisons, 2002, pp. 414–422 and references therein.
155. McConnell, H.: Blood 100:768–773, 2002.
156. Billaud, E. M.: Therapie 55(1):177–183, 2000.
157. Ponticelli, C., et al.: Drugs 1(1):55–60, 1999.
158. Kirkman, R. L.: Transplant. Proc. 31(1–2):1234–1235, 1999.
159. Vincenti, F.: N. Engl. J. Med. 338:161–165, 1998.
160. Oberholzer, J., et al.: Transplant. Int. 14(2):169–171, 2000.
161. Chan, G. L. C., Gruber, S. A., et al.: Crit. Care Clin. 6:841–892, 1990.
162. Hooks, M. A., Wade, C. S., and Milliken, W. J.: Pharmacotherapy 11:26–37, 1991.
163. Todd, P. A., and Brogden, R. N.: Drugs 37:871–899, 1989.
164. Topol, E. J., and Serruys, P. W.: Circulation 98:1802–1820, 1998.
165. Grabenstein, J. D. (ed.): Immunofacts: Vaccines and Immunologic Drugs. St. Louis, MO, Facts and Comparisons, 2002, pp. 455–462 and references therein.
166. Gelmon, K., Arnold, A., et al.: Proc. Am. Soc. Clin. Oncol. 20(69a):Abstr. 271, 2001.
167. Slamon, D. J., Leyland–Jones, B., et al.: N. Engl. J. Med. 344(11):783–792, 2000.
168. Grabenstein, J. D. (ed.): Immunofacts: Vaccines and Immunologic Drugs. St. Louis, MO, Facts and Comparisons, 2002, pp. 473–482 and references therein.
169. Hanauer, S. B.: N. Engl. J. Med. 334:841, 1996.
170. Bogard, W. C., Jr., et al.: Semin. Nucl. Med. 19(3):202–220, 1989.
171. Kassis, A. I.: J. Nucl. Med. 32(9):1751–1753, 1991.
172. Reilly, R. M.: Clin. Pharmacol. Ther. 10(5):359–375, 1991.
173. Reilly, R. M., et al.: Clin. Pharmacokinet. 28:126–142, 1995.
174. Grabenstein, J. D. (ed.): Immunofacts: Vaccines and Immunologic Drugs. St. Louis, MO, Facts and Comparisons, 2002, pp. 535–543 and references therein.
175. Grabenstein, J. D. (ed.): Immunofacts: Vaccines and Immunologic Drugs. St. Louis, MO, Facts and Comparisons, 2002, pp. 544–554 and references therein.
176. Quattrocchi, E., and Hove, I.: US Pharm. 23(4):54–63, 1998.
177. Rios, M.: Pharm. Tech. 25(1):34–40, 2000.
178. Ramsey, G.: Nat. Biotech. 16:40–44, 1998.
179. Khan, J., et al.: Biochim. Biophys. Acta 1423:17–28, 1999.
180. Persidis, A.: Nat. Biotech. 16:393–394, 1998.
181. Borman, S.: Chem. Eng. News 78:31–37, 2000.
182. Lau, K. F., and Sakul, H.: Annu. Rep. Med. Chem. 36:261–269, 2000.

CHAPTER 5

Immunobiologicals

JOHN M. BEALE, JR.

CHAPTER OVERVIEW

The immune system constitutes the body's defense against infectious agents. It protects the host by identifying and eliminating or neutralizing agents that are recognized as nonself. The entire range of immunological responses affects essentially every organ, tissue, and cell of the body. Immune responses include, in part, antibody (Ab) production, allergy, inflammation, phagocytosis, cytotoxicity, transplant and tumor rejection, and the many signals that regulate these responses.[1] At its most basic, the human immune system can be described in terms of the cells that compose it. Every aspect of the immune system, whether innate and nonspecific or adaptive and specific, is controlled by a set of specialized cells. Thus, this discussion of some of the fundamentals of immunology begins with the cells of the immune system.

CELLS OF THE IMMUNE SYSTEM

All immune cells derive from *pluripotent* stem cells in the bone marrow. These are cells that can differentiate into any other cell type, given the right kind of stimulus (Scheme 5.1). Various modes of differentiation beyond the stem cell give rise to unique cellular types, each with a specific function in the immune system. The first stage of differentiation gives rise to two intermediate types of stem cells and creates a branch point.[2] These cells are the myeloid cells (myeloid lineage) and the lymphoid cells (lymphoid lineage). Carrying the lineage further leads to additional branching. The myeloid cells differentiate into erythrocytes and platelets and also monocytes and granulocytes. The lymphoid cell differentiates into B cells and T cells, the cells that are at the center of adaptive immunity. The switching system for each pathway and cell type is governed by several colony-stimulating factors, stem cell factors, and interleukins. These control proliferation, differentiation, and maturation of the cells.

Major Histocompatibility Antigens: Self versus Nonself

The development of most immune responses depends on the recognition of what is *self* and what is *not self*. This determination must be clear and must be done in a very general way. This recognition is achieved by the expression of specialized surface markers on human cells. The major group of markers involved in this recognition consists of surface proteins. These are referred to as the *major histocompatibility complex*[3] (MHC) or *major histocompatibility antigens*. Proteins expressed on the cell surfaces are class I MHCs and class II MHCs. Both classes are highly polymorphic and so are highly specific to each individual. Class I MHCs can be found on virtually all nucleated cells in the human body, whereas class II MHC molecules are associated only with B lymphocytes and macrophages. Class I MHCs are markers that are recognized by natural killer cells and cytotoxic T lymphocytes. When a class I MHC is coexpressed with viral antigens on virus-infected cells, cytotoxic target cells are signaled. Class II MHC molecules are markers indicating that a cooperative immune state exists between immunocompetent cells, such as between an antigen-presenting cell (APC) and a T-helper cell during the induction of Ab formation.

Granulocytes[4]

If one views a granulocyte under a microscope, one can observe dense intracytoplasmic granules. The granules contain inflammatory mediators and digestive enzymes that destroy invading pathogens, control the rate and pathway of migration of chemotactic cells, and cause dilation of blood vessels at the infected site. The increased blood flow ensures that an ample supply of granulocytes and inflammatory mediators reaches the site of infection. There is a family of granulocytic cells, each member with its own specialized function. Under microscopic examination, some granulocytes are seen to be multinuclear and some mononuclear. The configuration of the nuclear region and the staining behavior provide ways of classifying granulocytes.

Neutrophils[4]

Neutrophils are the primary innate defense against pathogenic bacteria. They make up most (50%–75%) of the leukocyte fraction in the blood. Microscopically, neutrophils have multilobed nuclei. They respond to chemical motility factors, such as complement mediators released from infected or inflamed tissues, and migrate to a site of infection by the process of chemotaxis. There, they recognize, adhere to, and phagocytose invading microbes.

Phagocytes

The phagocytic process is initiated by contact and adhesion of an invading cell with a phagocyte cell membrane. Adhesion triggers a process whereby the phagocytic cell extrudes pseudopodia that surround the adhering microbe. As this process progresses, the microbe is actually surrounded by the phagocyte cell membrane. Then, invagination of the membrane fully engulfs the particle, and the membrane is

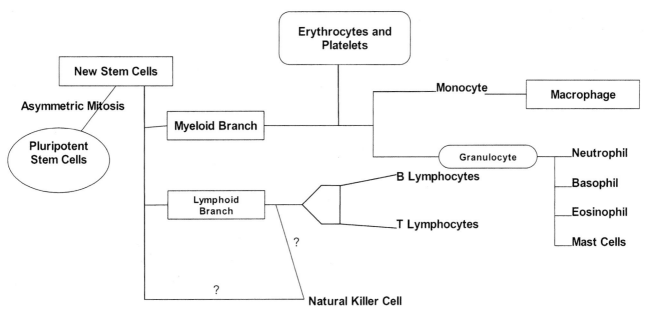

Scheme 5.1 ● Lineages of blood cells. All blood cells derive from a pluripotent stem cell. Various cytokines direct the cells into their specific populations.

resealed with the particle encased inside an intracellular vacuolar body called a *phagosome*. Lysosomes in the cytoplasm then fuse with the phagosome to form *phagolysosomes*. The antimicrobial compounds in the phagosomes and lysosomes kill the engulfed pathogen and enzymatically cleave its remains into smaller pieces.

Eosinophils[5]

Eosinophils are granulocytes that can function as phagocytes, but much less efficiently than neutrophils can. They are present as 2% to 4% of blood leukocytes. Their name derives from the intense staining reaction of their intracellular granules with the dye eosin. Eosinophil granules contain inflammatory mediators such as histamine and leukotrienes, so it makes sense that these cells are associated with the allergic response. Clues to the functions of eosinophils come from their behavior in certain disease states. Eosinophil counts are elevated above normal in the tissues in many different diseases, but they are recognized primarily for their diagnostic role in parasitic infections and in allergies. Eosinophils have a unique mode of action that lends to their extreme importance. Unlike neutrophils, eosinophils need not phagocytose a parasite to kill it. Indeed, some parasites are too large to allow phagocytosis. Eosinophils can physically surround a large parasite, forming a cell coat around the invader. Eosinophil granules release oxidative substances capable of destroying even large, multicellular parasites. Hence, even when phagocytosis fails, a mechanism exists to destroy large parasites.

Mast Cells and Basophils

Mast cells and basophils also release the inflammatory mediators commonly associated with allergy. Mast cells are especially prevalent in the skin, lungs, and nasal mucosa; their granules contain histamine. Basophils, present at only 0.2% of the leukocyte fraction in the blood, also contain histamine granules, but basophils are found circulating in the blood

and not isolated in connective tissue. Both mast cells and basophils have high-affinity immunoglobulin E (IgE) receptors. Complexes of antigen molecules with IgE receptors on the cell surface lead to cross-linking of IgE and distortion of the cell membrane. The distortion causes the mast cell to degranulate, releasing mediators of the allergic response. Because of its association with hypersensitivity, IgE has been called "reagin" in the allergy literature. Diagnostically, IgE levels are elevated in allergy, systemic lupus erythematosus, and rheumatoid arthritis. Cromolyn sodium is a drug that prevents mast cell degranulation and thus blocks the allergic response. Cromolyn is used in asthma.

Macrophages and Monocytes[4,5]

Macrophages and monocytes are mononuclear cells that are capable of phagocytosis. In addition to their phagocytic capabilities, they biosynthesize and release soluble factors (complement, monokines) that govern the acquired immune response. The half-life of monocytes in the bloodstream is about 10 hours, during which time they migrate into tissues and differentiate into macrophages. A macrophage is a terminally differentiated monocyte. Macrophages possess a true anatomical distribution because they develop in the tissues to have specialized functions. Special macrophages are found in tissues such as the liver, lungs, spleen, gastrointestinal (GI) tract, lymph nodes, and brain. These specific macrophages are called either *histiocytes* (generic term) or by certain specialized names (*Kupffer cells* in liver, *Langerhans cells* in skin, *alveolar macrophages* in lung) (Table 5.1). The entire macrophage network is called the *reticuloendothelial system*. Other macrophages exist free in the tissues, where they carry out more nonspecific functions. Macrophages kill more slowly than neutrophils but have a much broader spectrum. It has been estimated that more than 100 soluble inflammatory substances are produced by macrophages. These substances account for macrophages' prolific abilities to direct, modulate, stimulate, and retard the immune response.

TABLE 5.1 The Reticuloendothelial System

Tissue	Cell
Liver	Kupffer cells
Lung	Alveolar macrophages (dust cells)
Peritoneum	Peritoneal macrophages
Spleen	Dendritic cells
Skin	Langerhans cells
Brain	Microglial cells

Macrophages possess a very specialized function; they act as APCs (Fig. 5.1). APCs are responsible for the preprocessing of antigens, amplifying the numbers of antigenic determinant units, and presenting these determinant structures to the programming cells of the immune system. APCs in-

ternalize an organism or particle and digest it into small fragments still recognizable as antigen. The fragments are conjugated with molecules of the major histocompatibility complex 2 (MHC-II). These complexes are responsible for self or nonself cell recognition and ascertain that cells being processed are not self. MHCs also direct the binding of the antigenic determinant with immunoreactive cells. Once the antigen–MHC-II complex forms, it undergoes transcytosis to the macrophage's cell surface, where B lymphocytes and T-helper cells recognize the antigen via the B surface Ab and T-cell receptors. It is this step that transfers specificity and memory information from the determinant into the immune system through the modulation of B-cell differentiation. Under the regulatory influence of the T-helper cells, B cells are stimulated to differentiate into plasma cells that produce Ab. The T-helper cells accelerate and retard the

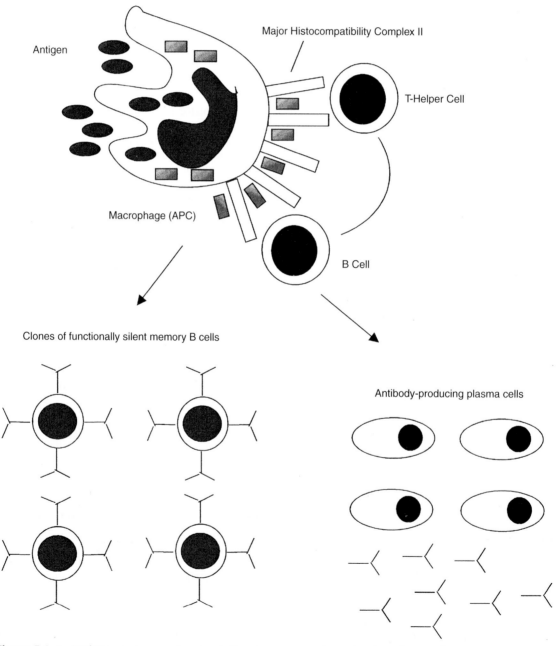

Figure 5.1 • Antigen capture and presentation by a macrophage lead to clones of Ab-producing plasma cells and memory B cells.

process as necessary. Thus, unlike the granulocytes, which have only destructive functions, monocytes and macrophages regulate and program the immune response.

The Lymphoid Cell Line: B and T Cells[2]

The lymphoid cell line differentiates into two types of lymphocytes, the B lymphocytes and the T lymphocytes. These cells constitute only about 20% to 45% of blood leukocytes. They are small cells, only slightly larger than an erythrocyte, but B and T cells can be identified microscopically by large nuclei that occupy most of the cytoplasmic volume. The nuclei are large to contain enough DNA to enable the T and B cells to biosynthesize massive amounts of protein needed to carry out their immune functions. T lymphocytes are involved in cell-mediated immunity (CMI); B lymphocytes differentiate into Ab-producing plasma cells. B lymphocytes express antibodies on their surfaces that bind antigens. T lymphocytes express specialized T-cell receptors on their surfaces that bind major histocompatibility complex 1 (MHC-I) and 2 (MHC-II) complexed with antigenic peptide fragments.

⬡ IMMUNITY

Immunity in humans can be conceptualized in several different ways. If just the type and specificity of the immune response are considered, the ideas of *innate* and *acquired* immunity are used. If only the components that are involved in the immune response are considered, the processes can be divided into *humoral* and *cellular* immunity. If the location of the immune response is considered, we find that the immune system consists of *serosal* (in the serum) immunity and *mucosal* (on mucosal epithelium surfaces) immunity.

Innate Immunity

Innate immunity is the most basic form of immunity and includes immune systems that are present in a human from birth. A clear distinction must be made between innate immunity and acquired (adaptive) immunity, which develops after birth, and then only after an antigenic challenge (Table 5.2). Innate immunity is the first line of defense against invasion by microbes and can be characterized as fast in response, nonspecific, and lacking in memory of the challenge. Acquired immunity develops through a complex system of reactions that are triggered by invasion with an infectious agent. It is slow in response to an infection, is *highly specific*, and has memory of previous infections. The memory, or anamnestic response, is responsible for the extremely rapid development of the immune response with subsequent challenges and is a hallmark of acquired immunity.

There are three separate components of innate immunity that work in concert to provide the whole response. There are physical barriers, cellular barriers, and soluble factors. The physical barriers include the largest, most exposed organ of the body (the skin), the mucosa, and its associated mucus. The keratinized layer of protein and lipid in the stratum corneum of the skin protects physically against various environmental, biological, and chemical assaults. The protection afforded by mucosal surfaces, such as those that are found in the throat, mouth, nose, and GI tract, is due to a surface epithelium. The epithelium consists of single or multiple layers of epithelial cells with tight gap junctions between them. This type of structure provides an impermeable physical barrier to microorganisms. Most of the time, epithelium is further protected by the secretion of mucus, such as from goblet cells in the GI mucosa. Mucus is a viscous layer consisting of glycopeptide and an acidic glycoprotein called *mucin*. Mucus can prevent penetration of microbial cells into the epithelium, significantly decreasing the possibility of infection by the mucosal route. Other components of the physical barriers in innate immunity are the tears (containing lysozyme), the acidic pH of the stomach, the low pH and flow of the urine, and the cilia in the lungs that constantly beat upward to remove inspired particulates and microbes.

Two components of the cellular innate immune response have already been discussed, granulocytes in the blood and tissue macrophages. When an infection occurs in the tissues, chemotactic factors liberated at the site migrate down a concentration gradient to the surrounding area. These agents make the capillary beds porous. Neutrophils follow the concentration gradient across the endothelium to the site of infection. There are three types of chemotactic factors: (a) formylmethionyl (f-Met) peptides released from the invading bacteria, (b) leukotrienes secreted by phagocytes, and (c) peptide fragments released from activated complement proteins such as C_{3a} and C_{5a}. Neutrophils and macrophages engulf and destroy microorganisms by phagocytosis. Nonphagocytic cells are also involved in the innate immune response, providing soluble chemical factors that enhance the innate response.

Soluble factors of innate immunity include (a) bactericidal factors, (b) complement, and (c) interferon. A bactericidal factor (Table 5.3) is an agent that kills bacteria. Perhaps the most fundamental bactericidal factor is the acid in the stomach. Secreted by goblet cells in the mucosal epithelial lining, stomach acid is responsible for disposing of most of the microbes that are consumed orally. Phagocytes or hepatocytes produce the other bactericidal factors. Most of these are directed toward the phagosome, where the predigested, phagocytically encapsulated

TABLE 5.2 Characteristics of Innate versus Acquired Immunity

Innate Immunity	Acquired Immunity
Present from birth	Develops later
Rapid	Slow
Nonspecific	Specific
No memory	Memory

TABLE 5.3 Bactericidal Factors

Factor	Formation	Site of Action
Oxygen ions and radicals	Induced	Phagosomes
Acid hydrolases	Preformed	Lysosomes
Cationic proteins	Preformed	Phagosomes
Defensins	Preformed	Phagosomes or extracellular
Lactoferrin	Preformed	Phagosomes

TABLE 5.4 Acute Phase Factors

Acute Phase Factor	Function/Activity
C-reactive protein	Chemotaxis and enhancement of phagocytosis
α_1-Antitrypsin	Inhibition of proteases
Complement factors	Control of the complement cascade
Fibrinogen	Blood coagulation

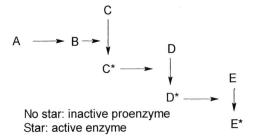

No star: inactive proenzyme
Star: active enzyme

bacterial cell is enclosed. The antimicrobial factors kill the immobilized microbes.

There are two types of antimicrobial factors, those that are preformed inside the phagocyte and one that is *induced* in response to the phagocytic process. The most important of the antimicrobial mechanisms is the respiratory burst, which generates oxygen radicals—superoxide, hydroxyl radicals, and hydrogen peroxide. The respiratory burst is the only induced mechanism. All of the active oxygen species are highly destructive to bacterial as well as host cells, so they are not produced until they are needed. The defensins are arginine- or cysteine-rich bactericidal peptides that exhibit an extremely broad spectrum of antimicrobial activity. The defensins will kill bacteria (Gram-positive and Gram-negative), fungi, and even some viruses. The mechanism of action of the defensins is unknown, but because the peptides are highly charged in an opposite sense to bacterial cell membranes, an electrostatic, membrane-disruptive interaction might be involved. Bacteria have an absolute requirement for iron, and to compete with the host for this element, they secrete high-affinity siderophore factors that scavenge iron from the host's stores. Lactoferrin is a substance produced by the host that binds iron more tightly than the bacterial chelator, preventing the invading organism's access to a critical nutrient. Lysozyme is an important component of the antimicrobial system. This enzyme hydrolyzes [1–4]-glycosidic bonds, as in the peptidoglycan of bacterial cell walls. Lysozyme is present in almost all body fluids, including tears and saliva.

Hepatocytes produce an array of *acute phase proteins* (Table 5.4) that are released into the serum during inflammation or infection. These proteins do not act directly on bacteria, but they augment the bactericidal activity of other antimicrobial factors.

COMPLEMENT

Complement is a system of at least 20 separate proteins and cofactors that continuously circulate in the bloodstream. Complement acts to kill bacterial cells that are missed by the neutrophils and the macrophages. There are actually two separate complement pathways. One, the *classical pathway*, operates in the adaptive or acquired immune response. The classical pathway has an absolute requirement for an Ab–antigen complex as a trigger. The other, the *alternative pathway*, requires no Ab or antigen to initiate and is operative in innate immunity. Both pathways operate in a tightly regulated cascade fashion. The proteins normally circulate as inactive proenzymes. When the pathways are activated, the product of each step activates the subsequent step.

THE ALTERNATIVE COMPLEMENT PATHWAY

In the alternative pathway, C3 is the initiating peptide (Fig. 5.2). In the serum, C3 is somewhat unstable (it is sensitive to proteases) and spontaneously decomposes into a large, active C3b fragment and a smaller, catalytically inactive

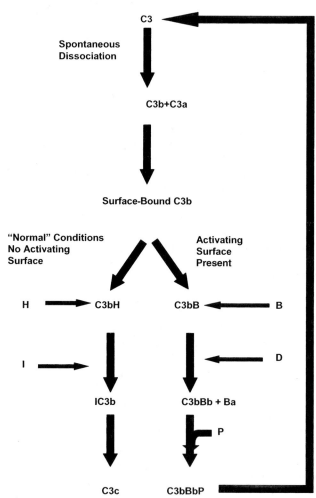

Figure 5.2 • Control of the alternative complement pathway by activating surfaces. When complement component C3b binds to a surface, there exist two possible outcomes. Under normal conditions, when no activating surface is present (e.g., if C3b has contacted normal tissue), sequential addition of blood cofactors H and I converts C3b into C3c, inactivating the complement protein. If an activating surface such as a microbe or damaged tissue is encountered, sequential addition of factors B and D drives the alternative pathway to the normal properdin (P) intermediate, and the complement cascade is triggered. The properdin-containing component (C3bBbP) feeds back to the beginning of the pathway, generating more C3.

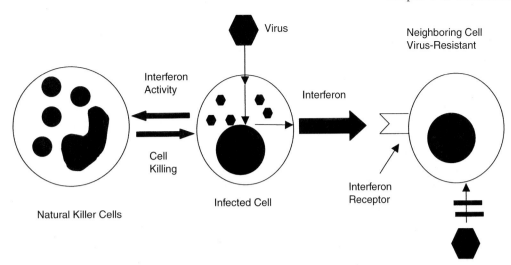

Figure 5.3 ● The function of interferon. When a virus infects a host cell, the cell expresses interferon. Interferon activates natural killer cells, causing killing of the infected host cells and elimination of the reservoir of infection. At the same time, interferon induces an antiviral state in neighboring cells, effectively breaking the cycle of infection.

C3a fragment. C3b now becomes bound to a surface, and it has two fates. We can define two types of surfaces. One, the nonactivating surface, is a surface that contains sialic acid or other acidic polysaccharides. The other, an activating surface, contains none of the acidic polysaccharides or sialic acid. This type conforms to a bacterial cell surface. Under normal circumstances, C3b will bind to a nonactivating surface. On binding, the C3b fragment becomes associated with factor H, a β-globulin that associates with an α chain on C3b. Sialic acid increases the affinity for factor H 100-fold. Factor H alters the shape of C3b in such a way that it becomes susceptible to attack by factor I, a serine esterase that cleaves the α chain of C3b, producing inactive iC3b. Attack by another protease produces a fragment designated C3c. In this pathway, factor H accelerates the decay of C3b. When factors H and I work together, they destroy C3b as fast as it is produced and shut down the pathway.

If C3b binds to an activating surface, the ability to bind to factor H is reduced, and C3b binds to a protein called factor B, forming C3bB. Bound factor B is cleaved by factor D into a fragment called Bb. The complex C3bBb has high C3-convertase activity and stimulates the pathway further. Factor P (properdin) binds to the complex, extending the half-life of C3bBbP. This fragment binds to the terminal complement components (C5–C9), creating a membrane attack complex and thus lysing the cell.

THE CLASSICAL COMPLEMENT PATHWAY

The classical complement pathway differs from the alternative pathway in that it requires a trigger in the form of an antigen–Ab complex. Only two antibodies can fix complement—IgG and IgM. The classical pathway is shown in Figure 5.3. The small fragments that are cleaved from the proenzymes have activities such as chemotactic stimulation and anaphylaxis. The *bar* over the names of some components of the pathway denotes an active complex. Note that the classical pathway does not operate with C1 to C9 in sequence. Rather, the sequence is C1, C4, C2, C3, C5, C6, C7, C8, and C9.

INTERFERONS

An important antiviral system is provided by the interferons (Table 5.5 and Fig. 5.4). The interferons are peptides that, when viral infection occurs, carry out three distinct functions. First, they send a signal to a natural killer cell that essentially leads to the self-destruction of the infected cell. Second, they induce an antiviral state in neighboring cells, limiting the viral infection. Third, when interferon receptors are bound on a target cell, the induction of the formation of antiviral proteins occurs. One such protein is the enzyme $2',5'$-oligoadenylate synthetase. This enzyme catalyzes the reaction that converts ATP into $2',5'$-oligoadenylate. This compound activates ribonuclease R, which possesses the specificity to hydrolyze viral RNA and thus can stop propagation of the virus inside the cell.

Acquired (Adaptive) Immunity

When the host is exposed to an antigen or organism that has been contacted previously, the *adaptive immune response* ensues. The adaptive immune response works through the B and T lymphocytes, which possess surface

TABLE 5.5 **Interferons**

Interferon	Producing Cells	Producing Mechanism	Isotypes	Molecular Mass	Receptor
Type 1					
IFN-α	Leukocytes		17	16–27 kDa	95–110 kDa
IFN-β	Fibroblasts	Viral infection	1	20 kDa	95–110 kDa
Type 2					
IFN-γ	T lymphocytes	Mitogen stimulation	1	20–24 kDa	90–95 kDa

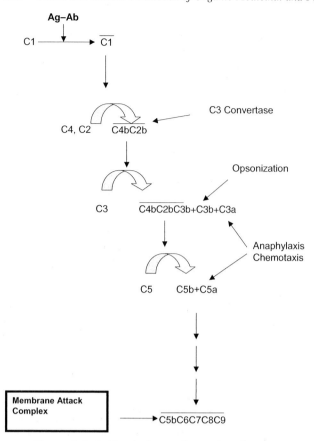

Figure 5.4 ● Classical complement pathway.

receptors specific for each invading organism. To account for all possible permutations of antigenic structure, natural and synthetic, that the host might encounter, the adaptive immune system uses genetic recombination of DNA and RNA splicing as a way of encoding its antibodies. Lymphocytes can recognize an estimated 10^7 different types of antigens through this genetic recombination mechanism, far more than a person is likely to encounter during a lifetime. Adaptive immunity is Ab-mediated immunity, based on circulating pools of antibodies that react with, and inactivate, antigens. These antibodies are found in the globulin fraction of the serum. Consequently, antibodies are also referred to as *immunoglobulins* (Ig). The adaptive immune response has the property of *memory*. The sensitivity, specificity, and memory for a particular antigen are retained, and subsequent exposures stimulate an enhanced response. Hence, the adaptive immune response differs from the innate in two respects: *specificity* and *memory*.

The adaptive immune response, like the innate, can be divided into two branches: humoral immunity and CMI. Humoral immunity is circulating immunity and is mediated by B lymphocytes and differentiated B lymphocytes known as plasma cells. CMI is controlled by the T lymphocytes. The immune function of T lymphocytes cannot be transferred by serum alone; the T cells must be present, whereas the immunity of the humoral system can be isolated from the serum and transferred. T cells are specially tailored to deal with intracellular infections (such as virus-infected cells), whereas B cells secrete soluble antibodies that can neutralize pathogens before their entry into host cells. Both B and T cells possess specific receptors on their surfaces to recognize unique stimulatory antigens. When B cells are stimulated, they express specific Ig or surface antibodies that are capable of binding to the antigen. A fraction of the B-cell population does not differentiate into Ab-producing cells but forms a pool of cells that retain the immunological memory. T cells express a specific antigen receptor, the T-cell receptor, similar in structure to the surface Ig receptor of B cells. This receptor is activated by a piece of processed antigen (presented with MHC-II). Activated T cells release soluble factors such as interleukins, cytokines, interferons, lymphokines, and colony-stimulating factors, all of which regulate the immune response. Interactions with some of these help to regulate the B-cell activity, directing the innate immune response.

IMMUNOGLOBULIN STRUCTURE AND FUNCTION

An Ab or Ig is composed of peptide chains with carbohydrate pendant groups. A schematic of the Ab IgG is shown in Figure 5.5. The peptide chains form the quaternary structure of the Ig, while the carbohydrate moieties serve

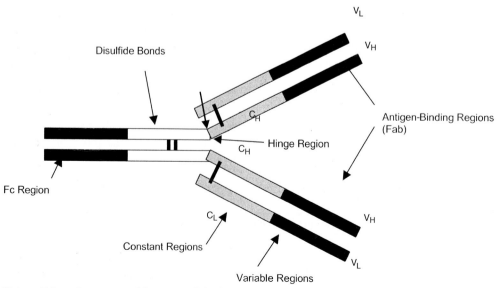

Figure 5.5 ● Structure of immunoglobulin G (IgG), showing antigen-binding regions and key elements of the molecule.

as antigen-recognition groups and probably as conformation-stabilizing units. The general structure of the Ig looks something like a Y, with the antigen-binding regions at the bifurcated end. In this area are peptide sequences that are "programmable" by the immune system to allow the Ig to recognize a large number of antigens.

Treatment with either of two enzymes, papain or pepsin, digests an Ab into fragments that are useful in understanding its molecular structure. Papain clips the Ab into two fragments that contain the antigen-binding regions. These fragments have been termed the *Fab*, or *antigen-binding, fragment*. The remaining part of the Ab after papain digestion contains two peptide chains linked by a disulfide bond. Treatment of the same Ab with pepsin yields the two Fab units joined by the disulfide bond, plus two of the distal peptide chains. These distal units have been crystallized and, hence, are termed the *Fc fragment* (for "crystallizable"). The disulfide bond, therefore, provides a demarcation between the two molecular regions. The nomenclature of an Ab includes a high–molecular weight, or heavy, chain on the inside and a low–molecular weight, or light, chain on the outside.

IMPORTANT FEATURES OF ANTIBODY MOLECULAR STRUCTURE[4,6]

As stated previously, the tip end of the Fab region binds antigen. There are two of these regions, so we say that the Ab is *bivalent* and can bind two antigen molecules. The overall amino acid sequence of the Ab dictates its conformation. The peptide sequence for most antibodies is similar, except for the hypervariable regions. The amino acid sequence at the end of the heavy chain (Fc) determines the class of the Ig (i.e., IgG, IgM, etc.). All antibodies resemble each other in basic shape, but each has a unique amino acid sequence that is complementary to the antigen in a "lock-and-key" interaction (antigen–Ab specificity). Some, such as IgM, are pentamers of IgG (Fig. 5.6). In reality, the lock-and-key model is too simplistic, and an induced fit model is preferred.

ANTIBODY PRODUCTION AND PROGRAMMING OF THE IMMUNE SYSTEM

The main element of the programming portion of the immune system is the macrophage. A common property of macrophages is *phagocytosis*, the capacity to engulf a particle or cell through invagination and sealing off of the cell membrane. The macrophages involved in the immune response set in motion a unique amplification process, so that a large response is obtained relative to the amount of antigen processed. The macrophages engulf antigenic particles and incorporate them into their cytoplasm, where the antigens are fragmented. The fragments are then combined with MHC-II, displayed on the cell membrane of the macrophage, and presented to the immune system. The presented antigens interact with B cells, causing differentiation to plasma cells and Ab secretion. T-helper cells also interact with the presented antigen and are stimulated to cause the B cells to proliferate and mature. Plasma cells are monoclonal (genetically identical) and produce monoclonal Ab. The process, from the pluripotent stem cell, to the B and T cells, to the plasma cells, is shown in Figure 5.1.

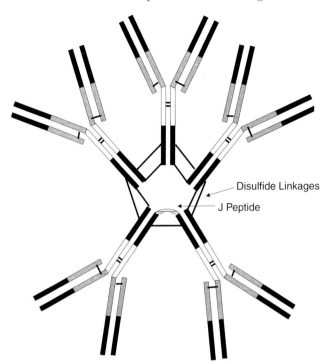

Figure 5.6 ● Pentameric structure of immunoglobulin M (IgM).

ANTIBODY FORMATION[5]

Figure 5.1 also indicates the actual Ab-producing steps. Plasma cells are clones of Ab-producing cells, which amplify the Ab response by their sheer numbers. The plasma cells can easily be regenerated if called on to do so by the memory functions. A population of plasma cells is shown at the bottom of the diagram. These are identical and amplify and produce large quantities of Ab, proportionally much greater than the amount of antigen that was initially processed.

THE ANAMNESTIC RESPONSE[5]

Because the programmed immune system has the property of memory, subsequent exposures to the same antigen are immediately countered. The actual memory response is referred to as the *anamnestic response*, a secondary response of high Ab titer to a particular antigen. This is due to "memory cell" formation as a result of the initial antigen stimulus (sensitization or immunization). The anamnestic response is demonstrated in Figure 5.7.

ANTIGEN–ANTIBODY REACTIONS[4]

An Ab is bivalent, and an antigen is multivalent, so lattice formation can occur (Fig. 5.8). The complex may be fibrous, particulate, matrixlike, soluble, or insoluble. These characteristics dictate the means of its disposal. Four fundamental reactions describe these processes: neutralization, precipitation, agglutination, and bacteriolysis.

Neutralization

Neutralization is an immunological disposal reaction for bacteria and for toxins (which are small and soluble). Once they bind the Ab, they are no longer toxic because their active site structures are covered and they cannot bind their

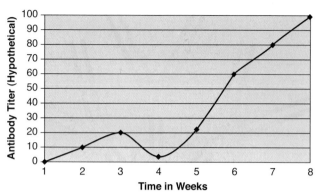

Figure 5.7 • Diagram of the time course of the anamnestic (memory) response. After the first immunization (week 1), the titer of Ab increases slowly to a low level and wanes. A challenge with the same antigen (shown in the diagram at week 4) elicits rapid development of a high titer of Ab in the blood.

targets. Examples of toxins are tetanospasmin (tetanus toxin; *Clostridium tetani*) and diphtheria toxin. Both react with specific receptors in the inhibitory interneurons of the nervous system, causing spastic paralysis or flaccid paralysis, respectively. When an Ab blocks the toxin's receptor-binding region, it can no longer bind to the neural receptors and is rendered harmless. The toxin–Ab complex is soluble and requires no further processing. The complex can then

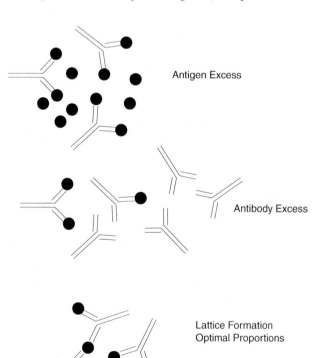

Figure 5.8 • Combining ratios of Ab and antigen. Because the Ab is bivalent, there exist a set of conditions under which optimal proportions yield a stable lattice structure, neutralizing the antigen. If antigen or Ab is in excess, the lattice will not form.

be eliminated by the kidneys. Bacteria are immobilized by neutralization.

Precipitation

When a soluble antigen reacts with an Ab, it may form an insoluble particulate precipitate. Such a complex cannot remain in the bloodstream in its insoluble state. These species must be removed by the spleen or through the reticuloendothelial system by phagocytosis.

Agglutination

Bacterial cells may be aggregated by binding to antibodies that mask negative ionic surface charges and cross-link cellular structures (Fig. 5.8). The bacteria are thus immediately immobilized. This limits their ability to maintain an infection, but it forms a particulate matrix. This type of complex must also undergo elimination through the reticuloendothelial system.

Bacteriolysis

Bacteriolysis is a complement-mediated reaction. The last five proteins in the cascade self-assemble to produce a membrane attack complex that disrupts the cell membranes of bacteria, acting like bacitracin or amphotericin B. The cell membranes lose integrity, cell contents leak out, membrane transport systems fail, and the cell dies. This type of reaction yields products that require no special treatment.

ANTIBODY TYPES AND REACTIONS

Ab types and reactions are classified on the basis of variations in a common section of the Fc fragment that governs biological activity in a general way.

IgG

IgG (Fc = γ) (Fig. 5.5) participates in precipitation reactions, toxin neutralizations, and complement fixation. IgG is the major (70%) human Ig. The Fab tip fixes antigen, and the Fc fragment can fix complement to yield agglutination or lysis. IgG is the only immunoglobulin that crosses the transplacental barrier and the neonatal stomach, so it provides maternal protection. IgG constitutes about 75% of the total Ab in the circulation. It is present at a concentration of about 15 mg/mL and has a half-life of 3 weeks, the longest of any of the Ab types. The light chains of IgG can possess either κ or λ variants. These slight differences in structure are called *isotypes*, and the phenomenon is termed *isotypic variation*.

IgM

IgM (Fc = μ) (Fig. 5.6) is present at a concentration of about 1.5 mg/mL and has a half-life of less than 1 week. This Ab participates in opsonization, agglutination reactions, and complement fixation. Opsonization, as stated previously, is a "protein coating" or tagging of a bacterium that renders it more susceptible to phagocytosis. A complex of the Fc portion of IgM plus C3b of complement is that protein. IgM is the first immunoglobulin formed during immunization, but it wanes and gives way to IgG. IgM is a pentamer, and its agglutination potency is about 1,000 times that of IgG. IgM is also responsible for the A, B, and O blood groups. The fundamental monomeric IgM structure is much like that of IgG. The pentamer is held together by disulfide bonds and a single J (joining) peptide. The affinity of an IgM monomer for antigen is less than that of IgG, but the multimeric structure raises the *avidity* of the molecule for an antigen.

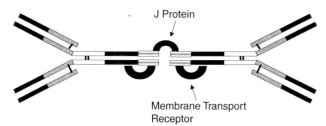

Figure 5.9 ● Structure of immunoglobulin A (IgA), the mucosal Ab that protects the GI tract and the respiratory mucosa.

IgA

IgA (Fc = α) (Fig. 5.9) is found in exocrine gland secretions (milk, saliva, tears), where it protects mucous membranes (e.g., in the respiratory tract). It is present in the serum as a monomer at a concentration of 1 to 2 mg/mL, but humans secrete about 1 g of the dimer per day in the mucosal fluids. Secretory IgA consists of two IgG-like units linked together at the Fc regions by a peptide known as the secretory fragment and a J fragment. The secretory fragment is actually part of the membrane receptor for IgA. The IgA molecule on the mucosal side of the membrane binds antigen, then binds to the receptor. By a process of transcytosis, the IgA–antigen complex is moved from the mucosa to the bloodstream, where IgG and IgM can react. Because it is distributed on the mucosa, IgA has an anatomically specific distribution, unlike the other antibodies. IgA is the mediator of oral polio vaccination (the mucosal reaction gives way to systemic protection).

IgD

IgD (Fc = δ) is present on the surface of B cells and, along with monomeric surface IgM, is an antigen receptor that activates Ig production. There is less than 0.1 mg/mL in the bloodstream, and the half-life is only 3 days.

IgE

IgE (Fc = ε) is the Ab responsible for hypersensitivity reactions. IgE complexes have a high affinity for host cell surfaces and can damage the host. High levels of IgE are found in persons with allergies of various types, as well as in autoimmune diseases. The Fc fragment is responsible for the Ig–cell reactivity. An Ab-plus-antigen reaction yields the typical Ab–antigen complex. The Fc portion of the Ab is actually part of the mast cell. When antigen binds to the Fab portion of the Ab, the IgE molecules become cross-linked. This probably distorts the membrane of the mast cells and stimulates them to release histamine, which causes bronchial constriction, itching, redness, and anaphylaxis.

⬡ ACQUISITION OF IMMUNITY

Several types of immunity must be considered when describing vaccines and other immunobiologicals. Some are artificial and some are natural. *Natural immunity* is endowed by phagocytic white blood cells, lysozyme in tears, the skin, and so on. *Acquired immunity* is acquired after birth (or by passage from mother to fetus). Thus, immunity may be classified as follows:

- *Active acquired immunity*: The host produces his or her own Ab.

- *Naturally acquired active immunity*: Occurs on recovery from a disease (or from antigen exposure).
- *Artificially acquired active immunity*: Occurs as a response to sensitization by a vaccine or toxoid.
- *Passive acquired immunity*: The subject receives Ab from an outside source, such as a γ-globulin injection, or by transplacental transfer.
- *Naturally acquired passive immunity*: Temporary neonatal protection from maternal IgG passes to the fetus in utero; this type of immunity is not long-lasting.
- *Artificially acquired passive immunity*: An Ab is given by injection (e.g., by an antitoxin or a γ-globulin injection).

Definitions of Immunobiologicals

Immunobiologicals include antigenic substances, such as vaccines and toxoids, or Ab-containing preparations, such as globulins and antitoxins, from human or animal donors. These products are used for active or passive immunization or therapy. All of the following are examples of immunobiologicals:

- *Vaccine*: A suspension of live (usually attenuated) or inactivated microorganisms (e.g., bacteria, viruses, or rickettsiae) or fractions thereof, administered to induce immunity and prevent infectious disease or its sequelae. Some vaccines contain highly defined antigens (e.g., the polysaccharide of *Haemophilus influenzae* type b [Hib] or the surface antigen of hepatitis B), others have antigens that are complex or incompletely defined (e.g., killed *Bordetella pertussis* or live attenuated viruses).
- *Toxoid*: A modified bacterial toxin that has been made nontoxic but retains the ability to stimulate the formation of antitoxin.
- *Immune globulin (IG)*: A sterile solution containing antibodies from human blood. It is obtained by cold ethanol fractionation of large pools of blood plasma and contains 15% to 18% protein. Intended for intramuscular administration, IG is primarily intended for routine maintenance of immunity in certain immunodeficient persons and for passive immunization against measles and hepatitis A. IG does not transmit hepatitis B virus (HBV), human immunodeficiency virus (HIV), or other infectious diseases.
- *Intravenous immune globulin (IGIV)*: A product derived from blood plasma from a donor pool similar to the IG pool but prepared so it is suitable for intravenous use. IGIV does not transmit infectious diseases. It is primarily used for replacement therapy in primary Ab deficiency disorders and for the treatment of Kawasaki disease, immune thrombocytopenia purpura, hypogammaglobulinemia in chronic lymphocytic leukemia, and some cases of HIV infection.
- *Specific immune globulin*: Special preparations obtained from blood plasma from donor pools preselected for a high Ab content against a specific antigen (e.g., hepatitis B immune globulin, varicella-zoster immune globulin [VZIG], rabies immune globulin, tetanus immune globulin, vaccinia immune globulin, and cytomegalovirus immune globulin). Like IG and IGIV, these preparations do not transmit infectious disease.
- *Antitoxin*: A solution of antibodies (e.g., diphtheria antitoxin and botulinum antitoxin) derived from the serum of animals immunized with specific antigens. Antitoxins are used to confer passive immunity and for treatment.

Vaccination denotes the physical act of administering a vaccine or toxoid. *Immunization* is a more inclusive term denoting the process of inducing or providing immunity artificially by administering an immunobiological. Immunization may be active or passive.

Immunobiologicals (Vaccines and Toxoids)[6–10]

A *vaccine* may be defined as a solution or suspension of killed or live/attenuated virus, killed rickettsia, killed or live/attenuated bacteria, or antigens derived from these sources, which are used to confer active, artificially acquired immunity against that organism or related organisms. When administered, the vaccine represents the initial exposure, resulting in the acquisition of immunity. A subsequent exposure or challenge (a disease) results in the anamnestic, or memory, response.

METHODS OF VACCINE PRODUCTION

Vaccine production methods have varied greatly over the years and are best discussed according to a parallel chronological and sophistication approach.

Killed (Inactivated) Pathogen

In this method, the normal pathogen is treated with a strong, denaturing disinfectant like formaldehyde or phenol. The process denatures the proteins and carbohydrates that are essential for the organism to live and infect a host, but if treated properly, the surface antigens are left intact. The process must be done carefully to control the unwinding of proteins or carbohydrates by denaturation, because the preparation must be recognized as the original antigen. The main problems with killed pathogen vaccines are the following: (a) if the vaccine is not inactivated totally, disease can result; (b) if the preparation is overtreated, vaccine failure usually results because of denaturation; (c) the production laboratory must grow the pathogen in large quantities to be commercially useful, putting laboratory technicians at risk; and (d) the patient may experience abnormal and harmful responses, such as fever, convulsions, and death. These vaccines typically are viewed as "dirty" vaccines, and some, like the pertussis vaccine, have been associated with problems serious enough to warrant their temporary removal from the market.

Live/Attenuated Pathogens

The word *attenuated* for our purposes simply means "low virulence." The true pathogen is altered phenotypically so that it cannot invade the human host and cannot get ahead of the host's immune system. Low-pathogenicity strains such as these were originally obtained by passage of the microbes through many generations of host animals. The idea was that the animal and the pathogen, if both were to survive, needed to adapt to live with each other without either partner being killed. Poliovirus is attenuated in this fashion in monkey kidney tissue. In a live/attenuated vaccine, antigenicity is still required, as is infectivity (polio vaccine yields an infection), but the host's immune system must be able to stay ahead of the infection. The key problems are the following: (a) the vaccine cannot be used if the patient is immunocompromised, has fever or malignancy, or is taking immunosuppressive drugs; (b) these vaccines should not be used during pregnancy; and (c) the attenuated organism commonly reverts to the virulent strain, which was the reason for the failure of some early polio vaccines. Today, biological quality control is very stringent, and these problems have been eliminated.

Live/Attenuated Related Strain

The live/attenuated related strain is antigenically related so that it can provide cross-immunity to the pathogen. For example, cowpox virus can be used in place of smallpox virus. The strains are antigenically similar enough so that the host's immune system reacts to the related strain to provide protection against the normal pathogen. The main advantage is that a true pathogen is not being used so that the chance of contracting the actual disease is zero. The problem with such vaccines is that they cause an infection. Cowpox is known to spread to the central nervous system in 1 in 10^5 cases, causing a potentially fatal form of meningitis.

Cellular Antigen from a Pathogen

The surface antigen (i.e., what is recognized as foreign) is harvested from the pathogen, purified, and reconstituted into a vaccine preparation. These antigens can take several forms, including the carbohydrate capsule, as in *Neisseria meningitidis*; pili, as in *N. gonorrhoeae*; flagella from motile bacteria (the basis for an experimental cholera vaccine); or the viral protein coat, as in the vaccine for hepatitis B. Advantages of the method are that there is virtually no chance of disease, contamination, or reversion and there are no storage problems. This method is currently as close to a "perfect approach" as we have. A problem is that the pathogen must be grown under careful control or an unsure source must be relied on. For example, hepatitis B vaccine was originally prepared from the serum of a controlled population of human carriers. Imagine the impact if one of the carriers developed another blood-borne disease. Additionally, these are strain-specific antigens (e.g., *N. gonorrhoeae* may require 1,500 different pilar antigens). Acellular vaccines may exhibit lower antigenicity in the very young and may require several injections for full immunological competence. To be safe and consistent, the antigenic component must be identified. Given the complex nature of biological materials, this is not always easy or even possible.

Genetically Engineered Pathogens[5]

The techniques of genetic engineering have allowed the pharmaceutical industry to prepare absolutely pure surface antigens while totally eliminating the pathogenic organism from the equation. As shown in Figure 5.10, the virus contains surface antigens (designated by *filled circles*). Inside the viral capsule is a circular piece of deoxyribonucleic acid (DNA) containing genes for the various biological molecules of the virus. The diagram shows, at about 3 o'clock, a small piece of DNA that codes for the surface antigen. The strategy is to isolate this piece of DNA and insert it into a rapidly growing expression vector for production of the surface protein. In this case, *Escherichia coli* serves as an excellent vector. It contains a plasmid that can be removed, clipped open, and used as a cassette to carry the viral DNA. Additionally, *E. coli* can be grown in batch to produce the viral surface antigen. To begin, the DNA is removed from the virus and the plasmid is removed from the vector. Viral and bacterial nucleic acid is treated with a restriction

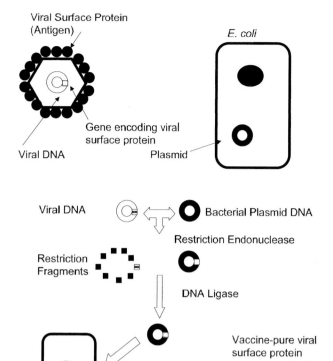

Figure 5.10 ● Preparation of a genetically engineered Ab.

endonuclease, which cleaves the DNA and plasmid at designated restriction sites. The viral DNA is cleaved into several fragments, each of which is ligated into the *E. coli* plasmid with a ligase enzyme. Plasmids are inserted into *E. coli*, and the organism is grown in batch fermentation. The organisms containing the gene for the viral surface protein can be separated by screening and purified to serve as the ultimate antigen producer—free of contamination or pathogenic viral particles. The pure antigen may then be constituted into a vaccine and used in human hosts.

USE OF VACCINES IN COMBINATION: DOSING[5,11]

Types of Vaccines

There are three basic types of vaccine preparations that are used clinically:

1. A *simple* vaccine contains one strain of a disease-causing organism (e.g., plague vaccine, *Pasteurella pestis*, and smallpox vaccine).
2. A *multivalent* vaccine is prepared from two or more strains of an organism that cause the same disease (e.g., polio is trivalent). Administration of the multiple strains is required for full protection because their antigens are not cross-immunizing. The immune system must mount a separate immune response to each strain.
3. A *polyvalent* vaccine is prepared from two or more organisms that cause different diseases. Polyvalent vaccines are given for convenience, primarily so that a child can be given one shot rather than several. The measles–mumps–rubella (MMR) vaccine is of the polyvalent type.

Types of Dosing

Vaccines can be administered according to various dosing regimens, depending on the vaccine type and the purpose of the injection:

1. A *single-dose vaccine* is usually assumed to confer, with one shot, "lifetime immunity." The smallpox vaccine was a single-dose vaccine.
2. In a *multiple-dosing* regimen, several doses are given, spaced weeks or months apart, to get maximum immunogenicity. Multiple dosing is usually done with inactivated vaccines, which are less antigenic. Multiple dosing is not the same as a booster dose.
3. A *booster dose* is administered years after the initial immunization schedule (regardless of single or multiple first dose). As a patient ages, Ab levels may wane. A booster is used to bolster immunity. Also, boosters are used if a patient is known or suspected to have been exposed to a pathogen (e.g., tetanus).
4. A *coadministered vaccine* is possible only if one vaccine does not interfere with another.
5. There are two physical forms of vaccines: A *fluid vaccine* is a solution or a suspension of the vaccine in saline of an aqueous buffer; the solution or suspension in an *adsorbed vaccine* is adsorbed on a matrix of aluminum or calcium phosphate. Like a sustained-release dosage form, in theory, there is longer exposure via a depot injection. The higher surface area of the matrix will be exposed to the immune system. Generally, adsorbed vaccines are preferred.

Pharmaceutical Principles of Vaccines

As expected for a live biological preparation, heat destroys live viral and bacterial vaccines. If the agent is not killed, the antigen may be altered. Like many biologicals, lyophilized vaccines are unstable after reconstitution. Ice crystals formed inside the protein structure during freeze-drying expand during thawing and disrupt the structure of the vaccine. Live vaccines can be inactivated by minute amounts of detergent. Detergent residue adhering to glassware is concentrated enough to act as a disinfectant. It is safe to use only plastic implements specified for the vaccine. The suspending medium may be sterile water, saline, or more complex systems containing protein or other constituents derived from the medium in which the vaccine is produced (e.g., serum proteins, egg antigens, and cell culture-derived antigens). Concentrated Ab suspensions (γ-globulins) are typical amphiphilic proteins and aggregate on storage. If injected, the particulates may cause anaphylaxis. Preservatives may be components of vaccines, antitoxins, and globulins. These components are present to inhibit or prevent bacterial growth in viral cultures or the final product or to stabilize the antigens or antibodies. Allergic reactions can occur if the recipient is sensitive to one of these additives (e.g., mercurial compounds [thimerosal], phenols, albumin, glycine, or neomycin).

Storage and Handling of Immunobiologicals

Failure to follow the exact recommendations for storage and handling of immunobiologicals can lead to an impotent preparation. During reconstituting, storing, and handling of immunobiologicals, the most important recommendation is to follow the package insert exactly. Vaccines should always be stored at their recommended temperature. Certain vaccines, such as polio vaccine, are sensitive to increased temperature. Other vaccines, such as oral polio vaccine, diphtheria and tetanus toxoids, and acellular pertussis vaccine, hepatitis B vaccine, influenza vaccine, and Hib conjugate vaccine (Hib-CV; among others), are sensitive to freezing.

Viral Vaccines[12]

SMALLPOX VACCINE (DRYVAX)

Smallpox vaccine is live *vaccinia* (cowpox) virus grown on the skin of a bovine calf. Smallpox is a highly lethal and disfiguring disease that was common throughout history. Smallpox vaccine was used routinely in the United States but today is no longer recommended. (There have been no reported cases of smallpox since the 1940s.) In 1982, smallpox was declared eradicated worldwide. With smallpox, the risks of the vaccine outweigh the benefits; the vaccine penetrates the central nervous system and potentially fatal encephalitis occurs in 1 of 10^5 patients. After exposure to smallpox, the vaccine can be injected to lessen the severity of the disease.

INFLUENZA VACCINE[13-17]

Influenza vaccine is a multivalent inactivated influenza virus or viral subunits (split vaccine). The virus is grown on chick embryo and inactivated by exposure to ultraviolet (UV) light or formaldehyde. The antigen type is protein. The vaccine in the United States contains thimerosal, a mercurial, as a preservative. *Influenza* is a respiratory tract infection with a 2-day incubation period. The disease may be devastating and can lead to pneumonia. Without the vaccine, influenza is common in epidemics and pandemics. To clarify, the *flu* is a GI infection with diarrhea and vomiting. Influenza requires weeks of incubation. Influenza is caused by two main genetic strains each year (A and B): type A is most common in humans; type B is less common. The virus mutates very rapidly, and vaccines must be tailored yearly. The World Health Organization (WHO) and the Centers for Disease Control and Prevention (CDC) monitor the migration of the disease from Southeast Asia, type the strains causing the occurrences, and order a vaccine to counter the organisms most likely to enter the United States. Influenza A viruses are categorized according to two cell surface protein antigens: hemagglutinin (H) and neuraminidase (N). Each of these is divided further into subtypes (H1, H2; N1, N2). Individual strains within a subtype are named for the location, isolation sequence number, and year of isolation (e.g., A/Beijing/2/90 [H1N1]). For example, the WHO-recommended formula for 2001 to 2002 included the following antigens: A/New Caledonia/20/99 (H1N1), A/Moscow/10/99 (H3N2), B/Sichuan/379/99, 15 μg each per 0.5 mL. A typical vaccine will be a mixture of three strains. Strains are selected each year in the spring on the basis of the disease trends observed and are released in the autumn. In general, those patients who are at high risk for complications from influenza are the following:

- Persons 65 years of age or older
- Residents of nursing homes and other chronic-care facilities that house persons of any age who have chronic medical conditions
- Adults and children who have chronic disorders of the pulmonary or cardiovascular systems, including asthma
- Adults and children who have required medical follow-up or hospitalization during the preceding year because

of chronic metabolic diseases (including diabetes mellitus), renal dysfunction, hemoglobinopathies, or immunosuppression (including immunosuppression caused by medications or HIV infection)
- Children and teenagers (aged 6 months–18 years) who are receiving long-term aspirin therapy and, therefore, might be at risk for developing Reye syndrome after influenza infection
- Women who will be in the second or third trimester of pregnancy during the influenza season
- Healthcare workers and those in close contact with persons at high risk, including household members
- Household members (including children) of persons in groups at high risk, including persons with pulmonary disorders, such as asthma, and healthcare workers who are at higher risk because of close contact

It is impossible to contract influenza from the vaccine. The only side effects may be local pain and tenderness at the injection site, with low-grade fever in 3% to 5% of patients. Aspirin and acetaminophen are effective in combating these symptoms. Allergic reactions are rare but may be seen in persons allergic to eggs. Immunity to influenza vaccine takes 2 weeks to develop. Some people fear the vaccine because of reports of a strange paralysis and lack of nerve sensation associated with the 1976 swine flu vaccine. This problem, Guillain-Barré syndrome, was associated only with this 1976 vaccine and has not been associated with vaccines since.[17]

POLIO VACCINES[18-20]

Polio is a dangerous viral infection that affects both muscle mass and the spinal cord. Some children and adults who contract polio become paralyzed, and some may die because of respiratory paralysis. Polio was the cause of the "infantile paralysis" epidemic of 1950 to 1953, which led to many paralyzed children and the specter of patients spending their lives in an iron lung. Serious cases of polio cause muscle pain and may make movement of the legs and/or arms difficult or impossible and, as stated previously, may make breathing difficult. Milder cases last a few days and may cause fever, sore throat, headache, and nausea. Interest in polio has increased because of recent local outbreaks; large numbers of people are unimmunized. There are no drugs or special therapies to cure polio; treatment is only supportive. The symptoms of polio may reappear 40 to 50 years after a severe infection. This phenomenon is known as postpolio muscle atrophy (PPMA). PPMA is not a reinfection or reactivation of the virus but is probably a form of rapid aging in polio survivors. There are two types of polio vaccines.

Inactivated Polio Vaccine (IPV)

There are several synonyms for the IPV vaccine: IPV, e-IPV, ep-IPV, and the Salk vaccine (1954 [IPOL, Aventis-Pasteur]). e-IPV is an enhanced potency poliovirus, more potent and immunogenic than any of the previous IPV formulations. e-IPV is recommended for all four infant doses because of the incidence of rare cases of oral polio vaccine (OPV)–associated paralytic poliomyelitis. e-IPV is also preferred for adults for the same reason. IPV is a trivalent (strains 1, 2, 3) vaccine grown in monkey kidney culture and subjected to elaborate precautions to ensure inactivation (typically, formaldehyde is used). The antigen form is whole virus. The antigen type is protein. The vaccine is injected to cause induction of active systemic immunity from polio but does not stop polio carriers, who shed the virus from the oral and nasal cavities.

Trivalent Oral Polio Vaccine (TOPV)

TOPV (Sabin vaccine, 1960) is a live attenuated whole virus vaccine (antigen type, protein) containing polio strains 1, 2, and 3. The virus culture is grown on monkey kidney tissue with the use of an elaborate attenuation protocol. Oral administration of the vaccine yields a local GI infection, and the initial immune response is via IgA (mucosal, local to the GI tract). The IgA–antigen complex undergoes transcytosis across the mucosal membrane, and systemic immunity is induced as IgM and IgG form. A major caution with TOPV is that it is a live vaccine and must never be injected. Indications are the following:

- Mass vaccination campaigns to control outbreaks of paralytic polio.
- Unvaccinated children who will travel in less than 4 weeks to areas where polio is endemic.
- Children of parents who do not accept the recommended number of vaccine injections. These children may receive OPV only for the third or fourth dose or both. In such cases, the healthcare provider should administer OPV only after discussing the risk of OPV-associated paralytic poliomyelitis with parents or caregivers.
- e-IPV is recommended for routine use in all four immunizing doses in infants and children.
- The WHO has advocated giving children e-IPV instead of TOPV to prevent exposure of others to virus shed through the nose and mouth.[21,22]

RUBELLA VACCINE[23]

German measles is a disease that was once called the "3-day measles" and was considered a normal childhood illness. It is a mild disease with few consequences, except in the first trimester of pregnancy. In these mothers, rubella causes birth defects in 50% of cases. Defects may include heart disease, deafness, blindness, learning disorders, and spontaneous abortion of the fetus. Symptoms of rubella are a low-grade fever, swollen neck glands, and a rash that lasts for about 3 days. About 1 of every 10 women of childbearing age in the United States is not protected against rubella. Also, 20% of all adults escaped this normal childhood disease or are not vaccinated.

Rubella vaccine (German measles vaccine, live, Meruvax II, Merck) is a live, attenuated rubella virus produced in human diploid cell culture. The antigen form of the vaccine is whole virus. The antigen type is protein. The vaccine is administered as part of the normal immunization schedule at 15 months. Side effects are minimal, but there may be some soreness and pain at the site of injection and stiffness of the joints.

A problem with the vaccine is that administration of a live virus is contraindicated in pregnancy. Indications are the following:

- Persons aged 12 months to puberty should be immunized routinely.
- Previously unimmunized children of susceptible pregnant women should receive the MMR vaccine. The trivalent vaccine is preferred for persons likely to be susceptible to mumps and rubella.

- Immunization of susceptible nonpregnant adolescent or adult women of childbearing potential is called for if precautions to avoid pregnancy are observed.
- Almost all children and some adults require more than one dose of MMR vaccine.
- On the first routine visit to the obstetrician/gynecologist, the immune status should be checked. If the woman is not immunized against rubella, the physician should administer the vaccine and stress avoiding pregnancy for 3 months.
- If the patient is already pregnant, the physician should not administer the vaccine.
- If exposure is suspected, the cord blood should be monitored for the presence of rubella antibodies.
- All unimmunized women should be vaccinated immediately after delivery of the baby.

MEASLES VACCINE (ATTENUVAX, MERCK)[23]

Measles is a very serious, highly contagious disease. It causes a high fever, rash, and a cough lasting 1 to 2 weeks. Some patients experience extreme sensitivity to light. The rash may occur inside the eyelids, producing a very painful condition. In the United States, between 3,000 and 28,000 cases occur each year, depending on factors such as weather and localized outbreaks. Outbreaks are very common in neighborhoods and schools. One of ten children contracting measles will develop an ear infection or pneumonia. Measles may infect the brain (encephalitis) and lead to convulsions, hearing loss, and mental disability. In the United States, 1 of every 500 to 10,000 children contracting measles dies from it. Severe sickness and death are more common in babies and adults than in elementary schoolchildren or teenagers. Measles has been linked to multiple sclerosis. In 1977, a severe epidemic occurred in the United States, and 50,000 cases were reported. Only 60% of the population was vaccinated.

Measles vaccine is composed of live/attenuated measles virus that is grown on chick embryo culture with an attenuation protocol. Indications are the following:

- Selective induction of active immunity against measles virus.
- Trivalent MMR vaccine is the preferred immunizing form for most children and many adults.
- Almost all children and many adults require more than one dose of MMR.
- Prior to international travel, persons susceptible to any of the three viruses should receive the single-antigen vaccine or the trivalent vaccine, as appropriate.
- Most persons born before 1956 are likely to have contracted the disease naturally and are not considered susceptible.
- Persons born after 1956 or those who lack adequate documentation of having had the disease should be vaccinated.

The vaccine is required by law at 15 months and again at 11 to 12 years of age. The vaccine can be administered after exposure to measles to lessen the disease severity. This is because Ab to the vaccine develops in 7 days, while the incubation period for the disease is 11 days. The vaccine should not be administered in pregnancy and should always be administered with great care to women of childbearing age. Because measles vaccine is cultivated in egg medium, care must be used in patients who are allergic to eggs and egg products. For this reason, a test dose regimen is used. The administration protocol is shown in Figure 5.11.

MUMPS VACCINE[24,25]

Mumps virus causes fever, headache, and a painful swelling of the parotid glands under the jaw. Mumps can be serious and is highly contagious. Prior to the vaccine, the disease was passed from child to child with ease. The disease runs its course over several days. Between 4,500 and 13,000 cases of mumps occur as outbreaks in the United States every year. In severe cases, mumps may cause inflammation of the coverings of the brain and spinal cord (meningitis); this occurs in about 10% of infected persons. Swelling of the brain itself occurs in 1 of 200 patients. Men may experience a painful swelling of the testicles (orchitis), which may presage sterility. Women may experience a corresponding infection of the ovaries. Male teens are often sicker than other groups of either sex. Mumps early in childhood has been linked to the development of juvenile diabetes.

The mumps vaccine (Mumpsvax, Merck) is a live, attenuated virus grown on chick embryo culture with attenuation protocols. The antigen form is whole virus. The antigen type is protein. Indications are the following:

- Induction of artificially acquired active immunity against mumps.
- Before international travel, immunize any susceptible individuals with the single-antigen vaccine or the trivalent MMR vaccine, as appropriate.
- Most children and some adults need more than one dose of MMR vaccine.
- Persons born prior to 1956 are generally considered immune.

Caution. Mumps vaccine is supplied with a diluent. Use only this diluent for reconstitution. Addition of a diluent with an antimicrobial preservative can render the vaccine inactive. The vaccine is normally administered to children at 15 months of age and again at 11 to 12 years. Because mumps vaccine is cultivated in egg medium, care used to be advised in patients allergic to eggs and egg products. Recent data show that persons who are allergic to egg and egg products fail to react to the mumps vaccine.

COMBINATION PRODUCTS (POLYVALENT VIRAL VACCINES)

If two or more vaccines are free of interference with each other, they can be administered as a mixture (polyvalent) for convenience. Examples of polyvalent viral vaccines are measles–rubella (MR), rubella–mumps (RM), and MMR. MMR is indicated for routine immunization at 15 months (not given at <1 year unless the child has been exposed or lacks immunocompetence). This is because maternal Abs interfere with development of vaccine immunity in small children. If the MMR is given at less than 1 year, revaccination is needed at 15 months of age.

CHICKENPOX VACCINE[21,26–30]

Chickenpox is caused by varicella-zoster virus. Every year, about 3.5 million people in the United States, mostly children, contract chickenpox. The incidence peaks between 3 and 9 years of age. Chickenpox causes a generalized rash, with 300 to 500 blisterlike lesions occurring on the scalp, face, and trunk. Symptoms include loss of appetite, malaise, and headache. The disease is usually benign but can lead to bacterial superinfection, pneumonia, encephalitis, and Reye syndrome. About 50 to 100 previously healthy children die of the disease. About 2% of all cases occur in adults, who have more serious symptoms than children have.

Varicella vaccine (Varivax, Merck) is derived from live virus from a child with natural varicella. The virus has been attenuated by passage through a series of guinea pig and human cell cultures. The final preparation is a lyophilized live, attenuated virus. The antigen form is whole virus. The antigen type is protein. The vaccine is well tolerated, with pain and redness at the injection site as the only side effects. The vaccine has shown tremendous success in reducing infections. Indications are the following:

- The vaccine is recommended for children 12 months to 12 years old as a single dose.
- Adults who are exposed to chickenpox should continue to receive VZIG.
- In elderly persons, varicella vaccine can boost immunity to varicella-zoster virus and may prevent or attenuate herpes zoster (shingles) attacks.

HEPATITIS VACCINES[30–40]

Hepatitis is a complex of diseases that causes fever, nausea, abdominal pain, jaundice, liver failure, and death. There are five clinically recognized types (A, B, C, D, and E).

Hepatitis A Vaccine

Hepatitis A virus (HAV; infectious hepatitis) causes an acute disease with an abrupt onset. About 15 to 50 days of incubation are required before the disease becomes clinically noticeable. The primary sign is jaundice. The disease lasts several weeks and is followed by complete recovery. Hepatitis A is transmitted when the virus is taken in by mouth. The fecal–oral route and close contact, unwashed food, and contaminated water account for most of the routes of transmission. The sexual anal–oral route is also a route of spread. Children under the age of 3 frequently have no symptoms but can transmit the disease to adults in child care centers. An injection of hepatitis A immune globulin is one way of preventing the disease but is only effective for about 30 days.

The hepatitis A vaccine (Havrix) is an inactivated preparation that is produced by propagation of the virus in cultured human diploid cells and then is inactivated with formalin. The antigen form is lysed whole viruses. The antigen type is protein. The course of immunization involves two injections over a 4-week period and a booster 12 months after the first injection. Indications are the following:

- Persons traveling outside the United States, except to Australia, Canada, Japan, New Zealand, and Western Europe
- Persons with chronic liver disease
- Persons living in an outbreak zone
- Persons who inject medications
- Persons engaging in high-risk sexual activity
- Child care workers caring for children younger than 2 years of age
- Developing countries with poor sanitation

Side effects are minor and usually limited to soreness at the injection site and fever.

Hepatitis B Vaccine

HBV, the cause of serum hepatitis, is a much more insidious, chronic disease, transmitted by needles, mucosal contact, blood, or high-risk sexual activity. The highest risk for contraction of hepatitis B is among intravenous drug abusers. The disease is linked to cirrhosis and liver cancer. There are about 200,000 new cases reported per year in the United States; of these, 10% become carriers, one fifth die from cirrhosis, and 1,000 die from liver cancer. The hepatitis B vaccine was first introduced in 1981. Initially, it was prepared as an inactivated vaccine from the plasma of carefully screened human, high-titer carriers/donors. In 1986, the recombinant DNA (rDNA) vaccine (Engerix B, Recombivax) was introduced to the market. The rDNA vaccine contains only viral subunits and may be used with hepatitis B immune globulin in a postexposure setting to boost the ability of the host to resist the infection. In adults, three doses should be given, at 0, 1, and 6 months. In children, the vaccine is given at birth, 1 month, and 9 months. Administration may be delayed in premature infants whose immune systems are not fully developed. If not immunized at birth, a child should receive three doses by 18 months. If the mother tests positive for hepatitis B, the vaccine plus the immune globulin must be given at or shortly after birth. The vaccine is 95% effective and is typically without side effects. Several high-risk groups have been identified: healthcare workers, student healthcare workers, people living in high-risk environments, and dentists. They should receive a three-dose course of the vaccine. In most other cases, a physician can judge whether a patient is at high risk or not. Side effects of the vaccine are minor.

Hepatitis C Vaccine

Hepatitis C virus (HCV) was once called hepatitis non-A, non-B but has been recognized as a separate entity. HCV infection is spread primarily by the parenteral route (transfusions), and unlike HBV, maternal–fetal and sexual transmission are uncommon. Acute infection may show few symptoms; fewer than 25% of patients develop full-blown hepatitis. Administration of interferon alpha (IFN-α) during the early acute phase can cure most patients. Unfortunately, 50% to 60% of those with HCV infection develop chronic hepatitis. This is often manifested by periodic increases in hepatic enzyme levels. Cirrhosis develops in 20% of chronic infectees; this usually requires 15 to 20 years to develop. Patients with HCV are at risk for hepatocellular carcinoma. Estimates are that 150,000 to 170,000 new cases occur in the United States per year. Intravenous drug users, transfusion patients, and healthcare workers are at highest risk.

Development of an HCV vaccine proved difficult but was accomplished in 1998. There are 15 genotypes, and the virus can modulate its antigens within the host's body. A new approach using genetic material from the virus, analogous to the approach to the influenza vaccine, is said to be promising.[41]

Hepatitis E

Hepatitis E virus (HEV) causes disease clinically indistinguishable from hepatitis A. Symptoms include malaise, anorexia, abdominal pain, arthritis-like symptoms, and fever. Distinguishing HEV from HAV must be done genetically. The incubation period is 2 to 9 weeks. The disease is usually mild and resolves in 2 weeks, with no sequelae. The fatality rate is 0.1% to 1%, except in pregnant women where the rate soars to 20%. No outbreaks have been reported in the United States as of 1996. There is currently no vaccine against HEV.

ROTAVIRUS VACCINE

There is a rotavirus vaccine included in the Recommended Childhood Immunization Schedule. This vaccine is used to provide immunity against rotavirus, the most common cause of severe diarrhea in children in the United States. All children have at least one rotavirus infection in the first 5 years of life, and there are about 20 deaths per year in this country. Children between the ages of 3 and 24 months of age have the highest rates of severe disease and hospitalization. The rotavirus vaccine is an oral vaccine, given as a series of three doses. It is recommended that the vaccine be administered at 2, 4, and 6 months of age. The most common side effect seems to be fever.

HUMAN PAPILLOMAVIRUS VACCINE

Human papillomavirus (HPV) is a sexually transmitted virus. It is passed through genital contact (such as vaginal and anal sex). The virus is also able to be transmitted by skin-to-skin contact. At least 50% of people who have had sex will have HPV at some time in their lives. Most contractees do not display any signs, and HPV may resolve on its own without causing any health problems.

Anyone who has ever had genital contact with another person may have HPV. Both men and women may contract and pass the virus often without knowing it. Because there may not be any signs, a person may have HPV even if years have passed since he or she had sex. A person is more likely to contract HPV if he or she has sex at an early age, has multiple sex partners, or has sex with a person who has had many partners.

There are many varieties of HPV. Not all of them cause health problems. Some strains of HPV cause genital warts or cervical cancer. HPV types 16 and 18 cause approximately 70% of cervical cancers. HPV types 6 and 11 cause approximately 90% of genital warts. There is no cure for the virus itself. There are treatments for genital warts, cervical changes, and cervical cancers. In a patient with genital warts, even if treated, the virus may still be present and may be passed onto sex partners. Even if not treated, warts may resolve, stay the same, increase in size, or increase in number. Warts such as these will not become cancerous. All women should get regular Pap tests. The Pap test looks for cell changes caused by HPV. The test finds cell changes early—so the cervix can be treated before the cells become cancerous. The test can also find cancer in its early stages, so it can be treated before it becomes too serious. Only rarely will a patient die from cervical cancer if the disease is caught early. There is a diagnostic test for HPV. This test is approved by the U.S. Food and Drug Administration (FDA) for HPV testing in women 30 years old or older. This test may be able locate HPV even before there are changes to the cervix. One can lower one's chances of getting HPV by abstinence, limiting the number of partners and using condoms.

There is a vaccine for HPV. This vaccine, marketed as Gardasil, prevents infection with HPV by virus subtypes 6, 11, 16, and 18. The vaccine is highly safe, and the only side effect in a patient might be a slight fever. Redness and irritation at the site of injection is also possible. The vaccine contains no live HPV virus, so it is impossible to get the disease from the vaccine. Gardasil is between 95% and 100%

efficacious against HPV types 6, 11, 16, and 18. The vaccine is approved by the FDA for girls and women with the age of 9 to 26 years. It is best to get the vaccine before becoming sexually active. The vaccine is given in a three-shot regimen after the first injection. The second injection is given 2 months later, and followed by a third injection 6 months after the first injection. The vaccine will not treat or cure HPV. It may help people who have one type of HPV from being infected with other types. For example, if the patient has type 6 HPV, it may protect that patient from contracting type 16.

Bacterial Vaccines[41–44]

PERTUSSIS VACCINE

Pertussis, also known as whooping cough, is a highly communicable infection caused by *B. pertussis*. *B. pertussis* produces an endotoxin that causes a spectrum of symptoms in a host. Pertussis occurs mainly in children, and there is no effective treatment once the disease becomes manifest. *Bordetella* endotoxin attacks the tracheal mucosa and causes extreme irritation. The inflammatory responses produce the characteristic "whooping inspiration" associated with pertussis. The swollen and irritated tissues may lead to choking in children. The cough may last for months and is often called the "hundred-day cough." About 4,200 cases of pertussis occur yearly in the United States. Pertussis is most dangerous to babies (younger than 1 year old). Even with the best supportive medical care, complications occur. At least 50% of pertussis patients must be hospitalized, 16% get pneumonia, 2% develop convulsions, and 1 in 200 babies dies or has lifelong complications.

Pertussis vaccine has been highly controversial in recent years. The original vaccine consisted of killed pertussis bacilli (*B. pertussis*) and was considered somewhat "dirty." Side effects such as fever and convulsions were common, and health authorities in the United States, Japan, and the United Kingdom decided that the risk of the vaccine outweighed the risk of contracting the disease. In all three of these countries, pertussis vaccine was removed from the routine immunization schedules. Almost immediately, pertussis, which had been held in check, began to occur in epidemics. In 1992, a new vaccine was developed that consists of bacterial fractions, combined with tetanus and diphtheria toxoids. This vaccine, called Acell-Immune, or diphtheria–tetanus–acellular pertussis (DTaP), is safe and highly effective and has been added to the routine immunization schedule. The vaccine is adsorbed and is used for routine immunization as the polyvalent preparation diphtheria–tetanus–pertussis (DTP) (at 2, 4, 6, and 15 months and at 4–6 years). Pertussis vaccination is recommended for most children. There is also a diphtheria–tetanus whole-cell pertussis (DTwP) vaccine on the market, but it is considered to be higher in side effects than DTaP. Lastly, a DTaP/Hib vaccine preparation is on the market and is recommended for use only as the fourth dose of the series. At present, the only indication is induction of active immunity against diphtheria and tetanus toxins and pertussis from age 6 weeks up to the seventh birthday.

HAEMOPHILUS INFLUENZA TYPE B CONJUGATE VACCINE

Hib causes the most common type of bacterial meningitis and is a major cause of systemic disease in children younger than 6 years old. The chances of contracting the disease are about 1 in 200. Of these contractees, 60% of all patients develop meningitis, while 40% display systemic signs. Hib is a tremendous problem in daycare centers, where the risk of contracting the disease is 400 times greater than in the general population. Hib has approximately a 10% mortality rate, and one third of all survivors have some sort of permanent damage, such as hearing loss, blindness, or impaired vision. Hib can also cause a throat inflammation that results in fatal choking or ear, joint, and skin infections.

Hib-CV is a sterile, lyophilized capsular polysaccharide from Hib vaccine, conjugated to various protein fragments. The antigen type is polysaccharide (phosphoribosyl ribitol phosphate) conjugated to protein. The conjugation produces a stronger, longer-lasting response through the adjuvant effect. Hib-CV is safe and almost completely effective and is a mandatory part of the childhood immunization schedule. The various forms of Hib-CV on the market are not generically equivalent. Indications are the following:

- Induction of artificially acquired active immunity against invasive disease caused by encapsulated Hib
- Routine immunization of all infants beginning at 2 months of age, recommended in the United States
- Immunization of risk groups, including children attending daycare centers, persons of low socioeconomic status, and household contacts of Hib cases

TUBERCULOSIS VACCINE

Tuberculosis (TB) is a serious disease caused by *Mycobacterium tuberculosis*. The organism becomes established in the lungs and forms walled-off abscesses that shield the bacterium from the immune system. The disease is diagnosed by a chest radiograph. Until the 1940s, persons with TB were sent to sanatoria, special hospitals to isolate TB patients. The vaccine is referred to as the bacillus Calmette-Guérin (BCG) vaccine and is a live/attenuated strain of *Mycobacterium bovis*. The antigenic form is the whole bacterium, and the antigen type is protein. The vaccine is of questionable efficacy and has been judged only 50% to 77% effective. The duration of protection is highly questionable. The incidence of TB in the United States is so low that the vaccine is not indicated in most cases. Indications are:

- Induction of artificially acquired active immunity against *M. tuberculosis* var. *hominis* to lower the risk of serious complications from TB
- Recommended for purified protein derivative of tuberculin (PPD) skin test—negative infants and children at high risk of intimate and prolonged exposure to persistently treated or ineffectively treated patients with infectious pulmonary TB
- Persons who are continuously exposed to TB patients who have mycobacteria resistant to isoniazid and rifampin and who cannot be removed from the source of exposure
- Healthcare workers in an environment where a high proportion of *M. tuberculosis* isolates are resistant to both isoniazid (INH) and rifampin, where there is a strong possibility of transmission of infection, and where infection control procedures have failed

An adverse effect of the BCG vaccine includes a positive TB skin test. A red blister forms within 7 to 10 days, then ulcerates and scars within 6 months. BCG is a live vaccine, so it cannot be administered to immunosuppressed patients, burn patients, or pregnant women unless exposed (and even then not in the first trimester).

CHOLERA VACCINE

Cholera is a disease caused by *Vibrio cholerae* that presents as severe, watery diarrhea caused by an enterotoxin secreted by the 01-serotype of *V. cholerae*. The disease occurs in pandemics in India, Bangladesh, Peru, and Latin America. The organisms never invade the enteric epithelium; instead, they remain in the lumen and secrete their enterotoxin. There are about 17 known virulence-associated genes necessary for colonization and toxin secretion. Secretory diarrhea is caused by release of an enterotoxin called *cholera toxin*, which is nearly identical with *E. coli* enterotoxin. It is composed of five binding peptides B and a catalytic peptide A. The peptides B bind to ganglioside GM_1 on the surface of the epithelial cells, setting in motion a series of events that causes diarrhea. The vaccine consists of whole cells of *V. cholerae* 01 that have been inactivated. The antigen form of the vaccine is whole bacterium, and the antigen type is protein toxin and lipopolysaccharide. Indications are the following:

- Induction of active immunity against cholera, such as in individuals traveling to or residing in epidemic or endemic areas
- Individuals residing in areas where cholera is endemic

MENINGOCOCCAL POLYSACCHARIDE VACCINE[45]

Meningococcal vaccine is an inactivated vaccine composed of capsular polysaccharide fragments of *Neisseria meningitidis*. There are four polysaccharide serotypes represented in the vaccine: A, C, Y, and W-135. The type A polysaccharide consists of a polymer of *N*-acetyl-*O*-mannosamine phosphate; the group C polysaccharide is mostly *N*-acetyl-*O*-acetylneuraminic acid. The antigens are conjugated to diphtheria toxoid carrier. Indications are the following:

- Induction of active immunity against selected strains of *N. meningitidis*
- Military recruits during basic training
- College freshmen and those living in dormitories
- Travelers to countries with epidemic meningococcal disease
- Household or institutional contacts of those with meningococcal disease
- Immunosuppressed persons (HIV, *Streptococcus pneumoniae*)
- To stop certain meningococcal group C outbreaks
- Persons aged 2 through 55 years of age at risk for invasive meningococcal disease

PNEUMOCOCCAL VACCINE

Pneumococcus is also known as *S. pneumoniae* or diplococcus. The microorganism protects itself from the immune system by producing a capsular polysaccharide that is highly antigenic. This polysaccharide is used to prepare the vaccine. The antigen form of pneumococcal vaccine is capsular polysaccharide fragments, and the antigen type is a polysaccharide mixture. The antigen is 23-valent. The following are indications:

- Induction of active immunity against pneumococcal disease caused by the pneumococcal antigen types included in the vaccine (the vaccine protects against pneumococcal pneumonia, pneumococcal bacteremia, and other pneumococcal infections)
- All adults at least 65 years old
- All immunocompetent individuals who are at increased risk of the disease because of pathological conditions
- Children at least 2 years old with chronic illness associated with increased risk of pneumococcal disease or its complications

Toxoids

Toxoids are detoxified toxins used to initiate active immunity (i.e., create an antitoxin). They are typically produced by formaldehyde treatment of the toxin. They are safe and unquestionably efficacious.

DISEASE STATES

All of these diseases are produced not by a bacterium but by an exotoxin produced by that organism. For example, powerful exotoxins are produced by *Corynebacterium diphtheriae* and *C. tetani*. The exotoxins are the most serious part of the disease. In both of the previously described disease states, survival does not confer immunity to subsequent infections, so lifelong vaccine boosters are needed.

In diphtheria, the exotoxin causes production of a pseudomembrane in the throat; the membrane then adheres to the tonsils. The organism releases a potent exotoxin that causes headache, weakness, fever, and adenitis. Severe diphtheria carries a 10% fatality rate. Only a few cases per year are reported in the United States.

Tetanus is caused by a skin wound with anaerobic conditions at the wound site. A potent exotoxin (tetanospasmin) is produced that attacks the nervous system. The first sign of disease is jaw stiffness; eventually, the jaw becomes fixed (lockjaw). The disease is essentially a persistent tonic spasm of the voluntary muscles. Fatality from tetanus is usually through asphyxia. Even with supportive treatment, tetanus is about 30% fatal in the United States. Recovery requires prolonged hospitalization. There have been 50 to 90 reported cases per year in the United States since 1975. There is no natural immunity to the exotoxin. The general rule of thumb is to follow the childhood immunization schedule carefully and immunize all persons of questionable immunization status. Adults require a booster every 10 years; patients who cannot remember their last one are due for another.

CLINICALLY USED TOXOIDS

Adsorbed Tetanus Toxoid
Tetanus is a disease that is also known as lockjaw. The causative organism is the anaerobic spore-forming bacterium *C. tetani*. The organism in the toxoid, adsorbed tetanus toxoid (T, adsorbed), is designated inactivated. The antigen form is toxoid, and the antigen type is protein. This toxoid lasts approximately 10 years. A booster is recommended if injured or every 5 years. Reactions other than pain at the site of injection are rare. Fluid tetanus toxoid is recommended only for the rare individual who is hypersensitive to the aluminum adjuvant.

Adsorbed Diphtheria and Tetanus Toxoid
This is recommended for children younger than 7 years old who should not get pertussis vaccine (designated DT).

Recommended Immunization Schedule for Persons Aged 0 Through 6 Years—United States • 2009
For those who fall behind or start late, see the catch-up schedule

Vaccine ▼ Age ►	Birth	1 month	2 months	4 months	6 months	12 months	15 months	18 months	19–23 months	2–3 years	4–6 years
Hepatitis B[1]	HepB	HepB		see footnote1		HepB					
Rotavirus[2]			RV	RV	RV[2]						
Diphtheria, Tetanus, Pertussis[3]			DTaP	DTaP	DTaP	see footnote3	DTaP				DTaP
Haemophilus influenzae type b[4]			Hib	Hib	Hib[4]	Hib					
Pneumococcal[5]			PCV	PCV	PCV	PCV				PPSV	
Inactivated Poliovirus			IPV	IPV		IPV					IPV
Influenza[6]						Influenza (Yearly)					
Measles, Mumps, Rubella[7]						MMR		see footnote7			MMR
Varicella[8]						Varicella		see footnote8			Varicella
Hepatitis A[9]						HepA (2 doses)				HepA Series	
Meningococcal[10]										MCV	

Range of recommended ages

Certain high-risk groups

Figure 5.11 ● Recommended immunization schedule for persons aged 0 to 6 years—United States, 2009. (Available at: http://www.cdc.gov/vaccines/recs/schedules/child-schedule.htm#printable. Accessed January 23, 2009.)

Adsorbed Tetanus and Diphtheria Toxoid for Adults

Adsorbed tetanus and diphtheria toxoid for adults (designated Td) is for children older than 7 years and for adults. It has a lower level of diphtheria toxoid (1/15) because older children are much more sensitive to "D." It is used for immunization of schoolchildren.

DTP

DTP is D and T toxoids with pertussis vaccine.

DTP Adsorbed

DTP adsorbed is used for early vaccination of infants in repeated doses, starting at 2 to 3 months.

The Routine Childhood Immunization Schedule

Figures 5.11, 5.12, and 5.13 show the Routine Childhood Immunization Schedule formulated by the Advisory Committee on Immunization Practices (2009). This schedule should be followed for all children and young adults regardless of economic circumstances. The three charts show the schedule for children aged birth to 6 years (Fig. 5.11), 7 to 18 years (Fig. 5.12), and the catch-up schedule when doses of vaccine are missed (Fig. 5.13).

⬡ NEW VACCINE TECHNOLOGIES: ADJUVANT TECHNOLOGY

In spite of the long history of vaccines, only a few adjuvants and vaccine delivery systems have been licensed for human use. There are several reasons for this. Vaccines based on live-attenuated organisms are invasive and are efficiently delivered to APCs. Pattern-recognized components of the cellular pathogens are recognized by the innate immune system and trigger an innate response. With the trend of using subunit vaccines and isolated antigens, immune potentiators and delivery systems have become major issues in vaccine technology.

Recommended Immunization Schedule for Persons Aged 7 Through 18 Years—United States • 2009
For those who fall behind or start late, see the schedule below and the catch-up schedule

Vaccine ▼ Age ►	7–10 years	11–12 years	13–18 years
Tetanus, Diphtheria, Pertussis[1]	see footnote 1	Tdap	Tdap
Human Papillomavirus[2]	see footnote 2	HPV (3 doses)	HPV Series
Meningococcal[3]	MCV	MCV	MCV
Influenza[4]	Influenza (Yearly)		
Pneumococcal[5]	PPSV		
Hepatitis A[6]	HepA Series		
Hepatitis B[7]	HepB Series		
Inactivated Poliovirus[8]	IPV Series		
Measles, Mumps, Rubella[9]	MMR Series		
Varicella[10]	Varicella Series		

Range of recommended ages

Catch-up immunization

Certain high-risk groups

Figure 5.12 ● Recommended immunization schedule for persons aged 7 through 18 years—United States, 2009. (Available at: http://www.cdc.gov/vaccines/recs/schedules/child-schedule.htm#printable. Accessed January 23, 2009.)

Catch-up Immunization Schedule for Persons Aged 4 Months Through 18 Years
Who Start Late or Who Are More Than 1 Month Behind—United States • 2009

The table below provides catch-up schedules and minimum intervals between doses for children whose vaccinations have been delayed. A vaccine series does not need to be restarted, regardless of the time that has elapsed between doses. Use the section appropriate for the child's age.

Vaccine	Minimum Age for Dose 1	Minimum Interval Between Doses			
		Dose 1 to Dose 2	Dose 2 to Dose 3	Dose 3 to Dose 4	Dose 4 to Dose 5
CATCH-UP SCHEDULE FOR PERSONS AGED 4 MONTHS THROUGH 6 YEARS					
Hepatitis B[1]	Birth	4 weeks	8 weeks (and at least 16 weeks after first dose)		
Rotavirus[2]	6 wks	4 weeks	4 weeks[2]		
Diphtheria, Tetanus, Pertussis[3]	6 wks	4 weeks	4 weeks	6 months	6 months[3]
Haemophilus influenzae type b[4]	6 wks	4 weeks if first dose administered at younger than age 12 months / 8 weeks (as final dose) if first dose administered at age 12-14 months / No further doses needed if first dose administered at age 15 months or older	4 weeks[4] if current age is younger than 12 months / 8 weeks (as final dose)[4] if current age is 12 months or older and second dose administered at younger than age 15 months / No further doses needed if previous dose administered at age 15 months or older	8 weeks (as final dose) This dose only necessary for children aged 12 months through 59 months who received 3 doses before age 12 months	
Pneumococcal[5]	6 wks	4 weeks if first dose administered at younger than age 12 months / 8 weeks (as final dose for healthy children) if first dose administered at age 12 months or older or current age 24 through 59 months / No further doses needed for healthy children if first dose administered at age 24 months or older	4 weeks if current age is younger than 12 months / 8 weeks (as final dose for healthy children) if current age is 12 months or older / No further doses needed for healthy children if previous dose administered at age 24 months or older	8 weeks (as final dose) This dose only necessary for children aged 12 months through 59 months who received 3 doses before age 12 months or for high-risk children who received 3 doses at any age	
Inactivated Poliovirus[6]	6 wks	4 weeks	4 weeks	4 weeks[6]	
Measles, Mumps, Rubella[7]	12 mos	4 weeks			
Varicella[8]	12 mos	3 months			
Hepatitis A[9]	12 mos	6 months			
CATCH-UP SCHEDULE FOR PERSONS AGED 7 THROUGH 18 YEARS					
Tetanus, Diphtheria/ Tetanus, Diphtheria, Pertussis[10]	7 yrs[10]	4 weeks	4 weeks if first dose administered at younger than age 12 months / 6 months if first dose administered at age 12 months or older	6 months if first dose administered at younger than age 12 months	
Human Papillomavirus[11]	9 yrs	Routine dosing intervals are recommended[11]			
Hepatitis A[9]	12 mos	6 months			
Hepatitis B[1]	Birth	4 weeks	8 weeks (and at least 16 weeks after first dose)		
Inactivated Poliovirus[6]	6 wks	4 weeks	4 weeks	4 weeks[6]	
Measles, Mumps, Rubella[7]	12 mos	4 weeks			
Varicella[8]	12 mos	3 months if the person is younger than age 13 years / 4 weeks if the person is aged 13 years or older			

Figure 5.13 ● Catch-up immunization schedule for persons aged 4 months through 18 years who start late or who are more than 1 month behind. (Available at: http://www.cdc.gov/vaccines/recs/schedules/child-schedule.htm#printable. Accessed January 23, 2009.)

There are a series of significant hurdles to the development of modern vaccines. Poor optimized vaccines must be improved. New vaccines for immunizing against diseases for which no vaccines exist are imperative. It is necessary to be able to respond quickly with vaccines to newly developing pathogenic organisms. The primary elements of useful vaccines are the antigen (against which the adaptive immune response is elicited), immunostimulants that activate the innate immune system, and delivery systems that target the vaccines to the appropriate site in a timely fashion.

Antigens
• Whole inactivated or attenuated organisms or a mixture of various strains
• Isolated and purified proteins, glycoproteins, and carbohydrates
• Recombinant proteins and glycoproteins

Immune Potentiators
• Bacterial products
• Toxins and lipids
• Nucleic acids
• Peptidoglycans
• Carbohydrates, peptides
• Cytokines and hormones
• Small molecules

Delivery Systems
• Mineral salts
• Surfactants
• Synthetic microparticles
• Oil-in-water emulsions
• Liposome

In designing a vaccine, first, an antigen is required. The antigen is the species against which an anamnestic immune response is targeted. In many cases, antigen selection is confounded by a multiplicity providing many potential antigens to choose from. Bacterial pathogens, often display this multiplicity. The manner in which the antigen is presented is also important. It may be necessary to maintain a specific three-dimensional tertiary structure for the antigen to be recognized.

It hasn't always been appreciated at the innate immune system, must be stimulated to modulate the adaptive immune response. Adjuvants, which stimulate early innate immune responses, aid in stimulating a strong and extended adaptive immune response. The nature of the vaccine delivery systems that target the vaccines to the appropriate immune cells is important to gain the necessary stimulation of the immune system.

The functional immune system is composed of two primary components. The innate immune system has evolved to respond within minutes, primarily to molecular patterns found in microbial pathogens. The adaptive immune response develops slowly, over days or weeks and generates highly specific responses based on antibodies targeted against a pathogen's antigens. The innate response is the first line of defense. Adaptive immunity uses selection and clonal expansion of immune cells containing specific, somatically rearranged receptor genes (T- and B-cell receptors) that recognize antigen from the pathogen. This response is specific and long-lasting (immunological memory). The innate immune responses lead to a fast burst of inflammatory cytokines and activation of APCs such as macrophages and dendritic cells (DCs). These responses are not clonal and lead to a conditioning of the immune system for later development of specific adaptive immune responses.

The innate immune response must be able to distinguish pathogenic microbes from self-components. To do this, the innate immune system depends on some fairly constant receptors that detect specific signatures from pathogens. These signatures have been highly conserved throughout evolution. The signatures are referred to as pathogen-associated molecular patterns (PAMPs). It has been shown that when one includes PAMP substances in experimental vaccines, a strong and long-lasting adaptive immune response develops. PAMPs are recognized by specific pattern recognition receptors. A number of such receptors have been identified. They are expressed on neutrophils, macrophages, DCs, and natural killer cells, as well as B cells in nonimmunological cells such as epithelial and endothelial cells. When PAMPs bind to pattern recognition receptors cells bearing the pattern recognition receptors are activated and begin to secrete chemokines and cytokines, and induce maturation and chemotaxis of other immune cells. Taken together, and inflammatory environment is created. This inflammation supports development of the adaptive immune responses.

What are pattern recognition receptors? Basically, they are receptors that do not induce phagocytosis such as Toll-like receptors (TLRs) and nucleotide oligomerization domain (NOD) proteins. They can also be receptors that induce phagocytosis such as mannose receptors, scavenger receptors, and β-glucan receptors. These receptors directly recognized ligands on the surface of pathogenic microbes and cause them to be engulfed by phagocytosis capable cells such as macrophages. The nonphagocytic receptors that recognized PAMPs can be extracellular (TLRs) or intracellular (NOD proteins). Activation of these receptors leads to a signal transduction cascade that activates transcription factors that result in expression of inflammatory cytokines and other cellular activation processes. These processes have been reviewed previously. It is now known that signaling of the innate immune system involves a highly complex effect of transmembrane and intracellular proteins. It is these that provide an extensive set of possible targets for vaccine adjuvants.

How does innate immunity lead to the conditioning of the adaptive immune response? Pattern recognition receptors signaling causes the activation of transcription factors such as NF-κB and IRF3 (interferon regulatory factor 3). Activation of these pattern recognition receptors produces the necessary inflammatory environment that supports fast development of host defenses. NF-κB controls the expression of proinflammatory cytokines such as IL-1β and TNF-α, while IRF3 causes production of antiviral type 1 interferon (IFN-α and IFN-β). It has been shown that portions of the innate immune response are absolutely essential for development of antigen-specific immunity. Therefore, elements of the innate immune response are potential targets for vaccine antigens.

A suitable adjuvant can enhance the effectiveness of a vaccine by accelerating the generation of a formidable immune response. Additionally, the adjuvant can cause veined responses for longer duration and can induce local mucosal immune responses all of which generate antibodies with increased avidity and neutralization capacity. An adjuvant also can elicit cytotoxic T lymphocytes, enhancing immune responses in people with weakened immune systems, such as children, elderly, or immunocompromised adults. Adjuvants can be important in commercial production of vaccines by reducing the amount of antigen that is required to generate a robust immune response, thus reducing the cost of the vaccine. A good functional definition of an adjuvant is a component added to a vaccine and enhances the immunogenicity of the antigens in vivo. It is very common to categorize adjuvants in terms of two types of systems. Immune potentiators tend to activate innate immunity directly. A good immune potentiator might facilitate the development of cytokines or react through pattern recognition receptors (which can be bacterial cell wall components). A delivery system such as an emulsion or microparticle can target vaccine antigens selectively to APCs and may put the antigens and immune potentiators in the same location where they can do the most good. It has been shown that the choice of a good immune potentiators and delivery system can enhance antigen-specific immune responses in vivo. This can be very important in the development of subunit vaccines, which typically generate a low-level immunity. A mixture of the immune potentiators, the delivery system, and the antigen, can optimize the immune response.

Current adjuvants that are licensed for use in humans are the mineral salts such as aluminum and calcium. Several bacterial and viral antigens have been adsorbed onto aluminum and calcium salts. Other types of adjuvants include emulsion and surfactant adjuvants, particulate delivery vehicles, microbial derivatives such as lipid A, and DCs and cytokines. These latter agents have not been licensed for use in humans at the present time, but many of these are being used in clinical trials at the present time. Indeed, vaccine development has historically focused on enhancing Ab responses and not the innate immune system. So most of the commonly used antigens elevate serum Ab titers, but do little to elicit the innate immune response. The requirement for vaccines against chronic illnesses such as HIV, HCV, TB, and herpes simplex virus as well as cancer, has caused researchers to focus their efforts on generation of cellular immune responses. Adjuvants that elicit this effect are being developed and clinically tested at the present time. A new recognition of the immunobiology of TLRs and pattern recognition receptors in general, immunoregulatory cells, and cells of innate and active immunity and their roles in responding and clearing specific diseases provides the background for their development.

Most of the research in vaccine development to the present time has been aimed at finding new antigens that can be used for protection against disease and ways that they can be presented to the immune system. Because of this, only a few delivery systems such as aluminum salts and oil and water emulsions have been investigated. At the present time, no immune potentiators have been approved for human use in prophylactic vaccines. There are several reasons for this situation, but the main one seems to be concern over the toxicity of these agents. Research over the last few years has centered on developing strategies for immune potentiator discovery. Indeed, the methods of high throughput screening that are used in the development of new drugs are being applied to immune potentiators and in the development of vaccine adjuvants.

While it is true that most natural PAMPs are based on polysaccharides, nucleic acids, or lipids, it has been shown that peptides can activate various pattern recognition receptors. Therefore, immune modulators can be based on simple peptides. This recognition opens the possibility of screening peptide libraries produced by combinatorial peptide synthesis for generation of new peptide ligands of pattern recognition receptors. Of course, using peptides is not without difficulty. Peptides display for pharmacokinetic profiles, low bioavailability, and degradation in vivo. As with other biological peptides that are being tested as drugs, widespread use might be restricted.

Another possibility for development of an adjuvant centers on using DCs, which are known to provide potency lymphocyte responses. DCs are being investigated in vaccines against various cancers. The difficulty and cost involved in preparing cell-based vaccine adjuvants probably will restrict their use in prophylactic vaccines. They will, however, likely be used in therapeutic vaccinations. Several TLR ligands such as lipopolysaccharide, have been tested for their ability to activate DCs to produce stimulatory molecules and chemotaxis. DCs have been shown to increase T-cell responses and can block inhibitory effects of regulatory cells. DCs also produce migration and recruitment of natural killer cells to the lymph nodes to provide stimulation of interferon γ necessary for T-helper cell polarization.

There are many barriers to be overcome in the development of adjuvants for vaccination. Because of the need for qualitatively specific immune responses, no single adjuvant will be broadly useful. Indeed, it will be necessary to use antigens on a tailor-made basis for different conditions. Dosing of the adjuvants according to one of the currently available routes of administration may not work for small molecules, and it may be required that specialized formulations be developed for delivery of the adjuvant into the cells and for retention at the site of injection. The highly potent activation of the innate immune response may cause toxic side effects, and hence may require methods to prevent diffusion from the injection site. Because some of the targets for the innate immune system are intracellular potentiators may be required to be membrane permeable and metabolically stable. Lastly, regulatory guidelines for licensing of new adjuvants are still being developed. It is not known what the scope of three clinical testing and toxicity testing will be required for adjuvant approval.

Although there is a growing acceptance by regulatory agencies and commercial vaccine producers that improved vaccine adjuvants are needed to meet the infectious disease challenges in future, new technologies carry the uncertainty of unknown risks and present the safety and regulatory hurdles that will be encountered with the additional novel immune potentiators and delivery systems the final vaccine formulations may be significant and are still largely ill-defined. The key focus should be on separating the potential increases in immune toxicity from improved immunogenicity provided by vaccine adjuvants.

⬡ NEW VACCINE TECHNOLOGIES: NUCLEIC ACID VACCINES

Naked nucleic acids (divested of any component of protein, carbohydrate, or lipid) are immunostimulatory and in principle can be used as vaccines. Short molecules of DNA and RNA are relatively simple to synthesize and can be tailored to immunize against bacterial and viral infections and cancers. Following administration (from a "gene gun" or by injection into the skin or muscle in solution or suspension like conventional vaccines) the genetic vaccines are taken up and translated into protein by the host cells. The protein, generated in situ, acts as an antigen and triggers the immune system. Because the naked nucleic acids lack coat protein such as would be present in viruses, they are not susceptible to neutralizing Ab reactions that could decrease their efficacy.

Entry into host cells presents a problem. On one hand, DNA can be spontaneously taken up by the cells, then transcribed and translated to produce protein. The uptake process may be inefficient. Cationic lipids have been tested to facilitate movement of DNA (as a complex) across the cell and nuclear membranes. These have been found to work fairly well in some cases. Other avenues of administration focus on mucosal surfaces of the lungs, digestive tract, and reproductive systems. Because mucosal surfaces are important barriers to infection and transmission of infectious diseases, they offer important possibilities for genetic vaccine administration.

A typical description of how a genetic vaccine works involves the specialized, bone marrow–derived DCs. DCs are the immune system's most powerful APCs. Antigen can be acquired by DCs in three principal ways. They can be directly transfected by nucleic acid vaccines. DCs are also known to acquire soluble antigen from the interstitial spaces that has been secreted or released by transfected cells. DCs can also engulf entire cells that have been injured or killed as a result of the vaccine or its function. Once the antigen has been taken up by the DCs, it is presented on their cell surfaces. DCs then express and elaborate surface adhesion molecules and chemokine receptors that cause them to migrate to the lymphatic organs. It is in these organs that the DCs are most effective at activating immune responses. It has been proposed that cell death induced by transfection of host cells by vaccines is the signal for activation of DCs by providing "danger signals" to those cells. The effect of these danger signals more strongly modulates the immune response.

New research has suggested that α-virus replicon-based naked DNA provides a stronger, more significant activation of the immune system than does naked DNA or RNA itself.

Despite a host of attractive possibilities presented by nucleic acid vaccines, no naked nucleic acid vectors have been approved for use in humans. Human data is lacking, and nucleic acid vaccines have not been unequivocally demonstrated to have significant efficacy in prevention or treatment (as therapeutic vaccines) of infectious diseases or cancers. Immunization with naked nucleic acids is relatively inefficient, and virus vectors generally induce a much greater immune response than do nucleic acid vaccines. The viral coat protein dramatically increases the virus's replication efficiency. Naked nucleic acids do not possess this feature. Despite being unproven in humans at the present time, genetic vaccines represent a fertile area for vaccine research. Presumably, as research proceeds the problems with using nucleic acid vaccines will be surmounted.

◆ R E V I E W   Q U E S T I O N S ◆

1. What is the chemical nature of an antigen?

2. What is an "antigenic determinant"?

3. What is the difference between T cells and B cells?

4. What are the functions of the major histocompatibility complexes (MHC-I and MHC-II) in programming the immune system?

5. What is the anamnestic response? How does the anamnestic response evolve with repeated challenges of vaccine or antigen?

6. Describe the various types of vaccines.

7. Describe the various ways that vaccines can be prepared.

8. Why is smallpox vaccine no longer recommended for general use?

9. How do nucleic acid vaccines work?

10. What is an adjuvant? How do adjuvants modify the immune response to an antigen?

REFERENCES

1. Grabenstein, J. D.: Immunofacts. St. Louis, MO, Facts and Comparisons, 2002, pp. 3–8.
2. Shen, W. G., and Louie, S. G.: Immunology for Pharmacy Students. Newark, NJ, Harwood Academic Publishers, 2000, p. 2.
3. Shen, W. G., and Louie, S. G.: Immunology for Pharmacy Students. Newark, NJ, Harwood Academic Publishers, 2000, pp. 10–11.
4. Hall, P. D., and Tami, J. A.: Function and evaluation of the immune system. In Di Piro, J. T., et al. (eds.). Pharmacotherapy, a Pathophysiologic Approach, 3rd ed. Norwalk, CT, Appleton & Lange, 1997, pp. 1647–1660 (and references therein).
5. Cremers, N.: Antigens, antibodies, and complement: Their nature and interaction. In Burrows, W. (ed.). Textbook of Microbiology, 20th ed. Philadelphia, W. B. Saunders, 1973, pp. 303–347.
6. Leder, P.: Sci. Am. 247:72–83, 1982.
7. Gilbert, P.: Fundamentals of immunology. In Hugo, W. B., and Russell, A. D. (eds.). Pharmaceutical Microbiology, 4th ed. London, Blackwell, 1987.
8. Bussert, P. D.: Sci. Am. 246:82–95, 1981.
9. Hood, L.: The immune system. In Alberts, B., et al. (eds.). The Molecular Biology of the Cell. New York, Garland, 1983, pp. 95–1012.
10. Sprent, J.: Cell 76:315–322, 1994.
11. Plotkin, S. L., and Plotkin, S. A.: A short history of vaccination. In Plotkin, S. A., and Mortimer, E. A., Jr. (eds.). Vaccines. Philadelphia, W. B. Saunders, 1988.
12. Hopkins, D. R.: Princes and Peasants: Smallpox in History. Chicago, University of Chicago Press, 1983, p. 1.
13. CDC: MMWR 43:1–3, 1994.
14. CDC: MMWR 44:937–943, 1996.
15. CDC: MMWR 41:103–107, 1992.
16. Barker, W. H., and Mullolly, J. P.: JAMA 244:2547–2549, 1980.
17. CDC: MMWR 40:700–708; 709–711, 1991.
18. CDC: Immunization Information. Polio, March 9, 1995.
19. CDC: MMWR 40:1–94, 1991.
20. CDC: MMWR 43:3–12, 1994.
21. Hadler, S. C.: Ann. Intern. Med. 108:457–458, 1988.
22. Revelle, A.: FDA Electronic Bull. Board, March 17, 1995, p. 95.
23. CDC: MMWR 45:304–307, 1996.
24. CDC: MMWR 31:617–625, 1982.
25. CDC: MMWR 39:11–15, 1991.
26. Varivax varicella virus vaccine live (OKA/Merck) prescribing information. Darmstadt, Germany, Merck & Co., 1995.
27. Varivax (recombinant OKA varicella zoster) vaccine ready for prescribing. Merck & Co. Recommendations and Procedures. Merck & Co. House Organ, 1996.
28. White, C. J.: Pediatr. Infect. Dis. 11:19–23, 1992.
29. Lieu, T. A., et al.: JAMA 271:375–381, 1980.
30. Halloran, M. E.: Am. J. Epidemiol. 140:81–104, 1994.
31. Grabenstein, J. D.: Immunofacts. St. Louis, MO, Facts and Comparisons, 2002, pp. 152–169.
32. Innis, B. L.: JAMA 271:1328–1334, 1994.
33. Revelle, M.: FDA Electronic Bull. Board, Feb. 22, 1995. FDA Reports, Feb. 27, 1995, pp. 5–6.
34. Alter, M. J., et al.: JAMA 263:1218–1222, 1990.
35. Interferon treatment for hepatitis B and C. American Liver Foundation. http://www.gastro.com.
36. Hepatitis C virus. Bug Bytes Newsletter 1, Dec. 27, 1994.
37. Mast, E. E., and Alter, M. J.: Semin. Virol. 4:273–283, 1993.
38. Hodder, S. L., and Mortimer, E. A.: Epidemiol. Rev. 14:243–267, 1992.
39. Rappuoli, R., et al.: Vaccine 10:1027–1032, 1992.
40. Englund, J., et al.: Pediatrics 93:37–43, 1994.
41. CDC: MMWR CDC Surveill. Summ. 41:1–9, 1992.
42. Fine, P., and Chen, R.: Am. J. Epidemiol. 136:121–135, 1992.
43. American Academy of Pediatrics Committee on Infectious Diseases: Pediatrics 92:480–488, 1993.
44. Rietschel, E. T., and Brade, H.: Sci. Am. 257:54–61, 1992.
45. Grabenstein, J.: Immunofacts. St. Louis, MO, Facts and Comparisons, 2009, pp. 147–159.

CHAPTER 6

Anti-infective Agents

JOHN M. BEALE, JR.

CHAPTER OVERVIEW

The history of work on the prevention of bacterial infection can be traced back to the 19th century when Joseph Lister (in 1867) introduced antiseptic principles for use in surgery and posttraumatic injury.[1] He used phenol (carbolic acid) as a wash for the hands, as a spray on an incision site, and on bandages applied to wounds. Lister's principles caused a dramatic decrease in the incidence of postsurgical infections.

Around 1881 and continuing to 1900, microbiologist Paul Ehrlich, a disciple of Robert Koch, began work with a set of antibacterial dyes and antiparasitic organic arsenicals. His goal was to develop compounds that retained antimicrobial activity at the expense of toxicity to the human host; he called the agents that he sought "magic bullets." At the time that Ehrlich began his experiments, there were only a few compounds that could be used in treating infectious diseases, and none was very useful in the treatment of severe Gram-positive and Gram-negative infections. Ehrlich discovered that the dyes and arsenicals could stain target cells *selectively* and that the antimicrobial properties of the dyes paralleled the staining activity. This discovery was the first demonstration of *selective toxicity*, the property of certain chemicals to kill one type of organism while not harming another. Selective toxicity is the main tenet of modern antimicrobial chemotherapy, and Ehrlich's seminal discovery paved the way for the development of the sulfonamides and penicillins and the elucidation of the mechanisms of *their* selective toxicity. Prior to Ehrlich's studies, the *local* antimicrobial properties of phenol and iodine were well known, but the only useful *systemic* agents were the herbal remedies cinchona for malaria and ipecac for amebic dysentery. Ehrlich's discovery of compound 606, the effective antisyphilitic drug Salvarsan,[2,3] was a breakthrough in the treatment of a serious, previously untreatable disease.

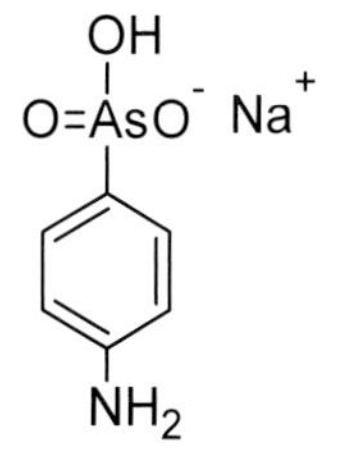

Atoxyl

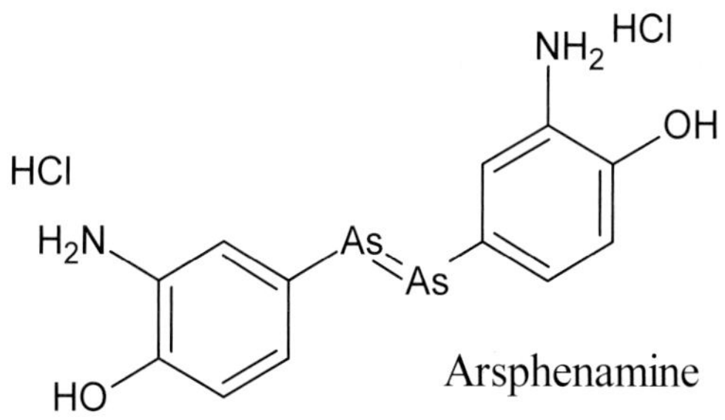

Arsphenamine

Until the 1920s, most successful anti-infective agents were based on the group-IIB element mercury and the group-VA elements arsenic and antimony. Atoxyl (sodium arsanilate and arsphenamine) was used for sleeping sickness.[4] Certain dyes, such as gentian violet and methylene blue, were also found to be somewhat effective, as were a few chemical congeners of the quinine molecule. Some of these agents represented significant achievements in anti-infective therapy, but they also possessed some important limitations. Heavy metal toxicity after treatment with mercury, arsenic, and antimony severely limited the usefulness of agents containing these elements.

Just prior to 1950, great strides were made in anti-infective therapy. The sulfonamides and sulfones (this chapter), more effective phenolic compounds such as hexachlorophene,

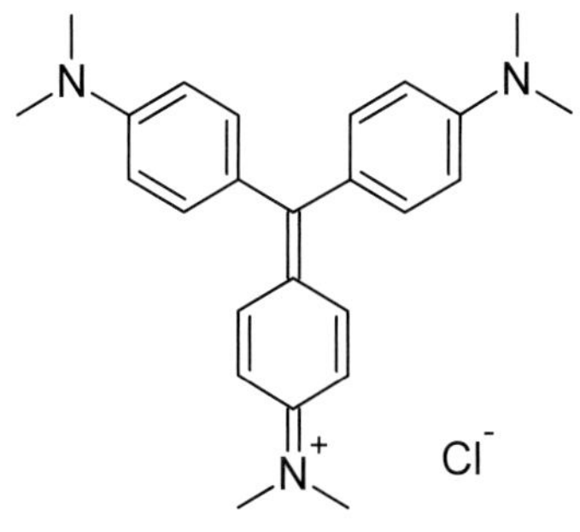

Gentian Violet

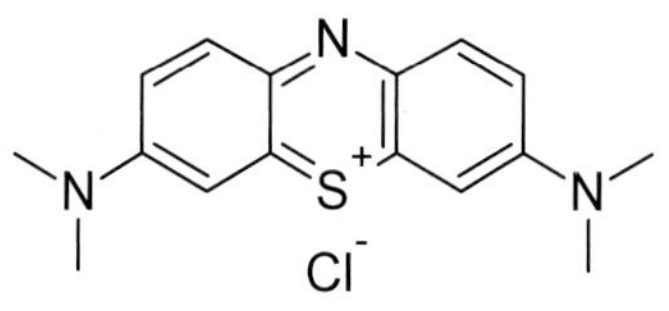

Methylene Blue

179

synthetic antimalarial compounds (Chapter 7), and several antibiotics (Chapter 8) were introduced to the therapeutic armamentarium.

Anti-infective agents may be classified according to various schemes. The chemical type of the compound, the biological property, and the therapeutic indication may be used singly or in combination to describe the agents. In this textbook, a combination of these classification schemes is used to organize the anti-infective agents. When several chemically divergent compounds are indicated for a specific disease or group of diseases, the therapeutic classification is used, and the drugs are subclassified according to chemical type. When the information is best unified and presented in a chemical or biological classification system, as for the sulfonamides or antibacterial antibiotics, then one of these classification systems is used.

This chapter addresses an extremely broad base of anti-infective agents, including the local compounds (alcohols, phenols, oxidizing agents, halogen-containing compounds, cationic surfactants, dyes, and mercurials), preservatives, antifungal agents, synthetic antibacterial drugs, antitubercular and antiprotozoal agents, and anthelmintics. Other chapters in this text are devoted to antibacterial antibiotics (Chapter 8), antiviral agents (Chapter 9), and antineoplastic antibiotics (Chapter 10).

Anti-infective agents that are used locally are called *germicides*, and within this classification, there are two primary subtypes (see Table 6.1) and several other definitions of sanitization. Antiseptics are compounds that kill (*-cidal*) or prevent the growth of (*-static*) microorganisms when applied to *living tissue*. This caveat of use on living tissue points to the properties that the useful antiseptic must have. The ideal antiseptic must have low-enough toxicity that it can be used directly on skin or wounds; it will exert a rapid and sustained lethal action against microorganisms (the spectrum may be narrow or broad depending on the use). The agent should have a low surface tension so that it will spread into the wound; it should retain activity in the presence of body fluids (including pus), be nonirritating to tissues, be nonallergenic, lack systemic toxicity when applied to skin or mucous membranes, and not interfere with healing. No antiseptic available today meets all of these criteria. A few antibiotics, such as bacitracin, polymyxin, silver sulfadiazine, and neomycin, are poorly absorbed through the skin and mucous membranes and are used topically for the treatment of local infections; they have been found very effective against infections such as these. In general, however, the topical use of antibiotics has been restricted by concern about the development of resistant microbial strains and possible allergic reactions. These problems can reduce the usefulness of these antibiotics for more serious infections.

A *disinfectant* is an agent that prevents transmission of infection by the destruction of pathogenic microorganisms when applied to *inanimate objects*. The ideal disinfectant exerts a rapidly lethal action against all potentially pathogenic microorganisms and spores, has good penetrating properties into organic matter, shares compatibility with organic compounds (particularly soaps), is not inactivated by living tissue, is noncorrosive, and is aesthetically pleasing (nonstaining and odorless). Locally acting anti-infective drugs are widely used by the lay public and are prescribed by members of the medical profession (even though the effectiveness of many of the agents has not been established completely). The germicide may be harmful in certain cases (i.e., it may retard healing). Standardized methods for evaluating and comparing the efficacy of germicides have only recently been developed.

Numerous classes of chemically divergent compounds possess local anti-infective properties. Some of these are outlined in Table 6.2.

The most important means of preventing transmission of infectious agents from person to person or from regions of high microbial load, such as the mouth, nose, or gut, to potential sites of infection is simply *washing the hands*. In fact, one of the breakthroughs in surgical technique in the 1800s was the finding that the incidence of postsurgical infection decreased dramatically if surgeons washed their hands before operating. Regular hand washing is properly done without disinfection to minimize drying, irritation, and sensitization of the skin. Simple soap and warm water remove bacteria efficiently. Skin disinfectants along with soap and water are usually used as preoperative surgical scrubs and sterilants for surgical incisions.

TABLE 6.1 Definitions and Standards for Removing Microorganisms

Antisepsis	Application of an agent to living tissue for the purpose of preventing infection
Decontamination	Destruction or marked reduction in the number or activity of microorganisms
Disinfection	Chemical or physical treatment that destroys most vegetative microbes or viruses, but not spores, in or on inanimate surfaces
Sanitization	Reduction of microbial load on an inanimate surface to a level considered acceptable for public health purposes
Sterilization	A process intended to kill or remove all types of microorganisms, including spores, and usually including viruses with an acceptably low probability of survival
Pasteurization	A process that kills nonsporulating microorganisms by hot water or steam at 65°C–100°C

⬡ EVALUATION OF THE EFFECTIVENESS OF A STERILANT

Evaluation of the effectiveness of antiseptics, disinfectants, and other sterilants (Table 6.1), although seemingly simple in principle, is an extremely complex task. One must consider the intrinsic resistance of the microbe, the microbial load, the mixture of the population of microorganisms present, the amount and nature of organic material present (e.g., blood, feces, tissue), the concentration and stability of the disinfectant or sterilant, the time and temperature of exposure, the pH, and the hydration and binding of the agent to surfaces. In summary, a host of parameters must be considered for each sterilant, and experimental assays may be difficult. Specific, standardized assays of activity are defined for each use. Toxicity for human subjects must also be evaluated. The Environmental Protection Agency (EPA)

TABLE 6.2 Common Sterilants and Their Range of Use

	Bacteria			Viruses			Other		
	Gram-positive	Gram-negative	Acid-fast	Spores	Lipophilic	Hydrophilic	Fungi	Amebic Cysts	Prions
Alcohols (isopropanol, ethanol)	+++	+++	+	−	+	+/−	N/A	N/A	−
Aldehydes (glutaraldehyde, formaldehyde)	+++	+++	++	+	+	++	+	N/A	−
Chlorhexidine gluconate	+++	++	−	−	+/−	−	N/A	N/A	−
Sodium hypochlorite, chlorine dioxide	+++	+++	++	+ (pH 7.6)	+	+ (high conc.)	++	+	++ (high conc.)
Hexachlorophene	+	−	−	−	−	−	−	−	−
Povidone-Iodine	+++	+++	+	+ (high conc.)	+	−	+	+	−
Phenols, quaternary ammonium	+++	+++	+/−	−	+	−	N/A	N/A	−
Strong oxidizing agents, cresols	+++	++/−	−		+	−	−	−	−

regulates disinfectants and sterilants and the Food and Drug Administration (FDA) regulates antiseptics.

There are some problems with improper use of these agents. Antiseptics and disinfectants may become contaminated by resistant microorganisms (e.g., spores), *Pseudomonas aeruginosa*, or *Serratia marcescens* and may actually transmit infection. Most topical antiseptics interfere with wound healing to some degree, so they should be used according to the proper directions and for a limited length of time.

⬡ ALCOHOLS AND RELATED COMPOUNDS

Alcohols and aldehydes have been used as antiseptics and disinfectants for many years.[5] Two of the most commonly used antiseptics and disinfectants are ethyl and isopropyl alcohol.

The antibacterial potencies of the primary alcohols (against test cultures of *Staphylococcus aureus*) increase with molecular weight until the 8-carbon atom octanol is reached. In general, one oxygen atom is capable of solubilizing seven or eight carbon atoms in water. As the primary alcohol chain length increases, van der Waals interactions increase, and the ability to penetrate microbial membranes increases. As water solubility decreases, the apparent antimicrobial potency diminishes with molecular weight. Branching of the alcohol chain decreases antibacterial potency; weaker van der Waals forces brought about by branching do not penetrate bacterial cell membranes as efficiently. The isomeric alcohols' potencies decrease in the order primary > secondary > tertiary. Despite this fact, 2-propanol (isopropyl alcohol) is used commercially instead of *n*-propyl alcohol, because it is less expensive. Isopropyl alcohol is slightly more active than ethyl alcohol against vegetative bacterial growth, but both alcohols are largely ineffective against spores. The activity of alcohols against microorganisms is the result of their ability to denature important proteins and carbohydrates.

Alcohol

Ethanol (ethyl alcohol, wine spirit) is a clear, colorless, volatile liquid with a burning taste and a characteristic pleasant odor. It is flammable, miscible with water in all proportions, and soluble in most organic solvents. Commercial ethanol contains approximately 95% ethanol by volume. This concentration forms an azeotrope with water that distills at 78.2°C. Alcohol has been known for centuries as a product of fermentation from grain and many other carbohydrates. Ethanol can also be prepared synthetically by the sulfuric-acid–catalyzed hydration of ethylene

The commerce in, and use of, alcohol in the United States is strictly controlled by the Treasury Department, which has provided the following definition for "alcohol": "The term *alcohol* means that substance known as ethyl alcohol, hydrated oxide of ethyl, or spirit of wine, from whatever source or whatever process produced, having a proof of 160 or more and not including the substances commonly known as whiskey, brandy, rum, or gin."

Denatured alcohol is ethanol that has been rendered unfit for use in intoxicating beverages by the addition of other substances. *Completely denatured alcohol* contains added wood alcohol (methanol) and benzene and is unsuitable for either internal or external use. *Specially denatured alcohol* is ethanol treated with one or more substances so that its use may be permitted for a specialized purpose. Examples are iodine in alcohol for tincture of iodine, methanol, and other substances in mouthwashes and aftershave lotions, and methanol in alcohol for preparing plant extracts.

The primary medicinal use of alcohol is external, as an antiseptic, preservative, mild counterirritant, or solvent. Rubbing alcohol is used as an astringent, rubefacient, and a mild local anesthetic. The anesthetic effect is results from the evaporative refrigerant action of alcohol when applied to the skin. Ethanol has even been injected near nerves and ganglia to alleviate pain. It has a low narcotic potency and has been used internally in diluted form as a mild sedative, a weak vasodilator, and a carminative.

Alcohol is metabolized in the human body by a series of oxidations:

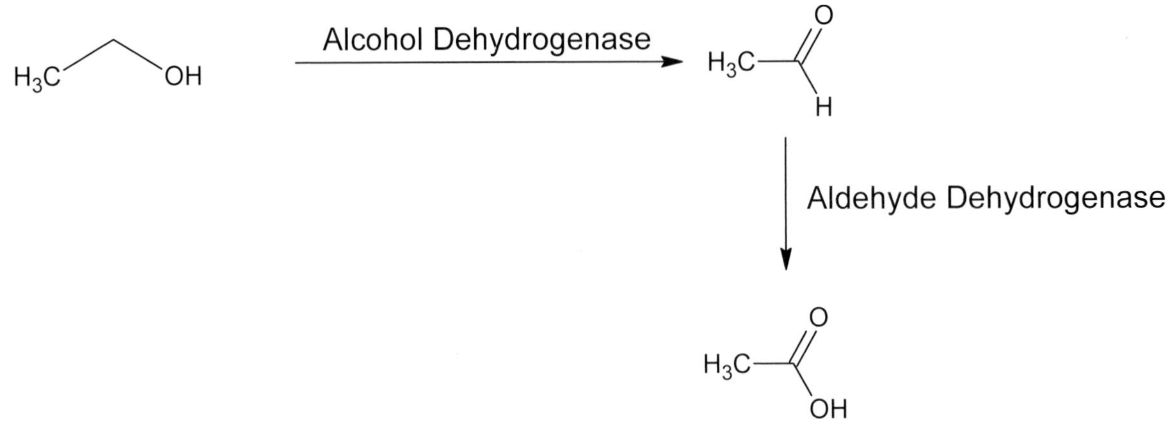

Acetaldehyde causes nausea, vomiting, and vasodilatory flushing. This fact has been used in aversion therapy with the drug disulfiram, which blocks aldehyde dehydrogenase, allowing acetaldehyde to accumulate.

Alcohol is used in the practice of pharmacy for the preparation of spirits, tinctures, and fluidextracts. *Spirits* are preparations containing ethanol as the sole solvent, whereas *tinctures* are hydroalcoholic mixtures. Many fluidextracts contain alcohol as a cosolvent.

The accepted bactericidal concentration of 70% alcohol is not supported by a study that discovered that the kill rates of microorganisms suspended in alcohol concentrations between 60% and 95% were not significantly different.[6] Concentrations below 60% are also effective, but longer contact times are necessary. Concentrations above 70% can be used safely for preoperative sterilization of the skin.[7] Alcohols are flammable and must be stored in cool, well-ventilated areas.

Dehydrated Ethanol

Dehydrated ethanol, or *absolute ethanol*, contains not less than 99% w/w of C_2H_5OH. It is prepared commercially by azeotropic distillation of an ethanol–benzene mixture, with provisions made for efficient removal of water. Absolute ethanol has a very high affinity for water and must be stored in tightly sealed containers. This form of ethanol is used primarily as a chemical reagent or solvent but has been injected for the local relief of pain in carcinomas and neuralgias. Absolute alcohol cannot be ingested because there is always some benzene remaining from the azeotropic distillation that cannot be removed.

Isopropyl Alcohol

Isopropanol (2-propanol) is a colorless, volatile liquid with a characteristic odor and a slightly bitter taste. It is considered a suitable substitute for ethanol in most cases but must not be ingested. Isopropyl alcohol is prepared commercially by the sulfuric-acid–catalyzed hydration of propylene:

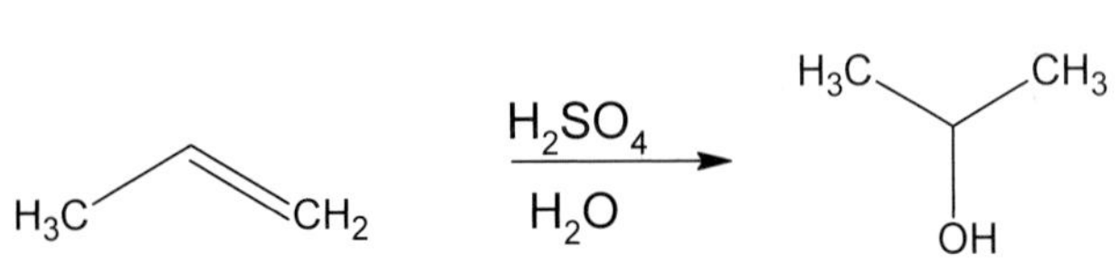

The alcohol forms a constant-boiling mixture with water that contains 91% v/v of 2-propanol. Isopropyl alcohol is used primarily as a disinfectant for the skin and for surgical instruments. The alcohol is rapidly *bactericidal* in the concentration

range of 50% to 95%. A 40% concentration is considered equal in antiseptic efficacy to a 60% ethanol in water solution. *Azeotropic isopropyl alcohol, United States Pharmacopeia (USP)*, is used on gauze pads for sterilization of the skin prior to hypodermic injections. Isopropyl alcohol is also used in pharmaceuticals and toiletries as a solvent and preservative.

Ethylene Oxide

Ethylene oxide, C_2H_4O, is a colorless, flammable gas that liquefies at 12°C. It has been used to sterilize temperature-sensitive medical equipment and certain pharmaceuticals that cannot be heat sterilized in an autoclave. Ethylene oxide diffuses readily through porous materials and very effectively destroys all forms of microorganisms at ambient temperatures.[8]

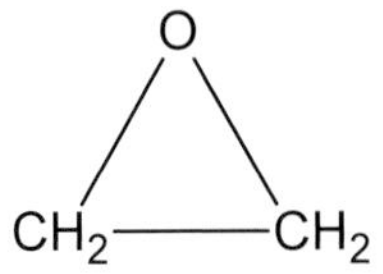

Ethylene oxide forms explosive mixtures in air at concentrations ranging from 3% to 80% by volume. The explosion hazard is eliminated when the gas is mixed with sufficient concentrations of carbon dioxide. *Carboxide* is a commercial sterilant containing 10% ethylene oxide and 90% carbon dioxide by volume that can be handled and released in air without danger of explosion. Sterilization is accomplished in a sealed, autoclave-like chamber or in gas-impermeable bags.

The mechanism of the germicidal action of ethylene oxide probably involves the alkylation of functional groups in nucleic acids and proteins by nucleophilic opening of the oxide ring. Ethylene oxide is a nonselective alkylating agent, and for that reason is extremely toxic and potentially carcinogenic. Exposure to skin and mucous membranes should be avoided, and inhalation of the gas should be prevented by use of an appropriate respiratory mask during handling and sterilization procedures.

Aldehydes

Formaldehyde Solution

Formalin is a colorless aqueous solution that officially contains not less than 37% w/v of formaldehyde (HCHO), with methanol added to retard polymerization. Formalin is miscible with water and alcohol and has a characteristic pungent aroma. Formaldehyde readily undergoes oxidation and polymerization, leading to formic acid and paraformaldehyde, respectively, so the preparation should be stored in tightly closed, light-resistant containers. Formalin must be stored at temperatures above 15°C to prevent cloudiness, which develops at lower temperatures.

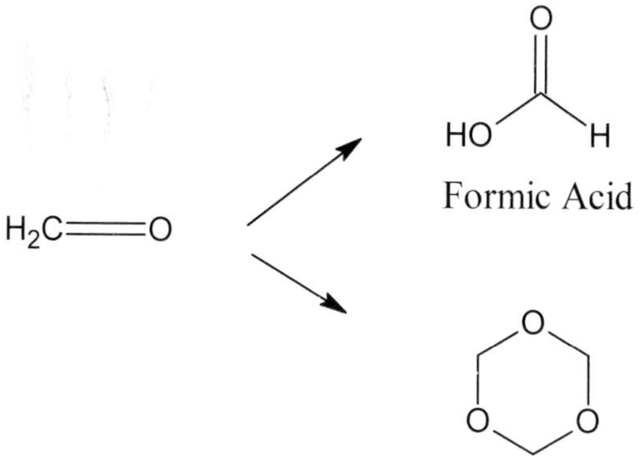

Formic Acid

Paraformaldehyde

The germicidal action of formaldehyde is slow but powerful. The mechanism of action is believed to involve direct, nonspecific alkylation of nucleophilic functional groups (amino, hydroxyl, and sulfhydryl) in proteins and nucleic acids to form carbinol derivatives. The action of formaldehyde is not confined to microorganisms. The compound is irritating to mucous membranes and causes hardening of the skin. Oral ingestion of the solution leads to severe gastrointestinal distress. Contact dermatitis is common with formalin, and pure formaldehyde is suspected to be a carcinogen.

Glutaraldehyde Disinfectant Solution
Glutaraldehyde (Cidex, a 5-carbon dialdehyde) is used as a dilute solution for sterilization of equipment and instruments that cannot be autoclaved. Commercial glutaraldehyde is stabilized in alkaline solution. The preparation actually consists of two components, glutaraldehyde and buffer, which are mixed together immediately before use. The activated solution contains 2% glutaraldehyde buffered at pH 7.5 to 8.0. Stabilized glutaraldehyde solutions retain more than 80% of their original activity 30 days after preparation,[9] whereas the nonstabilized alkaline solutions lose about 44% of their activity after 15 days. At higher pH (>8.5), glutaraldehyde rapidly polymerizes. Nonbuffered solutions of glutaraldehyde are acidic, possibly because of an acidic proton on the cyclic hemiacetal form. The acidic solutions are stable but lack sporicidal activity.

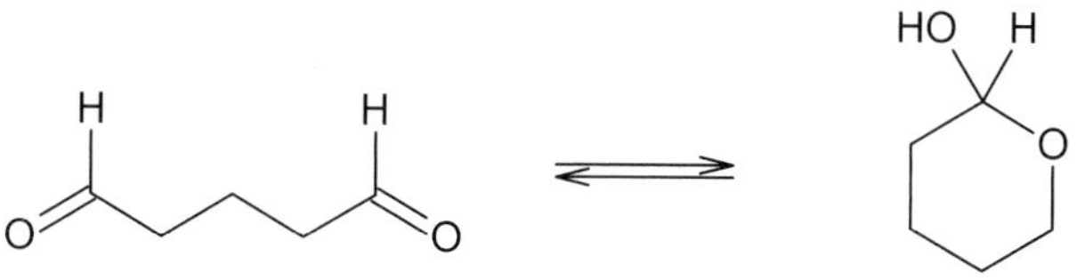

Glutaraldehyde

Glutaraldehyde Hemiacetal

⬡ PHENOLS AND THEIR DERIVATIVES

Phenol, *USP*, remains the standard to which the activity of most germicidal substances is compared. The *phenol coeffi-*

cient is defined as the ratio of a dilution of a given test disinfectant to the dilution of phenol that is required to kill (to the same extent) a strain of *Salmonella typhi* under carefully controlled time and temperature conditions. As an example, if the dilution of a test disinfectant is 10-fold greater than the dilution of phenol, the phenol coefficient is 10. Obviously, the phenol coefficient of phenol itself is 1. The phenol coefficient test has many drawbacks. Phenols and other germicides do not kill microorganisms uniformly, so variations in the phenol coefficient will occur. Moreover, the conditions used to conduct the test are difficult to reproduce exactly, so high variability between different measurements and laboratories is expected. Hence, the phenol coefficient may be unreliable.

Several phenols are actually more bactericidal than phenol itself. Substitution with alkyl, aryl, and halogen (especially in the *para* position) groups increases bactericidal activity. Straight-chain alkyl groups enhance bactericidal activity more than branched groups. Alkylated phenols and resorcinols are less toxic than the parent compounds while retaining bactericidal properties. Phenols denature bacterial proteins at low concentrations, whereas lysis of bacterial cell membranes occurs at higher concentrations.

Phenol
Phenol (carbolic acid) is a colorless to pale-pink crystalline material with a characteristic "medicinal odor." It is soluble to the extent of 1 part to 15 parts water, very soluble in alcohol, and soluble in methanol and salol (phenyl salicylate).

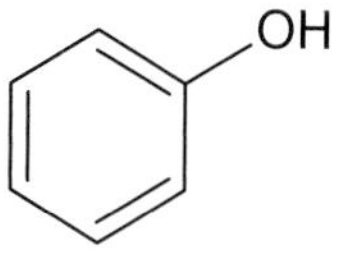

Phenol exhibits germicidal activity (general protoplasmic poison), is caustic to skin, exerts local anesthetic effects, and must be diluted to avoid tissue destruction and dermatitis.

Sir Joseph Lister introduced phenol as a surgical antiseptic in 1867, and it is still used occasionally as an antipruritic in phenolated calamine lotion (0.1%–1% concentrations). A 4% solution of phenol in glycerin has been used to cauterize small wounds. Phenol is almost obsolete as an antiseptic and disinfectant.

Liquified Phenol
Liquified phenol is simply phenol containing 10% water. The liquid form is convenient for adding phenol to various pharmaceutical preparations because it can be measured and transferred easily. The water content, however, precludes its use in fixed oils or liquid petrolatum, because the solution is not miscible with lipophilic ointment bases.

p-Chlorophenol
p-Chlorophenol is used in combination with camphor in liquid petrolatum as an external antiseptic and anti-irritant. The compound has a phenol coefficient of about 4.

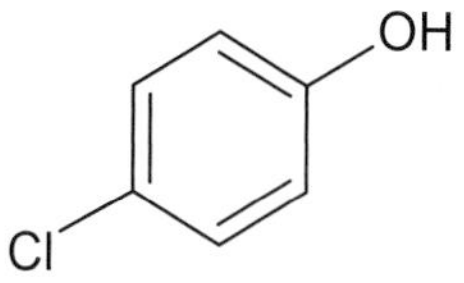

p-Chloro-m-xylenol

p-Chloro-*m*-xylenol (PC-MX; Metasep) is a nonirritating antiseptic agent with broad-spectrum antibacterial and antifungal properties. It is marketed in a 2% concentration as a shampoo. It has also been used topically for the treatment of tinea (ringworm) infections such as athlete's foot (tinea pedis) and jock itch (tinea cruris).

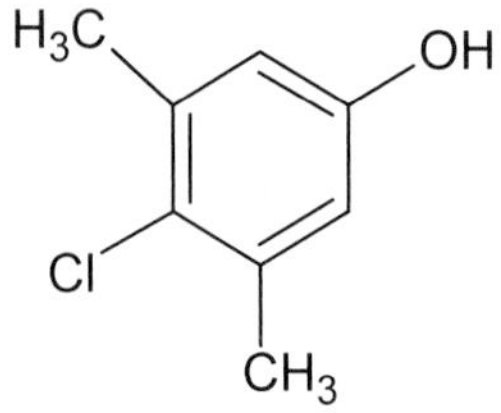

Hexachlorophene

Hexachlorophene, 2,2′-methylenebis (3,4,6-trichlorophenol); 2,2′-dihydroxy-3,5,6,3′,5′, 6′-hexachlorodiphenylmethane (Gamophen, Surgicon, pHisoHex) is a white to light-tan crystalline powder that is insoluble in water but is soluble in alcohol and most other organic solvents. A biphenol such as hexachlorophene will, in general, possess greater potency than a monophenol. In addition, as expected, the increased degree of chlorination of hexachlorophene increases its antiseptic potency further.

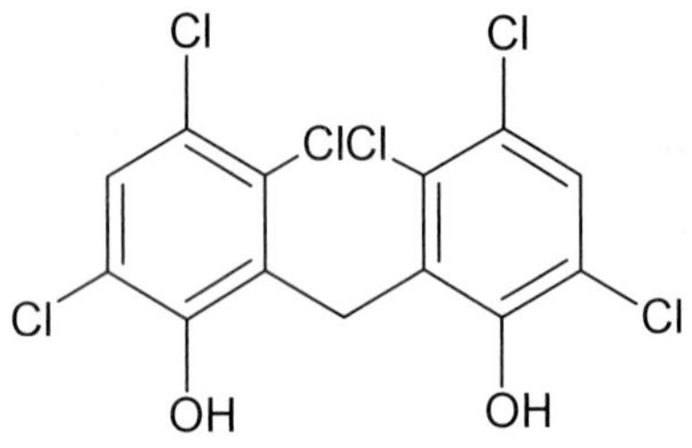

Hexachlorophene is easily adsorbed onto the skin and enters the sebaceous glands. Because of this, topical application elicits a prolonged antiseptic effect, even in low concentrations. Hexachlorophene is used in concentrations of 2% to 3% in soaps, detergent creams, lotions, and shampoos for various antiseptic uses. It is, in general, effective against Gram-positive bacteria, but many Gram-negative bacteria are resistant.

The systemic toxicity of hexachlorophene in animals after oral and parenteral administration had been known for some time, but in the late 1960s and early 1970s, reports of neurotoxicity in infants bathed in hexachlorophene and in burn patients cleansed with the agent prompted the FDA to ban its use in over-the-counter (OTC) antiseptic and cosmetic preparations.[10] Hexachlorophene is still available by prescription.

Cresol

Cresol is actually a mixture of three isomeric methylphenols:

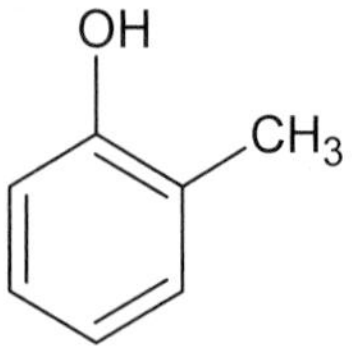

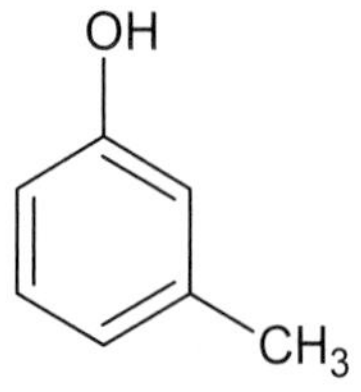

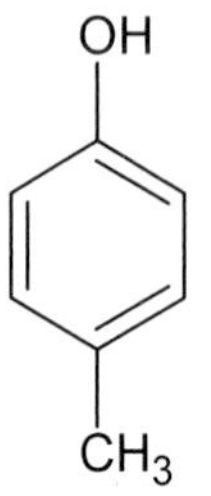

The mixture occurs as a yellow to brownish yellow liquid that has a characteristic odor of creosote. Cresol is obtained from coal tar or petroleum by alkaline extraction into aqueous medium, acidification, and fractional distillation. The mixture is an inexpensive antiseptic and disinfectant. It possesses a phenol coefficient of 2.5. Cresol is sparingly soluble in water, although alcohols and other organic solvents will solubilize it. The drawback to its use as an antiseptic is its unpleasant odor.

Chlorocresol

4-Chloro-3-methylphenol occurs as colorless crystals. Chlorocresol is only slightly soluble in water. At the low concentration that can be achieved in aqueous media, the compound is only useful as a preservative.

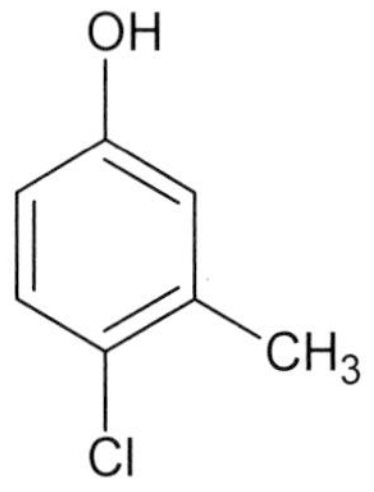

Thymol

Isopropyl *m*-cresol is extracted from oil of *Thymus vulgaris* (thyme, of the mint family) by partitioning into alkaline aqueous medium followed by acidification. The crystals obtained from the mother liquor are large and colorless, with a thymelike odor. Thymol is only slightly soluble in water, but it is extremely soluble in alcohols and other organic solvents. Thymol has mild fungicidal properties and is used in alcohol solutions and in dusting powders for the treatment of tinea (ringworm) infections.

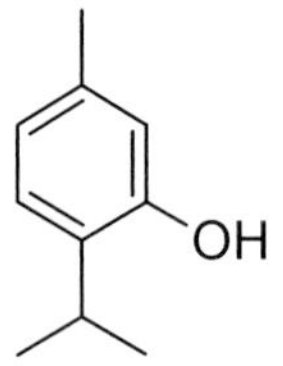

Eugenol

4-Allyl-2-methoxyphenol is obtained primarily from clove oil. It is a pale-yellow liquid with a strong aroma of cloves and a pungent taste. Eugenol is only slightly soluble in water but is miscible with alcohol and other organic solvents. Eugenol possesses both local anesthetic and antiseptic activity and can be directly applied on a piece of cotton to relieve toothaches. Eugenol is also used in mouthwashes because of its antiseptic property and pleasant taste. The phenol coefficient of eugenol is 14.4.

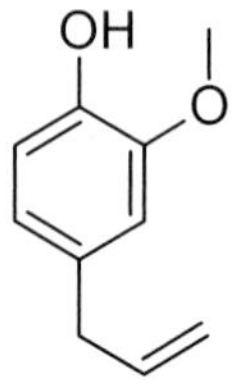

Resorcinol

m-Dihydroxybenzene (resorcin), or resorcinol, is prepared synthetically. It crystallizes as white needles or as an amorphous powder that is soluble in water and alcohol. Resorcinol is light sensitive and oxidizes readily, so it must be stored in tight, light-resistant containers. It is much less stable in solution, especially at alkaline pH. Resorcinol is only a weak antiseptic (phenol coefficient 0.4). Nevertheless, it is used in 1% to 3% solutions and in ointments and pastes in concentrations of 10% to 20% for the treatment of skin conditions such as ringworm, eczema, psoriasis, and seborrheic dermatitis. In addition to its antiseptic action, resorcinol is a *keratolytic* agent. This property causes the stratum corneum of the skin to slough, opening the barrier to penetration for antifungal agents.

Hexylresorcinol

4-Hexylresorcinol, or "hexylresorcinol," is a white crystalline substance with a faint phenolic odor. When applied to the tongue it produces a sensation of numbness. It is freely soluble in alcohol but only slightly soluble in water (1–20,000 parts). Hexylresorcinol is an effective antiseptic, possessing both bactericidal and fungicidal properties. The phenol coefficient of hexylresorcinol against *S. aureus* is 98. As is typical for alkylated phenols, hexylresorcinol possesses surfactant properties. The compound also has local anesthetic activity. Hexylresorcinol is formulated into throat lozenges because of its local anesthetic and antiseptic properties. These preparations are probably of little value. Hexylresorcinol (in the concentration in the lozenge) is probably not antiseptic, and the local anesthetic property can anesthetize the larynx, causing temporary laryngitis.

OXIDIZING AGENTS

In general, oxidizing agents that are of any value as germicidal agents depend on their ability to liberate oxygen in the tissues. Many of these agents are inorganic compounds, including hydrogen peroxide, several metal peroxides, and sodium perborate. All of these react in the tissues to generate oxygen and oxygen radicals. Other oxidizing agents, such as $KMnO_4$, denature proteins in microorganisms through a direct oxidation reaction. Oxidizing agents are especially effective against anaerobic bacteria and can be used in cleansing contaminated wounds. The bubbles that form during the liberation of oxygen help to dislodge debris. The effectiveness of the oxidizing agents is somewhat limited by their generally poor penetrability into infected tissues and organic matter. Additionally, the action of the oxidizers is typically transient.

Carbamide Peroxide Topical Solution

Carbamide peroxide (Gly-Oxide) is a stable complex of urea and hydrogen peroxide. It has the molecular formula $H_2NCONH_2 H_2O_2$. The commercial preparation is a solution of 12.6% carbamide peroxide in anhydrous glycerin. When mixed with water, hydrogen peroxide is liberated. Carbamide peroxide is used as both an antiseptic and disinfectant. The preparation is especially effective in the treatment of oral ulcerations or in dental care. The oxygen bubbles that are liberated remove debris.

Hydrous Benzoyl Peroxide

Hydrous benzoyl peroxide (Oxy-5, Oxy-10, Vanoxide) is a white granular powder. In its pure powder form, it is explosive. The compound is formulated with 30% water to make it safer to handle.

Compounded at 5% and 10% concentrations, benzoyl peroxide is both keratolytic and keratogenic. It is used in the treatment of acne. Benzoyl peroxide induces proliferation of epithelial cells, leading to sloughing and repair.[11]

HALOGEN-CONTAINING COMPOUNDS

IODOPHORS

Elemental iodine (I_2) is probably the oldest germicide still in use today. It was listed in 1830 in *USP*-II as a tincture and a liniment. Iodine tincture (2% iodine in 50% alcohol with sodium iodide), strong iodine solution (Lugol's solution, 5% iodine in water with potassium iodide), and iodine solution (2% iodine in water with sodium iodide) are currently official preparations in the *USP*. The iodide salt is admixed to increase the solubility of the iodine and to reduce its volatility. Iodine is one of the most effective and useful of the germicides. It probably acts to inactivate proteins by iodination of aromatic residues (phenylalanyl and tyrosyl) and oxidation (sulfhydryl groups). Mixing with several nonionic and cationic surfactants can solubilize iodine. Complexes form that retain the germicidal properties of the iodine while reducing its volatility and removing its irritant properties.[12] In some of the more active, nonionic surfactant complexes, it is estimated that approximately 80% of the dissolved iodine remains available in bacteriologically active form. These active complexes, called *iodophors,* are both bactericidal and fungicidal.

Povidone–Iodine

Povidone–iodine (Betadine, Isodine, polymer polyvinylpyrrolidone [PVP]–iodine) is a charge-transfer complex of iodine with the nonionic surfactant PVP. The complex is extremely water soluble and releases iodine very slowly. Hence, the preparation provides a nontoxic, nonvolatile, and nonstaining form of iodine that is not irritating to the skin or to wounds. Approximately 10% of the iodine in the complex is bioavailable. Povidone–iodine is used as an aqueous solution for presurgical disinfection of the incision site. It can also be used to treat infected wounds and damage to the skin, and it is effective for local bacterial and fungal infections. Several other forms of PVP–iodine are available, including aerosols, foams, ointments, surgical scrubs, antiseptic gauze pads, sponges, mouthwashes, and a preparation that disinfects whirlpool baths and hot tubs.

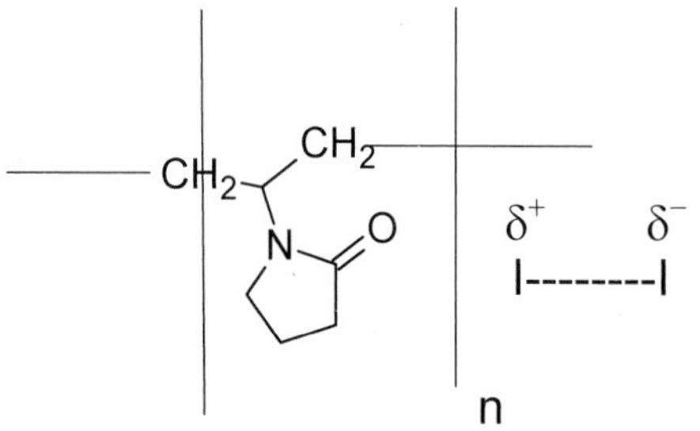

CHLORINE-CONTAINING COMPOUNDS

Chlorine and chlorine-releasing compounds have been used in the disinfection of water supplies for more than a century. The discovery that hypochlorous acid (HClO) is the active germicidal species that is formed when chlorine is dissolved in water led to the development and use of the first inorganic hypochlorite salts such as NaOCl and $Ca(OCl)_2$. Later, organic *N*-chloro compounds were developed as disinfectants. These compounds release hypochlorous acid when dissolved in water, especially in the presence of acid. Two equally plausible mechanisms have been proposed for the germicidal action of hypochlorous acid: the chlorination of amide nitrogen atoms and the oxidation of sulfhydryl groups in proteins. Organic compounds that form stable *N*-chloro derivatives include amides, imides, and amidines. *N*-Chloro compounds slowly release HOCl in water. The antiseptic effect of these agents is optimal at around pH 7.

Halazone

p-Dichlorosulfamoylbenzoic acid is a white, crystalline, photosensitive compound with a faint chlorine odor. Halazone is only slightly soluble in water at pH 7 but becomes very soluble in alkaline solutions. The sodium salt of halazone is used to disinfect drinking water.

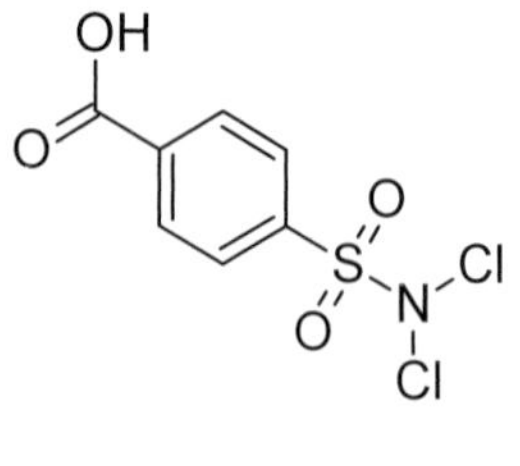

Chloroazodin

N,N-Dichlorodicarbonamidine (Azochloramid) is a bright yellow crystalline solid with a faint odor of chlorine. It is mostly insoluble in water and organic solvents and is unstable to light or heat. Chloroazodin will explode if heated above 155°C. The compound is soluble enough in water to be used in very dilute solution to disinfect wounds, as packing for dental caries, and for lavage and irrigation. A glyceryltriacetate solution is used as a wound dressing. The antiseptic action of chloroazodin is long lasting because of its extremely slow reaction with water.

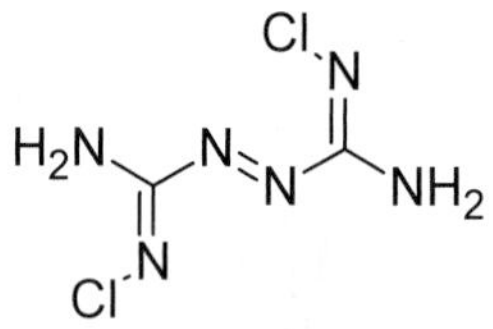

Oxychlorosene Sodium

Oxychlorosene (Clorpactin) is a complex of the sodium salt of dodecylbenzenesulfonic acid and hypochlorous acid. The complex slowly releases hypochlorous acid in solution.

Oxychlorosene occurs as an amorphous white powder that has a faint odor of chlorine. It combines the germicidal properties of HOCl with the emulsifying, wetting, and keratolytic actions of an anionic detergent. The agent has a marked and rapid-*cidal* action against most microorganisms, including both Gram-positive and Gram-negative bacteria, molds, yeasts, viruses, and spores. Oxychlorosene is used to treat localized infections (especially when resistant organisms are present), to remove necrotic tissue from massive infections or radiation necrosis, to counteract odorous discharges, to act as an irritant, and to disinfect cysts and fistulas. Oxychlorosene is marketed as a powder for reconstitution into a solution. A typical application uses a 0.1% to 0.5% concentration in water. Dilutions of 0.1% to 0.2% are used in urology and ophthalmology.

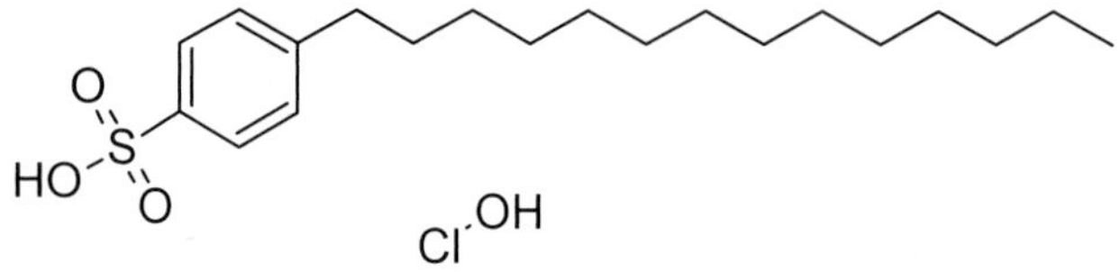

CATIONIC SURFACTANTS

All of the cationic surfactants are quaternary ammonium compounds (Table 6.3). For that reason, they are always ionized in water and exhibit surface-active properties. The compounds, with a polar head group and nonpolar hydrocarbon chain, form micelles by concentrating at the interface of immiscible solvents. The surface activity of these compounds, exemplified by lauryl triethylammonium sulfate, results from two structural moieties: (a) a cationic head group, which has a high affinity for water and (b) a long hydrocarbon tail, which has an affinity for lipids and nonpolar solvents.

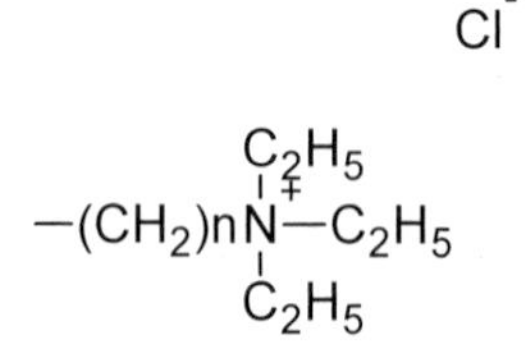

At the right concentration (the critical micelle concentration), the molecules concentrate at the interface between immiscible solvents, such as water and lipid, and water-in-oil or oil-in-water emulsions may be formed with the ammonium head group in the water layer and the nonpolar hydrocarbon chain associated with the oil phase. The synthesis and antimicrobial actions of the members of this class of com-

TABLE 6.3 Analogs of Dimethylbenzylammonium Chloride

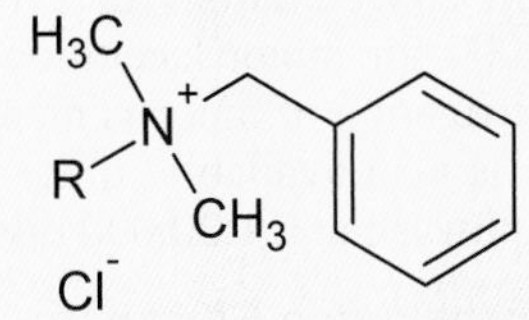

Head Group

Compound	R
Benzalkonium Chloride	$R = nC_8H_{17}$ to $C_{16}H_{33}$
Benzethonium Chloride	R= 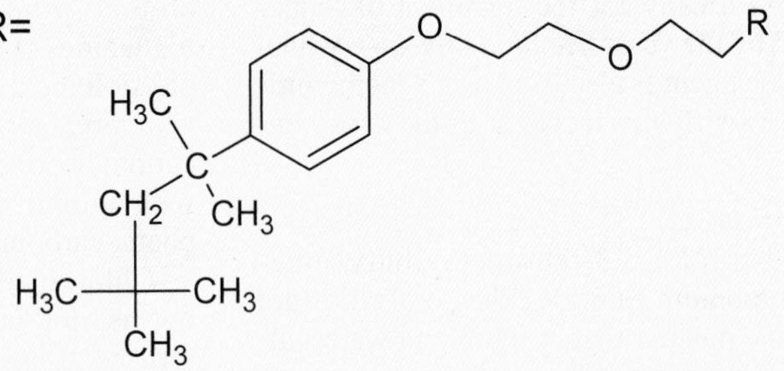
Methylbenzethonium Chloride	R= 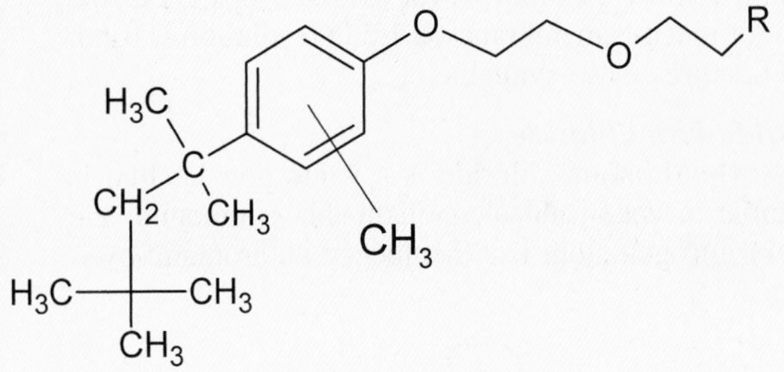

pounds were first reported in 1908, but it was not until the pioneering work of Gerhard Domagk in 1935[13] that attention was directed to their usefulness as antiseptics, disinfectants, and preservatives.

The cationic surfactants exert a bactericidal action against a broad spectrum of Gram-positive and Gram-negative bacteria. They are also active against several pathogenic species of fungi and protozoa. All spores resist these agents. The mechanism of action probably involves dissolution of the surfactant into the microbial cell membrane, destabilization, and subsequent lysis. The surfactants may also interfere with enzymes associated with the cell membrane.

The cationic surfactants possess several other properties. In addition to their broad-spectrum antimicrobial activity, they are useful as germicides. They are highly water soluble, relatively nontoxic, stable in solution, nonstaining, and noncorrosive. The surface activity causes a keratolytic action in the stratum corneum and, hence, provides good tissue penetration. In spite of these advantages, the cationic surfactants present several difficulties. Soaps and other anionic detergents inactivate them. All traces of soap must be removed from skin and other surfaces before they are applied. Tissue debris, blood, serum, and pus reduce the effectiveness of the surfactants. Cationic surfactants are also adsorbed on glass, talc, and kaolin to reduce or prevent their action. The bactericidal action of cationic surfactants is slower than that of iodine. Solutions of cationic surfactants intended for disinfecting surgical instruments, gloves, etc. should never be reused because they can harbor infectious microorganisms, especially *Pseudomonas* and *Enterobacter* spp.

Benzalkonium Chloride

Alkylbenzyldimethylammonium chloride (Zephiran) is a *mixture* of alkylbenzyldimethylammonium chlorides of the general formula $[C_6H_5CH_2N(CH_3)_2R]^+Cl^-$, where R represents a mixture of alkyl chains beginning with C_8H_{17} and extending to higher homologues with $C_{12}H_{25}$, $C_{14}H_{29}$, and $C_{16}H_{33}$. The higher–molecular-weight homologues compose the major fractions. Although variations in the physical and antimicrobial properties exist between individual members of the mixture, they are of little importance in the chemistry of the overall product. Benzalkonium chloride occurs as a white gel that is soluble in water, alcohol, and organic solvents. Aqueous solutions are colorless, slightly alkaline, and very foamy.

Benzalkonium chloride is a detergent, an emulsifier, and a wetting agent. It is used as an antiseptic for skin and mucous membranes in concentrations of 1:750 to 1:20,000. For irrigation, 1:20,000 to 1:40,000 concentrations are used. For storage of surgical instruments, 1:750 to 1:5,000 concentrations are used, with 0.5% $NaNO_3$ added as a preservative.

Methylbenzethonium Chloride

Benzyldimethyl[2-[2-[[4-(1,1,3,3-tetramethylbutyl) tolyl]oxy]ethoxy]ethyl]ammonium chloride (Diaparene) is a mixture of methylated derivatives of methylbenzethonium chloride. It is used specifically for the treatment of diaper rash in infants, caused by the yeast *Candida albicans*, which produces ammonia. The agent is also used as a general antiseptic. Its properties are virtually identical to those of benzethonium chloride.

Benzethonium Chloride

Benzyldimethyl[2-[2-[*p*-(1,1,3,3-tetramethylbutyl)phenoxy]ethoxy]ethyl]ammonium chloride (Phemerol chloride) is a colorless crystalline powder that is soluble in water, alcohol, and most organic solvents. The actions and uses of this agent are similar to those of benzalkonium chloride. It is used at a 1:750 concentration for skin antisepsis. For the irrigation of mucous membranes, a 1:5,000 solution is used. A 1:500 tincture is also available.

Cetylpyridinium Chloride

1-Hexadecylpyridinium chloride is a white powder that is very soluble in water and alcohol. In this compound, the quaternary nitrogen atom is a member of an aromatic pyridine ring.

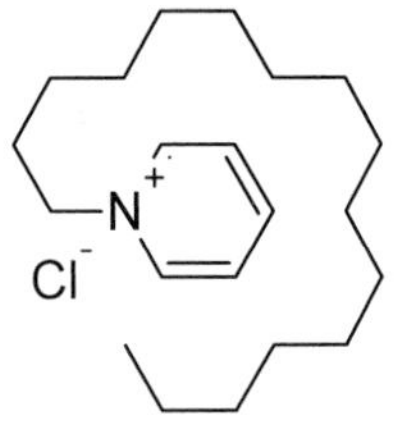

The cetyl derivative is the most active of a series of alkylpyridinium compounds. It is used as a general antiseptic in concentrations of 1:100 to 1:1,000 for intact skin, 1:1,000 for minor lacerations, and 1:2,000 to 1:10,000 for the irrigation of mucous membranes. Cetylpyridinium chloride is also available in the form of throat lozenges and a mouthwash at a 1:20,000 dilution.

Chlorhexidine Gluconate

1,6-Di(4'-chlorophenyldiguanido)hexane gluconate (Hibiclens) is the most effective of a series of antibacterial biguanides originally developed in Great Britain.[14]

The antimicrobial properties of the biguanides were discovered as a result of earlier testing of these compounds as possible antimalarial agents (Chapter 7). Although the biguanides are technically not bisquaternary ammonium compounds and, therefore, should probably be classified separately, they share many physical, chemical, and antimicrobial properties with the cationic surfactants. The biguanides are strongly basic, and they exist as dications at physiological pH. In chlorhexidine, the positive charges are counterbalanced by gluconate anions (not shown). Like cationic surfactants, these undergo inactivation when mixed with anionic detergents and complex anions such as phosphate, carbonate, and silicate.

Chlorhexidine has broad-spectrum antibacterial activity but is not active against acid-fast bacteria, spores, or viruses. It has been used for such topical uses as preoperative skin disinfection, wound irrigation, mouthwashes, and general sanitization. Chlorhexidine is not absorbed through skin or mucous membranes and does not cause systemic toxicity.

⬡ DYES

Organic dyes were used very extensively as anti-infective agents before the discovery of the sulfonamides and the antibiotics. A few cationic dyes still find limited use as anti-infectives. These include the triphenylmethane dyes gentian violet and basic fuchsin and the thiazine dye methylene blue. The dyes form colorless *leucobase* forms under alkaline conditions. Cationic dyes are active against Gram-positive bacteria and many fungi; Gram-negative bacteria are generally resistant. The difference in susceptibility is probably related to the cellular characteristics that underlie the Gram stain.

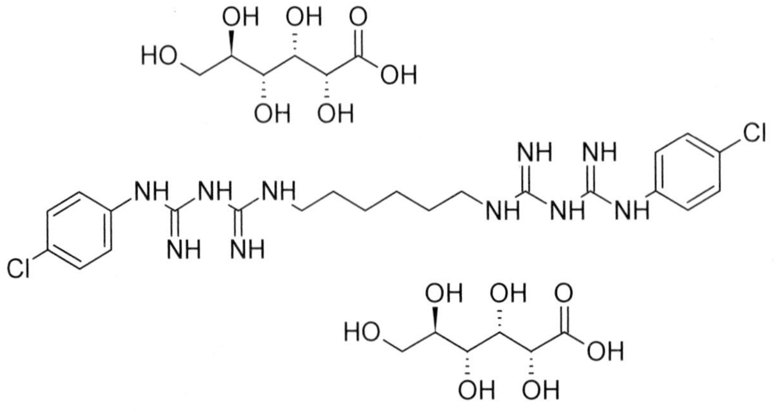

Chlorhexidine Gluconate

Gentian Violet

Gentian violet is variously known as hexamethyl-*p*-rosaniline chloride, crystal violet, methyl violet, and methylrosaniline chloride. It occurs as a green powder or green flakes with a metallic sheen. The compound is soluble in water (1:35) and alcohol (1:10) but insoluble in nonpolar organic solvents. Gentian violet is available in vaginal suppositories for the treatment of yeast infections. It is also used as a 1% to 3% solution for the treatment of ringworm and yeast infections. Gentian violet has also been used orally as an anthelmintic for strongyloidiasis (threadworm) and oxyuriasis.

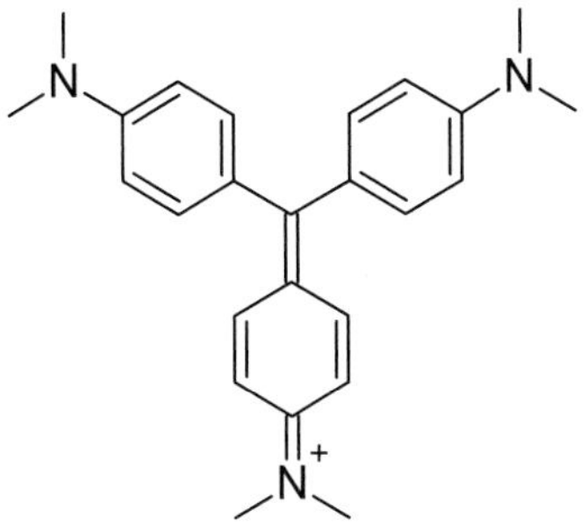

Basic Fuchsin

Basic fuchsin is a mixture of the chlorides of rosaniline and *p*-rosaniline. It exists as a green crystalline powder with a metallic appearance. The compound is soluble in water and in alcohol but insoluble in ether. Basic fuchsin is a component of carbol–fuchsin solution (Castellani's paint), which is used topically in the treatment of fungal infections, notably ringworm and athlete's foot.

Methylene Blue

Methylene blue is 3,7-bis(dimethylamino)-phenazathionium chloride (Urised). The compound occurs as a dark green crystalline powder with a metallic appearance that is soluble in water (1:25) and alcohol (1:65).

Methylene blue has weak antiseptic properties that make it useful for the treatment of cystitis and urethritis. The action of methylene blue is considered to be bacteriostatic. The compound colors the urine and stool blue green.

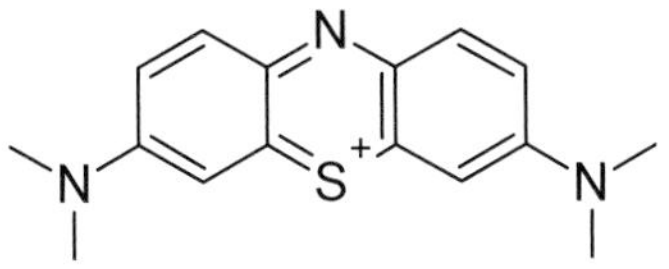

⬡ MERCURY COMPOUNDS (MERCURIALS)

Mercury and its derivatives have been used in medicine for centuries. Elemental mercury incorporated into ointment bases was used topically for the treatment of localized infections and syphilis. Several inorganic salts of mercury, such as mercuric chloride ($HgCl_2$) and mercurous chloride (calomel, Hg_2Cl_2) were at one time widely used as antiseptics. Ammoniated mercury [$Hg(NH_2)Cl$] is still occasionally used for skin infections such as impetigo, psoriasis, and ringworm. Mercuric oxide is sometimes used to treat inflammation resulting from infection of the eye. Although the potential interaction of mercuric ion with the tissues is greatly reduced by the low water solubility of these agents, they can be irritating and can cause hypersensitivity reactions; therefore, their use is not recommended.

The comparatively few organomercurials still in use are employed as antiseptics, preservatives, or diuretics. Organomercurials can be grouped into two general classes: (a) compounds with at least one carbon–mercury bond that does not ionize readily and (b) compounds with mercury bonded to heteroatoms (e.g., oxygen, nitrogen, sulfur) that ionize partially or completely. In addition to its effect on ionization, the organic moiety may increase the lipid solubility of an organomercurial compound, thereby facilitating its penetration into microorganisms and host tissues.

The antibacterial action of mercury compounds is believed to result from their reaction with sulfhydryl (-SH) groups in enzymes and other proteins to form covalent compounds of the type R-S-Hg-R′. This action is reversible by treatment with thiol-containing compounds such as cysteine and dimercaprol (BAL); hence, organomercurials, reacting reversibly, are largely bacteriostatic. The antibacterial activity of organomercurial antiseptics is greatly reduced in serum because of the presence of proteins that inactivate mercury compounds. Organomercurial antiseptics are not very effective against spores.

The disadvantages of mercurials for antiseptic and disinfectant uses far outweigh any possible advantages that they might have. Hence, other more effective and less potentially toxic agents are preferable.

Nitromersol

3-(Hydroxymercuri)-4-nitro-*o*-cresol inner salt (Metaphen) occurs as a yellow powder that is practically insoluble in

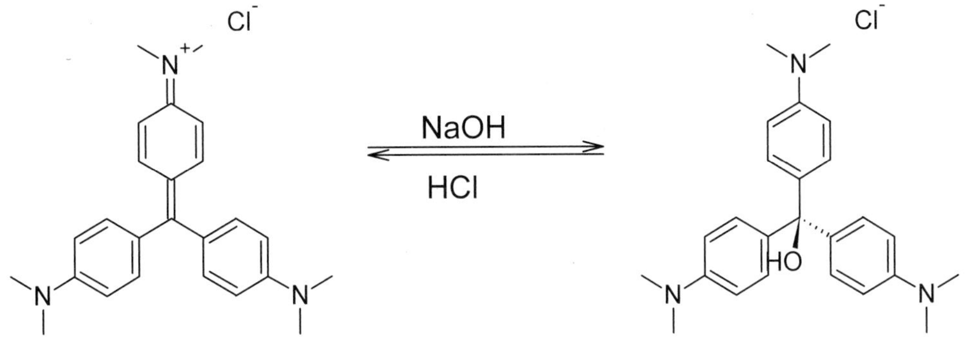

Hexamethyl p-Rosaniline

Chloride

Leucobase

water and is sparingly soluble in alcohol and most organic solvents. The sodium salt probably has the "inner salt" structure in which the inner shell electrons of mercury are occupied.[15] The bonding to mercury in this salt should be collinear, thus the following structure is somewhat improbable. Nevertheless, this structure is shown in the *USP* and the *Merck Index*.

Nitromersol is nonirritating to mucous membranes and is nonstaining. Therefore, at one time, it was a very popular antiseptic for skin and ocular infections. Nitromersol has largely been replaced by superior agents.

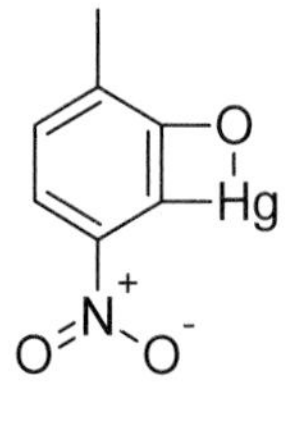

Thimerosal

[(*o*-Carboxyphenyl)-thio]ethylmercury sodium salt (Merthiolate) is a cream-colored, water-soluble powder. It is nonstaining and nonirritating to tissues. Thimerosal is a weakly bacteriostatic antiseptic that is applied topically in ointments or aqueous solutions.

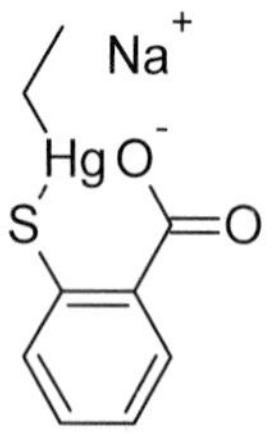

🛑 PRESERVATIVES

Preservatives are added to various dosage forms and cosmetic preparations to prevent microbial contamination. In parenteral and ophthalmic preparations, preservatives are used to maintain sterility in the event of accidental contamination during use. An ideal preservative would be effective at low concentrations against all possible microorganisms, be nontoxic and compatible with other constituents of the preparation, and be stable for the shelf life of the preparation. The ideal preservative does not exist, but there is quite a bit of experience with some of them. In some cases, combinations of preservative agents are used to approximate a mixture of ideal features.

p-Hydroxybenzoic Acid Derivatives

Esters of *p*-hydroxybenzoic acid (parabens) have distinct antifungal properties. Their toxicity to the human host is typically low because they undergo rapid hydrolysis in vivo to *p*-hydroxybenzoic acid, which is quickly conjugated and excreted. This property makes the parabens useful as preservatives for liquid dosage forms. The preservative activity generally increases with molecular weight, but the methyl ester is most effective against molds, whereas the propyl ester is most effective against yeasts. The more lipid-soluble propyl ester is the preferred preservative for drugs in oil or lipophilic bases.

Methylparaben

Methyl *p*-hydroxybenzoate, or methylparaben, is a white crystalline powder. It is soluble in water and alcohol but only slightly soluble in nonpolar organic solvents. Methylparaben is used as a safeguard against mold growth.

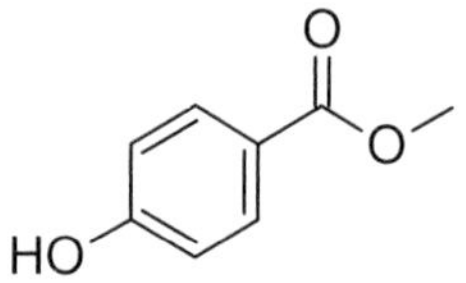

Propylparaben

Propyl *p*-hydroxybenzoate, or propylparaben, occurs as a white crystalline powder that is slightly soluble in water but soluble in most organic solvents. It is used as a preservative, primarily to retard yeast growth. Propylparaben sodium is a water-soluble sodium salt of the 4-phenol group. The pH of solutions of propylparaben sodium is basic (pH ~10).

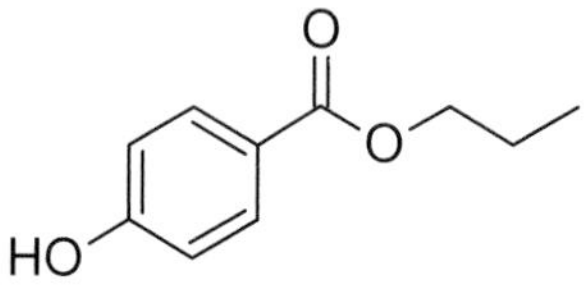

Butylparaben

n-Butyl *p*-hydroxybenzoate (butylparaben) occurs as a white crystalline powder that is sparingly soluble in water but very soluble in alcohols and in nonpolar organic solvents.

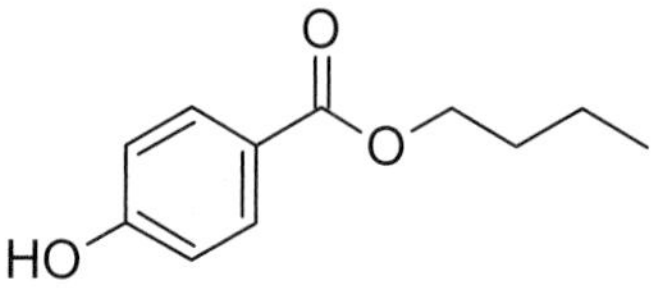

Ethylparaben

Ethyl *p*-hydroxybenzoate (ethylparaben) is a white crystalline powder that is slightly soluble in water but soluble in alcohol and most organic solvents.

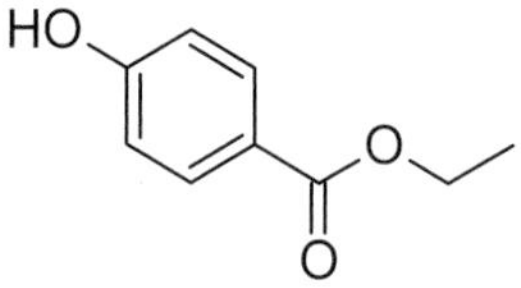

Other Preservatives

Chlorobutanol

1,1,1-Trichloro-2-methyl-2-propanol is a white crystalline solid with a camphorlike aroma. It occurs in an anhydrous form and a hemihydrate form, both of which sublime at room temperature and pressure. Chlorobutanol is slightly soluble in water and soluble in alcohol and in organic solvents.

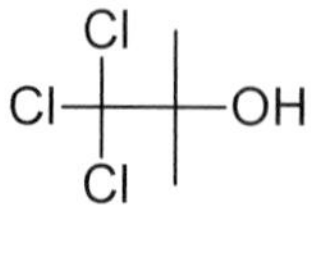

Chlorobutanol is used as a bacteriostatic agent in pharmaceuticals for injection, ophthalmic use, and intranasal administration. It is unstable when heated in aqueous solution, especially at pH greater than 7. Under these conditions, chlorobutanol undergoes elimination. Solutions with a pH of approximately 5 are reasonably stable at 25°C. Chlorobutanol is stable in oils and organic solvents.

Benzyl Alcohol

Benzyl alcohol (phenylcarbinol, phenylmethanol) occurs naturally as the unesterified form in oil of jasmine and in esters of acetic, cinnamic, and benzoic acids in gum benzoin, storax resin, Peru balsam, tolu balsam, and some volatile oils. It is soluble in water and alcohol and is a clear liquid with an aromatic odor.

Benzyl alcohol is commonly used as a preservative in vials of injectable drugs in concentrations of 1% to 4% in water or saline solution. Benzyl alcohol has the added advantage of having a local anesthetic action. It is commonly used in ointments and lotions as an antiseptic in the treatment of various pruritic skin conditions.

Phenylethyl Alcohol

Phenylethyl alcohol (2-phenylethanol, orange oil, rose oil, $C_6H_5CH_2CH_2OH$) is a clear liquid that is sparingly soluble in water ($\sim$2%). It occurs naturally in rose oil and pine-needle oil. It is used primarily in perfumery.

Benzoic Acid

Benzoic acid and its esters occur naturally in gum benzoin and in Peru and tolu balsams. It is found as a white crystalline solid that slowly sublimes at room temperature and is steam distillable. It is slightly soluble in water (0.3%) but more soluble in alcohol and in other polar organic solvents. It has a pK_a of 4.2. Benzoic acid is used externally as an antiseptic in lotions, ointments, and mouthwashes. It is more effective as a preservative in foods and pharmaceutical products at low pH (less than the pK_a). When used as a preservative in emulsions, its effectiveness depends on both pH and distribution into the two phases.[16]

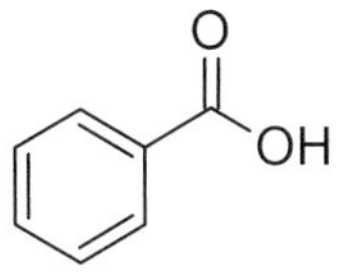

Sodium Benzoate

Sodium benzoate is a white crystalline solid that is soluble in water and alcohol. It is used as a preservative in acidic liquid preparations in which benzoic acid is released.

Sodium Propionate

Sodium propionate occurs as transparent colorless crystals that are soluble in water and alcohol. It is an effective antifungal agent that is used as a preservative. Sodium propionate is most effective at low pH.

Sorbic Acid

2,4-Hexadienoic acid is an effective antifungal preservative. It is sparingly soluble in water and has a pK_a of 4.8. Sorbic acid is used to preserve syrups, elixirs, ointments, and lotions containing components such as sugars that support mold growth.

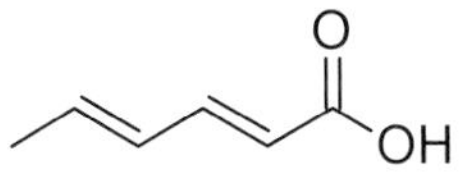

Potassium Sorbate

Potassium sorbate occurs as a white crystalline material that is soluble in water and alcohol. It is used in the same way as sorbic acid when greater water solubility is required.

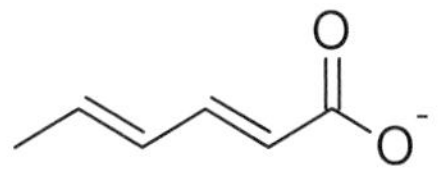

Phenylmercuric Nitrate

Phenylmercuric nitrate is a mixture of phenylmercuric nitrate and phenylmercuric hydroxide. It occurs as a white crystalline material that is sparingly soluble in water and slightly soluble in alcohol. It is used in concentrations of 1:10,000 to 1:50,000 to preserve injectable drugs against bacterial contamination. A disadvantage to organomercurials is that their bacteriostatic efficacy is reduced in the presence of serum.

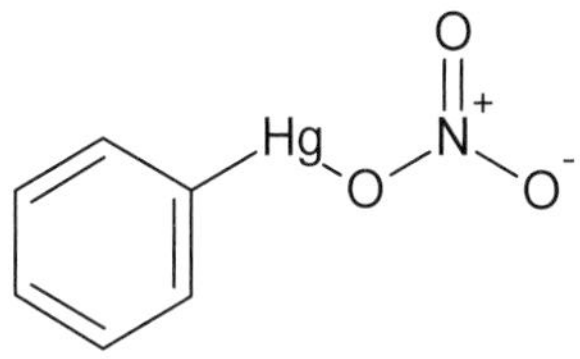

Phenylmercuric Acetate

Acetoxyphenylmercury occurs as white prisms that are soluble in alcohol but only slightly soluble in water. It is used as a preservative.

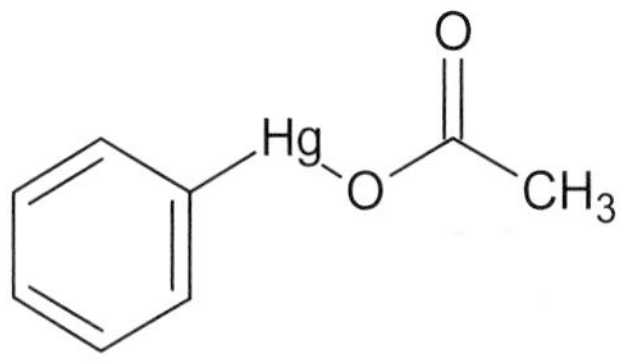

ANTIFUNGAL AGENTS

General Introduction to Fungi: Medical Mycology

The discovery that some infectious diseases could be attributed to fungi actually preceded the pioneering work of Pasteur and Koch with pathogenic bacteria by several years. Two microbiologists, Schönlein and Gruby, studied the fungus *Trichophyton schoenleinii* in 1839. In that same year, Langenbeck reported the yeastlike microorganism responsible for thrush (*C. albicans*). Gruby isolated the fungus responsible for favus on potato slices, rubbed it on the head of a child, and produced the disease. Hence, he fulfilled Koch's postulates 40 years before they were formulated.[17] In spite of its earlier beginnings, medical mycology was quickly overshadowed by bacteriology, and it has only recently begun to receive the serious attention that it deserves. This is perhaps attributable to the relatively benign nature of the common mycoses, the rarity of the most serious ones, and the need for a morphological basis for differential identification of these structurally complex forms.

Cursory examination shows that fungal infections fall into two well-defined groups: the superficial and the deep-seated mycoses.[18] The superficial mycoses are, by far, the most common and are caused, for the most part, by a relatively homogeneous group of fungi, the dermatophytes. These include the various forms of tinea, or ringworm, which are infections of the hair or hair follicles, the superficial infections of the intertriginous or flat areas of hairless skin, and infections of the nails. As a rule, these lesions are mild, superficial, and restricted. The causative microbes are specialized saprophytes with the unusual ability to digest keratin. They have their ultimate reservoir in the soil. Unlike the deep-seated mycoses, however, they are frequently transmitted from one host to another (e.g., athlete's foot). A species of yeast, *Candida*, also produces a dermatophyte-like disease.

Systemic Mycoses

The deep-seated, systemic mycoses have a sporadic distribution,[19] being common in some parts of the world and unknown in other geographical areas. These diseases have a heterogeneous etiology. Diseases caused by the systemic organisms include histoplasmosis, sporotrichosis, blastomycosis, coccidioidomycosis, cryptococcosis, and paracoccidioidomycosis. The causative agents for these diseases are soil-inhabiting saprophytes with the ability to adapt to the internal environment of their host. These organisms share a common route of infection. Fungal spores are inhaled into the lung, and a mild, coldlike condition may result. This may be the only symptom. In most cases, disease is inapparent. In asymptomatic disease, diagnosis is often made serendipitously. Sensitization, which reflects present or previous experience with the organism, may be detected by a skin test or other immunological procedure. The immune system deals with these infections by walling them off or by producing the giant cells that are common in type IV hypersensitivities. X-ray examination or autopsy frequently reveals these lesions. As stated previously, the causative organisms of the systemic infections are not typically transmitted from one host to another, but infection by the organism in an endemic area may be very common. Few infections develop into the severe, deep, spreading, and often-fatal disease seen in some persons. If the infection is symptomatic, the clinical signs may be those of a mild, self-limiting disease; or the infection may become progressive, with severe symptoms, tissue and organ damage, and, frequently, death. Recovery from a deep-seated infection of this type is accompanied by an uncertain anamnestic immune response.

Opportunistic Fungal Infections[20,21]

In recent years, because of overzealous use of antibacterial antibiotics, the use of immunosuppressive agents, cytotoxins, irradiation, and steroids, a new category of systemic mycoses has become prominent. These are the opportunistic fungal infections. There has been a precipitous rise in the incidence of these diseases. The patient, as a result of drug therapy, underlying disease, or medical manipulation, is deprived of the normal defenses conferred by microbial flora. This allows organisms of normally *low inherent virulence* to exploit the host. Such infections include systemic candidiasis, aspergillosis, and mucormycosis. Bacterial infections such as Gram-negative septicemia, nocardiosis, and *Pseudomonas* infection, fungal infections such as with *Pneumocystis carinii*, and viral opportunists such as

cytomegalovirus also attack such patients. Multiple infections with various microorganisms are common. *C. albicans* is a particularly common opportunist. This yeast is a member of the normal microbial flora of human hosts, especially in the vagina. Use of contraceptives often predisposes a patient to infection by *Candida* spp. Fungal flora that inhabit the bowel may develop into a superinfection with the use of antibiotics to sterilize the bowel before surgery. Oral candidiasis is common in poorly nourished persons, in patients on immunosuppressive drugs, and in persons with acquired immunodeficiency syndrome (AIDS). Opportunists can grow in nearly every circumstance in which a patient's immune system is compromised.

Cutaneous Infections (Dermatophytoses)[22-24]

By far, the most common types of human fungal disease are among the dermatophytoses. These are superficial infections of the keratinized epidermis and keratinized epidermal appendages (i.e., the hair and nails). The severity of an infection depends largely on the location of the lesion and the species of the fungus involved. Though certain other fungi, notably *Candida* spp., produce clinically similar diseases, a somewhat homogeneous group of fungi, termed the *dermatophytes*, is responsible for most cases. The ability of these organisms to invade and parasitize the cornified tissues of hair, skin, and nails is closely associated with, and dependent on, their common physiological characteristic—metabolic use of the highly insoluble scleroprotein keratin. The biochemical use of keratin is rare and is shared by the dermatophyte species of the family Gymnoascaceae, with only a few species of the family Onygenaceae, and certain tineae. In humans, the genera *Trichophyton* (notably *T. rubrum* [nails, beard, smooth skin], *T. tonsurans* [scalp, beard, nails], *T. violaceum* [scalp, skin nails], *T. mentagrophytes* [commonest cause of athlete's foot], *T. verrucosum* [scalp, beard], and *T. rubrum* [psoriasis-like lesions of smooth skin, infections of nails]), *Microsporum* (*M. gypseum* [scalp], *M. fulvum* [scalp, hairless skin], and *M. canis* [scalp, hairless skin]), and *Epidermophyton* (eczema) contain the most common dermatophytes. These organisms cause the conditions known as tinea (ringworm). Some of the common tinea infections are listed in Table 6.4. The fungus *Pityrosporum orbiculare* causes an additional type, tinea versicolor. This organism, called *Malassezia furfur* in older literature, causes yellow to brown patches or continuous scaling over the trunk and occasionally the legs, face, and neck. The affected areas may be identified by the inability to tan in the sun.

Regardless of the type of fungus that is causing an infection (Table 6.5), treatment is extremely difficult because fungi, like mammalians, are eukaryotes. Many biochemical structures, especially the cell membranes, are nearly identi-

TABLE 6.4 Locations of the Common Types of Tinea (Ringworm)

Type	Location
Tinea manuum	Hand
Tinea cruris	Groin
Tinea sycosis	Beard
Tinea capitis	Scalp
Tinea unguium	Nails

TABLE 6.5 Clinical Types of Fungal Infection

Type	Disease State	Causative Organism
Superficial infections	Tinea versicolor	*Pityrosporum orbiculare*
	Piedra	*Trichosporon cutaneum* (white)
		Piedraia hortae (black)
Cutaneous infections	Ringworm of scalp, hairless skin, nails	Dermatophytes, *Microsporum, Trichophyton, Epidermophyton*
	Candidosis of skin, mucous membranes, nails; sometimes generalized	*Candida albicans* and related forms
Subcutaneous infections	Chromomycosis	*Fonsecaea* and related forms
	Mycotic mycetoma	*Allescheria boydii, Madurella mycetoma,* etc.
	Entomophthoromycosis	*Basidiobolus haptosporus, Conidiobolus coronatus*
Systemic infections	Histoplasmosis	*Histoplasma capsulatum*
	Blastomycosis	*Blastomyces dermatiditis*
	Paracoccidioidomycosis	*Paracoccidioides brasiliensis*
	Coccidioidomycosis	*Coccidioides immitis*
	Cryptococcosis	*Cryptococcus neoformans*
	Sporotrichosis	*Sporothrix schenckii*
	Aspergillosis	*Aspergillus fumigates*
	Mucormycosis	*Mucor* spp., *Absidia* spp., *Rhizopus* spp.
	Histoplasmosis duboisii	*Histoplasma capsulatum* var. *duboisii*

cal, as are many biochemical reactions. Consequently, drugs that will kill a fungus will have a toxic effect on human cells at normal doses.

A slight difference exists in the cell membranes. Lipid bilayers by themselves are unstable and would be unable to hold their shape and support their functions. Sterols are embedded in the bilayers to act as stiffening agents. The 3-hydroxyl group represents the polar "head" group, and the nonpolar sterol skeleton and side chain align perfectly with the nonpolar chains of the bilayer. In human cells, the sterol in the membrane is cholesterol (Fig. 6.1). In fungi, the sterol is ergosterol (Fig. 6.2). This difference amounts to the only source of selectivity that we have in treating fungal infections. New antifungal drug development has focused on this difference as a way to achieve selectivity, creating highly potent antifungal drugs that are much less toxic to the human host.

Subcutaneous Fungal Infections[22]

Subcutaneous mycosis refers to a group of fungal diseases in which both the skin and subcutaneous tissue are involved but typically no dissemination to the internal organs occurs.

The causative agents are classified among several unrelated genera. They have the following characteristics in common: (a) they are primarily soil saprophytes of very low-grade virulence and invasive ability; and (b) in most human and animal infections, they gain access as a result of a trauma to the tissue. Many, if not all, organisms have the potential to establish local infections under certain circumstances, depending on their adaptability and the response of the host. The tissue reaction in most cases varies with the agent in question but usually remains a localized lesion similar to that elicited by a foreign body. The major disease types are chromomycosis, sporotrichosis, mycetoma, lobomycosis, and entomophthoromycosis. A type of dimorphism accompanies infection by agents of some of these groups. The organisms undergo a morphogenesis from their saprophytic form into a tissue or parasitic stage.

Tissue Reactions of Fungal Disease[23]

The tissue response of the host to the infecting fungus varies widely and depends somewhat on various invasive organisms. In dermatophyte infections, erythema is gener-

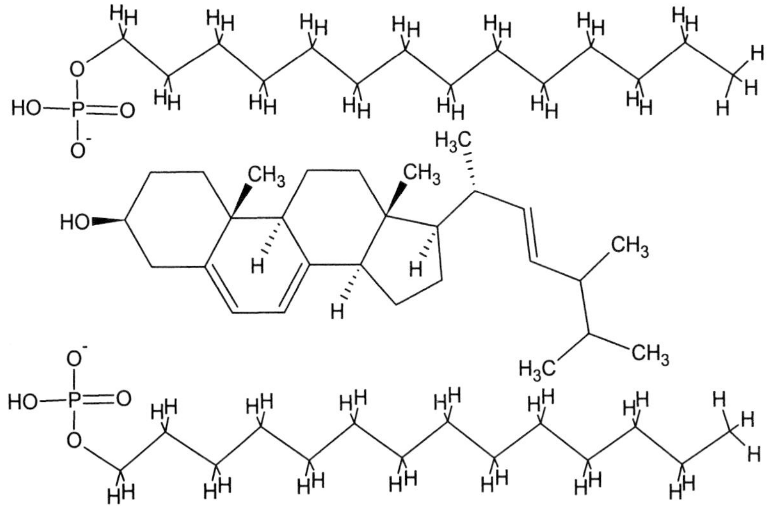

Figure 6.1 ● Cholesterol embedded in a lipid bilayer.

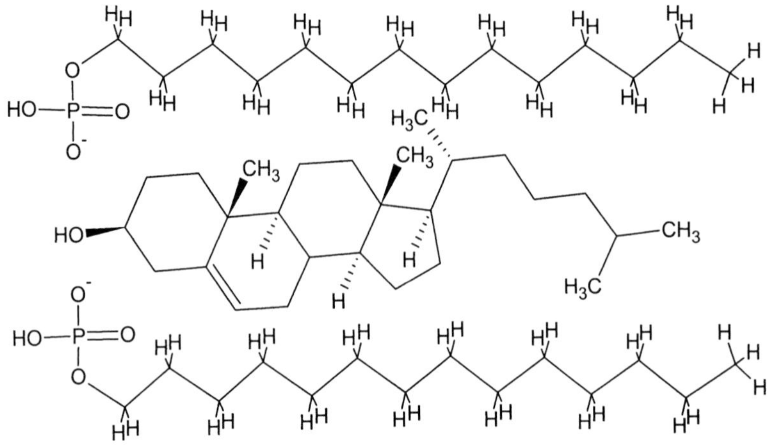

Figure 6.2 • Ergosterol embedded in a lipid bilayer.

ally produced and is a result of the irritation of the tissues by the organism. Sometimes, severe inflammation, followed by scar tissue and keloid formation, occurs. This results from an exaggerated inflammatory response and an allergic reaction to the organism and its products.

With organisms that invade living tissue, such as those responsible for subcutaneous and systemic disease, there is generally a uniform acute pyogenic reaction that gives way to various chronic disease outcomes. Granuloma with caseation and fibrocaseous pulmonary granuloma are potential outcomes of infection with *Histoplasma capsulatum*, and thrombotic arteritis, a thrombosis characterized by a purulent coagulative necrosis and invasion of blood vessels, may be caused during aspergillosis and mucormycosis. The large numbers of fungal species of many morphotypes, their disease etiology, and the diversity of outcomes make medical mycology a complex field.

Topical Agents for Dermatophytoses

Collectively, the dermatophytoses are called *tinea*, or *ringworm*. Since these infections tend to be topical, their treatment has been directed to surface areas of the skin. The skin is a formidable barrier to drug penetration, and many of the topical agents work best if an adjuvant is added that opens the barrier function of the skin. Keratolytic agents such as salicylic acid or other α-hydroxy compounds perform this function reasonably well.

FATTY ACIDS

Adults have an acidic, fatty substance in and on the skin called *sebum*. Sebum functions as a natural antifungal agent, part of the innate immune system. Fatty acids have been used for years with the idea that if a substance similar to sebum could be applied to the infected area, the effect of the sebum would be augmented and fungi could be eradicated. The application of fatty acids or their salts does in fact have an antifungal effect, albeit a feeble one.

The higher–molecular-weight fatty acids have the advantage of having lower volatility. Salts of fatty acids are also fungicidal and provide nonvolatile forms for topical application.

Propionic Acid
Propionic acid is an antifungal agent that is nonirritating and nontoxic. After application, it is present in perspiration

in low concentration (~0.01%). Salt forms with sodium, potassium, calcium, and ammonium are also fungicidal. Propionic acid is a clear, corrosive liquid with a characteristic odor. It is soluble in water and alcohol. The salts are usually used because they are nonvolatile and odorless.

Zinc Propionate
Zinc propionate occurs as an anhydrous form and as a monohydrate. It is very soluble in water but only sparingly soluble in alcohol. The salt is unstable to moisture, forming zinc hydroxide and propionic acid. Zinc propionate is used as a fungicide, particularly on adhesive tape.

Sodium Caprylate
Sodium caprylate is prepared from caprylic acid, which is a component of coconut and palm oils. The salt precipitates as cream-colored granules that are soluble in water and sparingly soluble in alcohol.

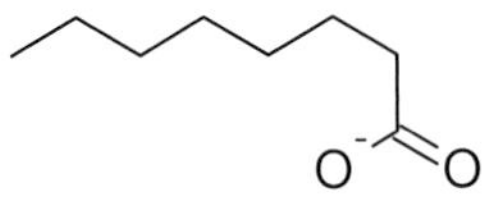

Sodium caprylate is used topically to treat superficial dermatomycoses caused by *C. albicans* and *Trichophyton*, *Microsporum*, and *Epidermophyton* spp. The sodium salt can be purchased in solution, powder, and ointment forms.

Zinc Caprylate
Zinc caprylate is a fine white powder that is insoluble in water or alcohol. The compound is used as a topical fungicide. The salt is highly unstable to moisture.

Undecylenic Acid
10-Undecenoic acid (Desenex, Cruex) obtained from the destructive distillation of castor oil. Undecylenic acid is a viscous yellow liquid. It is almost completely insoluble in water but is soluble in alcohol and most organic solvents.

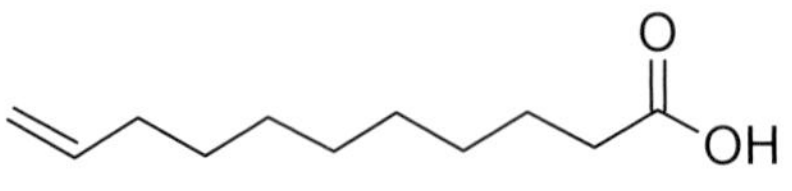

Undecylenic acid is one of the better fatty acids for use as a fungicide, although cure rates are low. It can be used in concentrations up to 10% in solutions, ointments, powders, and emulsions for topical administration. The preparation should never be applied to mucous membranes because it is a severe irritant. Undecylenic acid has been one of the agents traditionally used for athlete's foot (*tinea pedis*). Cure rates are low, however.

Triacetin

Glyceryl triacetate (Enzactin, Fungacetin) is a colorless, oily liquid with a slight odor and a bitter taste. The compound is soluble in water and miscible with alcohol and most organic solvents.

The activity of triacetin is a result of the acetic acid released by hydrolysis of the compound by esterases present in the skin. Acid release is a self-limiting process because the esterases are inhibited below pH 4.

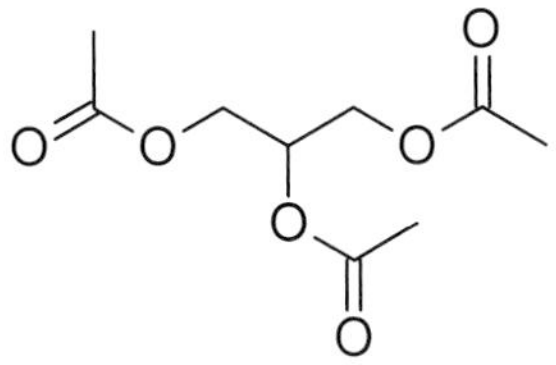

Salicylic Acid and Resorcinol

Salicylic acid is a strong aromatic acid (pK$_a$ 2.5) with both antiseptic and keratolytic properties. It occurs as white, needle-like crystals or a fluffy crystalline powder, depending on how the compound was brought out of solution. Salicylic acid is only slightly soluble in water but is soluble in most organic solvents. The greater acidity of salicylic acid and its lower solubility in water compared with *p*-hydroxybenzoic acid are the consequence of intramolecular hydrogen bonding.

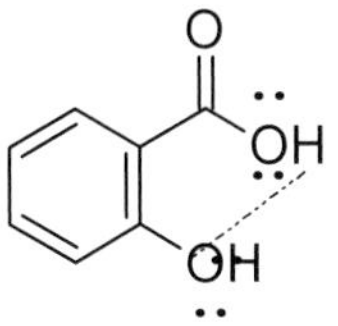

Salicylic acid is used externally in ointments and solutions for its antifungal and keratolytic properties. By itself, salicylic acid is a poor antifungal agent.

m-Hydroxyphenol (resorcinol) possesses antiseptic and keratolytic activity. It occurs as white, needlelike crystals and has a slightly sweet taste. Resorcinol is soluble in water, alcohols, and organic solvents.

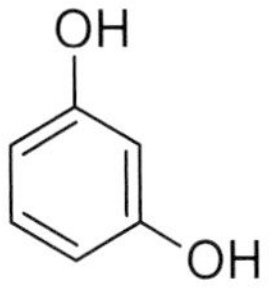

Benzoic Acid

Benzoic acid possesses appreciable antifungal effects, but it cannot penetrate the outer layer of the skin in infected areas. Therefore, benzoic acid when used as an antifungal agent must be admixed with a keratolytic agent. Suitable mixtures are benzoic acid and salicylic acid and benzoic acid and resorcinol. An old preparation that is still in use is Whitfield's Ointment, *USP*. This ointment contains benzoic acid, 6%, and salicylic acid, 6%, in a petrolatum base. The cure rates from preparations like these are low.

PHENOLS AND THEIR DERIVATIVES

Several phenols and their derivatives possess topical antifungal properties. Some of these, such as hexylresorcinols and parachlorometaxylenol have been used for the treatment of tinea infections. Two phenolic compounds, clioquinol and haloprogin, are still official in the *USP*. A third agent, ciclopirox olamine, is not a phenol but has properties like those of phenols. All of these agents appear to interfere with cell membrane integrity and function in susceptible fungi.

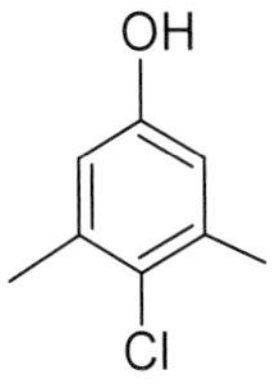

Haloprogin

3-Iodo-2-propynyl-2,4,5-trichlorophenyl ether (Halotex) crystallizes as white to pale yellow forms that are sparingly soluble in water and very soluble in ethanol. It is an ethereal derivative of a phenol. Haloprogin is used as a 1% cream for the treatment of superficial tinea infections.

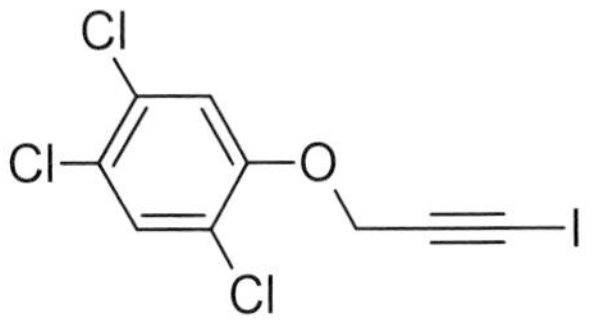

Formulations of haloprogin should be protected from light because the compound is photosensitive. Haloprogin is available as a solution and a cream, both in a 1% concentration. Haloprogin is probably not the first topical agent that should be recommended. Although the cure rates for topical fungal infections are relatively high, they come at a high price. The lesion typically worsens before it improves. Inflammation and painful irritation are common.

Clioquinol

5-Chloro-7-iodo-8-quinolinol, 5-chloro8-hydroxy-7-iodoquinoline, or iodochlorhydroxyquin (Vioform) occurs as a spongy, light-sensitive, yellowish white powder that is insoluble in water. Vioform was initially used as a substitute for iodoform in the belief that it released iodine in the tissues. It has been used as a powder for many skin conditions, such as atopic dermatitis, eczema, psoriasis, and impetigo. A 3% ointment or cream has been used vaginally as a treatment for *Trichomonas vaginalis* vaginitis. The best use for Vioform is in the topical treatment of fungal infections such as athlete's foot and jock itch. A combination with hydrocortisone (Vioform HC) is also available.

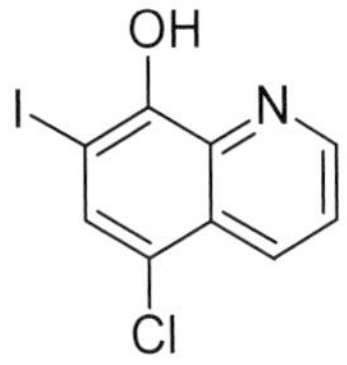

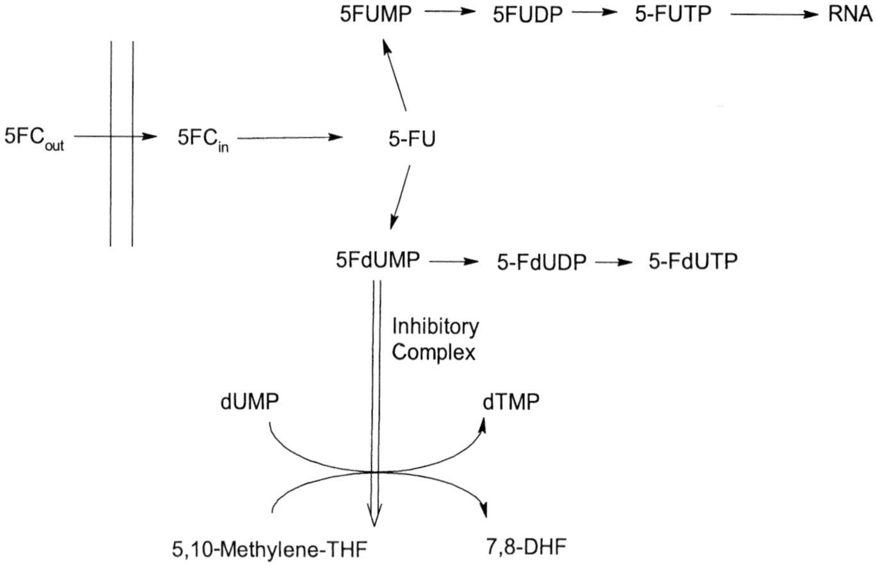

$$5\text{FUMP} \longrightarrow 5\text{FUDP} \longrightarrow 5\text{-FUTP} \longrightarrow \text{RNA}$$

$$5\text{FC}_{out} \quad \longrightarrow \quad 5\text{FC}_{in} \longrightarrow \quad 5\text{-FU}$$

$$5\text{FdUMP} \longrightarrow 5\text{-FdUDP} \longrightarrow 5\text{-FdUTP}$$

Inhibitory Complex

dUMP   dTMP

5,10-Methylene-THF   7,8-DHF

Figure 6.3 ● Mechanism of action of 5-fluorocytosine.

Ciclopirox Olamine[25]

6-Cyclohexyl-1-hydroxyl-4-methyl-2(1H)-pyridinone ethanolamine salt (Loprox) is a broad-spectrum antifungal agent intended only for topical use. It is active against dermatophytes as well as pathogenic yeasts (*C. albicans*) that are causative agents for superficial fungal infections.

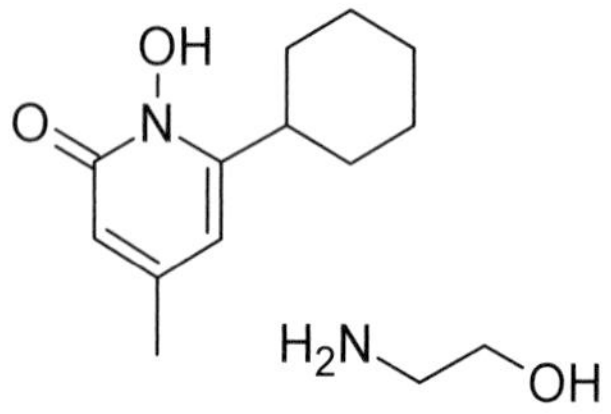

Ciclopirox is considered an agent of choice in the treatment of cutaneous candidiasis, tinea corporis, tinea cruris, tinea pedis, and tinea versicolor. It is a second-line agent for the treatment of onychomycosis (ringworm of the nails). Loprox is formulated as a cream and a lotion, each containing 1% of the water-soluble ethanolamine salt. Ciclopirox is believed to act on cell membranes of susceptible fungi at low concentrations to block the transport of amino acids into the cells. At higher concentrations, membrane integrity is lost, and cellular constituents leak out.

Nucleoside Antifungals

Flucytosine[26]

5-Fluorocytosine, 5-FC, 4-amino-5-fluoro-2(1H)-pyrimidinone, 2-hydroxy-4-amino-5-fluoropyrimidine (Ancobon). 5-Fluorocytosine is an orally active antifungal agent with a very narrow spectrum of activity. It is indicated only for the treatment of serious systemic infections caused by susceptible strains of *Candida* and *Cryptococcus* spp.

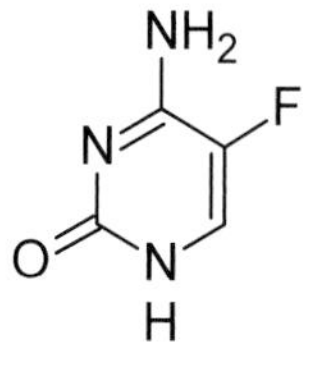

The mechanism of action of 5-fluorocytosine (5-FC) has been studied in detail and is presented in Figure 6.3. The drug enters the fungal cell by active transport on ATPases that normally transport pyrimidines. Once inside the cell, 5-fluorocytosine is deaminated in a reaction catalyzed by cytosine deaminase to yield 5-fluorouracil (5-FU). 5-Fluorouracil is the active metabolite of the drug. 5-Fluorouracil enters into pathways of both ribonucleotide and deoxyribonucleotide synthesis. The fluororibonucleotide triphosphates are incorporated into RNA, causing faulty RNA synthesis. This pathway causes cell death. In the deoxyribonucleotide series, 5-fluorodeoxyuridine monophosphate (F-dUMP) binds to 5,10-methylenetetrahydrofolic acid, interrupting the one-carbon pool substrate that feeds thymidylate synthesis. Hence, DNA synthesis is blocked.

Resistance to 5-FC is very common, and it occurs at several levels. A main one is at the step in which the drug is transported into the fungal cell. The transport system simply becomes impermeable to 5-FC. The cytosine deaminase step is another point at which resistance occurs, and the UMP pyrophosphorylase reaction is a third point at which fungal cells can become resistant. Regardless of which of these mechanisms operates, fungal resistance develops rapidly and completely when 5-FC is administered. After a few dosing intervals, the drug is essentially useless. One strategy used to decrease resistance and to prolong the effect of 5-FC is to administer it with the polyene antibiotic amphotericin B. The antibiotic creates holes in the fungal cell membrane, bypassing the transport step and allowing 5-FC to enter. Additionally, a lower dose of 5-FC can be used, preventing resistance by other mechanisms for a longer period.

Antifungal Antibiotics[27,28]

The antifungal antibiotics make up an important group of antifungal agents. All of the antibiotics are marked by their complexity. There are two classes: the polyenes, which contain a large number of agents with only a few being useful, and griseofulvin (one member of the class).

POLYENES

Several structurally complex antifungal antibiotics have been isolated from soil bacteria of the genus *Streptomyces*. The compounds are similar, in that they contain a system of conjugated double bonds in macrocyclic lactone rings. They differ from the erythromycin-type structures (macrolides; see Chapter 8), in that they are larger and contain the conjugated -*ene* system of double bonds. Hence, they are called the *polyene antibiotics*. The clinically useful polyenes fall into two groupings on the basis of the size of the macrolide ring. The 26-membered–ring polyenes, such as natamycin (pimaricin), form one group, whereas the 38-membered macrocycles, such as amphotericin B and nystatin, form the other group. Also common to the polyenes are (a) a series of hydroxyl groups on the acid-derived portion of the ring and (b) a glycosidically linked deoxyaminohexose called *mycosamine*. The number of double bonds in the macrocyclic ring differs also. Natamycin, the smallest macrocycle, is a pentaene; nystatin is a hexaene; and amphotericin B is a heptaene.

The polyenes have no activity against bacteria, rickettsia, or viruses, but they are highly potent, broad-spectrum antifungal agents. They do have activity against certain protozoa, such as *Leishmania* spp. They are effective against pathogenic yeasts, molds, and dermatophytes. Low concentrations of the polyenes in vitro will inhibit *Candida* spp., *Coccidioides immitis*, *Cryptococcus neoformans*, *H. capsulatum*, *Blastomyces dermatitidis*, *Mucor mucedo*, *Aspergillus fumigatus*, *Cephalosporium* spp., and *Fusarium* spp.

The use of the polyenes for the treatment of systemic infections is limited by the toxicities of the drugs, their low water solubilities, and their poor chemical stabilities. Amphotericin B, the only polyene useful for the treatment of serious systemic infections, must be solubilized with a detergent. The other polyenes are indicated only as topical agents for superficial fungal infections.

The mechanism of action of the polyenes has been studied in some detail. Because of their three-dimensional shape, a barrel-like nonpolar structure capped by a polar group (the sugar), they penetrate the fungal cell membrane, acting as "false membrane components," and bind closely with ergosterol, causing membrane disruption, cessation of membrane enzyme activity, and loss of cellular constituents, especially potassium ions. In fact, the first observable in vitro reaction upon treating a fungal culture with amphotericin B is the loss of potassium ions. The drug is fungistatic at low concentrations and fungicidal at high concentrations. This suggests that at low concentrations, the polyenes bind to a membrane-bound enzyme component, such as an ATPase.

Amphotericin B

The isolation of amphotericin B (Fungizone) was reported in 1956 by Gold et al.[29] The compound was purified from the fermentation beer of a soil culture of the actinomycete *Streptomyces nodosus*, which was isolated in Venezuela. The first isolate from the streptomycete was a separable mixture of two compounds, designated amphotericins A and B. In test cultures, compound B proved to be more active, and this is the one used clinically.[30] The structure and absolute stereochemistry are as shown.

Amphotericin B is believed to interact with membrane sterols (ergosterol in fungi) to produce an aggregate that forms a transmembrane channel. Intermolecular hydrogen bonding interactions among hydroxyl, carboxyl, and amino groups stabilize the channel in its open form, destroying symport activity and allowing the cytoplasmic contents to leak out. The effect is similar with cholesterol. This explains the toxicity in human patients. As the name implies, amphotericin B is an amphoteric substance, with a primary amino group attached to the mycosamine ring and a carboxyl group on the macrocycle. The compound forms deep yellow crystals that are sparingly soluble in organic solvents but insoluble in water. Although amphotericin B forms salts with both acids and bases, the salts are only slightly soluble in water (~0.1 mg/mL) and, hence, cannot be used systemically. To create a parenteral dosage form, amphotericin B is stabilized as a buffered colloidal dispersion in micelles with sodium deoxycholate.[31] The barrel-like structure of the antibiotic develops interactive forces with the micellar components, creating a soluble dispersion. The preparation is light, heat, salt, and detergent sensitive.

Parenteral amphotericin B is indicated for the treatment of severe, potentially life-threatening fungal infections, including disseminated forms of coccidioidomycosis and histoplasmosis, sporotrichosis, North American blastomycosis, cryptococcosis, mucormycosis, and aspergillosis.

The usefulness of amphotericin B is limited by a high prevalence of adverse reactions. Nearly 80% of patients treated with amphotericin B develop nephrotoxicity. Fever, headache, anorexia, gastrointestinal distress, malaise, and muscle and joint pain are common. Pain at the site of injection and thrombophlebitis are frequent complications of intravenous administration. The drug must never be administered intramuscularly. The hemolytic activity of amphotericin B may be a consequence of its ability to leach cholesterol from erythrocyte cell membranes.

For fungal infections of the central nervous system (CNS) (e.g., cryptococcosis), amphotericin B is mixed with cerebrospinal fluid (CSF) that is obtained from a spinal tap.

Amphotericin B

The solution of amphotericin B is then reinjected through the tap. For severe infections, this procedure may need to be repeated many times.

Amphotericin B for injection is supplied as a sterile lyophilized cake or powder containing 50 mg of antibiotic with 41 mg of sodium deoxycholate to be dispersed in 10 mL of water. The infusion, providing 0.1 mg/mL, is prepared by further dilution (1:50) with 5% dextrose for injection. Normal saline cannot be used because it will break the micelles. The suspension should be freshly prepared and used within 24 hours. Even the powder should be refrigerated and protected from light.

Several sterile dosage forms[32] with amphotericin B admixed with a lipid carrier have been developed with the goal of counteracting the dose-limiting toxicity of the drug following parenteral administration. These include amphotericin B colloidal dispersion (Amphocil, Amphocyte), which contains nearly equal parts of the drug and cholesterol sulfate in a suspension of disklike particles; Abelcet, a 1:1 combination of amphotericin B with L-α-dimyristoylphosphatidylcholine (7 parts) and L-α-dimyristoylphosphatidylglycerol (3 parts) to create a suspension of ribbonlike sheets; and liposomal amphotericin B (AmBisome), a small laminar vesicular preparation consisting of an approximately 1:10 molar ratio of amphotericin B and lipid (hydrogenated soy phosphatidyl choline, cholesterol, and distearoylphosphatidylcholine in a 10:5:4 ratio) for an aqueous suspension.

The rationale behind these lipid preparations is simple: amphotericin B should have a greater avidity for the lipid vehicle than for cholesterol in cell membranes. Hence, toxicity should be reduced. Lipid-associated amphotericin B should be drawn into the reticuloendothelial system, concentrating in the lymphatic tissues, spleen, liver, and lungs, where infectious fungi tend to locate. Lipases elaborated by the fungi and the host should release the drug from the lipid carrier, making it available to bind ergosterol in fungal cell membranes to exert its fungistatic and fungicidal activities.

Clinical use of each of the approved lipid preparations has shown reduced renal toxicity. Liposomal amphotericin B has been approved specifically for the treatment of pulmonary aspergillosis because of its demonstrated superiority to the sodium deoxycholate-stabilized suspension.

Amphotericin B is also used topically to treat cutaneous and mucocutaneous mycoses caused by *C. albicans*. The drug is supplied in various topical forms, including a 3% cream, a 3% lotion, a 3% ointment, and a 100-mg/mL oral

suspension. The oral suspension is intended for the treatment of oral and pharyngeal candidiasis. The patient should swish the suspension in his or her mouth and swallow it. The suspension has a very bad taste, so compliance may be a problem. A slowly developing resistance to amphotericin B has been described. This is believed to relate to alterations in the fungal cell membrane.

Nystatin

Nystatin (Mycostatin) is a polyene antibiotic that was first isolated in 1951 from a strain of the actinomycete *Streptomyces noursei* by Hazen and Brown.[33] It occurs as a yellow to light tan powder. Nystatin is very slightly soluble in water and sparingly soluble in organic solvents. The compound is unstable to moisture, heat, and light.

The aglycone portion of nystatin is called *nystatinolide*. It consists of a 38-membered macrolide lactone ring containing single tetraene and diene moieties separated by two methylene groups.[34] The aglycone also contains eight hydroxyl groups, one carboxyl group, and the lactone ester functionality. The entire compound is constructed by linking the aglycone to mycosamine. The complete structure of nystatin has been determined by chemical degradation and x-ray crystallography.[35]

Nystatin is not absorbed systemically when administered by the oral route. It is nearly insoluble under all conditions. It is also too toxic to be administered parenterally. Hence, it is used only as a topical agent. Nystatin is a valuable agent for the treatment of local and gastrointestinal monilial infections caused by *C. albicans* and other *Candida* species. For the treatment of cutaneous and mucocutaneous candidiasis, it is supplied as a cream, an ointment, and a powder. Vaginal tablets are available for the control of vaginal candidiasis. Oral tablets and troches are used in the treatment of gastrointestinal and oral candidiasis. Combinations of nystatin with tetracycline can be used to prevent monilial overgrowth caused by the destruction of bacterial microflora of the intestine during tetracycline therapy.

Although nystatin is a pure compound of known structure, its dosage is still expressed in terms of units. One milligram of nystatin contains not less than 2,000 *USP* units.

Natamycin[36,37]

Natamycin (pimaricin; Natacyn) is a polyene antibiotic obtained from cultures of *Streptomyces natalensis*.

The natamycin structure consists of a 26-membered lactone ring containing a tetraene chromophore, an α,β-unsaturated lactone carbonyl group, three hydroxyl groups, a carboxyl

Nystatin

group, a *trans* epoxide, and a glycosidically joined mycosamine. Like the other polyene antibiotics, natamycin is amphoteric.

The mechanism action of the smaller polyenes differs from that of amphotericin B and nystatin. The 26-membered–ring polyenes cause both potassium ion leakage and cell lysis at the same concentration, whereas the 38-membered–ring polyenes cause potassium leakage at low, fungistatic concentrations and cell lysis at high, fungicidal concentrations. The smaller polyenes are fungistatic and fungicidal within the same concentration range.

Natamycin possesses in vitro activity against several yeasts and filamentous fungi, including *Candida*, *Aspergillus*, *Cephalosporium*, *Penicillium*, and *Fusarium* spp. The drug is supplied as a 5% ophthalmic suspension intended for the treatment of fungal conjunctivitis, blepharitis, and keratitis.

Other Antifungal Antibiotics

Griseofulvin

Griseofulvin (Grisactin, Gris-PEG, Grifulvin) was first reported in 1939 by Oxford et al.[38] as an antibiotic obtained from the fungus *Penicillium griseofulvum*. It was isolated originally as a "curling factor" in plants. Application of extracts containing the antibiotic to fungus-infected leaf parts caused the leaf to curl up. The drug has been used for many years for its antifungal action in plants and animals. In 1959, griseofulvin was introduced into human medicine for the treatment of tinea infections by the systemic route.

Griseofulvin is an example of a rare structure in nature, a spiro compound. The structure of griseofulvin was determined by Grove et al.[39] to be 7-chloro-2′,4,6-trimethoxy-6′,β-methylspiro[benzofuran-2(3*H*)-1′-[2]cyclohexene]-3,4′-dione. The compound is a white, bitter, heat-stable powder or crystalline solid that is sparingly soluble in water but soluble in alcohol and other nonpolar solvents. It is very stable when dry.

Griseofulvin has been used for a long time for the systemically delivered treatment of refractory ringworm infections of the body, hair, nails, and feet caused by species of dermatophytic fungi including *Trichophyton*, *Microsporum*,

and *Epidermophyton*. After systemic absorption, griseofulvin is carried by the systemic circulation and capillary beds to the skin, nails, and hair follicles, where it concentrates in keratin precursor cells, which are gradually exfoliated and replaced by healthy tissue. Griseofulvin is a fungistatic agent, and as the new, healthy tissue develops, the drug prevents reinfection. Treatment must be continued until all of the infected tissue has been exfoliated, because old tissues will still support and harbor fungal growth. Therapy in slow-growing tissues, such as the nails, must be continued for several months. Compliance with the drug regimen is mandatory. In some cases, such as with the nails, it is possible to observe new, healthy tissue growing in to replace the infected tissue. Griseofulvin neither possesses antibacterial activity nor is effective against *P. obiculare*, the organism that causes tinea versicolor.

Few adverse effects have been reported for griseofulvin. The most common ones are allergic reactions such as rash and urticaria, gastrointestinal upset, headache, dizziness, and insomnia.

The oral bioavailability of griseofulvin is very poor. The compound is highly lipophilic with low water solubility. The most successful attempts at improving absorption have centered on creating micronized (ultramicrosized, microsized) griseofulvin. Reducing the particle size, in theory, should improve dissolution in the stomach and absorption. The efficiency of gastric absorption of griseofulvin ultramicrosized versus the microsized form is about 1.5, allowing a dosage reduction of one third. Several structural derivatives have been synthesized, but they have failed to improve absorption. Perhaps the best advice that the pharmacist can give a patient who is about to use griseofulvin is to take the drug with a fatty meal, as with salad dressing.

Griseofulvin is a mitotic spindle poison.[39,40] In vitro, it rapidly arrests cell division in metaphase. It causes a rapid, reversible dissolution of the mitotic spindle apparatus, probably by binding with the tubulin dimer that is required for microtubule assembly. The selective toxicity to fungi is probably because of the propensity of the drug to concentrate in tissues rich in keratin, where dermatophytes typically establish infections.

Allylamines and Related Compounds

The allylamine class of antifungal agents was discovered as a result of random screening of a chemical inventory for compounds with antifungal activity. Structure–activity studies in the series subsequently led to the discovery of compounds with enhanced potency and potential oral activity, such as terbinafine.[41,42] Investigation of the mechanism of action of the allylamines demonstrated that the compounds interfere with an early step in ergosterol biosynthesis, namely, the epoxidation of squalene catalyzed by squalene epoxidase. Squalene epoxidase[43] forms an epoxide at the C2–C3 position of squalene (Fig. 6.4). Opening of the epoxide under acid catalysis yields a carbocation that initiates the "squalene zipper" reaction that forms the steroid nucleus. Inhibition of squalene epoxidase shuts down the biosynthesis of ergosterol and causes an accumulation of squalene, which destabilizes the fungal cell membrane. The allylamines exert a fungicidal action against dermatophytes and other filamentous fungi, but their action against pathogenic yeasts, such as *Candida* spp., is largely fungistatic.

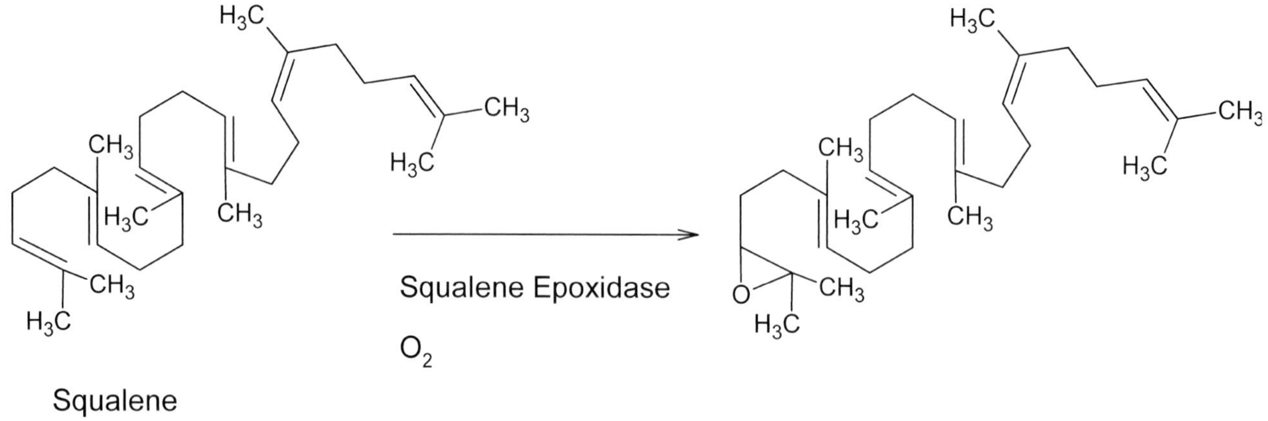

Figure 6.4 • Squalene epoxidase reaction.

Although mammalian squalene epoxidase is weakly inhibited by the allylamines, cholesterol biosynthesis does not appear to be altered.

Two allylamines, naftifine and terbinafine, have been approved as topical agents for the treatment of tinea pedis, tinea cruris, and tinea corporis caused by *Trichophyton rubrum*, *Trichophyton mentagrophytes*, or *Epidermophyton floccosum*, respectively. The topical agent tolnaftate, although not an allylamine, inhibits squalene epoxidase and has a spectrum of activity similar to that of the allylamines. Hence, tolnaftate is classified with the allylamines. The allylamines are weak bases that form hydrochloride salts that are slightly soluble in water.

Naftifine Hydrochloride

N-Methyl-*N*-(3-phenyl2-propenyl)-1-naphthalenemethanamine hydrochloride (Naftin) is a white crystalline powder that is soluble in polar solvents such as ethanol and methylene chloride. It is supplied in a 1% concentration in a cream and in a gel for the topical treatment of ringworm, athlete's foot, and jock itch. Although unapproved for these uses, naftifine has shown efficacy for treatment of ringworm of the beard, ringworm of the scalp, and tinea versicolor.

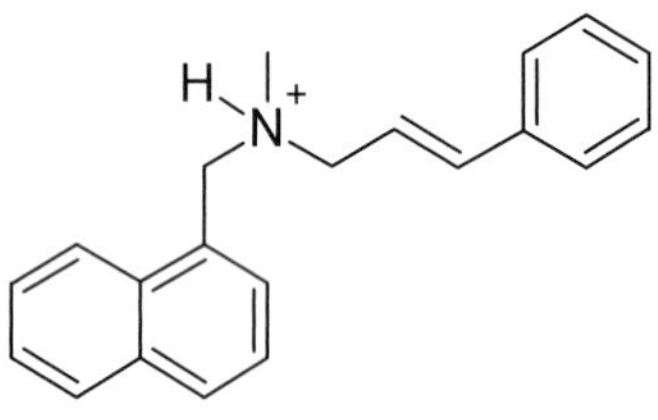

Terbinafine Hydrochloride

(*E*)-*N*-(6,6-dimethyl-2-hepten-4-ynyl)-*N*-methyl-1-naphthalene-methanamine hydrochloride (Lamisil) is an off-white crystalline material that is soluble in polar organic solvents such as methanol, ethanol, and methylene chloride but is only slightly soluble in water. The highly lipophilic free base is insoluble in water. Terbinafine hydrochloride is available in a 1% cream for topical administration for the treatment of tinea pedis, tinea corporis, and tinea cruris. Terbinafine is more potent than naftifine and has also demonstrated oral activity against onychomycosis (ringworm of the nails). It has not been approved in the United States for oral administration.

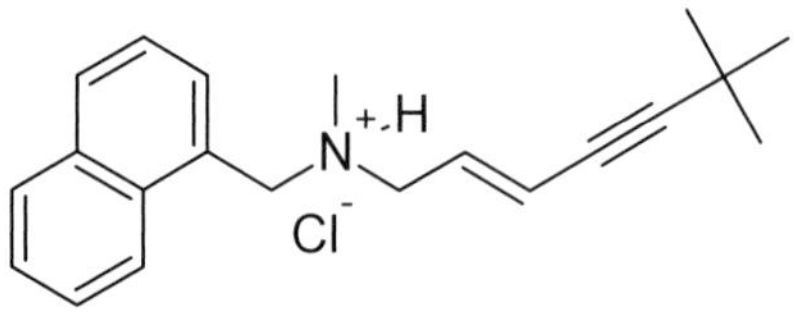

Tolnaftate

O,2-Naphthyl *m*,*N*-dimethylthiocarbanilate (Tinactin, Aftate, NP-27) is a white crystalline solid that is insoluble in water, sparingly soluble in alcohol, and soluble in most organic solvents. The compound, a thioester of β-naphthol, is fungicidal against dermatophytes, such as *Trichophyton*, *Microsporum*, and *Epidermophyton* spp., that cause superficial tinea infections. Tolnaftate is available in a concentration of 1% in creams, powders, aerosols, gels, and solutions for the treatment of ringworm, jock itch, and athlete's foot. Tolnaftate has been shown to act as an inhibitor of squalene epoxidase[44] in susceptible fungi, so it is classified with the allylamine antimycotics. Tolnaftate is formulated into preparations intended to be used with artificial fingernails to counteract the increased chance of ringworm of the nail beds.

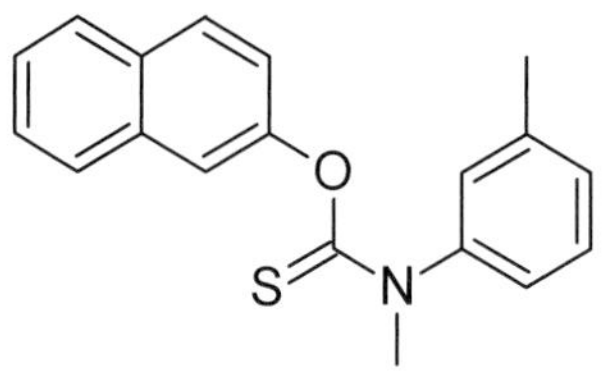

Azole Antifungal Agents

The azoles represent a class of synthetic antifungal agents that possess a unique mechanism of action. With these drugs, one can achieve selectivity for the infecting fungus over the host. Depending on the azole drug used, one can treat infections ranging from simple dermatophytoses to life-threatening, deep systemic fungal infections. Research currently under way in the United States is aimed at developing more potent azoles and compounds that penetrate the blood-brain barrier more effectively. The first members of the class were highly substituted imidazoles, such as clotrimazole and miconazole. Structure–activity studies revealed that the imidazole ring could be replaced with a bioisosteric 1,2,4-triazole ring without adversely affecting the antifungal properties of the molecule. Hence, the more generic term *azoles* refers to this class of antifungal agents.

ANTIFUNGAL SPECTRUM

The azoles tend to be effective against most fungi that cause superficial infections of the skin and mucous membranes, including the dermatophytes such as *Trichophyton*, *Epidermophyton*, and *Microsporum* spp. and yeasts such as *C. albicans*. On the other hand, they also exhibit activity against yeasts that cause systemic infections, including *C. immitis*, *C. neoformans*, *Paracoccidioides brasiliensis*, *Petriellidium boydii*, *B. dermatitidis*, and *H. capsulatum*.

MECHANISM OF ACTION

The effects of the azoles on fungal biochemistry have been studied extensively, but there is still much to be learned.[45] At

high in vitro concentrations (micromolar), the azoles are fungicidal; at low in vitro concentrations (nanomolar), they are fungistatic. The fungicidal effect is clearly associated with damage to the cell membrane, with the loss of essential cellular components such as potassium ions and amino acids. The fungistatic effect of the azoles at low concentration has been associated with inhibition of membrane-bound enzymes. A cytochrome P450-class enzyme, lanosterol 14α-demethylase, is the likely target for the azoles.[46] P450 possesses a heme moiety as part of its structure (Fig. 6.5), and the basic electron pairs of the azole rings can occupy a binding site on P450, preventing the enzyme from turning over. The function of lanosterol 14α-demethylase is to oxidatively remove a methyl group from lanosterol during ergosterol biosynthesis.

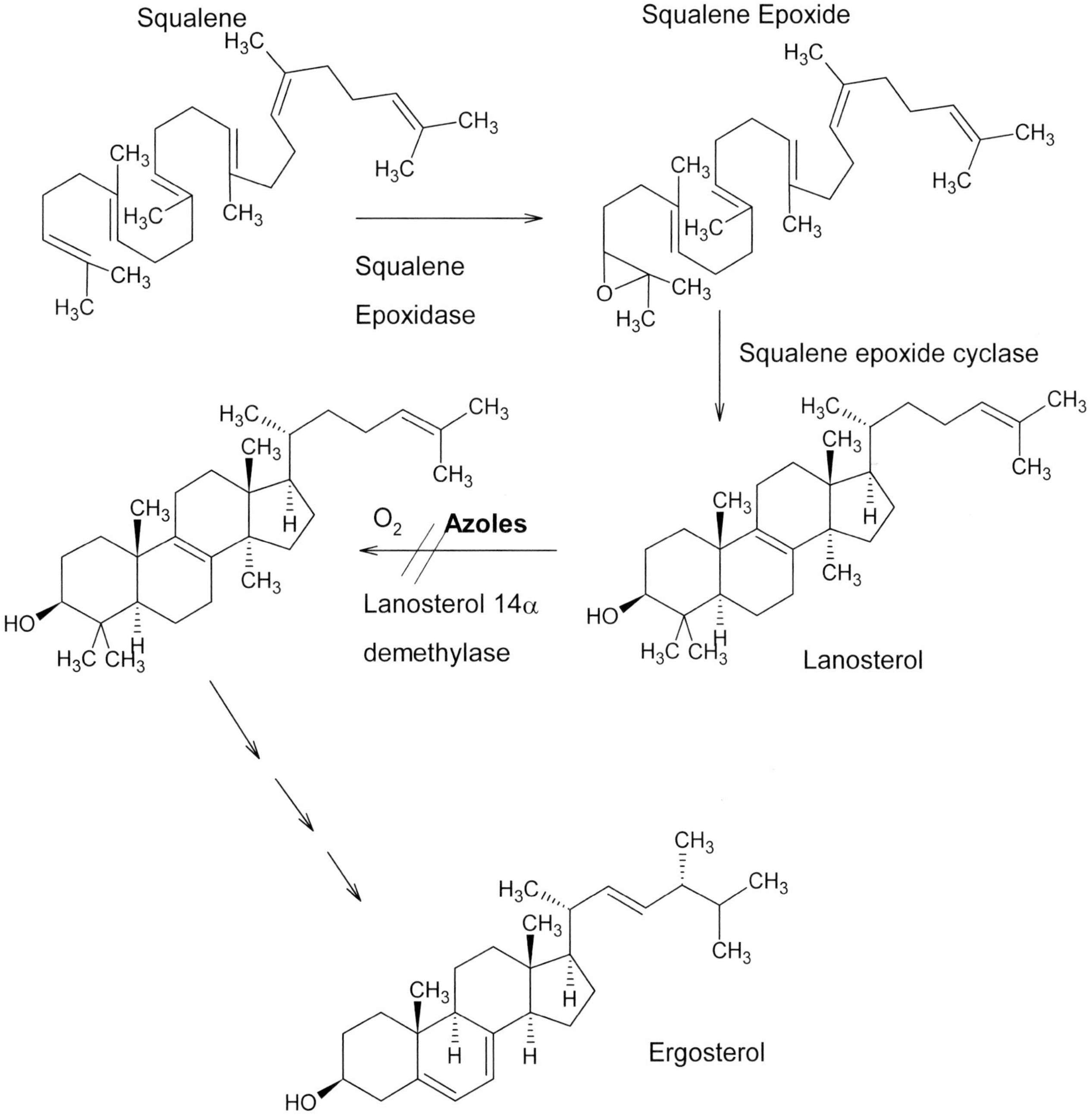

Figure 6.5 ● The inhibitory action of azole antifungal agents on the lanosterol 14-α-demethylase reaction.

When demethylation is inhibited, the 14α-sterol accumulates in the membrane, causing destabilization. As this happens, repair mechanisms, such as chitin synthesis, are initiated to patch the damage. This degrades membrane function further. Lanosterol 14α-demethylase is also required for mammalian biosynthesis of cholesterol, and the azoles are known to inhibit cholesterol biosynthesis.[47] In general, higher concentrations of the azoles are needed to inhibit the mammalian enzyme. This provides selectivity for antifungal action. The 1,2,4-triazoles appear to cause a lower incidence of endocrine effects and hepatotoxicity than the corresponding imidazoles, possibly because of a lower affinity for the mammalian cytochrome P450 enzymes involved.[48] The primary mode of resistance to the triazoles and imidazoles in *C. albicans* is the development of mutations in *ERG 11*, the gene coding for C14-α-sterol demethylase. These mutations appear to protect heme in the enzyme pocket from binding to azole but allow access of the natural substrate of the enzyme, lanosterol. Cross-resistance is conferred to all azoles. Increased azole efflux by the ATP-binding cassette (ABC-1, which normally transports cholesterol) and major facilitator superfamily transporters can add to fluconazole resistance in *C. albicans* and *C. glabrata*. Increased production of C14-α-sterol demethylase could be another cause of resistance.

STRUCTURE–ACTIVITY RELATIONSHIPS

The basic structural requirement for members of the azole class is a weakly basic imidazole or 1,2,4-triazole ring (pK$_a$ of 6.5–6.8) bonded by a nitrogen–carbon linkage to the rest of the structure. At the molecular level, the amidine nitrogen atom (N-3 in the imidazoles, N-4 in the triazoles) is believed to bind to the heme iron of enzyme-bound cytochrome P450 to inhibit activation of molecular oxygen and prevent oxidation of steroidal substrates by the enzyme. The most potent antifungal azoles possess two or three aromatic rings, at least one of which is halogen substituted (e.g., 2,4-dichlorophenyl, 4-chlorophenyl, 2,4-difluorophenyl), and other nonpolar functional groups. Only 2, and/or 2,4 substitution yields effective azole compounds. The halogen atom that yields the most potent compounds is fluorine, although functional groups such as sulfonic acids have been shown to do the same. Substitution at other positions of the ring yields inactive compounds. Presumably, the large nonpolar portion of these molecules mimics the nonpolar steroidal part of the substrate for lanosterol 14α-demethylase, lanosterol, in shape and size.

The nonpolar functionality confers high lipophilicity to the antifungal azoles. The free bases are typically insoluble in water but are soluble in most organic solvents, such as ethanol. Fluconazole, which possesses two polar triazole moieties, is an exception, in that it is sufficiently water soluble to be injected intravenously as a solution of the free base.

PRODUCTS

Clotrimazole

1-(*o*-Chloro-α,α-diphenylbenzyl)imidazole (Lotrimin, Gyne-Lotrimin, Mycelex) is a broad-spectrum antifungal drug that is used topically for the treatment of tinea infections and candidiasis. It occurs as a white crystalline solid that is sparingly soluble in water but soluble in alcohol and most organic solvents. It is a weak base that can be solubilized by dilute mineral acids.

Clotrimazole is available as a solution in polyethylene glycol 400, a lotion, and a cream in a concentration of 1%. These are all indicated for the treatment of tinea pedis, tinea cruris, tinea capitis, tinea versicolor, or cutaneous candidiasis. A 1% vaginal cream and tablets of 100 mg and 500 mg are available for vulvovaginal candidiasis. Clotrimazole is extremely stable, with a shelf life of more than 5 years.

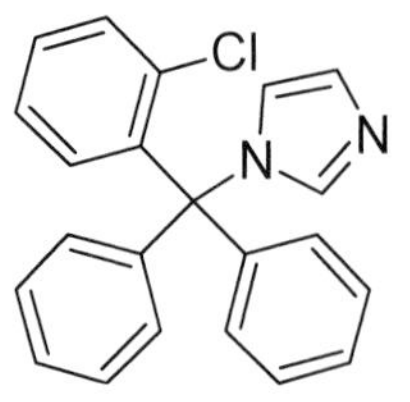

Although clotrimazole is effective against various pathogenic yeasts and is reasonably well absorbed orally, it causes severe gastrointestinal disturbances. It is also extensively protein bound and, hence, is not considered optimally bioavailable. Clotrimazole is not considered suitable for the treatment of systemic infections.

Econazole Nitrate

1-[2-[(4-Chlorophenyl)methoxy]-2-(2,4-dichlorophenyl)-ethyl]-1*H*-imidazole (Spectazole) is a white crystalline nitric acid salt of econazole. It is only slightly soluble in water and most organic solvents.

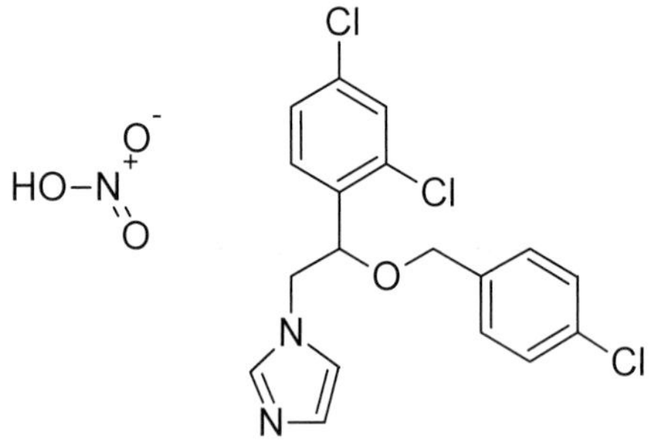

Econazole is used as a 1% cream for the topical treatment of local tinea infections and cutaneous candidiasis.

Butoconazole Nitrate

1-[4-(4-Chlorophenyl)-2-[(2,6-dichlorophenyl)-thio]butyl]-1*H*-imidazole (Femstat) is an extremely broad-spectrum antifungal drug that is specifically effective against *C. albicans*. It is supplied as a vaginal cream containing 2% of the salt. It is intended for the treatment of vaginal candidiasis.

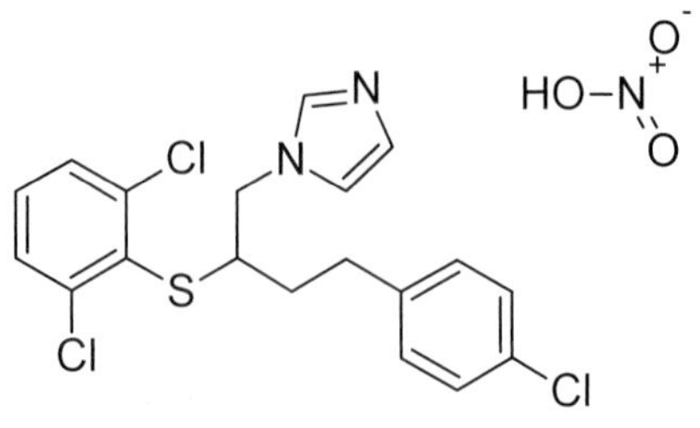

Sulconazole Nitrate

1-[2,4-Dichloro-β-[*p*-chlorobenzyl)thio]phenethyl]imidazole mononitrate (Exelderm) is the white crystalline nitric acid salt of sulconazole. It is sparingly soluble in water but soluble in ethanol. The salt is used in a solution and a cream in 1% concentration for the treatment of local tinea infections, such as jock itch, athlete's foot, and ringworm.

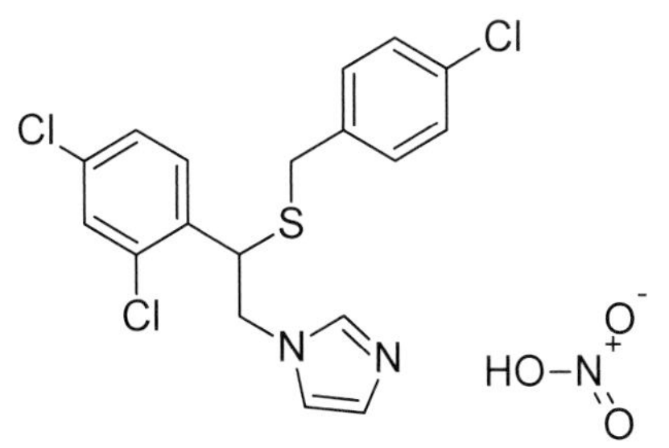

Oxiconazole Nitrate

(Z)-1-(2,4-dichlorophenyl)-2-(1*H*-imidazol-1-yl)ethanone-*O*-[2,4-dichlorophenyl)methyl]oxime mononitrate (Oxistat) is a white crystalline nitric acid salt. It is used in cream and lotion dosage forms in 1% concentration for the treatment of tinea pedis, tinea corporis, and tinea capitis.

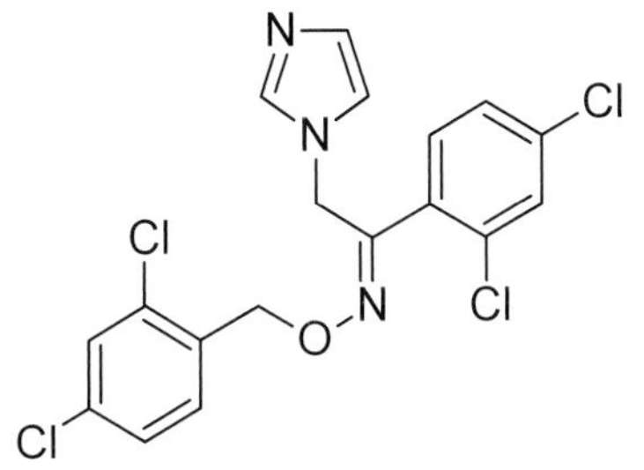

Tioconazole

1-[2-[(2-chloro-3-thienyl)methoxy]2-(2,4-dichlorophenyl)-ethyl]-1*H*-imidazole (Vagistat) is used for the treatment of vulvovaginal candidiasis. A vaginal ointment containing 6.5% of the free base is available. Tioconazole is more effective against *Torulopsis glabrata* than are other azoles.

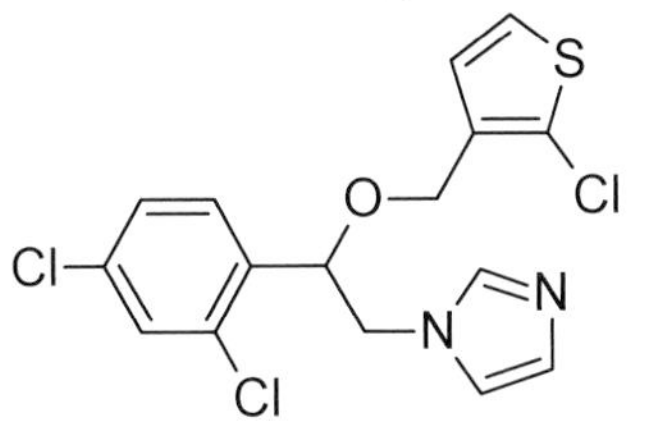

Miconazole Nitrate

1-[2-(2,4-Dichlorophenyl)-2-[2,4-dichlorophenyl]-methoxy]ethyl]-1*H*-imidazole mononitrate (Monistat, Micatin) is a weak base with a pK$_a$ of 6.65. The nitric acid salt occurs as white crystals that are sparingly soluble in water and most organic solvents.

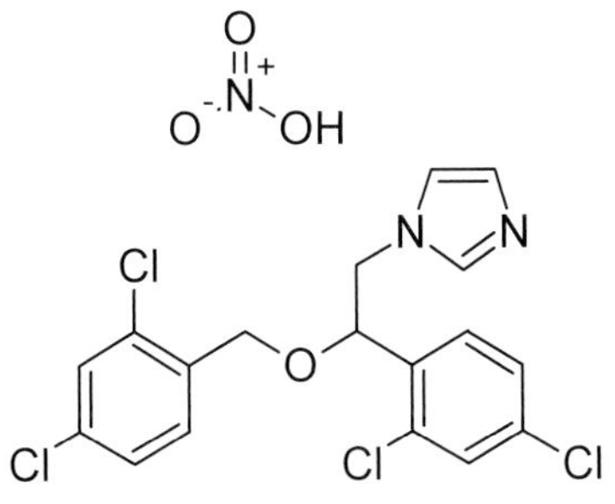

The free base is available in an injectable form, solubilized with polyethylene glycol and castor oil, and intended for the treatment of serious systemic fungal infections, such as candidiasis, coccidioidomycosis, cryptococcosis, petriellidiosis, and paracoccidioidomycosis. It may also be used for the treatment of chronic mucocutaneous candidiasis. Although serious toxic effects from the systemic administration of miconazole are comparatively rare, thrombophlebitis, pruritus, fever, and gastrointestinal upset are relatively common.

Miconazole nitrate is supplied in various dosage forms (cream, lotion, powder, and spray) for the treatment of tinea infections and cutaneous candidiasis. Vaginal creams and suppositories are also available for the treatment of vaginal candidiasis. A concentration of 2% of the salt is used in most topical preparations.

Ketoconazole

1-Acetyl-4-[4-[[2-(2,4-dichlorophenyl)-2(1*H*-imidazole-1-ylmethyl)-1,3-dioxolan-4-yl]methoxy]phenyl]piperazine (Nizoral) is a broad-spectrum imidazole antifungal agent that is administered orally for the treatment of systemic fungal infections. It is a weakly basic compound that occurs as a white crystalline solid that is very slightly soluble in water.

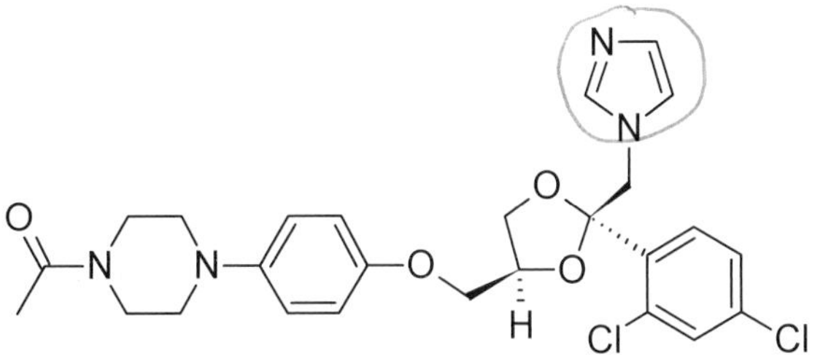

The oral bioavailability of ketoconazole depends on an acidic pH for dissolution and absorption. Antacids and drugs such as H$_2$-histamine antagonists and anticholinergics that inhibit gastric secretion interfere with its oral absorption. Ketoconazole is extensively metabolized to inactive metabolites, and the primary route of excretion is enterohepatic. It is estimated to be 95% to 99% bound to protein in the plasma.

Hepatotoxicity, primarily of the hepatocellular type, is the most serious adverse effect of ketoconazole. Ketoconazole is known to inhibit cholesterol biosynthesis,[47] suggesting that lanosterol 14α-demethylase is inhibited in mammals as well as in fungi. High doses have also been reported to lower testosterone and corticosterone levels, reflecting the inhibition of cytochrome P450-requiring enzymes involved in human steroid hormone biosynthesis.[48] Cytochrome P450 oxidases responsible for the metabolism of various drugs may also be inhibited by ketoconazole to cause enhanced effects. Thus, ketoconazole causes clinically significant increases in plasma concentrations of cyclosporine, phenytoin, and terfenadine. It may also enhance responses to sulfonylurea hypoglycemic and coumarin anticoagulant drugs.

Ketoconazole is a racemic compound, consisting of the *cis*-2*S*,4*R* and *cis*-2*R*,4*S* isomers. An investigation of the relative potencies of the four possible diastereomers of ketoconazole against rat lanosterol 14α-demethylase[49] indicated that the 2*S*,4*R* isomer was 2.5 times more active than its 2*R*,4*S* enantiomer. The *trans*-isomers, 2*S*,4*S* and 2*R*,4*R*, are much less active.[49]

Ketoconazole is recommended for the treatment of the following systemic fungal infections: candidiasis (including oral thrush and the chronic mucocutaneous form), coccidioidomycosis, blastomycosis, histoplasmosis, chromomycosis, and paracoccidioidomycosis. It is also used orally to treat severe refractory cutaneous dermatophytic infections not responsive to topical therapy or oral griseofulvin. The antifungal actions of ketoconazole and the polyene antibiotic amphotericin B are reported to antagonize each other.

Ketoconazole is also used topically in a 2% concentration in a cream and in a shampoo for the management of cutaneous candidiasis and tinea infections.

Terconazole

cis-1-[4-[[2-(2,4-Dichlorophenyl)-2-(1*H*-1,2,4-triazol-1-ylmethyl)-1,3-dioxolan-4-yl]methoxy]phenyl]-4-(1 methylethyl)piperazine (Terazol), or terconazole, is a triazole derivative that is used exclusively for the control of vulvovaginal moniliasis caused by *C. albicans* and other *Candida* species. It is available in creams containing 0.4% and 0.8% of the free base intended for 7-day and 3-day treatment periods, respectively. Suppositories containing 80 mg of the free base are also available.

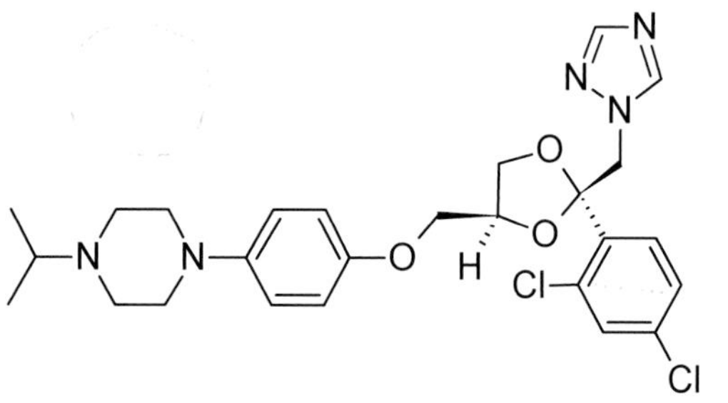

Itraconazole

4-[4-[4-[4-[[2-(2,4-Dichlorophenyl)-2-1*H*-1,2,4-triazol-1-ylmethyl)-1,3-dioxolan-4-yl]methoxy]phenyl]-1-piperazinyl]phenyl]-2,4-dihydro-2-(1-methylpropyl)-3*H*-1,2,4-triazol-3-one (Sporanox) is a unique member of the azole class that contains two triazole moieties in its structure, a weakly basic 1,2,4-triazole and a nonbasic 1,2,4-triazol-3-one.

Itraconazole is an orally active, broad-spectrum antifungal agent that has become an important alternative to ketoconazole. An acidic environment is required for optimum solubilization and oral absorption of itraconazole. Drugs such as H$_2$-histamine antagonists and antacids, which

reduce stomach acidity, reduce its gastrointestinal absorption. Food greatly enhances the absorption of itraconazole, nearly doubling its oral bioavailability. The drug is avidly bound to plasma proteins (nearly 99% at clinically effective concentrations) and extensively metabolized in the liver. Only one of the numerous metabolites, namely 1-hydroxyitraconazole, has significant antifungal activity. Virtually none of the unchanged drug is excreted in the urine. Thus, the dosage need not be adjusted in patients with renal impairment. The terminal elimination half-life of itraconazole ranges from 24 to 40 hours.

The primary indications for itraconazole are for the treatment of systemic fungal infections including blastomycosis, histoplasmosis (including patients infected with human immunodeficiency virus [HIV]), nonmeningeal coccidioidomycosis, paracoccidioidomycosis, and sporotrichosis. It may also be effective in the treatment of pergellosis, disseminated and deep organ candidiasis, coccidioidal meningitis, and cryptococcosis.

In general, itraconazole is more effective and better tolerated than is ketoconazole. Unlike ketoconazole, it is not hepatotoxic and does not cause adrenal or testicular suppression in recommended therapeutic doses.[14] Nonetheless, itraconazole can inhibit cytochrome P450 oxidases involved in drug and xenobiotic metabolism and is known to increase plasma levels of the antihistaminic drugs terfenadine and astemizole.

Fluconazole

α-(2,4-Difluorophenyl)-α-(1*H*-1,2,4-triazol-1-ylmethyl)-1*H*-1,2,4-triazole-1-ethanol or 2,4-difluoro-α,α-bis(1*H*-1,2,4-triazol-1-ylmethyl)benzyl alcohol (Diflucan) is a water-soluble bis-triazole with broad-spectrum antifungal properties that is suitable for both oral and intravenous administration as the free base. Intravenous solutions of fluconazole contain 2 mg of the free base in 1 mL of isotonic sodium chloride or 5% dextrose vehicle.

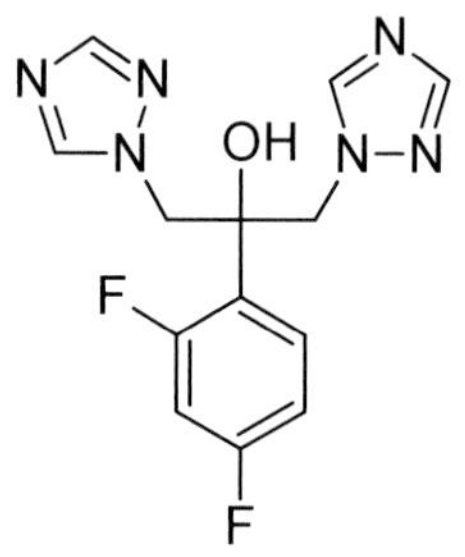

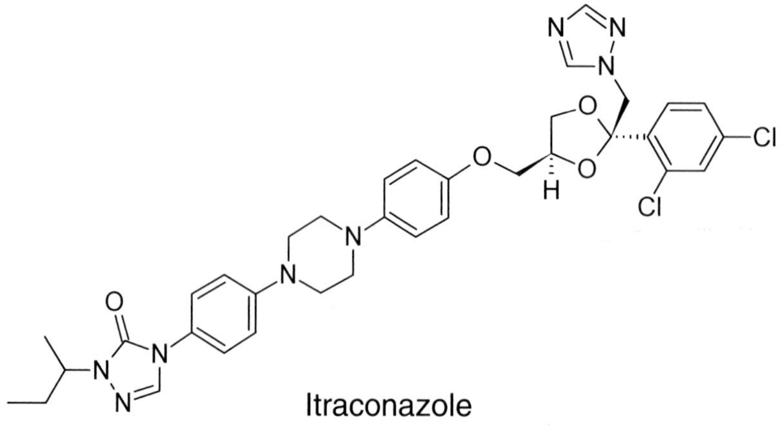

Itraconazole

The oral bioavailability of fluconazole, following administration of either tablet or oral suspension dosage forms, is excellent. Apparently, the presence of two weakly basic triazole rings in the molecule confers sufficient aqueous solubility to balance the lipophilicity of the 2,4-difluorophenyl group. The oral absorption of fluconazole, in contrast to the oral absorption of ketoconazole or itraconazole, is not affected by alteration in gastrointestinal acidity or the presence of food.

Fluconazole has a relatively long elimination half-life, ranging from 27 to 34 hours. It penetrates well into all body cavities, including the CSF. Plasma protein binding of fluconazole is less than 10%; the drug is efficiently removed from the blood by hemodialysis. Fluconazole experiences little or no hepatic metabolism and is excreted substantially unchanged in the urine. A small amount of unchanged fluconazole (~10%) is excreted in the feces. Side effects of fluconazole are largely confined to minor gastrointestinal symptoms. Inhibition of cytochrome P450 oxidases by fluconazole can give rise to clinically significant interactions involving increased plasma levels of cyclosporine, phenytoin, and the oral hypoglycemic drugs (tolbutamide, glipizide, and glyburide). Fluconazole does not appear to interfere with corticosteroid or androgen biosynthesis in dosages used to treat systemic fungal infections.

Fluconazole is recommended for the treatment and prophylaxis of disseminated and deep organ candidiasis. It is also used to control esophageal and oropharyngeal candidiasis. Because of its efficient penetration into CSF, fluconazole is an agent of choice for the treatment of cryptococcal meningitis and for prophylaxis against cryptococcosis in AIDS patients. Although fluconazole is generally less effective than either ketoconazole or itraconazole against nonmeningeal coccidioidomycosis, it is preferred therapy for coccidioidal meningitis. Fluconazole lends itself to one-dose therapies for vaginal candidiasis.

NEWER ANTIFUNGAL STRATEGIES

A newer azole is voriconazole.[50]

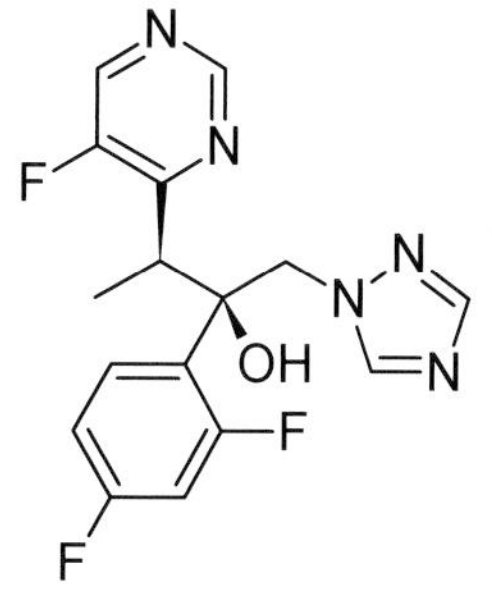

Unlike fluconazole, voriconazole has potent activity against a broad variety of fungi, including the clinically important pathogens. Several publications have substantiated the use of voriconazole against some of the newer and rarer fungal pathogens. Voriconazole is more potent than itraconazole against *Aspergillus* spp. and is comparable to posaconazole,[50] another azole that is in clinical trials, in its activity against *C. albicans*. In general, *Candida* spp. that are less susceptible to fluconazole possess higher MICs to voriconazole. The in vitro activity of posaconazole appears to be similar to that of voriconazole. Posaconazole is now in phase III clinical trials, and evidence of the efficacy of posaconazole against various fungal models, especially the rarer ones, continues to accumulate. Posaconazole exhibits high oral bioavailability, but its low water solubility makes its formulation into an intravenous solution impossible.

A search for potential prodrug forms of posaconazole has yielded a possible candidate, SCH 59884. The compound is inactive in vitro but is dephosphorylated in vivo to yield the active 4-hydroxybutyrate ester. This compound is hydrolyzed to the parent compound in the serum. Posaconazole undergoes extensive enterohepatic recycling, and most of the dose is eliminated in the bile and feces.

Syn2869 is a novel broad-spectrum compound that contains the piperazine-phenyl-triazolone side chain common to itraconazole and posaconazole, and it displays potency and an antifungal spectrum similar to those of the latter. Syn2869 demonstrates better activity than itraconazole in animal models of *C. albicans*, *C. glabrata*, and *C. neoformans*. The oral bioavailability (F) is 60%, and higher

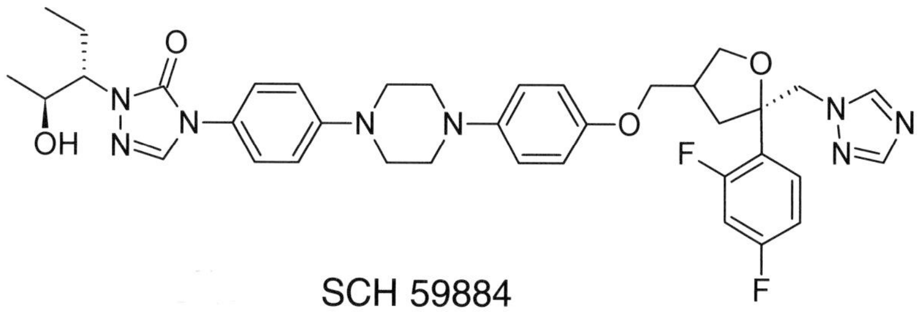

SCH 59884

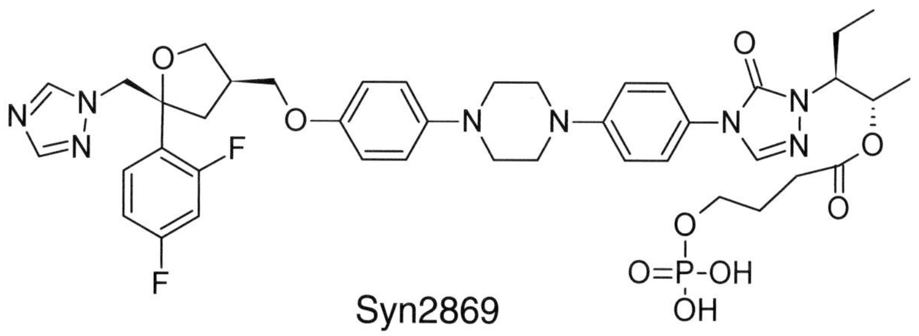

Syn2869

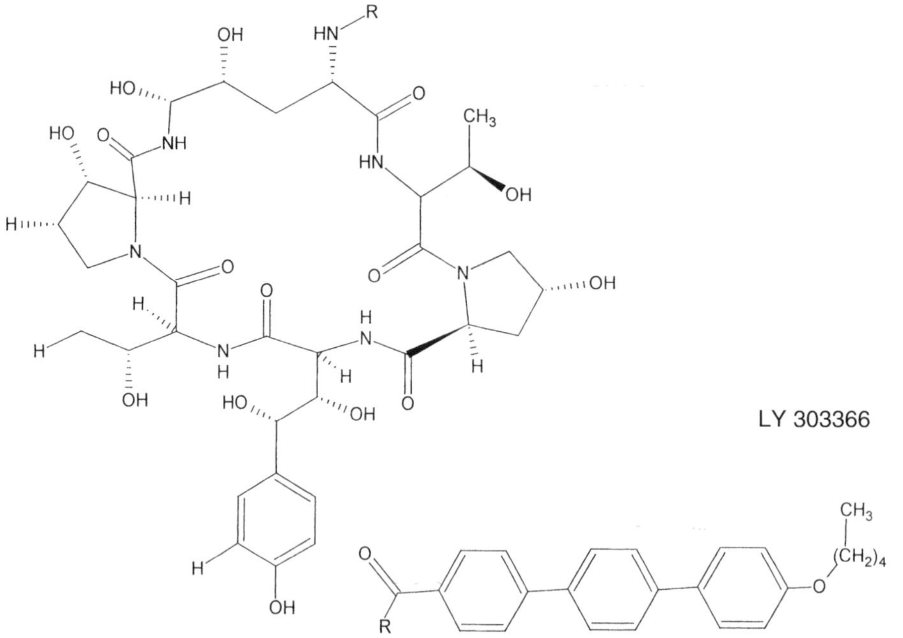

LY 303366

tissue-to-serum ratios than those found for itraconazole were claimed to contribute to the greater efficacy of the compound in a model of invasive pulmonary aspergillosis. Syn2869 also demonstrates considerable activity against the common mold pathogens.

ECHINOCANADINS AND PNEUMOCANADINS

Echinocanadins[51] and the closely related pneumocanadins[52] are natural products that were discovered in the 1970s. They act as noncompetitive inhibitors of (1,3)-β-d-glucan synthase,[53] an enzyme complex that forms stabilizing glucan polymers in the fungal cell wall. Three water-soluble derivatives of the echinocanadins and pneumocanadins are in endstage clinical development but have not yet been marketed.

LY 303366 is a pentyloxyterphenyl side chain derivative of echinocanadin B that was discovered at Eli Lilly. It was licensed for parenteral use in 2000. Studies have shown that the MICs of LY 303366 against *Candida* spp. range from 0.08 to 5.12 μg/mL, and similar activity was obtained against *Aspergillus* spp. Studies show highly potent activity of the compound in animal models of disseminated candidiasis, pulmonary aspergillosis, and esophageal candidiasis.

AUREOBASIDINS[54]

Aureobasidin A is a cyclic depsipeptide that is produced by fermentation in cultures of *Aureobasidium pullulan*. Aureobasidin A acts as a tight-binding noncompetitive inhibitor of the enzyme inositol phosphorylceramide synthase (IPC synthase[55]), which is an essential enzyme for fungal sphingolipid biosynthesis. A unique structural feature of the aureobasidins is the *N*-methylation of four of seven amide nitrogen atoms. The lack of tautomerism dictated by *N*-methylation may contribute to forming a stable solution conformer that is shaped somewhat like an arrowhead, the presumed biologically active conformation of aureobasidin-A.

The pradimycins and benanomycins are naphthacenequinones that bind mannan in the presence of Ca^{2+} to disrupt the cell membrane in pathogenic fungi. Both

demonstrate good in vitro and in vivo activity against *Candida* spp. and *C. neoformans* clinical isolates.

SYNTHETIC ANTIBACTERIAL AGENTS

Several organic compounds obtained by chemical synthesis on the basis of model compounds have useful antibacterial activity for the treatment of local, systemic, and/or urinary tract infections. Some chemical classes of synthetic antibacterial agents include the sulfonamides, certain nitroheterocyclic compounds (e.g., nitrofurans, metronidazole), and the quinolones. Some antibacterial agents that fail to achieve adequate concentrations in the plasma or tissues for the treatment of systemic infections following oral or parenteral administration are concentrated in the urine, where they can be effective for eradicating urinary tract infections. Nitrofurantoin (a nitrofuran), nalidixic acid (a quinolone), and methenamine are examples of such urinary tract antiinfectives.

Quinolones

The quinolones comprise a series of synthetic antibacterial agents patterned after nalidixic acid, a naphthyridine derivative introduced for the treatment of urinary tract infections in 1963. Isosteric heterocyclic groupings in this class include the quinolones (e.g., norfloxacin, ciprofloxacin, lomefloxacin), the naphthyridines (e.g., nalidixic acid, enoxacin), and the cinnolines (e.g., cinoxacin). Up to the present time, the clinical usefulness of the quinolones has been largely confined to the treatment of urinary tract infections. For urinary tract infections, good oral absorption, activity against common Gram-negative urinary pathogens, and comparatively higher urinary (compared with plasma and tissue) concentrations are the key useful properties. As a result of extensive structure–activity investigations leading to compounds with enhanced potency, extended spectrum of activity, and improved absorption and distribution properties, the class has evolved to the point that certain newer members

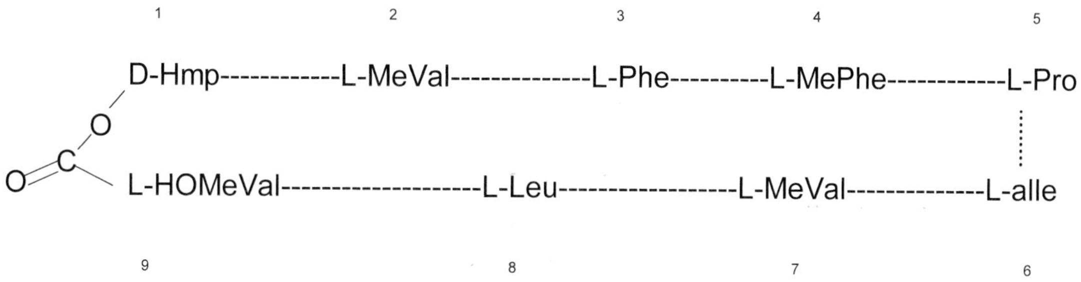

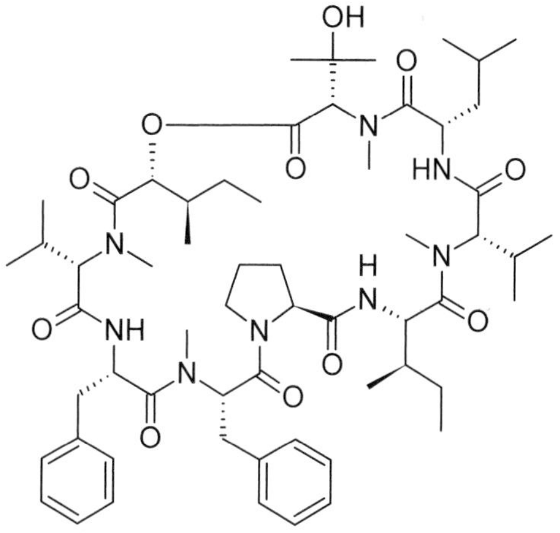

Aureobasidin A

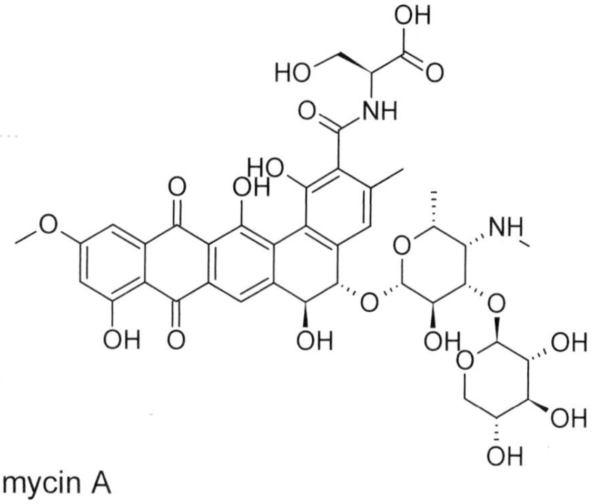

Pradimycin A

Benanomycin A

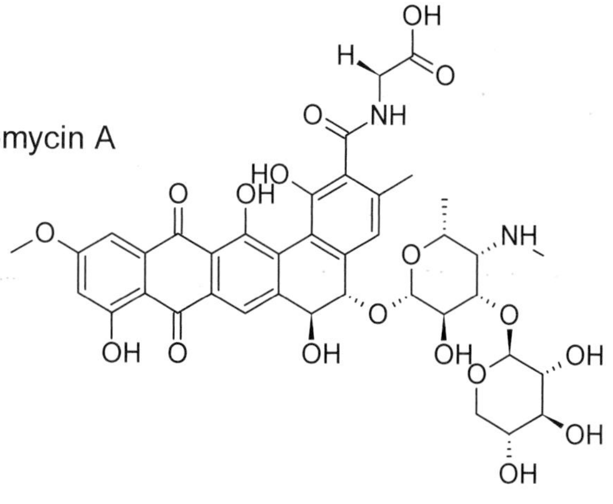

are useful for the treatment of various serious systemic infections. In fact, these more potent analogs are sometimes classified separately (from the urinary tract-specific agents) as the fluoroquinolones, because all members of the group have a 6-fluoro substituent in common.

Structure–activity studies have shown that the 1,4-dihydro-4-oxo-3-pyridinecarboxylic acid moiety is essential for antibacterial activity. The pyridone system must be annulated with an aromatic ring. Isosteric replacements of nitrogen for carbon atoms at positions 2 (cinnolines), 5 (1,5-napthyridines), 6 (1,6-naphthyridines), and 8 (1,8-naphthyridines) are consistent with retention of antibacterial activity. Although the introduction of substituents at position 2 greatly reduces or abolishes activity, positions 5, 6, 7 (especially), and 8 of the annulated ring may be substituted with good effects. For example, piperazinyl and 3-aminopyrrolidinyl substitutions at position 7 have been shown to convey enhanced activity on members of the quinolone class against *P. aeruginosa*. Fluorine atom substitution at position 6 is also associated with significantly enhanced antibacterial activity. Alkyl substitution at the 1-position is essential for activity, with lower alkyl (methyl, ethyl, cyclopropyl) compounds generally having progressively greater potency. Aryl substitution at the 1-position is also consistent with antibacterial activity, with a 2,4-difluorophenyl group providing optimal potency. Ring condensations at the 1,8-, 5,6-, 6,7-, and 7,8-positions also lead to active compounds.

The effective antibacterial spectrum of nalidixic acid and the earliest members of the quinolone class (e.g., oxolinic acid, cinoxacin) are largely confined to Gram-negative bacteria, including common urinary pathogens such as *Escherichia coli, Klebsiella, Enterobacter, Citrobacter,* and *Proteus* spp. *Shigella, Salmonella,* and *Providencia* are also susceptible. Strains of *P. aeruginosa, Neisseria gonorrhoeae,* and *Haemophilus influenzae* are resistant, as are the Gram-positive cocci and anaerobes. Newer members of the class possessing 6-fluoro and 7-piperazinyl substituents exhibit an extended spectrum of activity that includes effectiveness against additional Gram-negative pathogens (e.g., *P. aeruginosa, H. influenzae, N. gonorrhoeae*), Gram-positive cocci (e.g., *S. aureus*), and some streptococci. The quinolones generally exhibit poor activity against most anaerobic bacteria, including most *Bacteroides* and *Clostridium* species. In many cases, bacterial strains that have developed resistance to the antibacterial antibiotics, such as penicillin-resistant gonococci, methicillin-resistant *S. aureus*, and aminoglycoside-resistant *P. aeruginosa* are susceptible to the quinolones.

The bactericidal action of nalidixic acid and its congeners is known to result from the inhibition of DNA synthesis. This effect is believed to be caused by the inhibition of bacterial DNA gyrase (topoisomerase II), an enzyme responsible for introducing negative supercoils into circular duplex DNA.[56] Negative supercoiling relieves the torsional stress of helical DNA, facilitates unwinding, and, thereby, allows transcription and replication to occur. Although nalidixic acid inhibits gyrase activity, it binds only to single-stranded DNA and not to either the enzyme or double-helical DNA.[56] Bacterial DNA gyrase is a tetrameric enzyme consisting of two A and two B subunits, encoded by the *gyrA* and *gyrB* genes. Bacterial strains resistant to the quinolones have been identified, with decreased binding affinity to the enzyme because of amino acid substitution in either A or B subunits resulting from mutations in either *gyrA*[57] or *gyrB*[58] genes.

The highly polar quinolones are believed to enter bacterial cells through densely charged porin channels in the outer bacterial membrane. Mutations leading to altered porin proteins can lead to decreased uptake of quinolones and cause resistance.[59] Also, there is evidence for energy-dependent efflux of quinolones by some bacterial species. A quantitative structure–activity relationship (QSAR) study of bacterial cellular uptake of a series of quinolones[60] revealed an inverse relationship of uptake versus log *P* (a measure of lipophilicity) for Gram-negative bacteria, on the one hand, but a positive correlation of quinolone uptake to log *P* in Gram-positive bacteria, on the other. This result probably reflects the observed differences in outer envelope structures of Gram-negative and Gram-positive bacteria.[61]

The incidence (relatively low, <1%) of CNS effects associated with the quinolones (e.g., irritability, tremor, sleep disorders, vertigo, anxiety, agitation, convulsions) has been attributed to antagonism of γ-aminobutyric acid (GABA) receptors in the brain by the quinolones. Only fluoroquinolones having a 1-piperidino, a 3-amino-1-pyrrolidino, or similar basic moiety at the 7-position appear to have this property.[61] The low incidence of CNS effects for most quinolones is apparently because of their inability to penetrate the blood-brain barrier.

Another property of the quinolone class is phototoxicity, extreme sensitivity to sunlight. Quinolones possessing a halogen atom at the 8-position (e.g., lomefloxacin) have the highest incidence of phototoxicity, whereas those having an amino (e.g., sparfloxacin) or methoxy group at either the 5- or 8-position have the lowest incidence.[61]

The antibacterial quinolones can be divided into two classes on the basis of their dissociation properties in physiologically relevant conditions. The first class, represented by nalidixic acid, oxolinic acid (no longer marketed in the United States), and cinoxacin, possesses only the 3-carboxylic acid group as an ionizable functionality. The pK_a values for the 3-carboxyl group in nalidixic acid and other quinolone antibacterial drugs fall in the range of 5.6 to 6.4 (Table 6.6).[62] These comparatively high pK_a values relative to the pK_a of 4.2 for benzoic acid are attributed to the acid-weakening effect of hydrogen bonding of the 3-carboxyl group to the adjacent 4-carbonyl group.[62]

The second class of antibacterial quinolones embraces the broad-spectrum fluoroquinolones (namely, norfloxacin, enoxacin, ciprofloxacin, ofloxacin, lomefloxacin, and sparfloxacin), all of which possess, in addition to the 3-carboxylic acid group, a basic piperazino functionality at the 7-position and a 6-fluoro substituent. The pK_a values for the

pyridone

TABLE 6.6 Dissociation and Isoelectric Constants for Antibacterial Quinolones

Quinolone	$pK_1{}^a$	$pK_2{}^a$	pI^a	$QH^{+/-}/QH^0$
Nalidixic acid	6.03	—	—	—
Norfloxacin	6.39	8.56	7.47	118
Enoxacin	6.15	8.54	7.35	238
Ciprofloxacin	6.08	8.73	7.42	444
Ofloxacin	5.88	8.06	6.97	146
Lomefloxacin	5.65	9.04	7.35	3,018

Data are taken from Ross, D. L., and Riley, C. M.: J. Pharm. Biomed. Anal. 12: 1325, 1994.
[a]Each value represents an average of literature values.

more basic nitrogen atom of the piperazino group fall in the range of 8.1 to 9.3 (Table 6.6).[62] At most physiologically relevant pH values, significant dissociation of both the 3-carboxylic acid and the basic 7-(1-piperazino) groups occurs, leading to significant fractions of zwitterionic species. As an example, the dissociation equilibria for norfloxacin are illustrated in Figure 6.6.[62,63]

The tendency for certain fluoroquinolones (e.g., norfloxacin, ciprofloxacin) in high doses to cause crystalluria in alkaline urine is, in part, caused by the predominance of the comparatively less soluble zwitterionic form. Solubility data presented for ofloxacin in the 15th edition of the *USP* dramatically illustrate the effect of pH on water solubility of compounds of the fluoroquinolone class. Thus, the solubility of ofloxacin in water is 60 mg/mL at pH values ranging from 2 to 5, falls to 4 mg/mL at pH 7 (near the isoelectric point, pI), and rises to 303 mg/mL at pH 9.8.

The excellent chelating properties of the quinolones provide the basis for their incompatibility with antacids,

hematinics, and mineral supplements containing divalent or trivalent metals. The quinolones may form 1:1, 2:1, or 3:1 chelates with metal ions such as Ca^{+2}, Mg^{+2}, Zn^{+2}, Fe^{+2}, Fe^{+3}, and Bi^{+3}. The stoichiometry of the chelate formed depends on various factors, such as the relative concentrations of chelating agent (quinolone) and metal ion present, the valence (or charge) on the metal ion, and the pH. Since such chelates are often insoluble in water, coincidental oral administration of a quinolone with an antacid, a hematinic, or a mineral supplement can significantly reduce the oral bioavailability of the quinolone. As an example, the insoluble 2:1 chelate formed between ciprofloxacin and magnesium ion is shown in Figure 6.7. The presence of divalent ions (such as Mg^{+2}) in the urine may also contribute to the comparatively lower solubility of certain fluoroquinolones in urine than in plasma.

Nalidixic Acid

1-Ethyl-1,4-dihydro-7-methyl-4-oxo-1,8-naphthyridine-3-carboxylic acid (NegGram) occurs as a pale buff crystalline

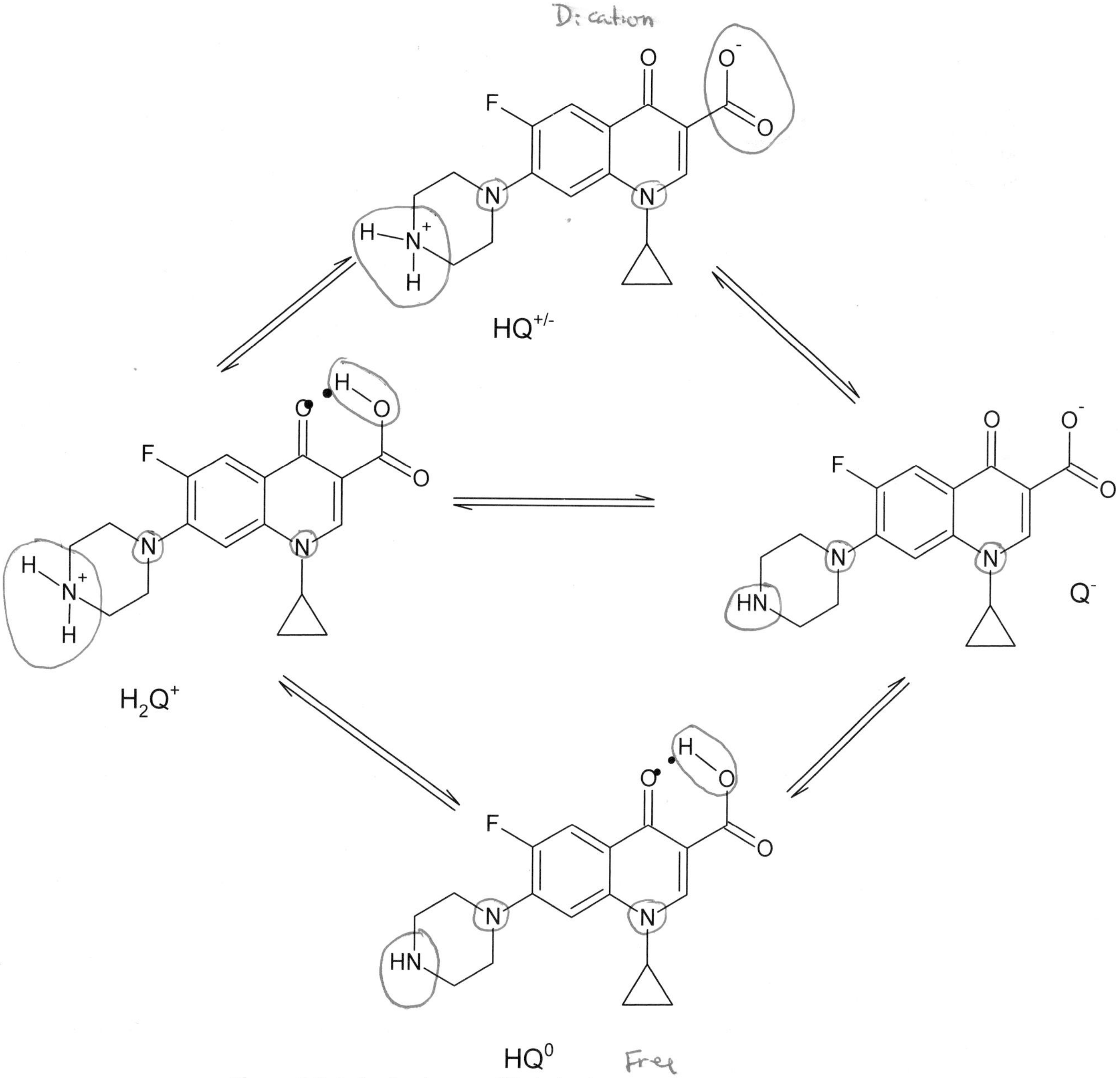

Figure 6.6 ● Ionization equilibria in the quinolone antibacterial drugs.

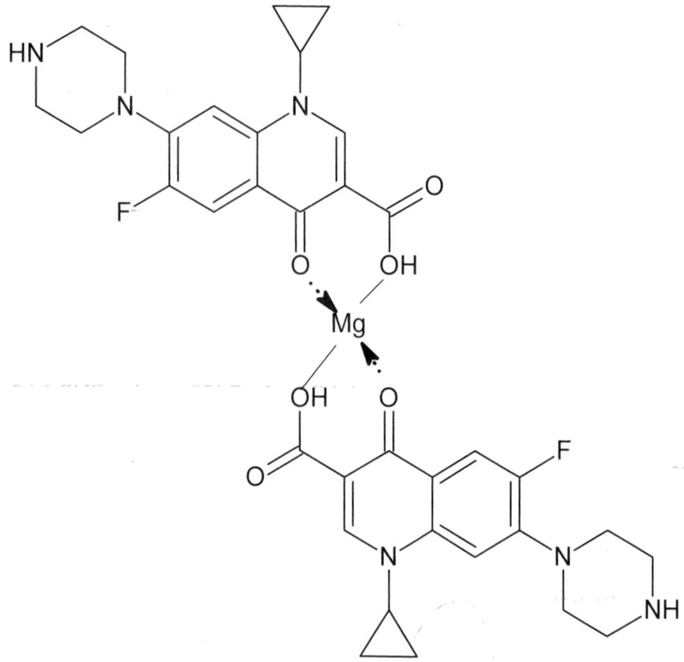

Figure 6.7 • A 2:1 chelate of a Mg^{2+} ion by ciprofloxacin.

powder that is sparingly soluble in water and ether but soluble in most polar organic solvents.

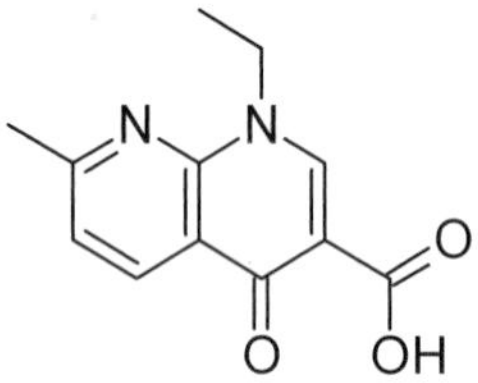

Nalidixic acid is useful in the treatment of urinary tract infections in which Gram-negative bacteria predominate. The activity against indole-positive *Proteus* spp. is particularly noteworthy, and nalidixic acid and its congeners represent important alternatives for the treatment of urinary tract infections caused by strains of these bacteria resistant to other agents. Nalidixic acid is rapidly absorbed, extensively metabolized, and rapidly excreted after oral administration. The 7-hydroxymethyl metabolite is significantly more active than the parent compound. Further metabolism of the active metabolite to inactive glucuronide and 7-carboxylic acid metabolites also occurs. Nalidixic acid possesses a $t_{1/2elim}$ of 6 to 7 hours. It is eliminated, in part, unchanged in the urine and 80% as metabolites.

Cinoxacin

1-Ethyl-1,4-dihydro-4-oxo[1,3]dioxolo[4,5g]cinnoline-3-carboxylic acid (Cinobac) is a close congener (isostere) of oxolinic acid (no longer marketed in the United States) and has antibacterial properties similar to those of nalidixic and oxolinic acids.

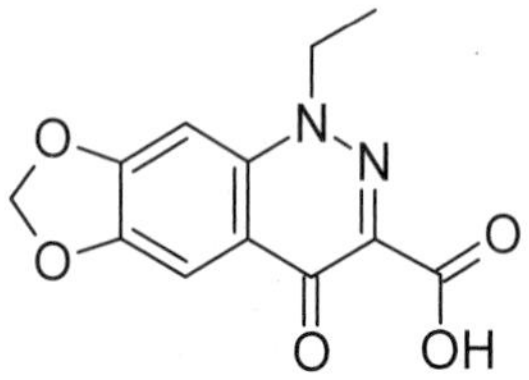

It is recommended for the treatment of urinary tract infections caused by strains of Gram-negative bacteria susceptible to these agents. Early clinical studies indicate that the drug possesses pharmacokinetic properties superior to those of either of its predecessors. Thus, following oral administration, higher urinary concentrations of cinoxacin than of nalidixic acid or oxolinic acid are achieved. Cinoxacin appears to be more completely absorbed and less protein bound than nalidixic acid.

Norfloxacin

1-Ethyl-6-fluoro-1,4-dihydro-4-oxo-7-(1-piperazinyl)-3-quinolinecarboxylic acid (Noroxin) is a pale yellow crystalline powder that is sparingly soluble in water. This quinoline has broad-spectrum activity against Gram-negative and Gram-positive aerobic bacteria. The fluorine atom provides increased potency against Gram-positive organisms, whereas the piperazine moiety improves antipseudomonal activity. Norfloxacin is indicated for the treatment of urinary tract infections caused by *E. coli*, *K. pneumoniae*, *Enterobacter cloacae*, *Proteus mirabilis*, indole-positive *Proteus* spp., including *P. vulgaris*, *Providencia rettgeri*, *Morganella morganii*, *P. aeruginosa*, *S. aureus*, and *S. epidermidis*, and group-D streptococci. It is generally not effective against obligate anaerobic bacteria. Norfloxacin in a single 800-mg oral dose has also been approved for the treatment of uncomplicated gonorrhea. The oral absorption of norfloxacin is about 40%. The drug is 15% protein bound and is metabolized in the liver. The $t_{1/2elim}$ is 4 to 8 hours. Approximately 30% of a dose is eliminated in the urine and feces.

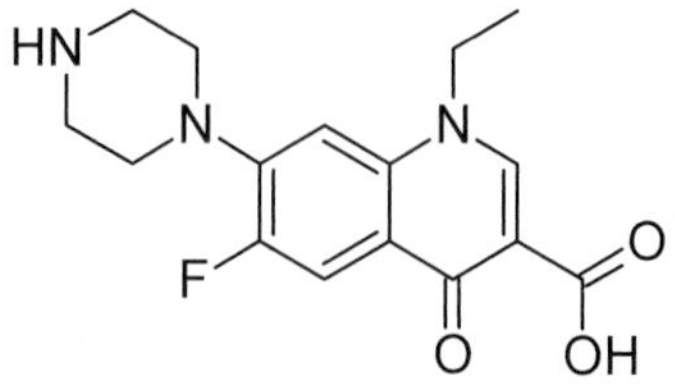

The oral absorption of norfloxacin is rapid and reasonably efficient. Approximately 30% of an oral dose is excreted in the urine in 24 hours, along with 5% to 8% consisting of less active metabolites. There is significant biliary excretion, with about 30% of the original drug appearing in the feces.

Enoxacin

1-Ethyl-6-fluoro-1,4-dihydro-4-oxo-7-(1-piperazinyl)-1,8-naphthyridine-3-carboxylic acid (Penetrex) is a quinolone with broad-spectrum antibacterial activity that is used primarily for the treatment of urinary tract infections and sexually transmitted diseases. Enoxacin has been approved for the treatment of uncomplicated gonococcal urethritis and has also been shown to be effective in chancroid caused by *Haemophilus ducreyi*. A single 400-mg dose is used for these indications. Enoxacin is also approved for the treatment of acute (uncomplicated) and chronic (complicated) urinary tract infections.

Enoxacin is well absorbed following oral administration. Oral bioavailability approaches 98%. Concentrations of the drug in the kidneys, prostate, cervix, fallopian tubes, and myometrium typically exceed those in the plasma. More than 50% of the unchanged drug is excreted in the urine. Metabolism, largely catalyzed by cytochrome P450 enzymes in the liver, accounts for 15% to 20% of the orally administered dose of enoxacin. The relatively short elimination half-life of enoxacin dictates twice-a-day dosing for the treatment of urinary tract infections.

Some cytochrome P450 isozymes, such as CYP 1A2, are inhibited by enoxacin, resulting in potentially important interactions with other drugs. For example, enoxacin has been reported to decrease theophylline clearance, causing increased plasma levels and increased toxicity. Enoxacin forms insoluble chelates with divalent metal ions present in antacids and hematinics, which reduce its oral bioavailability.

Ciprofloxacin

1-Cyclopropyl0-6-fluoro-1,4-dihydro-4-oxo-7-(1-piperazinyl)-3-quinolinecarboxylicacid (Cipro, Cipro IV) is supplied in both oral and parenteral dosage forms. The hydrochloride salt is available in 250-, 500-, and 750-mg tablets for oral administration. Intravenous solutions containing 200 mg and 400 mg are provided in concentrations of 0.2% in normal saline and 1% in 5% dextrose solutions.

The bioavailability of ciprofloxacin following oral administration is good, with 70% to 80% of an oral dose being absorbed. Food delays, but does not prevent, absorption. Significant amounts (20%–35%) of orally administered ciprofloxacin are excreted in the feces, in part because of biliary excretion. Biotransformation to less active metabolites accounts for about 15% of the administered drug. Approximately 40% to 50% of unchanged ciprofloxacin is excreted in the urine following oral administration. This value increases to 50% to 70% when the drug is injected intravenously. Somewhat paradoxically, the elimination half-life of ciprofloxacin is shorter following oral administration ($t_{1/2}$, 4 hours) than it is following intravenous administration ($t_{1/2}$, 5–6 hours). Ciprofloxacin inhibits the P450 species CYP 1A2.

The oral dose of this quinolone is typically 25% higher than the parenteral dose for a given indication. Probenecid significantly reduces the renal clearance of ciprofloxacin, presumably by inhibiting its active tubular secretion. Ciprofloxacin is widely distributed to virtually all parts of the body, including the CSF, and is generally considered to provide the best distribution of the currently marketed quinolones. This property, together with the potency and broad antibacterial spectrum of ciprofloxacin, accounts for the numerous therapeutic indications for the drug. Ciprofloxacin also exhibits higher potency against most Gram-negative bacterial species, including *P. aeruginosa*, than other quinolones.

Ciprofloxacin is an agent of choice for the treatment of bacterial gastroenteritis caused by Gram-negative bacilli such as enteropathogenic *E. coli, Salmonella* spp. (including *S. typhi*), *Shigella* spp., *Vibrio* spp., and *Aeromonas hydrophilia*. It is widely used for the treatment of respiratory tract infections and is particularly effective for controlling bronchitis and pneumonia caused by Gram-negative bacteria. Ciprofloxacin is also used for combating infections of the skin, soft tissues, bones, and joints. Both uncomplicated and complicated urinary tract infections caused by Gram-negative bacteria can be treated effectively with ciprofloxacin. It is particularly useful for the control of chronic infections characterized by renal tissue involvement. The drug also has important applications in controlling venereal diseases. A combination of ciprofloxacin with the cephalosporin antibiotic ceftriaxone is recommended as the treatment of choice for disseminated gonorrhea, whereas a single-dose treatment with ciprofloxacin plus doxycycline, a tetracycline antibiotic (Chapter 8), can usually eradicate gonococcal urethritis. Ciprofloxacin has also been used for chancroid. The drug has been approved for postexposure treatment of inhalational anthrax.

Injectable forms of ciprofloxacin are incompatible with drug solutions that are alkaline because of the reduced solubility of the drug at pH 7. Thus, intravenous solutions should not be mixed with solutions of ticarcillin sodium, mezlocillin sodium, or aminophylline. Ciprofloxacin may also induce crystalluria under the unusual circumstance that urinary pH rises above 7 (e.g., with the use of systemic alkalinizers or a carbonic anhydrase inhibitor or through the action of urease elaborated by certain species of Gram-negative bacilli).

Ofloxacin

9-Fluoro-2,3-dihydro-3-methyl-10(4-methyl-1-piperazin-yl)-7-oxo-7*H*-pyrido[1,2,3-de]-1,4,-benzoxazine-6-carboxylic acid (Floxin, Floxin IV) is a member of the quinolone class of antibacterial drugs wherein the 1- and 8-positions are joined in the form of a 1,4-oxazine ring.

Ofloxacin resembles ciprofloxacin in its antibacterial spectrum and potency. Like ciprofloxacin, this quinolone is also widely distributed into most body fluids and tissues. In fact, higher concentrations of ofloxacin are achieved in CSF than can be obtained with ciprofloxacin. The oral bioavailability of ofloxacin is superior (95%–100%) to that of ciprofloxacin, and metabolism is negligible (~3%). The amount of an administered dose of ofloxacin excreted in the urine in a 24- to 48-hour period ranges from 70% to 90%. There is relatively little biliary excretion of this quinolone. Although food can slow the oral absorption of ofloxacin, blood levels following oral or intravenous administration are comparable. The elimination half-life of ofloxacin ranges from 4.5 to 7 hours.

Ofloxacin has been approved for the treatment of infections of the lower respiratory tract, including chronic bronchitis and pneumonia, caused by Gram-negative bacilli. It is also used for the treatment of pelvic inflammatory disease and is highly active against both gonococci and chlamydia. In common with other fluoroquinolones, ofloxacin is not effective in the treatment of syphilis. A single 400-mg oral dose of ofloxacin in combination with the tetracycline antibiotic doxycycline is recommended by the Centers for Disease Control and Prevention (CDC) for the outpatient treatment of acute gonococcal urethritis. Ofloxacin is also used for the treatment of urinary tract infections caused by Gram-negative bacilli and for prostatitis caused by *E. coli*. Infections of the skin and soft tissues caused by staphylococci, streptococci, and Gram-negative bacilli may also be treated with ofloxacin.

Because ofloxacin has an asymmetric carbon atom in its structure, it is obtained and supplied commercially as a racemate. The racemic mixture has been resolved, and the enantiomers independently synthesized and evaluated for antibacterial activity.[64] The 3S(−) isomer is substantially more active (8–125 times, depending on the bacterial species) than the 3R(+) isomer and has recently been marketed as levofloxacin (Levaquin) for the same indications as the racemate.

Lomefloxacin

1-Ethyl-6,8-difluoro-1,4-dihydro-7-(3-methyl-1-piperazinyl)-4-oxo-3-quinolinecarboxylic acid (Maxaquin) is a difluorinated quinolone with a longer elimination half-life (7–8 hours) than other members of its class. It is the only quinolone for which once-daily oral dosing suffices. The oral bioavailability of lomefloxacin is estimated to be 95% to 98%. Food slows, but does not prevent, its oral absorption. The extent of biotransformation of lomefloxacin is only about 5%, and high concentrations of unchanged drug, ranging from 60% to 80%, are excreted in the urine. The comparatively long half-life of lomefloxacin is apparently because of its excellent tissue distribution and renal reabsorption and not

because of plasma protein binding (only ~10%) or enterohepatic recycling (biliary excretion is estimated to be ~10%).

Lomefloxacin has been approved for two primary indications. First, it is indicated for acute bacterial exacerbations of chronic bronchitis caused by *H. influenzae* or *Moraxella (Branhamella) catarrhalis*, but not if *Streptococcus pneumoniae* is the causative organism. Second, it is used for prophylaxis of infection following transurethral surgery. Lomefloxacin also finds application in the treatment of acute cystitis and chronic urinary tract infections caused by Gram-negative bacilli.

Lomefloxacin reportedly causes the highest incidence of phototoxicity (photosensitivity) of the currently available quinolones. The presence of a halogen atom (fluorine, in this case) at the 8-position has been correlated with an increased chance of phototoxicity in the quinolones.[40]

Sparfloxacin

Sparfloxacin, (*cis*)-5-amino-1-cyclopropyl-7-(3,5-dimethyl)-1-piperazinyl)-6,8-difluoro-1,4-dihydro-4-oxo-3-quinolinecarboxylic acid, is a newer fluoroquinolone.

This compound exhibits higher potency against Gram-positive bacteria, especially staphylococci and streptococci, than the fluoroquinolones currently marketed. It is also more active against chlamydia and the anaerobe *Bacteroides fragilis*. The activity of sparfloxacin against Gram-negative bacteria is also very impressive, and it compares favorably with ciprofloxacin and ofloxacin in potency against *Mycoplasma* spp., *Legionella* spp., *Mycobacteria* spp., and *Listeria monocytogenes*. Sparfloxacin has a long elimination half-life of 18 hours, which permits once-a-day dosing for most indications. The drug is widely distributed into most fluids and tissues. Effective concentrations of sparfloxacin are achieved for the treatment of skin and soft tissue infections, lower respiratory infections (including bronchitis and bacterial pneumonias), and pelvic inflammatory disease caused by gonorrhea and chlamydia. Sparfloxacin has also been recommended for the treatment of bacterial gastroenteritis and cholecystitis. The oral bioavailability of sparfloxacin is claimed to be good, and sufficient unchanged drug is excreted to be effective for the treatment of urinary tract infections. Nearly 20% of an orally administered dose is excreted as an inactive glucuronide.

The incidence of phototoxicity of sparfloxacin is the lowest of the fluoroquinolones, because of the presence of the 5-amino group, which counteracts the effect of the 8-fluoro substituent.

Levofloxacin

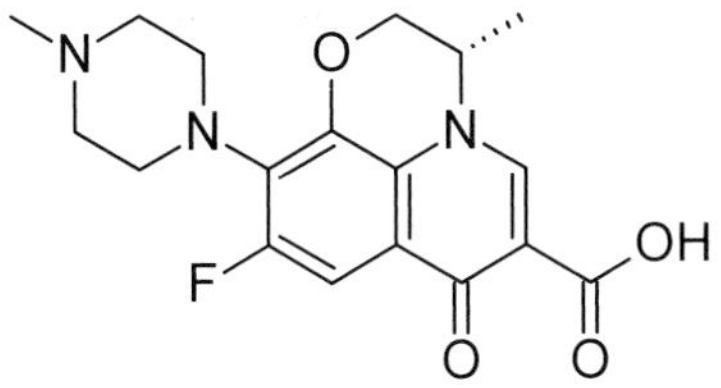

Nitrofurans

The first nitroheterocyclic compounds to be introduced into chemotherapy were the nitrofurans. Three of these compounds—nitrofurazone, furazolidone, and nitrofurantoin—have been used for the treatment of bacterial infections of various kinds for nearly 50 years. A fourth nitrofuran, nifurtimox, is used as an antiprotozoal agent to treat trypanosomiasis and leishmaniasis. Another nitroheterocyclic of considerable importance is metronidazole, which is an amebicide (a trichomonicide) and is used for the treatment of systemic infections caused by anaerobic bacteria. This important drug is discussed later in this chapter.

The nitrofurans are derivatives of 5-nitro-2-furaldehyde, formed on reaction with the appropriate hydrazine or amine derivative. Antimicrobial activity is present only when the nitro group is in the 5-position.

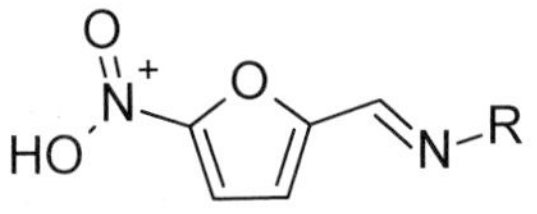

Nitrofurazone R=

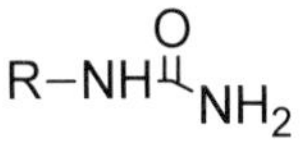

Furazolidone R=

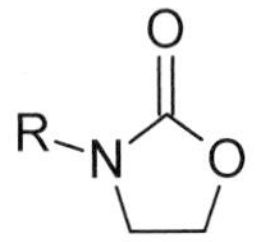

Nitrofurantoin R=

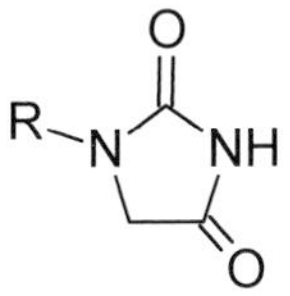

The mechanism of antimicrobial action of the nitrofurans has been extensively studied, but it still is not fully understood. In addition to their antimicrobial actions, the nitrofurans are known to be mutagenic and carcinogenic under certain conditions. It is thought that DNA damage caused by metabolic reaction products may be involved in these cellular effects.

Nitrofurazone

5-Nitro-2-furaldehyde semicarbazone (Furacin) occurs as a lemon-yellow crystalline solid that is sparingly soluble in water and practically insoluble in organic solvents. Nitrofurazone is chemically stable, but moderately light sensitive.

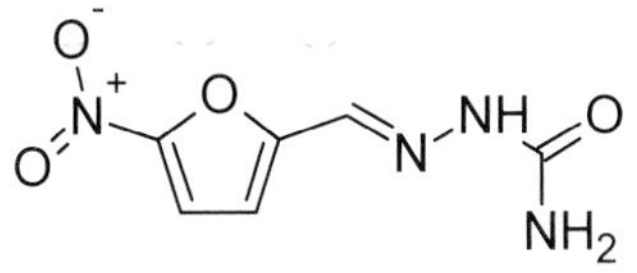

It is used topically in the treatment of burns, especially when bacterial resistance to other agents may be a concern. It may also be used to prevent bacterial infection associated with skin grafts. Nitrofurazone has a broad spectrum of activity against Gram-positive and Gram-negative bacteria, but it is not active against fungi. It is bactericidal against most bacteria commonly causing surface infections, including *S. aureus*, *Streptococcus* spp., *E. coli*, *Clostridium perfringens*, *Enterobacter* (*Aerobacter*) *aerogenes*, and *Proteus* spp.; however, *P. aeruginosa* strains are resistant.

Nitrofurazone is marketed in solutions, ointments, and suppositories in a usual concentration of 0.2%.

Furazolidone

3-[(5-Nitrofurylidene)amino]-2-oxazolidinone (Furoxone) occurs as a yellow crystalline powder with a bitter aftertaste. It is insoluble in water or alcohol. Furazolidone has bactericidal activity against a relatively broad range of intestinal pathogens, including *S. aureus*, *E. coli*, *Salmonella*, *Shigella*, *Proteus* spp., *Enterobacter*, and *Vibrio cholerae*. It is also active against the protozoan *Giardia lamblia*. It is recommended for the oral treatment of bacterial or protozoal diarrhea caused by susceptible organisms. The usual adult dosage is 100 mg 4 times daily.

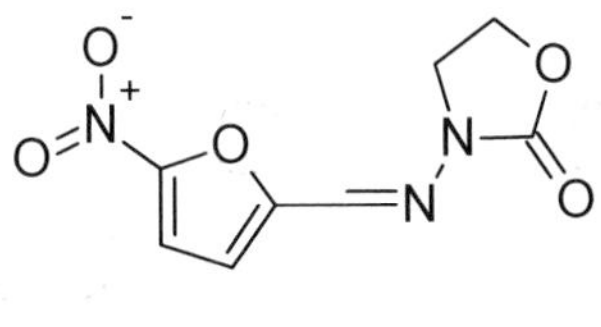

Only a small fraction of an orally administered dose of furazolidone is absorbed. Approximately 5% of the oral dose is detectable in the urine in the form of several metabolites. Some gastrointestinal distress has been reported with its use. Alcohol should be avoided when furazolidone is being used because the drug can inhibit aldehyde dehydrogenase.

Nitrofurantoin

Nitrofurantoin, 1-(5-nitro-2-furfurylidene)-1-aminohydantoin (Furadantin, Macrodantin), is a nitrofuran derivative that is suitable for oral use. It is recommended for the treatment of urinary tract infections caused by susceptible strains of *E. coli*, enterococci, *S. aureus*, *Klebsiella*, *Enterobacter*, and *Proteus* spp. The most common side effects are gastrointestinal (anorexia, nausea, and vomiting); however, hypersensitivity reactions (pneumonitis, rashes, hepatitis, and hemolytic anemia) have occasionally been observed. A macrocrystalline form (Macrodantin) is claimed to improve

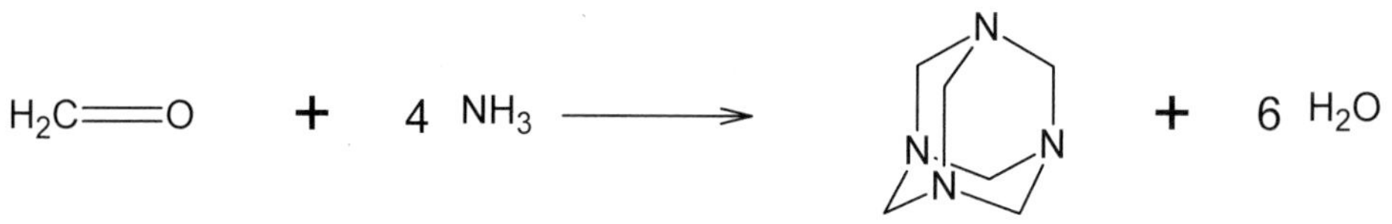

$$H_2C = O \quad + \quad 4 \ NH_3 \longrightarrow \quad + \quad 6 \ H_2O$$

gastrointestinal tolerance without interfering with oral absorption.

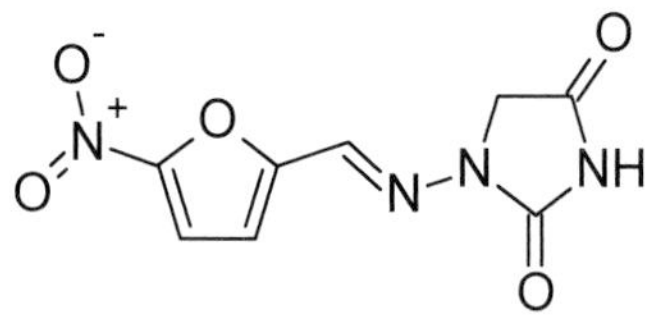

Methenamine and Its Salts

Methenamine

The activity of hexamethylenetetramine (Urotropin, Uritone) depends on the liberation of formaldehyde. The compound is prepared by evaporating a solution of formaldehyde and strong ammonia water to dryness.

The free base exists as an odorless, white crystalline powder that sublimes at about 260°C. It dissolves in water to form an alkaline solution and liberates formaldehyde when warmed with mineral acids. Methenamine is a weak base with a pK_a of 4.9.

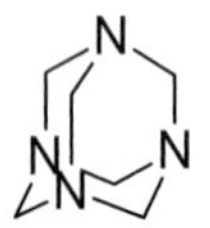

Methenamine is used internally as a urinary antiseptic for the treatment of chronic urinary tract infections. The free base has practically no bacteriostatic power; formaldehyde release at the lower pH of the kidney is required. To optimize the antibacterial effect, an acidifying agent such as sodium biphosphate or ammonium chloride generally accompanies the administration of methenamine.

Certain bacterial strains are resistant to the action of methenamine because they elaborate urease, an enzyme that hydrolyzes urea to form ammonia. The resultant high urinary pH prevents the activation of methenamine, rendering it ineffective. This problem can be overcome by the coadministration of the urease inhibitor acetohydroxamic acid (Lithostat).

Methenamine Mandelate

Hexamethylenetetramine mandelate (Mandelamine) is a white crystalline powder with a sour taste and practically no odor. It is very soluble in water and has the advantage of providing its own acidity, although in its use, the custom is to carry out a preliminary acidification of the urine for 24 to 36 hours before administration.

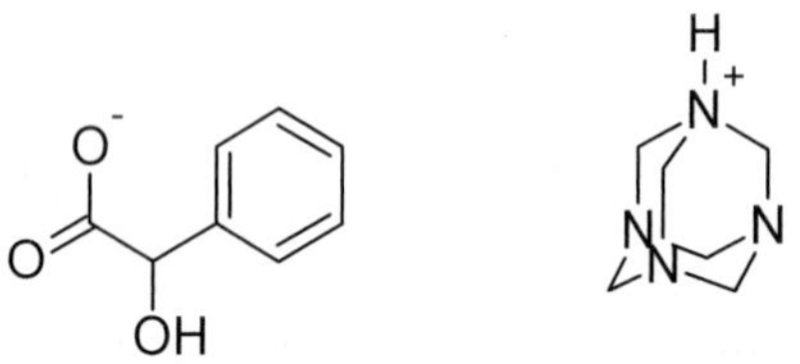

Methenamine Hippurate

Methenamine hippurate (Hiprex) is the hippuric acid salt of methenamine. It is readily absorbed after oral administration and is concentrated in the urinary bladder, where it exerts its antibacterial activity. Its activity is increased in acid urine.

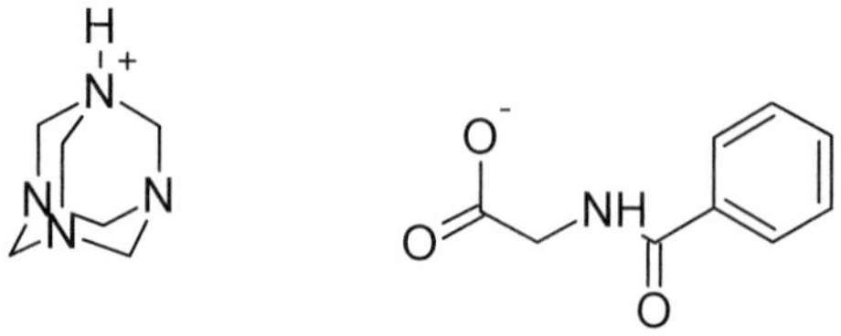

Urinary Analgesics

Pain and discomfort frequently accompany bacterial infections of the urinary tract. For this reason, certain analgesic agents, such as the salicylates or phenazopyridine, which concentrate in the urine because of their solubility properties, are combined with a urinary anti-infective agent.

Phenazopyridine Hydrochloride

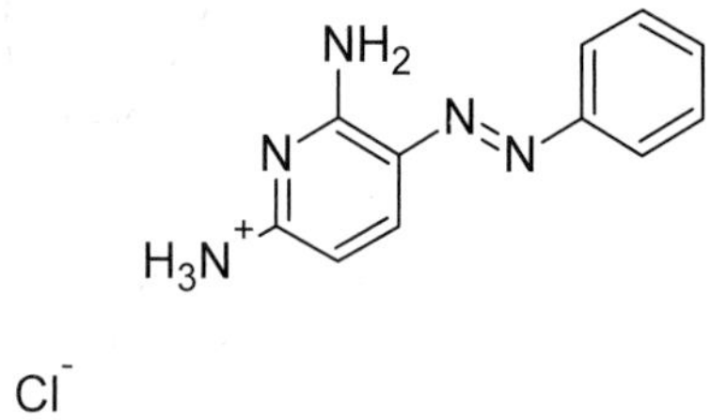

Phenazopyridine hydrochloride, 2,6-diamino-3-(phenylazopyridine hydrochloride (Pyridium), is a brick-red, fine crystalline powder. It is slightly soluble in alcohol, in chloroform, and in water.

Phenazopyridine hydrochloride was formerly used as a urinary antiseptic. Although it is active in vitro against staphylococci, streptococci, gonococci, and *E. coli*, it has no useful antibacterial activity in the urine. Thus, its present utility lies in its local analgesic effect on the mucosa of the urinary tract.

Usually, phenazopyridine is given in combination with urinary antiseptics. For example, it is available as Azo-Gantrisin, a fixed-dose combination with the sulfonamide antibacterial sulfisoxazole, and as Urobiotic, a combination with the antibiotic oxytetracycline and the sulfonamide sulfamethizole (Chapter 8). The drug is rapidly excreted in the urine, to which it gives an orange-red color. Stains in fabrics may be removed by soaking in a 0.25% solution of sodium dithionite.

Antitubercular Agents

Ever since Koch identified the tubercle bacillus, *Mycobacterium tuberculosis*, there has been keen interest in the development of antitubercular drugs. The first breakthrough in antitubercular chemotherapy occurred in 1938 with the observation that sulfanilamide had weak bacteriostatic properties. Later, the sulfone derivative dapsone (4,4′-diaminodiphenylsulfone) was investigated clinically. Unfortunately, this drug, which is still considered one of the most effective drugs for the treatment of leprosy and also has useful antimalarial properties, was considered too toxic because of the high dosages used. The discovery of the antitubercular activity of the aminoglycoside antibiotic streptomycin by Waksman et al. in 1944 ushered in the modern era of tuberculosis treatment. This development was quickly followed by discoveries of the antitubercular properties of *p*-aminosalicylic acid (PAS) first and then, in 1952, of isoniazid. Later, the usefulness of the synthetic drug ethambutol and, eventually, of the semisynthetic antibiotic rifampin was discovered.

Combination therapy, with the use of two or more antitubercular drugs, has been well documented to reduce the emergence of strains of *M. tuberculosis* resistant to individual agents and has become standard medical practice. The choice of antitubercular combination depends on various factors, including the location of the disease (pulmonary, urogenital, gastrointestinal, or neural), the results of susceptibility tests and the pattern of resistance in the locality, the physical condition and age of the patient, and the toxicities of the individual agents. For some time, a combination of isoniazid and ethambutol, with or without streptomycin, was the preferred choice of treatment among clinicians in this country. However, the discovery of the tuberculocidal properties of rifampin resulted in its replacement of the more toxic antibiotic streptomycin in most regimens. The synthetic drug pyrazinamide, because of its sterilizing ability, is also considered a first-line agent and is frequently used in place of ethambutol in combination therapy. Second-line agents for tuberculosis include the antibiotics cycloserine, kanamycin, and capreomycin and the synthetic compounds ethionamide and PAS.

A major advance in the treatment of tuberculosis was signaled by the introduction of the antibiotic rifampin into therapy. Clinical studies indicated that when rifampin is included in the regimen, particularly in combination with isoniazid and ethambutol (or pyrazinamide), the period required for successful therapy is shortened significantly. Previous treatment schedules without rifampin required maintenance therapy for at least 2 years, whereas those based on the isoniazid–rifampin combination achieved equal or better results in 6 to 9 months.

Once considered to be on the verge of worldwide eradication, as a result of aggressive public health measures and effective chemotherapy, tuberculosis has made a comeback of alarming proportions in recent years.[65] A combination of factors has contributed to the observed increase in tuberculosis cases, including the worldwide AIDS epidemic, the general relaxation of public health policies in many countries, the increased overcrowding and homelessness in major cities, and the increased emergence of multidrug-resistant strains of *M. tuberculosis*.

The development of drugs useful for the treatment of leprosy has long been hampered, in part, by the failure of the causative organism, *Mycobacterium leprae*, to grow in cell culture. However, the recent availability of animal models, such as the infected mouse footpad, now permits in vivo drug evaluations. The increasing emergence of strains of *M. leprae* resistant to dapsone, long considered the mainstay for leprosy treatment, has caused public health officials to advocate combination therapy.

Mycobacteria other than *M. tuberculosis* and *M. leprae*, commonly known as "atypical" mycobacteria, were first established as etiological agents of diseases in the 1950s. Atypical mycobacteria are primarily saprophytic species that are widely distributed in soil and water. Such organisms are not normally considered particularly virulent or infectious. Diseases attributed to atypical mycobacteria are on the increase, however, in large part because of the increased numbers of immunocompromised individuals in the population resulting from the AIDS epidemic and the widespread use of immunosuppressive agents with organ transplantation.

The most common disease-causing species are *Mycobacterium avium* and *Mycobacterium intracellulare*, which have similar geographical distributions, are difficult to distinguish microbiologically and diagnostically, and are thus considered a single complex (MAC). The initial disease attributed to MAC resembles tuberculosis, but skin and musculoskeletal tissues may also become involved. The association of MAC and HIV infection is dramatic. An overwhelming disseminated form of the disease occurs in severely immunocompromised patients, leading to high morbidity and mortality. Another relatively common atypical mycobacterium, *Mycobacterium kansasii*, also causes pulmonary disease and can become disseminated in immunocompromised patients. Patients infected with *M. kansasii* can usually be treated effectively with combinations of antitubercular drugs. MAC infections, in contrast, are resistant to currently available chemotherapeutic agents.

Isoniazid

Isonicotinic acid hydrazide, isonicotinyl hydrazide, or INH (Nydrazid) occurs as a nearly colorless crystalline solid that is very soluble in water. It is prepared by reacting the methyl ester of isonicotinic acid with hydrazine.

Isoniazid is a remarkably effective agent and continues to be one of the primary drugs (along with rifampin, pyrazinamide, and ethambutol) for the treatment of tuberculosis. It is not, however, uniformly effective against all forms of the disease. The frequent emergence of strains of the tubercle bacillus resistant to isoniazid during therapy was seen as the major shortcoming of the drug. This problem has been largely, but not entirely, overcome with the use of combinations.

The activity of isoniazid is manifested on the growing tubercle bacilli and not on resting forms. Its action, which is considered bactericidal, is to cause the bacilli to lose lipid content by a mechanism that has not been fully elucidated. The most generally accepted theory suggests that the principal effect of isoniazid is to inhibit the synthesis of mycolic acids,[66,67] high–molecular-weight, branched β-hydroxy fatty acids that constitute important components of the cell walls of mycobacteria.

A mycobacterial catalase–peroxidase enzyme complex is required for the bioactivation of isoniazid.[68] A reactive species, generated through the action of these enzymes on the drug, is believed to attack a critical enzyme required for mycolic acid synthesis in mycobacteria.[69] Resistance to INH, estimated to range from 25% to 50% of clinical isolates of INH-resistant strains, is associated with loss of catalase and peroxidase activities, both of which are encoded by a single gene, *katG*.[70] The target for the action of INH has recently been identified as an enzyme that catalyzes the NADH-specific reduction of 2-*trans*-enoylacyl carrier protein, an essential step in fatty acid elongation.[71] This enzyme is encoded by a specific gene, *inhA*, in *M. tuberculosis*.[72] Approximately 20% to 25% of INH-resistant clinical isolates display mutations in the *inhA* gene, leading to altered proteins with apparently reduced affinity for the active form of the drug. Interestingly, such INH-resistant strains also display resistance to ethionamide, a structurally similar antitubercular drug.[72] On the other hand, mycobacterial strains deficient in catalase–peroxidase activity are frequently susceptible to ethionamide.

Although treatment regimens generally require long-term administration of isoniazid, the incidence of toxic effects is remarkably low. The principal toxic reactions are peripheral neuritis, gastrointestinal disturbances (e.g., constipation, loss of appetite), and hepatotoxicity. Coadministration of pyridoxine is reported to prevent the symptoms of peripheral neuritis, suggesting that this adverse effect may result from antagonism of a coenzyme action of pyridoxal phosphate. Pyridoxine does not appear to interfere with the antitubercular effect of isoniazid. Severe hepatotoxicity rarely occurs with isoniazid alone; the incidence is much higher, however, when it is used in combination with rifampin.

Isoniazid is rapidly and almost completely absorbed following oral administration. It is widely distributed to all tissues and fluids within the body, including the CSF. Approximately 60% of an oral dose is excreted in the urine within 24 hours in the form of numerous metabolites as well as the unchanged drug. Although the metabolism of isoniazid is very complex, the principal path of inactivation involves acetylation of the primary hydrazine nitrogen. In addition to acetylisoniazid, the isonicotinyl hydrazones of pyruvic and α-ketoglutaric acids, isonicotinic acid, and isonicotinuric acid have been isolated as metabolites in humans.[73] The capacity to inactivate isoniazid by acetylation is an inherited characteristic in humans. Approximately half of persons in the population are fast acetylators (plasma half-life, 45–80 minutes), and the remainder slow acetylators (plasma half-life, 140–200 minutes).

Ethionamide

2-Ethylthioisonicotinamide (Trecator SC) occurs as a yellow crystalline material that is sparingly soluble in water. This nicotinamide has weak bacteriostatic activity in vitro but, because of its lipid solubility, is effective in vivo. In contrast to the isoniazid series, 2-substitution enhances activity in the thioisonicotinamide series.

Ethionamide is rapidly and completely absorbed following oral administration. It is widely distributed throughout the body and extensively metabolized to predominantly inactive forms that are excreted in the urine. Less than 1% of the parent drug appears in the urine.

Ethionamide is considered a secondary drug for the treatment of tuberculosis. It is used in the treatment of isoniazid-resistant tuberculosis or when the patient is intolerant to isoniazid and other drugs. Because of its low potency, the highest tolerated dose of ethionamide is usually recommended. Gastrointestinal intolerance is the most common side effect associated with its use. Visual disturbances and hepatotoxicity have also been reported.

Pyrazinamide

Pyrazinecarboxamide (PZA) occurs as a white crystalline powder that is sparingly soluble in water and slightly soluble in polar organic solvents. Its antitubercular properties were discovered as a result of an investigation of heterocyclic analogs of nicotinic acid, with which it is isosteric. Pyrazinamide has recently been elevated to first-line status in short-term tuberculosis treatment regimens because of its tuberculocidal activity and comparatively low short-term toxicity. Since pyrazinamide is not active against metabolically inactive tubercle bacilli, it is not considered suitable for long-term therapy. Potential hepatotoxicity also obviates long-term use of the drug. Pyrazinamide is maximally effective in the low pH environment that exists in macrophages (monocytes). Evidence suggests bioactivation of pyrazinamide to pyrazinoic acid by an amidase present in mycobacteria.[74]

Because bacterial resistance to pyrazinamide develops rapidly, it should always be used in combination with other drugs. Cross-resistance between pyrazinamide and either isoniazid or ethionamide is relatively rare. The mechanism of action of pyrazinamide is not known. Despite its structural similarities to isoniazid and ethionamide, pyrazinamide apparently does not inhibit mycolic acid biosynthesis in mycobacteria.

Pyrazinamide is well absorbed orally and widely distributed throughout the body. The drug penetrates inflamed meninges and, therefore, is recommended for the treatment of tuberculous meningitis. Unchanged pyrazinamide, the corresponding carboxylic acid (pyrazinoic acid), and the 5-hydroxy metabolite are excreted in the urine. The elimination half-life ranges from 12 to 24 hours, which allows the drug to be administered on either once-daily or even twice-weekly dosing schedules. Pyrazinamide and its metabolites are reported to interfere with uric acid excretion. Therefore, the drug should be used with great caution in patients with hyperuricemia or gout.

Ethambutol

Ethambutol, (+)-2,2′-(ethylenediimino)-di-1-butanol dihydrochloride, or EMB (Myambutol), is a white crystalline powder freely soluble in water and slightly soluble in alcohol.

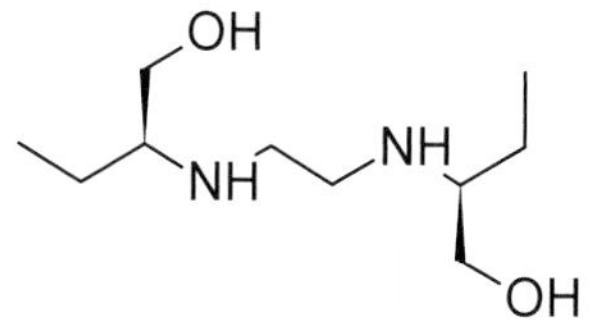

Ethambutol is active only against dividing mycobacteria. It has no effect on encapsulated or other nonproliferating forms. The in vitro effect may be bacteriostatic or bactericidal, depending on the conditions. Its selective toxicity toward mycobacteria appears to be related to the inhibition of the incorporation of mycolic acids into the cell walls of these organisms.

This compound is remarkably stereospecific. Tests have shown that, although the toxicities of the *dextro, levo,* and *meso* isomers are about equal, their activities vary considerably. The *dextro* isomer is 16 times as active as the *meso* isomer. In addition, the length of the alkylene chain, the nature of the branching of the alkyl substituents on the nitrogens, and the extent of *N*-alkylation all have a pronounced effect on the activity.

Ethambutol is rapidly absorbed after oral administration, and peak serum levels occur in about 2 hours. It is rapidly excreted, mainly in the urine. Up to 80% is excreted unchanged, with the balance being metabolized and excreted as 2,2′-(ethylenediimino)dibutyric acid and the corresponding dialdehyde.

Ethambutol is not recommended for use alone, but in combinations with other antitubercular drugs in the chemotherapy of pulmonary tuberculosis.

Aminosalicylic Acid

4-Aminosalicylic acid occurs as a white to yellowish white crystalline solid that darkens on exposure to light or air. It is slightly soluble in water but more soluble in alcohol. Alkali metal salts and the nitric acid salt are soluble in water, but the salts of hydrochloric acid and sulfuric acid are not. The acid undergoes decarboxylation when heated. An aqueous solution has a pH of approximately 3.2.

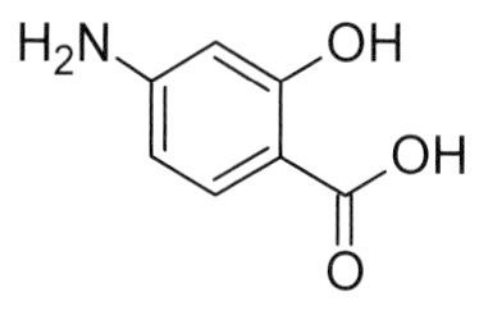

PAS is administered orally in the form of the sodium salt, usually in tablet or capsule form. Symptoms of gastrointestinal irritation are common with both the acid and the sodium salt. Various enteric-coated dosage forms have been used in an attempt to overcome this disadvantage. Other forms that are claimed to improve gastrointestinal tolerance include the calcium salt, the phenyl ester, and a combination with an anion exchange resin (Rezi-PAS). An antacid such as aluminum hydroxide is frequently prescribed.

The oral absorption of PAS is rapid and nearly complete, and it is widely distributed into most of the body fluids and tissues, with the exception of the CSF, in which levels are significantly lower. It is excreted primarily in the urine as both unchanged drug and metabolites. The *N*-acetyl derivative is the principal metabolite, with significant amounts of

the glycine conjugate also being formed. When administered with isoniazid (which also undergoes *N*-acetylation), PAS increases the level of free isoniazid. The biological half-life of PAS is about 2 hours.

The mechanism of antibacterial action of PAS is similar to that of the sulfonamides. Thus, it is believed to prevent the incorporation of *p*-aminobenzoic acid (PABA) into the dihydrofolic acid molecule catalyzed by the enzyme dihydrofolate synthetase. Structure–activity studies have shown that the amino and carboxyl groups must be *para* to each other and free; thus, esters and amides must readily undergo hydrolysis in vivo to be effective. The hydroxyl group may be *ortho* or *meta* to the carboxyl group, but optimal activity is seen in the former.

For many years, PAS was considered a first-line drug for the chemotherapy of tuberculosis and was generally included in combination regimens with isoniazid and streptomycin. However, the introduction of the more effective and generally better tolerated agents, ethambutol and rifampin, has relegated it to alternative drug status.

Aminosalicylate Sodium

Sodium 4-aminosalicylate (sodium PAS), a salt, occurs in the dihydrate form as a yellow-white powder or crystalline solid. It is very soluble in water in the pH range of 7.0 to 7.5, at which it is the most stable. Aqueous solutions decompose readily and darken. Two pH-dependent types of reactions occur: decarboxylation (more rapid at low pH) and oxidation (more rapid at high pH). Therefore, solutions should be prepared within 24 hours of administration.

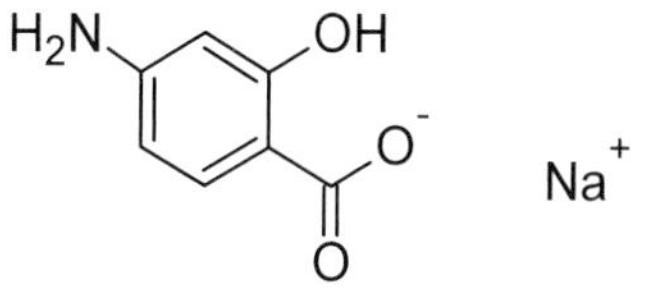

Clofazimine

Clofazimine (Lamprene) is a basic red dye that exerts a slow bactericidal effect on *M. leprae*, the bacterium that causes leprosy. It occurs as a dark red crystalline solid that is insoluble in water.

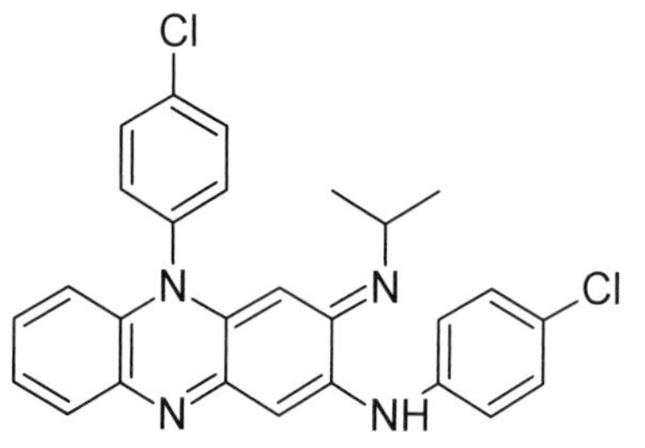

Clofazimine is used in the treatment of lepromatous leprosy, including dapsone-resistant forms of the disease. In addition to its antibacterial action, the drug appears to possess anti-inflammatory and immune-modulating effects that are of value in controlling neuritic complications and in suppressing erythema nodosum leprosum reactions associated with lepromatous leprosy. It is frequently used in combination with other drugs, such as dapsone or rifampin.

The mechanisms of antibacterial and anti-inflammatory actions of clofazimine are not known. The drug is known to bind to nucleic acids and concentrate in reticuloendothelial tissue. It can also act as an electron acceptor and may interfere with electron transport processes.

The oral absorption of clofazimine is estimated to be about 50%. It is a highly lipid-soluble drug that is distributed into lipoidal tissue and the reticuloendothelial system. Urinary excretion of unchanged drug and metabolites is negligible. Its half-life after repeated dosage is estimated to be about 70 days. Severe gastrointestinal intolerance to clofazimine is relatively common. Skin pigmentation, ichthyosis and dryness, rash, and pruritus also occur frequently.

Clofazimine has also been used to treat skin lesions caused by *Mycobacterium ulcerans*.

Antitubercular Antibiotics

RIFAMYCINS

The rifamycins are a group of chemically related antibiotics obtained by fermentation from cultures of *Streptomyces mediterranei*. They belong to a class of antibiotics called the *ansamycins* that contain a macrocyclic ring bridged across two nonadjacent positions of an aromatic nucleus. The term *ansa* means "handle," describing well the topography of the structure. The rifamycins and many of their semisynthetic derivatives have a broad spectrum of antimicrobial activity. They are most notably active against Gram-positive bacteria and *M. tuberculosis*. However, they are also active against some Gram-negative bacteria and many viruses. Rifampin, a semisynthetic derivative of rifamycin B, was released as an antitubercular agent in the United States in 1971. A second semisynthetic derivative, rifabutin, was approved in 1992 for the treatment of atypical mycobacterial infections.

The chemistry of rifamycins and other ansamycins has been reviewed.[75] All of the rifamycins (A, B, C, D, and E) are biologically active. Some of the semisynthetic derivatives of rifamycin B are the most potent known inhibitors of DNA-directed RNA polymerase in bacteria,[76] and their action is bactericidal. They have no activity against the mammalian enzyme. The mechanism of action of rifamycins as inhibitors of viral replication appears to differ from that for their bactericidal action. Their net effect is to inhibit the formation of the virus particle, apparently by preventing a specific polypeptide conversion.[77] Rifamycins bind to the β subunit of bacterial DNA-dependent RNA polymerases to prevent chain initiation.[78] Bacterial resistance to rifampin has been associated with mutations leading to amino acid substitution in the β subunit.[78] A high level of cross-resistance between various rifamycins has been observed.

Rifampin

Rifampin (Rifadin, Rimactane, Rifampicin) is the most active agent in clinical use for the treatment of tuberculosis. A dosage of as little as 5 μg/mL is effective against sensitive strains of *M. tuberculosis*. Rifampin is also highly active against staphylococci and *Neisseria, Haemophilus, Legionella*, and *Chlamydia* spp. Gram-negative bacilli are much less sensitive to rifampin. However, resistance to rifampin develops rapidly in most species of bacteria, including the tubercle bacillus. Consequently, rifampin is used only in combination with other antitubercular drugs, and it is ordinarily not recommended for the treatment of other

bacterial infections when alternative antibacterial agents are available.

Toxic effects associated with rifampin are relatively infrequent. It may, however, interfere with liver function in some patients and should neither be combined with other potentially hepatotoxic drugs nor used in patients with impaired hepatic function (e.g., chronic alcoholics). The incidence of hepatotoxicity was significantly higher when rifampin was combined with isoniazid than when either agent was combined with ethambutol. Allergic and sensitivity reactions to rifampin have been reported, but they are infrequent and usually not serious. Rifampin is a powerful inducer of hepatic cytochrome P450 oxygenases. It can markedly potentiate the actions of drugs that are inactivated by these enzymes. Examples include oral anticoagulants, barbiturates, benzodiazepines, oral hypoglycemic agents, phenytoin, and theophylline.

Rifampin is also used to eradicate the carrier state in asymptomatic carriers of *Neisseria meningitidis* to prevent outbreaks of meningitis in high-risk areas such as military facilities. Serotyping and sensitivity tests should be performed before its use because resistance develops rapidly. However, a daily dose of 600 mg of rifampin for 4 days suffices to eradicate sensitive strains of *N. meningitidis*. Rifampin has also been very effective against *M. leprae* in experimental animals and in humans. When it is used in the treatment of leprosy, rifampin should be combined with dapsone or some other leprostatic agent to minimize the emergence of resistant strains of *M. leprae*.

Other, nonlabeled uses of rifampin include the treatment of serious infections such as endocarditis and osteomyelitis caused by methicillin-resistant *S. aureus* or *S. epidermidis*, Legionnaires disease when resistant to erythromycin, and prophylaxis of *H. influenzae*–induced meningitis.

Rifampin occurs as an orange to reddish brown crystalline powder that is soluble in alcohol but only sparingly soluble in water. It is unstable to moisture, and a desiccant (silica gel) should be included with rifampin capsule containers. The expiration date for capsules stored in this way is 2 years. Rifampin is well absorbed after oral administration to provide effective blood levels for about 8 hours. Food, however, markedly reduces its oral absorption, and rifampin should be administered on an empty stomach. The drug is distributed in effective concentrations to all body fluids and tissues except the brain, despite the fact that it is 70% to 80% protein bound in the plasma. The principal excretory route is through the bile and feces, and high concentrations of rifampin and its primary metabolite, deacetylrifampin, are found in the liver and biliary system. Deacetylrifampin is also biologically active. Equally high concentrations of rifampin are found in the kidneys, and although substantial amounts of the drug are passively reabsorbed in the renal tubules, its urinary excretion is significant. Patients should be made aware that rifampin causes a reddish orange discoloration of the urine, stool, saliva, tears, and skin. It can also permanently discolor soft contact lenses.

Rifampin is also available in a parenteral dosage form consisting of a lyophilized sterile powder that, when reconstituted in 5% dextrose or normal saline, provides 600 mg of active drug in 10 mL for slow intravenous infusion. The parenteral form may be used for initial treatment of serious cases and for retreatment of patients who cannot take the drug by the oral route. Parenteral solutions of rifampin are stable for 24 hours at room temperature. Although rifampin is stable in the solid state, in solution it undergoes various chemical changes whose rates and nature are pH and temperature dependent.[79] At alkaline pH, it oxidizes to a quinone in the presence of oxygen; in acidic solutions, it hydrolyzes to 3-formyl rifamycin SV. Slow hydrolysis of the ester functions also occurs, even at neutral pH.

Rifabutin

Rifabutin, the spiroimidazopiperidyl derivative of rifamycin B was approved in the United States for the prophylaxis of disseminated MAC in AIDS patients on the strength of clinical trials establishing its effectiveness. The activity of rifabutin against MAC organisms greatly exceeds that of rifamycin. This rifamycin derivative is not effective, however, as monotherapy for existing disseminated MAC disease.

Rifabutin is a very lipophilic compound with a high affinity for tissues. Its elimination is distribution limited, with a half-life averaging 45 hours (range, 16–69 hours). Approximately 50% of an orally administered dose of rifabutin is absorbed, but the absolute oral bioavailability is only about 20%. Extensive first-pass metabolism and significant biliary excretion of the drug occur, with about 35% and 53% of the orally administered dose excreted, largely as metabolites, in the feces and urine, respectively. The 25-*O*-desacetyl and 31-hydroxy metabolites of rifabutin have been identified. The parent drug is 85% bound to plasma proteins in a concentration-independent manner. Despite its greater potency against *M. tuberculosis* in vitro, rifabutin is considered inferior to rifampin for the short-term therapy of tuberculosis because of its significantly lower plasma concentrations.

Although rifabutin is believed to cause less hepatotoxicity and induction of cytochrome P450 enzymes than rifampin, these properties should be borne in mind when the drug is used prophylactically. Rifabutin and its metabolites are highly colored compounds that can discolor skin, urine, tears, feces, etc.

Cycloserine

D-(+)-4-Amino-3-isoxazolidinone (Seromycin) is an antibiotic that has been isolated from the fermentation beer of three different *Streptomyces* species: *S. orchidaceus, S. garyphalus,* and *S. lavendulus.* It occurs as a white to pale yellow crystalline material that is very soluble in water. It is stable in alkaline, but unstable in acidic, solutions. The compound slowly dimerizes to 2,5-bis(aminoxymethyl)-3,6-diketopiperazine in solution or standing.

The structure of cycloserine was reported simultaneously by Kuehl et al.[80] and Hidy et al.[81] to be D-(+)-4-amino-3-isoxazolidinone. It has been synthesized by Stammer et al.[82] and by Smart et al.[83] Cycloserine is stereochemically related to D-serine. However, the L-form has similar antibiotic activity.

Cycloserine is presumed to exert its antibacterial action by preventing the synthesis of cross-linking peptide in the formation of bacterial cell walls.[84] Rando[85] has recently suggested that it is an antimetabolite for alanine, which acts as a suicide substrate for the pyridoxal phosphate-requiring enzyme alanine racemase. Irreversible inactivation of the enzyme thereby deprives the cell of the D-alanine required for the synthesis of the cross-linking peptide.

Although cycloserine exhibits antibiotic activity in vitro against a wide spectrum of both Gram-negative and Gram-positive organisms, its relatively weak potency and frequent toxic reactions limit its use to the treatment of tuberculosis. It is recommended for patients who fail to respond to other tuberculostatic drugs or who are known to be infected with organisms resistant to other agents. It is usually administered orally in combination with other drugs, commonly isoniazid.

Sterile Capreomycin Sulfate

Capastat sulfate, or capreomycin, is a strongly basic cyclic peptide isolated from *Streptomyces capreolus* in 1960 by Herr et al.[86] It was released in the United States in 1971 exclusively as a tuberculostatic drug. Capreomycin, which resembles viomycin (no longer marketed in the United States) chemically and pharmacologically, is a second-line agent used in combination with other antitubercular drugs. In particular, it may be used in place of streptomycin when either the patient is sensitive to, or the strain of *M. tuberculosis* is resistant to, streptomycin. Similar to viomycin, capreomycin is a potentially toxic drug. Damage to the eighth cranial nerve and renal damage, as with viomycin, are the more serious toxic effects associated with capreomycin therapy. There are, as yet, insufficient clinical data for a reliable comparison of the relative toxic potentials of capreomycin and streptomycin. Cross-resistance among strains of tubercle bacilli is rare between capreomycin and streptomycin.

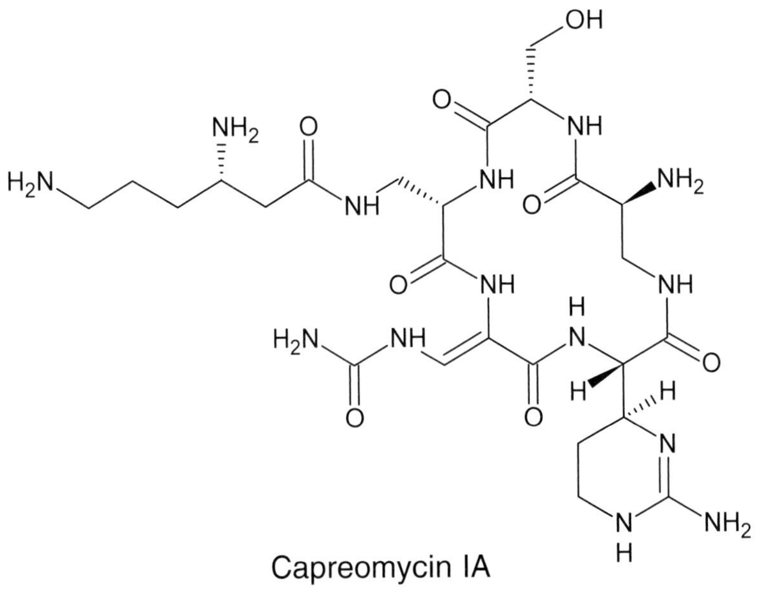

Capreomycin IA

Four capreomycins, designated IA, IB, IIA, and IIB, have been isolated from cultures of *S. capreolus*. The clinical agent contains primarily IA and IB. The close chemical relationship between capreomycins IA and IB and viomycin was established,[87] and the total synthesis and proof of structure of the capreomycins were later accomplished.[88] The structures of capreomycins IIA and IIB correspond to those of IA and IB but lack the β-lysyl residue. The sulfate salts are freely soluble in water.

⬡ ANTIPROTOZOAL AGENTS

In the United States and other countries of the temperate zone, protozoal diseases are of minor importance, whereas bacterial and viral diseases are widespread and are the cause of considerable concern. On the other hand, protozoal diseases are highly prevalent in tropical Third World countries, where they infect both human and animal populations, causing suffering, death, and enormous economic hardship. Protozoal diseases that are found in the United States are malaria, amebiasis, giardiasis, trichomoniasis, toxoplasmosis, and, as a direct consequence of the AIDS epidemic, *P. carinii* pneumonia (PCP).

Although amebiasis is generally thought of as a tropical disease, it actually has a worldwide distribution. In some areas with temperate climates in which sanitation is poor, the prevalence of amebiasis has been estimated to be as high as 20% of the population. The causative organism, *Entamoeba histolytica*, can invade the wall of the colon or other parts of the body (e.g., liver, lungs, skin). An ideal chemotherapeutic agent would be effective against both the intestinal and extraintestinal forms of the parasite.

Amebicides that are effective against both intestinal and extraintestinal forms of the disease are limited to the somewhat toxic alkaloids emetine and dehydroemetine, the nitroimidazole derivative metronidazole, and the antimalarial agent chloroquine (Chapter 7). A second group of amebicides that are effective only against intestinal forms of the disease includes the aminoglycoside antibiotic paromomycin, the 8-hydroxyquinoline derivative iodoquinol, the arsenical compound carbarsone, and diloxanide.

Other protozoal species that colonize the intestinal tract and cause enteritis and diarrhea are *Balantidium coli* and the flagellates, *G. lamblia* and *Cryptosporidium* spp. Balantidiasis responds best to tetracycline. Metronidazole and iodoquinol may also be effective. Giardiasis may be treated effectively with furazolidone, metronidazole, or the antimalarial drug quinacrine (Chapter 7). Cryptosporidiosis is normally self-limiting in immunocompetent patients and is not normally treated. The illness can be a serious problem in AIDS patients because no effective therapy is currently available.

Trichomoniasis, a venereal disease caused by the flagellated protozoan *T. vaginalis*, is common in the United States and throughout the world. Although it is not generally considered serious, this affliction can cause serious physical discomfort. Oral metronidazole provides effective treatment against all forms of the disease. It is also used to eradicate the organism from asymptomatic male carriers.

P. carinii is an opportunistic pathogen that may colonize the lungs of humans and other animals and, under the right conditions, can cause pneumonia. The organism has long been classified as a protozoan, but recent RNA evidence suggests that it may be more closely related to fungi. At one time, occasional cases of PCP were known to occur in premature, undernourished infants and in patients receiving immunosuppressant therapy. The situation changed with the onset of the AIDS epidemic. It is estimated that at least 60% and possibly as high as 85% of patients infected with HIV develop PCP during their lifetimes.

The combination of the antifolate trimethoprim and the sulfonamide sulfamethoxazole constitutes the treatment of choice for PCP. Other effective drugs include pentamidine, atovaquone, and a new antifolate, trimetrexate.

Toxoplasma gondii is an obligate intracellular protozoan that is best known for causing blindness in neonates. Toxoplasmosis, the disseminated form of the disease in which the lymphatic system, skeletal muscles, heart, brain, eye, and placenta may be affected, has become increasingly prevalent in association with HIV infection. A combination of the antifolate pyrimethamine and the sulfa drug sulfadiazine constitutes the most effective therapy for toxoplasmosis.

Various forms of trypanosomiasis, chronic tropical diseases caused by pathogenic members of the family Trypanosomidae, occur both in humans and in livestock. The principal disease in humans, sleeping sickness, can be broadly classified into two main geographic and etiological groups: African sleeping sickness caused by *Trypanosoma gambiense* (West African), *Trypanosoma rhodesiense* (East African), or *Trypanosoma congolense*; and South American sleeping sickness (Chagas disease) caused by *Trypanosoma cruzi*. Of the various forms of trypanosomiasis, Chagas disease is the most serious and generally the most resistant to chemotherapy. Leishmaniasis is a chronic tropical disease caused by various flagellate protozoa of the genus *Leishmania*. The more common visceral form caused by *Leishmania donovani*, called *kala-azar*, is similar to Chagas disease. Although these diseases are widespread in tropical areas of Africa and South and Central America, they are of minor importance in the United States, Europe, and Asia.

Chemotherapy of trypanosomiasis and leishmaniasis remains somewhat primitive and is often less than effective. In fact, it is doubtful that these diseases can be controlled by chemotherapeutic measures alone, without successful control of the intermediate hosts and vectors that transmit them. Heavy metal compounds, such as the arsenicals and antimonials, are sometimes effective but frequently toxic. The old standby suramin appears to be of some value in long- and short-term prophylaxis. The nitrofuran derivative nifurtimox may be a major asset in the control of these diseases, but its potential toxicity remains to be fully determined.

Metronidazole

2-Methyl-5-nitroimidazole-1-ethanol (Flagyl, Protostat, Metro IV) is the most useful of a group of antiprotozoal nitroimidazole derivatives that have been synthesized in various laboratories throughout the world. Metronidazole was first marketed for the topical treatment of *T. vaginalis* vaginitis. It has since been shown to be effective orally against both the acute and carrier states of the disease. The drug also possesses useful amebicidal activity and is, in fact, effective against both intestinal and hepatic amebiasis. It has also been found of use in the treatment of such other protozoal diseases as giardiasis and balantidiasis.

More recently, metronidazole has been found to possess efficacy against obligate anaerobic bacteria, but it is ineffective against facultative anaerobes or obligate aerobes. It is particularly active against Gram-negative anaerobes, such as *Bacteroides* and *Fusobacterium* spp. It is also effective against Gram-positive anaerobic bacilli (e.g., *Clostridium* spp.) and cocci (e.g., *Peptococcus*, *Peptidostreptococcus* spp.). Because of its bactericidal action, metronidazole has become an important agent for the treatment of serious infections (e.g., septicemia, pneumonia, peritonitis, pelvic infections, abscesses, meningitis) caused by anaerobic bacteria.

The common characteristic of microorganisms (bacteria and protozoa) sensitive to metronidazole is that they are anaerobic. It has been speculated that a reactive intermediate

formed in the microbial reduction of the 5-nitro group of metronidazole covalently binds to the DNA of the microorganism, triggering the lethal effect.[89] Potential reactive intermediates include the nitroxide, nitroso, hydroxylamine, and amine. The ability of metronidazole to act as a radiosensitizing agent is also related to its reduction potential.

Metronidazole is a pale yellow crystalline substance that is sparingly soluble in water. It is stable in air but is light sensitive. Despite its low water solubility, metronidazole is well absorbed following oral administration. It has a large apparent volume of distribution and achieves effective concentrations in all body fluids and tissues. Approximately 20% of an oral dose is metabolized to oxidized or conjugated forms. The 2-hydroxy metabolite is active; other metabolites are inactive.

Metronidazole is a weak base that possesses a pK_a of 2.5. Although it is administered parenterally only as the free base by slow intravenous infusion, metronidazole for injection is supplied in two forms: a ready-to-inject 100-mL solution containing 5 mg of base per mL; and a hydrochloride salt as 500 mg of a sterile lyophilized powder. Metronidazole hydrochloride for injection must first be reconstituted with sterile water to yield 5 mL of a solution having a concentration of 100 mg/mL and a pH ranging from 0.5 to 2.0. The resulting solution must then be diluted with either 100 mL of normal saline or 5% dextrose and neutralized with 5 mEq of sodium bicarbonate to provide a final solution of metronidazole base with an approximate concentration of 5 mg/mL and a pH of 6 to 7. Solutions of metronidazole hydrochloride are unsuitable for intravenous administration because of their extreme acidity. Reconstituted metronidazole hydrochloride solutions are stable for 96 hours at 30°C, whereas ready-to-use solutions of metronidazole base are stable for 24 hours at 30°C. Both solutions should be protected from light.

Diloxanide

Furamide, or eutamide, is the 2-furoate ester of 2,2-dichloro-4′-hydroxy-*N*-methylacetanilide. It was developed as a result of the discovery that various α,α-dichloroacetamides possessed amebicidal activity in vitro. Diloxanide itself and many of its esters are also active, and drug metabolism studies indicate that hydrolysis of the amide is required for the amebicidal effect. Nonpolar esters of diloxanide are more potent than polar ones. Diloxanide furoate has been used in the treatment of asymptomatic carriers of *E. histolytica*. Its effectiveness against acute intestinal amebiasis or hepatic abscesses, however, has not been established. Diloxanide furoate is a white crystalline powder. It is administered orally only as 500-mg tablets and may be obtained in the United States from the CDC in Atlanta, Georgia.

8-Hydroxyquinoline

Oxine, quinophenol, or oxyquinoline is the parent compound from which the antiprotozoal oxyquinolines have been derived. The antibacterial and antifungal properties of oxine and its derivatives, which are believed to result from the ability to chelate metal ions, are well known. Aqueous solutions of acid salts of oxine, particularly the sulfate (Chinosol, Quinosol), in concentrations of 1:3,000 to 1:1,000, have been used as topical antiseptics. The substitution of an iodine atom at the 7-position of 8-hydroxyquinolines yields compounds with broad-spectrum amebicidal properties.

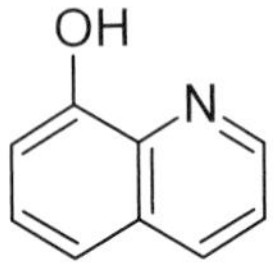

Iodoquinol

5,7-Diiodo-8-quinolinol, 5,7-diiodo-8-hydroxyquinoline, or diiodohydroxyquin (Yodoxin, Diodoquin, Diquinol) is a yellowish to tan microcrystalline, light-sensitive substance that is insoluble in water. It is recommended for acute and chronic intestinal amebiasis but is not effective in extraintestinal disease. Because a relatively high incidence of topic neuropathy has occurred with its use, iodoquinol should not be used routinely for traveler's diarrhea.

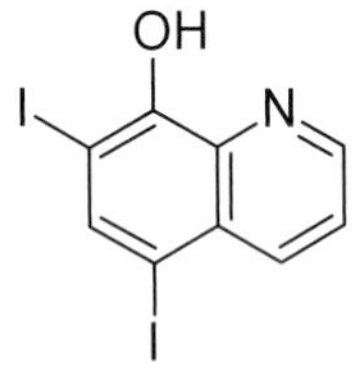

Emetine and Dehydroemetine

The alkaloids emetine and dehydroemetine are obtained by separation from extracts of ipecac. They occur as levorotatory, light-sensitive white powders that are insoluble in water. The alkaloids readily form water-soluble salts. Solutions of the hydrochloride salts intended for intramuscular injection should be adjusted to pH 3.5 and stored in light-resistant containers.

Emetine and dehydroemetine exert a direct amebicidal action on various forms of *E. histolytica*. They are protoplasmic poisons that inhibit protein synthesis in protozoal and mammalian cells by preventing protein elongation. Because their effect in intestinal amebiasis is solely symptomatic and the cure rate is only 10% to 15%, they should be used only in combination with other agents. The high concentrations of the alkaloids achieved in the liver and other tissues after intramuscular injection provide the basis for their high effectiveness against hepatic abscesses and

other extraintestinal forms of the disease. Toxic effects limit the usefulness of emetine. It causes a high frequency of gastrointestinal distress (especially nausea and diarrhea), cardiovascular effects (hypotension and arrhythmias), and neuromuscular effects (pain and weakness). A lower incidence of cardiotoxicity has been associated with the use of dehydroemetine (Mebadin), which is available from the CDC and is also amebicidal.

Emetine and dehydroemetine have also been used to treat balantidial dysentery and fluke infestations, such as fascioliasis and paragonimiasis.

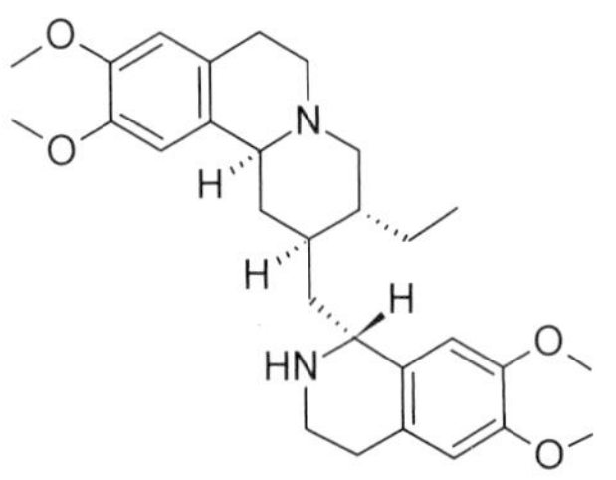

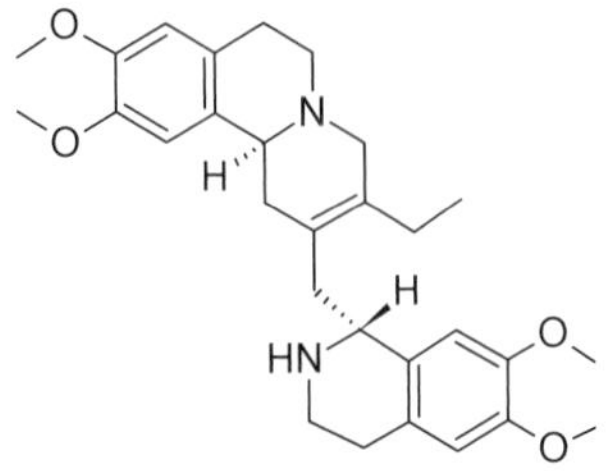

Pentamidine Isethionate

4,4′-(Pentamethylenedioxy)dibenzamidine diisethionate (NebuPent, Pentam 300) is a water-soluble crystalline salt that is stable to light and air. The principal use of pentamidine is for the treatment of pneumonia caused by the opportunistic pathogenic protozoan *P. carinii*, a frequent secondary invader associated with AIDS. The drug may be administered by slow intravenous infusion or by deep intramuscular injection for PCP. An aerosol form of pentamidine is used by inhalation for the prevention of PCP in high-risk patients infected with HIV who have a previous history of PCP infection or a low peripheral $CD4^+$ lymphocyte count.

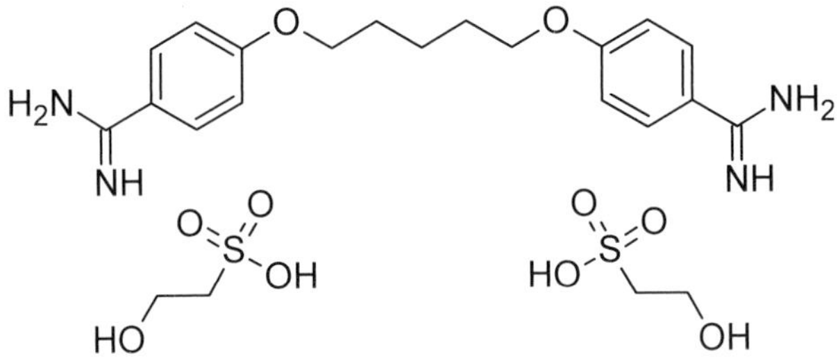

Both the inhalant (aerosol) and parenteral dosage forms of pentamidine isethionate are sterile lyophilized powders that must be made up as sterile aqueous solutions prior to use. Sterile water for injection must be used to reconstitute the aerosol, to avoid precipitation of the pentamidine salt. Adverse reactions to the drug are common. These include cough and bronchospasm (inhalation) and hypertension and hypoglycemia (injection).

Pentamidine has been used for the prophylaxis and treatment of African trypanosomiasis. It also has some value for treating visceral leishmaniasis. Pentamidine rapidly disappears from the plasma after intravenous injection and is distributed to the tissues, where it is stored for a long period. This property probably contributes to the usefulness of the drug as a prophylactic agent.

Atovaquone

3-[4-(4-Chlorophenyl)-cyclohexyl]-2-hydroxy-1,4-naphthoquinone (Mepron) is a highly lipophilic, water-insoluble analog of ubiquinone 6, an essential component of the mitochondrial electron transport chain in microorganisms. The structural similarity between atovaquone and ubiquinone suggests that the former may act as an antimetabolite for the latter and thereby interfere with the function of electron transport enzymes.

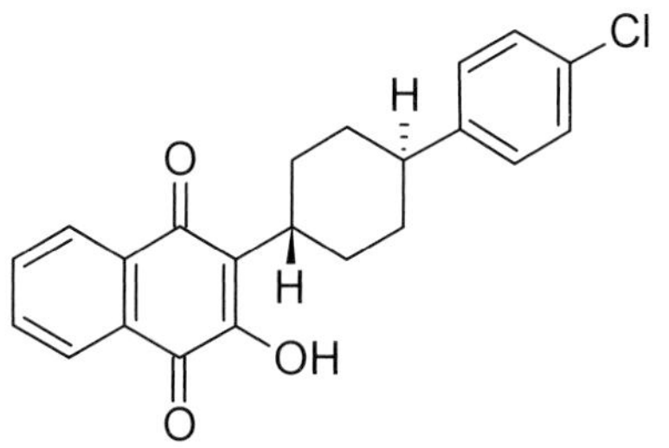

Atovaquone was originally developed as an antimalarial drug, but *Plasmodium falciparum* was found to develop a rapid tolerance to its action. More recently, the effectiveness of atovaquone against *P. carinii* was discovered. It is a currently recommended alternative to trimethoprim-sulfamethoxazole (TMP-SMX) for the treatment and prophylaxis of PCP in patients intolerant to this combination. Atovaquone was also shown to be effective in eradicating *T. gondii* in preclinical animal studies.

The oral absorption of atovaquone is slow and incomplete, in part because of the low water solubility of the drug. Aqueous suspensions provide significantly better absorption than do tablets. Food, especially if it has a high fat content, increases atovaquone absorption. Significant enterohepatic recycling of atovaquone occurs, and most (nearly 95%) of the drug is excreted unchanged in the feces. In vivo, atovaquone is largely confined to the plasma, where it is extensively protein bound (>99.9%). The half-life of the drug ranges from 62 to 80 hours. The primary side effect is gastrointestinal intolerance.

Eflornithine
Eflornithine is used for the treatment of West African sleeping sickness, caused by *Trypanosoma brucei gambiense*. It is specifically indicated for the meningoencephalitic stage of the disease. Eflornithine is a myelosuppressive drug that causes high incidences of anemia, leukopenia, and thrombocytopenia. Complete blood cell counts must be monitored during the course of therapy.

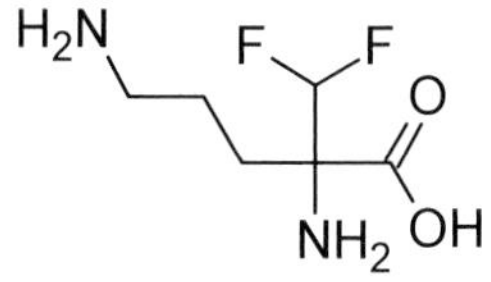

The irreversible inactivation of ornithine decarboxylase by eflornithine is accompanied by decarboxylation and release of fluoride ion from the inhibitor,[90] suggesting enzyme-catalyzed activation of the inhibitor. Only the (−) isomer, stereochemically related to L-ornithine, is active.

Eflornithine is supplied as the hydrochloride salt. It may be administered either intravenously or orally. Approximately 80% of the unchanged drug is excreted in the urine. Penetration of eflornithine into the CSF is facilitated by inflammation of the meninges.

Nifurtimox
Nifurtimox is 4-[(5-nitrofurfurylidene) amino]-3-methylthiomorpholine-1,1-dioxide, or Bayer 2502 (Lampit). The observation that various derivatives of 5-nitrofuraldehyde possessed, in addition to their antibacterial and antifungal

properties, significant and potentially useful antiprotozoal activity eventually led to discovery of particular nitrofurans with antitrypanosomal activity.

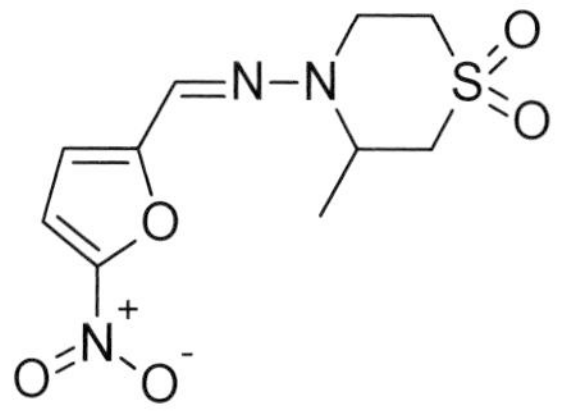

The most important of such compounds is nifurtimox because of its demonstrated effectiveness against *T. cruzi*, the parasite responsible for South American trypanosomiasis. In fact, use of this drug represents the only clinically proven treatment for both acute and chronic forms of the disease. Nifurtimox is available in the United States from the CDC.

Nifurtimox is administered orally. Oral bioavailability is high, but considerable first-pass metabolism occurs. The half-life of nifurtimox is 2 to 4 hours. The drug is poorly tolerated, with a high incidence of nausea, vomiting, abdominal pain, and anorexia reported. Symptoms of central and peripheral nervous system toxicity also frequently occur with nifurtimox.

Benznidazole
N-Benzyl-2-nitroimidazole-1-acetamide (Radanil, Rochagan) is a nitroimidazole derivative that is used for the treatment of Chagas disease. It is not available in the United States but is used extensively in South America. The effectiveness of benznidazole is similar to that of nifurtimox. Therapy for American trypanosomiasis with oral benznidazole requires several weeks and is frequently accompanied by adverse effects such as peripheral neuropathy, bone marrow depression, and allergic-type reactions.

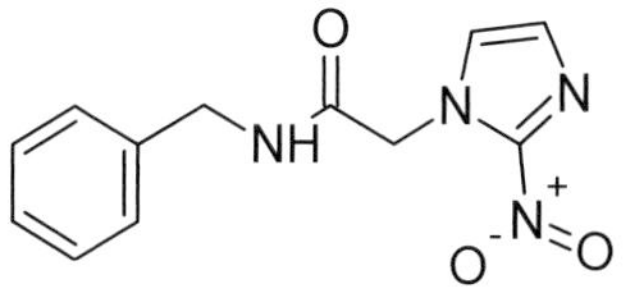

Melarsoprol
2-*p*-(4,6-Diamino-*s*-triazin-2-yl-amino)phenyl-4-hydroxymethyl-1,3,2-dithiarsoline (Mel B, Arsobal) is prepared by reduction of a corresponding pentavalent arsanilate to the trivalent arsenoxide followed by reaction of the latter with 2,3-dimercapto-1-propanol (British anti-Lewisite [BAL]). It has become the drug of choice for the treatment of the later stages of both forms of African trypanosomiasis. Melarsoprol has the advantage of excellent penetration into the CNS and, therefore, is effective against meningoencephalitic forms of *T. gambiense* and *T. rhodesiense*. Trivalent arsenicals tend to be more toxic to the host (as well as the parasites) than the corresponding pentavalent compounds. The bonding of arsenic with sulfur atoms tends to reduce host toxicity, increase chemical stability (to oxidation), and improve distribution of the compound to the arsenoxide. Melarsoprol shares the toxic properties of other

arsenicals, however, so its use must be monitored for signs of arsenic toxicity.

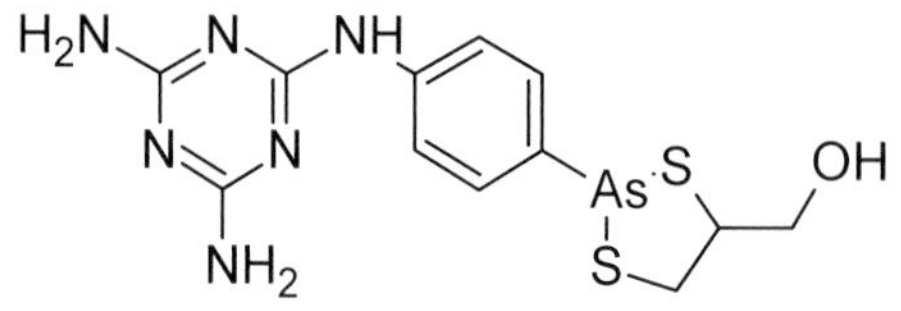

Sodium Stibogluconate

Sodium antimony gluconate (Pentostam) is a pentavalent antimonial compound intended primarily for the treatment of various forms of leishmaniasis. It is available from the CDC as the disodium salt, which is chemically stable and freely soluble in water. The 10% aqueous solution used for either intramuscular or intravenous injection has a pH of approximately 5.5. Like all antimonial drugs, this drug has a low therapeutic index, and patients undergoing therapy with it should be monitored carefully for signs of heavy metal poisoning. Other organic antimonial compounds are used primarily for the treatment of schistosomiasis and other flukes.

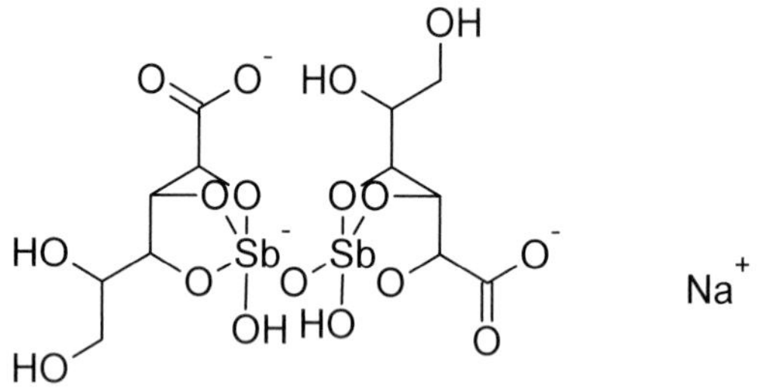

The antileishmanial action of sodium stibogluconate requires its reduction to the trivalent form, which is believed to inhibit phosphofructokinase in the parasite.

Dimercaprol

2,3-Dimercapto-1-propanol, BAL, or dithioglycerol is a foul-smelling, colorless liquid. It is soluble in water (1:20) and alcohol. It was developed by the British during World War II as an antidote for "Lewisite," hence the name British anti-Lewisite or BAL. Dimercaprol is effective topically and systematically as an antidote for poisoning caused by arsenic, antimony, mercury, gold, and lead. It can, therefore, also be used to treat arsenic and antimony toxicity associated with overdose or accidental ingestion of organoarsenicals or organoantimonials.

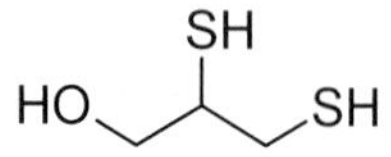

The antidotal properties of BAL are associated with the property of heavy metals to react with sulfhydryl (SH) groups in proteins (e.g., the enzyme pyruvate oxidase) and interfere with their normal function. 1,2-Dithiol compounds such as BAL compete effectively with such proteins for the metal by reversibly forming metal ring compounds of the following type:

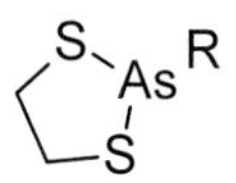

These are relatively nontoxic, metabolically conjugated (as glucuronides), and rapidly excreted.

BAL may be applied topically as an ointment or injected intramuscularly as a 5% or 10% solution in peanut oil.

Suramin Sodium

Suramin sodium is a high–molecular-weight bisurea derivative containing six sulfonic acid groups as their sodium salts. It was developed in Germany shortly after World War I as a byproduct of research efforts directed toward the development of potential antiparasitic agents from dyestuffs.

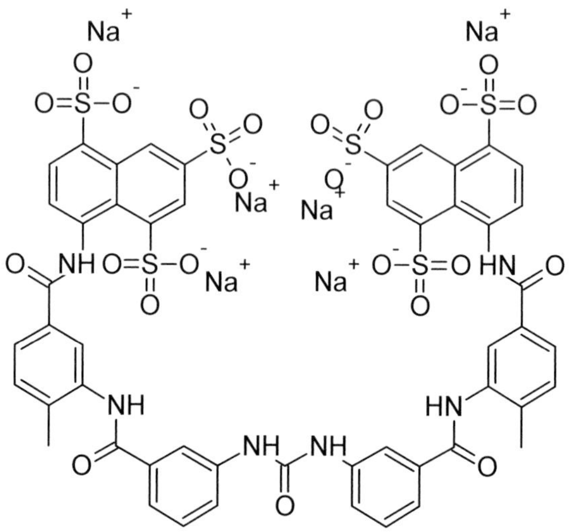

The drug has been used for more than half a century for the treatment of early cases of trypanosomiasis. Not until several decades later, however, was suramin discovered to be a long-term prophylactic agent whose effectiveness after a single intravenous injection is maintained for up to 3 months. The drug is tightly bound to plasma proteins, causing its excretion in the urine to be almost negligible.

Tissue penetration of the drug does not occur, apparently because of its high molecular weight and highly ionic character. Thus, an injected dose remains in the plasma for a very long period. Newer, more effective drugs are now available for short-term treatment and prophylaxis of African sleeping sickness. Suramin is also used for prophylaxis of onchocerciasis. It is available from the CDC.

⬡ ANTHELMINTICS

Anthelmintics are drugs that have the capability of ridding the body of parasitic worms or helminths. The prevalence of human helminthic infestations is widespread throughout the globe and represents a major world health problem, particularly in Third World countries. Helminths parasitic to humans and other animals are derived from two phyla, Platyhelminthes and Nemathelminthes. Cestodes (tapeworms) and trematodes (flukes) belong to the former, and nematodes or true roundworms belong to the latter. The helminth infestations of major concern on the North American continent are caused by roundworms (i.e., hookworm, pinworm, and *Ascaris* spp.). Human tapeworm and fluke infestations are rarely seen in the United States.

Several classes of chemicals are used as anthelmintics and include phenols and derivatives, piperazine and related compounds, antimalarial compounds (Chapter 7), various heterocyclic compounds, and natural products.

Piperazine

Hexahydropyrazine or diethylenediamine (Arthriticine, Dispermin) occurs as colorless, volatile crystals of the hexahydrate that are freely soluble in water. After the discovery of the anthelmintic properties of a derivative diethylcarbamazine, the activity of piperazine itself was established. Piperazine is still used as an anthelmintic for the treatment of pinworm (*Enterobius* [*Oxyuris*] *vermicularis*) and roundworm (*Ascaris lumbricoides*) infestations. It is available in various salt forms, including the citrate (official in the *USP*) in syrup and tablet forms.

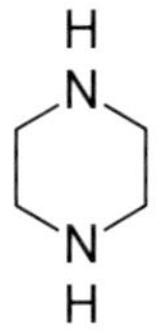

Piperazine blocks the response of the ascaris muscle to acetylcholine, causing flaccid paralysis in the worm, which is dislodged from the intestinal wall and expelled in the feces.

Diethylcarbamazepine Citrate

N,N-Diethyl-4-methyl-1-piperazinecarboxamide citrate or 1-diethylcarbamyl-4-methylpiperazine dihydrogen citrate (Hetrazan) is a highly water-soluble crystalline compound that has selective anthelmintic activity. It is effective against various forms of filariasis, including Bancroft, onchocerciasis, and laviasis. It is also active against ascariasis. Relatively few adverse reactions have been associated with diethylcarbamazine.

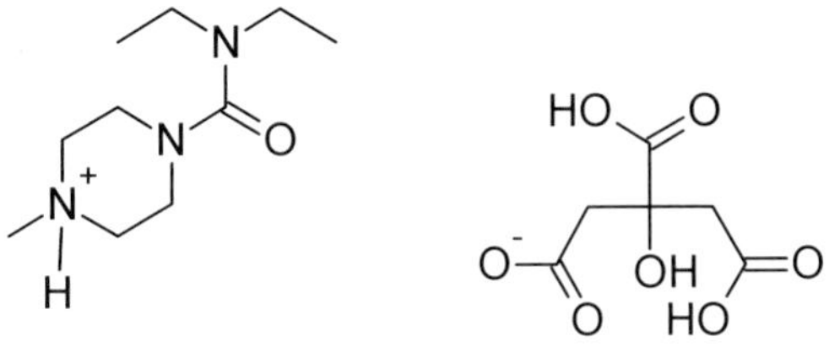

Pyrantel Pamoate

Trans-1,4,5,6,-Tetrahydro-1-methyl-2-[2-(2′-thienyl)ethenyl] pyrimidine pamoate (Antiminth) is a depolarizing neuromuscular blocking agent that causes spastic paralysis in susceptible helminths. It is used in the treatment of infestations caused by pinworms and roundworms (ascariasis). Because its action opposes that of piperazine, the two anthelmintics should not be used together. More than half of the oral dose is excreted in the feces unchanged. Adverse effects associated with its use are primarily gastrointestinal.

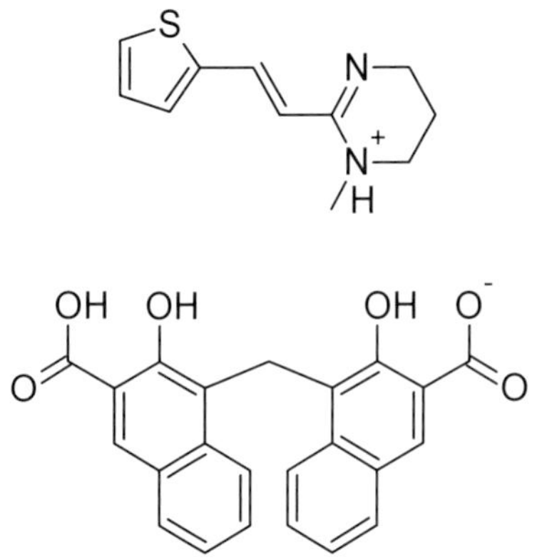

Thiabendazole

2-(4-Thiazolyl)benzimidazole (Mintezol) occurs as a white crystalline substance that is only slightly soluble in water but is soluble in strong mineral acids. Thiabendazole is a basic compound with a pK_a of 4.7 that forms complexes with metal ions.

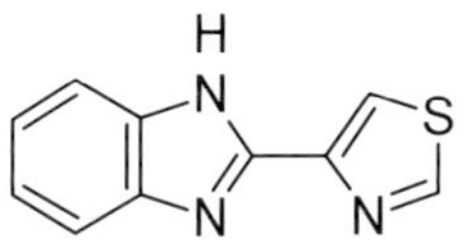

Thiabendazole inhibits the helminth-specific enzyme fumarate reductase.[91] It is not known whether metal ions are involved or if the inhibition of the enzyme is related to thiabendazole's anthelmintic effect. Benzimidazole anthelmintic drugs such as thiabendazole and mebendazole also arrest nematode cell division in metaphase by interfering with microtubule assembly.[92] They exhibit a high affinity for tubulin, the precursor protein for microtubule synthesis.

Thiabendazole has broad-spectrum anthelmintic activity. It is used to treat enterobiasis, strongyloidiasis (threadworm infection), ascariasis, uncinariasis (hookworm infection), and trichuriasis (whipworm infection). It has also been used to relieve symptoms associated with cutaneous larva migrans (creeping eruption) and the invasive phase of trichinosis. In addition to its use in human medicine, thiabendazole is widely used in veterinary practice to control intestinal helminths in livestock.

Mebendazole

Methyl 5-benzoyl-2-benzimidazolecarbamate (Vermox) is a broad-spectrum anthelmintic that is effective against various nematode infestations, including whipworm, pinworm, roundworm, and hookworm. Mebendazole irreversibly blocks glucose uptake in susceptible helminths, thereby depleting glycogen stored in the parasite. It apparently does not affect glucose metabolism in the host. It also inhibits cell division in nematodes.[71]

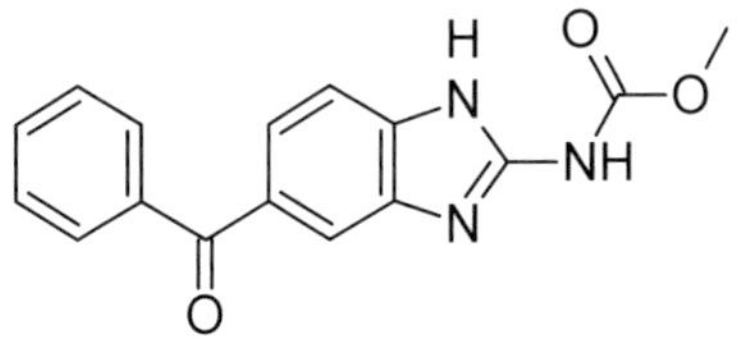

Mebendazole is poorly absorbed by the oral route. Adverse reactions are uncommon and usually consist of abdominal discomfort. It is teratogenic in laboratory animals and, therefore, should not be given during pregnancy.

Albendazole

Methyl 5-(propylthio)-2-benzimidazolecarbamate (Eskazole, Zentel) is a broad-spectrum anthelmintic that is not currently marketed in North America. It is available from the manufacturer on a compassionate use basis. Albendazole is widely used throughout the world for the treatment of intestinal nematode infection. It is effective as a single-dose treatment for ascariasis, New and Old World hookworm infections, and trichuriasis. Multiple-dose therapy with albendazole can eradicate pinworm, threadworm, capillariasis, clonorchiasis, and hydatid disease. The effectiveness of albendazole against tapeworms (cestodes) is generally more variable and less impressive.

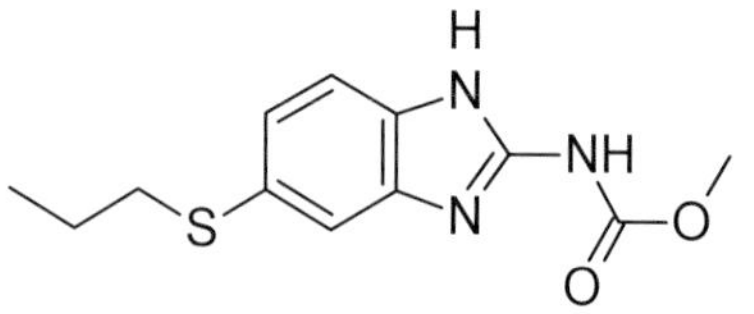

Albendazole occurs as a white crystalline powder that is virtually insoluble in water. The oral absorption of albendazole is enhanced by a fatty meal. The drug undergoes rapid and extensive first-pass metabolism to the sulfoxide, which is the active form in plasma. The elimination half-life of the sulfoxide ranges from 10 to 15 hours. Considerable biliary excretion and enterohepatic recycling of albendazole sulfoxide occurs. Albendazole is generally well tolerated in single-dose therapy for intestinal nematodes. The high-dose, prolonged therapy required for clonorchiasis or echinococcal disease therapy can result in adverse effects such as bone marrow depression, elevation of hepatic enzymes, and alopecia.

Niclosamide

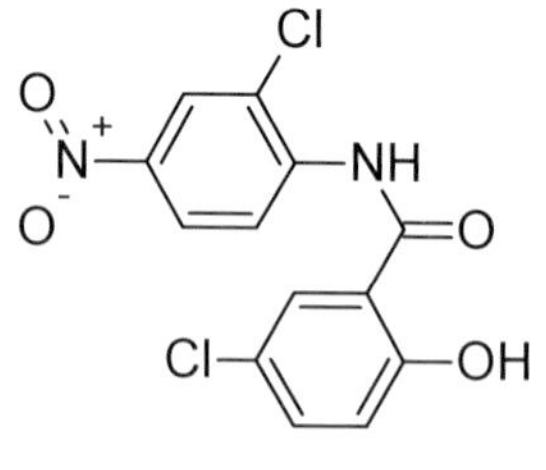

5-Chloro-*N*-(2-chloro-4-nitrophenyl)-2-hydroxybenzamide or 2,5′-dichloro-4′-nitrosalicylanilide (Cestocide, Mansonil, Yomesan) occurs as a yellowish white, water-insoluble powder. It is a potent taeniacide that causes rapid disintegration of worm segments and the scolex. Penetration of the drug into various cestodes appears to be facilitated by the digestive juices of the host, in that very little of the drug is absorbed by the worms in vitro. Niclosamide is well tolerated following oral administration, and little or no systemic absorption of it occurs. A saline purge 1 to 2 hours after ingestion of the taeniacide is recommended to remove the damaged scolex and worm segments. This procedure is mandatory in the treatment of pork tapeworm infestation to prevent possible cysticercosis resulting from release of live ova from worm segments damaged by the drug.

Bithionol

2,2′-Thiobis(4,6-dichlorophenol), or bis(2-hydroxy-3,5-dichlorophenyl)sulfide (Lorothidol, Bithin), a chlorinated bisphenol, was formerly used in soaps and cosmetics for its antimicrobial properties but was removed from the market for topical use because of reports of contact photodermatitis. Bithionol has useful anthelmintic properties and has been used as a fasciolicide and taeniacide. It is still considered the agent of choice for the treatment of infestations caused by the liver fluke *Fasciola hepatica* and the lung fluke *Paragonimus westermani*. Niclosamide is believed to be superior to it for the treatment of tapeworm infestations.

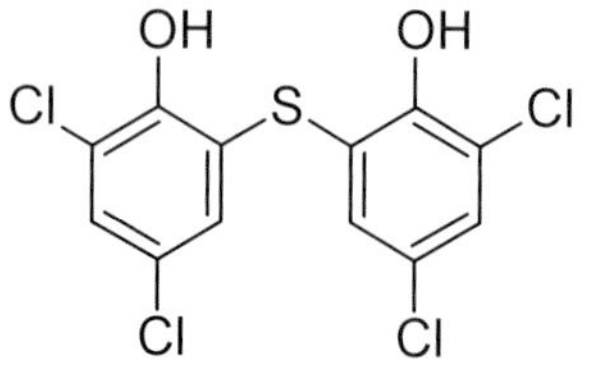

Oxamniquine

1,2,3,4-Tetrahydro-2-[(isopropylamino)methyl]-7-nitro-6-quinolinemethanol (Vansil) is an antischistosomal agent that is indicated for the treatment of *Schistosoma mansoni* (intestinal schistosomiasis) infection. It has been shown to inhibit DNA, RNA, and protein synthesis in schistosomes.[93] The 6-hydroxymethyl group is critical for activity; metabolic activation of precursor 6-methyl derivatives is critical. The oral bioavailability of oxamniquine is good; effective plasma levels are achieved in 1 to 1.5 hours. The plasma half-life is 1 to 2.5 hours. The drug is extensively metabolized to inactive metabolites, of which the principal one is the 6-carboxy derivative.

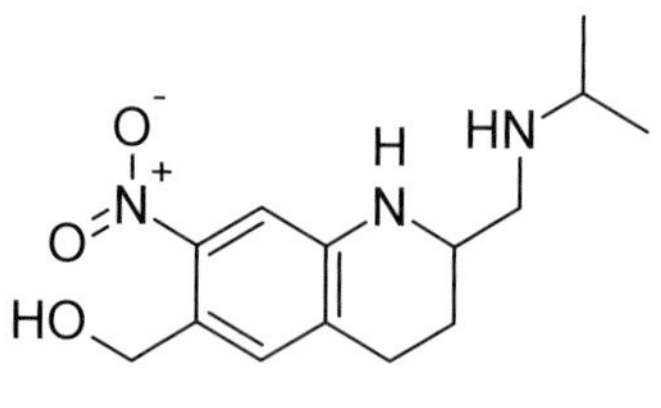

The free base occurs as a yellow crystalline solid that is slightly soluble in water but soluble in dilute aqueous mineral acids and soluble in most organic solvents. It is available in capsules containing 250 mg of the drug. Oxamniquine is generally well tolerated. Dizziness and drowsiness are common, but transitory, side effects. Serious reactions, such as epileptiform convulsions, are rare.

Praziquantel

2-(Cyclohexylcarbonyl)-1,2,3,6,7, 11b-hexahydro-4*H*-pyrazino[2,1-*a*]isoquinolin-4-one (Biltricide) is a broad-spectrum agent that is effective against various trematodes (flukes). It has become the agent of choice for the treatment of infections caused by schistosomes (blood flukes).

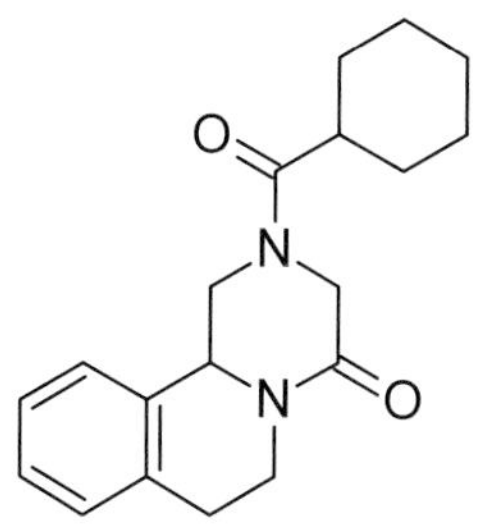

The drug also provides effective treatment for fasciolopsiasis (intestinal fluke), clonorchiasis (Chinese liver fluke), fascioliasis (sheep liver fluke), opisthorchosis (liver fluke), and paragonimiasis (lung fluke). Praziquantel increases cell membrane permeability of susceptible worms, resulting in the loss of extracellular calcium. Massive contractions and ultimate paralysis of the fluke musculature occurs, followed by phagocytosis of the parasite.

Following oral administration, about 80% of the dose is absorbed. Maximal plasma concentrations are achieved in 1 to 3 hours. The drug is rapidly metabolized in the liver in the first-pass. It is likely that some of the metabolites are also active. Praziquantel occurs as a white crystalline solid that is insoluble in water. It is available as 600-mg film-coated tablets. The drug is generally well tolerated.

Ivermectin

Ivermectin (Cardomec, Eqvalan, Ivomec) is a mixture of 22,23-dihydro derivatives of avermectins B_{1a} and B_{1b} prepared by catalytic hydrogenation. Avermectins are members of a family of structurally complex antibiotics produced by fermentation with a strain of *Streptomyces avermitilis*. Their discovery resulted from an intensive screening of cultures for anthelmintic agents from natural sources.[94] Ivermectin is active in low dosage against a wide variety of nematodes and arthropods that parasitize animals.[95]

The structures of the avermectins were established by a combination of spectroscopic[96] and x-ray crystallographic[97] techniques to contain pentacyclic 16-membered–ring aglycones glycosidically linked at the 3-position to a disaccharide

that comprises two oleandrose sugar residues. The side chain at the 25-position of the aglycone is *sec*-butyl in avermectin B_{1a}, whereas in avermectin B_{1b} it is isopropyl. Ivermectin contains at least 80% of 22,23-dihydroavermectin B_{1a} and no more than 20% 22,23-dihydroavermectin B_{1b}.

Ivermectin has achieved widespread use in veterinary practice in the United States and many countries throughout the world for the control of endoparasites and ectoparasites in domestic animals.[95] It has been found effective for the treatment of onchocerciasis ("river blindness") in humans,[98] an important disease caused by the roundworm *Oncocerca volvulus*, prevalent in West and Central Africa, the Middle East, and South and Central America. Ivermectin destroys the microfilariae, immature forms of the nematode, which create the skin and tissue nodules that are characteristic of the infestation and can lead to blindness. It also inhibits the release of microfilariae by the adult worms living in the host. Studies on the mechanism of action of ivermectin indicate that it blocks interneuron–motor neuron transmission in nematodes by stimulating the release of the inhibitory neurotransmitter GABA.[95] The drug has been made available by the manufacturer on a humanitarian basis to qualified treatment programs through the World Health Organization.

⬡ ANTISCABIOUS AND ANTIPEDICULAR AGENTS

Scabicides (antiscabious agents) are compounds used to control the mite *Sarcoptes scabiei*, an organism that thrives under conditions of poor personal hygiene. The incidence of scabies is believed to be increasing in the United States and worldwide and has, in fact, reached pandemic proportions.[99] Pediculicides (antipedicular agents) are used to eliminate head, body, and crab lice. Ideal scabicides and pediculicides must kill the adult parasites and destroy their eggs.

Benzyl Benzoate

Benzyl benzoate is a naturally occurring ester obtained from Peru balsam and other resins. It is also prepared synthetically from benzyl alcohol and benzoyl chloride. The ester is a clear colorless liquid with a faint aromatic odor. It is insoluble in water but soluble in organic solvents.

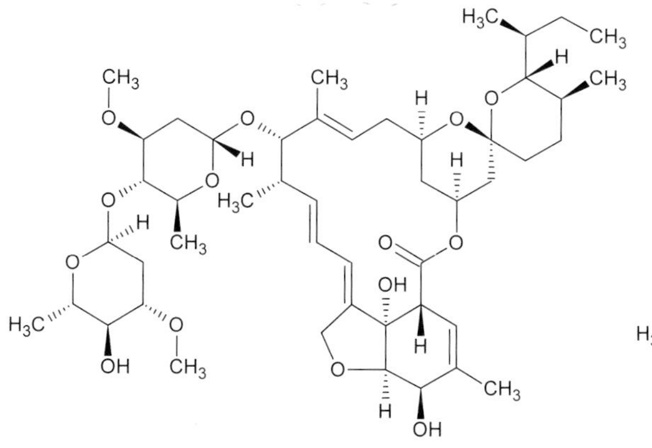

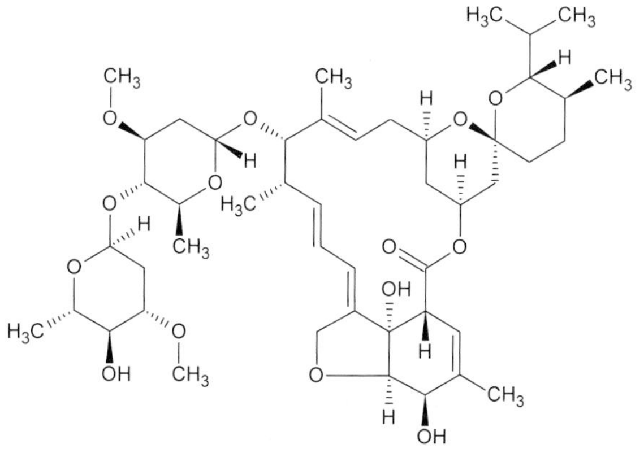

Benzyl benzoate is an effective scabicide when applied topically. Immediate relief from itching probably results from a local anesthetic effect; however, a complete cure is frequently achieved with a single application of a 25% emulsion of benzyl benzoate in oleic acid, stabilized with triethanolamine. This preparation has the additional advantage of being essentially odorless, nonstaining, and nonirritating to the skin. It is applied topically as a lotion over the entire dampened body, except the face.

Lindane

Lindane is 1,2,3,4,5,6-hexachlorocyclohexane, γ-benzene hexachloride, or benzene hexachloride (Kwell, Scabene, Kwildane, G-Well). This halogenated hydrocarbon is prepared by the chlorination of benzene. A mixture of isomers is obtained in this process, five of which have been isolated: α, β, γ, δ, and ε. The γ-isomer, present to 10% to 13% in the mixture, is responsible for the insecticidal activity. The γ-isomer may be separated by various extraction and chromatographic techniques.

Lindane occurs as a light buff to tan powder with a persistent musty odor, and it is bitter. It is insoluble in water but soluble in most organic solvents. It is stable under acidic or neutral conditions but undergoes elimination reactions under alkaline conditions.

The action of lindane against insects is threefold: it is a direct contact poison, it has a fumigant effect, and it acts as a stomach poison. The effect of lindane on insects is similar to that of DDT. Its toxicity in humans is somewhat lower than that of DDT. Because of its lipid solubility properties, however, lindane when ingested tends to accumulate in the body.

Lindane is used locally as a cream, lotion, or shampoo for the treatment of scabies and pediculosis.

CROTAMITON

N-Ethyl-*N*-(2-methylphenyl)-2-butenamide, or *N*-ethyl-*o*-crotonotoluidide (Eurax), is a colorless, odorless oily liquid. It is virtually insoluble in water but soluble in most organic solvents.

Crotamiton is available in 10% concentration in a lotion and a cream intended for the topical treatment of scabies.

Its antipruritic effect is probably because of a local anesthetic action.

Permethrin

Permethrin is 3-(2,2-Dichloroethenyl)-2,2-dimethylcyclopropanecarboxylic acid (3-phenoxyphenyl)methyl ester or 3-(phenoxyphenyl)methyl (±)-*cis*, *trans*-3-(2,2-dichloroethenyl)-2,2-dimethylcyclopropanecarboxylate (Nix). This synthetic pyrethrinoid compound is more stable chemically than most natural pyrethrins and is at least as active as an insecticide. Of the four isomers present, the 1(R),*trans* and 1(R),*cis*-isomers are primarily responsible for the insecticidal activity. The commercial product is a mixture consisting of 60% *trans* and 40% *cis* racemic isomers. It occurs as colorless to pale yellow low-melting crystals or as a pale yellow liquid and is insoluble in water but soluble in most organic solvents.

Permethrin exerts a lethal action against lice, ticks, mites, and fleas. It acts on the nerve cell membranes of the parasites to disrupt sodium channel conductance. It is used as a pediculicide for the treatment of head lice. A single application of a 1% solution effects cures in more than 99% of cases. The most frequent side effect is pruritus, which occurred in about 6% of the patients tested.

⬡ ANTIBACTERIAL SULFONAMIDES

The sulfonamide antimicrobial drugs were the first effective chemotherapeutic agents that could be used systemically for the cure of bacterial infections in humans. Their introduction led to a sharp decline in the morbidity and mortality of infectious diseases. The rapid development of widespread resistance to the sulfonamides soon after their introduction and the increasing use of the broader-spectrum penicillins in the treatment of infectious disease diminished the usefulness of sulfonamides. Today, they occupy a rather small place in the list of therapeutic agents that can be used for infectious disease. They are not completely outmoded, however. In the mid-1970s, the development of a combination of trimethoprim and sulfamethoxazole and the demonstration of its usefulness in the treatment and prophylaxis of certain opportunistic microbial infections led to resurgence in the use of some sulfonamides.

Fritz Mietzsch and Joseph Klarer of the I. G. Farbenindustrie laboratories systematically synthesized a series of azo dyes, each containing the sulfonamide functional group, as potential antimicrobial agents. Sulfonamide azo dyes were included in the test series because they were readily synthesized and possessed superior staining properties. The Bayer pathologist–bacteriologist who evaluated the new Mietzsch-Klarer dyes was a physician named Gerhard Domagk.[100–102] In 1932, Domagk began to study a brilliant red dye, later named Prontosil. Prontosil was found to protect against, and cure, streptococcal infections in mice.[100] Interestingly, Prontosil was inactive on bacterial cultures. Domagk and others continued to study Prontosil, and in 1933, the first of many cures of severe bacterial infections in humans was reported by Foerster,[103] who treated a 10-month-old infant suffering from staphylococcal septicemia and obtained a dramatic cure. The credit for most of the discoveries relating to Prontosil belongs to Domagk, and for his pioneering work in chemotherapy he was awarded the Nobel Prize in medicine and physiology in 1938. The Gestapo prevented him from actually accepting the award, but after the war, he received it in Stockholm in 1947.

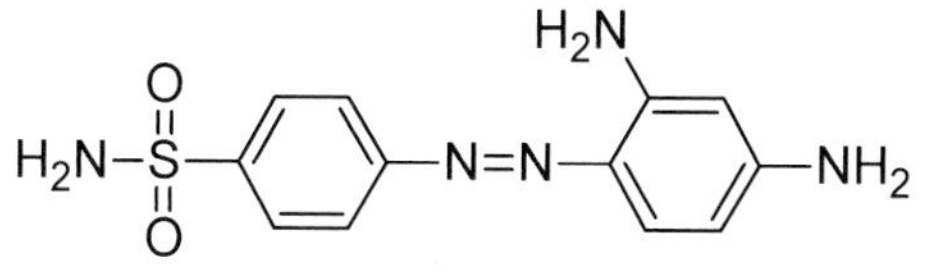

$$H_2N-\overset{\displaystyle O}{\underset{\displaystyle O}{\overset{\|}{\underset{\|}{S}}}}\text{—}\underset{}{\bigcirc}\text{—}N=N\text{—}\underset{NH_2}{\overset{H_2N}{\bigcirc}}$$

Prontosil is totally inactive in vitro but possesses excellent activity in vivo. This property of the drug attracted much attention and stimulated a large body of research activity into the sulfonamides. In 1935, Trefouel and coinvestigators[104] performed a structure–activity study on the sulfonamide azo dyes and concluded that the azo linkage was reductively cleaved to release the active antibacterial product, sulfanilamide. This finding was confirmed in 1937 when Fuller[105] isolated free sulfanilamide from the blood and urine of patients being treated with Prontosil. Favorable clinical results were reported with Prontosil and the active metabolite itself, sulfanilamide, in puerperal sepsis and meningococcal

infections. All of these findings ushered in the modern era of chemotherapy and the concept of the *prodrug.*

Following the dramatic success of Prontosil, a host of sulfanilamide derivatives was synthesized and tested. By 1948, more than 4,500 compounds[106] had been evaluated. Of these, only about two dozen have been used in clinical practice. In the late 1940s, broader experience with sulfonamides had begun to demonstrate toxicity in some patients, and resistance problems brought about by indiscriminate use of sulfonamides limited their use throughout the world. The penicillins were excellent alternatives to the sulfonamides, and they largely replaced the latter in antimicrobial chemotherapy.

Today, there are a few sulfonamides (Table 6.7) and especially sulfonamide-trimethoprim combinations that are used extensively for opportunistic infections in patients with AIDS.[107] A primary infection that is treated with the combination is PCP. The sulfonamide-trimethoprim combination can be used for treatment and prophylaxis. Additionally, cerebral toxoplasmosis can be treated in active infection or prophylactically. Urinary tract infections and burn therapy[107–111] round out the list of therapeutic applications. The sulfonamides are drugs of choice for a few other types of infections, but their use is quite limited in modern antimicrobial chemotherapy.[107–111]

The sulfonamides can be grouped into three classes on the basis of their use: oral absorbable agents, designed to give systemic distribution; *oral nonabsorbable agents* such as sulfasalazine; and topical agents such as sodium sulfacetamide ophthalmic drops.

TABLE 6.7 Therapy with Sulfonamide Antibacterials

Disease/Infection	Sulfonamides Commonly Used
Relatively Common Use	
Treatment and prophylaxis of *Pneumocystis carinii* pneumonia	Trimethoprim-sulfamethoxazole
Treatment and prophylaxis of cerebral toxoplasmosis	Pyrimethamine-sulfadiazine
First attack of urinary tract infection	Trimethoprim-sulfamethoxazole
Burn therapy: prevention and treatment of bacterial infection	Silver sulfadiazine and mafenide
Conjunctivitis and related superficial ocular infections	Sodium sulfacetamide
Chloroquine-resistant malaria (Chapter 9)	Combinations with quinine, others
	Sulfadoxine
	Sulfalene
Less Common Infections/Diseases	***Drugs of Choice or Alternates***
Nocardiosis	Trimethoprim-sulfamethoxazole
Severe traveler's diarrhea	Trimethoprim-sulfamethoxasole
Meningococcal infections	Sulfonamides, only if proved to be sulfonamide sensitive; otherwise, penicillin G, ampicillin, or (for penicillin-allergic patients) chloramphenicol should be used
Generally Not Useful	
Streptococcal infections	Most are resistant to sulfonamides
Prophylaxis of recurrent rheumatic fever	Most are resistant to sulfonamides
Other bacterial infections	The low cost of penicillin and the widespread resistance to sulfonamides limit their use; sulfonamides are still used in a few countries
Vaginal infections	The FDA and USP-DI find no evidence of efficacy
Reduction of bowel flora	Effectiveness not established
Ulcerative colitis	Corticosteroid therapy often preferred
	Relapses common with sulfonamides
	Salicylazosulfapyridine
	Side effects of the sulfanilamides sometimes mimic ulcerative colitis

Nomenclature of the Sulfonamides

Sulfonamide is a generic term that denotes three different cases:

1. Antibacterials that are *aniline-substituted sulfonamides* (the "sulfanilamides").

2. *Prodrugs* that react to generate active sulfanilamides (i.e., sulfasalazine).
3. *Nonaniline* sulfonamides (i.e., mafenide acetate).

There are also other commonly used drugs that are sulfonamides or sulfanilamides. Among these are the oral hypoglycemic drug tolbutamide, the diuretic furosemide, and the diuretic chlorthalidone.

In pharmaceutical chemistry, pK_b values are not used to compare compounds that are Lewis bases. Instead, if a pK_a of an amine is given, it refers to its salt acting as the conjugate acid. For example, aniline with a pK_a of 4.6 refers to

It does not refer to

A negative charge on a nitrogen atom is typically not stable unless it can be delocalized by resonance. This is what happens with the sulfanilamides. Therefore, the single pK_a usually given for sulfanilamides refers to the loss of an amide proton (Fig. 6.8)

Mechanism of Action of the Sulfonamides

Folinic acid (N^5-formyltetrahydrofolic acid), N^5,N^{10}-methylenetetrahydrofolic acid, and N^{10}-formyltetrahydrofolic acid are intermediates of several biosynthetic pathways that compose the one-carbon pool in animals, bacteria, and plants. A key reaction involving folate coenzymes is catalyzed by the enzyme thymidylate synthase, which transfers a methyl group from N^5,N^{10}-tetrahydrofolic acid to deoxyuridine monophosphate to form deoxythymidine monophosphate, an important precursor to DNA (Fig. 6.9).

Another key reaction is the generation of formyl groups for the biosynthesis of formylmethionyl tRNA units, the primary building blocks in protein synthesis. The sulfonamides are structural analogs of PABA that competitively inhibit the action of dihydropteroate synthase, preventing the addition of PABA to pteridine diphosphate and blocking the net biosynthesis of folate coenzymes. This action arrests bacterial growth and cell division. The competitive nature of the sulfonamides' action means that the drugs do no permanent damage to a microorganism; hence, they are bacteriostatic. The sulfonamides must be maintained at a minimum effective concentration to arrest the growth of bacteria long enough for the host's immune system to eradicate them.

Folate coenzymes are biosynthesized from dietary folic acid in humans and other animals. Bacteria and protozoa must biosynthesize them from PABA and pteridine diphosphate. Microbes cannot assimilate folic acid from the growth medium or from the host. The reasons for this are poorly understood,[102] but one possibility is that bacterial cell walls may be impermeable to folic acid.

Trimethoprim is an inhibitor of dihydrofolate reductase, which is necessary to convert dihydrofolic acid (FAH_2) into tetrahydrofolic acid (FAH_4) in bacteria (Fig. 6.10). Anand has reviewed this biochemistry.[102] Trimethoprim does not have a

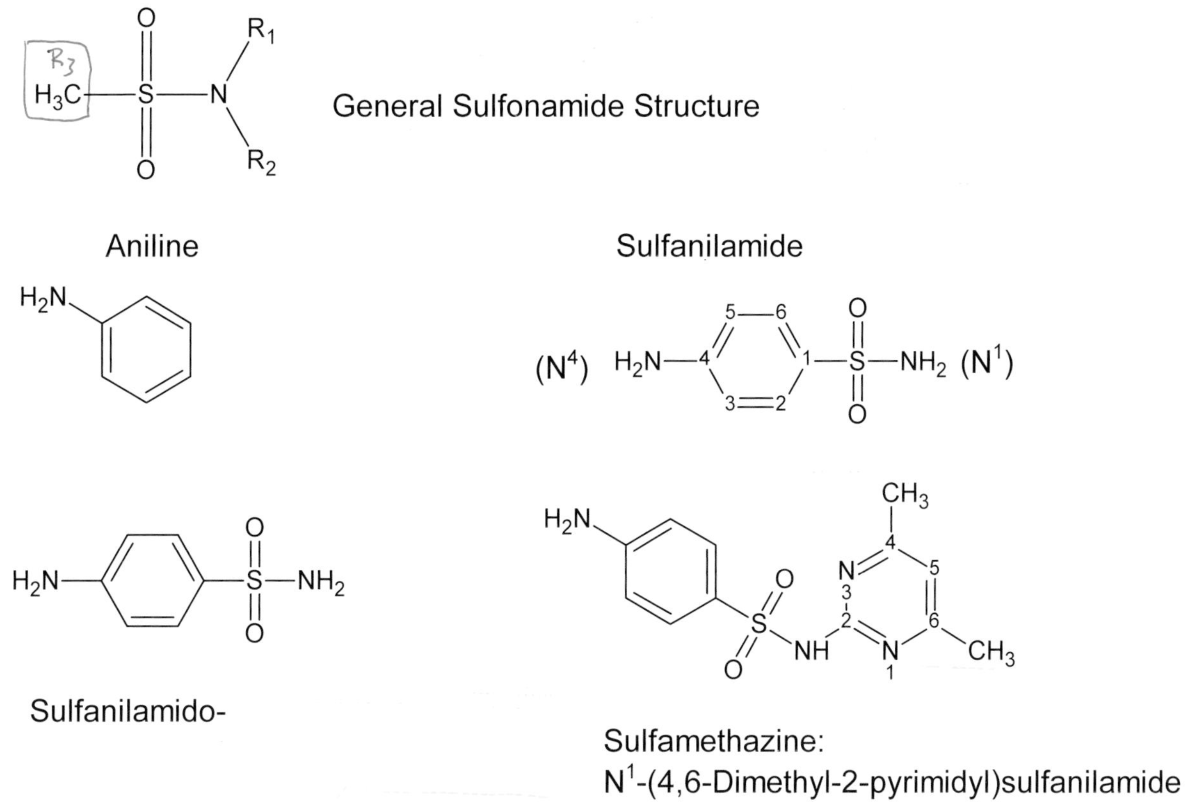

General Sulfonamide Structure

Aniline

Sulfanilamide

(N^4) H_2N—4   1—S—NH_2 (N^1)

Sulfanilamido-

H_2N—S—NH_2

Sulfamethazine:
N^1-(4,6-Dimethyl-2-pyrimidyl)sulfanilamide

Figure 6.8 ● General nomenclature of the sulfonamides.

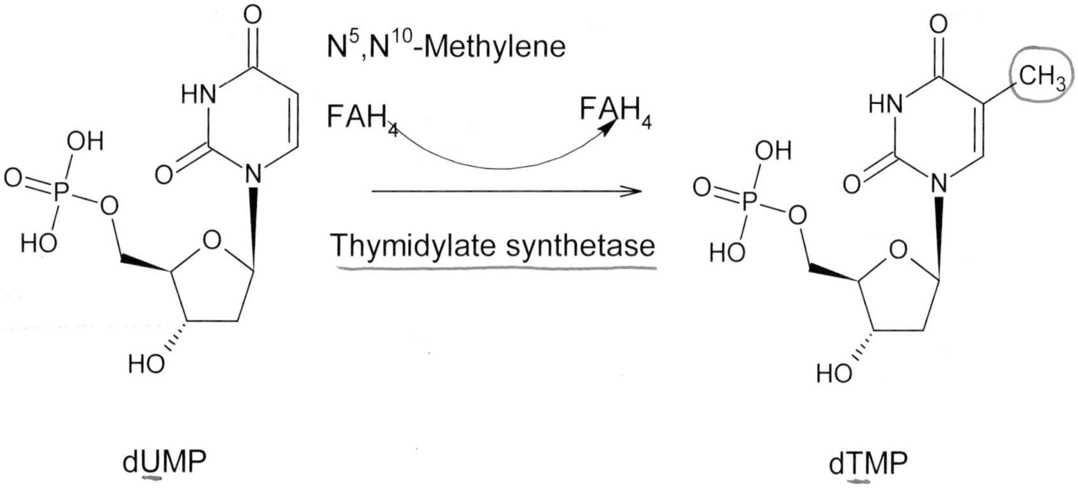

N^5,N^{10}-Methylene

FAH_4 FAH_4

Thymidylate synthetase

dUMP   dTMP

Other examples of folate-requiring one-carbon pool reactions:

Coenzyme	**Reaction**	
N^{10}-Formyl-FAH_4	Met-tRNA ⟶	Formyl-Met-tRNA
N^5N^{10}=Methylene-FAH_4	Glycine ⟶	Serine
N^5-Formyl-FAH_2	Homocysteine ⟶	Methionine

Figure 6.9 ● The thymidylate synthetase reaction and other reactions representing the one-carbon pool.

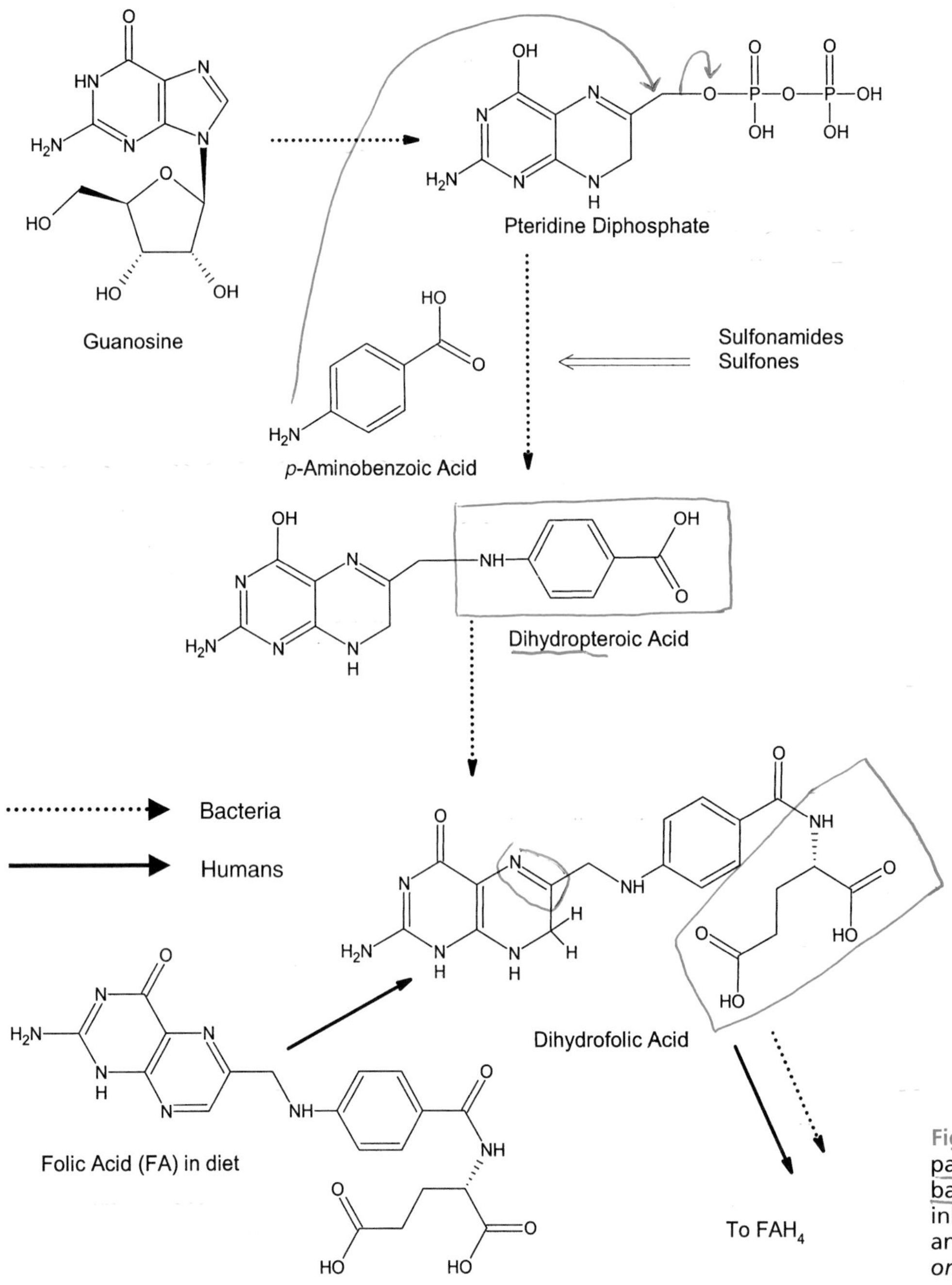

Figure 6.10 ● Folate pathways in humans and bacteria and the sites of inhibition by sulfonamides and trimethoprim. *(continues on next page)*

high affinity for the malaria protozoan's folate reductase, but it does have a high affinity for bacterial folate reductase.

The reverse situation exists for the antimalarial drug pyrimethamine.[112] Trimethoprim does have some affinity for human folate reductase, and this is the cause of some of the toxic effects of the drug.

Spectrum of Action of the Sulfonamides

Sulfonamides inhibit Gram-positive and Gram-negative bacteria, nocardia, *Chlamydia trachomatis*, and some protozoa. Some enteric bacteria, such as *E. coli* and *Klebsiella*, *Salmonella*, *Shigella*, and *Enterobacter* spp. are inhibited. Sulfonamides are infrequently used as single agents. Once drugs of choice for infections such as PCP, toxoplasmosis, nocardiosis, and other bacterial infections, they have been largely replaced by the fixed drug combination TMP–SMX and many

other antimicrobials. Many strains of once-susceptible species, including meningococci, pneumococci, streptococci, staphylococci, and gonococci are now resistant. Sulfonamides are, however, useful in some urinary tract infections because of their high excretion fraction through the kidneys.

Ionization of Sulfonamides (*acidic*)

The sulfonamide group, SO_2NH_2, tends to gain stability if it loses a proton, because the resulting negative charge is resonance stabilized.

Since the proton-donating form of the functional group is not charged, we can characterize it as an HA acid, along with carboxyl groups, phenols, and thiols. The loss of a proton can be associated with a pK_a for all of the compounds in the series. For example, the pK_a of sulfisoxazole (pK_a 5.0) indicates that the sulfonamide is a slightly weaker acid than acetic acid (pK_a 4.8). ≈ 5

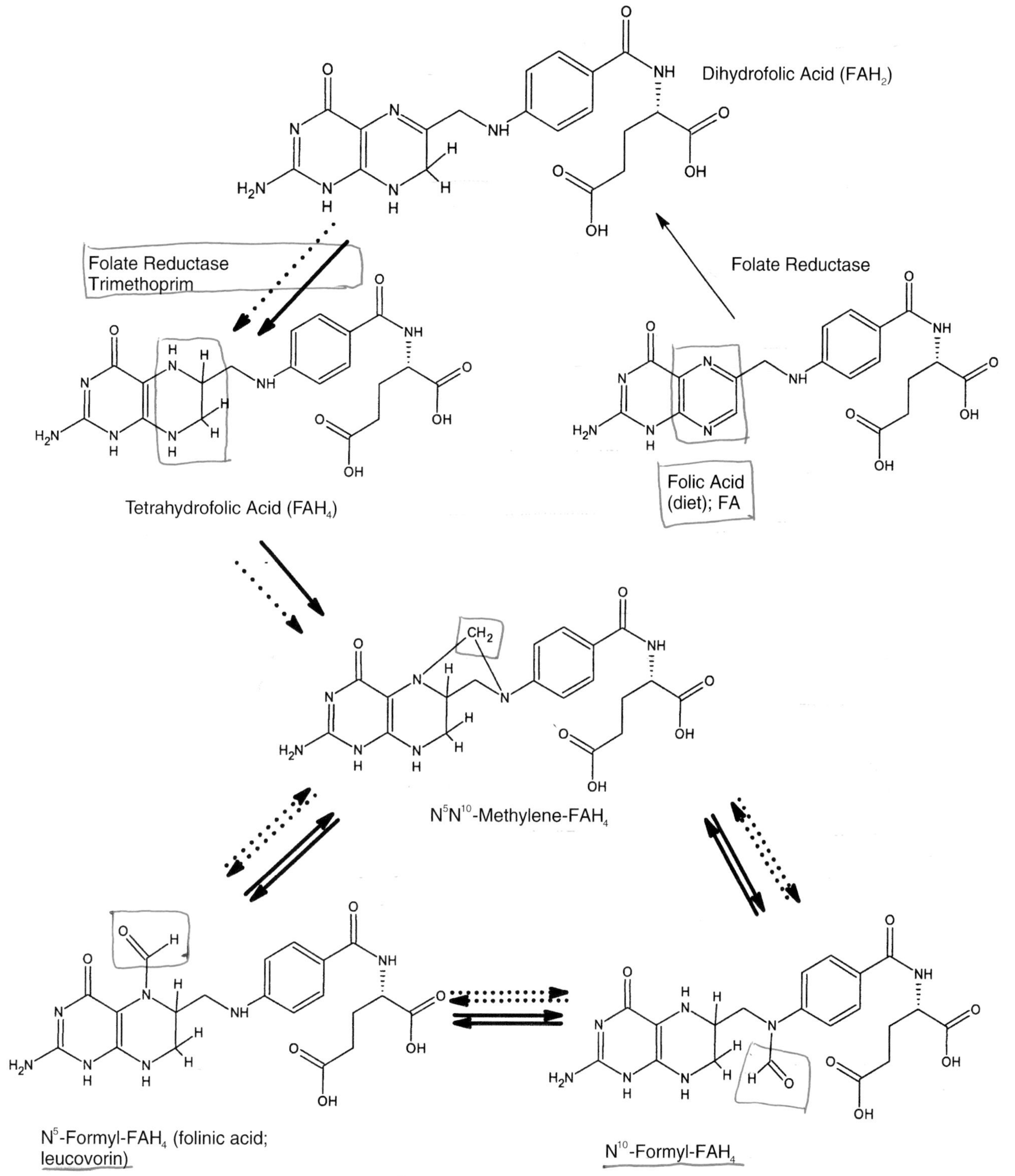

Dihydrofolic Acid (FAH$_2$)

Folate Reductase
Trimethoprim

Folate Reductase

Tetrahydrofolic Acid (FAH$_4$)

Folic Acid
(diet); FA

N^{5}N^{10}-Methylene-FAH$_4$

N^5-Formyl-FAH$_4$ (folinic acid;
leucovorin)

N^{10}-Formyl-FAH$_4$

Figure 6.10 ● *(Continued)*

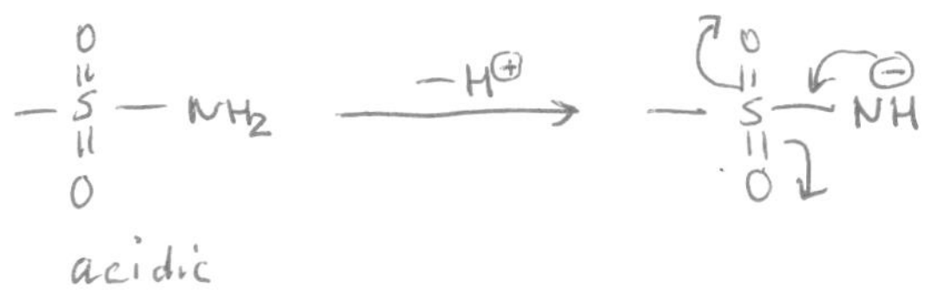

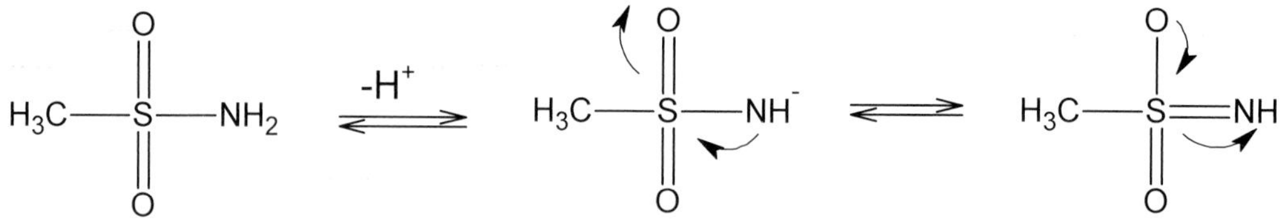

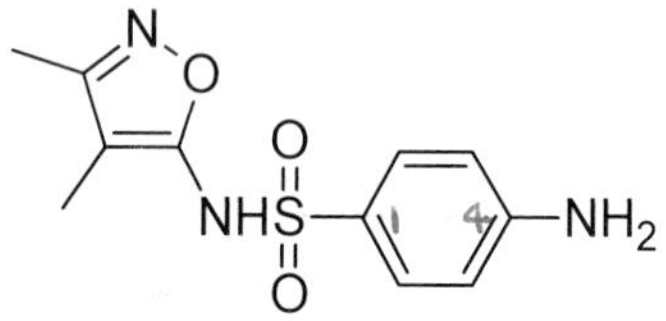

Crystalluria and the pK_a

Despite the tremendous ability of sulfanilamide to effect cures of pathogenic bacteria, its benefits were often offset by the propensity of the drug to cause severe renal damage by crystallizing in the kidneys. Sulfanilamides and their metabolites (usually acetylated at N^4) are excreted almost entirely in the urine. The pK_a of the sulfonamido group of sulfanilamide is 10.4, so the pH at which the drug is 50% ionized is 10.4. Obviously, unless the pH is above the pK_a, little of the water-soluble salt is present. Because the urine is usually about pH 6 (and potentially lower during bacterial infections), essentially all of the sulfanilamide is in the relatively insoluble, nonionized form in the kidneys. The sulfanilamide coming out of solution in the urine and kidneys causes crystalluria.

Early approaches to adjusting the solubility of sulfanilamide in the urine were the following:

1. Greatly increasing the urine flow. During the early years of sulfonamide use, patients taking the drugs were cautioned to "force fluids." The idea was that if the glomerular filtration rate could be increased, there would be less opportunity for seed crystals to form in the renal tubules.
2. Increasing the pH of the urine. The closer the pH of the urine is to 10.4 (for sulfanilamide itself), the more of the highly water-soluble salt form will be present. Oral sodium bicarbonate sometimes was, and occasionally still is, given to raise urine pH. The bicarbonate was administered before the initial dose of sulfanilamide and then prior to each successive dose.
3. Preparing derivatives of sulfanilamide that have lower pK_a values, closer to the pH of the urine. This approach has been taken with virtually all sulfonamides in clinical use today. Examples of the pK_a values of some ionizable sulfonamides are shown in Table 6.8.

4. Mixing different sulfonamides to achieve an appropriate total dose. The solubilities of the sulfonamides are independent of each other, and more of a mixture of sulfanilamides can stay in water solution at a given pH than can a single sulfonamide. Hence, trisulfapyrimidines, *USP* (triple sulfa), contain a mixture of sulfadiazine, sulfamerazine, and sulfamethazine. Such mixtures are seldom used today, however, because the individual agents have sufficiently low pK_a values to be partially ionized and adequately soluble in the urine, *providing that at least the normal urine flow is maintained.* Patients must be cautioned to maintain a normal fluid intake; forcing fluids, however, is no longer necessary.

The newer, semisynthetic sulfonamides possess lower pK_a values because electron-withdrawing, heterocyclic rings are attached to N^1, providing additional stability for the salt form. Hence, the drugs donate a proton more easily, and the pK_a values are lowered. Simpler electron withdrawing groups were extensively investigated but were found to be too toxic, poorly active, or both.

Metabolism, Protein Binding, and Distribution

Except for the poorly absorbed sulfonamides used for ulcerative colitis and reduction of bowel flora and the topical burn preparations (e.g., mafenide), sulfonamides and trimethoprim tend to be absorbed quickly and distributed well. As Mandell and Petri noted, sulfonamides can be found in the urine "within 30 minutes after an oral dose."[108]

The sulfonamides vary widely in plasma protein binding; for example, sulfisoxazole, 76%; sulfamethoxazole, 60%; sulfamethoxypyridazine, 77%; and sulfadiazine, 38%. (Anand[102] has published an excellent table comparing the percentage of protein binding, lipid solubility, plasma half-life, and N^4 metabolites.) The fraction that is protein bound is not active as an antibacterial, but because the binding is reversible, free, and therefore active, sulfonamide eventually becomes available. Generally, the more lipid soluble a sulfonamide is, at physiological pH, the more of it will be protein bound. Fujita and Hansch[113] have found that among sulfonamides with similar pK_a values, the lipophilicity of the

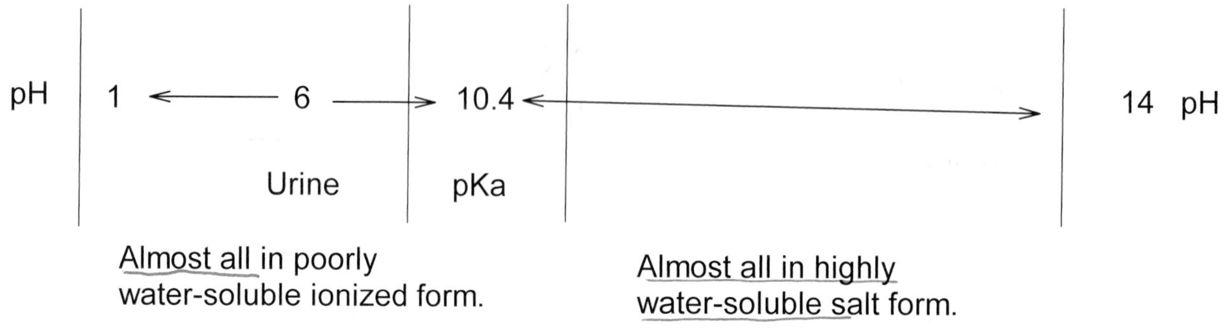

TABLE 6.8 pK$_a$ Values for Clinically Useful Sulfonamides

Sulfonamide	pK$_a$	protein bind (%)
Sulfadiazine	6.5	38
Sulfamerazine	7.1	
Sulfamethazine	7.4	
Sulfisoxazole	5.0	76
Sulfamethoxazole	6.1	60

N^1 group has the largest effect on protein binding. N^4-acetate metabolites of the sulfonamides are more lipid soluble and, therefore, more protein bound than the starting drugs themselves (which have a free 4-amino group that decreases lipid solubility). Surprisingly, the N^4-acetylated metabolites, although more strongly protein bound, are excreted more rapidly than the parent compounds.

Currently, the relationship between plasma protein binding and biological half-life is unclear. Many competing factors are involved, as reflected in sulfadiazine, with a serum half-life of 17 hours, which is much less protein bound than sulfamethoxazole, with a serum half-life of 11 hours.[102]

Sulfonamides are excreted primarily as mixtures of the parent drug, N^4-acetates, and glucuronides.[114] The N^4-acetates and glucuronides are inactive. For example, sulfisoxazole is excreted about 80% unchanged, and sulfamethoxazole is excreted 20% unchanged. Sulfadimethoxine is about 80% excreted as the glucuronide. The correlation between structure and route of metabolism has not yet been delineated, though progress has been made by Fujita.[113] Vree et al.,[114] however, have described the excretion kinetics and pK$_a$ values of N^1- and N^4-acetylsulfamethoxazole and other sulfonamides.

About 45% of trimethoprim and about 66% of sulfamethoxazole are partially plasma protein bound. Whereas about 80% of excreted trimethoprim and its metabolites are active as antibacterials, only 20% of sulfamethoxazole and its metabolites are active, with most of the activity coming from largely unmetabolized sulfamethoxazole. Six metabolites of trimethoprim are known.[115] It is likely, therefore, that sulfonamide-trimethoprim combinations using a sulfonamide with a higher active urine concentration will be developed in the future for urinary tract infections. Sulfamethoxazole and trimethoprim have similar half-lives, about 10 to 12 hours, but the half-life of the active fraction of sulfamethoxazole is shorter, about 9 hours.[115] (Ranges of half-lives have been summarized by Gleckman et al.,[116] and a detailed summary of pharmacokinetics has been made by Hansen.[115]) In patients with impaired renal function, concentrations of sulfamethoxazole and its metabolites may greatly increase in the plasma. A fixed combination of sulfamethoxazole and trimethoprim should not be used for patients with low creatinine clearances.

Mechanisms of Microbial Resistance to Sulfonamides

As noted previously, indiscriminate use of sulfonamides has led to the emergence of many drug-resistant strains of bacteria. Resistance is most likely a result of a compensatory increase in the biosynthesis of PABA by resistant bacteria,[117] although other mechanisms such as alterations in the binding strength of sulfonamides to the pathway enzymes, decreased permeability of the cell membrane, and active efflux of the sulfonamide may play a role.[102,116] As a rule, if a microbe is resistant to one sulfonamide, it is resistant to all. Of note is the finding that sulfonamide resistance can be quickly transferred from a resistant bacterial strain to a previously sensitive one in one or two generations. This resistance propagation is most likely a result of R-factor conjugation, as is the case for tetracycline resistance.

Several explanations have been reported to account for bacterial resistance to the dihydrofolate reductase inhibitor trimethoprim, including intrinsic resistance at the enzymatic level, the development of the ability by the bacteria to use the host's 5-deoxythymidine monophosphate (dTMP), and R-factor conjugation.

Synergistic Activities of Sulfonamides and Folate Reductase Inhibitors

If biosynthesis of bacterial (or protozoal) folate coenzymes is blocked at more than one point in the pathway, the result will be a synergistic antimicrobial effect. This is beneficial because the microbe will not develop resistance as readily as it would with a singly blocked pathway. The synergistic approach is used widely in antibacterial therapy with the combination of sulfamethoxazole and trimethoprim[102,118–120] (Septra, Bactrim, Co-Trimoxazole) and in antimalarial therapy with pyrimethamine plus a sulfonamide or quinine. Additional combinations with trimethoprim have been investigated (e.g., with rifampin).[121,122]

Toxicity and Side Effects

Various serious toxicity and hypersensitivity problems have been reported with sulfonamide and sulfonamide–trimethoprim combinations. Mandell and Petri[108] note that these problems occur in about 5% of all patients. Hypersensitivity reactions include fever, rash, Stevens-Johnson syndrome, skin eruptions, allergic myocarditis, photosensitization, and related conditions. Hematological side effects also sometimes occur, especially hemolytic anemia in individuals with a deficiency of glucose-6-phosphate dehydrogenase. Other reported hematological side effects include agranulocytosis and aplastic anemia. Crystalluria may occur, even with the modern sulfonamides, when the patient does not maintain normal fluid intake. Nausea and related gastrointestinal side effects are sometimes noted. Detailed summaries of incidences of side effects with trimethoprim-sulfamethoxazole have been published by Wormser and Deutsch[118] and by Gleckman et al.[116]

Structure–Activity Relationships

As noted previously in this chapter, several thousand sulfonamides have been investigated as antibacterials (and many as antimalarials). From these efforts, several structure–activity relationships have been proposed, as summarized by Anand.[102] The aniline (N^4) amino group is very important for activity because any modification of it other than to make prodrugs results in a loss of activity. For example, all of the N^4-acetylated metabolites of sulfonamide are inactive.

Various studies have shown that the active form of sulfonamide is the N^1-ionized salt. Thus, although many modern sulfonamides are much more active than unsubstituted sulfanilamide, they are only 2 to 6 times more active if equal amounts of N^1-ionized forms are compared.[123] Maximal

TABLE 6.9 Characteristics of Absorbable Short- and Intermediate-Acting Sulfonamides

Sulfonamide	Half-Life	Oral Absorption
Sulfisoxazole	Short (6 hours)	Prompt (peak levels in 1–4 hours)
Sulfamethizole	Short (9 hours)	Prompt
Sulfadiazine	Intermediate (10–17 hours)	Slow (peak levels in 4–8 hours)
Sulfamethoxazole	Intermediate (10–12 hours)	Slow
Sulfadoxine	Long (7–9 days)	Intermediate
Pyrimidine		
Trimethoprim	Intermediate (11 hours)	Prompt

activity seems to be exhibited by sulfonamides between pK_a 6.6 and 7.4.[123–126] This reflects, in part, the need for enough nonionized (i.e., more lipid soluble) drug to be present at physiological pH to be able to pass through bacterial cell walls.[127] Fujita and Hansch[113] also related pK_a, partition coefficients, and electronic (Hammett) parameters with sulfonamide activity (Table 6.9).

Sulfamethizole

4-Amino-*N*-(5-methyl-1,3,4-thiadiazole-2yl)benzenesulfonamide; *N*[1]-(5-methyl-1,3,4-thiadiazol-2-yl)sulfanilamide; 5-methyl-2-sulfanilamido-1,3,4-thiadiazole. Sulfamethizole's plasma half-life is 2.5 hours. This compound is a white crystalline powder soluble 1:2,000 in water.

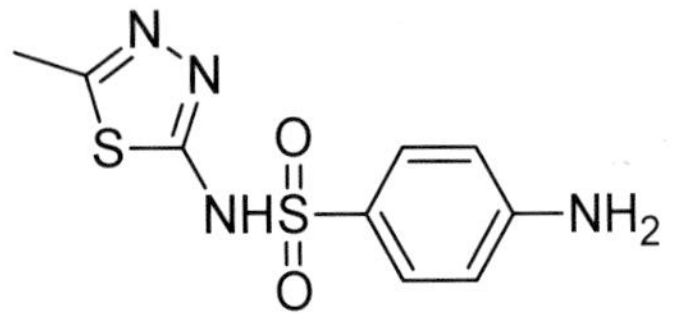

Sulfisoxazole (parent compd)

4-Amino-*N*-(3,4-dimethyl-5-isoxazolyl)benzenesulfonamide; *N*[1]-(3,4-dimethyl-5-isoxazolyl) sulfanilamide; 5-sulfanilamido-3,4-dimethylisoxazole. Sulfisoxazole's plasma half-life is 6 hours. This compound is a white, odorless, slightly bitter, crystalline powder. Its pK_a is 5.0. At pH 6, this sulfonamide has a water solubility of 350 mg in 100 mL, and its acetyl derivative has a solubility of 110 mg in 100 mL of water.

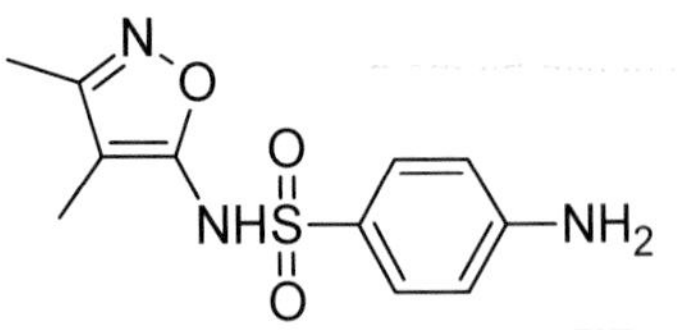

Sulfisoxazole possesses the action and the uses of other sulfonamides and is used for infections involving sulfonamide-sensitive bacteria. It is claimed to be effective in the treatment of Gram-negative urinary infections.

Sulfisoxazole Acetyl

N-[(4-Aminophenyl)sulfonyl]-*N*-(3,4-dimethyl-5-isoxazolyl)acetamide; *N*-(3,4-dimethyl-5-isoxazolyl)-*N*-sulfanily-lacetamide; *N*[1]-acetyl-*N*[1]-(3,4-dimethyl-5-isoxazolyl)sulfanilamide. Sulfisoxazole acetyl shares the actions and uses of the parent compound, sulfisoxazole. The acetyl derivative is tasteless and, therefore, suitable for oral administration, especially in liquid preparations. The acetyl compound is split in the intestinal tract and absorbed as sulfisoxazole; that is, it is a *prodrug* for sulfisoxazole.

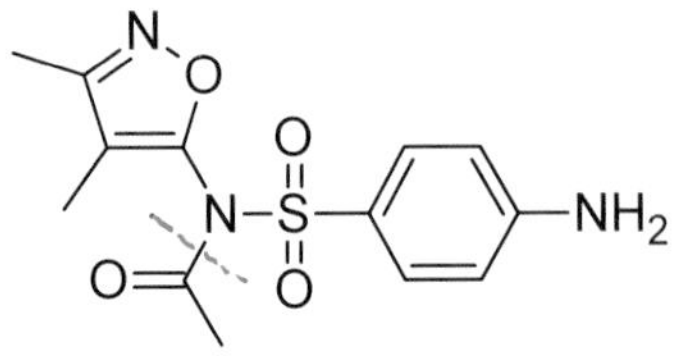

Sulfisoxazole Diolamine

4-Amino-*N*-(3,5-dimethyl-5-isoxazolyl)benzenesulfonamide compound with 2,2′-iminobis[ethanol](1:1); 2,2′-iminodiethanol salt of *N*[1]-(3,4-dimethyl-5-isoxazolyl)sulfanilamide. This salt is prepared by adding enough diethanolamine to a solution of sulfisoxazole to bring the pH to about 7.5. It is used as a salt to make the drug more soluble in the physiological pH range of 6.0 to 7.5 and is used in solution for systemic administration of the drug by slow intravenous, intramuscular, or subcutaneous injection when high enough blood levels cannot be maintained by oral administration alone. It also is used for instillation of drops or ointment in the eye for the local treatment of susceptible infections.

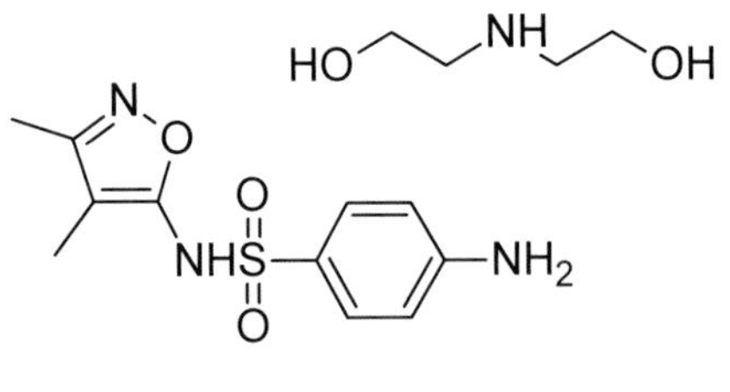

Sulfamethazine

4-Amino-*N*-(4,6-dimethyl-2-pyrimidinyl)benzenesulfonamide; *N*[1]-(4,6-dimethyl-2-pyrimidinyl)sulfanilamide; 2-sulfanilamido-4,6-dimethylpyrimidine. Sulfamethazine's plasma half-life is 7 hours. This compound is similar in chemical properties to sulfamerazine and sulfadiazine but does have greater water solubility than either. Its pK_a is 7.2. Because it is more soluble in acid urine than sulfamerazine is, the possibility of kidney damage from use of the drug is decreased. The human body appears to handle the drug unpredictably; hence, there is some disfavor to its use in this country except in combination sulfa therapy (in trisulfapyrimidines, *USP*) and in veterinary medicine.

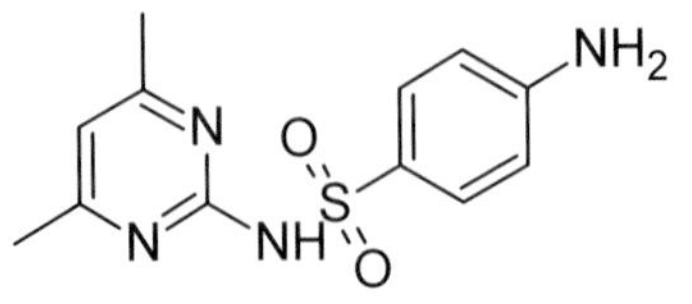

Sulfacetamide

N-[(4-Aminophenyl)sulfonyl]-acetamide; *N*-sulfanilylacetamide; *N*[1]-acetylsulfanilamide. Sulfacetamide's plasma half-life is 7 hours. This compound is a white crystalline powder, soluble in water (1:62.5 at 37°C) and in alcohol. It is very soluble in hot water, and its water solution is acidic. It has a pK$_a$ of 5.4.

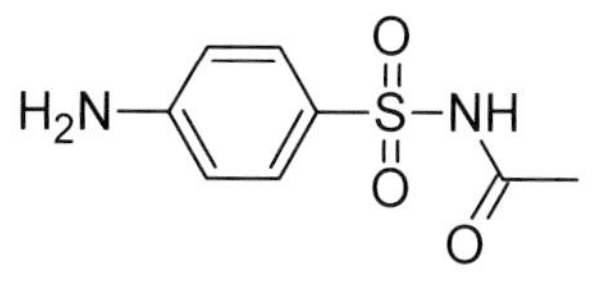

Sulfachloropyridazine

N^1-(6-Chloro-3-pyridazinyl) sulfanilamide. Sulfachloropyridazine's plasma half-life is 8 hours.

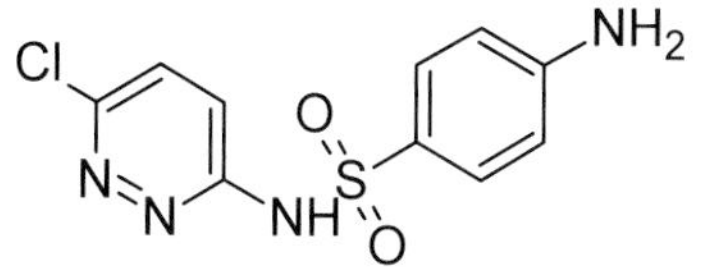

Sulfapyridine

4-Amino-N-2-pyridinylbenzenesulfonamide; N^1-2-pyridylsulfanilamide. Sulfapyridine's plasma half-life is 9 hours. This compound is a white, crystalline, odorless, and tasteless substance. It is stable in air but slowly darkens on exposure to light. It is soluble in water (1:3,500), in alcohol (1:440), and in acetone (1:65) at 25°C. It is freely soluble in dilute mineral acids and aqueous solutions of sodium and potassium hydroxide. The pK$_a$ is 8.4. Its outstanding effect in curing pneumonia was first recognized by Whitby; however, because of its relatively high toxicity, it has been supplanted largely by sulfadiazine and sulfamerazine. Several cases of kidney damage have resulted from acetylsulfapyridine crystals deposited in the kidneys. It also causes severe nausea in most patients. Because of its toxicity, it is used only for dermatitis herpetiformis.

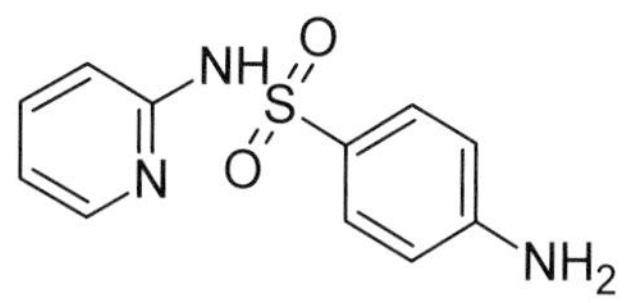

Sulfapyridine was the first drug to have an outstanding curative action on pneumonia. It gave impetus to the study of the whole class of N^1 heterocyclically substituted derivatives of sulfanilamide.

Sulfamethoxazole

4-Amino-N-(5-methyl-3-isoxazolyl)benzenesulfonamide; N^1-(5-methyl-3-isoxazolyl) sulfanilamide (Gantanol). Sulfamethoxazole's plasma half-life is 11 hours.

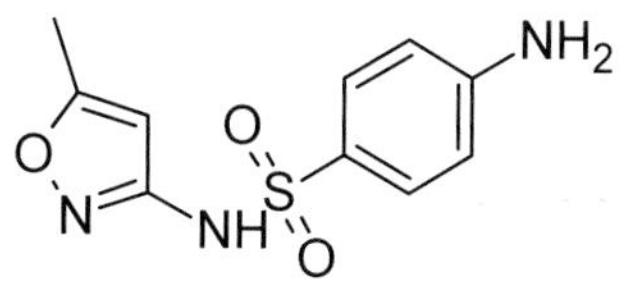

Sulfamethoxazole is a sulfonamide drug closely related to sulfisoxazole in chemical structure and antimicrobial activity. It occurs as a tasteless, odorless, almost white crystalline powder. The solubility of sulfamethoxazole in the pH range of 5.5 to 7.4 is slightly lower than that of sulfisoxazole

but higher than that of sulfadiazine, sulfamerazine, or sulfamethazine.

Following oral administration, sulfamethoxazole is not absorbed as completely or as rapidly as sulfisoxazole, and its peak blood level is only about 50% as high.

Sulfadiazine

4-Amino-N-2-pyrimidinyl-benzenesulfonamide; N^1-2-pyrimidinylsulfanilamide; 2-sulfanilamidopyrimidine. Sulfadiazine's plasma half-life is 17 hours. It is a white, odorless crystalline powder soluble in water to the extent of 1:8,100 at 37°C and 1:13,000 at 25°C, in human serum to the extent of 1:620 at 37°C, and sparingly soluble in alcohol and acetone. It is readily soluble in dilute mineral acids and bases. Its pK$_a$ is 6.3.

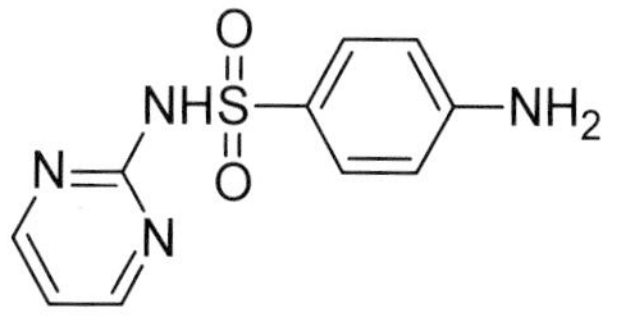

Sulfadiazine Sodium

Soluble sulfadiazine is an anhydrous, white, colorless, crystalline powder soluble in water (1:2) and slightly soluble in alcohol. Its water solutions are alkaline (pH 9–10) and absorb carbon dioxide from the air, with precipitation of sulfadiazine. It is administered as a 5% solution in sterile water intravenously for patients requiring an immediately high blood level of the sulfonamide.

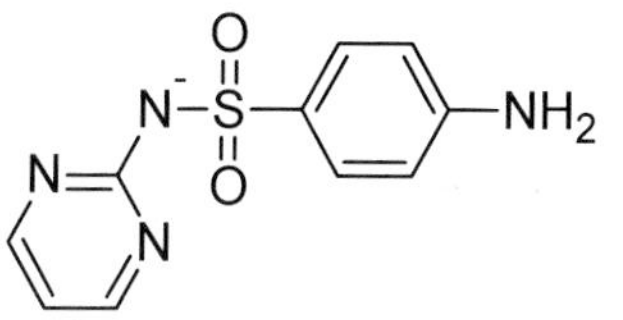

Mixed Sulfonamides

The danger of crystal formation in the kidneys from administration of sulfonamides has been greatly reduced through the use of the more soluble sulfonamides, such as sulfisoxazole. This danger may be diminished still further by administering mixtures of sulfonamides. When several sulfonamides are administered together, the antibacterial action of the mixture is the summation of the activity of the total sulfonamide concentration present, but the solubilities are independent of the presence of similar compounds. Thus, by giving a mixture of sulfadiazine, sulfamerazine, and sulfacetamide, the same therapeutic level can be maintained with much less danger of crystalluria, because only one third of the amount of any one compound is present. Descriptions of some of the mixtures used follow.

Trisulfapyrimidines, Oral Suspension

The oral suspension of trisulfapyrimidines contains equal weights of sulfadiazine, *USP*; sulfamerazine, *USP*; and sulfamethazine, *USP*, either with or without an agent to raise the pH of the urine.

Trisulfapyrimidines, Tablets

Trisulfapyrimidine tablets contain essentially equal quantities of sulfadiazine, sulfamerazine, and sulfamethazine.

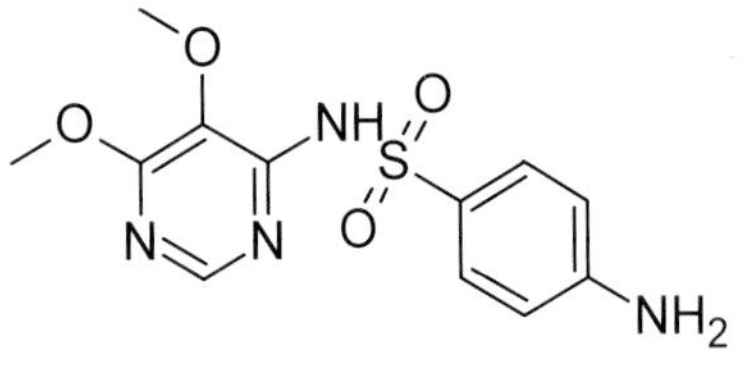

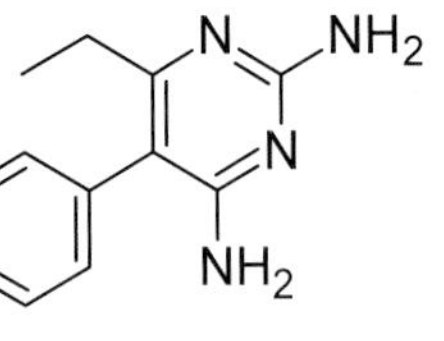

Sulfadoxine and Pyrimethamine

The mixture of sulfadoxine and pyrimethamine (Fansidar) is used for the treatment of *P. falciparum* malaria in patients in whom chloroquine resistance is suspected. It is also used for malaria prophylaxis for travelers to areas where chloroquine-resistant malaria is endemic.

Topical Sulfonamides

Sulfacetamide Sodium

N-Sulfanilylacetamide monosodium salt (Sodium Sulamyd) is obtained as the monohydrate and is a white, odorless, bitter, crystalline powder that is very soluble (1:2.5) in water. Because the sodium salt is highly soluble at the physiological pH of 7.4, it is especially suited, as a solution, for repeated topical applications in the local management of ophthalmic infections susceptible to sulfonamide therapy.

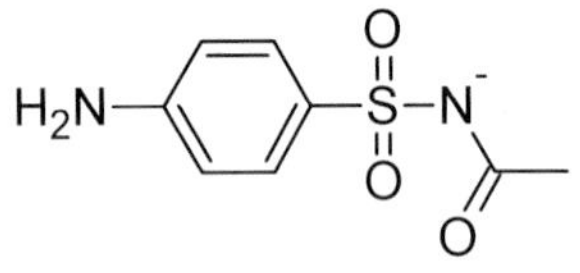

Sulfisoxazole Diolamine

Sulfisoxazole diolamine is described with the short- and intermediate-acting sulfonamides and also used in intravenous and intramuscular preparations.

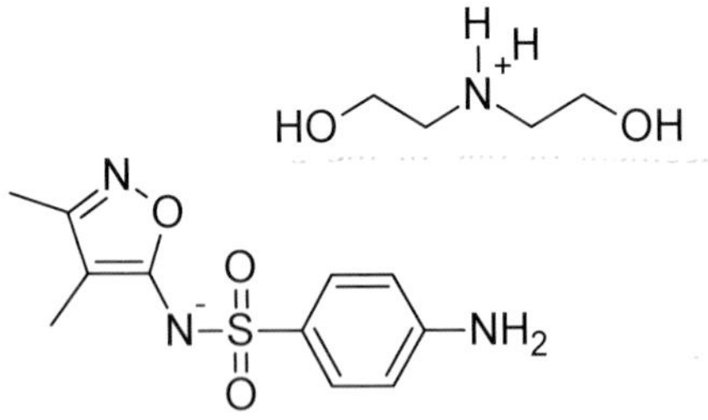

Triple Sulfa

Triple sulfa (sulfabenzamide, sulfacetamide, and sulfathiazole; Femguard) is used as a vaginal cream in the treatment of *Haemophilus vaginalis* vaginitis.

Nonabsorbable Sulfonamides

TOPICAL SULFONAMIDES FOR BURN THERAPY

Mafenide Acetate

4-(Aminomethyl)benzenesulfonamide acetate (Sulfamylon) is a homologue of the sulfanilamide molecule. It is not a true sulfanilamide-type compound, as it is not inhibited by PABA. Its antibacterial action involves a mechanism that differs from that of true sulfanilamide-type compounds.

This compound is particularly effective against *Clostridium welchii* in topical application and was used during World War II by the German army for prophylaxis of wounds. It is not effective orally. It is currently used alone or with antibiotics in the treatment of slow-healing, infected wounds.

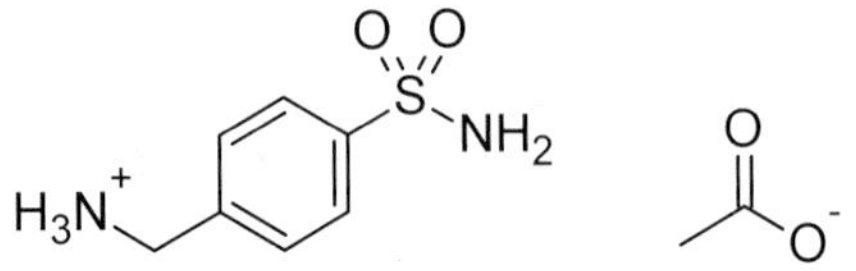

Some patients treated for burns with large quantities of this drug have developed metabolic acidosis. To overcome this adverse effect, a series of new organic salts was prepared.[16] The acetate in an ointment base proved to be the most efficacious.

Silver Sulfadiazine (Silvadene)

The silver salt of sulfadiazine applied in a water-miscible cream base has proved to be an effective topical antimicrobial agent, especially against *Pseudomonas* spp. This is particularly significant in burn therapy because pseudomonads are often responsible for failures in therapy. The salt is only slightly soluble and does not penetrate the cell wall but acts on the external cell structure. Studies using radioactive silver have shown essentially no absorption into body fluids. Sulfadiazine levels in the serum were about 0.5 to 2 mg/100 mL.

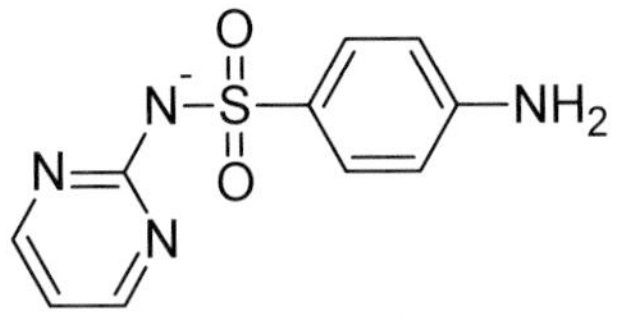

This preparation is reported to be easier to use than other standard burn treatments, such as application of freshly prepared dilute silver nitrate solutions or mafenide ointment.

Sulfonamides for Intestinal Infections, Ulcerative Colitis, or Reduction of Bowel Flora

Each of the sulfonamides in this group is a prodrug, which is designed to be poorly absorbable, though usually, in practice, a little is absorbed. Therefore, usual precautions with sulfonamide therapy should be observed. In the large intestine, the N^4-protecting groups are cleaved, releasing the free sulfonamide antibacterial agent. Today, only one example is used clinically, sulfasalazine.

Sulfasalazine

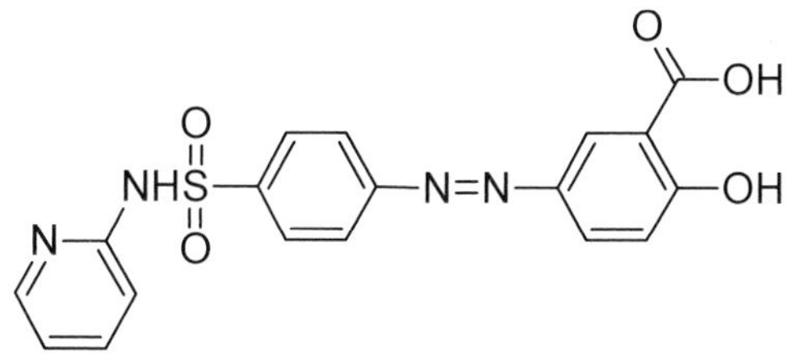

Sulfasalazine (2-hydroxy-5[[4-[(2-pyridinylamino)sulfonyl] phenyl]azo]benzoic acid or 5-[*p*-(2-pyridylsulfamoyl) phenylazo]salicylic acid) is a brownish yellow, odorless powder, slightly soluble in alcohol but practically insoluble in water, ether, and benzene.

Sulfasalazine is broken down in the body to *m*-aminosalicylic acid and sulfapyridine. The drug is excreted through the kidneys and is detectable colorimetrically in the urine, producing an orange-yellow color when the urine is alkaline and no color when the urine is acid.

⬡ DIHYDROFOLATE REDUCTASE (DR) INHIBITORS

Trimethoprim

Trimethoprim (5-[(3,4,5-trimethoxyphenyl)methyl]-2,4-pyrimidinediamine or 2,4-diamino-5-(3,4,5-trimethoxybenzyl)pyrimidine) is closely related to several antimalarials but does not have good antimalarial activity by itself; it is, however, a potent antibacterial. Originally introduced in combination with sulfamethoxazole, it is now available as a single agent.

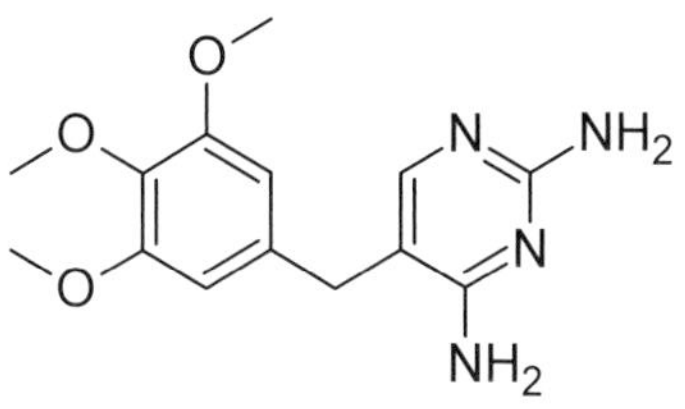

Approved by the FDA in 1980, trimethoprim as a single agent is used only for the treatment of uncomplicated urinary tract infections. The argument for trimethoprim as a single agent was summarized in 1979 by Wormser and Deutsch.[118] They point out that several studies comparing trimethoprim with TMP–SMX for the treatment of chronic urinary tract infections found no statistically relevant difference between the two courses of therapy. Furthermore, some patients cannot take sulfonamide products for the reasons discussed previously in this chapter. The concern is that when used as a single agent, bacteria now susceptible to trimethoprim will rapidly develop resistance. In combination with a sulfonamide, however, the bacteria will be less likely to do so. That is, they will not survive long enough to easily develop resistance to both drugs.

Sulfamethoxazole and Trimethoprim

The synergistic action of the combination of these two drugs is discussed previously in this chapter.

⬡ SULFONES

The sulfones are primarily of interest as antibacterial agents, though there are some reports of their use in the treatment of malarial and rickettsial infections. They are less effective than the sulfonamides. PABA partially antagonizes the action of many of the sulfones, suggesting that the mechanism of action is similar to that of the sulfonamides. Further, infections that arise in patients being treated with sulfones are cross-resistant to sulfonamides. Several sulfones have proved useful in the treatment of leprosy, but among them only dapsone is clinically used today.

It has been estimated that there are about 11 million cases of leprosy in the world, of which about 60% are in Asia (with 3.5 million in India alone). The first reports of dapsone resistance prompted the use of multidrug therapy with dapsone, rifampin, and clofazimine combinations in some geographic areas.[128]

The search for antileprotic drugs has been hampered by the inability to cultivate *M. leprae* in artificial media and by the lack of experimental animals susceptible to human leprosy. A method of isolating and growing *M. leprae* in the footpads of mice and in armadillos has been reported and has permitted a much wider range of research. Sulfones were introduced into the treatment of leprosy after it was found that sodium glucosulfone was effective in experimental tuberculosis in guinea pigs.

The parent sulfone, dapsone (4,4′-sulfonyldianiline), is the prototype for various analogs that have been widely studied. Four variations on this structure have given active compounds:

1. Substitution on both the 4- and 4′-amino functions
2. Monosubstitution on only one of the amino functions
3. Nuclear substitution on one of the benzenoid rings
4. Replacement of one of the phenyl rings with a heterocyclic ring

The antibacterial activity and the toxicity of the disubstituted sulfones are thought to be chiefly caused by the formation in vivo of dapsone. Hydrolysis of disubstituted derivatives to the parent sulfone apparently occurs readily in the acid medium of the stomach but only to a very limited extent following parenteral administration. Monosubstituted and nuclear-substituted derivatives are believed to act as entire molecules.

Dapsone

Dapsone (4,4′-sulfonylbisbenzeneamine; 4,4′-sulfonyldianiline; *p,p′*-diaminodiphenylsulfone; or DDS [Avlosulfon]) occurs as an odorless, white crystalline powder that is very slightly soluble in water and sparingly soluble in alcohol. The pure compound is light stable, but traces of impurities, including water, make it photosensitive and thus susceptible to discoloration in light. Although no chemical change is detectable following discoloration, the drug should be protected from light.

Dapsone is used in the treatment of both lepromatous and tuberculoid types of leprosy. Dapsone is used widely for all forms of leprosy, often in combination with clofazimine and rifampin. Initial treatment often includes rifampin with dapsone, followed by dapsone alone. It is also used to prevent the occurrence of multibacillary leprosy when given prophylactically.

Dapsone is also the drug of choice for dermatitis herpetiformis and is sometimes used with pyrimethamine for treatment of malaria and with trimethoprim for PCP.

Serious side effects can include hemolytic anemia, methemoglobinemia, and toxic hepatic effects. Hemolytic effects can be pronounced in patients with glucose-6-phosphate dehydrogenase deficiency. During therapy, all patients require frequent blood counts.

◆ R E V I E W Q U E S T I O N S ◆

1. What is the definition of an antiseptic?

2. What happens to the antimicrobial activity of alcohols as the carbon chain becomes more branched?

3. What kind of bond associates iodine with polyvinylpyrrolidone in PVP–iodine?

4. What is the most active agent for the clinical treatment of tuberculosis?

5. What is the function of dihydrofolate reductase in bacteria?

REFERENCES

1. Atlas, R. M.: Microbiology, Fundamentals and Applications. New York, Macmillan, 1984, p. 19.
2. Ehrlich, B.: United States Patent 986,148.
3. Christiansen, A.: J. Am. Chem. Soc. 42:2402, 1920.
4. Atlas, R. M.: Microbiology, Fundamentals and Applications. New York, Macmillan, 1984, p. 20.
5. Fleming, M., et al.: Ethanol. In Hardman, J. G., Limbird, L. E., and Gilman, A. G. (eds.). Goodman and Gilman's The Pharmacological Basis of Therapeutics. New York, McGraw-Hill, 2001.
6. DuMez, A. G.: J. Am. Pharm. Assoc. 28:416, 1939.
7. Gilbert, G. L.: Appl. Microbiol. 12:496, 1964.
8. Leech, P. N.: J. Am. Med. Assoc. 109:1531, 1937.
9. Miner, N. A., et al.: Am. J. Pharm. 34:376, 1977.
10. U.S. Food and Drug Administration: Hexachlorophene and Newborns. Bulletin, December 1971.
11. Vasarenesh, A.: Arch. Dermatol. 98:183, 1968.
12. Gershenfeld, L.: Milk Food Technol. 18:233, 1955.
13. Domagk, G.: Dtsch. Med. Wochenschr. 61:250, 1935.
14. Rose, F. L., and Swain, G. J.: J. Chem. Soc. 442, 1956.
15. Massey, A. G.: Main Group Elements. Chichester, England, Ellis Horwood Ltd., 1990, p. 160.
16. Garrett, E. R., and Woods, O. R.: J. Am. Pharm. Assoc. (Sci. Ed.) 42:736, 1953.
17. Rippon, J. W.: In Burrows, W. (ed.). Textbook of Microbiology. Philadelphia, W. B. Saunders, 1973, p. 683.
18. Friedman, L., et al.: J. Invest. Dermatol. 35:3–5, 1960.
19. Rippon, J. W.: In Burrows, W. (ed.). Textbook of Microbiology. Philadelphia, W. B. Saunders, 1973, p. 721.
20. Rippon, J. W.: In Burrows, W. (ed.). Textbook of Microbiology. Philadelphia, W. B. Saunders, 1973, p. 734.
21. Goldman, R. C., and Klein, L. L.: Annu. Rep. Med. Chem. 29:155, 1994.
22. Ajello, L.: Science 123:876, 1956.
23. Ajello, L.: Mycopathologia 17:315, 1962.
24. Rebell, G., and Taplin, D.: Dermatophytes. Miami, University of Miami Press, 1970.
25. Rieth, H.: Arzneim. Forsch. 31:1309, 1981.
26. Polak, A., and Scholer, H. J.: Chemotherapy 21:113, 1975.
27. Baginski, M., Resat, H., and McCammon, J. A.: Mol. Pharmacol. 52:560, 1997.
28. Baginski, M., Gariboldi, P., Bruni, P., et al.: Biophys. Chem. 65:91, 1997.
29. Gold, W., et al.: Antibiotics Annual 1955–1956. New York, Medical Encyclopedia, 1956.
30. Mechlinski, W., et al.: Tetrahedron Lett. 3873, 1970.
31. Graybill, J. R.: Ann. Intern. Med. 124:921, 1986.
32. Ianknegkt, R., et al.: Clin. Pharmacokinet. 23:279, 1992.
33. Hazen, E. L., and Brown, R.: Proc. Soc. Exp. Biol. Med. 76:93, 1951.
34. Pandey, R. C., and Rinehart, K. L.: J. Antibiot. 29:1035, 1976.
35. Lencelin, J. M., et al.: Tetrahedron Lett. 29:2827, 1988.
36. Struyk, A. P., Hoette, I., Orost, G., et al.: Antibiot. Ann. 878, 1957–1958.
37. Brik, H., et al.: Nystatin. In Florey, K. (ed.). Analytical Profiles of Drug Substances, vol. 10. New York, Academic Press, 1981, p. 513.
38. Oxford, A. E., et al.: Biochem. J. 33:240, 1939.
39. Grove, J. F., et al.: J. Chem. Soc. 3977, 1952.
40. Sloboda, R. D., Van Blaricom, G., Creasey, W. A., et al.: Biochem. Biophys. Res. Commun. 105:882, 1982.
41. Stütz, A., and Petranyi, G.: J. Med. Chem. 27:1539, 1984.
42. Ryder, N. S.: Antimicrob. Agents Chemother. 27:252, 1985.
43. Petranyi, G., et al.: Science 224:1239, 1984.
44. Gupta, M. P., et al.: J. Vet. Med. Mycol. 29:45, 1991.
45. Thomas, A. H.: Antimicrob. Chemother. 17:269, 1986.
46. Hitchcock, C. A.: Biochem. Soc. Trans. 19:782, 1991.
47. Pont, A., et al.: Arch. Intern. Med. 144:2150, 1984.
48. Vanden Bossche, H.: Drug Dev. Res. 8:287, 1986.
49. Rotstein, D. M., Kertesz, D. J., Walker, K. A. M., et al.: J. Med. Chem. 35:2818, 1992.
50. Dickinson, R. P., et al.: Med. Chem. Lett. 6:2031, 1996.
51. DeBono, M., et al.: J. Med. Chem. 38:3271, 1995.
52. Schwartz, R. E., Masurekar, P. S., and White, R. F.: Clin. Dermatol. 7:375, 1993.
53. Balkovec, J. M.: Annu. Rep. Med. Chem. 33:175, 1998.
54. Jao, E.: Tetrahedron Lett. 37:5661, 1996.
55. Nagiec, M. M., Nagiec, E. E., et al.: J. Biol. Chem. 272:9809, 1997.
56. Shen, L. L., Mitscher, L. A., Sharma, P. N., et al.: Biochemistry 28:3886, 1989.
57. Sreedharan, S., et al.: J. Bacteriol. 172:7260, 1990.
58. Yoshida, H., et al.: Antimicrob. Agents Chemother. 35:1647, 1991.
59. Yoshida, H., et al.: Antimicrob. Agents Chemother. 34:1273, 1990.
60. Bazile, S., et al.: Antimicrob. Agents Chemother. 36:2622, 1992.
61. Domagala, J. M.: J. Antimicrob. Chemother. 33:685, 1994.
62. Ross, D. L., and Riley, C. M.: J. Pharm. Biomed. Anal. 12:1325, 1994.
63. Lee, D. S., et al.: J. Pharm. Biomed. Anal. 12:157, 1994.
64. Mitscher, L. A., et al.: J. Med. Chem. 30:2283, 1987.
65. Bloom, B. R., and Murray, C. J. L.: Science 257:1055, 1992.
66. Winder, F. G., and Collins, P. B.: J. Gen. Microbiol. 63:41, 1970.
67. Quomard, A., Lacove, C., and LanPelle, G.: Antimicrob. Agents Chemother. 35:1035, 1991.
68. Youatt, J., and Tham, S. H.: Am. Rev. Respir. Dis. 100:25, 1969.
69. Johnsson, K., and Schultz, P. G.: J. Am. Chem. Soc. 116:7425, 1994.

70. Zhang, Y., et al.: Nature 358:591, 1992.
71. Dessen, A., et al.: Science 267:1638, 1995.
72. Banerjee, A., et al.: Science 263:227, 1994.
73. Boxenbaum, H. G., and Riegelman, S.: J. Pharm. Sci. 63:1191, 1974.
74. Heifets, L. B., Flory, M. A., and Lindholm-Levy, P. J.: Antimicrob. Agents Chemother. 33:1252, 1989.
75. Rinehart, K. L.: Acc. Chem. Res. 5:57, 1972.
76. Hartmann, G. R., et al.: Angew. Chem. Int. Ed. Engl. 24:1009, 1985.
77. Katz, E., and Moss, B.: Proc. Natl. Acad. Sci. U. S. A. 66:677, 1970.
78. Werli, W.: Rev. Infect. Dis. 5S:407, 1983.
79. Gallo, G. G., and Radaelli, P.: Rifampin. In Florey, K. (ed.). Analytical Profiles of Drug Substances. New York, Academic Press, 1976.
80. Kuehl, F. A., et al.: J. Am. Chem. Soc. 77:2344, 1955.
81. Hildy, P. H., et al.: J. Am. Chem. Soc. 77:2345, 1955.
82. Stammer, C. H., et al.: J. Am. Chem. Soc. 77:2346, 1955.
83. Smart, J., et al.: Experientia 13:291, 1957.
84. Neuhaus, F. C., and Lynch, J. L.: Biochemistry 3:471, 1964.
85. Rando, R. R.: Biochem. Pharmacol. 24:1153, 1975.
86. Herr, E. B., Pittenger, G. E., and Higgens, C. E.: Indiana Acad. Sci. 69:134, 1960.
87. Bycroft, B. W., et al.: Nature 231:301, 1971.
88. Nomoto, S., et al.: J. Antibiot. 30:955, 1977.
89. Knight, R. C., et al.: Biochem. Pharmacol. 27:2089, 1978.
90. Metcalf, B. W., et al.: J. Am. Chem. Soc. 100:2551, 1978.
91. Prichard, R. K.: Nature 228:684, 1970.
92. Friedman, P. A., and Platzer, E. G.: Biochim. Biophys. Acta 544: 605, 1978.
93. Pica-Mattoccia, L., and Cioli, D.: Am. J. Trop. Med. Hyg. 34:112, 1985.
94. Burg, R. W., et al.: Antimicrob. Agents Chemother. 15:361, 1979.
95. Campbell, W. C.: Science 221:823, 1983.
96. Albers-Schonberg, G., et al.: J. Am. Chem. Soc. 103:4216, 1981.
97. Springer, J. P., et al.: J. Am. Chem. Soc. 103:4221, 1981.
98. Aziz, M. A., et al.: Lancet 2:171, 1982.
99. Orkin, M., and Maibach, H. I.: N. Engl. J. Med. 298:496, 1978.
100. Domagk, G.: Dtsch. Med. Wochenschr. 61:250, 1935.
101. Baumler, E.: In Search of the Magic Bullet. London, Thames and Hudson, 1965.
102. Anand, N.: Sulfonamides and sulfones. In Wolff, M. E. (ed.). Burger's Medicinal Chemistry, vol. 2, 5th ed. New York, Wiley-Interscience, 1996, Chap. 33.
103. Foerster, J.: Z. Haut. Geschlechtskr. 45:459, 1933.
104. Trefouel, J., et al.: C. R. Seances Soc. Biol. 120:756, 1935.
105. Fuller, A. T.: Lancet 1:194, 1937.
106. Northey, E. H.: The Sulfonamides and Allied Compounds. ACS Monogr. Ser. Washington, DC, American Chemical Society, 1948.
107. MacDonald, L., and Kazanijan, P.: Formulary 31:470, 1996.
108. Petri, W. A.: Antimicrobial agents: Sulfonamides, trimethoprim-sulfamethoxazole, quinolones, and agents for urinary tract infection. In Gilman, A. G., et al. (eds.). The Pharmacological Basis of Therapeutics, 9th ed. New York, Macmillan, 1996.
109. Jawetz, E.: Principles of antimicrobial drug action. In Katzung, B. G. (ed.). Basic and Clinical Pharmacology, 6th ed. Norwalk, CT, Appleton & Lange, 1995.
110. Med. Lett. 30:33, 1988.
111. FDA Drug Bulletin, US Department of Health, Education and Welfare, Food and Drug Administration, Feb., 1980.
112. Med. Lett. 29:53, 1987.
113. Fujita, T., and Hansch, C.: J. Med. Chem. 10:991, 1967.
114. Vree, T. B., et al.: Clin. Pharmacokinet. 4:310, 1979.
115. Hansen, I.: Antibiot. Chemother. 25:217, 1978.
116. Gleckman, R., et al.: Am. J. Hosp. Pharm. 36:893, 1979.
117. Bushby, S. R., and Hitchings, G. H.: Br. J. Pharmacol. Chemother. 33:72, 1968.
118. Wormser, G. P., and Deutsch, G. T.: Ann. Intern. Med. 91:420, 1979.
119. Palminteri, R., and Sassella, D.: Chemotherapy 25:181, 1979.
120. Harvey, R. J.: J. Antimicrob. Chemother. 4:315, 1978.
121. Letters of Burchall, J. J., Then, R., and Poe, M.: Science 197:1300–1301, 1977.
122. Werlin, S. L., and Grand, R. J.: J. Pediatr. 92:450, 1978.
123. Fox, C. L., and Ross, H. M.: Proc. Soc. Exp. Biol. Med. 50:142, 1942.
124. Yamazaki, M., et al.: Chem. Pharm. Bull. (Tokyo) 18:702, 1970.
125. Bell, P. H., and Roblin, R. O.: J. Am. Chem. Soc. 64:2905, 1942.
126. Cowles, P. B.: Yale J. Biol. Med. 14:599, 1942.
127. Brueckner, A. H.: J. Biol. Med. 15:813, 1943.
128. Shepard, C. C.: N. Engl. J. Med. 307:1640, 1982.

SELECTED READING

Bloom, B. R. (ed.): Tuberculosis. Washington, DC, American Society for Microbiology Press, 1994.

Chu, D. T., and Fernandes, P. B.: Recent developments in the field of quinolone antibacterial agents. In Testa, B. (ed.). Advances in Drug Research, vol. 21. New York, Academic Press, 1991.

Como, J. A., and Dismukes, W. E.: Oral azoles as systemic antifungal chemotherapy. N. Engl. J. Med. 330:263, 1994.

Despommier, D. D., and Karapelou, J. W.: Parasitic Life Cycles. New York, Springer-Verlag, 1987.

Goldsmith, R. S., and Heyneman, D. (eds.): Tropical Medicine and Parasitology. New York, Appleton & Lange, 1989.

Hastings, R. C., and Franzblau, S. G.: Chemotherapy of leprosy. Annu. Rev. Pharmacol. Toxicol. 28:231, 1988.

Hooper, D. C., and Wolfson, J. S. (eds.): Quinolone Antimicrobial Agents, 2nd ed. Washington, DC, American Society for Microbiology Press, 1993.

Houston, S., and Fanning, A.: Current and potential treatment of tuberculosis. Drugs 48:689, 1994.

Jernigan, J. A., and Pearson, R. D.: Antiparasitic agents. In Mandell GL, Bennett J. E., and Dolin R. (eds.). Principles and Practice of Infectious Diseases, vol. 1, 4th ed. New York, Churchill-Livingstone, 1995.

Kreier, J. B., and Baker, J. R. (eds.): Parasitic Protozoa, 2nd ed. San Diego, Academic Press, 1991.

Reed, S.: Amebiasis: an update. Clin. Infect. Dis. 14:385, 1992.

Singh, S. K., and Sherma, S.: Current status of medical research in helminth disease. Med. Res. Rev. 11:581, 1991.

Wang, C. C.: Molecular mechanisms and therapeutic approaches to the treatment of African trypanosomiasis. Annu. Rev. Pharmacol. Toxicol. 35:93, 1995.

Yamaguchi, H., Kobazaski, G. S., and Takahashi, H. (eds.): Recent Advances in Antifungal Chemotherapy. New York, Marcel Dekker, 1992.

CHAPTER 7

Antimalarials

JOHN H. BLOCK

CHAPTER OVERVIEW

Malaria, one of the most widespread diseases, is caused by a *Plasmodium* parasite and is transmitted to humans by the *Anopheles* mosquito. It infects several hundred million people each year, results in several million deaths annually, and is a complex disease to treat. The causative agent is a group of parasitical protozoa of the *Plasmodium* genus transmitted by the female *Anopheles* mosquito. Its original treatment was quinine that became the prototypical molecule for the first generation of synthetic antimalarial drugs. The target for drug treatment and prophylaxis is the parasite, and each advance in the drug treatment of this disease has resulted in the parasite developing resistance. One of the most effective preventions is controlling the mosquito population that is the vector carrying the parasite to humans. The human immune system does respond to the parasite, but the development of an effective vaccine has been a challenge. Sequencing the plasmodium genome is providing information that may lead to other approaches to prevent and treat this debilitating disease.

History

Malaria's name is derived from "mala aria" or bad air, and has been called *ague*, *intermittent fever*, *marsh fever*, and *The Fever*.[1,2] The name is based on the early knowledge that malaria was associated with swamps and badly drained areas. The use of quinine for treating malaria has been known since the 17th century. Although malaria is an ancient disease, its upsurge seems to coincide with the advent of farming about 20,000 years ago. The clearing of land provided areas for ponds containing still water. The *Anopheles gambiae* mosquito uses still water that sits in ponds and containers to breed. The gathering of humans in farming communities provided the necessary concentration of people to form a reservoir of hosts for the parasite and "food" for the mosquitoes breeding in the ponds.[3–6]

Proof that the *Anopheles* mosquito is the carrier of the causative protozoa was obtained by Dr. Ronald Ross who was recognized in 1902 by receipt of the Nobel Prize in Medicine. In a scenario somewhat similar to that where definitive proof that yellow fever was transmitted by the *Aedes aegypti* mosquito was required, Dr. Ross strongly argued that malaria was transmitted by an insect vector and finally demonstrated that the parasite was carried in the stomach and salivary glands of the *Anopheles* mosquito. The latter discovery was important because it helped resolve the dispute whether malaria was spread by the bite of the mosquito or drinking water containing mosquito eggs and larvae.[7] The impact of malaria on the human species continues to be devastating. The role of diseases such as smallpox, plague, yellow fever, and polio on human history is fascinating, but, fortunately, is mostly historical. Although smallpox has been eliminated, the latter three diseases do reappear, but the cases are isolated. Plague is treated effectively with antibiotics, and there are vaccines for yellow fever and polio.

There are three potential ways to control malaria: elimination of the vector, drug therapy, and vaccination. Elimination of the vector is the simplest and most cost-effective. Drug therapy has the same challenges as those with development of antibiotics, resistance to the drug. The current antimalarial drugs, although reasonably effective, also have significant adverse reactions, and resistance is increasing. So far, no effective vaccine has been developed that is effective in vivo, but that may be changing because of a better understanding how the human immune system interacts with the parasite. The malaria parasite does elicit an immune response as evidenced by the fact that children with an initial exposure are more likely to die than adults who have recurring attacks.

Because malaria has been eliminated from North America, Europe, and parts of Asia, it becomes a potential problem when citizens from a malaria-free area travel into an area where malaria is endemic. It is common for these travelers going into areas where malaria is endemic to receive prescriptions for antimalarial drugs and use them prophylactically.[8] Many times, citizens of malaria-free countries returning from areas where malaria is endemic plus citizens of the latter countries who are coming to the malaria-free countries will have contracted malaria and will require antimalarial drugs for several months following their return. Also, there will be restriction on their ability to be blood donors. Most prescriptions for antimalarial drugs in North America are indicated for prophylaxis of travelers going to and coming from areas of the world where malaria is endemic.

Malaria

Malaria is caused by four species of the one-cell protozoan of the *Plasmodium* genus. They are:

Plasmodium falciparum: This species is estimated to cause approximately 50% of all malaria. It causes the most severe form of the disease and, because patients feel ill between acute attacks, debilitating form of the disease. One of the reasons it leaves the patient so weak is because it infects up to 65% of the patient's erythrocytes.

Plasmodium vivax: This species is the second most common species causing about 40% of all malarial cases. It can be very chronic in recurrence because it can reinfect liver cells.

Plasmodium malariae: Although causing only 10% of all malarial cases, relapses are very common.
Plasmodium ovale: This species is least common.

Figure 7.1 outlines the steps of the parasite as it is injected into the victim and where drug therapy might be effective. The mosquito stores the sporozoite form of the protozoan in its salivary glands. Upon biting the patient, the sporozoites are injected into the patient's blood. Ideally, this would be a good site for intervention before the parasite can infect the liver or erythrocyte. In the case of drug therapy, people living in areas endemic with malaria (and the mosquito vector) would need to take the drug constantly. Although this would be plausible for people living temporarily in these areas, it is not practical for the permanent residents. It is true that antimalarial drugs could be formulated into implanted depot dosage forms, but these are expensive, and many times require trained medical personnel to implant the drug.

Within minutes after being injected into the patient's blood, the sporozoites begin entering hepatocytes where they become primary schizonts and then merozoites. At this point, there are no symptoms. Depending on the *Plasmodium* species, the merozoites either rupture the infected hepatocytes and enter systemic circulation or infect other liver cells. The latter process is seen with *P. vivax*, *P. malariae*, and *P. ovale*, but not *P. falciparum*, and produces secondary schizonts.

This secondary infection of the liver can be very damaging and is one of the sites for possible drug intervention. Killing the secondary schizonts would accomplish two things, protect the liver from further damage and eliminate a reservoir of schizonts that can change to merozoites and enter systemic circulation. It needs to be noted that, as the protozoan changes from sporozoite to schizont to merozoites, its immunological character changes. Determination of the *Plasmodium* genome has shown that each form of the parasite produces a different set of proteins. At the same time, once the merozoites have left the hepatocyte and are in systemic circulation, they are susceptible to attack by the patient's immune system provided that it has "learned" to recognize the parasite. Therefore, another site for vaccine development is the merozoite stage. Depending on the *Plasmodium* species, a merozoite vaccine may or may not provide much protection to the liver, but it could reduce subsequent infection of the erythrocytes.

Merozoites in systemic circulation now infect the patient's erythrocytes where they reside for 3 to 4 days before reproducing. The reproduction stage in the erythrocyte can either produce more merozoites or another form called gametocytes. The latter has different immunological properties from the other forms. Either way, the newly formed merozoites or gametocytes burst out of the infected erythrocytes. The new merozoites infect additional erythrocytes and continue the cycle of reproducing, bursting out of the erythrocytes, and infecting more erythrocytes. The debris from the destroyed erythrocytes is one of the causes of severe fever and chills. Also, the patient's immune system will respond with repeated exposure to the parasite, and this will contribute to the patient's discomfort.

The conversion of merozoites results in male and female gametocytes. After entering the mosquito, they "mate," producing zygotes in the mosquito's stomach. The latter reside in the mosquito's stomach endothelium oocysts. Eventually, they migrate as sporozoites to the mosquito's salivary gland where the cycle begins again when the mosquito bites a

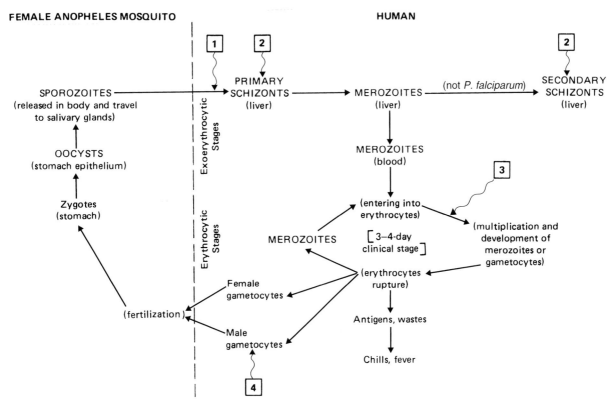

Figure 7.1 ● Stages of the parasite that causes malaria after injection into its victim. See discussion in the text. □ indicates site of antimalarial drug action in humans.

human. Note that, in effect, there are two reservoirs or vectors for the parasite: the mosquito that infects humans and humans that infect mosquitoes. Consistent with the latter, there have been some attempts at developing prophylactic agents that would be in the blood ingested by the mosquito. These drugs would stop further development of the parasite in the mosquito, preventing the insect from being a carrier.

There are at least two benefits to decoding the parasite's genome. One is to find a protein or biochemical reaction that is unique to *Plasmodium* species such that a drug can be designed that is selectively toxic to the protozoan. A second goal is to understand the genetic changes that lead to drug resistance. One of the main reasons for the increase in malaria since the late 1990s is the developing resistance to chloroquine, an antimalarial that has been widely used against *P. falciparum*. This resistance is blamed for the increasing mortality rates in Africa and to the resurgence of malaria.

The *P. falciparum* genome consists of the 30 million base pairs, forming 5,000 to 6,000 genes. It is nearly 80% adenine (A)-thymine (T) rich, making it difficult to tally base pairs on the parasites' 14 chromosomes.[9,10] (In contrast, the human genome is about 59% A-T.) The high A-T concentration made determination of the *Plasmodium* genome difficult to sequence because (a) it was more difficult to slice the chromosomal deoxyribonucleic acid (DNA) strands into smaller distinct segments that make it easier to sequence the nucleotides and then reassemble them into chromosome; and (b) the computer software would fail and had to be modified.[11] Because *P. vivax* is difficult to propagate in the laboratory, obtaining its genome has been a challenge. It turns out that although it resembles *P. falciparum*'s genome, it possesses novel gene families and potential alternative invasion pathways not previously recognized.[12]

Human Mutations that Protect against Malaria

There are at least six mutations in the human species that provide protection against malaria. These predominate in populations that historically lived and continue to live in areas endemic with malaria. The six mutations are sickling disease (formerly sickle cell anemia), glucose-6-phosphate dehydrogenase deficiency, hemoglobin C, various thalassemias, increased production of nitric oxide (NO), and pyruvate kinase deficiency. Sickling disease can be fatal in homozygotes although treatment has greatly improved. Heterozygotes usually are asymptomatic and show a 90% decrease in the chance of dying from *P. falciparum*.[13] Homozygotes with hemoglobin C usually are asymptomatic.[14] Erythrocyte glucose-6-phosphate dehydrogenase deficiency (actually 10%–15% of normal activity in the erythrocyte) can cause hemolytic anemia and prehepatic jaundice when the patient takes certain drugs or is exposed to some viral infections. Ironically, some of the antimalarial drugs must be used with caution in patients with erythrocyte glucose-6-phosphate dehydrogenase deficiency to minimize the risk of hemolytic anemia. The increased levels of oxidized glutathione in the erythrocyte that are deficient in this enzyme may prevent the parasite from maturing in the erythrocyte. The significance of thalassemia varies with the type of anemia and whether or not the patient is homozygote or heterozygote. The most recent identified mutation is pyruvate kinase deficiency. Because erythrocytes lack mitochondria, this enzyme is key to the formation of adenosine triphosphate (ATP) from phosphoenolpyruvate.[15] These mutations produce an erythrocyte such that the parasite has difficulty reproducing.

Another mutation is the ability of certain populations to increase their production of NO. The site is in the promoter region of the gene for nitric oxide synthase 2 that generates NO from arginine and involves a mutation where cytosine is replaced by thymine. The result is higher circulating levels of NO. Mechanistically, it is not known how increased NO provides this protection, because there appears to be no significant difference between blood levels of the parasite in individuals with the mutation compared with those with "normal" NO synthase. The protection may be from complications seen with malaria, giving the patient's immune system time to respond to the parasite.[16]

Controlling the Vector, the *Anopheles* Mosquito

The *Anopheles* mosquito has adapted very well to human habitats. As already pointed out, it requires still water to lay its eggs, wait for them to hatch, and then let the larvae, who feed on microscopic organisms in the still water, mature. Transient still water is ideal because it likely is not going to contain predators that will feed on the eggs and larvae. In general, mosquitoes need 1 to 2 weeks to develop into mature insects. This usually is enough time before predators begin to populate the still water.

Currently, there are two ways to control the mosquito carrier. One is to prevent contact between humans and the insect. Because the *Anopheles* mosquito is a nocturnal feeder, it is easier to control compared with the *Aedes aegypti* mosquito, which is a day feeder and carries both dengue and yellow fever. Putting screens on windows and using mosquito netting in bedrooms are very effective. The latter, when insecticide impregnated, has proven very effective.[17] As simple as the use of treated nets may seem, they produce a logistical challenge. It has been estimated that in 2007, 130 to 264 million treated nets are required to reach 80% coverage for 133 million children younger than 5 years and pregnant women living in 123 million households in risk areas in Africa.[18]

Second, elimination of the *Anopheles* mosquito, usually by application of insecticide and destroying its breeding areas, are the most effective ways to eliminate (as opposed to control) malaria. Areas that have been successful at eliminating infected mosquitoes include North America, Europe, and Russia. To do this, the adult female mosquito must be killed and breeding areas (still water) must be drained. One of the most effective insecticides has been dichlorodiphenyltrichloroethane (DDT). Dr. Paul Muller received the 1948 Nobel Prize in Medicine for discovering that DDT kills the malaria-carrying *Anopheles* mosquito. DDT is very long lasting and, unfortunately, accumulates in the environment. Although being long lasting is beneficial from the standpoint of mosquito control, it also means that these insecticides get into the food chain and can affect both animals, including birds, and humans. Indeed, use of DDT has been banned in most economically developed countries. Unfortunately, the areas of the world where malaria is endemic are economically poor and cannot (a) afford the newer insecticides that must be reapplied because they degrade, (b) fund and maintain the infrastructure to eliminate breeding areas, and (c) provide medical facilities, staff, and drugs to treat their citizens.

$$CCl_3$$

Cl—⟨ ⟩—CH—⟨ ⟩—Cl

DDT

POVERTY AND MALARIA

In general, malaria is endemic in areas of the world where poverty is rampant. There is not the infrastructure to eliminate the mosquito-breeding ponds, provide the insecticides to kill the mosquito and screens to separate the population from the mosquito, and provide the necessary drugs to treat the disease. In addition to pharmacological treatment, proper nutrition is important in surviving a malaria attack. The patient must replace the destroyed erythrocytes and, depending on the species of *Plasmodium*, hepatocytes. This requires calories from a high-quality diet that provides essential nutrients including amino acids, lipids, and trace minerals. The World Health Organization's 2008 Report (see Selected Reading) has scored countries based on the populations' lifestyles and availability of resources. Lack of proper food is one of those resources. In other words, just as the pathology of malaria is complex, so is its control and treatment.

Development of Vaccines

The complex nature of the parasite and its interactions with human red blood cells provide a large number of antigenic sites for the immune system.[19] A T-cell response that includes both CD4+ and CD8+ T cells and production of interferon and nitric oxide synthase induction is additional evidence that the human immune system does detect the parasite and responds accordingly.[20] An ideal vaccine should, at a minimum, be effective against both *P. falciparum* and *P. vivax*, the two species responsible for 90% of malarial cases. Currently, the RTS,S/AS01E vaccine is showing promise (see Selected Reading in the References at the end of the chapter). It contains surface proteins from the sporozoite stage, meaning it is designed for the immune system to stop the parasite as it enters the patient's blood from the mosquito and before the parasite can reach the liver where it matures and multiplies.

Development of Antimalarial Drugs

New antimalarial drugs must be developed constantly because the protozoa develop resistance by various mechanisms (see discussion of mechanisms with the different drugs), and there are a wide variety of adverse reactions. The combination of cost of drugs and their adverse reactions can make patient compliance difficult. Because there are four different species of protozoa that cause malaria, no one antimalarial drug is effective against all four species. There is a tremendous need for effective antimalarial agents.

◐ STIMULATION OF ANTIMALARIAL RESEARCH BY WAR

From 1941 to 1946 (World War II), more than 15,000 substances were synthesized and screened as possible antimalarial agents by the United States, Australia, and Great Britain. Activity increased again during the Vietnam War, especially because of the increasing problem of resistance to commonly used antimalarials. During the decade 1968 to 1978, more than 250,000 compounds were investigated as part of a U.S. Army search program.[21] Department of Defense funding of this research has continued.

Drugs Used to Prevent and Treat Malaria

There are four possible sites (Fig. 7.1) for drug therapy at this stage of the disease.

1. Kill the sporozoites injected by the mosquito and/or prevent the sporozoites from entering the liver.
2. Kill the schizonts residing in hepatocytes and/or prevent them from becoming merozoites.
3. Kill the merozoites in the blood and/or prevent them from developing into gametocytes.
4. Kill the gametocytes before they can enter the mosquito and reproduce into zygotes. Some have argued that the focus at this stage should be on the male gametocytes. This would block the female gametocytes from mating.

Antimalarial drugs (Table 7.1) are good examples of anti-infective agents with poor selective toxicity. Contrast them with the antibiotics (Chapter 8). Tetracyclines, chloramphenicol, and aminoglycosides act against bacterial ribosomes, but not mammalian. Penicillins and cyclosporins inhibit bacterial cell wall cross-linking, and mammals have cell membranes, not cell walls. The fluoroquinolones inhibit bacterial gyrase, but not mammalian topoisomerases. The biochemistry of the *Plasmodium* genus is similar to mammals, making it difficult to design drugs that will not adversely affect the patient. Some have indications beyond that of treating and preventing malaria. Nearly all of the antimalarial drugs currently in use are based on prototypical molecules isolated from plants (see Selected Reading).

◐ CINCHONA ALKALOIDS

The cinchona tree produces four alkaloids that function as prototypical molecules from which, until recently, most antimalarial drugs were based. These alkaloids (Fig. 7.2) are the enantiomeric pair quinine and quinidine and their desmethoxy analogs, cinchonidine (for quinine) and cinchonine (for quinidine). (Unfortunately, the nomenclature for the two series of alkaloids is inconsistent.) Their numbering system is based on rubane. The stereochemistry differs at positions 8 and 9 with quinine and cinchonidine being S,R and quinidine (cinchonine) being R,S. Historically, quinine has been the main treatment for malaria until the advent of World War II when battle in areas where malaria was endemic led to the search for more effective agents.

TABLE 7.1 Summary of Current Drugs Used to Prevent and Treat Malaria

Class	Generic Name	Indications for Malaria	Other Indications	Dosing Ranges for Treatment and Prophylaxis of Malaria
Cinchona alkaloids	Quinine	Chloroquine-resistant *P. falciparum*; combination with other antimalarials; not indicated for prophylaxis	Nocturnal leg cramps (see FDA restrictions on over-the-counter sales)	*Adults*: 260–650 mg t.i.d. for 6–12 days *Children*: 10 mg/kg every 8 hours for 5–7 days
	Quinidine	Not indicated for malaria in the United States	Cardiac arrhythmias	
4-Aminoquinolines	Chloroquine	Prophylaxis and treatment of *P. vivax*, *P. Malariae*, *P. ovale* malaria, and susceptible strains of *P. falciparum* malaria	Extraintestinal (liver) amebiasis The following indications are not approved in the United States Forms of hypercalcemia Rheumatoid arthritis Discoid and systemic lupus erythematosus Porphyria cutanea tarda Solar urticaria	Doses are expressed as chloroquine base equivalent *Prophylaxis for Children*: 5 mg/kg weekly up to a maximum of 300 mg *Prophylaxis for Adults*: 300 mg weekly See Centers for Disease Control and Prevention for current recommendations for treatment of acute attacks
	Hydroxy-chloroquine	Prophylaxis and treatment of *P. vivax*, *P. Malariae*, *P. ovale* malaria, and susceptible strains of *P. falciparum* malaria	Rheumatoid arthritis Discoid and systemic lupus erythematosus The following indications are not approved in the United States Forms of hypercalcemia Porphyria cutanea tarda Solar urticaria	Doses are expressed as hydroxy-chloroquine base equivalent *Prophylaxis for Children*: 5 mg/kg weekly up to a maximum adult dose *Prophylaxis for Adults*: 310 mg weekly on the same day; begin 1–2 weeks prior to exposure and continue for 4 weeks after leaving the endemic area See Centers for Disease Control and Prevention for current recommendations for treatment of acute attacks
	Mefloquine	Prophylaxis of *P. falciparum* (including chloroquine-resistant strains) and *P. vivax* malaria; treatment of *P. falciparum* and *P. vivax* malaria	None	*Prophylaxis (CDC) Children*: 62–250 mg weekly based on weight starting 1 week before travel and continuing for 4 weeks after leaving the endemic area *Prophylaxis for Adults*: 250 mg weekly for 4 weeks then 250 mg every other week starting 1 week before travel and continuing for 4 weeks after leaving the endemic area *Treatment for Adults*: 1,250 mg as a single dose taken with food and at least 240-mL water
8-Aminoquinolines	Primaquine	Prophylaxis and treatment of *P. vivax*	None	Begin treatment during the last 2 weeks or after stopping therapy with chloroquine or other antimalarial drug *Children*: 0.5 mg/kg/day for 14 days *Adults*: 26.3 mg daily for 14 days
Polycyclics	Doxycycline	Prophylaxis against *P. falciparum* strains resistant to chloroquine and sulfadoxine–pyrimethamine	Bacteria infections	*Prophylaxis*: begin only 1–2 days before travel and for 4 weeks after leaving the area; total use normally does not exceed 4 months *Children*: 2 mg/kg/day up to 100 mg/day *Adults*: 100 mg once daily
	Halfantrine	Treatment of *P. falciparum* and *P. vivax*	None	*Adults*: 500 mg every 6 hours for 3 doses (1,500 mg) repeated 7 days later *Children*: 250–375 mg based on body weight; follow the same schedule as adults

Class	Generic Name	Indications for Malaria	Other Indications	Dosing Ranges for Treatment and Prophylaxis of Malaria
Artemisinin family (usually used in combination with another antimalarial)	Artemisinin	Appears effective against all *Plasmodium* species including *P. falciparum* and *P. vivax*	None	*Adults*: 20 mg/kg on day 1 followed by 10 mg/kg for next 6 days
	Artemether	Similar profile as artemisinin	None	*Adults*: 4 mg/kg for 3 days followed by 1.6 mg/kg for 3 days
	Artesunate	Similar profile as artemisinin	None	*Adults*: 4 mg/kg for 3 days followed by 2 mg/kg for 2–4 days
	Dihydro-artemisinin	Similar profile as artemisinin	None	*Adults*: 4 mg/kg on day 1 followed by 2 mg/kg for 6 days
	Artemotil	Similar profile as artemisinin	None	*Adults*: 150 mg/kg by IM injection
Fixed combinations	Sulfadoxine and pyrimethamine	Prophylaxis and treatment of chloroquine-resistant *P. falciparum*	None	Each tablet contains 500-mg sulfadoxine and 25-mg pyrimethamine *Prophylaxis*: Begin 1–2 days prior to departure and continue for 4–6 weeks after return *Children*: ¼–1½ tablets based on age and whether administered once or twice weekly *Adults*: 1–2 tablets once or twice weekly *Treatment for Children*: ½–2 tablets based on age during an attack *Treatment for Adults*: 2–3 tablets during an attack
	Atovaquone and proguanil	Prophylaxis and treatment of *P. falciparum* resistant to other antimalarial drugs	None	*Adult Tablet*: 250-mg atovaquone & 100-mg proguanil *Pediatric Tablet*: 62.5-mg atovaquone & 25-mg proguanil *Prophylaxis*: Begin 1–2 days prior to departure and continue for 7 days after return *Children*: 1–3 pediatric tablets as a single daily dose based on weight *Adults*: 1 adult tablet daily *Treatment*: Take as a single dose for 3 consecutive days *Children*: 1–3 pediatric tablets as a single daily dose based on weight *Adults*: 4 tablets as a single daily dose for 3 consecutive days
	Artemether and lumefantrine	Treatment of *P. falciparum* resistant to other antimalarial drugs	None	*Adult Tablet*: 20-mg artemether & 120-mg lumefantrine; 4-dose regimen over 48 hrs or 6-dose regimen over 3 days *Pediatric Tablet*: 10-mg artemether & 60-mg lumefantrine; 4-dose regimen over 48 hrs or 6-dose regimen over 3 days

Quinine and Quinidine. Quinine has been used for "fevers" in South America since the 1600s. The pure alkaloids, quinine, and cinchonine were isolated in 1820. The stereoisomer, quinidine, is a more potent antimalarial, but it is also more toxic (less selectively toxic). Quinine is lethal for all *Plasmodium* schizonts (site 2 in Fig. 7.1) and the gametocites (site 4) from *P. vivax* and *P. malariae*, but not for *P. falciparum*. Today, quinine's spectrum of activity is considered too narrow for prophylactic use relative to the synthetic agents. The mechanism of action is discussed in the chloroquine section. The mechanism of resistance to quinine is poorly understood and varies with the susceptibility of the parasite to other aminoquinoline antimalarial drugs. Quinine is still indicated for malaria caused by *P. falciparum* resistant to other agents including chloroquine. Many times it is administered in combination with pyrimethamine and sulfadoxine, doxycycline, or mefloquine depending the specific form of malaria and geographical location.

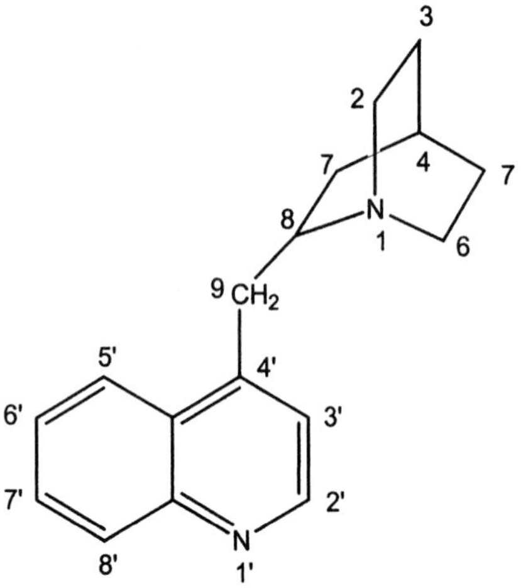

Rubane

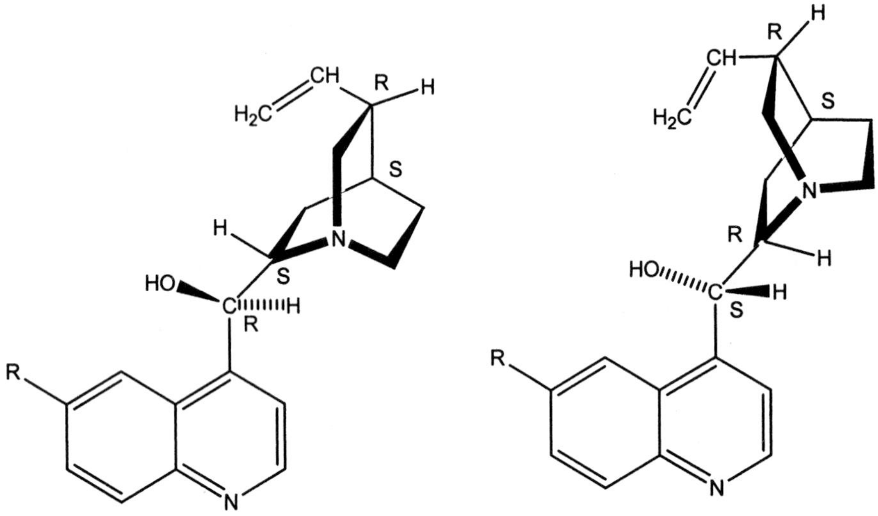

Quinine R = OCH₃
Cinchonidine R = H

Quinidine R = OCH₃
Cinchonine R = H

Figure 7.2 • Cinchona alkaloids.

A toxic syndrome is referred to as cinchonism. Symptoms start with tinnitus, headache, nausea, and disturbed vision. If administration is not stopped, cinchonism can proceed to involvement of the gastrointestinal tract, nervous and cardiovascular system, and the skin.

Quinine has also been used for nocturnal leg cramps, but pharmacists must remember that the Food and Drug Administration (FDA) ordered a stop to marketing quinine over the counter for this use because of a lack of proper studies proving its efficacy and possible adverse reactions.

The stereoisomer, quinidine, is a schizonticide, but its primary indication is cardiac arrhythmias. It is a good example where stereochemistry is important because it provides a significantly different pharmacological spectrum. Quinidine is discussed further in Chapter 19.

4-Aminoquinolines

The 4-aminoquinolines (Fig. 7.3) are the closest of the antimalarials that are based on the quinine structure. This group is substituted at the same position 4 as quinine and have an asymmetric carbon equivalent to quinine's C-9 position.

Just as with quinine, both isomers are active and the 4-aminoquinoline racemic mixtures are used. For the newest drug in this series, mefloquine, only the *R,S*-isomer is marketed. A significant difference from the commercial cinchona alkaloids is replacing the 6'-methoxy on quinine with a 7-chloro substituent on three of the 4-aminoquinolines. Amodiaquine is no longer used in the United States, and sontoquine has fallen into disuse.

Chloroquine and Chloroquine Phosphate. Chloroquine can be considered the prototypical structure that succeeded quinine and came into use in the mid-1940s. The phosphate salt is used in oral dosage forms (tablets), and the hydrochloride salt is administered parenterally. Until recently, chloroquine has been the main antimalarial drug used for both prophylaxis and treatment. Note that the list of indications for many of the other drugs in this chapter include *Plasmodium* resistant to chloroquine. It is indicated for *P. vivax*, *P. malariae*, *P. ovale*, and susceptible strains of *P. falciparum*. Chloroquine belongs to the 4-aminoquinoline series of which hundreds have been evaluated, but only about three to four are still in use.

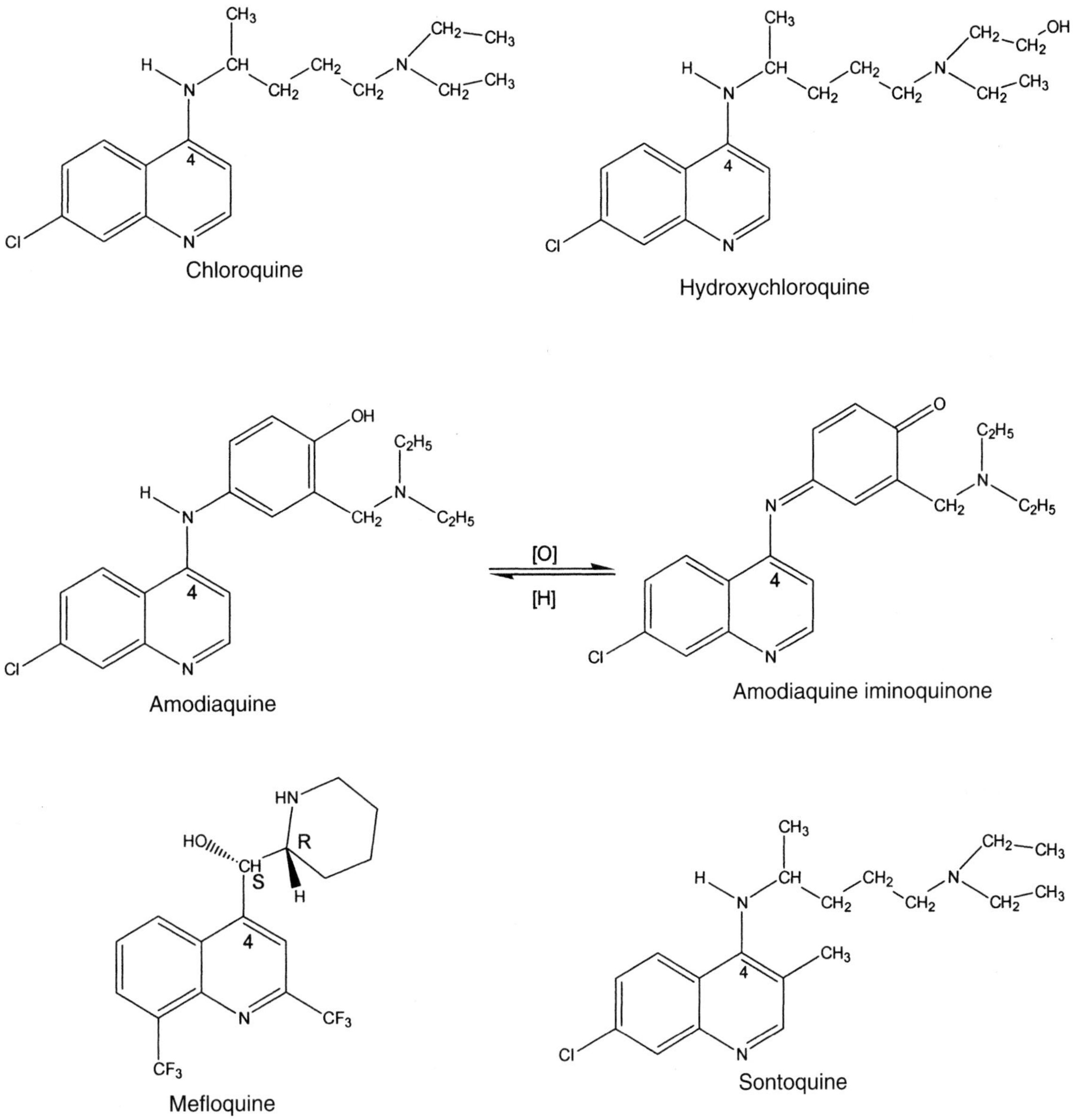

Figure 7.3 ● 4-Aminoquinolines.

Even though this drug has been used for many years, its mechanism of action is still not known. Its main site of action appears to be the parasite involving the erythrocyte's lysosome. The following actions have been suggested based on experimental evidence. A very complex mechanism is based on ferriprotoporphyrin IX, which is released by *Plasmodium* containing erythrocytes, acting as a chloroquine receptor. The combination of ferriprotoporphyrin IX and chloroquine causes lysis of the parasite's and/or the erythrocyte's membrane. Finally, there is evidence that chloroquine may interfere with *Plasmodium*'s ability to digest the erythrocyte hemoglobin or the parasite's nucleoprotein synthesis. The mechanism is based on the drug entering the erythrocyte's lysosome, which has an acid environment, where it becomes protonated. The protonated (positively charged) chloroquine is now trapped inside the lysosome because the pore that leads out of the lysosome is also positively charged. This leaves chloroquine bound to the patient's hemoglobin preventing the parasite from processing it properly.[24]

In general, chloroquine and the other 4-aminoquinolines are not effective against exoerythocytic parasites. Note that each of the mechanisms require that the parasite be inside the erythrocyte. Therefore, chloroquine does not prevent relapses of *P. vivax* or *P. ovale* malaria. The drug is also indicated for the treatment of extraintestinal amebiasis.

Effective such as chloroquine has been, it is a poor example of selective toxicity. Adverse reactions include retinopathy, hemolysis in patients with glucose-6-phosphate dehydrogenase deficiency (same mutation that confers resistance against malaria), muscular weakness, exacerbation of psoriasis and porphyria, and impaired liver function. Further examples of poor selective toxicity include off-label indications that include rheumatoid arthritis, systemic and discoid lupus erythemaosis (possibly as a immunosuppressant), and various dermatological conditions.

The increase in *P. falciparum* resistant to chloroquine is considered to be one of the main reasons for the increase in both the incidence and deaths from malaria. The key *Plasmodium* gene that confers resistance appears to be the *pfcrt* gene that codes for a transporter protein. The result of the changes in the gene is that the pore through which chloroquine might exit the lysosome is no longer positive charged, allowing protonated chloroquine to exit the lysosome.[35] There are at least eight mutations that have been identified in the *pfcrt* gene, and it is postulated that resistance occurs because of an accumulation of these mutations. Chloroquine remains effective when there are fewer mutations in the *pfcrt* gene. Once the critical number of mutations has occurred, the parasite spreads over a broad geographical area rendering chloroquine ineffective.[22–24]

Hydroxychloroquine. In most ways, hydroxychloroquine parallels chloroquine. Structurally, it differs solely with a hydroxy moiety on one of the *N*-ethyl groups. Like chloroquine, it remains in the body for over a month, and prophylactic dosing is once weekly. The other indications, both FDA approved and off-label, are very similar.

Amodiaquine. Amodiaquine is no longer marketed in the United States, but it is available in Africa. Mechanistically, it is very similar to chloroquine and does not have any advantages over the other 4-aminoquinoline drugs. When used for prophylaxis of malaria, it had a higher incidence of hepatitis and agranulocytosis than that was chloroquine. There is evidence that the hydroquinone (phenol) amine system readily oxidizes to a quinone imine (Fig. 7.3) either autoxidatively and/or metabolically, and this product may contribute to amodiaquine's toxicity.

Mefloquine HCl. The newest of the 4-aminoquinolines, mefloquine, is marketed as the *R,S*-isomer. It was developed in the 1960s as part of the U.S. Army's Walter Reed Institute for Medical Research antimalarial research program. It differs significantly from the other agents in this class by having two trifluromethyl moieties at positions 2' and 8' and no electronegative substituents at either positions 6' (quinine) or 7' (chloroquine). Mefloquine also differs from chloroquine and its analogs by being a schizonticide (site 2 in Fig. 7.1) acting before the parasite can enter the erythrocyte. There is some evidence that it acts by raising the pH in the parasite's vesicles interfering with its ability to process heme. Mefloquine-resistant strains of *P. falciparum* have appeared. Relapse can occur with acute *P. vivax* that has been treated with mefloquine because the drug does not eliminate the hepatic phase of this species, which can reinfect the liver.

Mefloquine is teratogenic in rats, mice, and rabbits. There is an FDA-required warning that this drug can cause exacerbate mental disorders and is contraindicated in patients with active depression, a recent history of depression, generalized anxiety disorder, psychosis, schizophrenia, and other major psychiatric disorders or a history of convulsions.

8-Aminoquinolines

The other major group of antimalarial drugs based on the cinchona alkaloid quinoline moiety is the substituted 8-aminoquinolines (Fig. 7.4). The first compound introduced in this series was pamaquine. During World War II, pentaquine, isopentaquine, and primaquine became available. Only primaquine, after being used during the Korean war, is in use today. All of the 8-aminoquinolines can cause hemolytic anemia in erythrocytic glucose-6-phosphate dehydrogenase-deficient patients. As pointed out in the introduction to this chapter, this is a common genetic trait found in populations living in areas endemic in malaria and provides some resistance to the parasite. Mechanism of action and spectrum of activity will be found in the primaquine section.

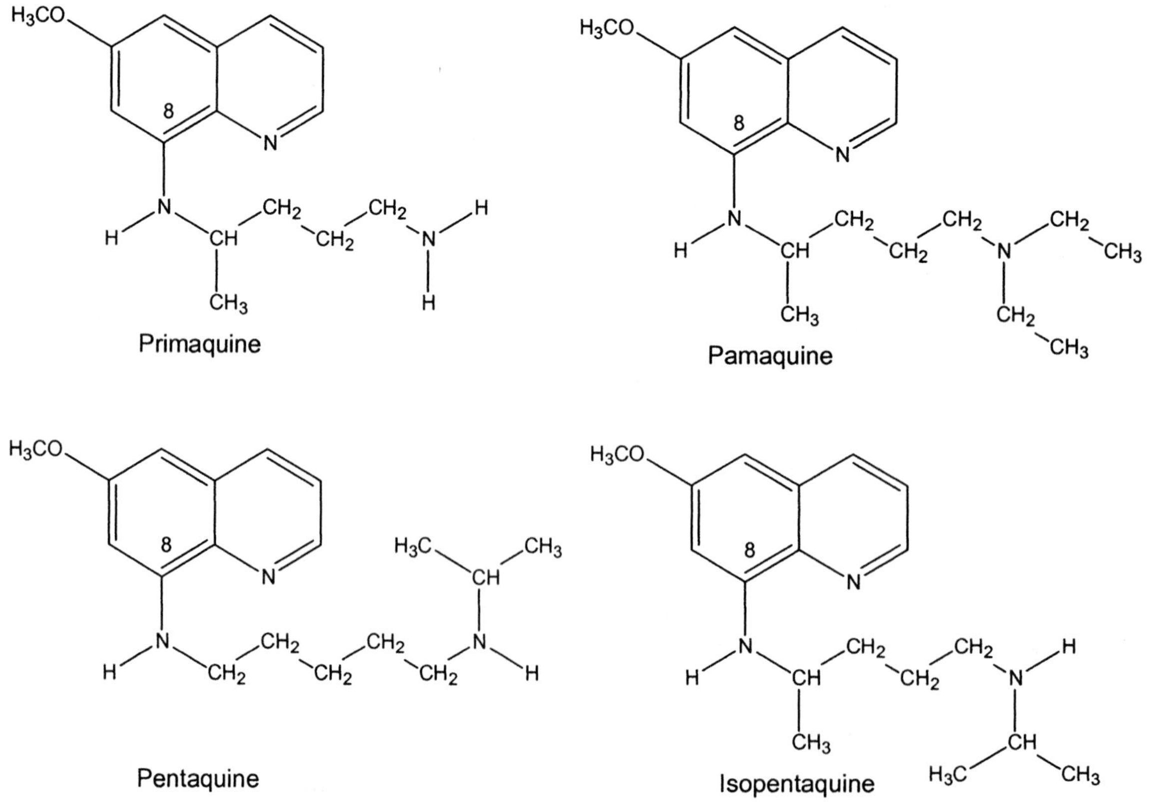

Figure 7.4 • 8-Aminoquinolines.

Very little variations are seen in the structure–activity relationships in this series. The four agents in Figure 7.4 all have a 6-methoxy moiety same as quinine, but the substituents are on the quinoline are located at position 8 rather than carbon-4 as found on the cinchona alkaloids. All agents in this series have a four to five carbon alkyl linkage or bridge between the two nitrogens. With the exception of pentaquine, the other three 8-aminoquinolines have one asymmetric carbon. Although some differences may be seen in the metabolism of each stereoisomer and type of adverse response, there is little difference in antimalarial activity based on the compounds stereochemistry.

Primaquine. Primaquine is the only 8-aminoquinoline currently in use for the treatment of malaria. It is not used for prophylaxis. Its spectrum of activity is one of the narrowest of the currently used antimalarial drugs being indicated only for exoerythrocytic *P. vivax* malaria (site 2 in Fig. 7.1). To treat endoerythrocytic *P. vivax*, chloroquine or a drug indicated for chloroquine-resistant *P. vivax* is used with primaquine. In addition to its approved indication, it is also active against the exoerythrocytic stages of *P. ovale* and primary exoerythrocytic stages of *P. falciparum*. Primaquine also inhibits the gameocyte stage (site 4 in Fig. 7.1) that eliminates the form required to infect the mosquito carrier. In vitro and in vivo studies indicate that the stereochemistry at the asymmetric is not important for antimalarial activity. There appears to be less toxicity with the levorotatory isomer, but this is dose dependent and may not be that important at the doses used to treat exoerythrocytic *P. vivax* malaria.

Although structurally related to the cinchona alkaloids, the 8-aminoquinolines act by a different mechanism of action. Primaquine appears to disrupt the parasite's mitochondria. The result is disruption of several processes including maturation into the subsequent forms. An advantage is destroying exoerythrocytic forms before the parasite can infect erythrocytes. It is the latter step in the infectious process that makes malaria so debilitating.

Polycyclic Antimalarial Drugs

There are three antimalarial drugs that have, in common, polycyclic ring systems (Fig.7.5). The first is the common tetracycline antibiotic, doxycycline. The second is halofantrine, and the third is the discontinued agent that was used in the South Pacific, quinacrine.

Doxycycline. Like the other tetracyclines, doxycycline (see Chapter 8) inhibits the pathogen's protein synthesis by reversibly inhibiting the 30S ribosomal subunit. Bacteria and *Plasmodium* ribosomal subunits differ significantly from mammalian ribosomes such that this group of antibiotics do not readily bind to mammalian ribosomes and, therefore, show good selective toxicity. Although doxycycline is a good antibacterial, its use for malaria is limited to prophylaxis against strains of *P. falciparumn* resistant to chloroquine and sulfadoxine–pyrimethamine. This use normally should not exceed 4 months. Because the tetracyclines chelate calcium, they can interfere with development of the permanent teeth in children. Therefore, their use in children definitely should be short term. Also,

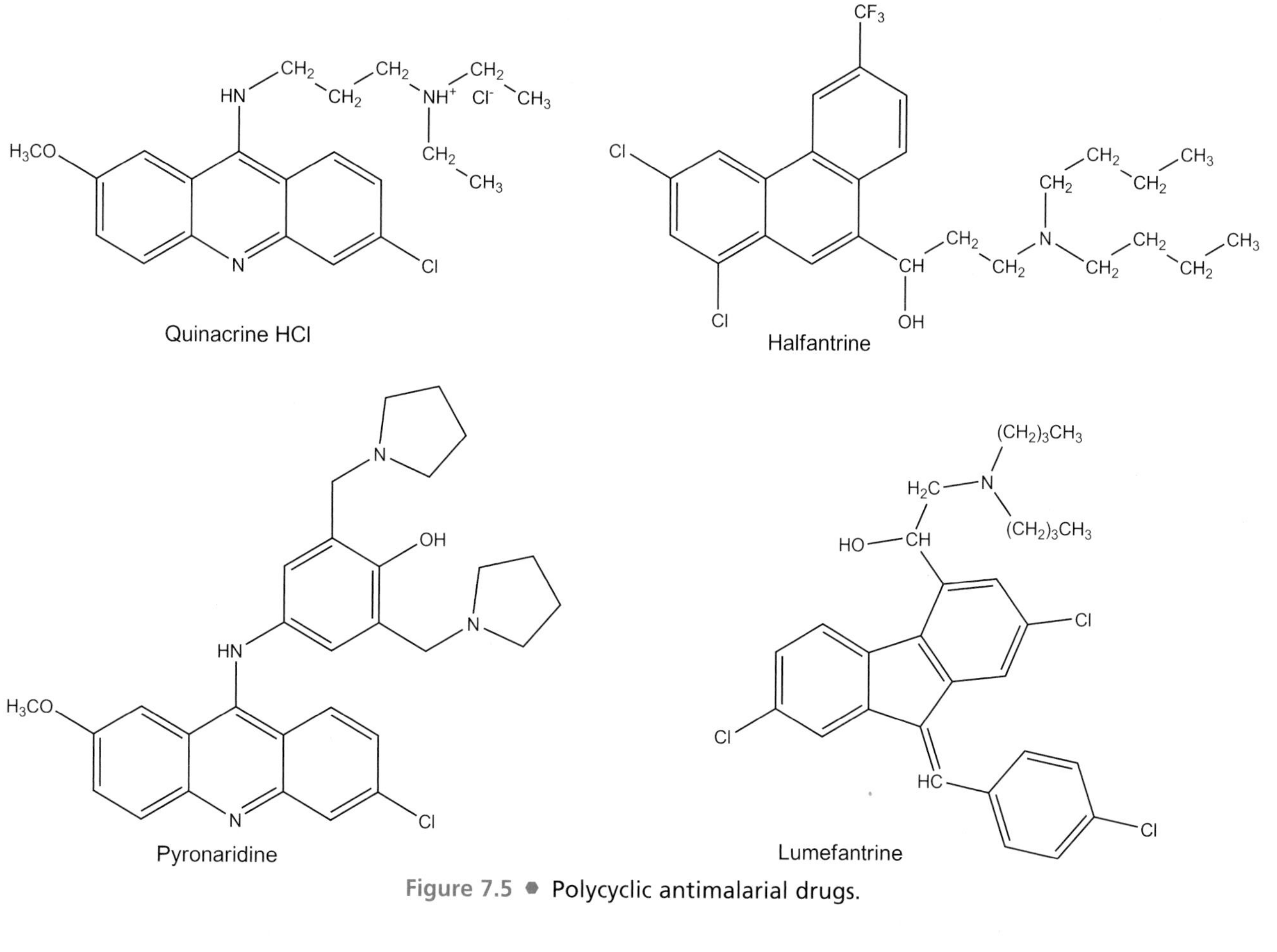

Figure 7.5 ● Polycyclic antimalarial drugs.

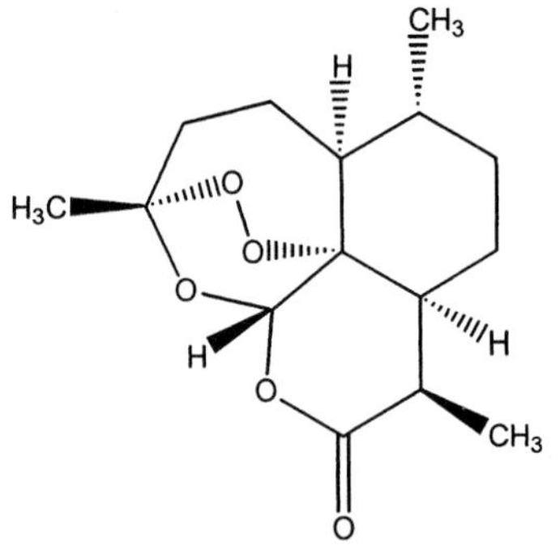

Figure 7.6 • Artemisinin and artemisinin-derived compounds.

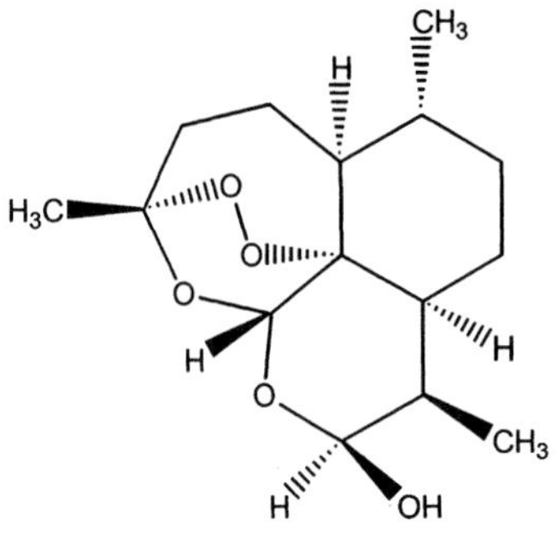

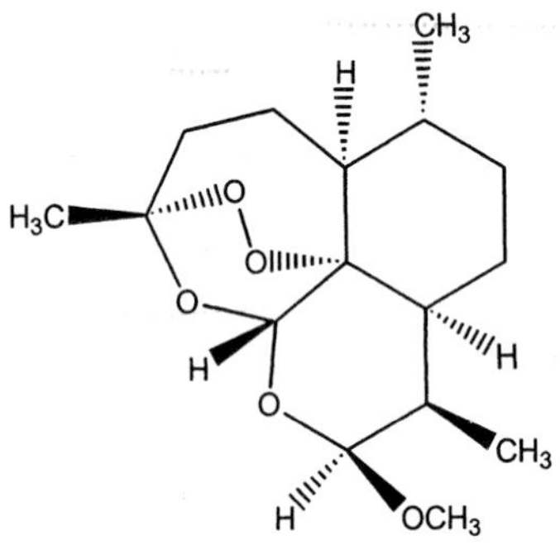

tetracycline photosensitivity must be kept in mind, particularly because areas where malaria is endemic are also the areas with the greatest sunlight.

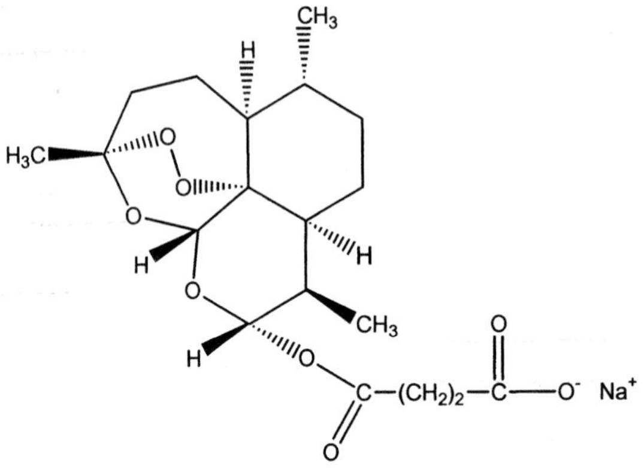

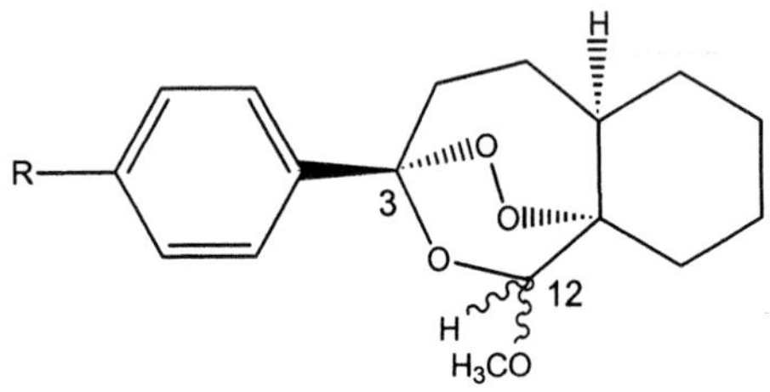

Halofantrine. Structurally, halofantrine differs from all other antimalarial drugs. It is a good example of drug design that incorporates bioisosteric principles as evidenced by the trifluromethyl moiety. Halofantrine is a schizonticide (sites 1 and 2 in Fig. 7.1) and has no affect on the sporozoite, gametocyte, or hepatic stages. Both the parent compound and *N*-desbutyl metabolite are equally active in vitro. Halfantrine's specific mechanism of action against the parasite is not known. There is contradictory evidence that its mechanism ranges from requiring heme to disrupting the mitochondria. There is a prominent warning that halfantrine can affect nerve conduction in cardiac tissue.

Lumefantrine. Lumefantrine was developed in China. Its mechanism of action is poorly understood. There is some evidence that it inhibits the formation of β-hematin by forming a complex with hemin. Lumefantrine is very lipophilic and is marketed in combination with the lipophilic artemesinin-derived artemether (Fig. 7.6).

Quinacrine HCl. Qunacrine is no longer available in the United States. It can be considered one of the most toxic of the antimalarial drugs even though, at one time, it was commonly used. It acts at many sites within the cell including intercalation of DNA strands, succinic dehydrogenase and mitochondrial electron transport, and cholinesterase. It may be tumorgenic and mutagenic and has been used as a sclerosing agent. Because it is an acridine dye, quinacrine can cause yellow discoloration of the skin and urine.

Artemisinin

The artemisinin series (Fig. 7.6) are the newest of the antimalarial drugs and are structurally unique when compared with the compounds previously and currently used. The parent compound, artemisinin, is a natural product extracted from the dry leaves of *Artemisia Annua* (sweet wormwood). The plant has to be grown each year from seed because mature plants may lack the active drug. The

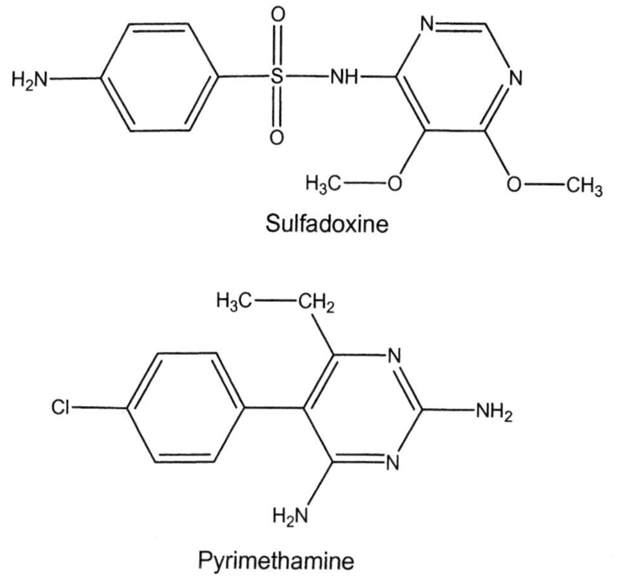

Sulfadoxine

Pyrimethamine

Figure 7.7 ● Sulfadoxine and pyrimethamine.

growing conditions are critical to maximize artemisinin yield. Thus far, the best yields have been obtained from plants grown in North Vietnam, Chongqing province in China, and Tanzania.[25]

All of the structures in Figure 7.6 are active against the *Plasmodium* genera that cause malaria. The key structure characteristic appears to be a "trioxane" consisting of the endoperoxide and dioxepin oxygens. This is shown by the somewhat simpler series of 3-aryltrioxanes at the bottom of Figure 7.6, which are active against the parasite. Note that the stereochemistry at position 12 is not critical.[26] Although in the victim's erythrocyte, the malaria parasite consumes the hemoglobin consisting of ferrous (Fe^{+2}) iron converting it to toxic hematin containing ferric (Fe^{+3}) and then reduced to heme with its ferrous iron. The heme iron reacts with the trioxane moiety releasing reactive oxygen and carbon radicals and the highly reactive $Fe^{IV} = O$ species. The latter is postulated to be lethal to the parasite.[27,28]

With the reduction of artemisinin to dihydroartemisinin, an asymmetic carbon forms and it is possible to form oil soluble and water soluble prodrugs. Both stereoisomers are active just as is seen in the simpler aryltrioxanes. The chemistry forming each of the artemisinin prodrugs results in the predominance of one isomer. The β-isomer predominates when producing the nonpolar methyl and ethyl ethers, whereas the α-isomer is the predominate product when forming the water-soluble hemisuccinate ester. The latter can be administered as 10-mg rectal capsules for patents who cannot take medication orally and parenteral treatment is not available.

Fixed Combinations

Because resistance is a frequent problem in the prophylaxis and treatment of malaria, combination therapies that use two distinctly different mechanisms have been developed. One combination inhibits folic acid biosynthesis and dihydrofolate reductase, and another combination acts on the parasite's mitochondria and its dihydrofolate reductase. Both drugs in the third combination act on hematin, but by two different mechanisms.

Sulfadoxine and Pyrimethamine. This combination (Fig. 7.7) uses a drug from the sulfonamide antibacterial group and a pyrimidinediamine similar to trimethoprim (see Chapter 8). The combination is considered to a schizontocide (site 2 in Fig. 7.1). The sulfonamide, sulfadoxine, interferes with the parasite's ability to synthesize folic acid, and the pyrimidinediamine, pyrimethamine, inhibits the reduction of folic acid to its active tetrahydrofolate coenzyme form. Sulfonamides block the incorporation of *p*-aminobenzoic acid (PABA) forming dihydropteroic acid. Note the structures of dihydrofolic acid and tetrahydrofolic acid and how PABA is the central part of the folate structure (see Chapter 28). Normally, sulfonamides exhibit excellent selective toxicity because humans do not synthesize the vitamin folic acid. Nevertheless, there are warnings of severe to fatal occurrences of erythema multiforme, Stevens-Johnson syndrome, toxic epidermal necrolysis, and serum-sickness syndromes attributed to the sulfadoxine.

Pyrimethamine, developed in the 1950s, inhibits the reduction of folic acid and dihydrofolic acid to the active tetrahydrofolate coenzyme form. Although the latter is required for many fundamental reactions involving pyrimidine biosynthesis, the focus in the parasite is regeneration of N^5,N^{10}-methylene tetrahydrofolate from dihydrofolate. The synthesis of thymidine 5′-monophosphate from deoxyuridine 5′-monophosphate is a universal reaction in all cells forming DNA. There are enough differences in this enzyme and dihydrofolate reductase found in mammalian, bacterial, and *Plasmodium* cells that folate reductase inhibitors can be developed that show reasonable selective toxicity. In the case of the malaria parasite, the intimate relationship between thymidylate synthase and

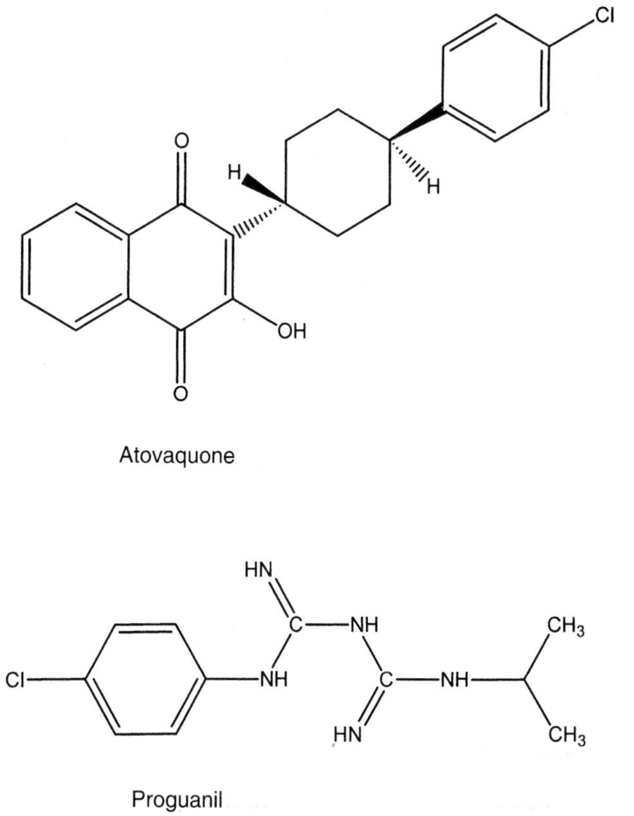

Atovaquone

Proguanil

Figure 7.8 ● Atovaquone and proguanil.

dihydrofolate reductase is such that pyrimethamine inhibits both enzymes.

This combination is indicated for prophylaxis and treatment of chloroquine resistance *P. falciparum* and may be used in combination with quinine. Although indicated only for *P. falciparum*, the combination is active against all the asexual erythocytic forms. It has no activity against the sexual gametocyte form. The fixed combination contains 500-mg sulfadoxine and 25-mg pyrimethamine. There is a wide number of sulfonamides that could be used in combination with pyrimethamine. The usual approach is to use a sulfonamide that has similar pharmacokinetic properties with the dihydrofolate reductase inhibitor. For this combination, the peak plasma sulfadoxine occurs in 2.5 to 6 hours and pyrimethamine 1.5 to 8 hours. Resistance has developed with much of it involving mutations in either or both of the genes coding for dihydrofolate reductase and thymidylate synthase.

Atovaquone and Proguanil HCl. Atovaquone and proguanil HCl (Fig. 7.8) are administered in combination in the ratio of 2.5 atovaquone to 1 proguanil HCl measured in mg (not mmoles). Proguanil, developed in 1945, is an early example of a prodrug. It is metabolized to cycloguanil

(Fig. 7.9), primarily by CYP2C19. The polymorphic nature of this hepatic enzyme explains why certain subpopulations do not respond to proguanil. These groups cannot convert proguanil to the active cycloguanil.

The basis for this combination is two distinct and unrelated mechanisms of action against the parasite. Atovaquone is a selective inhibitor of the *Plasmodium*'s mitochondrial electron transport system, and cycloguanil is a dihydrofolate reductase inhibitor. Atovaquone's chemistry is based on its being a naphthoquinone and participating in oxidation–reduction reactions as part of its quinone–hydroquinone system. It is patterned after Coenzyme Q found in the mitochondrial electron transport chains. The drug selectively interferes with mitochondrial electron transport, particularly at the parasite's cytochrome bc_1 site. This deprives the cell of needed ATP and could cause the cell to become anaerobic. Resistance to this drug comes from a mutation in the parasite's cytochrome.

Cycloguanil (Proguanil) interferes with deoxythymidylate synthesis by inhibiting dihydrofolate reductase. Resistance to proguanil/cycloguanil is attributed to amino acid changes near the dihydrofolate reductase binding site. Its elimination half-life (48–72 hour) is much shorter than the other antimalarial dihydrofolate reductase, pyrimethamine (mean

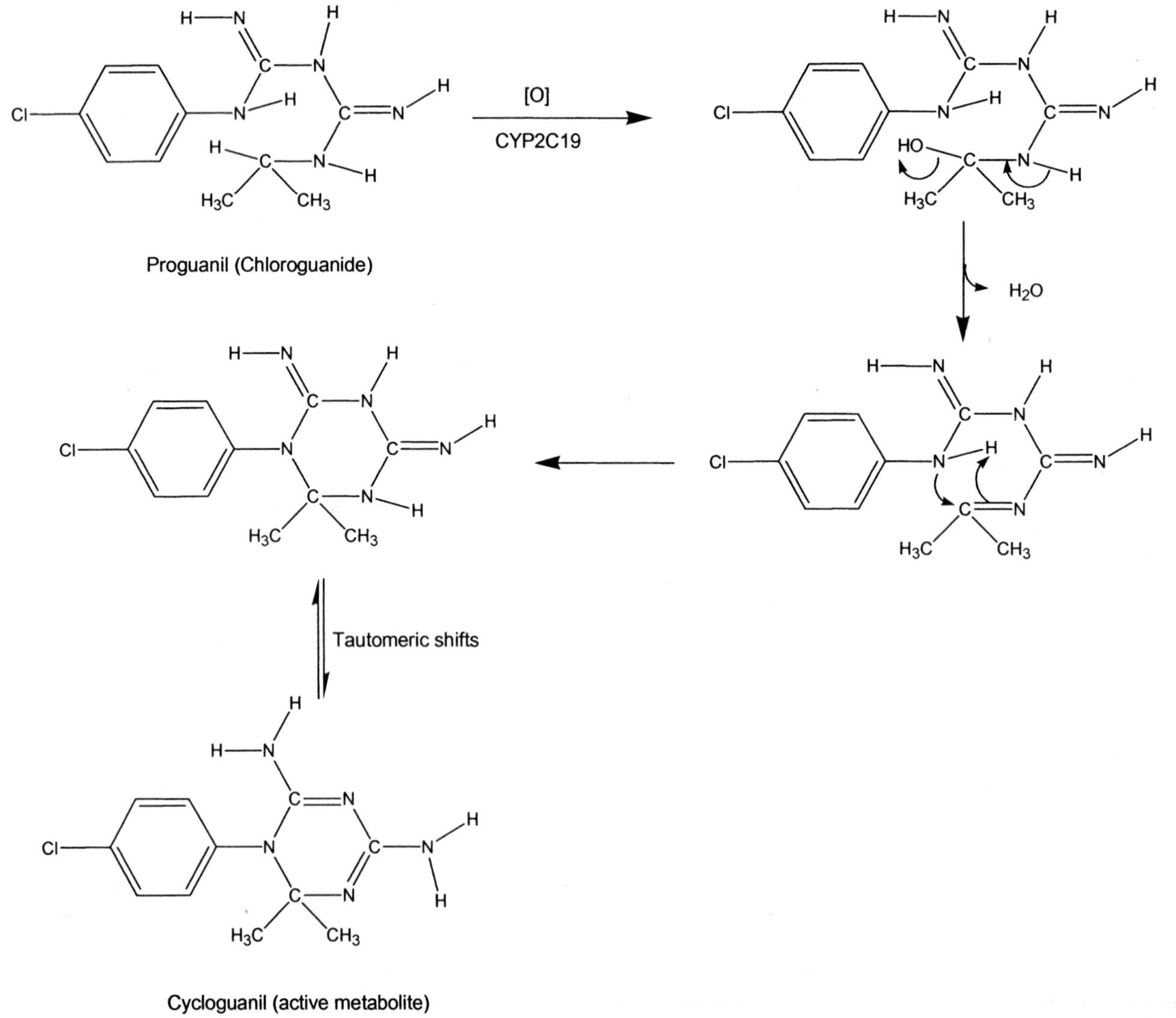

Proguanil (Chloroguanide)

Tautomeric shifts

Cycloguanil (active metabolite)

Figure 7.9 ● Conversion of proguanil to cycloguanil by CYP2C19.

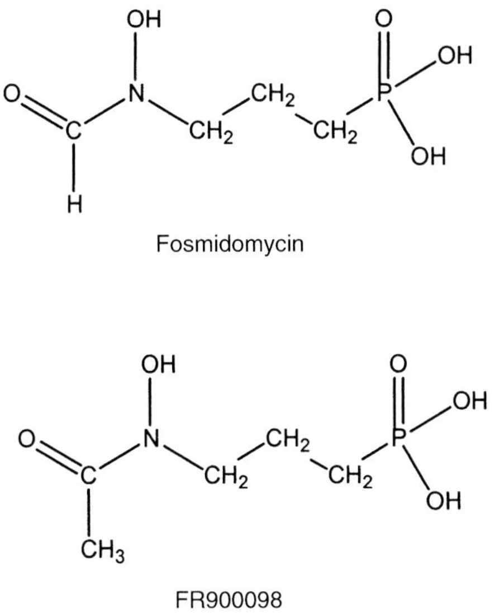

Fosmidomycin

FR900098

Figure 7.10 ● Fosmidomycin and a fosmidomycin analog.

elimination half-life of 111 hours). The combination is effective against both erythrocytic and exoerythrocytic *Plasmodium*. This drug combination is indicated for malaria resistant to chloroquine, halofantrine, mefloquine, and amodiaquine. Its main site is the sporozoite stage (site 1 in Fig. 7.1).

Artemether and Lumefantrine. These two antimalarials interfere with heme metabolism, thereby stopping development of the parasite in the erythrocyte states. Artemether, with its endoperoxide, acts oxidatively and lumefantrine may form a complex with hemin.

Future Trends

VACCINES

The development of an effective vaccine has been one of the most frustrating aspects in the prevention of malaria. There is no question that the *Plasmodium* parasite invokes an immune response. The problem seems to be identifying the antigenic component or components that cause a strong immune response. As already described, the RTS,S/AS01E vaccine is the only one showing promise.

NEW DRUG COMBINATIONS

Because of the general success of the artemisinin-based antimalarials, there have been several combinations evaluated. As mentioned previously, the artemether and lumefantrine combination has been approved. Undergoing phase III studies is a pyronaridine (Fig. 7.5) and artesunate (Fig. 7.6). Pyronaridine inhibits formation of hematin, possibly by a similar mechanism to that of chloroquine.[29]

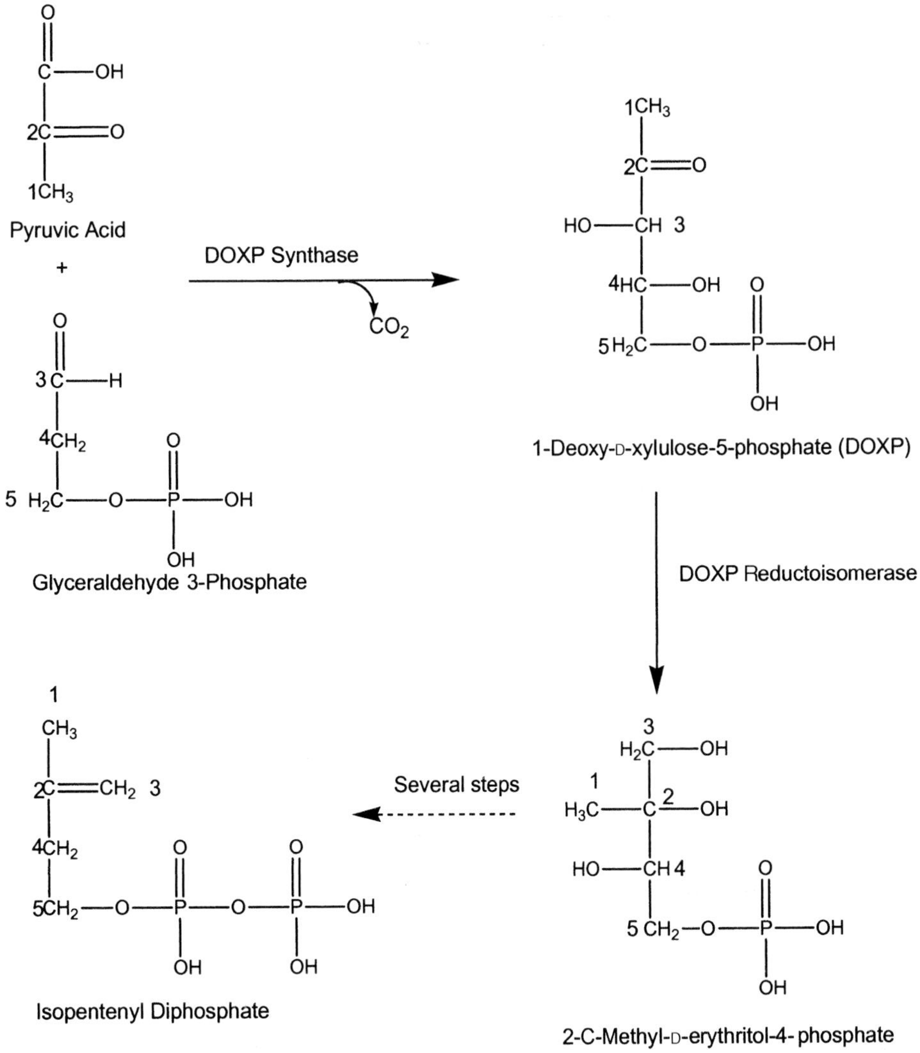

Figure 7.11 ● Nonmevalonate pathway.

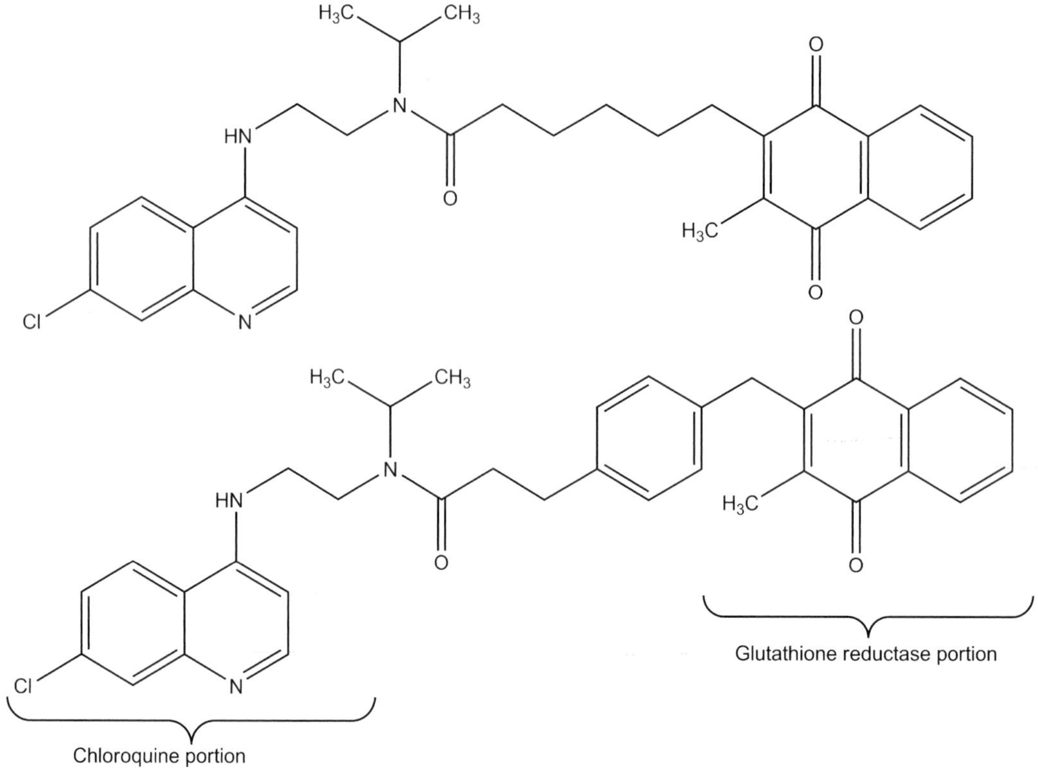

Figure 7.12 ● Possible glutathione reductase inhibitors.

NEW DRUG APPROACHES

Inhibition of the Nonmevalonate Pathway. Fosmidomycin (Fig. 7.10) was isolated from a Streptomyces fermentation broth in 1980. Its selective toxicity is based on inhibiting a biochemical pathway not found in humans and mammals in general. This is the nonmevalonate pathway to form isoprenoids. Mammals, including humans, form their isoprenoids solely by mevalonic acid pathway. Many microorganisms have both pathways. Whereas the mevalonate pathway starts with three molecules of acetyl Co forming 3-hydroxy-3-methylglutaryl coenzyme A (HMG-CoA) followed by reduction to mevalonic acid by HMG-CoA reductase (site of the statin drugs), the nonmevelonate pathway is carbohydrate based (Fig. 7.11). Condensation of pyruvate and glyceraldehyde-3-phosphate by DOXP synthase produces the five carbon 1-deoxy-D-xylulose-5-phosphate (DOXP), which undergoes a complex reduction and isomerization forming 2-C-methyl-D-erythritol-4-phosphate. The enzyme for this reaction, DOXP reductoisomerase, is inhibited by fosmidomycin. The basic five-carbon isoprene unit, isopentenyl diphosphate concludes the pathway. The atoms have been numbered to help follow the isomerization of the deoxy-xylulose intermediate to form the erythritol compound. The malaria parasite only has the nonmevalonate pathway, and initial studies show fosmidomycin to be relatively nontoxic in humans.[30] Replacement of fosmidomycin's *N*-aldehyde with an acetate produces a very active antimalarial agent that has been designated as FR900098.[31]

Inhibitors of Glutathione Reductase. The erythrocyte maintains a high oxygen environment and, therefore, has an elaborate reductase system to hold heme iron in the ferrous state. In contrast, the *Plasmodium* parasite lacks the antioxidant system to thrive in the erythrocyte's high oxygen environment and, therefore, has to rely on the erythrocyte's reductase pathways. This has led to development of compounds (Fig. 7.12) that inhibit erythrocytic glutathione reductase using chloroquine has the starting point for transport into the erythrocyte and naphthoquinone moiety to inhibit glutathione reductase.[32] These two molecules also are examples of the dual function approach in which the molecule attacks the parasite by two different mechanisms of action.

● R E V I E W   Q U E S T I O N S ●

1. Why is malaria seen in agricultural areas where humans live close to each other?

2. What nondrug methods are used to prevent humans from contracting malaria?

3. Why should it be possible to develop a vaccine against malaria?

4. Which two *Plasmodium* species are the preferable targets for antimalarial drug therapy because they account for nearly 90% of the cases?

5. Name the cells where the parasite resides.

6. Why is combination therapy becoming more common?

REFERENCES

1. Editors: Sci. Am. 286(6):8, 14, 38–45, 102–103, 2002.
2. Honigsbaum, M.: Men, Money and Malaria. New York, Farrar, Straus & Giroux, 2002.
3. Pennisi, E.: Science 293:416–417, 2001.
4. Tishkoff, S. A., Varkonyi, R., Cahinhinan, N., et al.: Science 293:455–462, 2001.
5. Luzzatto, L., and Notaro, R.: Science 293:442–443, 2001.
6. Volkman, S., Barry, A. E., Lyons, E. J., et al.: Science 293:482–484, 2001.
7. Bynum, W. F.: Science 295:47–48, 2002.
8. www.cdc.gov/travel.
9. Enserink, M., and Pennisi, E.: Science 295:1207, 2002.
10. Maher, B. A.: Scientist 16(6):28, 2002.
11. Pennisi, E.: Science 298:33, 2002.
12. Carlton, J. M., Adams, J. H., Silva, J. C., et al.: Nature 455:757–763, 2008, doi:10.1038/nature07327.
13. Hoffman, S. L.: Science 290:1509, 2000.
14. Pennisi, E.: Science 294:1439, 2001.
15. Ayi, K., Min-Oo, G., Serghides, L., et al.: N. Eng. J. Med. 358(17):1805, 2008.
16. Hobbs, M. R., Udhayakumar, V., Levesque, M. C., et al.: Lancet 360:1468, 2002.
17. Insecticide-Treated Mosquito Nets: a WHO Position Statement, http://www.who.int/malaria/docs/itn/ITNspospaperfinal.pdf.
18. Miller, J., Korenromp, E. L., Nahlen, B. L., et al.: J. Am. Med. Assoc. 297(20):2241, 2007.
19. Rodriguez, L. E., Curtidor, H., Urquiza, M., et al.: Chem. Rev. 108:3656, 2008.
20. Pombo, D. J., Lawrence, G., Hirunpetcharat, C., et al.: Lancet 360:610, 2002.
21. Van den Bossche, H.: Nature 273:626, 1978.
22. Hastings, I. M., Bray, P. G., and Ward, S. A.: Science 298:74, 2002.
23. Sidhu, A. B. S., Verider-Pinard, D., and Fidock, D. A.: Science 298:210, 2002.
24. Warhurst, D. C., Craig, J. C., and Adagu, I. S.: Lancet 360:(9345), 2002.
25. http://www.dafra.be/english/artemisinin.html.
26. Posner, G. H., Jeon, H. B., Parker, M. H., et al.: J. Med. Chem. 44:3054, 2001.
27. Posner, G. H., Cummings, J. N., Ploypradith, P., et al.: J. Am. Chem. Soc. 117:5885, 1995.
28. Posner, G. H., Park, S. B., González, L., et al.: J. Am. Chem. Soc. 118:3537, 1996.
29. Auparakkitanon, S., Chapoomram, S., Kuaha, K., et al.: Agents Chemother. 50:2197, 2006.
30. Jomaa, H., Wiesner, J., Sanderbrand, S., et al.: Science 285:1573, 1999.
31. Reichenberg, A., Wiesner, J., Weidemeyer, C., et al.: Bioorg. Med. Chem. Lett. 11:833, 2001.
32. Friebolin, W., Jannack, B., Wenzel, N., et al.: J. Med. Chem. 51:1260, 2008.

SELECTED READING

Honigsbaum, M.: The fever trail. In Search for the Cure for Malaria. New York, Farrar, Straux & Giroux, 2001.
Kaur, K., Jain, M., Kaur, T., et al.: Antimalarials from nature. Biorg. Med. Chem. 17:3229, 2009.
N. Engl. J. Med. 359(24):2521–2532, 2533–2544, 2545–2557, 2599–2601, 2601–2603, 2008. (These issues includes three articles and two editorials.)
Science 298(5591), 2002. (This issue reports the genome of the Anopheles gambiae mosquito and includes discussion on how this knowledge might be used to prevent malaria.)
World Health Organization (WHO): The World Health Report 2008, available as a downloadable PDF file at: http://www.who.int/malaria/wmr2008/. Additional information on malaria from the WHO at http://www.who.int/topics/malaria/en/

CHAPTER 8

Antibacterial Antibiotics

JOHN M. BEALE, JR.

CHAPTER OVERVIEW

Since Alexander Fleming accidentally discovered penicillin in 1929, the numbers of antibiotics that have been added to our therapeutic armamentarium has grown tremendously. Along with immunizing biologicals, antibiotics have turned the tide in terms of the treatment of infectious disease. They are truly medical miracles. Yet, because of the overuse of many of these agents and the biochemical fickleness of many bacteria, resistance to antibiotics has become a serious problem in the 21st century. Indeed, there are now organisms that cannot be arrested or killed by any of the common antibiotics. Clearly, new approaches are needed. This chapter will present each of the antibiotics as chemical classes, such as tetracyclines, aminoglycosides, macrolides, and β-lactam antibiotics. In each class, it is important to note the different ranges of bacteria that each will treat. Notably, it is difficult to define an absolute range for any antibiotic. Populations of bacteria differ in their characteristics among regions and hospitals in those region. So, sometimes, an antibiotic is listed as effective against a particular bacterial strain, but the concentration needed to kill the organism is too high. The bottom line is that when describing efficacy of an antibiotic against a particular organism, it is necessary to look at clinical results. This chapter will describe ranges of activity in a general sense. The history of the antibiotics is an interesting one and is well worth considering. Hence, the chapter will begin with a brief historical overview.

HISTORICAL BACKGROUND

Sir Alexander Fleming's accidental discovery of the antibacterial properties of penicillin in 1929[1] is largely credited with initiating the modern antibiotic era. Not until 1938, however, when Florey and Chain introduced penicillin into therapy, did practical medical exploitation of this important discovery begin to be realized. Centuries earlier, humans had learned to use crude preparations empirically for the topical treatment of infections, which we now assume to be effective because of the antibiotic substances present. As early as 500 to 600 BC, molded curd of soybean was used in Chinese folk medicine to treat boils and carbuncles. Moldy cheese had also been used for centuries by Chinese and Ukrainian peasants to treat infected wounds. The discovery by Pasteur and Joubert in 1877 that anthrax bacilli were killed when grown in culture in the presence of certain bacteria, along with similar observations by other microbiologists, led Vuillemin[2] to define antibiosis (literally "against life") as the biological concept of survival of the fittest, in which one organism destroys another to preserve itself. The word antibiotic was derived from this root. The use of the term by the lay public, as well as the medical and scientific communities, has become so widespread that its original meaning has become obscured.

In 1942, Waksman[3] proposed the widely cited definition that "an antibiotic or antibiotic substance is a substance produced by microorganisms, which has the capacity of inhibiting the growth and even of destroying other microorganisms." Later proposals[4-6] have sought both to expand and to restrict the definition to include any substance produced by a living organism that is capable of inhibiting the growth or survival of one or more species of microorganisms in low concentrations. The advances made by medicinal chemists to modify naturally occurring antibiotics and to prepare synthetic analogs necessitated the inclusion of semisynthetic and synthetic derivatives in the definition. Therefore, a substance is classified as an antibiotic if the following conditions are met:

1. It is a product of metabolism (although it may be duplicated or even have been anticipated by chemical synthesis).
2. It is a synthetic product produced as a structural analog of a naturally occurring antibiotic.
3. It antagonizes the growth or survival of one or more species of microorganisms.
4. It is effective in low concentrations.

The isolation of the antibacterial antibiotic tyrocidin from the soil bacterium *Bacillus brevis* by Dubois suggested the probable existence of many antibiotic substances in nature and provided the impetus for the search for them. An organized search of the order Actinomycetales led Waksman and associates to isolate streptomycin from *Streptomyces griseus*. The discovery that this antibiotic possessed in vivo activity against *Mycobacterium tuberculosis* in addition to numerous species of Gram-negative bacilli was electrifying. It was now evident that soil microorganisms would provide a rich source of antibiotics. Broad screening programs were instituted to find antibiotics that might be effective in the treatment of infections hitherto resistant to existing chemotherapeutic agents, as well as to provide safer and more effective chemotherapy. The discoveries of broad-spectrum antibacterial antibiotics such as chloramphenicol and the tetracyclines, antifungal antibiotics such as nystatin and griseofulvin (see Chapter 6), and the ever-increasing number of antibiotics that may be used to treat infectious agents that have developed resistance to some of the older antibiotics, attest to the spectacular success of this approach as it has been applied in research programs throughout the world.

CURRENT STATUS

Commercial and scientific interest in the antibiotic field has led to the isolation and identification of antibiotic substances that may be numbered in the thousands. Numerous semisynthetic and synthetic derivatives have been added to the total. Very few such compounds have found application in general medical practice, however, because in addition to the ability to combat infections or neoplastic disease, an antibiotic must possess other attributes. First, it must exhibit sufficient selective toxicity to be decisively effective against pathogenic microorganisms or neoplastic tissue, on the one hand, without causing significant toxic effects, on the other. Second, an antibiotic should be chemically stable enough to be isolated, processed, and stored for a reasonable length of time without deterioration of potency. The amenability of an antibiotic for oral or parenteral administration to be converted into suitable dosage forms to provide active drug in vivo is also important. Third, the rates of biotransformation and elimination of the antibiotic should be slow enough to allow a convenient dosing schedule, yet rapid and complete enough to facilitate removal of the drug and its metabolites from the body soon after administration has been discontinued. Some groups of antibiotics, because of certain unique properties, have been designated for specialized uses, such as the treatment of tuberculosis (TB) or fungal infections. Others are used for cancer chemotherapy. These antibiotics are described along with other drugs of the same therapeutic class: antifungal and antitubercular antibiotics are discussed in Chapter 6, and antineoplastic antibiotics are discussed in Chapter 10.

The spectacular success of antibiotics in the treatment of human diseases has prompted the expansion of their use into several related fields. Extensive use of their antimicrobial power is made in veterinary medicine. The discovery that low-level administration of antibiotics to meat-producing animals resulted in faster growth, lower mortality, and better quality has led to the use of these products as feed supplements. Several antibiotics are used to control bacterial and fungal diseases of plants. Their use in food preservation is being studied carefully. Indeed, such uses of antibiotics have necessitated careful studies of their long-term effects on humans and their effects on various commercial processes. For example, foods that contain low-level amounts of antibiotics may be able to produce allergic reactions in hypersensitive persons, or the presence of antibiotics in milk may interfere with the manufacture of cheese.

The success of antibiotics in therapy and related fields has made them one of the most important products of the drug industry today. The quantity of antibiotics produced in the United States each year may now be measured in several millions of pounds and valued at billions of dollars. With research activity stimulated to find new substances to treat viral infections that now are combated with only limited success and with the promising discovery that some antibiotics are active against cancers that may be viral in origin, the future development of more antibiotics and the increase in the amounts produced seem to be assured.

COMMERCIAL PRODUCTION

The commercial production of antibiotics for medicinal use follows a general pattern, differing in detail for each antibiotic. The general scheme may be divided into six steps: (a) preparation of a pure culture of the desired organism for use in inoculation of the fermentation medium; (b) fermentation, during which the antibiotic is formed; (c) isolation of the antibiotic from the culture medium; (d) purification; (e) assays for potency, sterility, absence of pyrogens, and other necessary data; and (f) formulation into acceptable and stable dosage forms.

SPECTRUM OF ACTIVITY

The ability of some antibiotics, such as chloramphenicol and the tetracyclines, to antagonize the growth of numerous pathogens has resulted in their designation as *broad-spectrum* antibiotics. Designations of spectrum of activity are of somewhat limited use to the physician, unless they are based on clinical effectiveness of the antibiotic against specific microorganisms. Many of the broad-spectrum antibiotics are active only in relatively high concentrations against some of the species of microorganisms often included in the "spectrum."

MECHANISMS OF ACTION

The manner in which antibiotics exert their actions against susceptible organisms varies. The mechanisms of action of some of the more common antibiotics are summarized in Table 8.1. In many instances, the mechanism of action is not fully known; for a few (e.g., penicillins), the site of action is known, but precise details of the mechanism are still under investigation. The biochemical processes of microorganisms are a lively subject for research, for an understanding of those mechanisms that are peculiar to the metabolic systems of infectious organisms is the basis for the future development of modern chemotherapeutic agents. Antibiotics that interfere with the metabolic systems found in microorganisms and not in mammalian cells are the most successful anti-infective agents. For example, antibiotics that interfere with the synthesis of bacterial cell walls have a high potential for selective toxicity. Some antibiotics structurally resemble some essential metabolites of microorganisms, which suggests that competitive antagonism may be the mechanism by which they exert their effects. Thus, cycloserine is believed to be an antimetabolite for D-alanine, a constituent of bacterial cell walls. Many antibiotics selectively interfere with microbial protein synthesis (e.g., the aminoglycosides, tetracyclines, macrolides, chloramphenicol, and lincomycin) or nucleic acid synthesis (e.g., rifampin). Others, such as the polymyxins and the polyenes, are believed to interfere with the integrity and function of microbial cell membranes. The mechanism of action of an antibiotic determines, in general, whether the agent exerts a bactericidal or a bacteriostatic

TABLE 8.1 Mechanisms of Antibiotic Action

Site of Action	Antibiotic	Process Interrupted	Type of Activity
Cell wall	Bacitracin	Mucopeptide synthesis	Bactericidal
	Cephalosporin	Cell wall cross-linking	Bactericidal
	Cycloserine	Synthesis of cell wall peptides	Bactericidal
	Penicillins	Cell wall cross-linking	Bactericidal
	Vancomycin	Mucopeptide synthesis	Bactericidal
Cell membrane	Amphotericin B	Membrane function	Fungicidal
	Nystatin	Membrane function	Fungicidal
	Polymyxins	Membrane integrity	Bactericidal
Ribosomes	Chloramphenicol	Protein synthesis	Bacteriostatic
50S subunit	Erythromycin	Protein synthesis	Bacteriostatic
	Lincomycins	Protein synthesis	Bacteriostatic
30S subunit	Aminoglycosides	Protein synthesis and fidelity	Bactericidal
	Tetracyclines	Protein synthesis	Bacteriostatic
Nucleic acids	Actinomycin	DNA and mRNA synthesis	Pancidal
	Griseofulvin	Cell division, microtubule assembly	Fungistatic
DNA and/or RNA	Mitomycin C	DNA synthesis	Pancidal
	Rifampin	mRNA synthesis	Bactericidal

action. The distinction may be important for the treatment of serious, life-threatening infections, particularly if the natural defense mechanisms of the host are either deficient or overwhelmed by the infection. In such situations, a bactericidal agent is obviously indicated. Much work remains to be done in this area, and as mechanisms of action are revealed, the development of improved structural analogs of effective antibiotics probably will continue to increase.

CHEMICAL CLASSIFICATION

The chemistry of antibiotics is so varied that a chemical classification is of limited value. Some similarities can be found, however, indicating that some antibiotics may be the products of similar mechanisms in different organisms and that these structurally similar products may exert their activities in a similar manner. For example, several important antibiotics have in common a macrolide structure (i.e., a large lactone ring). This group includes erythromycin and oleandomycin. The tetracycline family comprises a group of compounds very closely related chemically. Several compounds contain closely related amino sugar moieties, such as those found in streptomycins, kanamycins, neomycins, paromomycins, and gentamicins. The antifungal antibiotics nystatin and the amphotericins (see Chapter 6) are examples of a group of conjugated polyene compounds. The bacitracins, tyrothricin, and polymyxin are among a large group of polypeptides that exhibit antibiotic action. The penicillins and cephalosporins are β-lactam ring–containing antibiotics derived from amino acids.

MICROBIAL RESISTANCE

The normal biological processes of microbial pathogens are varied and complex. Thus, it seems reasonable to assume that there are many ways in which they may be inhibited and that different microorganisms that elaborate antibiotics antagonistic to a common "foe" produce compounds that are chemically dissimilar and that act on different processes. In fact, nature has produced many chemically different antibiotics that can attack the same microorganism by different pathways. The diversity of antibiotic structure has proved to be of real clinical value. As the pathogenic cell develops drug resistance, another antibiotic, attacking another metabolic process of the resisting cell, remains effective. The development of new and different antibiotics has been very important in providing the means for treating resistant strains of organisms that previously had been susceptible to an older antibiotic. More recently, the elucidation of biochemical mechanisms of microbial resistance to antibiotics, such as the inactivation of penicillins and cephalosporins by β-lactamase–producing bacteria, has stimulated research in the development of semisynthetic analogs that resist microbial biotransformation. The evolution of *nosocomial* (hospital-acquired) strains of staphylococci resistant to penicillin and of Gram-negative bacilli (e.g., *Pseudomonas* and *Klebsiella* spp., *Escherichia coli*, and others) often resistant to several antibiotics has become a serious medical problem. No doubt, the promiscuous and improper use of antibiotics has contributed to the emergence of resistant bacterial strains. The successful control of diseases caused by resistant strains of bacteria will require not only the development of new and improved antibiotics but also the rational use of available agents.

β-LACTAM ANTIBIOTICS

Antibiotics that possess the β-lactam (a four-membered cyclic amide) ring structure are the dominant class of agents currently used for the chemotherapy of bacterial infections. The first antibiotic to be used in therapy, penicillin (penicillin G or benzylpenicillin), and a close biosynthetic relative, phenoxymethyl penicillin (penicillin V), remain the agents of choice for the treatment of infections caused by most species of Gram-positive bacteria. The discovery of a second major group of β-lactam antibiotics, the cephalosporins, and chemical modifications of naturally occurring penicillins and cephalosporins have provided semisynthetic derivatives that are variously effective against bacterial species known to be resistant to penicillin, in particular, penicillinase-producing staphylococci and Gram-negative bacilli. Thus, apart from a few strains that have either inherent or acquired resistance, almost all bacterial species are sensitive to one or more of the available β-lactam antibiotics.

Mechanism of Action

In addition to a broad spectrum of antibacterial action, two properties contribute to the unequaled importance of β-lactam antibiotics in chemotherapy: a potent and rapid bactericidal action against bacteria in the growth phase and a very low frequency of toxic and other adverse reactions in the host. The uniquely lethal antibacterial action of these agents has been attributed to a selective inhibition of bacterial cell wall synthesis.[7] Specifically, the basic mechanism involved is inhibition of the biosynthesis of the dipeptidoglycan that provides strength and rigidity to the cell wall. Penicillins and cephalosporins acylate a specific bacterial D-transpeptidase,[8] thereby rendering it inactive for its role in forming peptide cross-links of two linear peptidoglycan strands by transpeptidation and loss of D-alanine. Bacterial D-alanine carboxypeptidases are also inhibited by β-lactam antibiotics.

Binding studies with tritiated benzylpenicillin have shown that the mechanisms of action of various β-lactam antibiotics are much more complex than previously assumed. Studies in *E. coli* have revealed as many as seven different functional proteins, each with an important role in cell wall biosynthesis.[9] These penicillin-binding proteins (PBPs) have the following functional properties:

- PBPs 1_a and 1_b are transpeptidases involved in peptidoglycan synthesis associated with cell elongation. Inhibition results in spheroplast formation and rapid cell lysis,[9,10] caused by *autolysins* (bacterial enzymes that create nicks in the cell wall for attachment of new peptidoglycan units or for separation of daughter cells during cell division[10]).
- PBP 2 is a transpeptidase involved in maintaining the rod shape of bacilli.[11] Inhibition results in ovoid or round forms that undergo delayed lysis.
- PBP 3 is a transpeptidase required for septum formation during cell division.[12] Inhibition results in the formation of filamentous forms containing rod-shaped units that cannot separate. It is not yet clear whether inhibition of PBP 3 is lethal to the bacterium.
- PBPs 4 through 6 are carboxypeptidases responsible for the hydrolysis of D-alanine–D-alanine terminal peptide bonds of the cross-linking peptides. Inhibition of these enzymes is apparently not lethal to the bacterium,[13] even though cleavage of the terminal D-alanine bond is required before peptide cross-linkage.

The various β-lactam antibiotics differ in their affinities for PBPs. Penicillin G binds preferentially to PBP 3, whereas the first-generation cephalosporins bind with higher affinity to PBP 1_a. In contrast to other penicillins and to cephalosporins, which can bind to PBPs 1, 2, and 3, amdinocillin binds only to PBP 2.

● THE PENICILLINS

Commercial Production and Unitage

Until 1944, it was assumed that the active principle in penicillin was a single substance and that variation in activity of different products was because of the amount of inert materials in the samples. Now we know that during the biological elaboration of the antibiotic, several closely related compounds may be produced. These compounds differ chemically in the acid moiety of the amide side chain. Variations in this moiety produce differences in antibiotic effect and in physicochemical properties, including stability. Thus, one can speak of penicillins as a group of compounds and identify each penicillin specifically. As each of the different penicillins was first isolated, letter designations were used in the United States; the British used Roman numerals.

Over 30 penicillins have been isolated from fermentation mixtures. Some of these occur naturally; others have been biosynthesized by altering the culture medium to provide certain precursors that may be incorporated as acyl groups. Commercial production of biosynthetic penicillins today depends chiefly on various strains of *Penicillium notatum* and *Penicillium chrysogenum*. In recent years, many more penicillins have been prepared semisynthetically and, undoubtedly, many more will be added to the list in attempts to find superior products.

Because the penicillin first used in chemotherapy was not a pure compound and exhibited varying activity among samples, it was necessary to evaluate it by microbiological assay. The procedure for assay was developed at Oxford, England, and the value became known as the *Oxford unit*: 1 Oxford unit is defined as the smallest amount of penicillin that will inhibit, in vitro, the growth of a strain of *Staphylococcus* in 50 mL of culture medium under specified conditions. Now that pure crystalline penicillin is available, the *United States Pharmacopoeia* (*USP*) defines *unit* as the antibiotic activity of 0.6 μg of penicillin G sodium reference standard. The weight–unit relationship of the penicillins varies with the acyl substituent and with the salt formed of the free acid: 1 mg of penicillin G sodium is equivalent to 1,667 units, 1 mg of penicillin G procaine is equivalent to 1,009 units, and 1 mg of penicillin G potassium is equivalent to 1,530 units.

The commercial production of penicillin has increased markedly since its introduction. As production increased, the cost dropped correspondingly. When penicillin was first available, 100,000 units sold for $20. Currently, the same quantity costs less than a penny. Fluctuations in the production of penicillins through the years have reflected changes in the relative popularity of broad-spectrum antibiotics and penicillins, the development of penicillin-resistant strains of several pathogens, the more recent introduction of semisynthetic penicillins, the use of penicillins in animal feeds and for veterinary purposes, and the increase in marketing problems in a highly competitive sales area.

Table 8.2 shows the general structure of the penicillins and relates the structure of the more familiar ones to their various designations.

Nomenclature

The nomenclature of penicillins is somewhat complex and very cumbersome. Two numbering systems for the fused bicyclic heterocyclic system exist. The *Chemical Abstracts* system initiates the numbering with the sulfur atom and assigns the ring nitrogen the 4-position. Thus, penicillins are named as 4-thia-l-azabicyclo[3.2.0]heptanes, according to this system. The numbering system adopted by the *USP* is the reverse of the *Chemical Abstracts* procedure, assigning

TABLE 8.2 Structure of Penicillins

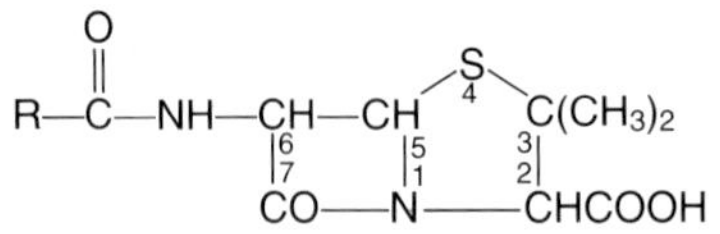

Generic Name	Chemical Name	R Group	Generic Name	Chemical Name	R Group
Penicillin G	Benzylpenicillin	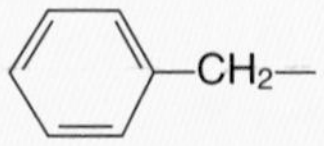	Amoxicillin	D-α-Amino-p-hydroxybenzylpenicillin	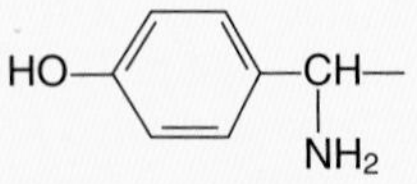
Penicillin V	Phenoxymethylpenicillin	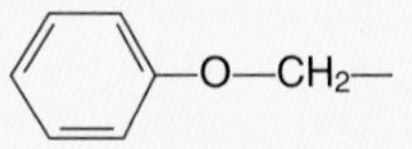	Cyclacillin	1-Aminocyclohexyl-penicillin	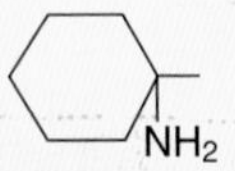
Methicillin	2,6-Dimethoxyphenyl-penicillin	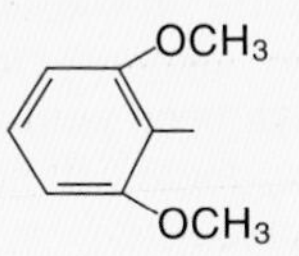	Carbenicillin	α-Carboxybenzyl-penicillin	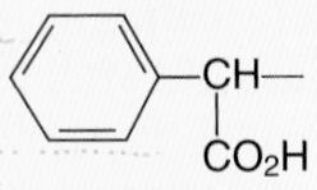
Nafcillin	2-Ethoxy-1-naphthyl-penicillin	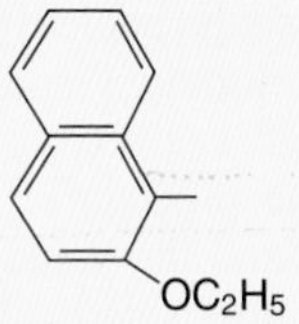	Ticarcillin	α-Carboxy-3-thienyl-penicillin	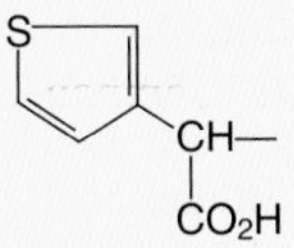
Oxacillin	5-Methyl-3-phenyl-4-isoxazolylpenicillin	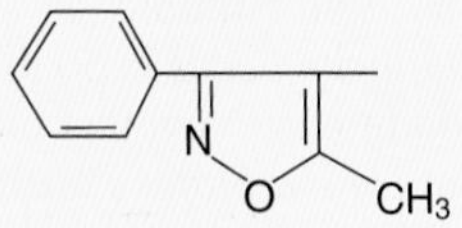	Piperacillin	α-(4-Ethyl-2,3-dioxo-1-piperazinylcarbonyl-amino)benzylpenicillin	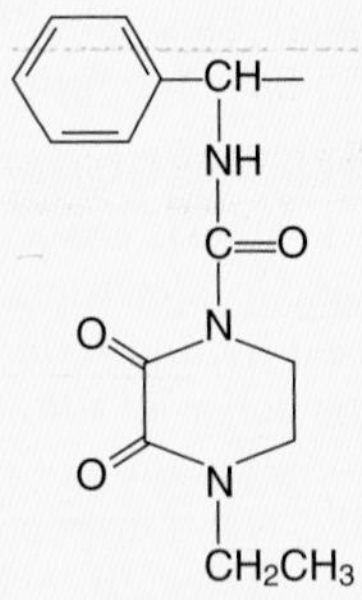
Cloxacillin	5-Methyl-3-(2-chlorophenyl)-4-isoxazolylpenicillin	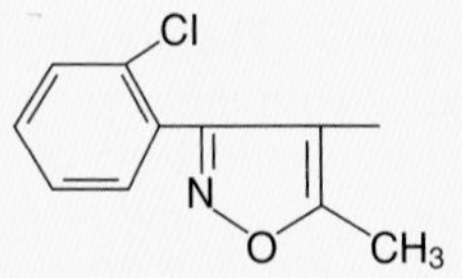	Mezlocillin	α-(1-Methanesulfonyl-2-oxoimidazolidino-carbonylamino)benzyl-penicillin	
Dicloxacillin	5-Methyl-3-(2,6-dichlorophenyl)-4-isoxazolylpenicillin	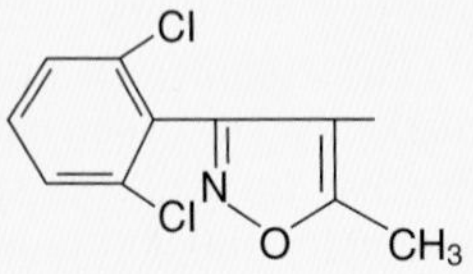			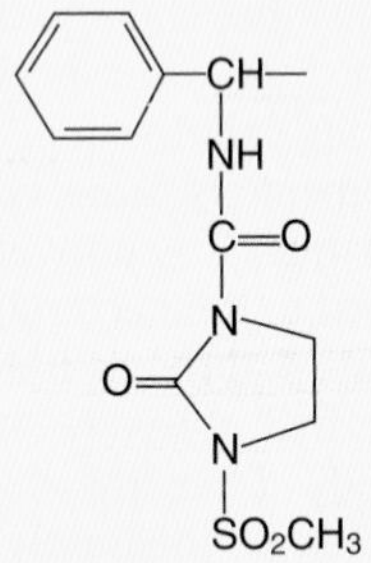
Ampicillin	D-α-Aminobenzyl-penicillin	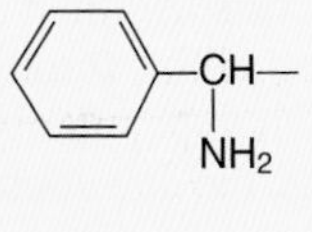			

number 1 to the nitrogen atom and number 4 to the sulfur atom. Three simplified forms of penicillin nomenclature have been adopted for general use. The first uses the name "penam" for the unsubstituted bicyclic system, including the amide carbonyl group, with one of the foregoing numbering systems as just described. Thus, penicillins generally are designated according to the *Chemical Abstracts* system as 5-acylamino-2,2-dimethylpenam-3-carboxylic acids. The second, seen more frequently in the medical literature, uses the name "penicillanic acid" to describe the ring system with substituents that are generally present (i.e., 2,2-dimethyl and 3-carboxyl). A third form, followed in this chapter, uses trivial nomenclature to name the entire 6-carbonylaminopenicillanic acid portion of the molecule penicillin and then distinguishes compounds on the basis of the R group of the acyl portion of the molecule. Thus, penicillin G is named benzylpenicillin, penicillin V is phenoxymethylpenicillin, methicillin is 2,6-dimethoxyphenylpenicillin, and so on. For the most part, the latter two systems serve well for naming and comparing closely similar penicillin structures, but they are too restrictive to be applied to compounds with unusual substituents or to ring-modified derivatives.

Stereochemistry

The penicillin molecule contains three chiral carbon atoms (C-3, C-5, and C-6). All naturally occurring and microbiologically active synthetic and semisynthetic penicillins have the same absolute configuration about these three centers. The carbon atom bearing the acylamino group (C-6) has the L configuration, whereas the carbon to which the carboxyl group is attached has the D configuration. Thus, the acylamino and carboxyl groups are *trans* to each other, with the former in the α and the latter in the β orientation relative to the penam ring system. The atoms composing the 6-aminopenicillanic acid (6-APA) portion of the structure are derived biosynthetically from two amino acids, L-cysteine (S-1, C-5, C-6, C-7, and 6-amino) and L-valine (2,2-dimethyl, C-2, C-3, N-4, and 3-carboxyl). The absolute stereochemistry of the penicillins is designated 3S:5R:6R, as shown below.

Synthesis

Examination of the structure of the penicillin molecule shows that it contains a fused ring system of unusual design, the β-lactam thiazolidine structure. The nature of the β-lactam ring delayed elucidation of the structure of penicillin, but its determination resulted from a collaborative research program involving groups in Great Britain and the United States during the years 1943 to 1945.[14] Attempts to synthesize these compounds resulted, at best, in only trace amounts until Sheehan and Henery-Logan[15] adapted techniques developed in peptide synthesis to the synthesis of penicillin V. This procedure is not likely to replace the established fermentation processes because the last step in the

reaction series develops only 10% to 12% penicillin. It is of advantage in research because it provides a means of obtaining many new amide chains hitherto not possible to achieve by biosynthetic procedures.

Two other developments have provided additional means for making new penicillins. A group of British scientists, Batchelor et al.[16] reported the isolation of 6-APA from a culture of *P. chrysogenum*. This compound can be converted to penicillins by acylation of the 6-amino group. Sheehan and Ferris[17] provided another route to synthetic penicillins by converting a natural penicillin, such as penicillin G potassium, to an intermediate (Fig. 8.1), from which the acyl side chain has been cleaved and which then can be treated to form biologically active penicillins with various new side chains. By these procedures, new penicillins, superior in activity and stability to those formerly in wide use, were found, and no doubt others will be produced. The first commercial products of these research activities were phenoxyethylpenicillin (phenethicillin) (Fig. 8.2) and dimethoxyphenylpenicillin (methicillin).

Chemical Degradation

The early commercial penicillin was a yellow-to-brown amorphous powder that was so unstable that refrigeration was required to maintain a reasonable level of activity for a short time. Improved purification procedures provided the white

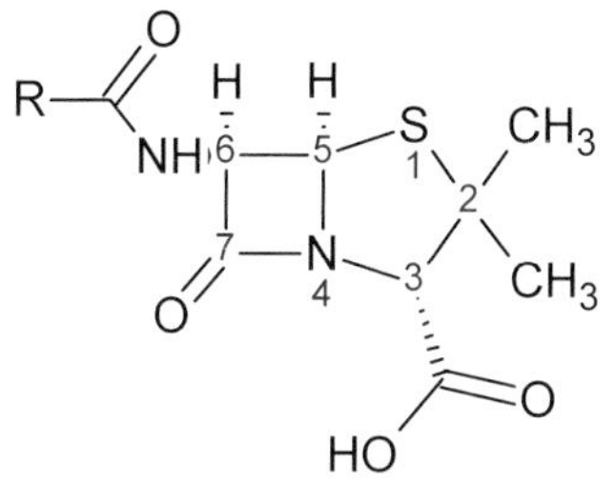

Chemical Abstracts

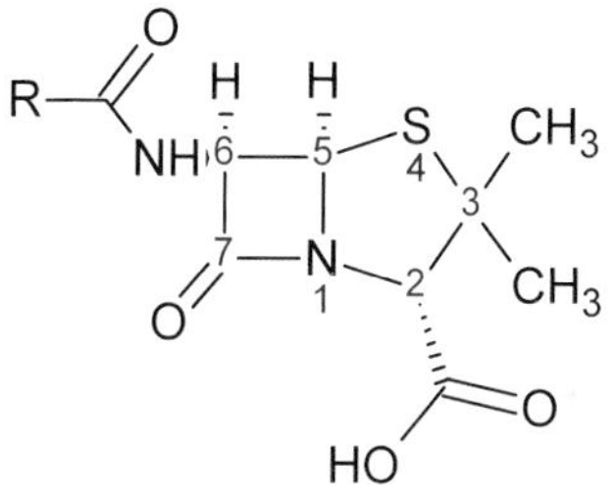

USP

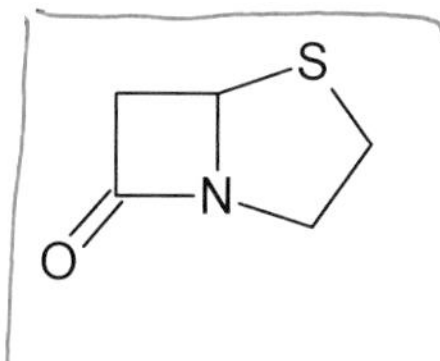

Penam

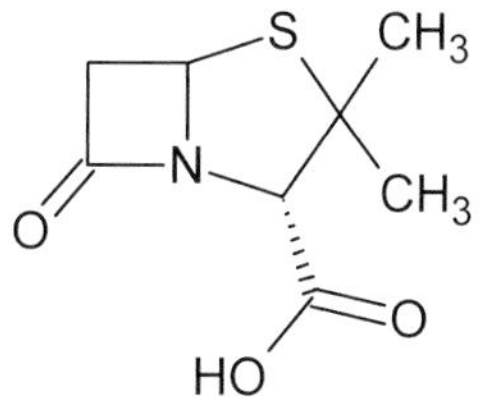

Penicillanic Acid

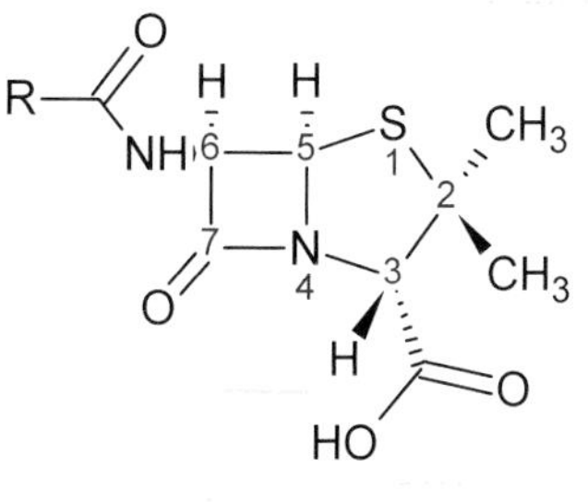

Chemical Abstracts

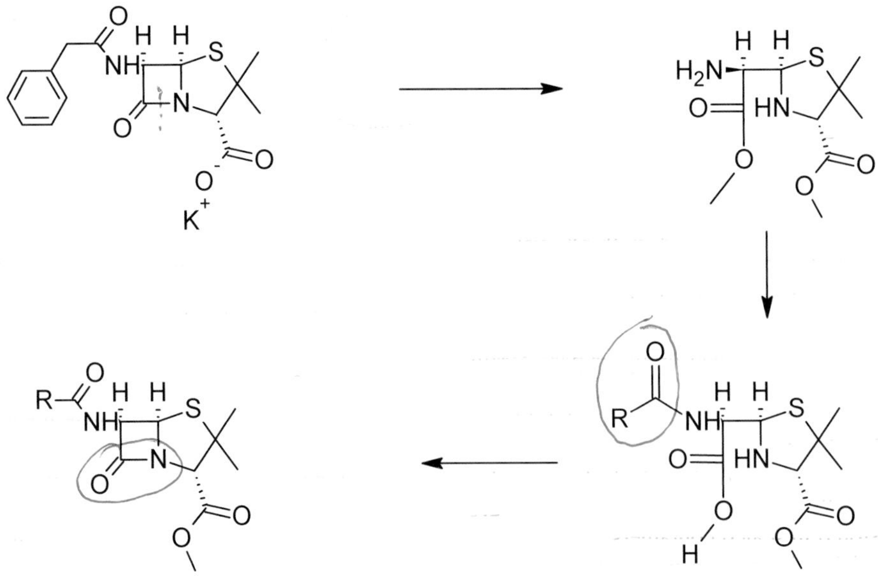

Figure 8.1 ● Conversion of natural penicillin to synthetic penicillin.

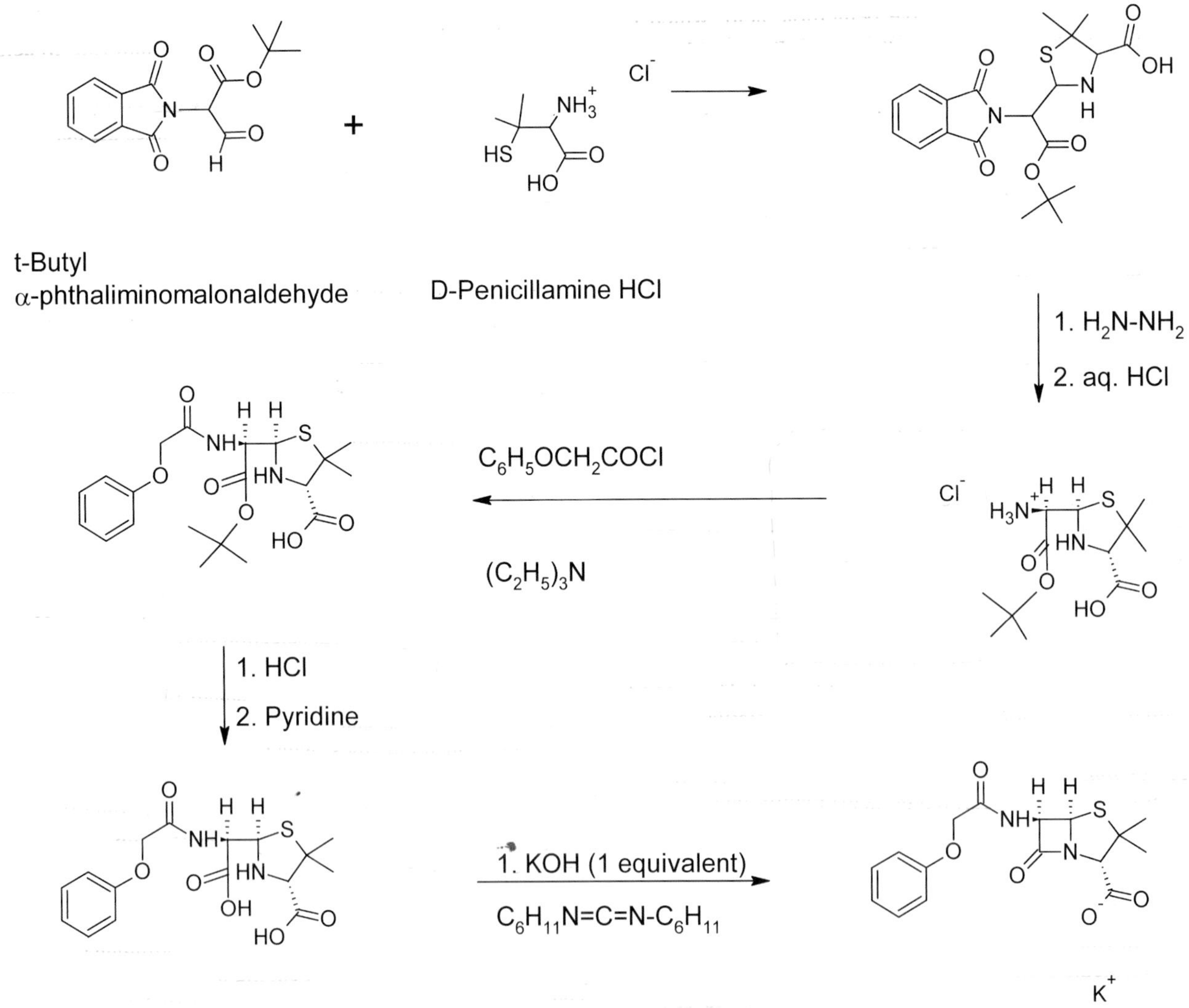

t-Butyl
α-phthaliminomalonaldehyde

D-Penicillamine HCl

Figure 8.2 ● Synthesis of phenoxymethylpenicillin.

crystalline material in use today. Crystalline penicillin must be protected from moisture, but when kept dry, the salts will remain stable for years without refrigeration. Many penicillins have an unpleasant taste, which must be overcome in the formation of pediatric dosage forms. All of the natural penicillins are strongly dextrorotatory. The solubility and other physicochemical properties of the penicillins are affected by the nature of the acyl side chain and by the cations used to make salts of the acid. Most penicillins are acids with pK_a values in the range of 2.5 to 3.0, but some are amphoteric. The free acids are not suitable for oral or parenteral administration. The sodium and potassium salts of most penicillins, however, are soluble in water and readily absorbed orally or parenterally. Salts of penicillins with organic bases, such as benzathine, procaine, and hydrabamine, have limited water solubility and are, therefore, useful as depot forms to provide effective blood levels over a long period in the treatment of chronic infections. Some of the crystalline salts of the penicillins are hygroscopic and must be stored in sealed containers.

The main cause of deterioration of penicillin is the reactivity of the strained lactam ring, particularly to hydrolysis. The course of the hydrolysis and the nature of the degradation products are influenced by the pH of the solution.[18,19] Thus, the β-lactam carbonyl group of penicillin readily undergoes nucleophilic attack by water or (especially) hydroxide ion to form the inactive penicilloic acid, which is reasonably stable in neutral to alkaline solutions but readily undergoes decarboxylation and further hydrolytic reactions in acidic solutions. Other nucleophiles, such as hydroxylamines, alkylamines, and alcohols, open the β-lactam ring to form the corresponding hydroxamic acids, amides, and esters. It has been speculated[20] that one of the causes of penicillin allergy may be the formation of antigenic penicilloyl proteins in vivo by the reaction of nucleophilic groups (e.g., ε-amino) on specific body proteins with the β-lactam carbonyl group. In strongly acidic solutions (pH <3), penicillin undergoes a complex series of reactions leading to various inactive degradation products (Fig. 8.3).[19] The first step appears to involve rearrangement to the penicillanic acid. This process is initiated by protonation of the β-lactam nitrogen, followed by nucleophilic attack of the acyl oxygen atom on the β-lactam carbonyl carbon. The subsequent opening of the β-lactam ring destabilizes the thiazoline ring, which then also suffers acid-catalyzed ring opening to form the penicillanic acid. The latter is very unstable and experiences two major degradation pathways. The most easily understood path involves hydrolysis of the oxazolone ring to form the unstable penamaldic acid. Because it is an enamine, penamaldic acid easily hydrolyzes to penicillamine (a major degradation product) and penaldic acid. The second path involves a complex rearrangement of penicillanic acid to a penillic acid through a series of intramolecular processes that remain to be elucidated completely. Penillic acid (an imidazoline-2-carboxylic acid) readily decarboxylates and suffers hydrolytic ring opening under acidic conditions to form a second major end product of acid-catalyzed penicillin degradation—penilloic acid. Penicilloic acid, the major product formed under weakly acidic to alkaline (as well as enzymatic) hydrolytic conditions, cannot be detected as an intermediate under strongly acidic conditions. It exists in equilibrium with penamaldic acid, however, and undergoes decarboxylation in acid to form penilloic acid. The third major product of the degradation is penicilloaldehyde,

formed by decarboxylation of penaldic acid (a derivative of malonaldehyde).

By controlling the pH of aqueous solutions within a range of 6.0 to 6.8 and refrigerating the solutions, aqueous preparations of the soluble penicillins may be stored for up to several weeks. The relationship of these properties to the pharmaceutics of penicillins has been reviewed by Schwartz and Buckwalter.[21] Some buffer systems, particularly phosphates and citrates, exert a favorable effect on penicillin stability, independent of the pH effect. Finholt et al.[22] showed that these buffers may catalyze penicillin degradation, however, if the pH is adjusted to obtain the requisite ions. Hydroalcoholic solutions of penicillin G potassium are about as unstable as aqueous solutions.[23] Because penicillins are inactivated by metal ions such as zinc and copper, it has been suggested that the phosphates and the citrates combine with these metals to prevent their existence as free ions in solution.

Oxidizing agents also inactivate penicillins, but reducing agents have little effect on them. Temperature affects the rate of deterioration; although the dry salts are stable at room temperature and do not require refrigeration, prolonged heating inactivates the penicillins.

Acid-catalyzed degradation in the stomach contributes strongly to the poor oral absorption of penicillin. Thus, efforts to obtain penicillins with improved pharmacokinetic and microbiological properties have focused on acyl functionalities that would minimize sensitivity of the β-lactam ring to acid hydrolysis while maintaining antibacterial activity.

Substitution of an electron-withdrawing group in the α position of benzylpenicillin markedly stabilizes the penicillin to acid-catalyzed hydrolysis. Thus, phenoxymethylpenicillin, α-aminobenzylpenicillin, and α-halobenzylpenicillin are significantly more stable than benzylpenicillin in acid solutions. The increased stability imparted by such electron-withdrawing groups has been attributed to decreased reactivity (nucleophilicity) of the side chain amide carbonyl oxygen atom toward participation in β-lactam ring opening to form penicillenic acid. Obviously, α-aminobenzylpenicillin (ampicillin) exists as the protonated form in acidic (as well as neutral) solutions, and the ammonium group is known to be powerfully electron-withdrawing.

Bacterial Resistance

Some bacteria, in particular most species of Gram-negative bacilli, are naturally resistant to the action of penicillins. Other normally sensitive species can develop penicillin resistance (either through natural selection of resistant individuals or through mutation). The best understood and, probably, the most important biochemical mechanism of penicillin resistance is the bacterial elaboration of enzymes that inactivate penicillins. Such enzymes, which have been given the nonspecific name *penicillinases*, are of two general types: β-lactamases and acylases. By far, the more important of these are the β-lactamases, enzymes that catalyze the hydrolytic opening of the β-lactam ring of penicillins to produce inactive penicilloic acids. Synthesis of bacterial β-lactamases may be under chromosomal or plasmid R factor control and may be either constitutive or inducible (stimulated by the presence of the substrate), depending on the bacterial species. The well-known resistance among strains of *Staphylococcus aureus* is apparently entirely because of the production of an inducible β-lactamase. Resistance among Gram-negative

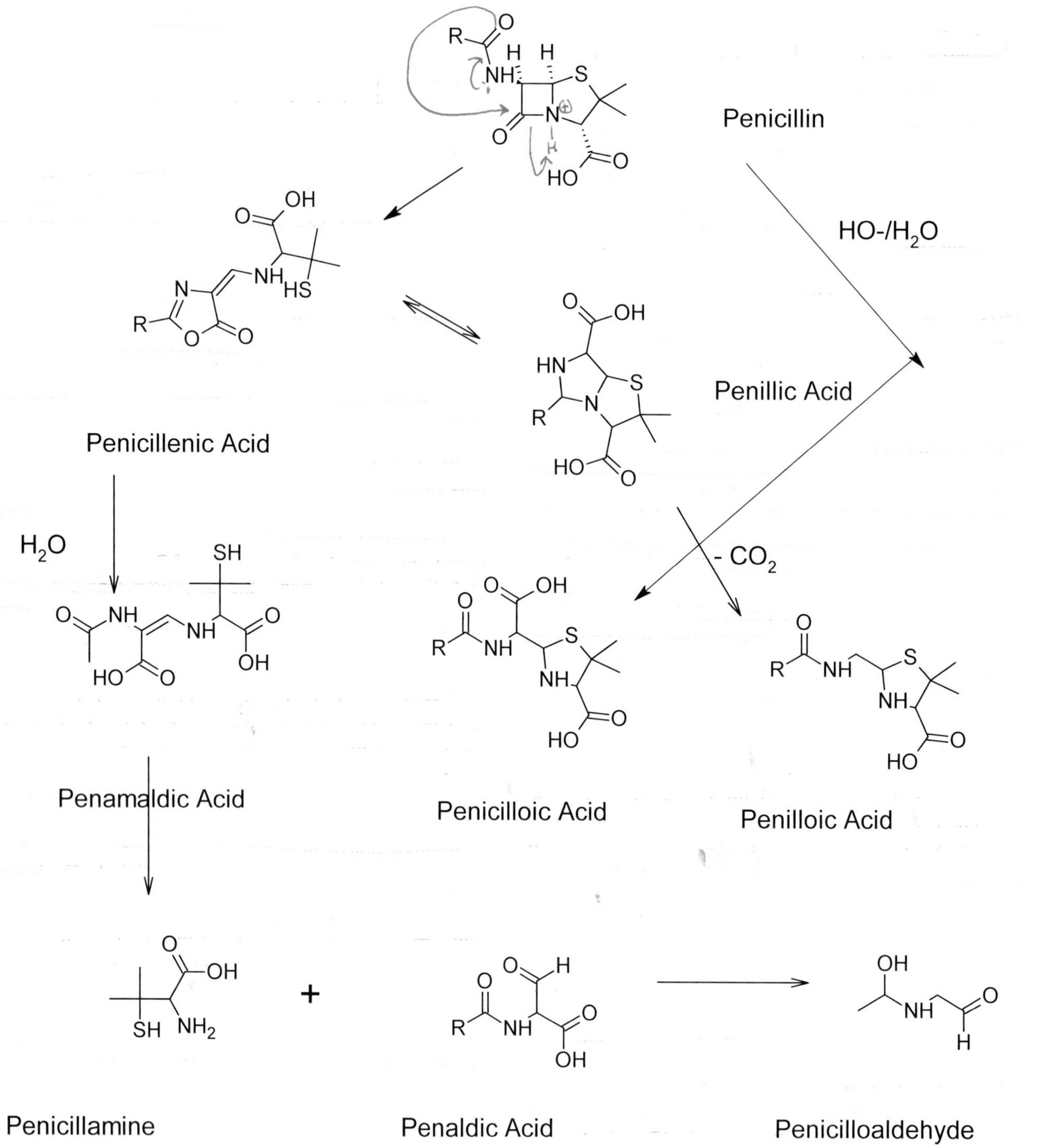

Figure 8.3 • Degradation of penicillins.

bacilli, however, may result from other poorly characterized "resistance factors" or constitutive β-lactamase elaboration. β-Lactamases produced by Gram-negative bacilli appear to be cytoplasmic enzymes that remain in the bacterial cell, whereas those elaborated by *S. aureus* are synthesized in the cell wall and released extracellularly. β-Lactamases from different bacterial species may be classified[24–26] by their structure, their substrate and inhibitor specificities, their physical properties (e.g., pH optimum, isoelectric point, molecular weight), and their immunological properties.

Specific acylases (enzymes that can hydrolyze the acyl-amino side chain of penicillins) have been obtained from several species of Gram-negative bacteria, but their possible role in bacterial resistance has not been well defined. These enzymes find some commercial use in the preparation of 6-APA for the preparation of semisynthetic penicillins. 6-APA is less active and hydrolyzed more rapidly (enzymatically and nonenzymatically) than penicillin.

Another important resistance mechanism, especially in Gram-negative bacteria, is decreased permeability to penicillins. The cell envelope in most Gram-negative bacteria is more complex than in Gram-positive bacteria. It contains an outer membrane (linked by lipoprotein bridges to the peptidoglycan cell wall) not present in Gram-positive bacteria, which creates a physical barrier to the penetration of antibiotics, especially those that are hydrophobic.[27] Small hydrophilic molecules, however, can traverse the outer membrane through pores formed by proteins called *porins*.[28] Alteration of the number or nature of porins in the cell envelope[28] also could be an important mechanism of antibiotic resistance. Bacterial resistance can result from changes in the affinity of PBPs for penicillins.[29] Altered PBP binding has been demonstrated in non–β-lactamase-producing strains of penicillin-resistant *Neisseria gonorrhoeae*[30] and methicillin-resistant *S. aureus* (MRSA).[31]

Certain strains of bacteria are resistant to the lytic properties of penicillins but remain susceptible to their growth-inhibiting effects. Thus, the action of the antibiotic has been converted from bactericidal to bacteriostatic. This mechanism of resistance is termed *tolerance* and apparently results from impaired autolysin activity in the bacterium.

Penicillinase-Resistant Penicillins

The availability of 6-APA on a commercial scale made possible the synthesis of numerous semisynthetic penicillins modified at the acylamino side chain. Much of the early work done in the 1960s was directed toward the preparation of derivatives that would resist destruction by β-lactamases, particularly those produced by penicillin-resistant strains of *S. aureus*, which constituted a very serious health problem at that time. In general, increasing the steric hindrance at the α-carbon of the acyl group increased resistance to staphylococcal β-lactamase, with maximal resistance being observed with quaternary substitution.[32] More fruitful from the standpoint of antibacterial potency, however, was the observation that the α-acyl carbon could be part of an aromatic (e.g., phenyl or naphthyl) or heteroaromatic (e.g., 4-isoxazolyl) system.[33] Substitutions at the *ortho* positions of a phenyl ring (e.g., 2,6-dimethoxy [methicillin]) or the 2-position of a 1-naphthyl system (e.g., 2-ethoxyl [nafcillin]) increase the steric hindrance of the acyl group and confer more β-lactamase resistance than shown by the unsubstituted compounds or those substituted at positions more distant from the α-carbon. Bulkier substituents are required to confer effective β-lactamase resistance among five-membered–ring heterocyclic derivatives.[34] Thus, members of the 4-isoxazolyl penicillin family (e.g., oxacillin, cloxacillin, and dicloxacillin) require both the 3-aryl and 5-methyl (3-methyl and 5-aryl) substituents for effectiveness against β-lactamase–producing *S. aureus*.

Increasing the bulkiness of the acyl group is not without its price, however, because all of the clinically available penicillinase-resistant penicillins are significantly less active than either penicillin G or penicillin V against most non–β-lactamase-producing bacteria normally sensitive to the penicillins. The β-lactamase–resistant penicillins tend to be comparatively lipophilic molecules that do not penetrate well into Gram-negative bacteria. The isoxazoyl penicillins, particularly those with an electronegative substituent in the 3-phenyl group (cloxacillin, dicloxacillin, and floxacillin), are also resistant to acid-catalyzed hydrolysis of the β-lactam, for the reasons described previously. Steric factors that confer β-lactamase resistance, however, do not necessarily also confer stability to acid. Accordingly, methicillin, which has electron-donating groups (by resonance) *ortho* to the carbonyl carbon, is even more labile to acid-catalyzed hydrolysis than is penicillin G because of the more rapid formation of the penicillenic acid derivative.

Extended-Spectrum Penicillins

Another highly significant advance arising from the preparation of semisynthetic penicillins was the discovery that the introduction of an ionized or polar group into the α-position of the side chain benzyl carbon atom of penicillin G confers activity against Gram-negative bacilli. Hence, derivatives with an ionized α-amino group, such as ampicillin and amoxicillin, are generally effective against such Gram-negative genera as *Escherichia*, *Klebsiella*, *Haemophilus*, *Salmonella*, *Shigella*, and non–indole-producing *Proteus*. Furthermore, activity against penicillin G–sensitive, Gram-positive species is largely retained. The introduction of an α-amino group in ampicillin (or amoxicillin) creates an additional chiral center. Extension of the antibacterial spectrum brought about by the substituent applies only to the D-isomer, which is 2 to 8 times more active than either the L-isomer or benzylpenicillin (which are equiactive) against various species of the aforementioned genera of Gram-negative bacilli.

The basis for the expanded spectrum of activity associated with the ampicillin group is not related to β-lactamase inhibition, as ampicillin and amoxicillin are even more labile than penicillin G to the action of β-lactamases elaborated by both *S. aureus* and various species of Gram-negative bacilli, including strains among the ampicillin-sensitive group. Hydrophilic penicillins, such as ampicillin, penetrate Gram-negative bacteria more readily than penicillin G, penicillin V, or methicillin. This selective penetration is believed to take place through the porin channels of the cell membrane.[35]

α-Hydroxy substitution also yields "expanded-spectrum" penicillins with activity and stereoselectivity similar to that of the ampicillin group. The α-hydroxybenzylpenicillins are, however, about 2 to 5 times less active than their corresponding α-aminobenzyl counterparts and, unlike the latter, not very stable under acidic conditions.

Incorporation of an acidic substituent at the α-benzyl carbon atom of penicillin G also imparts clinical effectiveness against Gram-negative bacilli and, furthermore, extends the spectrum of activity to include organisms resistant to ampicillin. Thus, α-carboxybenzylpenicillin (carbenicillin) is active against ampicillin-sensitive, Gram-negative species and additional Gram-negative bacilli of the genera *Pseudomonas*, *Klebsiella*, *Enterobacter*, indole-producing *Proteus*, *Serratia*, and *Providencia*. The potency of carbenicillin against most species of penicillin G-sensitive, Gram-positive bacteria is several orders of magnitude lower than that of either penicillin G or ampicillin, presumably because of poorer penetration of a more highly ionized molecule into these bacteria. (Note that α-aminobenzylpenicillins exist as zwitterions over a broad pH range and, as such, are considerably less polar than carbenicillin.) This increased polarity is apparently an advantage for the penetration of carbenicillin through the cell envelope of Gram-negative bacteria via porin channels.[35]

Carbenicillin is active against both β-lactamase–producing and non–β-lactamase-producing strains of Gram-negative bacteria. It is somewhat resistant to a few of the β-lactamases produced by Gram-negative bacteria, especially members of the Enterobacteriaceae family.[36] Resistance to β-lactamases elaborated by Gram-negative bacteria, therefore, may be an important component of carbenicillin's activity against some ampicillin-resistant organisms. β-Lactamases produced by *Pseudomonas* spp., however, readily hydrolyze carbenicillin. Although carbenicillin is also somewhat resistant to staphylococcal β-lactamase, it is considerably less so than methicillin or the isoxazoyl penicillins, and its inherent antistaphylococcal activity is less impressive than that of the penicillinase-resistant penicillins. The penicillinase-resistant penicillins, despite their resistance to most β-lactamases, however, share the lack of activity of penicillin G against Gram-negative bacilli, primarily because of an inability to penetrate the bacterial cell envelope.

Compared with the aminoglycoside antibiotics, the potency of carbenicillin against such Gram-negative bacilli as *Pseudomonas aeruginosa*, *Proteus vulgaris*, and *Klebsiella pneumoniae* is much less impressive. Large parenteral doses are required to achieve bactericidal concentrations in plasma and tissues. The low toxicity of carbenicillin (and the penicillins in general), however, usually permits (in the absence of allergy) the use of such high doses without untoward effects. Furthermore, carbenicillin (and other penicillins), when combined with aminoglycosides, exerts a synergistic bactericidal action against bacterial species sensitive to both agents, frequently allowing the use of a lower dose of the more toxic aminoglycoside than is normally required for treatment of a life-threatening infection. The chemical incompatibility of penicillins and aminoglycosides requires that the two antibiotics be administered separately; otherwise, both are inactivated. Iyengar et al.[37] showed that acylation of amino groups in the aminoglycoside by the β-lactam of the penicillin occurs.

Unlike the situation with ampicillin, the introduction of asymmetry at the α-benzyl carbon in carbenicillin imparts little or no stereoselectivity of antibacterial action; the individual enantiomers are nearly equally active and readily epimerized to the racemate in aqueous solution. Because it is a derivative of phenylmalonic acid, carbenicillin readily decarboxylates to benzylpenicillin in the presence of acid; therefore, it is not active (as carbenicillin) orally and must be administered parenterally. Esterification of the α-carboxyl group (e.g., as the 5-indanyl ester) partially protects the compound from acid-catalyzed destruction and provides an orally active derivative that is hydrolyzed to carbenicillin in the plasma. The plasma levels of free carbenicillin achieved with oral administration of such esters, however, may not suffice for effective treatment of serious infections caused by some species of Gram-negative bacilli, such as *P. aeruginosa*.

A series of α-acylureido–substituted penicillins, exemplified by azlocillin, mezlocillin, and piperacillin, exhibit greater activity against certain Gram-negative bacilli than carbenicillin. Although the acylureidopenicillins are acylated derivatives of ampicillin, the antibacterial spectrum of activity of the group is more like that of carbenicillin. The acylureidopenicillins are, however, superior to carbenicillin against *Klebsiella* spp., *Enterobacter* spp., and *P. aeruginosa*. This enhanced activity is apparently not because of β-lactamase resistance, in that both inducible and plasmid-mediated β-lactamases hydrolyze these penicillins. More facile penetration through the cell envelope of these particular bacterial species is the most likely explanation for the greater potency. The acylureidopenicillins, unlike ampicillin, are unstable under acidic conditions; therefore, they are not available for oral administration.

Protein Binding

The nature of the acylamino side chain also determines the extent to which penicillins are plasma protein bound.

Quantitative structure–activity relationship (QSAR) studies of the binding of penicillins to human serum[38,39] indicate that hydrophobic groups (positive π dependence) in the side chain appear to be largely responsible for increased binding to serum proteins. Penicillins with polar or ionized substituents in the side chain exhibit low-to-intermediate fractions of protein binding. Accordingly, ampicillin, amoxicillin, and cyclacillin experience 25% to 30% protein binding, and carbenicillin and ticarcillin show 45% to 55% protein binding. Those with nonpolar, lipophilic substituents (nafcillin and isoxazoyl penicillins) are more than 90% protein bound. The penicillins with less complex acyl groups (benzylpenicillin, phenoxymethylpenicillin, and methicillin) fall in the range of 35% to 80%. Protein binding is thought to restrict the tissue availability of drugs if the fraction bound is sufficiently high; thus, the tissue distribution of the penicillins in the highly bound group may be inferior to that of other penicillins. The similarity of biological half-lives for various penicillins, however, indicates that plasma protein binding has little effect on duration of action. All of the commercially available penicillins are secreted actively by the renal active transport system for anions. The reversible nature of protein binding does not compete effectively with the active tubular secretion process.

Allergy to Penicillins

Allergic reactions to various penicillins, ranging in severity from a variety of skin and mucous membrane rashes to drug fever and anaphylaxis, constitute the major problem associated with the use of this class of antibiotics. Estimates place the prevalence of hypersensitivity to penicillin G throughout the world between 1% and 10% of the population. In the United States and other industrialized countries, it is nearer the higher figure, ranking penicillin the most common cause of drug-induced allergy. The penicillins that are most frequently implicated in allergic reactions are penicillin G and ampicillin. Virtually all commercially available penicillins, however, have been reported to cause such reactions; in fact, cross-sensitivity among most chemical classes of 6-acylaminopenicillanic acid derivatives has been demonstrated.[40]

The chemical mechanisms by which penicillin preparations become antigenic have been studied extensively.[20] Evidence suggests that penicillins or their rearrangement products formed in vivo (e.g., penicillenic acids)[41] react with lysine ε-amino groups of proteins to form penicilloyl proteins, which are major antigenic determinants.[42,43] Early clinical observations with the biosynthetic penicillins G and V indicated a higher incidence of allergic reactions with unpurified, amorphous preparations than with highly purified, crystalline forms, suggesting that small amounts of highly antigenic penicilloyl proteins present in unpurified samples were a cause. Polymeric impurities in ampicillin dosage forms have been implicated as possible antigenic determinants and a possible explanation for the high frequency of allergic reactions with this particular semisynthetic penicillin. Ampicillin is known to undergo pH-dependent polymerization reactions (especially in concentrated solutions) that involve nucleophilic attack of the side chain amino group of one molecule on the β-lactam carbonyl carbon atom of a second molecule, and so on.[44] The high frequency of antigenicity shown by ampicillin polymers, together with

TABLE 8.3 Classification and Properties of Penicillins

Penicillin	Source	Acid Resistance	Oral Absorption (%)	Plasma Protein Binding (%)	β-Lactamase Resistance (*S. aureus*)	Spectrum of Activity	Clinical Use
Benzylpenicillin	Biosynthetic	Poor	Poor (20)	50–60	No	Intermediate	Multipurpose
Penicillin V	Biosynthetic	Good	Good (60)	55–80	No	Intermediate	Multipurpose
Methicillin	Semisynthetic	Poor	None	30–40	Yes	Narrow	Limited use
Nafcillin	Semisynthetic	Fair	Variable	90	Yes	Narrow	Limited use
Oxacillin	Semisynthetic	Good	Fair (30)	85–94	Yes	Narrow	Limited use
Cloxacillin	Semisynthetic	Good	Good (50)	88–96	Yes	Narrow	Limited use
Dicloxacillin	Semisynthetic	Good	Good (50)	95–98	Yes	Narrow	Limited use
Ampicillin	Semisynthetic	Good	Fair (40)	20–25	No	Broad	Multipurpose
Amoxicillin	Semisynthetic	Good	Good (75)	20–25	No	Broad	Multipurpose
Carbenicillin	Semisynthetic	Poor	None	50–60	No	Extended	Limited use
Ticarcillin	Semisynthetic	Poor	None	45	No	Extended	Limited use
Mezlocillin	Semisynthetic	Poor	Nil	50	No	Extended	Limited use
Piperacillin	Semisynthetic	Poor	Nil	50	No	Extended	Limited use

their isolation and characterization in some ampicillin preparations, supports the theory that they can contribute to ampicillin-induced allergy.[45]

Classification

Various designations have been used to classify penicillins, based on their sources, chemistry, pharmacokinetic properties, resistance to enzymatic spectrum of activity, and clinical uses (Table 8.3). Thus, penicillins may be biosynthetic, semisynthetic, or (potentially) synthetic; acid-resistant or not; orally or (only) parenterally active; and resistant to β-lactamases (penicillinases) or not. They may have a narrow, intermediate, broad, or extended spectrum of antibacterial activity and may be intended for multipurpose or limited clinical use. Designations of the activity spectrum as narrow, intermediate, broad, or extended are relative and do not necessarily imply the breadth of therapeutic application. Indeed, the classification of penicillin G as a "narrow-spectrum" antibiotic has meaning only relative to other penicillins. Although the β-lactamase–resistant penicillins have a spectrum of activity similar to that of penicillin G, they generally are reserved for the treatment of infections caused by penicillin G–resistant, β-lactamase–producing *S. aureus* because their activity against most penicillin G-sensitive bacteria is significantly inferior. Similarly, carbenicillin and ticarcillin usually are reserved for the treatment of infections caused by ampicillin-resistant, Gram-negative bacilli because they offer no advantage (and have some disadvantages) over ampicillin or penicillin G in infections sensitive to them.

Products

Penicillin G

For years, the most popular penicillin has been penicillin G, or benzylpenicillin. In fact, with the exception of patients allergic to it, penicillin G remains the agent of choice for the treatment of more different kinds of bacterial infection than any other antibiotic. It was first made available as the water-soluble salts of potassium, sodium, and calcium. These salts of penicillin are inactivated by the gastric juice and are not effective when administered orally unless antacids, such as calcium carbonate, aluminum hydroxide, and magnesium trisilicate; or a strong buffer, such as sodium citrate, is added. Also, because penicillin is absorbed poorly from the

intestinal tract, oral doses must be very large, about five times the amount necessary with parenteral administration. Only after the production of penicillin had increased enough to make low-priced penicillin available did the oral dosage forms become popular. The water-soluble potassium and sodium salts are used orally and parenterally to achieve high plasma concentrations of penicillin G rapidly. The more water-soluble potassium salt usually is preferred when large doses are required. Situations in which hyperkalemia is a danger, however, as in renal failure, require use of the sodium salt; the potassium salt is preferred for patients on salt-free diets or with congestive heart conditions.

The rapid elimination of penicillin from the bloodstream through the kidneys by active tubular secretion and the need to maintain an effective concentration in blood have led to the development of "repository" forms of this drug. Suspensions of penicillin in peanut oil or sesame oil with white beeswax added were first used to prolong the duration of injected forms of penicillin. This dosage form was replaced by a suspension in vegetable oil, to which aluminum monostearate or aluminum distearate was added. Today, most repository forms are suspensions of high–molecular weight amine salts of penicillin in a similar base.

Penicillin G Procaine

The first widely used amine salt of penicillin G was made with procaine. Penicillin G procaine (Crysticillin, Duracillin, Wycillin) can be made readily from penicillin G sodium by treatment with procaine hydrochloride. This salt is considerably less soluble in water than the alkali metal salts, requiring about 250 mL to dissolve 1 g. Free penicillin is released only as the compound dissolves and dissociates. It has an activity of 1,009 units/mg. A large number of preparations for injection of penicillin G procaine are commercially available. Most of these are either suspensions in water to which a suitable dispersing or suspending agent, a buffer, and a preservative have been added or suspensions in peanut oil or sesame oil that have been gelled by the addition of 2% aluminum monostearate. Some commercial products are mixtures of penicillin G potassium or sodium with penicillin G procaine; the water-soluble salt provides rapid development of a high plasma concentration of penicillin, and the insoluble salt prolongs the duration of effect.

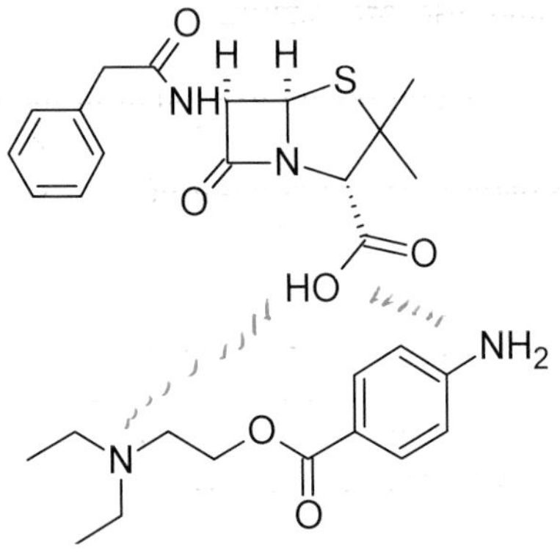

Penicillin G Benzathine

Since penicillin G benzathine, *N,N'*-dibenzylethylenediamine dipenicillin G (Bicillin, Permapen), is the salt of a diamine, 2 moles of penicillin are available from each molecule. It is very insoluble in water, requiring about 3,000 mL to dissolve 1 g. This property gives the compound great stability and prolonged duration of effect. At the pH of gastric juice, it is quite stable, and food intake does not interfere with its absorption. It is available in tablet form and in several parenteral preparations. The activity of penicillin G benzathine is equivalent to 1,211 units/mg.

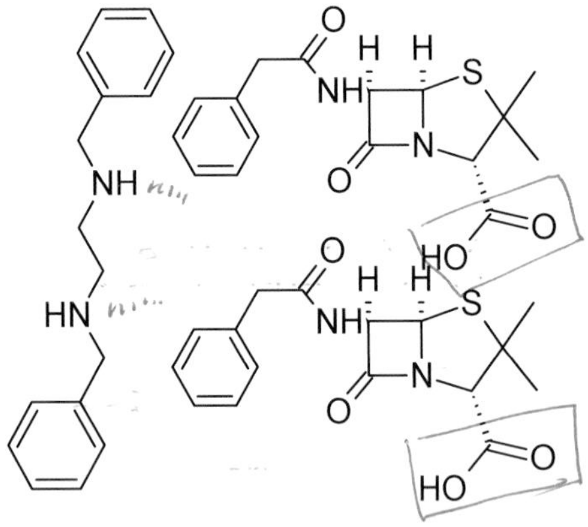

Several other amines have been used to make penicillin salts, and research is continuing on this subject. Other amines that have been used include 2-chloroprocaine; L-*N*-methyl-1,2-diphenyl-2-hydroxyethylamine (L-ephenamine); dibenzylamine; tripelennamine (Pyribenzamine); and *N,N'*-bis-(dehydroabietyl)ethylenediamine (hydrabamine).

Penicillin V

In 1948, Behrens et al.[46] reported penicillin V, phenoxymethylpenicillin (Pen Vee, V-Cillin) as a biosynthetic product. It was not until 1953, however, that its clinical value was recognized by some European scientists. Since then, it has enjoyed wide use because of its resistance to hydrolysis by gastric juice and its ability to produce uniform concentrations in blood (when administered orally). The free acid requires about 1,200 mL of water to dissolve 1 g,

and it has an activity of 1,695 units/mg. For parenteral solutions, the potassium salt is usually used. This salt is very soluble in water. Solutions of it are made from the dry salt at the time of administration. Oral dosage forms of the potassium salt are also available, providing rapid, effective plasma concentrations of this penicillin. The salt of phenoxymethylpenicillin with *N,N'*-bis(dehydroabietyl)ethylenediamine (hydrabamine, Compocillin-V) provides a very long-acting form of this compound. Its high water insolubility makes it a desirable compound for aqueous suspensions used as liquid oral dosage forms.

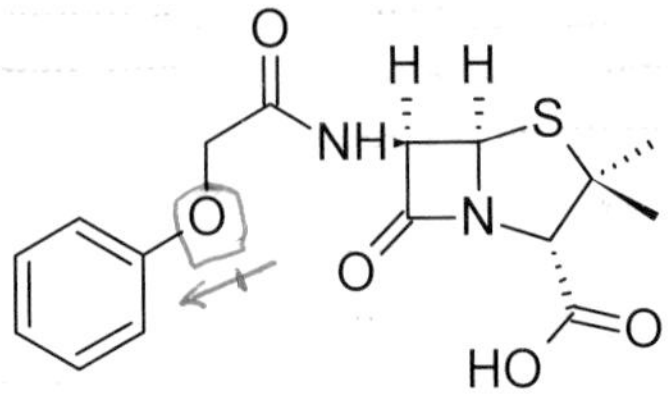

Methicillin Sodium

During 1960, methicillin sodium, 2,6-dimethoxyphenylpenicillin sodium (Staphcillin), the second penicillin produced as a result of the research that developed synthetic analogs, was introduced for medicinal use.

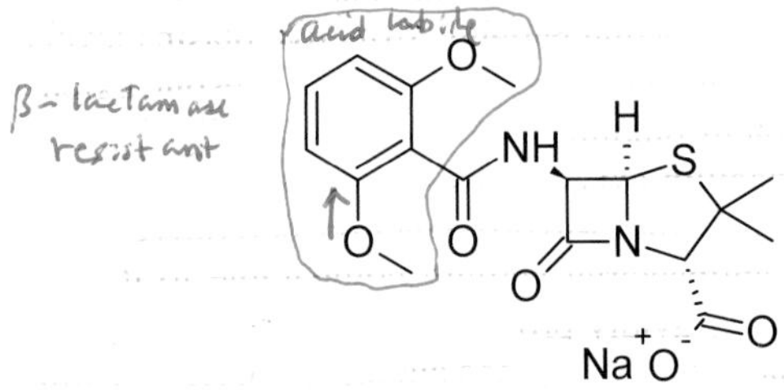

Reacting 2,6-dimethoxybenzoyl chloride with 6-APA forms 6-(2,6-dimethoxybenzamido)penicillanic acid. The sodium salt is a white, crystalline solid that is extremely soluble in water, forming clear, neutral solutions. As with other penicillins, it is very sensitive to moisture, losing about half of its activity in 5 days at room temperature. Refrigeration at 5°C reduces the loss in activity to about 20% in the same period. Solutions prepared for parenteral use may be kept as long as 24 hours if refrigerated. It is extremely sensitive to acid (a pH of 2 causes 50% loss of activity in 20 minutes); thus, it cannot be used orally.

Methicillin sodium is particularly resistant to inactivation by the penicillinase found in staphylococci and somewhat more resistant than penicillin G to penicillinase from *Bacillus cereus*. Methicillin and many other penicillinase-resistant penicillins induce penicillinase formation, an observation that has implications concerning use of these agents in the treatment of penicillin G-sensitive infections. Clearly, the use of a penicillinase-resistant penicillin should not be followed by penicillin G.

The absence of the benzyl methylene group of penicillin G and the steric protection afforded by the 2- and 6-methoxy groups make this compound particularly resistant to enzymatic hydrolysis.

Methicillin sodium has been introduced for use in the treatment of staphylococcal infections caused by strains resistant to other penicillins. It is recommended that it not be used in general therapy, to avoid the possible widespread development of organisms resistant to it.

The incidence of interstitial nephritis, a probable hypersensitivity reaction, is reportedly higher with methicillin than with other penicillins.

Oxacillin Sodium

Oxacillin sodium, (5-methyl3-phenyl-4-isoxazolyl)penicillin sodium monohydrate (Prostaphlin), is the salt of a semisynthetic penicillin that is highly resistant to inactivation by penicillinase. Apparently, the steric effects of the 3-phenyl and 5-methyl groups of the isoxazolyl ring prevent the binding of this penicillin to the β-lactamase active site and, thereby, protect the lactam ring from degradation in much the same way as has been suggested for methicillin. It is also relatively resistant to acid hydrolysis and, therefore, may be administered orally with good effect.

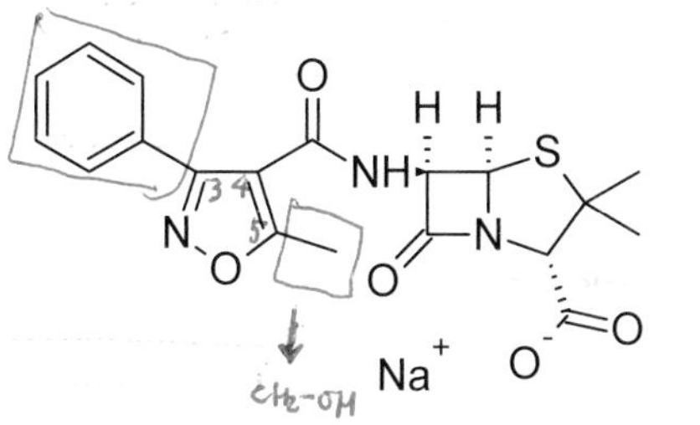

Oxacillin sodium, which is available in capsule form, is reasonably well absorbed from the gastrointestinal (GI) tract, particularly in fasting patients. Effective plasma levels of oxacillin are obtained in about 1 hour, but despite extensive plasma protein binding, it is excreted rapidly through the kidneys. Oxacillin experiences some first-pass metabolism in the liver to the 5-hydroxymethyl derivative. This metabolite has antibacterial activity comparable to that of oxacillin but is less avidly protein bound and more rapidly excreted. The halogenated analogs cloxacillin, dicloxacillin, and floxacillin experience less 5-methyl hydroxylation.

The use of oxacillin and other isoxazolylpenicillins should be restricted to the treatment of infections caused by staphylococci resistant to penicillin G. Although their spectrum of activity is similar to that of penicillin G, the isoxazolylpenicillins are, in general, inferior to it and the phenoxymethylpenicillins for the treatment of infections caused by penicillin G-sensitive bacteria. Because isoxazolylpenicillins cause allergic reactions similar to those produced by other penicillins, they should be used with great caution in patients who are penicillin sensitive.

Cloxacillin Sodium

The chlorine atom *ortho* to the position of attachment of the phenyl ring to the isoxazole ring enhances the activity of cloxacillin sodium, [3-(*o*-chlorophenyl)-5-methyl-4-isoxazolyl]penicillin sodium monohydrate (Tegopen), over that of oxacillin, not by increasing its intrinsic antibacterial activity but by enhancing its oral absorption, leading to higher plasma levels. In almost all other respects, it resembles oxacillin.

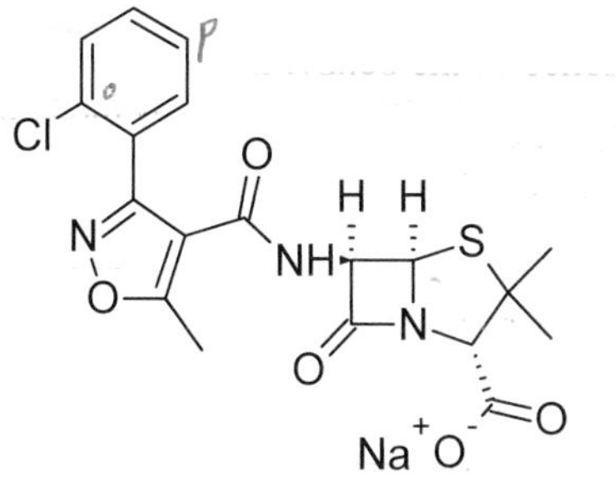

Dicloxacillin Sodium

The substitution of chlorine atoms on both carbons *ortho* to the position of attachment of the phenyl ring to the isoxazole ring is presumed to enhance further the stability of the oxacillin congener dicloxacillin sodium, [3-(2,6-dichlorophenyl)-5-methyl-4-isoxazolyl]penicillin sodium monohydrate (Dynapen, Pathocil, Veracillin) and to produce high plasma concentrations of it. Its medicinal properties and use are similar to those of cloxacillin sodium. Progressive halogen substitution, however, also increases the fraction bound to protein in the plasma, potentially reducing the concentration of free antibiotic in plasma and tissues. Its medicinal properties and use are the same as those of cloxacillin sodium.

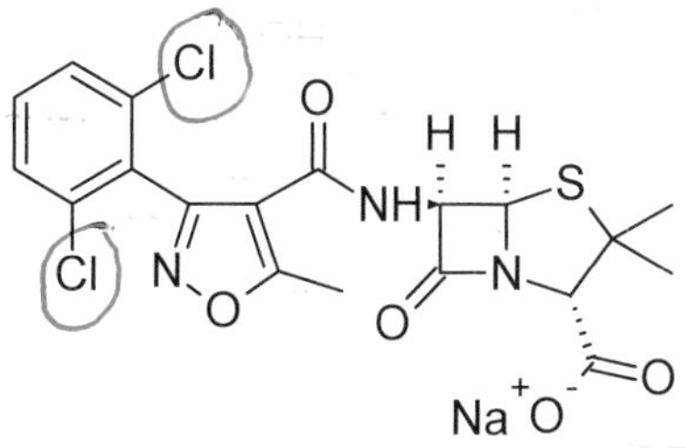

Nafcillin Sodium

Nafcillin sodium, 6-(2-ethoxy-1-naphthyl)penicillin sodium (Unipen), is another semisynthetic penicillin that resulted from the search for penicillinase-resistant compounds. Like methicillin, nafcillin has substituents in positions *ortho* to the point of attachment of the aromatic ring to the carboxamide group of penicillin. No doubt, the ethoxy group and the second ring of the naphthalene group play steric roles in stabilizing nafcillin against penicillinase. Very similar structures have been reported to produce similar results in some substituted 2-biphenylpenicillins.[33]

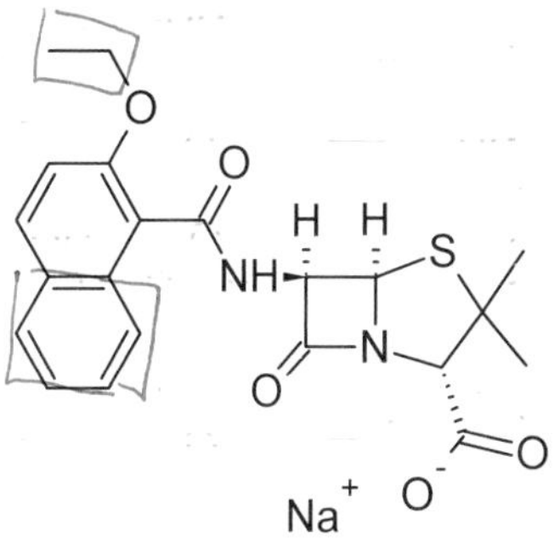

Unlike methicillin, nafcillin is stable enough in acid to permit its use by oral administration. When it is given orally, its absorption is somewhat slow and incomplete, but satisfactory plasma levels may be achieved in about 1 hour. Relatively small amounts are excreted through the kidneys; most is excreted in the bile. Even though some cyclic reabsorption from the gut may occur, nafcillin given orally should be readministered every 4 to 6 hours. This salt is readily soluble in water and may be administered intramuscularly or intravenously to obtain high plasma concentrations quickly for the treatment of serious infections.

Nafcillin sodium may be used in infections caused solely by penicillin G-resistant staphylococci or when streptococci are present also. Although it is recommended that it be used exclusively for such resistant infections, nafcillin is also effective against pneumococci and group A β-hemolytic streptococci. Because, like other penicillins, it may cause allergic side effects, it should be administered with care.

Ampicillin

Ampicillin, 6-[D-α-aminophenylacetamido]penicillanic acid, D-α-aminobenzylpenicillin (Penbritn, Polycillin, Omnipen, Amcill, Principen), meets another goal of the research on semisynthetic penicillins—an antibacterial spectrum broader than that of penicillin G. This product is active against the same Gram-positive organisms that are susceptible to other penicillins, and it is more active against some Gram-negative bacteria and enterococci than are other penicillins. Obviously, the α-amino group plays an important role in the broader activity, but the mechanism for its action is unknown. It has been suggested that the amino group confers an ability to cross cell wall barriers that are impenetrable to other penicillins. D-(−)-Ampicillin, prepared from D-(−)-α-aminophenylacetic acid, is significantly more active than L-(+)-ampicillin.

Ampicillin is not resistant to penicillinase, and it produces the allergic reactions and other untoward effects found in penicillin-sensitive patients. Because such reactions are relatively rare, however, it may be used to treat infections caused by Gram-negative bacilli for which a broad-spectrum antibiotic, such as a tetracycline or chloramphenicol, may be indicated but not preferred because of undesirable reactions or lack of bactericidal effect. Ampicillin is not so widely active, however, that it should be used as a broad-spectrum antibiotic in the same manner as the tetracyclines. It is particularly useful for the treatment of acute urinary tract infections caused by *E. coli* or *Proteus mirabilis* and is the agent of choice against *Haemophilus influenzae* infections. Ampicillin, together with probenecid, to inhibit its active tubular excretion, has become a treatment of choice for gonorrhea in recent years. β-Lactamase–producing strains of Gram-negative bacteria that are highly resistant to ampicillin, however, appear to be increasing in the world population. The threat from such resistant strains is particularly great with *H. influenzae* and *N. gonorrhoeae*, because there are few alternative therapies for infections caused by these organisms. Incomplete absorption and excretion of effective concentrations in the bile may contribute to the effectiveness of ampicillin in the treatment of salmonellosis and shigellosis.

Ampicillin is water soluble and stable in acid. The protonated α-amino group of ampicillin has a pK$_a$ of 7.3,[46] and thus it is protonated extensively in acidic media, which explains ampicillin's stability to acid hydrolysis and instability to alkaline hydrolysis. It is administered orally and is absorbed from the intestinal tract to produce peak plasma concentrations in about 2 hours. Oral doses must be repeated about every 6 hours because it is excreted rapidly and unchanged through the kidneys. It is available as a white,

crystalline, anhydrous powder that is sparingly soluble in water or as the colorless or slightly buff-colored crystalline trihydrate that is soluble in water. Either form may be used for oral administration, in capsules or as a suspension. Earlier claims of higher plasma levels for the anhydrous form than for the trihydrate following oral administration have been disputed.[47,48] The white, crystalline sodium salt is very soluble in water, and solutions for injections should be administered within 1 hour after being made.

Bacampicillin Hydrochloride

Bacampicillin hydrochloride (Spectrobid) is the hydrochloride salt of the 1-ethoxycarbonyloxyethyl ester of ampicillin. It is a prodrug of ampicillin with no antibacterial activity. After oral absorption, bacampicillin is hydrolyzed rapidly by esterases in the plasma to form ampicillin.

Oral absorption of bacampicillin is more rapid and complete than that of ampicillin and less affected by food. Plasma levels of ampicillin from oral bacampicillin exceed those of oral ampicillin or amoxicillin for the first 2.5 hours but thereafter are the same as for ampicillin and amoxicillin.[49] Effective plasma levels are sustained for 12 hours, allowing twice-a-day dosing.

Amoxicillin

Amoxicillin, 6-[D-(−)-α-amino-*p*- hydroxyphenylacetamido]penicillanic acid (Amoxil, Larotid, Polymox), a semisynthetic penicillin introduced in 1974, is simply the *p*-hydroxy analog of ampicillin, prepared by acylation of 6-APA with *p*-hydroxyphenylglycine.

Its antibacterial spectrum is nearly identical with that of ampicillin, and like ampicillin, it is resistant to acid, susceptible to alkaline and β-lactamase hydrolysis, and weakly protein bound. Early clinical reports indicated that orally administered amoxicillin possesses significant advantages over ampicillin, including more complete GI absorption to give higher plasma and urine levels, less diarrhea, and little or no effect of food on absorption.[50] Thus, amoxicillin has largely replaced ampicillin for the treatment of certain systemic and urinary tract infections for which oral administration is desirable. Amoxicillin is reportedly less effective than ampicillin in the treatment of bacillary dysentery, presumably because of its greater GI absorption. Considerable evidence suggests that oral absorption of α-aminobenzyl–substituted penicillins (e.g., ampicillin and amoxicillin) and cephalosporins is, at least in part, carrier mediated,[51] thus explaining their generally superior oral activity.

Amoxicillin is a fine, white to off-white, crystalline powder that is sparingly soluble in water. It is available in various oral dosage forms. Aqueous suspensions are stable for 1 week at room temperature.

Carbenicillin Disodium, Sterile

Carbenicillin disodium, disodium α-carboxybenzylpenicillin (Geopen, Pyopen), is a semisynthetic penicillin released in the United States in 1970, which was introduced in England and first reported by Ancred et al.[52] in 1967. Examination of its structure shows that it differs from ampicillin in having an ionizable carboxyl group rather than an amino group substituted on the α-carbon atom of the benzyl side chain. Carbenicillin has a broad range of antimicrobial activity, broader than any other known penicillin, a property attributed to the unique carboxyl group. It has been proposed that the carboxyl group improves penetration of the molecule through cell wall barriers of Gram-negative bacilli, compared with other penicillins.

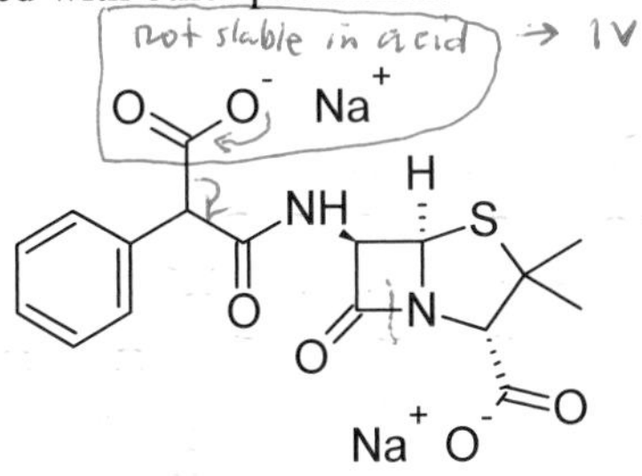

Carbenicillin is not stable in acids and is inactivated by penicillinase. It is a malonic acid derivative and, as such, decarboxylates readily to penicillin G, which is acid labile. Solutions of the disodium salt should be freshly prepared but, when refrigerated, may be kept for 2 weeks. It must be administered by injection and is usually given intravenously.

Carbenicillin has been effective in the treatment of systemic and urinary tract infections caused by *P. aeruginosa*, indole-producing *Proteus* spp., and *Providencia* spp., all of which are resistant to ampicillin. The low toxicity of carbenicillin, with the exception of allergic sensitivity, permits the use of large dosages in serious infections. Most clinicians prefer to use a combination of carbenicillin and gentamicin for serious pseudomonal and mixed coliform infections. The two antibiotics are chemically incompatible, however, and should never be combined in an intravenous solution.

Carbenicillin Indanyl Sodium

Efforts to obtain orally active forms of carbenicillin led to the eventual release of the 5-indanyl ester carbenicillin indanyl, 6-[2-phenyl-2-(5-indanyloxycarbonyl)acetamido]penicillanic acid (Geocillin), in 1972. Approximately 40% of the usual oral dose of indanyl carbenicillin is absorbed. After absorption, the ester is hydrolyzed rapidly by plasma and tissue esterases to yield carbenicillin. Thus, although the highly lipophilic and highly protein-bound ester has in vitro activity comparable with that of carbenicillin, its activity in vivo is due to carbenicillin. Indanyl carbenicillin thus provides an orally active alternative for the treatment of carbenicillin-sensitive systemic and urinary tract infections caused by *Pseudomonas* spp., indole-positive *Proteus* spp., and selected species of Gram-negative bacilli.

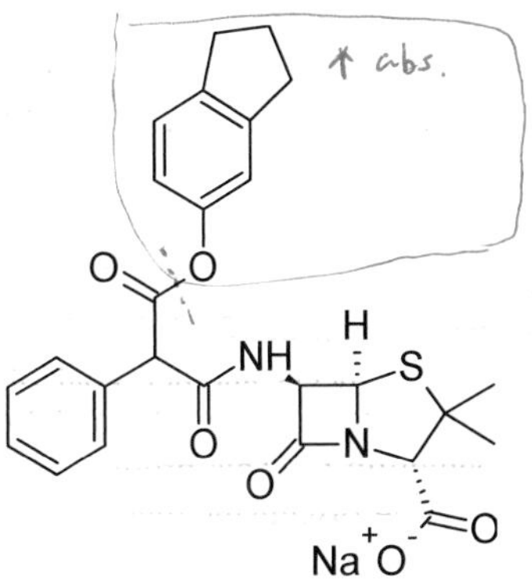

Clinical trials with indanyl carbenicillin revealed a relatively high frequency of GI symptoms (nausea, occasional vomiting, and diarrhea). It seems doubtful that the high doses required for the treatment of serious systemic infections could be tolerated by most patients. Indanyl carbenicillin occurs as the sodium salt, an off-white, bitter powder that is freely soluble in water. It is stable in acid. It should be protected from moisture to prevent hydrolysis of the ester.

Ticarcillin Disodium, Sterile

Ticarcillin disodium, α-carboxy-3-thienylpenicillin (Ticar), is an isostere of carbenicillin in which the phenyl group is replaced by a thienyl group. This semisynthetic penicillin derivative, like carbenicillin, is unstable in acid and, therefore, must be administered parenterally. It is similar to carbenicillin in antibacterial spectrum and pharmacokinetic properties. Two advantages for ticarcillin are claimed: (a) slightly better pharmacokinetic properties, including higher serum levels and a longer duration of action; and (b) greater in vitro potency against several species of Gram-negative bacilli, most notably *P. aeruginosa* and *Bacteroides fragilis*. These advantages can be crucial in the treatment of serious infections requiring high-dose therapy.

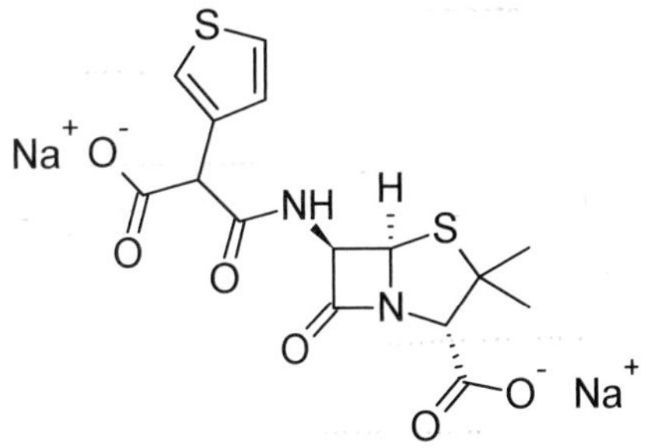

Mezlocillin Sodium, Sterile

Mezlocillin (Mezlin) is an acylureidopenicillin with an antibacterial spectrum similar to that of carbenicillin and ticarcillin; however, there are some major differences. It is much more active against most *Klebsiella* spp., *P. aeruginosa*, anaerobic bacteria (e.g., *Streptococcus faecalis* and *B. fragilis*), and *H. influenzae*. It is recommended for the treatment of serious infections caused by these organisms.

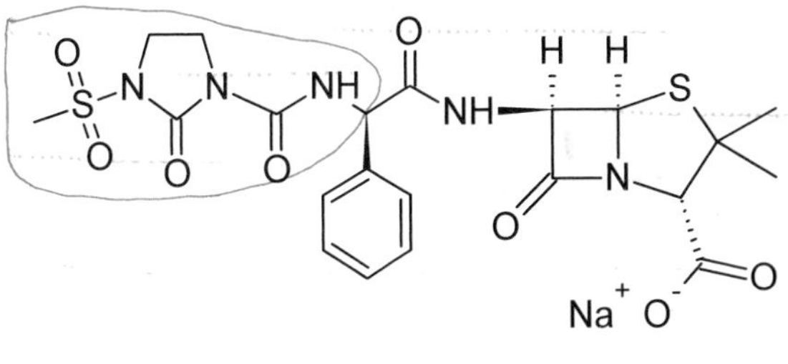

Mezlocillin is not generally effective against β-lactamase–producing bacteria, nor is it active orally. It is available as a white, crystalline, water-soluble sodium salt for injection. Solutions should be prepared freshly and, if not used within 24 hours, refrigerated. Mezlocillin and other acylureidopenicillins, unlike carbenicillin, exhibit nonlinear pharmacokinetics. Peak plasma levels, half-life, and area under the time curve increase with increased dosage. Mezlocillin has less effect on bleeding time than carbenicillin, and it is less likely to cause hypokalemia.

Piperacillin Sodium, Sterile

Piperacillin (Pipracil) is the most generally useful of the extended-spectrum acylureidopenicillins. It is more active than mezlocillin against susceptible strains of Gram-negative aerobic bacilli, such as *Serratia marcescens*, *Proteus*, *Enterobacter*, *Citrobacter* spp., and *P. aeruginosa*. Mezlocillin, however, appears to be more active against *Providencia* spp. and *K. pneumoniae*. Piperacillin is also active against anaerobic bacteria, especially *B. fragilis* and *S. faecalis* (enterococcus). β-Lactamase–producing strains of these organisms are, however, resistant to piperacillin, which is hydrolyzed by *S. aureus* β-lactamase. The β-lactamase susceptibility of piperacillin is not absolute because β-lactamase–producing, ampicillin-resistant strains of *N. gonorrhoeae* and *H. influenzae* are susceptible to piperacillin.

Piperacillin is destroyed rapidly by stomach acid; therefore, it is active only by intramuscular or intravenous administration. The injectable form is provided as the white, crystalline, water-soluble sodium salt. Its pharmacokinetic properties are very similar to those of the other acylureidopenicillins.

⬡ β-LACTAMASE INHIBITORS

The strategy of using a β-lactamase inhibitor in combination with a β-lactamase–sensitive penicillin in the therapy for infections caused by β-lactamase–producing bacterial strains has, until relatively recently, failed to live up to its obvious promise. Early attempts to obtain synergy against such resistant strains, by using combinations consisting of a β-lactamase–resistant penicillin (e.g., methicillin or oxacillin) as a competitive inhibitor and a β-lactamase– sensitive penicillin (e.g., ampicillin or carbenicillin) to kill the organisms, met with limited success. Factors that may contribute to the failure of such combinations to achieve synergy include (a) the failure of most lipophilic penicillinase-resistant penicillins to penetrate the cell envelope of Gram-negative bacilli in effective concentrations, (b) the reversible binding of

penicillinase-resistant penicillins to β-lactamase, requiring high concentrations to prevent substrate binding and hydrolysis, and (c) the induction of β-lactamases by some penicillinase-resistant penicillins.

The discovery of the naturally occurring, mechanism-based inhibitor clavulanic acid, which causes potent and progressive inactivation of β-lactamases (Fig. 8.4), has created renewed interest in β-lactam combination therapy. This interest has led to the design and synthesis of additional mechanism-based β-lactamase inhibitors, such as sulbactam and tazobactam, and the isolation of naturally occurring β-lactams, such as the thienamycins, which both inhibit β-lactamases and interact with PBPs.

The chemical events leading to the inactivation of β-lactamases by mechanism-based inhibitors are very complex. In a review of the chemistry of β-lactamase inhibition, Knowles[53] has described two classes of β-lactamase inhibitors: class I inhibitors that have a heteroatom leaving group at position 1 (e.g., clavulanic acid and sulbactam) and class II inhibitors that do not (e.g., the carbapenems). Unlike competitive inhibitors, which bind reversibly to the enzyme they inhibit, mechanism-based inhibitors react with the enzyme in much the same way that the substrate does. With the β-lactamases, an acyl-enzyme intermediate is formed by reaction of the β-lactam with an active-site serine hydroxyl group of the enzyme. For normal substrates, the acyl-enzyme intermediate readily undergoes hydrolysis, destroying the substrate and freeing the enzyme to attack more substrate. The acyl-enzyme intermediate formed when a mechanism-based inhibitor is attacked by the enzyme is diverted by tautomerism to a more stable imine form that hydrolyzes more slowly to eventually free the enzyme (transient inhibition), or for a class I inhibitor, a second group on the enzyme may be attacked to inactivate it. Because these inhibitors are also substrates for the enzymes that they inactivate, they are sometimes referred to as "suicide substrates."

Because class I inhibitors cause prolonged inactivation of certain β-lactamases, they are particularly useful in combination with extended-spectrum, β-lactamase–sensitive penicillins to treat infections caused by β-lactamase–producing bacteria. Three such inhibitors, clavulanic acid, sulbactam, and tazobactam, are currently marketed in the United States for this purpose. A class II inhibitor, the carbapenem derivative imipenem, has potent antibacterial activity in addition to its ability to cause transient inhibition of some β-lactamases. Certain antibacterial cephalosporins with a leaving group at the C-3 position can cause transient inhibition of β-lactamases by forming stabilized acyl-enzyme intermediates. These are discussed more fully later in this chapter.

The relative susceptibilities of various β-lactamases to inactivation by class I inhibitors appear to be related to the molecular properties of the enzymes.[25,54,55] β-Lactamases belonging to group A, a large and somewhat heterogenous group of serine enzymes, some with narrow (e.g., penicillinases or cephalosporinases) and some with broad (i.e., general β-lactamases) specificities, are generally inactivated by class I inhibitors. A large group of chromosomally encoded serine β-lactamases belonging to group C with specificity for cephalosporins are, however, resistant to inactivation by class I inhibitors. A small group of Zn^{2+}-requiring metallo-β-lactamases (group B) with broad substrate specificities[56] are also not inactivated by class I inhibitors.

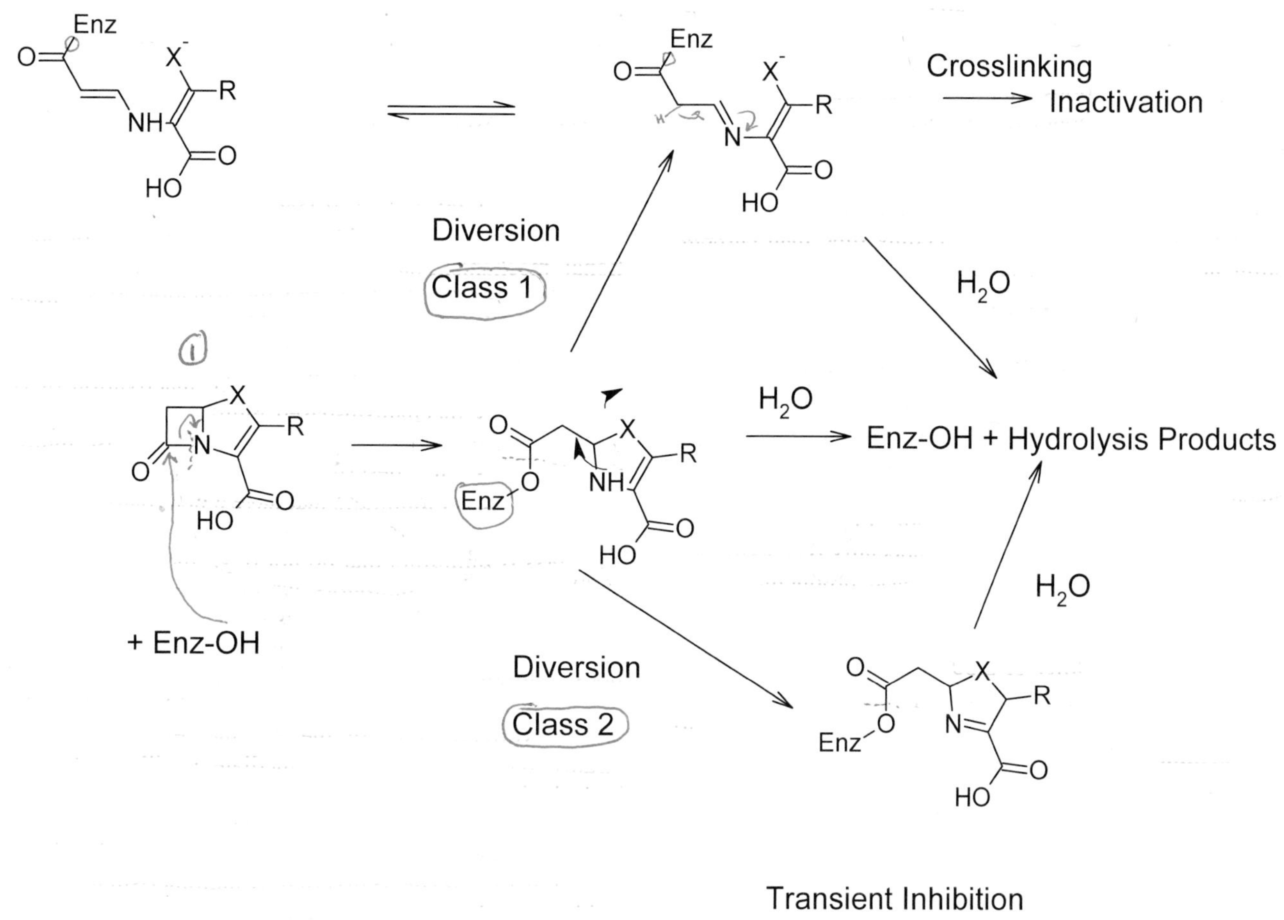

Figure 8.4 ● Mechanism-based inhibition of β-lactamases.

Products

Clavulanate Potassium

Clavulanic acid is an antibiotic isolated from *Streptomyces clavuligeris*. Structurally, it is a 1-oxopenam lacking the 6-acylamino side chain of penicillins but possessing a 2-hydroxyethylidene moiety at C-2. Clavulanic acid exhibits very weak antibacterial activity, comparable with that of 6-APA and, therefore, is not useful as an antibiotic. It is, however, a potent inhibitor of *S. aureus* β-lactamase and plasmid-mediated β-lactamases elaborated by Gram-negative bacilli.

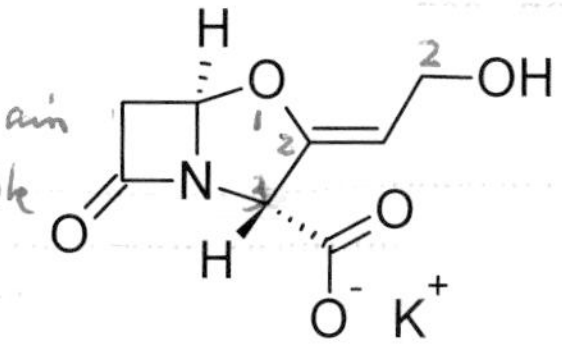

Combinations of amoxicillin and the potassium salt of clavulanic acid are available (Augmentin) in various fixed-dose oral dosage forms intended for the treatment of skin, respiratory, ear, and urinary tract infections caused by β-lactamase–producing bacterial strains. These combinations are effective against β-lactamase–producing strains of *S. aureus*, *E. coli*, *K. pneumoniae*, *Enterobacter*, *H. influenzae*, *Moraxella catarrhalis*, and *Haemophilus ducreyi*, which are resistant to amoxicillin alone. The oral bioavailability of amoxicillin and potassium clavulanate is similar. Clavulanic acid is acid-stable. It cannot undergo penicillanic acid formation because it lacks an amide side chain.

Potassium clavulanate and the extended-spectrum penicillin ticarcillin have been combined in a fixed-dose, injectable form for the control of serious infections caused by β-lactamase–producing bacterial strains. This combination has been recommended for septicemia, lower respiratory tract infections, and urinary tract infections caused by β-lactamase–producing *Klebsiella* spp., *E. coli*, *P. aeruginosa*, and other *Pseudomonas* spp., *Citrobacter* spp., *Enterobacter* spp., *S. marcescens*, and *S. aureus*. It also is used in bone and joint infections caused by these organisms. The combination contains 3 g of ticarcillin disodium and 100 mg of potassium clavulanate in a sterile powder for injection (Timentin).

Sulbactam

Sulbactam is penicillanic acid sulfone or 1,1-dioxopenicillanic acid. This synthetic penicillin derivative is a potent inhibitor of *S. aureus* β-lactamase as well as many β-lactamases elaborated by Gram-negative bacilli. Sulbactam has weak intrinsic antibacterial activity but potentiates the activity of ampicillin and carbenicillin against β-lactamase–producing *S. aureus* and members of the Enterobacteriaceae family. It does not, however, synergize with either carbenicillin or ticarcillin against *P. aeruginosa* strains resistant to these agents. Failure of sulbactam to penetrate the cell envelope is a possible explanation for the lack of synergy.

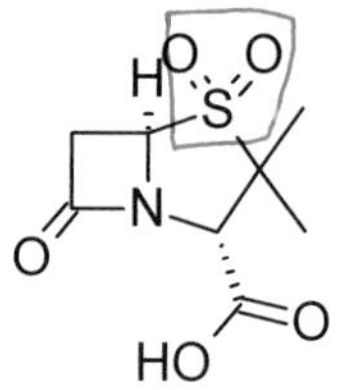

Fixed-dose combinations of ampicillin sodium and sulbactam sodium, marketed under the trade name *Unasyn* as sterile powders for injection, have been approved for use in the United States. These combinations are recommended for the treatment of skin, tissue, intra-abdominal, and gynecological infections caused by β-lactamase–producing strains of *S. aureus*, *E. coli*, *Klebsiella* spp., *P. mirabilis*, *B. fragilis*, and *Enterobacter* and *Acinetobacter* spp.

Tazobactam

Tazobactam is a penicillanic acid sulfone that is similar in structure to sulbactam. It is a more potent β-lactamase inhibitor than sulbactam[57] and has a slightly broader spectrum of activity than clavulanic acid. It has very weak antibacterial activity. Tazobactam is available in fixed-dose, injectable combinations with piperacillin, a broad-spectrum penicillin consisting of an 8:1 ratio of piperacillin sodium to tazobactam sodium by weight and marketed under the trade name *Zosyn*. The pharmacokinetics of the two drugs are very similar. Both have short half-lives ($t_{1/2}$ ~1 hour), are minimally protein bound, experience very little metabolism, and are excreted in active forms in the urine in high concentrations.

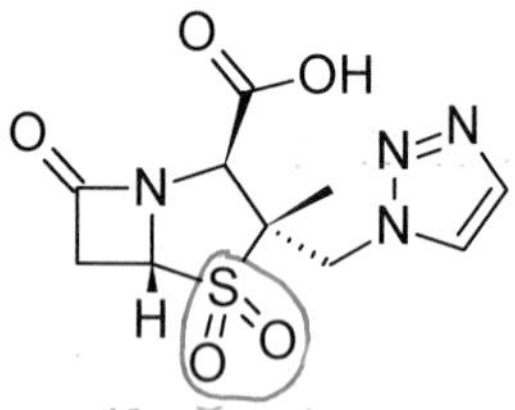

Approved indications for the piperacillin–tazobactam combination include the treatment of appendicitis, postpartum endometritis, and pelvic inflammatory disease caused by β-lactamase–producing *E. coli* and *Bacteroides* spp., skin and skin structure infections caused by β-lactamase–producing *S. aureus*, and pneumonia caused by β-lactamase–producing strains of *H. influenzae*.

CARBAPENEMS

Thienamycin

Thienamycin is a novel β-lactam antibiotic first isolated and identified by researchers at Merck[58] from fermentation of cultures of *Streptomyces cattleya*. Its structure and absolute configuration were established both spectroscopically and by total synthesis.[59,60] Two structural features of thienamycin are shared with the penicillins and cephalosporins: a fused bicyclic ring system containing a β-lactam and an equivalently attached 3-carboxyl group. In other respects, the thienamycins represent a significant departure from the established β-lactam antibiotics. The bicyclic system consists of a carbapenem containing a double bond between C-2 and C-3 (i.e., it is a 2-carbapenem, or Δ²-carbapenem, system). The double bond in the bicyclic structure creates considerable ring strain and increases the reactivity of the β-lactam to ring-opening reactions. The side chain is unique in two respects:

it is a simple 1-hydroxyethyl group instead of the familiar acylamino side chain, and it is oriented to the bicyclic ring system rather than having the usual β orientation of the penicillins and cephalosporins. The remaining feature is a 2-aminoethylthioether function at C-2. The absolute stereochemistry of thienamycin has been determined to be 5R:6S:8S. Several additional structurally related antibiotics have been isolated from various *Streptomyces* spp., including the four epithienamycins, which are isomeric to thienamycin at C-5, C-6, or C-8, and derivatives in which the 2-aminoethylthio side chain is modified.

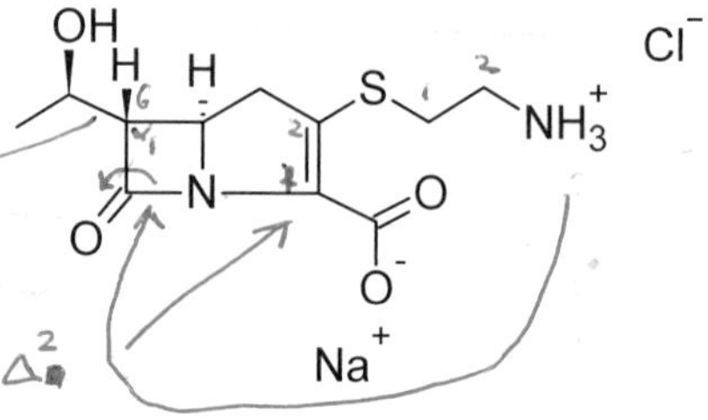

Thienamycin displays outstanding broad-spectrum antibacterial properties in vitro.[61] It is highly active against most aerobic and anaerobic Gram-positive and Gram-negative bacteria, including *S. aureus*, *P. aeruginosa*, and *B. fragilis*. Furthermore, it is resistant to inactivation by most β-lactamases elaborated by Gram-negative and Gram-positive bacteria and, therefore, is effective against many strains resistant to penicillins and cephalosporins. Resistance to lactamases appears to be a function of the α-1-hydroxyethyl side chain because this property is lost in the 6-nor derivative and epithienamycins with S stereochemistry show variable resistance to the different β-lactamases.

An unfortunate property of thienamycin is its chemical instability in solution. It is more susceptible to hydrolysis in both acidic and alkaline solutions than most β-lactam antibiotics, because of the strained nature of its fused ring system containing an endocyclic double bond. Furthermore, at its optimally stable pH between 6 and 7, thienamycin undergoes concentration-dependent inactivation. This inactivation is believed to result from intermolecular aminolysis of the β-lactam by the cysteamine side chain of a second molecule. Another shortcoming is its susceptibility to hydrolytic inactivation by renal dehydropeptidase-I (DHP-I),[62] which causes it to have an unacceptably short half-life in vivo.

Imipenem–Cilastatin

Imipenem is *N*-formimidoylthienamycin, the most successful of a series of chemically stable derivatives of thienamycin in which the primary amino group is converted to a nonnucleophilic basic function.[63] Cilastatin is an inhibitor of DHP-I. The combination (Primaxin) provides a chemically and enzymatically stable form of thienamycin that has clinically useful pharmacokinetic properties. The half-life of the drug is nonetheless short ($t_{1/2}$ ~1 hour) because of renal tubular secretion of imipenem. Imipenem retains the extraordinary broad-spectrum antibacterial properties of thienamycin. Its bactericidal activity results from the inhibition of cell wall synthesis associated with bonding to PBPs 1_b and 2. Imipenem is very stable to most β-lactamases. It is an inhibitor of β-lactamases from certain Gram-negative bacteria resistant to other β-lactam antibiotics (e.g., *P. aeruginosa*, *S. marcescens*, and *Enterobacter* spp.).

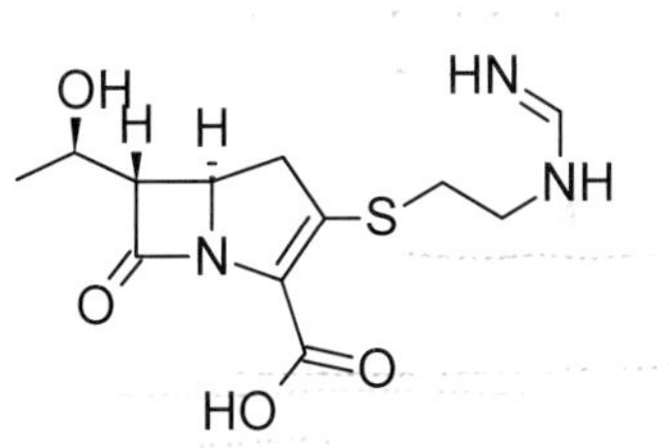

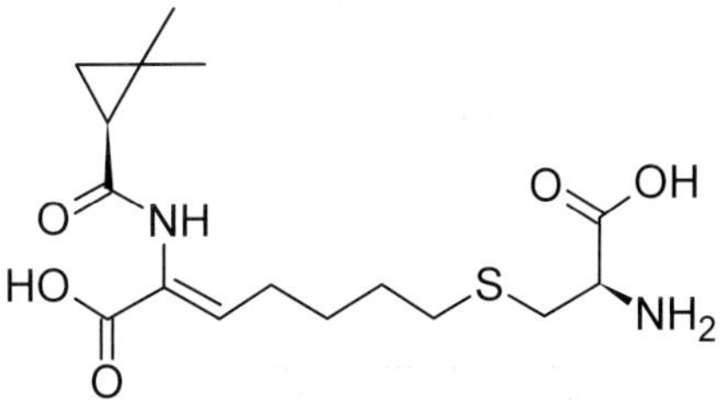

Imipenem is indicated for the treatment of a wide variety of bacterial infections of the skin and tissues, lower respiratory tract, bones and joints, and genitourinary tract, as well as of septicemia and endocarditis caused by β-lactamase–producing strains of susceptible bacteria. These include aerobic Gram-positive organisms such as *S. aureus, Staphylococcus epidermidis*, enterococci, and viridans streptococci; aerobic Gram-negative bacteria such as *E. coli, Klebsiella, Serratia, Providencia, Haemophilus, Citrobacter*, and indole-positive *Proteus* spp., *Morganella morganii, Acinetobacter* and *Enterobacter* spp., and *P. aeruginosa* and anaerobes such as *B. fragilis* and *Clostridium, Peptococcus, Peptidostreptococcus, Eubacterium*, and *Fusobacterium* spp. Some *Pseudomonas* spp. are resistant, such as *P. maltophilia* and *P. cepacia*, as are some methicillin-resistant staphylococci. Imipenem is effective against non–β-lactamase-producing strains of these and additional bacterial species, but other less expensive and equally effective antibiotics are preferred for the treatment of infections caused by these organisms.

The imipenem–cilastatin combination is marketed as a sterile powder intended for the preparation of solutions for intravenous infusion. Such solutions are stable for 4 hours at 25°C and up to 24 hours when refrigerated. The concomitant administration of imipenem and an aminoglycoside antibiotic results in synergistic antibacterial activity in vivo. The two types of antibiotics are, however, chemically incompatible and should never be combined in the same intravenous bottle.

NEWER CARBAPENEMS

The extended spectrum of antibacterial activity associated with the carbapenems together with their resistance to inactivation by most β-lactamases make this class of β-lactams an attractive target for drug development. In the design of new carbapenems, structural variations are being investigated with the objective of developing analogs with advantages over imipenem. Improvements that are particularly desired include stability to hydrolysis catalyzed by DHP-I,[62] stability to bacterial metallo-β-lactamases ("carbapenemases")[56] that hydrolyze imipenem, activity against MRSA,[31] and increased potency against *P. aeruginosa*, especially imipenem-resistant strains. Enhanced pharmacokinetic properties, such as oral bioavailability and a longer duration of action, have heretofore received little emphasis in carbapenem analog design.

Early structure–activity studies established the critical importance of the Δ^2 position of the double bond, the 3-carboxyl group, and the 6-α-hydroxyethyl side chain for both broad-spectrum antibacterial activity and β-lactamase stability in carbapenems. Modifications, therefore, have concentrated on variations at positions 1 and 2 of the carbapenem nucleus. The incorporation of a β-methyl group at the 1-position gives the carbapenem stability to hydrolysis by renal DHP-I.[64,65] Substituents at the 2-position, however, appear to affect

primarily the spectrum of antibacterial activity of the carbapenem by influencing penetration into bacteria. The capability of carbapenems to exist as zwitterionic structures (as exemplified by imipenem and biapenem), resulting from the combined features of a basic amine function attached to the 2-position and the 3-carboxyl group, may enable these molecules to enter bacteria via their charged porin channels.

Meropenem

Meropenem is a second-generation carbapenem that, to date, has undergone the most extensive clinical evaluation.[66] It has recently been approved as Merrem for the treatment of infections caused by multiply-resistant bacteria and for empirical therapy for serious infections, such as bacterial meningitis, septicemia, pneumonia, and peritonitis. Meropenem exhibits greater potency against Gram-negative and anaerobic bacteria than does imipenem, but it is slightly less active against most Gram-positive species. It is not effective against MRSA. Meropenem is not hydrolyzed by DHP-I and is resistant to most β-lactamases, including a few carbapenemases that hydrolyze carbapenem.

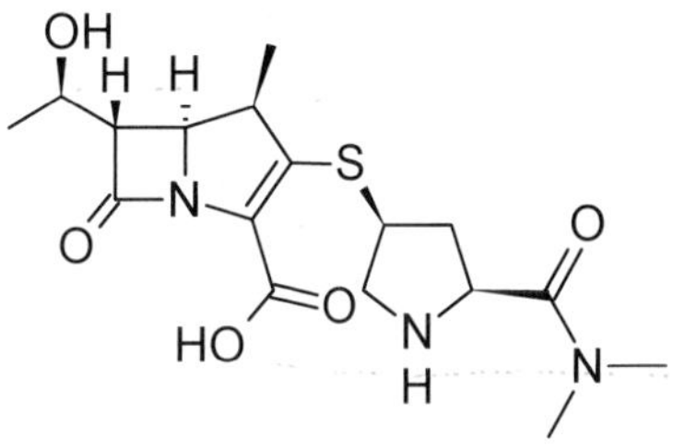

Meropenem

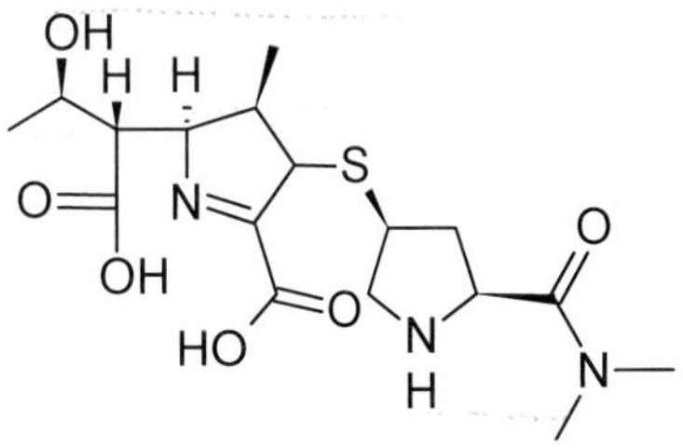

Meropenem metabolite

Like imipenem, meropenem is not active orally. It is provided as a sterile lyophilized powder to be made up in normal saline or 5% dextrose solution for parenteral administration. Approximately 70% to 80% of unchanged meropenem is excreted in the urine following intravenous or intramuscular administration. The remainder is the inactive metabolite formed by hydrolytic cleavage of the β-lactam ring. The lower incidence of nephrotoxicity of meropenem (compared with imipenem) has been correlated with its greater stability to DHP-I and the absence of the DHP-I inhibitor cilastatin in the preparation. Meropenem appears to be less epileptogenic than imipenem when the two agents are used in the treatment of bacterial meningitis.

Biapenem

Biapenem is a newer second-generation carbapenem with chemical and microbiological properties similar to those of meropenem.[67] Thus, it has broad-spectrum antibacterial activity that includes most aerobic Gram-negative and Gram-positive bacteria and anaerobes. Biapenem is stable to DHP-I[67] and resistant to most β-lactamases.[68] It is claimed to be less susceptible to metallo-β-lactamases than either imipenem or meropenem. It is not active orally.

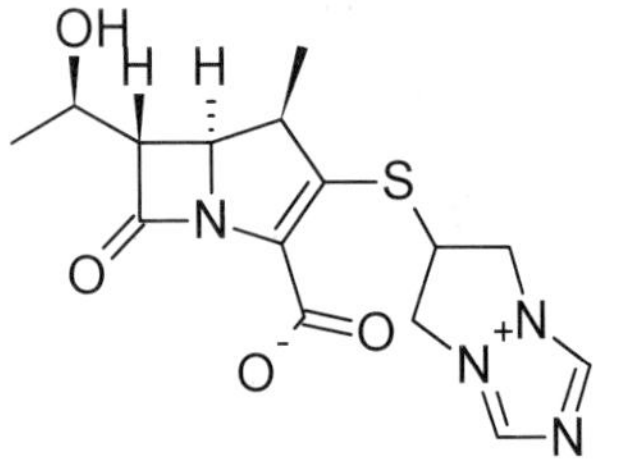

2 ⬡ CEPHALOSPORINS

Historical Background

The cephalosporins are β-lactam antibiotics isolated from *Cephalosporium* spp. or prepared semisynthetically. Most of the antibiotics introduced since 1965 have been semisynthetic cephalosporins. Interest in *Cephalosporium* fungi began in 1945 with Giuseppe Brotzu's discovery that cultures of *C. acremonium* inhibited the growth of a wide variety of Gram-positive and Gram-negative bacteria. Abraham and Newton[68a] in Oxford, having been supplied cultures of the fungus in 1948, isolated three principal antibiotic components: cephalosporin Pl, a steroid with minimal antibacterial activity; cephalosporin N, later discovered to be identical with synnematin N (a penicillin derivative now called penicillin N that had earlier been isolated from *C. salmosynnematum*); and cephalosporin C.

The structure of penicillin N was discovered to be D-(4-amino-4-carboxybutyl)penicillanic acid. The amino acid side chain confers more activity against Gram-negative bacteria, particularly *Salmonella* spp., but less activity against Gram-positive organisms than penicillin G. It has been used successfully in clinical trials for the treatment of typhoid fever but was never released as an approved drug.

Cephalosporin C turned out to be a close congener of penicillin N, containing a dihydrothiazine ring instead of the thiazolidine ring of the penicillins. Despite the observation that cephalosporin C was resistant to *S. aureus* β-lactamase,

early interest in it was not great because its antibacterial potency was inferior to that of penicillin N and other penicillins. The discovery that the α-aminoadipoyl side chain could be removed to efficiently produce 7-aminocephalosporanic acid (7-ACA),[69,70] however, prompted investigations that led to semisynthetic cephalosporins of medicinal value. The relationship of 7-ACA and its acyl derivatives to 6-APA and the semisynthetic penicillins is obvious. Woodward et al.[71] have prepared both cephalosporin C and the clinically useful cephalothin by an elegant synthetic procedure, but the commercially available drugs are obtained from 7-ACA as semisynthetic products.

Nomenclature

The chemical nomenclature of the cephalosporins is slightly more complex than even that of the penicillins because of the presence of a double bond in the dihydrothiazine ring. The fused ring system is designated by *Chemical Abstracts* as 5-thia-1-azabicyclo[4.2.0]oct-2-ene. In this system, cephalothin is 3-(acetoxymethyl)-7-[2-(thienylacetyl)amino]-8-oxo-5-thia-1-azabicyclo[4.2.0]oct-2-ene-2-carboxylic acid. A simplification that retains some of the systematic nature of the *Chemical Abstracts* procedure names the saturated bicyclic ring system with the lactam carbonyl oxygen *cepham* (cf., *penam* for penicillins). According to this system, all commercially available cephalosporins and cephamycins are named *3-cephems* (or Δ^3-cephems) to designate the position of the double bond. (Interestingly, all known 2-cephems are inactive, presumably because the β-lactam lacks the necessary ring strain to react sufficiently.) The trivialized forms of nomenclature of the type that have been applied to the penicillins are not consistently applicable to the naming of cephalosporins because of variations in the substituent at the 3-position. Thus, although some cephalosporins are named as derivatives of cephalosporanic acids, this practice applies only to the derivatives that have a 3-acetoxymethyl group.

Semisynthetic Derivatives

To date, the more useful semisynthetic modifications of the basic 7-ACA nucleus have resulted from acylations of the 7-amino group with different acids or nucleophilic substitution or reduction of the acetoxyl group. Structure–activity relationships (SARs) among the cephalosporins appear to parallel those among the penicillins insofar as the acyl group is concerned. The presence of an allylic acetoxyl function in the 3-position, however, provides a reactive site at which various 7-acylaminocephalosporanic acid structures can easily be varied by nucleophilic displacement reactions. Reduction of the 3-acetoxymethyl to a 3-methyl substituent to prepare 7-aminodesacetylcephalosporanic acid (7-ADCA)

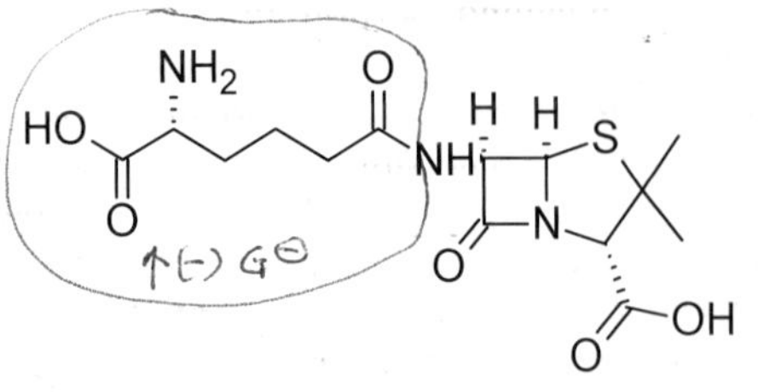

Penicillin N

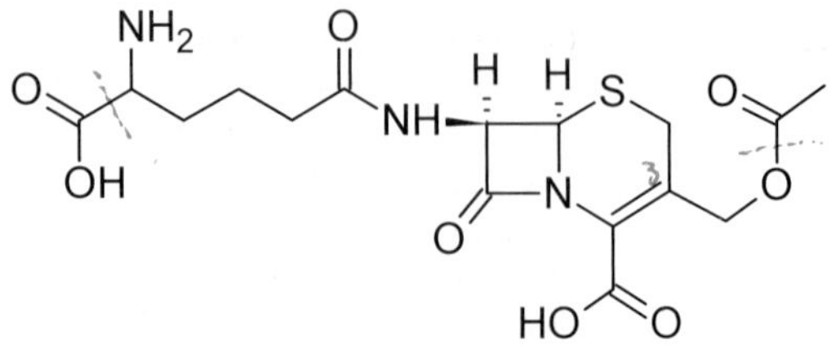

Cephalosporin C

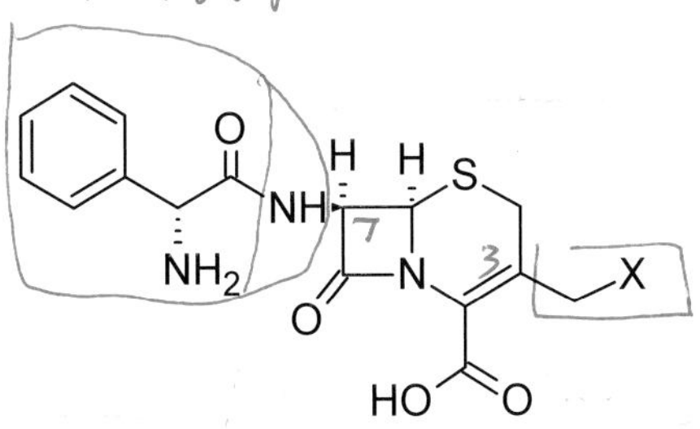

phenylglycyl = gly

Cephalosporin

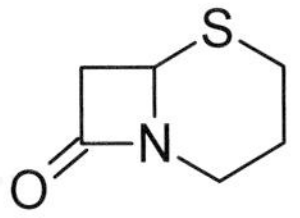

Cepham

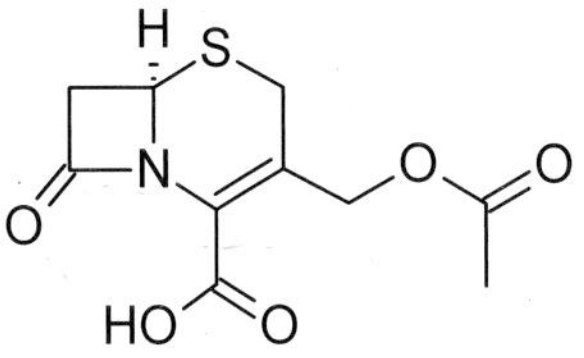

penam

Cephalosporanic Acid

derivatives can be accomplished by catalytic hydrogenation, but the process currently used for the commercial synthesis of 7-ADCA derivatives involves the rearrangement of the corresponding penicillin sulfoxide.[72] Perhaps the most noteworthy development thus far is the discovery that 7-phenylglycyl derivatives of 7-ACA and especially 7-ADCA are active orally.

In the preparation of semisynthetic cephalosporins, the following improvements are sought: (a) increased acid stability, (b) improved pharmacokinetic properties, particularly better oral absorption, (c) broadened antimicrobial spectrum, (d) increased activity against resistant microorganisms (as a result of resistance to enzymatic destruction, improved penetration, increased receptor affinity, etc.), (e) decreased allergenicity, and (f) increased tolerance after parenteral administration.

Structures of cephalosporins currently marketed in the United States are shown in Table 8.4.

Chemical Degradation

Cephalosporins experience various hydrolytic degradation reactions whose specific nature depends on the individual structure (Table 8.4).[73] Among 7-acylaminocephalosporanic acid derivatives, the 3-acetoxylmethyl group is the most reactive site. In addition to its reactivity to nucleophilic displacement reactions, the acetoxy function of this group readily undergoes solvolysis in strongly acidic solutions to form the desacetylcephalosporin derivatives. The latter lactonize to form the desacetylcephalosporin lactones, which are virtually inactive. The 7-acylamino group of some cephalosporins can also be hydrolyzed under enzymatic (acylases) and, possibly, nonenzymatic conditions to give 7-ACA (or 7-ADCA) derivatives. Following hydrolysis or solvolysis of the 3-acetoxymethyl group, 7-ACA also lactonizes under acidic conditions (Fig. 8.5).

The reactive functionality common to all cephalosporins is the β-lactam. Hydrolysis of the β-lactam of cephalosporins is believed to give initially cephalosporoic acids (in which the

R′ group is stable, [e.g., R′ = H or S heterocycle]) or possibly anhydrodesacetylcephalosporoic acids (7-ADCA, for the 7-acylaminocephalosporanic acids). It has not been possible to isolate either of these initial hydrolysis products in aqueous systems. Apparently, both types of cephalosporanic acid undergo fragmentation reactions that have not been characterized fully. Studies of the in vivo metabolism[74] of orally administered cephalosporins, however, have demonstrated arylacetylglycines and arylacetamidoethanols, which are believed to be formed from the corresponding arylacetylaminoacetaldehydes by metabolic oxidation and reduction, respectively. The aldehydes, no doubt, arise from nonenzymatic hydrolysis of the corresponding cephalosporoic acids. No evidence for the intramolecular opening of the β-lactam ring by the 7-acylamino oxygen to form oxazolones of the penicillanic acid type has been found in the cephalosporins. At neutral to alkaline pH, however, intramolecular aminolysis of the β-lactam ring by the α-amino group in the 7-ADCA derivatives cephaloglycin, cephradine, and cefadroxil occurs, forming diketopiperazine derivatives.[75,76] The formation of dimers and, possibly, polymers from 7-ADCA derivatives containing an α-amino group in the acylamino side chain may also occur, especially in concentrated solutions and at alkaline pH values.

Oral Cephalosporins

The oral activity conferred by the phenylglycyl substituent is attributed to increased acid stability of the lactam ring, resulting from the presence of a protonated amino group on the 7-acylamino portion of the molecule. Carrier-mediated transport of these dipeptide-like, zwitterionic cephalosporins[51] is also an important factor in their excellent oral activity. The situation, then, is analogous to that of the α-aminobenzylpenicillins (e.g., ampicillin). Also important for high acid stability (and, therefore, good oral activity) of the cephalosporins is the absence of the leaving group at the 3-position. Thus, despite the presence of the phenylglycyl side chain in its structure, the

(text continues on page 282)

zwitterionic = dipeptide + RNH₃⁺ → transport

3-bad LG + R-NH₃⁺ (EWG) → ↑ acid stable } → oral

TABLE 8.4 **Structure of Cephalosporins**

ORAL CEPHALOSPORINS

if α-NH₂⊕ then PO⊕

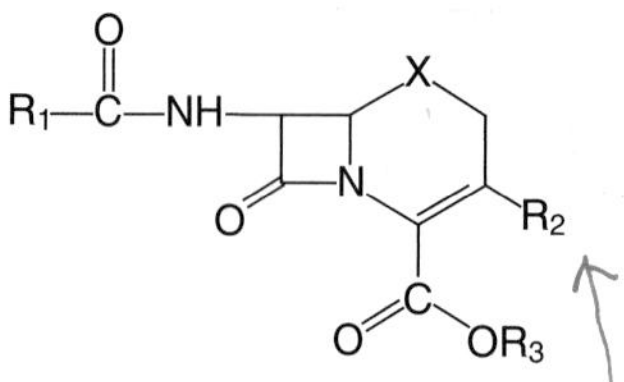

Generic Name	R₁	R₂	R₃	X
Cephalexin	(phenyl)–CH–(NH₂⁺)	—CH₃	—H	—S—
Cephradine *PO & parent.*	(phenyl)–CH–(NH₂⊕)	—CH₃	—H	—S—
Cefadroxil	HO–(phenyl)–CH–(NH₂⁺)	—CH₃	—H	—S—
Cefachlor	(phenyl)–CH–(NH₂⁺)	—Cl	—H	—S—
Cefprozil	HO–(phenyl)–CH–(NH₂⁺)	—CH=CHCH₃	—H	—S—
Loracarbef	(phenyl)–CH–(NH₂⁺)	—Cl	—H	—CH₂—
Cefuroxime axetil	(furan)–C–(NOCH₃) *resistance*	—CH₂OCNH₂ ($\overset{O}{\|}$)	—CHOCCH₃ ($\overset{O}{\|}$) / CH₃	—S—
Cefpodoxime proxetil	H₂N–(thiazole)–C–(NOCH₃)	—CH₂OCH₃	—CHOCOCH(CH₃)₂ ($\overset{O}{\|}$) / CH₃	—S—
Cefixime	H₂N–(thiazole)–C–(NOCH₂CO₂H)	—C=CH₂	—H	—S—

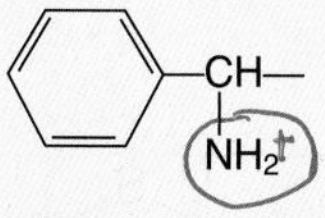

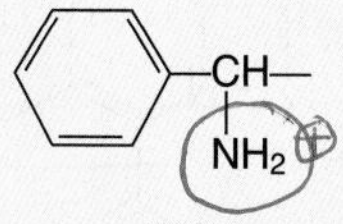

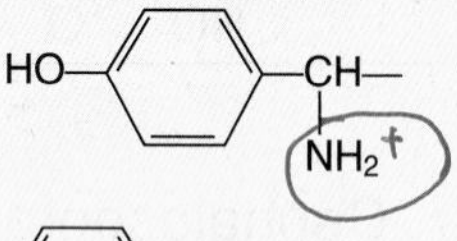

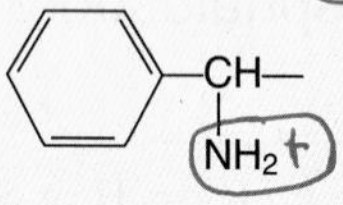

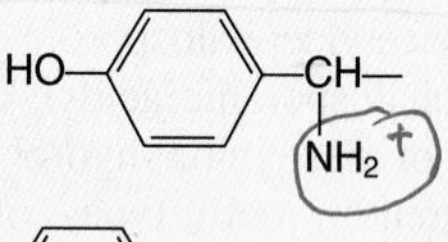

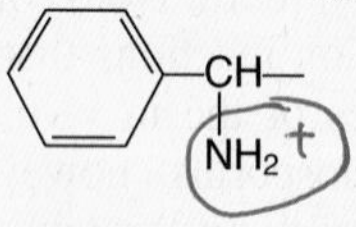

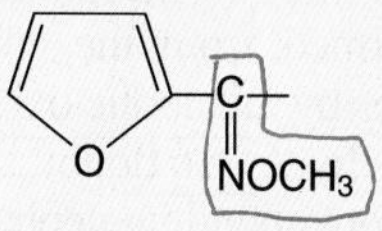

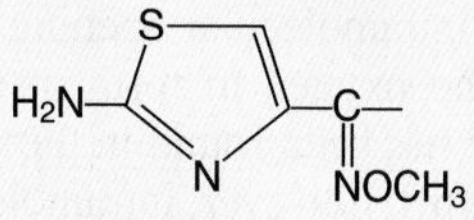

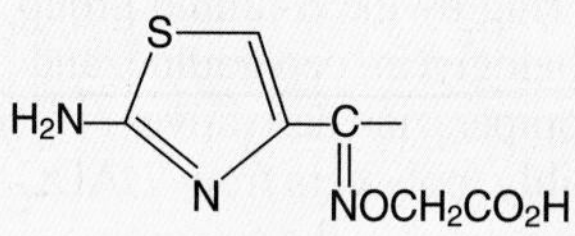

PARENTERAL CEPHALOSPORINS

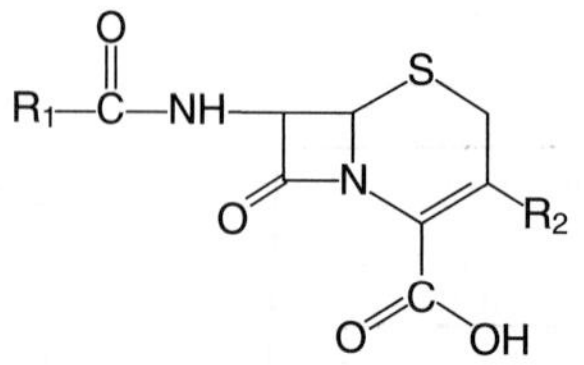

Generic Name	R₁	R₂
Cephalothin	(thiophene)–CH₂—	—CH₂OCCH₃ ($\overset{O}{\|}$) *PO⁻*
Cephapirin	(pyridine)–S–CH₂—	—CH₂OCCH₃ ($\overset{O}{\|}$) *PO⁻*

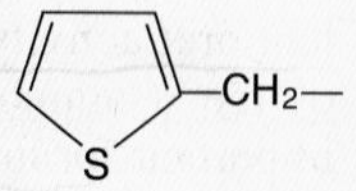

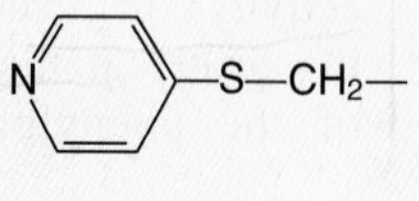

Generic Name	R₁	R₂ *MTT*

Cefazolin

(R₁ structure: 1,2,4-triazol-4-yl-CH₂–)

(R₂ structure: –CH₂S– thiadiazole with CH₃)

Cefamandole (underlined)

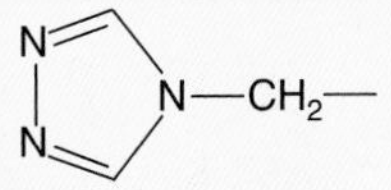

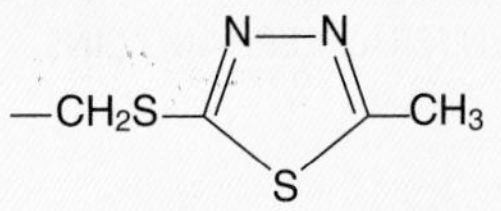

(R₁: phenyl-CH(OH)–)

} *Resistant to Lactamase*

(R₂: –CH₂S– tetrazole N-CH₃)

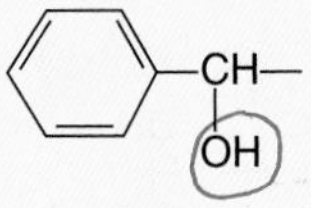

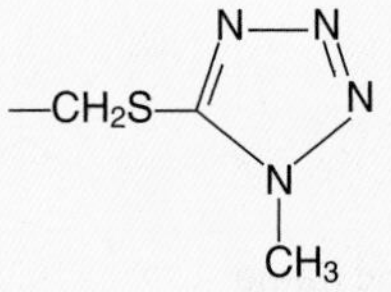

Cefonicid

(R₁: phenyl-CH(OH)–)

(R₂: –CH₂S– tetrazole N-CH₂SO₃H)

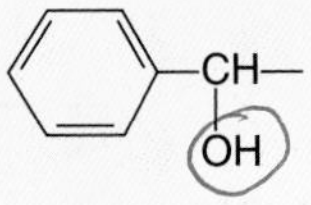

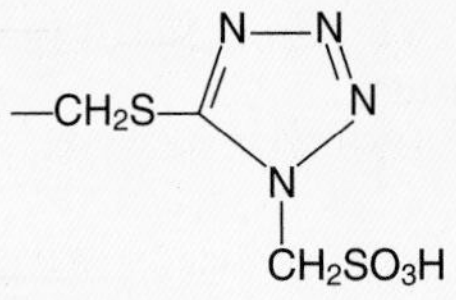

Ceforanide

(R₁: benzyl with CH₂NH₂)

(R₂: –CH₂S– tetrazole N-CH₂CO₂H)

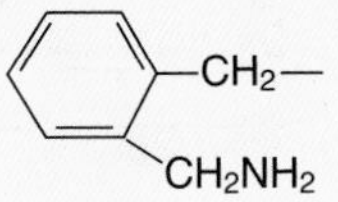

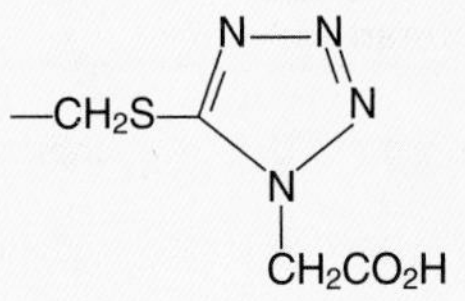

Cefuroxime

(R₁: furan-C(=NOCH₃)–)

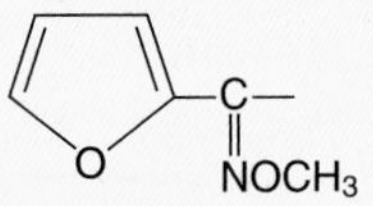

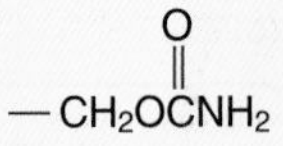

resistance

$-CH_2OCNH_2$ (C=O) *PO⁻*

Cefotaxime

resistant

(R₁: aminothiazole C(=NOCH₃)–)

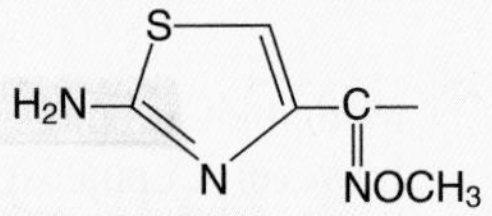

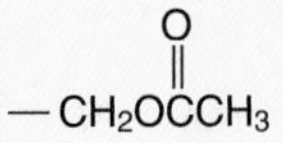

$-CH_2OCCH_3$ (C=O) *PO⁻*

Ceftizoxime

" "

(R₁: aminothiazole C(=NOCH₃)–)

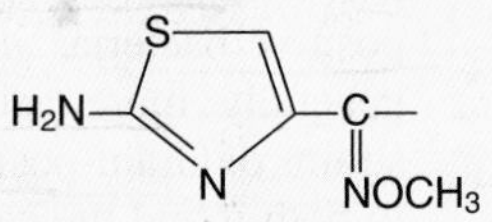

—H

Ceftriaxone

" "

(R₁: aminothiazole C(=NOCH₃)–)

(R₂: –CH₂S– triazinone with CH₃, OH, O)

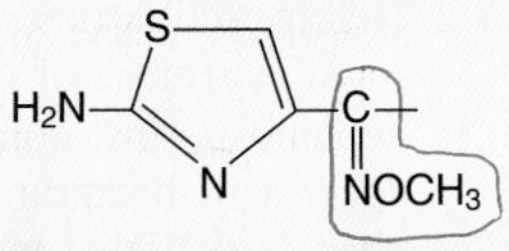

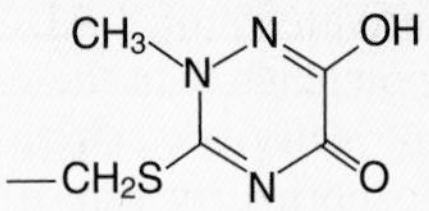

Ceftazidime

(R₁: aminothiazole C(=NO–C(CH₃)₂–CO₂H)–) → *polar*

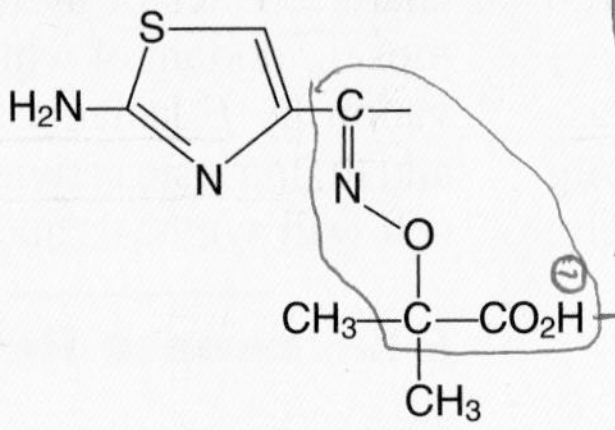

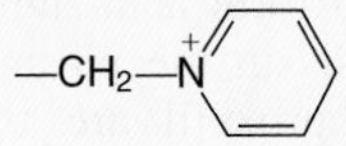

$-CH_2-$ pyridinium⁺

Cefoperazone

(R₁: HO-phenyl-CH(NH–C(=O)–piperazinedione-N-C₂H₅)–)

steric →
resistant to β-lactamase

MTT

(R₂: –CH₂S– tetrazole N-CH₃)

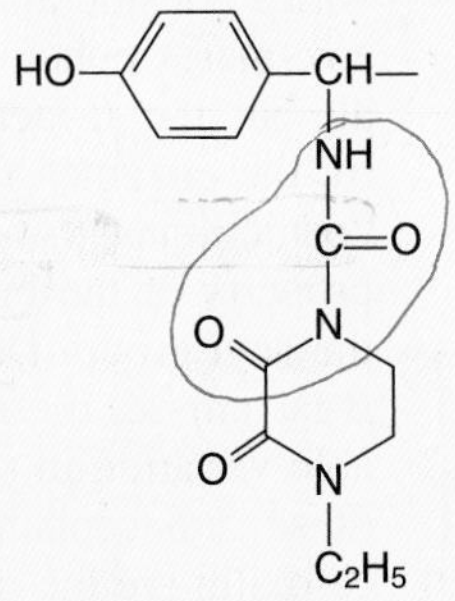

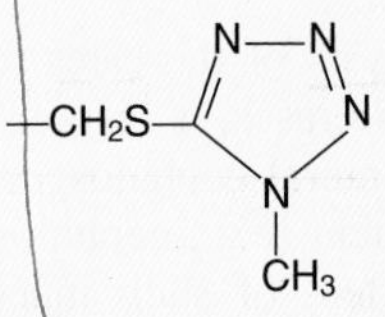

(table continues on page 282)

TABLE 8.4 **Structure of Cephalosporins** (continued)

PARENTERAL CEPHAMYCINS

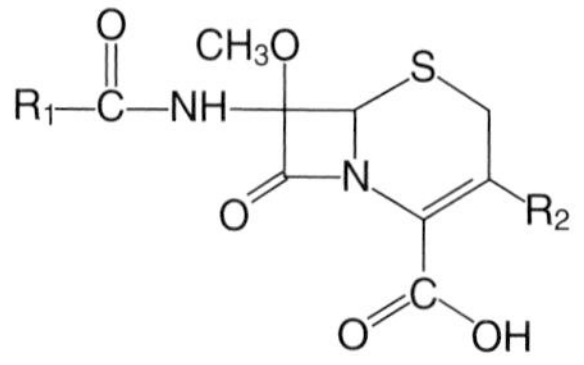

Generic Name	R$_1$	R$_2$
Cefoxitin	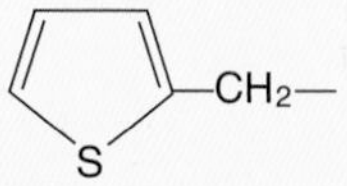	
Cefotetan	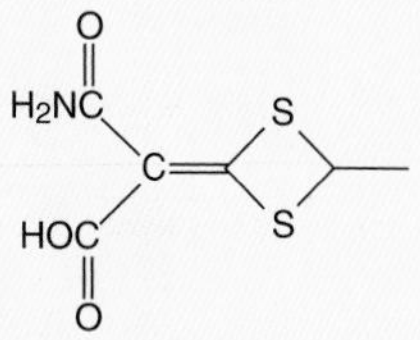	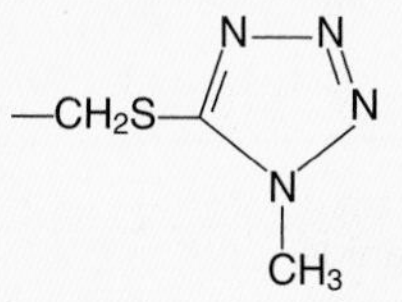
Cefmetazole	NCCH$_2$SCH$_2$—	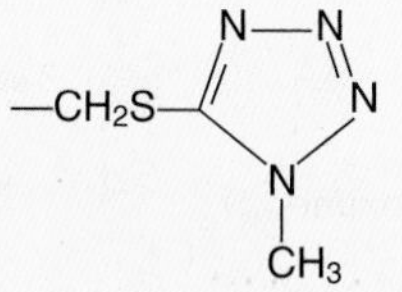

cephalosporanic acid derivative cephaloglycin is poorly absorbed orally, presumably because of solvolysis of the 3-acetoxyl group in the low pH of the stomach. The resulting 3-hydroxyl derivative undergoes lactonization under acidic conditions. The 3-hydroxyl derivatives and, especially, the corresponding lactones are considerably less active in vitro than the parent cephalosporins. Generally, acyl derivatives of 7-ADCA show lower in vitro antibacterial potencies than the corresponding 7-ACA analogs.

Oral activity can also be conferred in certain cephalosporins by esterification of the 3-carboxylic acid group to form acid-stable, lipophilic esters that undergo hydrolysis in the plasma. Cefuroxime axetil and cefpodoxime proxetil are two β-lactamase–resistant alkoximino-cephalosporins that are orally active ester prodrug derivatives of cefuroxime and cefpodoxime, respectively, based on this concept.

Parenteral Cephalosporins

Hydrolysis of the ester function, catalyzed by hepatic and renal esterases, is responsible for some in vivo inactivation of parenteral cephalosporins containing a 3-acetoxymethyl substituent (e.g., cephalothin, cephapirin, and cefotaxime). The extent of such inactivation (20%–35%) is not large enough to seriously compromise the in vivo effectiveness of acetoxyl cephalosporins. Parenteral cephalosporins lacking a hydrolyzable group at the 3-position are not subject to hydrolysis by esterases. Cephradine is the only cephalosporin that is used both orally and parenterally.

Spectrum of Activity

The cephalosporins are considered broad-spectrum antibiotics with patterns of antibacterial effectiveness comparable to that of ampicillin. Several significant differences exist, however. Cephalosporins are much more resistant to inactivation by β-lactamases, particularly those produced by Gram-positive bacteria, than is ampicillin. Ampicillin, however, is generally more active against non–β-lactamase-producing strains of Gram-positive and Gram-negative bacteria sensitive to both it and the cephalosporins. Cephalosporins, among β-lactam antibiotics, exhibit uniquely potent activity against most species of Klebsiella. Differential potencies of cephalosporins, compared with penicillins, against different species of bacteria have been attributed to several variable characteristics of individual bacterial species and strains, the most important of which probably are (a) resistance to inactivation by β-lactamases, (b) permeability of bacterial cells, and (c) intrinsic activity against bacterial enzymes involved in cell wall synthesis and cross-linking.

β-Lactamase Resistance

The susceptibility of cephalosporins to various lactamases varies considerably with the source and properties of these enzymes. Cephalosporins are significantly less sensitive than all but the β-lactamase–resistant penicillins to hydrolysis by the enzymes from *S. aureus* and *Bacillus subtilis*. The "penicillinase" resistance of cephalosporins appears to be a property of the bicyclic cephem ring system rather than of the acyl group. Despite natural resistance to staphylococcal β-lactamase, the different cephalosporins exhibit considerable variation in rates of hydrolysis by the enzyme.[77] Thus, of several cephalosporins tested in vitro, cephalothin and cefoxitin are the most resistant, and cephaloridine and cefazolin are the least resistant. The same acyl functionalities that impart β-lactamase resistance in the penicillins unfortunately render cephalosporins virtually inactive against *S. aureus* and other Gram-positive bacteria.

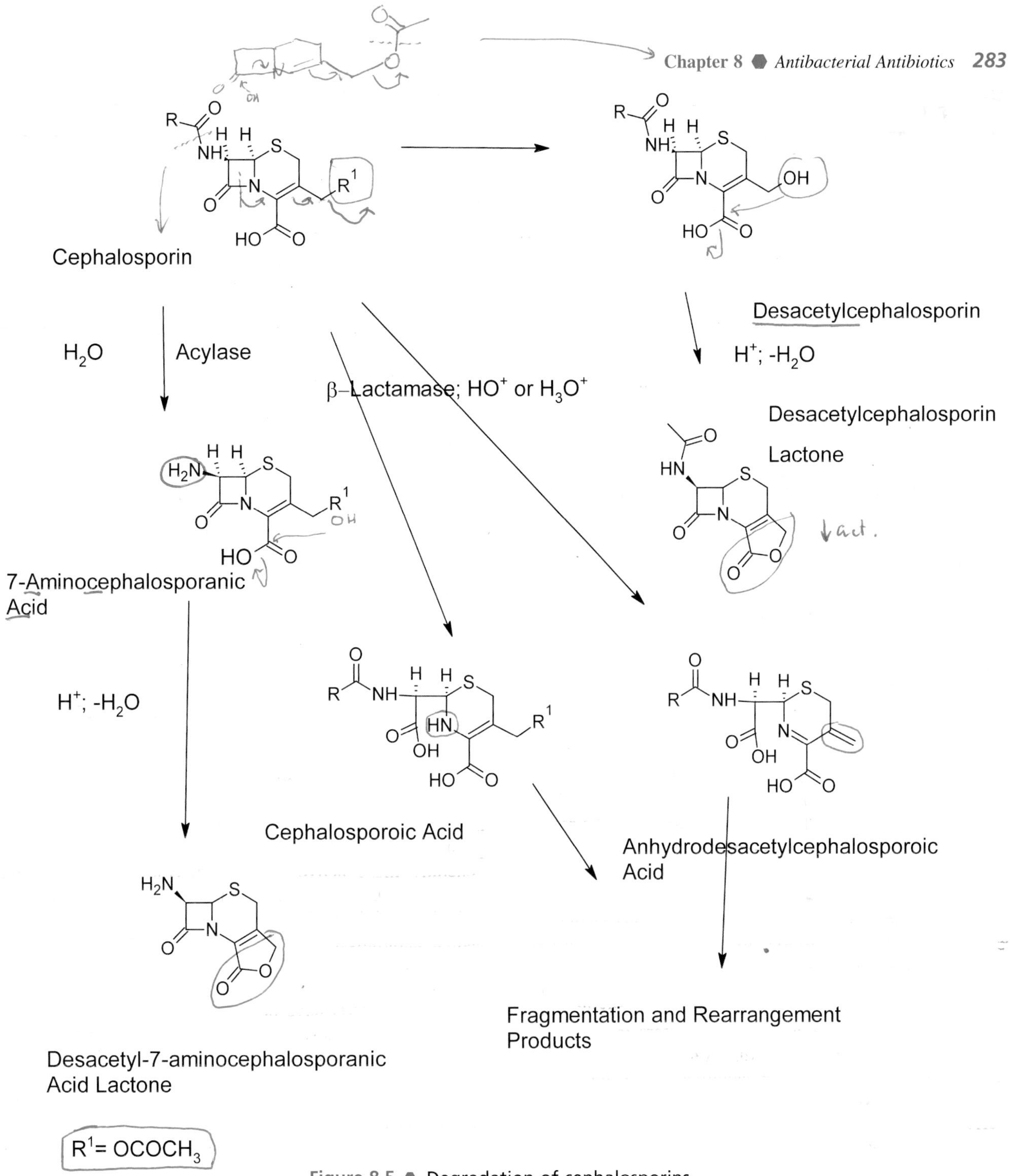

Figure 8.5 ● Degradation of cephalosporins.

β-Lactamases elaborated by Gram-negative bacteria present an exceedingly complex picture. Well over 100 different enzymes from various species of Gram-negative bacilli have been identified and characterized,[25] differing widely in specificity for various β-lactam antibiotics. Most of these enzymes hydrolyze penicillin G and ampicillin faster than the cephalosporins. Some inducible β-lactamases belonging to group C, however, are "cephalosporinases," which hydrolyze cephalosporins more rapidly. Inactivation by β-lactamases is an important factor in determining resistance to cephalosporins in many strains of Gram-negative bacilli.

The introduction of polar substituents in the aminoacyl moiety of cephalosporins appears to confer stability to some β-lactamases.[78] Thus, cefamandole and cefonicid, which contain an α-hydroxyphenylacetyl (or mandoyl) group, and

ceforanide, which has an *o*-aminophenyl acetyl group, are resistant to a few β-lactamases. Steric factors also may be important because cefoperazone, an acylureidocephalosporin that contains the same 4-ethyl-2,3-dioxo-1-piperazinylcarbonyl group present in piperacillin, is resistant to many β-lactamases. Oddly enough, piperacillin is hydrolyzed by most of these enzymes.

Two structural features confer broadly based resistance to β-lactamases among the cephalosporins: (a) an alkoximino function in the aminoacyl group and (b) a methoxyl substituent at the 7-position of the cephem nucleus having α stereochemistry. The structures of several β-lactamase–resistant cephalosporins, including cefuroxime, cefotaxime, ceftizoxime, and ceftriaxone, feature a methoximino acyl group. β-Lactamase resistance is enhanced modestly if the oximino substituent also features a polar function, as in ceftazidime, which has a 2-methylpropionic acid substituent on the oximino group. Both steric and electronic properties of the alkoximino group may contribute to the β-lactamase resistance conferred by this functionality since *syn*-isomers are more potent than *anti*-isomers.[78] β-Lactamase–resistant 7α-methoxylcephalosporins, also called cephamycins because they are derived from cephamycin C (an antibiotic isolated from *Streptomyces*), are represented by cefoxitin, cefotetan, cefmetazole, and the 1-oxocephalosporin moxalactam, which is prepared by total synthesis.

Base- or β-lactamase–catalyzed hydrolysis of cephalosporins containing a good leaving group at the 3-position is accompanied by elimination of the leaving group. The enzymatic process occurs in a stepwise fashion, beginning with the formation of a tetrahedral transition state, which quickly collapses into an acyl-enzyme intermediate (Fig. 8.6). This intermediate can then either undergo hydrolysis to free the enzyme (path 1) or suffer elimination of the leaving group to form a relatively stable acyl-enzyme with a conjugated imine structure (path 2). Because of the stability of the acyl-enzyme intermediate, path 2 leads to transient inhibition of the enzyme. Faraci

and Pratt[79,79a] have shown that cephalothin and cefoxitin inhibit certain β-lactamases by this mechanism, whereas analogs lacking a 3′ leaving group do not.

Antipseudomonal Cephalosporins

Species of *Pseudomonas*, especially *P. aeruginosa*, represent a special public health problem because of their ubiquity in the environment and their propensity to develop resistance to antibiotics, including the β-lactams. The primary mechanisms of β-lactam resistance appear to involve destruction of the antibiotics by β-lactamases and/or interference with their penetration through the cell envelope. Apparently, not all β-lactamase–resistant cephalosporins penetrate the cell envelope of *P. aeruginosa*, as only cefoperazone, moxalactam, cefotaxime, ceftizoxime, ceftriaxone, and ceftazidime have useful antipseudomonal activity. Two cephalosporins, moxalactam and cefoperazone, contain the same polar functionalities (e.g., carboxy and *N*-acylureido) that facilitate penetration into *Pseudomonas* spp. by the penicillins (see carbenicillin, ticarcillin, and piperacillin). Unfortunately, strains of *P. aeruginosa* resistant to cefoperazone and cefotaxime have been found in clinical isolates.

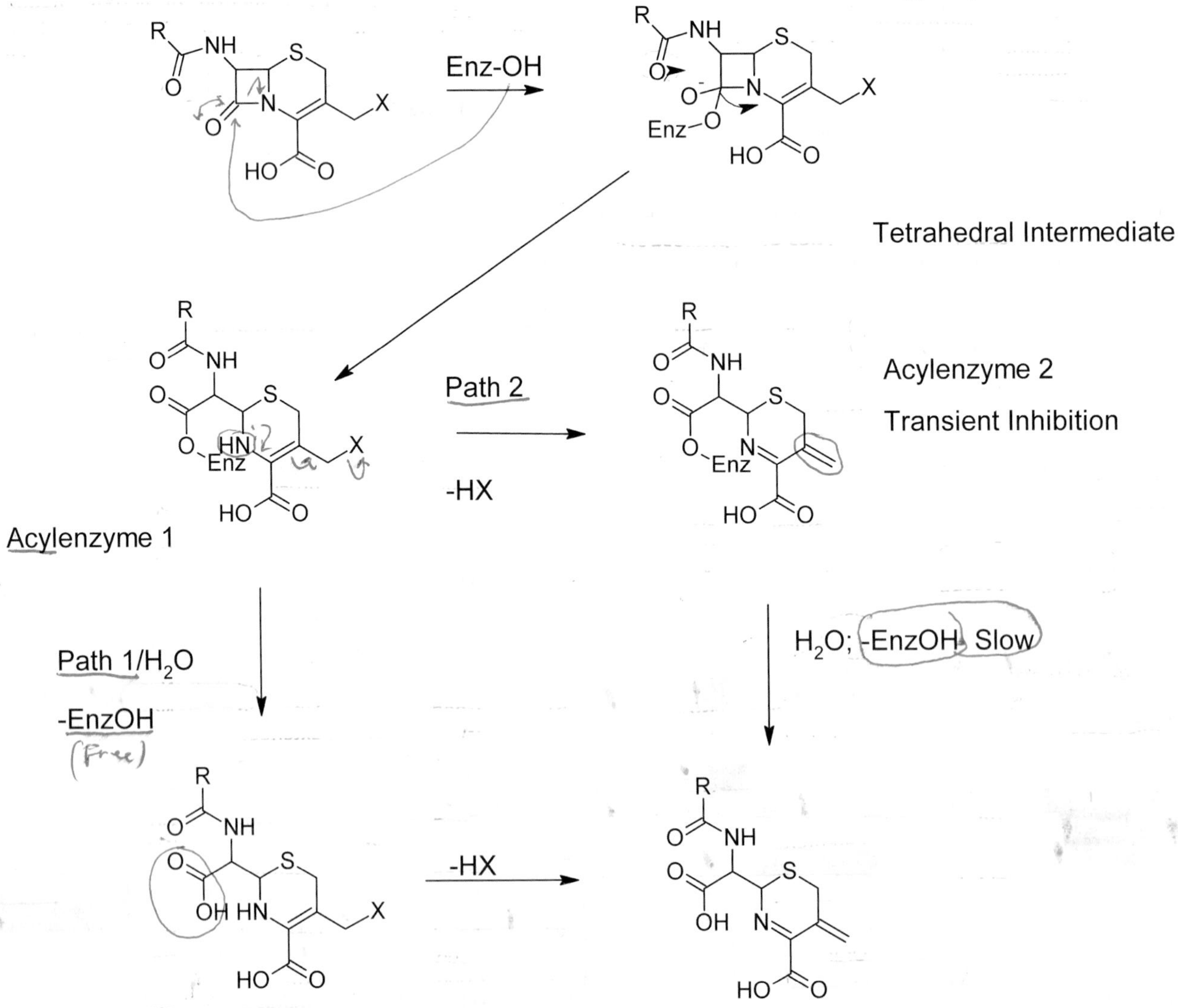

Figure 8.6 • Inhibition of β-lactamases by cephalosporins.

Adverse Reactions and Drug Interactions

Like their close relatives, the penicillins, the cephalosporin antibiotics are comparatively nontoxic compounds that, because of their selective actions on cell wall cross-linking enzymes, exhibit highly selective toxicity toward bacteria. The most common adverse reactions to the cephalosporins are allergic and hypersensitivity reactions. These vary from mild rashes to life-threatening anaphylactic reactions. Allergic reactions are believed to occur less frequently with cephalosporins than with penicillins. The issue of cross-sensitivity between the two classes of β-lactams is very complex, but the incidence is considered to be very low (estimated between 3% and 7%). The physician faced with the decision of whether or not to administer a cephalosporin to a patient with a history of penicillin allergy must weigh several factors, including the severity of the illness being treated, the effectiveness and safety of alternative therapies, and the severity of previous allergic responses to penicillins. Cephalosporins containing an *N*-methyl-5-thiotetrazole (MTT) moiety at the 3-position (e.g., cefamandole, cefotetan, cefmetazole, moxalactam, and cefoperazone) have been implicated in a higher incidence of hypoprothrombinemia than cephalosporins lacking the MTT group. This effect, which is enhanced and can lead to severe bleeding in patients with poor nutritional status, debilitation, recent GI surgery, hepatic disease, or renal failure, is apparently because of inhibition of vitamin K–requiring enzymes involved in the carboxylation of glutamic acid residues in clotting factors II, VII, IX, and X to the MTT group.[80] Treatment with vitamin K restores prothrombin time to normal in patients treated with MTT-containing cephalosporins. Weekly vitamin K prophylaxis has been recommended for high-risk patients undergoing therapy with such agents. Cephalosporins containing the MTT group should not be administered to patients receiving oral anticoagulant or heparin therapy because of possible synergism with these drugs.

The MTT group has also been implicated in the intolerance to alcohol associated with certain injectable cephalosporins: cefamandole, cefotetan, cefmetazole, and cefoperazone. Thus, disulfiram-like reactions, attributed to the accumulation of acetaldehyde and resulting from the inhibition of aldehyde dehydrogenase–catalyzed oxidation of ethanol by MTT-containing cephalosporins,[81] may occur in patients who have consumed alcohol before, during, or shortly after the course of therapy.

Classification

Cephalosporins are divided into first-, second-, third-, and fourth-generation agents, based roughly on their time of discovery and their antimicrobial properties (Table 8.5). In general, progression from first to fourth generation is associated with a broadening of the Gram-negative antibacterial spectrum, some reduction in activity against Gram-positive organisms, and enhanced resistance to β-lactamases. Individual cephalosporins differ in their pharmacokinetic properties, especially plasma protein binding and half-life, but the structural bases for these differences are not obvious.

TABLE 8.5 Classification and Properties of Cephalosporins

Cephalosporin	Generation	Route of Admin.	Acid Resistant	Plasma Protein Binding (%)	β-Lactamase Resistance	Spectrum of Activity	Antipseudomonal Activity
Cephalexin	First	Oral	Yes	5–15	Poor	Broad	No
Cephradine	First	Oral, parenteral	Yes	8–17	Poor	Broad	No
Cefadroxil	First	Oral	Yes	20	Poor	Broad	No
Cephalothin	First	Parenteral	No	65–80	Poor	Broad	No
Cephapirin	First	Parenteral	No	40–54	Poor	Broad	No
Cefazolin	First	Parenteral	No	70–86	Poor	Broad	No
Cefaclor	Second	Oral	Yes	22–25	Poor	Broad	No
Loracarbef	Second	Oral	Yes	25	Poor	Broad	No
Cefprozil	Second	Oral	Yes	36	Poor	Broad	No
Cefamandole	Second	Parenteral	No	56–78	Poor to avg.	Extended	No
Cefonicid	Second	Parenteral	No	99	Poor to avg.	Extended	No
Ceforanide	Second	Parenteral	No	80	Average	Extended	No
Cefoxitin	Second	Parenteral	No	13–22	Good	Extended	No
Cefotetan	Second	Parenteral	No	78–91	Good	Extended	No
Cefmetazole	Second	Parenteral	No	65	Good	Extended	No
Cefuroxime	Second	Oral, parenteral	Yes/No	33–50	Good	Extended	No
Cefpodoxime	Second	Oral	Yes	25	Good	Extended	No
Cefixime	Third	Oral	Yes	65	Good	Extended	No
Cefoperazone	Third	Parenteral	No	82–93	Avg. to good	Extended	Yes
Cefotaxime	Third	Parenteral	No	30–51	Good	Extended	Yes
Ceftizoxime	Third	Parenteral	No	30	Good	Extended	Yes
Ceftriaxone	Third	Parenteral	No	80–95	Good	Extended	Yes
Ceftazidime	Third	Parenteral	No	80–90	Good	Extended	Yes
Ceftibuten	Third	Oral	Yes	?	Good	Extended	No
Cefepime	Fourth	Parenteral	No	16–19	Good	Extended	Yes
Cefpirome	Fourth	Parenteral	No	–	Good	Extended	Yes

Products

Cephalexin

Cephalexin, 7α-(D-amino-α-phenylacetamido)-3-methyl-cephemcarboxylic acid (Keflex, Keforal), was designed purposely as an orally active, semisynthetic cephalosporin. The oral inactivation of cephalosporins has been attributed to two causes: instability of the β-lactam ring to acid hydrolysis (cephalothin and cephaloridine) and solvolysis or microbial transformation of the 3-methylacetoxy group (cephalothin, cephaloglycin). The α-amino group of cephalexin renders it acid stable, and reduction of the 3-acetoxymethyl to a methyl group circumvents reaction at that site.

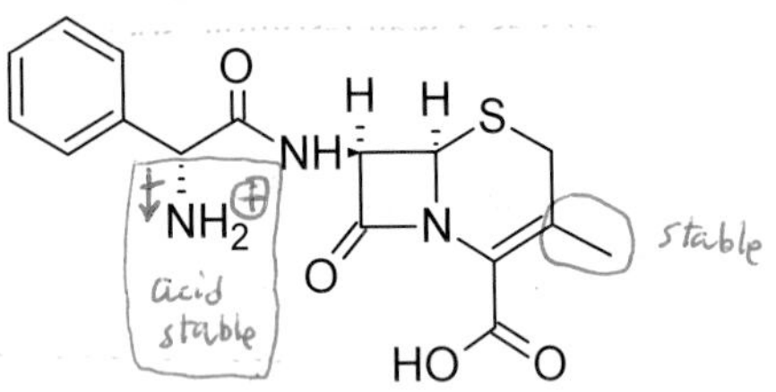

Cephalexin occurs as a white crystalline monohydrate. It is freely soluble in water, resistant to acid, and absorbed well orally. Food does not interfere with its absorption. Because of minimal protein binding and nearly exclusive renal excretion, cephalexin is recommended particularly for the treatment of urinary tract infections. It is also sometimes used for upper respiratory tract infections. Its spectrum of activity is very similar to those of cephalothin and cephaloridine. Cephalexin is somewhat less potent than these two agents after parenteral administration and, therefore, is inferior to them for the treatment of serious systemic infections.

Cephradine

Cephradine (Anspor, Velosef) is the only cephalosporin derivative available in both oral and parenteral dosage forms. It closely resembles cephalexin chemically (it may be regarded as a partially hydrogenated derivative of cephalexin) and has very similar antibacterial and pharmacokinetic properties.

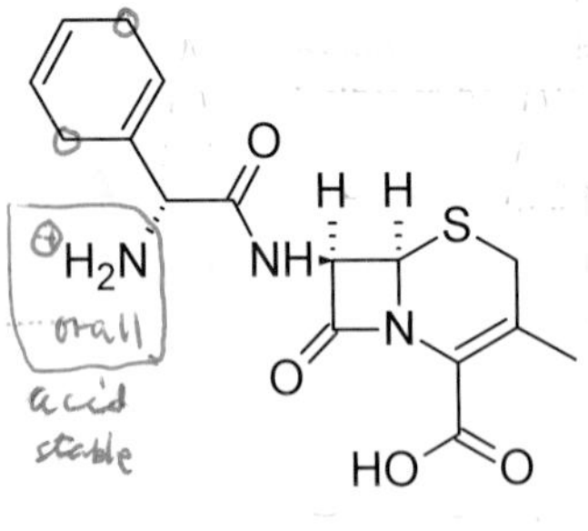

It occurs as a crystalline hydrate that is readily soluble in water. Cephradine is stable to acid and absorbed almost completely after oral administration. It is minimally protein bound and excreted almost exclusively through the kidneys. It is recommended for the treatment of uncomplicated urinary tract and upper respiratory tract infections caused by susceptible organisms. Cephradine is available in both oral and parenteral dosage forms.

Cefadroxil

Cefadroxil (Duricef) is an orally active semisynthetic derivative of 7-ADCA, in which the 7-acyl group is the D-hydroxylphenylglycyl moiety. This compound is absorbed well after oral administration to give plasma levels that reach 75% to 80% of those of an equal dose of its close structural analog cephalexin. The main advantage claimed for cefadroxil is its somewhat prolonged duration of action, which permits once-a-day dosing. The prolonged duration of action of this compound is related to relatively slow urinary excretion of the drug compared with other cephalosporins, but the basis for this remains to be explained completely. The antibacterial spectrum of action and therapeutic indications of cefadroxil are very similar to those of cephalexin and cephradine. The D-p-hydroxyphenylglycyl isomer is much more active than the L-isomer.

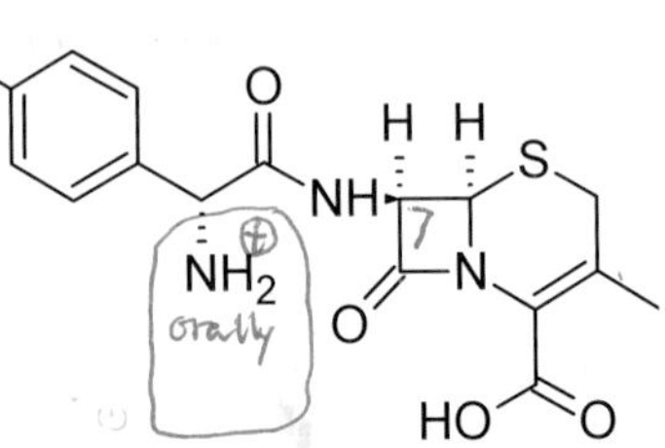

Cefaclor

Cefaclor (Ceclor) is an orally active semisynthetic cephalosporin that was introduced in the American market in 1979. It differs structurally from cephalexin in that the 3-methyl group has been replaced by a chlorine atom. It is synthesized from the corresponding 3-methylenecepham sulfoxide ester by ozonolysis, followed by halogenation of the resulting β-ketoester.[82] The 3-methylenecepham sulfoxide esters are prepared by rearrangement of the corresponding 6-acylaminopenicillanic acid derivative. Cefaclor is moderately stable in acid and achieves enough oral absorption to provide effective plasma levels (equal to about two-thirds of those obtained with cephalexin). The compound is apparently unstable in solution, since about 50% of its antimicrobial activity is lost in 2 hours in serum at 37°C.[83] The antibacterial spectrum of activity is similar to that of cephalexin, but it is claimed to be more potent against some species sensitive to both agents. Currently, the drug is recommended for the treatment of non–life-threatening infections caused by *H. influenzae*, particularly strains resistant to ampicillin.

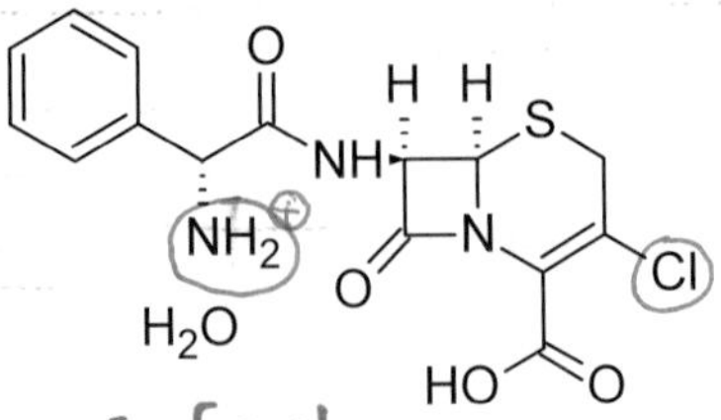

Cefaclor

Cefprozil

Cefprozil (Cefzil) is an orally active second-generation cephalosporin that is similar in structure and antibacterial spectrum to cefadroxil. Oral absorption is excellent (oral bioavailability is about 95%) and is not affected by antacids or histamine H_2-antagonists. Cefprozil exhibits greater in vitro activity against streptococci, *Neisseria* spp., and *S. aureus* than does cefadroxil. It is also more active than the first-generation cephalosporins against members of the Enterobacteriaceae family, such as *E. coli*, *Klebsiella* spp.,

P. mirabilis, and *Citrobacter* spp. The plasma half-life of 1.2 to 1.4 hours permits twice-a-day dosing for the treatment of most community-acquired respiratory and urinary tract infections caused by susceptible organisms.

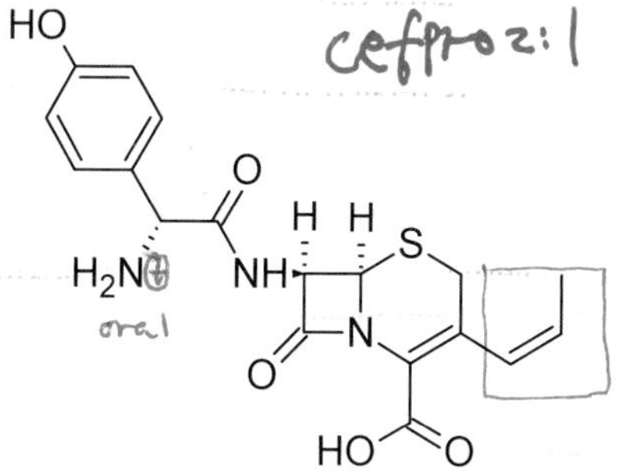

cefprozil
oral

Loracarbef

Loracarbef (Lorabid) is the first of a series of carbacephems prepared by total synthesis to be introduced.[84] Carbacephems are isosteres of the cephalosporin (or Δ^3-cephem) antibiotics in which the 1-sulfur atom has been replaced by a methylene (CH$_2$) group. Loracarbef is isosteric with cefaclor and has similar pharmacokinetic and microbiological properties. Thus, the antibacterial spectrum of activity resembles that of cefaclor, but it has somewhat greater potency against *H. influenzae* and *M. catarrhalis*, including β-lactamase-producing strains. Unlike cefaclor, which undergoes degradation in human serum, loracarbef is chemically stable in plasma. It is absorbed well orally. Oral absorption is delayed by food. The half-life in plasma is about 1 hour.

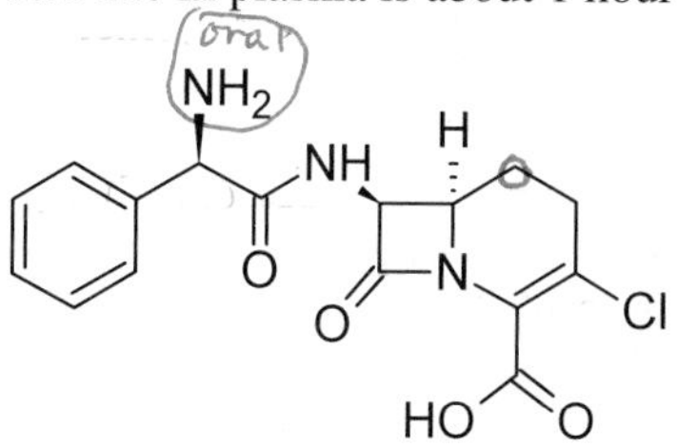

oral

Cephalothin Sodium

Cephalothin sodium (Keflin) occurs as a white to off-white, crystalline powder that is practically odorless. It is freely soluble in water and insoluble in most organic solvents. Although it has been described as a broad-spectrum antibacterial compound, it is not in the same class as the tetracyclines. Its spectrum of activity is broader than that of penicillin G and more similar to that of ampicillin. Unlike ampicillin, cephalothin is resistant to penicillinase produced by *S. aureus* and provides an alternative to the use of penicillinase-resistant penicillins for the treatment of infections caused by such strains.

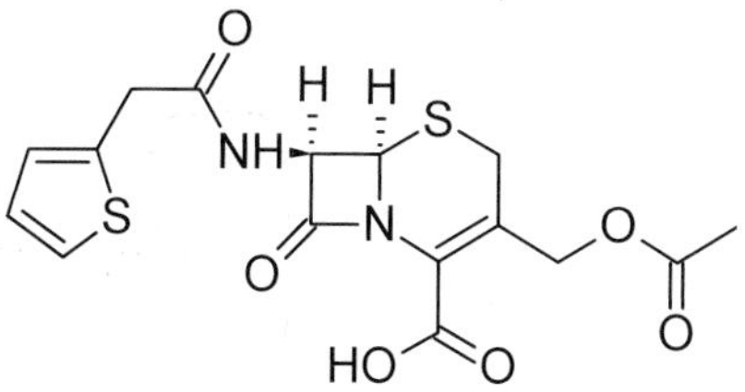

Cephalothin is absorbed poorly from the GI tract and must be administered parenterally for systemic infections. It

is relatively nontoxic and acid stable. It is excreted rapidly through the kidneys; about 60% is lost within 6 hours of administration. Pain at the site of intramuscular injection and thrombophlebitis following intravenous injection have been reported. Hypersensitivity reactions have been observed, and there is some evidence of cross-sensitivity in patients noted previously to be penicillin sensitive.

Cefazolin Sodium, Sterile (IV only)

Cefazolin (Ancef, Kefzol) is one of a series of semisynthetic cephalosporins in which the C-3 acetoxy function has been replaced by a thiol-containing heterocycle—here, 5-methyl-2-thio-1,3,4-thiadiazole. It also contains the somewhat unusual tetrazolylacetyl acylating group. Cefazolin was released in 1973 as a water-soluble sodium salt. It is active only by parenteral administration.

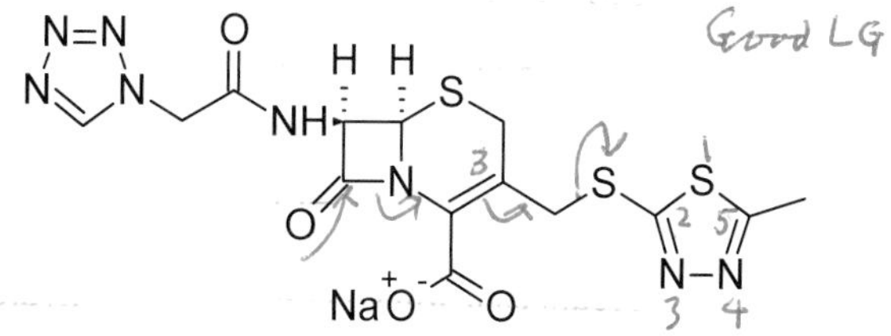

Good LG

Cefazolin provides higher serum levels, slower renal clearance, and a longer half-life than other first-generation cephalosporins. It is approximately 75% protein bound in plasma, a higher value than for most other cephalosporins. Early in vitro and clinical studies suggest that cefazolin is more active against Gram-negative bacilli but less active against Gram-positive cocci than either cephalothin or cephaloridine. Occurrence rates of thrombophlebitis following intravenous injection and pain at the site of intramuscular injection appear to be the lowest of the parenteral cephalosporins.

Cephapirin Sodium, Sterile

Cephapirin (Cefadyl) is a semisynthetic 7-ACA derivative released in the United States in 1974. It closely resembles cephalothin in chemical and pharmacokinetic properties. Like cephalothin, cephapirin is unstable in acid and must be administered parenterally in the form of an aqueous solution of the sodium salt. It is moderately protein bound (45%–50%) in plasma and cleared rapidly by the kidneys. Cephapirin and cephalothin are very similar in antimicrobial spectrum and potency. Conflicting reports concerning the relative occurrence of pain at the site of injection and thrombophlebitis after intravenous injection of cephapirin and cephalothin are difficult to assess on the basis of available clinical data.

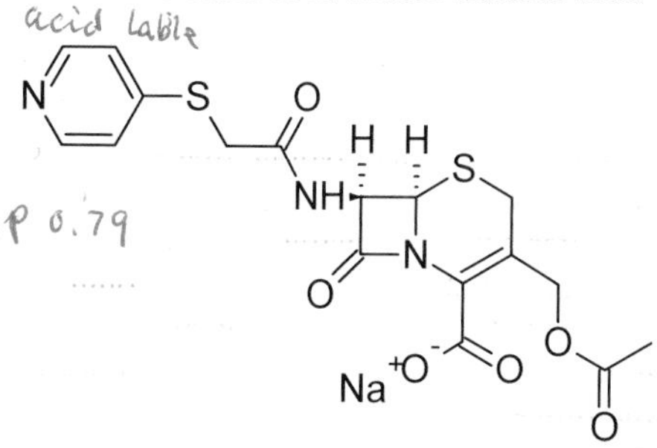

acid labile
Log P 0.79

Cefamandole Nafate

Cefamandole (Mandol) nafate is the formate ester of cefamandole, a semisynthetic cephalosporin that incorporates

D-mandelic acids as the acyl portion and a thiol-containing heterocycle (5-thio-1,2,3,4-tetrazole) in place of the acetoxy function on the C-3 methylene carbon atom. Esterification of the α-hydroxyl group of the D-mandeloyl function overcomes the instability of cefamandole in solid-state dosage forms[85] and provides satisfactory concentrations of the parent antibiotic in vivo through spontaneous hydrolysis of the ester at neutral to alkaline pH. Cefamandole is the first second-generation cephalosporin to be marketed in the United States.

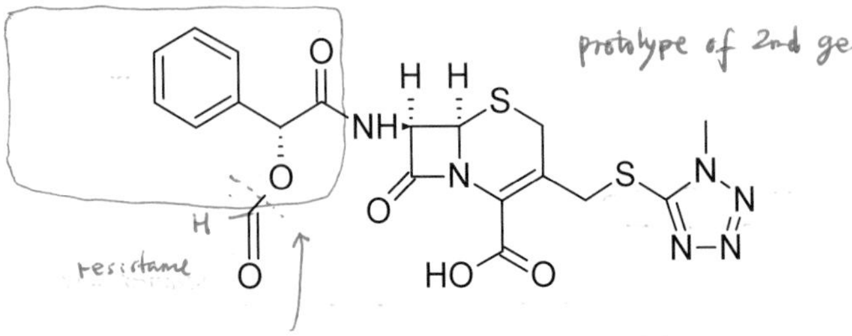

prototype of 2nd gen.

resistance

The D-mandeloyl moiety of cefamandole appears to confer resistance to a few β-lactamases, since some β-lactamase–producing, Gram-negative bacteria (particularly Enterobacteriaceae) that show resistance to cefazolin and other first-generation cephalosporins are sensitive to cefamandole. Additionally, it is active against some ampicillin-resistant strains of *Neisseria* and *Haemophilus* spp. Although resistance to β-lactamases may be a factor in determining the sensitivity of individual bacterial strains to cefamandole, an early study[86] indicated that other factors, such as permeability and intrinsic activity, are frequently more important. The L-mandeloyl isomer is significantly less active than the D-isomer.

Cefamandole nafate is very unstable in solution and hydrolyzes rapidly to release cefamandole and formate. There is no loss of potency, however, when such solutions are stored for 24 hours at room temperature or up to 96 hours when refrigerated. Air oxidation of the released formate to carbon dioxide can cause pressure to build up in the injection vial.

Cefonicid Sodium, Sterile

Cefonicid Sodium (Monocid) is a second-generation cephalosporin that is structurally similar to cefamandole, except that it contains a methane sulfonic acid group attached to the N-1 position of the tetrazole ring. The antimicrobial spectrum and limited β-lactamase stability of cefonicid are essentially identical with those of cefamandole.

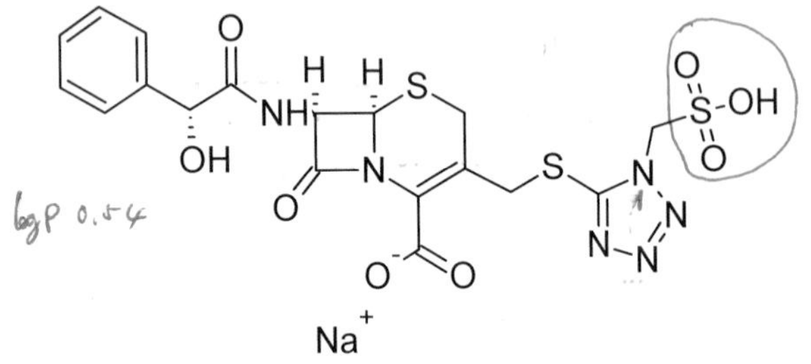

logP 0.54

Cefonicid is unique among the second-generation cephalosporins in that it has an unusually long serum half-life of approximately 4.5 hours. High plasma protein binding coupled with slow renal tubular secretion are apparently responsible for the long duration of action. Despite the high

fraction of drug bound in plasma, cefonicid is distributed throughout body fluids and tissues, with the exception of the cerebrospinal fluid.

Cefonicid is supplied as a highly water-soluble disodium salt, in the form of a sterile powder to be reconstituted for injection. Solutions are stable for 24 hours at 25°C and for 72 hours when refrigerated.

Ceforanide, Sterile

Ceforanide (Precef) was approved for clinical use in the United States in 1984. It is classified as a second-generation cephalosporin because its antimicrobial properties are similar to those of cefamandole. It exhibits excellent potency against most members of the Enterobacteriaceae family, especially *K. pneumoniae*, *E. coli*, *P. mirabilis*, and *Enterobacter cloacae*. It is less active than cefamandole against *H. influenzae*, however.

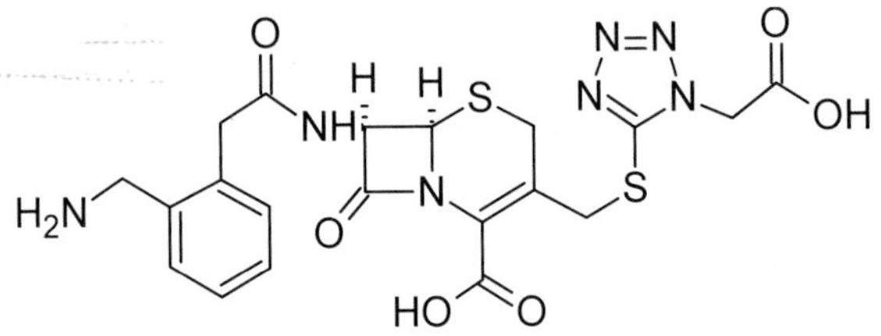

The duration of action of ceforanide lies between those of cefamandole and cefonicid. It has a serum half-life of about 3 hours, permitting twice-a-day dosing for most indications. Ceforanide is supplied as the sterile, crystalline disodium salt. Parenteral solutions are stable for 4 hours at 25°C and for up to 5 days when refrigerated.

Cefoperazone Sodium, Sterile

Cefoperazone (Cefobid) is a third-generation, antipseudomonal cephalosporin that resembles piperacillin chemically and microbiologically. It is active against many strains of *P. aeruginosa*, indole-positive *Proteus* spp., *Enterobacter* spp., and *S. marcescens* that are resistant to cefamandole. It is less active than cephalothin against Gram-positive bacteria and less active than cefamandole against most of the Enterobacteriaceae. Like piperacillin, cefoperazone is hydrolyzed by many of the β-lactamases that hydrolyze penicillins. Unlike piperacillin, however, it is resistant to some (but not all) of the β-lactamases that hydrolyze cephalosporins.

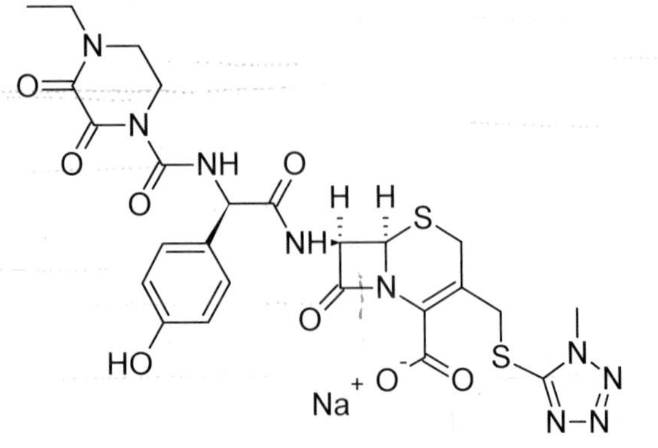

Cefoperazone is excreted primarily in the bile. Hepatic dysfunction can affect its clearance from the body. Although only 25% of the free antibiotic is recovered in the urine, urinary concentrations are high enough to be effective in the management of urinary tract infections caused by susceptible organisms. The relatively long half-life (2 hours) allows dosing twice a day. Solutions prepared from the crystalline sodium salt are stable for up to 4 hours at room temperature. If refrigerated, they will last 5 days without appreciable loss of potency.

Cefoxitin Sodium, Sterile

Cefoxitin (Mefoxin) is a semisynthetic derivative obtained by modification of cephamycin C, a 7α-methoxy-substituted cephalosporin isolated independently from various *Streptomyces* by research groups in Japan[87] and the United States. Although it is less potent than cephalothin against Gram-positive bacteria and cefamandole against most of the Enterobacteriaceae, cefoxitin is effective against certain strains of Gram-negative bacilli (e.g., *E. coli*, *K. pneumoniae*, *Providencia* spp., *S. marcescens*, indole-positive *Proteus* spp., and *Bacteroides* spp.) that are resistant to these cephalosporins. It is also effective against penicillin-resistant *S. aureus* and *N. gonorrhoeae*.

The activity of cefoxitin and cephamycins, in general, against resistant bacterial strains is because of their resistance to hydrolysis by β-lactamases conferred by the 7α-methoxyl substituent.[88] Cefoxitin is a potent competitive inhibitor of many β-lactamases. It is also a potent inducer of chromosomally mediated β-lactamases. The temptation to exploit the β-lactamase–inhibiting properties of cefoxitin by combining it with β-lactamase–labile β-lactam antibiotics should be tempered by the possibility of antagonism. In fact, cefoxitin antagonizes the action of cefamandole against *E. cloacae* and that of carbenicillin against *P. aeruginosa*.[89] Cefoxitin alone is essentially ineffective against these organisms.

The pharmacokinetic properties of cefoxitin resemble those of cefamandole. Because its half-life is relatively short, cefoxitin must be administered 3 or 4 times daily. Solutions of the sodium salt intended for parenteral administration are stable for 24 hours at room temperature and 1 week if refrigerated. 7α-Methoxyl substitution stabilizes, to some extent, the β-lactam to alkaline hydrolysis.

The principal role of cefoxitin in therapy seems to be for the treatment of certain anaerobic and mixed aerobic–anaerobic infections. It is also used to treat gonorrhea caused by β-lactamase–producing strains. It is classified as a second-generation agent because of its spectrum of activity.

Cefotetan Disodium

Cefotetan (Cefotan) is a third-generation cephalosporin that is structurally similar to cefoxitin. Like cefoxitin, cefotetan is resistant to destruction by β-lactamases. It is also a competitive inhibitor of many β-lactamases and causes transient

inactivation of some of these enzymes. Cefotetan is reported to synergize with β-lactamase–sensitive β-lactams but, unlike cefoxitin, does not appear to cause antagonism.[90]

The antibacterial spectrum of cefotetan closely resembles that of cefoxitin. It is, however, generally more active against *S. aureus*, and members of the Enterobacteriaceae family sensitive to both agents. It also exhibits excellent potency against *H. influenzae* and *N. gonorrhoeae*, including β-lactamase–producing strains. Cefotetan is slightly less active than cefoxitin against *B. fragilis* and other anaerobes. *Enterobacter* spp. are generally resistant to cefotetan, and the drug is without effect against *Pseudomonas* spp.

Cefotetan has a relatively long half-life of about 3.5 hours. It is administered on a twice-daily dosing schedule. It is excreted largely unchanged in the urine. Aqueous solutions for parenteral administration maintain potency for 24 hours at 25°C. Refrigerated solutions are stable for 4 days.

Cefotetan contains the MTT group that has been associated with hypoprothrombinemia and alcohol intolerance. Another cephalosporin that lacks these properties should be selected for patients at risk for severe bleeding or alcoholism.

Cefmetazole Sodium

Cefmetazole (Zefazone) is a semisynthetic, third-generation, parenteral cephalosporin of the cephamycin group. Like other cephamycins, the presence of the 7α-methoxyl group confers resistance to many β-lactamases. Cefmetazole exhibits significantly higher potency against members of the Enterobacteriaceae family but lower activity against *Bacteroides* spp. than cefoxitin. It is highly active against *N. gonorrhoeae*, including β-lactamase–producing strains. In common with other cephamycins, cefmetazole is ineffective against indole-positive *Proteus*, *Enterobacter*, *Providencia*, *Serratia*, and *Pseudomonas* spp. Cefmetazole has the MTT moiety associated with increased bleeding in certain high-risk patients. It has a plasma half-life of 1.1 hours.

Cefuroxime Sodium

Cefuroxime (Zinacef) is the first of a series of α-methoximinoacyl–substituted cephalosporins that constitute most of the third-generation agents available for clinical use. A *syn* alkoximino substituent is associated with β-lactamase stability in these cephalosporins.[78] Cefuroxime is classified as a second-generation cephalosporin because its spectrum of antibacterial activity more closely resembles that of cefamandole. It is, however, active against β-lactamase–producing strains that are resistant to cefamandole, such as *E. coli, K. pneumoniae, N. gonorrhoeae,* and *H. influenzae.* Other important Gram-negative pathogens, such as *Serratia,* indole-positive *Proteus* spp., *P. aeruginosa,* and *B. fragilis,* are resistant.

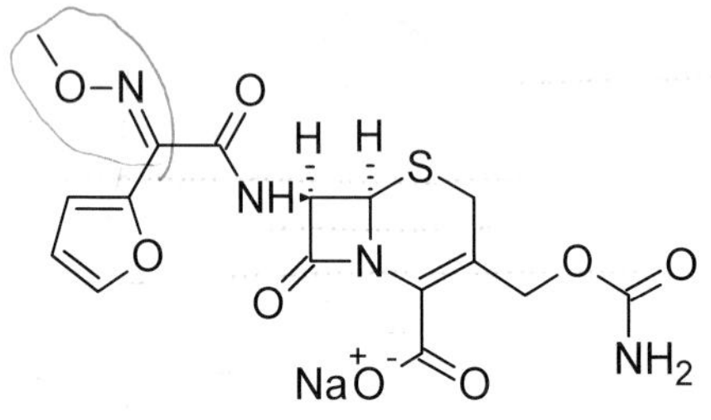

Cefuroxime is distributed throughout the body. It penetrates inflamed meninges in high enough concentrations to be effective in meningitis caused by susceptible organisms. Three-times-daily dosing is required to maintain effective plasma levels for most sensitive organisms, such as *Neisseria meningitidis, Streptococcus pneumoniae,* and *H. influenzae.* It has a plasma half-life of 1.4 hours.

Cefuroxime Axetil

Cefuroxime axetil (Ceftin) is the 1-acetyoxyethyl ester of cefuroxime. During absorption, this acid-stable, lipophilic, oral prodrug derivative of cefuroxime is hydrolyzed to cefuroxime by intestinal and/or plasma enzymes. The axetil ester provides an oral bioavailability of 35% to 50% of cefuroxime, depending on conditions. Oral absorption of the ester is increased by food but decreased by antacids and histamine H$_2$-antagonists. The latter effect may be because of spontaneous hydrolysis of the ester in the intestine because of the higher pH created by these drugs. Axetil is used for the oral treatment of non–life-threatening infections caused by bacteria that are susceptible to cefuroxime. The prodrug form permits twice-a-day dosing for such infections.

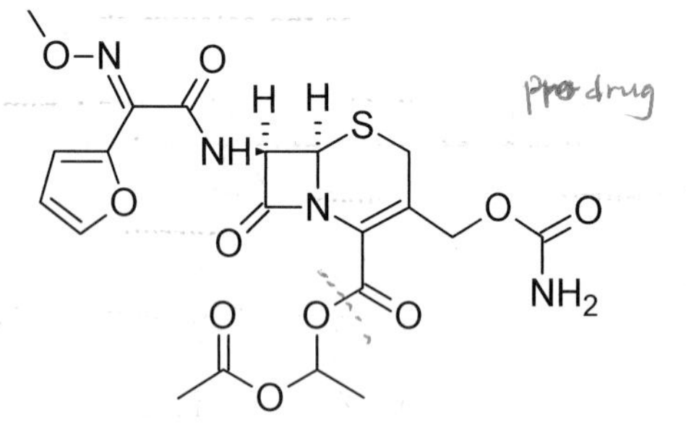

Cefpodoxime Proxetil

Cefpodoxime proxetil (Vantin) is the isopropyloxycarbonylethyl ester of the third-generation cephalosporin cefpodoxime. This orally active prodrug derivative is hydrolyzed by esterases in the intestinal wall and in the plasma to provide cefpodoxime. Tablets and a powder for the preparation of an aqueous suspension for oral pediatric administration are available. The oral bioavailability of cefpodoxime from the proxetil is estimated to be about 50%. Administration of the prodrug with food enhances its absorption. The plasma half-life is 2.2 hours, which permits administration on a twice-daily schedule.

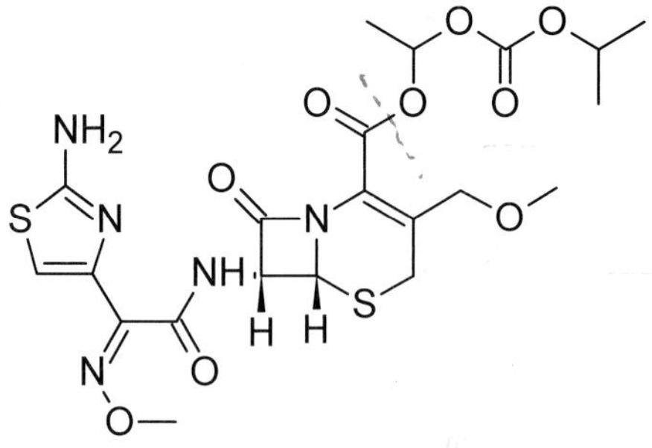

Cefpodoxime is a broad-spectrum cephalosporin with useful activity against a relatively wide range of Gram-positive and Gram-negative bacteria. It is also resistant to many β-lactamases. Its spectrum of activity includes *S. pneumoniae, Streptococcus pyogenes, S. aureus, H. influenzae, M. catarrhalis,* and *Neisseria* spp. Cefpodoxime is also active against members of the Enterobacteriaceae family, including *E. coli, K. pneumoniae,* and *P. mirabilis.* It thus finds use in the treatment of upper and lower respiratory infections, such as pharyngitis, bronchitis, otitis media, and community-acquired pneumonia. It is also useful for the treatment of uncomplicated gonorrhea.

Cefixime

Cefixime (Suprax) is the first orally active, third-generation cephalosporin that is not an ester prodrug to be approved for therapy in the United States. Oral bioavailability is surprisingly high, ranging from 40% to 50%. Facilitated transport of cefixime across intestinal brush border membranes involving the carrier system for dipeptides may explain its surprisingly good oral absorption.[91] This result was not expected because cefixime lacks the ionizable α-amino group present in dipeptides and β-lactams previously known to be transported by the carrier system.[51,91]

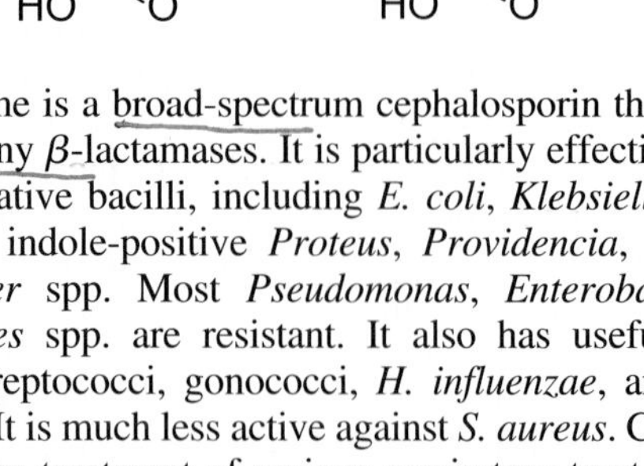

Cefixime is a broad-spectrum cephalosporin that is resistant to many β-lactamases. It is particularly effective against Gram-negative bacilli, including *E. coli, Klebsiella* spp., *P. mirabilis,* indole-positive *Proteus, Providencia,* and some *Citrobacter* spp. Most *Pseudomonas, Enterobacter,* and *Bacteroides* spp. are resistant. It also has useful activity against streptococci, gonococci, *H. influenzae,* and *M. catarrhalis.* It is much less active against *S. aureus.* Cefixime is used for the treatment of various respiratory tract infections (e.g., acute bronchitis, pharyngitis, and tonsillitis) and otitis media. It is also used to treat uncomplicated urinary tract infections and gonorrhea caused by β-lactamase–producing bacterial strains.

The comparatively long half-life of cefixime ($t_{1/2}$ is 3–4 hours) allows it to be administered on a twice-a-day schedule. Renal tubular reabsorption and a relatively high fraction of plasma protein binding (~65%) contribute to the long half-life. It is provided in two-oral dosage forms: 200- or 400-mg tablets and a powder for the preparation of an aqueous suspension.

Cefotaxime Sodium, Sterile

Cefotaxime (Claforan) was the first third-generation cephalosporin to be introduced. It possesses excellent broad-spectrum activity against Gram-positive and Gram-negative aerobic and anaerobic bacteria. It is more active than moxalactam against Gram-positive organisms. Many β-lactamase–producing bacterial strains are sensitive to cefotaxime, including *N. gonorrhoeae*, *Klebsiella* spp., *H. influenzae*, *S. aureus*, and *E. cloacae*. Some, but not all, *Pseudomonas* strains are sensitive. Enterococci and *Listeria monocytogenes* are resistant.

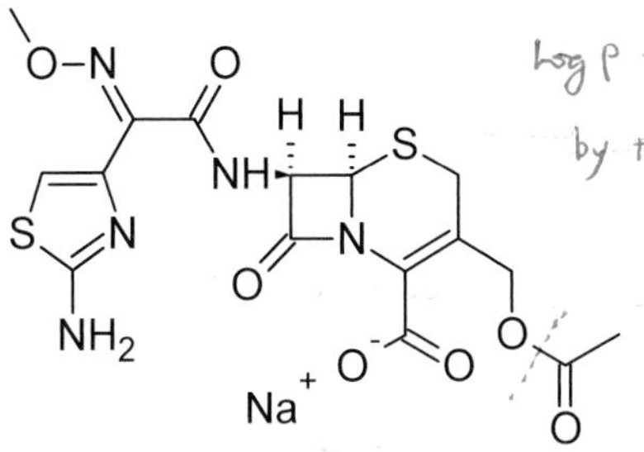

The *syn*-isomer of cefotaxime is significantly more active than the *anti*-isomer against β-lactamase–producing bacteria. This potency difference is, in part, because of greater resistance of the *syn*-isomer to the action of β-lactamases.[78] The higher affinity of the *syn*-isomer for PBPs, however, may also be a factor.[92]

Cefotaxime is metabolized in part to the less active desacetyl metabolite. Approximately 20% of the metabolite and 25% of the parent drug are excreted in the urine. The parent drug reaches the cerebrospinal fluid in sufficient concentration to be effective in the treatment of meningitis. Solutions of cefotaxime sodium should be used within 24 hours. If stored, they should be refrigerated. Refrigerated solutions maintain potency up to 10 days.

Ceftizoxime Sodium, Sterile

Ceftizoxime (Cefizox) is a third-generation cephalosporin that was introduced in 1984. This β-lactamase–resistant agent exhibits excellent activity against the Enterobacteriaceae, especially *E. coli*, *K. pneumoniae*, *E. cloacae*, *Enterobacter aerogenes*, indole-positive and indole-negative *Proteus* spp., and *S. marcescens*. Ceftizoxime is claimed to be more active than cefoxitin against *B. fragilis*. It is also very active against Gram-positive bacteria. Its activity against *P. aeruginosa* is somewhat variable and lower than that of either cefotaxime or cefoperazone.

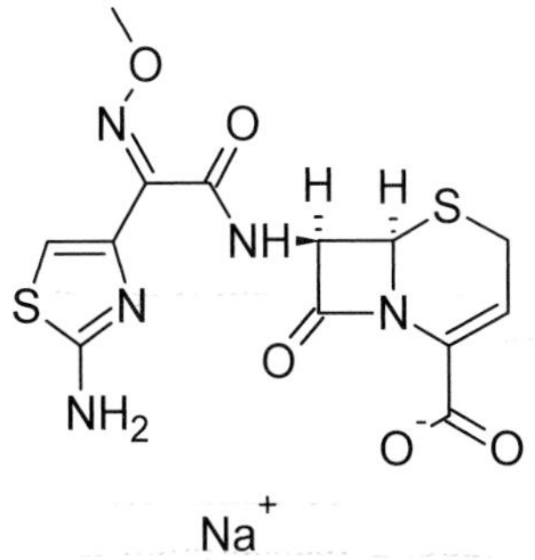

Ceftizoxime is not metabolized in vivo. It is excreted largely unchanged in the urine. Adequate levels of the drug are achieved in the cerebrospinal fluid for the treatment of Gram-negative or Gram-positive bacterial meningitis. It must be administered on a thrice-daily dosing schedule because of its relatively short half-life. Ceftizoxime sodium is very stable in the dry state. Solutions maintain potency for up to 24 hours at room temperature and 10 days when refrigerated.

Ceftriaxone Disodium, Sterile

Ceftriaxone (Rocephin) is a β-lactamase–resistant cephalosporin with an extremely long serum half-life. Once-daily dosing suffices for most indications. Two factors contribute to the prolonged duration of action of ceftriaxone: high protein binding in the plasma and slow urinary excretion. Ceftriaxone is excreted in both the bile and the urine. Its urinary excretion is not affected by probenecid. Despite its comparatively low volume of distribution, it reaches the cerebrospinal fluid in concentrations that are effective in meningitis. Nonlinear pharmacokinetics are observed.

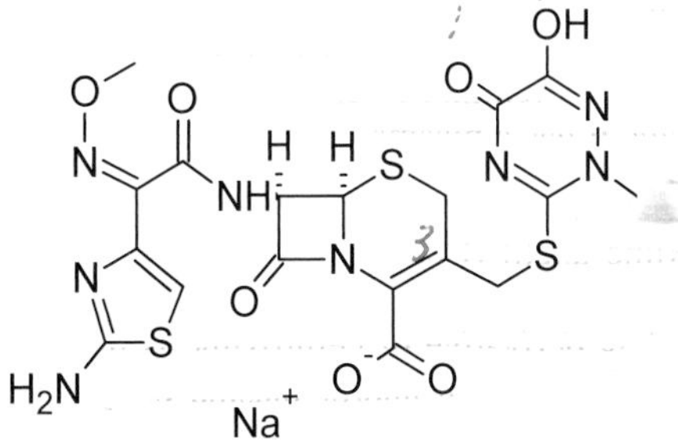

Ceftriaxone contains a highly acidic heterocyclic system on the 3-thiomethyl group. This unusual dioxotriazine ring system is believed to confer the unique pharmacokinetic properties of this agent. Ceftriaxone has been associated with sonographically detected "sludge," or pseudolithiasis, in the gallbladder and common bile duct.[93] Symptoms of cholecystitis may occur in susceptible patients, especially those on prolonged or high-dose ceftriaxone therapy. The culprit has been identified as the calcium chelate.

Ceftriaxone exhibits excellent broad-spectrum antibacterial activity against both Gram-positive and Gram-negative organisms. It is highly resistant to most chromosomally and plasmid-mediated β-lactamases. The activity of ceftriaxone against *Enterobacter*, *Citrobacter*, *Serratia*, indole-positive *Proteus*, and *Pseudomonas* spp. is particularly impressive. It is also effective in the treatment of ampicillin-resistant gonorrhea and *H. influenzae* infections but generally less active than cefotaxime against Gram-positive bacteria and *B. fragilis*.

Solutions of ceftriaxone sodium should be used within 24 hours. They may be stored up to 10 days if refrigerated.

Ceftazidime Sodium, Sterile

Ceftazidime (Fortaz, Tazidime) is a β-lactamase–resistant third-generation cephalosporin that is noted for its antipseudomonal activity. It is active against some strains of *P. aeruginosa* that are resistant to cefoperazone and ceftriaxone. Ceftazidime is also highly effective against β-lactamase–producing strains of the Enterobacteriaceae family. It is generally less active than cefotaxime against Gram-positive bacteria and *B. fragilis*.

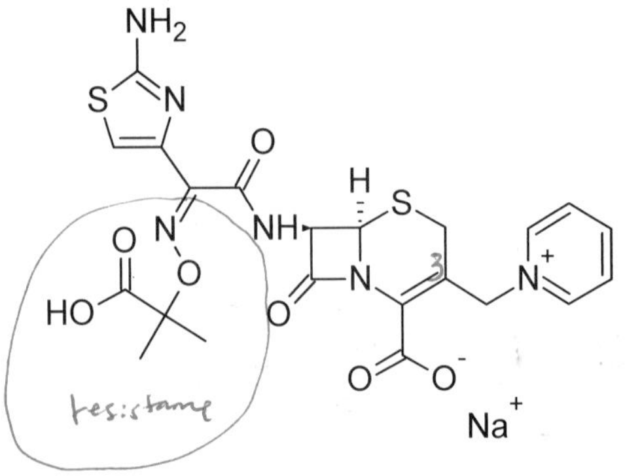

The structure of ceftazidime contains two noteworthy features: (a) a 2-methylpropionicoxaminoacyl group that confers β-lactamase resistance and, possibly, increased permeability through the porin channels of the cell envelope and (b) a pyridinium group at the 3-position that confers zwitterionic properties on the molecule.

Ceftazidime is administered parenterally 2 or 3 times daily, depending on the severity of the infection. Its serum half-life is about 1.8 hours. It has been used effectively for the treatment of meningitis caused by *H. influenzae* and *N. meningitidis*.

NEWER CEPHALOSPORINS

Cephalosporins currently undergoing clinical trials or recently being marketed in the United States fall into two categories: (a) orally active β-lactamase–resistant cephalosporins and (b) parenteral β-lactamase–resistant antipseudomonal cephalosporins. The status of some of these compounds awaits more extensive clinical evaluation. Nonetheless, it appears that any advances they represent will be relatively modest.

Ceftibuten

Ceftibuten (Cedax) is a recently introduced, chemically novel analog of the oximino cephalosporins in which an olefinic methylene group (C=CHCH₂-) with *Z* stereochemistry has replaced the *syn* oximino (C=NO-) group. This isosteric replacement yields a compound that retains resistance to hydrolysis catalyzed by many β-lactamases, has enhanced chemical stability, and is orally active. Oral absorption is rapid and nearly complete. It has the highest oral bioavailability of the third-generation cephalosporins.[94] Ceftibuten is excreted largely unchanged in the urine and has a half-life of about 2.5 hours. Plasma protein binding of this cephalosporin is estimated to be 63%.

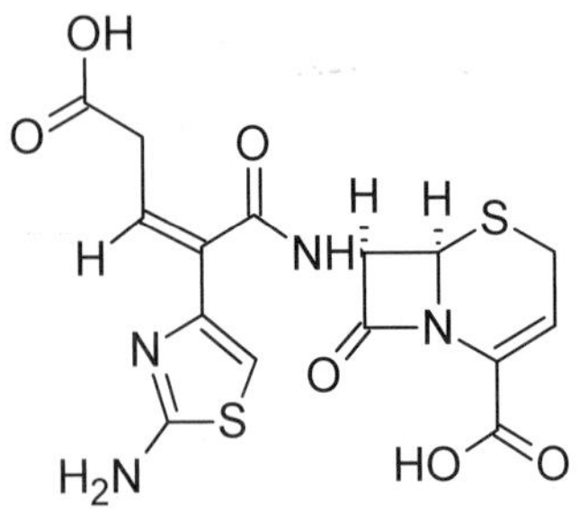

Ceftibuten possesses excellent potency against most members of the Enterobacteriaceae family, *H. influenzae*, *Neisseria* spp., and *M. catarrhalis*. It is not active against *S. aureus* or *P. aeruginosa* and exhibits modest antistreptococ-

cal activity. Ceftibuten is recommended in the management of community-acquired respiratory tract, urinary tract, and gynecological infections.

Cefpirome

Cefpirome (Cefrom) is a newer parenteral, β-lactamase–resistant cephalosporin with a quaternary ammonium group at the 3-position of the cephem nucleus. Because its potency against Gram-positive and Gram-negative bacteria rivals that of the first-generation and third-generation cephalosporins, respectively, cefpirome is being touted as the first fourth-generation cephalosporin.[95] Its broad spectrum includes methicillin-sensitive staphylococci, penicillin-resistant pneumococci, and β-lactamase–producing strains of *E. coli*, *Enterobacter*, *Citrobacter*, and *Serratia* spp. Its efficacy against *P. aeruginosa* is comparable with that of ceftazidime. Cefpirome is excreted largely unchanged in the urine with a half-life of 2 hours.

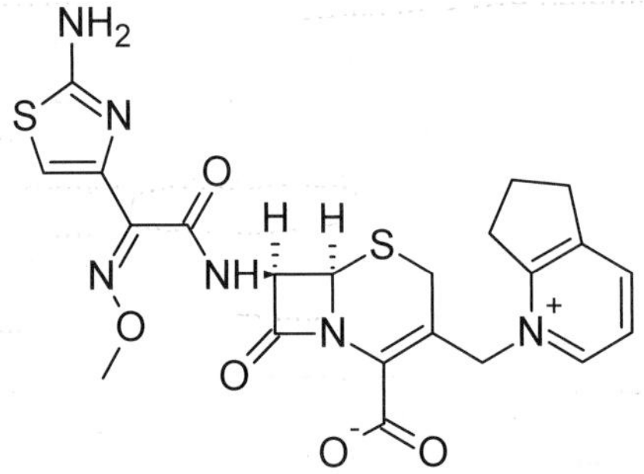

Cefepime

Cefepime (Maxipime, Axepin) is a parenteral, β-lactamase–resistant cephalosporin that is chemically and microbiologically similar to cefpirome. It also has a broad antibacterial spectrum, with significant activity against both Gram-positive and Gram-negative bacteria, including streptococci, staphylococci, *Pseudomonas* spp., and the Enterobacteriaceae. It is active against some bacterial isolates that are resistant to ceftazidime.[96] The efficacy of cefepime has been demonstrated in the treatment of urinary tract infections, lower respiratory tract infections, skin and soft tissue infections, chronic osteomyelitis, and intra-abdominal and biliary infections. It is excreted in the urine with a half-life of 2.1 hours. It is bound minimally to plasma proteins. Cefepime is also a fourth-generation cephalosporin.

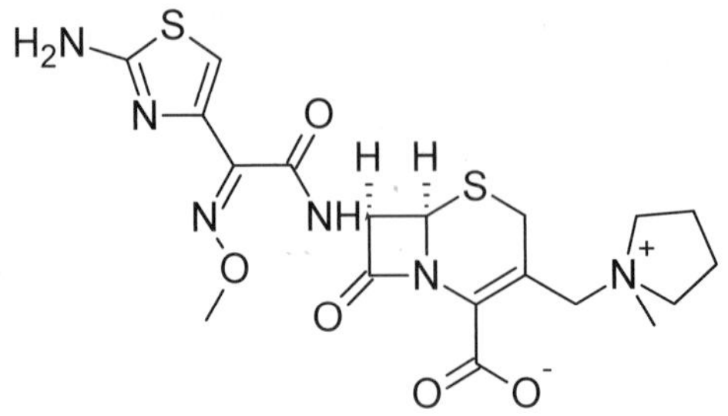

Future Developments in Cephalosporin Design

Recent research efforts in the cephalosporin field have focused primarily on two desired antibiotic properties: (a) increased permeability into Gram-negative bacilli, leading to

TOC-039

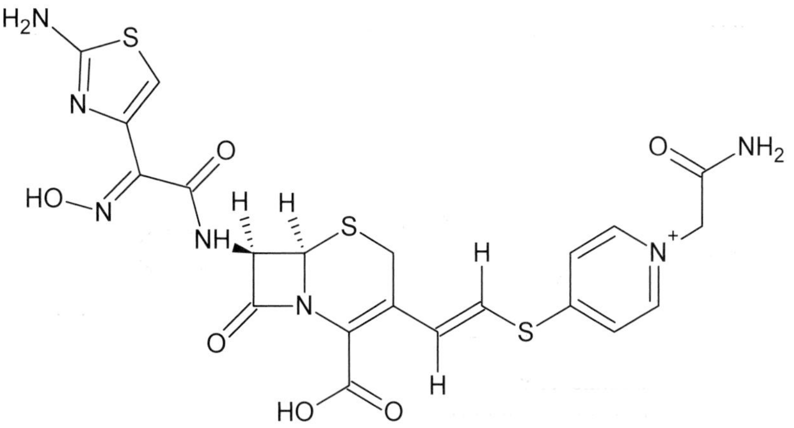

enhanced efficacy against permeability-resistant strains of Enterobacteriaceae and *P. aeruginosa*, and (b) increased affinity for altered PBPs, in particular the PBP 2a (or PBP 2′) of MRSA.[31]

The observation that certain catechol-substituted cephalosporins exhibit marked broad-spectrum antibacterial activity led to the discovery that such compounds and other analogs capable of chelating iron could mimic natural siderophores (iron-chelating peptides) and thus be actively transported into bacterial cells via the *tonB*-dependent iron-transport system.[97,98] This provides a means of attacking bacterial strains that resist cellular penetration of cephalosporins.

A catechol-containing cephalosporin that exhibits excellent in vitro antibacterial activity against clinical isolates and promising pharmacokinetic properties is GR-69153. GR-69153 is a parenteral β-lactamase–resistant cephalosporin with a broad spectrum of activity against Gram-positive and Gram-negative bacteria.

The antibacterial spectrum of GR-69153 includes most members of the Enterobacteriaceae family, *P. aeruginosa*, *H. influenzae*, *N. gonorrhoeae*, *M. catarrhalis*, staphylococci, streptococci, and *Acinetobacter* spp. It was not active against enterococci, *B. fragilis*, or MRSA. The half-life of GR-69153 in human volunteers was determined to be 3.5 hours, suggesting that metabolism by catechol-*O*-methyltransferase may not be an important factor. The relatively long half-life would permit once-a-day parenteral dosing for the treatment of many serious bacterial infections.

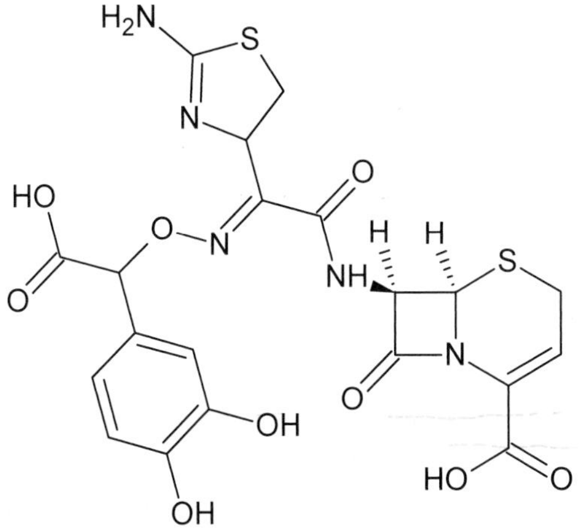

An experimental cephalosporin that has exhibited considerable promise against MRSA in preclinical evaluations is TOC-039.

TOC-039 is a parenteral, β-lactamase–resistant, hydroxyimino cephalosporin with a vinylthiopyridyl side chain attached to the 3-position of the cephem nucleus. It is a broad-spectrum agent that exhibits good activity against most aerobic Gram-positive and Gram-negative bacteria, including staphylococci, streptococci, enterococci, *H. influenzae*, *M. catarrhalis*, and most of the Enterobacteriaceae family.[99] A few strains of *P. vulgaris*, *S. marcescens*, and *Citrobacter freundii* are resistant, and TOC-039 is inactive against *P. aeruginosa*. Although the minimum inhibiting concentration (MIC) of TOC-039 against MRSA is slightly less than that of vancomycin, it is more rapidly bactericidal. Future clinical evaluations will determine if TOC-039 has the appropriate pharmacokinetic and antibacterial properties in vivo to be approved for the treatment of bacterial infections in humans.

MONOBACTAMS

The development of useful monobactam antibiotics began with the independent isolation of sulfazecin (SQ 26,445) and other monocyclic β-lactam antibiotics from saprophytic soil bacteria in Japan[100] and the United States.[101] Sulfazecin was found to be weakly active as an antibacterial agent but highly resistant to β-lactamases.

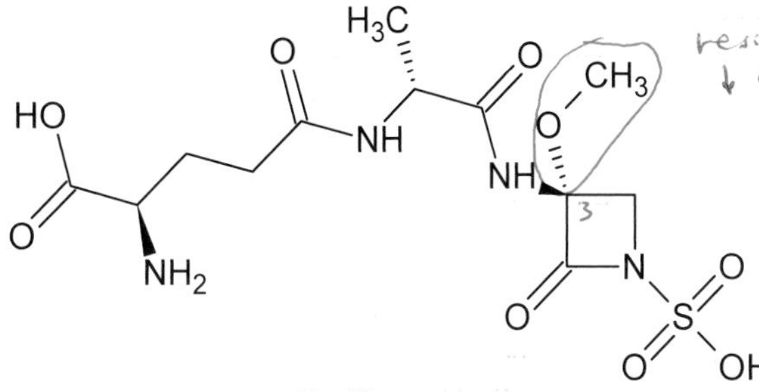

GR-69153

Sulfazecin

Extensive SAR studies[102] eventually led to the development of aztreonam, which has useful properties as an antibacterial agent. Early work established that the 3-methoxy group, which was in part responsible for β-lactamase stability in the series, contributed to the low antibacterial potency and poor chemical stability of these antibiotics. A 4-methyl group, however, increases stability to β-lactamases and activity against Gram-negative bacteria at the same time. Unfortunately, potency against Gram-positive bacteria decreases. 4,4-Gem-dimethyl substitution slightly decreases antibacterial potency after oral administration.

Products

Aztreonam Disodium

Aztreonam (Azactam) is a monobactam prepared by total synthesis. It binds with high affinity to PBP 3 in Gram-negative bacteria only. It is inactive against Gram-positive bacteria and anaerobes. β-Lactamase resistance is like that of ceftazidime, which has the same isobutyric acid oximinoacyl group. Aztreonam does not induce chromosomally mediated β-lactamases.

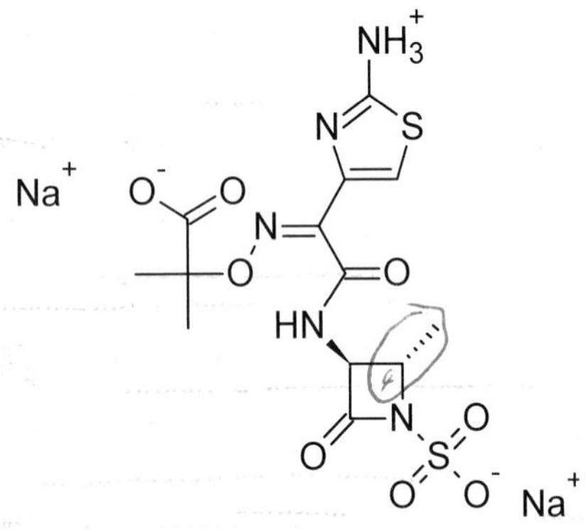

Aztreonam is particularly active against aerobic Gram-negative bacilli, including *E. coli*, *K. pneumoniae*, *Klebsiella oxytoca*, *P. mirabilis*, *S. marcescens*, *Citrobacter* spp., and *P. aeruginosa*. It is used to treat urinary and lower respiratory tract infections, intra-abdominal infections, and gynecological infections, as well as septicemias caused by these organisms. Aztreonam is also effective against, but is not currently used to treat, infections caused by *Haemophilus*, *Neisseria*, *Salmonella*, indole-positive *Proteus*, and *Yersinia* spp. It is not active against Gram-positive bacteria, anaerobic bacteria, or other species of *Pseudomonas*.

Urinary excretion is about 70% of the administered dose. Some is excreted through the bile. Serum half-life is 1.7 hours, which allows aztreonam to be administered 2 or 3 times daily, depending on the severity of the infection. Less than 1% of an orally administered dose of aztreonam is absorbed, prompting the suggestion that this β-lactam could be used to treat intestinal infections.

The disodium salt of aztreonam is very soluble in water. Solutions for parenteral administration containing 2% or less are stable for 48 hours at room temperature. Refrigerated solutions retain full potency for 1 week.

Tigemonam

Tigemonam is a newer monobactam that is orally active.[103] It is highly resistant to β-lactamases. The antibacterial spectrum of activity resembles that of aztreonam. It is very active against the Enterobacteriaceae, including *E. coli*, *Klebsiella*, *Proteus*, *Citrobacter*, *Serratia*, and *Enterobacter* spp. It also exhibits good potency against *H. influenzae* and *N. gonorrhoeae*. Tigemonam is not particularly active against Gram-positive or anaerobic bacteria and is inactive against *P. aeruginosa*.

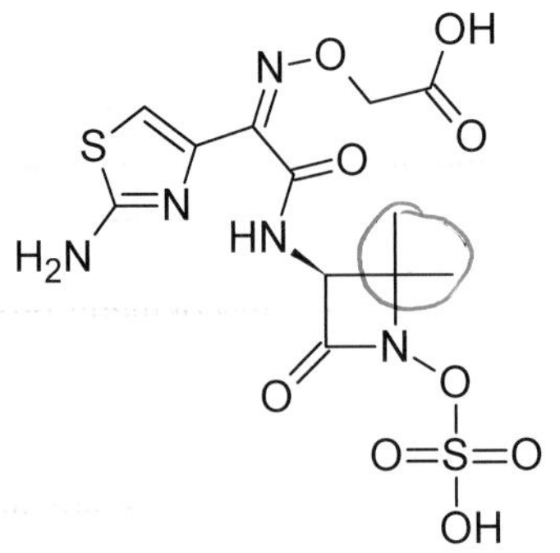

In contrast to the poor oral bioavailability of aztreonam, the oral absorption of tigemonam is excellent. It could become a valuable agent for the oral treatment of urinary tract infections and other non–life-threatening infections caused by β-lactamase–producing Gram-negative bacteria.

AMINOGLYCOSIDES

The discovery of streptomycin, the first aminoglycoside antibiotic to be used in chemotherapy, was the result of a planned and deliberate search begun in 1939 and brought to fruition in 1944 by Schatz and associates.[104] This success stimulated worldwide searches for antibiotics from the actinomycetes and, particularly, from the genus *Streptomyces*. Among the many antibiotics isolated from that genus, several are compounds closely related in structure to streptomycin. Six of them—kanamycin, neomycin, paromomycin, gentamicin, tobramycin, and netilmicin—currently are marketed in the United States. Amikacin, a semisynthetic derivative of kanamycin A, has been added, and it is possible that additional aminoglycosides will be introduced in the future.

All aminoglycoside antibiotics are absorbed very poorly (less than 1% under normal circumstances) following oral administration, and some of them (kanamycin, neomycin, and paromomycin) are administered by that route for the treatment of GI infections. Because of their potent broad-spectrum antimicrobial activity, they are also used for the treatment of systemic infections. Their undesirable side effects, particularly ototoxicity and nephrotoxicity, have restricted their systemic use to serious infections or infections caused by bacterial strains resistant to other agents. When administered for systemic infections, aminoglycosides must be given parenterally, usually by intramuscular injection. An additional antibiotic obtained from *Streptomyces*, spectinomycin, is also an aminoglycoside but differs chemically and microbiologically from other members of the group. It is used exclusively for the treatment of uncomplicated gonorrhea.

Chemistry

Aminoglycosides are so named because their structures consist of amino sugars linked glycosidically. All have at least one aminohexose, and some have a pentose lacking an amino group (e.g., streptomycin, neomycin, and paromomycin). Additionally, each of the clinically useful aminoglycosides contains a highly substituted 1,3-diaminocyclohexane central ring; in kanamycin, neomycin, gentamicin, and tobramycin, it is deoxystreptamine, and in streptomycin, it is streptadine. The aminoglycosides are thus strongly basic compounds that exist as polycations at physiological pH. Their inorganic acid salts are very soluble in water. All are available as sulfates. Solutions of the aminoglycoside salts are stable to autoclaving. The high water solubility of the aminoglycosides no doubt contributes to their pharmacokinetic properties. They distribute well into most body fluids but not into the central nervous system, bone, or fatty or connective tissues. They tend to concentrate in the kidneys and are excreted by glomerular filtration. Aminoglycosides are apparently not metabolized in vivo.

Spectrum of Activity

Although the aminoglycosides are classified as broad-spectrum antibiotics, their greatest usefulness lies in the treatment of serious systemic infections caused by aerobic Gram-negative bacilli. The choice of agent is generally between kanamycin, gentamicin, tobramycin, netilmicin, and amikacin. Aerobic Gram-negative and Gram-positive cocci (with the exception of staphylococci) tend to be less sensitive; thus, the β-lactams and other antibiotics tend to be preferred for the treatment of infections caused by these organisms. Anaerobic bacteria are invariably resistant to the aminoglycosides. Streptomycin is the most effective of the group for the chemotherapy of TB, brucellosis, tularemia, and *Yersinia* infections. Paromomycin is used primarily in the chemotherapy of amebic dysentery. Under certain circumstances, aminoglycoside and β-lactam antibiotics exert a synergistic action in vivo against some bacterial strains when the two are administered jointly. For example, carbenicillin and gentamicin are synergistic against gentamicin-sensitive strains of *P. aeruginosa* and several other species of Gram-negative bacilli, and penicillin G and streptomycin (or gentamicin or kanamycin) tend to be more effective than either agent alone in the treatment of enterococcal endocarditis. The two antibiotic types should not be combined in the same solution because they are chemically incompatible. Damage to the cell wall caused by the β-lactam antibiotic is believed to increase penetration of the aminoglycoside into the bacterial cell.

Mechanism of Action

Most studies concerning the mechanism of antibacterial action of the aminoglycosides were carried out with streptomycin. However, the specific actions of other aminoglycosides are thought to be qualitatively similar. The aminoglycosides act directly on the bacterial ribosome to inhibit the initiation of protein synthesis and to interfere with the fidelity of translation of the genetic message. They bind to the 30S ribosomal subunit to form a complex that cannot initiate proper amino acid polymerization.[105] The binding of streptomycin and other aminoglycosides to ribosomes also causes misreading mutations of the genetic code, apparently resulting from failure of specific aminoacyl RNAs to recognize the proper codons on messenger RNA (mRNA) and hence incorporation of improper amino acids into the peptide chain.[106] Evidence suggests that the deoxystreptamine-containing aminoglycosides differ quantitatively from streptomycin in causing misreading at lower concentrations than those required to prevent initiation of protein synthesis, whereas streptomycin is equally effective in inhibiting initiation and causing

misreading.[107] Spectinomycin prevents the initiation of protein synthesis but apparently does not cause misreading. All of the commercially available aminoglycoside antibiotics are bactericidal, except spectinomycin. The mechanism for the bactericidal action of the aminoglycosides is not known.

Microbial Resistance

The development of strains of Enterobacteriaceae resistant to antibiotics is a well-recognized, serious medical problem. Nosocomial (hospital acquired) infections caused by these organisms are often resistant to antibiotic therapy. Research has established clearly that multidrug resistance among Gram-negative bacilli to various antibiotics occurs and can be transmitted to previously nonresistant strains of the same species and, indeed, to different species of bacteria. Resistance is transferred from one bacterium to another by extrachromosomal R factors (DNA) that self-replicate and are transferred by conjugation (direct contact). The aminoglycoside antibiotics, because of their potent bactericidal action against Gram-negative bacilli, are now preferred for the treatment of many serious infections caused by coliform bacteria. A pattern of bacterial resistance to each of the aminoglycoside antibiotics, however, has developed as their clinical use has become more widespread. Consequently, there are bacterial strains resistant to streptomycin, kanamycin, and gentamicin. Strains carrying R factors for resistance to these antibiotics synthesize enzymes that are capable of acetylating, phosphorylating, or adenylylating key amino or hydroxyl groups of the aminoglycosides. Much of the recent effort in aminoglycoside research is directed toward identifying new, or modifying existing, antibiotics that are resistant to inactivation by bacterial enzymes.

Resistance of individual aminoglycosides to specific inactivating enzymes can be understood, in large measure, by using chemical principles. First, one can assume that if the target functional group is absent in a position of the structure normally attacked by an inactivating enzyme, then the antibiotic will be resistant to the enzyme. Second, steric factors may confer resistance to attack at functionalities otherwise susceptible to enzymatic attack. For example, conversion of a primary amino group to a secondary amine inhibits *N*-acetylation by certain aminoglycoside acetyl transferases. At least nine different types of aminoglycoside-inactivating enzymes have been identified and partially characterized.[108] The sites of attack of these enzymes and the biochemistry of the inactivation reactions is described briefly, using the kanamycin B structure (which holds the dubious distinction of being a substrate for all of the enzymes described) for illustrative purposes (Fig. 8.7).

Aminoglycoside-inactivating enzymes include (a) aminoacetyltransferases (designated AAC), which acetylate the 6'-NH$_2$ of ring I, the 3-NH$_2$ of ring II, or the 2'-NH$_2$ of ring I; (b) phosphotransferases (designated APH), which phosphorylate the 3'-OH of ring I or the 2″-OH of ring III; and (c) nucleotidyltransferases (ANT), which adenylate the 2″-OH of ring III, the 4'-OH of ring I, or the 4″-OH of ring III.

The gentamicins and tobramycin lack a 3'-hydroxyl group in ring I (see the section on the individual products for structures) and, consequently, are not inactivated by the phosphotransferase enzymes that phosphorylate that group in the kanamycins. Gentamicin C$_1$ (but not gentamicins C$_{1a}$

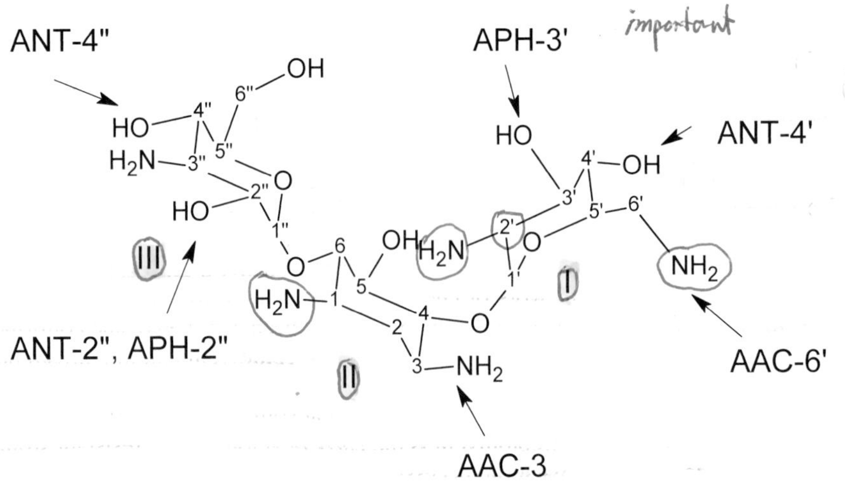

Figure 8.7 • Inactivation of kanamycin B by bacterial enzymes.

or C_2 or tobramycin) is resistant to the acetyltransferase that acetylates the 6'-amino group in ring I of kanamycin B. All gentamicins are resistant to the nucleotidyltransferase enzyme that adenylylates the secondary equatorial 4''-hydroxyl group of kanamycin B because the 4''-hydroxyl group in the gentamicins is *tertiary* and is oriented axially. Removal of functional groups susceptible to attacking an aminoglycoside occasionally can lead to derivatives that resist enzymatic inactivation and retain activity. For example, the 3'-deoxy-, 4'-deoxy-, and 3',4'-dideoxykanamycins are more similar to the gentamicins and tobramycin in their patterns of activity against clinical isolates that resist one or more of the aminoglycoside-inactivating enzymes.

The most significant breakthrough yet achieved in the search for aminoglycosides resistant to bacterial enzymes has been the development of amikacin, the 1-*N*-L-(-)-amino-α-hydroxybutyric acid (L-AHBA) derivative of kanamycin A. This remarkable compound retains most of the intrinsic potency of kanamycin A and is resistant to virtually all aminoglycoside-inactivating enzymes known, except the aminoacetyltransferase that acetylates the 6'-amino group and the nucleotidyltransferase that adenylylates the 4'-hydroxyl group of ring I.[108,109] The cause of amikacin's resistance to enzymatic inactivation is unknown, but it has been suggested that introduction of the L-AHBA group into kanamycin A markedly decreases its affinity for the inactivating enzymes. The importance of amikacin's resistance to enzymatic inactivation is reflected in the results of an investigation on the comparative effectiveness of amikacin and other aminoglycosides against clinical isolates of bacterial strains known to be resistant to one or more of the aminoglycosides.[110] In this study, amikacin was effective against 91% of the isolates (with a range of 87%–100%, depending on the species). Of the strains susceptible to other systemically useful aminoglycosides, 18% were susceptible to kanamycin, 36% to gentamicin, and 41% to tobramycin.

Low-level resistance associated with diminished aminoglycoside uptake has been observed in certain strains of *P. aeruginosa* isolated from nosocomial infections.[111] Bacterial susceptibility to aminoglycosides requires uptake of the drug by an energy-dependent active process.[112] Uptake is initiated by the binding of the cationic aminoglycoside to anionic phospholipids of the cell membrane. Electron transport–linked transfer of the aminoglycoside through the cell membrane then occurs. Divalent cations such as Ca^{2+} and

Mg^{2+} antagonize the transport of aminoglycosides into bacterial cells by interfering with their binding to cell membrane phospholipids. The resistance of anaerobic bacteria to the lethal action of the aminoglycosides is apparently because of the absence of the respiration-driven active-transport process for transporting the antibiotics.

Structure–Activity Relationships

Despite the complexity inherent in various aminoglycoside structures, some conclusions on SARs in this antibiotic class have been made.[113] Such conclusions have been formulated on the basis of comparisons of naturally occurring aminoglycoside structures, the results of selective semisynthetic modifications, and the elucidation of sites of inactivation by bacterial enzymes. It is convenient to discuss sequentially aminoglycoside SARs in terms of substituents in rings I, II, and III.

Ring I is crucially important for characteristic broad-spectrum antibacterial activity, and it is the primary target for bacterial inactivating enzymes. Amino functions at 6' and 2' are particularly important as kanamycin B (6'-amino, 2'-amino) is more active than kanamycin A (6'-amino, 2'-hydroxyl), which in turn is more active than kanamycin C (6'-hydroxyl, 2'-amino). Methylation at either the 6'-carbon or the 6'-amino positions does not lower appreciably antibacterial activity and confers resistance to enzymatic acetylation of the 6'-amino group. Removal of the 3'-hydroxyl or the 4'-hydroxyl group or both in the kanamycins (e.g., 3',4'-dideoxykanamycin B or dibekacin) does not reduce antibacterial potency. The gentamicins also lack oxygen functions at these positions, as do sisomicin and netilmicin, which also have a 4',5'-double bond. None of these derivatives is inactivated by phosphotransferase enzymes that phosphorylate the 3'-hydroxyl group. Evidently, the 3'-phosphorylated derivatives have very low affinity for aminoglycoside-binding sites in bacterial ribosomes.

Few modifications of ring II (deoxystreptamine) functional groups are possible without appreciable loss of activity in most of the aminoglycosides. The 1-amino group of kanamycin A can be acylated (e.g., amikacin), however, with activity largely retained. Netilmicin (1-*N*-ethylsisomicin) retains the antibacterial potency of sisomicin and is resistant to several additional bacteria-inactivating enzymes. 2''-Hydroxysisomicin is claimed to be resistant to bacterial strains that adenylate the 2″-hydroxyl group of ring III, whereas 3-deaminosisomicin exhibits good activity against bacterial strains that elaborate 3-acetylating enzymes.

Ring III functional groups appear to be somewhat less sensitive to structural changes than those of either ring I or ring II. Although the 2″-deoxygentamicins are significantly less active than their 2″-hydroxyl counterparts, the 2″-amino derivatives (seldomycins) are highly active. The 3″-amino group of gentamicins may be primary or secondary with high antibacterial potency. Furthermore, the 4″-hydroxyl group may be *axial* or *equatorial* with little change in potency.

Despite improvements in antibacterial potency and spectrum among newer naturally occurring and semisynthetic aminoglycoside antibiotics, efforts to find agents with improved margins of safety have been disappointing. The potential for toxicity of these important chemotherapeutic agents continues to restrict their use largely to the hospital environment.

The discovery of agents with higher potency/toxicity ratios remains an important goal of aminoglycoside research. In a now somewhat dated review, however, Price[114] expressed doubt that many significant clinical breakthroughs in aminoglycoside research would occur in the future.

Products

Streptomycin Sulfate, Sterile

Streptomycin sulfate is a white, odorless powder that is hygroscopic but stable toward light and air. It is freely soluble in water, forming solutions that are slightly acidic or nearly neutral. It is very slightly soluble in alcohol and is insoluble in most other organic solvents. Acid hydrolysis yields streptidine and streptobiosamine, the compound that is a combination of L-streptose and N-methyl-L-glucosamine.

Streptomycin acts as a triacidic base through the effect of its two strongly basic guanidino groups and the more weakly basic methylamino group. Aqueous solutions may be stored at room temperature for 1 week without any loss of potency, but they are most stable if the pH is between 4.5 and 7.0. The solutions decompose if sterilized by heating, so sterile solutions are prepared by adding sterile distilled water to the sterile powder. The early salts of streptomycin contained impurities that were difficult to remove and caused a histamine-like reaction. By forming a complex with calcium chloride, it was possible to free the streptomycin from these impurities and to obtain a product that was generally well tolerated.

The organism that produces streptomycin, *S. griseus*, also produces several other antibiotic compounds: hydroxystreptomycin, mannisidostreptomycin, and cycloheximide (q.v.).

Of these, only cycloheximide has achieved importance as a medicinally useful substance. The term *streptomycin A* has been used to refer to what is commonly called streptomycin, and mannisidostreptomycin has been called *streptomycin B*. Hydroxystreptomycin differs from streptomycin in having a hydroxyl group in place of one of the hydrogen atoms of the streptose methyl group. Mannisidostreptomycin has a mannose residue attached in glycosidic linkage through the hydroxyl group at C-4 of the N-methyl-L-glucosamine moiety. The work of Dyer et al.[115,116] to establish the stereochemical structure of streptomycin has been completed, and confirmed with the total synthesis of streptomycin and dihydrostreptomycin by Japanese scientists.[117]

Clinically, a problem that sometimes occurs with the use of streptomycin is the early development of resistant strains of bacteria, necessitating a change in therapy. Other factors that limit the therapeutic use of streptomycin are chronic toxicities. Neurotoxic reactions have been observed after the use of streptomycin. These are characterized by vertigo, disturbance of equilibrium, and diminished auditory perception. Additionally, nephrotoxicity occurs with some frequency. Patients undergoing therapy with streptomycin should have frequent checks of renal monitoring parameters. Chronic toxicity reactions may or may not be reversible. Minor toxic effects include rashes, mild malaise, muscular pains, and drug fever.

As a chemotherapeutic agent, streptomycin is active against numerous Gram-negative and Gram-positive bacteria. One of the greatest virtues of streptomycin is its effectiveness against the tubercle bacillus, *M. tuberculosis*. By itself, the antibiotic is not a cure, but it is a valuable adjunct to other treatment modalities for TB. The greatest drawback to the use of streptomycin is the rather rapid development of resistant strains of microorganisms. In infections that may be because of bacteria sensitive to both streptomycin and penicillin, the combined administration of the two antibiotics has been advocated. The possible development of damage to the otic nerve by the continued use of streptomycin-containing preparations has discouraged the use of such products. There has been an increasing tendency to reserve streptomycin products for the treatment of TB. It remains one of the agents of choice, however, for the treatment of certain "occupational" bacterial infections, such as brucellosis, tularemia, bubonic plague, and glanders. Because streptomycin is not absorbed when given orally or destroyed significantly in the GI tract, at one time it was used rather widely in the treatment of infections of the intestinal tract. For systemic action, streptomycin usually is given by intramuscular injection.

Neomycin Sulfate

In a search for antibiotics less toxic than streptomycin, Waksman and Lechevalier[118] isolated neomycin (Mycifradin, Neobiotic) in 1949 from *Streptomyces fradiae*. Since then, the importance of neomycin has increased steadily, and today, it is considered one of the most useful antibiotics for the treatment of GI infections, dermatological infections, and acute bacterial peritonitis. Also, it is used in abdominal surgery to reduce or avoid complications caused by infections from bacterial flora of the bowel. It has broad-spectrum activity against various organisms and shows a low incidence of toxic and hypersensitivity reactions. It is absorbed very slightly from the digestive tract, so its oral use ordinarily does not produce any systemic effect. The development of neomycin-resistant strains of pathogens is rarely reported in those organisms against which neomycin is effective.

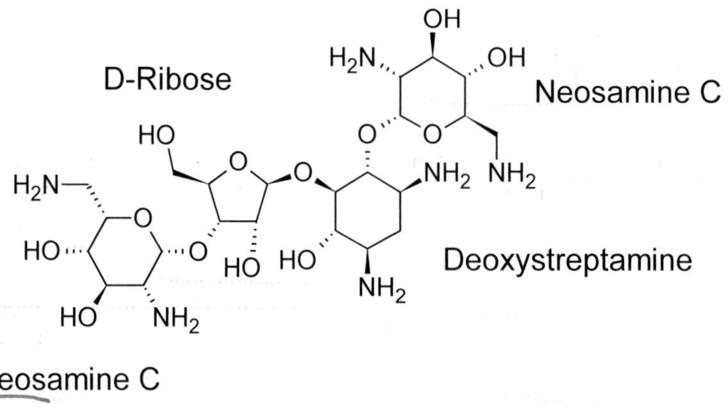

Neomycin as the sulfate salt is a white to slightly yellow, crystalline powder that is very soluble in water. It is hygroscopic and photosensitive (but stable over a wide pH range and to autoclaving). Neomycin sulfate contains the equivalent of 60% of the free base.

Neomycin, as produced by *S. fradiae*, is a mixture of closely related substances. Included in the "neomycin complex" is neamine (originally designated *neomycin A*) and neomycins B and C. *S. fradiae* also elaborates another antibiotic, the fradicin, which has some antifungal properties but no antibacterial activity. This substance is not present in "pure" neomycin.

The structures of neamine and neomycins B and C are known, and the absolute configurational structures of neamine and neomycin were reported by Hichens and Rinehart.[119] Neamine may be obtained by methanolysis of neomycins B and C, during which the glycosidic link between deoxystreptamine and D-ribose is broken. Therefore, neamine is a combination of deoxystreptamine and neosamine C, linked glycosidically (α) at the 4-position of deoxystreptamine. According to Hichens and Rinehart, neomycin B differs from neomycin C by the nature of the sugar attached terminally to D-ribose. That sugar, called *neosamine B*, differs from neosamine C in its stereochemistry. Rinehart et al.[120] have suggested that in neosamine the configuration is 2,6-diamino-2,6-dideoxy-L-idose, in which the orientation of the 6-aminomethyl group is inverted to the 6-amino-6-deoxy-D-glucosamine in neosamine C. In both instances, the glycosidic links were assumed to be α. Huettenrauch[121] later suggested, however, that both of the diamino sugars in neomycin C have the D-glucose configuration and that the glycosidic link is β in the one attached to D-ribose. The latter stereochemistry has been confirmed by the total synthesis of neomycin C.[122]

Paromomycin Sulfate

The isolation of paromomycin (Humatin) was reported in 1956 from a fermentation with a *Streptomyces* sp. (PD 04998), a strain said to resemble *S. rimosus* very closely. The parent organism had been obtained from soil samples collected in Colombia. Paromomycin, however, more closely resembles neomycin and streptomycin in antibiotic activity than it does oxytetracycline, the antibiotic obtained from *S. rimosus*.

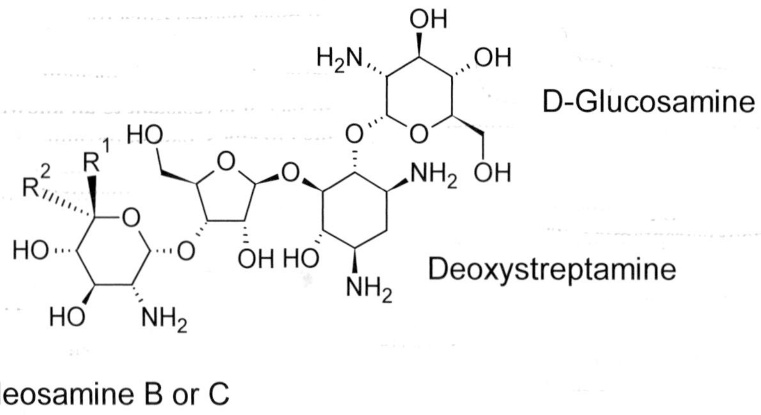

Paromomycin I: R^1=H; R^2=CH$_2$NH$_2$

Paromomycin II: R^1=CH$_2$NH$_2$; R^2= H

The general structure of paromomycin was reported by Haskell et al.[123] as one compound. Subsequently, chromatographic determinations have shown paromomycin to consist of two fractions, paromomycin I and paromomycin II. The absolute configurational structures for the paromomycins, as shown in the structural formula, were suggested by Hichens and Rinehart[119] and confirmed by DeJongh et al.[124] by mass spectrometric studies. The structure of paromomycin is the same as that of neomycin B, except that paromomycin contains D-glucosamine instead of the 6-amino-6-deoxy-D-glucosamine found in neomycin B. The same structural relationship is found between paromomycin II and neomycin C. The combination of D-glucosamine and deoxystreptamine is obtained by partial hydrolysis of both paromomycins and is called *paromamine* [4-(2-amino-2-deoxy-α-4-glucosyl)deoxystreptamine].

Paromomycin has broad-spectrum antibacterial activity and has been used for the treatment of GI infections caused by *Salmonella* and *Shigella* spp., and enteropathogenic *E. coli*. Currently, however, its use is restricted largely to the treatment of intestinal amebiasis. Paromomycin is soluble in water and stable to heat over a wide pH range.

Kanamycin Sulfate

Kanamycin (Kantrex) was isolated in 1957 by Umezawa and coworkers[125] from *Streptomyces kanamyceticus*. Its activity against mycobacteria and many intestinal bacteria, as well as several pathogens that show resistance to other antibiotics, brought a great deal of attention to this antibiotic. As a result, kanamycin was tested and released for medical use in a very short time.

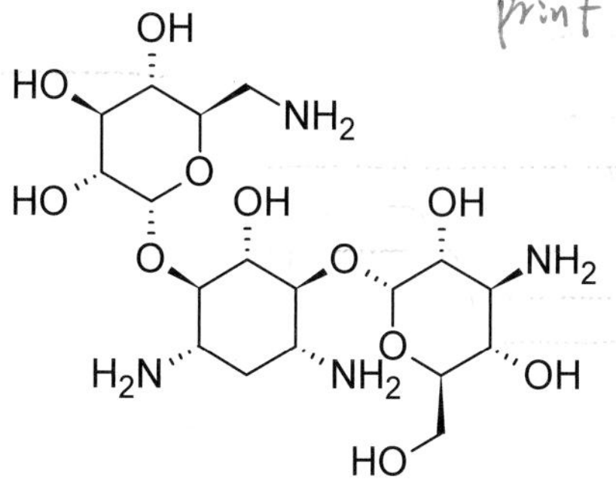

Research activity has been focused intensively on determining the structures of the kanamycins. Chromatography showed that *S. kanamyceticus* elaborates three closely related structures: kanamycins A, B, and C. Commercially available kanamycin is almost pure kanamycin A the least toxic of the three forms. The kanamycins differ only in the sugar moieties attached to the glycosidic oxygen on the 4-position of the central deoxystreptamine. The absolute configuration of the deoxystreptamine in kanamycins reported by Tatsuoka et al.[126] is shown above. The chemical relationships among the kanamycins, the neomycins, and the paromomycins were reported by Hichens and Rinehart.[119] The kanamycins do not have the D-ribose molecule that is present in neomycins and paromomycins. Perhaps this structural difference is related to the lower toxicity observed with kanamycins. The kanosamine fragment linked glycosidically to the 6-position of deoxystreptamine is 3-amino-3-deoxy-D-glucose (3-D-glucosamine) in all three kanamycins. The structures of the kanamycins have been proved by total synthesis.[127,128] They differ in the substituted D-glucoses attached glycosidically to the 4-position of

the deoxystreptamine ring. Kanamycin A contains 6-amino-6-deoxy-D-glucose; kanamycin B contains 2,6-diamino-2,6-dideoxy-D-glucose; and kanamycin C contains 2-amino-2-deoxy-D-glucose (see preceding diagram).

Kanamycin is basic and forms salts of acids through its amino groups. It is water soluble as the free base, but it is used in therapy as the sulfate salt, which is very soluble. It is stable to both heat and chemicals. Solutions resist both acids and alkali within the pH range of 2.0 to 11.0. Because of possible inactivation of either agent, kanamycin and penicillin salts should not be combined in the same solution.

The use of kanamycin in the United States usually is restricted to infections of the intestinal tract (e.g., bacillary dysentery) and to systemic infections arising from Gram-negative bacilli (e.g., *Klebsiella*, *Proteus*, *Enterobacter*, and *Serratia* spp.) that have developed resistance to other antibiotics. It has also been recommended for preoperative antisepsis of the bowel. It is absorbed poorly from the intestinal tract; consequently, systemic infections must be treated by intramuscular or (for serious infections) intravenous injections. These injections are rather painful, and the concomitant use of a local anesthetic is indicated. The use of kanamycin in the treatment of TB has not been widely advocated since the discovery that mycobacteria develop resistance very rapidly. In fact, both clinical experience and experimental work[129] indicate that kanamycin develops cross-resistance in the tubercle bacilli with dihydrostreptomycin, viomycin, and other antitubercular drugs. Like streptomycin, kanamycin may cause decreased or complete loss of hearing. On development of such symptoms, its use should be stopped immediately.

Amikacin

Amikacin, 1-N-amino-α-hydroxybutyrylkanamycin A (Amikin), is a semisynthetic aminoglycoside first prepared in Japan. The synthesis formally involves simple acylation of the 1-amino group of the deoxystreptamine ring of kanamycin A with L-AHBA. This particular acyl derivative retains about 50% of the original activity of kanamycin A against sensitive strains of Gram-negative bacilli. The L-AHBA derivative is much more active than the D-isomer.[130] The remarkable feature of amikacin is that it resists attack by most bacteria-inactivating enzymes and, therefore, is effective against strains of bacteria that are resistant to other aminoglycosides,[110] including gentamicin and tobramycin. In fact, it is resistant to all known aminoglycoside-inactivating enzymes, except the aminotransferase that acetylates the 6′-amino group[109] and the 4′-nucleotidyl transferase that adenylates the 4′-hydroxyl group of aminoglycosides.[108]

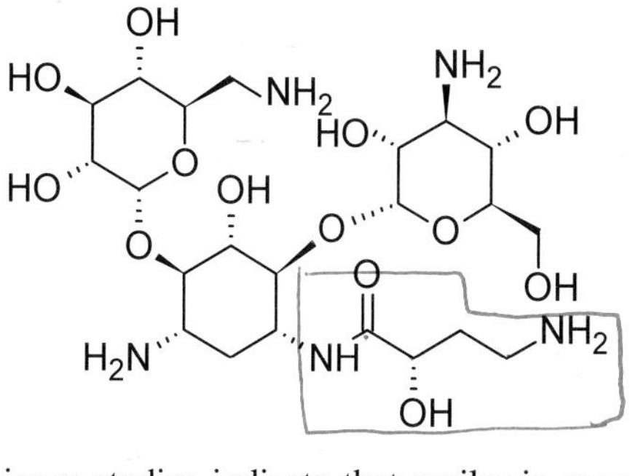

Preliminary studies indicate that amikacin may be less ototoxic than either kanamycin or gentamicin.[131] Higher dosages of amikacin are generally required, however, for the treatment of most Gram-negative bacillary infections. For this reason, and to discourage the proliferation of bacterial strains resistant to it, amikacin currently is recommended for the treatment of serious infections caused by bacterial strains resistant to other aminoglycosides.

Gentamicin Sulfate (prototype)

Gentamicin (Garamycin) was isolated in 1958 and reported in 1963 by Weinstein et al.[132] to belong to the streptomycinoid (aminocyclitol) group of antibiotics. It is obtained commercially from *Micromonospora purpurea*. Like the other members of its group, it has a broad spectrum of activity against many common pathogens, both Gram-positive and Gram-negative. Of particular interest is its strong activity against *P. aeruginosa* and other Gram-negative enteric bacilli.

Gentamicin is effective in the treatment of various skin infections for which a topical cream or ointment may be used. Because it offers no real advantage over topical neomycin in the treatment of all but pseudomonal infections, however, it is recommended that topical gentamicin be reserved for use in such infections and in the treatment of burns complicated by pseudomonemia. An injectable solution containing 40 mg of gentamicin sulfate per milliliter may be used for serious systemic and genitourinary tract infections caused by Gram-negative bacteria, particularly *Pseudomonas*, *Enterobacter*, and *Serratia* spp. Because of the development of strains of these bacterial species resistant to previously effective broad-spectrum antibiotics, gentamicin has been used for the treatment of hospital-acquired infections caused by such organisms. Resistant bacterial strains that inactivate gentamicin by adenylylation and acetylation, however, appear to be emerging with increasing frequency.

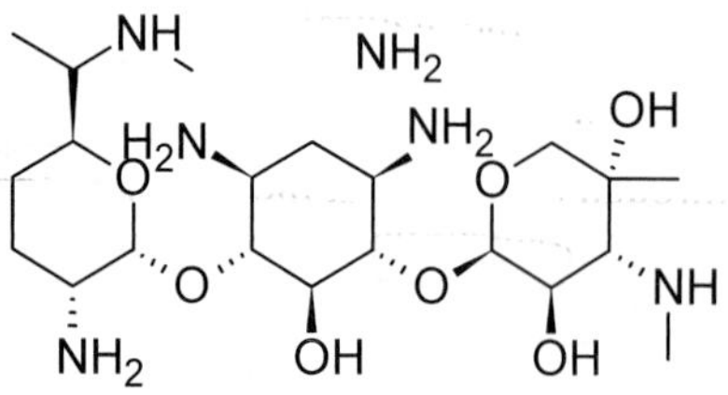

Gentamicin sulfate is a mixture of the salts of compounds identified as gentamicins C_1, C_2, and C_{1a}. These gentamicins were reported by Cooper et al.[133] to have the structures shown in the diagram. The absolute stereochemistries of the sugar components and the geometries of the glycosidic linkages have also been established.[134]

Coproduced, but not a part of the commercial product, are gentamicins A and B. Their structures were reported by Maehr and Schaffner[135] and are closely related to those of the gentamicins C. Although gentamicin molecules are similar in many ways to other aminocyclitols such as streptomycins, they are sufficiently different that their medical effectiveness is significantly greater. Gentamicin sulfate is a white to buff substance that is soluble in water and insoluble in alcohol, acetone, and benzene. Its solutions are stable over a wide pH range and may be autoclaved. It is chemically incompatible with carbenicillin, and the two should not be combined in the same intravenous solution.

Tobramycin Sulfate

Introduced in 1976, tobramycin sulfate (Nebcin) is the most active of the chemically related aminoglycosides called *nebramycins* obtained from a strain of *Streptomyces tenebrar-*

ius. Five members of the nebramycin complex have been identified chemically.[136]

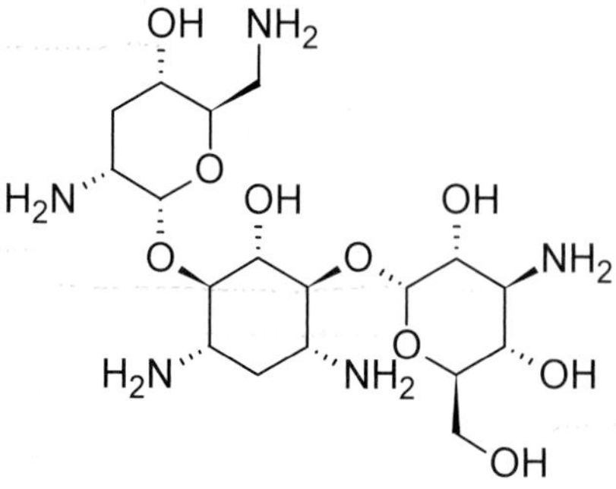

Factors 4 and 4′ are 6″-*O*-carbamoylkanamycin B and kanamycin B, respectively; factors 5′ and 6 are 6″-*O*-carbamoyltobramycin and tobramycin; and factor 2 is apramycin, a tetracyclic aminoglycoside with an unusual bicyclic central ring structure. Kanamycin B and tobramycin probably do not occur in fermentation broths per se but are formed by hydrolysis of the 6-*O*″-carbamoyl derivatives in the isolation procedure.

The most important property of tobramycin is its activity against most strains of *P. aeruginosa*, exceeding that of gentamicin by twofold to fourfold. Some gentamicin-resistant strains of this troublesome organism are sensitive to tobramycin, but others are resistant to both antibiotics.[137] Other Gram-negative bacilli and staphylococci are generally more sensitive to gentamicin. Tobramycin more closely resembles kanamycin B in structure (it is 3′-deoxykanamycin B).

Netilmicin Sulfate

Netilmicin sulfate, 1-*N*-ethylsisomicin (Netromycin), is a semisynthetic derivative prepared by reductive ethylation[138] of sisomicin, an aminoglycoside antibiotic obtained from *Micromonospora inyoensis*.[139] Structurally, sisomicin and netilmicin resemble gentamicin C_{1a}, a component of the gentamicin complex.

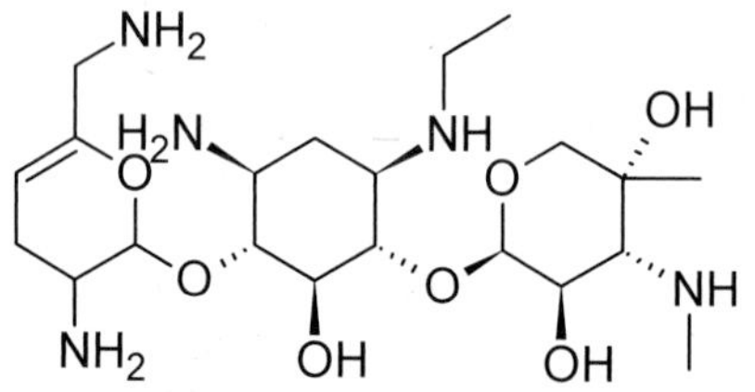

Against most strains of Enterobacteriaceae, *P. aeruginosa*, and *S. aureus*, sisomicin and netilmicin are comparable to gentamicin in potency.[140] Netilmicin is active, however, against many gentamicin-resistant strains, in particular among *E. coli*, *Enterobacter*, *Klebsiella*, and *Citrobacter* spp. A few strains of gentamicin-resistant *P. aeruginosa*, *S. marcescens*, and indole-positive *Proteus* spp. are also sensitive to netilmicin. Very few gentamicin-resistant bacterial strains are sensitive to sisomicin, however. The potency of netilmicin against certain gentamicin-resistant bacteria is attributed to its resistance to inactivation by bacterial enzymes that adenylylate or phosphorylate gentamicin and sisomicin. Evidently, the introduction of a 1-ethyl group in sisomicin markedly decreases the affinity of these enzymes for the molecule in a manner similar to that observed in the 1-*N*-ε-amino-α-hydroxybutyryl amide of kanamycin A (amikacin). Netilmicin, however, is inactivated by most of the bacterial enzymes that acetylate aminoglycosides, whereas amikacin is resistant to most of these enzymes.

The pharmacokinetic and toxicological properties of netilmicin and gentamicin appear to be similar clinically, though animal studies have indicated greater nephrotoxicity for gentamicin.

Sisomicin Sulfate

Although sisomicin has been approved for human use in the United States, it has not been marketed in this country. Its antibacterial potency and effectiveness against aminoglycoside-inactivating enzymes resemble those of gentamicin. Sisomicin also exhibits pharmacokinetics and pharmacological properties similar to those of gentamicin.

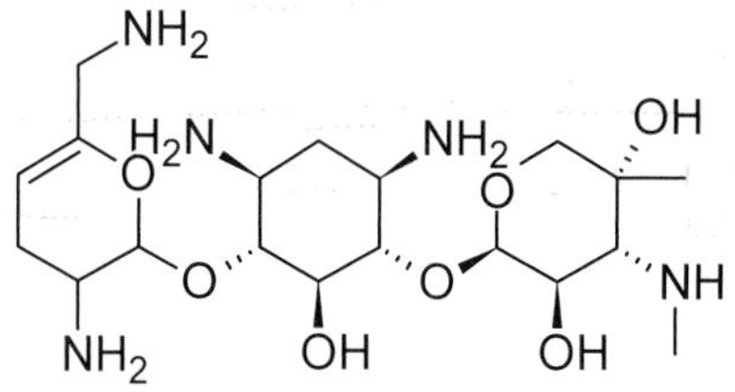

Spectinomycin Hydrochloride, Sterile

The aminocyclitol antibiotic spectinomycin hydrochloride (Trobicin), isolated from *Streptomyces spectabilis* and once called actinospectocin, was first described by Lewis and Clapp.[141] Its structure and absolute stereochemistry have been confirmed by x-ray crystallography.[142] It occurs as the white, crystalline dihydrochloride pentahydrate, which is stable in the dry form and very soluble in water. Solutions of spectinomycin, a hemiacetal, slowly hydrolyze on standing and should be prepared freshly and used within 24 hours. It is administered by deep intramuscular injection.

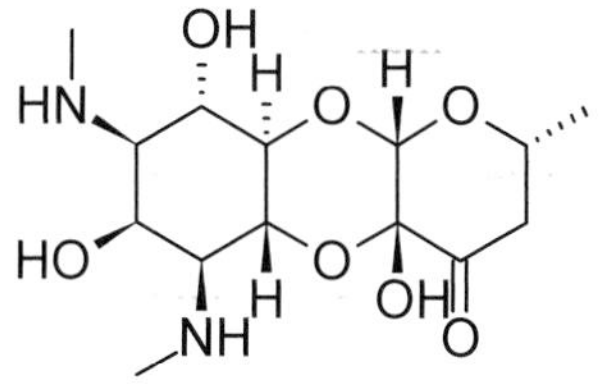

Spectinomycin is a broad-spectrum antibiotic with moderate activity against many Gram-positive and Gram-negative bacteria. It differs from streptomycin and the streptamine-containing aminoglycosides in chemical and antibacterial properties. Like streptomycin, spectinomycin interferes with the binding of transfer RNA (tRNA) to the ribosomes and thus with the initiation of protein synthesis. Unlike streptomycin or the streptamine-containing antibiotics, however, it does not cause misreading of the messenger. Spectinomycin exerts a bacteriostatic action and is inferior to other aminoglycosides for most systemic infections. Currently, it is recommended as an alternative to penicillin G salts for the treatment of uncomplicated gonorrhea. A cure rate of more than 90% has been observed in clinical studies for this indication. Many physicians prefer to use a tetracycline or erythromycin for prevention or treatment of suspected gonorrhea in penicillin-sensitive patients because, unlike these agents, spectinomycin is ineffective against syphilis. Furthermore, it is considerably more expensive than erythromycin and most of the tetracyclines.

TETRACYCLINES

Chemistry

Among the most important broad-spectrum antibiotics are members of the tetracycline family. Nine such compounds—tetracycline, rolitetracycline, oxytetracycline, chlortetracycline, demeclocycline, meclocycline, methacycline, doxycycline, and minocycline—have been introduced into medical use. Several others possess antibiotic activity. The tetracyclines are obtained by fermentation procedures from *Streptomyces* spp. or by chemical transformations of the natural products. Their chemical identities have been established by degradation studies and confirmed by the synthesis of three members of the group, oxytetracycline,[143,144] 6-demethyl-6-deoxytetracycline,[145] and anhydrochlortetracycline,[146] in their (α) forms. The important members of the group are derivatives of an octahydronaphthacene, a hydrocarbon system that comprises four annulated six-membered rings. The group name is derived from this tetracyclic system. The antibiotic spectra and chemical properties of these compounds are very similar but not identical.

The stereochemistry of the tetracyclines is very complex. Carbon atoms 4, 4a, 5, 5a, 6, and 12a are potentially chiral, depending on substitution. Oxytetracycline and doxycycline, each with a 5α-hydroxyl substituent, have six asymmetric centers; the others, lacking chirality at C-5, have only five. Determination of the complete, absolute stereochemistry of the tetracyclines was a difficult problem. Detailed x-ray diffraction analysis[147–149] established the stereochemical formula shown in Table 8.6 as the orientations found in the natural and semisynthetic tetracyclines. These studies also confirmed that conjugated systems exist in the structure from C-10 through C-12 and from C-1 through C-3 and that the formula represents only one of several canonical forms existing in those portions of the molecule.

Structure of the Tetracyclines

The tetracyclines are amphoteric compounds, forming salts with either acids or bases. In neutral solutions, these substances exist mainly as zwitterions. The acid salts, which are formed through protonation of the enol group on C-2, exist as crystalline compounds that are very soluble in water. These amphoteric antibiotics will crystallize out of aqueous solutions of their salts, however, unless stabilized by an excess of acid. The hydrochloride salts are used most commonly for oral administration and usually are encapsulated because they are bitter. Water-soluble salts may be obtained also from bases, such as sodium or potassium hydroxides, but they are not stable in aqueous solutions. Water-insoluble salts are formed with divalent and polyvalent metals.

The unusual structural groupings in the tetracyclines produce three acidity constants in aqueous solutions of the acid salts (Table 8.7). The particular functional groups responsible for each of the thermodynamic pK_a values were determined by Leeson et al.[150] as shown in the diagram that follows. These groupings had been identified previously by Stephens et al.[151] as the sites for protonation, but their earlier assignments, which produced the values responsible for

TABLE 8.6   Structures of Tetracyclines

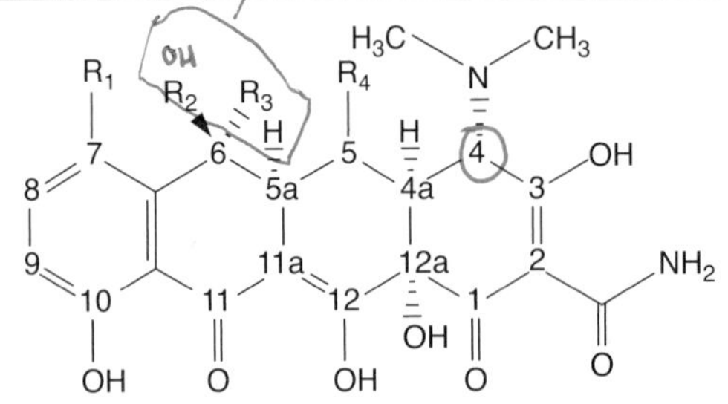

	R_1	R_2	R_3	R_4
Tetracycline	H	OH	CH₃	H
Chlortetracycline	Cl	OH	CH₃	H
Oxytetracycline	H	OH	CH₃	OH
Demeclocycline	Cl	OH	H	H
Methacycline	H	CH₂	H	OH
Doxycycline	H	CH₃	H	OH
Minocycline	N(CH₃)₂	H	H	H

pK_{a2} and pK_{a3}, were opposite those of Leeson et al.[150] This latter assignment has been substantiated by Rigler et al.[152]

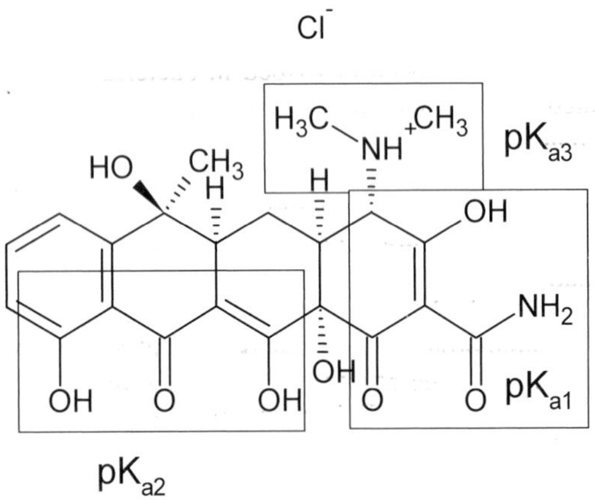

The approximate pK_a values for each of these groups in the six tetracycline salts in common use are shown (Table 8.7). The values are taken from Stephens et al.,[151] Benet and Goyan,[153] and Barringer et al.[154] The pK_a of the 7-dimethyl-amino group of minocycline (not listed) is 5.0.

An interesting property of the tetracyclines is their ability to undergo epimerization at C-4 in solutions of intermediate pH range. These isomers are called *epitetracyclines*.

Under acidic conditions, an equilibrium is established in about 1 day and consists of approximately equal amounts of the isomers. The partial structures below indicate the two forms of the epimeric pair. The 4-epitetracyclines have been isolated and characterized. They exhibit much less activity than the "natural" isomers, thus accounting for the decreased therapeutic value of aged solutions.

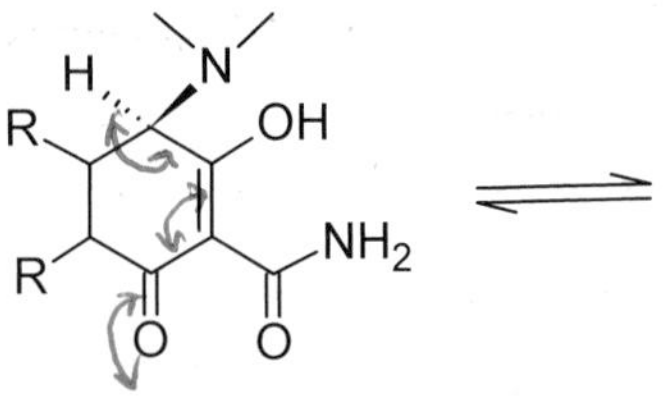

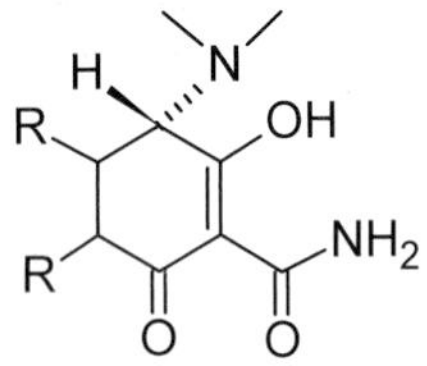

Epi   Natural

Strong acids and strong bases attack tetracyclines with a hydroxyl group on C-6, causing a loss in activity through modification of the C ring. Strong acids produce dehydration through a reaction involving the 6-hydroxyl group and the 5a-hydrogen. The double bond thus formed between positions 5a and 6 induces a shift in the position of the double bond between C-11a and C-12 to a position between C-11 and C-11a, forming the more energetically favored resonant system of the naphthalene group found in the inactive anhydrotetracyclines. Bases promote a reaction between the 6-hydroxyl group and the ketone group at the 11-position, causing the bond between the 11 and 11a atoms to cleave, forming the lactone ring found in the inactive isotetracycline. These two unfavorable reactions stimulated research that led to the development of the more stable and longer-acting compounds 6-deoxytetracycline, methacycline, doxycycline, and minocycline.

TABLE 8.7 pK_a Values (of Hydrochlorides) in Aqueous Solution at 25°C

	pK_{a1}	pK_{a2}	pK_{a3}
Tetracycline	3.3	7.7	9.5
Chlortetracycline	3.3	7.4	9.3
Demeclocycline	3.3	7.2	9.3
Oxytetracycline	3.3	7.3	9.1
Doxycycline	3.4	7.7	9.7
Minocycline	2.8	7.8	9.3

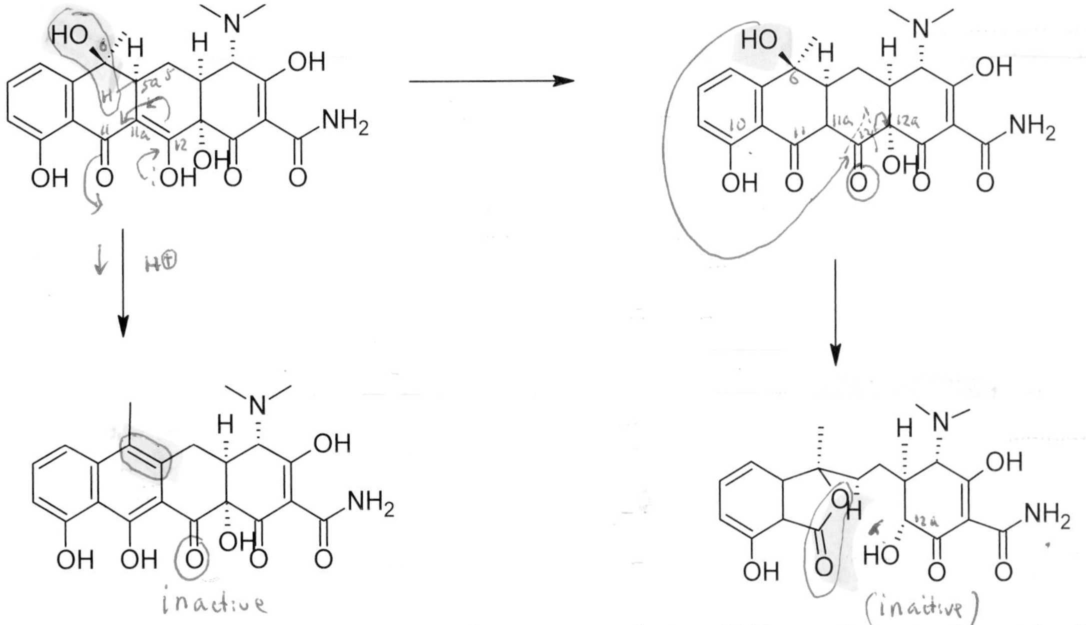

inactive

(inactive)   Isotetracycline

Stable chelate complexes are formed by the tetracyclines with many metals, including calcium, magnesium, and iron. Such chelates are usually very insoluble in water, accounting for the impaired absorption of most (if not all) tetracyclines in the presence of milk; calcium-, magnesium-, and aluminum-containing antacids; and iron salts. Soluble alkalinizers, such as sodium bicarbonate, also decrease the GI absorption of the tetracyclines.[155] Deprotonation of tetracyclines to more ionic species and the observed instability of these products in alkaline solutions may account for this observation. The affinity of tetracyclines for calcium causes them to be incorporated into newly forming bones and teeth as tetracycline–calcium orthophosphate complexes. Deposits of these antibiotics in teeth cause a yellow discoloration that darkens (a photochemical reaction) over time. Tetracyclines are distributed into the milk of lactating mothers and will cross the placental barrier into the fetus. The possible effects of these agents on the bones and teeth of the child should be considered before their use during pregnancy or in children younger than 8 years of age.

Mechanism of Action and Resistance

The strong binding properties of the tetracyclines with metal ions caused Albert[156] to suggest that their antibacterial properties may be because of an ability to remove essential metal ions as chelated compounds. Elucidation of details of the mechanism of action of the tetracyclines,[157] however, has defined more clearly the specific roles of magnesium ions in molecular processes affected by these antibiotics in bacteria. Tetracyclines are specific inhibitors of bacterial protein synthesis. They bind to the 30S ribosomal subunit and, thereby, prevent the binding of aminoacyl tRNA to the mRNA–ribosome complex. Both the binding of aminoacyl tRNA and the binding of tetracyclines at the ribosomal binding site require magnesium ions.[158] Tetracyclines also bind to mammalian ribosomes but with lower affinities, and they apparently do not achieve sufficient intracellular concentrations to interfere with protein synthesis. The selective toxicity of the tetracyclines toward bacteria depends strongly on the self-destructive capacity of bacterial cells to concentrate these

agents in the cell. Tetracyclines enter bacterial cells by two processes: passive diffusion and active transport. The active uptake of tetracyclines by bacterial cells is an energy-dependent process that requires adenosine triphosphate (ATP) and magnesium ions.[159]

Three biochemically distinct mechanisms of resistance to tetracyclines have been described in bacteria[160]: (a) efflux mediated by transmembrane-spanning, active-transport proteins that reduces the intracellular tetracycline concentration; (b) ribosomal protection, in which the bacterial protein synthesis apparatus is rendered resistant to the action of tetracyclines by an inducible cytoplasmic protein; and (c) enzymatic oxidation. Efflux mediated by plasmid or chromosomal protein determinants *tet*-A, -E, -G, -H, -K, and -L, and ribosomal protection mediated by the chromosomal protein determinants *tet*-M, -O, and -S are the most frequently encountered and most clinically significant resistance mechanisms for tetracyclines.

Spectrum of Activity

The tetracyclines have the broadest spectrum of activity of any known antibacterial agents. They are active against a wide range of Gram-positive and Gram-negative bacteria, spirochetes, mycoplasma, rickettsiae, and chlamydiae. Their potential indications are, therefore, numerous. Their bacteriostatic action, however, is a disadvantage in the treatment of life-threatening infections such as septicemia, endocarditis, and meningitis; the aminoglycosides and/or cephalosporins usually are preferred for Gram-negative and the penicillins for Gram-positive infections. Because of incomplete absorption and their effectiveness against the natural bacterial flora of the intestine, tetracyclines may induce superinfections caused by the pathogenic yeast *Candida albicans*. Resistance to tetracyclines among both Gram-positive and Gram-negative bacteria is relatively common. Superinfections caused by resistant *S. aureus* and *P. aeruginosa* have resulted from the use of these agents over time. Parenteral tetracyclines may cause severe liver damage, especially when given in excessive dosage to pregnant women or to patients with impaired renal function.

Structure–Activity Relationships

The large amount of research carried out to prepare semi-synthetic modifications of the tetracyclines and to obtain individual compounds by total synthesis revealed several interesting SARs. Reviews are available that discuss SARs among the tetracyclines in detail,[161–163] their molecular and clinical properties,[164] and their synthesis and chemical properties.[162,163,165,166] Only a brief review of the salient structure–activity features is presented here. All derivatives containing fewer than four rings are inactive or nearly inactive. The simplest tetracycline derivative that retains the characteristic broad-spectrum activity associated with this antibiotic class is 6-demethyl-6-deoxytetracycline. Many of the precise structural features present in this molecule must remain unmodified for derivatives to retain activity. The integrity of substituents at carbon atoms 1, 2, 3, 4, 10, 11, 11a, and 12, representing the hydrophilic "southern and eastern" faces of the molecule, cannot be violated drastically without deleterious effects on the antimicrobial properties of the resulting derivatives.

A-ring substituents can be modified only slightly without dramatic loss of antibacterial potency. The enolized tricarbonylmethane system at C-1 to C-3 must be intact for good activity. Replacement of the amide at C-2 with other functions (e.g., aldehyde or nitrile) reduces or abolishes activity. Monoalkylation of the amide nitrogen reduces activity proportionately to the size of the alkyl group. Aminoalkylation of the amide nitrogen, accomplished by the Mannich reaction, yields derivatives that are substantially more water soluble than the parent tetracycline and are hydrolyzed to it in vivo (e.g., rolitetracycline). The dimethylamino group at the 4-position must have the α orientation; 4-epitetracyclines are very much less active than the natural isomers. Removal of the 4-dimethylamino group reduces activity even further. Activity is largely retained in the primary and N-methyl secondary amines but rapidly diminishes in the higher alkylamines. A cis-A/B-ring fusion with a β-hydroxyl group at C-12a is apparently also essential. Esters of the C-12a hydroxyl group are inactive, with the exception of the formyl ester, which readily hydrolyzes in aqueous solutions. Alkylation at C-11a also leads to inactive compounds, demonstrating the importance of an enolizable β-diketone functionality at C-11 and C-12. The importance of the shape of the tetracyclic ring system is illustrated further by substantial loss in antibacterial potency resulting from epimerization at C-5a. Dehydrogenation to form a double bond between C-5a and C-11a markedly decreases activity, as does aromatization of ring C to form anhydrotetracyclines.

In contrast, substituents at positions 5, 5a, 6, 7, 8, and 9, representing the largely hydrophobic "northern and western" faces of the molecule, can be modified with varying degrees of success, resulting in retention and, sometimes, improvement of antibiotic activity. A 5-hydroxyl group, as in oxytetracycline and doxycycline, may influence pharmacokinetic properties but does not change antimicrobial activity. 5a-Epitetracyclines (prepared by total synthesis), although highly active in vitro, are unfortunately much less impressive in vivo. Acid-stable 6-deoxytetracyclines and 6-demethyl-6-deoxytetracyclines have been used to prepare various monosubstituted and disubstituted derivatives by electrophilic substitution reactions at C-7 and C-9 of the D ring. The more useful results have been achieved with the

introduction of substituents at C-7. Oddly, strongly electron-withdrawing groups (e.g., chloro [lortetracycline] and nitro) and strongly electron-donating groups (e.g., dimethylamino [minocycline]) enhance activity. This unusual circumstance is reflected in QSAR studies of 7- and 9-substituted tetracyclines,[162,167] which indicated a squared (parabolic) dependence on σ, Hammet's electronic substituent constant, and in vitro inhibition of an E. coli strain. The effect of introducing substituents at C-8 has not been studied because this position cannot be substituted directly by classic electrophilic aromatic substitution reactions; thus, 8-substituted derivatives are available only through total synthesis.[168]

The most fruitful site for semisynthetic modification of the tetracyclines has been the 6-position. Neither the 6α-methyl nor the 6β-hydroxyl group is essential for antibacterial activity. In fact, doxycycline and methacycline are more active in vitro than their parent oxytetracycline against most bacterial strains. The conversion of oxytetracycline to doxycycline, which can be accomplished by reduction of methacycline,[169] gives a 1:1 mixture of doxycycline and epidoxycycline (which has a β-oriented methyl group); if the C-11a α-fluoro derivative of methacycline is used, the β-methyl epimer is formed exclusively.[170] 6-Epidoxycycline is much less active than doxycycline. 6-Demethyl-6-deoxytetracycline, synthesized commercially by catalytic hydrogenolysis of the 7-chloro and 6-hydroxyl groups of 7-chloro-6-demethyltetracycline, obtained by fermentation of a mutant strain of Streptomyces aureofaciens,[171] is slightly more potent than tetracycline. More successful from a clinical standpoint, however, is 6-demethyl-6-deoxy-7-dimethylaminotetracycline (minocycline)[172] because of its activity against tetracycline-resistant bacterial strains.

6-Deoxytetracyclines also possess important chemical and pharmacokinetic advantages over their 6-oxy counterparts. Unlike the latter, they are incapable of forming anhydrotetracyclines under acidic conditions because they cannot dehydrate at C-5a and C-6. They are also more stable in base because they do not readily undergo β-ketone cleavage, followed by lactonization, to form isotetracyclines. Although it lacks a 6-hydroxyl group, methacycline shares the instability of the 6-oxytetracyclines in strongly acetic conditions. It suffers prototropic rearrangement to the anhydrotetracycline in acid but is stable to β-ketone cleavage followed by lactonization to the isotetracycline in base. Reduction of the 6-hydroxyl group also dramatically changes the solubility properties of tetracyclines. This effect is reflected in significantly higher oil/water partition coefficients of the 6-deoxytetracyclines than of the tetracyclines (Table 8.8).[173,174] The greater lipid solubility of the 6-deoxy compounds has important pharmacokinetic consequences.[162,164] Hence, doxycycline and minocycline are absorbed more completely following oral administration, exhibit higher fractions of plasma protein binding, and have higher volumes of distribution and lower renal clearance rates than the corresponding 6-oxytetracyclines.

Polar substituents (i.e., hydroxyl groups) at C-5 and C-6 decrease lipid versus water solubility of the tetracyclines. The 6-position is, however, considerably more sensitive than the 5-position to this effect. Thus, doxycycline (6-deoxy-5-oxytetracycline) has a much higher partition coefficient than either tetracycline or oxytetracycline. Nonpolar substituents (those with positive σ values; see Chapter 2),

Good

TABLE 8.8 Pharmacokinetic Properties[a] of Tetracyclines

Tetracycline	K_{pc} Octanol/ Water pH 5.6[b]	Absorbed Orally (%)	Excreted in Feces (%)	Excreted in Urine (%)	Protein Bound (%)	Volume of Distribution (% body weight)	Renal Clearance (mL/min/ 1.73 m²)	Half-life (h)
Tetracycline	0.056	58	20–50	60	24–65	156–306	50–80	10
Oxytetracycline	0.075	77–80	50	70	20–35	180–305	99–102	9
Chlortetracycline	0.41	25–30	>50	18	42–54	149	32	7
Demeclocycline	0.25	66	23–72	42	68–77	179	35	15
Doxycycline	0.95	93	20–40	27–39	60–91	63	18–28	15
Minocycline	1.10	100	40	5–11	55–76	74	5–15	19

[a]Values taken from Brown, J. R., and Ireland, D. S.: Adv. Pharmacol. Chemother. 15:161, 1978.
[b]Values taken from Colazzi, J. L., and Klink, P. R.: J. Pharm. Sci. 58:158, 1969.

for example, 7-dimethylamino, 7-chloro, and 6-methyl, have the opposite effect. Accordingly, the partition coefficient of chlortetracycline is substantially greater than that of tetracycline and slightly greater than that of demeclocycline. Interestingly, minocycline (5-demethyl-6-deoxy-7-dimethyl-aminotetracycline) has the highest partition coefficient of the commonly used tetracyclines.

The poorer oral absorption of the more water-soluble compounds tetracycline and oxytetracycline can be attributed to several factors. In addition to their comparative difficulty in penetrating lipid membranes, the polar tetracyclines probably experience more complexation with metal ions in the gut and undergo some acid-catalyzed destruction in the stomach. Poorer oral absorption coupled with biliary excretion of some tetracyclines is also thought to cause a higher incidence of superinfections from resistant microbial strains. The more polar tetracyclines, however, are excreted in higher concentrations in the urine (e.g., 60% for tetracycline and 70% for oxytetracycline) than the more lipid-soluble compounds (e.g., 33% for doxycycline and only 11% for minocycline). Significant passive renal tubular reabsorption coupled with higher fractions of protein binding contributes to the lower renal clearance and longer durations of action of doxycycline and minocycline compared with those of the other tetracyclines, especially tetracycline and oxytetracycline. Minocycline also experiences significant *N*-dealkylation catalyzed by cytochrome P450 oxygenases in the liver, which contributes to its comparatively low renal clearance. Although all tetracyclines are distributed widely into tissues, the more polar ones have larger volumes of distribution than the nonpolar compounds. The more lipid-soluble tetracyclines, however, distribute better to poorly vascularized tissue. It is also claimed that the distribution of doxycycline and minocycline into bone is less than that of other tetracyclines.[175]

↑ lipophilic → ↑ protein bound → ↓ D_v

Products

Tetracycline

Chemical studies on chlortetracycline revealed that controlled catalytic hydrogenolysis selectively removed the 7-chloro atom and so produced tetracycline (Achromycin, Cyclopar, Panmycin, Tetracyn). This process was patented by Conover[176] in 1955. Later, tetracycline was obtained from fermentations of *Streptomyces* spp., but the commercial supply still chiefly depends on hydrogenolysis of chlortetracycline.

Tetracycline is 4-dimethyl amino-1,4,4a,5,5a,6,11,12a-octahydro-3,6,10,12,12a-pentahydroxy-6-methyl-1,11-dioxo-2-naphthacenecarboxamide. It is a bright yellow, crystalline salt that is stable in air but darkens on exposure to strong sunlight. Tetracycline is stable in acid solutions with a pH above 2. It is somewhat more stable in alkaline solutions than chlortetracycline, but like those of the other tetracyclines, such solutions rapidly lose potency. One gram of the base requires 2,500 mL of water and 50 mL of alcohol to dissolve it. The hydrochloride salt is used most commonly in medicine, though the free base is absorbed from the GI tract about equally well. One gram of the hydrochloride salt dissolves in about 10 mL of water and in 100 mL of alcohol. Tetracycline has become the most popular antibiotic of its group, largely because its plasma concentration appears to be higher and more enduring than that of either oxytetracycline or chlortetracycline. Also, it is found in higher concentration in the spinal fluid than the other two compounds.

Several combinations of tetracycline with agents that increase the rate and the height of plasma concentrations are on the market. One such adjuvant is magnesium chloride hexahydrate (Panmycin). Also, an insoluble tetracycline phosphate complex (Tetrex) is made by mixing a solution of tetracycline, usually as the hydrochloride, with a solution of sodium metaphosphate. There are various claims concerning the efficacy of these adjuvants. The mechanisms of their actions are not clear, but reportedly[177,178] these agents enhance plasma concentrations over those obtained when tetracycline hydrochloride alone is administered orally. Remmers et al.[179,180] reported on the effects that selected aluminum–calcium gluconates complexed with some tetracyclines have on plasma concentrations when administered orally, intramuscularly, or intravenously. Such complexes enhanced plasma levels in dogs when injected but not when given orally. They also observed enhanced plasma levels in experimental animals when complexes of tetracyclines with aluminum metaphosphate, aluminum pyrophosphate, or aluminum–calcium phosphinicodilactates were administered orally. As noted previously, the tetracyclines can form stable chelate complexes with metal ions such as calcium and magnesium, which retard absorption from the GI tract. The complexity of the systems involved has not permitted unequivocal substantiation of the idea that these adjuvants compete with the tetracyclines for substances in the alimentary tract that would otherwise be free to complex with these antibiotics and thereby retard their absorption. Certainly, there is no evidence that the metal ions per se act as buffers, an idea alluded to sometimes in the literature.

Tetracycline hydrochloride is also available in ointments for topical and ophthalmic administration. A topical solution is used for the management of acne vulgaris.

Rolitetracycline

Rolitetracycline, *N*-(pyrrolidinomethyl)tetracycline (Syntetrin), was introduced for use by intramuscular or intravenous injection. This derivative is made by condensing tetracycline with pyrrolidine and formaldehyde in the presence of *tert*-butyl alcohol. It is very soluble in water (1 g dissolves in about 1 mL) and provides a means of injecting the antibiotic in a small volume of solution. It has been recommended for cases when the oral dosage forms are not suitable, but it is no longer widely used.

Chlortetracycline Hydrochloride

Chlortetracycline (Aureomycin hydrochloride) was isolated by Duggar[181] in 1948 from *S. aureofaciens*. This compound, which was produced in an extensive search for new antibiotics, was the first of the group of highly successful tetracyclines. It soon became established as a valuable antibiotic with broad-spectrum activities.

It is used in medicine chiefly as the acid salt of the compound whose systematic chemical designation is 7-chloro-4-(dimethylamino)-1,4,4a,5,5a,6,11,12a-octahydro-3,6,10,12,12a-pentahydroxy-6-methyl-1,11-dioxo-2-naphthacenecarboxamide. The hydrochloride salt is a crystalline powder with a bright yellow color, which suggested its brand name, *Aureomycin*. It is stable in air but slightly photosensitive and should be protected from light. It is odorless and bitter. One gram of the hydrochloride salt will dissolve in about 75 mL of water, producing a pH of about 3. It is only slightly soluble in alcohol and practically insoluble in other organic solvents.

Oral and parenteral forms of chlortetracycline are no longer used because of the poor bioavailability and inferior pharmacokinetic properties of the drug. It is still marketed in ointment forms for topical and ophthalmic use.

Oxytetracycline Hydrochloride

Early in 1950, Finlay et al.[182] reported the isolation of oxytetracycline (Terramycin) from *S. rimosus*. This compound was soon identified as a chemical analog of chlortetracy-

cline that showed similar antibiotic properties. The structure of oxytetracycline was elucidated by Hochstein et al.[183] and this work provided the basis for the confirmation of the structure of the other tetracyclines.

Oxytetracycline hydrochloride is a pale yellow, bitter, crystalline compound. The amphoteric base is only slightly soluble in water and slightly soluble in alcohol. It is odorless and stable in air but darkens on exposure to strong sunlight. The hydrochloride salt is a stable yellow powder that is more bitter than the free base. It is much more soluble in water, 1 g dissolving in 2 mL, and more soluble in alcohol than the free base. Both compounds are inactivated rapidly by alkali hydroxides and by acid solutions below pH 2. Both forms of oxytetracycline are absorbed rapidly and equally well from the digestive tract, so the only real advantage the free base offers over the hydrochloride salt is that it is less bitter. Oxytetracycline hydrochloride is also used for parenteral administration (intravenously and intramuscularly).

Methacycline Hydrochloride

The synthesis of methacycline, 6-deoxy-6-demethyl-6-methylene-5-oxytetracycline hydrochloride (Rondomycin), reported by Blackwood et al.[184] in 1961, was accomplished by chemical modification of oxytetracycline. It has an antibiotic spectrum like that of the other tetracyclines but greater potency; about 600 mg of methacycline is equivalent to 1 g of tetracycline. Its particular value lies in its longer serum half-life; doses of 300 mg produce continuous serum antibacterial activity for 12 hours. Its toxic manifestations and contraindications are similar to those of the other tetracyclines.

The greater stability of methacycline, both in vivo and in vitro, results from modification at C-6. Removal of the 6-hydroxy group markedly increases the stability of ring C to both acids and bases, preventing the formation of isotetracyclines by bases. Anhydrotetracyclines still can form, however, by acid-catalyzed isomerization under strongly acidic conditions. Methacycline hydrochloride is a yellow to dark yellow, crystalline powder that is slightly soluble in water and insoluble in nonpolar solvents. It should be stored in tight, light-resistant containers in a cool place.

Demeclocycline

Demeclocycline, 7-chloro-6-demethyltetracycline (Declomycin), was isolated in 1957 by McCormick et al.[171] from a mutant strain of *S. aureofaciens*. Chemically, it is 7-chloro-4-(dimethylamino)1,4,4a,5,5a,6, 11, 12a-octahydro-3, 6, 10, 12, 12a-pentahydroxy1, 11-dioxo2-naphthacenecarboxamide. Thus, it differs from chlortetracycline only in the absence of the methyl group on C-6.

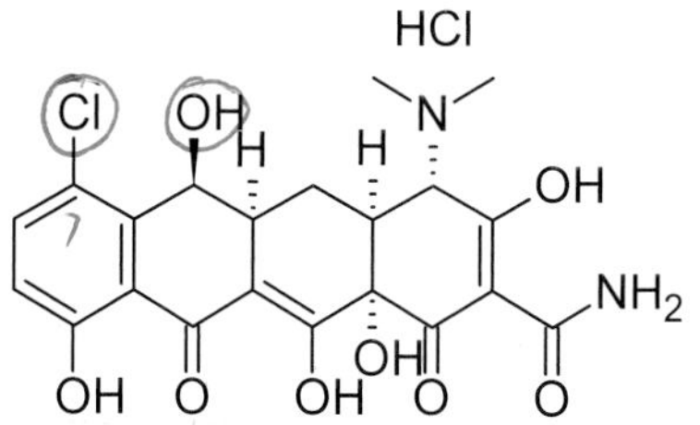

Demeclocycline is a yellow, crystalline powder that is odorless and bitter. It is sparingly soluble in water. A 1% solution has a pH of about 4.8. It has an antibiotic spectrum like that of other tetracyclines, but it is slightly more active than the others against most of the microorganisms for which they are used. This, together with its slower rate of elimination through the kidneys, makes demeclocycline as effective as the other tetracyclines, at about three fifths of the dose. Like the other tetracyclines, it may cause infrequent photosensitivity reactions that produce erythema after exposure to sunlight. Demeclocycline may produce this reaction somewhat more frequently than the other tetracyclines. The incidence of discoloration and mottling of the teeth in youths from demeclocycline appears to be as low as that from other tetracyclines.

Meclocycline Sulfosalicylate

Meclocycline, 7-chloro-6-deoxy-6-demethyl-6-methylene-5-oxytetracycline sulfosalicylate (Meclan), is a semisynthetic derivative prepared from oxytetracycline.[184] Although meclocycline has been used in Europe for many years, it became available only relatively recently in the United States for a single therapeutic indication, the treatment of acne. It is available as the sulfosalicylate salt in a 1% cream.

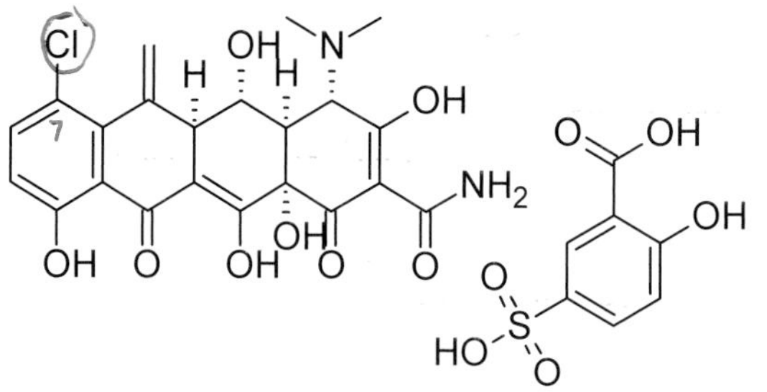

Meclocycline sulfosalicylate is a bright yellow, crystalline powder that is slightly soluble in water and insoluble in organic solvents. It is light sensitive and should be stored in light-resistant containers.

Doxycycline ✗

A more recent addition to the tetracycline group of antibiotics available for antibacterial therapy is doxycycline, α-6-deoxy-5-oxytetracycline (Vibramycin), first reported by Stephens et al.[185] in 1958. It was obtained first in small yields by a chemical transformation of oxytetracycline, but it is now produced by catalytic hydrogenation of methacycline or by reduction of a benzyl mercaptan derivative of methacycline with Raney nickel. The latter process produces a nearly pure form of the 6α-methyl epimer. The 6α-methyl epimer is more than 3 times as active as its β-epimer.[169] Apparently, the difference in orientation of the methyl groups, which slightly affects the shapes of the molecules, causes a substantial difference in biological

effect. Also, absence of the 6-hydroxyl group produces a compound that is very stable in acids and bases and that has a long biological half-life. In addition, it is absorbed very well from the GI tract, thus allowing a smaller dose to be administered. High tissue levels are obtained with it, and unlike other tetracyclines, doxycycline apparently does not accumulate in patients with impaired renal function. Therefore, it is preferred for uremic patients with infections outside the urinary tract. Its low renal clearance may limit its effectiveness, however, in urinary tract infections.

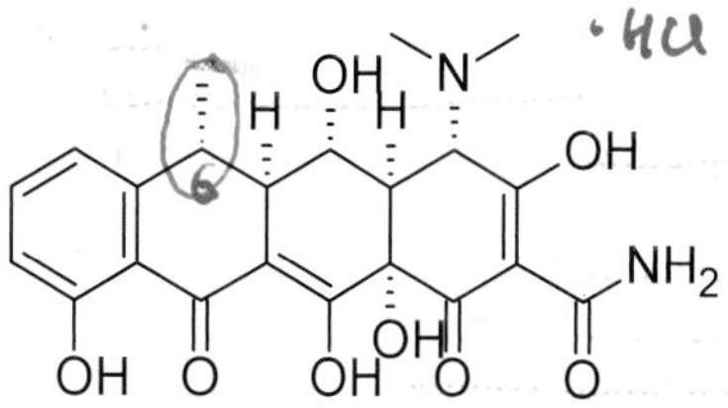

Doxycycline is available as a hydrate salt, a hydrochloride salt solvated as the hemiethanolate hemihydrate, and a monohydrate. The hydrate form is sparingly soluble in water and is used in a capsule; the monohydrate is water insoluble and is used for aqueous suspensions, which are stable for up to 2 weeks when kept in a cool place.

Minocycline Hydrochloride ✱

Minocycline, 7-dimethylamino-6-demethyl-6-deoxytetracycline (Minocin, Vectrin), the most potent tetracycline currently used in therapy, is obtained by reductive methylation of 7-nitro-6-demethyl-6-deoxytetracycline.[172] It was released for use in the United States in 1971. Because minocycline, like doxycycline, lacks the 6-hydroxyl group, it is stable in acids and does not dehydrate or rearrange to anhydro or lactone forms. Minocycline is well absorbed orally to give high plasma and tissue levels. It has a very long serum half-life, resulting from slow urinary excretion and moderate protein binding. Doxycycline and minocycline, along with oxytetracycline, show the least in vitro calcium binding of the clinically available tetracyclines. The improved distribution properties of the 6-deoxytetracyclines have been attributed to greater lipid solubility.

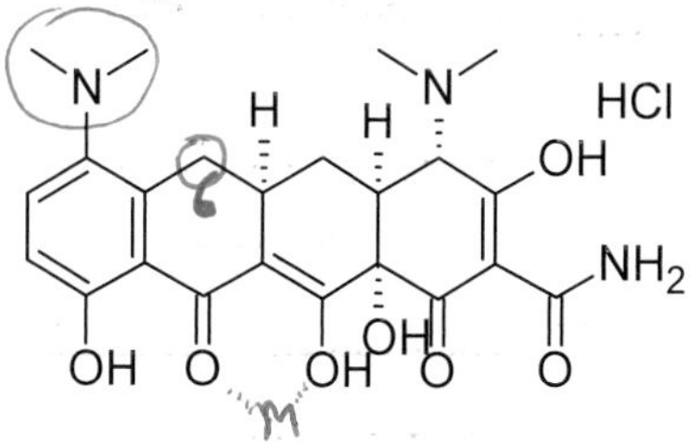

Perhaps the most outstanding property of minocycline is its activity toward Gram-positive bacteria, especially staphylococci and streptococci. In fact, minocycline has been effective against staphylococcal strains that are resistant to methicillin and all other tetracyclines, including doxycycline.[186] Although it is doubtful that minocycline will replace bactericidal agents for the treatment of life-threatening staphylococcal infections, it may become a useful alternative for the treatment of less serious tissue infections. Minocycline has been recommended for the treatment of chronic bronchitis and other upper respiratory tract infections. Despite its relatively low renal clearance, partially compensated for by high serum and tissue levels, it has been recommended for the treatment of urinary tract infections. It has been effective in the eradication of *N. meningitidis* in asymptomatic carriers.

NEWER TETRACYCLINES

The remarkably broad spectrum of antimicrobial activity of the tetracyclines notwithstanding, the widespread emergence of bacterial genes and plasmids encoding tetracycline resistance has increasingly imposed limitations on the clinical applications of this antibiotic class in recent years.[164] This situation has prompted researchers at Lederle Laboratories to reinvestigate SARs of tetracyclines substituted in the aromatic (D) ring in an effort to discover analogs that might be effective against resistant strains. As a result of these efforts, the glycylcyclines, a class of 9-dimethylglycylamino-(DMG)-substituted tetracyclines exemplified by DMG-minocycline (DMG-MINO), and DMG-6-methyl-6-deoxytetracycline (DMG-DMDOT) were discovered.[187–189]

The first of these to be marketed was tigecycline.

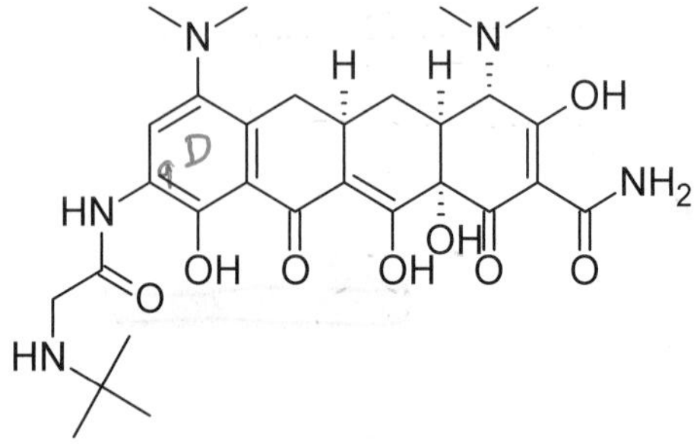

The glycylcyclines retain the broad spectrum of activity and potency exhibited by the original tetracyclines against tetracycline-sensitive microbial strains and are highly active against bacterial strains that exhibit tetracycline resistance mediated by efflux or ribosomal protection determinants. If ongoing clinical evaluations of the glycylcyclines establish favorable toxicological and pharmacokinetic profiles for these compounds, a new class of "second-generation" tetracyclines could be launched.

⬡ MACROLIDES

Among the many antibiotics isolated from the actinomycetes is the group of chemically related compounds called the *macrolides.* In 1950, picromycin, the first of this group to be identified as a macrolide compound, was first reported. In 1952, erythromycin and carbomycin were reported as new antibiotics, and they were followed in subsequent years by other macrolides. Currently, more than 40 such compounds are known, and new ones are likely to appear in the future. Of all of these, only two, erythromycin and oleandomycin, have been available consistently for medical use in the United States. In recent years, interest has shifted away from novel macrolides isolated from soil samples (e.g., spiramycin, josamycin, and rosamicin), all of which thus far have proved to be clinically inferior to erythromycin and semisynthetic derivatives of erythromycin (e.g., clarithromycin and azithromycin), which have superior pharmacokinetic properties because of their enhanced acid stability and improved distribution properties.

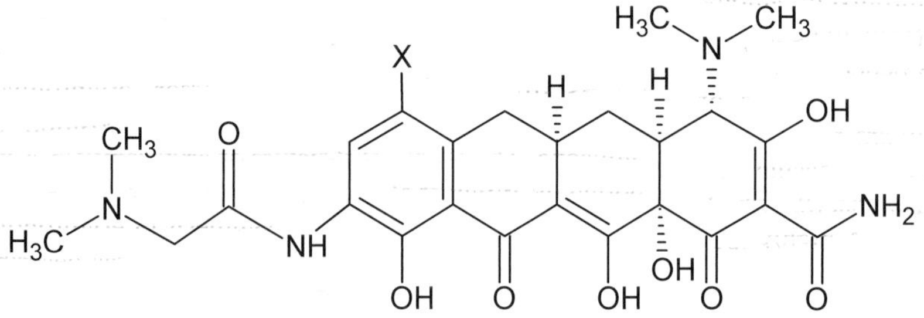

X = N(CH₃)₂   9-(Dimethylglycylamino)minocycline (DMG-MINO)

X = H   9-(Dimethylglycylamino)-6-demethyl-6-deoxytetracycline (DMG-DMDOT)

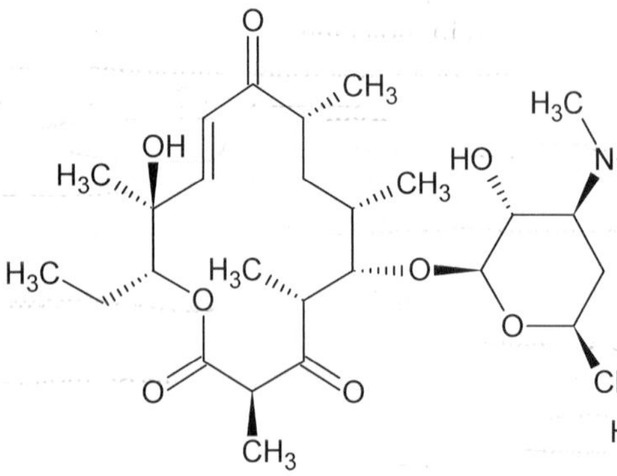

Picromycin

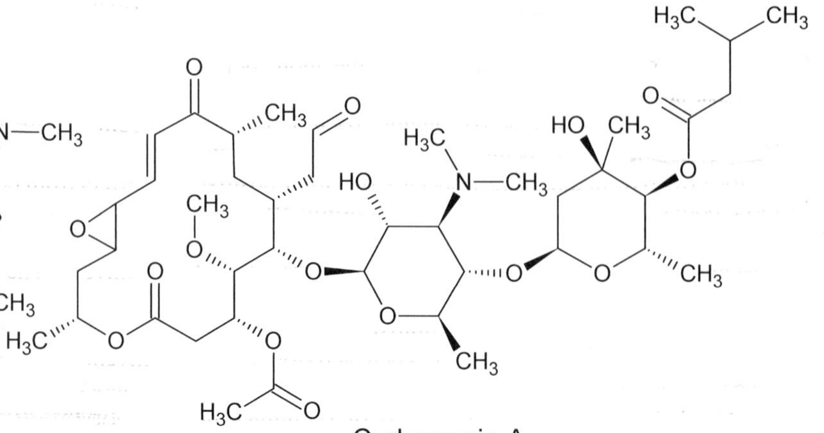

Carbomycin A

Chemistry

The macrolide antibiotics have three common chemical characteristics: (a) a large lactone ring (which prompted the name *macrolide*), (b) a ketone group, and (c) a glycosidically linked amino sugar. Usually, the lactone ring has 12, 14, or 16 atoms in it, and it is often unsaturated, with an olefinic group conjugated with the ketone function. (The polyene macrocyclic lactones, such as natamycin and amphotericin B; the ansamycins, such as rifampin; and the polypeptide lactones generally are not included among the macrolide antibiotics.) They may have, in addition to the amino sugar, a neutral sugar that is linked glycosidically to the lactone ring (see discussion that follows under "Erythromycin"). Because of the dimethylamino group on the sugar moiety, the macrolides are bases that form salts with pK$_a$ values between 6.0 and 9.0. This feature has been used to make clinically useful salts. The free bases are only slightly soluble in water but dissolve in somewhat polar organic solvents. They are stable in aqueous solutions at or below room temperature but are inactivated by acids, bases, and heat. The chemistry of macrolide antibiotics has been the subject of several reviews.[190,191]

Mechanism of Action and Resistance

Some details of the mechanism of antibacterial action of erythromycin are known. It binds selectively to a specific site on the 50S ribosomal subunit to prevent the translocation step of bacterial protein synthesis.[192] It does not bind to mammalian ribosomes. Broadly based, nonspecific resistance to the antibacterial action of erythromycin among many species of Gram-negative bacilli appears to be largely related to the inability of the antibiotic to penetrate the cell walls of these organisms.[193] In fact, the sensitivities of members of the Enterobacteriaceae family are pH dependent, with MICs decreasing as a function of increasing pH. Furthermore, protoplasts from Gram-negative bacilli, which lack cell walls, are sensitive to erythromycin. A highly specific resistance mechanism to the macrolide antibiotics occurs in erythromycin-resistant strains of *S. aureus*.[194,195] Such strains produce an enzyme that methylates a specific adenine residue at the erythromycin-binding site of the bacterial 50S ribosomal subunit. The methylated ribosomal RNA remains active in protein synthesis but no longer binds erythromycin. Bacterial resistance to the lincomycins apparently also occurs by this mechanism.

Spectrum of Activity

The spectrum of antibacterial activity of the more potent macrolides, such as erythromycin, resembles that of penicillin. They are frequently active against bacterial strains that are resistant to the penicillins. The macrolides are generally effective against most species of Gram-positive bacteria, both cocci and bacilli, and exhibit useful effectiveness against Gram-negative cocci, especially *Neisseria* spp. Many of the macrolides are also effective against *Treponema pallidum*. In contrast to penicillin, macrolides are also effective against *Mycoplasma*, *Chlamydia*, *Campylobacter*, and *Legionella* spp. Their activity against most species of Gram-negative bacilli is generally low and often unpredictable, though some strains of *H. influenzae* and *Brucella* spp. are sensitive.

Products

Erythromycin

Early in 1952, McGuire et al.[196] reported the isolation of erythromycin (E-Mycin, Erythrocin, Ilotycin) from *Streptomyces erythraeus*. It achieved rapid early acceptance as a well-tolerated antibiotic of value for the treatment of various upper respiratory and soft-tissue infections caused by Gram-positive bacteria. It is also effective against many venereal diseases, including gonorrhea and syphilis, and provides a useful alternative for the treatment of many infections in patients allergic to penicillins. More recently, erythromycin was shown to be effective therapy for Eaton agent pneumonia (*Mycoplasma pneumoniae*), venereal diseases caused by *Chlamydia*, bacterial enteritis caused by *Campylobacter jejuni*, and Legionnaires disease.

The commercial product is erythromycin A, which differs from its biosynthetic precursor, erythromycin B, in having a hydroxyl group at the 12-position of the aglycone. The chemical structure of erythromycin A was reported by Wiley et al.[197] in 1957 and its stereochemistry by Celmer[198] in 1965. An elegant synthesis of erythronolide A, the aglycone present in erythromycin A, was described by Corey et al.[199]

The amino sugar attached through a glycosidic link to C-5 is desosamine, a structure found in several other macrolide antibiotics. The tertiary amine of desosamine (3,4,6-trideoxy-3-dimethylamino-D-*xylo*-hexose) confers a basic character to erythromycin and provides the means by which acid salts may be prepared. The other carbohydrate structure linked as a glycoside to C-3 is called *cladinose* (2,3,6-trideoxy-3-methoxy-3-C-methyl-L-*ribo*-hexose) and is unique to the erythromycin molecule.

As is common with other macrolide antibiotics, compounds closely related to erythromycin have been obtained from culture filtrates of *S. erythraeus*. Two such analogs have been found, erythromycins B and C. Erythromycin B differs from erythromycin A only at C-12, at which a hydrogen has replaced the hydroxyl group. The B analog is more acid stable but has only about 80% of the activity of erythromycin. The C analog differs from erythromycin by the replacement of the methoxyl group on the cladinose moiety with a hydrogen atom. It appears to be as active as erythromycin but is present in very small amounts in fermentation liquors.

Erythromycin is a very bitter, white or yellow-white, crystalline powder. It is soluble in alcohol and in the other common organic solvents but only slightly soluble in water. The free base has a pK_a of 8.8. Saturated aqueous solutions develop an alkaline pH in the range of 8.0 to 10.5. It is extremely unstable at a pH of 4 or below. The optimum pH for stability of erythromycin is at or near neutrality.

Erythromycin may be used as the free base in oral dosage forms and for topical administration. To overcome its bitterness and irregular oral absorption (resulting from acid destruction and adsorption onto food), various enteric-coated and delayed-release dose forms of erythromycin base have been developed. These forms have been fully successful in overcoming the bitterness but have solved only marginally problems of oral absorption. Erythromycin has been chemically modified with primarily two different goals in mind: (a) to increase either its water or its lipid solubility for parenteral dosage forms and (b) to increase its acid stability (and possibly its lipid solubility) for improved oral absorption. Modified derivatives of the antibiotic are of two types: acid salts of the dimethylamino group of the desosamine moiety (e.g., the glucoheptonate, the lactobionate, and the stearate) and esters of the 2'-hydroxyl group of the desosamine (e.g., the ethylsuccinate and the propionate, available as the lauryl sulfate salt and known as the estolate).

The stearate salt and the ethylsuccinate and propionate esters are used in oral dose forms intended to improve absorption of the antibiotic. The stearate releases erythromycin base in the intestinal tract, which is then absorbed. The ethylsuccinate and the estolate are absorbed largely intact and are hydrolyzed partially by plasma and tissue esterases to give free erythromycin. The question of bioavailability of the antibiotic from its various oral dosage and chemical forms has caused considerable concern and dispute over the past two decades.[200–205] It is generally believed that the 2'-esters per se have little or no intrinsic antibacterial activity[206] and, therefore, must be hydrolyzed to the parent antibiotic in vivo. Although the ethylsuccinate is hydrolyzed more efficiently than the estolate in vivo and, in fact, provides higher levels of erythromycin following intramuscular administration, an equal dose of the estolate gives higher levels of the free antibiotic following oral administration.[201,205] Superior oral absorption of the estolate is attributed to its both greater acid stability and higher intrinsic absorption than the ethylsuccinate. Also, oral absorption of the estolate, unlike that of both the stearate and the ethylsuccinate, is not affected by food or fluid volume content of the gut. Superior bioavailability of active antibiotic from oral administration of the estolate over the ethylsuccinate, stearate, or erythromycin base cannot necessarily be assumed, however, because the estolate is more extensively protein bound than erythromycin itself.[207] Measured fractions of plasma protein binding for erythromycin-2'-propionate and erythromycin base range from 0.94 to 0.98 for the former and from 0.73 to 0.90 for the latter, indicating a much higher level of free erythromycin in the plasma. Bioavailability studies comparing equivalent doses of the enteric-coated base, the stearate salt, the ethylsuccinate ester, and the estolate ester in human volunteers[203,204] showed delayed but slightly higher bioavailability for the free base than for the stearate, ethylsuccinate, or estolate.

One study, comparing the clinical effectiveness of recommended doses of the stearate, estolate, ethylsuccinate, and free base in the treatment of respiratory tract infections, failed to demonstrate substantial differences among them.[208] Two other clinical studies, comparing the effectiveness of the ethylsuccinate and the estolate in the treatment of streptococcal pharyngitis, however, found the estolate to be superior.[209,210]

The water-insoluble ethylsuccinate ester is also available as a suspension for intramuscular injection. The glucoheptonate and lactobionate salts, however, are highly water-soluble derivatives that provide high plasma levels of the active antibiotic immediately after intravenous injection. Aqueous solutions of these salts may also be administered by intramuscular injection, but this is not a common practice.

Erythromycin is distributed throughout the body water. It persists in tissues longer than in the blood. The antibiotic is concentrated by the liver and excreted extensively into the bile. Large amounts are excreted in the feces, partly because of poor oral absorption and partly because of biliary excretion. The serum half-life is 1.4 hours. Some cytochrome P450-catalyzed oxidative demethylation to a less active metabolite may also occur. Erythromycin inhibits cytochrome P450-requiring oxidases, leading to various potential drug interactions. Thus, toxic effects of theophylline, the hydroxycoumarin anticoagulants, the benzodiazepines alprazolam and midazolam, carbamazepine, cyclosporine, and the antihistaminic drugs terfenadine and astemizole may be potentiated by erythromycin.

The toxicity of erythromycin is comparatively low. Primary adverse reactions to the antibiotic are related to its actions on the GI tract and the liver. Erythromycin may stimulate GI motility following either oral or parenteral administration.[211] This dose-related, prokinetic effect can cause abdominal cramps, epigastric distress, and diarrhea, especially in children and young adults. Cholestatic hepatitis occurs occasionally with erythromycin, usually in adults and more frequently with the estolate.

Erythromycin Stearate

Erythromycin stearate (Ethril, Wyamycin S, Erypar) is the stearic acid salt of erythromycin. Like erythromycin base, the stearate is acid labile. It is film coated to protect it from acid degradation in the stomach. In the alkaline pH of the duodenum, the free base is liberated from the stearate and absorbed. Erythromycin stearate is a crystalline powder that is practically insoluble in water but soluble in alcohol and ether.

Erythromycin Ethylsuccinate

Erythromycin ethylsuccinate (EES, Pediamycin, EryPed) is the ethylsuccinate mixed ester of erythromycin in which the 2′-hydroxyl group of the desosamine is esterified. It is absorbed as the ester and hydrolyzed slowly in the body to form erythromycin. It is somewhat acid labile, and its absorption is enhanced by the presence of food. The ester is insoluble in water but soluble in alcohol and ether.

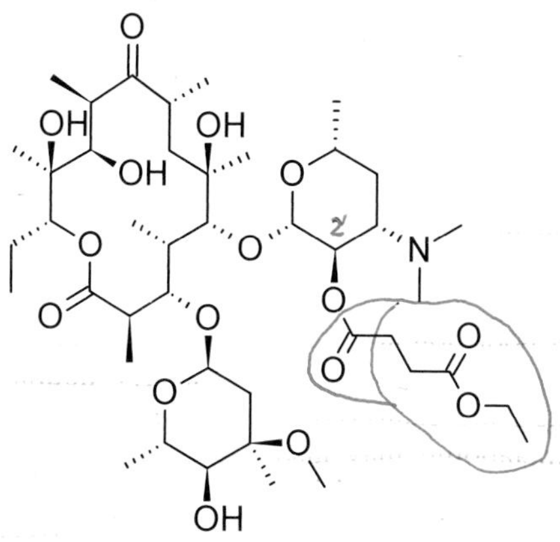

Erythromycin Estolate

Erythromycin estolate, erythromycin propionate lauryl sulfate (Ilosone), is the lauryl sulfate salt of the 2′-propionate ester of erythromycin. Erythromycin estolate is acid stable and absorbed as the propionate ester. The ester undergoes slow hydrolysis in vivo. Only the free base binds to bacterial ribosomes. Some evidence, however, suggests that the ester is taken up by bacterial cells more rapidly than the free base and undergoes hydrolysis by bacterial esterases within the cells. The incidence of cholestatic hepatitis is reportedly higher with the estolate than with other erythromycin preparations.

Erythromycin estolate occurs as long needles that are sparingly soluble in water but soluble in organic solvents.

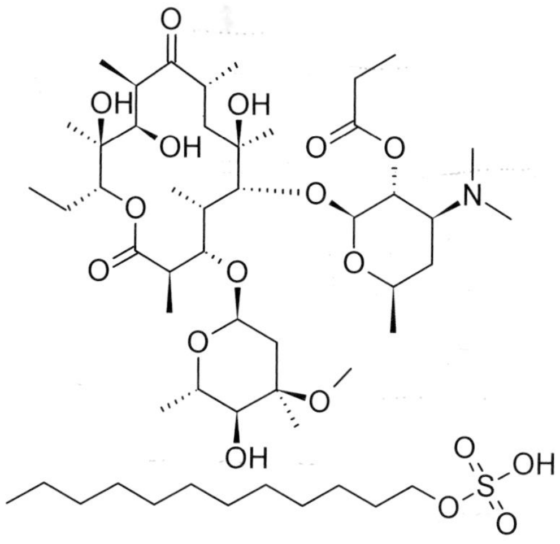

Erythromycin Gluceptate, Sterile

Erythromycin gluceptate, erythromycin glucoheptonate (Ilotycin Gluceptate), is the glucoheptonic acid salt of erythromycin. It is a crystalline substance that is freely soluble in water and practically insoluble in organic solvents. Erythromycin gluceptate is intended for intravenous administration for the treatment of serious infections, such as Legionnaires disease, or when oral administration is not possible. Solutions are stable for 1 week when refrigerated.

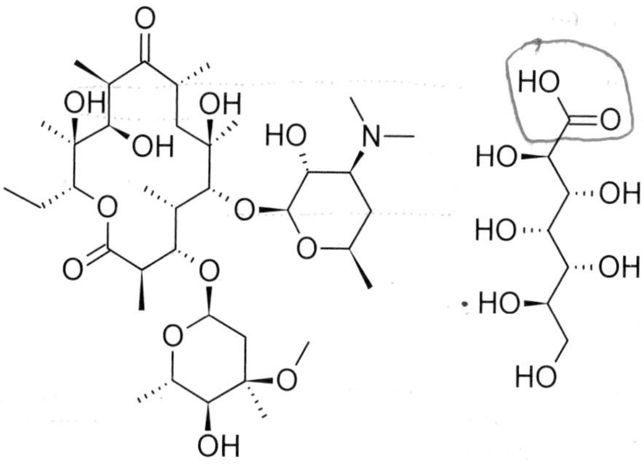

Erythromycin Lactobionate

Erythromycin lactobionate is a water-soluble salt prepared by reacting erythromycin base with lactobiono-σ-lactone. It occurs as an amorphous powder that is freely soluble in water and alcohol and slightly soluble in ether. It is intended, after reconstitution in sterile water, for intravenous administration to achieve high plasma levels in the treatment of serious infections.

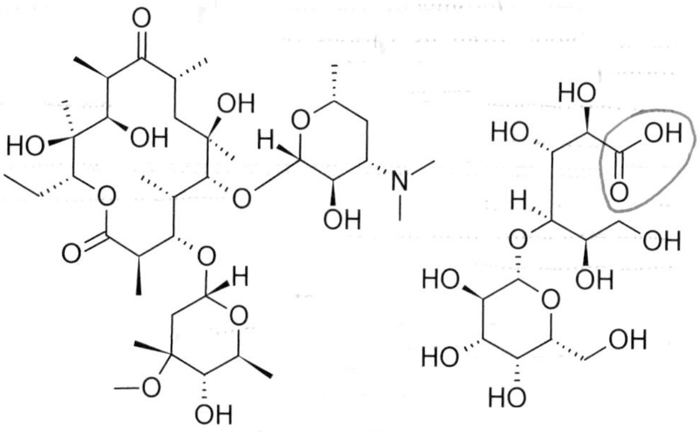

Clarithromycin

Clarithromycin (Biaxin) is the 6-methyl ether of erythromycin. The simple methylation of the 6-hydroxyl group of erythromycin creates a semisynthetic derivative that fully retains the antibacterial properties of the parent antibiotic, with markedly increased acid stability and oral bioavailability and reduced GI side effects associated with erythromycin.[212] Acid-catalyzed dehydration of erythromycin in the stomach initiates as a sequence of reactions, beginning with $\Delta^{6,7}$-bond migration followed by formation of an 8,9-anhydro-6,9-hemiketal and terminating in a 6,9:9,12-spiroketal. Since neither the hemiketal nor the spiroketal exhibits significant antibacterial activity, unprotected erythromycin is inactivated substantially in the stomach. Furthermore, evidence suggests that the hemiketal may be largely responsible for the GI (prokinetic) adverse effects associated with oral erythromycin.[211]

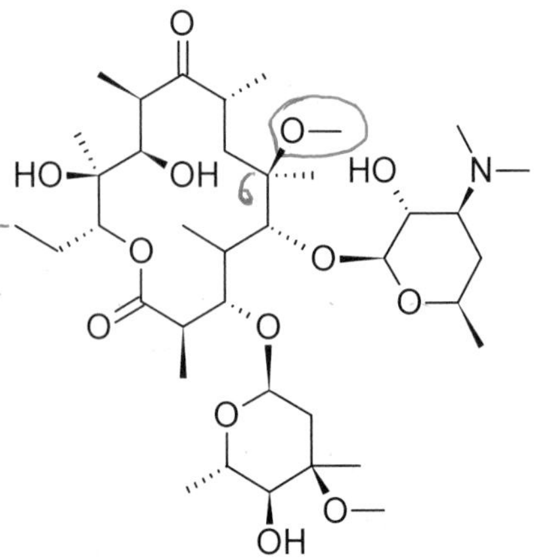

[handwritten annotations: "Log P"; "14-HO ← active"; near structure "6"; on right structure "Polar ↑ G⊖ act." "no liver metabolism" "no (-) P450 → no DDI"]

Clarithromycin is well absorbed following oral administration. Its oral bioavailability is estimated to be 50% to 55%. The presence of food does not significantly affect its absorption. Extensive metabolism of clarithromycin by oxidation and hydrolysis occurs in the liver. The major metabolite is the 14-hydroxyl derivative, which retains antibacterial activity. The amount of clarithromycin excreted in the urine ranges from 20% to 30%, depending on the dose, whereas 10% to 15% of the 14-hydroxy metabolite is excreted in the urine. Biliary excretion of clarithromycin is much lower than that of erythromycin. Clarithromycin is widely distributed into the tissues, which retain much higher concentrations than the plasma. Protein-binding fractions in the plasma range from 65% to 70%. The plasma half-life of clarithromycin is 4.3 hours.

Some of the microbiological properties of clarithromycin also appear to be superior to those of erythromycin. It exhibits greater potency against *M. pneumoniae*, *Legionella* spp., *Chlamydia pneumoniae*, *H. influenzae*, and *M. catarrhalis* than does erythromycin. Clarithromycin also has activity against unusual pathogens such as *Borrelia burgdorferi* (the cause of Lyme disease) and the *Mycobacterium avium* complex (MAC). Clarithromycin is significantly more active than erythromycin against group A streptococci, *S. pneumoniae*, and the viridans group of streptococci in vivo because of its superior oral bioavailability. Clarithromycin is, however, more expensive than erythromycin, which must be weighed against its potentially greater effectiveness.

Adverse reactions to clarithromycin are rare. The most common complaints relate to GI symptoms, but these seldom require discontinuance of therapy. Clarithromycin, like erythromycin, inhibits cytochrome P450 oxidases and, thus, can potentiate the actions of drugs metabolized by these enzymes.

Clarithromycin occurs as a white crystalline solid that is practically insoluble in water, sparingly soluble in alcohol, and freely soluble in acetone. It is provided as 250- and 500-mg oral tablets and as granules for the preparation of aqueous oral suspensions containing 25 or 50 mg/mL.

Azithromycin

Azithromycin (Zithromax) is a semisynthetic derivative of erythromycin, prepared by Beckman rearrangement of the corresponding 6-oxime, followed by *N*-methylation and reduction of the resulting ring-expanded lactam. It is a prototype of a series of nitrogen-containing 15-membered ring macrolides known as *azalides*.[213] Removal of the 9-keto group coupled with incorporation of a weakly basic tertiary

amine nitrogen function into the macrolide ring increases the stability of azithromycin to acid-catalyzed degradation. These changes also increase the lipid solubility of the molecule, thereby conferring unique pharmacokinetic and microbiological properties.[214]

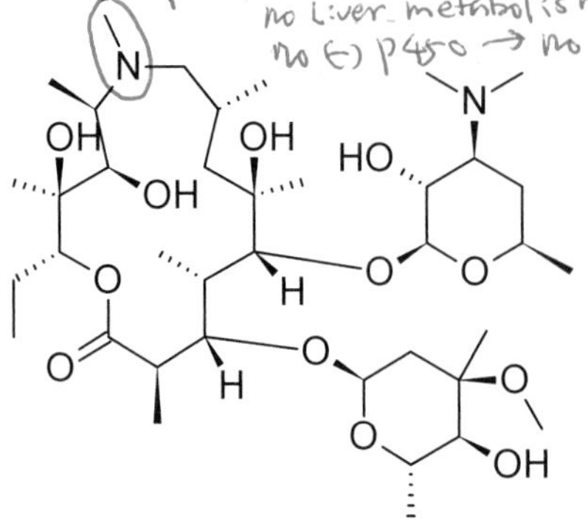

The oral bioavailability of azithromycin is good, nearly 40%, provided the antibiotic is administered at least 1 hour before or 2 hours after a meal. Food decreases its absorption by as much as 50%. The pharmacokinetics of azithromycin are characterized by rapid and extensive removal of the drug from the plasma into the tissues followed by a slow release. Tissue levels far exceed plasma concentrations, leading to a highly variable and prolonged elimination half-life of up to 5 days. The fraction of azithromycin bound to plasma proteins is only about 50% and does not exert an important influence on its distribution. Evidence indicates that azithromycin is largely excreted in the feces unchanged, with a small percentage appearing in the urine. Extensive enterohepatic recycling of the drug occurs. Azithromycin apparently is not metabolized to any significant extent. In contrast to the 14-membered ring macrolides, azithromycin does not significantly inhibit cytochrome P450 enzymes to create potential drug interactions.

The spectrum of antimicrobial activity of azithromycin is similar to that observed for erythromycin and clarithromycin but with some interesting differences. In general, it is more active against Gram-negative bacteria and less active against Gram-positive bacteria than its close relatives. The greater activity of azithromycin against *H. influenzae*, *M. catarrhalis*, and *M. pneumoniae* coupled with its extended half-life permits a 5-day dosing schedule for the treatment of respiratory tract infections caused by these pathogens. The clinical efficacy of azithromycin in the treatment of urogenital and other sexually transmitted infections caused by *Chlamydia trachomatis*, *N. gonorrhoeae*, *H. ducreyi*, and *Ureaplasma urealyticum* suggests that single-dose therapy with it for uncomplicated urethritis or cervicitis may have advantages over use of other antibiotics.

Dirithromycin

Dirithromycin (Dynabac) is a more lipid-soluble prodrug derivative of 9*S*-erythromycyclamine prepared by condensation of the latter with 2-(2-methoxyethoxy)acetaldehyde.[215] The 9*N*,11*O*-oxazine ring thus formed is a hemi-aminal that is unstable under both acidic and alkaline aqueous conditions and undergoes spontaneous hydrolysis to form erythromycyclamine. Erythromycyclamine is a semisynthetic derivative of erythromycin in which the 9-keto group of the erythronolide ring has been converted to an amino group. Erythromycyclamine retains the antibacterial properties of erythromycin in vitro but exhibits poor bioavailability following oral administration. The prodrug, dirithromycin, is provided as enteric-coated tablets to protect it from acid-catalyzed hydrolysis in the stomach.

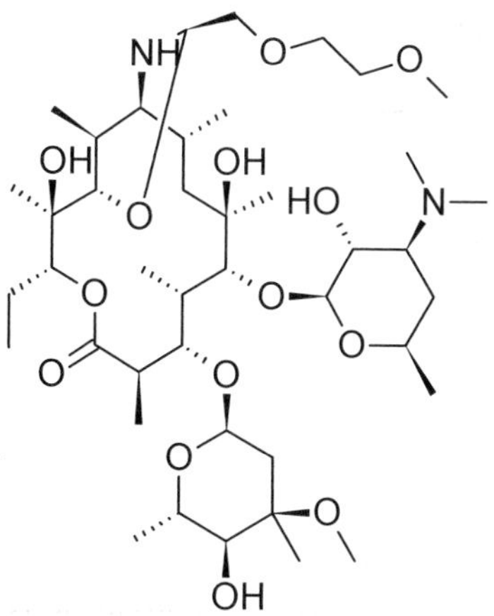

Orally administered dirithromycin is absorbed rapidly into the plasma, largely from the small intestine. Spontaneous hydrolysis to erythromycyclamine occurs in the plasma. Oral bioavailability is estimated to be about 10%, but food does not affect absorption of the prodrug.

The low plasma levels and large volume of distribution of erythromycyclamine are believed to result from its rapid distribution into well-perfused tissues, such as lung parenchyma, bronchial mucosa, nasal mucosa, and prostatic tissue. The drug also concentrates in human neutrophils. The elimination half-life is estimated to be 30 to 44 hours. Most of the prodrug and its active metabolite (62%–81% in normal human subjects) are excreted in the feces, largely via the bile, following either oral or parenteral administration. Urinary excretion accounts for less than 3%.

The incidence and severity of GI adverse effects associated with dirithromycin are similar to those seen with oral erythromycin. Preliminary studies indicate that dirithromycin and erythromycyclamine do not interact significantly with cytochrome P450 oxygenases. Thus, the likelihood of interference in the oxidative metabolism of drugs such as phenytoin, theophylline, and cyclosporine by these enzymes may be less with dirithromycin than with erythromycin. Dirithromycin is recommended as an alternative to erythromycin for the treatment of bacterial infections of the upper and lower respiratory tracts, such as pharyngitis, tonsillitis, bronchitis, and pneumonia, and for bacterial infections of other soft tissues and the skin. The once-daily dosing schedule for dirithromycin is advantageous in terms of better patient compliance. Its place in therapy remains to be fully assessed.[216]

Troleandomycin

Oleandomycin, as its triacetyl derivative troleandomycin, triacetyloleandomycin (TAO), remains available as an alternative to erythromycin for limited indications permitting use of an oral dosage form. Oleandomycin was isolated by Sobin et al.[217] The structure of oleandomycin was proposed by Hochstein et al.[218] and its absolute stereochemistry elucidated by Celmer.[219] The oleandomycin structure consists of two sugars and a 14-member lactone ring designated an *oleandolide*. One of the sugars is desosamine, also present in erythromycin; the other is L-oleandrose. The sugars are linked glycosidically to the positions 3 and 5, respectively, of oleandolide.

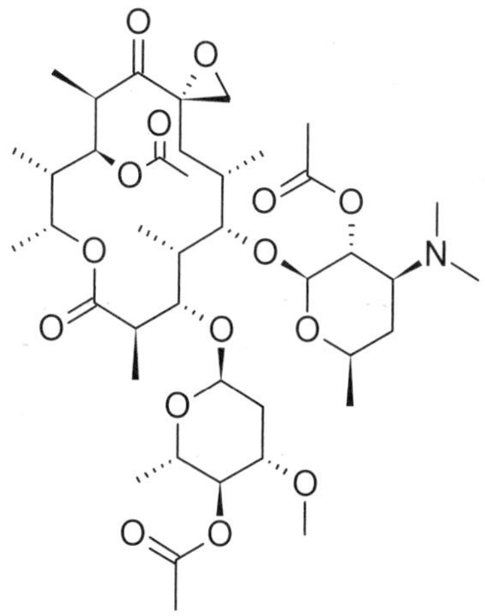

Oleandomycin contains three hydroxyl groups that are subject to acylation, one in each of the sugars and one in the oleandolide. The triacetyl derivative retains the in vivo antibacterial activity of the parent antibiotic but possesses superior pharmacokinetic properties. It is hydrolyzed in vivo to oleandomycin. Troleandomycin achieves more rapid and higher plasma concentrations following oral administration than oleandomycin phosphate, and it has the additional advantage of being practically tasteless. Troleandomycin occurs as a white, crystalline solid that is nearly insoluble in water. It is relatively stable in the solid state but undergoes chemical degradation in either aqueous acidic or alkaline conditions.

Because the antibacterial spectrum of activity of oleandomycin is considered inferior to that of erythromycin, the pharmacokinetics of troleandomycin have not been studied extensively. Oral absorption is apparently good, and detectable blood levels of oleandomycin persist up to 12 hours after a 500-mg dose of troleandomycin. Approximately 20% is recovered in the urine, with most excreted in the feces, primarily as a result of biliary excretion. There is some epigastric distress following oral administration, with an incidence similar to that caused by erythromycin. Troleandomycin is the most potent inhibitor of cytochrome P450 enzymes of the commercially available macrolides. It may potentiate the hepatic toxicity of certain anti-inflammatory steroids and oral contraceptive drugs as well as the toxic effects of theophylline, carbamazepine, and triazolam. Several allergic reactions, including cholestatic hepatitis, have also been reported with the use of troleandomycin.

Approved medical indications for troleandomycin are currently limited to the treatment of upper respiratory infections caused by such organisms as *S. pyogenes* and *S. pneumoniae*. It may be considered an alternative to oral forms of erythromycin. It is available in capsules and as a suspension.

LINCOMYCINS

The lincomycins are sulfur-containing antibiotics isolated from *Streptomyces lincolnensis*. Lincomycin is the most active and medically useful of the compounds obtained from fermentation. Extensive efforts to modify the lincomycin structure to improve its antibacterial and pharmacological properties resulted in the preparation of the 7-chloro-7-deoxy derivative clindamycin. Of the two antibiotics, clindamycin appears to have the greater antibacterial potency and better pharmacokinetic properties. Lincomycins resemble macrolides in antibacterial spectrum and biochemical mechanisms of action. They are primarily active against Gram-positive bacteria, particularly the cocci, but are also effective against non–spore-forming anaerobic bacteria, actinomycetes, mycoplasma, and some species of *Plasmodium*. Lincomycin binds to the 50S ribosomal subunit to inhibit protein synthesis. Its action may be bacteriostatic or bactericidal depending on various factors, including the concentration of the antibiotic. A pattern of bacterial resistance and cross-resistance to lincomycins similar to that observed with the macrolides has been emerging.[195]

Products

Lincomycin Hydrochloride

Lincomycin hydrochloride (Lincocin), which differs chemically from other major antibiotic classes, was isolated by Mason et al.[220] Its chemistry was described by Hoeksema et al.[221] who assigned the structure, later confirmed by Slomp and MacKellar,[222] given in the diagram below. Total syntheses of the antibiotic were accomplished independently in 1970 in England and the United States.[223,224] The structure contains a basic function, the pyrrolidine nitrogen, by which water-soluble salts with an apparent pK_a of 7.6 may be formed. When subjected to hydrazinolysis, lincomycin is cleaved at its amide bond into *trans*-L-4-*n*-propylhygric acid (the pyrrolidine moiety) and methyl α-thiolincosamide (the sugar moiety). Lincomycin-related antibiotics have been reported by Argoudelis[225] to be produced by *S. lincolnensis*. These antibiotics differ in structure at one or more of three positions of the lincomycin structure: (a) the *N*-methyl of the hygric acid moiety is substituted by a hydrogen; (b) the *n*-propyl group of the hygric acid moiety is substituted by an ethyl group; and (c) the thiomethyl ether of the α-thiolincosamide moiety is substituted by a thioethyl ether.

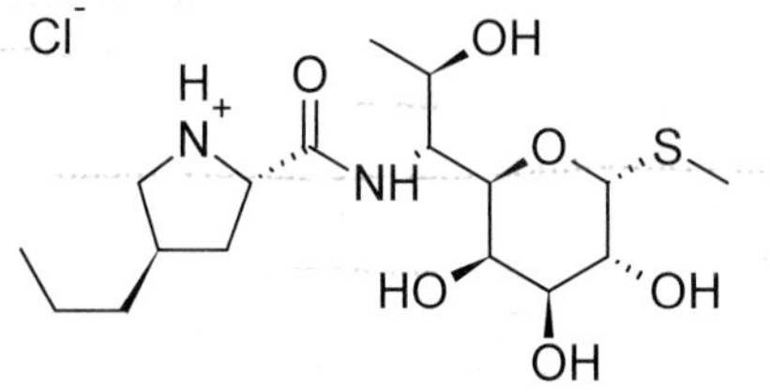

Lincomycin is used for the treatment of infections caused by Gram-positive organisms, notably staphylococci, β-hemolytic streptococci, and pneumococci. It is absorbed moderately well orally and distributed widely in the tissues. Effective concentrations are achieved in bone for the treatment of staphylococcal osteomyelitis but not in the cerebrospinal fluid for the treatment of meningitis. At one time, lincomycin was considered a nontoxic compound, with a low incidence of allergy (rash) and occasional GI complaints (nausea, vomiting, and diarrhea) as the only adverse effects. Recent reports of severe diarrhea and the development of pseudomembranous colitis in patients treated with lincomycin (or clindamycin), however, have necessitated reappraisal of the role of these antibiotics in therapy. In any event, clindamycin is superior to lincomycin for the treatment of most infections for which these antibiotics are indicated.

Lincomycin hydrochloride occurs as the monohydrate, a white, crystalline solid that is stable in the dry state. It is readily soluble in water and alcohol, and its aqueous solutions are stable at room temperature. It is degraded slowly in acid solutions but is absorbed well from the GI tract. Lincomycin diffuses well into peritoneal and pleural fluids and into bone. It is excreted in the urine and the bile. It is available in capsule form for oral administration and in ampules and vials for parenteral administration.

Clindamycin Hydrochloride

In 1967, Magerlein et al.[226] reported that replacement of the 7(*R*)-hydroxy group of lincomycin by chlorine with inversion of configuration resulted in a compound with enhanced antibacterial activity in vitro. Clinical experience with this semisynthetic derivative, clindamycin, 7(*S*)-chloro-7-deoxylincomycin (Cleocin), released in 1970, has established that its superiority over lincomycin is even greater in vivo. Improved absorption and higher tissue levels of clindamycin and its greater penetration into bacteria have been attributed to a higher partition coefficient than that of lincomycin. Structural modifications at C-7 (e.g., 7(*S*)-chloro and 7(*R*)-OCH₃) and of the C-4 alkyl groups of the hygric acid moiety[227] appear to influence activity of congeners more through an effect on the partition coefficient of the molecule than through a stereospecific binding role. Changes in the α-thiolincosamide portion of the molecule seem to decrease activity markedly, however, as evidenced by the marginal activity of 2-deoxylincomycin, its anomer, and 2-*O*-methyllincomycin.[227,228] Exceptions to this are fatty acid and phosphate esters of the 2-hydroxyl group of lincomycin and clindamycin, which are hydrolyzed rapidly in vivo to the parent antibiotics.

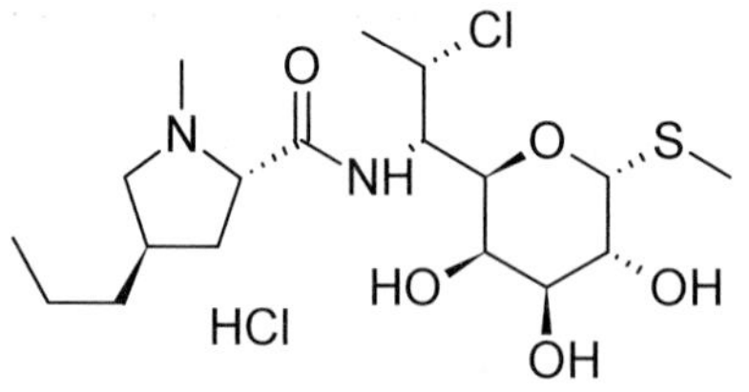

Clindamycin is recommended for the treatment of a wide variety of upper respiratory, skin, and tissue infections caused by susceptible bacteria. Its activity against streptococci, staphylococci, and pneumococci is indisputably high, and it is one of the most potent agents available against some non–spore-forming anaerobic bacteria, the *Bacteroides* spp. in particular. An increasing number of reports of clindamycin-associated GI toxicity, which range in severity from diarrhea to an occasionally serious pseudomembranous colitis, have, however, caused some clinical experts to call for a reappraisal of the role of this antibiotic in therapy. Clindamycin- (or lincomycin)-associated colitis may be particularly dangerous in elderly or debilitated patients and has caused deaths in such individuals. The colitis, which is usually reversible when the drug is discontinued, is now believed to result from an overgrowth of a clindamycin-resistant strain of the anaerobic intestinal bacterium *Clostridium difficile*.[229] The intestinal lining is damaged by a glycoprotein endotoxin released by lysis of this organism.

The glycopeptide antibiotic vancomycin has been effective in the treatment of clindamycin-induced pseudomembranous colitis and in the control of the experimentally induced bacterial condition in animals. Clindamycin should be reserved for staphylococcal tissue infections, such as cellulitis and osteomyelitis, in penicillin-allergic patients and for severe anaerobic infections outside the central nervous system. Ordinarily, it should not be used to treat upper respiratory tract infections caused by bacteria sensitive to other safer antibiotics or in prophylaxis.

Clindamycin is absorbed rapidly from the GI tract, even in the presence of food. It is available as the crystalline, water-soluble hydrochloride hydrate (hyclate) and the 2-palmitate ester hydrochloride salts in oral dosage forms and as the 2-phosphate ester in solutions for intramuscular or intravenous injection. All forms are chemically very stable in solution and in the dry state.

Clindamycin Palmitate Hydrochloride

Clindamycin palmitate hydrochloride (Cleocin Pediatric) is the hydrochloride salt of the palmitic acid ester of cleomycin. The ester bond is to the 2-hydroxyl group of the lincosamine sugar. The ester serves as a tasteless prodrug form of the antibiotic, which hydrolyzes to clindamycin in the plasma. The salt form confers water solubility to the ester, which is available as granules for reconstitution into an oral solution for pediatric use. Although absorption of the palmitate is slower than that of the free base, there is little difference in overall bioavailability of the two preparations. Reconstituted solutions of the palmitate hydrochloride are stable for 2 weeks at room temperature. Such solutions should not be refrigerated because thickening occurs that makes the preparation difficult to pour.

Clindamycin Phosphate

Clindamycin phosphate (Cleocin Phosphate) is the 2-phosphate ester of clindamycin. It exists as a zwitterionic structure that is very soluble in water. It is intended for parenteral (intravenous or intramuscular) administration for the treatment of serious infections and instances when oral administration is not feasible. Solutions of clindamycin phosphate are stable at room temperature for 16 days and for up to 32 days when refrigerated.

⬡ POLYPEPTIDES

Among the most powerful bactericidal antibiotics are those that possess a polypeptide structure. Many of them have been isolated, but unfortunately, their clinical use has been limited by their undesirable side reactions, particularly renal toxicity. Another limitation is the lack of systemic activity of most peptides following oral administration. A chief source of the medicinally important members of this class has been *Bacillus* spp. The antitubercular antibiotics capreomycin and viomycin (see Chapter 6) and the antitumor antibiotics actinomycin and bleomycin are peptides isolated from *Streptomyces* spp. The glycopeptide antibiotic vancomycin, which has become the most important member of this class, is isolated from a closely related actinomycete, *Amycolatopsis orientalis*.

Polypeptide antibiotics variously possess several interesting and often unique characteristics: (a) they frequently consist of several structurally similar but chemically distinct entities isolated from a single source; (b) most of them are cyclic, with a few exceptions (e.g., the gramicidins); (c) they frequently contain D-amino acids and/or "unnatural" amino acids not found in higher plants or animals; and (d) many of them contain non–amino acid moieties, such as heterocycles, fatty acids, sugars, etc. Polypeptide antibiotics may be acidic, basic, zwitterionic, or neutral depending on the number of free carboxyl and amino or guanidino groups in their structures. Initially, it was assumed that neutral compounds, such as the gramicidins, possessed cyclopeptide structures. Later, the gramicidins were determined to be linear, and the neutrality was shown to be because of a combination of the formylation of the terminal amino group and the ethanolamine amidation of the terminal carboxyl group.[230]

Antibiotics of the polypeptide class differ widely in their mechanisms of action and antimicrobial properties. Bacitracin and vancomycin interfere with bacterial cell wall synthesis and are effective only against Gram-positive bacteria. Neither antibiotic apparently can penetrate the outer envelope of Gram-negative bacteria. Both the gramicidins and the polymyxins interfere with cell membrane functions in bacteria. However, the gramicidins are effective primarily against Gram-positive bacteria, whereas the polymyxins are effective only against Gram-negative species. Gramicidins are neutral compounds that are largely incapable of penetrating the outer envelope of Gram-negative bacteria. Polymyxins are highly basic compounds that penetrate the outer membrane of Gram-negative bacteria through porin channels to act on the inner cell membrane.[231] The much thicker cell wall of Gram-positive bacteria apparently bars penetration by the polymyxins.

Vancomycin Hydrochloride ✳

The isolation of the glycopeptide antibiotic vancomycin (Vancocin, Vancoled) from *Streptomyces orientalis* (renamed *A. orientalis*) was described in 1956 by McCormick et al.[232] The organism originally was obtained from cultures of an Indonesian soil sample and subsequently has been obtained from Indian soil. Vancomycin was introduced in 1958 as an antibiotic active against Gram-positive cocci, particularly streptococci, staphylococci, and pneumococci. It is not active against Gram-negative bacteria, with the exception of *Neisseria* spp. Vancomycin is recommended for use when infections fail to respond to treatment with the more common antibiotics or when the infection is known to be caused by a resistant organism. It is particularly effective for the treatment of endocarditis caused by Gram-positive bacteria.

Vancomycin hydrochloride is a free-flowing, tan to brown powder that is relatively stable in the dry state. It is very soluble in water and insoluble in organic solvents. The salt is quite stable in acidic solutions. The free base is an amphoteric substance, whose structure was determined by a combination of chemical degradation and nuclear magnetic resonance (NMR) studies and x-ray crystallographic analysis of a close analog.[233] Slight stereochemical and conformational revisions in the originally proposed structure were made later.[234,235] Vancomycin is a glycopeptide containing two glycosidically linked sugars, glucose and vancosamine, and a complex cyclic peptide aglycon containing aromatic residues linked together in a unique resorcinol ether system.

Vancomycin inhibits cell wall synthesis by preventing the synthesis of cell wall mucopeptide polymer. It does so by binding with the D-alanine-D-alanine terminus of the uridine diphosphate-N-acetylmuramyl peptides required for mucopeptide polymerization.[236] Details of the binding were elucidated by the elegant NMR studies of Williamson

et al.[237] The action of vancomycin leads to lysis of the bacterial cell. The antibiotic does not exhibit cross-resistance to β-lactams, bacitracin, or cycloserine, from which it differs in mechanism. Resistance to vancomycin among Gram-positive cocci is rare. High-level resistance in clinical isolates of enterococci has been reported, however. This resistance is in response to the inducible production of a protein, encoded by vancomycin A, that is an altered ligase enzyme that causes the incorporation of a D-alanine-D-lactate depsipeptide instead of the usual D-alanine-D-alanine dipeptide in the peptidoglycan terminus.[238] The resulting peptidoglycan can still undergo cross-linking but no longer binds vancomycin.

Vancomycin hydrochloride is always administered intravenously (never intramuscularly), either by slow injection or by continuous infusion, for the treatment of systemic infections. In short-term therapy, the toxic side reactions are usually slight, but continued use may lead to impaired auditory acuity, renal damage, phlebitis, and rashes. Because it is not absorbed or significantly degraded in the GI tract, vancomycin may be administered orally for the treatment of staphylococcal enterocolitis and for pseudomembranous colitis associated with clindamycin therapy. Some conversion to aglucovancomycin likely occurs in the low pH of the stomach. The latter retains about three fourths of the activity of vancomycin.

Teicoplanin

Teicoplanin (Teichomycin A_2, Targocid) is a mixture of five closely related glycopeptide antibiotics produced by the actinomycete *Actinoplanes teichomyceticus*.[239,240] The teicoplanin factors differ only in the acyl group in the northernmost of two glucosamines glycosidically linked to the cyclic peptide aglycone. Another sugar, D-mannose, is common to all of the teicoplanins. The structures of the teicoplanin factors were determined independently by a combination of chemical degradation[241] and spectroscopic[242,243] methods in three different groups in 1984.

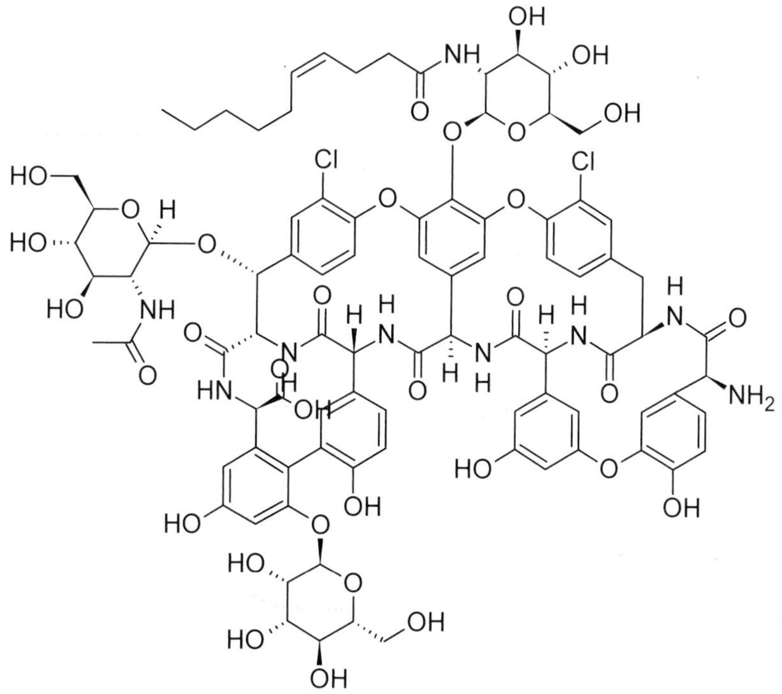

The teicoplanin complex is similar to vancomycin structurally and microbiologically but has unique physical properties that contribute some potentially useful advantages.[244] While retaining excellent water solubility, teicoplanin has significantly greater lipid solubility than vancomycin. Thus, teicoplanin is distributed rapidly into tissues and penetrates phagocytes well. The complex has a long elimination half-life, ranging from 40 to 70 hours, resulting from a combination of slow tissue release and a high fraction of protein binding in the plasma (~90%). Unlike vancomycin, teicoplanin is not irritating to tissues and may be administered by intramuscular or intravenous injection. Because of its long half-life, teicoplanin may be administered on a once-a-day dosing schedule. Orally administered teicoplanin is not absorbed significantly and is recovered 40% unchanged in the feces.

Teicoplanin exhibits excellent antibacterial activity against Gram-positive organisms, including staphylococci, streptococci, enterococci, *Clostridium* and *Corynebacterium* spp., *Propionibacterium acnes*, and *L. monocytogenes*. It is not active against Gram-negative organisms, including *Neisseria* and *Mycobacterium* spp. Teicoplanin impairs bacterial cell wall synthesis by complexing with the terminal D-alanine-D-alanine dipeptide of the peptidoglycan, thus preventing cross-linking in a manner entirely analogous to the action of vancomycin.

In general, teicoplanin appears to be less toxic than vancomycin. Unlike vancomycin, it does not cause histamine release following intravenous infusion. Teicoplanin apparently also has less potential for causing nephrotoxicity than vancomycin.

Bacitracin

The organism from which Johnson et al.[245] produced bacitracin in 1945 is a strain of *B. subtilis*. The organism had been isolated from debrided tissue from a compound fracture in 7-year-old Margaret Tracy, hence the name "bacitracin." Bacitracin is now produced from the licheniformis group (*B. subtilis*). Like tyrothricin, the first useful antibiotic obtained from bacterial cultures, bacitracin is a complex

mixture of polypeptides. So far, at least 10 polypeptides have been isolated by countercurrent distribution techniques: A, A^1, B, C, D, E, F$_1$, F$_2$, F$_3$, and G. The commercial product known as bacitracin is a mixture of principally A, with smaller amounts of B, D, E, and F$_{1-3}$.

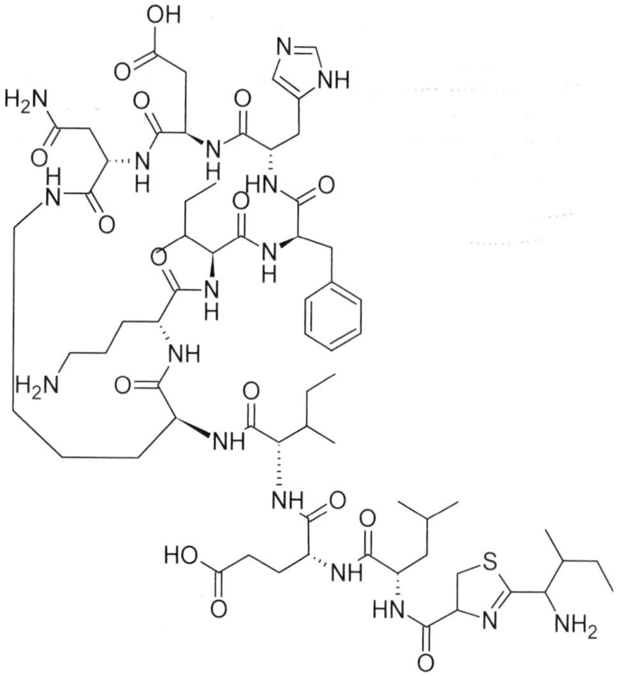

The official product is a white to pale buff powder that is odorless or nearly so. In the dry state, bacitracin is stable, but it rapidly deteriorates in aqueous solutions at room temperature. Because it is hygroscopic, it must be stored in tight containers, preferably under refrigeration. The stability of aqueous solutions of bacitracin is affected by pH and temperature. Slightly acidic or neutral solutions are stable for as long as 1 year if kept at a temperature of 0 to 5°C. If the pH rises above 9, inactivation occurs very rapidly. For greatest stability, the

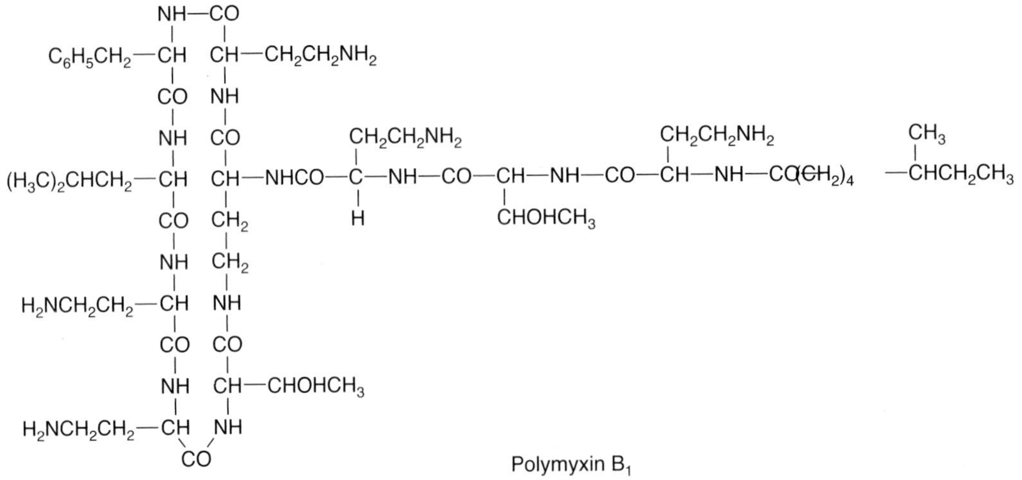

Polymyxin B₁ structure:

$$C_6H_5CH_2-CH \begin{array}{c} NH-CO \\ | \quad | \end{array} CH-CH_2CH_2NH_2$$

Polymyxin B₁

pH of a bacitracin solution is best adjusted to 4 to 5 by the simple addition of acid. The salts of heavy metals precipitate bacitracin from solution, with resulting inactivation. Ethylenediaminetetraacetic acid (EDTA) also inactivates bacitracin, which led to the discovery that a divalent ion (i.e., Zn^{2+}) is required for activity. In addition to being water soluble, bacitracin is soluble in low-molecular-weight alcohols but insoluble in many other organic solvents, including acetone, chloroform, and ether.

The principal work on the chemistry of the bacitracins has been directed toward bacitracin A, the component in which most of the antibacterial activity of crude bacitracin resides. The structure shown in the diagram was proposed by Stoffel and Craig[246] and subsequently confirmed by Ressler and Kashelikar.[247]

The activity of bacitracin is measured in units per milligram. The potency per milligram is not less than 40 units/mg except for material prepared for parenteral use, which has a potency of not less than 50 units/mg. It is a bactericidal antibiotic that is active against a wide variety of Gram-positive organisms, very few Gram-negative organisms, and some others. It is believed to exert its bactericidal effect through inhibition of mucopeptide cell wall synthesis. Its action is enhanced by zinc. Although bacitracin has found its widest use in topical preparations for local infections, it is quite effective in several systemic and local infections when administered parenterally. It is not absorbed from the GI tract; accordingly, oral administration is without effect, except for the treatment of amebic infections within the alimentary canal.

Polymyxin B Sulfate

Polymyxin (Aerosporin) was discovered in 1947 almost simultaneously in three separate laboratories in the United States and Great Britain.[248–250] As often happens when similar discoveries are made in widely separated laboratories, differences in nomenclature, referring to both the antibiotic-producing organism and the antibiotic itself, appeared in references to the polymyxins. Because the organisms first designated as *Bacillus polymyxa* and *B. aerosporus* Greer were found to be identical species, the name *B. polymyxa* is used to refer to all of the strains that produce the closely related polypeptides called *polymyxins*. Other organisms (e.g., see "Colistin" later) also produce polymyxins. Identified so far are polymyxins A, B₁,

B₂, C, D₁, D₂, M, colistin A (polymyxin E₁), colistin B (polymyxin E₂), circulins A and B, and polypeptin. The known structures of this group and their properties have been reviewed by Vogler and Studer.[251] Of these, polymyxin B as the sulfate usually is used in medicine because, when used systemically, it causes less kidney damage than the others.

Polymyxin B sulfate is a nearly odorless, white to buff powder. It is freely soluble in water and slightly soluble in alcohol. Its aqueous solutions are slightly acidic or nearly neutral (pH 5–7.5) and, when refrigerated, stable for at least 6 months. Alkaline solutions are unstable. Polymyxin B was shown to be a mixture by Hausmann and Craig,[252] who used countercurrent distribution techniques to obtain two fractions that differ in structure only by one fatty acid component. Polymyxin B₁ contains (+)-6-methyloctan-1-oic acid (isopelargonic acid), a fatty acid isolated from all of the other polymyxins. The B₂ component contains an isooctanoic acid, $C_8H_{16}O_2$, of undetermined structure. The structural formula for polymyxin B has been proved by the synthesis by Vogler et al.[253]

Polymyxin B sulfate is useful against many Gram-negative organisms. Its main use in medicine has been in topical applications for local infections in wounds and burns. For such use, it frequently is combined with bacitracin, which is effective against Gram-positive organisms. Polymyxin B sulfate is absorbed poorly from the GI tract; therefore, oral administration is of value only in the treatment of intestinal infections such as pseudomonal enteritis or infections caused by *Shigella* spp. It may be given parenterally by intramuscular or intrathecal injection for systemic infections. The dosage of polymyxin is measured in units. One milligram contains not less than 6,000 units. Some additional confusion on nomenclature for this antibiotic exists because Koyama et al.[254] originally named the product colimycin, and that name is used still. Particularly, it has been the basis for variants used as brand names, such as Coly-Mycin, Colomycin, Colimycin-E, and Colimicin-A.

Colistin Sulfate

In 1950, Koyama et al.[254] isolated an antibiotic from *Aerobacillus colistinus* (*B. polymyxa* var. *colistinus*) that was given the name *colistin* (Coly-Mycin S). It was used in Japan and in some European countries for several years before it was made available for medicinal use in the United States. It is recommended especially for the treatment of

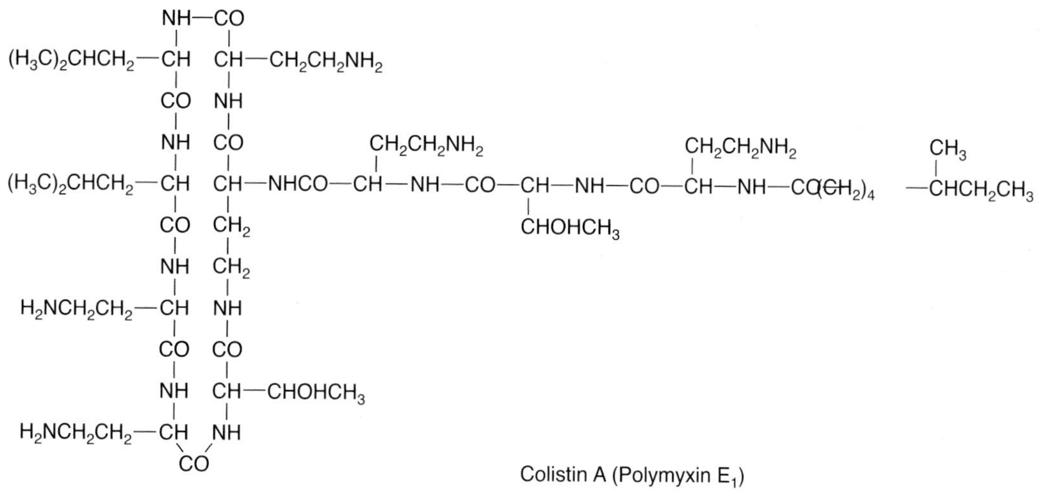

Colistin A (Polymyxin E₁)

refractory urinary tract infections caused by Gram-negative organisms such as *Aerobacter, Bordetella, Escherichia, Klebsiella, Pseudomonas, Salmonella,* and *Shigella* spp.

Chemically, colistin is a polypeptide, reported by Suzuki et al.[255] whose major component is colistin A. They proposed the structure shown below for colistin A, which differs from polymyxin B only by the substitution of D-leucine for D-phenylalanine as one of the amino acid fragments in the cyclic portion of the structure. Wilkinson and Lowe[256] have corroborated the structure and have shown that colistin A is identical with polymyxin E₁.

Two forms of colistin have been prepared, the sulfate and methanesulfonate, and both forms are available for use in the United States. The sulfate is used to make an oral pediatric suspension; the methanesulfonate is used to make an intramuscular injection. In the dry state, the salts are stable, and their aqueous solutions are relatively stable at acid pH from 2 to 6. Above pH 6, solutions of the salts are much less stable.

Colistimethate Sodium, Sterile

In colistin, five of the terminal amino groups of the α-aminobutyric acid fragment may be readily alkylated. In colistimethate sodium, pentasodium colistinmethanesulfonate, sodium colistimethanesulfonate (Coly-Mycin M), the

methanesulfonate radical is the attached alkyl group, and a sodium salt may be made through each sulfonate. This provides a highly water-soluble compound that is very suitable for injection. In the injectable form, it is given intramuscularly and is surprisingly free from toxic reactions compared with polymyxin B. Colistimethate sodium does not readily induce the development of resistant strains of microorganisms, and there is no evidence of cross-resistance with the common broad-spectrum antibiotics. It is used for the same conditions mentioned for colistin.

Gramicidin

Gramicidin is obtained from tyrothricin, a mixture of polypeptides usually obtained by extraction of cultures of *B. brevis.* Tyrothricin was isolated in 1939 by Dubos[257] in a planned search to find an organism growing in soil that would have antibiotic activity against human pathogens. With only limited use in therapy now, it is of historical interest as the first in the series of modern antibiotics. Tyrothricin is a white to slightly gray or brown-white powder, with little or no odor or taste. It is practically insoluble in water and is soluble in alcohol and dilute acids. Suspensions for clinical use can be prepared by adding an alcoholic solution to calculated amounts of distilled water or isotonic saline solutions.

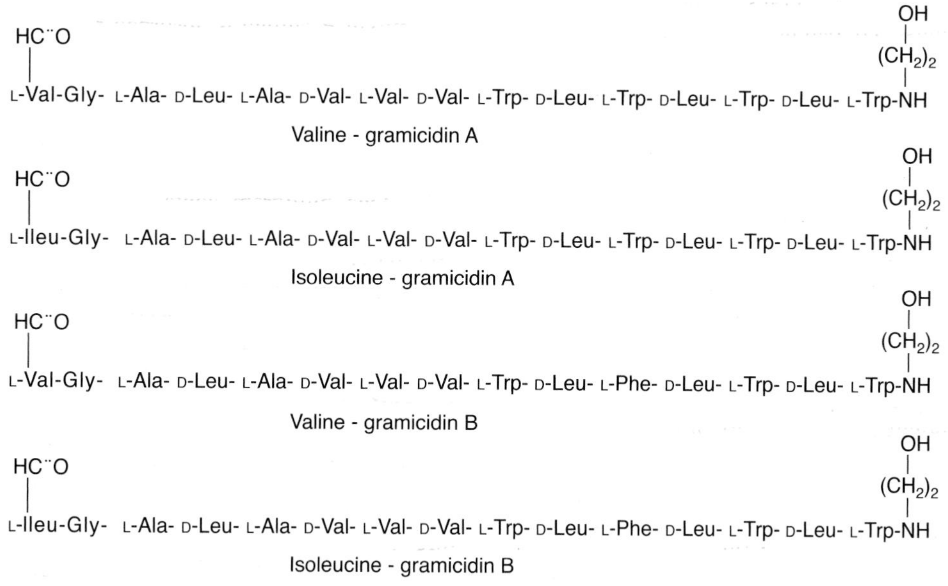

L-Val-Gly- L-Ala- D-Leu- L-Ala- D-Val- L-Val- D-Val- L-Trp- D-Leu- L-Trp- D-Leu- L-Trp- D-Leu- L-Trp-NH

Valine - gramicidin A

L-Ileu-Gly- L-Ala- D-Leu- L-Ala- D-Val- L-Val- D-Val- L-Trp- D-Leu- L-Trp- D-Leu- L-Trp- D-Leu- L-Trp-NH

Isoleucine - gramicidin A

L-Val-Gly- L-Ala- D-Leu- L-Ala- D-Val- L-Val- D-Val- L-Trp- D-Leu- L-Phe- D-Leu- L-Trp- D-Leu- L-Trp-NH

Valine - gramicidin B

L-Ileu-Gly- L-Ala- D-Leu- L-Ala- D-Val- L-Val- D-Val- L-Trp- D-Leu- L-Phe- D-Leu- L-Trp- D-Leu- L-Trp-NH

Isoleucine - gramicidin B

Tyrothricin is a mixture of two groups of antibiotic compounds, the gramicidins and the tyrocidines. Gramicidins are the more active components of tyrothricin, and this fraction, which is 10% to 20% of the mixture, may be separated and used in topical preparations for the antibiotic effect. Five gramicidins, A_2, A_3, B_1, B_2, and C, have been identified. Their structures have been proposed and confirmed through synthesis by Sarges and Witkop.[230] The gramicidins A differ from the gramicidins B by having a tryptophan moiety substituted by an L-phenylalanine moiety. In gramicidin C, a tyrosine moiety substitutes for a tryptophan moiety. In both of the gramicidin A and B pairs, the only difference is the amino acid located at the end of the chain, which has the neutral formyl group on it. If that amino acid is valine, the compound is either valine-gramicidin A or valine-gramicidin B. If that amino acid is isoleucine, the compound is isoleucine-gramicidin, either A or B.

Tyrocidine is a mixture of tyrocidines A, B, C, and D, whose structures have been determined by Craig et al.[258,259] The synthesis of tyrocidine A was reported by Ohno et al.[260]

L-Val → L-Orn → L-Leu → X → L-Pro

L-Tyr ← Glu ← L-Asp ← Z ← Y

Glu–NH₂, L-Asp–NH₂

	X	Y	Z
Tyrocidine A:	D-Phe	D-Phe	D-Phe
Tyrocidine B:	D-Phe	L-Tyr	D-Phe
Tyrocidine C:	D-Tyr	L-Tyr	D-Phe
Tyrocidine D:	D-Tyr	L-Tyr	D-Tyr

Gramicidin acts as an ionophore in bacterial cell membranes to cause the loss of potassium ion from the cell.[261] It is bactericidal.

Tyrothricin and gramicidin are effective primarily against Gram-positive organisms. Their use is restricted to local applications. Tyrothricin can cause lysis of erythrocytes, which makes it unsuitable for the treatment of systemic infections. Its applications should avoid direct contact with the bloodstream through open wounds or abrasions. It is ordinarily safe to use tyrothricin in troches for throat infections, as it is not absorbed from the GI tract. Gramicidin is available in various topical preparations containing other antibiotics, such as bacitracin and neomycin.

UNCLASSIFIED ANTIBIOTICS

Among the many hundreds of antibiotics that have been evaluated for activity, several have gained significant clinical attention but do not fall into any of the previously considered groups. Some of these have quite specific activities against a narrow spectrum of microorganisms. Some have found a useful place in therapy as substitutes for other antibiotics to which resistance has developed.

Chloramphenicol

The first of the widely used broad-spectrum antibiotics, chloramphenicol (Chloromycetin, Amphicol) was isolated by Ehrlich et al.[262] in 1947. They obtained it from *Streptomyces venezuelae*, an organism found in a sample of soil collected in Venezuela. Since then, chloramphenicol has been isolated as a product of several organisms found in soil samples from widely separated places. More importantly, its chemical structure was established quickly, and in 1949, Controulis et al.[263] reported its synthesis. This opened the way for the commercial production of chloramphenicol by a totally synthetic route. It was the first and still is the only therapeutically important antibiotic to be so produced in competition with microbiological processes. Diverse synthetic procedures have been developed for chloramphenicol. The commercial process generally used starts with *p*-nitroacetophenone.[264]

Chloramphenicol is a white, crystalline compound that is very stable. It is very soluble in alcohol and other polar organic solvents but only slightly soluble in water. It has no odor but has a very bitter taste.

Chloramphenicol possesses two chiral carbon atoms in the acylamidopropanediol chain. Biological activity resides almost exclusively in the D-*threo* isomer; the L-*threo* and the D- and L-*erythro* isomers are virtually inactive.

Chloramphenicol is very stable in the bulk state and in solid dosage forms. In solution, however, it slowly undergoes various hydrolytic and light-induced reactions.[265] The rates of these reactions depend on pH, heat, and light. Hydrolytic reactions include general acid–base-catalyzed hydrolysis of the amide to give 1-(*p*-nitrophenyl)-2-aminopropan-1,3-diol and dichloroacetic acid and alkaline hydrolysis (above pH 7) of the α-chloro groups to form the corresponding α,α-dihydroxy derivative.

The metabolism of chloramphenicol has been investigated thoroughly.[266] The main path involves formation of the 3-*O*-glucuronide. Minor reactions include reduction of the *p*-nitro group to the aromatic amine, hydrolysis of the amide, and hydrolysis of the α-chloracetamido group, followed by reduction to give the corresponding α-hydroxyacetyl derivative.

Strains of certain bacterial species are resistant to chloramphenicol by virtue of the ability to produce chloramphenicol acetyltransferase, an enzyme that acetylates the hydroxy groups at the positions 1 and 3. Both the 3-acetoxy and the 1,3-diacetoxy metabolites lack antibacterial activity.

Numerous structural analogs of chloramphenicol have been synthesized to provide a basis for correlation of structure to antibiotic action. It appears that the *p*-nitrophenyl group may be replaced by other aryl structures without appreciable loss in activity. Substitution on the phenyl ring with several different types of groups for the nitro group, a very unusual structure in biological products, does not greatly decrease activity. All such compounds yet tested are less active than chloramphenicol. As part of a QSAR study, Hansch et al.[267] reported that the 2-NHCOCF₃ derivative is

1.7 times as active as chloramphenicol against *E. coli*. Modification of the side chain shows that it possesses high specificity in structure for antibiotic action. Conversion of the alcohol group on C-1 of the side chain to a keto group causes appreciable loss in activity. The relationship of the structure of chloramphenicol to its antibiotic activity will not be seen clearly until the mode of action of this compound is known. Brock[268] reports on the large amount of research that has been devoted to this problem. Chloramphenicol exerts its bacteriostatic action by a strong inhibition of protein synthesis. The details of such inhibition are as yet undetermined, and the precise point of action is unknown. Some process lying between the attachment of amino acids to sRNA and the final formation of protein appears to be involved.

The broad-spectrum activity of chloramphenicol and its singular effectiveness in the treatment of some infections not amenable to treatment by other drugs made it an extremely popular antibiotic. Unfortunately, instances of serious blood dyscrasias and other toxic reactions have resulted from the promiscuous and widespread use of chloramphenicol in the past. Because of these reactions, it is recommended that it not be used in the treatment of infections for which other antibiotics are as effective and less hazardous. When properly used, with careful observation for untoward reactions, chloramphenicol provides some of the very best therapy for the treatment of serious infections.[269]

Chloramphenicol is recommended specifically for the treatment of serious infections caused by strains of Gram-positive and Gram-negative bacteria that have developed resistance to penicillin G and ampicillin, such as *H. influenzae*, *Salmonella typhi*, *S. pneumoniae*, *B. fragilis*, and *N. meningitidis*. Because of its penetration into the central nervous system, chloramphenicol is a particularly important alternative therapy for meningitis. It is not recommended for the treatment of urinary tract infections because 5% to 10% of the unconjugated form is excreted in the urine. Chloramphenicol is also used for the treatment of rickettsial infections, such as Rocky Mountain spotted fever.

Because it is bitter, this antibiotic is administered orally either in capsules or as the palmitate ester. Chloramphenicol palmitate is insoluble in water and may be suspended in aqueous vehicles for liquid dosage forms. The ester forms by reaction with the hydroxyl group on C-3. In the alimentary tract, it is hydrolyzed slowly to the active antibiotic. Chloramphenicol is administered parenterally as an aqueous suspension of very fine crystals or as a solution of the sodium salt of the succinate ester of chloramphenicol. Sterile chloramphenicol sodium succinate has been used to prepare aqueous solutions for intravenous injection.

Chloramphenicol Palmitate

Chloramphenicol palmitate is the palmitic acid ester of chloramphenicol. It is a tasteless prodrug of chloramphenicol intended for pediatric use. The ester must hydrolyze in vivo following oral absorption to provide the active form. Erratic serum levels were associated with early formulations of the palmitate, but the manufacturer claims that the bioavailability of the current preparation is comparable to that of chloramphenicol itself.

Chloramphenicol Sodium Succinate

Chloramphenicol sodium succinate is the water-soluble sodium salt of the hemisuccinate ester of chloramphenicol. Because of the low solubility of chloramphenicol, the sodium succinate is preferred for intravenous administration. The availability of chloramphenicol from the ester following intravenous administration is estimated to be 70% to 75%; the remainder is excreted unchanged.[269,270] Poor availability of the active form from the ester following intramuscular injection precludes attaining effective plasma levels of the antibiotic by this route. Orally administered chloramphenicol or its palmitate ester actually gives higher plasma levels of the active antibiotic than does intravenously administered chloramphenicol sodium succinate.[270,271] Nonetheless, effective concentrations are achieved by either route.

Novobiocin Sodium

In the search for new antibiotics, three different research groups independently isolated novobiocin, streptonivicin (Albamycin) from *Streptomyces* spp. It was reported first in 1955 as a product of *S. spheroides* and *S. niveus*. Currently, it is produced from cultures of both species. Until the common identity of the products obtained by the different research groups was ascertained, the naming of this compound was confused. Its chemical identity was established as 7-[4-(carbamoyloxy)tetrahydro-3-hydroxy-5-methoxy-6,6-dimethylpyran-2-yloxyl-4-hydroxy-3-[4-hydroxy-3-(3-methyl-2-butenyl)benzamido]-8-methylcoumarin by Shunk et al.[272] and Hoeksema et al.[273] and confirmed by Spencer et al.[274,275]

Chemically, novobiocin has a unique structure among antibiotics, though, like several others, it possesses a glycosidic sugar moiety. The sugar in novobiocin, devoid of its carbamate ester, has been named *noviose* and is an aldose with the configuration of L-lyxose. The aglycon moiety has been termed *novobiocic acid*.

Novobiocin is a pale yellow, somewhat photosensitive compound that crystallizes in two chemically identical forms with different melting points (polymorphs). It is soluble in methanol, ethanol, and acetone but is quite insoluble in less polar solvents. Its solubility in water is affected by pH. It is readily soluble in basic solutions, in which it deteriorates, and is precipitated from acidic solutions. It behaves as a diacid, forming two series of salts.

The enolic hydroxyl group on the coumarin moiety behaves as a rather strong acid (pKa 4.3) and is the group by which the commercially available sodium and calcium salts are formed. The phenolic -OH group on the benzamido moiety also behaves as an acid but is weaker than the former, with a pKa of 9.1. Disodium salts of novobiocin have been prepared. The sodium salt is stable in dry air but loses activity in the presence of moisture. The calcium salt is quite water insoluble and is used to make aqueous oral suspensions. Because of its acidic characteristics, novobiocin combines to form salt complexes with basic antibiotics. Some of these salts have been investigated for their combined antibiotic effect, but none has been placed on the market, as they offer no advantage.

The action of novobiocin is largely bacteriostatic. Its mode of action is not known with certainty, though it does inhibit bacterial protein and nucleic acid synthesis. Studies indicate that novobiocin and related coumarin-containing antibiotics bind to the subunit of DNA gyrase and possibly interfere with DNA supercoiling[276] and energy transduction in bacteria.[277] The effectiveness of novobiocin is confined largely to Gram-positive bacteria and a few strains of *P. vulgaris*. Its low activity against Gram-negative bacteria is apparently because of poor cellular penetration.

Although cross-resistance to other antibiotics is reported not to develop with novobiocin, resistant *S. aureus* strains are known. Consequently, the medical use of novobiocin is reserved for the treatment of staphylococcal infections resistant to other antibiotics and sulfas and for patients allergic to these drugs. Another shortcoming that limits the usefulness of novobiocin is the relatively high frequency of adverse reactions, such as urticaria, allergic rashes, hepatotoxicity, and blood dyscrasias.

Mupirocin

Mupirocin (pseudomonic acid A, Bactroban) is the major component of a family of structurally related antibiotics, pseudomonic acids A to D, produced by the submerged fermentation of *Pseudomonas fluorescens*. Although the antimicrobial properties of *P. fluorescens* were recorded as early as 1887, it was not until 1971 that Fuller et al.[278] identified the metabolites responsible for this activity. The structure of the major and most potent metabolite, pseudomonic acid A (which represents 90%–95% of the active fraction from *P. fluorescens*), was later confirmed by chemical synthesis[279] to be the 9-hydroxynonanoic acid ester of monic acid.

The use of mupirocin is confined to external applications.[280] Systemic administration of the antibiotic results in rapid hydrolysis by esterases to monic acid, which is inactive in vivo because of its inability to penetrate bacteria. Mupirocin has been used for the topical treatment of impetigo, eczema, and folliculitis secondarily infected by susceptible bacteria, especially staphylococci and β-hemolytic streptococci. The spectrum of antibacterial activity of mupirocin is confined to Gram-positive and Gram-negative cocci, including staphylococci, streptococci, *Neisseria* spp., and *M. catarrhalis*. The activity of the antibiotic against most Gram-negative and Gram-positive bacilli is generally poor, with the exception of *H. influenzae*. It is not effective against enterococci or anaerobic bacteria.

Mupirocin interferes with RNA synthesis and protein synthesis in susceptible bacteria.[281,282] It specifically and reversibly binds with bacterial isoleucyl tRNA synthase to prevent the incorporation of isoleucine into bacterial proteins.[282] High-level, plasmid-mediated mupirocin resistance in *S. aureus* has been attributed to the elaboration of a modified isoleucyl tRNA that does not bind mupirocin.[283] Inherent resistance in bacilli is likely because of poor cellular penetration of the antibiotic.[284]

Mupirocin is supplied in a water-miscible ointment containing 2% of the antibiotic in polyethylene glycols 400 and 3350.

Quinupristin/Dalfopristin

Quinupristin/dalfopristin (Synercid) is a combination of the streptogramin B quinupristin with the streptogramin A dalfopristin in a 30:70 ratio.

Both of these compounds are semisynthetic derivatives of two naturally occurring pristinamycins produced in fermentations of *Streptomyces pristinaspiralis*. Quinupristin and dalfopristin are solubilized derivatives of pristinamycin Ia and pristinamycin IIa, respectively, and therefore are suitable for intravenous administration only.

The spectrum of activity of quinupristin/dalfopristin is largely against Gram-positive bacteria. The combination is active against Gram-positive cocci, including *S. pneumoniae*, β-hemolytic and α-hemolytic streptococci, *Enterococcus faecium*, and coagulase-positive and coagulase-negative staphylococci. The combination is mostly inactive against Gram-negative organisms, although *M. catarrhalis* and *Neisseria* spp. are susceptible. The combination is bactericidal against streptococci and many staphylococci, but bacteriostatic against *E. faecium*.

Quinupristin and dalfopristin are protein synthesis inhibitors that bind to the 50S ribosomal subunit. Quinupristin, a type B streptogramin, binds at the same site as the macrolides and has a similar effect, resulting in inhibition of polypeptide elongation and early termination of protein synthesis. Dalfopristin binds to a site near that of quinupristin. The binding of dalfopristin results in a conformational change in the 50S ribosomal subunit, synergistically enhancing the binding of quinupristin at its target site. In most bacterial species, the cooperative and synergistic binding of these two compounds to the ribosome is bactericidal.

Synercid should be reserved for the treatment of serious infections caused by multidrug-resistant Gram-positive organisms such as vancomycin-resistant *E. faecium*.

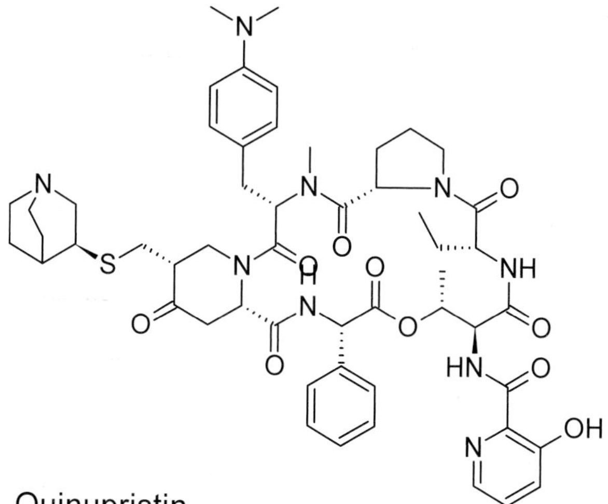

Quinupristin

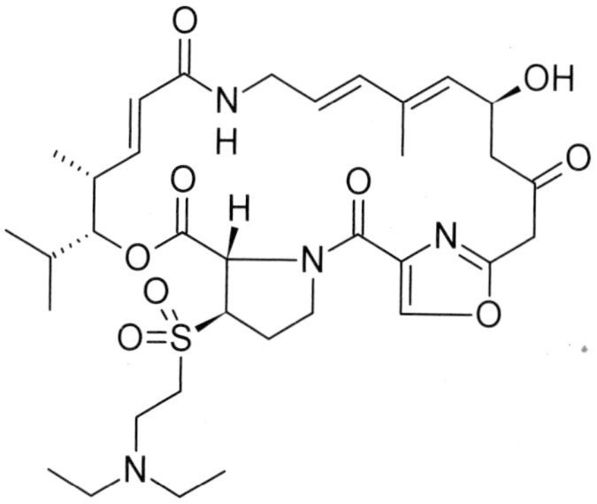

Dalfopristin

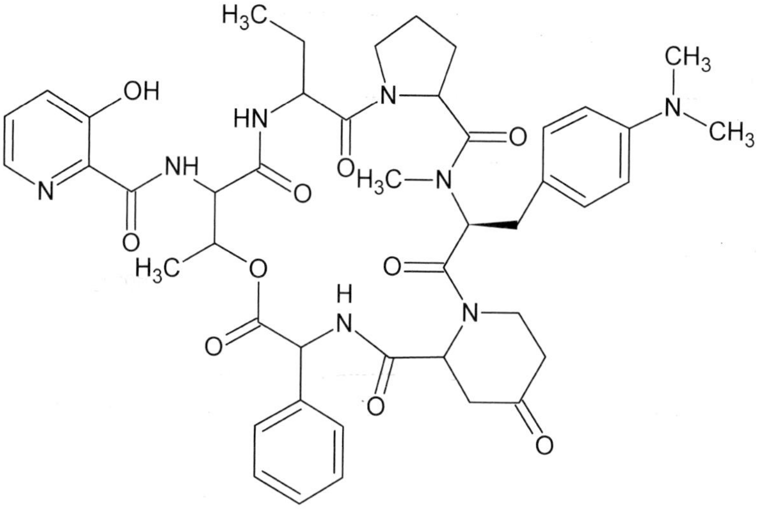

Pristinamycin 1A

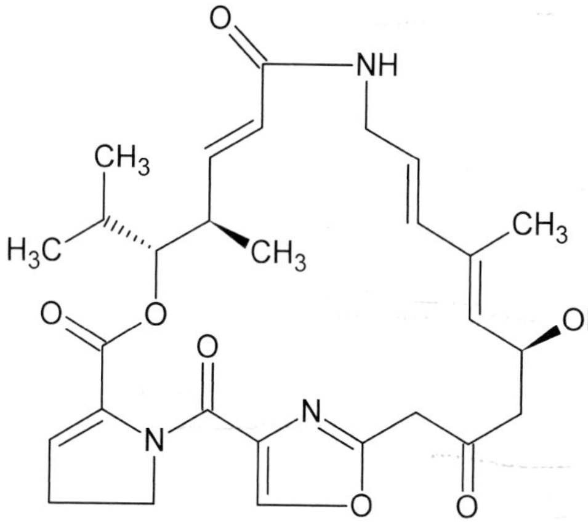

Pristinamycin 2A

Linezolid

Linezolid (Zyvox) is an oxazolidinedione-type antibacterial agent that inhibits bacterial protein synthesis. It acts in the early translation stage, preventing the formation of a functional initiation complex. Linezolid binds to the 30S and 70S ribosomal subunits and prevents initiation complexes involving these subunits. Collective data suggest that the oxazolidindiones partition their ribosomal interaction between the two subunits. Formation of the early tRNA^{fMet}-mRNA-70S or 30S is prevented. Linezolid is a newer synthetic agent, and hence, cross-resistance between the antibacterial agent and other inhibitors of bacterial protein synthesis has not been seen.

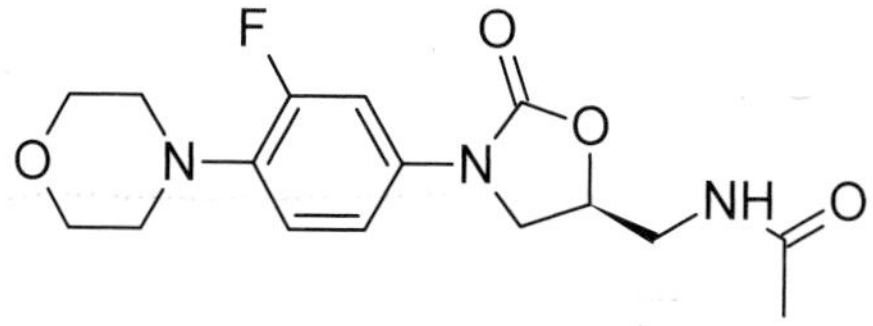

Linezolid possesses a wide spectrum of activity against Gram-positive organisms, including MRSA, penicillin-resistant pneumococci, and vancomycin-resistant *Enterococcus faecalis* and *E. faecium*. Anaerobes such as *Clostridium*, *Peptostreptococcus*, and *Prevotella* spp. are sensitive to linezolid.

Linezolid is a bacteriostatic agent against most susceptible organisms but displays bactericidal activity against some strains of pneumococci, *B. fragilis*, and *Clostridium perfringens*.

The indications for linezolid are for complicated and uncomplicated skin and soft-tissue infections, community- and hospital-acquired pneumonia, and drug-resistant Gram-positive infections.

Fosfomycin Tromethamine

Fosfomycin tromethamine (Monurol) is a phosphonic acid epoxide derivative that was initially isolated from fermentations of *Streptomyces* spp. The structure of the drug is shown next. Making the tromethamine salt greatly expanded the therapeutic utility of this antibacterial because water solubility increased enough to allow oral administration.

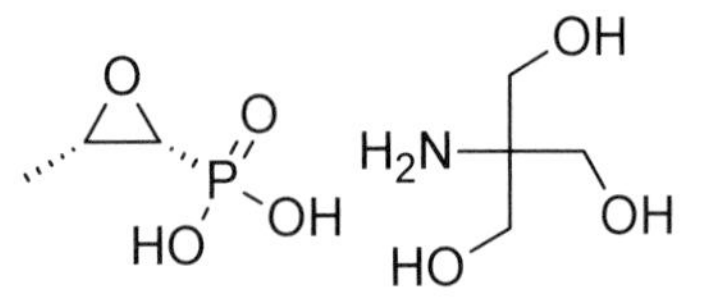

Fosfomycin is a broad-spectrum, bactericidal antibacterial that inhibits the growth of *E. coli*, *S. aureus*, and *Serratia*, *Klebsiella*, *Citrobacter*, *Enterococcus*, and *Enterobacter* spp. at a concentration less than 64 mg/L. Currently fosfomycin is recommended as single-dose therapy for uncomplicated urinary tract infections. It possesses in vitro efficacy similar to that of norfloxacin and trimethoprim-sulfamethoxazole.

Fosfomycin covalently inactivates the first enzyme in the bacterial cell wall biosynthesis pathway, UDP-*N*-acetylglucosamine enolpyruvyl transferase (MurA) by alkylation of the cysteine-115 residue. The inactivation reaction occurs through nucleophilic opening of the epoxide ring. Resistance to fosfomycin can occur through chromosomal mutations that result in reduced uptake or reduced MurA affinity for the inhibitor. Plasmid-mediated resistance mechanisms involve conjugative bioinactivation of the antibiotic with glutathione. The frequency of resistant mutants in in vitro studies has been low, and there appears to be little cross-resistance between fosfomycin and other antibacterials.

NEWER ANTIBIOTICS

Tigecycline

Tigecycline (Tygacil) is a first-in-class (a glycylcycline) intravenous antibiotic that was designed to circumvent many important bacterial resistance mechanisms. It is not affected by resistance mechanisms such as ribosomal protection, efflux pumps, target site modifications, β-lactamases, or DNA gyrase mutations. Tigecycline binds to the 30S ribosomal subunit and blocks peptide synthesis. The glycylcyclines bind to the ribosome with five times the affinity of common tetracyclines. Tigecycline also possesses a novel mechanism of action, interfering with the mechanism of ribosomal protection proteins. Tigecycline, unlike common tetracyclines, is not expelled from the bacterial cell by efflux pumping processes.

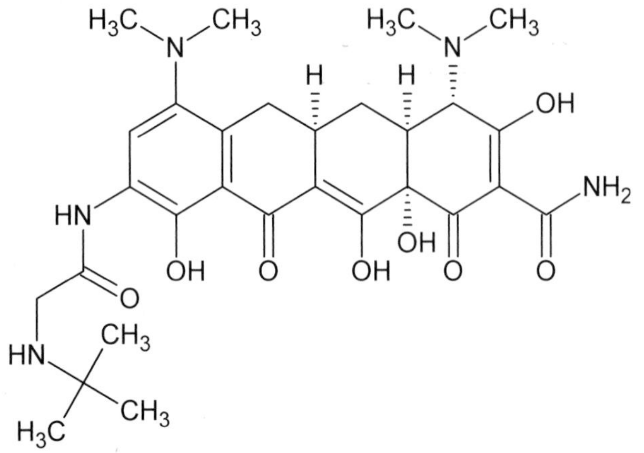

Tigecycline is recommended for the treatment of complicated skin and skin structure infections caused by *E. coli*, *E. faecalis* (vancomycin-susceptible isolates), *S. aureus* (methicillin-susceptible and methicillin-resistant isolates), *S. pyogenes*, and *B. fragilis* among others. Tigecycline is also indicated for complicated intra-abdominal infections caused by strains of *Clostridium*, *Enterobacter*, *Klebsiella*, and *Bacteroides*. To reduce the development of resistance to tigecycline, it is recommended that this antibiotic be used only for those infections caused by proven susceptible bacteria.

Glycylcyclines are structurally similar to tetracyclines, and appear to have similar adverse effects. These may include photosensitivity, pancreatitis, and pseudotumor cerebri. Nausea and vomiting have been reported.

Aztreonam

Azactam (aztreonam for injection, intravenous or intramuscular) contains the active ingredient aztreonam, which is a member of the monobactam class of antibiotics. A true antibiotic, aztreonam was originally isolated from cultures of the bacterium *Chromobacterium violaceum*. Now, the antibiotic is prepared by total synthesis. Monobactams possess a unique monocyclic β-lactam nucleus, and are structurally unlike other β-lactams like the penicillins, cephalosporins, carbapenems, and cephamycins. The β-lactam arrangement of aztreonam is unique, possessing an *N*-sulfonic acid functionality. This group activates the β-lactam ring toward attack. The side chain (3-position) aminothiazolyl oxime moiety and the 4-methyl group specify the antibacterial spectrum and β-lactamase resistance.

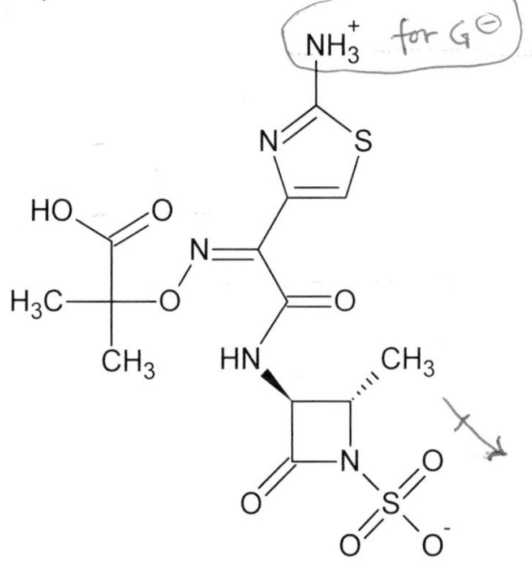

The mechanism of action of aztreonam is essentially identical to that of other β-lactam antibiotics. The action of aztreonam is inhibition of cell wall biosynthesis resulting from a high affinity of the antibiotic for penicillin binding protein 3 (PBP-3). Unlike other β-lactam antibiotics, aztreonam does not induce bacterial synthesis of β-lactamases. The structure of aztreonam confers resistance to hydrolysis by penicillinases and cephalosporinases synthesized by most Gram-negative and Gram-positive pathogens. Because of these properties, aztreonam is typically active against Gram-negative aerobic microorganisms that resist antibiotics hydrolyzed by β-lactamases. Aztreonam is active against strains that are multiply-resistant to antibiotics such as cephalosporins, penicillins, and aminoglycosides. The antibacterial activity is maintained over a broad pH range (6–8) in vitro, as well as in the presence of human serum and under anaerobic conditions.

Aztreonam for injection is indicated for the treatment of infections caused by susceptible Gram-negative microorganism, such as urinary tract infections (complicated and uncomplicated), including pyelonephritis and cystitis (initial and recurrent) caused by *E. coli*, *K. pneumoniae*, *P. mirabilis*, *P. aeruginosa*, *E. cloacae*, *K. oxytoca*, *Citrobacter* sp., and *S. marcescens*. Aztreonam is also indicated for lower respiratory tract infections, including pneumonia and bronchitis caused by *E. coli*, *K. pneumoniae*, *P. aeruginosa*, *H. influenzae*, *P. mirabilis*, *S. marcescens*, and *Enterobacter* species. Aztreonam is also indicated for septicemia caused by *E. coli*, *K. pneumoniae*, *P. aeruginosa*, *P. mirabilis*, *S. marcescens*, and *Enterobacter* spp. Other infections responding to aztreonam include skin and skin structure infections, including those associated with postoperative wounds and ulcers and burns. These may be caused by *E. coli*, *P. mirabilis*, *S. marcescens*, *Enterobacter* species, *P. aeruginosa*, *K. pneumoniae*, and *Citrobacter* species. Intra-abdominal infections, including peritonitis caused by *E. coli*, *Klebsiella* species including *K. pneumoniae*, *Enterobacter* species including *E. cloacae*, *P. aeruginosa*, *Citrobacter* species including *C. freundii*, and *Serratia* species including *S. marcescens*. Some gynecologic infections, including endometritis and pelvic cellulitis caused by *E. coli*, *K. pneumoniae*, *Enterobacter* species including *E. cloacae*, and *P. mirabilis* also respond to aztreonam.

Ertapenem

Ertapenem (Invanz, for injection) is a synthetic 1-β-methyl carbapenem that is structurally related to β-lactam antibiotics, particularly the thienamycin group. Its mechanism of action is the same as that of other β-lactam antibiotics. The structure resists β-lactamases and dehydropeptidases.

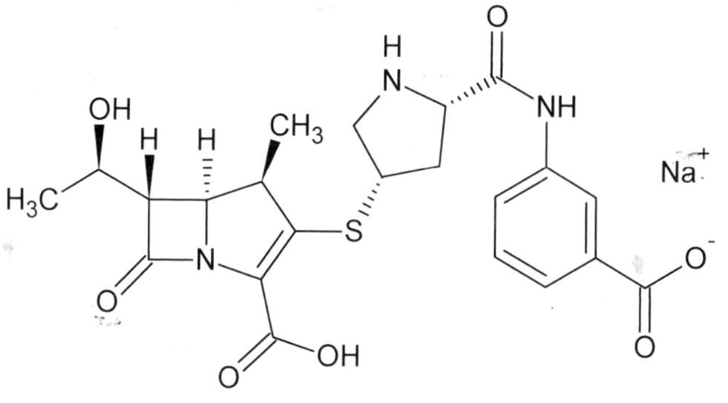

Ertapenem is indicated for the treatment of moderate to severe infections caused by susceptible strains causing complicated intra-abdominal infections such as *Escherichia*, *Clostridium*, *Peptostreptococcus*, and *Bacteroides*. The antibiotic is also indicated for complicated skin and skin structure infections including diabetic foot infections (without osteomyelitis). Treatable strains include *Staphylococcus* (MSSA), *Streptococcus*, *Escherichia*, *Klebsiella*, *Proteus*, and *Bacteroides*. Ertapenem is also indicated for community-acquired pneumonia caused by *S. pneumoniae*, *Haemophilus infljuenzae*, and *M. catarrhalis*. Complicated urinary tract infections and acute pelvic infections round out the indications for ertapenem.

Telithromycin ✶

Telithromycin (Ketek) is an orally bioavailable macrolide. The antibiotic is semisynthetic. Telithromycin is classified as a *ketolide*, and it differs chemically from the macrolide group of antibacterials by the lack of α-L-cladinose at 3-position of the erythronolide A ring, resulting in a 3-keto function. It is further characterized by imidazolyl and pyridyl rings inked to the macrolide nucleus through a butyl chain. The mechanism of action of telithromycin is the same as that of the macrolide class.

Telithromycin causes a blockade of protein synthesis by binding to domains II and V of 23S rRNA of the 50S ribosomal subunit. Because telithromycin binds at domain II, activity against Gram-positive cocci is retained in the presence of resistance mediated by methylases that alter the domain V binding site. The antibiotic is also believed to inhibit the assembly of ribosomes. Resistance to telithromycin occurs because of riboprotein mutations.

Telithromycin is active against aerobic Gram-positive microorganisms such as *S. pneumoniae* (including multidrug-resistant isolates), aerobic Gram-negative organisms such as *H. influenzae* and *M. catarrhalis*, and *M. pneumoniae*. Ketek is recommended for use in patients 18 years of age or older.

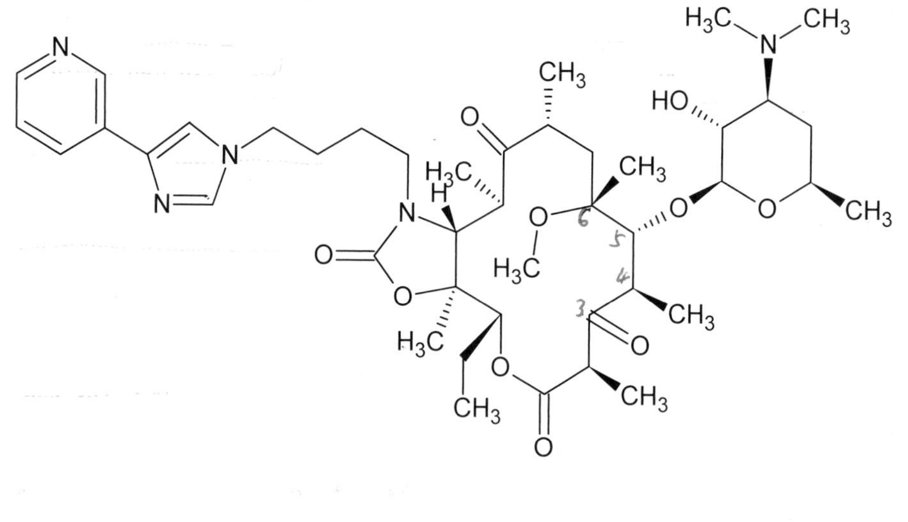

Telithromycin is metabolized by cytochrome P450. It therefore possesses several drug–drug interactions because of its ability to interact with various P450 isoforms. CYP3A4 inhibitors such as itraconazole caused the C_{max} of telithromycin to increase by 22% and the area under the curve (AUC) to increase by 54%. Ketoconazole and grapefruit juice demonstrated similar patterns. CYP3A4 substrates such as cisapride caused a dramatic increase in telithromycin plasma concentration. Simvastatin and midazolam also demonstrated increases in AUC when telithromycin was added. CYP2D6 substrates showed no effect on drug kinetics when administered with telithromycin. Other drug–drug interactions with telithromycin include digoxin (plasma peak and trough levels increased by 73% and 21%, respectively), theophylline (16% and 17% in steady-state C_{max} and AUC, respectively), and some oral contraceptives.

NEW DIRECTIONS IN ANTIBIOTIC DISCOVERY

Considering the rapid development of multidrug resistance to the antibiotics currently in our armamentarium, research into new agents is crucial. Multidrug resistant bacteria have become a major public health crisis because existing antibiotics are no longer effective in many cases. Antibiotics like vancomycin that have traditionally been drugs of last resort are becoming the first line of treatment of resistant infections. Unfortunately, in recent times very few novel antibiotics have been reported, and the development of new compounds by the pharmaceutical industry has been slow. Some consider that the reason for this situation is that industry is more concerned with developing drugs for chronic use in patients, instead of agents like antibiotics that are used acutely. The situation may be getting better. The Pharmaceutical Research and Manufacturing Association reports that in 2008, there are about 80 new antibiotics and antibacterial agents in various stages of development (it wasn't specified how many of these 80 agents are actually antibiotics). It is safe to assume that screening in nature for novel antibiotics is proceeding. Unfortunately, many agents that are isolated from nature are compounds that are mechanistically the same as antibiotics currently on the market.

It is essential to discover antibiotics that act through the disruption of a novel target. One success story is found in the research of scientists at Merck, who conducted high-throughput screenings of specialized metabolites against FabF, an enzyme that is involved in bacterial fatty acid biosynthesis. These screenings led to the discovery of a new antibiotic hitting a new target, platensimycin. Isolated from *Streptomyces platensis* cultures, platensimycin[285,286] represents a new structural class of antibiotics with very potent broad-spectrum activity against Gram-positive bacteria. It is interesting that to date, no cross-resistance has been observed. This feature is probably because of platensimycin's unique mechanism of action.

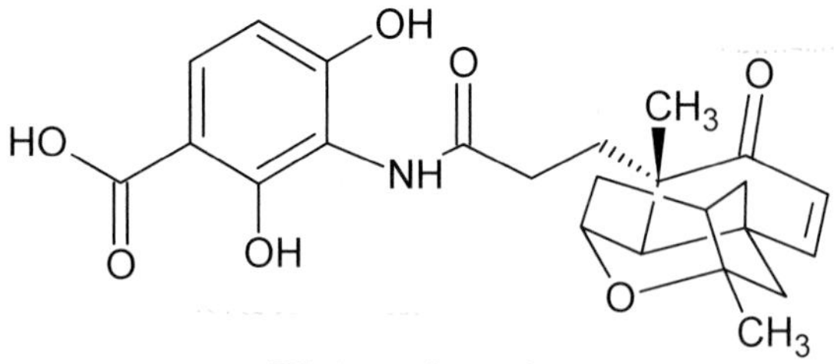

Platensimycin

In nature there are two distinct types of fatty acid biosynthesis pathways. Type 1 is referred to as the *associated system*, whereas type 2 is referred to as the *dissociated system*. Associated systems are found in higher organisms. These are composed of a large multidomain protein that is capable of catalyzing all of the steps of fatty acid biosynthesis. Dissociated systems are found in plants and bacteria. In these systems a set of discrete enzymes each catalyze a single step in the biosynthetic pathway, Hence, type 2 biosynthesis represents a good target for novel antibiotics. Moreover, two enzymes of the dissociated pathway, FabH and FabF/B, are well-conserved across many bacterial strains. This fact goes hand in hand with broad spectrum activity.

In vitro, platensimycin compares favorably with linezolid. No cross-resistance to MRSA, vancomycin-intermediate *S. aureus*, and vancomycin-resistant enterococci has been observed. An efflux mechanism arrears to preclude platensimycin's activity in Gram-negative bacteria.

The total synthesis of platensimycin has been reported[287] and a congener, carbaplatensimycin,[288] has been synthesized as well. The activity of carbaplatensimycin is similar to that of the parent platensimycin.

It is safe to assume that if any success is to be had against the rapidly developing multidrug-resistant bacteria, novel targets will have to be found. The platensimycin story is just the first case of this kind of antibiotic development.

● R E V I E W   Q U E S T I O N S ●

1. Compare and contrast the mechanisms of action of the tetracyclines and the macrolides.

2. Give the correct definition of an "antibiotic."

3. Can penicillins and aminoglycosides be used synergistically? If so, how?

4. What are "PBPs"? How do they work in the mechanism of action of the penicillins?

5. What is an aglycone?

6. How does spectinomycin differ from the other aminoglycoside antibiotics?

7. What bacterial genus synthesizes most of the clinically used antibiotics?

8. What are multidrug-resistant bacteria? Why are they of concern to medicine?

9. What is the unique mechanism of action of platensimycin?

10. Why do we say that cephalosporins possess "intrinsic β-lactamase resistance"?

REFERENCES

1. Fleming, A.: Br. J. Exp. Pathol. 10:226, 1929.
2. Vuillemin, P.: Assoc. Fr. Avance Sc.: 2:525, 1889.
3. Waksman, S. A.: Science 110:27, 1949.
4. Benedict, R. G., and Langlykke, A. F.: Annu. Rev. Microbiol. 1:193, 1947.
5. Baron, A. L.: Handbook of Antibiotics. New York, Reinhold, 1950, p. 5.
6. Lancini, G., Parenti, F., and Gallo, G. G.: Antibiotics: An Interdisciplinary Approach, 3rd ed. New York, Plenum Press, 1995, p. 1.
7. Yocum, R. R., et al.: J. Biol. Chem. 255:3977, 1980.
8. Waxman, D. J., and Strominger, J. L.: Annu. Rev. Pharmacol. 52:825, 1983.
9. Spratt, B. G.: Proc. Natl. Acad. Sci. U. S. A. 72:2999, 1975.
10. Spratt, B. G.: Eur. J. Biochem. 72:341, 1977.
11. Tomasz, A.: Annu. Rev. Microbiol. 33:113, 1979.
12. Spratt, B. G., and Pardee A. B.: Nature 254:516, 1975.
13. Suzuki, H., et al.: Proc. Natl. Acad. Sci. U. S. A. 75:664, 1978.
14. Clarke, H. T., et al.: The Chemistry of Penicillin. Princeton, NJ, Princeton University Press, 1949, p. 454.
15. Sheehan, J. C., and Henery-Logan, K. R.: J. Am. Chem. Soc. 81:3089, 1959.
16. Batchelor, F. R., et al.: Nature 183:257, 1959.
17. Sheehan, J. C., and Ferris, J. P.: J. Am. Chem. Soc. 81:2912, 1959.
18. Hou, J. P., and Poole, J. W.: J. Pharm. Sci. 60:503, 1971.
19. Blaha, J. M., et al.: J. Pharm. Sci. 65:1165, 1976.
20. Schwartz, M. A.: J. Pharm. Sci. 58:643, 1969.
21. Schwartz, M. A., and Buckwalter, F. H.: J. Pharm. Sci. 51:1119, 1962.
22. Finholt, P., Jurgensen, G., and Kristiansen, H.: J. Pharm. Sci. 54:387, 1965.
23. Segelman, A. B., and Farnsworth, N. R.: J. Pharm. Sci. 59:725, 1970.
24. Sykes, R. B., and Matthew, M.: J. Antimicrob. Chemother. 2:115, 1976.
25. Bush, K., Jacoby, G. A., and Medeiros, A. A.: Antimicrob. Agents Chemother. 39:1211, 1995.
26. Ambler, R. P.: Phil. Trans. R. Soc. Lond. [B] 289:321, 1980.
27. Zimmerman, W., and Rosselet, A.: Antimicrob. Agents Chemother. 12:368, 1977.
28. Yoshimura, F., and Nikaido, H.: Antimicrob. Agents Chemother. 27:84, 1985.
29. Malouin, F., and Bryan, L. E.: Antimicrob. Agents Chemother. 30:1, 1986.
30. Dougherty, T. J., et al.: Antimicrob. Agents Chemother. 18:730, 1980.
31. Hartman, B., and Tomasz, A.: Antimicrob. Agents Chemother. 19:726, 1981.
32. Brain, E. G., et al.: J. Chem. Soc. 1445, 1962.
33. Stedman, R. J., et al.: J. Med. Chem. 7:251, 1964.
34. Nayler, J. H. C.: Adv. Drug Res. 7:52, 1973.
35. Nikaido, H., Rosenberg, E. Y., and Foulds, J.: J. Bacteriol. 153:232, 1983.
36. Matthew, M.: J. Antimicrob. Chemother. 5:349, 1979.
37. Iyengar, B. S., et al.: J. Med. Chem. 29:611, 1986.
38. Hansch, C., and Deutsch, E. W.: J. Med. Chem. 8:705, 1965.
39. Bird, A. E., and Marshall, A. C.: Biochem. Pharmacol. 16:2275, 1967.
40. Stewart, G. W.: The Penicillin Group of Drugs. Amsterdam, Elsevier, 1965.
41. Corran, P. H., and Waley, S. G.: Biochem. J. 149:357, 1975.
42. Batchelor, F. R., et al.: Nature 206:362, 1965.
43. DeWeck, A. L.: Int. Arch. Allergy 21:20, 1962.
44. Smith, H., and Marshall, A. C.: Nature 232:45, 1974.
45. Monroe, A. C., et al.: Int. Arch. Appl. Immunol. 50:192, 1976.
46. Behrens, O. K., et al.: J. Biol. Chem. 175:793, 1948.
47. Mayersohn, M., and Endrenyi, L.: Can. Med. Assoc. J. 109:989, 1973.
48. Hill, S. A., et al.: J. Pharm. Pharmacol. 27:594, 1975.
49. Neu, H. C.: Rev. Infect. Dis. 3:110, 1981.
50. Neu, H. C.: J. Infect. Dis. 12S:1, 1974.
51. Westphal, J. F., et al.: Clin. Pharmacol. Ther. 57:257, 1995.
52. Ancred, P., et al.: Nature 215:25, 1967.
53. Knowles, J. R.: Acc. Chem. Res. 18:97, 1985.
54. Bush, K., et al.: Antimicrob. Agents Chemother. 37:429, 1993.
55. Payne, D. J., et al.: Antimicrob. Agents Chemother. 38:767, 1994.
56. Payne, D. J.: J. Med. Microbiol. 39:93, 1993.
57. Micetich, R. G., et al.: J. Med. Chem. 30:1469, 1987.
58. Merck & Co., Inc.: U.S. Patent 3,950,357 (April 12, 1976).
59. Johnston, D. B. R., et al.: J. Am. Chem. Soc. 100:313, 1978.
60. Albers-Schonberg, G., et al.: J. Am. Chem. Soc. 100:6491, 1978.
61. Kahan, J. S., et al.: 16th Conference on Antimicrobial Agents and Chemotherapy, Chicago, 1976, Abstr. 227.
62. Kropp, H., et al.: Antimicrob. Agents Chemother. 22:62, 1982.
63. Leanza, W. J., et al.: J. Med. Chem. 22:1435, 1979.
64. Shih, D. H., et al.: Heterocycles 21:29, 1984.
65. Hikida, M., et al.: J. Antimicrob. Chemother. 30:129, 1992.
66. Wiseman, L. R., et al.: Drugs 50:73, 1995.
67. Petersen, P. J., et al.: Antimicrob. Agents Chemother. 35:203, 1991.
68. Felici, A., et al.: Antimicrob. Agents Chemother. 39:1300, 1995.
68a. Abraham, E. P., and Newton, G. G.: Biochem. J. 79:377, 1961.
69. Morin, R. B., et al.: J. Am. Chem. Soc. 84:3400, 1962.
70. Fechtig, B., et al.: Helv. Chim. Acta 51:1108, 1968.
71. Woodward, R. B., et al.: J. Am. Chem. Soc. 88:852, 1966.
72. Morin, R. B., et al.: J. Am. Chem. Soc. 85:1896, 1963.
73. Yamana, T., and Tsuji, A.: J. Pharm. Sci. 65:1563, 1976.
74. Sullivan, H. R., and McMahon, R. E.: Biochem. J. 102:976, 1967.
75. Indelicato, J. M., et al.: J. Med. Chem. 17:523, 1974.
76. Tsuji, A., et al.: J. Pharm. Sci. 70:1120, 1981.
77. Fong, I. W., et al.: Antimicrob. Agents Chemother. 9:939, 1976.
78. Cimarusti, C. M.: J. Med. Chem. 27:247, 1984.
79. Faraci, W. S., and Pratt, R. F.: Biochemistry 24:903, 1985.
79a. Faraci, W. S., and Pratt, R. F.: Biochemistry 25:2934, 1986.
80. Bechtold, H., et al.: Thromb. Haemost. 51:358, 1984.
81. Buening, M. K., et al.: JAMA 245:2027, 1981.
82. Kukolja, S.: Synthesis of 3-methylenecepham, a key and general intermediate in the preparation of 3-substituted cephalosporins. In Elks, J. (ed.). Recent Advances in the Chemistry of Beta-Lactam Antibiotics. Chichester, Burlington House, 1977, p. 181.
83. Gillett, A. P., et al.: Postgrad. Med. 55(Suppl. 4):9, 1979.
84. Cooper, R. G. D.: Am. J. Med. 92(Suppl. 6A):2S, 1992.
85. Indelicato, J. M., et al.: J. Pharm. Sci. 65:1175, 1976.
86. Ott, J. L., et al.: Antimicrob. Agents Chemother. 15:14, 1979.
87. Nagarajan, R., et al.: J. Am. Chem. Soc. 93:2308, 1971.
88. Stapley, E. O., et al.: Antimicrob. Agents Chemother. 2:122, 1972.
89. Goering, R. V., et al.: Antimicrob. Agents Chemother. 21:963, 1982.
90. Grassi, G. G., et al.: J. Antimicrob. Chemother. 11(Suppl. A): 45, 1983.
91. Tsuji, A., et al.: J. Pharm. Pharmacol. 39:272, 1987.
92. Labia, R., et al.: Drugs Exp. Clin. Res. 10:27, 1984.
93. Park, H. Z., Lee, S. P., and Schy, A. L.: Gastroenterology 100:1665, 1991.
94. Fassbender, M., et al.: Clin. Infect. Dis. 16:646, 1993.
95. Schafer, V., et al.: J. Antimicrob. Chemother. 29(Suppl A):7, 1992.
96. Sanders, C. C.: Clin. Infect. Dis. 17:369, 1993.
97. Watanabe, N. A., et al.: Antimicrob. Agents Chemother. 31:497, 1987.
98. Erwin, M. E., et al.: Antimicrob. Agents Chemother. 35:927, 1991.
99. Hanaki, H., et al.: Antimicrob. Agents Chemother. 39:1120, 1995.
100. Imada, A., et al.: Nature 289:590, 1981.
101. Sykes, R. B., et al.: Nature 291:489, 1981.
102. Bonner, D. B., and Sykes, R. B.: J. Antimicrob. Chemother. 14:313, 1984.
103. Tanaka, S. N., et al.: Antimicrob. Agents Chemother. 31:219, 1987.
104. Schatz, A., et al.: Proc. Soc. Exp. Biol. Med. 55:66, 1944.
105. Weisblum, B., and Davies, J.: Bacteriol. Rev. 32:493, 1968.
106. Davies, J., and Davis, B. D.: J. Biol. Chem. 243:3312, 1968.
107. Lando, D., et al.: Biochemistry 12:4528, 1973.
108. Shaw, K. J., et al.: Microbiol. Rev. 57:138, 1993.
109. Chevereau, P. J. L., et al.: Biochemistry 13:598, 1974.
110. Price, K. E., et al.: Antimicrob. Agents Chemother. 5:143, 1974.
111. Bryan, L. E., et al.: J. Antibiot. (Tokyo) 29:743, 1976.
112. Hancock, R. E. W.: J. Antimicrob. Chemother. 8:249, 1981.
113. Cox, D. A., et al.: The aminoglycosides. In Sammes, P. G. (ed.). Topics in Antibiotic Chemistry, vol. 1. Chichester, Ellis Harwood, 1977, p. 44.
114. Price, K. E.: Antimicrob. Agents Chemother. 29:543, 1986.
115. Dyer, J. R., and Todd, A. W.: J. Am. Chem. Soc. 85:3896, 1963.
116. Dyer, J. R., et al.: J. Am. Chem. Soc. 87:654, 1965.
117. Umezawa, S., et al.: J. Antibiot. (Tokyo) 27:997, 1974.
118. Waksman, S. A., and Lechevalier, H. A.: Science 109:305, 1949.
119. Hichens, M., and Rinehart, K. L., Jr.: J. Am. Chem. Soc. 85:1547, 1963.
120. Rinehart, K. L., Jr., et al.: J. Am. Chem. Soc. 84:3218, 1962.
121. Huettenrauch, R.: Pharmazie 19:697, 1964.
122. Umezawa, S., and Nishimura, Y.: J. Antibiot. (Tokyo) 30:189, 1977.
123. Haskell, T. H., et al.: J. Am. Chem. Soc. 81:3482, 1959.

124. DeJongh, D. C., et al.: J. Am. Chem. Soc. 89:3364, 1967.
125. Umezawa, H., et al.: J. Antibiot. [A] 10:181, 1957.
126. Tatsuoka, S., et al.: J. Antibiot. [A] 17:88, 1964.
127. Nakajima, M.: Tetrahedron Lett. 623, 1968.
128. Umezawa, S., et al.: J. Antibiot. (Tokyo) 21:162, 367, 424, 1968.
129. Morikubo, Y.: J. Antibiot. [A] 12:90, 1959.
130. Kawaguchi, H., et al.: J. Antibiot. (Tokyo) 25:695, 1972.
131. Paradelis, A. G., et al.: Antimicrob. Agents Chemother. 14:514, 1978.
132. Weinstein, M. J., et al.: J. Med. Chem. 6:463, 1963.
133. Cooper, D. J., et al.: J. Infect. Dis. 119:342, 1969.
134. Cooper, D. J., et al.: J. Chem. Soc. C 3126, 1971.
135. Maehr, H., and Schaffner, C. P.: J. Am. Chem. Soc. 89:6788, 1968.
136. Koch, K. F., et al.: J. Antibiot. [A] 26:745, 1963.
137. Lockwood, W., et al.: Antimicrob. Agents Chemother. 4:281, 1973.
138. Wright, J. J.: J. Chem. Soc. Chem. Commun. 206, 1976.
139. Wagman, G. H., et al.: J. Antibiot. (Tokyo) 23:555, 1970.
140. Braveny, I., et al.: Arzneimittelforschung 30:491, 1980.
141. Lewis, C., and Clapp, H. W.: Antibiot. Chemother. 11:127, 1961.
142. Cochran, T. G., and Abraham, D. J.: J. Chem. Soc. Chem. Commun. 494, 1972.
143. Muxfeldt, H., et al.: J. Am. Chem. Soc. 90:6534, 1968.
144. Muxfeldt, H., et al.: J. Am. Chem. Soc. 101:689, 1979.
145. Korst, J. J., et al.: J. Am. Chem. Soc. 90:439, 1968.
146. Muxfeldt, H., et al.: Angew. Chem. Int. Ed. 12:497, 1973.
147. Hirokawa, S., et al.: Z. Krist. 112:439, 1959.
148. Takeuchi, Y., and Buerger, M. J.: Proc. Natl. Acad. Sci. U. S. A. 46:1366, 1960.
149. Cid-Dresdner, H.: Z. Krist. 121:170, 1965.
150. Leeson, L. J., Krueger, J. E., and Nash, R. A.: Tetrahedron Lett. 1155, 1963.
151. Stephens, C. R., et al.: J. Am. Chem. Soc. 78:4155, 1956.
152. Rigler, N. E., et al.: Anal. Chem. 37:872, 1965.
153. Benet, L. Z., and Goyan, J. E.: J. Pharm. Sci. 55:983, 1965.
154. Barringer, W., et al.: Am. J. Pharm. 146:179, 1974.
155. Barr, W. H., et al.: Clin. Pharmacol. Ther. 12:779, 1971.
156. Albert, A.: Nature 172:201, 1953.
157. Jackson, F. L.: Mode of action of tetracyclines. In Schnitzer, R. J., and Hawking, F. (eds.). Experimental Chemotherapy, vol. 3. New York, Academic Press, 1964, p. 103.   old
158. Bodley, J. W., and Zieve, F. J.: Biochem. Biophys. Res. Commun. 36:463, 1969.
159. Dockter, M. E., and Magnuson, A.: Biochem. Biophys. Res. Commun. 42:471, 1973.
160. Speer, B. S., Shoemaker, N. B., and Salyers, A. A.: Clin. Microbiol. Rev. 5:387, 1992.
161. Durckheimer, W.: Angew. Chem. Int. Ed. 14:721, 1975.
162. Brown, J. R., and Ireland, D. S.: Adv. Pharmacol. Chemother. 15:161, 1978.
163. Mitscher, L. A.: The Chemistry of the Tetracycline Antibiotics. New York, Marcel Dekker, 1978.
164. Chopra, I., Hawkey, P. M., and Hinton, M.: J. Antimicrob. Chemother. 29:245, 1992.
165. Clive, D. L. J.: Q. Rev. 22:435, 1968.
166. Hlavka, J. J., and Boothe, J. H. (eds.): The Tetracyclines. New York, Springer-Verlag, 1985.
167. Cammarata, A., and Yau, S. J.: J. Med. Chem. 13:93, 1970.
168. Glatz, B., et al.: J. Am. Chem. Soc. 101:2171, 1979.
169. Schach von Wittenau, M., et al.: J. Am. Chem. Soc. 84:2645, 1962.
170. Stephens, C. R., et al.: J. Am. Chem. Soc. 85:2643, 1963.
171. McCormick, J. R. D., et al.: J. Am. Chem. Soc. 79:4561, 1957.
172. Martell, M. J., Jr., and Boothe, J. H.: J. Med. Chem. 10:44, 1967.
173. Colazzi, J. L., and Klink, P. R.: J. Pharm. Sci. 58:158, 1969.
174. Schumacher, G. E., and Linn, E. E.: J. Pharm. Sci. 67:1717, 1978.
175. Schach von Wittenau, M.: Chemotherapy 13S:41, 1968.
176. Conover H.: U.S. Patent 2,699,054 (Jan. 11, 1955).
177. Bunn, P. A., and Cronk, G. A.: Antibiot. Med. 5:379, 1958.
178. Gittinger, W. C., and Wiener, H.: Antibiot. Med. 7:22, 1960.
179. Remmers, E. G., et al.: J. Pharm. Sci. 53:1452, 1534, 1964.
180. Remmers, E. G., et al.: J. Pharm. Sci. 54:49, 1965.
181. Duggar, B. B.: Ann. N. Y. Acad. Sci. 51:177, 1948.
182. Finlay, A. C., et al.: Science 111:85, 1950.
183. Hochstein, F. A., et al.: J. Am. Chem. Soc. 75:5455, 1953.
184. Blackwood, R. K., et al.: J. Am. Chem. Soc. 83:2773, 1961.
185. Stephens, C. R., et al.: J. Am. Chem. Soc. 80:5324, 1958.
186. Minuth, J. N.: Antimicrob. Agents Chemother. 6:411, 1964.
187. Goldstein, F. W., Kitzis, M. D., and Acar, J. F.: Antimicrob. Agents Chemother. 38:2218, 1994.
188. Sum, P. K., et al.: J. Med. Chem. 37:184, 1994.
189. Tally, F. T., Ellestad, G. A., and Testa, R. T.: J. Antimicrob. Chemother. 35:449, 1995.
190. Kirst, H.: Prog. Med. Chem. 31:265, 1994.
191. Lartey, P. A., Nellans, H. N., and Tanaka, S. K.: Adv. Pharmacol. 28:307, 1994.
192. Wilhelm, J. M., et al.: Antimicrob. Agents Chemother. 236, 1967.
193. Leclercq, R., and Courvalin, P.: Antimicrob. Agents Chemother. 35:1273, 1991.
194. Lai, C. J., and Weisblum, B.: Proc. Natl. Acad. Sci. U. S. A. 68:856, 1971.
195. Leclercq, R., and Courvalin, P.: Antimicrob. Agents Chemother. 35:1267, 1991.
196. McGuire, J. M., et al.: Antibiot. Chemother. 2:821, 1952.
197. Wiley, P. F.: J. Am. Chem. Soc. 79:6062, 1957.
198. Celmer, W. D.: J. Am. Chem. Soc. 87:1801, 1965.
199. Corey, E. J., et al.: J. Am. Chem. Soc. 101:7131, 1979.
200. Stephens, C. V., et al.: J. Antibiot. (Tokyo) 22:551, 1969.
201. Bechtol, L. D., et al.: Curr. Ther. Res. 20:610, 1976.
202. Welling, P. G., et al.: J. Pharm. Sci. 68:150, 1979.
203. Yakatan, G. J., et al.: J. Clin. Pharmacol. 20:625, 1980.
204. Tjandramaga, T. B., et al.: Pharmacology 29:305, 1984.
205. Croteau, D., Bergeron, M. G., and Lebel, M.: Antimicrob. Agents Chemother. 32:561, 1989.
206. Tardrew, P. L., et al.: Appl. Microbiol. 18:159, 1969.
207. Janicki, R. S., et al.: Clin. Pediatr. (Phila.) 14:1098, 1975.
208. Nicholas, P.: N. Y. State J. Med. 77:2088, 1977.
209. Derrick, C. W., and Dillon, H. C.: Am. J. Dis. Child. 133:1146, 1979.
210. Ginsburg, C. M., et al.: Pediatr. Infect. Dis. 1:384, 1982.
211. Itoh, Z., et al.: Am. J. Physiol. 11:G320, 1985.
212. Sturgill, M. C., and Rapp, R. P.: Ann. Pharmacother. 26:1099, 1992.
213. Bright, G. M., et al.: J. Antibiot. (Tokyo) 41:1029, 1988.
214. Peters, D. H., Friedel, H. A., and McTavish, D.: Drugs 44:750, 1992.
215. Counter, F. T., et al.: Antimicrob. Agents Chemother. 35:1116, 1991.
216. Brogden, R. N., and Peters, D. H.: Drugs 48:599, 1994.
217. Sobin, B. A., et al.: Antibiotics Annual 1954–1955. New York, Medical Encyclopedia, 1955, p. 827.
218. Hochstein, F. A., et al.: J. Am. Chem. Soc. 82:3227, 1960.
219. Celmer, W. D.: J. Am. Chem. Soc. 87:1797, 1965.
220. Mason, D. J., et al.: Antimicrob. Agents Chemother. 544, 1962.
221. Hoeksema, H., et al.: J. Am. Chem. Soc. 86:4223, 1964.
222. Slomp, G., and MacKellar, F. A.: J. Am. Chem. Soc. 89:2454, 1967.
223. Howarth, G. B., et al.: J. Chem. Soc. C 2218, 1970.
224. Magerlein, B. J.: Tetrahedron Lett. 685, 1970.
225. Argoudelis, A. D., et al.: J. Am. Chem. Soc. 86:5044, 1964.
226. Magerlein, B. J., et al.: J. Med. Chem. 10:355, 1967.
227. Bannister, B.: J. Chem. Soc. Perkin Trans. I:1676, 1973.
228. Bannister, B.: J. Chem. Soc. Perkin Trans. I:3025, 1972.
229. Bartlett, J. G.: Rev. Infect. Dis. 1:370, 1979.
230. Sarges, R., and Witkop, B.: J. Am. Chem. Soc. 86:1861, 1964.
231. Storm, D. R., Rosenthal, K. S., and Swanson, P. E.: Annu. Rev. Biochem. 46:723, 1977.
232. McCormick, M. H., et al.: Antibiotics Annual 1955–1956. New York, Medical Encyclopedia, 1956, p. 606.
233. Sheldrick, G. M., et al.: Nature 27:233, 1978.
234. Williamson, M. P., and Williams, D. H.: J. Am. Chem. Soc. 103:6580, 1981.
235. Harris, C. M., et al.: J. Am. Chem. Soc. 105:6915, 1983.
236. Perkins, H. R., and Nieto, M.: Ann. N. Y. Acad. Sci. 235:348, 1974.
237. Williamson, M. P., et al.: Tetrahedron Lett. 40:569, 1984.
238. Walsh, C. T.: Science 261:308, 1993.
239. Parenti, F., et al.: J. Antibiot. (Tokyo) 31:276, 1978.
240. Bardone, M. R., Paternoster, M., and Coronelli, C.: J. Antibiot. (Tokyo) 31:170, 1978.
241. Coronelli, C., et al.: J. Antibiot. (Tokyo) 37:621, 1984.
242. Hunt, A. H., et al.: J. Am. Chem. Soc. 106:4891, 1984.
243. Barna, J. C. J., et al.: J. Am. Chem. Soc. 106:4895, 1984.
244. Brogden, R. N., and Peters, D. H.: Drugs 47:823, 1994.
245. Johnson, B. A., et al.: Science 102:376, 1945.
246. Stoffel, W., and Craig, L. C.: J. Am. Chem. Soc. 83:145, 1961.
247. Ressler, C., and Kashelikar, D. V.: J. Am. Chem. Soc. 88:2025, 1966.
248. Benedict, R. G., and Langlykke, A. F.: J. Bacteriol. 54:24, 1947.
249. Stansly, P. G., et al.: Bull. Johns Hopkins Hosp. 81:43, 1947.
250. Ainsworth, G. C., et al.: Nature 160:263, 1947.
251. Vogler, K., and Studer, R. O.: Experientia 22:345, 1966.
252. Hausmann, W., and Craig, L. C.: J. Am. Chem. Soc. 76:4892, 1952.

253. Vogler, K., et al.: Experientia 20:365, 1964.
254. Koyama, Y., et al.: J. Antibiot. [A] 3:457, 1950.
255. Suzuki, T., et al.: J. Biochem. 54:41, 1963.
256. Wilkinson, S., and Lowe, L. A.: J. Chem. Soc. 4107, 1964.
257. Dubos, R. J.: J. Exp. Med. 70:1, 1939.
258. Paladini, A., and Craig, L. C.: J. Am. Chem. Soc. 76:688, 1954.
259. King, T. P., and Craig, L. C.: J. Am. Chem. Soc. 77:627, 1955.
260. Ohno, M., et al.: Bull. Soc. Chem. Jpn. 39:1738, 1966.
261. Finkelstein, A., and Anderson, O. S.: J. Membr. Biol. 59:155, 1981.
262. Ehrlich, J., et al.: Science 106:417, 1947.
263. Controulis, J., et al.: J. Am. Chem. Soc. 71:2463, 1949.
264. Long, L. M., and Troutman, H. D.: J. Am. Chem. Soc. 71:2473, 1949.
265. Szulcewski, D., and Eng, F.: Anal. Profiles Drug Subst. 4:47, 1972.
266. Glazko, A.: Antimicrob. Agents Chemother. 655, 1966.
267. Hansch, C., et al.: J. Med. Chem. 16:917, 1973.
268. Brock, T. D.: Chloramphenicol. In Schnitzer, R. J., and Hawking, F. (eds.). Experimental Chemotherapy, vol. 3. New York, Academic Press, 1964, p. 119.
269. Shalit, I., and Marks, M. I.: Drugs 28:281, 1984.
270. Kauffman, R. E., et al.: J. Pediatr. 99:963, 1981.
271. Kramer, W. G., et al.: J. Clin. Pharmacol. 24:181, 1984.
272. Shunk, C. H., et al.: J. Am. Chem. Soc. 78:1770, 1956.
273. Hoeksema, H., et al.: J. Am. Chem. Soc. 78:2019, 1956.
274. Spencer, C. H., et al.: J. Am. Chem. Soc. 78:2655, 1956.
275. Spencer, C., et al.: J. Am. Chem. Soc. 80:140, 1958.
276. Gellert, M., et al.: Proc. Natl. Acad. Sci. U. S. A. 73:4474, 1976.
277. Sugino, A., et al.: Proc. Natl. Acad. Sci. U. S. A. 75:4842, 1978.
278. Fuller, A. T., et al.: Nature 134:416, 1971.
279. Chain, E. B., and Mellows, G.: J. Chem. Soc. Perkin Trans. I:294, 1977.
280. Pappa, K. A.: J. Am. Acad. Dermatol. 22:873, 1990.
281. Hughes, J., and Mellows, G.: J. Antibiot. (Tokyo) 31:330, 1978.
282. Hughes, J., and Mellows, G.: Biochem. J. 176:305, 1978.
283. Gilbart, J., Perry, C. R., and Slocombe, B.: Antimicrob. Agents Chemother. 37:32, 1993.
284. Capobianco, J. O., Doran, C. C., and Goldman, R. C.: Antimicrob. Agents Chemother. 33:156, 1989.
285. Wang, J., et. al.: Nature 441: 358 (2006).
286. Singh, S. B., Jayasuriya, H., Ondeyka, J. G., et. al.: J. Am. Chem. Soc. 128, 11916, 2006.
287. Nicolaou, K. C., Li, A., and Edmonds, D. J.: Angew. Chem. Int. Ed. 45, 7086, 2006.
288. Nicolaou, K. C., Tang, Y., Wang, J., et. al.: J. Am. Chem. Soc. 129, 14850, 2007.

SELECTED READING

Conte, J. E.: Manual of Antibiotics and Infectious Diseases, 8th ed. Baltimore, Williams & Wilkins, 1995.
Franklin, T. J., and Snow, G. A.: Biochemistry of Antimicrobial Action, 4th ed. London, Chapman & Hall, 1989.
Jawetz, E., et al.: Medical Microbiology, 20th ed. Norwalk, CT, Appleton & Lange, 1995.
Lambert, H. P., and O'Grady, W. D. (eds.): Antibiotic and Chemotherapy, 6th ed. New York, Churchill-Livingstone, 1992.
Lancini, G., Parenti, F., and Gallo, G. G.: Antibiotics, A Multidisciplinary Approach. New York, Plenum Press, 1995.
Mandell, G. L., Bennett, J. E., and Dolin, R. (eds.): Principles and Practice of Infectious Diseases, vol. 1, 4th ed. New York, Churchill-Livingstone, 1995.
Neu, H. C.: The crisis of antibiotic resistance. Science 257:1064, 1992.
Page, M. I. (ed.): The Chemistry of Beta Lactams. New York, Chapman & Hall, 1992.
Silver, L. L., and Bostian, K. A.: Discovery and development of new antibiotics: The problem of drug resistance. Antimicrob. Agents Chemother. 37:377, 1993.

CHAPTER 9

Antiviral Agents

JOHN M. BEALE, JR.

CHAPTER OVERVIEW

Viral diseases constitute a set of difficult-to-treat conditions. Over the years, many different antiviral agents have been discovered and synthesized, and these have provided various means of treatment of viral conditions. This chapter will begin with some concepts of viral taxonomy and the steps in the infectious cycle of viruses, as well as biochemical steps that can be used as targets in antiviral therapy. We will then move into the arena of prevention of viral infection through the use of chemoprophylaxis. Chemoprophylaxis is accomplished through the use of immunization with vaccines, agents such as amantadine and rimantidine for influenza prophylaxis, and the neuraminidase inhibitors zanamivir and oseltamivir. Interferons (IFNs) will then be discussed as chemoprophylactic agents. Nucleoside antimetabolites will be discussed as compounds that inhibit polymerases and are incorporated into viral nucleic acids, causing these macromolecules to become unstable. An extended discussion of reverse transcriptase (RT) inhibitors and nonnucleoside reverse transcriptase inhibitors (NNRTIs) follows. The chapter concludes with a discussion of human immunodeficiency virus (HIV), protease inhibitors (PIs), combination therapy, and short-interfering RNA (siRNA) and RNA interference.

Objectives of this chapter are to understand the biochemistry of viruses, to learn the mechanisms of action of the antiviral agents, and to develop a knowledge of which antiviral agent should be used in any given infection.

THE CLASSIFICATION AND BIOCHEMISTRY OF VIRUSES

Viruses are unique organisms. They are the smallest of all self-replicating organisms, able to pass through filters that retain the smallest bacteria.[1] The simplest viruses contain a small amount of DNA or RNA surrounded by an uncomplicated protein coat. Some of the more complex viruses have a lipid bilayer membrane surrounding the nucleic acid.[2] Viruses must replicate in living cells, which has led many to argue that viruses are not even living organisms but that they somehow exist at the interface of the living and the nonliving.[1] The most basic requirement is for the virus to induce either profound or subtle changes in the host cell, so that viral genes are replicated and viral proteins are expressed. This will result in the formation of new viruses, usually many more than the number that infected the cell initially. Viruses conduct no metabolic processes on their own; they depend totally on a host cell, which they invade and parasitize to subvert subcellular machinery. They use part of the cell's equipment for replication of viral nucleic acids and expression of viral genes, all of the cell's protein synthesis machinery, and all of the cell's energy stores that are generated by its own metabolic processes. The virus turns the biochemical systems of the host cell to its own purposes, completely subverting the infected cell. An infection that results in the production of more viruses than initiation of infection is called a *productive infection*. The actual number of infectious viruses produced in an infected cell is termed the *burst size*. This number can range from 10 to more than 10,000, depending on the type of cell infected, the nature of the virus, and other factors.[3]

Viruses are known to infect every form of life.[1] A typical DNA virus will enter the nucleus of the host cell, where viral DNA is transcribed into messenger RNA (mRNA) by host cell RNA polymerase. mRNA is then translated into virus-specific proteins that facilitate assembly, maturation, and release of newly formed virus into surrounding tissues. RNA viruses are somewhat different, in that their replication relies on enzymes in the virus itself to synthesize mRNA.

An adult virus possesses only one type of nucleic acid (either a DNA or an RNA genome). This feature differentiates viruses from other intracellular parasites, such as *Chlamydia* (which possesses both DNA and RNA when replicating within a cell) and the *Rickettsiae* (which, in addition to DNA and RNA, have autonomous energy-generating systems). Viruses are very different from these other intracellular parasites. Another unique feature of viruses is that their organized structure is completely lost during replication within the host cell; the nucleic acid and proteins exist dispersed in the cytoplasm.

CLASSIFICATION OF VIRUSES

Viruses are classified on the basis of several features:

- Nucleic acid content (DNA or RNA)
- Viral morphology (helical, icosahedral)
- Site of replication in cell (cytoplasm or nucleus)
- Coating (enveloped or nonenveloped)
- Serological typing (antigenic signatures)
- Cell types infected (B lymphocytes, T lymphocytes, monocytes)

The Baltimore Classification Scheme[4] (Table 9.1) gives an alternate means of relating the different virus types.

TABLE 9.1 Baltimore Classification Scheme for Viruses

I) Single-stranded RNA viruses
  A) Positive sense (virion RNA-like cellular mRNA)
    1) Nonenveloped
      (a) Icosahedral
        (i) Picornaviruses (polio, hepatitis A, rhinovirus)
        (ii) Calicivirus
        (iii) Plant virus relatives of Picornavirus
        (iv) MS2 bacteriophage
    2) Enveloped
      (a) Icosahedral
        (i) Togaviruses (rubella, equine encephalitis, Sindbis)
        (ii) Flaviviruses (yellow fever, dengue fever)
      (b) Helical
        (i) Coronavirus
  B) Positive sense but requires RNA to be converted to DNA via a virion-associated enzyme (reverse transcriptase)
    1) Enveloped
      (a) Retroviruses
        (i) Oncornaviruses
        (ii) Lentiviruses
  C) Negative-sense RNA (opposite polarity to cellular mRNA, requires a virion-associated enzyme to begin the replication cycle)
    1) Enveloped
      (a) Helical
        (i) Mononegaviruses (rabies, vesicular stomatitis virus, paramyxovirus, filovirus)
        (ii) Segmented genome (orthomyxovirus-influenza, bunyavirus, arenavirus)
II) Double-stranded RNA viruses
  A) Nonenveloped
    1) Icosahedral
      (a) Reovirus
      (b) Rotavirus
III) Single-stranded DNA viruses
  A) Nonenveloped
    1) Icosahedral
      (a) Parvoviruses (canine distemper, adeno-associated virus)
      (b) Bacteriophage ΦX174
IV) Double-stranded DNA viruses
  A) Nuclear replication
    1) Nonenveloped
      (a) Icosahedral
        (i) Small circular DNA genome (papoviruses, SV40, polyomaviruses, papillomaviruses)
        (ii) "Medium" sized, complex morphology, linear DNA (adenovirus)
    2) Enveloped-nuclear replicating
      (a) Icosahedral
        (i) Herpesviruses (linear DNA)
        (ii) Hepadnavirus (virion encapsidates RNA that is converted to DNA by reverse transcriptase)
  B) Cytoplasmic replication
    1) Icosahedral
      (a) Iridovirus
    2) Complex symmetry
      (a) Poxvirus
  C) Bacterial viruses
    1) Icosahedral with tail
      (a) T-series bacteriophages
      (b) Bacteriophage λ

The following lists some virus types together with diseases that they cause:

- RNA viruses: picornaviruses (polio, hepatitis A, rhinovirus); togavirus (rubella, equine encephalitis); flavivirus (yellow fever, dengue fever, St. Louis encephalitis); bunyaviruses (encephalitis, hemorrhagic fever); rhabdoviruses (vesicular stomatitis); myxoviruses (mumps, measles); reoviruses or rotaviruses (diarrhea); filovirus (Ebola, Marburg); arenaviruses (lymphocytic choriomeningitis); retroviruses (HIV)
- DNA viruses: herpesviruses (herpes, cold sores); papovaviruses (polyoma, warts); adenoviruses (respiratory complaints); poxvirus (smallpox); parvovirus (canine distemper)

It has been estimated that viruses cause more than 60% of the infectious diseases that occur in the developing countries. Bacterial infections account for only 15%. Table 9.2 provides a synopsis of virus types with their possible therapeutic modalities.

TARGETS FOR THE PREVENTION OF VIRAL INFECTIONS—CHEMOPROPHYLAXIS

Immunization

Prevention of viral infections by conferring artificially acquired active immunity with vaccines is the main approach for preventing most viral diseases. Safe and highly

TABLE 9.2 Classification of Viruses Causing Disease in Humans

Family Agent	Disease	Vaccine	Chemotherapy
RNA Viruses			
Picornavirus			
Enterovirus	Polio; three serotypes cause meningitis, paralysis	Live and killed vaccines (very effective)	None
Coxsackie viruses	Variety of symptoms	None	None
Rhinovirus	Common cold, pneumonia (more than 10 serotypes)	None	None
Hepatitis A virus	Hepatitis (usually mild and rarely chronic)	Inactivated virus (effective)	None
Calicivirus			
Norwalk virus	Gastroenteritis	None	None
Togavirus			
Alphaviruses (group A arboviruses)	Encephalitis, hemorrhagic fevers	Attenuated virus (generally effective)	None
Rubivirus	Rubella (German measles)	Attenuated virus	None
Flavivirus			
Flaviviruses (group B arboviruses)	Yellow fever, dengue, encephalitis, hemorrhagic fevers	Attenuated virus (generally effective)	None
Hepatitis C virus	Hepatitis	None	None
Coronavirus	Respiratory infection	None	None
Rhabdovirus			
Rabies virus	Rabies	Inactivated virus (effective)	None
Vesicular stomatitis virus		None	None
Filovirus			
Marburg virus	Marburg disease	None	None
Ebola virus	Hemorrhagic fever	None	None
Paramyxovirus			
Parainfluenza virus	Respiratory infection	None	None
Respiratory syncytial virus	Respiratory infection	Attenuated virus (effectiveness uncertain)	Ribavirin
Morbillivirus	Measles (rubeola)	Attenuated virus (90% effective)	None
Mumps virus	Mumps	Attenuated virus	None
Orthomyxovirus			
Influenza virus	Influenza (A, B, C serotypes)	Attenuated virus (70% effective)	Amantadine
Bunyavirus			
Hantavirus	Fever, renal failure	None	None
Arboviruses	Encephalitis, hemorrhagic fever	None	None
Arenavirus			
Lymphocytic choriomeningitis virus	Meningitis	None	None
Junin, Machupo viruses	Hemorrhagic fever	None	None
Lassa virus	Hemorrhagic fever	None	Ribavirin
Reovirus			
Human rotavirus	Gastroenteritis in infants	None	None
Orbivirus	Colorado tick fever	Inactivated virus (effectiveness unknown)	None
Retrovirus			
Human immunodeficiency viruses (HIV-1, HIV-2)	AIDS and AIDS-related complex (ARC)	None	AZT, ddI, ddC, stavudine
Human T-cell lymphotropic viruses (HTLV-1, HTLV-2)	T-cell leukemia, lymphoma	None	None
DNA Viruses			
Herpesvirus			
Herpes simplex 1	Stomatitis, eye infections, encephalitis	Inactivated virus (efficacy uncertain)	Iudr, ara-A
Herpes simplex 2	Genital herpes, skin eruptions	None	Acyclovir
Varicella zoster	Chickenpox (children), shingles (adults)	None	Acyclovir
Cytomegalovirus	Infections in the immunocompromised, neonates	None	Ganciclovir, foscarnet
Epstein-Barr virus	Infectious mononucleosis, Burkitt's lymphoma	None	None
Papovavirus			
Papillomavirus	Warts	None	Podophyllin
Polyomavirus (JC virus)	Progressive leukoencephalopathy		None
Adenovirus			
Human adenovirus	Upper respiratory tract and eye infections	None	None
Hepadnavirus			
Hepatitis B virus	Hepatitis (may become chronic)	Inactivated subunit (very effective)	None
Poxvirus			
Variola	Smallpox	Vaccinia (cowpox) (very effective)	Methisazone
Parvovirus			
Human parvovirus B19	Erythema, hemolytic anemia	None	None

effective vaccines are available for the prevention of polio, rubella, measles, mumps, influenza, yellow fever, encephalitis, rabies, smallpox (now considered to be eradicated worldwide, but still of interest from a biological warfare standpoint), and hepatitis B. Vaccines developed to prevent infection with herpesvirus, Epstein-Barr virus, cytomegalovirus (CMV), respiratory syncytial virus (RSV), and HIV have so far proved ineffective or unreliable. The development of a new vaccine that is effective against a chronic disease–causing virus such as HIV (acquired immunodeficiency syndrome [AIDS]) can be a daunting task. The primary principles of vaccine development apply: the vaccine must be sufficiently antigenic to induce an effective antibody response, even in very young patients; the vaccine must not cause the disease that it is designed to prevent or cause some other toxic manifestation as the early killed vaccines did; and, ideally, the vaccine should produce a lasting form of immunity, with a minimum requirement for booster doses. These requirements are difficult enough to meet for viruses that cause acute infections. The chronic cases are much more complicated. It is difficult to overcome the tendency of some viruses to undergo rapid mutation, leading to multiple antigenic epitopes; this makes development of a broadly effective vaccine much more difficult.

Biochemical Targets for Antiviral Therapy

With the discovery of antibiotics and anti-infective agents, the science of treating bacterial infections moved forward at a rapid rate. The development of useful antiviral agents (antibiotics and antiviral agents), in contrast, has historically lagged behind. There are several reasons for this. Unlike bacteria, viruses will not grow in simple synthetic culture media. They must infect human or animal cells to propagate.[5] For example, the most commonly used cell cultures in virology derive from primates (including humans and monkeys), rodents (including hamsters and mice), and birds (especially chickens). These culture methods are very reliable[6] and are in widespread use for the propagation of virus particles, but they are more difficult to perform than their bacterial counterparts. Hence, drug-screening techniques with viruses have taken longer to catch up with those in bacteria. Another possible reason for the lag in antiviral drug development lies in the comparative biochemical simplicity of viruses vis-à-vis bacteria and their use of the biochemical processes of a host cell. There are fewer specialized targets for potential attack by chemotherapeutic agents. The rapid, spectacular successes of immunization procedures for the prevention of certain viral diseases may have contributed to a relative lack of interest in antiviral chemotherapy. Another feature of mild viral infections, such as the common cold, is that clinical symptoms do not appear until the infection is well established and the immune processes of the host have begun to mount a successful challenge. Thus, for many common viral infections, chemotherapy is simply not an appropriate choice of treatment. Chemotherapeutic agents are needed, however, to combat viruses that cause severe or chronic infections, such as encephalitis, AIDS, and herpes, particularly in patients with compromised immune systems.

THE INFECTIOUS PROCESS FOR A VIRUS

Despite their simplicity relative to bacteria, viruses still possess various biochemical targets for potential attack by chemotherapeutic agents. An appropriate chemical compound may interrupt each of these. Hence, a thorough understanding of the specific biochemical events that occur during viral infection of the host cell should guide the discovery of site-specific antiviral agents. The process of viral infection can be sequenced in seven stages:

1. *Adsorption,* attachment[7] of the virus to specific receptors on the surface of the host cells, a specific recognition process.
2. *Entry*, penetration[7] of the virus into the cell.
3. *Uncoating*, release[7] of viral nucleic acid from the protein coat.
4. *Transcription*, production of viral mRNA from the viral genome.[8]
5. *Translation*, synthesis[8] of viral proteins (coat proteins and enzymes for replication) and viral nucleic acid (i.e., the parental genome or complimentary strand). This process uses the host cell processes to express viral genes, resulting in a few or many viral proteins involved in the replication process. The viral proteins modify the host cell and allow the viral genome to replicate by using host and viral enzymes. The mechanisms by which this occurs are complex. This is often the stage at which the cell is irreversibly modified and eventually killed.
6. *Assembly* of the viral particle. New viral coat proteins assemble into capsids (the protein envelope that surrounds nucleic acid and associated molecules in the core) and viral genomes.[8]
7. *Release* of the mature virus from the cell by budding from the cell membrane or rupture of the cell and repeat of the process, from cell to cell or individual to individual.[8] Enveloped viruses typically use budding on the plasma membrane, endoplasmic reticulum, or Golgi membranes. Nonenveloped viruses typically escape by rupture of the host cell.

Life cycles of different viruses provide many different possible schemes. To show the typical complexity, the life cycle of the influenza type A virus is shown in Figure 9.1.

Step 1: The virion attaches to the host cell membrane via hemagglutinin and enters the cytoplasm via receptor-mediated endocytosis, forming an *endosome*. A cellular trypsinlike enzyme cleaves HA into products HA1 and HA2 (not shown). HA2 promotes fusion of the virus envelope and the endosomal membranes. A minor virus envelope protein M2 acts as an ion channel, thereby making the interior of the virion more acidic. As a result, major envelope M1 dissociates from the nucleocapsid.

Step 2: In Step 2, viral nucleoproteins are translated into the nucleus by interaction between the nucleoproteins and cellular transport machinery.

Step 3: In the nucleus, the viral polymerase complexes transcribe (Step 3a) and replicate (Step 3b) the viral RNAs.

Step 4: Newly synthesized mRNAs migrate to cytoplasm where they are translated.

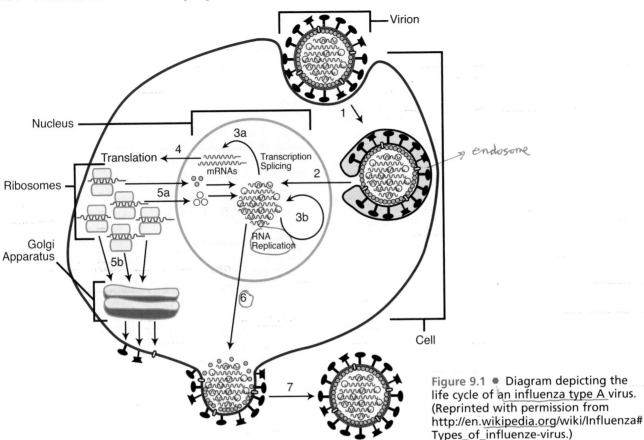

Figure 9.1 ● Diagram depicting the life cycle of an influenza type A virus. (Reprinted with permission from http://en.wikipedia.org/wiki/Influenza#Types_of_influenze-virus.)

Step 5: Posttranslational processing of HA, NA, and M2 includes transport via the Golgi apparatus to the cell membrane (Step 5b). Structural regulatory proteins and nuclear export proteins move to the nucleus (Step 5a).

Step 6: The newly formed nucleocapsids migrate into the cytoplasm in a nuclear export protein-dependent process and eventually interact via M1 with a region of the cell membrane where neuraminidase, hemagglutinin, and M2 have been inserted.

Step 7: The newly synthesized virions bud from the infected cell. Neuraminidase destroys the sialic acid moiety of cellular receptors, thereby releasing the progeny virions.

The initial attachment of viral particles to cells probably involves multiphasic interactions between viral attachment protein(s) and host cell surface receptors. For instance, in the case of the alphaherpesviruses, internalization involves a cascade of events that involve different glycoproteins and different cell surface molecules at different stages. Different cell surface proteins may be used for the initial attachment and entry into target cells and for cell-to-cell spread across closely apposed populations of cells.[9] The pattern of systemic illness produced during an acute viral infection in large part depends on the specific organs infected and, in many cases, on the capacity of the viruses to infect discrete populations of cells within these organs. This property is called *tissue tropism*.[10,11] The tissue tropism of a virus is influenced by the interaction between various hosts and viral factors.

Although the specific viral attachment proteins and specific receptors on target cells are important, a variety of other virus–host interactions can play an important role in determining the tropism of a virus. Increasing attention is being focused on *coreceptors* in mediating viral binding. For instance, entry of HIV-1 into target cells requires the presence of both CD4+ and a second coreceptor protein that belongs to the G-protein–coupled seven-transmembrane receptor family, including the chemokine receptor proteins CCR5 and CXCR4. Cells that express CD4+ but not the coreceptor are resistant to HIV infection. Host cellular receptors can be integrins, heparans, sialic acids, gangliosides, ceramides, phospholipids, and major histocompatibility antigens (to name a few). There is substantial evidence that the cellular receptor for influenza viruses is the peptidoglycan component *N*-acetylmuramic acid, which binds a protein molecule, hemagglutinin, projecting from the viral surface.[12] The binding of *N*-acetylmuramic acid and hemagglutinin sets in motion a sequence of events, whereby the viral envelope and the host cell membrane dissolve into each other, and the viral contents enter the cell. Initiation of HIV-1 infection involves the interaction of specific glycoprotein molecules (gp120) that stud the viral cell surface with an antigenic CD4+ receptor molecule on helper T lymphocytes along with a cytokine coreceptor.[13–16] Substantial evidence indicates that viruses enter cells by *endocytosis*, a process that involves fusion of the viral envelope with the cell membrane, intermixing of components, and dissolution of the membranes of virus and cell. Various receptors and coreceptors facilitate this reaction.[17–19]

Before a virus can begin a replication cycle within a host cell, its outer envelope and capsid must be removed to release its nucleic acid genome. For complex DNA viruses such as vaccinia (its binding receptor is the epidermal growth factor receptor), the uncoating process occurs in two stages[17]:

1. Host cell enzymes partially degrade the envelope and capsid to reveal a portion of the viral DNA, which serves as a template for mRNA synthesis.
2. mRNAs code for the synthesis of viral enzymes, which complete the degradation of the protein coat, allowing the virus to fully enter the host.

The proteins of the viral envelope and capsule are the primary targets for antibodies synthesized in response to immunization techniques. Protein synthesis inhibitors such as cycloheximide and puromycin inhibit the uncoating process, but they are not selective enough to be as useful as antiviral agents.

In the critical fourth and fifth stages of infection, the virus usurps the energy-producing and synthetic functions of the host cell to replicate its own genome and to synthesize viral enzymes and structural proteins.[20] Simple RNA viruses conduct both replication and protein synthesis in the cytoplasm of the host cell. These contain specific RNA polymerases (RNA replicases) responsible for replication of the genome. Some single-stranded RNA viruses, such as poliovirus, have a (+)-RNA genome that serves the dual function of messenger for protein synthesis and template for the synthesis of a complementary strand of (−)-RNA, from which the (+)-RNA is replicated. In poliovirus (a picornavirus), the message is translated as a single large open reading frame whose product is cleaved enzymatically into specific viral enzymes and structural proteins.[18,21] Other RNA viruses, such as influenza viruses, contain (−)-RNA, which serves as the template for the synthesis of a complementary strand of (+)-RNA. The (+)-RNA strand directs viral protein synthesis and provides the template for the replication of the (−)-RNA genome. Certain antibiotics, such as the rifamycins, inhibit viral RNA polymerases in vitro, but none has yet proved clinically useful. Bioactivated forms of the nucleoside analog ribavirin variously inhibit ribonucleotide synthesis, RNA synthesis, or RNA capping in RNA viruses. Ribavirin has been approved for aerosol treatment of severe lower respiratory infections caused by RSV.

Retroviruses constitute a special class of RNA viruses that possess an RNA-dependent DNA polymerase (*reverse transcriptase*) required for viral replication. In these viruses, a single strand of complementary DNA (cDNA) is synthesized on the RNA genome (*reverse transcription*), duplicated, and circularized to a double-stranded proviral DNA. The proviral DNA is then integrated into the host cell chromosomal DNA to form the template (*apovirus* or *virogene*) required for the synthesis of mRNAs and replication of the viral RNA genome. During the process of cDNA biosynthesis, a ribonuclease (RNase) degrades the RNA strand, leaving only DNA. *Oncogenic* (cancer-causing) viruses, such as the human T-cell leukemia viruses (HTLV) and the related HIV, are retroviruses. Retroviral RT is a good target for chemotherapy, being inhibited by the triphosphates of certain dideoxynucleosides, such as 2′,3′-deoxy-3′azidothymidine (AZT, zidovudine), 2′,3′-dideoxycytidine (ddCyd, zalcitabine), and 2′,3′-dideoxy-2′,3′-didehydrothymidine (D4T, stavudine), all of which have been approved for the treatment of AIDS. The nomenclature of these agents is straightforward. A 2′,3′-dideoxynucleoside is referred to as ddX, whereas the unsaturated 2′,3′-dideoxy-2′,3′-didehydronucleosides are named

d4X. The dideoxynucleoside triphosphates are incorporated into viral DNA in place of the corresponding 2′-deoxynucleoside (i.e., 2′-deoxythymidine, 2′-deoxycytidine, or 2′-deoxyadenosine) triphosphate.[22,23] This reaction terminates the viral DNA chain, because the incorporated dideoxynucleoside lacks the 3′-hydroxyl group required to form a 3′,5′-phosphodiester bond with the next 2′-deoxynucleotide triphosphate to be incorporated.

The DNA viruses constitute a heterogeneous group whose genome is composed of DNA. They replicate in the nucleus of a host cell. Some of the DNA viruses are simple structures, consisting of a single DNA strand and a few enzymes surrounded by a capsule (e.g., parvovirus) or a lipoprotein envelope (e.g., hepatitis B virus). Others, such as the herpesviruses and poxviruses, are large, complex structures with double-stranded DNA genomes and several enzymes encased in a capsule and surrounded by an envelope consisting of several membranes. DNA viruses contain DNA-dependent RNA polymerases (*transcriptases*), DNA polymerases, and various other enzymes (depending on the complexity of the virus) that may provide targets for antiviral drugs. The most successful chemotherapeutic agents discovered thus far are directed against replication of herpesviruses. The nucleoside analogs idoxuridine, trifluridine, and vidarabine block replication in herpesviruses by three general mechanisms: first, as the monophosphates, they interfere with the biosynthesis of precursor nucleotides required for DNA synthesis; second, as triphosphates, they competitively inhibit DNA polymerase; and third, the triphosphates are incorporated into the growing DNA itself, resulting in DNA that is brittle and does not function normally. Acyclonucleosides (e.g., acycloguanosine) are bioactivated sequentially by viral and host cell kinases to the acyclonucleotide monophosphate and the acyclonucleoside triphosphate, respectively. The latter inhibits viral DNA polymerase and terminates the viral DNA strand, since no 3′-hydroxyl group is available for the subsequent formation of a 3′,5′-phosphodiester bond with the next nucleoside triphosphate. The structure of acyclovir with the acyclosugar chain rotated into a pentose configuration shows clearly the absence of the 3′-hydroxyl group.

Late stages in viral replication require important virus-specific processing of certain viral proteins by viral or cellular proteases. Retroviruses, such as HIV, express three genes as precursor polyproteins. Two of these gene products, designated the p55gag and p160gag-pol proteins for their location on the genome, undergo cleavage at several sites by a virally encoded protease to form structural (viral coat) proteins (p17, p24, p8, and p7) and enzymes required for replication (RT, integrase, and protease). The demonstration that HIV protease, a member of the aspartyl protease family of enzymes, is essential for the maturation and infectivity of HIV particles[24] has stimulated major research efforts to develop effective inhibitors of this step. These efforts have led to several candidates, some that are on the market and many that are in clinical trials.

To complete the replication cycle, the viral components are assembled into the mature viral particle, or *virion.* For simple, nonenveloped viruses (e.g., the picornavirus poliovirus), the genome and only a few enzymes are encased by capsid proteins to complete the virion. Other, more complex viruses are enveloped by one or more membranes containing carbohydrate and lipoprotein components derived from the host cell membrane.

Once the mature virion has been assembled, it is ready for release from the cell. The release of certain viruses (e.g., poliovirus) is accompanied by lysis of the host cell membrane and cell death. Some of the enveloped viruses, however, are released by *budding* or *exocytosis,* a process involving fusion between the viral envelope and the cell membrane. This process is nearly a reversal of the entry process; the host cell membrane remains intact under these conditions, and the cell may survive.

Chemoprophylaxis is an alternative to active immunization for the prevention of viral infection. With chemoprophylaxis, one uses a chemical agent that interferes with a step in early viral infectivity. The immune system is not directly stimulated by the drug but is required to respond to any active infection. It would seem that the most successful chemoprophylactic agents would be those that prevent penetration of the virus into the host cell. In principle, this can be achieved by blocking any of three steps prior to the start of the replication cycle: (a) attachment of the virion to the host cell via its receptor complex, (b) its entry into the cell via endocytosis, or (c) release of the viral nucleic acid from the protein coat. At present, only a single class of agents affects these early stages of replication.[13-16] The adamantanamines (amantadine and rimantadine) have been approved for controlling influenza type A infection. These drugs appear to interfere with two stages of influenza type A viral replication: preventing the early stage of viral uncoating and disturbing the late stage of viral assembly. Clinical studies have shown that amantadine and rimantadine are effective in both prophylaxis and treatment of active influenza type A infection.

Chemoprophylaxis Influenza

Amantadine and Rimantadine (-) A, not B

Amantadine and rimantadine are both drugs that interfere with penetration of host cells by viruses and block early-stage replication. Amantadine, 1-adamantanamine hydrochloride (Symmetrel), and its α-methyl derivative rimantadine, α-methyl-1-adamantane methylamine hydrochloride (Flumadine), are unusual caged tricyclic amines with the following structures:

Amantadine has been used for years as a treatment for Parkinson disease. Both of these agents will specifically inhibit replication of the influenza type A viruses at low concentrations. Rimantadine is generally 4 to 10 times more active than amantadine. The adamantanamines have two mechanisms in common: (a) they inhibit an early step in viral replication, most likely viral uncoating,[25] and (b) in some strains, they affect a later step that probably involves viral assembly, possibly by interfering with hemagglutinin processing. The main biochemical locus of action is the influenza type A virus M2 protein, which is an integral membrane protein that functions as an ion channel. The M2 channel is a proton transport system. By interfering with the function of the M2 protein, the adamantanamines inhibit acid-mediated dissociation of the ribonucleoprotein complex early in replication. They also interfere with transmembrane proton pumping, maintaining a high intracellular proton concentration relative to the extracellular concentration and enhancing acidic pH-induced conformational changes in the hemagglutinin during its intracellular transport at a later stage. The conformational changes in hemagglutinin prevent transfer of the nascent virus particles to the cell membrane for exocytosis.

Resistant variants of influenza type A have been recovered from amantadine- and rimantadine-treated patients. Resistance with inhibitory concentrations increased more than 100-fold have been associated with single nucleotide changes that lead to amino acid substitutions in the transmembrane domain of M2. Amantadine and rimantadine share cross-susceptibility and resistance.[25,26]

Amantadine and rimantadine are approved in the United States for prevention and treatment of influenza type A virus infections. Seasonal prophylaxis with either drug is about 70% to 90% protective[27] against influenza type A. The drugs have no effect on influenza type B. The primary side effects are related to the central nervous system and are dopaminergic. This is not surprising, because amantadine is used in the treatment of Parkinson disease. Rimantadine has significantly fewer side effects, probably because of its extensive biotransformation. Less than 50% of a dose of rimantadine is excreted unchanged, and more than 20% appears in the urine as metabolites.[28] Amantadine is excreted largely unchanged in the urine.

(NMI)

NEURAMINIDASE INHIBITORS: ZANAMIVIR AND (-) A & B   OSELTAMIVIR

Sheathing the protein coat of the influenza virus is a lipid envelope. Two macromolecules, surface glycoproteins, are embedded in the lipid envelope: hemagglutinin and neuraminidase. These glycoproteins fulfill separate functions in the viral cycle. Hemagglutinin is important for binding of the virus to the host cell membrane by a terminal sialic acid residue. Neuraminidase is an enzyme. It functions in several of the early activation steps of the virus and occurs in both influenza A and B viruses. Neuraminidase is believed to be a sialidase, cleaving a bond between a terminal sialic acid unit and a sugar. This action is important in enhancing the penetration of viruses into host cells, and hence enhances the infectivity of the virus. If the sialic acid–sugar bond is prevented from being cleaved, the viruses tend to aggregate and the migration of viruses into host cells is inhibited. Hence, drugs that inhibit neuraminidase should be useful in interfering with infection caused by influenza virus type A and B.

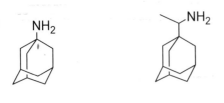

Amantadine   Rimantadine

The importance of neuraminidase in the infectivity of influenza types A and B suggests that it should be a good target for the development of antiviral drugs. Indeed, neuraminidase inhibitors are clinically useful agents in blocking the spread of the viruses. The x-ray crystal structure of neuraminidase has been determined, and it shows that the sialic acid–binding site of neuraminidase is nearly identical in influenza types A and B. The transition state of sialic acid cleavage is believed to proceed through a stabilized carbonium ion. Drug molecules that have been developed strongly resemble the transition state. The first of these, 2-deoxy-2,3-dehydro-*N*-acetylneuraminic acid, is a highly active neuraminidase inhibitor but it is not specific for the viral enzyme. This compound has served as a starting point for the development for virus-specific agents. These molecules, zanamivir and oseltamivir, are effective agents in interfering with infection and spread of influenza virus types A and B (recall that amantadine and rimantadine are only effective against type A).

2-deoxy-2,3-dehydro-N-acetylneuraminic acid

DANA: lead compd.
(NMI)

Zanamivir

X-ray crystallography of 2-deoxy-2,3-dehydro-*N*-acetyl-neuraminic acid bound to neuraminidase showed the three-dimensional structure of the receptor site at which the sialic acid units on the virus bind. Zanamivir is identical to 2-deoxy-2,3-dehydro-*N*-acetylneuraminic acid except that it possesses a guanidino group at position 4 instead of a hydroxyl group. At positions 119 and 227 of the receptor site, there exist glutamic acid residues. Zanamivir has been shown to form a salt bridge with the guanidine and Glu-119 and a charge transfer interaction with Glu-227. These interactions increase the interaction strength with the enzyme and create an excellent competitive inhibitor and an effective antiviral agent for influenza types A and B.

Human studies have shown that zanamivir is effective when administered before or after exposure to the influenza virus. If administered before exposure to the virus, the drug reduced viral propagation, infectivity, and disease symptoms. If administered after exposure, the drug reduces propagation, viral titer, and illness. Zanamivir is marketed as a dry powder for oral inhalation. It is used in adolescents and adults who

have been exposed and are symptomatic for not more than 2 days. Zanamivir is also indicated for prophylactically treating family members of a person who has developed influenza.

Oseltamivir Phosphate

The x-ray crystal structures of neuraminidase and the viral receptor site showed clearly that additional binding sites exist for the C-5 acetamido carbonyl group and the arginine residue at position 152 of the receptor site. In addition, the C-2 carboxyl group of sialic acid binds to Arg 118, Arg 292, and Arg 371. Position C-6 is capable of undergoing a hydrophobic interaction with various amino acids, including Glu, Ala, Arg, and Ile. Maximum binding to neuraminidase occurs when the C-6 substituent is substituted with a nonpolar chain. In oseltamivir, this nonpolar group is 3-pentyl. An important feature of oseltamivir is the ethyl ester, which makes the drug orally efficacious. This drug is the first orally active agent for use against influenza A and B. It is also indicated for the treatment of acute illness. If administered within 2 days after the onset of influenza symptoms, the drug is effective.

Oseltamivir is actually a prodrug in its ethyl ester form. Ester hydrolysis releases the active oseltamivir molecules.

INTERFERONS: INTERFERON ALFA (INTRON A, ROFERON A) AND INTERFERON BETA (BETASERON)

IFNs are extremely potent cytokines that possess antiviral, immunomodulating, and antiproliferative actions.[29] IFNs are synthesized by infected cells in response to various inducers (Fig. 9.2) and, in turn, elicit either an antiviral state in neighboring cells or a natural killer cell response that destroys the initially infected cell (Fig. 9.3). There are three classes of human IFNs that possess significant antiviral activity. These are IFN-α (more than 20 subtypes), IFN-β (2 subtypes), and IFN-γ. IFN-α is used clinically in a recombinant form (called *interferon alfa*). IFN-β (Betaseron) is a recombinant form marketed for the treatment of multiple sclerosis.

IFN-α and IFN-β are produced by almost all cells in response to viral challenge. However, interferon production is not limited to viral stimuli. Various other triggers, including cytokines such as interleukin-1, interleukin-2, and tumor necrosis factor, will elicit the production of IFNs. Both IFN-α and IFN-β are elicited by exposure of a cell to double-stranded viral RNA. IFN-α is produced by lymphocytes and macrophages, whereas IFN-β is biosynthesized in fibroblasts and epithelial cells. IFN-γ production is restricted to T lymphocytes and natural killer cells responding to antigenic stimuli, mitogens, and specific cytokines. IFN-α and IFN-β bind to the same receptor, and the genes for both are encoded on chromosome 9. The receptor for IFN-γ is unique,

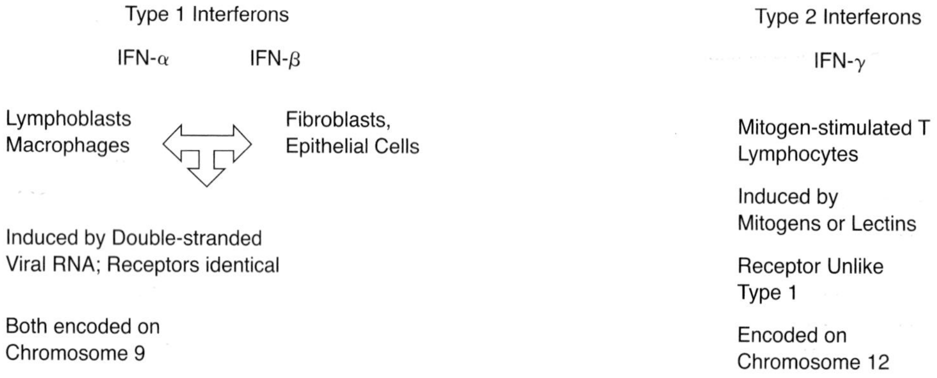

Type 1 Interferons		Type 2 Interferons
IFN-α IFN-β		IFN-γ

Lymphoblasts, Macrophages	Fibroblasts, Epithelial Cells	Mitogen-stimulated T Lymphocytes
Induced by Double-stranded Viral RNA; Receptors identical		Induced by Mitogens or Lectins
		Receptor Unlike Type 1
Both encoded on Chromosome 9		Encoded on Chromosome 12

Figure 9.2 ● Types of interferon.

and only one subtype has been identified. The genes for this molecule are encoded on chromosome 12. IFN-γ has less antiviral activity than IFN-α and IFN-β but more potent immunoregulatory effects. IFN-γ is especially effective in activating macrophages, stimulating cell membrane expression of class II major histocompatibility complexes (MHC-II), and mediating the local inflammatory responses. Most animal viruses are sensitive to the antiviral actions of IFNs. The instances in which a virus is insensitive to IFN typically involve DNA viruses.[13]

On binding to the appropriate cellular receptor, the IFNs induce the synthesis of a cascade of antiviral proteins that contribute to viral resistance. The antiviral effects of the IFNs are mediated through inhibition of[30]:

• Viral penetration or uncoating
• Synthesis of mRNA
• Translation of viral proteins
• Viral assembly and release

With most viruses, the IFNs predominantly inhibit protein synthesis. This takes place through the intermediacy of IFN-induced proteins such as $2',5'$-oligoadenylate ($2',5'$-OA) synthetases (Fig. 9.4) and a protein kinase, either of which can inhibit viral protein synthesis in the presence of double-stranded RNA. $2',5'$-OA activates a cellular endoribonuclease (RNase) (Fig. 9.5) that cleaves both cellular and viral RNA. The protein kinase selectively phosphorylates and inactivates eukaryotic initiation factor 2 (eIF2), preventing initiation of the mRNA–ribosome complex. IFN also induces a specific phosphodiesterase that cleaves a portion of

transfer RNA (tRNA) molecules and thereby interferes with peptide elongation.[30] The infection sequence for a given virus may be inhibited at one or several steps. The principal inhibitory effect differs among virus families. Certain viruses can block the production or activity of selected IFN-inducible proteins and thus counter the IFN effect.

IFNs cannot be absorbed orally; to be used therapeutically, they must be given intramuscularly or subcutaneously. The biological effects are quite long, so pharmacokinetic parameters are difficult to determine. The antiviral state in peripheral blood mononuclear cells typically peaks 24 hours after a dose of IFN-α and IFN-β, then decreases to baseline in 6 days.[31] Both recombinant and natural INF-α and INF-β are approved for use in the United States for the treatment of condyloma acuminatum (venereal warts), chronic hepatitis C, chronic hepatitis B, Kaposi sarcoma in HIV-infected patients, other malignancies, and multiple sclerosis.

Attempts have been made to produce drugs that selectively induce interferon production. One such molecule, tilorone induces interferon in murine models but is not effective in humans.

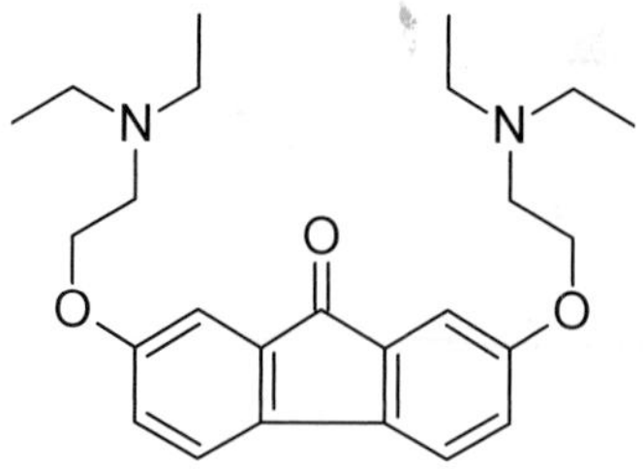

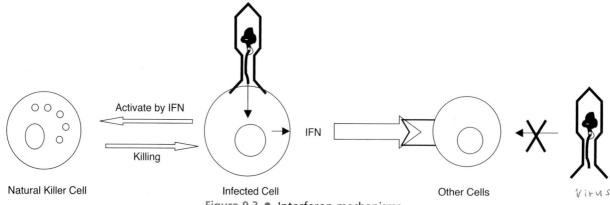

Figure 9.3 ● Interferon mechanisms.

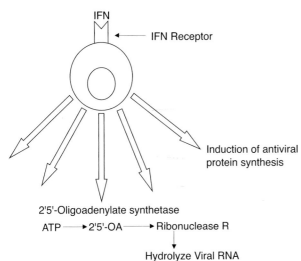

Figure 9.4 ● IFNs predominantly inhibit protein synthesis.

⬡ NUCLEOSIDE ANTIMETABOLITES: INHIBITING VIRAL REPLICATION

Inhibitors of DNA Polymerase

Idoxuridine

Idoxuridine, 5-iodo-2′-deoxyuridine (Stoxil, Herplex), was introduced in 1963 for the treatment of herpes simplex keratitis.[32] The drug is an iodinated analog of thymidine that inhibits replication of several DNA viruses in vitro. The

susceptible viruses include the herpesviruses and poxviruses (vaccinia).

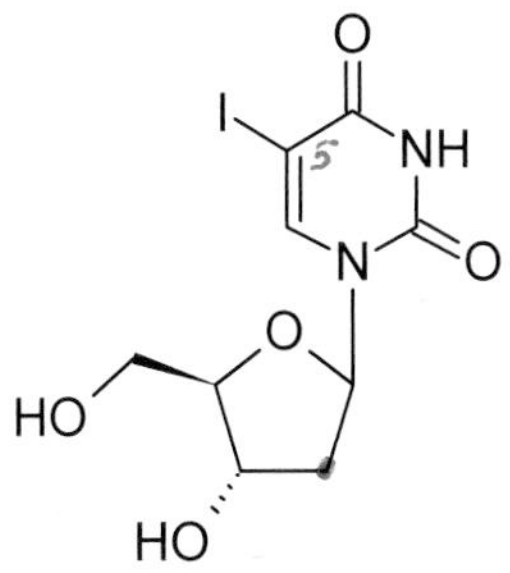

The mechanism of action of idoxuridine has not been completely defined, but several steps are involved in the activation of the drug. Idoxuridine enters the cell and is phosphorylated at O-5 by a viral thymidylate kinase to yield a monophosphate, which undergoes further biotransformation to a triphosphate. The triphosphate is believed to be both a substrate and an inhibitor of viral DNA polymerase, causing inhibition of viral DNA synthesis and facilitating the synthesis of DNA that contains the iodinated pyrimidine. The altered DNA is more susceptible to strand breakage and leads to faulty transcription. When the iodinated DNA is transcribed, the results are miscoding errors in RNA and faulty protein synthesis. The ability of idoxuridylic acid to substitute for deoxythymidylic acid in the synthesis of DNA may be a result of the similar van der Waals radii of iodine (2.15 Å) and the thymidine methyl group (2.00 Å).

In the United States, idoxuridine is approved only for the topical treatment of herpes simplex virus (HSV) keratitis;

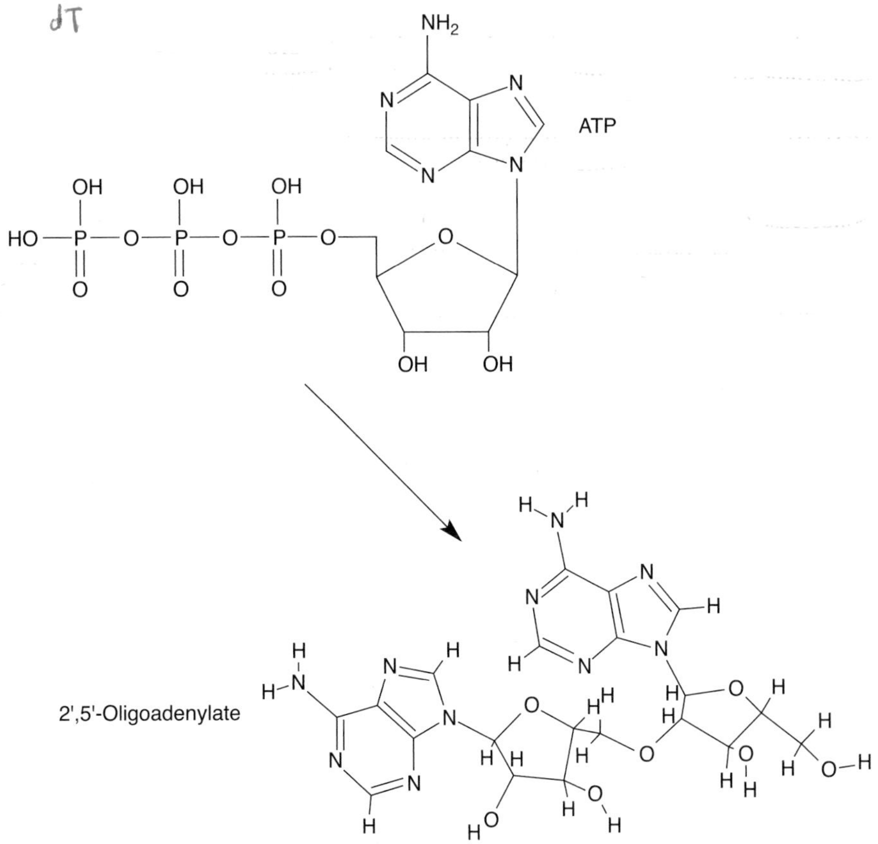

Figure 9.5 ● Structure of 2′,5′-oligoadenylate.

although outside the United States, a solution of idoxuridine in dimethyl sulfoxide is available for the treatment of herpes labialis, genitalis, and zoster. The use of idoxuridine is limited because the drug lacks selectivity; low, subtherapeutic concentrations inhibit the growth of uninfected host cells. The effective concentration of idoxuridine is at least 10 times greater than that of acyclovir.

Idoxuridine occurs as a pale yellow, crystalline solid that is soluble in water and alcohol but poorly soluble in most organic solvents. The compound is a weak acid, with a pK_a of 8.25. Aqueous solutions are slightly acidic, yielding a pH of about 6.0. Idoxuridine is light and heat sensitive. It is supplied as a 0.1% ophthalmic solution and a 0.5% ophthalmic ointment.

Cytarabine

Cytarabine is a pyrimidine nucleoside drug that is related to idoxuridine. This agent is primarily used as an anticancer agent for Burkitt lymphoma and myeloid and lymphatic leukemias. Cytarabine blocks the cellular utilization of deoxycytidine, hence inhibiting the replication of viral DNA. Before it becomes active, the drug is converted to monophosphates, diphosphates, and triphosphates, which block DNA polymerase and the C-2 reductase that converts cytidine diphosphate into the deoxy derivative.

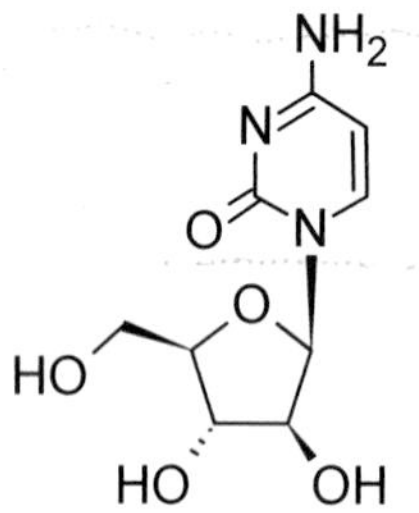

The antiviral use of cytarabine is in the treatment of herpes zoster (shingles), herpetic keratitis, and viral infections that resist idoxuridine. Cytarabine is usually administered topically. Toxicity occurs on bone marrow, the gastrointestinal (GI) tract, and the kidneys.

Trifluridine

Trifluridine, 5-trifluoromethyl-29-deoxyuridine (Viroptic), is a fluorinated pyrimidine nucleoside that demonstrates in vitro inhibitory activity against HSV-1 and HSV-2, CMV, vaccinia, and some adenoviruses.[33] Trifluridine possesses a trifluoromethyl group instead of an iodine atom at the 5-position of the pyrimidine ring. The van der Waals radius of the trifluoromethyl group is 2.44 Å, somewhat larger than that of the iodine atom.

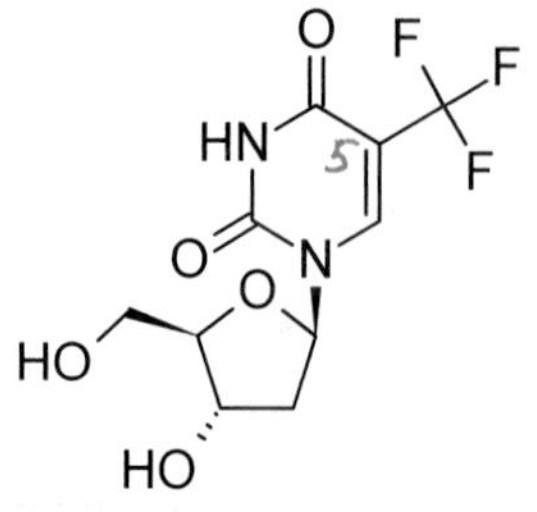

Like idoxuridine, the antiviral mechanism of trifluridine involves inhibition of viral DNA synthesis. Trifluridine monophosphate is an irreversible inhibitor of thymidylate

synthetase, and the biologically generated triphosphate competitively inhibits thymidine triphosphate incorporation into DNA by DNA polymerase. In addition, trifluridine in its triphosphate form is incorporated into viral and cellular DNA, creating fragile, poorly functioning DNA.

Trifluridine is approved in the United States for the treatment of primary keratoconjunctivitis and recurrent epithelial keratitis caused by HSV types 1 and 2. Topical trifluridine shows some efficacy in patients with acyclovir-resistant HSV cutaneous infections. Trifluridine solutions are heat sensitive and require refrigeration.

Vidarabine

Chemically, vidarabine (Vira-A), is 9-β-D-arabinofuranosyl-ladenine. The drug is the 2' epimer of natural adenosine. Introduced in 1960 as a candidate anticancer agent, vidarabine was found to have broad-spectrum activity against DNA viruses.[34] The drug is active against herpesviruses, poxviruses, rhabdoviruses, hepadnavirus, and some RNA tumor viruses. Vidarabine was marketed in the United States in 1977 as an alternative to idoxuridine for the treatment of HSV keratitis and HSV encephalitis. Although the agent was initially prepared chemically, it is now obtained by fermentation with strains of *Streptomyces antibioticus*.

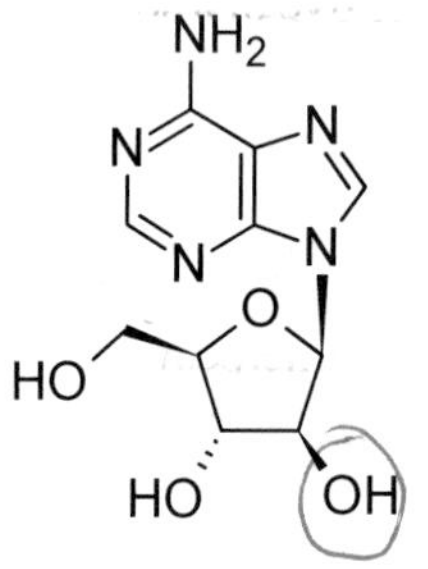

The antiviral action of vidarabine is completely confined to DNA viruses. Vidarabine inhibits viral DNA synthesis. Enzymes within the cell phosphorylate vidarabine to the triphosphate, which competes with deoxyadenosine triphosphate for viral DNA polymerase. Vidarabine triphosphate is also incorporated into cellular and viral DNA, where it acts as a chain terminator. The triphosphate form of vidarabine also inhibits a set of enzymes that are involved in methylation of uridine to thymidine: ribonucleoside reductase, RNA polyadenylase, and S-adenosylhomocysteine hydrolase.

At one time in the United States, intravenous vidarabine was approved for use against HSV encephalitis, neonatal herpes, and herpes or varicella zoster in immunocompromised patients. Acyclovir has supplanted vidarabine as the drug of choice in these cases.

In the treatment of viral encephalitis, vidarabine had to be administered by constant flow intravenous infusion because of its poor water solubility and rapid metabolic conversion to a hypoxanthine derivative in vivo. These problems, coupled with the availability of less toxic and more effective agents, have caused intravenous vidarabine to be withdrawn from the U. S. market.

Vidarabine occurs as a white, crystalline monohydrate that is soluble in water to the extent of 0.45 mg/mL at 25°C. The drug is still available in the United States as a 3% ointment for the treatment of HSV keratitis.

Adefovir Dipivoxil

Adefovir is an orally active prodrug that is indicated for the treatment of the chronic form of hepatitis B. The dipivoxil moieties are hydrolyzed by ubiquitous esterases to yield adefovir, which is phosphorylated by adenylate kinase to yield adefovir diphosphate. This compound is inhibitory at HBV DNA polymerase. In addition, adefovir undergoes incorporation into viral DNA and causes chain termination. Adefovir is poorly absorbed by the oral route, but the dipivoxil ester groups cause the bioavailability to increase to approximately 60%.

Acyclovir*

Acyclovir, 9-[2-(hydroxyethoxy)methyl]-9H-guanine (Zovirax), is the most effective of a series of acyclic nucleosides that possess antiviral activity. In contrast with true nucleosides that have a ribose or a deoxyribose sugar attached to a purine or a pyrimidine base, the group attached to the base in acyclovir is similar to an open chain sugar, albeit lacking in hydroxyl groups. The clinically useful antiviral spectrum of acyclovir is limited to herpesviruses. It is most active (in vitro) against HSV type 1, about two times less against HSV type 2, and 10 times less potent against varicella–zoster virus (VZV). An advantage is that uninfected human cells are unaffected by the drug.

The ultimate effect of acyclovir is the inhibition of viral DNA synthesis. Transport into the cell and monophosphorylation are accomplished by a thymidine kinase that is encoded by the virus itself.[35] The affinity of acyclovir for the viral thymidine kinase is about 200 times that of the corresponding mammalian enzyme. Hence, some selectivity is attained. Enzymes in the infected cell catalyze the conversion of the monophosphate to acyclovir triphosphate, which is present in 40 to 100 times greater concentrations in HSV-infected than uninfected cells. Acyclovir triphosphate competes for endogenous deoxyguanosine triphosphate (dGTP); hence, acyclovir triphosphate competitively inhibits viral DNA polymerases. The triphosphorylated drug is also incorporated into viral DNA, where it acts as a chain terminator. Because it has no 3′-hydroxyl group, no 3′,5′-phosphodiester bond can form. This mechanism is essentially a suicide inhibition because the terminated DNA template containing acyclovir as a ligand binds to, and irreversibly inactivates, DNA polymerase. Resistance to acyclovir can occur, most often by deficient thymidine kinase activity in HSV isolates. Acyclovir

resistance in vesicular stomatitis virus (VSV) isolates is caused by mutations in VSV thymidine kinase or, less often, by mutations in viral DNA polymerase.

Two dosage forms of acyclovir are available for systemic use: oral and parenteral. Oral acyclovir is used in the initial treatment of genital herpes and to control mild recurrent episodes. It has been approved for short-term treatment of shingles and chickenpox caused by VZV. Intravenous administration is indicated for initial and recurrent infections in immunocompromised patients and for the prevention and treatment of severe episodes. The drug is absorbed slowly and incompletely from the GI tract, and its oral bioavailability is only 15% to 30%. Nevertheless, acyclovir is distributed to virtually all body compartments. Less than 30% is bound to protein. Most of the drug is excreted unchanged in the urine, about 10% excreted as the carboxy metabolite.

Acyclovir occurs as a chemically stable, white, crystalline solid that is slightly soluble in water. Because of its amphoteric properties (pK$_a$ values of 2.27 and 9.25), solubility is increased by both strong acids and bases. The injectable form is the sodium salt, which is supplied as a lyophilized powder, equivalent to 50 mg/mL of active acyclovir dissolved in sterile water for injection. Because the solution is strongly alkaline (pH ~ 11), it must be administered by slow, constant intravenous infusion to avoid irritation and thrombophlebitis at the injection site.

Adverse reactions are few. Some patients experience occasional GI upset, dizziness, headache, lethargy, and joint pain. An ointment composed of 5% acyclovir in a polyethylene glycol base is available for the treatment of initial, mild episodes of herpes genitalis. The ointment is not an effective preventer of recurrent episodes.

Valacyclovir Hydrochloride *

Valacyclovir (Valtrex) is the hydrochloride salt of the L-valyl ester of acyclovir. The compound is a water-soluble crystalline solid, and it is a prodrug intended to increase the bioavailability of acyclovir by increasing lipophilicity. Valacyclovir is hydrolyzed rapidly and almost completely to acyclovir following oral administration. Enzymatic hydrolysis of the prodrug is believed to occur during enterohepatic cycling. The oral bioavailability of valacyclovir is three to five times that of acyclovir, or about 50%.[36]

Valacyclovir has been approved for the treatment of herpes zoster (shingles) in immunocompromised patients. The side effect profile observed in valacyclovir is comparable with bioequivalent doses of acyclovir. Less than 1% of an administered dose of valacyclovir is recovered in the urine. Most of the dose is eliminated as acyclovir.

Ganciclovir

Ganciclovir, 9-[(1,3-dihydroxy-2-propoxy) methyl]guanine) or DHPG (Cytovene), is an analog of acyclovir, with an additional hydroxymethyl group on the acyclic side chain.

This structural modification, while maintaining the activity against HSV and VSV possessed by acyclovir, greatly enhances the activity against CMV infection.

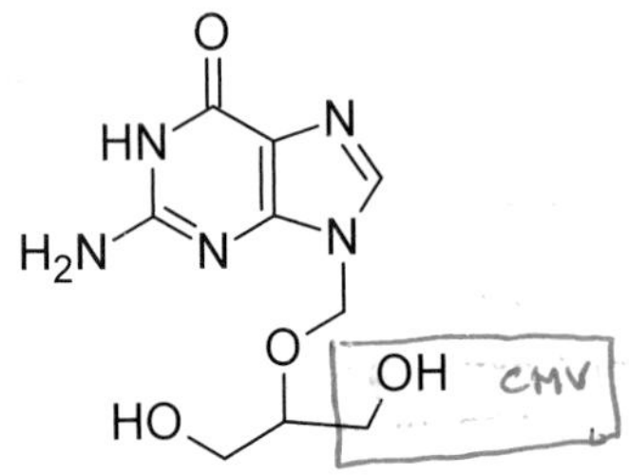

After administration, similar to acyclovir, ganciclovir is phosphorylated inside the cell by a virally encoded protein kinase to the monophosphate.[37] Host cell enzymes catalyze the formation of the triphosphate, which reaches more than 10-fold higher concentrations in infected cells than in uninfected cells. This selectivity is caused by the entry and monophosphorylation step. Further phosphorylation with cellular enzymes occurs, and the triphosphate that is formed selectively inhibits viral DNA polymerase. Ganciclovir triphosphate is also incorporated into viral DNA causing strand breakage and cessation of elongation.[38]

The clinical usefulness of ganciclovir is limited by the toxicity of the drug. Ganciclovir causes myelosuppression, producing neutropenia, thrombocytopenia, and anemia. These effects are probably associated with inhibition of host cell DNA polymerase.[39] Potential central nervous system side effects include headaches, behavioral changes, and convulsions. Ganciclovir is mutagenic, carcinogenic, and teratogenic in animals.

Toxicity limits its therapeutic usefulness to the treatment and suppression of sight-threatening CMV retinitis in immunocompromised patients and to the prevention of life-threatening CMV infections in at-risk transplant patients.[21]

Oral and parenteral dosage forms of ganciclovir are available, but oral bioavailability is poor. Only 5% to 10% of an oral dose is absorbed. Intravenous administration is preferable. More than 90% of the unchanged drug is excreted in the urine. Ganciclovir for injection is available as a lyophilized sodium salt for reconstitution in normal saline, 5% dextrose in water, or lactated Ringer solution. These solutions are strongly alkaline (pH ~11) and must be administered by slow, constant, intravenous infusion to avoid thrombophlebitis.

Famciclovir and Penciclovir

Famciclovir is a diacetyl prodrug of penciclovir.[40] As a prodrug, it lacks antiviral activity. Penciclovir, 9-[4-hydroxy-3-hydroxymethylbut-1-yl] guanine, is an acyclic guanine

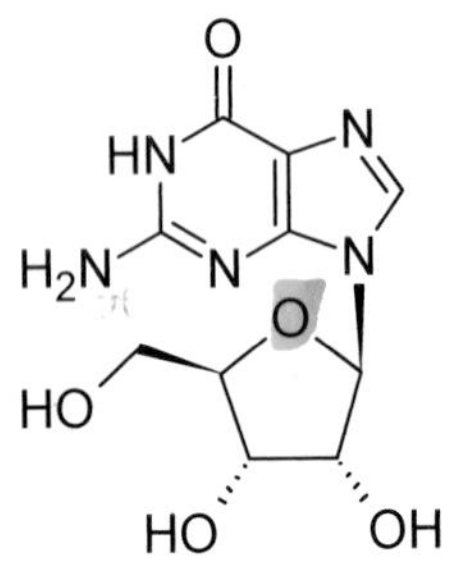

Guanosine

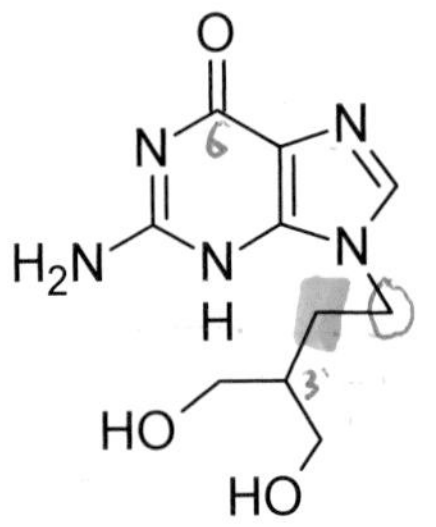

Penciclovir

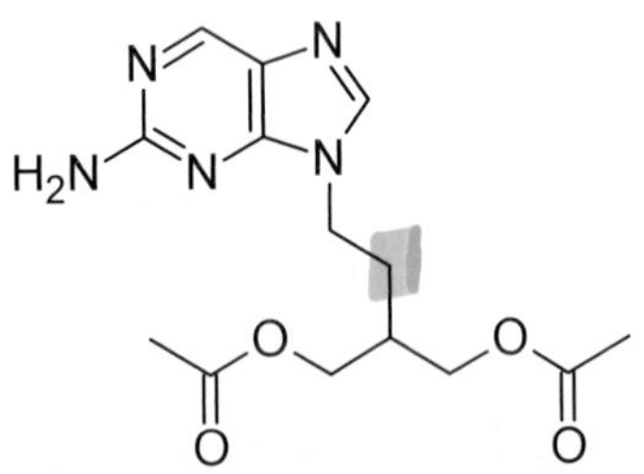

Famciclovir

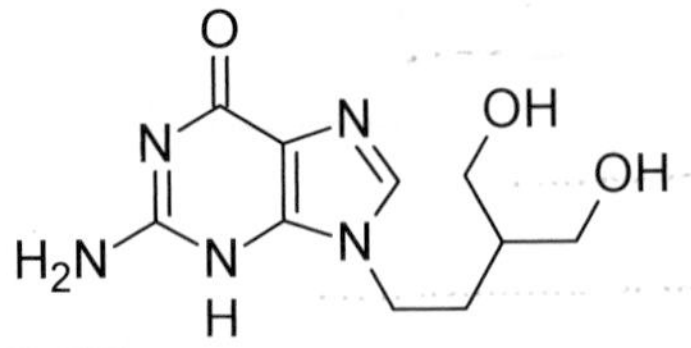

Penciclovir

nucleoside analog. The structure is similar to that of acyclovir, except in penciclovir, a side chain oxygen has been replaced by a carbon atom and an extra hydroxymethyl group is present. Inhibitory concentrations for HSV and VSV are typically within twice that of acyclovir. Penciclovir also inhibits the growth of hepatitis B virus.

Penciclovir inhibits viral DNA synthesis. In HSV- or VSV-infected cells, penciclovir is first phosphorylated by viral thymidine kinase[41] and then further elaborated to the triphosphate by host cell kinases. Penciclovir triphosphate is a competitive inhibitor of viral DNA polymerase. The pharmacokinetic parameters of penciclovir are quite different from those of acyclovir. Although penciclovir triphosphate is about 100-fold less potent in inhibiting viral DNA polymerase than acyclovir triphosphate, it is present in the tissues for longer periods and in much higher concentrations than acyclovir. Because it is possible to rotate the side chain of penciclovir into a pseudopentose, the triphosphorylated metabolite possesses a 3'-hydroxyl group. This relationship is shown on page 342 with guanosine. Penciclovir is not an obligate chain terminator,[41] but it does competitively inhibit DNA elongation. Penciclovir is excreted mostly unchanged in the urine.

Penciclovir (Denvir) has been approved for the topical treatment of recurrent herpes labialis (cold sores) in adults. It is effective against HSV-1 and HSV-2.[42] It is available as a cream containing 10% penciclovir.

Cidofovir

Cidofovir, (*S*)-3-hydroxy-2-phosphonomethoxypropyl cytosine (HPMPC, Vistide), is an acyclonucleotide analog that possesses broad-spectrum activity against several DNA viruses. Unlike other nucleotide analogs that are activated to nucleoside phosphates, Cidofovir is a phosphonic acid derivative. The phosphonic acid is not hydrolyzed by phosphatases in vivo but is phosphorylated by cellular kinases to yield a diphosphate. The diphosphate acts as an antimetabolite to deoxycytosine triphosphate (dCTP). Cidofovir diphosphate is a competitive inhibitor of viral DNA[43] polymerase and can be incorporated into the growing viral DNA strand, causing DNA chain termination.

Cidofovir possesses a high therapeutic index against CMV and has been approved for treating CMV retinitis in patients with AIDS. Cidofovir is administered by slow, constant intravenous infusion in a dose of 5 mg/kg over a 1-hour period once a week for 2 weeks. This treatment is followed by a maintenance dose every 2 weeks. About 80% of a dose of Cidofovir is excreted unchanged in the urine, with a $t_{1/2elim}$ of 2 to 3 hours. The diphosphate antimetabolite, in contrast, has an extremely long half-life (17–30 hours).

The main dose-limiting toxicity of cidofovir involves renal impairment. Renal function must be monitored closely. Pretreatment with probenecid and prehydration with intravenous normal saline can be used to reduce the nephrotoxicity of the drug. Patients must be advised that cidofovir is not a cure for CMV retinitis. The disease may progress during or following treatment.

Foscarnet Sodium

Trisodium phosphonoformate is an inorganic pyrophosphate analog that inhibits replication in herpesviruses (CMV, HSV, and VSV) and retroviruses (HIV).[44] Foscarnet (Foscavir) is taken up slowly by the cells and does not undergo significant intracellular metabolism. Foscarnet is a reversible, noncompetitive inhibitor at the pyrophosphate-binding site of the viral DNA polymerase and RT. The ultimate effect is inhibition of the cleavage of pyrophosphate from deoxynucleotide triphosphates and a cessation of the incorporation of nucleoside triphosphates into DNA (with the concomitant release of pyrophosphate).[45] Because the inhibition is noncompetitive with respect to nucleoside triphosphate binding, foscarnet can act synergistically with nucleoside triphosphate antimetabolites (e.g., zidovudine and didanosine triphosphates) in the inhibition of viral DNA synthesis. Foscarnet does not require bioactivation by viral or cellular enzymes and, hence, can be effective against resistant viral strains that are deficient in virally encoded nucleoside kinases.[45]

Foscarnet is a second-line drug for the treatment of retinitis caused by CMV in patients with AIDS. The drug causes metabolic abnormalities including increases or decreases in blood Ca^{2+} levels. Nephrotoxicity is common, and this side effect precludes the use of foscarnet in other infections caused by herpesvirus or as single-agent therapy for HIV infection. Foscarnet is an excellent ligand for metal ion binding, which undoubtedly contributes to the electrolyte imbalances observed with the use of the drug.[46] Hypocalcemia, hypomagnesemia, hypokalemia, and hypophosphatemia and hyperphosphatemia are observed in patients treated with foscarnet. Side effects such as paresthesias, tetani, seizures, and cardiac arrhythmias may result. Because foscarnet is nephrotoxic, it may augment the toxic effects of other nephrotoxic drugs, such as amphotericin B and pentamidine, which are frequently used to control opportunistic infections in patients with AIDS.

Foscarnet sodium is available as a sterile solution intended for slow intravenous infusion. The solution is compatible with normal saline and 5% dextrose in water but is incompatible with calcium-containing buffers such as lactated Ringer solution and total parenteral nutrition (TPN) preparations. Foscarnet reacts chemically with acid salts such as midazolam, vancomycin, and pentamidine. Over 80% of an injected dose of foscarnet is excreted unchanged in the urine.[44] The long elimination half-life of foscarnet is thought to result from its reversible sequestration into bone.[46]

Reverse Transcriptase Inhibitors

An early event in the replication of HIV-1 is reverse transcription, whereby genomic RNA from the virus is converted into a cDNA–RNA complex, then into double-stranded DNA ready for integration into the host chromosome. The enzyme that catalyzes this set of reactions is *reverse tran-*

scriptase. RT actually operates twice prior to the integration step. Its first function is the creation of the cDNA–RNA complex; RT acts alone in this step. In the second step, the RNA chain is digested away by RNase H, whereas RT creates the double-stranded unintegrated DNA.

All of the classical antiretroviral agents are 2′,3′-dideoxynucleoside analogs. These compounds share a common mechanism of action in inhibiting the RT of HIV. Because RT acts early in the viral infection sequence, inhibitors of the enzyme block acute infection of cells but are only weakly active in chronically infected ones. Even though the RT inhibitors share a common mechanism of action, their pharmacological and toxicological profiles differ dramatically.

Zidovudine

Zidovudine, 3′-azido-3′-deoxythymidine or AZT, is an analog of thymidine that possesses antiviral activity against HIV-1, HIV-2, HTLV-1, and several other retroviruses. This nucleoside was synthesized in 1978 by Lin and Prusoff[47] as an intermediate in the preparation of amino acid analogs of thymidine. A screening program directed toward the identification of agents potentially effective for the treatment of patients with AIDS led to the discovery of its unique antiviral properties 7 years later.[48] The next year, the clinical effectiveness of AZT in patients with AIDS and AIDS-related complex (ARC) was demonstrated.[49] AZT is active against retroviruses, a group of RNA viruses responsible for AIDS and some kinds of leukemia. Retroviruses possess a RT or an RNA-directed DNA polymerase that directs the synthesis of a DNA copy (proviral DNA) of the viral RNA genome that is duplicated, circularized, and incorporated into the DNA of an infected cell. The drug enters the host cells by diffusion and is phosphorylated by cellular thymidine kinase. Thymidylate kinase then converts the monophosphate into diphosphates and triphosphates. The rate-determining step is conversion to the diphosphate, so high levels of monophosphorylated AZT accumulate in the cell. Low levels of diphosphate and triphosphate are present. Zidovudine triphosphate competitively inhibits RT with respect to thymidine triphosphate. The 3′-azido group prevents formation of a 5′,3′-phosphodiester bond, so AZT causes DNA chain termination, yielding an incomplete proviral DNA.[50] Zidovudine monophosphate also competitively inhibits cellular thymidylate kinase, thus decreasing intracellular levels of thymidine triphosphate. The antiviral selectivity of AZT is caused by its greater $(100\times)$[51] affinity for HIV RT than for human DNA polymerases. The human γ-DNA polymerase of mitochondria is more sensitive to zidovudine; this may contribute to the toxicity associated with the drug's use. Resistance is common and is a result of point mutations at multiple sites in RT, leading to a lower affinity for the drug.[52]

Zidovudine is recommended for the management of adult patients with symptomatic HIV infection (AIDS or ARC) who have a history of confirmed *Pneumocystis carinii* pneumonia or an absolute $CD4^+$ (T4 or T_H cell) lymphocyte count below 200/mm^3 before therapy. The hematological toxicity of the drug precludes its use in asymptomatic patients. Anemia and granulocytopenia are the most common toxic effects associated with AZT.

For oral administration, AZT is supplied as 100-mg capsules and as a syrup containing 10 mg AZT per mL. The injectable form of AZT contains 10 mg/mL and is injected intravenously. AZT is absorbed rapidly from the GI tract and distributes well into body compartments, including the cerebrospinal fluid (CSF). It is metabolized rapidly to an inactive glucuronide in the liver. Only about 15% is excreted unchanged. Because AZT is an aliphatic azide, it is heat and light sensitive. It should be protected from light and stored at 15°C to 25°C.

Didanosine

Didanosine (Videx, ddI) is 2′,3′-dideoxyinosine (ddI), a synthetic purine nucleoside analog that is bioactivated to 2′,3′-dideoxy-ATP (ddATP) by host cellular enzymes.[53] The metabolite, ddATP, accumulates intracellularly, where it inhibits RT and is incorporated into viral DNA to cause chain termination in HIV-infected cells. The potency of didanosine is 10- to 100-fold less than that of AZT with respect to antiviral activity and cytotoxicity, but the drug causes less myelosuppression than AZT causes.[54]

Didanosine is recommended for the treatment of patients with advanced HIV infection who have received prolonged treatment with AZT but have become intolerant to, or experienced immunosuppression from, the drug. AZT and ddI act synergistically to inhibit HIV replication in vitro, and ddI is effective against some AZT-resistant strains of HIV.[55] Painful peripheral neuropathy (tingling, numbness, and pain in the hands and feet) and pancreatitis (nausea, abdominal pain, elevated amylase) are the major dose-limiting toxicities of didanosine. Didanosine is given orally in the form of buffered chewable tablets or as a solution prepared from the powder. Both oral dosage forms are buffered to prevent acidic decomposition of ddI to hypoxanthine in the stomach. Despite the buffering of the dosage forms, oral bioavailability is quite low and highly variable. Less than 20% of a dose is excreted in the urine, which suggests extensive metabolism.[56] Food interferes with absorption, so the oral drug must be given at least 1 hour before or 2 hours after meals. High-dose therapy can cause hyperuricemia in some patients because of the increased purine load.

Zalcitabine

Zalcitabine, 2′,3′-dideoxycytidine or ddCyd, is an analog of cytosine that demonstrates activity against HIV-1 and HIV-2, including strains resistant to AZT. The potency (in peripheral blood mononuclear cells) is similar to that of AZT, but the drug is more active in populations of monocytes and macrophages as well as in resting cells.

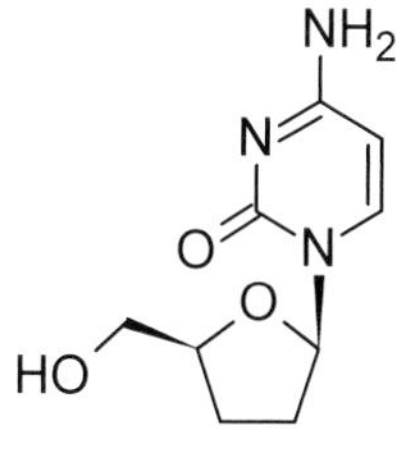

Zalcitabine enters human cells by carrier-facilitated diffusion and undergoes initial phosphorylation by deoxycytidine kinase. The monophosphorylated compound is further metabolized to the active metabolite, dideoxycytidine-5′-triphosphate (ddCTP), by cellular kinases.[57] ddCTP inhibits RT by competitive inhibition with dCTP. Most likely, ddCTP causes termination of the elongating viral DNA chain.

Zalcitabine inhibits host mitochondrial DNA synthesis at low concentrations. This effect may contribute to its clinical toxicity.[58]

The oral bioavailability of zalcitabine is over 80% in adults and less in children.[59] The major dose-limiting side effect is peripheral neuropathy, characterized by pain, paresthesias, and hypesthesia, beginning in the distal lower extremities. These side effects are typically evident after several months of therapy with zalcitabine. A potentially fatal pancreatitis is another toxic effect of treatment with ddC. The drug has been approved for the treatment of HIV infection in adults with advanced disease who are intolerant to AZT or who have disease progression while receiving AZT. ddC is combined with AZT for the treatment of advanced HIV infection.

Stavudine

Stavudine, 2′3′-didehydro-2′-deoxythymidine (D4T, Zerit), is an unsaturated pyrimidine nucleoside that is related to thymidine. The drug inhibits the replication of HIV by a mechanism similar to that of its close congener, AZT.[60] Stavudine is bioactivated by cellular enzymes to a triphosphate. The triphosphate competitively inhibits the incorporation of thymidine triphosphate (TTP) into retroviral DNA by RT.[61] Stavudine also causes termination of viral DNA elongation through its incorporation into DNA.

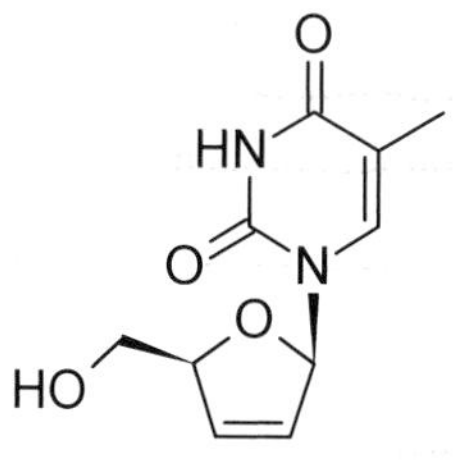

Stavudine is available as capsules for oral administration. The drug is acid stable and well absorbed (about 90%) following oral administration. Stavudine has a short half-life (1–2 hours) in plasma and is excreted largely unchanged (85%–90%) in the urine.[62] As with ddC, the primary dose-limiting effect is peripheral neuropathy. At the recommended dosages, approximately 15% to 20% of patients experience symptoms of peripheral neuropathy. Stavudine is recommended for the treatment of adults with advanced HIV infection who are intolerant of other approved therapies or who have experienced clinical or immunological deterioration while receiving these therapies.

Abacavir

Abacavir is a nucleoside reverse transcriptase inhibitor NRTI that has been approved for use in combination therapies for the treatment of HIV and AIDS. Once in the tissues, it is metabolized by stepwise phosphorylation to the monophosphate, diphosphate, and triphosphate. Abacavir is highly bioavailable (>75%) and is effective by the oral route. It penetrates the blood-brain barrier efficiently. Abacavir has been reported to produce life-threatening hypersensitivity reactions in some patients.

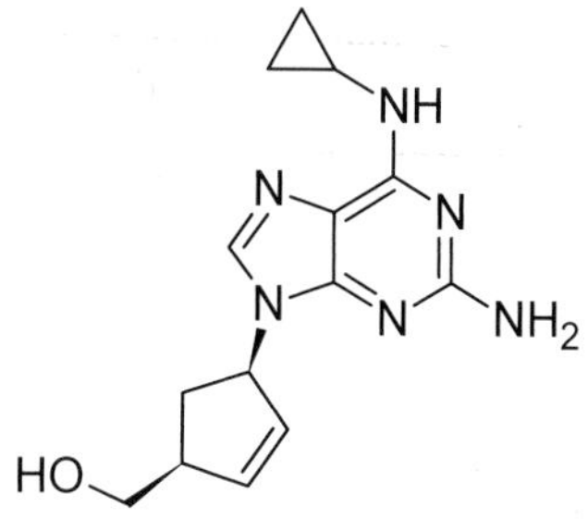

Tenofovir Disoproxil

Tenofovir disoproxil is a prodrug analogously with abacavir. Plasma and tissue esterases cleave the phosphate protecting groups, releasing the active drug. The bioavailability of tenofovir is about 35% when administered with food. The drug is approved by the Food and Drug Administration (FDA) for the treatment of HIV infections in adult patients. Recommendations are for the drug to be administered with other RT inhibitors or PIs to achieve synergism.

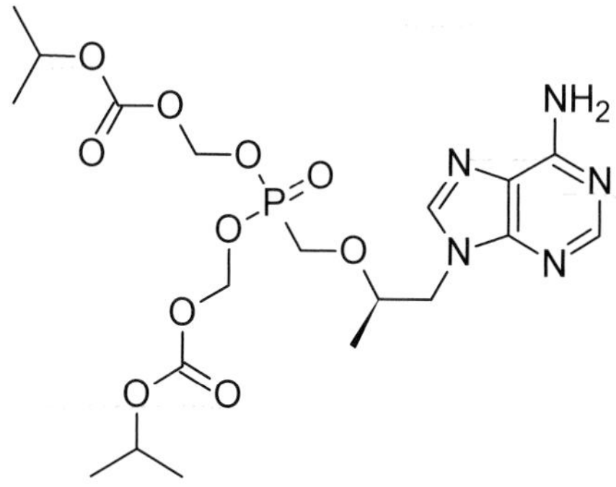

Lamivudine

Lamivudine is (−)-2′,3′-dideoxy-3′-thiacytidine, (−)-β-L-(2R,5S)-1,3-oxathiolanylcytosine, 3TC, or (−)-(S)-ddC. Lamivudine is a synthetic nucleoside analog that differs from 2′,3′-dideoxycytidine (ddC) by the substitution of a sulfur atom in place of a methylene group at the 3′-position of the ribose ring. In early clinical trials, lamivudine exhibited highly promising antiretroviral activity against HIV and low toxicity in the dosages studied.[63,64] Preliminary pharmacokinetic studies indicated that it exhibited good oral bioavailability (F = ~80%) and a plasma half-life of 2 to 4 hours.[63]

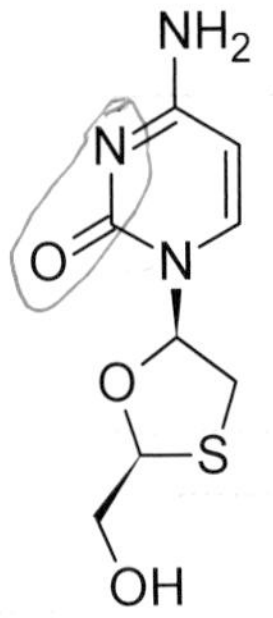

It is interesting that the unnatural stereoisomer $(-)$-(S)-ddC exhibits greater antiviral activity against HIV than the natural enantiomer $(+)$-(S)-ddC.[65] Both enantiomers are bioactivated by cellular kinases to the corresponding triphosphates.[66] Both SddCTP isomers inhibit HIV RT and are incorporated into viral DNA to cause chain termination. $(+)$-S-ddCTP inhibits cellular DNA polymerases much more strongly than $(-)$-SddCTP, explaining the greater toxicity associated with $(+)$-(S)-ddC. Initial metabolic comparison of SddCTP isomers has failed to explain the greater potency of the $(-)$-isomer against HIV. Therefore, although the intracellular accumulation of $(-)$-S-ddCTP was twice that of $(+)$-S-ddCTP, the latter was one and a half times more potent as an inhibitor of HIV RT, and the two isomers were incorporated into viral DNA at comparable rates. The puzzle was solved with the discovery of a cellular $3',5'$-exonuclease, which was found to cleave terminal $(+)$-S-ddCMP incorporated into viral DNA 6 times faster than $(-)$-S-ddCMP from the viral DNA terminus.

Resistance to lamivudine develops rapidly as a result of a mutation in codon 184 of the gene that encodes HIV-RT when the drug is used as monotherapy for HIV infection.[64] When combined with AZT, however, lamivudine caused substantial increases in $CD4^+$ counts. The elevated counts were sustained over the course of therapy.[67] The codon mutation that causes resistance to lamivudine suppresses AZT resistance,[67] thus increasing the susceptibility of the virus to the drug combination.

Emtricitabine

Emtricitabine is an orally active NRTI whose pharmacokinetics are favorable for once-daily administration.

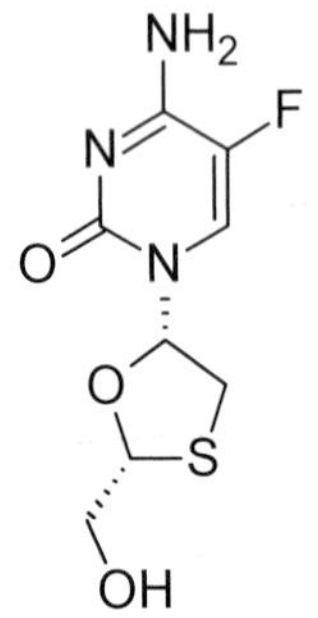

Miscellaneous Nucleoside Antimetabolites

Ribavirin

Ribavirin is 1-β-D-ribofuranosyl-1,2,4-thiazole-3-carboxamide. The compound is a purine nucleoside analog with a modified base and a D-ribose sugar moiety.

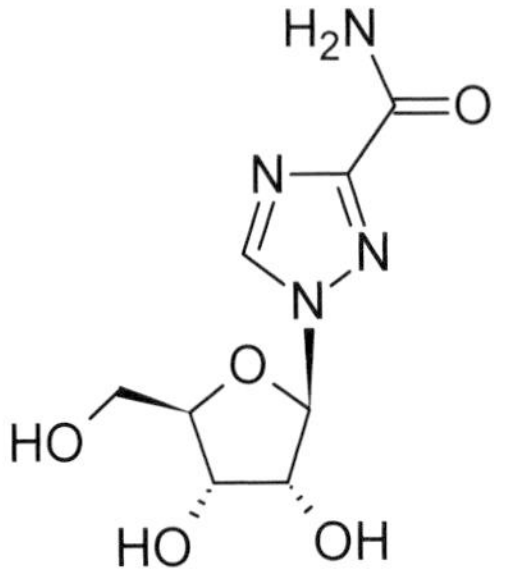

Ribavirin inhibits the replication of a very wide variety of RNA and DNA viruses,[68] including orthomyxoviruses, paramyxoviruses, arenaviruses, bunyaviruses, herpesviruses, adenoviruses, poxvirus, vaccinia, influenza virus (types A and B), parainfluenza virus, and rhinovirus. In spite of the broad spectrum of activity of ribavirin, the drug has been approved for only one therapeutic indication—the treatment of severe lower respiratory infections caused by RSV in carefully selected hospitalized infants and young children.

The mechanism of action of ribavirin is not known. The broad antiviral spectrum of ribavirin, however, suggests multiple modes of action.[69] The nucleoside is bioactivated by viral and host cellular kinases to give the monophosphate (RMP) and the triphosphate (RTP). RMP inhibits inosine monophosphate (IMP) dehydrogenase, thereby preventing the conversion of IMP to xanthine monophosphate (XMP). XMP is required for guanosine triphosphate (GTP) synthesis. RTP inhibits viral RNA polymerases. It also prevents the end capping of viral mRNA by inhibiting guanyl-N'-methyltransferase. Emergence of viral resistance to ribavirin has not been documented.

Ribavirin occurs as a white, crystalline, polymorphic solid that is soluble in water and chemically stable. It is supplied as a powder to be reconstituted in an aqueous aerosol containing 20 mg/mL of sterile water. The aerosol is administered with a small-particle aerosol generator (SPAG). Deterioration in respiratory function, bacterial pneumonia, pneumothorax, and apnea have been reported in severely ill infants and children with RSV infection. The role of ribavirin in these events has not been determined. Anemia, headache, abdominal pain, and lethargy have been reported in patients receiving oral ribavirin.

Unlabeled uses of ribavirin include aerosol treatment of influenza types A and B and oral treatment of hepatitis, genital herpes, and Lassa fever. Ribavirin does not protect cells against the cytotoxic effects of the AIDS virus.

NEWER AGENTS FOR THE TREATMENT OF HIV INFECTION

When HIV-1 was characterized and identified as the causative agent of AIDS in 1983,[70,71] scientists from all over the world joined in the search for a prevention or cure for the disease. Mapping the HIV-1 genome and elucidating the replication cycle of the virus have supplied key information.[72] Biochemical targets, many of which are proteins involved in the replication cycle of the virus, have been cloned and sequenced. These have been used to develop rapid, mechanism-based assays for the virus to complement tissue culture screens for whole virus. Several of the biochemical steps that have been characterized have served as targets for clinical candidates as well as for successfully licensed drugs.[73,74]

Despite the many advances in the understanding of the HIV virus and its treatment, there is not yet a cure for the infection. Emergent resistance[75] to clinically proven drugs such as the RT inhibitors and the PIs has complicated the picture of good therapeutic targets. The idea of using a vaccine as a therapeutic tool has been complicated by the fact that the vaccine apparently can modulate its antigenic structures in its chronic infectious state.[76]

Vaccines

The chronology of vaccine development and use in the 20th century is nothing short of a medical miracle. Diseases such as smallpox and polio, which once ravaged large populations, have become distant memories. The technique of sensitizing a human immune system by exposure to an antigen so that an anamnestic response is generated on subsequent exposure seems quite simple on the surface. Hence, it is natural that a vaccine approach to preventing AIDS be tried. The successes achieved so far have involved live/attenuated or killed whole-cell vaccines and, in more recent times, recombinant coat proteins.

Successes with vaccines of the live/attenuated (low-virulence), killed whole virus or the recombinant coat protein types have primarily involved acute viral diseases in which a natural infection and recovery lead to long-term immunity.

This type of immunity is of the humoral or antibody-mediated type, and it is the basis for successes in immunizing the human population. Causative organisms of chronic infections do not respond to vaccines. The AIDS virus causes a chronic disease in which infection persists despite a strong antibody response to the virus (at least initially, HIV can circumvent the humoral response to infection by attacking and killing CD4$^+$ T cells). These T cells, also known as *T-helper cells*, upregulate the immune response. By eradicating the CD4$^+$ cells, the HIV virus effectively destroys the immune system. Cell-mediated immune responses are critical to the prevention and treatment of HIV infection. To be effective, a vaccine against HIV must elicit an appropriate cellular immune response in addition to a humoral response. In other words, the vaccine must have the potential to act on both branches of the immune system.

The initial work on vaccine development focused on isotypic variants of the HIV envelope glycoprotein gp120 obtained by recombinant DNA techniques. This target was chosen because of concerns about the safety of live/attenuated vaccines. The gp120 glycoprotein is a coat protein, and if great care is taken, a virus-free vaccine is obtainable. Moreover, glycoprotein gp120 is the primary target for neutralizing antibodies associated with the first (attachment) step in HIV infection.[77] Early vaccines were so ineffective that the National Institutes of Health suspended plans for massive clinical trials in high-risk individuals.[78] There are several reasons why the vaccine failed.[79] There are multiple subtypes of the virus throughout the world; the virus can infect by means of both cell-free and cell-associated forms; the virus has demonstrated its own immunosuppressive, immunopathological, and infection-enhancing properties of parts of the envelope glycoprotein; and vaccines have not been able to stimulate and maintain high enough levels of immunity to be effective.

The failure of the first generation of AIDS vaccines led to a reexamination of the whole AIDS vaccine effort.[79] As a guide for research efforts, several criteria for an "ideal" AIDS vaccine have been developed. The ideal AIDS vaccine should (a) be safe, (b) elicit a protective immune response in a high proportion of vaccinated individuals, (c) stimulate both cellular and humoral branches of the immune system, (d) protect components against all major HIV subtypes, (e) induce long-lasting protection, (f) induce local immunity in both genital and rectal mucosa, and (g) be practical for worldwide delivery and administration. It is not yet known how well the second-generation AIDS vaccines will satisfy the previously described criteria or when one might receive approval for widespread use in humans.

A new era in the treatment of AIDS and ARC was ushered in with the advent of some clinically useful, potent inhibitors of HIV. For the first time in the history of AIDS, the death rate reversed itself. There are several different classes of drugs that can be used to treat HIV infection. These are the NRTIs, the NNRTIs, the HIV PIs, the HIV entry inhibitors, and the HIV integrase inhibitors (IN). At present, at least 14 antiretroviral agents belonging to three distinct classes (NRTIs, NNRTIs, PIs) have been licensed for use in patients in the United States. All of these agents are limited by rapid development of resistance and cross-resistance; so commonly, three drugs are used at the same time, each acting at a different point in HIV replication. These drugs can effect dramatic reductions in viral load, but eventually, as resistance develops, the virus reasserts itself.

Nonnucleoside Reverse Transcriptase Inhibitors

Cloned HIV-1 RT facilitates the study of the effects of a novel compound on the kinetics of the enzyme. Random screening of chemical inventories by the pharmaceutical industry has led to the discovery of several NNRTIs of the enzyme. These inhibitors represent several structurally distinct classes. The NNRTIs share several common biochemical and pharmacological properties.[74,80,81] Unlike the nucleoside antimetabolites, the NNRTIs do not require bioactivation by kinases to yield phosphate esters. They are not incorporated into the growing DNA chain. Instead, they bind to an allosteric site that is distinct from the substrate (nucleoside triphosphate)-binding site of RT. The inhibitor can combine with either free or substrate-bound enzyme, interfering with the action of both. Such binding distorts the enzyme, so that it cannot form the enzyme–substrate complex at its normal rate, and once formed, the complex does not decompose at the normal rate to yield products. Increasing the substrate concentration does not reverse these effects. Hence, NNRTIs exhibit a classical noncompetitive inhibition pattern with the enzyme.

The NNRTIs are extremely potent in in vitro cell culture assays and inhibit HIV-1 at nanomolar concentrations. NNRTIs inhibit RT selectively; they do not inhibit the RTs of other retroviruses, including HIV-2 and simian immunodeficiency virus (SIV). The NNRTIs have high therapeutic indices (in contrast to the nucleosides) and do not inhibit mammalian DNA polymerases. The NRTIs and NNRTIs are expected to exhibit a synergistic effect on HIV, because they interact with different mechanisms on the enzyme. The chief problem with the NNRTIs is the rapid emergence of resistance among HIV isolates.[75] Resistance is a result of point mutations in the gene coding for the enzyme. Cross-resistance between structurally different NNRTIs is more common than between NNRTIs and NRTIs. In the future, clinical use of the NNRTIs is expected to use combinations with the nucleosides to reduce toxicity to the latter, to take advantage of additive or synergistic effects, and to reduce the emergence of viral resistance.[75,80] The tricyclic compound nevirapine (Viramune),[82] the bis(heteroacyl)piperazine (BHAP) derivative delavirdine (Rescriptor),[83] and efavirenz[84] have been approved for use in combination with NRTIs such as AZT for the treatment of HIV infection. Numerous others, including the quinoxaline derivative GW-420867X,[84] the tetrahydroimidazobenzodiazpinone (TIBO) analog R-82913,[85] and calanolide-A[84] are in clinical trials.

Nevirapine

Nevirapine (Viramune)[82] is more than 90% absorbed by the oral route and is widely distributed throughout the body. It distributes well into breast milk and crosses the placenta. Transplacental concentrations are about 50% those of serum. The drug is extensively transformed by cytochrome P450 (CYP) to inactive hydroxylated metabolites; it may undergo enterohepatic recycling.

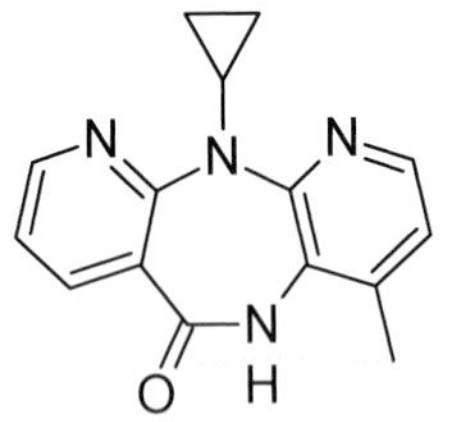

The half-life decreases from 45 to 23 hours over a 2- to 4-week period because of autoinduction. Elimination occurs through the kidney, with less than 3% of the parent compound excreted in the urine.[82] Dosage forms are supplied as a 50 mg/5 mL oral suspension and a 200-mg tablet.

Delavirdine

Delavirdine (Rescriptor)[83] must be used with at least two additional antiretroviral agents to treat HIV-1 infections. The oral absorption of delavirdine is rapid, and peak plasma concentrations develop in 1 hour. Extensive metabolism occurs in the liver by CYP isozyme 3A (CYP3A) or possibly CYP2D6. Bioavailability is 85%. Unlike nevirapine, which is 48% protein bound, delavirdine is more than 98% protein bound. The half-life is 2 to 11 hours, and elimination is 44% in feces, 51% in urine, and less than 5% unchanged in urine. Delavirdine induces its own metabolism.[83] Oral dosage forms are supplied as a 200-mg capsule and a 100-mg tablet.

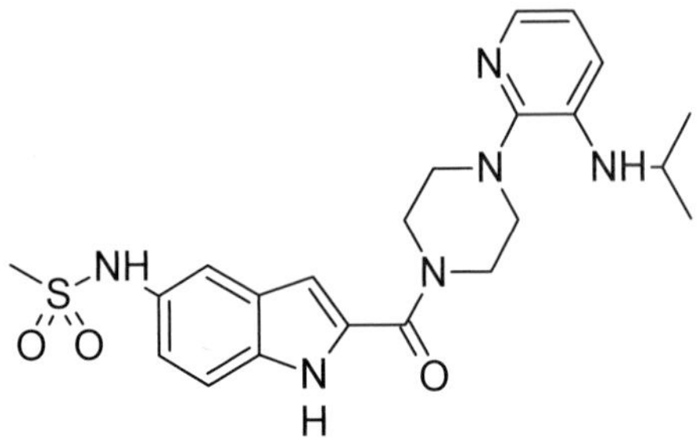

Efavirenz

Efavirenz (Sustiva)[84] is also mandated for use with at least two other antiretroviral agents. The compound is more than 99% protein bound, and CSF concentrations exceed the free fraction in the serum. Metabolism occurs in the liver. The half-life of a single dose of efavirenz is 52 to 76 hours, and 40 to 55 after multiple doses (the drug induces its own metabolism). Peak concentration is achieved in 3 to 8 hours. Elimination is 14% to 34% in urine (as metabolites) and 16% to 41% in feces (primarily as efavirenz).[84] The oral dosage form is supplied as a capsule.

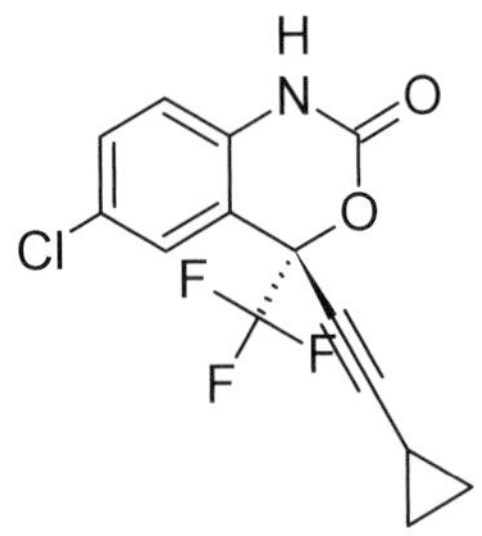

HIV Protease Inhibitors

A unique biochemical target in the HIV-1 replication cycle was revealed when HIV protease was cloned and expressed[86,87] in *Escherichia coli*. HIV protease is an enzyme that cleaves gag-pro propeptides to yield active enzymes that function in the maturation and propagation of new virus. The catalytically active protease is a symmetric dimer of two identical 99 amino acid subunits, each contributing the triad Asp-Thr-Gly to the active site.[86,87] The homodimer is unlike monomeric aspartyl proteases (renin, pepsin, cathepsin D), which also have different substrate specificities. The designs of some inhibitors[86,87] for HIV-1 protease exploit the C_2 symmetry of the enzyme. HIV-1 protease has active site specificity for the triad Tyr-Phe-Pro in the unit Ser-(Thr)-Xaa-Xaa-Tyr-Phe-Pro, where Xaa is an arbitrary amino acid.

HIV PIs are designed to mimic the transition state of hydrolysis at the active site; these compounds are called *analog inhibitors*. Hydrolysis of a peptide bond proceeds through a transition state that is sp^3 hybridized and, hence, tetrahedral. The analog inhibitors possess a preexisting sp^3 hybridized center that will be drawn into the active site (one hopes with high affinity) but will not be cleavable by the enzyme. This principle has been used to prepare hundreds of potentially useful transition state inhibitors.[86,87] Unfortunately, very few of these are likely to be clinically successful candidates for the treatment of HIV infection. Because HIV PIs are aimed at arresting replication of the virus at the maturation step to prevent the spread of cellular infection, they should possess good oral bioavailability and a relatively long duration of action. A long half-life is also desirable because of the known development of resistance by HIV under selective antiviral pressure.[74,75] Resistance develops by point mutations.

Most of the early PIs are high–molecular-weight, dipeptide- or tripeptide-like structures, generally with low water solubility. The bioavailability of these compounds is low, and the half-life of elimination is very short because of hydrolysis or hepatic metabolism.[88] Strategies aimed at increasing water solubility and metabolic stability have led to the development of several highly promising clinical candidates. Saquinavir (Invirase),[81] indinavir (Crixivan),[89] ritonavir (Norvir),[90] nelfinavir (Viracept),[91] and amprenavir (Agenerase)[92] have been approved for the treatment of HIV-infected patients. Several others are in clinical trials.

There is an important caution for the use of PIs. As a class, they cause dyslipidemia, which includes elevated cholesterol and triglycerides and a redistribution of body fat centrally to cause the "protease paunch" buffalo hump, facial atrophy, and breast enlargement. These agents also cause hyperglycemia.

Saquinavir

Saquinavir (Invirase)[89] is well tolerated following oral administration. Absorption of saquinavir is poor but is increased with a fatty meal. The drug does not distribute into the CSF, and it is approximately 98% bound to plasma proteins. Saquinavir is extensively metabolized by the first-pass effect. Bioavailability is 4% from a hard capsule and 12% to 15% from a soft capsule. Saquinavir lowers p24 antigen levels in HIV-infected patients, elevates $CD4^+$ counts, and exerts a synergistic antiviral effect when combined with RT inhibitors such as AZT and ddC.[93–95] Although HIV-1 resistance to saquinavir and other HIV PIs occurs in vivo, it is believed to be less stringent and less frequent than resistance to the RT inhibitors.[96] Nevertheless, cross-resistance between different HIV PIs appears to be common and additive,[97] suggesting that using combinations of inhibitors from this class would not constitute rational prescribing. The drug should be used in combination with at least two other antiretroviral drugs to minimize resistance. Dosage forms are Invirase (hard capsule) and Fortovase (soft capsule).

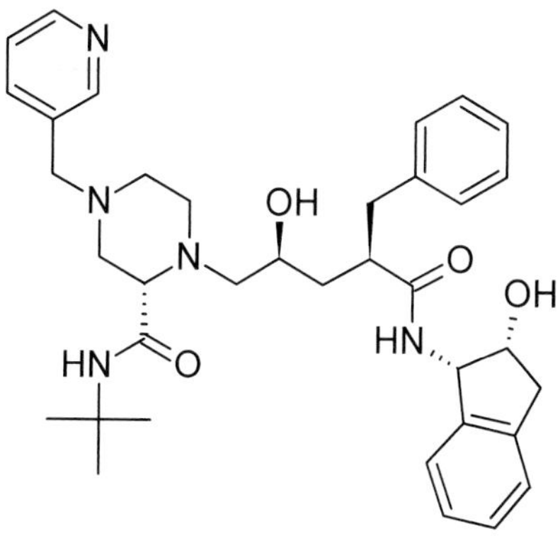

Ritonavir, Amprenavir, and Nelfinavir

Ritonavir (Norvir),[98] amprenavir (Agenerase),[99] and nelfinavir (Viracept)[100] have similar properties and cautionary statements. All cause dyslipidemia, and they have a host of drug interactions, mainly because they inhibit CYP3A4. These agents must always be used with at least two other antiretroviral agents. Used properly, the PIs are an important part of HIV therapy.

Lopinavir

Lopinavir is a protease inhibitor that has been approved for use in combination with ritonavir for patients with HIV who have not responded to other treatment modalities. Lopinavir is used in excess over ritonavir. Ritonavir at amounts given has no antiretroviral activity, Ritonavir inhibits lopinavir's metabolism by CYP3A4, causing a higher level of lopinavir in the system. The combination is the first protease inhibitor approved for patients as young as 6 months of age.

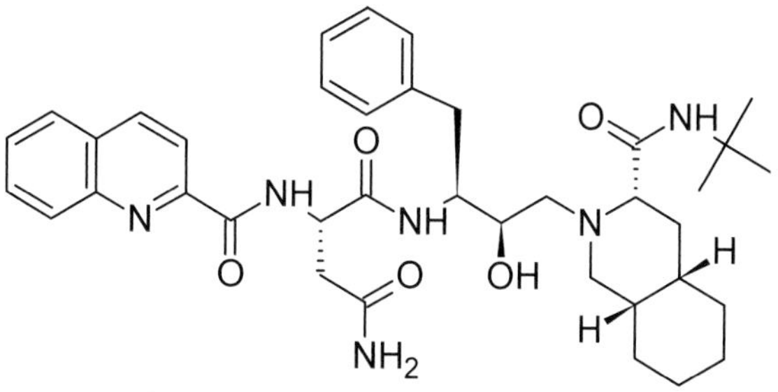

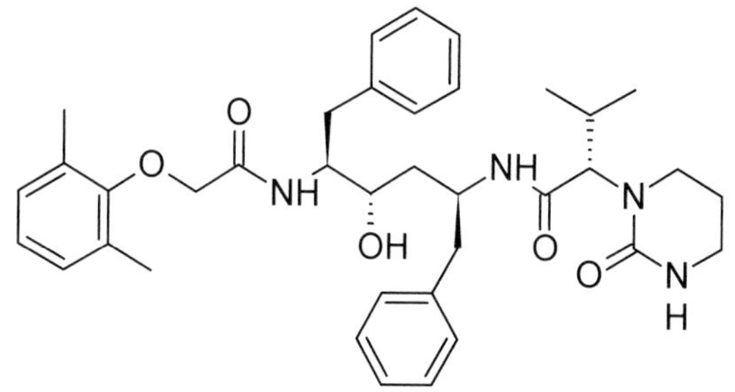

Indinavir

When administered with a high-fat diet, indinavir (Crixivan)[90] achieves a maximum serum concentration of 77% of the administered dose. The drug is 60% bound in the plasma. It is extensively metabolized by CYP3A4, and seven metabolites have been identified. Oral bioavailability is good, with a t_{max} of 0.8 ± 0.3 hour. The half-life of elimination is 1.8 hour, and the elimination products are detectable in feces and urine. Indinavir also causes dyslipidemia. The available dosage forms are capsules of 200 mg, 333 mg, and 400 mg.

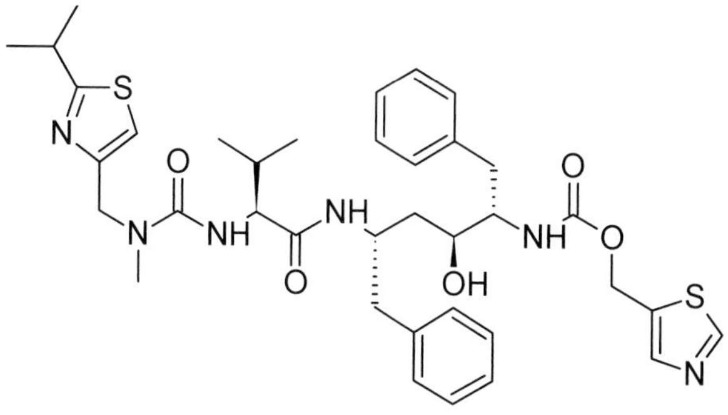

Ritonavir

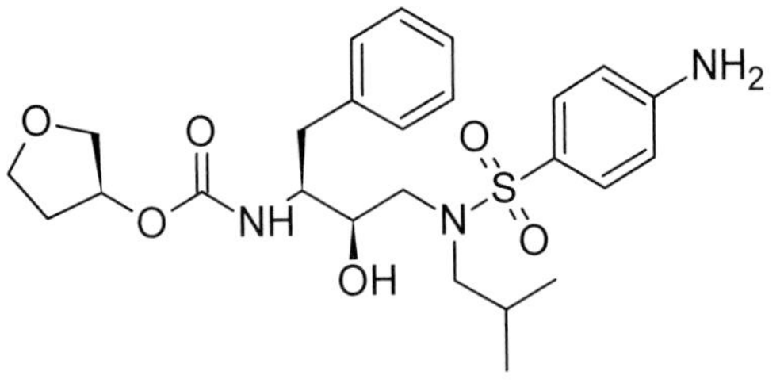

Amprenavir

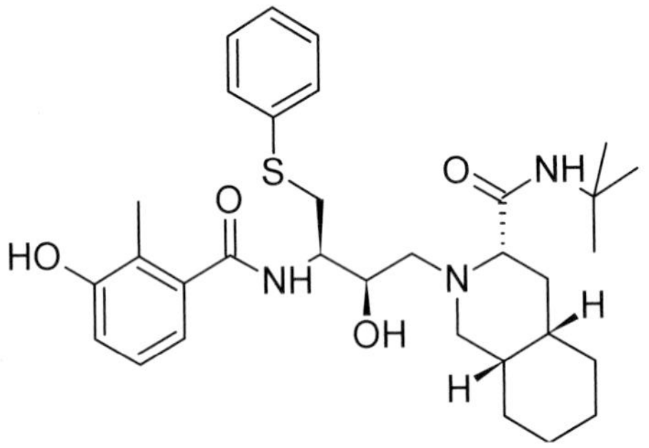

Nelfinavir

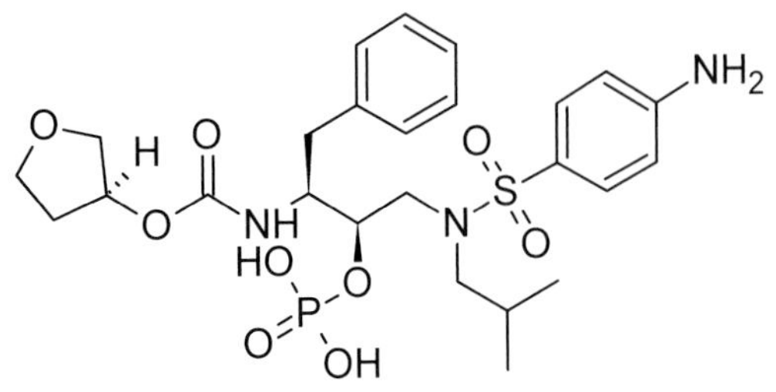

Tipranavir

Tipranavir is unique among the PIs because it is not a peptidomimetic compound. It does appear to bind to the active site of HIV-1 protease the same as the peptidomimetics do. The benefit of this agent is that, because it is a different chemical structure, cross-resistance does not develop to the same extent as seen with the peptidomimetics. The drug is administered with a booster dose of ritonavir. This protocol inhibits CYP3A4, causing the levels of tipranavir to increase.

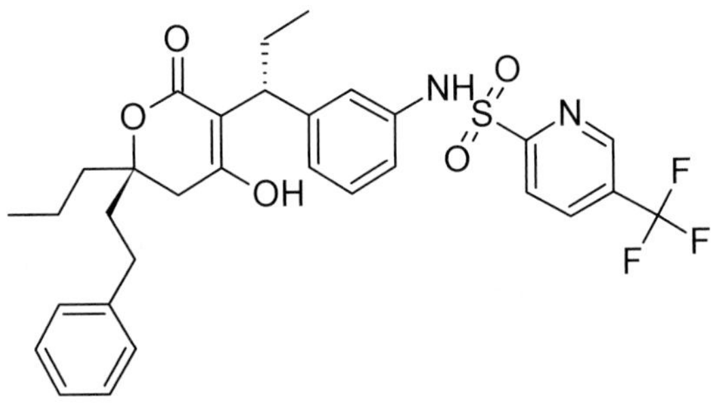

Atazanavir

Atazanavir is an antiretroviral agent that has been approved by the FDA for use in combination with other anti-RT agents for the treatment of HIV infections. The drug is always used in combination with RT inhibitors.

Several other nonpeptide inhibitors of HIV protease have been developed as a result of two very different approaches. For example, the C_2 symmetry of the active site of the enzyme was exploited in the structure-based design of the symmetric cyclic urea derivative DMP-323.[101] This inhibitor exhibited potent activity against the protease in vitro, excellent anti-HIV activity in cell culture, and promising bioavailability in experimental animals. In phase I clinical trials, however, the bioavailability of DMP-323 was poor and highly variable, possibly because of its low water solubility and a high fraction of hepatic metabolism. Subsequent synthesis of nonsymmetric derivatives DMP-850[101] (page 351) and DMP-851[101] yielded in vitro antiviral potency comparable with that of the already-approved PIs. These were selected as clinical candidates on the basis of their favorable pharmacokinetics in dogs. In a second approach, random screening of chemical inventories yielded the 5,6-dihydropyran-2-one–based inhibitor[102] PD-178390 (page 351). This compound, in addition to having good potency against HIV protease and good anti-HIV activity in cell culture, exhibits high bioavailability in experimental animals. PD-178390 appears not to share the resistance profile of the other PIs, and no virus resistant to the compound emerged, even during the prolonged in vitro selection.

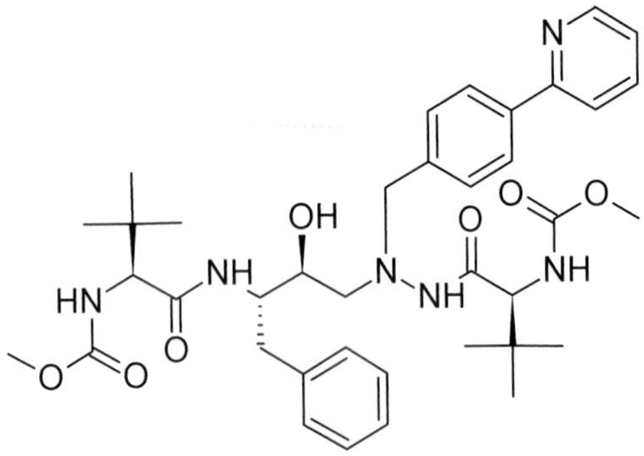

Fosamprenavir

Fosamprenavir is used in combination with other HIV drugs in adult patients. Like the other PIs, this compound is a prodrug that produces the active drug upon hydrolysis. In this case, the active drug is amprenavir, a peptidomimetic transition state inhibitor. Fosamprenavir is typically administered in combination with RT inhibitors.

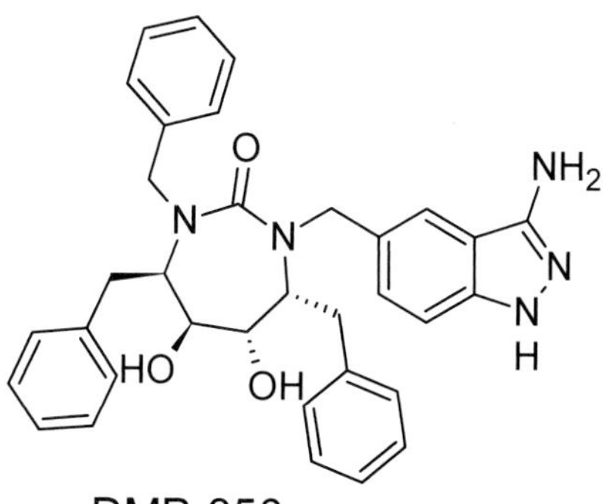

DMP-850

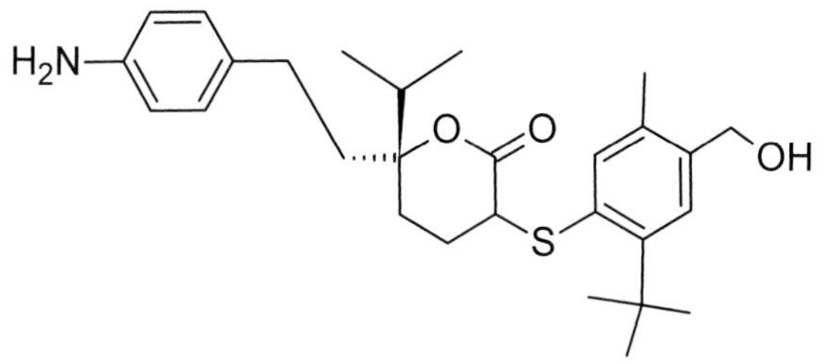

PD-178390

Dipeptide PIs containing 2-hydroxy-3-amino-4-arylbu-tanoic acid in their scaffold showed promising preclinical results. JE-2147[103], containing the allophenylnorstatin moiety, exhibited potent in vitro anti-HIV activity. JE-2147 appears to fully retain its susceptibility against various HIV strains resistant to multiple approved PIs and exhibits good oral bioavailability and a good pharmacokinetic profile in two animal species. Also, emergence of resistance was considerably delayed with JE-2147.

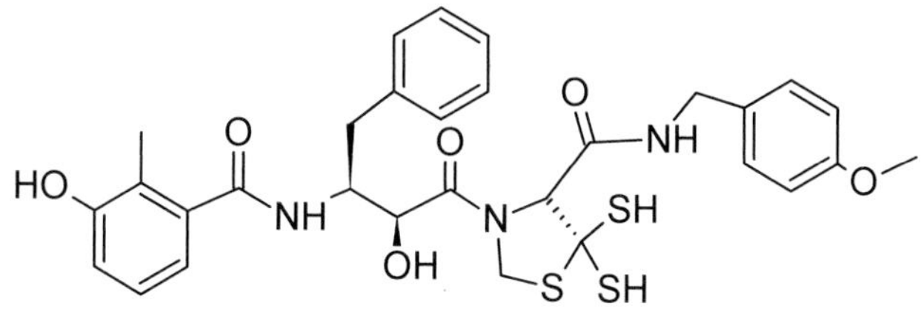

JE-2147

HIV Entry Inhibitors

Entry of HIV into a cell is a complex process that involves several specific membrane protein interactions. Initially, viral glycoprotein gp120 mediates the virus attachment via its binding to at least two host membrane receptors, CD4$^+$ and the chemokine coreceptor. This bivalent interaction induces a conformational change in the viral fusion protein gp41. Protein gp41 acts as the anchor for gp120 in the virus. With the conformational change, the viral envelope fuses with the host cell membrane. In addition to gp120–chemokine receptor interaction, the fusion activity of gp41 is currently being explored as a novel target for antiretroviral therapy. At least one agent from each class is in clinical testing.

Chemokine Receptor Binders

Most HIV-1 isolates rely on the CCR5 coreceptor for entry (R5 strains). In later stages of the disease, however, more pathogenic selection variants of the virus emerge in about 40% of individuals, which use the CXCR4 coreceptor in addition to CCR5 (R5X4 strains) or the CXCR4 receptor only (X4 strains). Bicyclam compound AMD-3100[104] was the first compound identified as a CXCR4-specific inhibitor that interferes with the replication of X4 but not R5 viruses. The compound is currently in phase II clinical evaluations. It is used as an injectable agent because of its limited bioavailability.

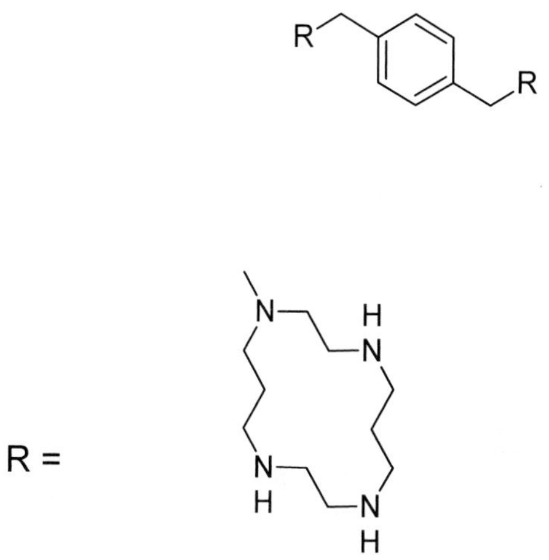

AMD-3100

Several positively charged 9- to14-mer peptides have been described as capable of blocking the CXCR4 coreceptor. A small molecule, TAK-779,[105] exhibits high-affinity binding to the CCR5 coreceptor, specifically blocking R5 isolates.

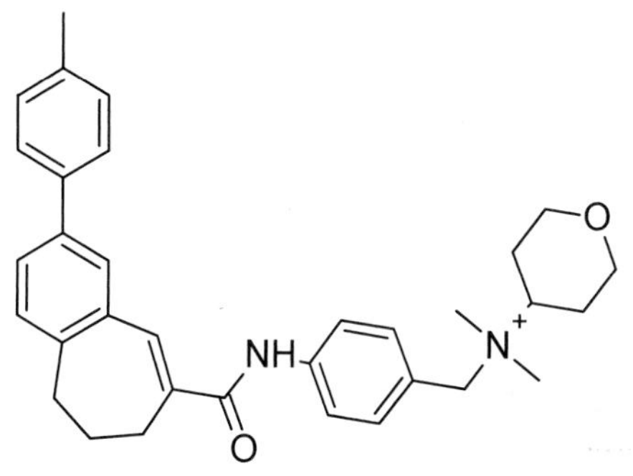

TAK-779

Inhibitors of GP41 Fusion Activity

The fusion of the HIV-1 viral envelope with host plasma membrane is mediated by gp41, a transmembrane subunit of the HIV-1 glycoprotein subunit complex. Pentafuside[106] (T-20) is a 36-mer peptide that is derived from the C-terminal repeat of gp41. Pentafuside appears to inhibit the formation of the fusion-competent conformation of gp41 by interfering with the interaction between its C- and N-terminal repeat. Pentafuside is a potent inhibitor of HIV-1 clinical isolates, and it is currently in clinical trials.

Integrase Inhibitors

Two closely related types of small molecules that block strand transfer catalyzed by recombinant integrase have been identified. Both types show in vitro antiviral activity. The diketo acids[107] inhibit strand transfer catalyzed by recombinant integrase with an IC_{50} less than 0.1 μm. Mutations that conferred resistance to the diketo acids mapped near conserved residues in the IN enzyme. This finding demonstrates that the compounds have a highly specific mechanism of action. X-ray crystallography of the bound tetrazole[108] derivative revealed that the inhibitor was centered in the active site of IN near acidic catalytic residues.

Short-Interfering RNA

RNA interference is a phenomenon that has been recently used as a way to silence genes that are part of viral replication cycles. The siRNAs very specifically interrupt gene function and switch off some aspect of a disease. The siRNAs are found in higher organisms (eukaryotes) and are typically double-stranded duplexes of RNA of about 21 base pairs. In nature, these siRNAs are produced by excision from a parent duplex RNA molecule. The siRNAs instruct the cell to split specific mRNAs that have identical sequences as the siRNAs. As antiviral therapy, the idea would be for the siRNAs to stop synthesis of mRNAs of a pathogenic organism. Antiviral siRNA therapies can be tailored for any given pathogen. The use of siRNAs as potential therapeutic modalities is a highly active area of research at the present time.

Combination Antiviral Therapy

Combination antiviral therapy, in which a mixture of drugs possessing different mechanisms of action, has been shown to be advantageous for several reasons. The antiviral effect of the combination is excellent, toxicities are decreased, and resistance to any drug in the combination is slow to develop. Resistance to single drugs such as amantadine, ganciclovir, and acyclovir is problematic. Administered of a given agent in combination with other types of drugs retards the development of such resistance. Combination treatment is especially important in antiretroviral therapy.

Typical antiretroviral therapy, as exemplified by HIV treatment, includes combinations of NRTI or NNRTI along with PIs. The key that makes the combination work is that the drugs act to inhibit HIV virus replication at different stages of the viral infective cycle. The RT inhibitors (NRTIs or NNRTIs) prevent RNA formation or viral protein synthesis or inactivate the catalytic site of RT (NNRTIs). The PIs act once the provirus integrates into the host's genes. Protease is necessary to split viral precursor polypeptides into new virus. The combination of RTs and PIs is synergistic. There are many two- and three-drug combinations that have been reported to be useful in various viral infections.

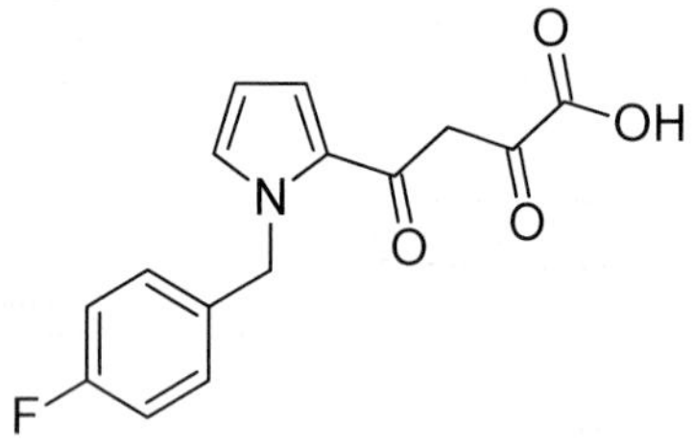

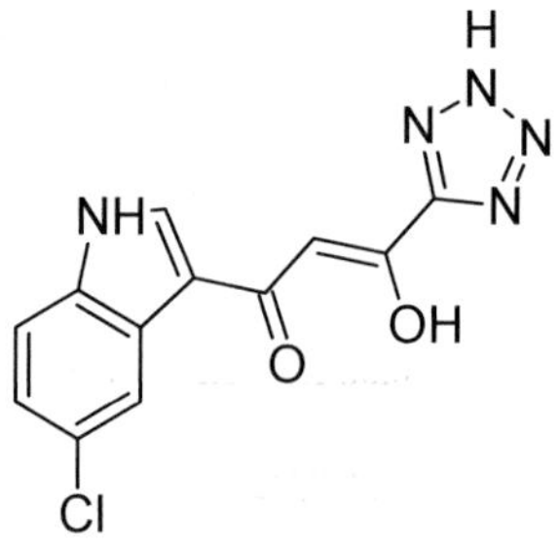

Tetrazole

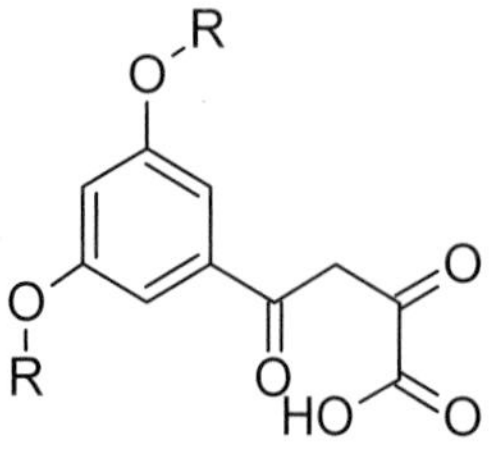

R= Benz   Diketo

● R E V I E W   Q U E S T I O N S ●

1. What is the difference between the lytic cycle and the lysogenic cycle in viruses?

2. What is an RNA virus? What is a DNA virus?

3. What is the mechanism of action of an antimetabolite antiviral drug?

4. What is chemoprophylaxis? How might you exercise chemoprophylaxis against the influenza virus?

5. What is the mechanism of action of amantadine?

6. Describe the mechanism of action of the IFNs as antiviral agents.

7. Describe the class of agents that we call NRRTIs.

8. What kinds of drugs are typically used in combination therapy of HIV?

9. Describe the HIV entry inhibitors.

10. How do the HIV protease inhibitors exert their mechanism of action?

REFERENCES

1. Condit, R. C.: Principles of virology. In Knipe, D. M., and Howley, P. M. (eds.). Fundamental Virology, 4th ed. New York, Lippincott Williams & Wilkins, 2001, p. 19.
2. Harrison, S. C.: Principles of viral structure. In Knipe, D. M., and Howley, P. M. (eds.). Fundamental Virology, 4th ed. New York, Lippincott Williams & Wilkins, 2001, p. 53.
3. Wagner, E. K., and Hewlett, M. J. (eds.): Basic Virology. Malden, MA, Blackwell Science, 1999, p. 12.
4. Wagner, E. K., and Hewlett, M. J. (eds.): Basic Virology. Malden, MA, Blackwell Science, 1999, p. 61.
5. Beale, J. M., Jr.: Immunobiologicals. In Block, J. H., and Beale, J. M., Jr. (eds.). Wilson and Gisvold's Textbook of Organic Medicinal and Pharmaceutical Chemistry, 11th ed. Baltimore, Lippincott Williams & Wilkins, 2004, p. 10.
6. Freshney, R. I.: Culture of Animal Cells, 3rd ed. New York, Wiley-Liss, 1994.
7. Young, J. A. T.: Virus entry and uncoating. In Knipe, D. M., and Howley, P. M. (eds.). Fundamental Virology, 4th ed. New York, Lippincott Williams & Wilkins, 2001, p. 87.
8. Hunter, E.: Virus assembly. In Knipe, D. M., and Howley, P. M. (eds.). Fundamental Virology, 4th ed. New York, Lippincott Williams & Wilkins, 2001, p. 171.
9. Lamb, R. A., and Choppin, R. W.: Annu. Rev. Biochem. 52:467, 1983.
10. Cann, A. J.: Principles of Molecular Virology, 3rd ed. New York, Academic Press, 2001, p. 114.
11. Tyler, K. L., and Nathanson, N.: Pathogenesis of viral infections. In Knipe, D. M., and Howley, P. M. (eds.). Fundamental Virology, 4th ed. New York, Lippincott Williams & Wilkins, 2001, pp. 214–220.
12. Dimitrov, R. S.: Cell 91:721, 1997.
13. Dingwell, K. S., Brunetti, C. R., Hendricks, R. L., et al.: J. Virol. 68:834, 1994.
14. Haywood, A. M.: J. Virol. 68:1, 1994.
15. Norkin, L. C.: Clin. Microbiol. Rev. 8:298–315, 1995.
16. Chesebro, B., Buller, R., Portis, J., et al.: J. Virol. 64:215, 1990.
17. Clapham, P. R., Blanc, D., and Weiss, R. A.: Virology 181:703, 1991.
18. Harrington, R. D., and Geballe, A. P.: J. Virol. 67:5939, 1993.
19. Haywood, A. M.: J. Virol. 68:1, 1994.
20. Young, J. A. T.: Virus entry and uncoating. In Knipe, D. M., and Howley, P. M. (eds.). Fundamental Virology, 4th ed. New York, Lippincott Williams & Wilkins, 2001, p. 96
21. Wagner, E. K., and Hewlett, M. J. (eds.): Basic Virology. Malden, MA, Blackwell Science, 1999, p. 257
22. Mitsuya, H., and Broder, S.: Proc. Natl. Acad. Sci. U. S. A. 83:1911, 1986.
23. Johnson, M. A., et al.: J. Biol. Chem. 263:1534, 1988.
24. Kohl, N. E., et al.: Proc. Natl. Acad. Sci. U. S. A. 85:4686, 1988.
25. Hay, A. J.: Semin. Virol. 3:21, 1992.
26. Hayden, F. G., Belsche, R. B., Clover, R. D., et al.: N. Engl. J. Med. 321:1696, 1989.
27. Douglas, R. G.: N. Engl. J. Med. 322:443, 1990.
28. Capparelli, E. V., Stevens, R. C., and Chow, M. S.: Clin. Pharmacol. Ther. 43:536, 1988.

29. Baron, S., et al.: Introduction to the interferon system. In Baron, S., Dianzani, F., Stanton, G., et al. (eds.). Interferon: Principles and Medical Applications. Galveston, University of Texas, Texas Medical Branch, 1992, pp. 1–15.
30. Sen, G. C., and Ransohoff, R. M.: Adv. Virus Res. 42:57, 1993.
31. Bocci, V.: HIV proteases. In Baron, S., Dianzani, F., Stanton, G., et al. (eds.). Interferon: Principles and Medical Applications. Galveston, University of Texas, Texas Medical Branch, 1992, pp. 417–425.
32. Prusoff, W. H.: Idoxuridine or how it all began. In DeClerq, E. (ed.). Clinical Use of Antiviral Drugs. Norwell, MA, Martinus Nijhoff, 1988, pp. 15–24.
33. Birch, et al.: J. Infect. Dis. 166:108, 1992.
34. Pavin-Langston, D., et al.: Adenosine Arabinoside: An Antiviral Agent. New York, Raven Press, 1975.
35. Schaeffer, H. J., et al.: Nature 272:583, 1978.
36. Weller, S., et al.: Clin. Pharmacol. Ther. 54:595, 1993.
37. Sullivan, V., et al.: Nature 358:162, 1992.
38. Clair, M. H., et al.: Antimicrob. Agents Chemother. 25:191, 1984.
39. Faulds, D., and Heel, R. C.: Drugs 39:597, 1990.
40. Vere Hodge, R. A.: Antiviral Chem. Chemother. 4:67, 1993.
41. Earnshaw, D. L., et al.: Antimicrob. Agents Chemother. 36:2747, 1992.
42. Alrabiah, F. A., and Sachs, S. L.: Drugs 52:17, 1996.
43. Xiong, X., et al.: Biochem. Pharmacol. 51:1563, 1996.
44. Chrisp, P., and Chessold, S. P.: Drugs 41:104, 1991.
45. Crumpacker, C. S.: Am. J. Med. 92(Suppl. 2A):25, 1992.
46. Jacobson, M. A., et al.: J. Clin. Endocrinol. Metab. 72:1130, 1991.
47. Lin, T. S., and Prusoff, W. H.: J. Med. Chem. 21:109, 1978.
48. Mitsuya, H., et al.: Proc. Natl. Acad. Sci. U. S. A. 82:7096, 1985.
49. Yarchoan, R., et al.: Lancet 1:575, 1986.
50. Furman, P. A., et al.: Proc. Natl. Acad. Sci. U. S. A. 873:8333, 1986.
51. St. Clair, M. H., et al.: Antimicrob. Agents Chemother. 31:1972, 1987.
52. Richman, D. D., et al.: J. Infect. Dis. 164:1075, 1991.
53. Johnson, M. A., and Fridland, A.: Mol. Pharmacol. 36:291, 1989.
54. McLaren, C., et al.: Antiviral Chem. Chemother. 2:321, 1991.
55. Johnson, V. A., et al.: J. Infect. Dis. 164:646, 1991.
56. Knupp, C. A., et al.: Clin. Pharmacol. Ther. 49:523, 1991.
57. Yarchoan, R., et al.: N. Engl. J. Med. 321:726, 1989.
58. Chen, C., Vazquez-Padua, M., and Cheng, Y.: Mol. Pharmacol. 39:625, 1991.
59. Broder, S.: Am. J. Med. 88(Suppl. 5B):25, 1990.
60. Ho, H. T., and Hitchcock, M. J. M.: Antimicrob. Agents Chemother. 33:844, 1989.
61. Huang, P., Farquhar, D., and Plunkett, W.: J. Biol. Chem. 267:2817, 1992.
62. Browne, M. J., et al.: J. Infect. Dis. 167:21, 1993.
63. Van Leeuwen, R., et al.: J. Infect. Dis. 171:1166, 1995.
64. Pluda, J. M., et al.: J. Infect. Dis. 171:1438, 1995.
65. Coates, J. A. V., et al.: Antimicrob. Agents Chemother. 36:202, 1992.
66. Skalski, V., et al.: J. Biol. Chem. 268:23234, 1993.
67. Larder, B. A., et al.: Science 269:696, 1995.
68. Sidwell, R. W., et al.: Science 177:705, 1972.
69. Robins, R. K.: Chem. Eng. News Jan. 27:28, 1986.
70. Gallo, R. C., et al.: Science 220:865, 1983.

71. Barré-Sinoussi, F., et al.: Science 220:868, 1983.
72. Haseltine, W. A.: FASEB J. 5:2349, 1991.
73. Yarchoan, R., Mitsuya, H., and Broder, S.: Trends Pharmacol. Sci. 14:196, 1993.
74. DeClerq, E.: J. Med. Chem. 38:2491, 1995.
75. Richman, D. D.: Annu. Rev. Pharmacol. Toxicol. 32:149, 1993.
76. Cease, K. B., and Berzofsky, J. A.: Annu. Rev. Immunol. 12:923, 1994.
77. Lasky, L. A., et al.: Science 23:209, 1986.
78. Cohen, J.: Science 264:1839, 1994.
79. Koff, W. C.: Science 266:1335, 1994.
80. Spence, R. A., et al.: Science 267:988, 1995.
81. Vacca, J. P., et al.: Proc. Natl. Acad. Sci. U. S. A. 91:4096, 1994.
82. Merluzzi, U. T., et al.: Science 250:1411, 1990.
83. Romero, D. L.: Drugs Future 19:7, 1994.
84. Pedersen, O., and Pedersen, E.: Antiviral Chem. Chemother. 10:285, 1999.
85. Pialoux, G., et al.: Lancet 338:140, 1991.
86. Wlodawer, R., and Erickson, J. W.: Annu. Rev. Biochem. 62:543, 1993.
87. Chow, Y. K., et al.: Nature 361:650, 1993.
88. Roberts, N. A., et al.: Science 248:358, 1990.
89. Kun, E. E., et al.: J. Am. Chem. Soc. 117:1181, 1995.
90. Kempf, D. J., et al.: Proc. Natl. Acad. Sci. U. S. A. 92:2484, 1995.
91. Nelfinavir. St. Louis, Facts and Comparisons, 2000, p. 1431.
92. Kageyama, S., et al.: Antimicrob. Agents Chemother. 37:810, 1993.
93. Reich, S. H., et al.: Proc. Natl. Acad. Sci. U. S. A. 92:3298, 1995.
94. Johnson, V. A., Merrill, D. P., Chou, T.-C., et al.: J. Infect. Dis. 166:1143, 1992.
95. Craig, J. C., et al.: Antiviral Chem. Chemother. 4:161, 1993.
96. Craig, J. C., et al.: Antiviral Chem. Chemother. 4:335, 1993.
97. Condra, J. H., et al.: Nature 374:569, 1995.
98. Wei, X., et al.: Nature 373:117, 1995.
99. Ho, D. D., et al.: Nature 373:123, 1995.
100. Kageyama, S., et al.: Antimicrob. Agents Chemother. 37:810, 1993.
101. DeLucca, G., et al.: Pharm. Biotechnol. 11:257, 1998.
102. Prasad, J., et al.: Bioorg. Med. Chem. 7:2775, 1999.
103. Yoshimura, K., et al.: Proc. Natl. Acad. Sci. U. S. A. 96:8675, 1999.
104. Hendrix, C., et al.: 6th Conference on Retroviruses and Opportunistic Infections, Abstr. 610, 1999.
105. Baba, M., et al.: Proc. Natl. Acad. Sci. U. S. A. 96:5698, 1999.
106. Wild, C., et al.: Proc. Natl. Acad. Sci. U. S. A. 91:9770, 1994.
107. Hazuda, D., et al.: Science 287:646, 2000.
108. Goldgur, Y., et al.: Proc. Natl. Acad. Sci. U. S. A. 96:13040, 1999.

C H A P T E R **10**

Antineoplastic Agents

FORREST T. SMITH AND C. RANDALL CLARK

C H A P T E R   O V E R V I E W

Antineoplastic agents describe the chemistry, use, metabolism, and adverse effect profiles for the alkylating agents, antibiotics, natural products, antimetabolites, and tyrosine kinase (TK) inhibitors used in the treatment of cancer. Emphasis has been placed on understanding how cell division and cell death are regulated and how drugs may influence these processes as well as how cancer cells may become resistant to the actions of the antineoplastics. Topics such as apoptosis, DNA alkylation, reactive oxygen species (ROS), and the role of growth factors in controlling transcription and translation are especially important in the discussion of antineoplastic agents; however, in a wider sense, it is important for pharmacists to appreciate the role of these subjects in several other areas such as neurodegenerative diseases, mutagenicity, cardiovascular toxicity, and cell signaling.

INTRODUCTION

The American Cancer Society defines cancer as a group of diseases characterized by uncontrolled growth, and the spread of abnormal cells that left untreated may lead to death. Related to this definition is the term *neoplasia*, which is the uncontrolled growth of new tissue, the product of which is known as a *tumor*, and these tumors may be either malignant or benign. Malignant tumors have the capability of invading surrounding tissues and moving to distant locations in the body in a process known as *metastasis*; characteristics that benign tumors do not possess. Treatment of malignant tumors or cancer has generally involved initially surgical removal followed by radiation and/or chemotherapy, if necessary. In those cases where complete surgical removal is not feasible, radiation and chemotherapy become the only available options. The term *chemotherapy*, in the strictest sense, refers to drugs that are used to kill cells and includes both antibiotics and agents used in the treatment of cancer, but it is often used to refer exclusively to anticancer agents also known as *antineoplastics*. Traditional chemotherapy has been based on the principle of selective toxicity; however, this has been difficult to achieve in the case of cancer cells because these cells utilize the biochemical pathways used by normal cells. In many cases, the agents have attempted to exploit the increased proliferative rates of cancer cells compared with normal cells. This has been difficult to achieve even in a relative sense because, in part, of the fact that not all normal tissue is slowly proliferative and, conversely, not all cancer cells are highly proliferative.

Increased knowledge of intercellular and intracellular communication has led to the development of several newer agents that have shown some effectiveness in treating several cancers, especially when used in combination with more traditional agents. These have included several monoclonal antibodies that target the overproduction of growth factor receptors and TK inhibitors that target the transduction process involved in growth factor stimulation.

Progress against neoplastic disease has also been greatly aided by early detection resulting from increased public awareness and improved diagnostics. As a result, neoplasms are often detected before they have a chance to metastasize and become more difficult to treat. Surgery followed by chemotherapy is often effective in accomplishing a 5-year survival in cancers that are discovered early and have not metastasized. The approach to treatment depends on the extent of the disease and the so-called stage. There are several methods of staging including the commonly used TNM system, where T—tumor, N—lymph node involvement, and M—metastasis. In this system, T and N are followed by numbers (1, 2, 3, etc.) to indicate the size of the tumor and the extent of lymph node involvement, respectively, where higher numbers are associated with more advanced disease. M is followed by either "0" to indicate metastasis has not occurred or "1" to indicate that it has. An alternative system utilizes stage 0 through stage IV designations, with higher numbers indicating progression of the disease. In this system, stage IV indicates that the primary tumor has metastasized.

Even with all the advancements, progress in many cases has been very slow. In comparing 5-year survival rates for patients with pancreatic cancer diagnosed between 1975 and 1977, with those diagnosed between 1996 and 2003, the rate increased from 2% to only 5%. Five-year survival rates for lung cancer patients increased from 13% to 16% during the same interval. It is obvious that these results do not represent tremendous progress in these types of cancer, and some of the increase may be ascribed to increased public awareness and better diagnostic methods that have allowed for earlier detection. This is important because the starting date in calculating a 5-year survival rate is the day of initial detection. This lack of progress in lung cancer is especially ominous since the American Cancer Society estimates that lung cancer will account for the greatest percentage of cancer deaths in 2008.[1]

As part of the definition, cancer is a group of diseases and these have been traditionally grouped together based on the organ in which the cancer originated. Even this grouping is somewhat misleading, because all cancers of a particular organ may not be caused by the same genetic alterations. This has important consequences for therapy, because the ability to respond to a chemotherapeutic agent is partly dependent on the genetic abnormality occurring in the cell.

The primary risk factor for most cancers is age. There are certainly other risk factors such as exposure to environmental toxins, but generally, as aging occurs, the chance of developing cancer increases. This is related to the genetic component of cancer so that every time a cell divides, there is a small chance that an aberrant cancer cell may arise as a result of mutation or translocation of DNA. This is cumulative so that the chances increase with an increasing number of cell divisions and, hence, age.

Normal cellular growth and proliferation are generally driven by factors external to the cell. Mitogenic signals such as hormones and growth factors direct the cell to undergo mitosis and are generally released from other tissues setting up a system of checks and balances where any one cell type is not allowed to proliferate in an uncontrolled manner. In cancer cells, this system may become disrupted in several ways. For example, some cells may acquire the ability to synthesize their own growth factors in a process known as *autocrine signaling*. It is also possible for cells to lose the requirements for growth factors altogether and still be capable of proliferating. There are numerous ways in which this may come about. For example, the signal transduction processes in which the interaction of a growth factor and its receptor is translated into cellular division may become permanently activated at any one point along the chain or at multiple points. Central to this idea is the concept of oncogenes or cancer-producing genes, the products of which may be responsible for these types of alterations. Oncogenes themselves are not normally present in the genome; however, precursors known as *proto-oncogenes* are commonly seen. Alterations in these proto-oncogenes by mutation or translocation may result in their transformation to an oncogene and the development of cancer. Several of these are listed in Table 10.1, but it should be kept in mind that although conversion of any particular proto-oncogene to an oncogene may be associated with a particular cancer, it is not seen in all patients that develop this type of cancer.

The process of cell division occurs through a series of phases that collectively are known as the *cell cycle*. Starting in the G_1 for gap 1 or growth 1 phase, the enzymes necessary for the replication of DNA are synthesized (Fig. 10.1). Alternatively, cells may enter the G_0 phase in which they do not prepare for cell division but carry on normal metabolic processes. Entry into G_0 (sometimes referred to as *senescence*) is not an irreversible process; however, some

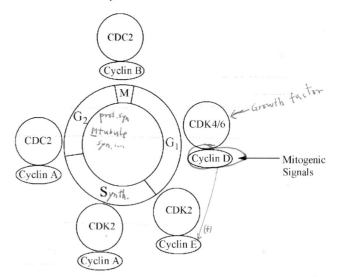

Figure 10.1 • Cyclins and the cell cycle.

cells such as nerve cells never divide. If the cell is to undergo division, it will progress to the S phase where DNA is replicated. This is followed by the G_2 phase, during which additional protein synthesis occurs including the formation of the microtubules. The M phase, which is further subdivided into prophase, metaphase, anaphase, and telophase, follows in which the DNA is segregated and cell division occurs. During the entire cycle, movement from one phase to the next is driven by proteins known as *cyclins* and their associated cyclin-dependent kinases (CDKs). There are several subtypes of cyclins with their CDKs, the concentrations of which change or cycle as the cell moves from G_1 through M phase, and this concentration change is associated with moving the cell into the next phase. The D-type cyclins paired with CDK4/6 are in high concentration during the G_1 phase, and their formation is under the control of external growth factors. Subsequent to this, the D-type cyclins help drive the formation of cyclin E with its CDK2, which drives the cell from the G_1 to the S phase. This is followed by formation of A- and B-type cyclins with their CDKs, which push the cell into G_2 and subsequently into M, respectively.

The progression through the cell cycle is a highly regulated process, and the cell is constantly monitoring itself to make sure that the necessary enzymes are present and the genome is intact. If problems are encountered, the cell may be slowed from progressing or undergo programmed cell death also known as *apoptosis*. Regulation of the cell through the cell cycle is the function of the tumor suppressor proteins such as retinoblastoma protein (Rb), p21[Cip1], and p53.[2] Especially important in this regard is p53, sometimes referred to as the guardian of the cell, it functions as a transcription factor and may activate genes, the products of which are involved in the repair of DNA. When damage becomes too severe to be repaired, p53 may direct the cell to die. One of the best examples of this is seen during overexposure to the sun. The UV damage that the skin has suffered is detected by p53 and the cells undergo apoptosis with the resulting peeling away of the dead skin.[3] Activation of p53 may occur in response to various stresses that cause damage to the genome, but it has been found that in many cancer cells, p53 and other tumor suppressor genes are not

TABLE 10.1 Selected Oncogenes and the Associated Human Cancer

Oncogene	Oncogene Product	Associated Human Cancer
ETS	Transcription factor	Leukemia
RAS	G-protein	Ovarian, bladder, lung
RAF	Serine-threonine kinase	Bladder
KIT	Receptor tyrosine kinase	Colon
SIS	Growth factor	Various
TP53	Transcription factor (p53)	Various

functioning. Although a normal cell would undergo apoptosis in this situation, the cancerous cells continue to survive and may mutate more readily because the system of genetic checks and balances is no longer in place.

The process of apoptosis can occur by both an intrinsic and extrinsic pathway (Fig. 10.2). The intrinsic pathway begins when cytochrome c is released from the mitochondria via channels present in the mitochondrial membrane. The state of this channel is controlled by several different proteins such that opening is stimulated by the proapoptotic p53 products Bad, Bax, and Bid and closure is stimulated by the antiapoptotic Bcl-2 and Bcl-X$_L$ proteins. Opening of the channel releases cytochrome c into the cytoplasm where it combines with apoptotic protease activating factor-1 (apaf-1) molecules to form a wheel-like structure of seven spokes known as the *apoptosome*. This then binds and activates caspase-9, which activates additional caspase enzymes in a cascade fashion. The caspase enzymes cleave numerous proteins within the cell, leading to profound morphological changes and cell death.

The extrinsic pathway is activated when ligands of the tumor necrosis factor family of proteins (TNF-α, FasL, TRAIL) interact with the so-called death receptors (FAS, DR3-5, TNFR1) present on the cell surface. This interaction serves to covert procaspase to active caspase-8/10, which is capable of activating the executioner caspases directly, and in this process, the proapoptotic Bid is activated by caspase-8, which opens the mitochondrial channel allowing for the release of cytochrome c. This then functions as it had in the intrinsic pathway to form the apoptosome.

The ability of drugs to kill cancer cells is generally believed to be because of their ability to induce the process of apoptosis. In high-dose therapy, cell death may occur by necrosis but this is also toxic to the patient. In a general sense, the antineoplastics target DNA or the process of DNA replication and stimulate apoptosis but the exact mechanisms by which this stimulation occurs are not known with certainty. The effectiveness of the agents is reduced in cells where apoptosis fails to occur properly, and this is a property of many cancer cells. Normal cells with fully functioning apoptotic

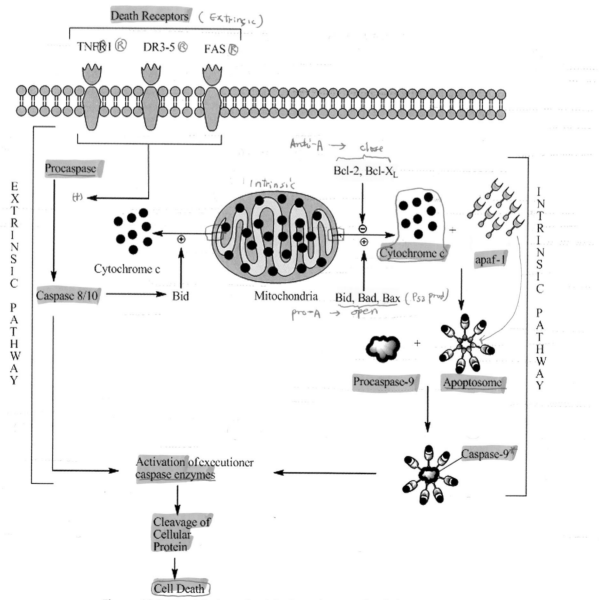

Figure 10.2 ● Intrinsic and extrinsic pathways of cellular apoptosis.

mechanisms may then become susceptible to the action of the antineoplastics increasing the toxicity of the agents.

DRUG CLASSES

Alkylating Agents

The alkylating agents are a class of drugs that are capable of forming covalent bonds with important biomolecules. The major targets of drug action are nucleophilic groups present on DNA (especially the 7-position of guanine); however, proteins and RNA among others may also be alkylated. Alkylation of DNA is thought to lead to cell death, although the exact mechanism is uncertain. Potential mechanisms of cell death include activation of apoptosis caused by p53 activation and disruption of the template function of DNA. In many cases, however, the cancer cells have dysfunctional p53 so that even though the cell has been unable to replicate DNA error free, cell death via apoptosis does not occur. In this way, cancer cells may become resistant to the effects of alkylating agents. Another possibility is that the cancer cells, like normal cells, have various mechanisms by which alkylated DNA bases can be excised.

Disruption of the template function of DNA may have several effects. There are several potential nucleophilic sites on DNA, which are susceptible to electrophilic attack by an alkylating agent (N-2, N-3, and N-7 of guanine, N-1, N-3, and N-7 of adenine, 0–6 of thymine, N-3 of cytosine). The most important of these for many alkylating agents is the N-7 position of guanine whose nucleophilicity may be enhanced by adjacent guanine residues. Alkylation converts the base to an effective leaving group so that attack by water leads to depurination and the loss of genetic information if the resulting depurination is not repaired by the cell (Scheme 10.1). Additionally, alkylation has been proposed to result in altered base pairing away from the normal G-C: A-T hydrogen bonds because of alterations in tautomerization.[4] The alkylation also leads to increased acidity of the N-1 nitrogen reducing the pK_a from 9 to 7 to 8 giving rise to a zwitterionic form that may also mispair. For those agents that possess two reactive functionalities, both interstrand and intrastrand cross-linking becomes possible. When interstrand links occur, separation of the two strands during replication is prevented and therefore replication is blocked.

Most of the currently used alkylating agents are nonselective regarding the sequence of DNA with which they react. Therefore, it is uncertain whether alkylation will lead to a cytotoxic event. Some alkylation reactions may lead to inconsequential results, and others may be easily repaired by the cell. Recent efforts have been directed at producing more sequence-selective alkylators that could be used at lower concentrations in an effort to reduce the significant side effects associated with this group of agents.

The general mechanism for alkylation involves nucleophilic attack by —N=, —NH_2, —OH, —O—PO_3H of DNA and RNA, while additional nucleophiles (—SH, COOH, etc.) present on proteins may also react (Scheme 10.2). Anion

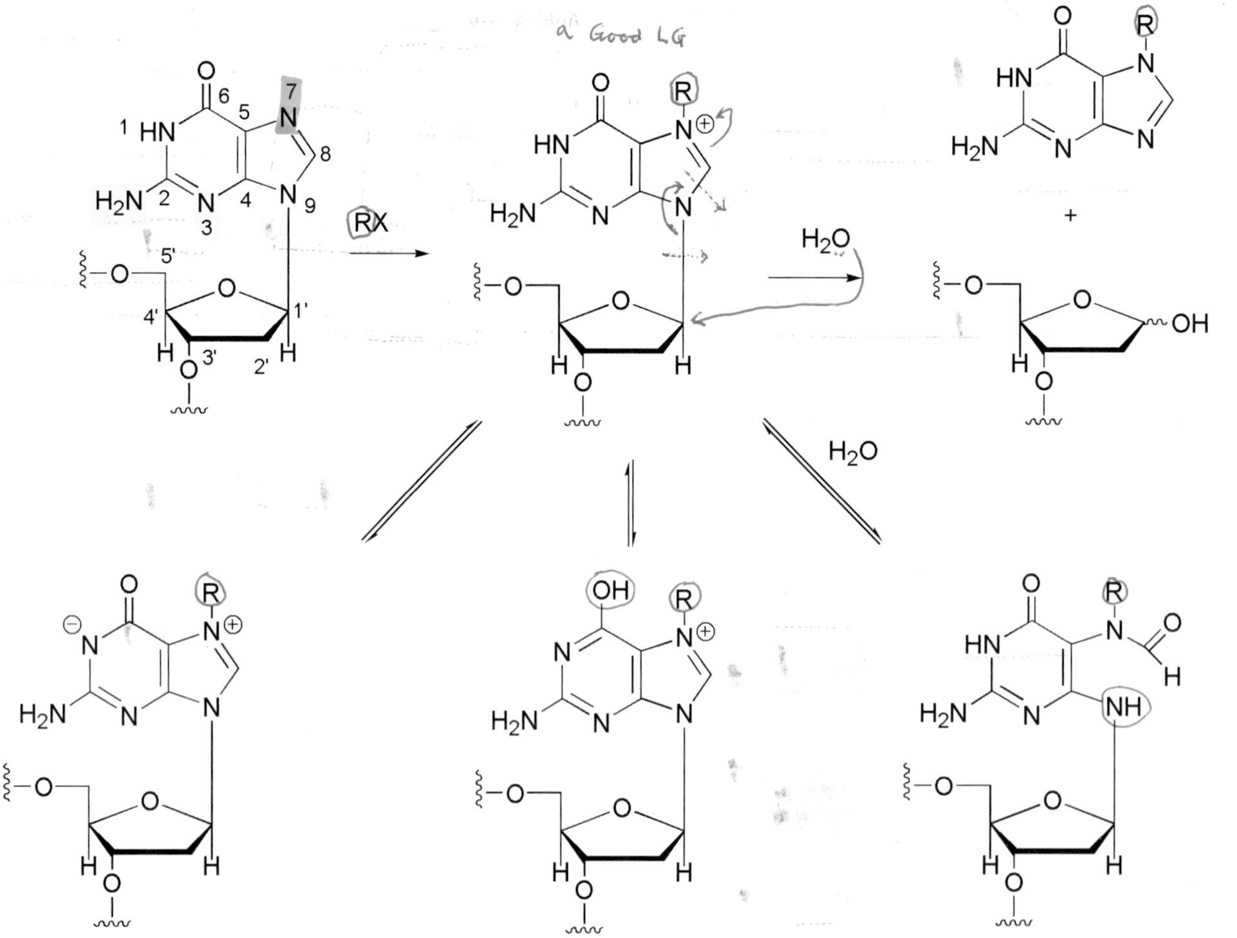

Scheme 10.1 ● Alkylation of guanine N-7 and subsequent depurination of DNA.

DNA-Nuc-H + R-X $\xrightarrow{\text{Alkylation}}$ DNA-Nuc-R + $H^{\oplus}$ + $X^{\ominus}$

Scheme 10.2 ● General reaction for alkylation and inactivation of alkylating agents.

H_2O + R-X $\xrightarrow{\text{Inactivation}}$ H_2O + $H^{\oplus}$ + $X^{\ominus}$

Where X = a leaving group

formation increases the reactivity of the nucleophile compared with the un-ionized form (—O⁻ is more nucleophilic than OH). Reaction with water is also possible, because it represents the nucleophile in greatest abundance in the body and this becomes more likely as the electrophile becomes more reactive. Reaction involves displacement of a leaving group on the electrophile by the nucleophile. The reactivity of the electrophile is dependent in part on the ability of the leaving group to stabilize a negative charge.

Along with a common mechanism, there are other characteristics that the alkylating agents share. Mechanisms by which cells may become resistant to these agents are thought to be similar and include decreased cellular uptake, increased inactivation by detoxifying nucleophilic thiols such as glutathione, increased DNA repair processes, and decreased drug activation when this is necessary for generation of an alkylating species. Functioning apoptotic mechanisms are thought to be important for the effectiveness of these agents at normal doses, and those cells that do not possess these mechanisms may not respond. In high-dose therapy involving bone marrow transplants, the cell may be overwhelmed by the damage caused by these agent and die because of necrosis. The alkylating agents are thought to be effective from G_0-M and are, therefore, not considered cell cycle–specific agents. Many of the toxicities seen with the various agents are similar. Myelosuppression and gastrointestinal (GI) disruption, which often present as nausea and vomiting are commonly seen and are caused by the highly proliferative nature of these tissues, and therefore susceptibility to the effects of the alkylating agents. It is interesting to note that although cancer cells may develop resistance to the alkylating agents, this is not generally seen for cells of the bone marrow and GI tract because of

the genetic stability and functioning DNA repair mechanisms present in these cells. However, an additional long-term consequence of the administration of these agents is the emergence of secondary cancers that are associated with the mutagenic effects of the alkylating agents themselves.

NITROGEN MUSTARDS

The nitrogen mustards are compounds that are chemically similar to sulfur mustard or mustard gas developed and used in World War I. The term "mustard" comes from the similarity in the blisters produced by the compound and those seen upon exposure to the oil of black mustard seeds. Investigation of sulfur mustard revealed that it possessed antineoplastic properties but because the compound existed as a gas at room temperature, handling and administration of the material were difficult. Conversion of the sulfide to a tertiary amine allowed for the formation of salts, which exist as solids at room temperature allowing for easier handling and dosing. The term mustard was then extended to the nitrogen analogs (nitrogen mustards) given their chemical similarity.

Mustards such as mechlorethamine are classified as dialkylating agents in that one mustard molecule can alkylate two nucleophiles.[5] The initial acid–base reaction is necessary to release the lone pair of electrons on nitrogen, which subsequently displaces chloride to give the highly reactive aziridinium cation (Scheme 10.3). Nucleophilic attack can then occur at the aziridinium carbon to relieve the small ring strain and neutralize the charge on nitrogen. This process can then be repeated provided a second leaving group is present.[6]

Mechlorethamine is highly reactive, in fact, too reactive and therefore nonselective, making it unsuitable for oral

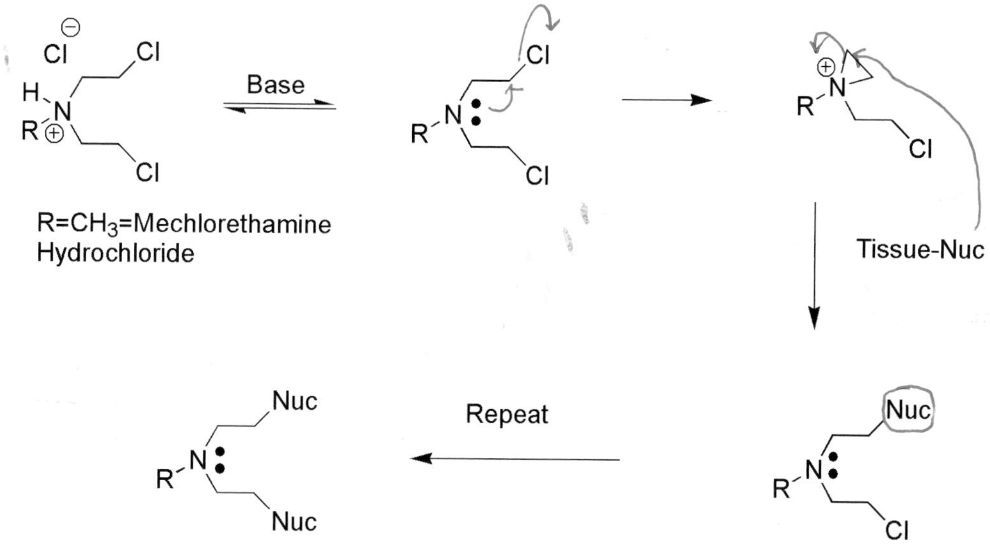

myelo = marrow

R=CH$_3$=Mechlorethamine
Hydrochloride

Tissue-Nuc

Scheme 10.3 ● Alkylation of nucleophilic species by nitrogen mustards.

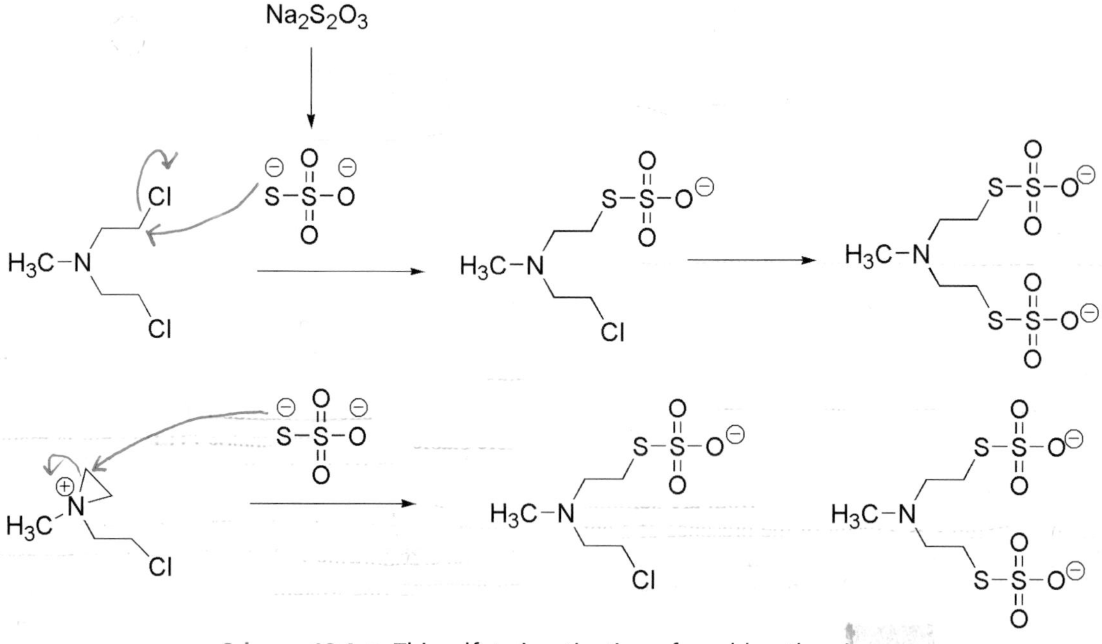

Scheme 10.4 ● Thiosulfate inactivation of mechlorethamine.

administration and necessitating direct injection into the tumor. In cases of extravasation (drug escapes from the tumor into the underlying tissue), the antidote sodium thiosulfate ($Na_2S_2O_3$), a strong nucleophile, may be administered. It is capable of reacting with electrophilic sites on the mustard, and once reaction has occurred, the resulting adduct has increased water solubility and may be readily eliminated (Scheme 10.4). Cancer patients are at an increased risk of extravasation because of the fragility of their veins resulting from radiation, previous chemotherapy treatments, or malnutrition.

The lack of selectivity of mechlorethamine led to attempts to improve on the agent. One rationale was to reduce the reactivity by reducing the nucleophilicity of nitrogen, thereby slowing aziridinium cation formation. This could be accomplished by replacement of the weakly electron-donating methyl group with groups that were electron withdrawing (-I). This is seen in the case of chlorambucil and melphalan by attachment of nitrogen to a phenyl ring (Fig. 10.3).[7] Reactivity was reduced such that these compounds could be administered orally. In the case of melphalan, attachment of the mustard functionality to a phenylalanine moiety was not only an attempt to reduce reactivity but also an attempt to increase entry into cancer cells by utilization of carrier-mediated uptake.[8] Melphalan was found to utilize active transport to gain entry into cells, but selective uptake by cancer cells has not been demonstrated. [9]

Attachment of more highly electron-withdrawing functionalities was utilized in the case of cyclophosphamide and ifosfamide (Fig. 10.4). In these cases, aziridinium cation formation is not possible until the electron-withdrawing

function has been altered. In the case of cyclophosphamide, it was initially believed that the drug could be selectively activated in cancer cells because they were believed to contain high levels of phosphoramidase enzymes. This would remove the electron-withdrawing phosphoryl function and allow aziridine formation to occur. However, it turned out that the drug was activated by cytochrome P450 (CYP) isozymes CYP2B6 and CYP3A4/5 to give a carbinolamine that could undergo ring opening to give the aldehyde.[10,11] The increased acidity of the aldehyde α-hydrogen facilitates a retro-Michael decomposition (Scheme 10.5). The ionized phosphoramide is now electron-releasing via induction and allows aziridinium cation formation to proceed. Acrolein is also formed as a result of this process, which may itself act as an electrophile that has been associated with bladder toxicity. Alternatively, the agent may be inactivated by alcohol dehydrogenase–mediated oxidation of the carbinolamine to give the amide or by further oxidation of the aldehyde intermediate to give the acid by aldehyde dehydrogenase.

To decrease the incidence of kidney and bladder toxicity, the sulfhydryl (—SH) containing agent mesna may be administered and functions to react with the electrophilic species that may be present in the kidney. The sulfonic acid functionality serves to help concentrate the material in the urine, and the nucleophilic sulfhydryl group may react with the carbinolamine, aziridinium cation, the chloro substituents of cyclophosphamide, or via conjugate addition with acrolein (Scheme 10.6). This inactivation and detoxification may also be accomplished by other thiol-containing proteins such as

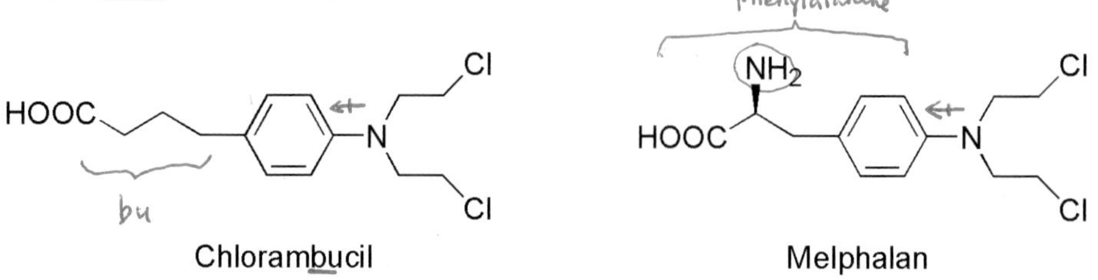

Figure 10.3 ● Structure of chlorambucil and melphalan.

Chlorambucil

Melphalan

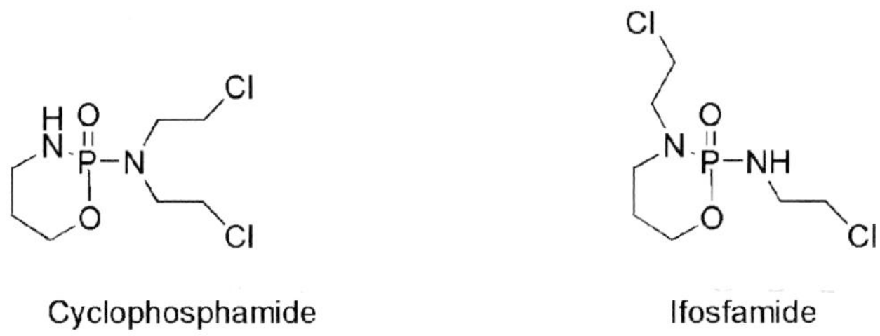

Figure 10.4 ● Structures of cyclophosphamide and ifosfamide.

glutathione. Increased levels of these proteins may occur as cancer cells become resistant to these alkylating agents.

Ifosfamide contains similar functionality and also requires activation by CYP2B6 and CYP3A4/5 (Scheme 10.7). Although the agents are similar, there are differences in the metabolism and activity of the agents.[12,13] Both are administered as racemic mixtures as a result of the presence of a chiral phosphorus atom. There appears to be little difference in the metabolic fate of the *R*- and *S*-isomers of cyclophosphamide, but in the case of ifosfamide, the *R*-isomer is converted to the required 4-hydroxy-ifosfamide 2 to 3 times faster than the *S*-isomer.[14] The *S*-isomer undergoes preferential oxidation of the side chain to give *N*-dechloroethylation, which removes the ability of the agent to cross-link DNA and also produces the neurotoxic and urotoxic chloroacetaldehyde. An additional difference between cyclophosphamide and ifosfamide is the larger alkylating species that ultimately

results after metabolic activation of ifosfamide. This results in the reactive form of ifosfamide having a higher affinity for DNA than the analogous form of cyclophosphamide and differences in the interstrand and intrastrand links that ultimately result. The differential metabolism also results in increased formation of the urotoxic chloroacetaldehyde in the case of ifosfamide such that bladder toxicity that normally presents as hemorrhagic cystitis becomes dose limiting with this agent.

THIOTEPA

The early success of the nitrogen mustards led researchers to investigate other compounds that contained a preformed aziridine ring, and thiotepa resulted from this work. Thiotepa containing the thiophosphoramide functionality was found to be more stable than the oxa-analog (TEPA) but is metabolically converted to TEPA by desulfuration in vivo.[15] Thiotepa incorporates a less reactive aziridine ring compared with that formed in mechlorethamine. The adjacent thiophosphoryl is electron withdrawing and, therefore, reduces the reactivity of the aziridine ring system. Although thiotepa is less reactive than many other alkylating agents, it has been shown to form cross-links. This is believed to occur by sequential reactions of thiotepa itself with DNA (Scheme 10.8).[16] Monoalkylation is also possible as a result of aziridine formation via hydrolysis of thiotepa. Thiotepa is also metabolized by oxidative desulfurization mediated by CYP2B1 and CYP2C11.[17] The decreased stability of the resulting TEPA undergoes hydrolysis to give aziridine, which may function to monoalkylate

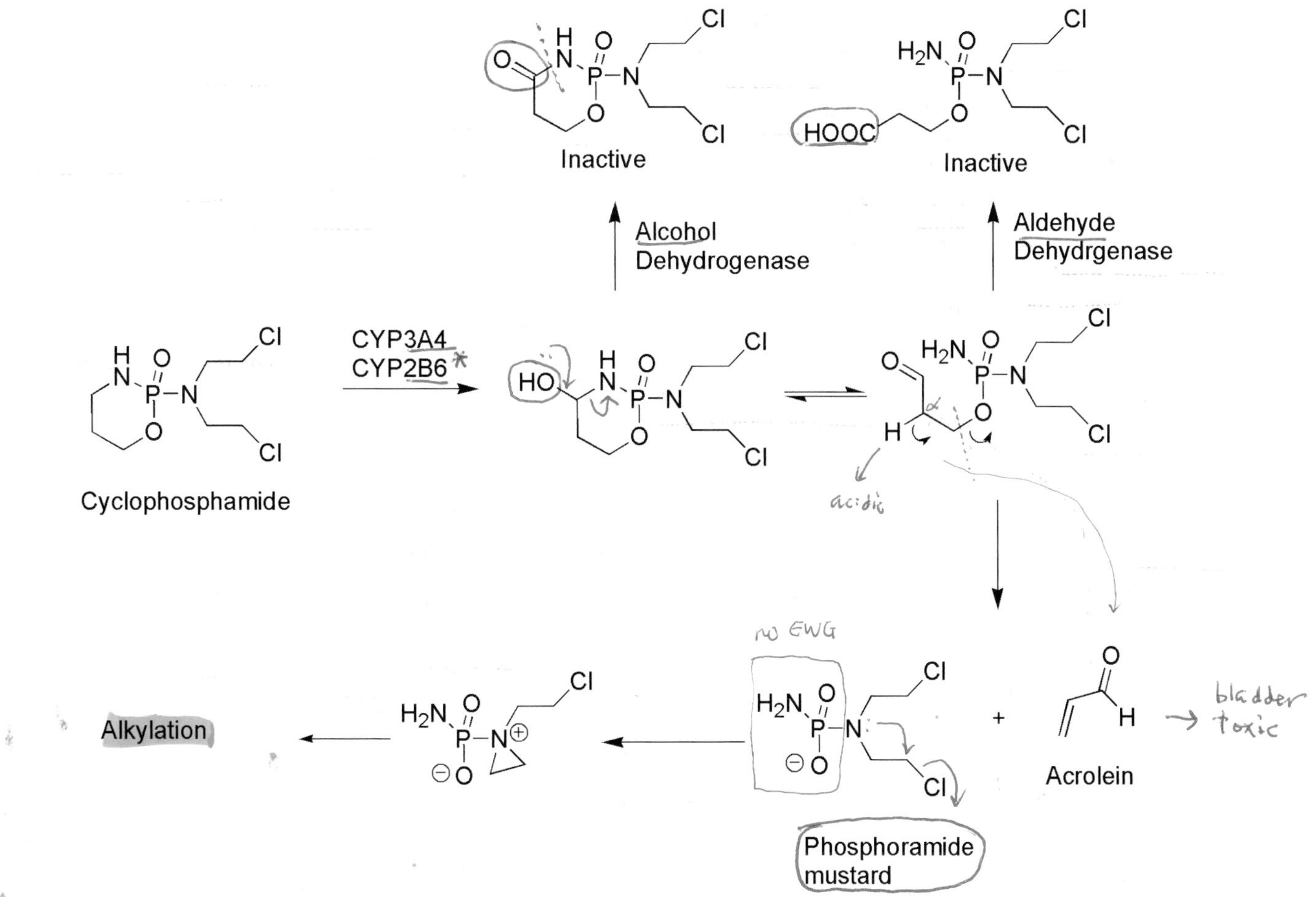

Scheme 10.5 ● Metabolic and chemical activation of cyclophosphamide.

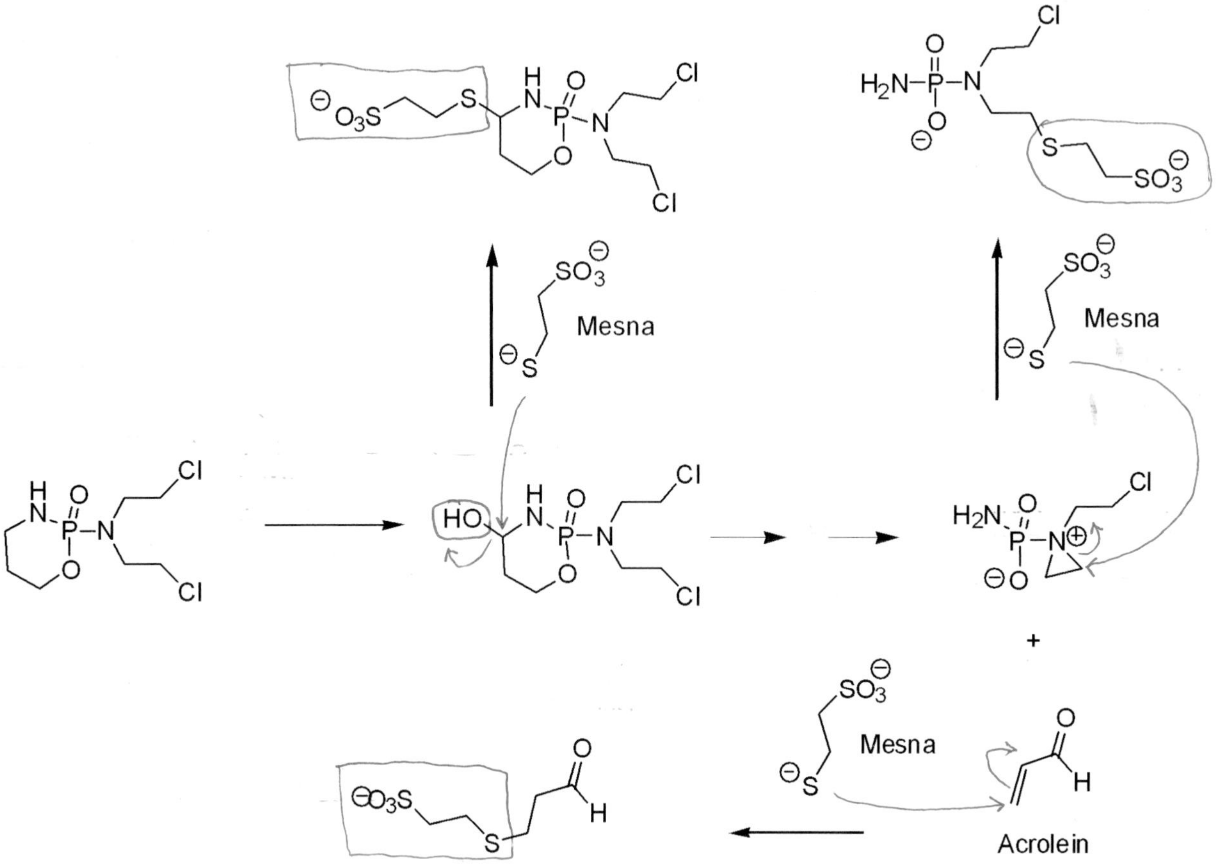

Scheme 10.6 ● Detoxification of cyclophosphamide by mesna.

DNA.[18] The conclusion that aziridine is the active alkylating agent once thiotepa has been converted to TEPA is based on the fact that when TEPA is incubated with DNA, no cross-links are formed and only monoadducts are generated. The reactivity of aziridine generated by either route may be somewhat enhanced within cancer cells, where the pH is normally reduced 0.2 to 0.4 pH units resulting in an increase in reactivity toward nucleophilic attack.

BUSULFAN

As an alternative to utilizing aziridines as electrophilic species, it was found that simply utilizing a carbon chain terminated at both ends by leaving groups gave compounds capable of acting as cross-linking agents (Scheme 10.9).[19] Busulfan utilizes two sulfonate functionalities as leaving groups separated by a four-carbon chain that reacts with DNA to primarily form intrastrand cross-link at 5′-GA-3′ sequences.[20] The sulfonates are also subject to displacement by the sulfhydryl functions found in cysteine and glutathione, and metabolic products are formed as a result of nucleophilic attack by these groups to generate sulfonium species along with methane sulfonic acid.[21] This is followed by conversion to tetrahydrothiophene, and further oxidation products are subsequently produced to give the sulfoxide and sulfone. The cyclic sulfone known as *sulfolane* may be further oxidized to give 3-hydroxysulfolane.

ORGANOPLATINUM COMPOUNDS

There are several organometallic compounds based on platinum that play a central role in many cancer treatment

protocols (Fig. 10.5). The first of these, cisplatin, was discovered by Barnett Rosenberg as a result of experiments investigating the role of electrical current on cell division. *Escherichia coli* cells in an ammonium chloride solution had an electrical current applied through platinum electrodes.[22] It was subsequently found that cell division was inhibited but not as a result of the current but from the reaction of the ammonium chloride with what was thought to be an inert platinum electrode. Further investigation led to the identification of *cis*-$[PtCl_2(NH_3)_2]$ as the active species and mechanistic studies revealed that after administration of the agent to mammals, the dichloro species is maintained in the blood stream as a result of the relatively high chloride concentration (Scheme 10.10).[23] Movement into the tumor cells is accomplished by passive diffusion or carrier-mediated transport. Once inside the tumor cell, the drug encounters a lower chloride concentration and one chloro group is substituted by a water molecule in a process known as *aquation*. This serves to "trap" the molecule in the cell as a result of ionization. Reaction with DNA occurs preferentially at the N-7 of guanine of two adjacent guanine residues resulting in primarily (95%) intrastrand cross-links.[24]

Platinum (II) is considered to be a "soft" electrophile and as a result, its complexes are subject to attack by "soft" nucleophiles such as thiol groups found on proteins. This can result in significant protein binding (88%–95%) and inactivation caused by the presence of thiols in albumin, glutathione, and other proteins.[25] Cisplatin administration is also associated with significant nephrotoxicity and neurotoxicity that is dose limiting. These factors lead to the development of less

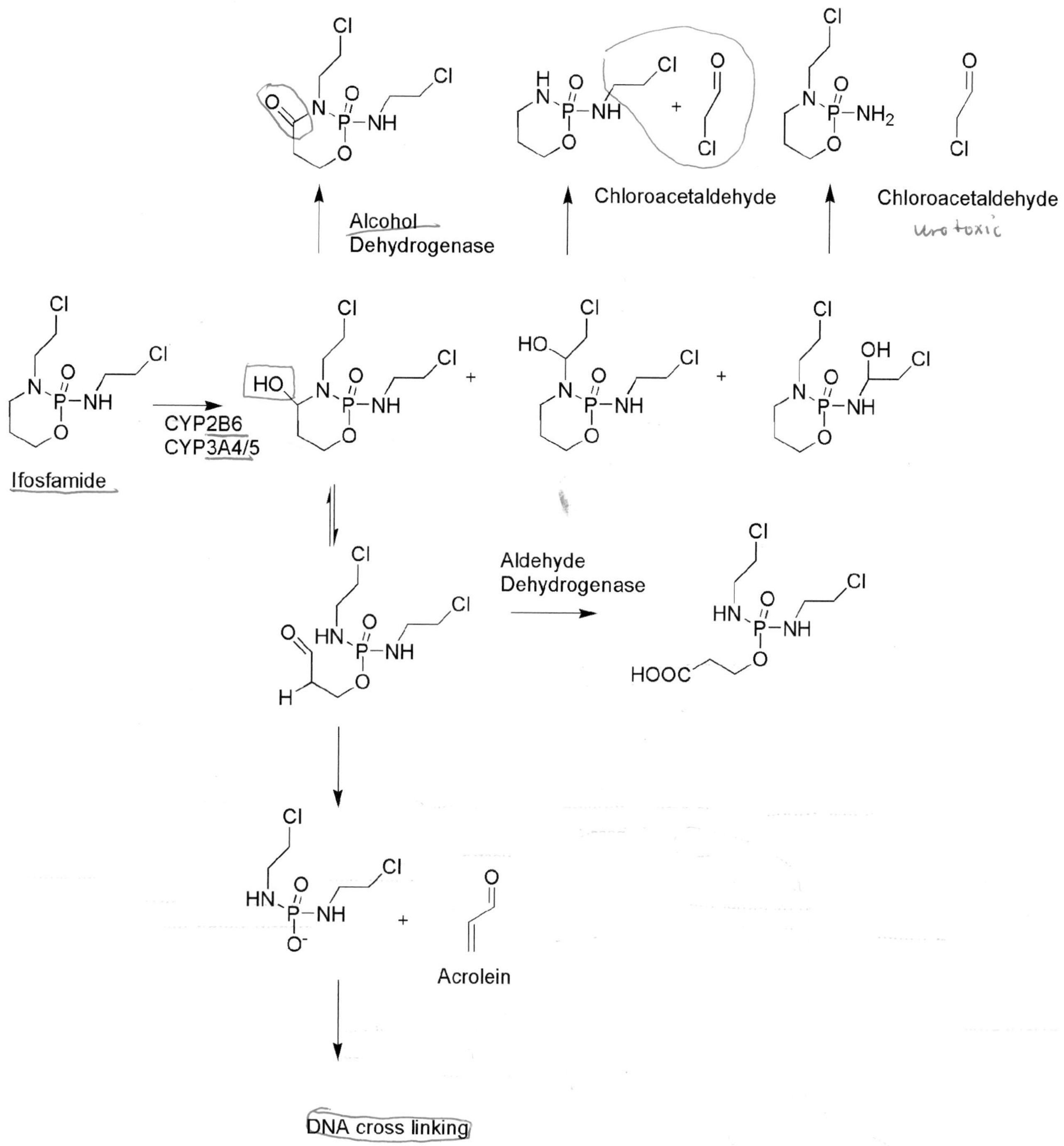

Scheme 10.7 ⬤ Metabolic and chemical activation of ifosfamide.

reactive platinum compounds such as carboplatin and oxaliplatin in which the leaving group was incorporated into a chelate. More recently, there has been interest in the development of Pt(IV) compounds, which are much less reactive and believed to function as prodrugs requiring reduction to the Pt(II) species prior to reaction with nucleophiles. One such agent, satraplatin is currently in clinical trials. One advantage of these agents is the possibility of oral administration. Satraplatin has shown similar activity when given orally to that of cisplatin given by injection.

Tumor cells may become resistant to the platins by mechanisms that are seen with other chemotherapeutic agents such as decreased uptake, increased inactivation by thiol-containing proteins and increased DNA repair. However, a deficiency in a type of DNA repair known as *mismatch repair* (MMR) has also been implicated in resistance to cisplatin and carboplatin.[26] The process of MMR involves several enzymes that are responsible for maintaining the integrity of the genome, and interest has focused on the interaction of these enzymes with repeating units found throughout DNA known as *microsatellites*. When MMR processes are not operating, these microsatellites may become longer or shorter and this is known as *microsatellite instability*. This can result in frame shift errors such that tumor suppressor genes may become less effective, and the tumor cells therefore fail to undergo apoptosis even if

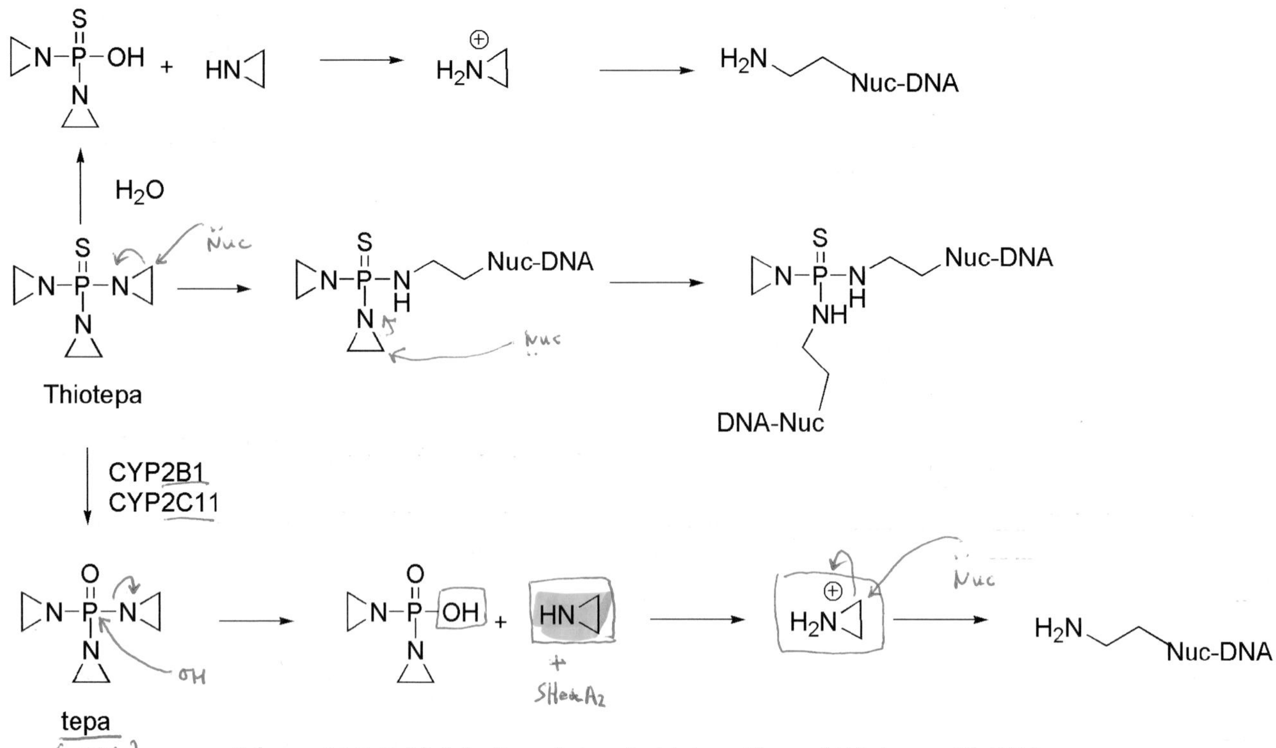

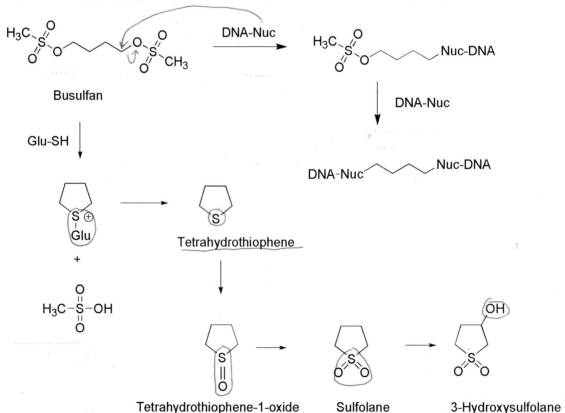

Scheme 10.8 ● Metabolic and chemical interactions of thiotepa with DNA.

alkylation has occurred. The binding of cisplatin- and carboplatin-DNA adducts by the MMR enzymes results in increased cytotoxicity of these agents. Several rationales have been put forward as to why this occurs, including the involvement of MMR enzymes in downstream signaling that activates apoptosis. A second rationale involves the ability

of MMR enzymes to remove replication errors that occur past the point of adduct formation, and in the process of removing these errors, gaps in the DNA are created, which lead to cell death. When there is a deficiency in the MMR enzymes, cells may be resistant to cisplatin and carboplatin because both of these agents produce the same DNA adduct.

Scheme 10.9 ● Metabolic and chemical reactions of busulfan.

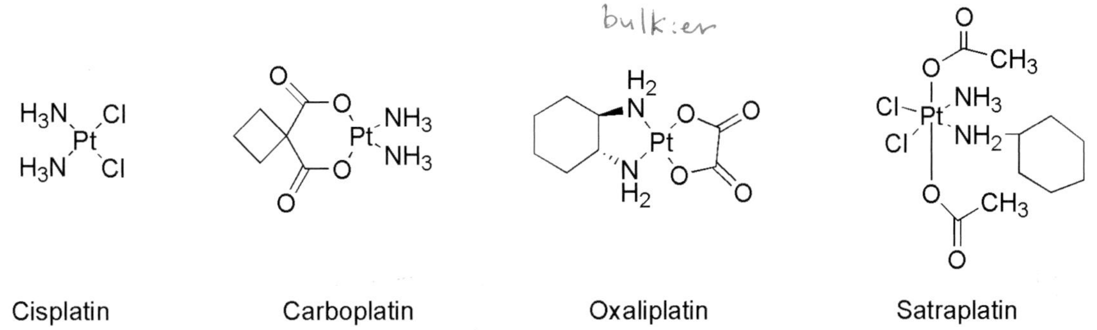

bulkier

| Cisplatin | Carboplatin | Oxaliplatin | Satraplatin |

Figure 10.5 ● Platinum-containing antineoplastics.

The bulkier oxaliplatin-DNA adduct does not seem to be recognized by the same enzymes and does not depend on MMR enzymes for its cytotoxicity, and several cell lines that are resistant to cisplatin and carboplatin are still susceptible to oxaliplatin. In addition, several DNA polymerases are unable to replicate past cisplatin-DNA adducts but are able to replicate past oxaliplatin-DNA adducts.[27] This difference has been used to explain the greater mutagenicity that is seen with cisplatin compared with oxaliplatin. These two compounds both form primarily intrastrand links between adjacent guanine residues or adjacent guanine–adenine residues; however, nuclear magnetic resonance (NMR) analysis has recently shown that the amount of DNA bending is much greater, and the minor groove is widened for the cisplatin-DNA adduct compared with the oxaliplatin-DNA adduct. The greater bending associated with cisplatin-DNA adducts is recognized by MMR enzymes possibly explaining the differential effects of cisplatin and oxaliplatin on these enzymes.

NITROSOUREAS

The nitrosoureas were discovered as a result of drug screening by the Cancer Chemotherapy National Service Center, which identified N-methyl-N'-nitroguanidine as having activity against L1210 leukemia.[28] Further development of this lead compound was based on the idea that its chemical decomposition was leading to the formation of diazomethane (CH_2N_2) and subsequent alkylation of DNA. This led to the nitrosoureas, where it was found that activity could be enhanced by attachment of a 2-haloethyl substituent to both nitrogens (Fig. 10.6).

These compounds are reasonably stable at pH = 4.5 but undergo both acid and base catalyzed decomposition at lower and higher pH, respectively. There are several pathways of decomposition that are possible for these compounds, but the one that appears to be most important for alkylation of DNA involves abstraction of the NH proton, which is relatively acidic (pK_a = 8–9), followed by rearrangement to give an isocyanate and a diazohydroxide. The diazohydroxide, upon protonation followed by loss of water, yields a diazo species that decomposes to a reactive carbocation (Scheme 10.11).[22] The isocyanate functions to carbamylate proteins and RNA, whereas the carbocation is believed to be the agent responsible for DNA alkylation.[29–31] Alternative mechanisms of decomposition have also been proposed involving formation of chlorovinyl carbocations. In those cases where there is a chloroethyl moiety attached to the N-nitroso urea functionality, crosslinking of DNA occurs. Alkylation occurs preferentially at the N-7 position of guanine with minor amounts of alkylation at guanine O-6.[32]

Detoxification pathways of the nitrosoureas are also possible and can play a role in resistance to this group of agents. Two major routes of inactivation have been identified and are indicated in Scheme 10.12. The first of these involves dechlorination, which is facilitated by CYP participation and involves cyclization to give 4,5-dihydro-[1,2,3]oxadiazole and the isocyanate, which is still capable of carbamylating proteins.[33] The oxadiazole can be further degraded by hydrolysis to give several inactive products. The second route involves denitrosation, which in the case of BCNU (carmustine) has been shown to be catalyzed by CYP monooxygenases and glutathione-S-reductase.[34]

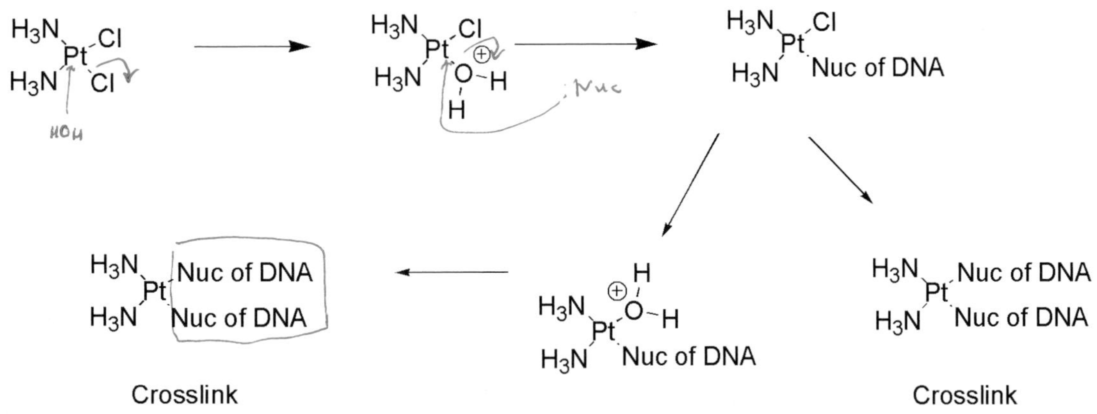

Scheme 10.10 ● Mechanism of cisplatin activation and formation of DNA adducts.

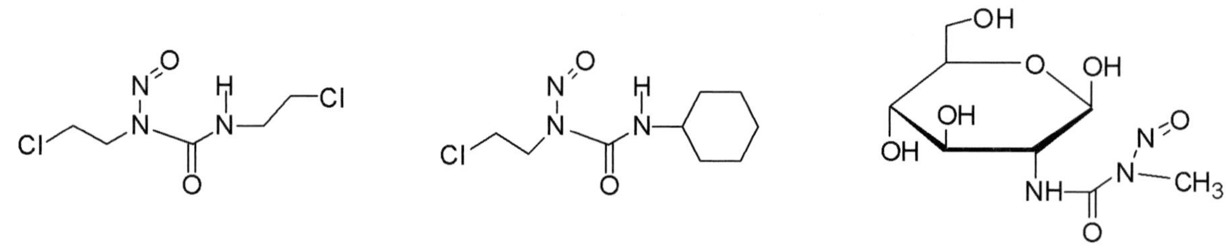

Carmustine (BCNU)   Lomustine (CCNU)   Streptozocin

Figure 10.6 ● Nitrosoureas antineoplastics.

PROCARBAZINE, DACARBAZINE, AND TEMOZOLOMIDE

Procarbazine is an antineoplastic agent that was originally developed as a result of efforts to find new inhibitors of monoamine oxidase. Subsequent screening revealed antineoplastic activity.[35] It was initially believed that the cytotoxicity was related to the ability of the compound to undergo auto-oxidation to give hydrogen peroxide, which in the presence of Fe^{+2} would produce hydroxide radicals capable of cleaving DNA.[36,37] Subsequent work showed that although this did occur, sufficient amounts of hydrogen peroxide were not produced to account for the observed effects. Metabolism studies revealed that oxidation of procarbazine does occur in the liver and is mediated by CYP and monoamine oxidase to give azo-procarbazine. This compound may also be generated nonenzymatically in an aerobic environment (Scheme 10.13).[38–40] There are several chemical and metabolic pathways that azo-procarbazine may then undergo, and there is some disagreement regarding the exact structure of the active alkylating species. One such route involves CYP-mediated oxidation of the benzylic methylene carbon with subsequent decomposition to give methyldiazine and the aldehyde. The methyldiazine may then decompose by homolytic bond cleavage to give methyl and hydrogen radicals along with nitrogen gas or be further oxidized to give the diazo compound, which can decompose to give the methyl carbocation. Methyldiazine may also be produced by a minor route involving isomerization of

azo-procarbazine to give the hydrazone, which subsequently undergoes hydrolysis to give the aldehyde and methylhydrazine. Methylhydrazine may react with oxygen to give methyldiazine, which then decomposes as before. Studies utilizing radiolabeled procarbazine indicated that the terminal methyl group was found covalently bound to the N-7 position of guanine especially on tRNA disrupting its function and preventing protein, RNA, and DNA synthesis.[41] There was also a small amount of methylation at the O-6 position of guanine.[42] Hydrazines are also capable of inhibiting monoamine oxidase as seen with isocarboxazid and phenelzine; however, procarbazine is only a weak inhibitor of this enzyme. The agent is also capable of inhibiting aldehyde dehydrogenase and producing a disulfiram-like reaction. Given the involvement of the CYP system in its activation, the action of procarbazine is subject to drug interactions with both inducers and inhibitors of this system.

Somewhat related is dacarbazine, which was initially thought to act as an inhibitor of purine biosynthesis, but later was shown to be an alkylating agent.[43] Activation of the agent occurs through the action of CYP (isozymes 1A1, 1A2, and 2E1) to give the demethylated product monomethyl triazeno imidazole carboxamide (MTIC) (Scheme 10.14).[44] Tautomerization allows for decomposition to give the aminocarboxamido-imidazole and diazomethane, which is capable of alkylating DNA.[45] An alternative pathway involves acid catalyzed or photoinduced loss of dimethylamine to give an alternative diazo compound (diazo-IC), which may not only

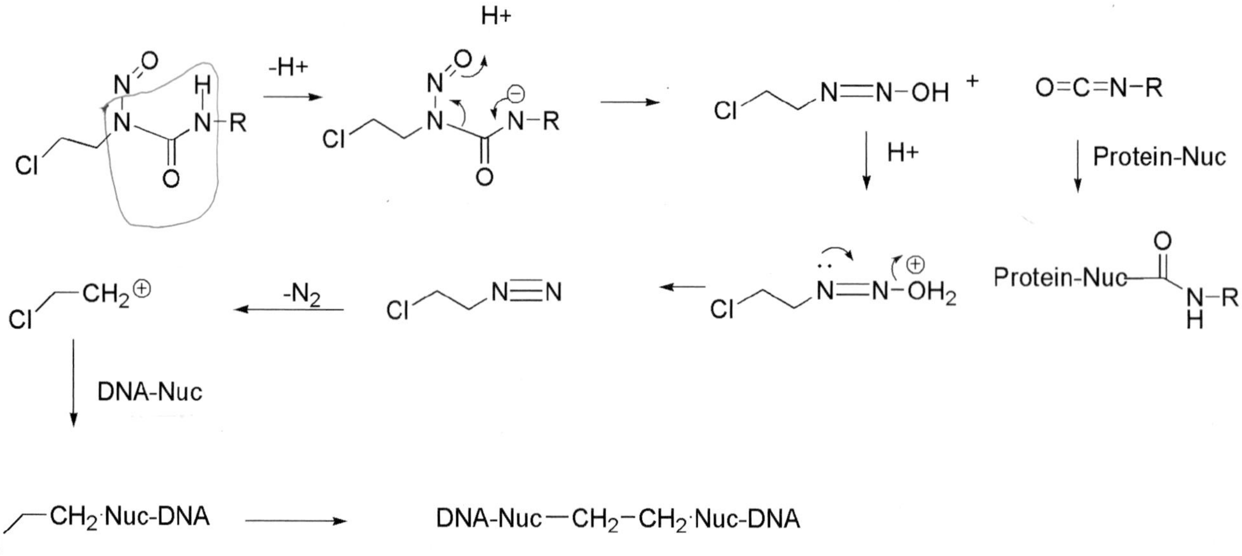

Scheme 10.11 ● Mechanism of DNA alkylation by nitrosoureas.

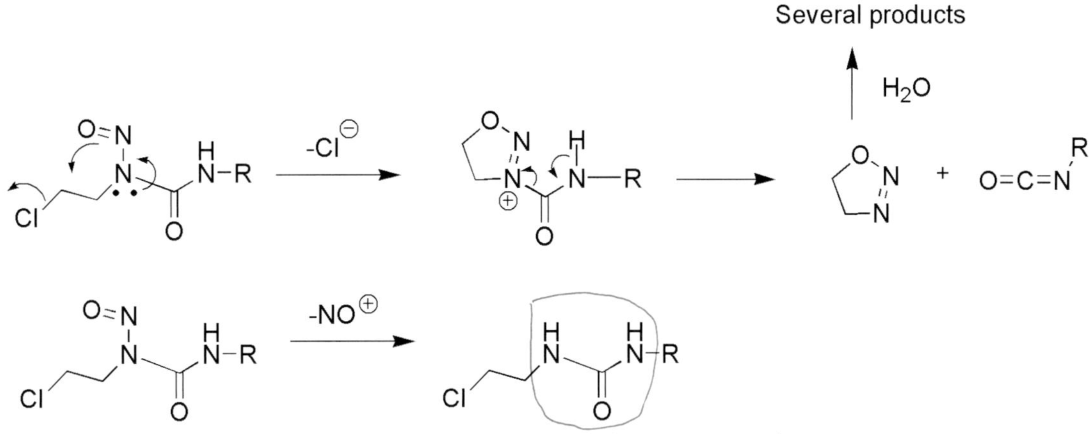

Several products

Scheme 10.12 ● Metabolic and chemical inactivation of nitrosoureas.

generate a carbocation but also undergoes internal cyclization to give 2-azo-hypoxanthine.[46] Formation of diazo-IC has been associated with pain at the injection site, which is often seen during dacarbazine administration.[47] Methylation of DNA occurs at N-7, N-3 and O-6 of guanine among other sites.[48] Dacarbazine proved to be more active against murine tumors than against human tumors. This was attributed to the enhanced ability of mice to metabolize the agent to MTIC

and the subsequent conversion to a methylating species.[49] Building on this idea was temozolomide, which undergoes conversion to the same intermediate, MTIC, as dacarbazine, but it does not require metabolic activation to do so.[50,51] Hydrolysis of temozolomide gives the carboxy-triazene, which spontaneously loses CO_2 to give MTIC. Dacarbazine must be administered intravenously; however, the related temozolomide may be administered orally.

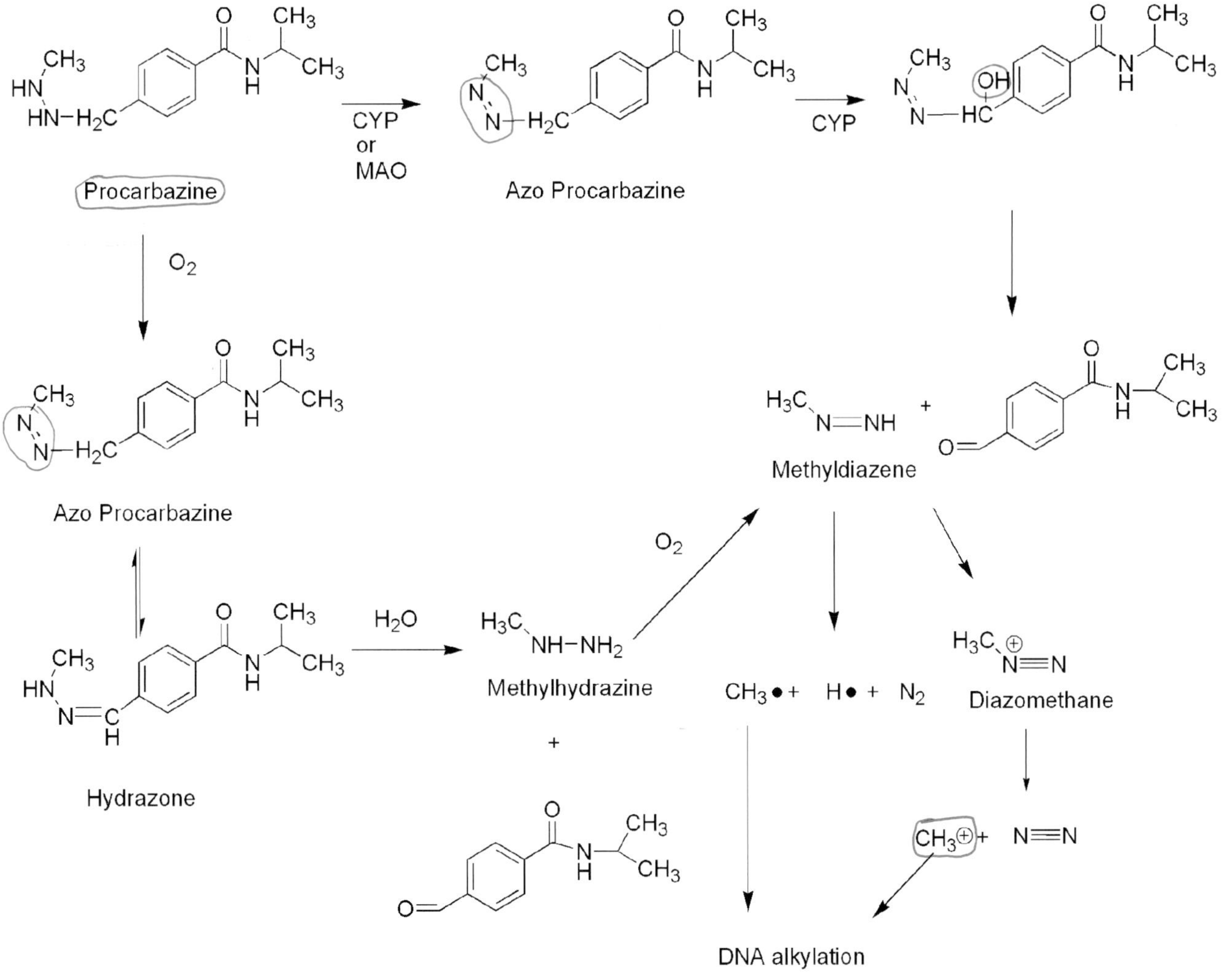

Scheme 10.13 ● Metabolic and chemical activation of procarbazine.

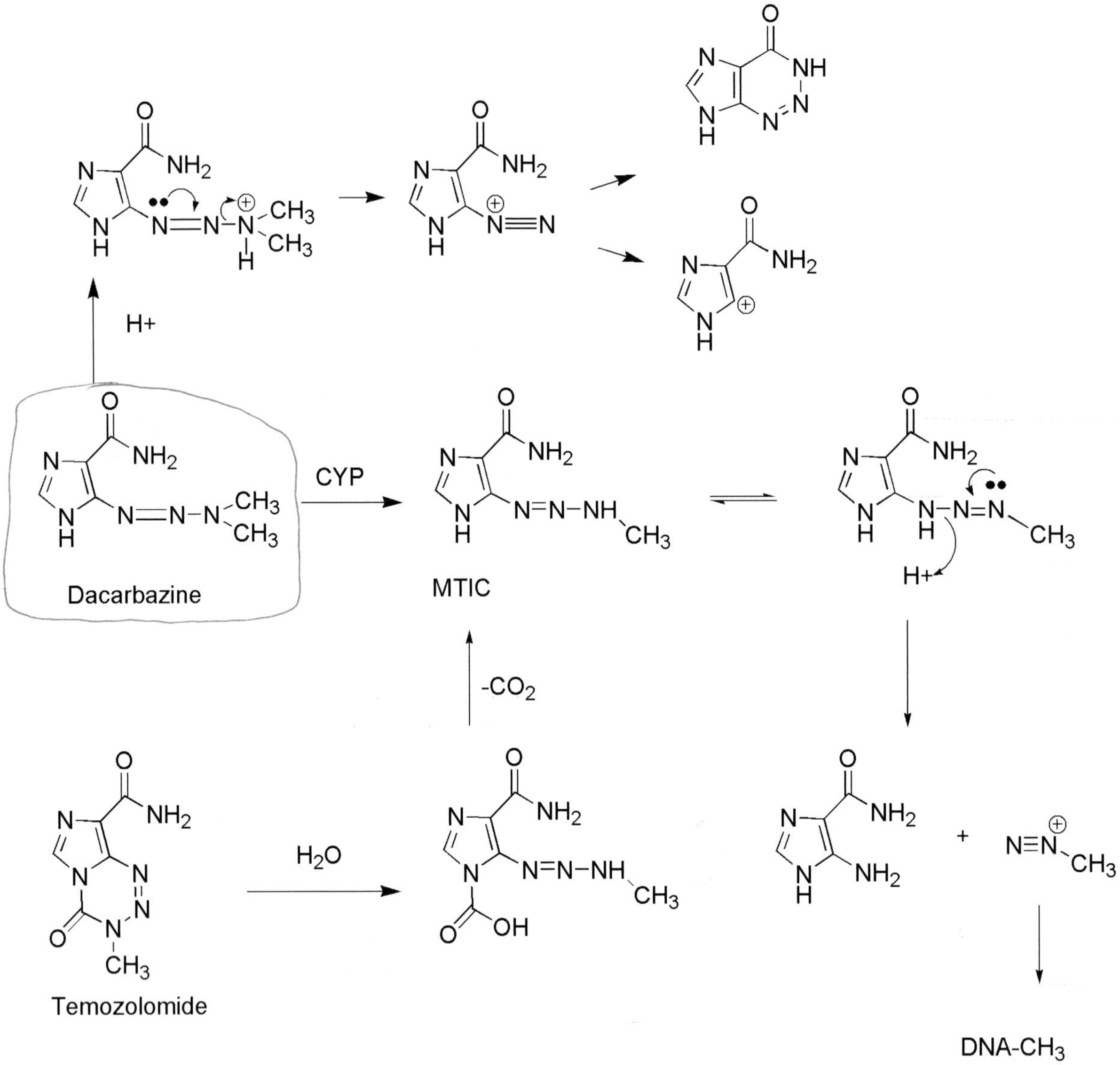

Scheme 10.14 ● Metabolic and chemical activation of dacarbazine and temozolomide.

Individual Agents

MECHLORETHAMINE HYDROCHLORIDE (NH2, MUSTARGEN)

Mechlorethamine is available in 10-mg vials for intravenous (IV) administration in the treatment of Hodgkin's lymphoma. It is part of the MOPP regimen used in treating this condition, which is comprised of *m*echlorethamine, vincristine (*O*ncovin), *p*rocarbazine, and *p*rednisone. The agent is also used topically in the treatment of mycosis fungoides, a rare type of cancer but the most common type of cutaneous T-cell lymphoma. Additional uses have included treatment of cancers that have resulted in pleural effusion. Although the compound is a potent alkylating agent, resistance may develop as a result of increased inactivation by sulfhydryl containing proteins such as glutathione and increased expression of DNA repair mechanisms. Adverse effects include dose-limiting myelosuppression and nausea/vomiting. There is a significant risk of extravasation upon IV administration, and the agent may produce pain at the injection site. Additional adverse effects include alopecia, azoospermia, amenorrhea, hyperuricemia, and an increased risk of secondary cancers.

CHLORAMBUCIL (AMBOCHLORIN, ABMOCLORIN, LEUKERAN)

Chlorambucil is available as 2-mg tablets for oral administration in the treatment of Hodgkin's lymphoma, and chronic lymphocytic leukemia in combination with prednisone and as a single agent. The mechanisms of resistance are the same as those seen for other agents of the class such as mechlorethamine. The agent is well absorbed (75%) upon oral administration and highly protein bound. Metabolism is mediated by CYP and occurs extensively to give several metabolites, including the active phenylacetic acid–nitrogen mustard. The drug is eliminated via the kidneys with a terminal elimination half-life of 1.5 hours. Adverse effects include dose-limiting myelosuppression, which are seen as both leucopenia and thrombocytopenia. Nausea and vomiting occur less often than for mechlorethamine. Additional adverse effects include hyperuricemia, azoospermia, amenorrhea, seizures, pulmonary fibrosis, and skin rash.

MELPHALAN (L-PAM, ALKERAN, L-PHENYLALANINE MUSTARD)

Melphalan is available in 2-mg tablets and 50-mg vials for oral and IV administration, respectively in the treatment of multiple myeloma, breast and ovarian cancer, and in high-dose therapy when bone marrow transplant is being utilized. The mechanisms of resistance are the same as those seen for mechlorethamine. The agent is poorly absorbed when given by the oral route. Melphalan is highly plasma protein bound (80%–90%) and inactivated in the blood by water to give the hydroxy metabolites. Elimination occurs primarily in the feces with an elimination half-life of 38 to 108 minutes. The commonly seen adverse effects are myelosuppression, nausea, and vomiting. Nausea is normally mild with normal doses but becomes severe when high doses are used during bone marrow transplant. Less commonly seen adverse effects are hypersensitivity reactions, skin rash, and alopecia. Secondary cancers are also of concern with the use of the agent.

CYCLOPHOSPHAMIDE (CTX, CPM, CPA, CLAFEN, CYTOXAN, NEOSAR)

Cyclophosphamide is available in 25- and 50-mg tablets for oral administration and 100-, 200-, 500-, 1,000-, and 2,000-mg vials for IV use in the treatment of a wide variety of cancers, including breast cancer, non-Hodgkin's lymphoma, chronic lymphocytic leukemia, ovarian cancer, bone and soft tissue sarcoma, rhabdomyosarcoma, neuroblastoma, and Wilms tumor. Coadministration of mesna is recommended. The alkylating agent is cell cycle–nonspecific, and mechanisms of resistance are similar to those seen for other alkylating agents including decreased uptake and activation and increased inactivation by glutathione and oxidase enzymes (aldehyde dehydrogenase and alcohol dehydrogenase) as well as increased DNA repair mechanisms. The agent is well absorbed when given orally. Metabolism by CYP2B6 and 3A4/5 is required for activation of the agent, and metabolites are formed as a result of this activation by subsequent reactions that are shown in Scheme 10.5. The major metabolite seen in plasma is the phosphoramide mustard, although there is a small amount of material (10%) arising from the dechloroethylation, which is primarily mediated by 3A4/5. This metabolic pathway gives rise to a small amount of chloroacetaldehyde, which is both neurotoxic and nephrotoxic. The parent compound and metabolites are eliminated in the urine with an elimination half-life of 4 to 6 hours. Adverse effects include dose-limiting myelosuppression, which normally presents as leucopenia. Bladder toxicity, which presents as hemorrhagic cystitis, is related to the formation of electrophilic species in the kidney including acrolein and may be treated by administration of mesna and increased water intake. Additionally, amenorrhea may be seen and sterility may be permanent. Other effects include alopecia, cardiotoxicity, inappropriate secretion of antidiuretic hormone, and an increased risk of secondary cancers.

IFOSFAMIDE (IPHOSPHAMIDE, IFO, CYFOS, IFEX, IFOSFAMIDUM)

Ifosfamide is available in 1- and 3-g vials for IV administration as Food and Drug Administration (FDA)-approved third-line therapy in the treatment of testicular cancer. It has also been utilized (although not FDA approved) in the treatment of a wide variety of cancers including Hodgkin's and non-Hodgkin's lymphoma, soft tissue sarcoma, germ cell tumors, small cell lung cancer, non–small cell lung cancer (NSCLC), cancers of the head and neck, bladder cancer, cervical cancer, and Ewing sarcoma. Coadministration of mesna is recommended. The mechanisms of resistance are identical to those seen with cyclophosphamide. The drug is widely distributed with a low extent of protein binding (20%). Metabolism primarily by CYP3A4/5 and CYP2B6 is required for activation of the compound (Scheme 10.7). The agent is administered as the racemic mixture as a result of the presence of the chiral phosphorus atom, and differential metabolism of the *R*- and *S*-isomers has been observed. In contrast to cyclophosphamide, there is a greater amount of deactivation of the agent by *N*-dechloroethylation and subsequently more chloroacetaldehyde is produced, which may result in a greater amount of neurotoxicity and nephrotoxicity than seen with cyclophosphamide. The *N*-dechloroethylated metabolites are the predominate species seen in the plasma. The parent and metabolites are eliminated in the urine with an elimination half-life of 3 to 10 hours. The major components found in the urine are the dechlorethylated metabolites. Dose-limiting toxicities include myelosuppression and bladder toxicity. Other adverse effects include nausea, alopecia, amenorrhea, inappropriate secretion of antidiuretic hormone, as well as the production of secondary cancers. Neurotoxicity, which is associated with the production of chloroacetaldehyde presents as confusion, seizure, weakness, and hallucination, and coma may occur.

THIOTEPA (TRIETHYLENETHIOPHOSPHORAMIDE, GIROSTAN, STEPA, TESPA, THIOPLEX, TIFOSYL)

Thiotepa is available in 15-mg vials for IV administration in the treatment of bladder cancer, ovarian cancer, and breast cancer. It has been used in the past in the treatment of lymphomas such as Hodgkin's and non-Hodgkin's lymphoma but has now mostly been replaced by other agents. The agent is widely distributed after infusion, and 40% is bound to plasma proteins. Metabolism mediated by CYP2B1 and CYP2C11 effects desulfurization to give TEPA from which aziridine may arise. Metabolites have also been identified as arising from glutathione conjugation of thiotepa followed by formation of the mercapturic acid derivative. However, the excretion profile has only accounted for a small percentage (10%–22%) of the administered dose. The elimination half-life of the compound is 2 to 3 hours. Adverse effects include dose-limiting myelosuppression and mucositis. Additionally, nausea, vomiting, skin rash, hemorrhagic cystitis, and secondary cancers may occur.

BUSULFAN (BUSULFEX, MYLERAN)

Busulfan is available as 2-mg tablets for oral administration and 10-mL vials for IV administration in the treatment of chronic myelogenous leukemia (CML) and in high-dose therapy for refractory leukemia with bone marrow transplant. The agent is well absorbed when given orally, well distributed into tissues, and crosses the blood-brain barrier. Metabolism occurs in the liver as shown in Scheme 10.9 to give mainly methane sulfonic acid by the action of glutathione-*S*-transferase. Other identified metabolites in humans have included tetrahydrothiophene-1-oxide, sulfalene, and 3-hydroxysulfolane. The metabolites are excreted primarily in the urine, and the terminal elimination half-life is 2.5 hours. Adverse effects include dose-limiting myelosuppression; nausea and vomiting that occur commonly but are generally mild; and pulmonary symptoms including interstitial pulmonary fibrosis, which is referred to as "busulfan lung," occurs belatedly (1–10 years posttreatment) and although rare, it is severe. Other adverse effects include mucositis, skin rash, impotence, amenorrhea, infertility, hepatoxicity, insomnia, anxiety, and an increased risk of secondary malignancies. At normal doses, the agent is well tolerated except for the myelosuppression that occurs. This has allowed for high-dose therapy with the agent when accompanied by bone marrow transplant to counter the myelosuppressive effects.

CISPLATIN (CIS-DIAMINEDICHLOROPLATINUM, DDP, PLATINOL, PLATINOL-AQ)

Cisplatin is available in 10- and 50-mg vials for IV administration in the treatment of a wide variety of cancers including non-Hodgkin's lymphoma, bladder cancer, ovarian cancer, testicular cancer, and cancers of the head and neck. A liposomal form is also available as well as an injectable collagen matrix gel containing cisplatin. Compared with other platins, cisplatin is the most reactive and therefore the most effective in platinating DNA. After IV administration, the agent is widely distributed, highly protein bound (90%), and concentrates in the liver and kidney. After infusion, covalent attachment to plasma proteins occurs such that after 4 hours, 90% of drug is protein bound. The elimination of platinum from the blood is a slow process with a terminal elimination half-life of 5 to 10 days. Metabolism involves aquation, which occurs to a greater extent once distribution out of the plasma has occurred. Additional metabolites have been seen resulting from reaction with glutathione and cysteine. The greater reactivity of cisplatin gives rise to significant toxicities compared with other platins. These include dose-limiting nephrotoxicity, which normally presents as elevated blood urea nitrogen (BUN) and creatinine. This effect is cumulative upon repeated dosing and may progress further to necrosis, altered epithelial cells, cast formation, and thickening of the tubular basement membranes but is generally reversible upon discontinuation of drug treatment. Sodium thiosulfate may be given to reduce the nephrotoxicity. Neurotoxicity may also be dose limiting, normally presenting initially as numbness but may progress to seizure. Other adverse effects include myelosuppression, nausea, vomiting, alopecia, ototoxicity, ocular toxicity, azoospermia, impotence, myocardial infarction, thrombotic events, and inappropriate secretion of antidiuretic hormone.

CARBOPLATIN (CBDCA, PARAPLAT, PARAPLATIN)

Carboplatin is available in 50-, 150-, and 450-mg vials for IV administration in the treatment of ovarian cancer, bladder cancer, germ cell tumors, head and neck cancers, small cell lung cancer, and NSCLC. Activation of the agent occurs by aquation in a manner similar to that seen for cisplatin. The presence of the chelating 1,1-cyclobutane-dicarboxylate slows this reaction 100-fold and reduces the toxicity of the agent. The sites of alkylation and mechanisms of resistance are like those seen for cisplatin, and the two agents show cross-resistance. The agent is widely distributed upon IV administration but, because of its greater stability, it binds slowly to plasma proteins, requiring 24 hours to reach 90% bound drug compared with 4 hours for cisplatin. The agent is eliminated in the urine with a terminal elimination half-life of 2 to 6 hours. Adverse effects include myelosuppression, which is dose limiting. Other adverse effects include renal toxicity, nausea, vomiting, and peripheral neuropathy, but these occur much less frequently than with cisplatin.

OXALIPLATIN (DIAMINOCYCLOHEXANE PLATINUM, DACH-PLATINUM, ELOXATIN)

Oxaliplatin is available in 50- and 100-mg vials for IV administration in the treatment of ovarian cancer, metastatic colorectal cancer, and early stage colon cancer in combination with 5-fluorouracil/leucovorin. The activation of the agent occurs in low-chloride environments to give the aquated species, which subsequently reacts with DNA in a manner similar to cisplatin. The mechanisms of resistance are similar for the two agents; however, oxaliplatin is not recognized by MMR enzymes and does not show cross-resistance with cisplatin. The agent is widely distributed, highly protein bound (85%–88%), and irreversibly binds to erythrocytes. Numerous metabolites have been identified many of which are produced as a result of nonenzymatic processes and include chloro-, dichloro-, monoaquo-, and diaquo-species. The parent and metabolites are eliminated primarily in the urine with a long terminal elimination half-life of 240 hours. Neurotoxicity is dose limiting and normally presents as peripheral neuropathy, which may be exacerbated by exposure to low temperatures. The neurotoxicity is normally reversible in contrast to that seen with cisplatin, which may be irreversible. Other adverse effects include nausea, vomiting, diarrhea, myelosuppression, and hypersensitivity reactions. Ototoxicity and renal toxicity occur only rarely in contrast to cisplatin.

CARMUSTINE (BIS-CHLOROETHYL-NITROSOUREA, BCNU, BECENUM, CARMUBRIS, BICNU, GLIADEL)

Carmustine is available in a 100-mg vial for IV administration in the treatment of several types of brain tumors, Hodgkin's and non-Hodgkin's disease, and multiple myeloma. The agent is also available as an implantable wafer containing 7.7 mg of drug for intracavity implantation in the treatment of glioblastoma multiforme. Cytotoxicity is associated with cross-linking of DNA and RNA and carbamoylation of glutathione reductase. Cross-resistance is not seen with other alkylating agents. The agent is very lipid soluble and easily crosses the blood-brain barrier, achieving concentrations greater than 50% of those seen in plasma. Metabolism involves both the nonenzymatic formation of reactive intermediates that may react with glutathione and other thiol-containing proteins, as well as enzymatic reductive denitrosation and dechlorination. The half-life of the agent in plasma is short (15–20 minutes) because of rapid decomposition. Myelosuppression is dose limiting and may present as thrombocytopenia, leucopenia, or more rarely as anemia. This is generally seen 24 to 48 days after treatment. Pulmonary toxicity occurs rarely at low doses but at high doses such as those seen during bone marrow transplant may present as dyspnea, cough, pulmonary infiltrates, and progress to respiratory failure. This may be seen years after the completion of therapy. Other toxicities include nausea, vomiting, pain at the injection site, impotence, sterility, amenorrhea, and infertility. Hepatotoxicity may initially present as elevations in serum transaminase levels. There is also an increased risk of secondary cancers as is often seen with the alkylating agents.

LOMUSTINE (CHLOROETHYL-CYCLOHEXYL-NITROSOUREA, CCNU, CEENU)

Lomustine is available in 10-, 40-, and 100-mg capsules for oral administration in the treatment of primary and metastatic brain cancers and Hodgkin's lymphoma. This lipophilic agent is well absorbed, widely distributed, and crosses the blood-brain barrier. Lomustine undergoes extensive hepatic metabolism, which is mediated by CYP3A4 to give several hydroxylated metabolites, which arise as a result of oxidation of the cyclohexyl ring. Several of these are more active than the parent compound. Denitrosation and dechlorination have also been demonstrated to occur for lomustine as well. The intact drug was not found in plasma when the agent was administered orally. Elimination occurs primarily in the urine with an elimination half-life of 16 to 72 hours. Myelosuppression is dose limiting and presents in a manner similar to that seen with carmustine. Other toxicities include nausea, vomiting, anorexia, impotence, sterility, amenorrhea, and infertility. Pulmonary and renal toxicity are rarely seen during standard-dose therapy but increase during high-dose therapy.

STREPTOZOCIN (STREPTOZOTOCIN, STZ, ZANOSAR)

Streptozocin is available in 1-g vials for IV administration in the treatment of metastatic islet cell carcinoma of the pancreas, colon cancer, and Hodgkin's disease. Activation results in the formation of methyl carbonium ions, which alkylate DNA, but the agent is less effective in alkylating DNA and carbamylating proteins than other nitrosoureas, which is because in part of an intramolecular carbamoylation. The internal carbamate group migration occurs via the hydroxyl groups of the glucose portion of the molecule. There is a reduced effect on RNA function compared with other nitrosoureas as well. The hydrophilic agent is rapidly cleared from the plasma with an elimination half-life of 35 minutes. The presence of the glucose moiety allows for utilization of glucose transporters, which concentrate the compound in the β-cells of the pancreas. The metabolism of the agent has not been well characterized. Renal toxicity is dose limiting and may present initially as proteinuria and azotemia but may progress to renal failure. Nausea and vomiting may be severe with the agent, whereas myelosuppression is generally mild. Normal glucose metabolism may be altered so that hypoglycemia or hyperglycemia may be seen. In some animal species, streptozocin produces diabetes but much milder effects are seen in man.

PROCARBAZINE HYDROCHLORIDE (PCZ, PCB, MATULANE)

Procarbazine is available in 50-mg tablets for oral administration in the treatment of Hodgkin's (part of MOPP) and non-Hodgkin's disease, brain cancer, and mycosis fungoides. The major mechanisms of resistance appear to be enhanced activity of DNA-repair enzymes including enhanced *O*-6-alkylguanine DNA transferase (AGAT),

which removes the methyl group from the O-6 of guanine. The agent is rapidly and completely absorbed after oral administration and extensively metabolized in the liver to give azo-procarbazine followed by further oxidation to methyldiazine and the aldehyde. The parent drug and metabolites cross the blood-brain barrier. Elimination occurs in the urine mostly as metabolites with an elimination half-life of 1 hour. Myelosuppression is dose limiting, generally presenting as thrombocytopenia that may be followed by leucopenia. Glucose-6-phosphate dehydrogenase deficient patients may develop hemolytic anemia during procarbazine therapy. Other adverse effects include nausea, vomiting, hypersensitivity, flulike symptoms, amenorrhea, and azoospermia. Central nervous symptom effects may be seen, including lethargy, confusion, neuropathies, and seizure.

DACARBAZINE (DTIC, DTIC-DOME)

Dacarbazine is available in 100- and 200-mg vials for IV administration in the treatment of Hodgkin's disease, malignant melanoma, carcinoid cancer, neuroblastoma, and soft tissue sarcoma. Resistance to dacarbazine has been primarily attributed to enhanced activity of AGAT. The volume of distribution exceeds the amount of water in the body suggesting the compound distributes into body tissues possibly the liver. The agent is not highly protein bound (20%) and is metabolized in the liver by CYP to give MTIC and 4-amino-5-imidazole-carboxamide (AIC). The demethylation reaction is mediated by isozymes CYP1A1/2 and CYP2E1. Elimination occurs via the urine with 40% to 50% occurring as unchanged drug. Dose-limiting myelosuppression presents as both leucopenia and thrombocytopenia. Other adverse effects include nausea, vomiting, flulike symptoms, photosensitivity, and pain at the injection site.

ALTRETAMINE (HMM, HEXALEN, HEXAMETHYLMELAMINE)

Altretamine (Fig. 10.7) is available in 50-mg capsules for oral administration as a second-line treatment for ovarian cancer. The mechanism of action has not been firmly established, although the spectrum of activity is similar to that for other alkylating agents; however, cross-resistance is not seen. Cytotoxicity has been correlated with metabolism to give the carbinolamines, which may form imines capable of cross-linking, or decompose to give formaldehyde, which may react with nucleophiles on DNA or proteins. The agent is well absorbed upon oral administration, well distributed, and highly (90%) plasma protein bound. The agent is extensively metabolized in the liver by CYP to give demethylated metabolites

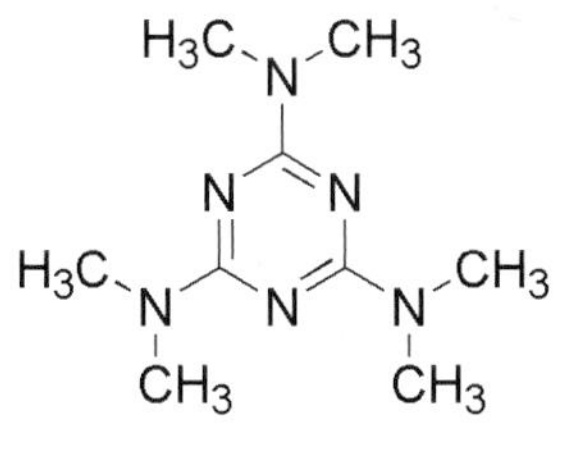

Altretamine

Figure 10.7 ● Chemical structure of altretamine.

via the previously mentioned carbinolamines. Elimination occurs primarily in the urine as mostly demethylated metabolites with a terminal elimination half-life of 4 to 10 hours. Myleosuppression and nausea/vomiting are dose-limiting toxicities. Other adverse effects include lethargy, agitation, hallucinations, skin rash, and elevations in transaminase levels, flulike symptoms, abdominal cramps, and diarrhea.

◉ ANTIMETABOLITES

Antimetabolites are compounds closely related in structure to a cellular precursor molecule, yet these imposter substances are capable of preventing the proper use or formation of the normal cellular product. These antimetabolites are similar enough in structure in many cases to interact with the normal cellular process but differ in a manner sufficient to alter the outcome of that pathway. Most antimetabolites are effective cancer chemotherapeutic agents via interaction with the biosynthesis of nucleic acids. Therefore, several of the useful drugs used in antimetabolite therapy are purines, pyrimidines, folates, and related compounds. The antimetabolite drugs may exert their effects by several individual mechanisms involving enzyme inhibition at active, allosteric, or related sites. Most of these targeted enzymes and processes are involved in the regulatory steps of cell division and cell/tissue growth. Often the administered drug is actually a prodrug form of an antimetabolite and requires activation in vivo to yield the active inhibitor. The administration of many purine and pyrimidine antimetabolites requires the formation of the nucleoside and finally the corresponding nucleotide for antimetabolite activity. An antimetabolite and its transformation products may inhibit several different enzymes involved in tissue growth. These substances are generally cell cycle specific with activity in the S phase.

The purine and pyrimidine antimetabolites are often compounds incorporated into nucleic acids and the nucleic acid polymers (DNA, RNA, etc.). The antifolates are compounds designed to interact at cofactor sites for enzymes involved in the biosynthesis of nucleic acid bases. The biosynthesis of these nucleic acid bases depend heavily on the availability of folate cofactors, hence antimetabolites of the folates find utility as antineoplastic agents. The antitumor effects of all these compounds attempting to masquerade as the natural precursor compound may occur because of a malfunction in the biosynthesis of the corresponding macromolecules. Classic examples of pyrimidine and purine antimetabolites are 5-fluorouracil and 6-mercaptopurine, respectively, and the classic antifolate is methotrexate.

The purine analog 6-mercaptopurine and its bioactivation products interact with many enzymes in the various stages of cell division.[52] The activity of 6-mercaptopurine requires bioactivation to its ribonucleotide, 6-thioinosinate, by the enzyme hypoxanthine-guanine phosphoribosyl transferase (HGPRT). 6-Thioinosinate is a potent inhibitor of the conversion of 5-phosphoribosylpyrophosphate into 5-phosphoribosylamine. The ribose diphosphate and triphosphates of 6-mercaptopurine are active enzyme inhibitors, and the triphosphate can be incorporated into DNA and RNA to inhibit chain elongation.

The pyrimidine analog 5-fluorouracil was designed based on the observation that in certain tumors, uracil was used for nucleic acid pyrimidine biosynthesis.[53] Fluorine, at the 5-position of uracil, blocks the conversion of uridylate to thymidylate, thus diminishing DNA biosynthesis. The fluorine induced increase in acidity (inductive effect) was expected to cause the molecule to bind more strongly to enzymes of the various stages of pyrimidine biosynthesis. Thymidine is a logical target, because it is only found in DNA and not in RNA. 5-Fluorouracil is activated by anabolism to 5-fluoro-2-deoxyuridylic acid, and this activated species is a strong inhibitor of thymidylate synthetase, the enzyme that converts 2′-deoxyuridylic acid to thymidylic acid.

Methotrexate inhibits the binding of the substrate folic acid to the enzyme dihydrofolate reductase (DHFR), resulting in reductions in the synthesis of nucleic acid bases, perhaps most importantly, the conversion of uridylate to thymidylate as catalyzed by thymidylate synthetase, which requires folate cofactors.

The pathways for the normal biosynthesis of the pyrimidine and purine bases are summarized in Schemes 10.15 and 10.16, respectively. The biosynthesis of pyrimidine and purine monomers is a central component for DNA and RNA formation in mammalian cells. The process of cell division and tissue growth is a very complex set of biochemical events with many feedback controls. Thus, antimetabolite drugs based on pyrimidine, purine, and related structures may exert their effects by altering many metabolic processes and pathways. The final step in Figure 10.15 illustrates the conversion of ribonucleotides to deoxyribonucleotides catalyzed by ribonucleotide reductase. The substrate for this enzyme is the ribonucleotide diphosphate, and the process is the same for both purine and pyrimidine bases.

Pyrimidine Drugs

The anticancer drugs based on pyrimidine structure are shown in Figure 10.8. The pyrimidine derivative 5-fluorouracil (5-FU) was designed to block the conversion of uridine to thymidine. The normal biosynthesis of thymidine involves methylation of the 5-position of the pyrimidine ring of uridine. The replacement of the hydrogen at the 5-position of uracil with a fluorine results in an antimetabolite drug, leading to the formation of a stable covalent ternary complex composed of 5-FU, thymidylate synthase (TS), and cofactor (a tetrahydrofolate species). The normal pathway for the formation of thymidine from uridine catalyzed by the enzyme TS is shown in Scheme 10.17. Anticancer drugs targeting this enzyme should selectively inhibit the formation of DNA because thymidine is not a normal component of RNA.

TS is responsible for the reductive methylation of deoxyuridine monophosphate (dUMP) by 5,10-methylenetetrahydrofolate to yield dTMP and dihydrofolate.[54] Because thymine is unique to DNA, the TS enzyme system plays an important role in replication and cell division. The tetrahydrofolate cofactor species serves as both the one-carbon donor and the hydride source in this system. The initial step of the process involves the nucleophilic attack by a sulfhydryl group of a cystine residue at the 6-position of dUMP. The resulting enolate adds to the methylene of 5,10-CH_2-THF perhaps activated via the very reactive N-5-iminium ion (see Scheme 10.17). The iminium ion likely forms at N-5 and only after 5,10-CH_2-THF binds to TS.[54]

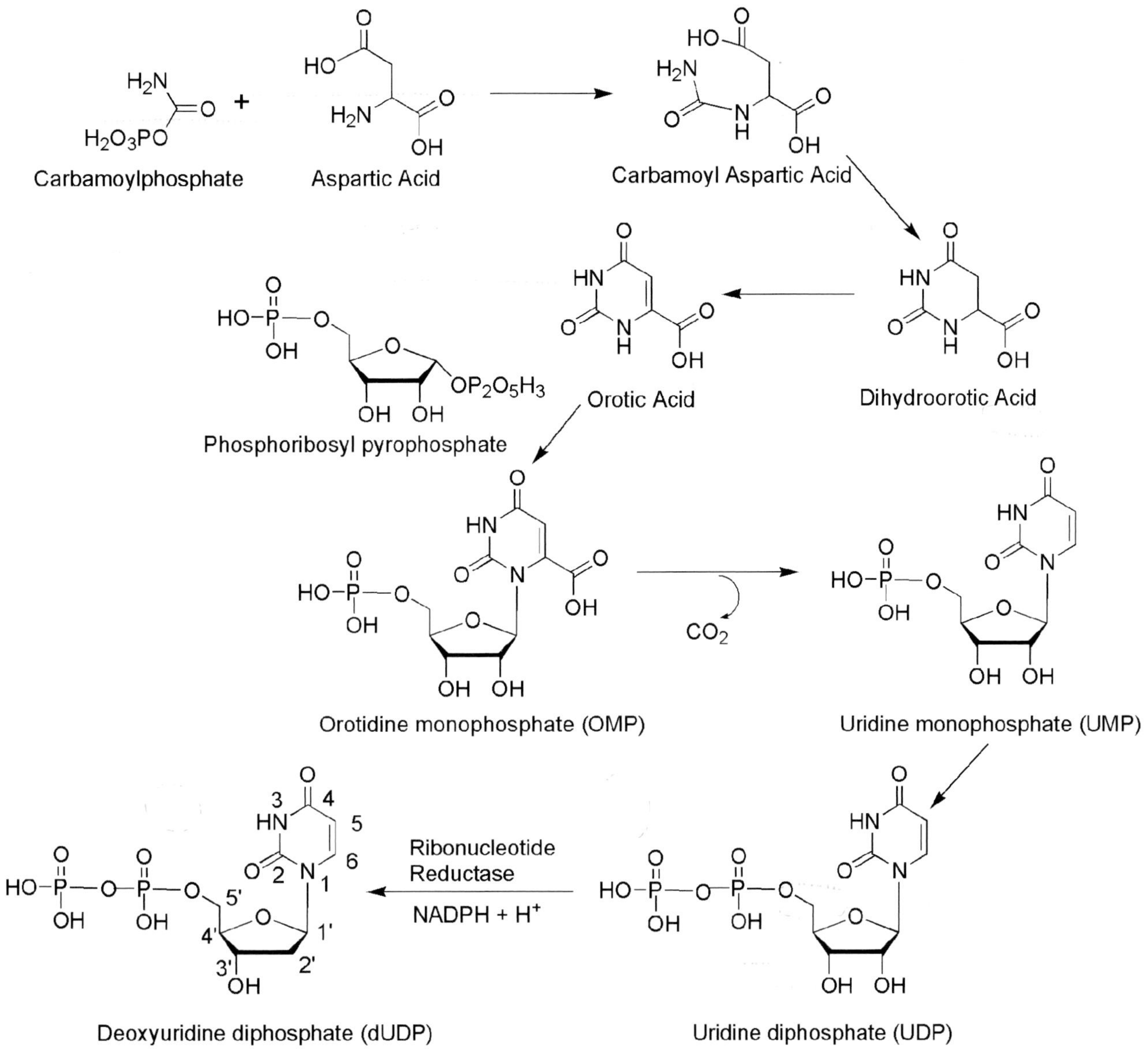

Scheme 10.15 ● Biosynthetic pathway for pyrimidine nucleotides.

The iminium ion is likely formed at N-5 because it is the more basic of the two nitrogens, whereas N-10 is the better leaving group. The loss of the proton at the 5-position of dUMP and elimination of folate yields the exocyclic methylene uracil species. The final step involves hydride transfer from THF and elimination to yield the enzyme, DHF, and dTMP.

5-Fluorouracil is activated by conversion to the corresponding nucleotide species,[53] 5-fluoro-2-deoxyuridylic acid (see Scheme 10.18). The resulting 5-fluoro-2′-deoxyuridylic acid is a powerful inhibitor of thymidylate synthetase, the enzyme that converts 2′-deoxyuridylic acid to thymidylic acid. In the inhibiting reaction, the sulfhydryl group of TS adds via conjugate addition to the 6-position of the fluorouracil moiety (Scheme 10.19). The carbon at the 5-position then binds to the methylene group of 5,10-methylenetetrahydrofolate following initial formation of the more electrophilic form of folate the N-5-iminium ion. In the normal process, this step is followed by the elimination of dihydrofolate from the ternary complex, regeneration of

the active enzyme species, and the product thymidine. Central to this process is the loss of the proton at the 5-position of uracil to form the exocyclic methylene uracil species. The 5-fluorine is stable to elimination, and a terminal product results, involving the enzyme, cofactor, and substrate, all covalently bonded (Scheme 10.19).

The chemical mechanism of inhibition of thymidylate synthetase by 5-fluorouracil is shown in Scheme 10.19. This process clearly shows that in order to inactivate the TS enzyme, both 5-FU and the tetrahydrofolate species are required to form the ternary complex. Some clinical studies have shown that administration of a tetrahydrofolate source prior to treatment with 5-FU results in greater inhibition of total TS activity. The administered source of active 5,10-methylenetetrahydrofolate is leucovorin, *N*-5-formyl-tetrahydrofolate.

TS is the most obvious and well-documented mechanism of action for 5-FU cytotoxic activity. However, other mechanisms may play a role in the overall value of this drug in the treatment of human cancer. The triphosphate of 5-FU

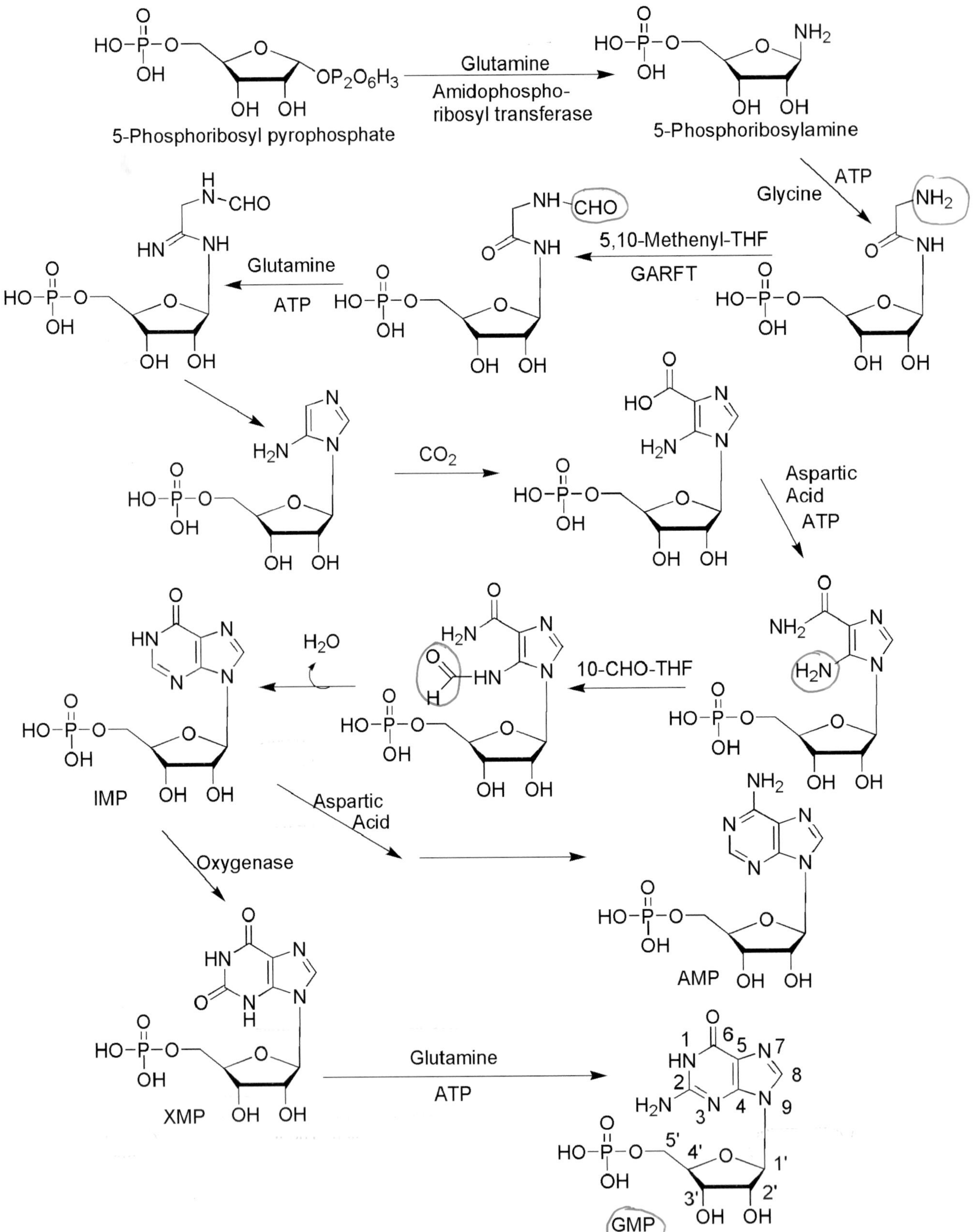

Scheme 10.16 ● Biosynthetic pathway for purine nucleotides. (THF, tetrahydrofolate.)

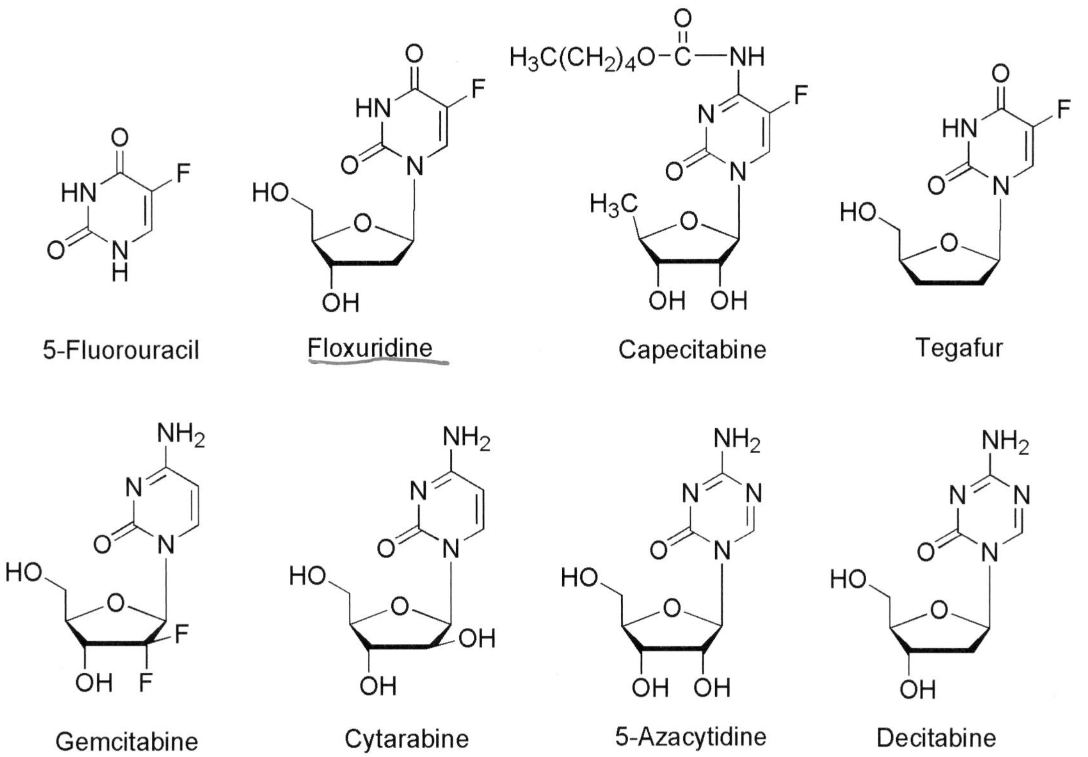

Figure 10.8 ● Anticancer drugs based on pyrimidine and related compounds.

nucleotide is a substrate for RNA polymerases, and 5-FU is incorporated into the RNA of some cell lines. The incorporation of 5-FU into DNA via DNA polymerase occurs in some tissue lines even though uracil is not a common component of human DNA. The 5-FU in DNA likely serves as substrate for the editing and repair enzymes involved in DNA processing for cell division and tissue growth. The actual addition of 5-FU into RNA and/or DNA may not be the direct cytotoxic event, but the incorporation may lead to less efficient utilization of cellular resources. The significance of these various mechanisms on the overall cytotoxic effects of 5-FU may vary with cell line and tissue.

The metabolic activation (anabolism) of 5-FU required to produce the anticancer effects accounts for no more than 20% of the administered amount of drug in most patients. Catabolic inactivation via the normal pathways for uracil consumes the remaining approximate 80% of the dose. The major enzyme of pyrimidine catabolism is dihydropyrimidine dehydrogenase (DPD), and 5-FU is a substrate for this enzyme.[55] The DPD catabolism of 5-FU is shown in Scheme 10.20. The formation of dihydro-5-FU (5-FU-H$_2$) occurs very rapidly and accounts for the majority of the total 5-FU dose in most patients. Thus, α-fluoro-β-alanine is the major human metabolite of 5-FU.[56] Uracil is a substrate for this enzyme system also and has been dosed with 5-FU and 5-FU prodrugs in an attempt to saturate DPD and conserve active drug species. Variability in the levels of DPD activity among the patient population is a major factor in the bioavailability of 5-FU. Inhibitors of DPD such as uracil or 5-chloro-2,4-dihydroxypyridine (CDHP)[53] increase the plasma concentration–time curve of 5-FU by preventing 5-FU catabolism. One mechanism of drug resistance in 5-FU–treated patients may be caused by increased levels of DPD in the target tissue. The observed low bioavailability of 5-FU as a result of the catabolic efficiency of DPD and other enzymes has lead to the development of unique dosing routes and schedules as well as the development of prodrug forms of 5-FU.[53]

Attempts at chemical modification of 5-FU to protect from catabolic events have produced several prodrug forms, which are converted via in vivo metabolic and/or chemical transformation to the parent drug 5-FU.[57] Figure 10.8 shows the structure of the more common prodrug forms of 5-FU. The carbamate derivative of 5′-deoxy-5-fluorocytidine is known as *capecitabine*, and it is converted to 5-FU through a series of activation steps. The activation sequence is shown in Scheme 10.21. The initial step is carbamate hydrolysis followed by deamination, then hydrolysis of the sugar moiety to yield 5-FU. Some of these activation steps take place at a higher rate in tumor tissue leading to selective accumulation in those cells.[53] The last step in the sequence shown in Scheme 10.21 is catalyzed by phosphorolases, and these enzymes occur in higher levels in colorectal tumors. Despite this complex activation process, capecitabine still exhibits some of the significant toxicities of 5-fluorouracil. The tetrahydrofuran derivative tegafur is slowly converted to 5-FU but requires quite high doses to reach therapeutic plasma concentrations. Esters of the *N*-hydroxymethyl derivative of tegafur show greater anticancer activity than tegafur.[58]

Pyrimidine analogs as antimetabolites for cancer therapy have been developed based on the cytosine structure as well. Modification of the normal ribose or deoxyribose moiety has produced useful drug species such as cytarabine (ara-C) and gemcitabine, see Figure 10.8. Cytosine arabinoside (ara-C or cytarabine) is simply the arabinose sugar instead

(text continues on page 378)

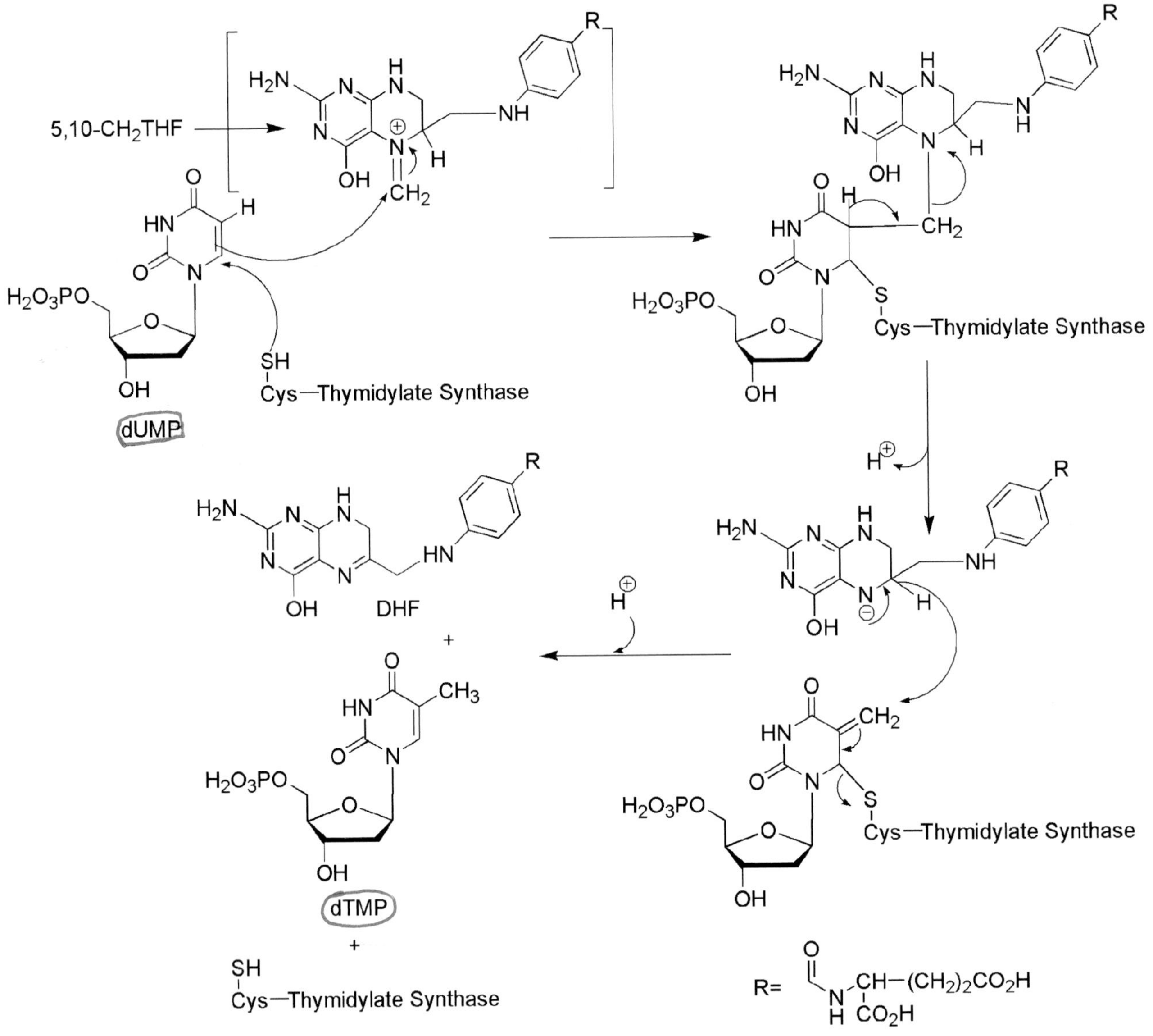

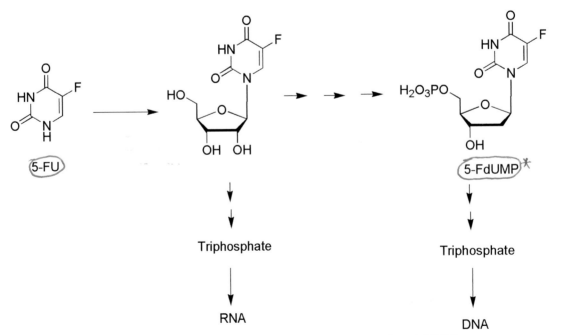

Scheme 10.17 ● Biochemical conversion of uridine to thymidine.

Scheme 10.18 ● Metabolic activation of 5-fluorouracil to 5-FdUMP.

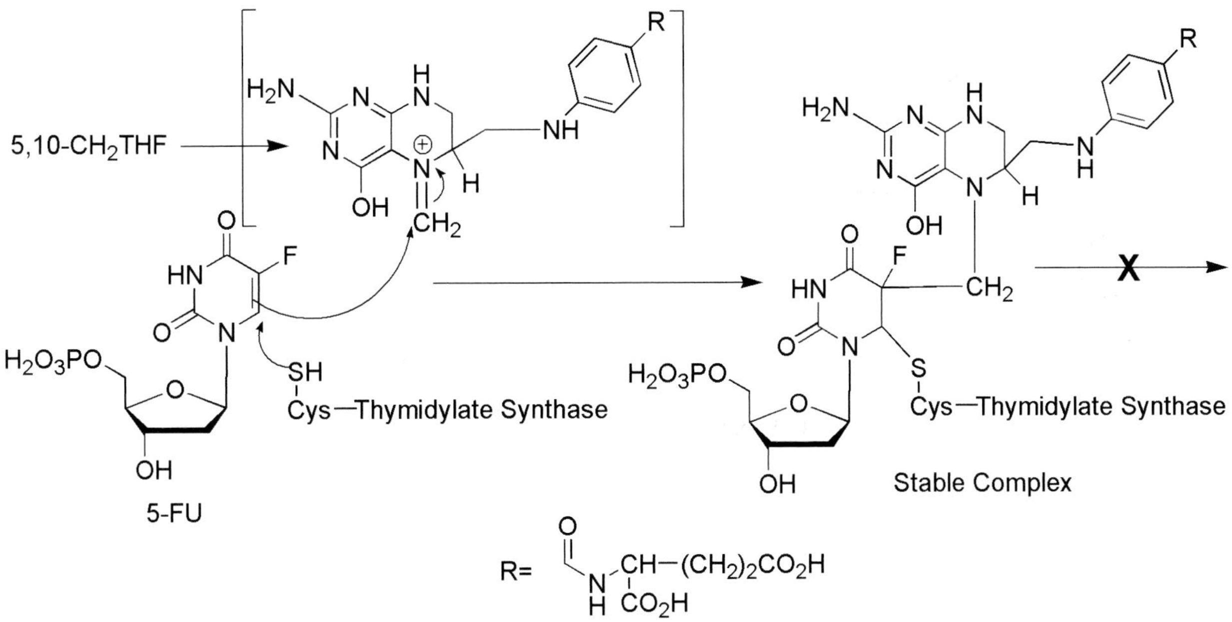

Scheme 10.19 ● Mechanism of inhibition of TS by 5-fluorouracil.

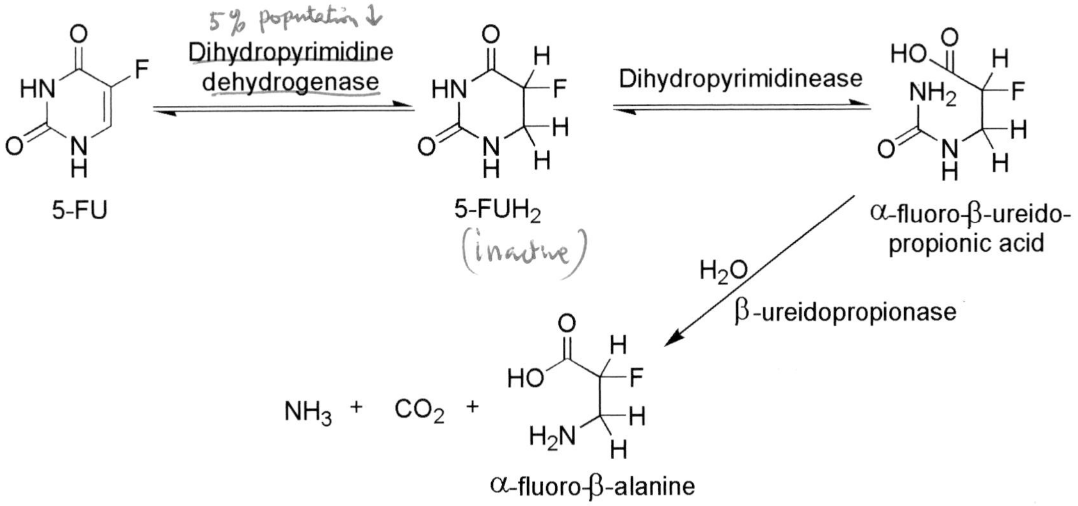

Scheme 10.20 ● Catabolic inactivation of 5-FU by dihydropyrimidine dehydrogenase.

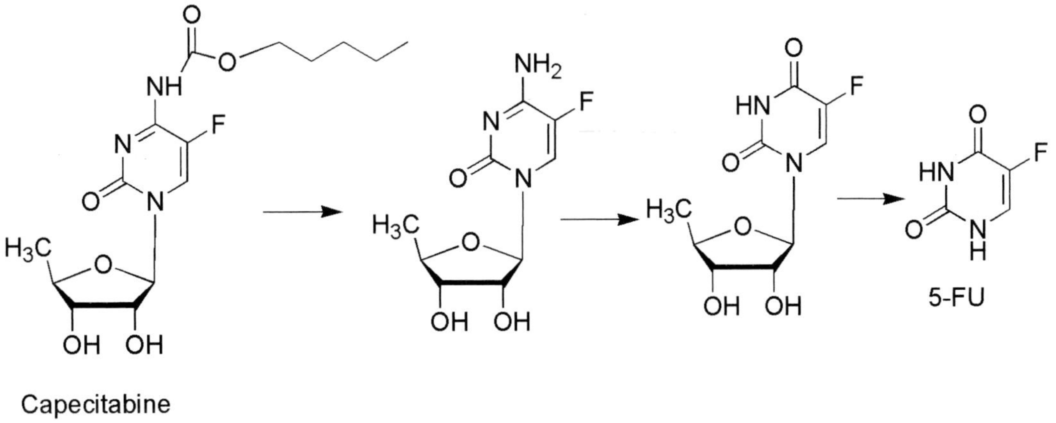

Scheme 10.21 ● Metabolic activation of capecitabine to 5-FU.

of ribose, and the only difference in structure is the epimeric hydroxyl group at the 2'-position of the pentose sugar. This epimeric sugar is similar enough to the natural ribose to allow ara-C to be incorporated into DNA, and its mechanism of action may include a slowing of the DNA chain elongation reaction via DNA polymerase or cellular inefficiencies in DNA processing or repair after incorporation.

Gemcitabine[59] is the result of fluorination of the 2'-position of the sugar moiety. Gemcitabine is the 2',2'-difluoro deoxycytidine species and after its anabolism to diphosphate and triphosphate metabolites, it inhibits ribonucleotide reductase and competes with 2'-deoxycytidine triphosphate for incorporation into DNA. The mechanism of action for gemcitabine is likely similar to that of ara-C including alteration of the rate of incorporation into DNA as well as the rate of DNA processing and repair.

Modification of the pyrimidine ring has also been explored for the development of potential anticancer drugs based on antimetabolite theory. Several pyrimidine nucleoside analogs have one more or one less nitrogen in the heterocyclic ring. They are known as *azapyrimidine* or *deazapyrimidine nucleosides*. 5-Azacytidine is an example of a drug in this category (see Fig. 10.8). This compound was developed via organic synthesis and later found as a natural product of fungal metabolism. The mode of action of this compound is complex involving reversible inhibition of DNA methyltransferase, and this lack of methylated DNA activates tumor suppressor genes. In certain tumor systems, it is incorporated into nucleic acids, which may result in misreading or processing errors.

Purine Drugs

The anticancer drugs based on purine structure are shown in Figure 10.9. The design of antimetabolites based on purine structure began with isosteric thiol/sulfhydryl group to replace the 6-hydroxyl group of hypoxanthine and guanine. One of the early successes was 6-mercaptopurine (6-MP), the thiol analog of hypoxanthine.[60] This purine requires bioactivation to its ribonucleotide, 6-thioinosinate (6-MPMP), by the enzyme HGPRT. The resulting nucleotide (Scheme 10.22) is a potent inhibitor of an early step in basic purine biosynthesis, the conversion of 5-phosphoribosylpyrophosphate into 5-phosphoribosylamine (see Scheme 10.16). The ribose diphosphate and triphosphates of 6-mercaptopurine are active enzyme inhibitors, and the triphosphate can be incorporated into DNA and RNA to inhibit chain elongation.[61] However, the major antineoplastic action of 6-MP appears to be related to the inhibition of purine biosynthesis.

Thioguanine (6-TG) is the 6-mercapto analog of guanine, analogous to 6-MP. Thioguanine is converted into its ribonucleotide by the same enzyme that acts on 6-mercaptopurine. It is converted further into the diphosphates and triphosphates. These species inhibit most of the same enzymes that are inhibited by 6-mercaptopurine.[62] Thioguanine is also incorporated into RNA, and its 2'-deoxy metabolite is incorporated into DNA. The incorporation into RNA and DNA and the subsequent disruption of these polymers may account for a greater portion of the antineoplastic activity of thioguanine compared with 6-MP.[63]

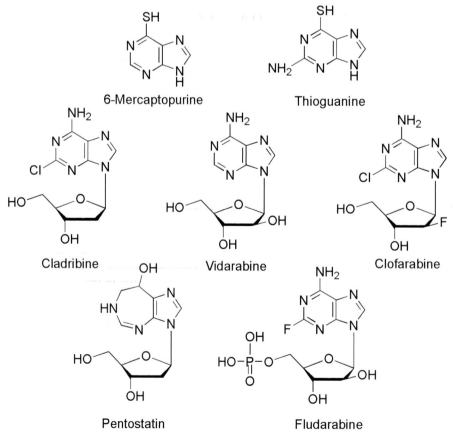

Figure 10.9 ● Anticancer drugs based on purines and related compounds.

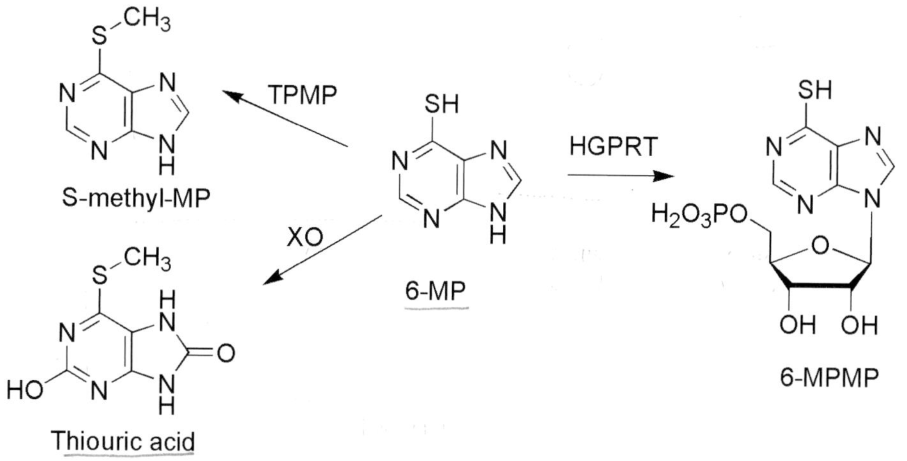

Scheme 10.22 ● Conversion of 6-MP to active 6-thioinosine-5-monophosphate (6-MPMP) by HPGRT and inactivation by xanthine oxidase and thiopurine methyl transferase.

The antineoplastic activity of these purines as well as most antimetabolites depends on the relative rates of enzymatic activation and inactivation of these compounds in various tissues and cells. Drug resistance in certain cell lines may be caused by lower activity of activating enzymes or higher activity of catabolic enzymes.[64] For the classic purine antimetabolites 6-MP major pathways of inactivation (see Scheme 10.22) include *S*-methylation via thiopurine-*S*-methyl-transferase (TPMT) and oxidation by the enzyme xanthine oxidase (XO).[62] Xanthine oxidase converts the drugs to the inactive thiouric acid, and inhibition of the enzymes responsible for the catabolic breakdown of the purine drugs can potentiate the drug's antineoplastic activity. Allopurinol is a potent inhibitor of xanthine oxidase and is often used as an adjuvant in purine anticancer drug therapy. Allopurinol increases both the potency and the toxicity of 6-mercaptopurine. Its main importance is that it prevents the uric acid kidney toxicity caused by the release of purines from destroyed cancer cells.

Heterocyclic derivatives of 6-mercaptopurine, such as azathioprine, were designed to protect it from catabolic reactions. Although azathioprine has antitumor activity, it is not significantly better than 6-mercaptopurine. It has an important role, however, as an immunosuppressive agent in organ transplants. Adenine arabinoside (Vidarabine) contains the sugar, D-arabinose, which is epimeric with D-ribose at the 2′-position. This structural change makes it a competitive inhibitor of DNA polymerase, and this activity accounts for its antineoplastic activity as well as its antiviral action. Adenine arabinoside and some of its derivatives are limited in their antitumor effect by susceptibility to adenosine deaminase. This enzyme converts them into the inactive hypoxanthine arabinoside derivatives. High levels of adenosine deaminase accounts for resistance of certain tumors to the action of adenine arabinoside.

The addition of fluorine to the sugar moiety has produced some purine-based drugs with resistance to the catabolic activity of adenosine deaminase. In contrast to the susceptibility of adenosine arabinoside to adenosine deaminase, its 2-fluoro derivative, fludarabine, is stable to this enzyme. The antineoplastic activity of fludarabine depends on its anabolic conversion to the corresponding triphosphate. 2-Chloro-2′-deoxyadenosine (cladribine) also is resistant to adenosine deaminase. It is phosphorylated in cells to the

triphosphate by cytidine kinase, and the triphosphate inhibits enzymes required for DNA repair.

Folates

Folic acid and the structures of the major antifolate anticancer drugs are shown in Figure 10.10. Methotrexate is the classic antimetabolite of folic acid structurally derived by *N*-methylation of the para-aminobenzoic acid residue (PABA) and replacement of a pteridine hydroxyl by the bioisosteric amino group. The conversion of —OH to —NH$_2$ increases the basicity of N-3 and yields greater enzyme affinity. This drug competitively inhibits the binding of the substrate folic acid to the enzyme DHFR, resulting in reductions in the synthesis of nucleic acid bases, perhaps most importantly, the conversion of uridylate to thymidylate as catalyzed by thymidylate synthetase.[65] In addition, purine synthesis is inhibited because the *N*-10-formyl tetrahydrofolic acid is a formyl donor involved in purine synthesis. The interconversion of the various folate species is shown in Scheme 10.23. Recall that in Scheme 10.16, THFs are cofactors in at least two key steps in the normal biosynthesis of purines.

Methotrexate[66] is a broad-spectrum antineoplastic agent commonly used in the treatment of acute lymphoblastic and myeloblastic leukemia and other lymphomas and sarcomas. The major side effects seen are bone marrow suppression, pulmonary fibrosis, and GI ulceration. Leucovorin is often given 6 to 24 hours after methotrexate to prevent the long-term effects on normal cells by preventing the inhibition of DNA synthesis. Related to this is Pemetrexed, but its scope is greater in that it not only inhibits DHFR but also TS and glycinamide ribonucleotide formyltransferase (GARFT), which is involved in purine biosynthesis (see Fig. 10.16). The material is taken into tumor cells by the reduced folate-carrier systems and subsequently converted to the polyglutamate, which is retained in the cell.

Products

5-FLUOROURACIL (5-FU, EFUDEX, ADRUCIL, FLUOROPLEX)

The drug is available in a 500-mg or 10-mL vial for IV use and as a 1% and 5% topical cream. 5-FU is used in the treatment of several carcinoma types including breast cancer,

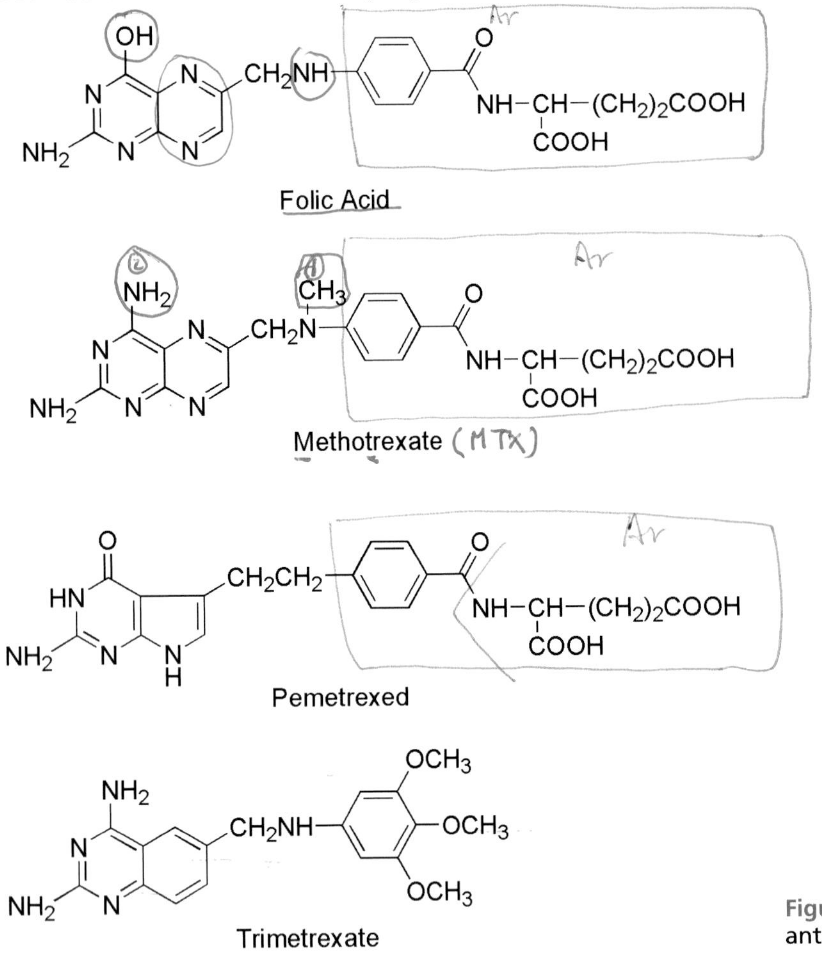

Figure 10.10 ● Structures of folic acid and antifolate anticancer drugs.

colorectal cancer, stomach cancer, pancreatic cancer, and topical use in basal cell cancer of the skin. The mechanism of action includes inhibition of the enzyme TS by the deoxyribose monophosphate metabolite, 5-FdUMP. The triphosphate metabolite is incorporated into DNA and the ribose triphosphate into RNA. These incorporations into growing chains result in inhibition of synthesis and function of DNA and RNA. Resistance can occur as a result of increased expression of TS, decreased levels of reduced folate substrate 5,10-methylenetetrahydrofolate, or increased levels of dihydropyrimidine dehydrogenase. Dihydropyrimidine dehydrogenase is the main enzyme responsible for 5-FU catabolism.

Bioavailability following oral absorption is erratic. Administration of 5-FU by IV yields high drug concentrations in bone marrow and liver. The drug does distribute into the central nervous system (CNS). Significant drug interactions include enhanced toxicity and antitumor activity of 5-FU following pretreatment with leucovorin. Toxicities include dose-limiting myelosuppression, mucositis, diarrhea, and hand–foot syndrome (numbness, pain, erythema, dryness, rash, swelling, increased pigmentation, nail changes, pruritus of the hands and feet).

CAPECITABINE (XELODA)

The drug is available in a 150- and 500-mg tablets for oral use. This drug is a fluoropyrimidine carbamate prodrug form of 5-fluorouracil (5-FU). It is used to treat breast cancer and colorectal cancer. The drug is converted to 5-FU by the enzyme thymidine phosphorylase following esterase ac-

tivity to hydrolyze the carbamate moiety and deamination. Capecitabine is readily absorbed by the GI tract, and peak plasma levels of 5-FU occur about 2 hours after oral administration. Indications, drug interactions, and toxicities are equivalent to those of 5-FU.

CYTARABINE (CYTOSINE ARABINOSIDE, ARA-C, CYTOSAR-U, TARABINE)

The drug is available in 100-, 500-, 1,000-, and 2,000-mg multidose vials for IV use. Cytarabine is used in the treatment of acute myelogenous leukemia and CML. This drug is a deoxycytidine analog originally isolated from the sponge *Cryptothethya crypta*. It is active following intracellular activation to the nucleotide metabolite ara-CTP. The resulting ara-CTP is incorporated into DNA resulting in chain termination and inhibition of DNA synthesis and function. Resistance can occur because of decreased activation or transport and increased catabolic breakdown. Metabolic breakdown within the GI tract leads to poor bioavailability. The drug distributes rapidly into tissues and total body water with cerebrospinal fluid (CSF) levels reaching 20% to 40% of those in plasma. Cytidine deaminase is the primary catabolic enzyme involved in the inactivation of cytarabine. Drug interactions include antagonism of the effects of gentamicin, decreasing the oral bioavailability of digoxin, as well as enhancing the cytotoxicity of various alkylating agents, cisplatin, and ionizing radiation. Pretreatment with methotrexate enhances the formation of ara-CTP metabolites resulting in enhanced cytotoxicity.

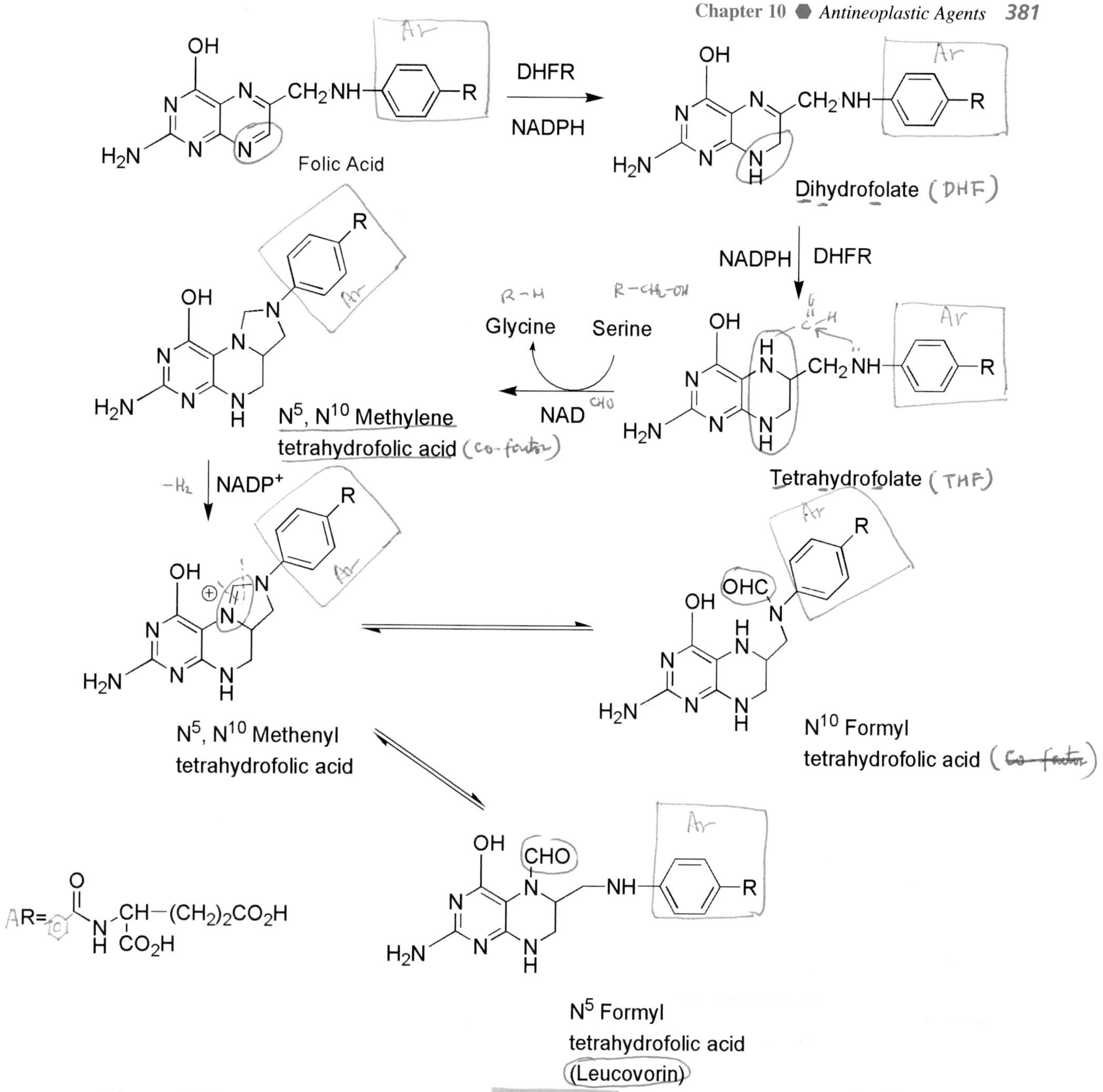

Scheme 10.23 ● Interconversion of various folate species. (DHFR, dihydrofolate reductase.)

Toxicities include myelosuppression, leukopenia and thrombocytopenia, nausea and vomiting anorexia, diarrhea, and mucositis. Neurotoxicity is usually expressed as ataxia, lethargy, and confusion. An allergic reaction often described in pediatric patients includes fever, myalgia, malaise, bone pain, skin rash, conjunctivitis, and chest pain.

FLOXURIDINE (FLUORODEOXYURIDINE, FUDR)

The drug is available as a 500-mg vial of lyophilized powder. The drug is used to treat metastatic GI adenocarcinoma. The mechanism of action of this fluoropyrimidine deoxynucleoside analog involves metabolic conversion to 5-fluorouracil (5-FU) metabolites resulting in inhibition of TS thus disrupting DNA synthesis, function, and repair. Resistance can occur because of increased expression of TS,

decreased levels of reduced folate 5,10-methylenetetrahydrofolate, increased activity of DNA repair enzymes, and increased expression of dihydropyrimidine dehydrogenase (the major catabolic enzyme). The drug is poorly absorbed from the GI tract and is extensive metabolized to 5-FU and 5-FU metabolites. Dihydropyrimidine dehydrogenase is the main enzyme responsible for 5-FU catabolism, and it is present in liver, GI mucosa, white blood cells, and kidney. The drug interaction and toxicity profiles are equivalent to those of 5-FU.

GEMCITABINE (DFDC, GEMZAR)

The drug is available as the hydrochloride salt in 200- and 1,000-mg lyophilized single-dose vials for IV use. Gemcitabine is used to treat bladder cancer, breast cancer, pancreatic cancer, and NSCLC. Gemcitabine is a potent radiosensitizer, and it increases the cytotoxicity of cisplatin. The mechanism of action of this fluorine-substituted deoxycytidine analog involves inhibition of DNA synthesis and function via DNA chain termination. The triphosphate metabolite is incorporated into DNA inhibiting several DNA polymerases and incorporated into RNA inhibiting proper function of mRNA. Resistance can occur because of decreased expression of the activation enzyme deoxycytidine kinase or decreased drug transport as well as increased expression of catabolic enzymes. Drug oral bioavailability is low because of deamination within the GI tract, and the drug does not cross the blood-brain barrier. Metabolism by deamination to 2′, 2′-difluorouridine (dFdU) is extensive. Drug toxicity includes myelosuppression, fever, malaise, chills, headache, myalgias, nausea, and vomiting.

CLADRIBINE (2-CHLORODEOXYADENOSINE, 2-CDA, LEUSTATIN)

The drug is available in a 10-mg or 10-mL single-use vial for IV use. Cladribine is used for chronic lymphocytic leukemia, hairy cell leukemia, and non-Hodgkin's lymphoma. The mechanism of action of this purine deoxyadenosine analog involves incorporation into DNA resulting in inhibition of DNA chain extension and inhibition of DNA synthesis and function. This incorporation into DNA occurs via the triphosphate metabolite active species. The 2-chloro group on the adenine ring produces resistance to breakdown by adenosine deaminase. Resistance to the anticancer effects can occur because of decreased expression of the activating enzyme or overexpression of the catabolic enzymes. Oral bioavailability is variable and averages about 50%. The drug crosses the blood-brain barrier; however, CSF concentrations reach only 25% of those in plasma. The drug is selectively activated inside the cell, and intracellular concentrations of phosphorylated metabolites exceed those in plasma. Toxicities include myelosuppression, neutropenia, immunosuppression, fever, nausea, and vomiting.

FLUDARABINE (2-F-ARA-AMP, FLUDARA)

The drug is available as the phosphate salt in a 50-mg vial for IV use. Fludarabine is used to treat chronic lymphocytic leukemia and non-Hodgkin's lymphoma. The mechanism of action involves the triphosphate metabolite and its inhibition of DNA chain elongation. The 2-fluoro group on the adenine ring renders fludarabine resistant to breakdown by adenosine deaminase. The drug is rapidly dephosphorylated to 2-fluoro-ara-adenosine (F-ara-A) after administration. F-ara-A is taken into the cell and subsequently re-phosphorylated to yield the triphosphate (F-ara-ATP), the active drug species. Resistance can occur via decreased expression of the activating enzymes and decreased drug transport. Fludarabine is orally bioavailable and is distributed throughout the body reaching high levels in liver, kidney, and spleen. The drug is metabolized to F-ara-A, which enters cells via the nucleoside transport system and is rephosphorylated by deoxycytidine kinase to fludarabine monophosphate and finally fludarabine triphosphate, the active species. About 25% of F-ara-A is excreted unchanged in urine. Drug interactions include an increased incidence of fatal pulmonary toxicity when fludarabine is used in combination with pentostatin. Additionally, fludarabine may potentiate the effects of several other anticancer drugs including cytarabine, cyclophosphamide, and cisplatin. Toxicities include myelosuppression, immunosuppression, fever, nausea, and vomiting.

MERCAPTOPURINE (6-MP, MERCAPTOPURINUM, PURINETHOL)

The drug is available as a 50-mg tablet for oral use. The primary uses of mercaptopurine are in the treatment of lymphoblastic leukemia, acute lymphocytic leukemia, and Crohn disease. The mechanism of action includes incorporation of mercaptopurine into DNA and RNA via the triphosphate metabolite. This incorporation inhibits synthesis and function of the resulting modified DNA or RNA. The parent drug is inactive and requires phosphorylation for activity. Resistance can occur via decreased expression of the activating enzymes or increased expression of the major catabolic enzymes. Oral absorption is generally incomplete (about 50%) and the drug does not enter the CNS in therapeutic quantities. Mercaptopurine is metabolized by methylation, and the methylated product has anticancer activity. Oxidation by xanthine oxidase yields inactive metabolites. The concurrent use of xanthine oxidase inhibitors such as allopurinol can enhance the potency of mercaptopurine by inhibiting its catabolic breakdown. The toxicities for mercaptopurine include myelosuppression, immunosuppression, nausea, vomiting, diarrhea, dry skin, urticaria, and photosensitivity.

THIOGUANINE (6-THIOGUANINE, 6-TG, TABLOID)

The drug is available in 40-mg tablets for oral use. Thioguanine is used to treat acute nonlymphocytic leukemia. The mechanism of action involves incorporation of the triphosphate into DNA and RNA, resulting in inhibition of processing and function. Intracellular phosphorylation is required for activity and inhibition of purine biosynthesis. Resistance can include decreased expression of the activating enzyme, decreased drug transport, and/or increased expression of catabolic enzymes. The oral absorption of thioguanine is poor, and the drug does not appear to cross the blood-brain barrier. Major metabolic pathways involve deamination or methylation. Thioguanine is not a substrate for the enzyme xanthine oxidase in contrast to mercaptopurine. Toxicities include myelosuppression, immunosuppression, nausea, vomiting, mucositis, and diarrhea.

PENTOSTATIN (2′-DEOXYCOFORMYCIN, DCF, NIPENT)

The drug is available in 10-mg vials for IV use. The drug is used to treat leukemias such as hairy cell leukemia, chronic lymphocytic leukemia, and lymphoblastic leukemia. The mechanism of action involves inhibition of the enzyme adenosine deaminase yielding increased cellular levels of deoxyadenosine and deoxyadenosine triphosphate (dATP). The increased levels of dATP are cytotoxic to lymphocytes. Pentostatin is a fermentation product of Streptomyces antibioticus. Resistance appears to involve decreased cellular transport or increased expression of catabolic enzymes. Acid instability prevents oral administration, and the drug is only administered by IV. The drug is distributed in total body water but does not enter the CNS. The majority of the dosage is excreted unchanged in the urine. Fatal pulmonary toxicity has occurred when pentostatin and fludarabine are used in combination. Toxicities include myelosuppression, immunosuppression, nausea, vomiting, headache, lethargy, and fatigue.

METHOTREXATE (MTX, ABITREXATE, MEXATE, FOLEX)

The drug is available in 50-, 100-, 200-, and 1,000-mg vials for IV use. Methotrexate is used to treat several cancer types including breast cancer, bladder cancer, colorectal cancer, and head and neck cancer. The mechanism of action of methotrexate involves inhibition of DHFR leading to a depletion of critical reduced folates. The reduced folates are necessary for biosynthesis of several purines and pyrimidines. Resistance to methotrexate can occur because of decreased carrier-mediated transport of drug into cells or increased expression of the target enzyme DHFR. Oral bioavailability varies with dose because of saturable uptake processes, and high doses are required to reach therapeutic levels in the CNS. The majority of drug dosage is excreted unchanged in the urine. The renal excretion of methotrexate is inhibited by several carboxylic acid drugs such as penicillins, probenecid, nonsteroidal anti-inflammatory agents, and aspirin. Methotrexate enhances 5-FU antitumor effects when given 24 hours prior to the fluoropyrimidine. Methotrexate toxicity includes myelosuppression, mucositis, nausea, vomiting, severe headaches, renal toxicity, acute cerebral dysfunction, skin rash, and hyperpigmentation.

PEMETREXED (MTA, ALIMTA)

The drug is available in a 100-mg sterile vial for IV use. The drug appears to be effective against a range of tumors including mesothelioma, NSCLC, colorectal cancer, bladder cancer, and lung cancer. The mechanism of action involves inhibition of TS resulting in inhibition of thymidylate and DNA synthesis. This drug is a pyrrolopyrimidine analog of folate with antifolate activity. Resistance can occur by increased expression of TS, decreased binding affinity for TS, or decreased drug transport into cells. The drug is administered only via the IV route and distributes to all tissues. Cellular activation to the more potent polyglutamated forms occurs, and the majority of the dose is excreted unchanged in the urine. The drug interaction and toxicity profiles are similar to that of methotrexate.

TRIMETREXATE (TMTX, NEUTREXIN)

The drug is available as a lyophilized powder in 5- or 30-mg vials for IV use. The drug is used to treat colorectal cancer, head and neck cancer as well as NSCLC. The mechanism of action of trimetrexate involves folate antagonism and inhibition of thymidylate synthesis. Trimetrexate does not form intracellular polyglutamate adducts as does methotrexate and other related compounds. Resistance can occur by increased expression of the target enzyme, decreased binding affinity for the target enzyme, or decreased intracellular drug transport. Trimetrexate is administered only by the IV route and distributed throughout the body with extensive binding to plasma proteins. The major catabolic pathways involve *O*-demethylation followed by glucuronide conjugation. The drug interaction and toxicity profiles are similar to those for methotrexate.

HYDROXYUREA (DROXIA, HYDREA)

$HONH-CO-NH_2$. The drug is available in a 500-mg capsule for oral use. Hydroxyurea is often considered an antimetabolite drug, and it is used to treat myelogenous leukemia, ovarian cancer, and essential thrombocytosis. The mechanism of action of hydroxyurea involves inhibition of DNA biosynthesis by inhibition of the enzyme ribonucleotide reductase (see Fig. 10.15). Resistance can occur via increased expression of ribonucleotide reductase. The oral bioavailability is quite high approaching 100% and the drug is distributed to all tissues. Hydroxyurea readily enters the CNS and distributes to human breast milk. A major portion of the total dose is excreted unchanged in the urine. The drug has been shown to increase the toxicity of 5-FU, and hydroxyurea may increase the effectiveness of some antimetabolite HIV drugs. The toxicity profile includes myelosuppression, leucopenia, nausea, vomiting, pruritus hyperpigmentation, headache, drowsiness, and confusion.

⬡ ANTIBIOTICS AND NATURAL PRODUCTS

A variety of the anticancer agents available today are derived from natural sources with several of these being obtained from microbial sources (antibiotics). Many of the antineoplastic antibiotics are produced by the soil fungus *Streptomyces*. Both the antibiotic and natural product classes have multiple inhibitory effects on cell growth; however, they primarily act to disrupt DNA function and cell division.

There are several mechanisms by which these agents target DNA, including intercalation, alkylation, and strand breakage either directly or as a result of enzyme inhibition. Intercalation is a process by which a planar molecule of the appropriate size inserts itself between adjacent base pairs of DNA and in so doing, it causes a local unwinding that may disrupt the normal template function of DNA. Intercalation requires that the drug induce a cavity between base pairs so that insertion may occur. The interaction of the intercalator and the adjacent base pairs occurs by the overlap of *p*-orbitals of the intercalator and the base pairs. The *p*-orbitals of the intercalation species are provided by a combination of aromatic and conjugated systems that impart the planarity required for intercalation. The drug–DNA interaction is further stabilized by side chains attached to the intercalation species. The side chains often include a cationic moiety, which may form ionic bonds with the anionic phosphate backbone. Alternative modes of stabilization may occur through a combination of van der Waals interaction or hydrogen bonds. The overall result of these interactions is to cause a local bend or kink in DNA resulting in a local shape distortion. This may produce several effects but is often associated with inhibition of normal DNA function.

By virtue of their ability to induce bends or kinks in DNA, intercalators may also result in inhibition of topoisomerase enzymes. In order for the cell to store the nearly 2 m of DNA that it contains, it is necessary to fold the genetic material into a more compact form and in the process, knots and tangles are produced. Topoisomerase enzymes are responsible for the unwinding and relaxation of DNA so that transcription may occur.[67] There are two major types of topoisomerase enzymes, which are important sites of action for antineoplastics. Topoisomerase I makes a single-strand break in DNA and subsequently allows the other strand to spin, relieving any tension associated with the packing process and subsequently reseals the broken strand. Topoisomerase II makes double-strand breaks in DNA allowing an intact chain to pass through and then subsequently reseals the double-strand break. In this way, it can relieve the knotting that occurs upon folding of the DNA. Both enzymes are believed to recognize sequences of DNA, bind and function by formation of a transient phosphodiester bond between the DNA strand and a tyrosine residue present on the protein. Inhibition may occur at different steps in the process such that if there is stabilization of the cleavable complex, the resealing step may be delayed or prevented resulting in strand breakage. This may then activate the apoptotic cascade.

There are several natural products that are capable of disrupting the formation and function of the mitotic spindle. These include the epipodophyllotoxins, the taxanes, and the vinca alkaloids. The mitotic spindle forms during the M phase of the cell cycle and is responsible for moving the replicated DNA to opposite ends of the cell in preparation for cell division. During prophase, the cytoskeleton made of proteins, which gives the cell its shape, begins to breakdown providing the building blocks for the mitotic spindle. The cell then progresses to prometaphase, where the nuclear membrane begins to disappear and the spindle begins to form attaching the centrosomes to the kinetochores, which are proteins joining the two sister chromatids. Tension is then applied to the spindle so that during metaphase, the chromatids align near the center of the cell. In anaphase, a further increase in tension separates the sister chromatids at the kinetochore, and they are pulled to opposite ends of the cell. Ultimately, the microtubules will disintegrate and reform the cytoskeleton. The process is highly controlled and there are several proteins including "motor proteins," which are involved in coordinating the process.

Actinomycins

The actinomycins are a group of compounds that are isolated from various species of Streptomyces, all of which contain the same phenoxazone chromophore but differ in the attached peptide portion. Originally, these materials were investigated for use as antibiotics, but they proved to be too toxic. From this group emerged actinomycin D, which is known as *dactinomycin* and contains identical pentapeptides bound through an amide linkage utilizing the amino group of L-threonine with carbonyls at positions 1 and 9.[68] The pentapeptides namely L-threonine, D-valine, L-proline, sarcosine, and L-methylvaline form a lactone via the side chain hydroxyl of L-threonine and the carboxyl group of L-methylvaline (Fig. 10.11).

Dactinomycin binds noncovalently to double-stranded DNA by partial intercalation between adjacent guanine-cytosine bases resulting in inhibition of DNA function. The structural feature of dactinomycin important for its mechanism of cytotoxicity is the planar phenoxazone ring, which facilitates intercalation between DNA base pairs. The peptide loops are located within the minor groove and provide for additional interactions (Fig. 10.12). The preference for GpC base pairs is thought to be partly related to the formation of a hydrogen bond between the 2-amino groups of

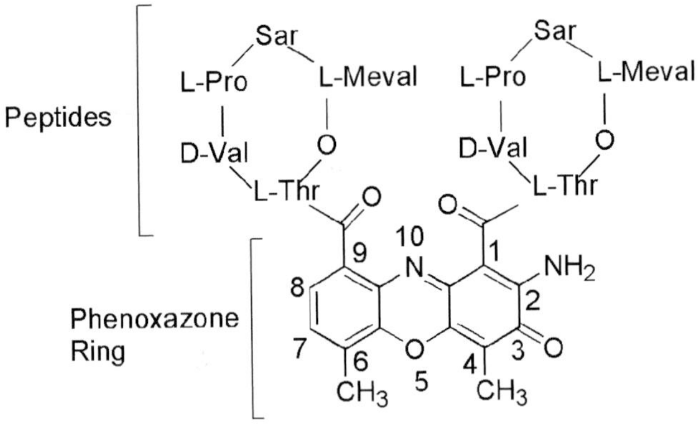

Figure 10.11 • Structure of dactinomycin.

guanine and the carbonyls of the L-threonine residues.[69] Additional hydrophobic interactions and hydrogen bonds are proposed to form between the peptide loops and the sugars and base pairs within the minor groove. In all, actinomycin D spans four to five DNA base pairs (Fig. 10.12). This results in high affinity with the molecule only slowly dissociating from DNA. Additional modes of binding are also possible for the molecule. The primary effect of this interaction is the inhibition of DNA-directed RNA synthesis and specifically RNA polymerase. DNA synthesis may also be inhibited, and the agent is considered cell cycle specific for the G_1 and S phases. The drug has been found to bind to single-stranded DNA and double-stranded DNA without adjacent GpC sequences.[70] It has been suggested that binding to single-stranded DNA may occur as the strands separate during transcription, and this may be responsible for the inhibition of RNA polymerase.[71] Those genes that were being actively transcribed, which would require strand separation, would be more susceptible to this type of binding. Inhibition of topoisomerase II also occurs such that the enzyme-DNA complex is stabilized and strand breakage may be seen. Resistance is caused by a decreased ability of tumor cells to take up the drug and P-glycoprotein (Pgp)-mediated efflux.

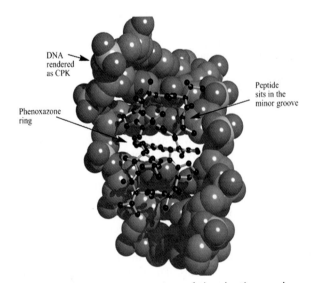

Figure 10.12 • Representation of the dactinomycin–DNA complex. (Reprinted with permission from Hou, M. H., et al.: Nucleic Acids Res. 30:4910, 2002.)

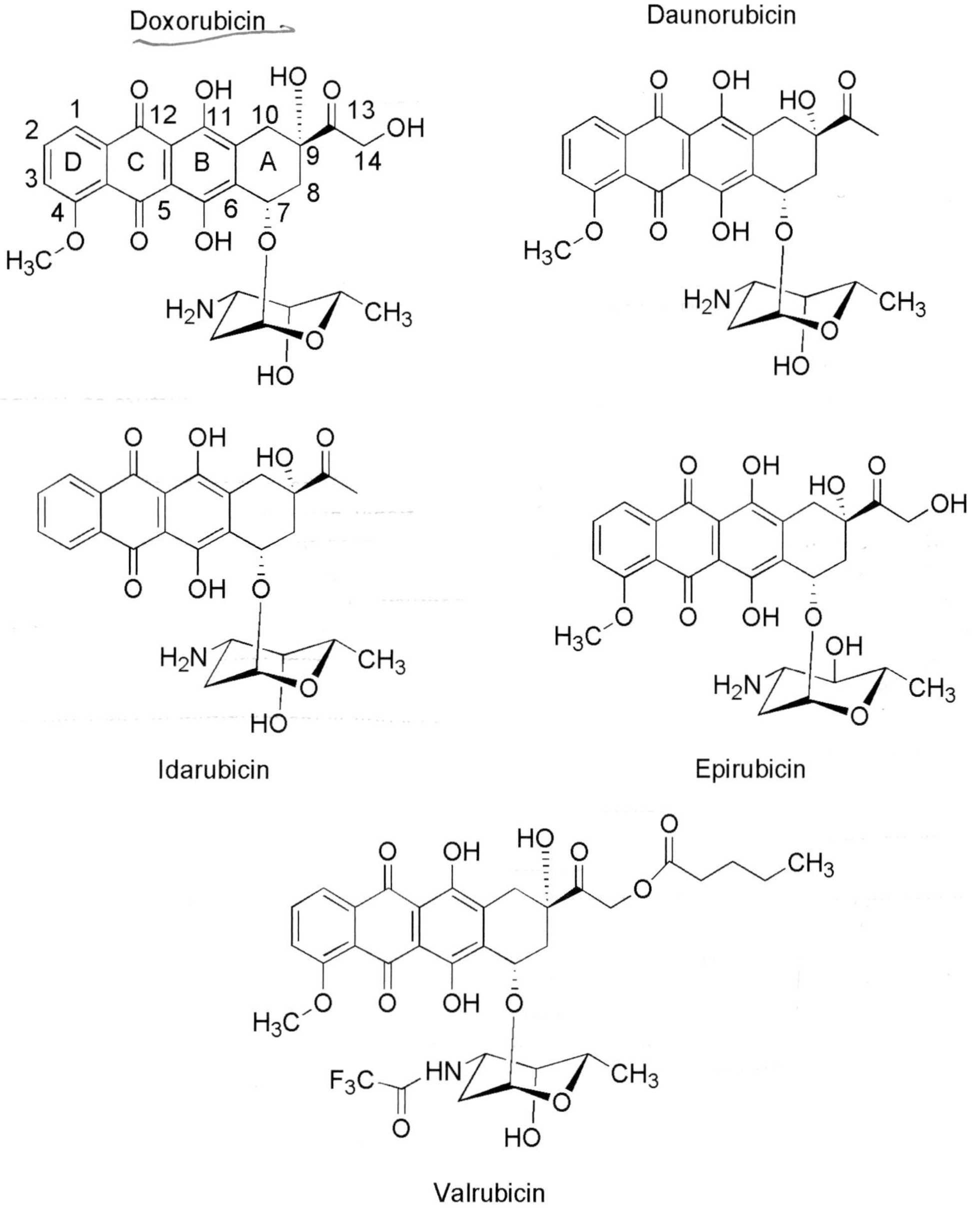

Figure 10.13 ● Structure of the anthracycline antibiotics.

Anthracyclines

The anthracycline antibiotics (Fig. 10.13) are characterized by a planar oxidized anthracene nucleus fused to a cyclohexane ring that is subsequently connected via a glycosidic linkage to an amino sugar. Initially discovered in the early 1960s when they were isolated from *Streptomyces peucetius*, hundreds of compounds belonging to this class have subsequently been discovered of which five are used clinically in the United States (doxorubicin, daunorubicin, idarubicin, epirubicin, and valrubicin). The conjugated systems found in these molecules impart a red color, which is reflected in the name.

Studies of the mechanism by which the anthracyclines exhibit their cytotoxic effects initially focused on the ability of the compounds to associate with DNA resulting from intercalation of their planar ring system reinforced by auxiliary binding of the amino sugar. Subsequent work focused on the ability of these compounds to generate free radicals.

Although free radical generation is thought to be important in the toxicity, it was not shown to occur in the nucleus and therefore not likely associated with their antiproliferative effects. Currently, the accepted mechanism involves intercalation followed by inhibition of topoisomerase II resulting in strand breakage leading to apoptosis.[72] The anthracyclines are considered specific for the S phase of the cell cycle. There is data to support increased binding of p53 with DNA when anthracyclines are administered, which would stimulate the apoptotic process, although some studies have failed to confirm this.[73,74] Several of these agents have been cocrystallized with B-DNA oligomers and the three-dimensional structure determined by x-ray crystallography. The general features show rings B and C intercalating between CpG base pairs and ring D protruding into the major groove. The sugar moiety lies within the minor groove and along with ring A is important for interaction and inhibition of topoisomerase II by stabilization of the cleavable complex. The amino sugar seems to play an especially important role and compounds lacking this functionality failed to inhibit the enzyme. In the case of doxorubicin and daunorubicin, specificity is provided by the hydrogen bonding between O-9 of the anthracycline and N-2 and N-3 of guanine. The x-ray data also suggested that the interaction with DNA is stabilized by the formation of several hydrogen bonds through bridging water molecules.[75] The formation of covalent bonds between anthracyclines and DNA also is supported by several studies in which formaldehyde is produced by oxidation of cellular components or other anthracycline molecules. This oxidation results from the production of ROS such as H_2O_2, which are generated during redox cycling of anthracyclines (Scheme 10.24). The generated formaldehyde may then form a methylene bridge between the 4'-amino group of the anthracycline and the 2-amino group of guanine in DNA.[76]

Although the anthracyclines produce several adverse effects that are typical for antineoplastics, cardiotoxicity is a special concern with this class of agents. The associated cardiomyopathies and congestive heart failure (CHF) have been related to the ability of these compounds to undergo redox cycling.[77] This is most notable in the case of daunorubicin and doxorubicin and less of a problem in the newer derivatives, idarubicin and epirubicin. The C ring of the anthracy-

clines is subject to a one or two electron reduction by several different enzymes including NAD(P)H-oxidoreductases and CYP reductases to give the semiquinone or hydroquinone. The case of the one electron reduction is shown in Scheme 10.25. This may undergo reversion to the starting quinone in futile redox cycling accompanied by the production of superoxide radical. The radical is normally converted to H_2O_2 by superoxide dismutase and H_2O_2 is then converted to H_2O and O_2 by catalase. However, the production of superoxide ($O_2^{-\cdot}$) is also associated with the release of iron from intracellular stores, which may be chelated by the anthracycline. The iron then diverts the normal detoxification pathway by catalase so that more potent radicals such as hydroxyl radical ($\cdot OH$) are produced. Myocardial cells possess lower levels of catalase and therefore are less able to detoxify the H_2O_2 that results from redox cycling. This results in increasing levels of $\cdot OH$ for which a detoxification pathway does not exist and therefore cellular damage occurs. Materials such as $O_2^{-\cdot}$, $\cdot OH$, and H_2O_2 are known as *reactive oxygen species* or ROS and in sufficiently high concentration produce cellular damage. Hydroxyl radicals cause single-strand breaks in DNA, which would activate p53 and enhance apoptosis in cardiac cells. Studies have also shown that doxorubicin administration stimulates both the intrinsic and extrinsic pathways of

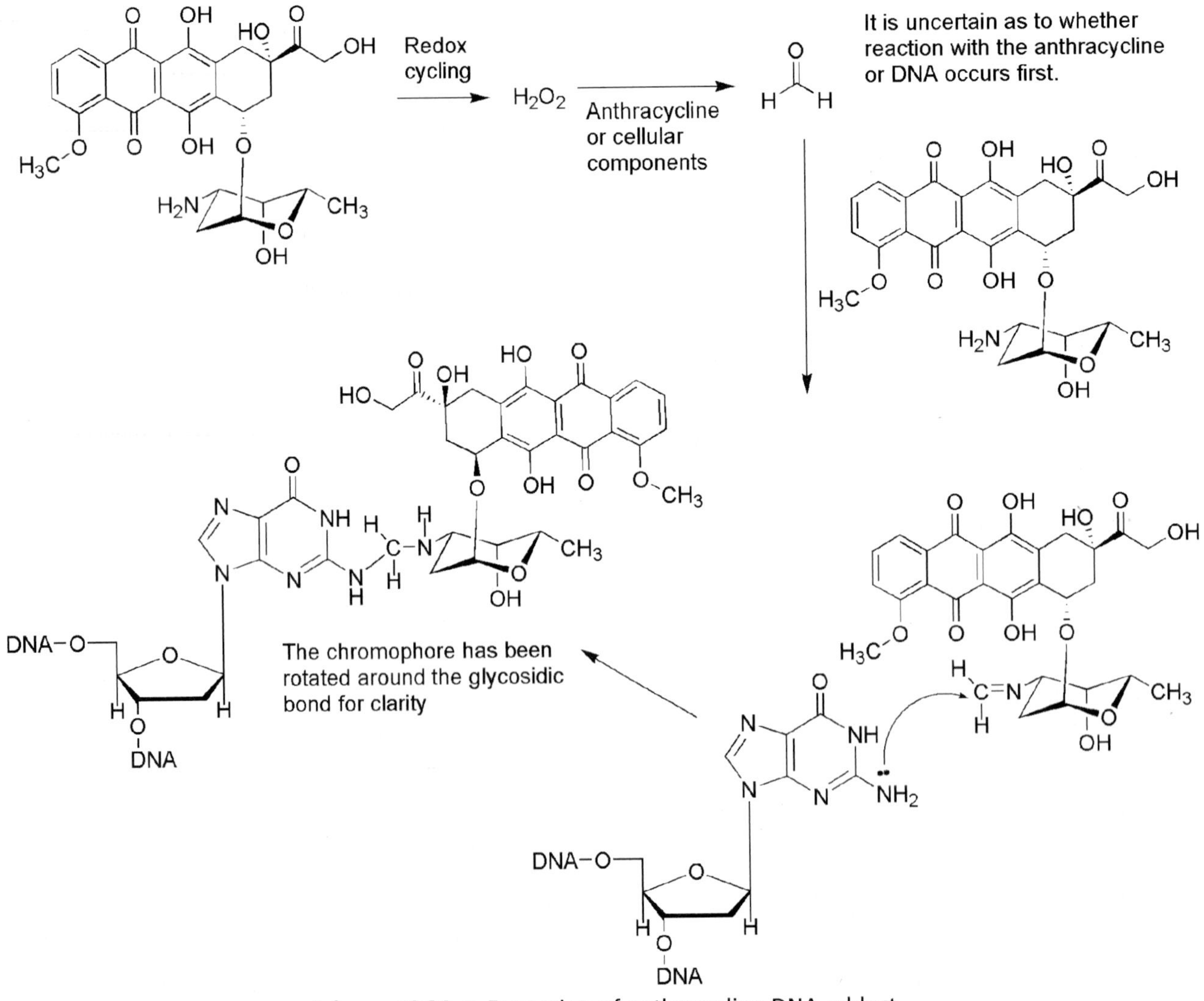

Scheme 10.24 • Formation of anthracycline-DNA adduct.

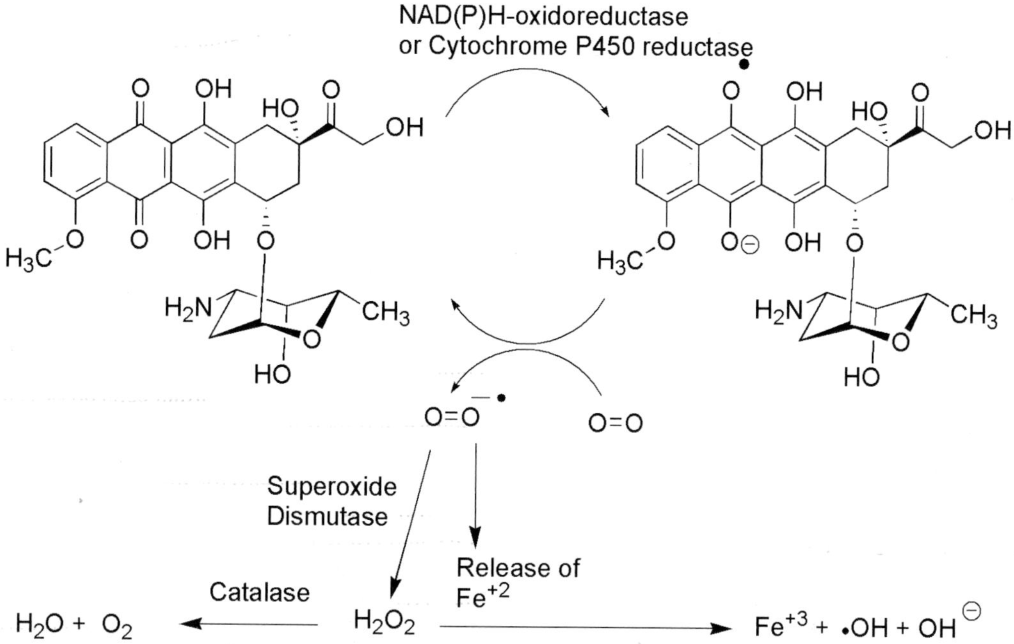

Scheme 10.25 ● Process of anthracycline redox cycling.

apoptosis in numerous ways, and this has been linked to the increased production of H_2O_2 and hydroxyl radical. One proposed mechanism involves damage to the mitochondrial membrane by H_2O_2 and ·OH resulting in the release of cytochrome c, which would activate the intrinsic pathway (Fig. 10.2).[78] This sequence of events would be desirable in a cancer cell but not in a normal cardiac cell.

Additional mechanisms of cardiotoxicity have been proposed, which involve the metabolic reduction of the anthracycline C-13 ketone to the alcohol.[79] Several pharmacological effects have been associated with the resulting alcohols including loss of Ca^{+2} homeostasis and inhibition of Na^+/K^+-ATPase in cardiac cells. The formation of doxorubicin C-13 alcohol, doxorubicinol has been associated with conversion of iron regulatory protein-1 (IRP-1) into a null protein that is no longer able to maintain iron homeostasis.[80] It has been proposed that the loss of iron regulation may contribute to the cardiotoxicity seen with doxorubicin. However, compared with doxorubicin, daunorubicin and idarubicin form greater amounts of the alcohol metabolites and exhibit similar and reduced cardiotoxicity, respectively. This suggests that metabolism to the alcohols is not solely responsible for the cardiotoxicity.

Several strategies have been developed to reduce the cardiotoxicity associated with the anthracyclines. Slow infusion over 48 to 96 hours versus administration of a bolus given over 15 minutes was implemented in the 1980s and has proven to be effective in reducing the toxicity without adversely affecting the antineoplastic effects. Given the proposed mechanism of toxicity, it is not surprising that several antioxidants have been investigated including vitamins A, C, and E and also thiol-containing reducing agents such as acetylcysteine. These, however, have not proved effective in large measure. An alternative strategy is to chelate the iron required for the activation of H_2O_2, and for this, dexrazoxane (Totect) is used.[81] Radiolabeling experiment have shown that dexrazoxane is rapidly taken up into myocardial cells, where it is subsequently hydrolyzed by a two-step

process to yield the diamide acid (Scheme 10.26), which chelates free iron and iron bound to the anthracycline and is similar to the chelating agent ethylenediaminetetraacetic acid (EDTA). This has been proven effective and has allowed patients to tolerate higher doses and increased numbers of cycles of the anthracyclines. Dexrazoxane is also an inhibitor of topoisomerase II that, unlike the anthracyclines, does not result in strand breaks.[82] This additional property is important in its utility as antidote in cases of anthracycline extravasation.[83] The anthracyclines are often administered with other antineoplastics such as the taxanes and trastuzumab, which may have cardiotoxicities themselves leading to an increased risk despite the precautions mentioned.

Related to the anthracyclines is mitoxantrone, which is shown in Figure 10.14. Although mitoxantrone is a synthetic agent, it is included with the natural products because it is mechanistically similar to the anthracyclines. Produced in the late 1970s, it is a derivative of a synthetic dye and is classified as an anthracenedione.[84] The mechanism involves intercalation by the chromophore, which is stabilized by the 2-[(2-aminoethyl)amino]ethanol side chain presumably as a

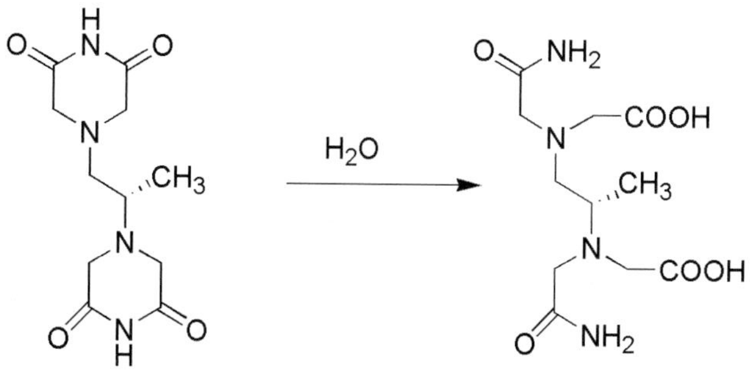

Dexrazoxane

Scheme 10.26 ● Aqueous hydrolysis of dexrazoxane to yield the iron-chelating metabolite.

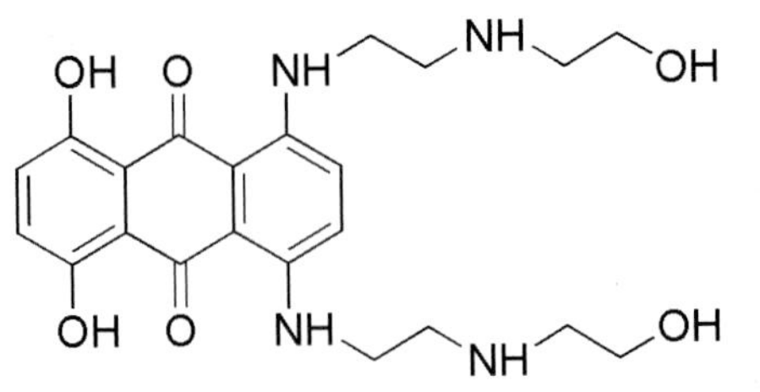

Mitoxantrone

Figure 10.14 • Structure of mitoxantrone.

result of an ionic interaction of the protonated amines with the phosphate backbone of DNA. The formation of covalent adducts with DNA have also been demonstrated to occur in a manner similar to the anthracyclines. In this case, however, other enzymes such as myeloperoxidase are responsible for the generation of formaldehyde.[85] Topoisomerase II is inhibited, and strand breakage occurs similar to that seen with the anthracyclines. In contrast to the anthracyclines, mitoxantrone is not a substrate for the reductase enzymes responsible for the conversion to the semiquinone so that ROS are not generated by this process.[86] This lack of activation has been attributed to the presence of the side chains. This has the effect of reducing the cardiotoxicity but not completely eliminating it, and caution should be used especially in those patients with existing cardiovascular problems.

Individual Agents

DACTINOMYCIN-D (ACT-D, ACTINOMYCIN-D, COSMEGEN, LYOVAC COSMEGEN)

Dactinomycin is available in vials containing 0.5 mg of drug for reconstitution in sterile water for IV administration This antibiotic is most effective in the treatment of rhabdomyosarcoma and Wilms tumor in children as well as in the treatment of choriocarcinoma, Ewing sarcoma, Kaposi sarcoma, and testicular carcinoma. The pharmacokinetics of dactinomycin has not been well characterized, but it appears to concentrate in nucleated blood cells. The agent is 5% to 15% plasma protein bound and is excreted mostly unchanged in urine and bile. Other metabolites have not been characterized. The terminal elimination half-life is 30 to 40 hours. Myelosuppression is dose limiting with both leucopenia and thrombocytopenia being the most likely presentation. Nausea and vomiting occur shortly (2 hours) after treatment and may be severe. Mucositis and diarrhea also result from irritation of the GI tract. Hair loss is commonly associated with the agent as is hyperpigmentation of the skin and erythema.

DOXORUBICIN HYDROCHLORIDE (ADM, ADR, ADRIA, ADRIAMYCIN)

Doxorubicin is available as both the conventional dosage form and a liposomal preparation, both of which are administered by infusion. Doxorubicin HCl powder is available in 10-, 20-, 50-, and 150-mg vials and is widely used in treating various cancers, including leukemias, soft and bone tissue sarcomas, Wilms tumor, neuroblastoma, small cell lung cancer, and ovarian and testicular cancer. Resistance to the agent involves decreased expression of topoisomerase II and

mutations in this enzyme that decrease binding of the drug. The agent may also be actively secreted from cancer cells by Pgp. The agent is rapidly taken up into tissues following injection with a distributive half-life of 5 minutes followed by a slow elimination half-life of 20 to 48 hrs. The primary route of elimination is in the bile and feces. Metabolism involves reduction of the C-13 ketone to yield doxorubicinol (active) along with cleavage of the amino sugar to give the aglycone. The aglycones are also capable of undergoing redox cycling and producing ROS.

The toxicities associated with doxorubicin include dose-limiting cardiotoxicity and myelosuppression. Most patients will experience alopecia and nausea. Cardiotoxicity is a limiting factor in the administration of doxorubicin, which, in its most severe form, may progress to CHF. This may occur during therapy or during months or years following the termination of therapy. The percentage of patients that progress to CHF increases with increasing cumulative dose.

The liposomal form of doxorubicin (Doxil) offers several advantages including an improved pharmacokinetic profile with slower plasma clearance giving a distributive half-life of 45 hours versus 5 minutes for doxorubicin and a smaller volume of distribution of 4 L versus 254 L for doxorubicin.[87] There is also reportedly an increased uptake of doxorubicin in tumor cells, which has been attributed to the ability of the liposomes to break down in the more acidic environment associated with tumor cells or by the release of enzymes from the tumor cells that degrade the liposomes. The liposomes decrease uptake by myocardial tissue, so cardiotoxicity is less common. The liposomes also reduce conversion to doxorubicinol, which has been implicated in the cardiotoxicity of doxorubicin. Additionally, there is a decrease in the incidence of extravasation. Other adverse effects are also decreased including less nausea, alopecia, and stomatitis although skin toxicity, which is normally seen as a rash on the feet and hands, may occur frequently.

DAUNORUBICIN HYDROCHLORIDE (DAUNOMYCIN, DNM, DNR, CERUBIDINE, RUBIDOMYCIN)

Daunorubicin is available in 20- and 100-mg vials for reconstitution. The agent is given intravenously for the treatment of acute nonlymphocytic and lymphocytic leukemia. Other unlabeled uses include CML and Kaposi sarcoma. In general, its use is more limited than that of doxorubicin. Daunorubicin lacks the hydroxyl groups found at C-14 of doxorubicin. This leads to an increase in the amount of the alcohol metabolite daunorubicinol (active) arising as a result of reduction of the side chain ketone. This, however, does not appear to lead to a significant increase in the occurrence of cardiotoxicity compared with doxorubicin. The mechanisms of resistance and toxicities of daunorubicin are similar to that of doxorubicin; the major difference between the two agents being the spectrum of cancers that they are used treat.

A liposomal form of daunorubicin is also available known as *DaunoXome*. The drug offers the same advantages as those seen for the liposomal form of doxorubicin.

EPIRUBRICIN HYDROCHLORIDE (4'-EPIADRIAMYCIN, EPI-ADR, ELLENCE)

Epirubicin is available in 50- and 200-mg vials for IV administration for the treatment of breast cancer. It also has several unlabeled uses in various cancers in combination with other agents including therapy for small cell lung cancer, NSCLC, Hodgkin's lymphoma, and non-Hodgkin's lymphoma. Epirubicin is the 4'-epimer of doxorubicin, which exhibits a lower level of cardiotoxicity compared with doxorubicin. The reduced cardiotoxicity has been attributed to the epimerization of 4'-OH, which places this –OH function in an equatorial position resulting in increased glucuronidation, faster clearance, and reduced metabolic reduction to epirubicinol, the C-13 alcohol (compared with doxorubicin). The glucuronide, which forms via glucuronidation of the 4'-alcohol, is the major metabolite found in plasma and urine.[88] Epirubicinol that does form has little cytotoxic activity. Other minor metabolites that are seen are the aglycones of epirubicin and epirubicinol. These factors have allowed epirubicin to be used in larger doses than doxorubicin with less cardiotoxicity. Other toxicities typical of the class are also seen with epirubicin. Like doxorubicin, it has a short distributive half-life of 5 minutes; however, plasma levels are 20% to 30% lower with an increased volume of distribution. The agent has an elimination half-life of 16 hours, which is shorter than that of doxorubicin. Epirubicin is eliminated primarily by biliary excretion.

IDARUBICIN HYDROCHLORIDE (4-DEMETHOXYDAUNOMYCIN, DMDR, IDAMYCIN)

Idarubicin is available in 5-, 10-, and 20-mL vials for IV administration in the treatment of acute myeloid leukemia and acute nonlymphocytic leukemia. The compound lacks the 4-methoxy group and terminal side-chain alcohol of doxorubicin making it the most lipophilic of the four major anthracyclines (doxorubicin, daunorubicin, epirubicin, idarubicin), and it is considered less cardiotoxic than doxorubicin. The removal of the 4-methoxy group also increases inhibition of topoisomerase II. The drug has a fast distributive phase and a high volume of distribution reflecting binding to tissue. Concentrations in blood and bone marrow cells are 100 times higher than those found in plasma, reflecting its use in treating leukemias. Metabolism of the agent primarily occurs by conversion to idarubicinol via reduction of the side chain ketone to the alcohol, which retains activity as an antineoplastic. Elimination occurs primarily in the bile. Adverse effects are similar to those found for doxorubicin; however, there is a lower incidence of cardiotoxicity.

VALRUBICIN (AD 32, VALSTAR)

Valrubicin is available in 200-mg vials for intravesicular administration in the treatment of bladder cancer (orphan drug status). The increased lipophilicity associated with the valeric acid ester and trifluoro acetate functionalities increases tissue penetration and remains intact because, in large measure, of the lack of exposure to hydrolyzing enzymes caused by direct delivery into the bladder followed by voiding of the instilled solution. This local action also minimizes cardiotoxicity and other adverse effects seen with other anthracyclines. The major adverse effects that are seen are bladder irritation and reddening of the urine.

MITOXANTRONE HCL (DHAD, NOVANTRONE)

Mitoxantrone is supplied as a blue aqueous solution in 10- and 20-mg vials for IV administration in the treatment of acute lymphoid leukemia, acute myeloid leukemia, breast cancer, prostate cancer, non-Hodgkin's lymphoma, and multiple sclerosis. The mechanisms of resistance are the same as those seen for the anthracyclines. The distribution half-life is 1.1 to 3.1 hours, and the drug has a large volume of distribution (11 L/kg). The elimination half-life ranged from 23 to 215 hours, and elimination was primarily via the bile. Metabolism of the agent involves oxidation of the side-chain alcohols to give the monocarboxylic and dicarboxylic acids.[89] Other toxicities are those seen for the anthracyclines and include myelosuppression, nausea, vomiting, mucositis, diarrhea, and alopecia. The intense color of the parent drug and metabolites may turn the urine blue.

Epipodophyllotoxins

The epipodophyllotoxins (Fig. 10.15) are semisynthetic derivatives of podophyllotoxin, which is isolated from the mayapple (mandrake) root and functions as an inhibitor of microtubule function.[90,91] Chemical modification has led to compounds with a different mechanism of action, which involves inhibition of topoisomerase enzymes.[92,93] The change in mechanism was associated with removal of the 4'-methyl group of podophyllotoxin. Further alteration in podophyllotoxin involved the addition of the glycosidic portion of the molecules.

Etoposide acts on topoisomerase II stabilizing the cleavable complex leading to single- and double-strand breaks. If enough breaks are initiated, apoptosis is activated. Etoposide is believed to bind to topoisomerase II in the absence of DNA, because it shows little tendency to interact with DNA alone.[94,95] The etoposide-topoisomerase II complex then binds DNA, and strand cleavage occurs; however, the ligation step is inhibited. Binding of the drug occurs near the site at which the cleaved phosphodiester bond is held by the enzyme. One etoposide molecule stabilizes the cleavable complex of one chain, and therefore two etoposide molecules are necessary to mediate double-strand breaks.[96] The concentration of the agent will then determine whether single- or double-strand breaks occur. The resulting breaks in normal cells may lead to mutations and translocations that have been associated with the development of leukemias posttreatment. The agents are considered cell cycle specific and act in the late S and G_2 phases of the cell cycle.

The glycosidic moiety of the epipodophyllotoxins, which is lacking in podophyllotoxin, is associated with converting these compounds from tublin binders to topoisomerase inhibitors. Replacement of the glycosidic 8-methyl group with thiophene gives tenoposide, which is 10-fold more potent than etoposide. The glycosidic moiety is not an absolute requirement for activity, and other more active compounds are known in which it has been replaced. The 4'-OH group is important for the activity of the compounds, and loss of this functionality results in greatly reduced levels of strand breaks. Removal of one of the adjacent methoxy groups by CYP3A4 mediated oxidative-*O*-dealkylation gives the catechol analogs, which are more potent than the parent molecules.[97,98] The catechol analogs may be further oxidized to give the quinones, which are also more active than the parent (Scheme 10.27). There are several mechanisms by which cells become resistant to the epipodophyllotoxins including increased efflux by Pgp as seen for many of the other natural products. Additionally, topoisomerase II levels may decrease

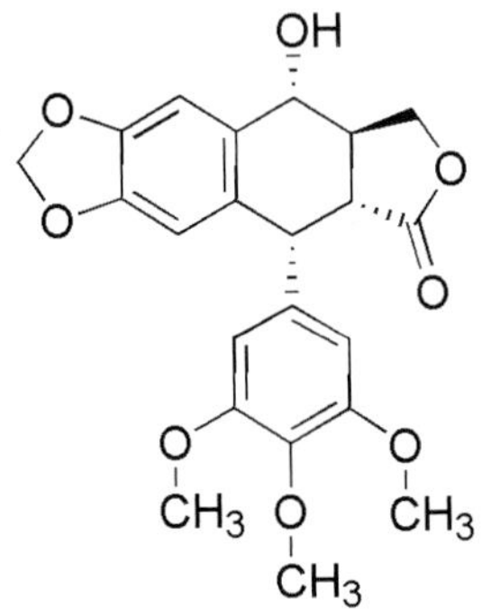

Figure 10.15 ● Structures of the epipodophyllotoxins.

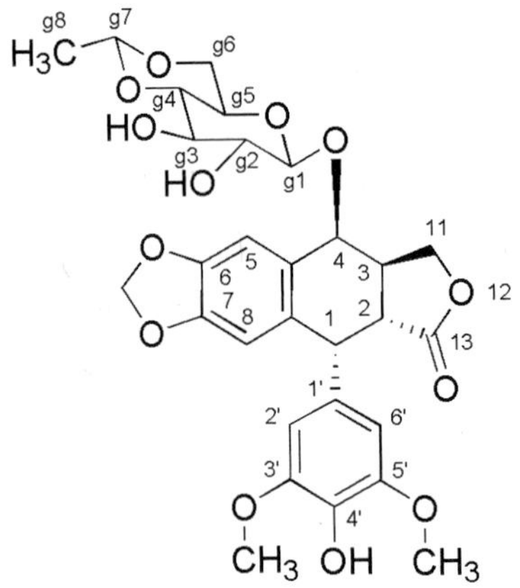

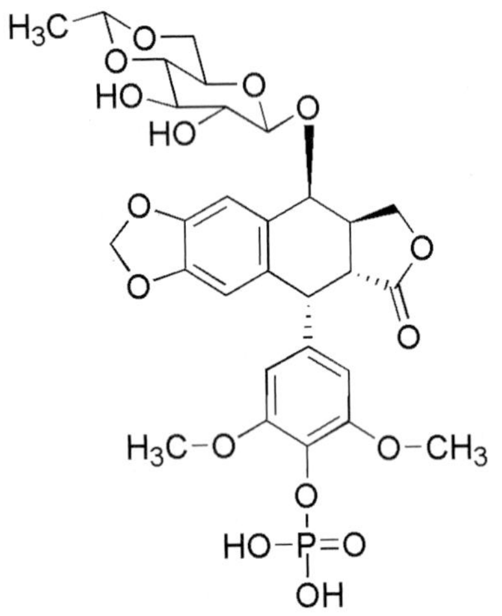

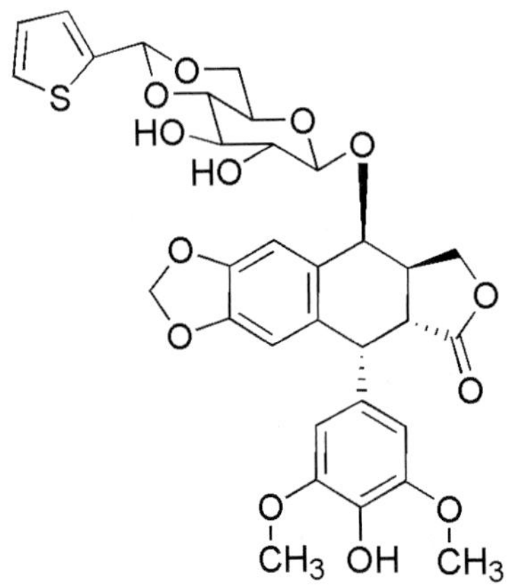

or develop altered binding sites with lower affinity for these agents. Increased DNA repair mechanisms may also decrease the effectiveness of these agents. There are mechanisms by which double-strand breaks in DNA can be repaired. If for example a strand break occurs in the late portion of the S phase or in the G_2 phase after DNA has been replicated, the sister chromatid can be utilized as a template to make the repair in a process known as *homologous recombination* without the loss of genetic material. However, if a sister chromatid is not available, then a process known as *nonhomologus end joining* may be utilized. In this process, after a double-strand break has occurred, exonucleases remove additional base pairs from each strand creating overhangs. If complementary sequences are present in the overhangs, the strands can associate and the missing bases can be filled in. This process, however, results in the loss of some genetic material.

ETOPOSIDE (VP-16, VEPESID, TOPOSAR)

Etoposide is available in 50- and 100-mg capsules for oral use and in 100-mg vials for IV use. The agent is approved for use in testicular cancer and small cell lung cancer. It has also been used in a wide variety of cancers including NSCLC,

Hodgkin's and non-Hodgkin's disease, Kaposi sarcoma, acute lymphocytic leukemia, neuroblastoma, choriocarcinoma, and epithelial, ovarian, testicular, gastric, endometrial, and breast cancers. Etoposide is one of the few natural product derivatives that can be administered orally. When given by this route, bioavailability is 50%. Administration by the IV route is also utilized, and the drug is widely distributed when given by either route. The agent is highly protein bound (90%) primarily to albumin. Low albumin levels may lead to an increase in free drug and require a lowering of the dose. The drug does not penetrate the blood-brain barrier at normal doses but does during high-dose therapy. Elimination occurs primarily in the urine with 30% to 40% of an IV dose appearing as unchanged drug. The elimination half-life is 5 to 10 hours. Metabolism involves opening of the lactone ring to give the hydroxy acid as the major metabolite. Epimerization occurs at C-3 to give the *cis*-lactone, which may also undergo hydrolysis to give the hydroxy acid. Glucuronidation and sulfation of the 4'-OH give products that are inactive. Active metabolites are formed as a result of CYP3A4 mediated oxidative-*O*-demethylation of the 3'-methoxy group to give the catechol followed by oxidation to give the quinone. The toxicities of etoposide include dose-limiting myelosuppression,

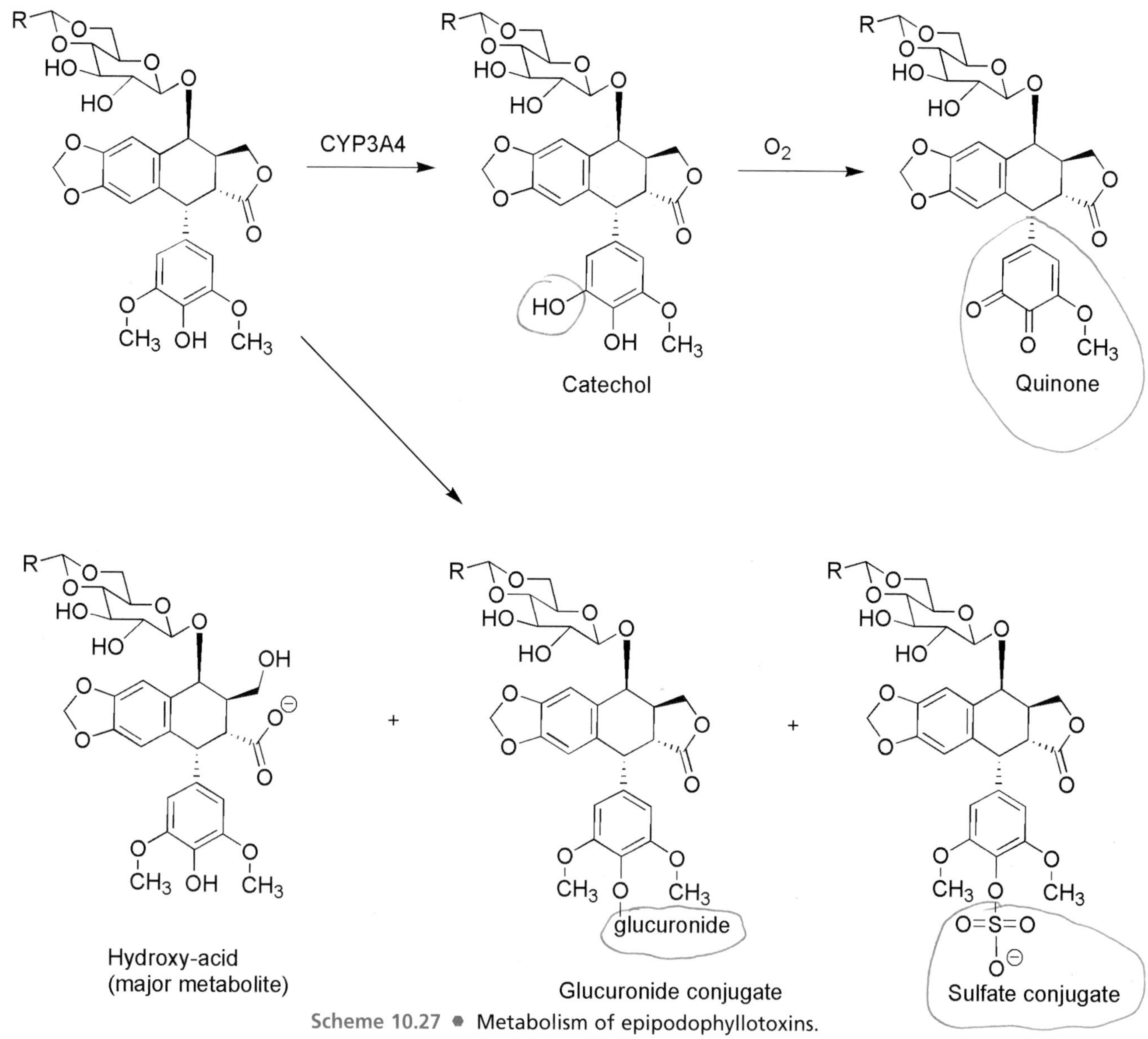

Scheme 10.27 ● Metabolism of epipodophyllotoxins.

which normally presents as leucopenia. In addition, the drug produces nausea and vomiting in 30% to 40% of patients, which is more commonly seen when the drug is administered orally. The agent also produces anorexia, alopecia, mucositis, and hypersensitivity reactions that may be caused by etoposide or Cremophor EL (polyoxyethylated castor oil), which is used as a vehicle for IV administration of the drug. Leukemia, especially acute myelogenous leukemia, has been associated with the drugs' ability to produce strand breaks with resultant translocation of genetic material. The leukemias are generally seen 5 to 8 years posttreatment and have been associated with translocation of several different genes resulting in breakpoints around the mixed lineage leukemia (*MLL*) gene. Transcription and translation of this altered DNA gives chimeric proteins, which form partly from the translocated gene and partly from the *MLL* gene. Exactly how these chimeric proteins lead to leukemia is not known, but similar alterations are seen with other topoisomerase inhibitors.

Etoposide phosphate is a prodrug of etoposide and is converted to the parent by the action of phosphatases. The increased water solubility does not require Cremophor EL or

other vehicles to be used. The agent is administered IV and used in the treatment of germ cell tumors, small cell lung cancers, and NSCLCs.

TENIPOSIDE (VM-26, VUMON)

Teniposide is available in 50-mg ampules with Cremophor EL for IV administration in the treatment of acute lymphoblastic leukemia (ALL). The agent is more potent as an inhibitor of topoisomerase II. The pharmacokinetics of teniposide is similar to that of etoposide; however, the more lipophilic teniposide is more highly protein bound (99%) and less is excreted unchanged in the urine (10%–20%). There is also greater overall metabolism of teniposide; however, CYP3A4-mediated conversion to the active catechol is slower compared with etoposide. Elimination occurs primarily in the urine with a terminal elimination half-life of 5 hours.

Camptothecins

The camptothecins (Fig. 10.16) are inhibitors of topoisomerase I and are used clinically for the treatment of various

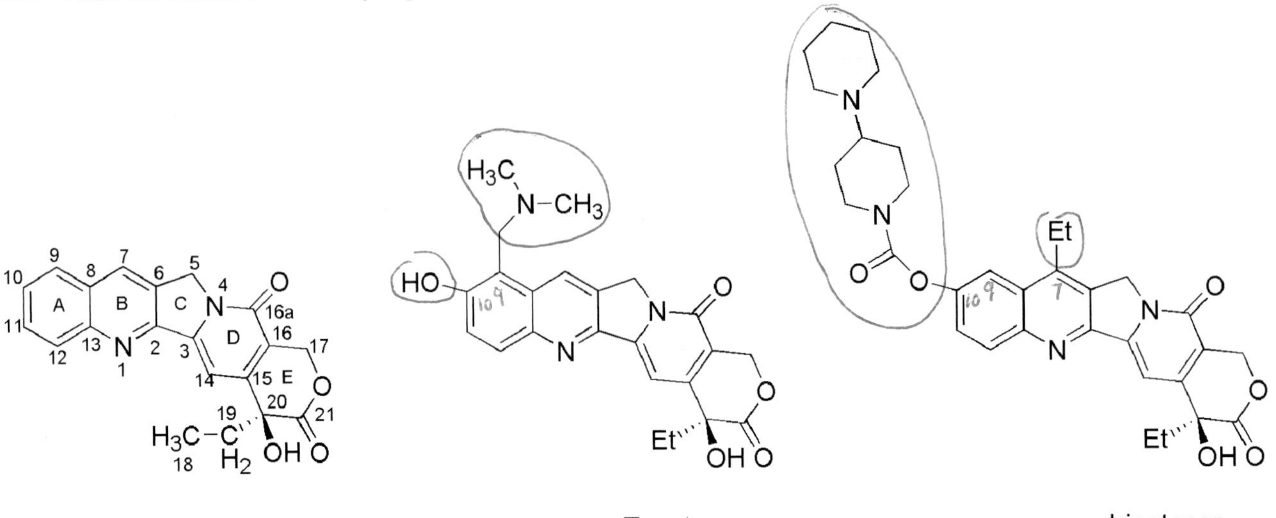

Figure 10.16 ● Structures of topoisomerase I inhibitors.

cancers.[99] The lead drug for this class of agents was camptothecin, which was discovered in the 1960s by Wani and Wall[100] who isolated the material from *Camptotheca acuminata*, an ornamental tree found in China. Initial testing of the isolated material revealed promising antitumor activity, but testing in phase II trials gave disappointing results. The reason for this outcome was that camptothecin had low water solubility, and to overcome this, the sodium salt had been prepared and used during the trials. This was accomplished by hydrolysis of the E-ring lactone to give the carboxylate salt (Scheme 10.28). The resulting ring-opened material was 10 times less active and more toxic producing inflammation of the small intestines, blood in the urine, and myelosuppression.[101,102] Interest in the material subsided until it was revealed that the mechanism of antitumor action was inhibition of topoisomerase I.[103] Subsequently, the incorporation of side chains containing basic amines led to the more water-soluble derivatives, topotecan and irinotecan (Fig. 10.16).[104,105] These agents could be administered as the lactone giving better clinical results. Topoisomerase I produces single-strand breaks in DNA, utilizing a similar mechanism to topoisomerase II.[106,107] The enzyme binds to supercoiled DNA and cleaves a single strand resulting in the formation of a cleavable complex with formation of a transient phosphodiester bond between DNA and a tyrosine residue of topoisomerase I. The complementary strand of the double helix then passes through the break, and the enzyme then reseals the initial strand break. In this way, local supercoils are removed from DNA. The camptothecin analogs bind to the enzyme DNA complex after strand cleavage has occurred, such that the planar structure of the drug can intercalate between DNA base pairs and and then

stabilize the cleavable complex. The binding site for this intercalation is only formed after the enzyme is bound to DNA, and once this site is occupied by the drug, it prevents the realignment necessary for resealing of the initial strand break.

X-ray crystal structures have been solved for several camptothecin analogs bound to DNA and topoisomerase I.[108] In the case of topotecan, the results indicate that the planar portion of the drug intercalates between base pairs at the DNA cleavage site. In this process, the 5'-OH of the cleaved strand is shifted away from the phosphotyrosine bond formed between the enzyme and DNA. This shift prevents the 5'-OH from attacking the phosphotyrosine bond and resealing the strands after supercoiling has been removed. The result is strand breakage. Other key interactions involve a direct hydrogen bond between Asp-533 of topoisomerase I and the 20-OH of topotecan. There is a water-bridged hydrogen bond between the lactone carbonyl at C-21of the drug and the phosphotyrosine of the covalent topoisomerase I-DNA adduct. An additional water-bridged hydrogen bond forms between Asn-722 and the pyridine carbonyl at C-16a of topotecan. Arg-364 is located in proximity to the quinoline nitrogen at N-1, although the interatomic distance was not close enough to allow for a specific interaction in the case of topotecan. Subsequent work with camptothecin, which binds with a slight twist of the planar ring system relative to topetecan, allowed for the formation of a hydrogen bond between Arg-364 and the N-1 nitrogen.[109] The drugs orient such that C-7, C-9, and C-10 are directed into the major groove so that bulky substituents can be tolerated at these positions. These interactions are summarized in Figure 10.17. The result of

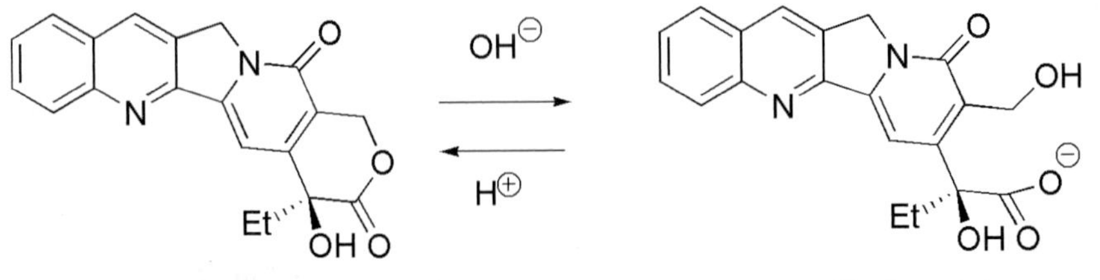

Scheme 10.28 ● Chemical hydrolysis of camptothecin lactone.

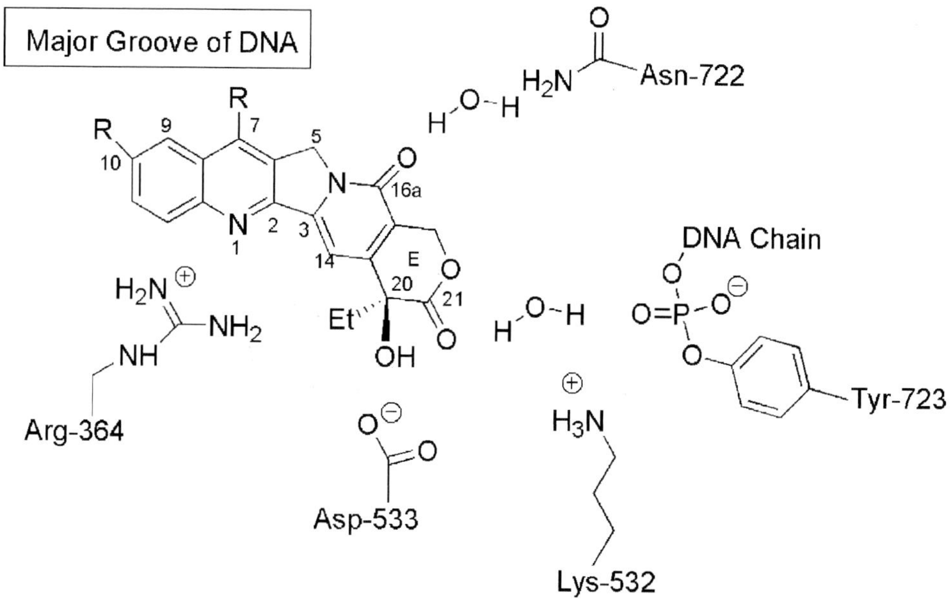

Figure 10.17 ● Interactions between camptothecins and topoisomerase I.

this binding is the formation of single-strand breaks most notably at replication forks that occur during the S phase. Strand breakage of the leading strand of DNA during replication results in double-strand breakage and ultimately leads to cell death.

Several mechanisms of resistance to the camptothecin analogs are known. Different neoplasms express different levels of topoisomerase I, and this is thought to explain the susceptibility of any specific cancer to these agents. It is also possible for cells to decrease their expression of this enzyme or develop altered forms to which these compounds can no longer bind. Increased DNA-repair enzymes may limit the damage to DNA, and these agents are susceptible to Pgp-mediated efflux. The agents have also been shown to activate nuclear factor-κB (NF-κB), which has an antiapoptotic effect so that strand breaks may not initiate apoptosis.

Irinotecan undergoes hydrolysis of its carbamate moiety by irinotecan-converting enzyme to give SN-38, which is 1,000 times more potent than the parent compound (Scheme 10.29).[110] There is wide interpatient variability in the extent of this transformation, which may explain differential responses to the agent. Further metabolism involves the glucuronidation (isozyme UGT1A1) of the resulting phenolic function of SN-38 to give SN-38G, which is inactive. An additional metabolite forms as a result of CYP3A4-mediated conversion to [4-*N*-(5-aminopentanoic acid)-1-piperidino]carbonylcamptothecin (APC), which is 100 times less active than SN-38. There is also the additional complication that the parent and metabolites may exist as the lactones or as the inactive hydroxy acid forms.

IRINOTECAN HYDROCHLORIDE (CPT-11, CAMPTOSAR)

Irinotecan is available in 100-mg or 5-mL vials for IV administration and is used in combination with 5-FU and leucovorin as first-line treatment of metastatic colon cancer. The agent may also be used as a single agent in colorectal cancer as a second-line therapy when 5-FU therapy has failed. Additional uses include small cell lung cancer, NSCLC, cervical cancer, esophageal cancer, and gastric can-

cer. Irinotecan is 30% to 60% plasma protein bound, whereas the active metabolite SN-38 is 95% protein bound. Binding of SN-38 as the lactone stabilizes the material to ring opening. The elimination of the agent occurs primarily in the bile with a minor amount of renal elimination. The excretion of active metabolites or inactive metabolites such as the glucuronide SN-38G, which may be converted back to SN-38 in the bile, has been associated with severe diarrhea. Irinotecan and SN-38 have half-lives of 8 and 14 hours, respectively. Irinotecan has two dose-limiting toxicities, myelosuppression and diarrhea. The diarrhea occurs in two forms, early and late. The early form occurs within the first 24 hours after administration. It has been associated with inhibition of acetylcholinesterase, which results in increased gut motility. This early phase is also associated with flushing, abdominal pain, and excessive sweating. Atropine can be used to relieve these symptoms but it is not recommended for prophylactic use unless there has been a prior episode. The late-phase diarrhea occurs after 24 hours and has been associated with the presence of active material, particularly SN-38 in the gut, and may last 3 to 10 days. The prolonged nature may lead to dehydration and electrolyte imbalances. Loperamide therapy is recommended at the first appearance of a loose stool. If the diarrhea persists, additional agents may be used including antibiotics that decrease β-glucosidase–producing bacteria in the gut and prevent the overgrowth of pathogenic bacteria.[111] Other toxicities include emesis and alopecia.

TOPOTECAN HYDROCHLORIDE (HYCAMPTAMINE, TOPO, HYCAMTIN)

Topotecan is supplied in 4-mg vials and administered IV for the treatment of ovarian cancer, cervical cancer, and small cell lung cancer in those patients who did not respond to first-line therapy. Following IV administration, the drug is widely distributed with 10% to 35% of the agent bound to plasma proteins. There is evidence that the agent may cross the blood-brain barrier to some extent. In plasma, an equilibrium is established between the lactone and the less active hydroxy acid with 20% of the drug present as the lactone 1 hour after the infusion is complete. In contrast to irinotecan,

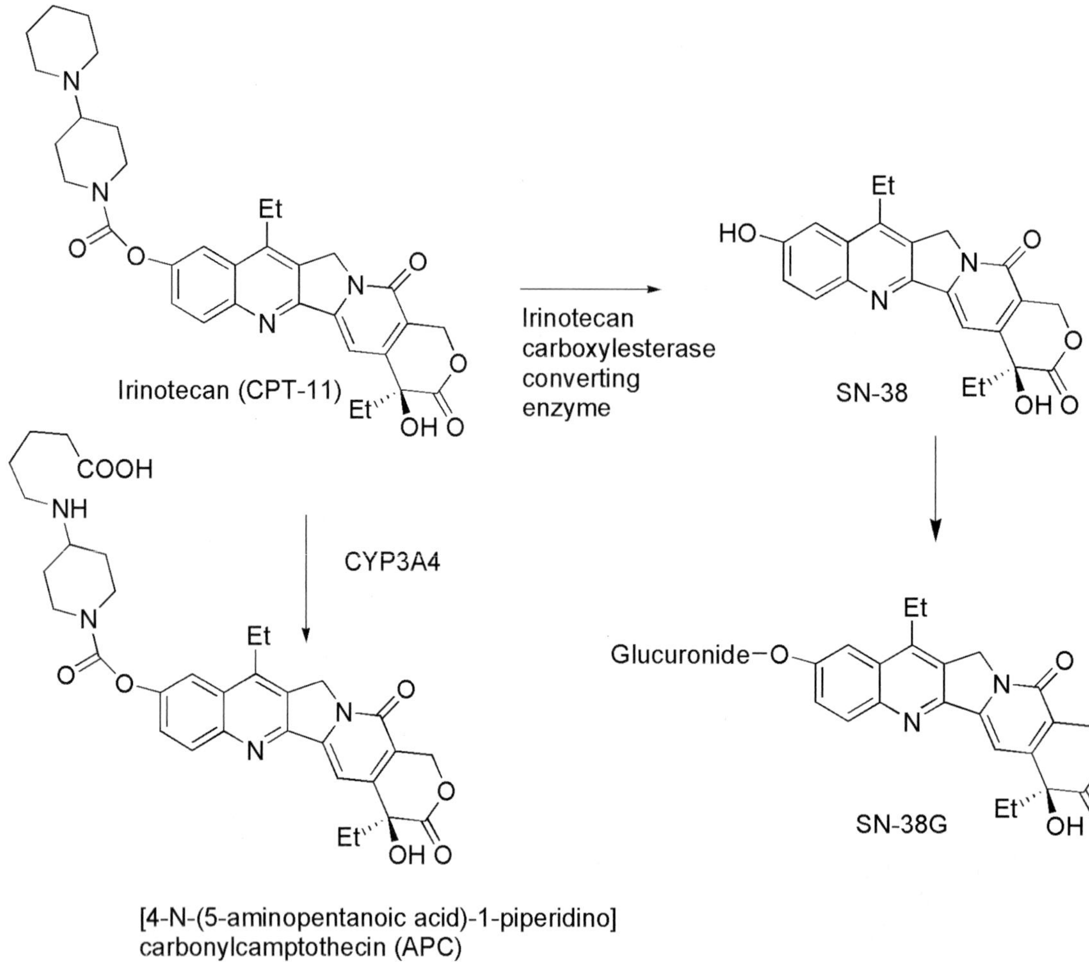

Scheme 10.29 ● Metabolism of irinotecan.

both the lactone and the hydroxy acid bind equally well to human serum albumin. *N*-Demethylation of the tertiary amine to give the secondary amine is mediated by CYP3A4 and represents a minor route of metabolism. Glucuronidation of the parent and the phase I metabolites also occurs to a limited (10%) extent.[112] Elimination occurs primarily in the urine, with 30% of the dose being recovered as unchanged drug. The terminal elimination half-life is 2 to 3 hours. The major toxicity seen for topotecan is dose-limiting myelosuppression. Nausea and vomiting are seen in most (70%–80%) patients, along with diarrhea and abdominal pain. Other toxicities include headache myalgias, alopecia and elevation of serum transaminases, alkaline phosphatases, and bilirubin. Microscopic hematuria (blood in the urine) may also be seen.

Bleomycin

Bleomycin is a glycopeptide antibiotic complex isolated from *Streptomyces verticillus* initially by Umezawa.[113] At least 13 different fractions of bleomycin have been isolated with the clinically used product (Blenoxane) being a mixture of predominantly A_2 (55%–70%) and B_2 (25%–32%) fractions (Fig. 10.18). Of these fractions, A_2 appears to possess the greatest antineoplastic activity. Copper is found in the naturally occurring material, and its removal is important for the material used clinically because it significantly reduces activity.

Bleomycin binds Fe^{+2} through multiple interactions with the amino terminal end of the peptide chain (Fig. 10.19).[114] Bleomycin may itself initiate the release of iron necessary for this complexation. Interaction with DNA subsequently occurs through the bithiazole portion of the molecule, which intercalates between G-C base pairs with a preference for genes undergoing transcription. Held in proximity to DNA by this interaction, in an aerobic environment, Fe^{+2} is oxidized to Fe^{+3} in a one-electron process with the electron being transferred to molecular oxygen.[115] This gives the activated form of bleomycin, which has been formulated as $HOO^-Fe(III)$-bleomycin, which is believed to possess square bipyramidal geometry. This then results in the production of ROS in the form of superoxide and hydroxide radical, which initiate single-strand breakage of the phosphodiester backbone and release of DNA bases by oxidative cleavage of the 3′-4′ bond of the deoxyribose moiety.[116] This activity may be enhanced in the presence of mercaptans such as glutathione, which can facilitate the action of reductase enzymes in reducing the Fe^{+3} that is generated back to Fe^{+2} so that the process may continue. The agent is most active in the G_2 and M phases of the cell cycle.

NMR studies of bleomycin complexed with cobalt have confirmed the intercalation of the bithiazole with adjacent G-C base pairs with the dimethylsulfonium chain (bleomycin A_2) projecting into the major groove where the sulfonium cation may interact with the phosphate backbone

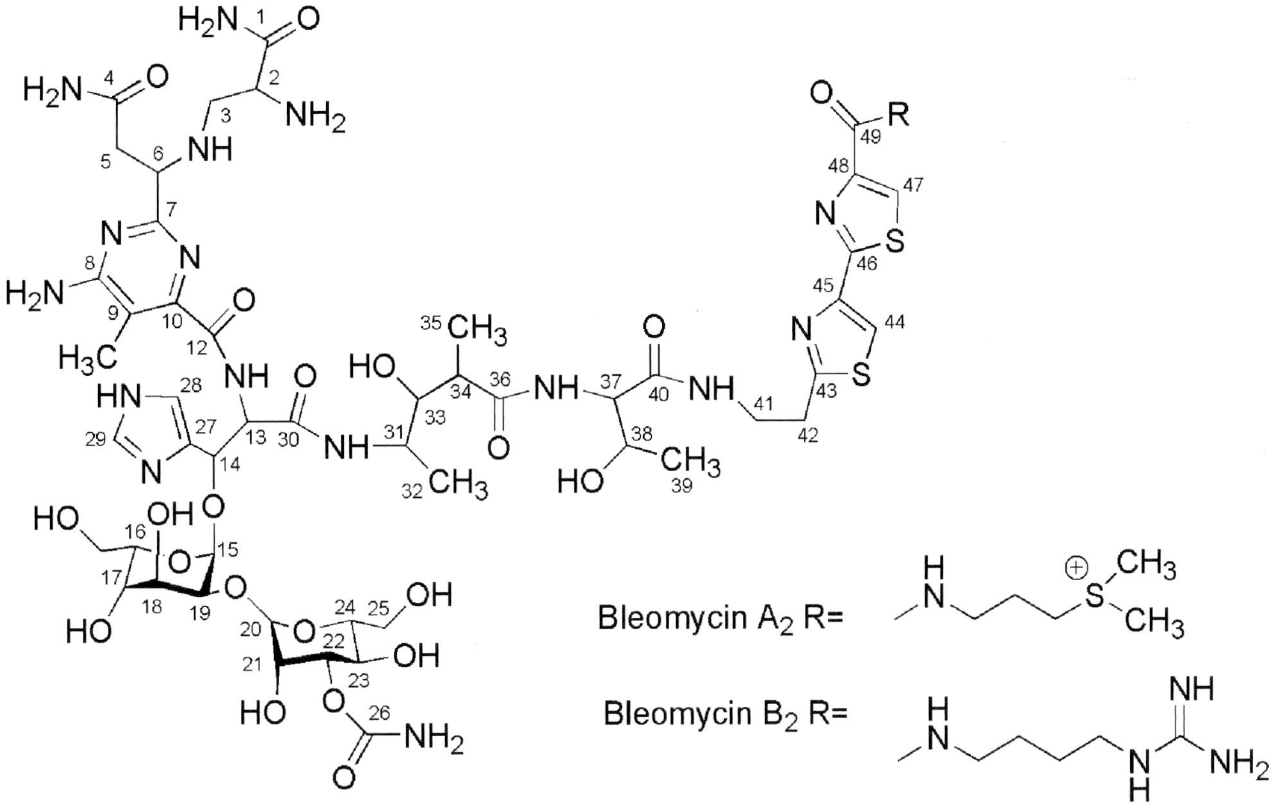

Figure 10.18 ● Structure of bleomycins.

or N-7 of a purine base adjacent to the site of intercalation (Fig. 10.20).[117,118] Additional stabilization is provided by hydrogen bonding of the amino-pyrimidine ring with a guanine residue in the minor groove. This also serves to orient the coordinated metal and the hydroperoxide ligand toward the minor groove.

Bleomycin is notable for its lack of myelotoxicity, and this allows it to be combined with other myelosuppressants without a resulting additive effect. The acute toxicities seen with bleomycin are erythema (reddening of the skin), hyperpigmentation (skin darkening) found predominately on the extremities, and pulmonary toxicity. The pulmonary toxicity may first occur as pneumonitis (inflammation of lung tissue), which normally responds to glucocorticosteroid therapy. Chronic pulmonary toxicity is expressed as pulmonary fibrosis, which is irreversible and limits utility of the agent.

The toxicity profile of bleomycin is explained by its route of inactivation. Hydrolysis of the N-terminal amide to the carboxylic acid increase the pK_a of the amine at C-2 from 7.3 to 9.4, resulting in a greater degree of ionization and decreased binding to DNA.[119] The enzyme responsible for this conversion is known as *bleomycin hydrolase*, and it is present in most tissue but found in low concentration in skin and lung tissue. Tumor cells that are resistant to bleomycin may contain high levels of this enzyme.

BLEOMYCIN SULFATE (BLEO, BLM, BLENOXANE)

Bleomycin occurs as a white powder and is available in 15- and 30-U vials for reconstitution in water. It may be given intravenously, intramuscularly, or subcutaneously. It is used

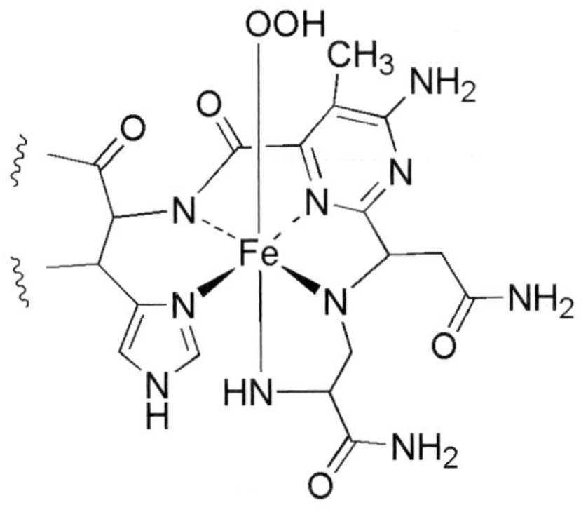

Figure 10.19 ● Structure of the bleomycin-Fe-O₂ complex.

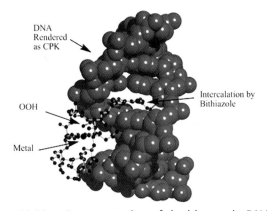

Figure 10.20 ● Representation of the bleomycin-DNA complex. (Reprinted with permission from Zhao, C., et al.: J. Inorgan. Biochem. 91:259, 2002.)

in the treatment of squamous cell carcinoma of the head neck, cervix, penis, and vulva. It is also used in Hodgkin's and non-Hodgkin's lymphoma as well as testicular carcinoma. Unlabeled uses include the treatment of mycosis fungoides, osteosarcoma, and AIDS-related Kaposi sarcoma.

Bleomycin given intravenously has a distribution half-life of 10 to 20 minutes with a small volume of distribution of 20 L. The major metabolite results from hydrolysis of the amide at C-1 to give the inactive carboxylic acid. The drug is primarily eliminated in the kidneys with 60% to 70% of the drug recovered in the urine as unchanged drug. The serum elimination is related to glomerular filtration rate, such that those patients with a creatinine clearance greater than 35 mL/min have a serum total elimination half-life of 115 minutes, and in those with a creatinine clearance less than 35 mL/min, the serum total elimination half-life exponentially increases with decreasing creatinine clearance.

Dermatological reactions are the most commonly seen adverse effect with erythema, hyperpigmentation, rash, and tenderness occurring in 50% of the patients taking the drug. The most serious adverse effect is the pulmonary fibrosis previously mentioned. Treatment with bleomycin can increase the risk of pulmonary toxicity that may occur if the patient is subsequently administered oxygen during surgery.

Vinca Alkaloids

The vinca alkaloids (Fig. 10.21) are extracted from the leaves of *Catharanthus roseus* (periwinkle), and were originally investigated for their hypoglycemic properties but latter found to possess antineoplastic actions.[120] The alkaloids are composed of a catharanthine moiety containing the indole subunit and the vindoline moiety containing the dihydroindole subunit joined by a carbon–carbon bond. Vincristine and vin-

blastine differ only in the group attached to the dihydroindole nitrogen, which is a methyl group in vinblastine and a formyl group in vincristine. Vinorelbine is a semisynthetic material resulting from loss of water across the 3',4' bond and first prepared by the use of a modified Polonovski reaction of vinblastine followed by hydrolysis.[121]

The vinca alkaloids were initially believed to gain entry into the cell by an energy-dependent process, but more recent work suggests that entry occurs by an energy- and temperature-independent mechanism similar to passive diffusion. The agents then begin to accumulate in cells with intracellular concentrations 5- to 500-fold higher than extracellular concentrations. Once in the cell, the vincas bind to tubulin disrupting formation and function of the mitotic spindle.

The mitotic spindle is composed of the microtubules, which function as part of the cell's cytoskeleton and are important in maintaining cellular shape. They are also involved in transport within the cell and cell signaling as well as playing a pivotal role in the movement of chromosomes during mitosis. The microtubules are composed of heterodimers of α-tubulin and β-tubulin, which may arrange as alternating heterodimers around a hollow axis to form the protofilaments of the microtubule. The behavior of the microtubules are regulated in part by microtubule-associated proteins (MAPs), which may bind to soluble tubulin or the microtubules themselves.[122] As part of the mitotic process, the length of the microtubule will change because of polymerization and depolymerization of the associated tubulin. Tubulin is capable of binding guanosine-5'-triphosphate (GTP) and hydrolyzing it to guanosine diphosphate (GDP) and inorganic phosphate (P_i). When this hydrolysis occurs and P_i dissociates another tubulin-GTP complex adds to the microtubule. This forms the GTP cap and as long as tubulin-GTP or tubulin-GDP with associated P_i is present at the end

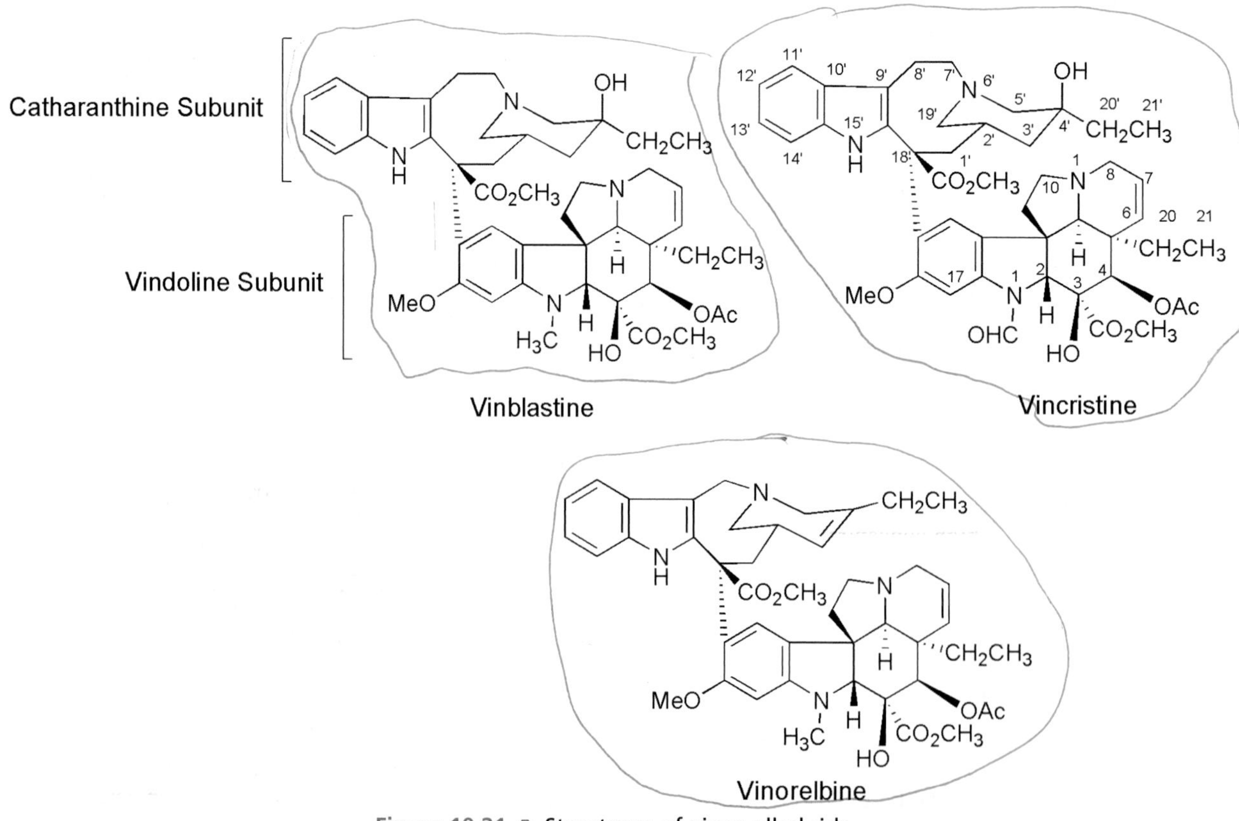

Figure 10.21 • Structures of vinca alkaloids.

of the microtubule, shortening or depolymerization is prevented. The ends of the microtubules are differentiated by the activity that is occurring and are designated as plus and minus. When the microtubule elongates and shortens, it does so primarily at the plus end. The minus end undergoes less pronounced changes in length and is normally attached to a microtubule-organizing center. In a process known as "dynamic instability," the ends go through phases of slow prolonged growth and rapid shortening, such that the overall length changes. In the process of treadmilling, there is growth at one end counterbalanced by shortening at the other, such that the overall length does not change appreciably. Both of these processes are important for the cell to successfully complete mitosis.[123]

As the cell prepares for mitosis, the microtubules that make up the cytoskeleton are degraded and reassembled into the mitotic spindle. During prometaphase, the microtubules grow out from the spindle poles to connect to the kinetochores of the individual chromosomes. This involves both polymerization of tubulin and depolymerization as the microtubule seeks out the chromosome representing a period of dynamic instability. These processes continue as the chromosomes are aligned at the metaphase plate, and during this alignment, treadmilling occurs.[124] Chromosomes are subsequently moved to the spindle poles during anaphase as microtubules attached to the spindle poles shorten and other microtubules known as *intepolar microtubules* lengthen.

The vincas bind to tubulin in a reversible manner at sites different from those at which other inhibitors of spindle function bind including the podophyllotoxins and the taxanes. Combinations of these agents may give synergistic effects because of their unique binding sites. X-ray studies indicate that vinblastine binds between the α- and β-tubulin heterodimers and other studies have shown that there are both high-affinity binding sites located at the end of the spindle and low-affinity sites located along the intact spindle.[125,126] Binding at the high-affinity sites prevents both lengthening and shortening of the spindle and thereby disrupts its function. Both dynamic instability and treadmilling are inhibited by the vinca alkaloids. Binding at low-affinity sites, which occurs at higher drug concentration, leads to breakdown of the spindle as tubulin depolymerizes. Initial binding at these low-affinity sites leads to an alteration in structure that exposes additional vinca-binding sites. The intracellular concentration of the drug then determines which of these effects is seen. As a result of these actions, the mitotic spindle fails to form properly, chromosomes do not move to the metaphase plate, anaphase fails to occur, and the cell undergoes apoptosis.[127] The agents are considered specific for the M phase of the cell cycle. Other activities have been observed including antimetabolite activity, inhibition of protein synthesis, and altered lipid metabolism, but these are only seen at very high concentrations of the drugs. Inhibition of angiogenesis has also been associated with the vinca alkaloids.[128]

Microtubules also play important roles in axons or nerve fibers, and disruption of this function is thought to be responsible for the neuropathies seen with this group of compounds. This seems to be most pronounced for vincristine and presumably represents a greater affinity for this type of microtubule. The specific effects the vincas have on axonal microtubules is not as well defined as it is for the mitotic spindle.

Resistance to the vinca alkaloids occurs by several different mechanisms that are also associated with resistance to several high–molecular-weight molecules with diverse mechanisms of action also used in treating cancer.[129] This multidrug resistance (MDR) is also seen with the taxanes, epipodophyllotoxins, and the anthracyclines although the resistance is usually greatest to the principal agent to which the patient was exposed. The MDR has been associated with several proteins including permeability glycoprotein (Pgp) and multidrug resistance protein (MRP1), which function to actively secrete the molecules from the cell. There are several inhibitors of Pgp such as calcium channel blockers and cyclosporine, which have been investigated to decrease drug efflux; however, these first-generation inhibitors were not successful in reducing drug efflux. There are several newer agents that have proven to be more potent inhibitors of Pgp, but none is currently approved. An additional mechanism of resistance involves altered forms of tubulin to which the vincas fail to bind.

VINBLASTINE SULFATE (VLB, VELBAN, VELSAR)

Vinblastine sulfate is available as a powder in 10-mg vials and as a solution in 10- and 25-mL vials for IV administration in the treatment of various cancers including Hodgkin's disease, lymphocytic lymphoma, histiocytic lymphoma, advanced mycosis fungoides, advanced testicular carcinoma, and Kaposi sarcoma. It has also been used in treating choriocarcinoma and breast cancer when other therapies have failed. Vinblastine is part of the ABVD (adriamycin, bleomycin, vinblastine, and dacarbazine) regimen used in the treatment of Hodgkin's lymphoma. This may be alternated with the MOPP regimen. Extravasation is a concern with the vincas and is treated by administration of hyaluronidase and application of heat. Hyaluronidase hydrolyzes hyaluronic acid, a polysaccharide component of the connective tissue. In so doing, the drug may increase diffusion out of the area of extravasation more quickly, preventing the buildup of toxic levels. Vinblastine is highly protein bound and metabolized by CYP to the 4-*O*-desacetyl metabolite, which has been shown to be active although only small amounts have been recovered in the bile and feces. The metabolism of the vinca alkaloids has not been well characterized. Vinblastine is eliminated primarily in the feces; however, little of the unchanged drug has been recovered. Metabolism appears to involve CYP3A but other than the desacetyl derivative, other metabolites have not been characterized. The elimination half-life for vinblastine is 25 hours. Like vinorelbine, myelosuppression is commonly seen with vinblastine and is dose limiting. Inflammation of the GI tract is more commonly seen with vinblastine than vincristine. Nausea and vomiting may also occur. Other adverse effects include alopecia, secretion of antidiuretic hormone, headache, and depression. Neurotoxicity is mild compared with vincristine, but peripheral neuropathy may be seen. An additional manifestation of this neurotoxicity is hypertension related to disruption of autonomic function.

VINCRISTINE SULFATE (LCR, VCR, LEUROCRISTINE, ONCOVIN)

Vincristine sulfate is available as a 1-mg/mL solution in 1-, 2-, and 5-mL vials for IV administration in acute leukemia and as part of a multidrug regime for Hodgkin's and

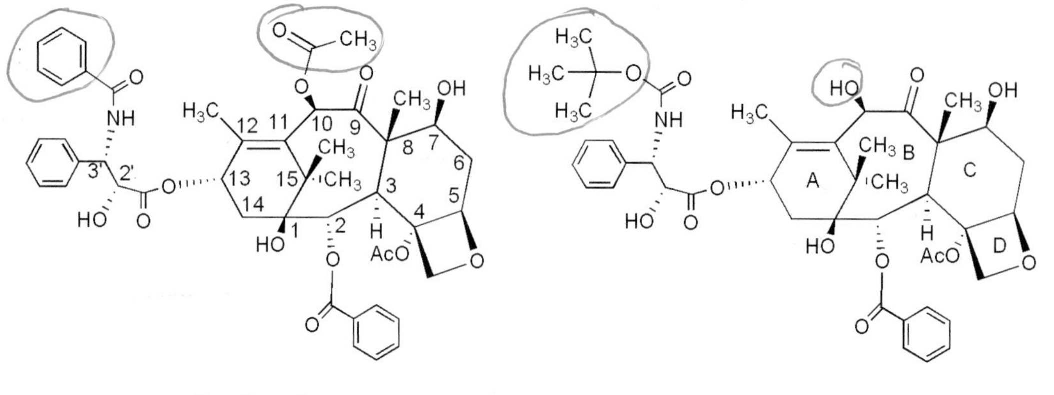

Paclitaxel

Docetaxel

Figure 10.22 • Structures of the taxanes.

non-Hodgkin's lymphoma as well as rhabdomyosarcoma, neuroblastoma, Ewing sarcoma, Wilms tumor, soft tissue sarcoma, testicular cancer, liver cancer, and head and neck cancers. It has also been utilized in treating pediatric cancer. Vincristine is highly protein bound (75%) and may also bind to platelets that contain large amounts of tubulin. Numerous metabolites have been detected and several have been identified, one of which is the 4-O-desacetyl derivative. The metabolism that does occur is believed to largely be mediated by CYP3A. Elimination occurs primarily in the bile with a terminal elimination half-life of 23 to 85 hours. The most commonly seen toxicity for vincristine is a dose-limiting neurotoxicity caused by effects on axonal microtubules. Symptoms are variable and include peripheral neuropathy, ataxia, seizure, bone pain, and coma. Constipation is also a commonly seen toxicity, and laxatives may be used prophylactically. Other toxicities include alopecia, skin rash, mild myelosuppression, secretion of antidiuretic hormone, azospermia, and amenorrhea.

VINORELBINE DITARTRATE (VNB, VRL, NAVELBINE)

Vinorelbine ditartrate is available in 1- and 5-mL vials at a concentration of 10 mg/mL for IV use. It is FDA approved for the treatment of NSCLC. The agent has also been used in treating metastatic breast cancer, cervical cancer, uterine cancer, and lung cancer especially in older patients or those with physical difficulties. Vinorelbine is the most lipophilic of the vinca alkaloids because of modifications of the catharanthine ring system and dehydration of the piperidine ring. This allows the agent to be quickly taken up into cells including lung tissue where concentrations are 300-fold higher than plasma concentrations. This is 3 to 13 times higher than the lung concentrations seen with vincristine. The agent is highly protein bound (80%–91%) and metabolized by CYP3A. The major metabolite seen is the 4-O-desacetyl derivative, which is equally active with the parent but only formed in small quantities. The agent is eliminated primarily (33%–88%) in the bile with some appearing in the urine (16%–30%). The elimination half-life is 27 to 43 hours. The toxicities seen for vinorelbine include myelosuppression, which is dose limiting but ceases upon discontinuation of drug. This is most commonly seen as a neutropenia, and patient's neutrophil count should be monitored prior to and during therapy to decrease the chance of infection. Additional toxicities include nausea/vomiting, elevation of liver function tests, alopecia, generalized fatigue, and inappropriate secretion of antidiuretic hormone. Neurotoxicity is seen with vinorelbine but occurs to a lesser degree compared with other vinca alkaloids because of its decreased affinity for axonal microtubules.

Taxanes

The taxanes, specifically, taxol (or paclitaxel) was discovered in the 1960s as part of a large-scale screening program conducted by the National Cancer Institute on plant extracts.[130] Taxol (Fig. 10.22), isolated from the bark of the pacific yew tree, proved to be active against various cancer models; however, interest in the material waned because of the lack of available material and formulation problems. Interest was renewed as the mechanism of action was elucidated, new sources of material were identified, and the formulation problems were resolved.

The formulation problems seen in the early development of paclitaxel were caused by poor water solubility, which was addressed by the use of Cremophor EL and ethanol as vehicles. Cremophor EL is a polyoxyethylated castor oil, and early experience with this formulation resulted in a high percentage of hypersensitivity reactions including rash, bronchospasm, and hypotension, which were associated with the ability of Cremophor EL to cause histamine release. Administration of antihistamines and corticosteroids prior to paclitaxel administration reduces the percentage of patients experiencing hypersensitivity reactions to 1% to 3%.[131]

The taxanes bind to tubulin at a site distinct from the vinca alkaloids. In the absence of x-ray crystal structures of bound drug, photoaffinity probes of paclitaxel have identified two sites at which binding may occur to β-tubulin. The first site was located at the N-terminus and involved residues 1 to 31. The second site involved residues 217 to 231 of β-tubulin and although these two sites are widely separated in the primary structure, they are close to each other in the tertiary structure.[132] The binding site is located on the luminal side of the microtubule and located in the middle of the β-tubulin subunit. Docetaxel binds to the same site with greater affinity. Binding of taxanes at low concentration results in stabilization of the microtubule and prevents depolymerization. At higher concentrations, polymerization is enhanced, and the normal equilibrium between free tubulin and polymer is modified. The taxanes inhibit both treadmilling and dynamic instability, and cells are most affected in the M phase when microtubule dynamics are undergoing the greatest change. Mitosis is blocked at the metaphase anaphase boundary, and cells undergo apoptosis.[133] Paclitaxel has also been shown to enhance phosphorylation of a serine residue of Bcl-2, an antiapoptotic protein resulting in inhibition of Bcl-2's ability to block apoptosis. The proapoptotic proteins Bad and Bax are stimulated and in a similar manner, docetaxel has been shown to induce apoptosis by activation of caspase enzymes.[134]

Resistance to the taxanes is like that seen for the vinca alkaloids and other agents and involves Pgp-mediated efflux. Alterations in the structure of β-tubulin may also occur and result in decreased binding of taxanes to the microtubules and therefore reduced cytotoxicity.

PACLITAXEL (TAX, TAXOL)

Paclitaxel is available in single-dose vials of 30 mg/5 mL and 100 mg/16.7 mL for IV administration in the treatment of breast, ovarian, NSCLC, and AIDS-related Kaposi sarcoma. Other uses have included treatment of head, neck, esophageal, cervical, prostate, and bladder cancers.

Paclitaxel is highly plasma protein bound (>90%) and does not penetrate the CNS. Metabolism involves CYP-mediated oxidation to give 6α-hydroxypaclitaxel (CYP2C8) and para hydroxylation of the phenyl group attached to the 3'-position (CYP3A4). The 6α-hydroxy metabolite normally predominates, but the para hydroxy metabolite may occur to a greater degree in those patients with liver disease or when CYP3A4 has been induced. Both metabolites are less active than the parent and do not undergo phase II conjugation reactions. Elimination occurs primarily in the feces, and the elimination half-life is 9 to 50 hours depending on the infusion period.

The major toxicity seen with paclitaxel is a dose-limiting myelosuppression that normally presents as neutropenia. The previously mentioned hypersensitivity reactions occur but are greatly reduced by antihistamine pretreatment. Interaction with the axonal microtubules such as that seen for the vincas also occurs and leads to numbness and paresthesias (abnormal touch sensations including burning and prickling). The agent is also available as an albumin-bound formulation (Abraxane) to eliminate the need for the solubilizing agents associated with the hypersensitivity reactions. Other adverse effects include bradycardia, which may progress to heart block, alopecia, mucositis, and/or diarrhea. Paclitaxel produces moderate nausea and vomiting that is short-lived.

DOCETAXEL (TXT, TAXOTERE)

Docetaxel is available in single-dose vials of 20 mg/0.5 mL and 80 mg/2 mL for IV administration in the treatment of breast, NSCLC, and prostate cancers. It has also been utilized in non–FDA-approved treatment of head, neck, gastric, bladder, and refractory ovarian cancers.

Docetaxel is highly plasma protein bound (80%) and widely distributed with the highest concentration in the hepatobiliary system, but it does not appear to cross the blood-brain barrier. The metabolism of docetaxel has been less well studied than that of paclitaxel. The use of human liver microsomes has indicated that metabolism involves oxidation of one of the *tert*-butyl methyl groups of the C-13 side chain to initially give the alcohol. Further oxidation to the aldehyde and carboxylic acid both of which may cyclize with the carbamate nitrogen to give stereoisomeric hydroxyoxazolidinones and an oxazolidinedione, respectively. No active metabolites have been identified. The major enzyme involved is CYP3A4. The drug is primarily eliminated in the feces with a terminal half-life of 11 hours.

The adverse effects profile for docetaxel is similar to that of paclitaxel but also includes reversible fluid retention that is dose related. This has been associated with an initial increase in capillary permeability followed by a decrease in lymphatic drainage later in the therapy. Restriction of sodium intake and pretreatment with corticosteroids is usually successful in minimizing this adverse effect. Peripheral neuropathy is seen with docetaxel but occurs less often than with paclitaxel. Fatigue and muscle pain are commonly seen, and fever may occur in up to 30% of patients who are infection free.

IXABEPILONE (AZAEPOTHILONE B, IXEMPRA)

The epothilones are macrocyclic lactones that have a mechanism of action similar to that of the taxanes but offer several advantages (Fig. 10.23).[135] Ixabepilone is the semisynthetic amide analog of epothilone B that is isolated from the myxobacterium *Sorangium cellulosum*. The epothilones showed potent in vitro activity but greatly decreased activity in vivo caused by metabolic instability via hydrolysis of the macrocyclic lactone. Conversion to the lactam increased stability and maintained in vivo activity. Ixabepilone has been recently (2007) approved for the treatment of metastatic breast cancer that is resistant to the taxanes. The agent is believed to bind to the same site occupied by the taxanes. Molecular modeling studies have been utilized to identify a common pharmacophore between the taxanes and epothilones.[136] Key structural components that assume comparable relative position are indicated in Table 10.2. Like the taxanes, ixabepilone binds to β-tubulin and stabilizes microtubules resulting in cell death. The agent is useful in cancers that have become resistant to the taxanes, because it is not removed by Pgp and is still capable of binding

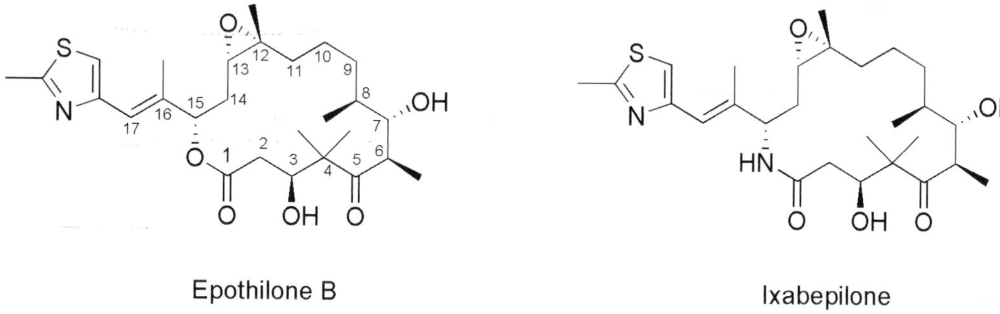

Epothilone B

Ixabepilone

Figure 10.23 ● Structures of epithilones.

TABLE 10.2 **Functional Groups Yielding Analogous Microtubule Binding in Paclitaxel and Epothilone B**

Paclitaxel	Epothilone B
C-15 gem-dimethyl	C-4 gem-dimethyl
C-1 OH	C-3 OH
C-9 carbonyl	C-7 OH
C-5 oxetane-oxygen	C-12,13 epoxide oxygen
C-3′ phenyl ring	C-17 thiazole ring

to altered beta tubulin to which the taxanes no longer bind. Increased water solubility also allows the agent to be administered without the need for Cremophor EL, reducing the chance of hypersensitivity reactions. The current indications for the agent are in metastatic breast cancer in combination with capecitabine after the failure of an anthracycline and a taxane and as monotherapy in metastatic breast cancer after failure of an anthracycline, a taxane, and capecitabine. The agent is extensively metabolized in the liver primarily by CYP3A4 to give over 30 different metabolites. Elimination occurs primarily in the feces (65%) with a smaller amount (21%) occurring in the urine. The terminal elimination half-life is 52 hours. Major toxicities associated with the use of ixabepilone have included peripheral neuropathy and myelosuppression occurring as neutropenia. Occurring less frequently are alopecia, nausea, vomiting, mucositis, diarrhea, and muscle pain.

MITOMYCIN C

Mitomycin C (Fig. 10.24) was isolated from *Streptomyces caespitosus* in 1958 by Japanese workers and is considered the prototype of the bioreductive alkylating agents.[137–139] Mitomycin is sometimes included as an alkylating agent but is included here because it is a naturally occurring material. The drug contains what would appear to be reactive functionalities, including the quinone and aziridine functionalities, both or which would be thought to be susceptible to nucleophilic attack; however, the reactivity of these functionalities is reduced because of steric and electronic effects in the parent molecule. It was reasoned that selective activation could be achieved in a reductive environment such as that found in an area of low oxygen content. This is known to occur in tumors where the fast-growing cells often grow beyond the blood supply that would normally provide oxygen.[140] A normal cell would undergo apoptosis under these conditions, but because cancer cells often have their apoptotic mechanisms inhibited they continue to survive with little or no oxygen available. Mitomycin C is capable of being activated and alkylating DNA in an anaerobic environ-

ment, but there is actually little selectivity for hypoxic cells. Activation can occur enzymatically by both one- and two-electron processes. Reductive enzymes such as NADPH-CYP reductase and DT-diaphorase have been implicated in these processes.[141] Involvement of one-electron processes such as those seen for the anthracylines result in redox cycling and the production of ROS that may result in DNA damage, but the cytotoxicity of mitomycin C is primarily associated with its ability to alkylate DNA. The hydroquinone can result from a single two-electron process or a one-electron process followed by disproportionation to give the hydroquinone (Scheme 10.30).[142–144] The electrons of the amine are no longer withdrawn by the quinone system and are now free to expel methoxide followed by loss of a proton to give the leuco-aziridinomitosene. This reduction renders positions C-1 and C-10 reactive to nucleophilic attack because of the fact that there are leaving groups attached, and they are now benzylic positions so that the intermediate carbocations can be stabilized. Several pathways are possible from this point, and the specific route is dependent on the conditions in the cell. Shown in Scheme 10.30 is one possible pathway that occurs under more acidic conditions and results in the formation of interstrand and intrastrand cross-links. Protonation of the aziridine is followed by ring opening to give the carbocation, which can be stabilized by resonance involving the hydroquinone system. Nucleophiles on DNA may attack at C-1 with concomitant electron movement. This can be repeated in a similar manner at C-10, which allows for cross-linking. There are several other possibilities under different conditions. DNA is alkylated by mitomycin C at both the N-2 and N-7 positions of guanine

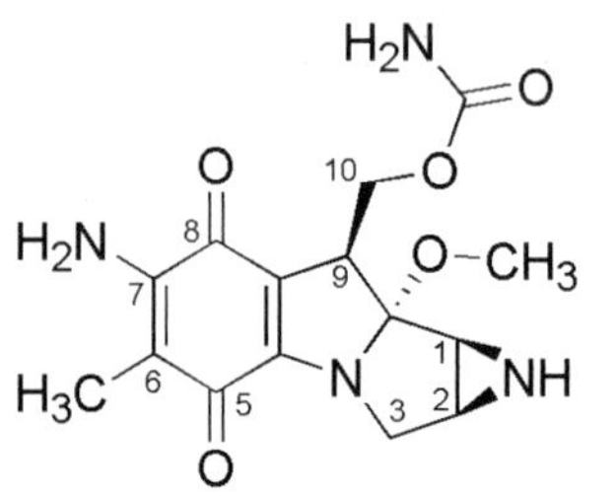

MITOMYCIN C (MITC, MTC, MUTAMYCIN)

Mitomycin C is available in 5-, 20-, and 40-mg vials for IV administration in the treatment of cancers of the stomach and pancreas when other treatments have failed. Other uses have included breast, NSCLC, cervical, bladder, and head and neck cancers. Mechanisms of resistance include increased synthesis of nucleophilic detoxifying compounds such as glutathione, decreased expression of activating enzymes such as DT-diaphorase, and increased efflux by Pgp. The drug is rapidly cleared from the plasma after administration and widely distributed but does not cross the blood-brain barrier. The parent and metabolites are excreted mainly in the feces with an elimination half-life of 50 minutes. Adverse effects include dose-limiting myelosuppression, mild nausea and vomiting, mucositis, anorexia, fatigue, and interstitial pneumonitis.

⬡ PROTEIN KINASE INHIBITORS

In the last several years, several new treatment options have become available based on increased knowledge of growth factors and cell signaling. Although these agents have provided great benefit in some cases and their utility is still being determined, it is important to remember that in many cases they are used in combination with more traditional chemotherapeutic agents to achieve a better outcome. The traditional agents are often used in combination as well in attempts to increase success and prevent resistance.

Figure 10.24 ● Structure of mitomycin C.

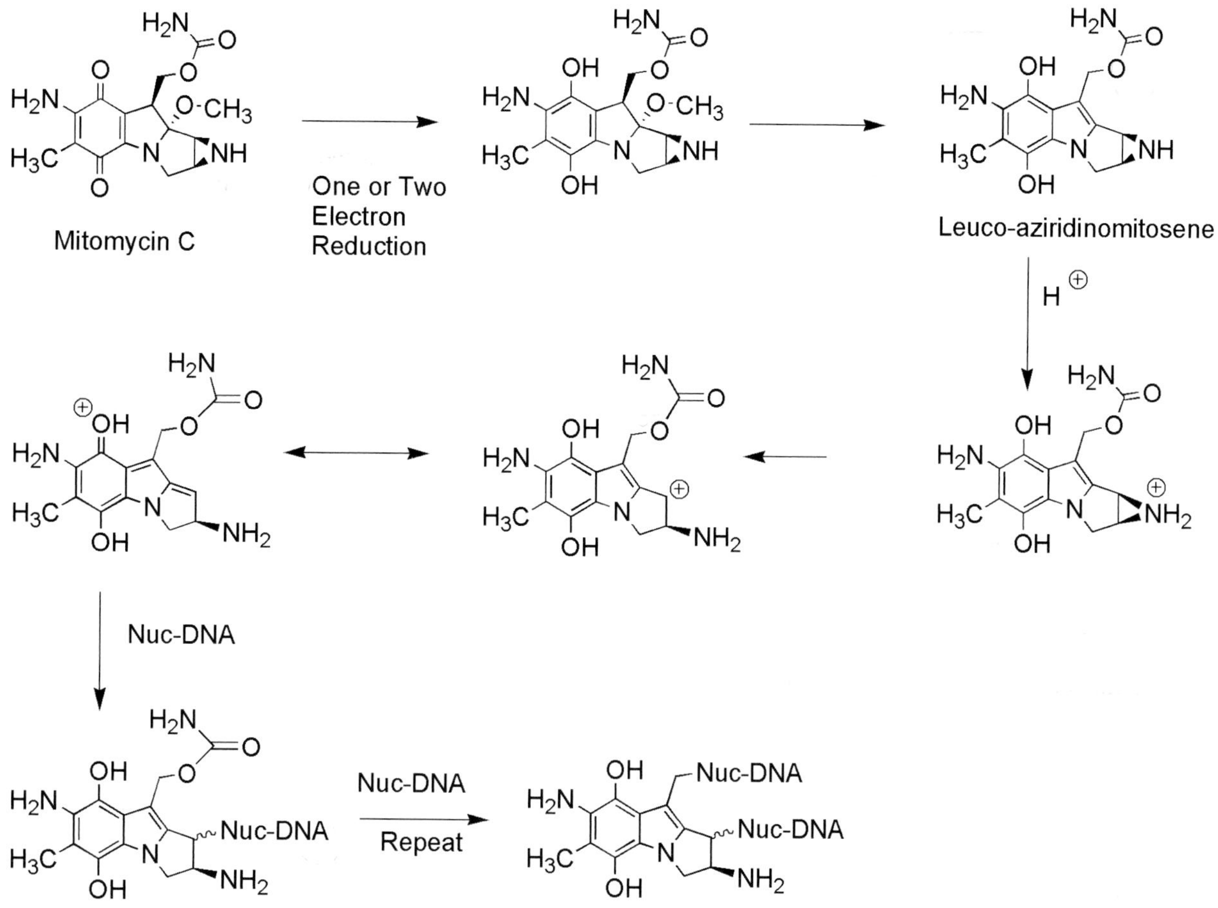

Scheme 10.30 ● Alkylation of DNA by mitomycin C.

It was realized early on that the growth and proliferation of many tissues was under the control of the endocrine system, in which endocrine glands secreted hormones and that hormones or their antagonists were useful in controlling the overgrowth of these tissues. It was found later that other growth factors, many of which were secreted by nearby cells, were also involved in controlling the growth and proliferation of the target tissue and this became known as *paracrine control*. Many of these growth factors have been identified and several along with their receptors are indicated in Table 10.3.[144]

These receptors have become targets for several different monoclonal antibodies that have been recently introduced.

TABLE 10.3 Growth Factors and Receptors of Paracrine Origin

Growth Factor	Designation	Receptor
Epidermal growth factor	EGF	EGF-R
Platelet-derived growth factor	PDGF	PDGF-R
Nerve growth factor	NGF	Trk
Vascular endothelial growth factor	VEGF	VEGF-R
Stem cell factor	SCF	Kit
Glial cell line–derived neurotropic factor	GFL	RET

Further work identified the pathways by which interaction with these cell surface receptors resulted in growth and proliferation of cells. There are various mechanisms by which these processes occur, but a generalized pathway involves interaction of a growth factor with a growth factor receptor occurring as a monomer present in the phospholipid bilayer of the cell membrane, which results in dimerization of the receptors (Scheme 10.31). The receptors themselves possess an extracellular-binding domain for interaction with the growth factors, an intracellular domain, and a connecting transmembrane region. The intracellular domain of these receptor proteins often function as kinases, many of which are TKs that phosphorylate residues on the other monomer receptor. The resulting phosphorylated residues are recognized by the Src homology 2 domain (SH2) of cytoplasmic proteins such as Shc, Grb-2, and Sos, which activate Ras. These cytoplasmic proteins then serve to transmit the growth signals from the growth factor receptors to Ras (Fig. 10.25). Ras is a G protein tethered to the cytoplasmic membrane, which may bind GTP resulting in activation of Ras or bind GDP resulting in Ras inactivation. Ras also normally has the ability to hydrolyze GTP to inactivate itself. Many cancers are found to have altered forms of Ras, which is present in a hyperactive state. Ras, in its activated form activates a series of kinases, many of which are TKs with various effects on cells. Notable is the Ras-Raf-MEK-ERK pathway also known as the *mitogen-activated protein kinase* (MAPK) pathway. This is a

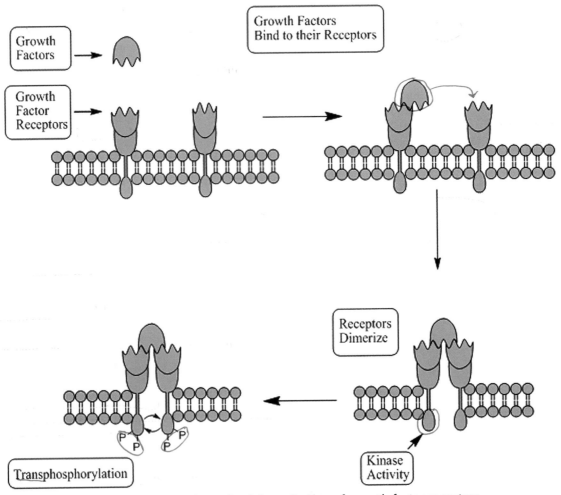

Scheme 10.31 ● Schematic of the activation of growth factor receptors.

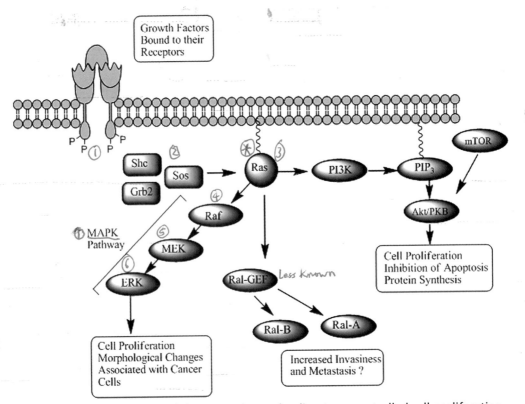

Figure 10.25 ● Schematic of the Ras pathways leading to uncontrolled cell proliferation.

cascade effect, whereby one kinase phosphorylates and activates more of the next kinase in the pathway amplifying the signal in the process. Stimulation of this pathway results in the activation of several transcription factors involved in the expression of growth factors, cyclin D1 (involved in controlling cell division, see Fig. 10.1), and transcription factors Fos and Jun, which were first discovered as viral oncogenes and are known to be elevated in several human cancers. In addition, overactivation of this pathway may result in loss of contact inhibition, loss of anchorage dependence, and changes in cell shape, all of which are characteristic of cancer cells.

The second major pathway activated by Ras is PI3K-PIP3-Akt/PKB whose activation increases cell proliferation but perhaps most importantly, inhibits apoptosis. When Ras is activated, phosphatidylinositol(4,5)-diphosphate (PIP_2) is further phosphorylated to give phosphatidylinositol(3,4,5)-triphosphate PIP_3, which remains embedded in the plasma membrane but attracts and activates other kinases namely protein kinase B (PKB), a serine-threonine kinase. Overactivity of this pathway results in decreased apoptosis, increased proliferation and increased cell size. Specific effects include inactivation of the proapoptotic protein Bad (Fig. 10.2) and activation of antiapoptotic NF-κB.

The third pathway involves Ras-mediated activation of Ral-GEF (Guanine nucleotide exchange factor), which acts on Ral-A and Ral-B to stimulate their exchange of GDP for GTP and hence their activation. The activation of this pathway, although less well understood, seems to allow cancer cells to metastasize and invade.

Overactivity of these pathways is present in several different cancers, and consequently, several agents have been developed to correct this. One such approach is the inhibition of kinases whose normal activity has been amplified.

Working in Philadelphia in the 1960s, scientists discovered a genetic abnormality present in 95% of patients with CML.[145] The abnormality was a translocation between chromosomes 22 and 9 in which the *ABL* gene (analogous to the Abelson proto-oncogene found in mice) originally on chromosome 9 was translocated to chromosome 22, such that it was fused with BCR gene (breakpoint cluster region). The new chromosome was designated as the Philadelphia translocation or the Philadelphia chromosome (Ph[1]).[146] The fusion of these two genes resulted in a protein that encoded the entire ABL gene and as many as three additional proteins from BCR. The product of this fusion was found to be a TK that was always activated. This altered TK utilizes ATP to phosphorylate and activate numerous pathways including MAPK and Akt/PKB along with several others. This leads to proliferation of white cells that normally lasts about a year, when the disease becomes more difficult to treat and eventually to the terminal blast phase lasting several months.

Imatinib (Fig. 10.26) was developed to specifically inhibit this unique TK and does so rather selectively by binding to the ATP-binding pocket and stabilizing an inactive form of the enzyme. Protein kinases have similar structures and consist of C- and N-terminal lobes with the active site formed by a cleft between the two lobes. The activity of the enzyme is regulated by an activation loop that is extended in the active form of the enzyme and provides for substrate binding. X-ray crystal studies of imatinib binding to Abl show that the drug binds in the cleft formed by the two lobes of the enzyme through the formation of several hydrogen bonds and hydrophobic interactions with the pyridine ring assuming the postion occupied by ATP in the active enzyme.[147] Imatinib binding locks the enzyme in a conformation in which the activation loop is oriented so as to block substrate binding. Specificity for the BCR-ABL kinase is not complete because of structural similarity of TKs, and those associated with the PDGF receptor and the receptor for SCF known as KIT are also inhibited (Table 10.3). The agent has been found to be effective in 90% of patients in the chronic stage (the chronic stage last 4–6 years and precedes the proliferation stage mentioned previously). Blast-phase patients respond at a rate of 60% but usually relapse after several months.[148]

The tremendous success of imatinib led to other agents that could be used in the case of resistance. Specifically, dasatinib can bind to either an active or inactive form of the enzyme and is 100 times more potent compared with imatinib. It has the ability to overcome resistance associated with amino acid alterations that leads to decreased affinity for imatinib. As the structure is altered, binding to other TKs (BCR-ABL, PDGF, SRC, KIT) is manifested, which may eventually lead to other indications but at this time, it is used primarily in those cases when patients fail to respond to imatinib.[149]

This general idea of targeting TKs was extended to the EGF receptor. It was hoped that by targeting EGF TKs the inhibitors would be applicable to a wide range of cancers. Recall that after the receptors dimerize, they transphosphorylate each other and act as TKs. Currently, there are two structurally similar agents in use, gefitinib and erlotinib, which bind to the ATP-binding site and thereby inhibit the resulting cascade that would normally occur from activation of the EGF receptor.[150,151] The benefit of the agents was hoped to be caused by inhibition to the Ras pathway so that ultimately, all three arms could be affected (MAPK, Akt/PKB, and Ral-GEF). The agents are modestly selective for this kinase. Currently both compounds have indications for NSCLC generally as alternatives after the failure of more traditional therapy, and gefitinib has an additional indication against pancreatic cancer. Initial results have not been as dramatic as that seen with imatinib. There are also several known mutations and deletions in the EGF receptor of cancer patients and this may affect the activity of these compounds. Specifically, point mutations in the *KRAS* gene (a member of the Ras family) have been associated with resistance to these agents and tests have become available to detect this prior to initiating therapy.

The activation of numerous tyrosine and serine-threonine kinases offers many theoretical targets for drug intervention when these pathways become overactive as is often the case in neoplastic cells. These kinase enzymes are all thought to have evolved from a common ancestor and as such possess a great deal of structural similarity that complicates the development of agents, which are selective for a single kinase. This has led to the strategy of simultaneously inhibiting numerous kinase enzymes, and consequently there are several multikinase inhibitors now available. Sorafenib was originally developed using high-throughput testing and parallel synthesis as an inhibitor of the serine-threonine kinase Raf.[152] It proved to be a potent inhibitor of this enzyme with an $IC_{50} = 6$ nM and acted by stabilizing an inactive form of

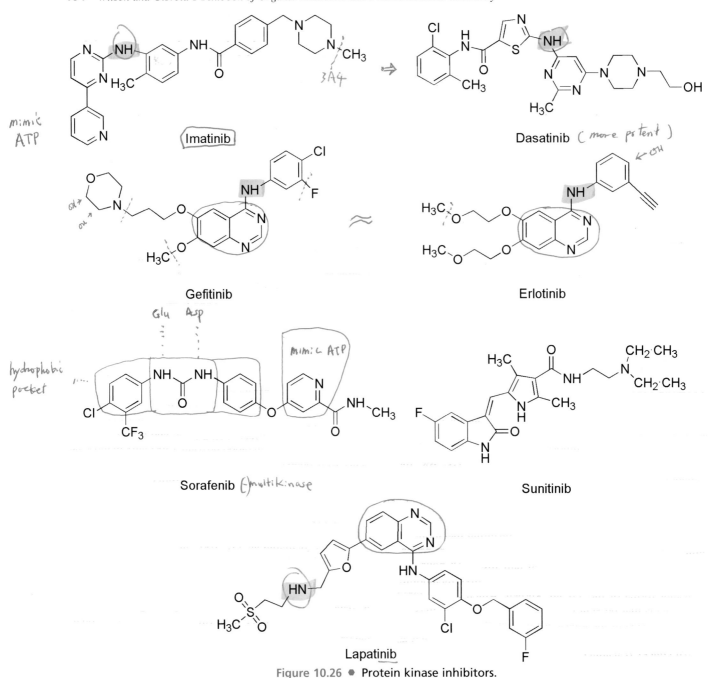

Figure 10.26 ● Protein kinase inhibitors.

the enzyme similar to imatinib. Subsequent x-ray analysis of the drug receptor complex showed that the pyridine ring occupied the ATP-binding site of Raf, whereas the trifluoromethyl-chloro–substituted phenyl ring occupied a hydrophobic pocket in the cleft formed by the two lobes of the protein.[153] The urea moiety forms two hydrogen bonds, one through interaction of the amide proton with the carboxylate of Glu500 and the second through interaction of the carbonyl oxygen with the peptide amide N-H of Asp593. The compound also has the capacity to inhibit several other TKs associated with growth factor receptors including PDGF-R, VEGF-R, RET-kinase, and c-Kit with IC50s in the range of 20 to 90 nM. In some cancer models, the compound has been shown to be effective even though the MAPK pathway was not inhibited and this has been explained by the compounds inhibition of angiogenesis. This has been attributed to the effects on inhibition of PDGF-R and VEGF-R phosphorylation and the role these growth factor receptors play in the creation of new blood vessels. The agent was investigated and subsequently approved for use in renal cell carcinoma (RCC) because of the fact that this particular cancer is often associated with increased activity of the targets inhibited by sorafenib and the high level of neoangiogenesis that is seen in this cancer.

As a group of agents, the protein kinase inhibitors have the advantage of oral administration and better patient tolerability. The major adverse effects include a skin rash that normally appears early in therapy on the upper torso and is generally mild but may become more serious in some cases. Mild diarrhea and nausea are also commonly seen but are generally controlled with the administration of antiemetics and antidiarrheals. Mild myelosuppression is also seen with several of these agents. There has been concern about cardiotoxicity associated with protein kinase inhibitors because of the fact that multiple kinases may be inhibited. This could potentially have several effects on signaling processes in cardiac tissue. For example if the Akt/PKB pathway was blocked, apoptosis may become activated and cardiac cells would die (Table 10.3). There has been some evidence for cardiotoxicity in this class and the agents have been ranked with imatinib, dasatinib, sorafenib, and sunitinib having known or likely cardiotoxicity and gefitinib, erlotinib, and lapatinib having low cardiotoxicity. Concern of cardiotoxicity is also a result of the fact that other drugs such as the anthracyclines and several of the monoclonal antibodies directed against the EGF-R are known to have cardiotoxicity associated with their use.[154] Therefore, patients who have already been exposed to these agents may experience additional adverse effects to their cardiovascular system if a protein kinase inhibitor were utilized and it also produced significant cardiotoxicity. Studies for the most part have not evaluated the cardiotoxicity of these agents and the given ranking is based on preliminary data, but there is concern about the cardiovascular effects of this class of agents.

IMATINIB MESYLATE (STI-571, GLEEVEC)

Imatinib is available in 100- and 400-mg capsules for oral administration and is indicated for the treatment of CML, gastrointestinal stromal tumors (GIST) that express Kit and acute lymphoplastic leukemia that is positive for the Philadelphia chromosome.

Bioavailability of the agent is nearly 100% by the oral route. The agent is highly protein bound and metabolized to the *N*-desmethyl derivative by CYP3A4-mediated removal of the piperazinyl methyl group. The resulting metabolite is similar to the parent in activity. Elimination occurs primarily in the feces, and the terminal half-life is 18 hours for the parent and 40 hours of the *N*-desmethyl metabolite. Resistant forms of the TK are known, which have altered amino acids that prevent binding. In addition, there may be increased levels of the kinase itself. The drug is also a substrate for Pgp and an additional efflux transporter known as *breast cancer resistance protein* (BCRP), both of which remove the drug from the cell. These transporters are also inhibited by the agent as well. Severe side effects include ascites, neutropenia, thrombocytopenia, skin rash, and pulmonary edema. Less serious side effects include nausea/vomiting, heartburn, and headache but overall, the agent is better tolerated than most other medications used in treating the disease.

DASATINIB (BMS-354825, SPRYCEL)

Dasatinib is available in 20-, 50-, and 70-mg tablets for oral administration in the treatment of CML and ALL that are Ph[1] positive. Although dasatinib is more potent than imatinib, bioavailability is much lower with values ranging between 14% to 34%. The agent is extensively metabolized with as many as 29 metabolites seen as result of oxidation by primarily CYP3A4 and phase II conjugation. The agent may act as an inhibitor of CYP3A4 and CYP2C8. Metabolism does give an active metabolite, but

this accounts for only 5% of the total and is not believed to be important for the overall activity of the agent. Dasatinib is 95% protein bound with a terminal half-life of 3 to 5 hours. The majority of the drug and metabolites are eliminated in the feces. The most common side effects are skin rash, nausea, diarrhea, and fatigue. Serious side effects include myelosuppression appearing as neutropenia and thrombocytopenia, bleeding of the brain and GI tract, and fluid retention.

GEFITINIB (ZD1839, IRESSA)

Geftinib is available as 250-mg tablets for oral administration in the treatment of NSCLC for those patients who have failed to respond to platinum-based therapies and docetaxel and has also been used against squamous cell cancers of the head and neck. The agent is an inhibitor of the TK of EGF-R and possibly other TKs as well. Gefitinib is both a substrate and inhibitor of Pgp and BCRP. The agent is absorbed slowly after being administered orally with 60% bioavailability. Metabolism occurs in the liver and is mediated primarily by CYP3A4 to give eight identified metabolites resulting from defluorination of the phenyl ring, oxidative-*O*-demethylation, and multiple products arising as a result of oxidation of the morpholine ring. The *O*-demethylated product represents the predominate metabolite and is 14-fold less active compared with the parent. The parent and metabolites are eliminated in the feces with a terminal elimination half-life of 48 hours. The drug appears to be well tolerated with the most commonly reported side effects being rash and diarrhea. It may also cause elevations in blood pressure especially in those patients with preexisting hypertension, elevation of transaminase levels, and mild nausea and mucositits.

ERLOTINIB HYDROCHLORIDE (CP-358,774, TARCEVA)

Erlotinib is available as 25-, 100-, and 150-mg tablets for oral administration and is used after failure of first-line therapy in metastatic NSCLC and as first-line therapy in combination with gemcitabine in the treatment of metastatic pancreatic cancer, and in treating malignant gliomas. The structural similarity to gefitnib imparts similar pharmacokinetic behavior with bioavailability of 60% and protein binding of 93%. The agent is extensively metabolized primarily by CYP3A4. Three major metabolic pathways have been identified, involving oxidative-*O*-demethylation of the side chains followed by further oxidation to give the carboxlic acids, oxidation of the acetylene functionality to give a carboxylic acid, and aromatic hydroxylation of the phenyl ring para to the electron-donating nitrogen. The metabolites are primarily eliminated in the feces, and the terminal half-life is 36 hours.[155] The major toxicities seen with the agent are dose-limiting skin rash and diarrhea. Other common adverse effects include shortness of breath, fatigue, and nausea.

SORAFENIB TOSYLATE (BAY 43-9006, NEXAVAR)

Sorafenib is available in 200-mg tablets for oral administration and is used in the treatment of RCC and colon cancer. The agent is classified as a multikinase inhibitor because of its action on numerous kinase enzymes including the PDGF-R, VEGF-R, Kit, and Raf. Sorafenib is 39% to 48%

bioavailable and CYP3A4-mediated metabolism gives eight identified metabolites including the N-oxide, which is equally active with the parent. However, the majority of the drug in plasma is present as the parent compound. Sorafenib is highly protein bound (99.5%). The drug is eliminated primarily in the feces (77%) with 19% appearing in the urine as glucuronides (UGT1A1) and has a elimination half-life of 24 to 48 hours. The most commonly seen toxicity is skin rash that normally occurs within the first 6 weeks of therapy. Other adverse effects include hypertension, fatigue, increased wound healing time, and increased risk of bleeding.

LAPATINIB DITOSYLATE (GSK572016, TYKERB)

Lapatinib is available in 250-mg tablets for oral administration and is used in combination with cabecitabine in the treatment of breast cancer for those patients that over express the type 2 EGF-R and who have previously received taxane, anthracycline, and trastuzumab therapy. The type 2 EGF-R is one subtype of this receptor and is also known as HER2 or ErbB-2. The agent is a receptor TK inhibitor targeting the ErbB-1 and ErbB-2 subtypes. Binding occurs at the ATP-binding site and thereby prevents phosphorylation and the subsequent activation of other kinase enzymes. ErbB-1 overexpression occurs in approximately 27% to 30% of breast cancers, while ErbB-2 is over expressed in 20% to 25% of cases.[156] The agent has demonstrated IC_{50} values of <0.2 μM against ErbB-1 and 2 from several different cancer cell lines and dissociates slowly ($t_{1/2} = 300$ min) from these receptor TKs.[157] The drug is both a substrate and an inhibitor of the efflux transporters Pgp and BCRP. It is also an inhibitor of the hepatic uptake transporter OATP1B1, which is an organic anion transporter.[158] The absorption of lapatinib is incomplete and variable after oral administration. The agent is extensively metabolized by CYP3A4 and CYP3A5, with minor contributions from CYP2C19 and CYP2C8. Lapatinib inhibits CYP3A and CYP2C8 at clinically relevant concentrations. The agent is highly (99%) protein bound and eliminated primarily in the feces. The half-life of the agent increase upon repeated dosing, taking 6 days to reach steady state that gives an effective half-life of 24 hours. The most commonly seen adverse effects of lapatinib therapy are skin rash and diarrhea. Skin rash is commonly seen with many of the other TK inhibitors and agents that target ErbB-1. Lapatinib-induced diarrhea is usually mild to moderate. There have been reports of decreases in left ventricular ejection fraction associated with the agent, although this appears to occur only rarely and is reversible upon discontinuation of therapy.

SUNITINIB MALATE (SU11248, SUTENT)

Sunitinib is available in 12.5-, 25-, and 50-mg capsules for oral administration for the treatment of advanced RCC and GIST upon the failure of imatinib. The agent is a multikinase inhibitor and has been shown to inhibit PDGF-R, VEGF-R, Kit, RET, and the colony-stimulating factor receptor (CSR-1R). The result of this spectrum of activity is a slowing of tumor progression and inhibition of angiogenesis both of which are useful in the highly vascularized cancers, RCC and GIST. The median TTP (time to tumor progression) was 27.3 weeks for sunitinib and 6.4 weeks

for placebo. Progression-free survival was also significant with a median time of 24.1 weeks for sunitinib and 6 weeks for placebo. The agent is well absorbed upon oral administration, and both the parent and major metabolite are highly (90%–95%) protein bound. Metabolism is mediated primarily by CYP3A4 to give the N-desethyl derivative, which is the major metabolite (23%–37%), equally active with the parent and undergoes further metabolism by CYP3A4. The terminal elimination half-life for the parent and N-desethyl derivative are 40 to 60 hours and 80 to 110 hours, respectively. Elimination occurs primarily via the feces. Common adverse effects of sunitinib include fatigue, diarrhea, yellow skin discoloration, anorexia, nausea, and mucositis. Mild myelosuppression has been reported in patients with GIST including neutropenia, lymphopenia, thrombocytopenia, and anemia. There have been reports of cardiotoxicity including decreases in left ventricular ejection fraction, which occurred in 11% of patients during a GIST study.

MISCELLANEOUS COMPOUNDS

TEMSIROLIMUS (CCI-779, TORISEL)

Temsirolimus (Fig. 10.27) is an esterified derivative of rapamycin and in a similar manner binds initially to the protein FKBP-12(FK506-binding protein).[159] This complex then acts to inhibit the mammalian target of rapamycin (mTOR), a serine-threonine kinase that plays a crucial role in cell division. It is somewhat unique in its method of kinase inhibition, because it actually binds to an allosteric modulator of the kinase rather than just binding to the ATP-binding site like most other kinase inhibitors. Binding of temsirolimus inhibits the phosphorylating activity of mTOR. As shown in Table 10.3, mTOR regulates the Akt/PKB pathway, and therefore, one way in which the agent acts is to inhibit this pathway. An additional mechanism involves the ability of mTOR to initiate protein synthesis independent of the Akt/PKB pathway. Blockade of mTOR results in inhibition of protein synthesis and prevents the cell from moving past the G_1 phase into the S phase. More specifically, mTOR is prevented from phosphorylating 4E-binding protein-1(4E-BP1) an initiating factor and 40S ribosomal protein S6 kinase (p70S6 kinase), both of which are involved in initiating protein synthesis necessary for the cell cycle. In addition, mTOR is involved in the control of several growth factors such VEGF, PDGF, and TGF, which are involved in cell growth and angiogenesis. Temsirolimus is available as a 25-mg/mL injection for IV administration in the treatment of advanced RCC. The agent is extensively metabolized and undergoes rapid hydrolysis of the ester function to give rapamycin that retains activity.[160] Additional metabolism is mediated primarily by CYP3A4 to give several hydroxylated and demethylated metabolites that are inactive. The agent and metabolites are eliminated primarily in the feces with half-lives of 17 and 55 hours for temsirolimus and rapamycin, respectively. This agent, like rapamycin, possesses immunosuppressant properties and there is an increased risk of infection. The most serious side effects are interstitial lung disease, perforation of the bowel, and acute renal failure although these occur only rarely. The most commonly seen side

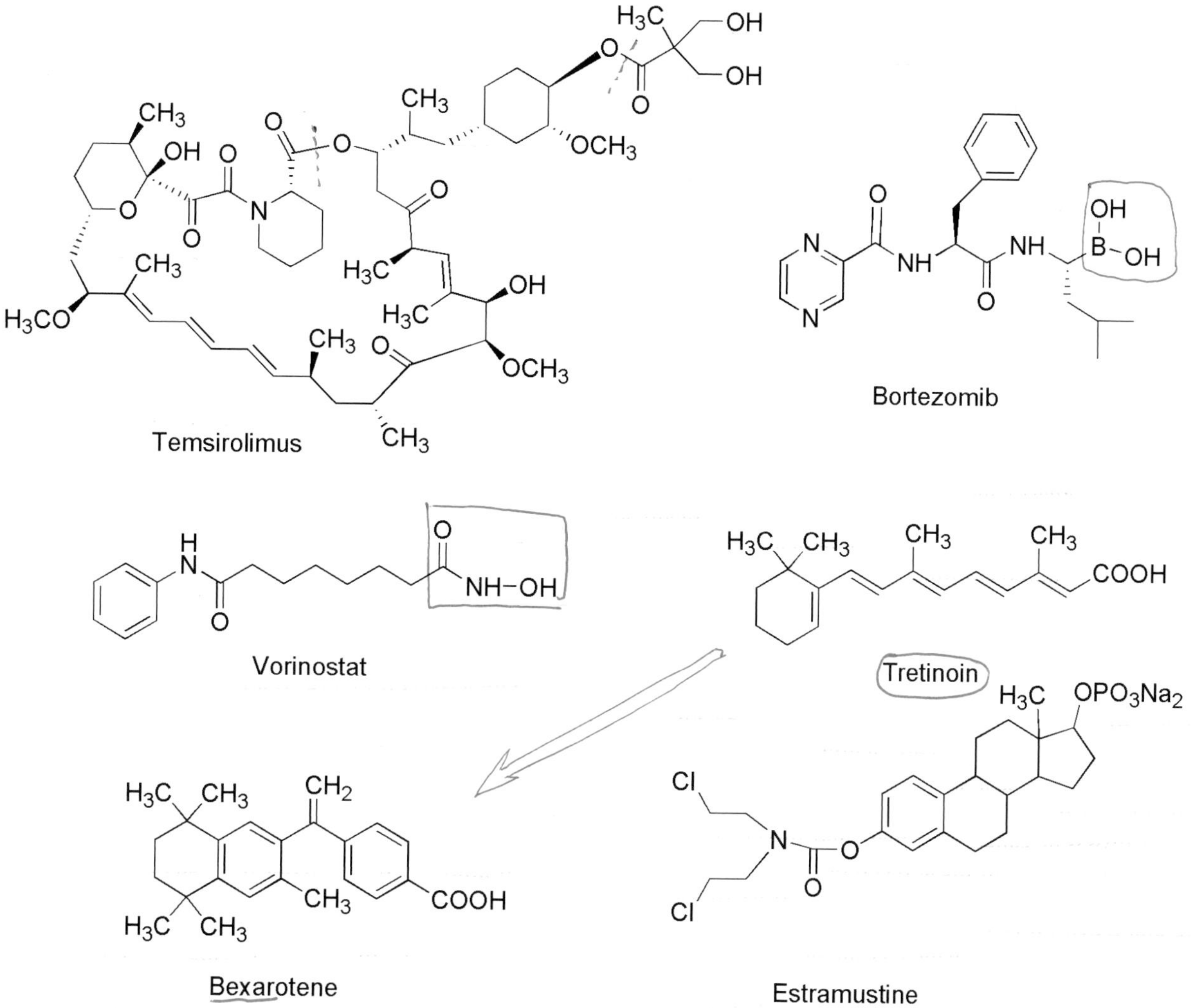

Figure 10.27 ● Miscellaneous antineoplastic agents.

effects are rash, weakness, mucositis, nausea, edema, and anorexia.

BORTEZOMIB (VELCADE)

Proteasomes normally function to degrade proteins that are no longer needed by the cell. Such proteins are normally marked by the addition of ubiquitin, a 76 amino acid protein that is added to the ε-amino group of lysine residues on the target proteins. The marked proteins are then hydrolyzed by the large barrel-shaped proteasomes to give peptides of 7 to 8 residues that may be further hydrolyzed and reutilized by the cell. This process serves to regulate protein levels within the cell, remove defective proteins, and becomes important in maintaining normal signal transduction. Inhibition of the proteasomes results in the build up of ubiquitylated proteins, which disrupts cell-signaling processes and cell growth (Fig. 10.28). The signaling by transcription factor NF-κB (nuclear factor κB) appears to be especially sensitive to bortezomib. NF-κB is associated with the transcription of antiapoptotic and proliferative genes but is under the control of IκB (inhibitor of NF-κB). IκB can itself be phosphorylated by IKK (IκB kinase), which marks IκB for ubiquitylation and destruction allowing NF-κB to mediate its antiapoptotic and proliferative ef-

fects. In the presence of the competitive inhibitor bortezomib ($IC_{50} = 0.6$ nM), the 26S proteasome is inhibited and the ubiquitylated IκB is still capable of inhibiting NF-κB, preventing its effects.[161]

The agent is used primarily in treating multiple myeloma, where NF-κB is thought to be especially important because of its regulation of VEGF and adhesion molecules, which play important roles in this cancer. The agent is also used in treating non-Hodgkin's lymphoma.

Bortezomib is available in 10-mL vials containing 3.5 mg that is administered intravenously for the treatment of multiple myeloma. The agent contains the unique boronic acid group, which serves as a bioisosteric replacement for an aldehyde functionality and forms a tetrahedral complex with a threonine hydroxyl group present on the proteasome. Several aldehydes were known to be proteasome inhibitors, but their incorporation resulted in racemization of the α-carbon. The boronic acids were not susceptible to the same racemization, and stereochemistry was preserved in vivo giving maximal inhibition. The agent has a half-life of 9 to 15 hours with the major metabolizing enzymes being CYP3A4 and CYP2C19.[162] Metabolism involves the oxidative removal of boron from the agent to give two diastereomeric carbinolamines. Both of the metabolites are inactive, the boronic acid functionality

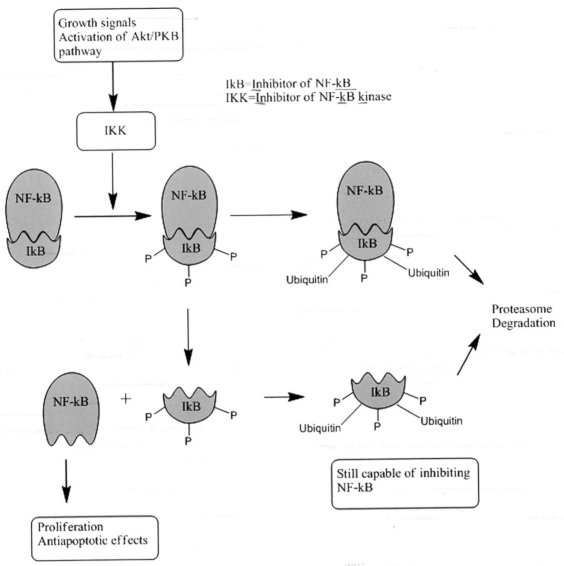

IkB=Inhibitor of NF-kB
IKK=Inhibitor of NF-kB kinase

Figure 10.28 ● Actions of proteasomes on NF-κB.

being necessary for binding of the proteasome. The elimination of the agent has not been well characterized.

The major toxicities seen with the agent are generalized weakness, nausea, vomiting, diarrhea, peripheral neuropathy, fever, and orthostatic hypotension. Myelosuppression also occurs normally as thrombocytopenia and neutropenia.

VORINOSTAT (SUBEROYLANILIDE HYDROXAMIC ACID, SAHA, ZOLINZA)

Histones are proteins around which DNA is wound in the process of packing DNA into the nucleus. They also have a role in regulating the transcription of genes, and this is controlled by the covalent modifications acetylation, phosphorylation, and methylation to which they are subject. The specific modifications present on the histones or histone code has been proposed to determine which transcription factors associate with specific genes and result in their replication.[163] Acetylation occurs at the ε-amino group of lysine and is accomplished by histone acetyltransferase enzymes, whereas deacetyltion is accomplished by histone deacetylase enzymes. The result of inhibition of histone deacetylase is hyperacetylation of lysine residues of the histone proteins. The positively charged ε-amino groups of the lysine residues are believed to interact with the negatively charged phosphate backbone of DNA. Once acetylation has occurred, this interaction is prevented, and the binding of transcription factors is favored. Therefore, the inhibition of deacetylation by vorinostat, a histone deacetylase inhibitor (HDACis), results in the increased transcription of certain genes. Specifically, this has been associated with upregulation of a regulatory protein known as p21, which serves to inhibit progression past the G_1 phase of the cell cycle. Other genes and their proteins are also effected by vorionostat such as Hsp90 (heat shock protein 90) and BCL6.

Vorinostat fits the basic pharmacophore for the HDACis (Fig. 10.29), which consists of a hydrophobic cap region connected to a zinc coordinating functionality by a hydrophobic linker.[164] The hydroxamic acid functionality is capable of bidendate binding to zinc present in the enzyme and is a major factor in the overall binding of the compound. The compound inhibits HDAC1, 2, 3, and 6 classes of this enzyme with nanomolar (<86 nM) IC_{50} values.[165]

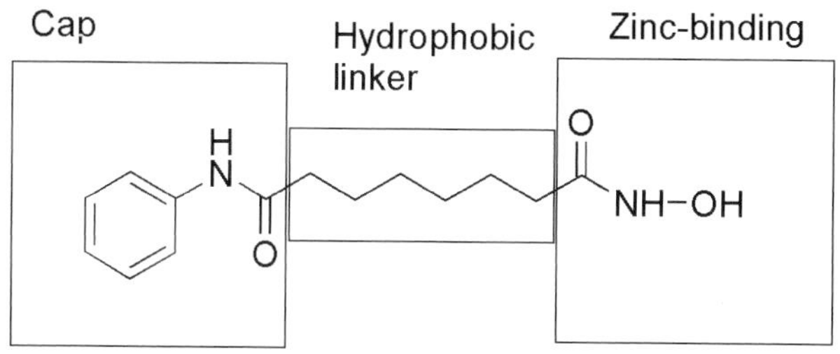

Figure 10.29 ● Pharmacophore for histone deacetylase inhibitors.

The agent is given orally and is available in 100-mg capsules for the treatment of cutaneous T-cell lymphoma. The bioavailability is 43%, and the agent is 71% bound to plasma proteins. Extensive metabolism of the agent occurs to give the *O*-glucuronide of the hydroxamic acid function and 4-anilino-4-oxobutanoic acid with minimal involvement of isozymes of CYP. The metabolites, both of which are inactive, are eliminated in the urine and the drug has a terminal elimination half-life of 2 hours. The most commonly reported adverse effects are fatigue, diarrhea, and nausea. Elevations in glucose and triglyceride levels are commonly seen with the agent. The agent has been associated with thrombocytopenia, an increased risk of clotting resulting in pulmonary embolism and possibly prolongation of the QTc interval.

ARSENIC TRIOXIDE (AS2O3, TRISENOX)

Arsenic trioxide is available in 10-mL vials for IV administration as second-line therapy in the treatment of acute promyelocytic leukemia (APL). The mechanism of the agent has not been well characterized; however, work has indicated that the agent may cause the degradation of a protein that blocks myeloid differentiation. Acute lymphocytic leukemia is associated with a translocation in which the promyelocytic leukemia (PML) gene is fused with the retinoic acid receptor gene (RARα), and the protein that results from this genetic rearrangement prevents myeloid differentiation.[166] Arsenic trioxide is capable of degrading this protein and allowing the cells to differentiate. Additional effects have included stimulation of apoptosis by decreasing Bcl-2 activity and stimulation of caspase enzymes and p53. Angiogenesis is inhibited by the inhibition of VEGF at the protein level.[167] The agent is widely distributed after IV administration; however, the pharmacokinetics of the agent have not been well characterized. Metabolism studies have shown that the agent undergoes reduction to trivalent arsenic followed by methylation to give monomethylarsonic and dimethylarsinic acids, which are eliminated in the urine. Unlike most other antineoplastic agents, myelosuppression does not occur in fact many patients (50%–60%) experience leukocytosis in which white blood cell count increases. APL differentiation syndrome is seen in many patients (30%) and presents as fever, shortness of breath, weight gain, pulmonary infiltrates, and pleural or pericardial effusions. This may be fatal and is commonly treated with high-dose dexamethasone upon initial suspicion. The presentation of APL differentiation syndrome are identical for arsenic trioxide and retinoic acid. Additional adverse effects include fatigue, a prolonged QT interval, dizziness, mild hyperglycemia, and mild nausea and vomiting.

TRETINOIN (ALL-TRANS-RETINOC ACID, ATRA, RETIN-A, VESANOID)

Tretinoin is available in 10-mg capsules for oral administration in the treatment of APL. The mechanism of action involves passive diffusion through the cell membrane and then movement to the nucleus where it interacts with the retinoic acid receptor (RAR) portion of the PML-RARα fusion protein. Binding of tretinoin allows the cell to differentiate and has also been shown to result in the destruction of the PML-RARα fusion protein. Resistance to tretinoin is problematic and associated with an increase in cellular retinoic acid–binding proteins (CRAPBs) located in the cytosol. The complexation with tretinoin prevents movement into the nucleus and may present the drug to metabolizing enzymes that inactivate it. Amino acid mutation of the PML-RARα protein has also been established as a mechanism of resistance. The agent is well absorbed upon oral administration and highly (95%) protein bound. Metabolism occurs in the liver and several inactive metabolites have been identified including 13-*cis*-retinoic acid, 4-oxo *cis*-retinoic, 4-oxo *trans*-retinoic acid and 4-oxo *trans*-retinoic acid glucuronide. Elimination occurs in the urine (63%) and feces (31%) with an elimination half-life of 40 to 120 minutes. Vitamin A toxicity is seen in nearly all patients and presents as headache, fever, dryness of the skin, skin rash, mucositis, and peripheral edema. APL differentiation syndrome such as that seen for arsenic trioxide also occurs. Cardiovascular effects include flushing, hypotension, CHF, stroke, and myocardial infarction have been reported but occur only rarely. There are also several CNS and GI effects that have been associated with the agent as well.

BEXAROTENE (TARGRETIN)

Bexarotene is available in 75-mg capsules for oral administration in the treatment of refractory cutaneous T-cell lymphoma. The agent is also available as a gel that may be used topically. The mechanism of action has not been fully established but is thought to involve binding to retinoid receptors resulting ultimately in the formation of transcription factors that promote cell differentiation and regulate cellular proliferation.[168] Bexarotene has been demonstrated to activate apoptosis as a result of stimulation of caspase 3 and inhibition of survivin, an antiapoptotic protein that would normally inhibit caspase activity.[169] Apoptosis is also stimulated because of cleavage of poly(ADP-Ribose) polymerase, which is antiapoptotic. Reduced expression of the retinoid receptor subtypes RXRα and RARα has also been demonstrated for the agent. Absorption is nearly complete after oral administration and plasma protein binding is high (<99%).[170] There is extensive metabolism in the liver to give 6- and 7-hydroxy-bexarotene and 6- and 7-oxo-bexarotene as well as glucuronides of these metabolites and the parent. Elimination occurs via the feces with an elimination half-life of 7 hours. Adverse effects include hypercholesterolemia, hypertriglyceridemia, hypothyroidism, myelosuppression, nausea, and skin rash.

ASPARAGINASE (L-ASPARAGINASE, ELSPAR, L-ASNASE, CRISTANASPASE)

Asparaginase is available in 10-mL vials for intramuscular and IV use in the treatment of acute lymphocytic leukemia.

Tumor cells are unable to synthesize asparagine, and therefore must utilize what is available in the extracellular environment. The agent acts by hydrolyzing extracellular asparagine to aspartate and ammonia. The tumor cells are then deprived of a necessary nutrient, and protein synthesis is inhibited leading to cell death. The agent is specific for the G_1 phase of the cell cycle. Resistance occurs because of the development of the tumor cells ability to produce asparagine synthetase that allows them to synthesize the required amino acid. Antibody production directed at asparaginase may be stimulated by the agent as well. The agent remains in the extracellular space after parental administration and is 30% protein bound. The metabolism of the agent has not been well characterized and the plasma half-life depends on the formulation of the drug. The *E. coli*-derived agent has a plasma half-life of 40 to 50 hours, whereas polyethylene glycol-asparaginase's half-life is 3 to 5 days. Adverse effects include hypersensitivity reactions, fever, chills, nausea, lethargy, confusion, hallucinations, and possibly coma. Myelosuppression is not generally seen. An increased risk of bleeding and clotting is seen in half of the patients taking the agent.

ESTRAMUSTINE PHOSPHATE SODIUM (EM, EMCYT)

Estramustine as the phosphate is available in 140-mg capsules for the treatment of prostate cancer. Although originally designed as an alkylating agent, it has been shown to be devoid of alkylating activity and functions as an inhibitor of microtubule function by binding to microtubule associate proteins (MAPs) and also binds to tubulin at a site that is distinct from that of the vinca alkaloids but thought to partially overlap with that of pacilataxel.[171] The major mechanism by which cells become resistant to the agent involves increased efflux, although this is not mediated by Pgp as is the case with other microtubule inhibitors such as the taxanes and vinca alkaloids. Therefore, the agent does not show cross-resistance with these agents. As an inhibitor of microtubules, it is cell cycle specific acting in the M phase. The agent is well absorbed upon oral administration with hydrolysis of the water solubilizing phosphate beginning to occur in the GI tract. Metabolism involves the formation of the active estromustine, which arises from oxidation of the C17 alcohol to give the ketone. Additional inactive metabolites result from carbamate hydrolysis to give estradiol and estrone. The parent and metabolites are primarily eliminated in the feces with a terminal elimination half-life of 20 hours. The adverse effects of the agent are nausea and vomiting, which is generally mild but the severity may increase upon prolonged administration. Gynecomastia also commonly occurs, and diarrhea may also be seen. Less commonly seen effects include myelosuppression, skin rash, and cardiovascular abnormalities including CHF.

There are several agents that manipulate the endocrine system to inhibit cell growth that are used in treating cancers that are endocrine dependent. Additionally, there are also several monoclonal antibodies that have been developed and are currently used in treating cancer. Both of these groups of agents are discussed elsewhere in this text.

● R E V I E W   Q U E S T I O N S ●

1. The agent shown is most likely to result from which of these agents?

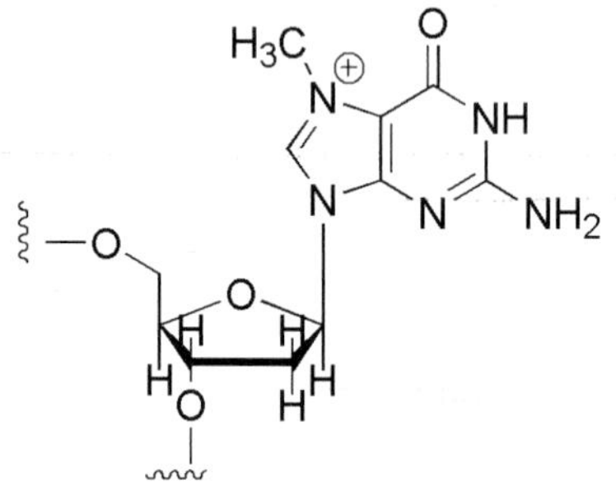

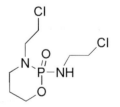

   a. methotrexate and temozolomide
   b. temozolomide and streptozocin
   c. streptozocin and cyclophosphamide
   d. cyclophosphamide and methotrexate
   e. 5-fluorouracil and streptozocin

2. The following agent is capable of chelating iron and generating ROS. It has been associated with pulmonary toxicity, which is related to reduced levels of an enzyme in lung tissue that normally inactivates the compound.
   a. bleomycin
   b. doxorubicin
   c. mitoxantrone
   d. procarbazine

3. The following agent is an inhibitor of a topoisomerase enzyme and binds to both DNA and the enzyme itself. It has been associated with the production of cardiotoxicity that may progress to CHF related to the production of ROS.
   a. mitoxantrone
   b. mechlorethamine
   c. daunorubicin
   d. epirubicin
   e. topotecan

4. For the agent shown below, what would be the effect of coadministration of a CYP inducer and an inhibitor of alcohol dehydrogenase?

Ifosfamide

   a. increased cytotoxicity and bladder toxicity
   b. increased cytotoxicity and decreased bladder toxicity
   c. decreased cytotoxicity and increased bladder toxicity
   d. decreased cytotoxicity and decreased bladder toxicity

REFERENCES

1. Ries, L. A. G., et al.: SEER Cancer Statistics Review, 1975–2005, National Cancer Institute. Bethesda, MD, 2007
2. Weinberg, R. A.: The Biology of Cancer, Garland Science, 2007, Chapters 8 and 9, pp. 209–356.
3. Ziegler, A. M., et al.: Nature 372:773, 2002.
4. Topal, M. D., and Fresco, J. R.: Nature 263:285, 1976.
5. Gilman, A., and Phillips, F. S.: Science 103:409, 1946.
6. Kohn, S., et al.: J. Mol. Biol. 19:266, 1966.
7. Everett, R. L., et al.: J. Chem. Soc. 2386, 1953.
8. Bergel, F., and Stock, J. A.: J. Chem. Soc. 76:2409, 1954.
9. Dufor, M., et al.: Cancer Chemother. Pharmacol. 15:125, 1985.
10. Engle, T. W., et al.: J. Med. Chem. 22:897, 1979.
11. Chen, C. S., et al.: Mol. Pharmacol. 65:1278, 2004.
12. Huang, Z., et al.: Biochem. Pharmacol. 59:961, 2000.
13. Zhang, J., et al.: Curr. Drug Ther. 1:55, 2006.
14. Chen, C. S., et al.: Drug Metab. Dispos. 33:1261, 2005.
15. Chang, T. K. H., et al.: J. Pharm. Exp. Ther. 274:270, 1995.
16. McCann, J. J., et al.: Cancer Res. 31:1573, 1971
17. Teicher, B. A., et al.: Cancer Res. 49: 4996, 1989.
18. van Maanen, M. J., et al.: Cancer Treat. Rev. 26:257, 2000.
19. Haddow, A., and Timmis, G. M.: Lancet 1:207, 1953.
20. Iwamoto, T., et al.: Cancer Sci. 95:454, 2004.
21. Hassan, M., et al.: Eur. J. Clin. Pharm. 36:525, 1989.
22. Rosenberg, B.: In Lippert, B. (ed.). Cisplatin: Chemistry and Biochemistry of a Leading Anticancer Drug. Verlag Helvetica Chimica Acta: Zurich. Weinheim, Germany, Wiley-VCH, 1999, pp. 3–27.
23. Eastman, A.: In Lippert, B. (ed.). Cisplatin: Chemistry and Biochemistry of a Leading Anticancer Drug. Verlag Helvetica Chimica Acta: Zurich. Weinheim, Germany, Wiley-VCH, 1999, pp. 111–134.
24. Eastman, A.: Biochemistry 25:3912, 1986.
25. Esposito, B. P., and Najjar, R.: Coord. Chem. Rev. 232:137, 2002.
26. Nehmé, A., et al.: Br. J. Cancer 79:1104, 1999.
27. Chaney, S. G., et al.: Crit. Rev. Oncol. Hematol. 53:3, 2005.
28. Wheeler, G. P.: A Review on the Mechanism of Action of Nitrosoureas in Cancer Chemotherapy, 30, Sartorelli, A symposium sponsored by the Division of Medicinal Chemistry at 169th Meeting of the American Chemical Society, Philadelphia, PA April, 1975, pp. 87–114.
29. Gnewuch, C. T., and Sosnovsky, G.: Chem. Rev. 97:829, 1997.
30. Wheeler, G. P., and Chumley, S.: J. Med. Chem. 10:259, 1967.
31. Wheeler, G. P.: Cancer Res. 35:2974. 1975.
32. Eisenbrand, G., et al.: Cancer Res. Clin. Oncol. 112:196, 1986.
33. Lemoine, A., et al.: Xenobiotica 21:775, 1991.
34. Potter, D. W., and Reed D. J.: Arch. Biochem. Biophys. 216:158, 1982
35. Zeller, P., et al.: Experientia 19:129, 1963.
36. Berneis, K. M., et al.: Experientia 19:132, 1963.
37. Renschler, M. F.: Eur. J. Cancer 40:1934, 2004.
38. Wienkam, R. J., and Shiba, D. A.: Life Sci. 22:937, 1978
39. Dunn, D. L., et al.: Cancer Res. 39:4555, 1979.
40. Tweedie, D. J., et al.: Drug Metab. Dispos. 19:793, 1991.
41. Souliotis, Y. L., et al.: Cancer Res. 50:2759, 1990.
42. Wiestler, O. D., et al.: J. Cancer Res. Clin. Oncol. 108:56, 1984.
43. Montgomery, J. A.: Cancer Treat. Rep. 60:125, 1976.
44. Reid, J. M., et al.: Clin. Cancer Res. 5:2192, 1999.
45. Clark, A. S., et al.: J. Med. Chem. 38:1493, 1996.
46. Saunder, P. P., and Shulz, G. A.: Biochem. Pharmacol. 19:911, 1970.
47. Kawahara, K., et al.: Jpn. J. Clin. Pharmacol. Ther. 32:15, 2001.
48. Gibson, N. W., et al.: Carcinogenisis 7:259, 1986.
49. Rutty, C. J., et al.: Br. J. Cancer 48:140, 1983.
50. Stevens, M. F. G., et al.: Cancer Res. 47:5846, 1987.
51. Lowe, P. R., et al.: J. Med. Chem. 35:3377, 1992.
52. Ordentlich, P., et al.: J. Biol. Chem. 278:24791, 2003.
53. Malet-Martino, M., and Martino, R.: Oncologist 7:288, 2002.
54. Carreras, C. W., and Santi, D. V.: Annu. Rev. Biochem. 64:721, 1995.
55. Diasio, R. B., and Johnson, M. R.: Clin. Cancer Res. 5:2672, 1999.
56. Porter, D. J. Y., et al.: Biochem. Pharmacol. 50:1475, 1995.
57. Cunningham, D., and James, R. D.: Eur. J. Cancer 37:826, 2001.
58. Engel, D., et al.: J. Med. Chem. 51:314, 2008.
59. Burris, H. A., III, et al.: J. Clin. Oncol. 15: 2403, 1997.
60. Hitchings, G. H., and Elion, G. B.: Acc. Chem. Res. 2:202, 1969.
61. Innocenti, F., et al.: Ther. Drug Monit. 22:375, 2000.
62. Dervieux, T., et al.: Leukemia 15:1706, 2001.
63. Aarbakke, J., et al.: Trends Pharmacol. Sci. 18:3, 1997.
64. Rowland, K., et al.: Xenobiotica 29:615, 1999.
65. Schiffer, C. A., et al.: Biochem. 34:16279, 1995.
66. De Angelis, P. M., et al.: Mol. Cancer, 5:20, 2006.
67. Champoux, J. J.: Annu. Rev. Biochem. 70: 369, 2001.
68. Selman, A., et al.: Proc. Natl. Acad. Sci. U. S. A. 44:602, 1958.
69. Hou, M. H., et al.: Nucleic Acids Res. 30:4910, 2002.
70. Wadkins, R. M., et al.: Biochemistry. 37:11915, 1998.
71. Wadkins, R. M., et al.: J. Mol. Biol. 262:53, 1996.
72. Minotti, G., et al.: Pharmacol. Rev. 56:185, 2004.
73. Inoue, A., et al.: Cancer Lett. 157:105, 2000.
74. Perego, P., et al.: Curr. Med. Chem. 8:31, 2001.
75. Christine, A., and Frederick, C. A., et al.: Biochemistry 29: 2538, 1990.
76. Taatjes, D. J., et al.: J. Med. Chem. 40:1276, 1997.
77. Gutierrez, P. L.: Front. Biosci. 5:629, 2000.
78. Clementi, M. E., et al.: Anticancer Res. 23:2445, 2003.
79. Sacco, G., et al.: Br. J. Pharmacol. 139:641, 2003.
80. Brazzolotto, X., et al.: Biochim. Biophys. Acta 1593:209, 2003.
81. Hasinoff, B. B., et al.: Curr. Med. Chem. 5:1, 1998.
82. Hasinoff, B. B., et al.: Biochem. Pharmacol. 50:953, 1995.
83. Seppo, W., et al.: Clin. Cancer Res. 6:3680, 2000.
84. Zee-Cheng, R. K., et al.: J. Med. Chem. 21:291, 1978.
85. Panousis, C., et al.: Anticancer Drug Des. 10:593, 1995.
86. Fisher, G. R., and Patterson, L. H.: Cancer Chemother. Pharmacol. 30:451, 1992.
87. Gabizon, A., et al.: J. Control. Release 53:275, 1998.
88. Weenen, H., et al.: Eur. J. Cancer Clin. Oncol. 20:919, 1984.
89. Joachim Mian, J., et al.: Cancer Res. 51: 3427, 1991.
90. Stahelin, H. F., and von Wartburg, A.: Cancer Res. 51: 5, 1991.
91. Hande, K. R.: Eur. J. Cancer 34:1514, 1998.
92. Chen, G. L., et al.: J. Biol. Chem. 259:13560, 1984.
93. Yang, L., et al.: Cancer Res. 45:5872, 1985.
94. Chow, K. C., et al.: Mol. Pharmacol. 34:467, 1988.
95. Baldwin, E. L., and Osheroff, N.: Curr. Med. Chem. Anticancer Agents 5:363, 2005.
96. Bromberg, K. D., et al.: J. Biol. Chem. 278:7406, 2003.
97. Mans, D. R., et al.: Br. J. Cancer 62:54, 1990.
98. Relling, M. V., et al.: Mol. Pharmacol. 45:352, 1994.
99. Li, Q. Y., et al.: Curr. Med. Chem. 13:2021, 2006.
100. Wall, M. E., et al.: J. Am. Chem. Soc. 88:3888, 1966.
101. Burke, T. G., and Mi, Z.: Anal. Biochem. 212:285, 1993.
102. Gottlieb, J. A., and Luce, J. K.: Cancer Chemother. Rpt. 56:103, 1972.
103. Hsiang, Y. H., et al.: J. Biol.Chem. 260:14873, 1986.
104. Hecht, S. M., et al.: J. Med. Chem. 34:98, 1991.
105. Negoro, S., et al.: J. Natl. Cancer Inst. 83:1164, 1991.
106. James, J., and Champoux, J. J.: Annu. Rev. Biochem. 70:369, 2001.
107. Watt, P. M., and Hickson, I. D.: Biochem. J. 303:681, 1994.
108. Staker, B. L.: Proc. Natl. Acad. Sci. U. S. A. 99:15387, 2002.
109. Staker, B. L., et al.: J. Med. Chem. 48:2336, 2005.
110. Abigerges, D., et al.: J. Clin. Oncol. 13:210, 1995.
111. Yang, X., et al.: Curr. Med. Chem. 12:1343, 2005.
112. Rosing, H., et al.: Anticancer Drugs 9:587, 1998.
113. Umezawa, H., et al.: J. Antibiot. Ser. A 19:200, 1966.
114. Stubbe, J., and Kozarich, J. W.: Chem. Rev. 87:107, 1987.
115. Sausville, E. A., et al.: Biochemistry 17: 2746, 1978.
116. Giloni, L., et al.: J. Biol. Chem. 256:8608, 1981.
117. Zhao, C., et al.: J. Inorgan. Biochem. 91:259, 2002.
118. Wu, W., et al.: J. Am. Chem. Soc. 118:1281, 1996.
119. Argoudelis, Al A., et al.: J. Antibiot. 24:543, 1971.
120. Noble, R. L., et al.: Ann. N. Y. Acad. Sci. 76:882, 1958.
121. Mangeney, P., et al.: Tetrahedron 35:2175, 1979.
122. Pellegrini, F., and Budman, D. R.: Cancer Invest. 23:264, 2005.
123. Jordan, M. A.: Curr. Med. Chem. Anticancer Agents 2:17, 2002.
124. Jordan, M. A.: Nat. Rev. Cancer 4:253, 2004.
125. Gigant, B., et al.: Nature 435:519, 2005.
126. Jordan, M. A., et al.: Cancer Res. 51:2212, 1991.
127. Tucker, R. W., et al.: Cancer Res. 37:4346, 1977.
128. Vacca, A., et al.: Blood 94:4143, 1999.
129. Lockhart, A., et al.: Mol. Ther. 2:685, 2003.
130. Wani, M. C., et al.: J. Am. Chem. Soc. 93:2325, 1971.
131. Dye, D., and Watkins, J.: Br. Med. J. 280:1353, 1980.
132. Rao, S., et al.: J. Biol. Chem. 270:20235, 1995.
133. Jordan, M. A., et al.: Proc. Natl. Acad. Sci. U. S. A. 90:9552, 1993.
134. Blagosklonny, M. V.: Leukemia 15:869, 2001.
135. Bollag, D. M., et al.: Cancer Res. 55:2325, 1995.

136. Giannakakou, P., et al.: Proc. Natl. Acad. Sci. U. S. A. 97:2904, 1999.
137. Wakaki, S., et al.: Antibiot. Chemother. 8:228, 1958.
138. Webb, J. S., et al.: J. Am. Chem. Soc. 84:3185, 1962.
139. Lin, A. J., et al.: Cancer Chemother. Rep. 4:23, 1974.
140. Borowy-Borowski, H., et al.: Biochemistry 29:2999, 1990.
141. Saurajyoti, B., et al.: Inter. J. Cancer 109:703, 2004.
142. Han, I., and Kohn, H.: J. Org. Chem. 56:4648, 1991.
143. Cummings, J., et al.: Biochem. Pharm. 56:405, 1998.
144. Weinberg, R. A.: The Biology of Cancer, Garland Science, 2007, Chapters 5 and 6, pp. 119–207.
145. Rowley, J. D.: Nature 243:290, 1973.
146. deKlein, A., et al.: Nature 300:765, 1982.
147. Nagar, B., et al.: Cancer Res. 6:4236, 2002.
148. Druker, B. J., et al.: N. Engl. J. Med. 344:1038, 2001.
149. Talpaz, M., et al.: N. Engl. J. Med. 354:2531, 2006.
150. Dowell J., et al.: Nat. Rev. Drug Discov. 4:13, 2005.
151. Tedesco, K. L., et al.: Curr. Treat. Options Oncol. 5:393, 2004
152. Scott Wilhelm, S., et al.: Nat. Rev. Drug Disc. 5:835, 2006.
153. Wan, P. T., et al.: Cell 116:855, 2004.
154. Force, T., et al.: Nature 7:335, 2007.
155. Ling, J., et al.: Drug Met. Dispos 34:420, 2006
156. Moy, B., and Goss, P. E.: Oncologist 11:1047, 2006.
157. Konecny, G. E., et al.: Cancer Res. 66:1630, 2006.

158. Polli, J. W., et al.: Drug Metab. Dispos. 36:695, 2008.
159. Hidalgo, M., et al.: Clin. Cancer Res. 12:5755, 2006
160. Cai, P., et al.: Drug Met. Dispos. 35:1554, 2007.
161. McCormack, T., et al.: J. Biol. Chem. 272:26103, 1997.
162. Pekol, T., et al.: Drug Metab. Dispos. 33:771, 2005.
163. Brittain, H., et al.: Annu. Rev. Med. Chem. 42:337, 2007.
164. Jung, M., et al.: Bioorg. Med. Chem. Lett. 7:1655, 1997.
165. Miller, W. H., et al.: Cancer Res. 62:3893, 2002.
166. Xiao, Y. F., et al.: World J. Gastroenterol. 12:5780, 2006.
167. Zhu, J., et al.: Proc. Natl. Acad. Sci. U. S. A. 94:3978, 1997.
168. Zhang, C., et al.: Clin. Cancer Res. 8:1234, 2002.
169. Esteva, F. J., et al.: J. Clin. Oncol. 21:999, 2003.
170. Howell, S. R., et al.: Drug Metab. Dispos. 29:990, 2001.
171. Dahllof, B., et al.: Cancer Res. 53:4573, 1993.

SELECTED READING

Chu, E., and DeVita, V. T.: Physician's Cancer Chemotherapy Drug Manual 2004, Sudbury, MA, Jones and Bartlett, 2003.
Grochow, L. B., and Ames, M. M.: A Clinician's Guide to Chemotherapy Pharmacokinetics and Pharmacodynamics, Baltimore, MD, Williams and Wilkins, 1998.
Holland, J. F., et al.: Cancer Medicine 7. London, BC Decker Inc., 2006.
Weinberg, R. A.: The Biology of Cancer. Garland Science, 2007.

CHAPTER 11

Agents for Diagnostic Imaging

JEFFREY J. CHRISTOFF

CHAPTER OVERVIEW

Diagnostic medical imaging encompasses a group of techniques often used in the diagnosis and subsequent treatment of disease. Medical imaging procedures are typically considered low-risk events in comparison to direct surgical visualization and often provide information or treatment methods that are simply not available by any other means. Medical imaging techniques use electromagnetic radiation to pass through tissue and convey the internal information necessary to create an image of the tissue or organ. The different types of medical imaging techniques diverge in their physical means, methods, and the information that they can provide. All of the techniques can provide anatomical and/or functional information that is often displayed as an image for interpretation by a physician trained to evaluate the meaning of the image in the context of the disease state.

Medical imaging began with Roentgen's discovery of x-rays in 1895, and it has been the domain of diagnostic radiology ever since. In its earliest days, the specialty of radiology used x-rays to produce images of the chest and skeleton. At the present time, diagnostic imaging uses decaying radioactive tracers (nuclear medicine), ionizing radiation (x-rays and computed tomography [CT]), radio waves (magnetic resonance imaging [MRI]), and high-frequency sound waves (ultrasound) to produce diagnostic images of the body. Today, radiologists and other physicians can use these imaging techniques to facilitate interventional procedures, such as organ biopsy or abscess drainage.

Nuclear medicine procedures utilize radioactive tracers, (i.e., radiopharmaceuticals) and specialized radiation detectors to follow these compounds as they distribute to various organs or tissues. The other imaging modalities, x-rays, CT, MRI, and ultrasound, often utilize contrast agents to enhance information obtained about the organs or organ systems during imaging. This chapter is a discussion of the chemistry and physics of selected agents used in various medical imaging procedures.

◆ RADIOPHARMACEUTICALS

Radioactivity and Nuclear Medicine

Atomic nuclei are either stable or radioactive. Stable nuclei generally have a proton-to-neutron ratio near 1:1. As this ratio deviates significantly away from unity, atomic nuclei become unstable and have a greater amount of internal nuclear energy. Such unstable nuclei are radioactive and obtain stability by emitting energy in the form of particulate and/or electromagnetic radiation that propagates through space or matter. Selected radioactive nuclei are present in nature, while many other radioactive nuclei are produced by bombarding stable nuclei with high-energy particles.

Ionizing radiation is radiation, that when interacting with matter, can cause changes in the atomic or nuclear structure. The first type of ionizing radiation is particulate radiation, which includes alpha (α), beta (β^- or β^+), proton (p), and neutron (n) particles. Particulate radiation is energy in the form of mass with kinetic energy. On the atomic scale, energy is usually measured in electron volts (eV). By definition, an *electron volt* is the energy needed to accelerate an electron across a potential difference of 1 V. The second type of ionizing radiation is called *electromagnetic radiation*. Electromagnetic radiation is an electric and magnetic disturbance that is propagated through space at the speed of light.

Electromagnetic radiation is unaffected by either an electrical or magnetic field because it has no charge. These properties are shared by radio waves (10^{-10}–10^{-6} eV), microwaves (10^{-6}–10^{-2} eV), infrared (10^{-2}–1 eV), visible light (1–2 eV), ultraviolet (2–100 eV), x-rays (100–10^4 eV) and gamma (γ) rays (100–10^6 eV). The various forms of electromagnetic radiation differ in their frequency and, therefore, their energy. The energy of electromagnetic radiation can be calculated in electron volts from the following equation:

$$E = hv = hc / \lambda$$

where h is Planck constant (4.13×10^{-15} eV*sec), v is the frequency (hertz), c is the speed of light (cm/sec), and λ is the wavelength (cm). The difference between x-rays and γ-rays is based on where they originate; x-rays come from outside the nucleus via the electron orbitals, whereas γ-rays originate in the nucleus via nuclear transformations. These highly energetic x-rays and γ-rays have properties resembling both waves and particles. Therefore, x-rays and γ-rays are often referred to as *photons*.

Radionuclides are unstable nuclei that undergo processes called *decay*. In many cases, the composition of the nucleus transforms from one element into another element. A nucleus may undergo a single transformation or several decays before finally reaching a stable configuration. Nuclear particles, either a proton or a neutron, are called *nucleons*. A species of atom with a specified number of neutrons and protons in its nucleus is called a *nuclide*. Nuclides with the same number of protons and a different number of neutrons are called *isotopes*. Nuclides with the same number of neutrons and a different number of protons are called *isotones*. Nuclides with same atomic mass are called *isobars*. Nuclides with the same number of protons and atomic mass but at two energy levels are called *isomers*.

The atomic nucleus has discrete energy levels. In a stable atom, the energy level is called the *ground (g) state*. An unstable, high-energy nucleus or a stable nucleus that is excited to a higher level by interaction with high-speed particles can emit this excess energy by decaying to the ground state. If this decay process is delayed, the excited state may be referred to as a *metastable (m) state*. During decay, energy is released from the nucleus. Depending on the properties of the nuclide, this may occur by simply releasing the energy in the form of a γ-ray or ejecting an energetic particle from the nucleus with or without γ-ray emission.

Nuclides are characterized by the following notation:

$$_Z^A X_N^{(valence)} \quad \text{Example } _{53}^{131} I_{78}^{-1}$$

where X is the symbol of the chemical element to which the nuclide belongs, A represents the atomic mass (number of neutrons plus the number of protons), and Z represents the atomic number (number of protons). The right side of the element is reserved for the oxidation state (valence), and N represents the number of neutrons. In most medical references, various notations indicating the element and mass number are used (e.g., ^{131}I, I-131, or iodine-131).

The nuclide at the beginning of the decay sequence is referred to as the *parent*. The nuclide produced by decay is referred to as the *daughter*. Daughter nuclei may be stable or unstable. There are five types of radioactive decay processes described below that are distinguished according to the nature of the primary radiation event. A particular radioactive nucleus may decay by more than one process. The type of decay that occurs for a particular isotope generally depends on the balance of protons and neutrons in the nucleus.

1. **Isomeric transition (IT)**. IT is a decay process where the nucleus simply changes from a higher energy level to a lower energy level by emitting γ-rays. Therefore, both mass number and atomic number remain unchanged. The daughter nucleus is the same chemical element as the original nucleus. The original nucleus, before the transition, is said to be in a metastable (m) state if the transition from the higher energy level to the lower level is delayed by a measurable period of time. Depending on the decaying nuclide, this delay could last from fractions of a second to months. The predominant isotope used in nuclear medicine procedures, Tc-99m, has a half-life of 6 hours. Since no particles are emitted during this nuclear transformation, Tc-99m is considered a pure gamma emitter.

   Example: $^{99m}Tc \rightarrow ^{99}Tc + \gamma - ray$ (140 keV)

2. **Electron capture (EC)**. The nucleus captures an electron (e^-) from the electron cloud of the atom (mainly the K shell). This electron combines with a proton (p) to produce a neutron (n). The excess energy from this transformation can be liberated in the form of a γ-ray and/or a neutrino (v, a highly energetic, chargeless particle of extremely small mass). Therefore, no charged nuclear particles are emitted during this transformation. Other events occurring within the vacant electron orbital can lead to the production of secondary x-rays.

   $$p^+ + e^- \rightarrow n + v + \gamma - ray$$

   Example: $^{123}I \xrightarrow{EC} ^{123}Te + \gamma - ray$ (159 keV)

3. **Positron emission (β^+)**. An alternative decay process in a proton rich nucleus is the conversion of a proton to a neutron with the subsequent ejection of an energetic *positron* and a neutrino. Positrons are considered antimatter and exist only for very short periods of time. The positron loses its kinetic energy, by interacting with surrounding atoms. The positron ultimately combines with a free electron from one of the surrounding atoms in an interaction in which the rest masses of both particles are converted to two γ-rays of 511 keV emitted approximately 180° to each other. This combination is called *annihilation radiation*. This characteristic decay process is utilized for the specialized imaging technique called *positron emission tomography* (PET).

   $$p^+ \rightarrow n + \beta^+ + v$$

   $$\beta^+ + e^- \rightarrow 2\,\gamma - rays \text{ (511 keV)}$$

   Example: $^{18}F \rightarrow ^{18}O + \beta^+ + 2\,\gamma - rays$ (511 keV)

4. **Negatron emission (β^-)**. A neutron-rich nucleus decays by the conversion of a neutron to a proton with subsequent emission of an energetic *negatron* and an antineutrino ($\bar{v}$, a highly energetic, chargeless particle of extremely small mass) with or without γ-ray emission.

   $$n \rightarrow p^+ + \beta^- + \bar{v} + \gamma - ray$$

   Example: $^{99}Mo \rightarrow ^{99m}Tc + \beta^- + \gamma - ray$ (740 keV)

5. **Alpha-particle emission ($_2^4 He^{+2}$)**. A heavy, unstable nucleus may decay to a daughter nuclide and an *alpha particle* consisting of two protons and two neutrons, essentially the equivalent to a charged helium nucleus. If the particle has sufficient energy, it may escape the nucleus in an excited energy state with/without the emission of excess energy in the form of a γ-ray.

   Example: $^{226}Ra \rightarrow ^{222}Rn + _2^4 He^{+2}$ (4.59 MeV)
   $+ \gamma - ray$ (187 keV)

These decay processes are random events. It is impossible to predict when an individual atom of a particular radionuclide will spontaneously decay. In quantitative terms, however, this process follows first-order kinetics. The *radioactive decay law* is the number of atoms that decay per unit time. Radioactive decay is proportional to the number of atoms (N) present and a decay constant (λ) characteristic for the particular radionuclide.

$$\frac{-dN}{dt} = \lambda N$$

To obtain the number of decaying atoms for a measurable period of time, the differential equation must be integrated. Therefore, the basic equation for radioactive decay is expressed as follows in terms of atoms:

$$N_t = N_0 e^{-\lambda t}$$

where N_t (number of atoms at time t) and N_0 (number of atoms at time 0). Activity (A) of a radionuclide is also expressed as the number of atoms disintegrating per unit of time ($A = \lambda N$). With the substitution of A/λ into the equation above for N and simplifying the result,

$$A_t = A_0 e^{-\lambda t}$$

where A_t is the activity at time t, A_0 is the original activity, and λ is the decay constant.

A radionuclide's decay is routinely expressed as its physical half-life, the time in which one half of the atoms decay. Mathematically, this is expressed as

$$t_{1/2} = \frac{\ln 2}{\lambda}$$

where $t_{1/2}$ is the physical half-life and λ is the decay constant. Substitution into the previous equation for the decay constant, λ, provides

$$A_t = A_0\, e^{-(\ln 2)t/t_{1/2}}$$

which is simplified to

$$A_t = A_0(0.5)^{t/t_{1/2}}$$

where A_t is the activity at time t, A_0 is the original activity, t is the elapsed time interval, and $t_{1/2}$ is the physical half-life of the radionuclide of interest. This equation is frequently utilized directly or indirectly in daily operations of a nuclear pharmacy or nuclear medicine department.

The activity (A) of radionuclides can be expressed in the following three ways: (a) in disintegrations per unit time (usually disintegrations per second [dps] or disintegrations per minute [dpm]), (b) in curies (Ci), and (c) in becquerels (Bq; 1 Bq = 1 dps). A *curie* is defined as the quantity of any radionuclide that decays at a rate of 3.7×10^{10} dps, a number closely approximating the historically calculated number of dps in 1 g of pure radium. More recently, the International System of Units (SI) has adopted the becquerel as the official unit of radioactivity. The curie is still traditionally utilized in clinical practice, and the relevant conversion factor to remember is the following:

1 millicurie (mCi) = 37 megabequerels (MBq)

An example of a routine radioactive decay calculation follows:

A sample of sodium iodide (^{123}I) is calibrated by the manufacturer at 200 μCi on May 14 at 12 PM C.S.T. What is the activity remaining on May 15 at 3 PM E.S.T.? The $t_{1/2}$ of ^{123}I is 13.2 hours. (Note: Calculations of elapsed time must also indicate variations in time zones incurred during transport).

$$(t_{1/2} = 13.2 \text{ hours})$$

$$A = (200\ \mu\text{Ci})\,(0.5)^{(26/13.2)}$$

$$A = (200\ \mu\text{Ci})\,(0.255)$$

$$A = 51.1\ \mu\text{Ci}$$

Radionuclide Production

Radionuclides utilized in nuclear medicine are artificially produced. This is accomplished when small charged or uncharged particles bombard atomic nuclei and initiate a process of nuclear change. The artificial production of a radionuclide requires preparation of target nuclei (parent), irradiation of the target, and chemical separation of the daughter radionuclide produced from the nuclear reaction. The daughter radionuclide is converted to the desired radiopharmaceutical form. Quality assurance tests of the physical, chemical, and pharmaceutical qualities (i.e., sterility and apyrogenicity) of the final product are per-

formed. The systems used for practical production of radionuclides are a nuclear reactor, cyclotron, or radioisotope generator.

The shorthand nuclear physics notation of artificial nuclear transformation reaction is as follows:

$$^{112}\text{Cd(p,2n)}^{111}\text{In}$$

where Cd-112 is the stable target nuclei, a proton (p) is the bombarding particle, two neutrons (2n) are emitted from the nucleus during the transformation, and In-111 is the daughter radionuclide produced.

The introduction of radionuclide generators into nuclear medicine arose from the need to administer larger doses of a short half-life radionuclide to obtain higher quality images. The general principle of the radionuclide generator is that a long-lived parent is bound to some adsorbent material in a chromatographic ion exchange column and the daughter is eluted from the column with some solvent or gas. When considering potential radioactive parent and daughter pairs, two scenarios can be envisioned depending on the magnitude of difference in half-lives between the long-lived parent and the short-lived daughter. If the parent nuclide has a sufficiently longer half-life than the daughter nuclide (10-fold to 100-fold), a state of transient equilibrium is ultimately reached when the daughter nuclide is being produced from the parent at the same rate as the daughter decays. In the situation where the parent half-life is much longer than that of the daughter ($>$1,000-fold), a state of secular equilibrium is reached when the daughter nuclide is being produced from the parent at the same rate as the parent decays

There are many possible parent–daughter generator systems for clinical use, but there is only one in routine use in nuclear medicine, the molybdenum-99/technetium-99m system. All of the molybdenum-99 at the present time is obtained as a fission product of uranium-235 from nuclear reactors.

$$^{235}\text{U(n, fission)}^{236}\text{U} \rightarrow {}^{99}\text{Mo} + \text{other radionuclides}$$

Inorganic radiochemistry techniques separate molybdenum-99 from the other radionuclides. Molybdenum-99 ($t_{1/2} = 66$ hours) decays by negatron emission to technetium-99m ($t_{1/2} = 6$ hours), which decays by IT to technetium-99 by emitting a γ-ray (140 keV). Anionic molybdate ($^{99}\text{MoO}_4^{-2}$) is loaded on a column of alumina (Fig. 11.1). The molybdate ions adsorb firmly to the alumina, and the generator column is autoclaved to sterilize the system. Then the rest of the generator is assembled under aseptic conditions into its final form in a lead-shielded container. Each generator is eluted with sterile normal saline (0.9% sodium chloride). The alumina column is an inorganic ion exchange column where chloride ions (Cl^-) exchange for pertechnetate ions ($^{99\text{m}}\text{TcO}_4^-$) but not molybdate ions (MoO_4^{-2}). The column eluate contains sodium pertechnetate as well as sodium chloride. Elution efficiency of contemporary molybdenum-99/technetium-99m generators is approximately 80% to 90% per elution.

The method for calculating how much daughter ion present on the column at any given time is complex because it must consider the decay rates of parent and daughter nuclides, the abundance daughter nuclide produced from the parent, as well as any daughter nuclide initially present or remaining on the column after previous elution

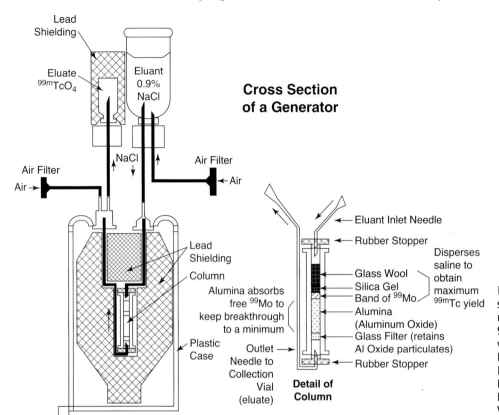

Figure 11.1 • Cross-sectional diagram of a molybdenum-99/technetium-99m generator. (Reprinted with permission from Bushberg, J. T., et al.: The Essential Physics of Medical Imaging, 2nd ed. Philadelphia: Lippincott Williams and Wilkins, 2002.)

(Fig. 11.2). In the case of Mo-99 ($t_{1/2}$ = 66 hours), only 86% of the atoms decay to Tc-99m ($t_{1/2}$ = 6 hours). Typical elution efficiencies of commercially available generators are approximately 80% to 90%. The equation for the theoretical activity of the daughter nuclide present at any time (t) after a previous elution is as follows:

$$A_d^t = (A_p^0)\lambda_d[(e^{-\lambda_p t} - e^{-\lambda_d t})/(\lambda_d - \lambda_p)] + A_d^0 e^{-\lambda_d t}$$

where A_p^0 is the activity of the parent at the time of the previous elution, A_d^0 is the activity of the daughter at the time of the previous elution, λ_p and λ_d are their respective decay constants, and t is the time since the last elution of the generator. The generator system can be eluted several times each day to obtain collective radioactivity because Tc-99m is constantly produced by Mo-99 decay. The time interval since the last elution will determine the maximal amount of Tc-99m available for elution. Approximately 40% of maximal Tc-99m is available after 6 hours, whereas maximal Tc-99m activity is achieved in 23 hours.[1]

Biological Effects of Radiation

The absorption of ionizing radiation by living cells always produces effects potentially harmful to the irradiated organism. An undesirable aspect to the medical use of radiation is that a small number of the atoms in the body tissues will have electrons removed as a result of the photons. Radiation that does this is called *ionizing radiation* and is potentially damaging to body tissues. Therefore, in using ionizing radiation, as in using other pharmaceutical agents, the risks must be balanced with the medical benefits provided for the patient.

The amount of radiation energy absorbed by tissue is called *radiation absorbed dose* and is specified in rads or millirads. A dose of 1 rad implies 100 ergs of energy absorbed

per gram of any tissue. The unit of exposure for x-rays and γ radiation in air, the *roentgen*, is used to specify radiation levels in the environment. One roentgen is the amount of radiation that produces 1 electrostatic unit (ESU) of charge of either sign per 0.001293 g of air at standard temperature and pressure (STP). The SI has adopted the gray (Gy) to replace the rad (1 Gy = 100 rads). Again, the more traditional unit is still used in clinical medicine. In the case of electromagnetic radiation such as x-rays or γ-rays, the roentgen and rad are equivalent.

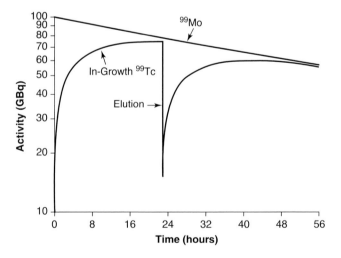

Figure 11.2 • Time–activity curve of a molybdenum-99/technetium-99m generator system demonstrating the in-growth of technetium-99m and subsequent elution. (Reprinted with permission from Bushberg, J. T., et al.: The Essential Physics of Medical Imaging, 2nd ed. Philadelphia: Lippincott Williams and Wilkins, 2002.)

The major difference between electromagnetic radiation (x-rays or γ-rays) and particulate radiation (β^+, β^-, and α particles) lies in the ability of electromagnetic rays to penetrate matter. Whereas particles travel only a few millimeters before expending all their energy, x-rays and γ-rays distribute their energy more diffusely and can travel through several centimeters of tissue.

Particle emitters deliver highly localized radiation doses to biological molecules. Damage results from the direct absorption of this radiation energy. This is known as the *direct effect* of radiation damage. The radiation dose of particle emitters is generally clinically useful for therapeutic use, with limited benefits for diagnostic use.

X-rays and γ-rays deliver more uniform doses in a less concentrated way throughout the irradiated volume of tissue. Damage is indirectly produced by formation of free radicals (atoms or molecules with an unpaired electron). The *indirect effect* of radiation damage generally involves aqueous free radicals as intermediaries in the transfer of radiation energy to the biological molecules.

All biological systems contain water as the most abundant molecule ($\sim$80%). Radiolysis of water is the most likely event in the initiation of biological damage from diagnostic x-rays and γ-rays. The absorption of energy by a water molecule results in the ejection of an electron with the formation of a free radical ion ($H_2O^{\cdot+}$). The free radical ion dissociates to yield a hydrogen ion (H^+) and a hydroxyl free radical ($HO^\cdot$). The hydroxyl free radicals combine to form hydrogen peroxide (H_2O_2), which is an oxidizing agent. In addition, hydrogen free radicals ($H^\cdot$) can form, which can combine with oxygen (O_2) and form a hydroperoxy-free radical ($HO_2^\cdot$). These free radical intermediates are very reactive chemically and can attack and alter chemical bonds.

The only significant "target" molecule for biological damage is DNA. Types of DNA damage include single- and double-chain breakage as well as intermolecular or intramolecular cross-linking of double-stranded DNA. With the direct effect of radiation, the damage makes cell replication impossible. Cell death occurs. For the indirect effect of radiation, if the damage is not lethal but changes the genetic sequence or structure, mutations occur that may lead to cancer or birth of genetically damaged offspring. Some effects of radiation may develop within a few hours; others may take years to become apparent. Consequently, the effects of ionizing radiation on human beings may be classified as somatic (affecting the irradiated person) or genetic (affecting progeny).

Radiation dose can only be estimated, and its "measurement" is called *radiation dosimetry*. In the case of x-ray exposure, most radiation "doses" in the literature are described as the entrance exposure (in roentgens per minute) to the patient. In diagnostic nuclear medicine procedures, patients are irradiated by radiopharmaceuticals localized in certain organs or distributed throughout their bodies. Because the radionuclides are taken internally, there are many variables, and the radiation absorbed dose (rad) to individual patients cannot be measured. It can only be estimated by calculation. Under normal circumstances, no radiation worker or patient undergoing diagnostic investigation by radiopharmaceutical or radiographic procedures should ever suffer from any acute or long-term injury. Typical radiation doses to patients from radiopharmaceuticals are similar to, or less than, those from radiographic procedures.

Radiopharmaceuticals

Medical science provides a framework or paradigm in which to understand disease and to maintain health. Nuclear medicine is the branch of medical science that contributes to medicine by the use of the radiotracer method for diagnosis, and the use of in vivo radioactivity for therapy.

Nuclear medicine generally involves the administration of radioactively labeled compounds to *trace* a biological process. This process may be mechanical (gastric emptying, blood flow, cardiac wall motion) or a variety of other physiological functions. Within the concept of a "radiotracer" is the implication that the agent administered will not disturb the functional aspects of the process you wish to examine. In nuclear medicine, this concept is used to trace physiological processes in vivo and then compare them with known normal images or levels. These images are interpreted within the context of relevant pathophysiology to allow diagnosis of disease. The information obtained from diagnostic images can also be used to follow the patient for improvement following treatment. In clinical practice, nuclear medicine also makes use of in vitro diagnostic methods (radioimmunoassay) as well as in vivo radiopharmaceutical therapy.

The most common application of nuclear medicine is to image the distribution of radiopharmaceuticals in specific tissues or organ systems with a scintillation (Anger) camera for diagnostic purposes. Fundamentally, these instruments or cameras allow in vivo detection and localization of radiotracers. The purpose of the gamma camera is to record the location and intensity of the radiation within the imaging field (Fig. 11.3).

Radiation in the form of gamma photons (occasionally x-rays) initially enters the camera through the collimator, which usually is a sheet of lead with multiple small, precisely made holes. The collimator covers the detector's crystal. The purpose of the collimator is to decrease scattered radiation and to increase the overall resolution of the system. Photons that are not blocked by the collimator then enter a large sodium iodide (with a small amount of thallium) crystal that absorbs γ-rays. The absorbed energy in the crystal is emitted as a flash of light (called a *scintillation*), which is proportional to the

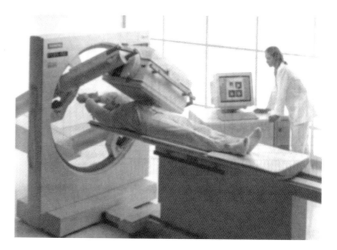

Figure 11.3 ● Patient being imaged with a scintillation (Anger) camera. (Reprinted with permission from Bushberg, J. T., et al.: The Essential Physics of Medical Imaging, 2nd ed. Philadelphia: Lippincott Williams and Wilkins, 2002.)

energy of the γ-ray. Coupled to the back of the NaI(Tl) crystal are photomultiplier (PM) tubes that convert the light flashes to electrical pulses proportional to the amount of light. To localize the original source of the photon (and create an image), a computer assigns *x–y* spatial coordinates to the various γ-rays coming from the patient and stores this information in a matrix. After data collection, the image is converted into a signal for display on a video monitor. The images obtained with the scintillation camera are called *scintigrams*, *scintigraphs*, or *scans*.

Nuclear medicine imaging studies involve the generation of images that represent the functional status of various organs in the body. When interfaced with computer systems, information regarding dynamic physiological parameters such as organ perfusion, metabolism, excretion, and the presence or absence of obstruction can be obtained. Images can be focused on a portion of the body, or an image of the whole body can be acquired by moving the camera from head to toe.

Cross-sectional images of organs can be obtained by rotating a position-sensitive scintillation camera detector about the patient. This type of procedure is called *single photon emission computed tomography* (SPECT), which is the counterpart of CT or computed axial tomography (CAT) scans in diagnostic radiology. Most SPECT systems (Fig. 11.4) use one to three scintillation detectors that rotate about the patient.

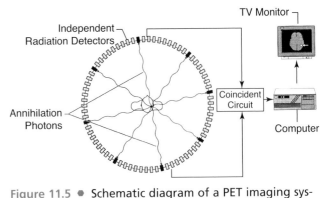

Figure 11.5 ● Schematic diagram of a PET imaging system with multiple scintillation detectors that localize positron decay by coincident detection of annihilation photons.

SPECT is routinely used when imaging the brain or heart to demonstrate three-dimensional distribution of radioactivity in these organs.

A newer modality for imaging uses multiple detector heads to image positron-emitting radiopharmaceuticals by PET (Fig. 11.5). The physics associated with annihilation radiation allow PET cameras to utilize coincident circuitry to facilitate the acquisition of high resolution images for the two photons emitted approximately 180 degrees from each during positron decay. When the photon pair is detected by two detectors, it is known that a decay event took place along a straight line between those detectors. Computer models will calculate a three-dimensional image of the subsequent data set to prepare PET images of the area of interest. Although various positron emitting nuclides can be covalently attached to numerous biologically important molecules for development of PET radiopharmaceuticals, *[18]F-fluorodeoxyglucose* (^{18}F-FDG) is by far, the major clinical PET agent.

The incidence of adverse reactions to radiopharmaceuticals is very low. Most adverse events are allergic reactions and occur within minutes of intravenous injection. In the case of radiolabeled murine antibodies, an anaphylactic reaction may occur on rare occasions.

Fluorine Radiochemistry

The clinically useful radioisotope of fluorine for organ imaging is fluorine-18. Fluorine-18 is produced in a cyclotron according to the $^{18}O(p,n)^{18}F$ nuclear reaction. Fluorine-18 ($t_{1/2}$ = 110 min) decays predominantly by positron emission to oxygen-18 with γ-ray emissions of 511 keV (194%). Fluorine-18 can be attached to several physiologically active molecules and, with the great strength of the C–F bond, appears to be a very useful label for radiopharmaceuticals.[2] Radiotracer production involves relatively complicated synthetic pathways, and the preparation of high–specific-activity compounds presents many problems. The short half-life of fluorine-18 makes it necessary to complete the synthetic and purification procedure quickly.

FLOURINE RADIOPHARMACEUTICALS

2-Fluoro-2-Deoxy-D-Glucose (^{18}F). The only F-18 radiopharmaceutical presently available is fluorine ^{18}F-FDG, the structure of which is shown on next page. Synthesis of ^{18}F-FDG by nucleophilic displacement of a protected

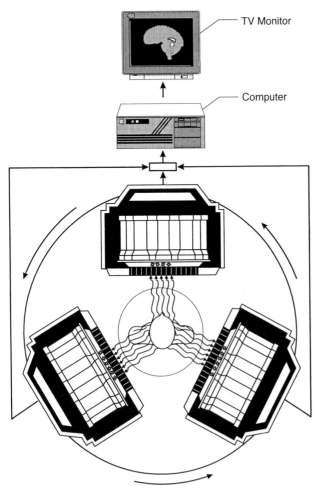

Figure 11.4 ● Schematic diagram of a rotating triple-detector scintillation camera system for single photon emission computed tomography (SPECT).

mannose triflate derivative, hydrolysis of the protecting groups, and purification by solid phase extraction is the typical method of production.[3] The synthetic cascade and subsequent purification is routinely accomplished in about 50 minutes by an automated synthesizer.[4,5]

The high glycolytic rate of many neoplasms compared with that of the surrounding tissues facilitates tumor imaging with this glucose analog. Both glucose and ^{18}F-FDG are transported into the cell and phosphorylated; however, ^{18}F-FDG does not get catabolized as an energy source, nor is it effectively degraded by glucose-6-phosphatase. Thus, energetically active tissues accumulate ^{18}F-FDG. Because of the widespread anatomical distribution of metastases, a whole-body imaging technique using a tumor-specific radiopharmaceutical, such as ^{18}F-FDG, is very useful for tumor detection and mapping to evaluate the extent and relative metabolic activity of the disease.

^{18}F-FDG can also be used for diagnostic imaging of myocardial viability and in the evaluation of seizure disorders.[6]

(^{18}F)-2-Fluoro-2-deoxy-D-glucose

Gallium Radiochemistry

The only radioisotope of gallium that is presently used is gallium-67, which is produced in a cyclotron by proton bombardment of a zinc metal target according to the ^{68}Zn(p,2n)^{67}Ga nuclear reaction. Gallium-67 ($t_{1/2} = 78.2$ hours) decays by EC to stable zinc-67 with principal γ-ray emissions of 93 keV (38%), 185 keV (24%), and 300 keV (16%). The radiotracer is isolated by dissolution of the target in hydrochloric acid followed by isopropyl ether extraction of the gallium-67 from the zinc and other impurities. Gallium-67 is back-extracted from the isopropyl ether into 0.2 M hydrochloric acid, evaporated to dryness, and dissolved in sterile, pyrogen-free 0.05 M hydrochloric acid.[7] Gallium is an amphoteric element that acts as a metal at low pH but forms insoluble hydroxides when the pH is raised above 2 in the absence of chelating agents. At high pH, gallium hydroxide acts as a nonmetal and dissolves in ammonia to form gallates. Gallium forms compounds of oxidation states $+1$, $+2$, and $+3$; however, only the Ga^{+3} state is stable in aqueous solutions.

GALLIUM RADIOPHARMACEUTICALS

Gallium Citrate (^{67}Ga). The gallium (III)–citrate complex is formed by adding the required amount of sodium citrate (0.15 M) to gallium (III) chloride and adjusting the pH to 4.5 to 8.0 with sodium hydroxide. Recent studies have proposed a 1:2 gallium:citrate complex.[8,9]

The patient receives an intravenous injection of 5 to 10 mCi (185–370 MBq) of gallium (^{67}Ga) citrate, and whole-body images are then obtained 24, 48, and 72 hours after injection. Gallium localizes at sites of inflammation or infection as well as various tumors. It is used in clinical practice in the staging

and evaluation of recurrence of lymphomas. Gallium localizes normally in the liver and spleen, bone, nasopharynx, lacrimal glands, and breast tissue. There is also some secretion in the bowel; consequently, the patient may require a laxative and/or enemas to evacuate enteric radioactivity prior to the 48-hour image. As more specific radiotracers have been developed, the nonspecific normal localization of gallium radioactivity has limited its clinical use.

Gallium (^{67}Ga) Citrate

Indium Radiochemistry

The most commonly used radioisotope of indium is indium-111, which is produced in a cyclotron by proton bombardment of a cadmium target according to the ^{112}Cd(p,2n)^{111}In nuclear reaction. Indium-111 ($t_{1/2} = 67.3$ hours) decays by EC to stable cadmium-111 with principal γ-ray emissions of 171 keV (91%) and 245 keV (94%). The radiotracer is isolated by dissolution in hydrochloric acid to form indium chloride (^{111}In). In aqueous solution, lower valence states of indium have been described, but they are unstable and are rapidly oxidized to the trivalent state. In acid solution, indium hexaaqua complexes $[In(H_2O)_6]^{+3}$ are stable at low pH but are hydrolyzed (above pH 3.5) to form a precipitate of indium hydroxide $In(OH)_3$.[5] Indium is stabilized in solution above pH 3.5 if it is complexed with a weak chelating agent such as sodium citrate and stronger chelating agents such as 8-hydroxyquinoline (oxine) or diethylenetriamine pentaacetic acid (DTPA). Monoclonal antibodies and peptides are radiolabeled with indium by using compounds called *bifunctional chelating agents*. Bifunctional chelating agents are molecules that can be attached to the antibody or peptide as well as to the radionuclide.

INDIUM RADIOPHARMACEUTICALS

Indium (^{111}In) Capromab (ProstaScint). Capromab pendetide is a murine monoclonal immunoglobulin G (IgG) antibody conjugated to the linker-chelator, glycyl-tyrosyl-(N,-diethylenetriamine pentaacetic acid)-lysine hydrochloride (Gly-Tyr-Lys-DTPA·HCl). This conjugated antibody is directed against the glycoprotein expressed on prostate epithelium, prostate-specific membrane antigen. It is indicated in the evaluation of newly diagnosed patients with biopsy-proven prostate cancer who are at high risk for pelvic lymph

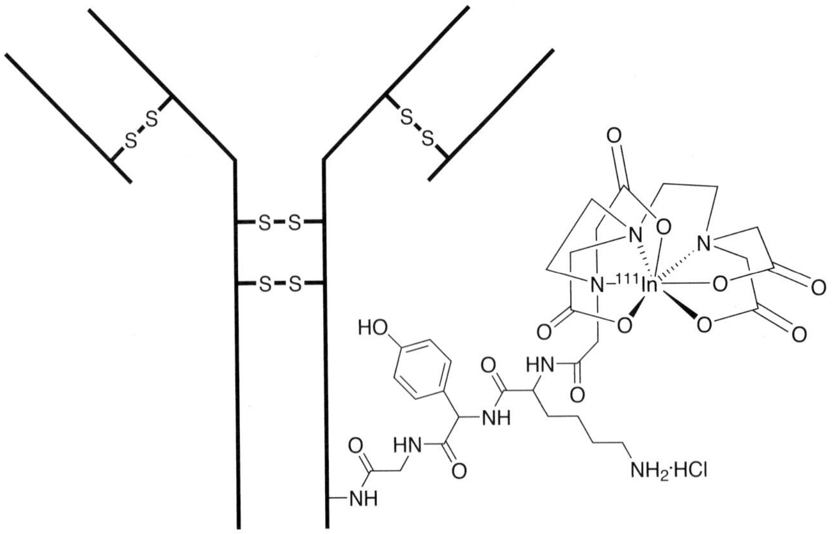

Indium (^{111}In) Capromab Pendetide

node metastases as well as postprostatectomy patients with a rising prostate-specific antigen (PSA), whom there is a high clinical suspicion of metastatic disease.

The kit utilized to prepare this radiotracer contains capromab pendetide, sodium acetate buffer, and a 0.22-μm filter. A portion of the sodium acetate buffer is added to a vial of indium (In-111) chloride to stabilize the radiolabel as an indium (In-111) acetate complex for subsequent reaction with the conjugated antibody. The buffered indium (In-111) acetate complex is added to the capromab pendetide and allowed to incubate for 30 minutes at room temperature. After incubation is complete, the remaining sodium acetate buffer is added to the capromab (In-111) pendetide mixture. The patient dose is drawn into a syringe that was fitted with the 0.22-μm filter. The tagged product must be used within 8 hours of preparation. A schematic representing the bifunctional IgG antibody modified is shown.

The patient receives an intravenous injection of 5 mCi (185 MBq). Since the radiotracer accumulates in both the bladder and bowel, patient preparation includes a cathartic laxative the night before imaging, an enema 1 hour prior to imaging, and the patient is likely to be catheterized. Images of the pelvis are taken 30 minutes after the injection to assess the blood pool distribution, and whole-body or spot images as well as specific pelvic/abdomen images are acquired between 72 and 120 hours after administration.

Indium Chloride (^{111}In). Indium (III) chloride is a sterile, colorless solution that is isolated from the production of radiolabeled indium-111 from cadmium-112 by dissolution in hydrochloric acid solution (0.05 M) and has a pH of 1.4. It is primarily used to radiolabel pharmaceuticals such as monoclonal antibodies and peptides that are used for cancer imaging.

Indium (^{111}In) Oxyquinoline. Indium (^{111}In) oxyquinoline (Indium [^{111}In] oxine) is formed by adding the required amount of 8-hydroxyquinoline sulfate to indium (III) chloride (^{111}In). Other ingredients include polysorbate 80 as a stabilizer and HEPES buffer to adjust the pH range to 6.5 to 7.5. The structure of indium (^{111}In) oxyquinoline is shown.[10]

This radiochemical is indicated for the preparation of patient-specific radiolabeled leukocytes to assess the presence or absence of a suspected infection that is unable to be confirmed by other imaging modalities. Approximately 50 mL of a patient's blood is drawn. The blood will be processed to separate the leukocytes from the plasma and other cellular components. The leukocytes will be incubated with indium (^{111}In) oxyquinoline for 20 minutes, washed with saline, resuspended in the patient's own plasma, and reinfused to the patient within 5 hours of the initial blood draw. The goal in leukocyte preparation is to achieve 200 to 500 μCi of activity in the tagged cells. Images are acquired 2 to 48 hours after reinjection of the radiolabeled cells, allowing the cells to localize at the suspected site of infection.

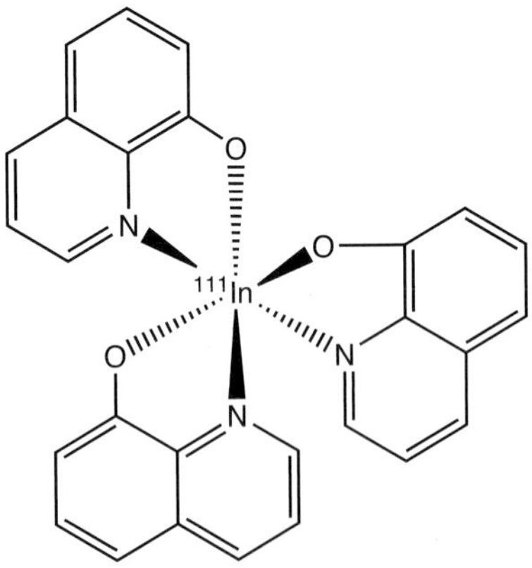

Indium (^{111}In) Oxyquinoline

Indium (^{111}In) Pentetate. Indium (^{111}In) pentetate is formed by adding the required amount of calcium or sodium pentetate (DTPA) to the indium (^{111}In) chloride and adjusting the pH to 7 to 8 with sodium hydroxide and/or hydrochloric acid. A proposed structure of ^{111}In-DTPA is shown on next page.[11,12]

This tracer is indicated for use in cisternography. The patient undergoes a lumbar puncture under sterile conditions and receives an intrathecal injection of 0.5 mCi (18.5 MBq) of indium (^{111}In) pentetate, which distributes into the cerebrospinal fluid (CSF). Initial images are obtained to ensure a good intrathecal injection. Images of the spinal canal and CSF spaces of the brain are acquired intermittently to assess CSF flow or leakage from the normal CSF space.

Another use for ^{111}In-DTPA is in dual isotope gastric emptying studies. After a 6-hour fast, the patient ingests a solid meal of oatmeal or scrambled egg mixed with 1 mCi (37 MBq) of ^{99m}Tc-sulfur colloid along with a liquid meal of water mixed with 0.5 mCi (18.5 MBq) of ^{111}In-DTPA. The patient's stomach is imaged 5 minutes after the meal as the initial gastric image utilizing appropriate camera settings to detect each isotope separately. Imaging continues every 5 to 15 minutes until the recorded activity is reduced to one half the initial gastric activity. Normal values are 50 to 80 minutes for solid meals and 10 to 15 minutes for liquid meals[4]; however, these values can vary based on the size and composition of the meal.[5]

Indium (^{111}In) Pentetate

Indium (^{111}In) Pentetreotide (OctreoScan). Pentetreotide is a modified peptide hormone that consists of a bifunctional chelating agent, DTPA, linked to octreotide, a long-acting analog of the endogenous hormone somatostatin. Somatostatin is a 14–amino acid peptide hormone that binds to the somatostatin receptor. These receptors have been found on many cells of neuroendocrine origin and are expressed in large numbers on nearly all tumors of such origin. The drug is indicated in the imaging of primary and metastatic neuroendocrine tumors bearing somatostatin receptors.

The kit utilized to prepare this radiotracer contains pentetreotide, a solution of indium (^{111}In) chloride/ferric chloride, and a transfer needle. The addition of ferric chloride and the use of the transfer needle are necessary to increase the labeling yield. The radiolabeled solution is added to the pentetreotide vial and incubated at room temperature for 30 minutes. The tagged product must be used within 6 hours of preparation. The structure of labeled radiopharmaceutical, indium (^{111}In) pentetreotide, is shown.[13]

The patient receives an intravenous injection of 3 to 6 mCi (111–222 MBq) of indium (^{111}In) pentetreotide depending on the type of imaging camera that will be used to obtain images. Whole-body images are obtained 4 to 48 hours after injection to localize the primary tumor and sites of metastases.

Indium (In-111) Pentetreotide

Iodine Radiochemistry

Iodine is in group VIIB with the other halogens (fluorine, chlorine, bromine, and astatine). In aqueous solution, compounds of iodine are known with at least five different oxidation states; however, in nuclear medicine, the -1 and $+1$ oxidation states are the most significant. The -1 oxidation state represented as sodium iodide (NaI) is important for thyroid studies and, when obtained in a reductant-free solution (no sodium thiosulfate), is a starting material for the radiolabeling of iodinated radiopharmaceuticals. The common methods for introducing radioiodine into organic compounds are isotope exchange reactions, electrophilic substitution of hydrogen in activated aromatic systems, nucleophilic substitution, and addition to double bonds.[14] Electrophilic substitution on tyrosine side chains is commonly used for protein labeling, The electrophilic species (I^+) can be generated from iodide (I^-) by various oxidizing agents, including (a) chloramine-T (*N*-chloro-*p*-toluene sulfonamide) sodium, (b) enzyme oxidation of (lactoperoxidase), and (c) Iodo-Gen (1,3,4,6-tetrachlora-3α-6α-diphenylglycoluril).

The useful radioisotopes of iodine for organ imaging are iodine-123 and iodine-131. Iodine-123 is produced in a cyclotron by bombarding a xenon-124 target with a proton according to the ^{124}Xe (p,2n)^{123}Cs→^{123}Xe→^{123}I sequence. Iodine-123 is isolated in the iodide form. Cesium-123 ($t_{1/2}$ = 5.9 min) decays by EC to xenon-123 ($t_{1/2}$ = 2.1 hours), which decays to iodine-123. Iodine-123 ($t_{1/2}$ = 13.3 hours) decays by EC to tellurium-123, with a principal γ-ray emission of 159 keV (83%), which makes it the ideal radioisotope of iodine for organ imaging because of increased detection efficiency and reduced radiation burden to the patient. The main disadvantage of I-123 is the need for daily delivery from commercial suppliers because of its short half-life.

Iodine-131 is obtained from a reactor by production of tellurium-131. It is prepared by nuclear bombardment of ^{235}U(n,fission)^{131}Te→^{131}I or ^{130}Te(n,γ)^{131}Te→^{131}I. I-131 is isolated in the iodide form. Tellurium-131 ($t_{1/2}$ = 25 minutes) decays by β^- emission to iodine-131. Iodine-131 ($t_{1/2}$ = 8.04 days) decays by β^- emission to stable xenon-131, with five significant γ-ray emissions ranging from 80 to 723 keV. The major γ-ray of 364 keV (82%) provides good tissue penetration for organ imaging. I-131 properties are either desirable or undesirable based on one's perspective. The high radiation dose from the β^- particles may be undesirable when used for diagnostic purposes, but highly desirable for therapeutic use. The long half-life provides sufficient time for radiolabeling syntheses, but can be problematic in terms of waste disposal. Finally, poor quality images are obtained by current gamma cameras because the high-energy γ-rays are not efficiently recorded by the detector.

IODINE PHARMACEUTICALS

Sodium Iodide (^{123}I). The major indications for thyroid imaging with sodium iodide (^{123}I) are for evaluation of thyroid function (uptake) and/or morphology (imaging). The patient fasts before receiving the oral dose of 0.1 to 0.4 mCi (3.7–14.8 MBq) of sodium iodide (^{123}I) typically in an encapsulated dosage form. Images are obtained of the thyroid and surrounding area 4 to 6 hours after ingestion.

Sodium Iodide (^{131}I). Diagnostic use of sodium iodide (^{131}I) with microcurie doses for evaluating thyroid function and/or morphology is no longer preferred because of the higher radiation dose associated with particle decay from this isotope. Doses from 1 to 10 mCi (37–370 MBq) are used for whole-body imaging to detect metastatic thyroid cancer and/or residual thyroid tissue following thyroidectomy. Whole-body images are obtained 48 to 72 hours later.

Therapeutic use of sodium iodide (^{131}I) occurs in hyperthyroidism or differentiated types of thyroid cancers. A patient with hyperthyroidism will receive an oral dose of 5 to 10 mCi (185–370 MBq) of sodium iodide (^{131}I). The dose could be higher for patients with toxic nodular goiter or other special situations. Treatment doses for differentiated thyroid carcinoma with or without metastases range from 30 to 200 mCi (1,110–7,400 MBq). Seven days after the therapeutic dose, a whole-body scan is performed in an effort to detect metastases not seen on the pretherapy diagnostic images. Thyroid hormone medication will be discontinued for several weeks prior to radiotherapy and thyroid-stimulating hormone (TSH) levels must be evaluated to ensure maximal uptake of the radiotracer for therapy.[15]

Iodine (^{131}I) Tositumomab (Bexxar). Tositumomab is a murine IgG monoclonal antibody directed against the CD20 antigen found on the surface of normal and malignant B lymphocytes. Iodine tositumomab (^{131}I) is a radioiodinated derivative of the antibody indicated for the treatment of patients with CD20 antigen-expressing relapsed or refractory, non-Hodgkin lymphoma. A schematic representing an IgG antibody labeled with covalently linked I-131 is shown. The exact number and position of the covalently linked I-131 is not described.

The treatment regimen occurs in two discrete steps: the dosimetric (diagnostic distribution) and therapeutic steps. Each step consists of a sequential infusion of unlabeled Tositumomab followed by iodine (^{131}I) tositumomab. The patient is premedicated with a thyroid protective agent (either potassium iodide or Lugol solution) for at least 24 hours, and will also receive acetaminophen and diphenhydramine shortly before the infusions begin. The dosimetric step administers 450-mg unlabeled tositumomab followed by 5 mCi (185 MBq) of iodine (^{131}I) tositumomab.

The patient is imaged three times over the next 7 days to assess the biodistribution of the radiolabeled antibody. Imaging occurs within 1 hour following the radiolabeled antibody infusion, 2 to 4 days after the infusion, and also 6 to 7 days after the infusion. If the dosimetric dose's biodistribution is altered, no further drug will be administered. If the dosimetric dose's biodistribution is as expected, the thera-

peutic dose can be administered 7 to 14 days after the dosimetric infusion.

The therapeutic dose is calculated based on the assessment of the patient's biodistribution and elimination of the dosimetric infusion as well as the patient's platelet count. Clinical studies have reported calculated therapeutic doses of 450-mg unlabeled tositumomab followed by 50 to 200 mCi (1,300–5,900 MBq) of iodine (^{131}I) tositumomab. Thyroid protective agents are administered daily until 2 weeks after the last radioiodine dose.[16]

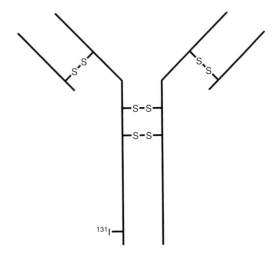

Iodine (I-131) Tositumomab

Technetium Radiochemistry

The most commonly used radioisotope of technetium is technetium-99m, which is produced by molybdenum-99 β^- decay in a molybdenum-99/technetium-99m generator. Technetium-99m ($t_{1/2} = 6$ hours) decays by IT to technetium-99 ($t_{1/2} = 2.1 \times 10^5$ years) with principal γ-ray emissions of 140 keV (100%). The radiotracer is collected as pertechnetate ions ($^{99m}TcO_4^-$) from the generator by elution from the alumina column with sterile normal saline (0.9% sodium chloride). Long-lived radioactive impurities such as molybdate ions ($^{99}MoO_4$) that coelute from the generator column with pertechnetate ions ($^{99m}TcO_4^-$) theoretically may shorten the manufacturer's recommended expiration time of each elution since the Nuclear Regulatory Commission (NRC) and *United States Pharmacopeia* (*USP*) limits molybendum-99 breakthrough to no more than 0.15 μCi of ^{99}Mo per 1 mCi of ^{99m}Tc in the preparation.[5] In clinical practice, molybendum-99 breakthrough is a rare occurrence.

Technetium, is a transition state metal and is the only "artificial" element with a lower atomic number than uranium. No stable isotopes exist in nature. All known isotopes of technetium are radioactive, and as such, has hindered the study of technetium's chemistry. However, milligram quantities of Tc-99 (a weak β^- emitter; $t_{1/2} = 2.1 \times 10^5$ years) are now available for characterization of technetium complexes. Technetium can exist in eight oxidation states, from -1 to $+7$. The $+7$ ($^{99m}TcO_4^-$) and $+4$ state ($^{99m}TcO_2$, or hydrolyzed-reduced technetium-99m) are the most stable forms.[4]

The chemistry of technetium is similar to that of rhenium and is dominated by forming compounds by bonding between the electron-deficient metal and electronegative groups, which are capable of donating electron pairs. Some examples of these electronegative groups include amines, carboxylic acids, hydroxyls, isonitriles, oximes, phosphates, phosphines, and sulfhydryls. Various oxidation states (e.g., +1, +3, +5, etc.) are prepared in the presence of the reducing agent and stabilized by complexation with available ligands.

Tc-99m radiopharmaceuticals are by far the most commonly used radiotracers in day-to-day diagnostic nuclear medicine practice. Almost all technetium radiopharmaceuticals are metal–electron donor complexes. Compounds that contain two or more electron donor groups and bind to a metal are called *chelating agents*. As the pertechnetate ($^{99m}TcO_4{}^-$) ion, technetium will not form metal−donor complexes. However, the pertechnetate ion can be reduced by a stannous salt or other methods to an oxidation state that will complex with various monodentate, bidentate, or polydentate ligands. The most common reducing agent used in clinical practice is the stannous ion.

Technetium-99m radiopharmaceuticals are prepared by combining sodium pertechnetate ($Na^{99m}TcO_4$) with nonradioactive components in a sterile reaction vial. The primary chemical substances in the vial are the complexing agent (ligand) and a stannous salt-reducing agent (stannous chloride, stannous fluoride, or stannous tartrate). The oxidation state of technetium in various complexes as well as the actual chemical structure of many radiopharmaceuticals has yet to be characterized. Several reviews of technetium chemistry are available for further study.[17–20]

After preparation of the radiopharmaceutical, tests for radiochemical purity should be carried out to ensure that the radiotracer is in the correct radiochemical form. Analytical quality control methods include paper and thin-layer chromatography, column chromatography, and solvent extraction. Likely, radiochemical impurities include unreacted sodium pertechnetate ($Na^{99m}TcO_4$), hydrolyzed-reduced technetium ($^{99m}TcO_2$) colloid, technetium–tin colloid, and possibly radiochemical complexes different from the one expected (e.g., ^{99m}Tc-monodentate rather than ^{99m}Tc-bidentate ligand, etc.). The sterile vials containing the stannous salt and the ligand are lyophilized under a sterile inert gas atmosphere (i.e., nitrogen or argon). The ligand in the reaction vial determines the final chemical structure of the ^{99m}Tc-complex and the biological fate after intravenous injection of the radiopharmaceutical.

TECHNETIUM RADIOPHARMACEUTICALS

Sodium Pertechnetate (^{99m}Tc). Sodium pertechnetate (^{99m}Tc) is a sterile, colorless solution in normal saline (0.9% NaCl), obtained by elution of the sterile Mo–99/Tc-99m generator. The major use of sodium pertechnetate (^{99m}Tc) is the preparation of various technetium-99m radiopharmaceuticals either in a nuclear pharmacy or nuclear medicine department. On-site preparation of radiolabeled red blood cells (RBCs) requires the availability of sodium pertechnetate since the radiolabeled cells must be reinfused to the patient within 30 minutes of preparation.

The pertechnetate ion ($^{99m}TcO_4{}^-$), which has an ionic radius and charge similar to the iodide ion (I^-) and is concentrated in the thyroid, salivary glands, kidneys, stomach, and choroid plexus in the brain. It can be used in a diluted solution from the Mo–99/Tc-99m generator elution to image the

thyroid, Meckel's diverticulum (stomach tissue in the intestine), salivary glands, and to detect processes that disrupt the blood-brain barrier (i.e., tumors, abscesses, strokes).

Like iodide, pertechnetate is trapped by the thyroid. Pertechnetate, however, cannot be utilized to prepare thyroid hormone. The patient receives an intravenous injection of 5 to 10 mCi (185–370 MBq) of Tc-99m pertechnetate, and thyroid images are obtained 20 to 30 minutes after injection. The usual dose for other imaging procedures such as Meckel's diverticulum and salivary gland imaging is also 5 to 10 mCi (185–370 MBq), whereas 20 mCi (740 MBq) is used for blood-brain barrier imaging.

Sodium Pertechnetate (^{99m}Tc)

Technetium (^{99m}Tc) Bicisate (Neurolite). Technetium (^{99m}Tc) bicisate is a neutral, lipophilic complex that crosses the blood-brain barrier and is selectively retained in the brain.

The kit used to prepare the product contains two vials. Vial "A" contains the ligand, tin, and other components that must be protected from light, whereas vial "B" contains a buffer solution. The radiopharmaceutical is prepared by adding sodium pertechnetate (^{99m}Tc) to the shielded "B" vial containing the buffer. The vial A containing lyophilized bicisate, EDTA, mannitol, and stannous chloride is reconstituted with 3 mL of normal saline (0.9% NaCl). Within 30 seconds, 1 mL of the saline solution from vial A is transferred to vial B and allowed to incubate at room temperature for 30 minutes. The tagged product must be used within 6 hours of preparation. The structure of the technetium complex is [N,N′-ethylene-di-L-cysteinato(3−)]oxo [^{99m}Tc]technetium(V) diethyl ester.[21]

After intravenous injection of 20 mCi (740 MBq) of Tc-99m bicisate, about 5% of the injected dose is localized within the brain cells 5 minutes after injection. Ester hydrolysis traps the radiotracer within the brain. This radiotracer is indicated for the evaluation of stroke, but it is used off-label to clinically evaluate various brain disorders, especially brain perfusion ("brain death").

Technetium (^{99m}Tc) Bicisate

Technetium (^{99m}Tc) Disofenin (Hepatolite). Technetium (^{99m}Tc) disofenin is a 2:1 complex of ligand:metal that is rapidly eliminated via the hepatobiliary system. Clearance from the blood is delayed by high bilirubin levels. The primary clinical indication for this product is possible acute cholecystitis. In acute cholecystitis, there is

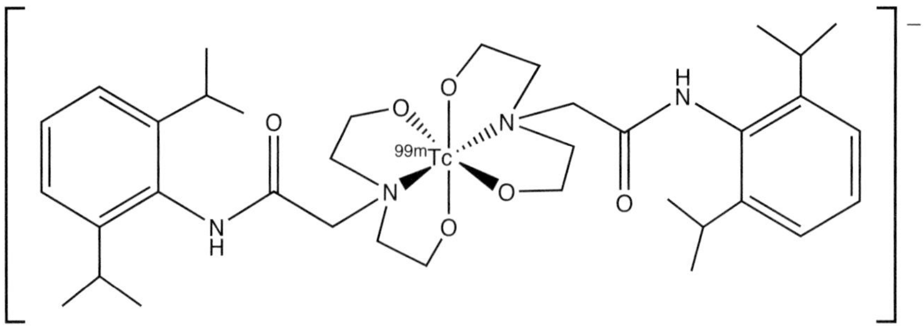

Technetium (^{99m}Tc) Disofenin

obstruction of the cystic duct leading to the gallbladder. The gallbladder is not visualized because the radiotracer cannot enter it. Some other clinical conditions that can be diagnosed by biliary images are common bile duct obstruction, biliary leak following surgery, biliary atresia, and a choledochal cyst.

The product is prepared by adding sodium pertechnetate (^{99m}Tc) to the shielded vial containing disofenin and stannous chloride. The preparation is allowed to incubate for 4 minutes. The product should be used within 6 hours of preparation. The structure of the technetium complex is shown.[22,23] Hepatobiliary agents are commonly referred to as *HIDA agents*, or *hepatobiliary aminodiacetic acids*.

The fasting patient receives an intravenous injection of 5 mCi (185 MBq), which is taken up by the hepatocytes in the liver by active anionic transport. Patients with bilirubin levels greater than 5 mg/dL require an 8 mCi (296 MBq) dose. Then the radiopharmaceutical is excreted in bile, via the biliary canaliculus, into the bile ducts, with accumulation in the gallbladder and finally excretion via the common bile duct into the small bowel. The normal patient exhibits early accumulation of the radiopharmaceutical in the liver and the gallbladder.

Technetium (^{99m}Tc) Exametazime (Ceretec). Technetium (^{99m}Tc) exametazime[5] is a mixture of unstable lipophilic enantiomers that rapidly cross the blood-brain barrier and is trapped in the tissues. The proposed trapping mechanism for localization includes reduction by glutathione. A similar diffusion and trapping process occurs with autologous lymphocytes in vitro.

Exametazime is also known as *hexamethylpropyleneamine oxime* or HMPAO. The radiolabeled complex is indicated for cerebral perfusion in stroke, but is most commonly used for the radiolabeling of autologous leukocytes as an adjunct in the localization of intra-abdominal infection and inflammatory bowel disease.

Each kit includes several components: (a) reaction vials containing a mixture of exametazime, stannous chloride, and sodium chloride; (b) vials of 1% methylene blue; (c) vials of phosphate buffer in 0.9% NaCl; and (d) 0.45-μm syringe filters. Product preparation depends on the intended use.

For use as a cerebral perfusion agent, the kit can be prepared with or without stabilizer. Shelf life is 4 hours with stabilizer, but only 30 minutes without stabilizer. Stabilizer is prepared by injecting 0.5 mL of 1% methylene blue in the phosphate buffer vial. Fresh sodium pertechnetate (^{99m}Tc) elution (<2 hours old) is added to the shielded vial containing exametazime. The vial is gently agitated for 10 seconds and used immediately because this unstabilized complex has a shelf life of approximately 30 minutes. For stabilization, 2 mL of the methylene blue/phosphate buffer mixture is added to the reconstituted exametazime vial within 2 minutes of the technetium (^{99m}Tc) exametazime vial reconstitution. Since the stabilized product is dark blue, a syringe filter is utilized to prevent inadvertent administration of particulate matter. Unstabilized product should be visually inspected for a clear, colorless appearance prior to administration. The patient receives an intravenous dose of 10 to 20 mCi (370–740 MBq). Dynamic imaging begins immediately following injection for up to 10 minutes. Static imaging may be performed from 15 minutes to 6 hours after injection.

For the radiolabeling of autologous leukocytes, approximately 50 mL of a patient's blood is drawn. The blood will be processed to separate the leukocytes from the

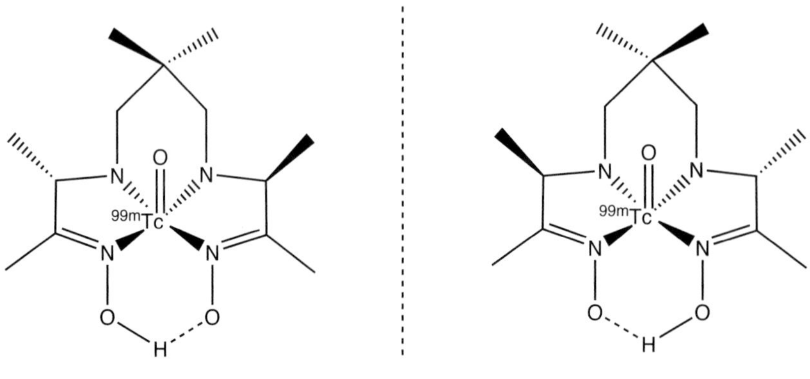

Technetium (^{99m}Tc) Exametazime

plasma and other cellular components. Fresh sodium pertechnetate (^{99m}Tc) elution (<2 hours old) is added to the shielded vial containing exametazime. The vial is gently agitated for 10 seconds and used immediately. The leukocytes will be incubated with technetium (^{99m}Tc) exametazime for 15 minutes, washed with saline, resuspended in the patient's own plasma, and reinfused to the patient as soon as possible. The goal in leukocyte preparation is to achieve 7 to 25 mCi of activity in the tagged cells. Images are acquired 2 to 4 hours after reinjection of the radiolabeled cells, allowing the cells to localize at the suspected site of infection.

Technetium (^{99m}Tc) Macroaggregated Albumin. Technetium (^{99m}Tc) macroaggregated albumin (^{99m}Tc-MAA) is a sterile white suspension of human albumin aggregates formed by denaturing human albumin at 80°C for 30 minutes at pH 5 (isoelectric point of albumin).[4] The particle size and number of particles can be estimated with a hemocytometer grid. The particle composition within the suspension should be between 10 and 100 μm, with no particles greater than 150 μm. Commercial manufacturing practices provide a consistent range for the number of particles per vial as well as a consistent range of particle size. This primary use of this agent is for the imaging of the pulmonary microcirculation to assess potential pulmonary emboli. Another much less common indication is to evaluate peritoneovenous (LeVeen) shunt patency.

In general, the kit is prepared by adding sodium pertechnetate (^{99m}Tc) to the shielded vial containing albumin, aggregated albumin, and stannous chloride, gently inverting the reconstituted suspension (to prevent foaming), and allowing the mixture to incubate at room temperature for 15 minutes. Gentle inversion of the vial is recommended to provide a uniform suspension prior to withdrawing a patient dose into a syringe. If the syringe is not used immediately, it should be gently inverted to resuspend the particles prior to injection. The tagged product is to be used within 12 hours of preparation. The precise structure of the radiolabeled complex is unknown at this time.

The patient receives an intravenous injection of 2 to 5 mCi (74–185 MBq) of the Tc-99m albumin aggregates, which lodge in some of the small pulmonary arterioles and capillaries. The number of aggregates recommended for good image quality and patient safety is 100,000 to 500,000 particles; thus, only a small fraction of the 280 billion capillaries are occluded. Multiple images of the lung are obtained to assess lung perfusion. The distribution of the particles in the lung is a function of regional blood flow; consequently,

in the normal lung, the particles are distributed uniformly throughout the lung. When blood flow is occluded because of emboli, multiple segmental "cold" (decreased radioactivity) defects are seen. This procedure is almost always combined with a xenon-133 gas or technetium-99m DTPA aerosol lung ventilation scan (should be normal in pulmonary embolism) and same-day chest radiograph x-ray (should be normal).

Technetium (^{99m}Tc) Mebrofenin (Choletec). Technetium (^{99m}Tc) mebrofenin[22,23] is a 2:1 complex of ligand:metal that is rapidly eliminated via the hepatobiliary system. The presence of bromine within the structure of mebrofenin makes the drug more lipophilic, and thus it has higher hepatic extraction than other hepatobiliary iminodiacetic acids (HIDA). Clearance from the blood is also affected by bilirubin levels, but generally to a much lesser extent because of the higher hepatic extraction. The clinical indication for this product is hepatobiliary imaging.

The product is prepared by adding sodium pertechnetate (^{99m}Tc) to the shielded vial containing mebrofenin, stannous fluoride and preservatives, and allowing the mixture to incubate for 15 minutes. The presence of preservatives allows this kit to be used for up to 18 hours after preparation.

The fasting patient receives an intravenous injection of 5 mCi (185 MBq), which is taken up by the hepatocytes in the liver by active anionic transport. Patients with bilirubin levels greater than 1.5 mg/dL may require a 10 mCi (370 MBq) dose.

Technetium (^{99m}Tc) Medronate. Technetium (^{99m}Tc) Medronate (^{99m}Tc-MDP)[24] is a diphosphonate complex with technetium-99m indicated for bone imaging to identify areas of altered osteogenesis. The clinical use of this agent is for investigation of skeletal problems such as metastatic disease to the bones, osteomyelitis, Paget disease, fractures, primary bone tumors, avascular necrosis, metabolic bone disease, and loose or infected hip prostheses. Stress fractures can be diagnosed by bone imaging when x-rays are completely normal. Bone radioscintigraphy is one of the most commonly performed nuclear medicine diagnostic procedures because the whole-body survey allows evaluation of the entire skeleton, which cannot be done as cost-effectively by any other imaging modality.

The relatively weak complex is prepared by adding sodium pertechnetate (^{99m}Tc) to the shielded vial containing medronic acid, a stannous salt (varies among manufacturers) with or without an antioxidant stabilizer. Radiolabeling

Technetium (^{99m}Tc) Mebrofenin

requires an incubation of 1 to 2 minutes, and the recommended shelf life is 6 hours.

The patient receives an intravenous injection of 10 to 20 mCi (370–740 MBq) of Tc-99m medronate, which localizes in bone according to the degree of metabolic activity. Tc-99m medronate is absorbed onto hydroxyapatite crystals at sites of new bone formation with about 50% to 60% of the injected dose distributed throughout the skeleton within 3 hours; the rest is excreted by the kidneys. The patient should void immediately prior to imaging to minimize interference from the bladder. Images are obtained 1 to 4 hours postinjection.

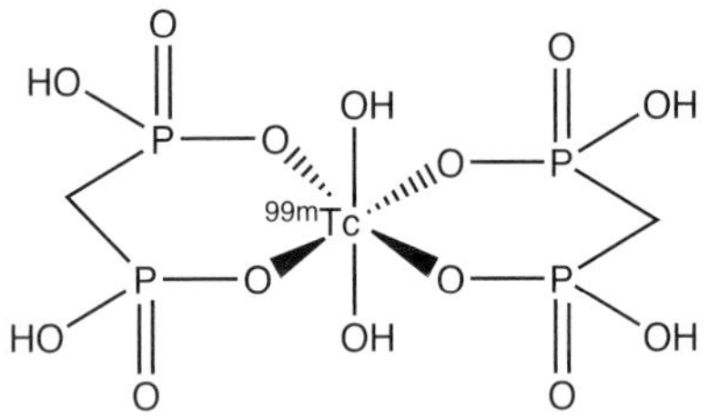

Technetium (^{99m}Tc) Medronate

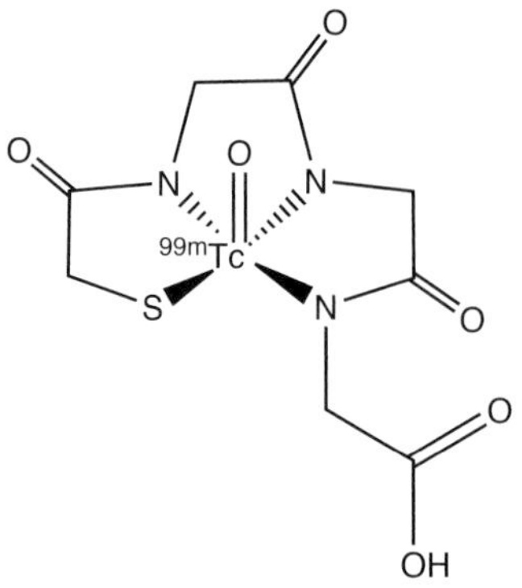

Technetium (^{99m}Tc) Mertiatide (TechneScan MAG3).
Technetium (^{99m}Tc) mertiatide complex is the radiopharmaceutical agent of choice to provide information about relative function of the kidneys and urine outflow because of its high renal extraction efficiency. Indications include renal artery stenosis in nonperfused kidneys, renal transplant assessment, and outflow obstruction.

The kit includes a reaction vial containing betiatide (a mertiatide prodrug), stannous chloride dihydrate, sodium tartrate, and lactose monohydrate sealed under argon. A filter-containing vented needle is also included. Betiatide must be protected from light. The generator elution utilized for the preparation of this complex should be no more than 6 hours old. The complex is prepared by inserting the venting needle through the shielded reaction vial's rubber stopper and then adding sodium pertechnetate (^{99m}Tc) to the shielded reaction vial. Before the pertechnetate syringe is removed, the plunger should be pulled back so that 2 mL of room air replaces the argon in the vial. Room air is required to for oxidation of excess stannous ion to ensure high radiochemical purity. The reaction vial is heated at 100°C for 10 minutes and then allowed to cool for 15 minutes. Initially, a weak ^{99m}Tc-tartrate complex is formed followed by ligand exchange with mertiatide (formed by the hydrolysis of betiatide) to form the desired technetium (^{99m}Tc) mertiatide complex.[25]

The patient receives a bolus intravenous injection of 10 mCi (370 MBq) and dynamic images are obtained every 3 to 5 seconds to study blood flow to the kidneys. Sequential static images are then obtained for 20 to 30 minutes to evaluate renal cortical uptake, excretion, and tubular clearance. Delayed images may be required to evaluate patients with obstruction or renal failure. Normally, there is prompt symmetric bilateral perfusion, good bilateral cortical accumulation with visualization of the collecting systems by 3 to 5 minutes post injection, and rapid excretion into the bladder, with no delay to indicate partial or complete obstruction.

Technetium (^{99m}Tc) Mertiatide

Technetium (^{99m}Tc) Oxidronate Injection.
Technetium (^{99m}Tc) oxidronate (^{99m}Tc-HDP)[24] is a hydroxylated diphosphonate complex with technetium-99m also indicated for bone imaging to identify areas of altered osteogenesis. The additional hydroxyl group on the methylene spacer connecting the phosphonate groups of medronate provides higher binding affinity for hydroxyapatite crystals in bone; however, subjective criteria indicate no advantage to use of this agent.

The relatively weak complex is prepared by adding sodium pertechnetate (^{99m}Tc) to the shielded vial containing oxidronate sodium, stannous chloride, sodium chloride, and gentisic acid. Radiolabeling requires an incubation of 30 to 60 seconds, and the recommended shelf life is 8 hours.

The recommended dose is an intravenous injection of 10 to 20 mCi (370–740 MBq). The patient should void immediately prior to imaging to minimize interference from the bladder. Images are obtained 1 to 4 hours postinjection.

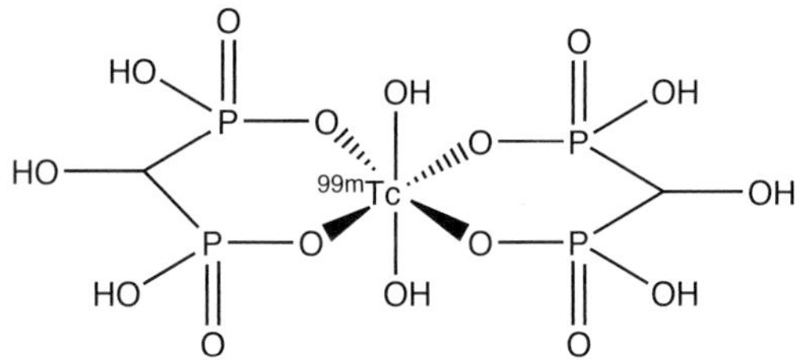

Technetium (^{99m}Tc) Oxidronate

Technetium (^{99m}Tc) Pentetate.
Technetium (^{99m}Tc) pentetate (^{99m}Tc DTPA) is a complex between DTPA and technetium-99m. The precise structure of Tc-99m pentetate is unknown; evidence suggests the central metal atom may be at a +4 oxidation state.[5,12] The clinical indications for this agent are renal imaging, renal functional studies (perfusion and GFR), and brain imaging. An additional clinical use of ^{99m}Tc DTPA is as an aerosol for pulmonary studies.

The complex is formed when sodium pertechnetate (^{99m}Tc) is added to a shielded vial containing DTPA (or a pentasodium or a calcium trisodium salt thereof) with or without an antioxidant and a stannous salt. Recommended incubations times vary from a few minutes up to 15 minutes in length, and the shelf life is between 6 and 12 hours depending on the absence or presence of an antioxidant, respectively.

For renal imaging and GFR studies, the patient receives an intravenous injection of 3 to 5 mCi (111–185 MBq) and the kidneys are imaged for 20 to 30 minutes. The GFR is calculated by a quantitative method using a combination of imaging and counting the radioactivity in serum and urine samples. Renal and brain perfusion studies use doses from 10 to 20 mCi (370–740 MBq). Both dynamic and static images are usually acquired for perfusion studies. For lung studies, 30 to 50 mCi (1.11–1.85 GBq) is placed in a closed, disposable nebulizer system. After 5 to 10 minutes of inhalation by the patient, the nebulizer is detached and patient images from various projections are obtained. Images are comparable to those obtained with xenon-133.

Technetium (^{99m}Tc) Pyrophosphate

Technetium (^{99m}Tc) Pentetate

Technetium (^{99m}Tc) Pyrophosphate.

Technetium (^{99m}Tc) pyrophosphate (^{99m}Tc-PYP)[20] is a pyrophosphate complex with technetium-99m indicated for bone, cardiac, and blood pool imaging. The primary current clinical uses are for cardiac and blood pool imaging.

For cardiac imaging, the complex is prepared by adding sodium pertechnetate (^{99m}Tc) to the shielded vial containing sodium pyrophosphate and stannous fluoride. Radiolabeling requires an incubation of 30 to 60 seconds, and the recommended shelf life is 6 hours. For blood pool imaging, the vial is reconstituted with normal saline (0.9% NaCl) and used within the next 30 minutes without further processing. The unlabeled pyrophosphate/stannous fluoride solution is administered to the patient intravenously 15 to 60 minutes prior to sodium pertechnetate (^{99m}Tc) for in vivo labeling of RBCs.

The recommended dose for cardiac imaging is an intravenous injection of 10 to 15 mCi (370–555 MBq) of technetium (^{99m}Tc) pyrophosphate within 24 to 144 hours after the onset of symptoms. The mechanism of radiotracer accumulation in damaged myocardium is unclear, but it is assumed that the radiotracer may bind to an ongoing calcification process that occurs in the damaged cells. For blood pool imaging (gated cardiac blood pool or gastrointestinal [GI] bleeding), the stannous salt is administered and allowed to accumulate by binding to hemoglobin in the RBCs. Then, 20 to 30 mCi (740–1,110 MBq) of sodium pertechnetate (^{99m}Tc) is administered. The pertechnetate ion also penetrates the RBC, but encounters the stannous salt for in vivo reduction and entrapment within the RBCs.

Technetium (^{99m}Tc) Red Blood Cells (UltraTag RBC Kit).

An in vitro method is available to radiolabel a patient's donated RBCs for use in blood pool imaging (gated cardiac blood pool or GI bleeding) studies. A sterile reaction vial containing stannous chloride is used to radiolabel a patient's own RBCs with sodium pertechnetate (^{99m}Tc). Briefly, the patient's blood (1–3 mL) is drawn with acid citrate dextrose (ACD) or heparin (100 units) used as an anticoagulant. The blood is labeled with the patient's name and hospital number and added to the sterile reaction vial. After mixing and incubation for 5 minutes, sodium hypochlorite (6 mg) is added to the vial to oxidize excess stannous ions (Sn^{+2}) to stannic ions (Sn^{+4}). Then, a citrate buffer is added to adjust the pH to about 7.4. Finally, 30 mCi (1,110 MBq) of sodium pertechnetate (^{99m}Tc) is added to the vial, mixed and incubated for 20 minutes. Without further preparation, the patient receives an intravenous injection of 25 mCi (925 MBq) of his or her own radiolabeled RBCs.

Technetium (^{99m}Tc) Sestamibi (Cardiolite and Miraluma).

Technetium (^{99m}Tc) sestamibi is a lipophilic cation complex represented as ^{99m}Tc-(MIBI)$_6^+$, where MIBI is 2-methoxyisobutyl isonitrile.[26] It is clinically indicated as a myocardial perfusion agent for detecting coronary artery disease and evaluation of myocardial function (accomplished by imaging during rest and during cardiovascular stress with either exercise or pharmacologic stress) as well as a second line diagnostic drug after mammography to assist in the evaluation of breast lesions in patients with an abnormal mammogram or a palpable breast mass. An additional clinical use is the evaluation of hyperparathyroidism.

Preparation of ^{99m}Tc sestamibi begins with the addition of sodium pertechnetate (^{99m}Tc) to shielded reaction vial containing tetrakis (2methoxyisobutyl isonitrile) copper (I) tetrafluoroborate, sodium citrate, L-cysteine hydrochloride, mannitol, and stannous chloride. Initially, the reduced technetium-99m forms a weak complex with citrate, which undergoes a ligand exchange with the isonitrile during a 10-minute heating period in a boiling water bath. The reaction vial requires cooling for 15 minutes before use. The recommended shelf life is 6 hours.

Technetium (^{99m}Tc) sestamibi accumulates in the myocardium by facilitated diffusion from the Na^+/H^+ antiporter.[27] There is no "redistribution," or movement of the tracer out of the myocardium and back into the bloodstream. This tracer has several advantages as a myocardial perfusion agent when compared with thallous (^{201}Tl) chloride. The shorter half-life of technetium-99m (6 hours) when compared with thallium-201 (73 hours) allows administration of a larger dose for shorter imaging times. The

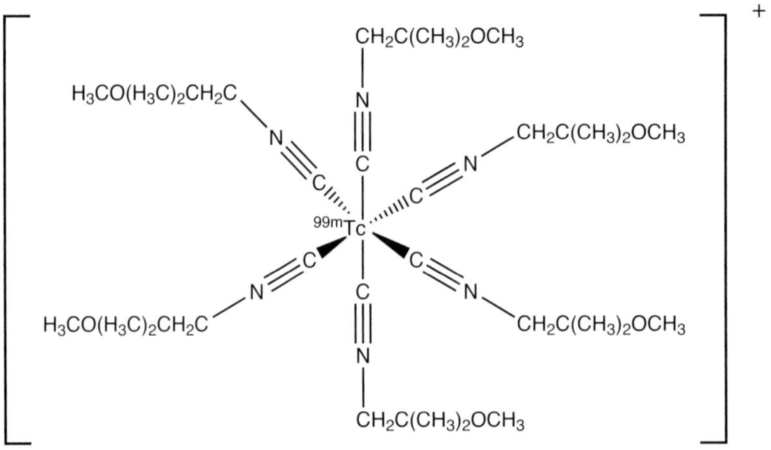

Technetium (^{99m}Tc) Sestamibi

higher energy γ-ray (140 keV) also provides better quality images with contemporary gamma cameras.

Myocardial perfusion imaging is, by far, the most common nuclear medicine procedure. Various myocardial perfusion protocols utilize ^{99m}Tc sestamibi for one or both procedures: 1-day rest first, stress second, 1-day stress first, rest second, 1-day stress first, rest if ischemia is present, 2-day protocols, and dual-isotope studies. The 1-day rest first, stress second protocol utilizes 8 to 10 mCi (296–370 MBq) while the patient is at rest (normal blood flow). Imaging occurs 30 to 60 minutes later. Sufficient time is needed for the radiotracer to clear the liver before imaging. One to four hours after the rest study, 25 to 30 mCi (925–1,110 MBq) is injected at peak stress (treadmill or pharmacologic stress with increased blood flow demand), and imaging occurs 15 to 60 minutes later. Two-day protocols typically utilize 20 to 25 mCi (740–925 MBq) doses for both the rest and stress images. Dual-isotope protocols typically perform a thallium rest study first, followed shortly thereafter with a ^{99m}Tc stress study.[15]

The recommended dose for ^{99m}Tc sestamibi when used for breast imaging is 20 to 30 mCi (740–1,110 MBq). When used for parathyroid imaging, the recommended dose is 25 to 30 mCi (925–1,110 MBq).

Technetium (^{99m}Tc) Succimer Injection. 2,3-dimercaptosuccinic acid (DMSA, succimer) forms a hydrophilic complex when labeled with technetium-99m that is useful in evaluating renal function, especially in children.

The pH-dependent preparation of ^{99m}Tc-DMSA begins with the addition of sodium pertechnetate (^{99m}Tc) to shielded reaction vial containing 2,3-dimercaptosuccinic acid, stannous chloride, ascorbic acid, and inositol at a pH range of 2 to 3. Various metal-DMSA complexes are initially formed, but over the 10-minute incubation period at this acidic pH, the hexacoordinate complex[28] of three carboxylic acids and three sulfhydryls produces a tracer with the highest renal uptake.[5] Localization of such a complex prepared at a certain pH is not altered if the environmental pH is subsequently changed.[29] This complex has a shelf life of 4 hours.

The patient is injected with 2 to 6 mCi (74–222 MBq) of ^{99m}Tc-DMSA and images are taken 1 to 2 hours later.

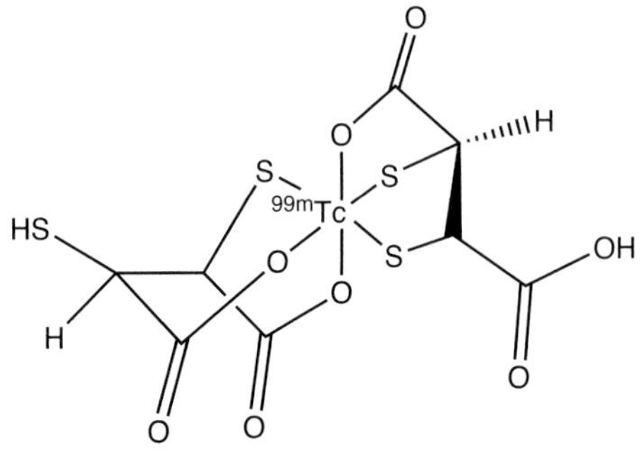

Technetium (^{99m}Tc) Succimer

Technetium (^{99m}Tc) Sulfur Colloid. Technetium (^{99m}Tc) sulfur colloid (^{99m}Tc-SC) is a dispersion of particles larger than those found in solution, but small enough to remain suspended in the delivery matrix for a very long time. It is indicated for use by injection to assess functional capacity of reticuloendothelial cells of the liver, spleen, and bone marrow, to evaluate peritoneovenous (LeVeen) shunt patency. It is indicated orally to assess gastric emptying. Another use involves the intralymphatic or peritumoral administration for radioguided sentinel lymph node biopsy.

Kits for the preparation of ^{99m}Tc-SC include the following three vials: (a) a reaction vial containing sodium thiosulfate, edentate disodium, and gelatin; (b) "vial A," which is an aqueous solution of dilute hydrochloric acid; and (c) "vial B," which is an aqueous solution of sodium biphosphate and sodium hydroxide. Sodium pertechnetate (^{99m}Tc) solution is added to the shielded reaction vial followed by the addition of the dilute hydrochloric acid. Upon heating in a water bath, the acid reacts with the thiosulfate and ^{99m}TcO$_4^-$ to form the colloidal metal sulfide, ^{99m}Tc$_2$S$_7$. Short heating periods provide a higher population of smaller colloid particles in the final preparation,[30] whereas extended heating periods produce larger particles with increasing amounts of colloidal sulfur.[18] After the heating period has ended, the reaction vial is cooled for a brief period, and then the chemical reaction is quenched by the addition of the aqueous solution of sodium biphosphate and sodium hydroxide to the reaction vial. The inclusion of gelatin as an ingredient prevents colloid particles from clumping together. Particle sizes range from 0.1 to 1 μm, with a mean size of 0.3 μm.[4]

After intravenous injection of 1 to 12 mCi (37–444 MBq) of ^{99m}Tc-SC, the tracer is rapidly cleared from the blood by the reticuloendothelial cells of the liver, spleen, and bone marrow. Uptake depends on the relative blood perfusion rate and the functional capacity of the cells. In the normal patient, 85% of the radiocolloid is phagocytized by Kupffer cells in the liver, 7.5% by the spleen, and the remainder by the bone marrow, lungs, and kidneys. Liver-spleen images can be acquired within 20 minutes of administration. Bone marrow imaging studies are performed 1 hour after injection of 10 mCi (370 MBq) of ^{99m}Tc-SC. Normal bone marrow will take up the radiocolloid, but diseased bone marrow appears as "cold" defects in patients with tumor deposits in the marrow.

Technetium (^{99m}Tc) sulfur colloid use for GI studies includes gastroesophageal reflux (GER) and gastric emptying of solid food. Gastroesophageal reflux imaging is performed after having the patient swallow acidified orange juice mixed with 1 mCi (37 MBq) of ^{99m}Tc-SC. Normal patients do not demonstrate reflux. Gastric emptying imaging is performed after the patient swallows solid food (i.e., scrambled eggs or pancakes) radiolabeled with 1 mCi (37 MBq) of ^{99m}Tc-SC. In general, the normal gastric emptying half-time is less than 90 minutes for solid food.[15] Imaging begins shortly after administration and monitors the migration of the colloid particles.

Identification of sentinel lymph nodes for subsequent biopsy in breast cancer[31] and melanoma[32] patients is accomplished by the administration of several injections totaling 0.5 to 1.5 mCi (19–56 MBq) of filtered (0.22-μm filter) or unfiltered ^{99m}Tc-SC. Smaller colloid particles may translocate more readily into the lymphatic system, whereas larger particles remain at the injection site.[15,30] Imaging begins shortly after administration and monitors the migration of the colloid particles.

Technetium (^{99m}Tc) Tetrofosmin (Myoview). Technetium (^{99m}Tc) tetrofosmin is a lipophilic cation complex[33] clinically indicated as a myocardial perfusion agent for detecting regions of reversible myocardial ischemia in the presence or absence of infracted myocardium, identifying changes in perfusion induced by pharmacologic stress in patients with coronary artery disease, and assessing left ventricular dysfunction.

Preparation of technetium (^{99m}Tc) tetrofosmin begins with the addition of sodium pertechnetate (^{99m}Tc) to shielded reaction vial containing tetrofosmin [6,9-bis(2-ethoxyethyl)-3,12-dioxa-6,9-diphosphatetradecane], stannous chloride, disodium sulphosalicylate, sodium D-gluconate, and sodium hydrogen carbonate. Initially, the reduced technetium-99m forms a weak complex with gluconate which undergoes a ligand exchange with tetrofosmin during a 15-minute incubation period at room temperature. The recommended shelf life is 8 hours.

Technetium (^{99m}Tc) tetrofosmin accumulates in the myocardium by facilitated diffusion from the Na$^+$/H$^+$ antiporter.[27] There is essentially no "redistribution," or movement of the tracer out of the myocardium back into the bloodstream. Heart:liver ratios are somewhat higher for technetium (^{99m}Tc) tetrofosmin as compared with technetium (^{99m}Tc) sestamibi and allows for a shorter interval between injection and imaging for technetium (^{99m}Tc) tetrofosmin.[34]

Various myocardial perfusion protocols utilize technetium (^{99m}Tc) tetrofosmin for 1-day, 2-day, and dual isotope studies. One day protocols should utilize 5 to 12 mCi (185–444 MBq) for the first dose (rest or stress). Imaging can commence as early as 15 minutes later. One to four hours after the first study, 15 to 33 mCi (555–1,221 MBq) is injected for the second study. Two-day protocols typically utilize 30 mCi (1,110 MBq) doses for both the rest and stress images. Dual-isotope protocols typically perform a thallium rest study first, followed shortly thereafter with a technetium-99m stress study.[15]

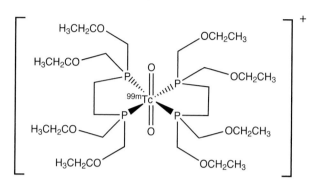

Technetium (^{99m}Tc) Tetrofosmin

Thallium Radiochemistry

The clinically useful radioisotope of thallium is thallium-201. This isotope is produced in a cyclotron by proton bombardment of a thallium metal target according to a ^{203}Tl(p,3n)^{201}Pb→^{201}Tl sequence. Lead-201 ($t_{1/2}$ = 9.4 hours) decays by EC to thallium-201. Thallium-201 ($t_{1/2}$ = 73 hours) decays by EC to stable mercury-201, with principal γ-ray emissions of 135 keV (3%) and 167 keV (10%), and mercury-201 daughter x-rays from 69 to 80 keV (94.5%), all of which can be used for organ imaging.

The irradiated thallium target is dissolved in nitric acid, and the Pb-201 is separated from the thallium-203 by sequential ion exchange column chromatography with an EDTA containing mobile phase. Unbound lead-201 is allowed to decay for approximately 24 hours and passed through another ion exchanged column. Resin-bound thallium-201 (III) is eluted with hydrazine sulfate to provide thallium-201 (I). The elute containing thallium-201 ions are converted to the chloride salt form. The pH is adjusted to 4.5 to 7.0 with sodium hydroxide, made isotonic with sodium chloride containing benzyl alcohol as a preservative, and sterilized by filtration.[4,35]

THALLIUM RADIOPHARMACEUTICALS

Thallous (^{201}Tl) Chloride. The most common clinical uses of this radiotracer are for the evaluation of myocardial perfusion and myocardial viability. It is also indicated for the localization of parathyroid hyperactivity. It is commercially available as a ready-to-use intravenous solution.

Thallous (^{201}Tl) chloride accumulates in viable myocardial tissue by Na$^+$/K$^+$ ATPase as well as Na$^+$/K$^+$/2Cl$^-$ symporter[27] much like potassium ions and is a dynamic exchange between the myocardial cell and the blood. Uptake is dependent on blood flow rates; at very high flow rates, extraction efficiency decreases. Thallous (^{201}Tl) chloride does not concentrate in scarred or infarcted myocardium.

These concepts are the basis for the stress/redistribution imaging strategy employed for the detection of coronary artery disease. To do this, the patient submits to either physiological "stress" (treadmill exercise) or pharmacological "stress" with an intravenous infusion of a vasodilator depending upon the patient's physical condition. At maximum stress, the patient is injected with 3 to 4 mCi (111–148 MBq) of thallous (^{201}Tl) chloride. The "stress test" accentuates the myocardial perfusion abnormality because areas of significant arterial narrowing cannot respond to the increased blood flow demands of the stress as well as normal arteries. Images of the heart are obtained immediately after stress. Damaged or ischemic myocardium show less thallous (^{201}Tl) chloride uptake than surrounding normal heart muscle. Three hours after stress, the resting patient may be imaged again or will be injected with another 1.0 to 1.5 mCi (37–56 MBq) of thallous (^{201}Tl) chloride prior to imaging to provide information under normal (rest) conditions. Ischemic tissues will "fill in" during rest images demonstrating normal uptake, whereas infarcted tissue continues to demonstrate reduced uptake.

Dual isotope perfusion studies utilize thallous (^{201}Tl) chloride to first acquire rest images. Later, a technetium-99m perfusion agent is used to acquire the stress images.[15,36]

Xenon Radiochemistry

The clinical radioisotope of xenon for organ imaging is xenon-133, a noble gas used in its elemental form. Xenon-133 is produced in a nuclear reactor as a byproduct of uranium fission by the nuclear reaction ^{235}U(n, fission)^{133}Xe. Xenon-133 ($t_{1/2}$ = 5.3 days) decays by β^- emission to cesium-133, with γ-ray emission of 81 keV (37%). Gases used in lung ventilation studies must be chemically and physiologically inert at the concentrations used for imaging studies. Xenon-133 is chemically inert and insoluble in water, which makes it insoluble in body fluids. Unfavorable physical characteristics of xenon-133 include poor image quality because of the low tissue penetration of the low-energy γ-ray, increased patient dose due to β^- emission, and the low γ-ray emission yield (36 γ-rays/100 disintegrations).

XENON RADIOPHARMACEUTICALS

Xenon (^{133}Xe). Radioactive xenon (^{133}Xe) gas is supplied at standard pressure and room temperature in a septum-sealed glass vial in doses of 10 to 20 mCi (370–740 MBq) in either stable xenon carrier mixed with atmospheric air or 5% xenon carrier mixed with 95% carbon dioxide suitable for inhalation by the patient for diagnostic evaluation of pulmonary function and imaging of the lungs. The shelf life of the vials is 14 days because of the more rapid decay of xenon (^{133}Xe) gas when compared with the subsequent build-up of slower decaying impurities.

The general procedure involves mixing the vial contents of xenon-133 gas in air or oxygen in a closed-circuit spirometer system that delivers the radioactive gas, allowing the patient to breath the gas mixture. The inhalation study consists of wash-in, equilibrium and washout phases, with the patient sitting or supine. The wash-in phase is the first breath of the xenon-133 bolus, the equilibrium phase consists of the patient breathing the mixture for 5 minutes, and for the washout phase, the patient exhales xenon-133 gas into an activated charcoal trap. Images are obtained continuously for approximately 10 minutes with the gamma (γ-ray) camera. In the wash-in study, the patient inspires the bolus and holds their breath for several seconds. In the equilibrium study, there is an initial distribution of the radioactive gas throughout the lungs. In the washout phase, the xenon-133 gas clears readily from the lungs. In the abnormal study, the initial flow into the lungs of xenon-133 gas is delayed, and the outflow is also delayed. These abnormal lung ventilation findings add significant information in the evaluation of pulmonary embolism (blood clots in the lungs) when combined with the results of a lung blood perfusion study with Tc-99m macroaggregated albumin.

⬡ CONTRAST AGENTS

Radiography and Computed Tomography

A photographic film containing a radiographic image is properly called a *radiograph*, although it is commonly referred to as an *x-ray* or a *film*. The relative difference between the light and dark areas on a radiographic image reflects what is called *radiographic contrast*. Traditional radiographic images of the body, such as skeletal, abdominal, and chest x-rays, have four radiographic densities: air, fat, water (organs, muscle, soft tissue), and bone/metal. Organs and tissues are made visible according to how well they attenuate x-rays. The attenuation of x-rays by tissues is a complex process that depends on many factors, including, but not limited to, the energy of the x-ray beam and the density of the tissue. Bone has an average density of about 1.16 g/cm^3, which accounts for its ability to absorb most of the radiation it encounters.

Whereas traditional radiological "film" studies have been used since 1895 and continue to be a mainstay of diagnostic medical imaging, they have their limitations. Many organs and tissues of the body are not easily discriminated from each other on traditional radiographic images. For example, the liver, spleen, kidneys, intestines, bladder, and abdominal musculature all have very similar radiographic densities and are difficult, if not impossible, to distinguish from each other.

To produce diagnostic x-rays, a very high voltage (20,000–150,000 volts) is applied to a glass vacuum tube that contains a cathode and a rotating anode (Fig. 11.6). The cathode is a filament that is heated to a very high temperature, which provides a copious source of electrons. These electrons are accelerated toward the positively charged anode. When the accelerated electrons strike the anode (called the *target*), x-rays are produced. The distribution of x-rays is as a continuous spectrum. Lower-energy x-rays are absorbed by an aluminum filter, while higher-energy x-rays travel through the patient, exposing the x-ray film, and producing a traditional radiograph. Digital radiography is the process of producing a digital radiographic image where a specialized phosphor plate is used in place of traditional film. Such digital images can be readily viewed on a monitor, stored, and transferred much like any other type of digital information.

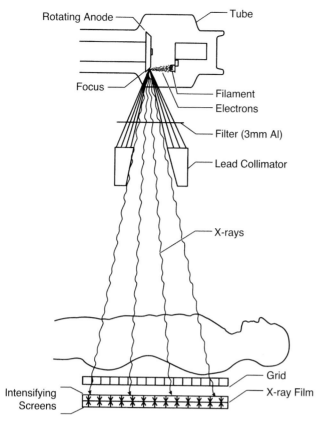

Figure 11.6 ● Schematic diagram of an x-ray tube for production of x-ray films.

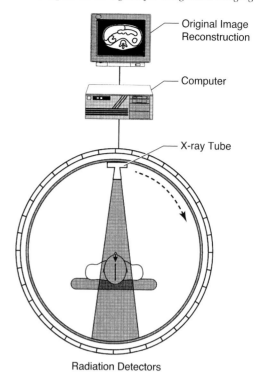

Figure 11.8 ● Schematic diagram of a computerized axial tomography (CAT) system for producing cross-sectional images of the body.

An invaluable modification of the x-ray system is fluoroscopy (Fig. 11.7). This modality allows one to visualize organs in motion, position the patient for spot film exposures, instill contrast media into hollow cavities, and insert catheters into arteries.

CT (sometimes called CAT, Fig. 11.8) uses ordinary x-ray energies for imaging and applies complex mathematical reconstructions to produce multiple images of the body in the axial and other planes. This technique typically provides more detailed information about the anatomical region of interest because the images obtained are numerous thin slices of the imaged area. With this process, the reconstructed images increase the visibility of small differences in the radiographic densities between tissues to a far greater extent than traditional radiographic film.

RADIOLOGICAL CONTRAST AGENTS

From the earliest days of radiology, considerable effort has been devoted to developing compounds that if swallowed or injected would increase the radiographic contrast between various tissues and organs. Injection of air or other gases into a GI tube in the esophagus, stomach, or duodenum or into a rectal tube in the colon provides increased radiographic contrast for evaluating the gut; however, the information obtained by this technique is limited, and more opaque substances have been developed.

Any agent or compound administered to a patient to improve the visualization of an organ or tissue is called a *contrast agent*. Contrast agents can be classified as negative or positive. Air and other gases are negative contrast agents because they render a structure, such as the gut, more translucent. An agent that increases the radiographic opacity of an organ or tissue is a positive contrast agent. Most contrast

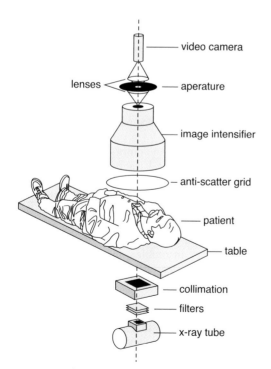

Figure 11.7 ● Schematic diagram of a fluoroscopic x-ray system for real-time imaging during medical procedures. (Reprinted with permission from Bushberg, J. T., et al.: The Essential Physics of Medical Imaging, 2nd ed. Philadelphia: Lippincott Williams and Wilkins, 2002.)

agents used in diagnostic radiology are positive contrast agents.

An ideal radiographic contrast agent should have the following properties: (a) readily available, (b) inexpensive, (c) excellent x-ray absorption characteristics at the x-ray energies used in diagnostic radiology, (d) minimal toxicity, (e) patient acceptance, (f) chemical stability, (g) high-water solubility with low viscosity and no significant osmotic effects, and (h) the ability to be administered for selective tissue uptake and excretion.

No compound has all of these characteristics. Barium sulfate and various iodine compounds, however, produce excellent radiological contrast with low patient toxicity and relatively low cost. The use of barium and iodine compounds as radiological contrast agents is based on their radiographic appearance, distribution, and elimination from the body. Contrast media are used in very large quantities and are usually administered over a brief period of time.

Barium sulfate is a nearly ideal contrast agent for oral and rectal studies of the GI tract. It produces a metal-like density on radiological studies, is inexpensive, and when properly utilized, has minimal patient morbidity and mortality. While various water-soluble barium compounds are quite toxic, barium sulfate is an insoluble white power that is a colloidal suspension in water.

Most intravenous contrast agents used to opacify blood vessels and increase contrast in solid organs, such as the liver, are water-soluble organic iodides. Iodine absorbs x-rays effectively at many energy levels and produces opacities similar to bone density during radiographic studies. While iodine's radiographic density is somewhat less than that of barium sulfate, it is still very useful for radiographic contrast.

Early water-soluble contrast agents consisted of triiodinated benzoic acid salts. In solution, these salts dissociate into two particles: (a) a triiodinated anion and (b) a cation, usually sodium or methylglucamine (meglumine). These compounds, known as *high-osmolar contrast medium* (HOCM), have in effect three iodine atoms for every two ions in solution, a 3:2 ratio. They are often called *conventional, ionic ratio 1.5 contrast agents*, or *triiodinated monomers* and are represented by diatrizoate and iothalamate.[37] Various fixed ratios of sodium diatrizoate and meglumine diatrizoate are also available in proprietary products.

These water-soluble iodinated salts are administered in fairly high volumes and concentrations to achieve satisfactory radiological contrast. It is not unusual to administer as much as 100 mL or more of a 30% to 70% solution intravenously.[38] The typical concentrations used for various studies have an osmolality of 5 times or more to that of normal plasma. Administration of these HOCM agents can be associated with osmotoxic effects. Initially, water shifts rapidly from the interstitial and cellular spaces into the plasma after injection of an HOCM. This is typically accompanied by vasodilatation, local pain and warmth, a metallic taste in the mouth, and flushing. Later, there is an osmotic diuresis as these agents are excreted by the kidneys.

Various nonionic water-soluble compounds with a higher ratio of iodine content per osmotic particle have been developed. These types of agents, known as *low-osmolar contrast medium or isotonic contrast media* (LOCM or ICM), produce far fewer osmotic effects. Various monomers such as iohexol, iopamidol, iopramide, ioversol, and ioxilan as well as dimers such as iodipamide, iodixanol, and ioxaglate have been described.[38]

All of the water-soluble iodinated contrast media are clear, colorless, viscous liquids. Even though they are clear liquids, they are often called "dyes" when their administration is being explained to patients. Sodium salts are slightly less viscous than the meglumine salts, which are typically less viscous than nonionic monomers, which are typically less viscous than nonionic dimers. Viscosity is a function of temperature and can be reduced by warming the contrast agent to body temperature prior to its administration.

Water-soluble iodinated contrast media have relatively small molecular sizes and low chemical reactivity with body fluids and tissues. Their pharmacodynamic characteristics are similar to those of extracellular tracers. They have low lipid solubility and distribute throughout extracellular spaces. They do not significantly penetrate into intracellular spaces. Special attention must be given to ensure that iodinated contrast agents are not administered intrathecally unless they are indicated for such use. Inadvertent intrathecal administration can cause serious outcomes such as convulsions, cerebral hemorrhage, brain edema, and death.

Water-soluble iodinated contrast agents are cleared from the body by glomerular filtration. They are neither reabsorbed nor secreted by the renal tubules. When renal function is compromised, these contrast agents are eliminated in part or totally through the liver and gut. This alternate elimination pathway occurs at a much slower rate than elimination when compared with glomerular filtration in a healthy person.

Water-soluble organic iodides are the largest group of radiological contrast agents. In addition to water-insoluble barium sulfate, there is an iodinated fatty acid derivative of poppy seed oil that is occasionally utilized in the clinic. Unsaturated fatty acids are monoiodicated or diiodinated before conversion to an ester. These substances are susceptible to light-induced decomposition, and the oily nature of the formulation excludes intravascular use.

Radiological contrast agents that are administered orally or intravascularly in large amounts infrequently report adverse effects. Nevertheless, any radiological contrast material may produce an untoward patient reaction, even sudden death.[39–42]

Events can occur when contrast material is aspirated or when it leaks from the GI tract. Hypertonic ionic water-soluble contrast agents are potentially dangerous if aspirated into the tracheobronchial tree. They are irritating and can cause pulmonary edema. Contrast material that leaks out of the bowel into the abdomen, pelvis, or chest is potentially quite dangerous, especially barium sulfate. Barium sulfate is insoluble, and its particulate nature means it is poorly cleared from the mediastinum, peritoneum, and retroperitoneum. Water-soluble agents, on the other hand, are rapidly absorbed from these areas almost as quickly as if they had been injected intravenously. In general, water-soluble agents that leak from the GI tract rarely cause significant problems beyond transient inflammation.

The intravenous or intra-arterial injection of iodinated contrast material can lead to a diverse assortment of contrast reactions, most of which are minor and easily treated. Minor reactions include injection pain, a feeling of general body warmth and discomfort, mild nausea and vomiting, a strong metallic taste in the mouth, and mild urticaria (hives). Minor reactions dissipate within a few minutes with patient reassurance and observation.

Intermediate or moderate reactions are those that require some form of therapy but are not life-threatening. These reactions include difficulty breathing, severe hives, severe nausea and vomiting, mild hypotension, wheezing, and other related reactions. Treatment ranges from administration of intravenous fluids to the use of intravenous diphenhydramine and/or corticosteroids. Epinephrine may be administered, and atropine is used if there is a vasovagal reaction with hypotension and bradycardia.

Severe reactions are those that are life-threatening. They include sudden cardiovascular collapse and death, as well as severe hypotension; severe shortness of breath, wheezing, or laryngoedema; loss of consciousness; massive hives and angioneurotic edema; ventricular cardiac arrhythmias; angina; and myocardial infarction. Treatment depends on the patient's signs and symptoms and includes intravenous fluids, oxygen, various drugs (including epinephrine, diphenhydramine, and atropine), and possible cardiopulmonary resuscitation (CPR).

Barium Sulfate. Commercial preparations of barium sulfate differ in their density and ability to coat the bowel wall. These characteristics are determined by the particle size of the barium suspension, its viscosity, and concentration of the contrast agent. Flavoring agents, suspending agents, and other additives may be utilized in preparing various products.

Barium sulfate preparations are given orally or rectally and are used to study the esophagus, stomach, duodenum, entire small bowel, colon, or the total bowel. Most patients find the taste of these flavored mixtures tolerable, but they dislike the heavy texture of the barium.

Concentrated barium suspensions ranging from 50% to 210% weight/volume (wt/vol) are frequently used for traditional radiographic imaging. Dilute suspensions ranging from 1.5% to 5% weight/volume (wt/vol) are typically used for CT studies.

The quantity and concentration of barium sulfate suspension administered to the patient will depend on the selected procedure. In general, upper GI studies will administer the contrast agent just prior to imaging, whereas lower GI studies recommend intake several hours prior to the procedure. For total bowel opacification, the patient should consume contrast agent the night preceding the examination, additional agent a few hours prior to examination, and a third dose approximately 15 minutes prior to examination.

Diatrizoate. Diatrizoate is a water-soluble, ionic monomer. It is commercially available as the meglumine salt, sodium salt, or as fixed combinations of the two salt forms. These triiodobenzoic acid salts contain 47% organically bound iodine.

Numerous products with various concentrations of one or two of the salt forms are available for various imaging procedures. Indicated uses include angiography, venography, excretory urography, retrograde cystourethrography, retrograde or ascending pyelography, operative, T-tube, or percutaneous transhepatic cholangiography, splenoportography, arthrography; discography, radiographic examination of the GI tract when barium sulfate is contraindicated (i.e., suspected perforation of the GI tract), adjunct contrast enhancement in CT of the torso (dual contrast study), and hysterosalpingography.

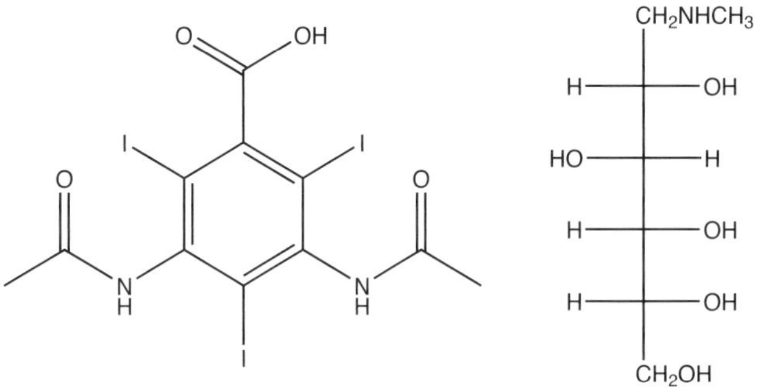

Diaztriazoate Meglumine

Ethiodized Oil (Ethiodol). This product is a mixture of iodinated fatty acid ethyl esters of poppy-seed oil, primarily as ethyl monoiodostearate and ethyl diiodostearate. It contains 37% organically bound iodine, has considerably reduced viscosity when compared with the triiodobenzoic acid derivatives, and is not miscible with plasma. Ethiodol is indicated for use as a radiopaque medium for hysterosalpingography and lymphography.

Iodipamide Meglumine. Iodipamide is a water-soluble, ionic dimer that is administered as the meglumine salt in combination with diatrizoate meglumine as the commercial product, Sinografin. Iodipamide has 50% bound iodine content. Intravenous use was associated with significant adverse effects, and the product is now indicated solely for use in hysterosalpingography.

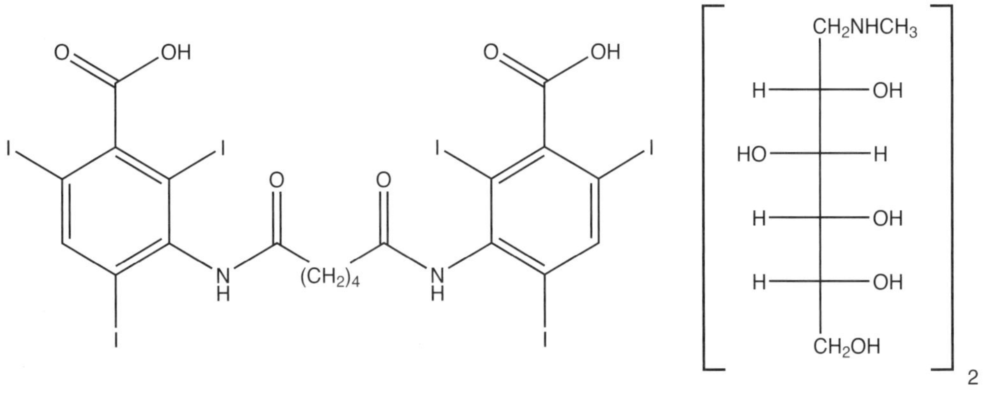

Iodipamide Meglumine

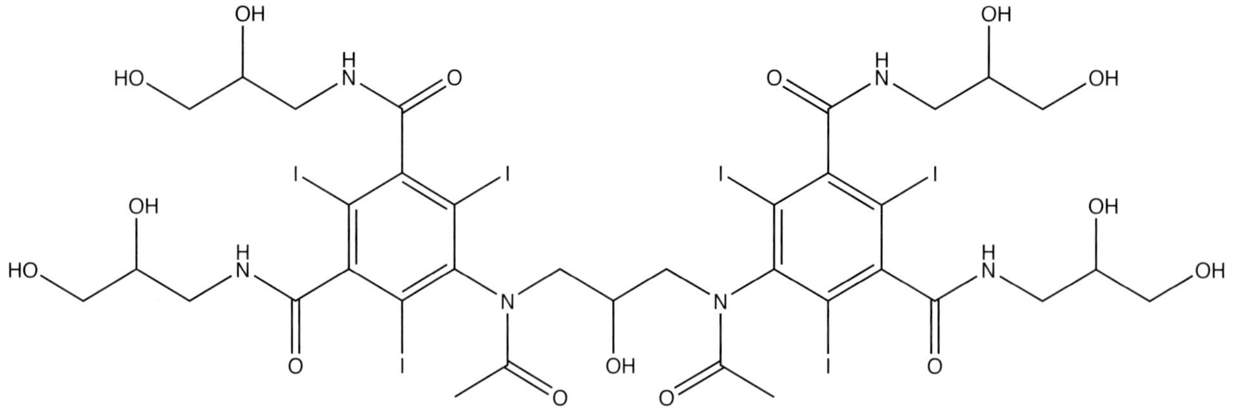

Iodixanol

Iodixanol (Visipaque). Iodixanol is a viscous, isosmolar, nonionic, water-soluble dimer with 49% iodine content. It is formulated as an isotonic solution for intravascular injection and indicated for excretory urography, angiography, and CT procedures.

Iohexol (Omnipaque). Iohexol is a low-osmolar, nonionic monomer with 46% iodine content. Iohexol is one of the few iodinated contrast agents indicated for intrathecal use (myelography). Only selected concentrations of the product have this indication. Besides myelography, iohexol finds widespread use in excretory urography, angiography, and CT procedures. Specific concentrations may have additional indications in adults and/or children for arthrography, hysterosalpingography, endoscopic retrograde pancreatography, cholangiopancreatography, herniography, voiding cystourethrography, oral pass-thru examination of the GI tract or CT of the abdomen.

Iopamidol (Isovue). Iopamidol is a low-osmolar, nonionic monomer with 49% organically bound iodine. It is indicated for use in angiography, excretory urography, and numerous CT procedures.

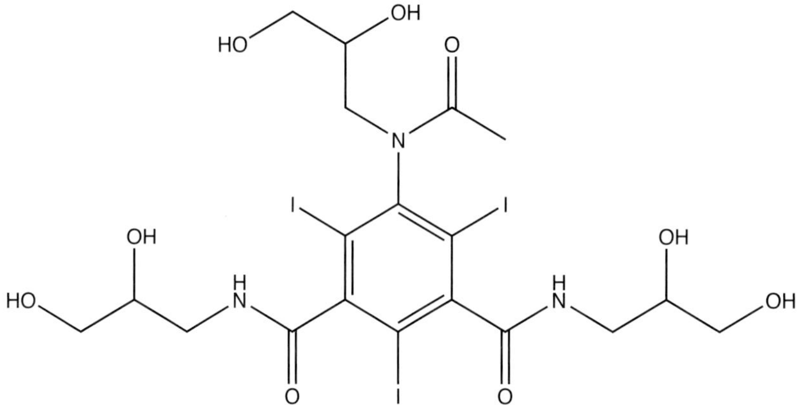

Iohexol

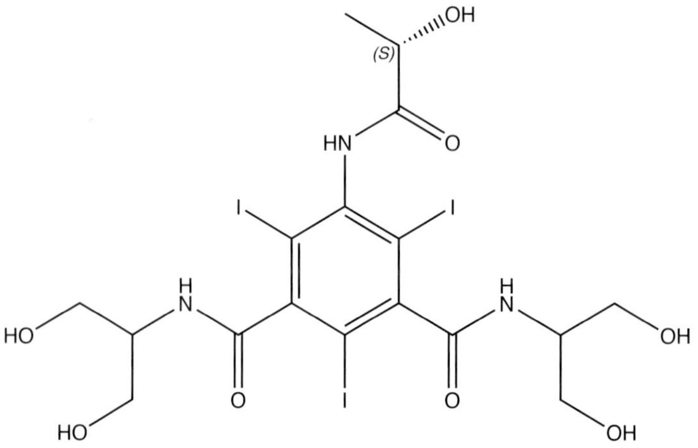

Iopamidol

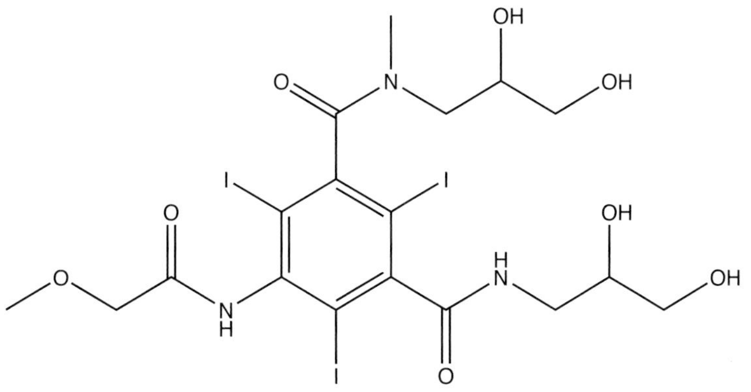

Iopromide

Iopromide (Ultravist).   Iopromide is a low-osmolar, nonionic monomer with 48% bound iodine content. It is indicated for use in angiography, excretory urography, and numerous CT procedures.

Iothalamate Meglumine (Conray).   Iothalamate meglumine is a high-osmolar, ionic monomer with 47% bound iodine content. Conray is indicated for use in angiography, excretory urography, arthrography, cholangiography, endoscopic retrograde cholangiopancreatography, and various CT procedures.

Ioversol (Optiray).   Ioversol is a low-osmolar, nonionic monomer with 47% bound iodine content. It is indicated for angiography, excretory urography, ventriculography, and various CT procedures.

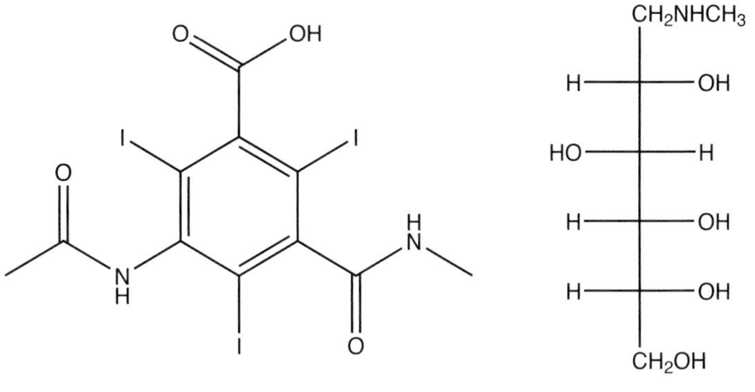

Iothalamate Meglumine

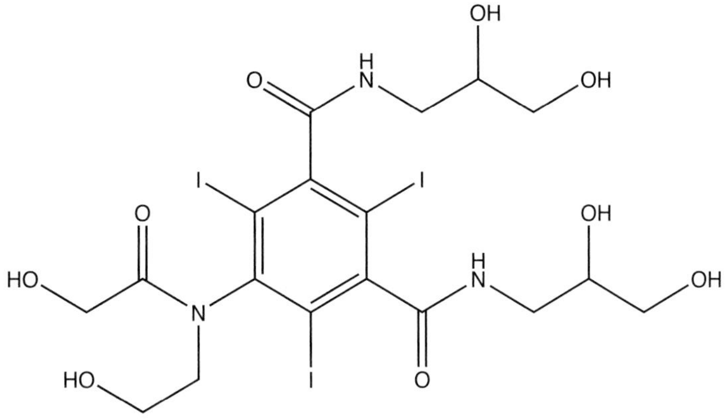

Ioversol

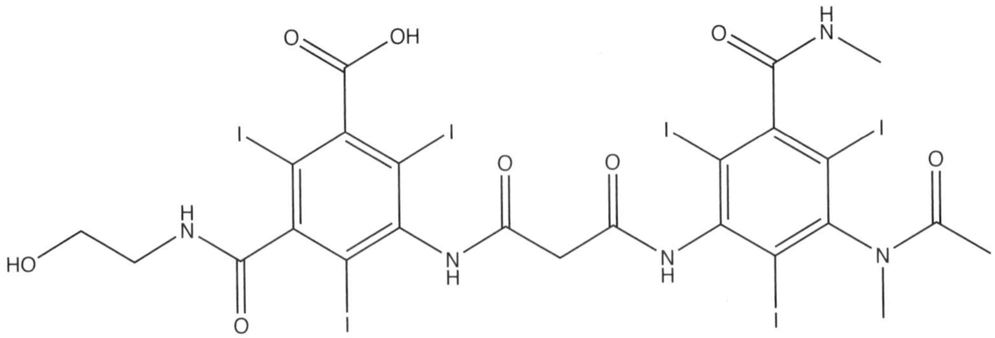

Ioxaglate

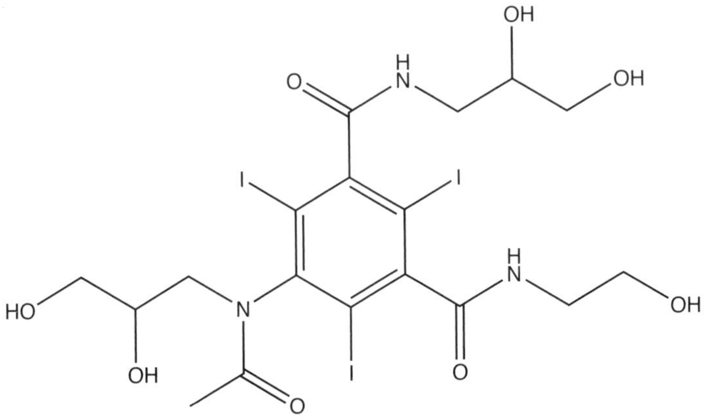

Ioxilan

Ioxaglate (Hexabrix). Ioxaglate is a high-osmolal, ionic dimer with 32% bound iodine content. It is commercially formulated as a mixture of its meglumine and sodium salts. Ioxaglate is indicated for angiography, excretory urography, and various CT procedures.

Ioxilan (Oxilan). Ioxilan is a low-osmolar, nonionic monomer with 48% bound iodine content. It is indicated for angiography, excretory urography, and various CT procedures.

Magnetic Resonance Imaging

MRI is a unique method of medical imaging. The strength of MRI as an imaging modality is its ability to detect small changes within soft tissues by using nonionizing radiation. The exquisite soft tissue images produced by MRI are analogous to the cross-sectional images of the body produced by CT with the benefit of MRI images being performed in any desired plane (coronal, axial, sagittal, oblique, etc.).

When a patient is placed in a large, strong, uniform magnetic field (Fig. 11.9), a population of hydrogen nuclei (protons) in all hydrogen-containing molecules align themselves with the magnetic field. Once aligned in the magnetic field, these nuclei will precess (spin like a gyroscope) with a characteristic spin frequency related to the magnetic field strength. The tesla (T) is the official unit of magnetic field strength, and MRI is normally performed between 0.5 to 1.5 T.

By directing low-energy, electromagnetic radiation to a defined region of the patient's body, the magnetized, process-

ing hydrogen nuclei can selectively absorb this energy to become excited. The excitation is accomplished by a complex series of radiofrequency pulses at the same frequency as the precessing hydrogen nuclei. Each burst of energy displaces the magnetic orientation of precessing nuclei. When the excitation energy field is removed, the displaced nuclei will lose the acquired energy, returning to magnetic equilibrium. These decaying (i.e., relaxing) nuclei emit a weak, but detectable, radio wave (i.e., signal), whose strength and manner of relaxation can be used to generate diagnostic medical images.

The timing of data acquisition from the relaxing nuclei is just as important as the number of nuclei that are excited in the observed tissues. Early receiver detection of emitted proton signals following discontinuance of the radiofrequency pulse is called a T1-weighted sequence (longitudinal or spin-lattice relaxation). T1 images have good resolution and are useful for gaining anatomic information. Late receiver detection of emitted signals is called a T2-weighted sequence (transverse or spin–spin relaxation). T2 images are useful in identifying pathologies because T2 images have better contrast between water (high proton density) and soft tissue (relatively less proton density).[43–45]

MAGNETIC RESONANCE CONTRAST AGENTS

When a molecule is placed in a magnetic field, it displays a certain susceptibility to becoming magnetized and an ability to alter the magnetic field of the immediate environment into which it has been placed. The ability of a substance to produce additional magnetism within a magnetic field is known as its *susceptibility*. A vacuum has a susceptibility defined as

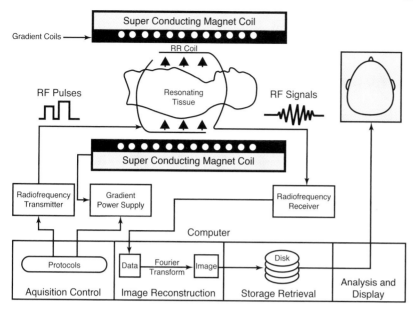

Figure 11.9 ● Schematic diagram of an MRI system demonstrating radiofrequency pulses and the strong magnetic field.

zero in comparison with water. Many nonmetallic materials are diamagnetic; they have negative susceptibility and induce weaker magnetic fields in the local environment. Such substances generally have fully paired electrons. Materials with unpaired orbiting electrons are said to be paramagnetic, because when placed in an applied magnetic field, they strengthen the magnetic fields within their vicinity. The magnitude of paramagnetic influence is proportional to the strength of the applied field. A substance with many unpaired electrons will be superparamagnetic, because it produces a stronger supplementary magnetic field. Ferromagnetic materials have very large numbers of unpaired electrons and produce a large, supplementary magnetization to the applied field that remains once the magnetic field has been removed.

Gadolinium-containing contrast agents rely on unpaired electrons to produce magnetic changes in nearby water molecules. These paramagnetic agents predominantly decrease tissue T1 relaxation time, which increases tissue intensity on T1-weighted images. Such agents are known as positive contrast agents because they brighten tissues associated with the nearby paramagnetic substance.

Many contrast agents used for MRI are extracellular paramagnetic agents. The primary paramagnetic metal ion used is gadolinium, a rare earth element. Gadolinium ions (Gd^{+3}) form when prepared in 0.05 M hydrochloric acid and are extremely effective for enhancing water proton relaxation rates. The ion itself, however, is toxic for human use. The ion quickly binds to ferric (Fe+3) protein-binding sites, most notably plasma transferrin, and has a long biological half-life of several weeks. In addition, the ion readily forms insoluble compounds by interacting with endogenous ions including phosphate, carbonate, and hydroxide.[46]

Consequently, the development of gadolinium MRI contrast agents has mainly focused on chelated compounds that clear rapidly from the body through the kidneys and exhibit minimal toxicity. These include gadobenate dimeglumine (MultiHance), gadodiamide (Omniscan), gadopentetate dimeglumine (Magnevist), gadoteridol (ProHance), and gadoversetamide (Optimark).[47]

All intravenous gadolinium complexes are hypertonic when compared with plasma. The most common side effects

are headache, nausea, dizziness, taste perversions, and vasodilation. A rare adverse event, nephrogenic systemic fibrosis, is more likely to occur in patients with severe acute or chronic renal insufficiency (<30 mL/min). Postmarketing reports identified such an event following single and multiple administrations of gadolinium-based contrast agents. These reports have not always identified a specific agent, and repetitive administration of the same or different agents carries similar risk if the time interval between the administrations precludes clearance of the contrast agent from the body.[48,49]

Manganese (Mn^{2+}) is strongly paramagnetic and can be used to form complexes used as MRI contrast agents. At this time, the only parenteral manganese compound used in humans is mangafodipir trisodium. This compound is delivered to tissues with active metabolism, such as the pancreas, renal cortex, GI tract, heart, and adrenal glands. The effect of mangafodipir trisodium is to decrease T1 relaxation time, which enhances signal intensity on T1-weighted images.

Superparamagnetic iron oxide colloids (SPIO) contain a crystalline core composed of iron oxide complexes. The core may be coated with dextran, siloxanes, or another large polysaccharide. The particles vary in size from 1 and 10 μm, and their biological characteristics can be altered by changing their coating. Large particles accumulate in the liver and spleen, whereas smaller particles remain in the circulation longer and tend to aggregate in lymph nodes. Ferumoxides and ferumoxsil are examples of such agents.

Because the main MRI effect of the iron oxide particles is on T2-weighted images, they decrease the signal intensity of the tissue in which they accumulate. Such iron oxide agents are known as negative contrast agents, because they darken tissues associated with the accumulation of ferromagnetic particles. Enhancement of T1-weighted images is less dramatic, but can be obtained. SPIO contrast agents provide enhancement of the liver and/or spleen when injected intravenously or the bowel when administered orally.[50]

Ferumoxides (Feridex). Ferumoxides is a black to reddish brown aqueous colloid of SPIO particles associated

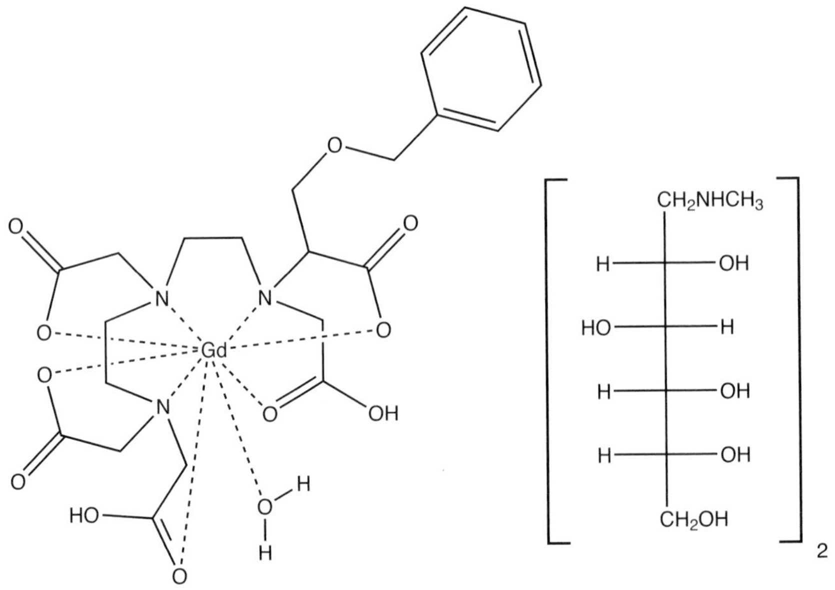

Gadobenate Dimeglumine

with dextran. It is administered intravenously and taken up by cells of the reticuloendothelial system (RES). It is indicated to enhance T2-weighted images used to assess lesions of the liver. Hepatic tissues with decreased RES function retain their usual signal intensity, so the contrast between abnormal and normal tissue is enhanced.

Ferumoxsil (GastroMARK). Ferumoxsil is a turbid, slightly viscous, dark brown to orange-brown aqueous suspension of silicone-coated, SPIO for oral administration. The suspension distributes to the stomach and small intestine within 30 to 45 minutes and passes distally to the large intestine within 4 to 7 hours after ingestion. It is indicated to enhance the delineation of the bowel and to distinguish it from organs and tissues that are adjacent to the upper regions of the GI tract. Its usefulness in the distal GI regions is limited by transit time and dilution. Both T1- and T2-weighted images may be enhanced with ferumoxsil.

Gadobenate Dimeglumine (MultiHance). Gadobenate dimeglumine is an ionic, clear, colorless, gadolinium-containing solution. This salt solution has 6.9 times the osmolality of plasma. It is indicated to enhance the visualization of central nervous system (CNS) lesions associated with an abnormal blood-brain barrier or abnormal vascularity of the brain, spine, or associated tissues when using T1-weighted sequences.

Gadodiamide (Omniscan). Gadodiamide is a clear, colorless to slightly yellow, gadolinium-based contrast agent indicated to visualize lesions with abnormal vascularity in the CNS and body. It is a nonionic gadolinium complex administered by intravenous injection with an osmolality of 2.8 times that of plasma. Gadodiamide decreases both the T1 and T2 relaxation times in tissues where it is distributed. In clinical MRI, the effect is prima-

rily on the T1 relaxation time resulting in an increase in T1-weighted sequence signal intensity.

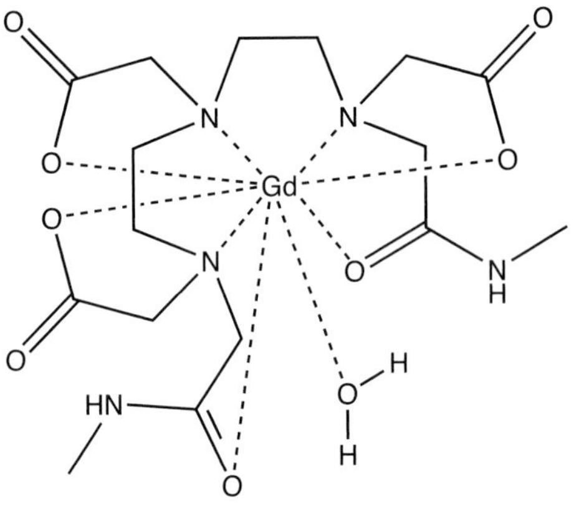

Gadodiamide

Gadopentetate Dimeglumine (Magnevist). Gadopentetate dimeglumine is an ionic, clear, colorless to slightly yellow, gadolinium-based contrast agent indicated to visualize lesions with abnormal vascularity in the CNS and body. This salt solution has 6.9 times the osmolality of plasma. Like other gadolinium-based contrast agents, the primary clinical effect is on T1 relaxation time.

Gadoteridol (ProHance). Gadoteridol is a nonionic clear, colorless to slightly yellow, gadolinium-based contrast agent indicated to visualize lesions with abnormal vascularity in the CNS, head, and neck. It is a hypertonic solution with an osmolality of 2.2 times that of plasma. Clinical enhancement of images occurs primarily when using T1-weighted sequences.

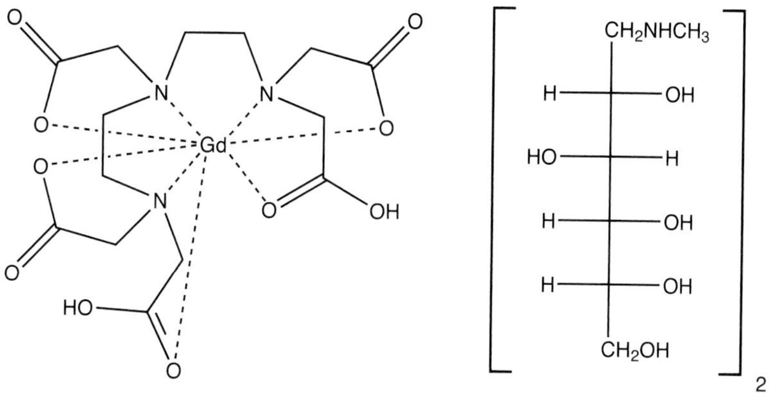

Gadopentetate dimeglumine

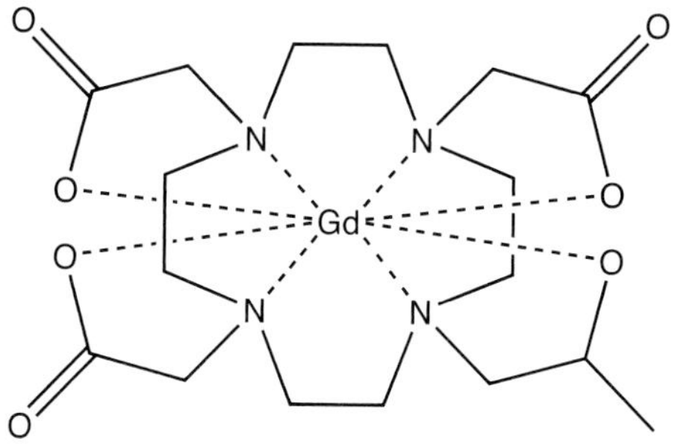

Gadoteridol

Gadoversetamide (OptiMARK). Gadoversetamide a nonionic clear, colorless to slightly yellow, gadolinium-based contrast agent indicated to visualize lesions with abnormal vascularity of the CNS or liver. It is a hypertonic solution with an osmolality of 3.9 times that of plasma. The primary clinical effect is on T1 relaxation time.

Mangafodipir Trisodium (Teslascan). Mangafodipir trisodium is a clear bright to dark yellow chelate of paramagnetic manganese for intravenous administration. Manganese is distributed to the liver and pancreas and shortens the T1-weighted relaxation time. It is indicated to detect metastatic lesions of the liver, focal pancreatic lesions, and hepatocellular carcinoma.

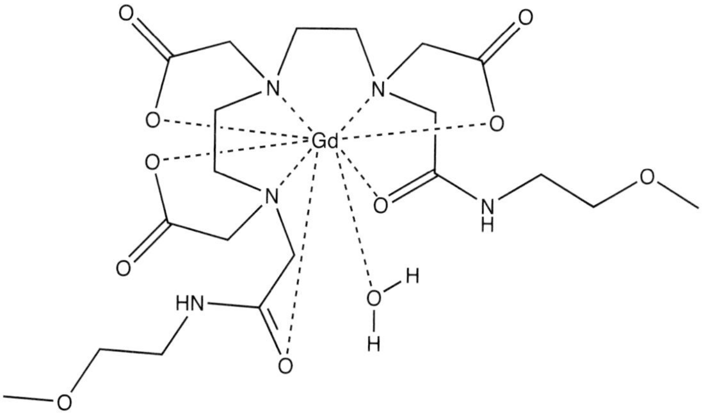

Gadoversetamide

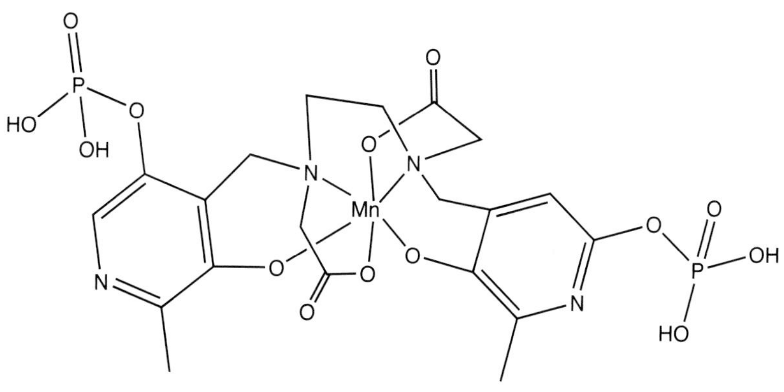

Mangafodipir

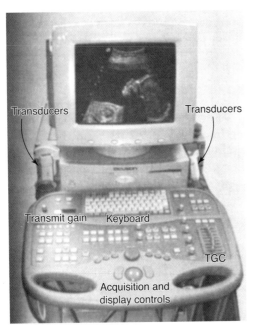

Figure 11.10 ● A portable ultrasound system. (Reprinted with permission from Bushberg, J. T., et al.: The Essential Physics of Medical Imaging, 2nd ed. Philadelphia: Lippincott Williams and Wilkins, 2002.)

Ultrasound Imaging

Diagnostic ultrasound imaging uses high-frequency sound waves from 1 to 20 MHz to produce cross-sectional images of the body. A small handheld transducer connected to a larger ultrasound unit is used to scan the body part of interest (e.g., the abdomen), and the resultant images are displayed on a monitor in real time (Fig. 11.10). Images may be stored digitally or printed later on film. Various body tissues reflect the sound waves in characteristic fashion, and diagnostic ultrasound is similar to the sonar imaging used by aquatic mammals and submarines. Differing tissues (e.g., the liver and the right kidney) have different acoustic properties. At the interface between tissues with different acoustic properties, the sound waves are reflected back to the transducer and are displayed on the screen, showing the tissues as well as the tissue interface. Unfortunately, gas-containing structures (lungs, bowel) as well as bones either absorb or scatter most of the sound waves and are not usually imaged satisfactorily by ultrasound. Solid organs (liver, spleen, kidneys), organs containing fluid (heart, gallbladder, urinary bladder), blood vessels, fatty tissue, and muscles, however, are usually amenable to diagnostic sonographic imaging.

Ultrasound finds widespread application in diagnostic radiology, obstetrics, gynecology, and cardiology because it produces diagnostic results comparable or even superior in some cases to other imaging techniques that require the use of ionizing radiation. Ultrasound machines are often portable and may be taken to the patient's bedside. Moreover, diagnostic ultrasound has no known harmful effects.

ULTRASOUND CONTRAST AGENTS

Contrast agents are not used for most diagnostic ultrasound examinations. Because ultrasound relies on the detection of sound waves reflected from tissue interfaces, gases can create prominent acoustic interfaces near body tissues and can be adapted for use as contrast agents. Microbubbles containing air or other gases that are introduced into the bloodstream, act by increasing the ultrasound signal reflected from the vessel contents or from the structures fed by the vessels. Ultrasound contrasts agents relying on microbubbles may be described as (a) encapsulated microbubbles, (b) gaseous liposomes, or (c) colloidal suspensions and emulsions. These agents allow visualization of small vessels, identification of tumor vascularity, improved contrast visualization of solid organs, and improved visualization of heart chambers and vascular grafts. Ultrasound contrast agents are generally very safe. They are designed so that no large bubbles form in the body (95% or more are $<10\ \mu m$), and they have relatively short life spans before breaking down and dissipating. Microbubble decomposition occurs during passage through the heart and lungs and limits the time of beneficial imaging enhancement. Recent warnings regarding severe cardiopulmonary reactions have led to a change in the label for ultrasound microspheres.[51]

Perflutren (Protein-Type A Microspheres—Optison or Lipid Microspheres—Definity). Perflutren (also known as octafluoropropane) is a volatile gas that efficiently reflects sound waves. This gas is encapsulated as a protein or lipid microsphere that is generated when a solution of protein or lipids is agitated with the gas immediately prior to use. The milky white suspension of microspheres must be injected shortly after activation for maximal contrast enhancement. Protein shells consist primarily of human albumin associated with small amounts of *N*-acetyltryptophan and caprylic acid. Lipid shells consist of a phospholipid mixture, one of which is a polyethylene glycol phospholipid. Perflutren microspheres are indicated in suboptimal echocardiograms to improve the delineation of left ventricular borders.

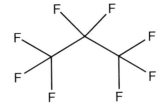

Perflutren

<hr />

● R E V I E W   Q U E S T I O N S ●

1. Describe two methods of radioactive decay that lack the production of charged nuclear particles. Why are such decay processes desirable for producing diagnostic images?

2. A physician requests a ventilation scan and a perfusion scan for a patient with a suspected pulmonary embolism. What radiopharmaceuticals will be used for this procedure and how do they localize in the region of interest?

3. What are the properties of the radioisotopes used in a dual isotope stress test?

4. A production lot of F-18 FDG is calibrated at 50 mCi/mL at 6 AM. What is the activity per milliliter by 10:30 AM later the same day?

5. What are the properties associated with x-ray, MRI, or ultrasound contrast agents that provide each class with the desirable characteristics for producing diagnostic images?

REFERENCES

1. Lamson III, M., Hotte, C. E., and Ice, R. D.: J. Nucl. Med. Technol. 4:21–26, 1976.
2. Palmer, A. J., Clark, J. C., and Goulding, R. W.: Int. J. Appl. Radiat. Isotopes 28:53–65, 1977.
3. Hamacher, K., Coenen, H. H., and Stocklin, G.: J. Nucl. Med. 27:235, 1986.
4. Saha, G. B.: Fundamentals of Nuclear Pharmacy, 5th ed. New York, Springer-Verlag, 2004.
5. Kowalsky, R. J., and Falen, S. W.: Radiopharmaceuticals in Nuclear Pharmacy and Nuclear Medicine, 2nd ed. Washington, DC, American Pharmacists Association, 2004.
6. Gambhir, S. S., Czernin, J., Schwimmer, J., et al.: J. Nucl. Med. 42:1S–93S, 2001.
7. Brown, L. C., Callahan, A. P., Skidmore, M. R., et al.: Int. J. Appl. Radiat. Isotopes 24(11):651–655, 1973.
8. O'Brien, P., Salacinski, H., and Motevalli, M.: J. Am. Chem. Soc. 119:12695–12696, 1997.
9. Matzapetakis, M., Kourgiantakis, M., Dakanali, M., et al.: Inorg. Chem. 40(8):1734–1744, 2001.
10. Green, M. A., and Huffman, J. C.: J. Nucl. Med. 29:417–420, 1988.
11. Maceke, H. R., Riesen, A., and Ritter, W.: J. Nucl. Med. 30:1235–1239, 1989.
12. Jurisson, S., Berning, D., Jia, W., et al.: Chem. Rev. 93:1137–1156, 1993.
13. Liu, S.: Chem. Soc. Rev. 33:445–461, 2004.
14. Baldwin, R. M.: Int. J. Radiat. Appl. Instru. Part A. Appl. Radiat. Isotopes 37:817–821, 1986.
15. Ziessman, H. A., O'Malley, J. P., and Thrall, J. H.: Nuclear Medicine: The Requisites in Radiology, 3rd ed. Philadelphia, PA, Elsevier Mosby, 2006.
16. Macklis, R. M.: Semin. Radiat. Oncol. 17(3):176–183, 2007.
17. Schwochau, K.: Angew. Chem. Int. Ed. Engl. 33(22):2231–2350, 1994.
18. Eckelman, W. C., Stiegman, J., and Paik, C. H.: Radiopharmaceutical chemistry. In Harbert, J. C., Eckelman, W. C., and Neumann, R. D. (eds.). Nuclear Medicine: Diagnosis and Therapy. New York, Thieme Medical Publishers, 1996, pp. 213–266.
19. Mazzi, U., Schibli, R., Pietzsch, H. J., et al.: Technetium in medicine. In Zolle, I. (ed.). Technetium-99m Pharmaceuticals: Preparation and Quality Control in Nuclear Medicine. New York, Springer Berlin Heidelberg, 2007, pp. 7–58.
20. Zolle, I., Bremer, P. O., and Jánoki, G.: Monographs of Tc-99m Pharmaceuticals. In Zolle, I. (ed.). Technetium-99m Pharmaceuticals: Preparation and Quality Control in Nuclear Medicine. Berlin, Springer, 2007, pp. 173–337.
21. Taylor, A., Hansen, L., Eshima, D., et al.: J. Nucl. Med. 38(5):821–826, 1997.
22. Loberg, M. D., and Fields, A. T.: Int. J. Appl. Radiat. Isotopes 29(3):167–173, 1978.
23. Costello, C. E., Brodack, J. W., Jones, A. G., et al.: J. Nucl. Med. 24(4):353–355, 1983.
24. Dewanjee, M. K.: Semin. Nucl. Med. 20(1):5–27, 1990.
25. Banerjee, S. R., Maresca, K. P., Francesconi, L., et al.: Nucl. Med. Biol. 32:1–20, 2005.
26. Hjelstuen, O. K.: Analyst 120:863–866, 1995.
27. Arbab, S. A., Koizumi, K., Toyama, K., et al.: J. Nucl. Med. 39(2):266–271, 1998.
28. Moretti, J. L., Rapin, J. R., Saccavini J. C., et al.: Int. J. Nucl. Med. Biol. 11(3–4):270–274, 1984.
29. Kubiatowicz, D. O., Bolles, T. F., Nora, J. C., et al.: J. Pharm. Sci. 68(5):621–623, 1979.
30. Williams, B. S., Hinkle, G. H., Douthit, R. A., et al.: J. Nucl. Med. Technol. 27(4):309–317, 1999.
31. Mariani, G., Moresco, L., Viale, G., et al.: J. Nucl. Med. 42:1198–1215, 2001.
32. Mariani, G., Gipponi, M., Moresco, L., et al.: J. Nucl. Med. 43:811–827, 2002.
33. Kelly, J. D., Forster, A. M., Higley, B., et al.: J. Nucl. Med. 34(2):222–227, 1993.
34. Jain, D.: Semin. Nucl. Med. 35(3):221–236, 1999.
35. Lebowitz, E., and Greene, M. W.: Production of high purity radiothallium. US Patent 3993538, 1976; http://www.freepatentsonline.com/3993538.html, accessed 10/15/2007.
36. Pandit-Taskar, N., Grewal, R. K., and Strauss, H. W.: Cardiovascular System. In Christian, P. E., and Waterstram-Rich, K. M. (eds.) Nuclear Medicine and PET/CT: Technology and Techniques, 6th ed. St. Louis, Mosby Elsevier, 2007, pp. 479–512.
37. Jacobsson, B. F., Jorulf, H., Kalantar, M. S., et al.: Radiology 167:601–605, 1988.
38. Krause, W., and Schneider, P. W.: Chemistry of x-ray contrast agents. In Krause, W. (ed.). Contrast Agents II: Optical, Ultrasound, X-Ray and Radiopharmaceutical Imaging. Berlin, Springer-Verlag, 2002, pp. 107–150.
39. Tramèr, M. R., von Elm, E., Loubeyre, P., et al.: BMJ 333:675, 2006 doi:10.1136/bmj.38905.634132.AE (published 31 July 2006).
40. Idée, J. M., Pinès, E., Prigent, P., et al.: Fundam. Clin. Pharmacol. 19(3):263–281, 2005.
41. Morcos, S. K., Dawson, P., Pearson, J. D., et al.: Eur. J. Radiol. 29(1):31–46, 1998.
42. Maddox, T. G.: Am. Fam. Physician 66(7):1229–1234, 2002.
43. Erkonen, W. E.: Radiography, computed tomography, magnetic resonance imaging, and ultrasonography: principles and indications. In Erkonen, W. E. (ed.). Radiology 101: The Basics and Fundamentals of Imaging. Philadelphia, Lippincott Williams & Wilkins, 2005, pp. 1–16.
44. Weissleder, R., Wittenberg, J., Harisinghani, M. G., et al.: Primer of Diagnostic Imaging, 4th ed. Philadelphia, Mosby, 2007.
45. Bushberg, J. T., Seibert, J. A., and Leidholdt, E. M., Jr.: The Essential Physics of Medical Imaging, 2nd ed. Philadelphia, Lippincott Williams & Wilkins, 2002.
46. Tweedle, M. F., Wedeking, P., and Kumar, K.: Invest. Radiol. 30:372–380, 1995.
47. Lin, S., and Brown, J. J.: J. Magn. Reson. Imaging 25:884–899, 2007.
48. Marckmann, P., Skov, L., Rossen, K., et al.: J. Am. Soc. Nephrol. 17(9):2359–2362, 2006.
49. US Food and Drug Administration, Important Drug Warning for Gadolinium-Based Contrast Agents; http://www.fda.gov/medwatch/safety/2007/gadolinium_DHCP.pdf, accessed 10/09/2007.
50. Bonnemain, B.: The superparamagnetic iron oxides. In Dawson, P., Cosgrove, D. O., and Grainger, R. G. (eds.). Textbook of Contrast Media. Oxford, UK, Isis Medical Media, 1999, pp. 373–378.
51. US Food and Drug Administration. Micro-bubble Contrast Agents (marketed as Definity (Perflutren Lipid Microsphere) Injectable Suspension and Optison (Perflutren Protein-Type A Microspheres for Injection), http://www.fda.gov/cder/drug/InfoSheets/HCP/microbubbleHCP.htm, accessed 10/15/2007.

SELECTED READING

Bushberg, J. T., Seibert, J. A., and Leidholdt, E. M., Jr.: The Essential Physics of Medical Imaging, 2nd ed. Philadelphia, Lippincott Williams & Wilkins, 2002.
Christian, P. E., and Waterstram-Rich, K. M.: Nuclear Medicine and PET/CT: Technology and Techniques, 6th ed. St. Louis, Mosby Elsevier, 2007.
Dawson, P., Cosgrove, D. O., and Grainger, R. G.: Textbook of Contrast Media. Oxford, UK, Isis Medical Media, 1999.
Erkonen, W. E.: Radiology 101: The Basics and Fundamentals of Imaging. Philadelphia, Lippincott Williams & Wilkins, 2005.
Hall, E. J., and Giaccia, A. J.: Radiobiology for the Radiologist, 6th ed. Philadelphia, Lippincott Williams & Wilkins, 2006.

Harbert, J. C., Eckelman, W. C., and Neumann, R. D.: Nucelar Medicine: Diagnosis and Therapy. New York, Thieme Medical Publishers, 1996.

Huda, W., and Slone, R. M.: Review of Radiologic Physics, 2nd ed. Philadelphia, Lippincott Williams & Wilkins, 2003.

Kowalsky, R. J., and Falen, S. W.: Radiopharmaceuticals in Nuclear Pharmacy and Nuclear Medicine, 2nd ed. Washington, DC, American Pharmacists Association, 2004.

Krause, W.: Contrast Agents I: Magnetic Resonance Imaging. Berlin, Springer-Verlag, 2002.

Krause, W.: Contrast Agents II: Optical, Ultrasound, X-Ray and Radiopharmaceutical Imaging. Berlin, Springer-Verlag, 2002.

Krause, W.: Contrast Agents III: Radiopharmaceuticals: From Diagnosis to Therapeutics. Berlin, Springer-Verlag, 2005.

Lombardi, M. H.: Radiation Safety in Nuclear Medicine, 2nd ed. Boca, Raton, CRC Press, 2007.

Saha, G. B.: Fundamentals of Nuclear Pharmacy, 5th ed. New York, Springer-Verlag, 2004.

Sandler, M. P., Coleman, R. E., Patton, J. A., et al.: Diagnostic Nuclear Medicine, 4th ed. Philadelphia, Lippincott Williams & Wilkins, 2003.

Weissleder, R., Wittenberg, J., Harisinghani, M. G., et al.: Primer of Diagnostic Imaging, 4th ed. Philadelphia, Mosby, 2007.

Ziessman, H. A., O'Malley, J. P., and Thrall, J. H.: Nuclear Medicine: The Requisites in Radiology, 3rd ed. Philadelphia, Elsevier Mosby, 2006.

Zolle, I.: Technetium-99m Pharmaceuticals: Preparation and Quality Control in Nuclear Medicine. Berlin: Springer, 2007.

WEB SITES OF INTEREST

Bracco Diagnostics,
http://www.bracco.com

Covidien Imaging,
http://www.imaging.mallinckrodt.com

DRAXIMAGE,
http://www.draximage.com

GE Healthcare,
http://md.gehealthcare.com

Lantheus Medical Imaging,
http://www.radiopharm.com

Pharmalucence,
http://www.pharmalucence.com

The Nuclear Pharmacy,
http://nuclearpharmacy.uams.edu

CHAPTER 12

Central Nervous System Depressants

SHENGQUAN LIU

CHAPTER OVERVIEW

Although the brain is undoubtedly the most wondrously complex organ, it is possible to distil the way it works into two opposing forces; excitation and inhibition (depressing). Central nervous system (CNS) depressants are drugs that can be used to slow down or "depress" the functions of the CNS. Although many agents have the capacity to depress the function of the CNS, CNS depressants discussed in this chapter include only anxiolytics, sedative–hypnotics, and antipsychotics.

There is some overlap between the first two groups. They often have several structural features in common and likewise often share at least one mode of action, positive modulation of the action of γ-aminobutyric acid (GABA) at $GABA_A$ receptor complex. The list of anxiolytic, sedative, and hypnotic drugs is a short one—benzodiazepines, Z-drugs, barbiturates, and a miscellaneous group.

Antipsychotic drugs—previously known as *neuroleptic drugs*, *antischizophrenic drugs*, or *major tranquilizers*—are used in the symptomatic treatment of thought disorders (psychoses), most notably the schizophrenias. Antipsychotics are grouped into typical and atypical categories. Both categories share a common feature, a dopamine (DA)-like structure, often hydrophobically substituted. This feature can be related to the most commonly cited action of these agents, competitive antagonism of DA at D_2 or occasionally D_3 or D_4 receptors in the limbic system. The fundamental differences between typical and atypical antipsychotics are that the atypical agents are (a) less prone to produce extrapyramidal symptoms (EPS), because they are less able to block striata D_2 receptors vis-à-vis limbic D_2 and D_3 receptors, and (b) more active against negative symptoms (social withdrawal, apathy, anhedonia).

ANXIOLYTIC, SEDATIVE, AND HYPNOTIC AGENTS

In addition to benzodiazepines, barbiturates, and a miscellaneous group, many drugs belonging to other pharmacological classes may possess one or more of the anxiolytic, sedative, and hypnotic activities. An arbitrary classification of these agents is as follows:

1. $GABA_A$ receptor modulators
   - Benzodiazepines are highly effective anxiolytic and hypnotic agents (e.g., diazepam, chlordiazepoxide, prazepam, clorazepate, oxazepam, alprazolam, flur- azepam, lorazepam, triazolam, temazepam, estazolam, and quazepam). They bind to benzodiazepine-binding sites on $GABA_A$ receptor (also known as benzodiazepine receptor [BzR]). They are sometimes called benzodiazepine receptor agonists (BzRAs).
   - Nonbenzodiazepine hypnotics (Z-drugs): Imidazopyridine (zolpidem), pyrazolopyrimidine (zaleplon), and cyclopyrrolone (zopiclone and its [S]-[+]-enantiomer eszopiclone).
   - Barbiturates including amobarbital, aprobarbital, butabarbital, pentobarbital, phenobarbital, and secobarbital are largely obsolete and superseded by benzodiazepines. Their use is now confined to anesthesia and treatment of epilepsy.
   - General anesthetics and ethanol.
2. Melatonin-1 receptor (MT_1) agonists. A new drug in this area is ramelteon (Rozerem).[1] Currently, 10 Food and Drug Administration (FDA)-approved drugs for insomnia include nine BzRAs (five benzodiazepines, four non-benzodiazepines) and ramelteon.
3. Atypical azaspirodecanediones: Buspirone is a partial 5-HT_{1A} receptor agonist and an anxiolytic. It is less sedative and has less abuse potential.
4. Miscellaneous drugs such as chloral hydrate, meprobamate, and glutethimide are no longer recommended, but occasionally used.
5. Antipsychotics and anticonvulsants. It has been proposed that DA has a facilitative and active role in the sleep–wakefulness cycle. Waking appears to be a state maintained by D_2 receptor activation, whereas blocking D_2 receptor appears to cause sedation.
6. Antidepressants: Many antidepressants cause sedation, of which trazodone, doxepin, and mirtazapine have been shown to be effective in the treatment of insomnia in patients with depression. Several selective serotonin reuptake inhibitors (SSRIs), including escitalopram, fluoxetine, fluvoxamine, paroxetine, and sertraline, became the first-line therapy for some anxiety disorders in 1990s because they are not as addictive as benzodiazepines.
7. Sedative H_1-antihistamines: diphenhydramine and doxylamine:
   Diphenhydramine is sometimes used as sleeping pills, particularly for wakeful children. It is proposed that histamine may have an involvement in wakefulness and rapid eye movement (REM) sleep. Histamine-related functions in the CNS are regulated at postsynaptic sites by both H_1 and H_2 receptors, whereas the H_3 receptors appear to be a presynaptic autoreceptor regulating the

synthesis and release of histamine. The H_1 receptor agonists and the H_3 receptor antagonists increase wakefulness, whereas the H_1 receptor antagonists and H_3 receptor agonists have the opposite effect. Another example of H_1-antihistamines is doxylamine.

8. β-Adrenoceptor antagonists (e.g., propranolol) are sometimes used by actors and musicians to reduce the symptoms of stage fright, but their use by snooker players to minimize tremor is banned as unsportsmanlike.

9. New areas explored for sleep-promoting agents:
   - Adenosine-2A receptor (A_{2A}) agonists (adenosine is a possible endogenous sleep-producing agent).
   - Linoleamide and 9,10-octadecenoamide are possible endogenous sleep-producing agents and are positive modulators of $GABA_A$ receptors.[2]
   - Anandamide is an endogenous cannabinoid that might be used as a lead to search for new hypnotics.

The properties and side effects of FDA-approved hypnotics and commonly used but not FDA-approved hypnotics are reviewed.[3,4] Older sedative–hypnotic drugs depress the CNS in a dose-dependent manner, progressively producing calming or drowsiness (sedation), sleep, unconsciousness, surgical anesthesia, coma, and eventually death from respiratory and cardiovascular depression. Although many factors influence the pharmacokinetic profile of sedatives and hypnotics, because most of them are in the nonionized form at physiological pH, their high lipophilicity is an important factor for following properties. (a) Most of them are absorbed well from the gastrointestinal (GI) tract, with good distribution to the brain. This property is responsible for the rapid onset of CNS effects of triazolam, thiopental, and newer hypnotics. (b) Many sedative–hypnotics cross the placental barrier during pregnancy. (c) They are also detectable in breast milk. (d) Some drugs with highest lipophilicity have short duration of action because of their redistribution. (e) Most drugs in this class are highly protein bond. (f) Metabolism to more water-soluble metabolites is necessary for their clearance from the body. Thus, the primary means of elimination of the benzodiazepines is metabolism, and most of them are extensively metabolized. Consequently, their duration of action depends mainly on the rate of metabolism and if their metabolites are active. Benzodiazepines are the most important drugs in both groups; therefore, the two groups are discussed together in the first section.

GABA$_A$ Receptors, Benzodiazepines, and Related Compounds

GABA system (deficiency of GABA activity in CNS) is important in the pathophysiology of anxiety and insomnia. GABA is the most common and major inhibitory neurotransmitter (NT) in the brain and it exerts its rapid inhibitory action mostly through GABA receptors. It is known to activate two types of receptors, the ionotropic $GABA_A$ and $GABA_C$ receptors and the metabotropic $GABA_B$ receptor. $GABA_A$ receptor is the target for many anxiolytics and sedative–hypnotic agents including benzodiazepines, barbiturates, zolpidem, zaleplon, eszopiclone, steroids, anticonvulsive agents, and many other drugs that bind to different binding sites of the $GABA_A$ receptors in neuronal membranes in the CNS.[5,6] It is a ligand-gated chloride ion channel. Upon activation, Cl^- influx is increased and the membrane becomes hyperpolarized, resulting in neuronal inhibition.

$GABA_A$ receptor exists as heteropentomeric transmembrane subunits arranged around a central chloride ion (Cl^-) channel. The five polypeptide subunits (each subunit has an extracellular N-terminal domain, four membrane-spanning domains, and an intracellular loop) that together make up the structure of $GABA_A$ receptors come from the subunit families α, β, γ, δ, ε, π, ρ, and ξ. There are six isoforms of the α-polypeptide (α_1–α_6), four of the β with two splice variants, and three of the γ with two variants. Most receptors consist of α, β, and γ combinations. Of these, α_1, β_2, and γ_2 are most common. The most common pentomeric GABA receptor combination includes two α_1, two β_2, and one γ_2 subunit. Other highly expressed combinations are α_2, β_2, γ_2 and α_2, β_3, γ_2.

The subunit composition of the receptors has great bearing on the response to benzodiazepines and other ligands. The multiplicity of subunits results in heterogeneity in $GABA_A$ receptors and is responsible, at least in part, for the pharmacological diversity in benzodiazepine effects. For example, α, β, and γ subunits confer benzodiazepine sensitivity to the receptors, whereas α and β subunits confer barbiturates sensitivity to the receptors. The benzodiazepine recognition site is in the extracellular N-terminus of the α_1, α_2, α_3, and α_5 subunits. Studies suggest that α_1 *subunits* are required for *hypnotic*, amnesic, and possibly anticonvulsant effects of benzodiazepines, whereas α_2 *subunits* are required for the *anxiolytic* and myorelaxant effects of benzodiazepines. The mutation to arginine of a histidine residue of the $GABA_A$ receptor α_1 subunit render receptors containing that subunit insensitive to the enhancing hypnotic effects of diazepam. Whereas, if arginine replaces histidine in an α_2 subunit, the anxiolytic effect of benzodiazepines is lost.[5] In addition, α_3 and α_5 subunits may be involved in other actions of benzodiazepines; α_4 or α_6 subunits do not respond to benzodiazepines.

Although the binding domain of the benzodiazepines is considered to be in the N-terminal domain of the α subunit, the benzodiazepines also require a γ_2 subunit for most positive allosteric effects. Amino acid residues in the α_1 subunit that have been identified as key binding sites within the benzodiazepine-binding site are His 101, Tyr 161, Thr 162, Gly 200, Ser 204, Thr 206, and Val 211. In the γ subunit, Phe 77 has been identified.[2,5,7–12]

When benzodiazepines bind to a benzodiazepine recognition site, one of several allosteric sites that modulate the effect of GABA binding to $GABA_A$ receptors located on GABA receptor complex, the benzodiazepines induce conformational (allosteric) changes in the GABA-binding site, thereby increasing the affinity of the receptor for GABA. As a result, the *frequency* of Cl^- channel openings is increased over that resulting from the binding of GABA alone, and the cell is further hyperpolarized, yielding a more pronounced decrease in cellular excitability. The benzodiazepines appear to have *no direct* effect on the $GABA_A$ complex or ionophore.

Several newer agents that have structural characteristics broadly related to the benzodiazepines, including imidazopyridines (zolpidem), pyrazolopyrimidines (zaleplon), and cyclopyrrolone (eszopiclone), can act as positive modulators at the benzodiazepine α_1 recognition site selectively with fewer side effects.

Benzodiazepines and related compounds can act as agonists, antagonists, or inverse agonists at the benzodiazepine-

β-Carboline

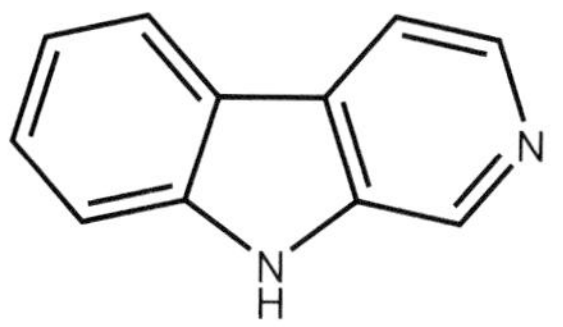

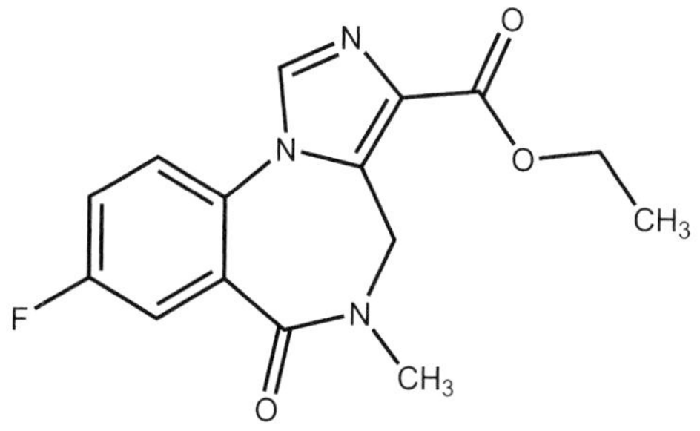

Flumazenil (Romazicon)
An imidazobenzodiazepinone
A BZR antagonist

binding site on $GABA_A$ receptor. Most classical benzodiazepines are positive modulators (*agonists*), many probably nonselectively for all the receptor subtypes that respond to benzodiazepines. Some have been claimed to be relatively selective as T-drugs and anticonvulsants. Some β-carbolines are negative modulators (*inverse agonists*) at benzodiazepine modulatory sites. Negative modulators diminish the positive effect of GABA on chloride flux. In whole animals, they appear to increase anxiety, produce panic attacks, and improve memory. There are also compounds that can occupy benzodiazepine modulatory sites, have no effect on chloride flux themselves, and block positive and negative modulators. They have been called variously *antagonists*, *zero modulators*, and *neutralizing allosteric modulators*. One such compound, flumazenil, is used clinically to counteract the sedative effect of benzodiazepines and benzodiazepine overdose.

In addition to benzodiazepine allosteric modulatory sites, there are other allosteric sites that recognize respectively, barbiturates, inhalation anesthetics, alcohols, propofol (separate sites), and neurosteroids. The convulsants picrotoxin and pentylenetetrazole have definite binding sites on GABA receptors.

The field of benzodiazepines was opened with the synthesis of chlordiazepoxide by Sternbach and the discovery of its unique pharmacological properties by Randall.[13] Chlordiazepoxide (see the discussion on individual compounds) is a 2-amino benzodiazepine, and other amino compounds have been synthesized. When it was discovered that chlordiazepoxide is rapidly metabolized to a series of active benzodiazepine-2-ones (see the general scheme of metabolic relationships), however, emphasis shifted to the synthesis and testing of the latter group. Most benzodiazepines are 5-aryl-1,4-benzodiazepines and contain a carboxamide group in the seven-membered diazepine ring structure. Empirical structure–activity relationships (SARs) for antianxiety activity have been tabulated for this group (analogous statements apply for the older 2-amino group).[13,14] The comparative quantitative SAR on nonbenzodiazepine compounds is also reviewed.[15] The following general structure helps to visualize it (Fig. 12.1).

Aromatic or heteroaromatic ring A is required for the activity that may participate in π-π stacking with aromatic amino acid residues of the receptor. An electronegative substituent at position 7 is required for activity, and the more electronegative it is, the higher the activity. Positions 6, 8, and 9 should not be substituted. A phenyl ring C at position 5 promotes activity. If this phenyl group is *ortho* (2′) or d*iortho* (2′,6′) substituted with electron-withdrawing groups, activity is increased. On the other hand, *para* substitution decreases activity greatly. In diazepine ring B, saturation of the 4,5-double bond or a shift of it to the 3,4-position decreases activity. Alkyl substitution at the 3-position decreases activity; substitution with a 3-hydroxyl does not. The presence or absence of the 3-hydroxyl group is important pharmacokinetically. Compounds without the 3-hydroxyl group are nonpolar, 3-hydroxylated in liver slowly to active 3-hydroxyl metabolites, and have long overall half-lives. In

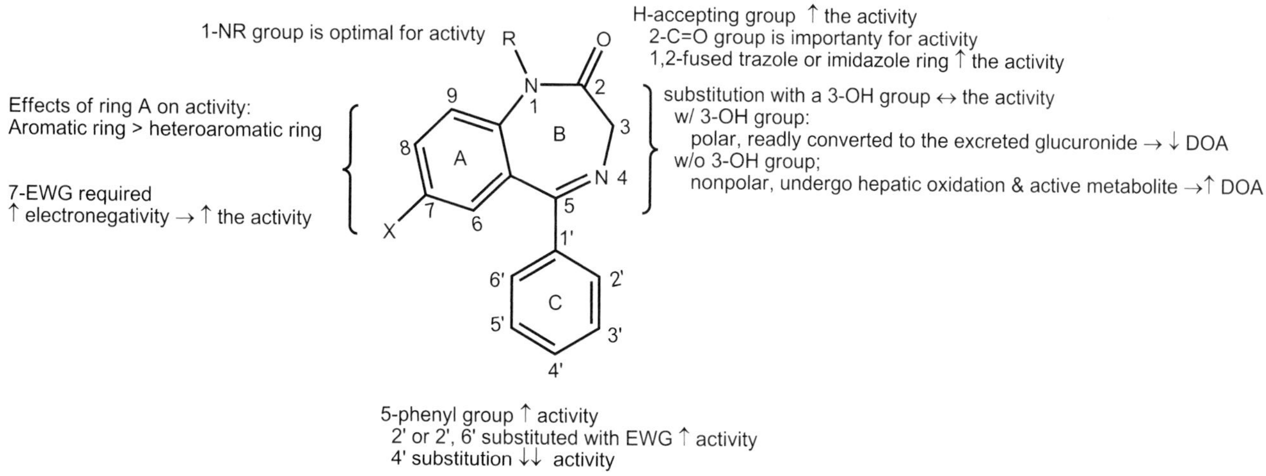

1-NR group is optimal for activity

Effects of ring A on activity:
Aromatic ring > heteroaromatic ring

7-EWG required
↑ electronegativity → ↑ the activity

H-accepting group ↑ the activity
2-C=O group is importanty for activity
1,2-fused trazole or imidazole ring ↑ the activity

substitution with a 3-OH group ↔ the activity
w/ 3-OH group:
    polar, readily converted to the excreted glucuronide → ↓ DOA
w/o 3-OH group;
    nonpolar, undergo hepatic oxidation & active metabolite → ↑ DOA

5-phenyl group ↑ activity
2′ or 2′, 6′ substituted with EWG ↑ activity
4′ substitution ↓↓ activity

Figure 12.1 ● General structure and SAR of benzodiazepines.

contrast, 3-hydroxyl compounds are much more polar, rapidly converted to inactive 3-glucuronides, which are excreted in urine and thus are short-lived (Fig. 12.1). The 2-carbonyl function is important for activity, as is the nitrogen atom at position 1. The N_1-alkyl side chains are tolerated. A proton-accepting group at C2 is required and may interact with histidine residue (as a proton donor) in benzodiazepine-binding site of $GABA_A$ receptor. Other triazole or imidazole rings capable of H-bonding can be fused on positions 1 and 2 and increase the activity.

Additional research yielded compounds with a fused triazolo ring, represented by triazolam and alprazolam. Midazolam, with a fused imidazolo ring, also followed. These compounds are short acting because they are metabolized rapidly by α-hydroxylation of the methyl substituent on the triazolo or imidazolo ring (analogs to benzylic oxidation). The resulting active α-hydroxylated metabolite is quickly inactivated by glucuronidation. The compounds are also metabolized by 3-hydroxylation of the benzodiazepine ring. Interestingly, an electron-attracting group at position 7 is not required for activity in some of these compounds.

The physicochemical and pharmacokinetic properties of the benzodiazepines greatly affect their clinical utility. Most benzodiazepines are lipophilic, in the nonionized form and thus well absorbed from the GI tract, whereas the more polar compounds (e.g., those with a 3-hydroxyl group) tend to be absorbed more slowly than the more lipophilic compounds.

These drugs tend to be highly bound to plasma proteins; in general, the more lipophilic the drug, the greater the binding. However, they do not compete with other protein-bound drugs. They are also very effectively distributed to the brain. Generally, the more lipophilic the compound, the greater is the distribution to the brain, at least initially. When diazepam is used as an anesthetic, it initially distributes to the brain and then redistributes to sites outside the brain. The benzodiazepines are extensively metabolized. The metabolism of benzodiazepines has received much study.[16,17] Some of the major metabolic relationships are shown in Figure 12.2. Metabolites of some benzodiazepines are not only active but also have long half-lives, thus these drugs are long acting. Many benzodiazepines are metabo-

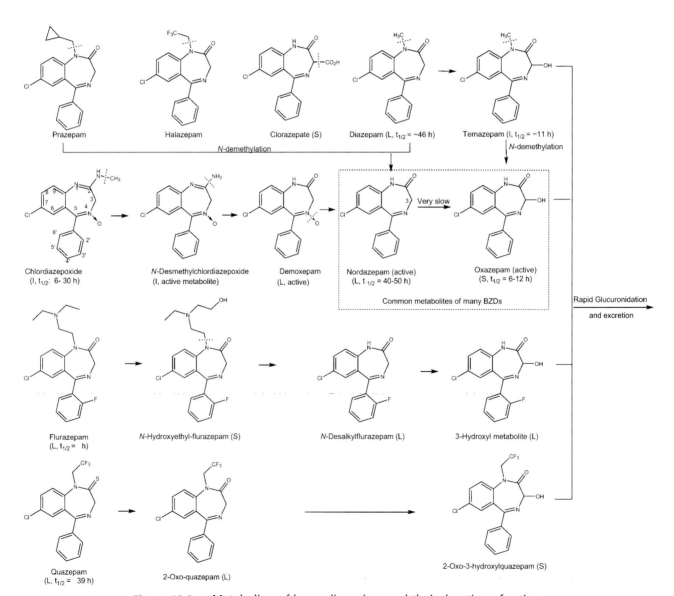

Figure 12.2 ● Metabolism of benzodiazepines and their duration of action.

lized by cytochrome P450 (CYP) 3A4 and CYP2C19. CYP3A4 inhibitors (erythromycin, clarithromycin, ritonavir, itraconazole, ketoconazole, nefazodone, and grapefruit juice) can affect their metabolism. However, they do not induce the metabolism of other drugs. Therefore, the drugs have fewer drug interactions than barbiturates. In addition, they have lower abuse potential and a much greater margin of safety than the barbiturates.

BENZODIAZEPINES

Chlordiazepoxide Hydrochloride, **United States Pharmacopeia (USP).** Chlordiazepoxide hydrochloride, 7-chloro-2-(methylamino)-5-phenyl-3*H*-1,4-benzodiazepine 4-oxide monohydrochloride (Librium), is well absorbed after oral administration. Peak plasma levels are reached in 2 to 4 hours. The half-life of chlordiazepoxide is 6 to 30 hours. *N*-demethylation and hydrolysis of the condensed amidino group are rapid and extensive, producing demoxepam as a major metabolite. Demoxepam can undergo four different metabolic fates. It is converted principally to its active metabolite nordazepam, which is also a major active metabolite of diazepam, clorazepate, and prazepam. Nordazepam, in turn, is converted principally to active oxazepam (marketed separately), which conjugated to the excreted glucuronide. Because of the long half-life of parent drug and its active metabolites, this drug is long acting and self-tapering. As with diazepam (vide infra), repeated administration of chlordiazepoxide can result in accumulation of parent drug and its active metabolites, and thus cause excessive sedation.

Diazepam, **USP.** Diazepam, 7-chloro-1,3-dihydro-1-methyl-5-phenyl-2*H*-1,4-benzodiazepine-2-one (Valium), is prototypical and was the first member of the benzodiazepine-2-one group to be introduced. It is very lipophilic and is thus rapidly and completely absorbed after oral administration. Maximum peak blood concentration occurs in 2 hours and elimination is slow, with a half-life of about ~46 hours. As with chlordiazepoxide, diazepam is metabolized by *N*-demethylation to active nordazepam, which is 3-hydroxylated to active oxazepam (vide infra) and then metabolized according to the general scheme (Fig. 12.2). Like chlordiazepoxide, repeated administration of diazepam leads to accumulation of an active nordazepam,

which can be detected in the blood for more than 1 week after discontinuation of the drug. This drug is a long acting for the same reason. Diazepam is metabolized to nordazepam by CYP2C19 and CYP3A4. Cimetidine, by inhibiting CYP3A4, decreases the metabolism and clearance of diazepam. Thus, drugs that affect the activity of CYP2C19 or CYP3A4 may alter diazepam kinetics. Because diazepam clearance is decreased in the elderly and in patients with hepatic insufficiency, a dosage reduction may be warranted. It is widely used for several anxiety states and has an additional wide range of uses (e.g., as an anticonvulsant, a premedication in anesthesiology, and in various spastic disorders).

Prazepam, **USP.** Prazepam, 7-chloro-1-(cyclopropylmethyl)-1,3-dihydro-5-phenyl-2*H*-1,4-benzodiazepine-2-one (Verstran), has a long overall half-life. Extensive *N*-dealkylation occurs to yield active nordazepam. 3-Hydroxylation of both prazepam and nordazepam occurs.

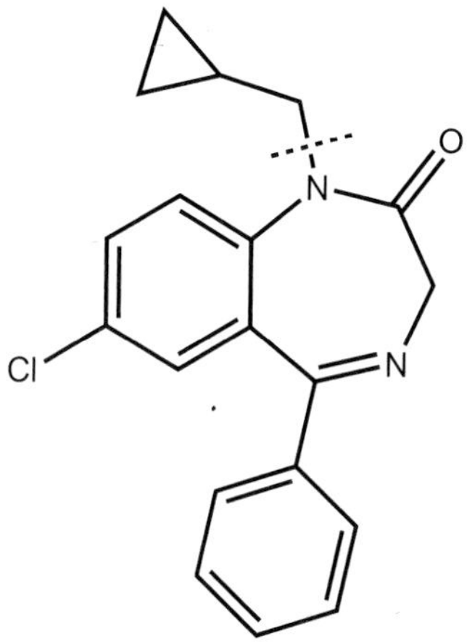

Prazepam

Halazepam, **USP.** Halazepam, 7-chloro-1,3-dihydro-5-phenyl-1(2,2,2-trifluoroethyl)-2*H*-1,4-benzodiazepine-2-one (Paxipam), is marketed as an anxiolytic and well absorbed. It is active and present in plasma, but much of its activity is caused by the major active metabolites nordazepam and oxazepam.

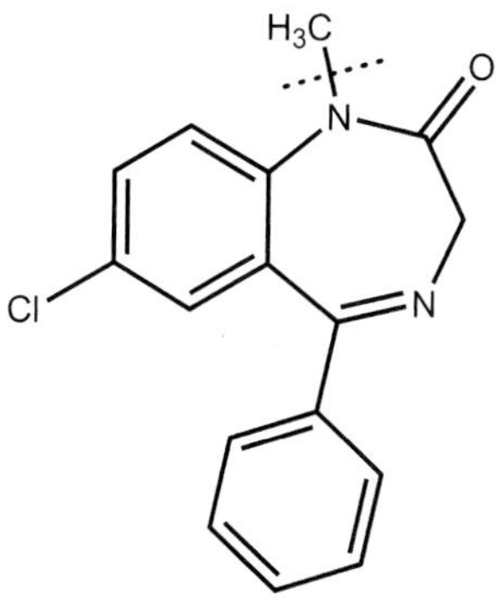

Diazepam: Log P = 3.86, t$_{1/2}$ = ~46 h

Long-acting, Protein binding = 99%

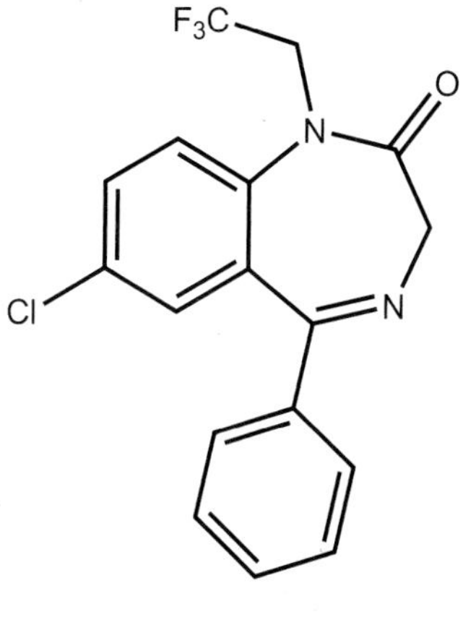

Halazepam

Flurazepam Hydrochloride, USP. Flurazepam hydrochloride, 7-chloro-1-[2-(diethylamino)ethyl]-5-(2-fluorophenyl)-1, 3-dihydro-2*H*-1, 4-benzodiazepine-2-one dihydrochloride (Dalmane), is notable as a benzodiazepine marketed almost exclusively for use in insomnia. Metabolism of the dialkylaminoalkyl side chain is extensive. A major metabolite is N^1-dealkyl flurazepam, which has a very long half-life and persists for several days after administration. Consequently, it produces cumulative clinical effects and side effects (e.g., excessive sedation) and residual pharmacologic activity, even after discontinuation.

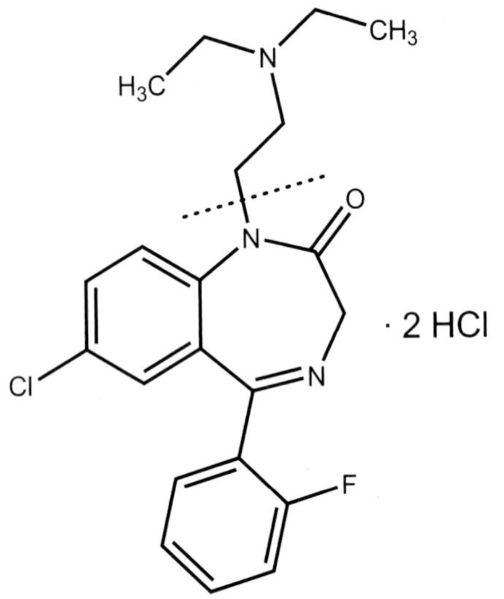

oxidation to the 2-oxo compound and then *N*-dealkylation. Both metabolites are active; the first reportedly is the more potent and selective. Thereafter, 3-hydroxylation and glucuronidation occur.

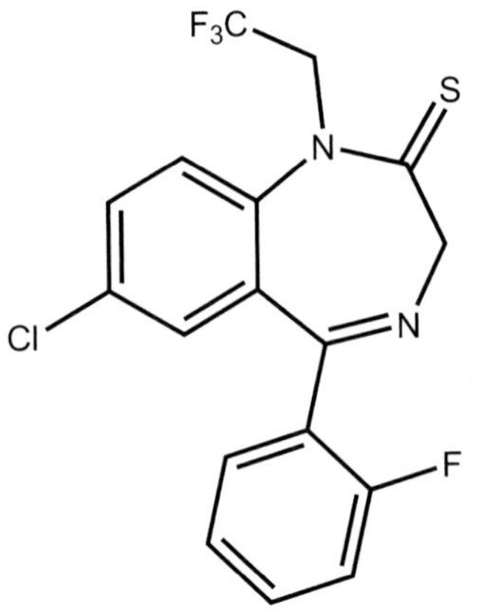

Quazepam
$t_{1/2} = 39$
long-acting

Flurazepam hydrochloride
$t_{1/2}$ = ~7 h,
$t_{1/2}$ of its active metabolite = 50 h
long-acting

Quazepam. Quazepam (Doral) and its active metabolites reportedly are relatively selective for the benzodiazepine modulatory site on GABA$_A$ receptors with α_1 subunit and are hypnotic agents. Quazepam is metabolized by

Clorazepate Dipotassium. Clorazepate dipotassium, 7-chloro-2,3-dihydro-2-oxo-5-phenyl-1*H*-1,4-benzodiazepine-3-carboxylic acid dipotassium salt monohydrate (Tranxene), can be considered a prodrug. Inactive itself, it undergoes rapid decarboxylation by the acidity of the stomach to nordazepam (a major active metabolite of diazepam), which has a long half-life and undergoes hepatic conversion to active oxazepam. Despite the polar character of the drug as administered, because it is quickly converted in the GI tract to an active nonpolar compound, it has a quick onset, overall long half-life, and shares similar clinical and pharmacokinetic properties to chlordiazepoxide and diazepam.

Oxazepam, USP. Oxazepam, 7-chloro-1,3-dihydro-3-hydroxy-5-phenyl-2*H*-1,4-benzodiazpin-2-one (Serax), is an active metabolite of both chlordiazepoxide and diazepam and can be considered a prototype for the 3-hydroxy benzo-

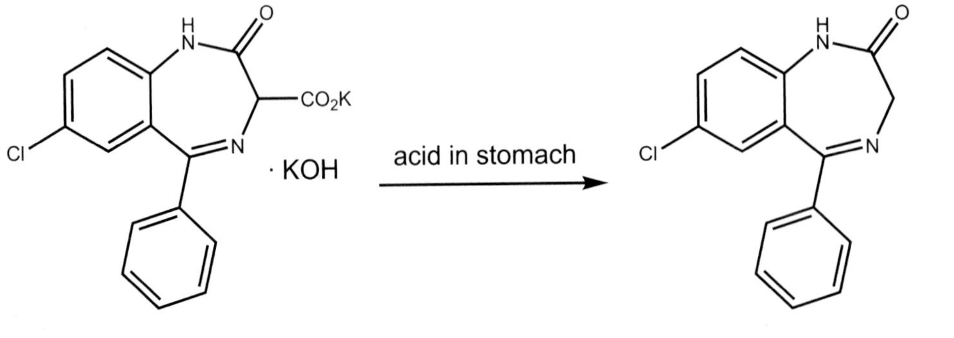

Clorazepate Dipotassium
(polar and inactive prodrug)

acid in stomach

Nordazepam (nonpolar and an active metabolite)
$t_{1/2}$ = 40-50 h

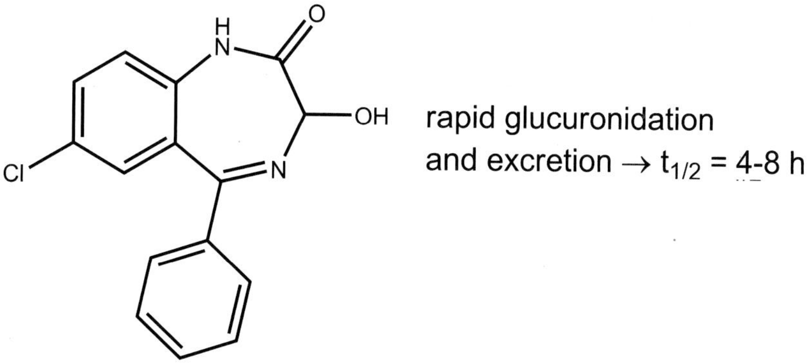

rapid glucuronidation
and excretion → t$_{1/2}$ = 4-8 h

Oxazepam, Log P = 2.31

diazepines. For the stereochemistry of this and other 3-hydroxy compounds, see the chapter dealing with metabolism. It is much more polar than diazepam. Oxazepam is rapidly inactivated to glucuronidated metabolites that are excreted in the urine. Thus, the half-life of oxazepam is about 4 to 8 hours, and it is marketed as a short-acting anxiolytic. As a result, its cumulative effects with chronic therapy are much less than with long-acting benzodiazepine such as chlordiazepoxide and diazepam.

Lorazepam, **USP.** Lorazepam, 7-chloro-5-(2-chlorophenyl)-3-dihydro-3-hydroxy-2*H*-1,4-benzodiazepine-2-one (Ativan), is the 2′-chloro derivative of oxazepam. In keeping with overall SARs, the 2′-chloro substituent increases activity. As with oxazepam, metabolism is relatively rapid and uncomplicated because of the 3-hydroxyl group in the compound. Thus, it also has short half-life (2–6 hours) and similar pharmacological activity.

Temazepam. Temazepam, 7-chloro-1,3-dihydro-3-hydroxy-1-methyl-5-phenyl -2*H*-1,4-benzodiazepine-2-one (Restoril), also occurs as a minor metabolite of diazepam. It can be visualized as *N*-methyl oxazepam, and indeed, a small amount of *N*-demethylation occurs slowly. However, metabolism proceeds mainly through glucuronidation of the 3-hydroxyl group, thus, it is intermediate acting and marketed as a hypnotic said to have little or no residual effect.

TRIAZOLOBENZODIAZEPINES

Alprazolam, **USP.** Alprazolam, 8-chloro-1-methyl-6-phenyl-4*H*-*s*-triazolo[4,3-*a*][1,4]benzodiazepine (Xanax), is rapidly absorbed from the GI tract. Protein binding is lower (~70%) than with most benzodiazepines because of its lower lipophilicity. α-Hydroxylation of the methyl group to the methyl alcohol (a reaction analogous to benzylic hydroxylation) followed by conjugation is rapid; consequently, the duration of action is short. The drug is a highly potent anxiolytic on a milligram basis.

Triazolam, **USP.** Triazolam, 8-chloro-6-(*o*-chlorophenyl)-1-methyl-4*H*-*s*-triazolo[4,3-a][1,4] benzodiazepine (Halcion), has all of the characteristic benzodiazepine pharmacological actions. It is an ultra–short-acting hypnotic because it is rapidly α-hydroxylated to the 1-methyl alcohol, which is then rapidly conjugated and excreted. Consequently, it has gained popularity as sleep inducers, especially in elderly patients, because it causes less daytime sedation. It is metabolically inactivated primarily by hepatic and intestinal CYP3A4; therefore, coadministration with grapefruit juice increases its peak plasma concentration by 30%, leading to increased drowsiness.

Midazolam. This drug is used intravenously as a short-acting sedative–hypnotic and as an induction anesthetic because of its short half-life for the same reason. Further information can be found in the section on anesthetics.

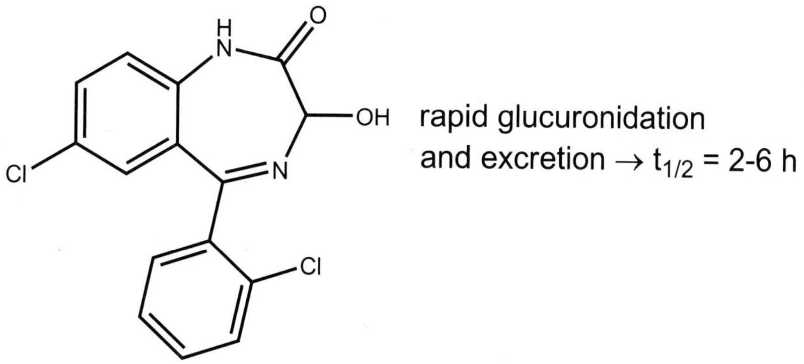

rapid glucuronidation
and excretion → t$_{1/2}$ = 2-6 h

Lorazepam

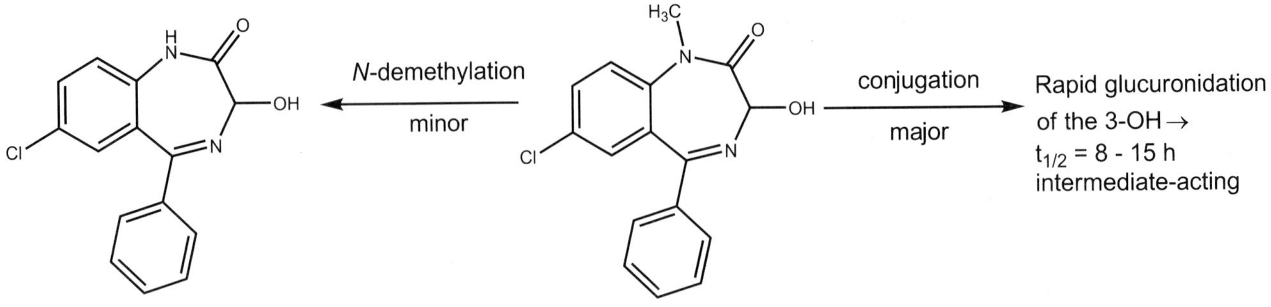

Oxazepam (active)

Temazepam

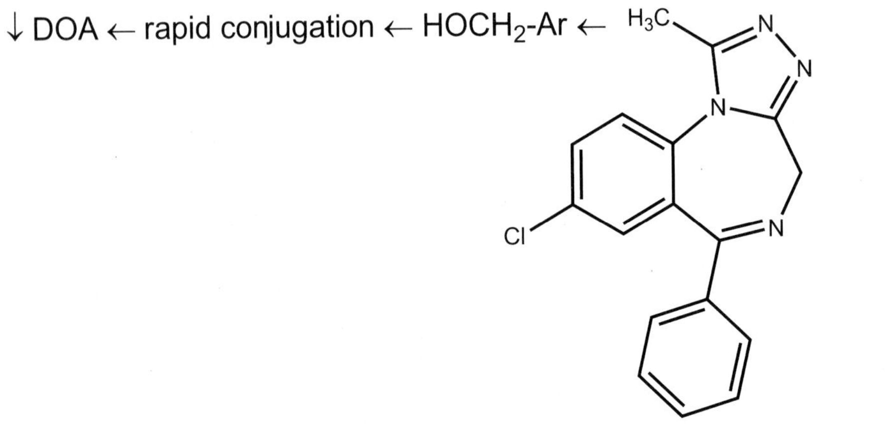

N-demethylation
minor

conjugation
major

Rapid glucuronidation
of the 3-OH →
$t_{1/2}$ = 8 - 15 h
intermediate-acting

↓ DOA ← rapid conjugation ← HOCH$_2$-Ar ←

Alprazolam
$t_{1/2}$ = ~12 h
Log P = 2.50
protein binding = ~70%

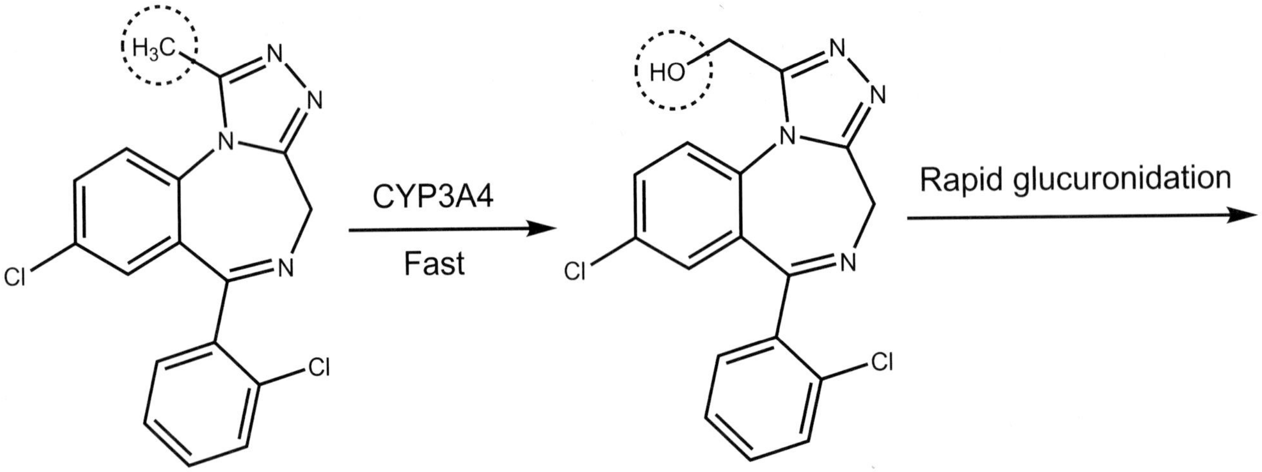

Triazolam
Fast metabolism
$t_{1/2}$ = ~ 4 h
short-acting
Less daytime sedation

CYP3A4
Fast

An α-hydroxylated metabolite
Eliminated as *O*-glucuronides

Rapid glucuronidation

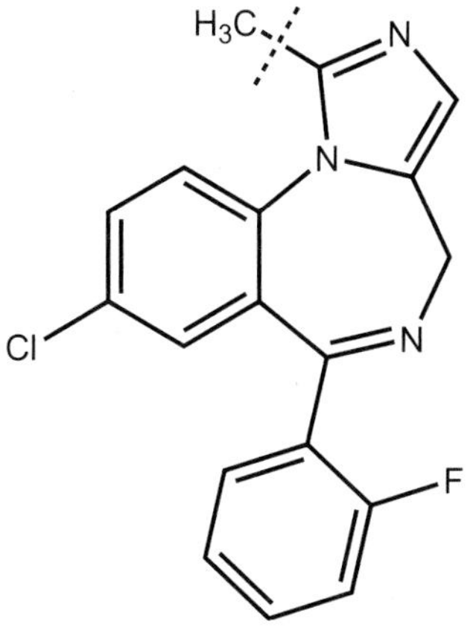

Midazolam
Log P = 3.67
$t_{1/2}$ = ~2 h

NONBENZODIAZEPINE BzRAs

Zolpidem (Ambien, an imidazopyridine) and eszopiclone (Lunesta, a cyclopyrrolone) are nonbenzodiazepines and have been introduced as short- and moderate-acting hypnotics, respectively. Zolpidem exhibits a high selectivity for the α_1 subunit of benzodiazepine-binding site on GABA$_A$ receptor complex, whereas eszopiclone is a "superagonist" at BzRs with the subunit composition $\alpha_1\beta_2\gamma_2$ and $\alpha_1\beta_2\gamma_3$. Zolpidem has a rapid onset of action of 1.6 hours and good bioavailability (72%), mainly because it is lipophilic and has no ionizable groups at physiological pH. Food can prolong the time to peak concentration without affecting the half-life probably for the same reason. It has short elimination half-life, because its aryl methyl groups is extensively α-hydroxylated to inactive metabolites by CYP3A4 followed by further oxidation by aldehyde dehydrogenase to the ionic carboxylic acid. The metabolites are inactive, short-lived, and eliminated in the urine. Its half-life in the elderly or the patients with liver disease is increased. Therefore, dosing should be modified in patients with hepatic insufficiency and the elderly. Because it has longer elimination half-life than zaleplon, it may be preferred for sleep maintenance. It was the most commonly prescribed drug for insomnia in 2001.

Zopiclone was originally marketed as a racemic mixture. Because its *S*-isomer is a primary active hypnotic, it is now marketed as eszopiclone in the United States. It is less selective for the α_1 subunit of GABA$_A$ receptor, and it has relatively longer elimination half-life (~6 hours) than zolpidem and zaleplon. Consequently, it may be used for patients who tend to awaken during the night.

Zaleplon. Zaleplon (Sonata, a pyrazolopyrimidine) is another short-acting nonbenzodiazepine hypnotic. Pharmacologically and pharmacokinetically, zaleplon is similar to zolpidem; both are hypnotic agents with short half-lives. It also has selective high affinity for α_1-subunit containing BzRs but produces effects at other BzR/GABA$_A$ subtypes as well. Zaleplon is well absorbed following oral administration with an absolute bioavailability of approximately 30% because of significant presystemic metabolism. It exhibits a mean half-life of approximately 1 hour, with less than 1% of the dose excreted unchanged in urine. It is primarily metabolized by aldehyde oxidase to 5-oxo-zaleplon and is also metabolized to a lesser extent by CYP3A4. *N*-demethylation yields desethylzaleplon, which is quickly converted, presumably by aldehyde oxidase, to 5-oxo-desethylzaleplon. These oxidative metabolites are then converted to glucuronides and eliminated in urine. All of zaleplon's metabolites are pharmacologically inactive. It may have a more rapid onset (about 1 hour) and termination of action than zolpidem, and therefore, it is good to initiate sleep instead of keeping sleep.

Melatonin Receptor Agonist: Ramelteon

In the brain, three melatonin receptors (MT$_1$, MT$_2$, and MT$_3$) have been characterized. Activation of the MT$_1$ receptor results in sleepiness, whereas the MT$_2$ receptor may be related to the circadian rhythm. MT$_3$ receptors may be related to intraocular pressure. Their endogenous ligand, melatonin (*N*-acetyl-5-methoxytryptamine), at times referred to as "the hormone of darkness," is *N*-acetylated and *O*-methylated product of serotonin found in the pineal gland and is biosynthesized and released at night and may play a role in the circadian rhythm of humans. It is promoted commercially as a sleep aid by the food supplement industry. However, it is a poor hypnotic drug because of its poor potency, poor absorption, poor oral bioavailability, rapid metabolism, and nonselective effects.

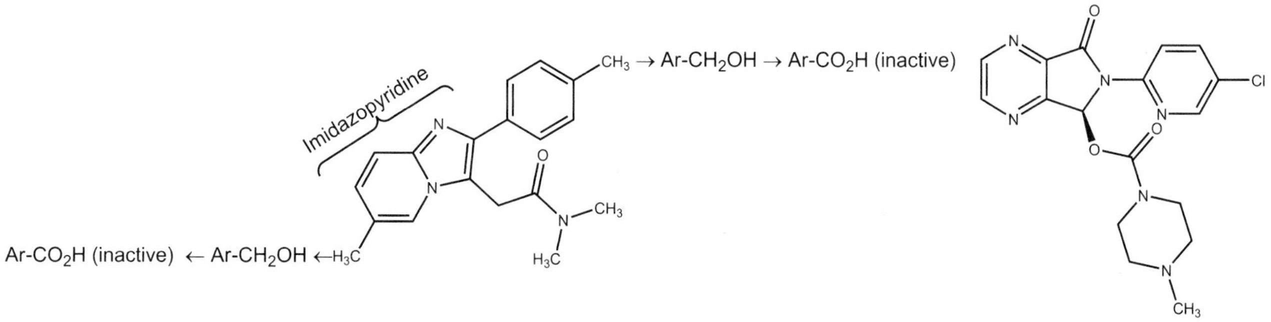

Zolpidem
Log P = 2.61
$t_{1/2}$ = 2.5
short-acting

Eszopiclone
$t_{1/2}$ = 5-6 h
moderate-acting

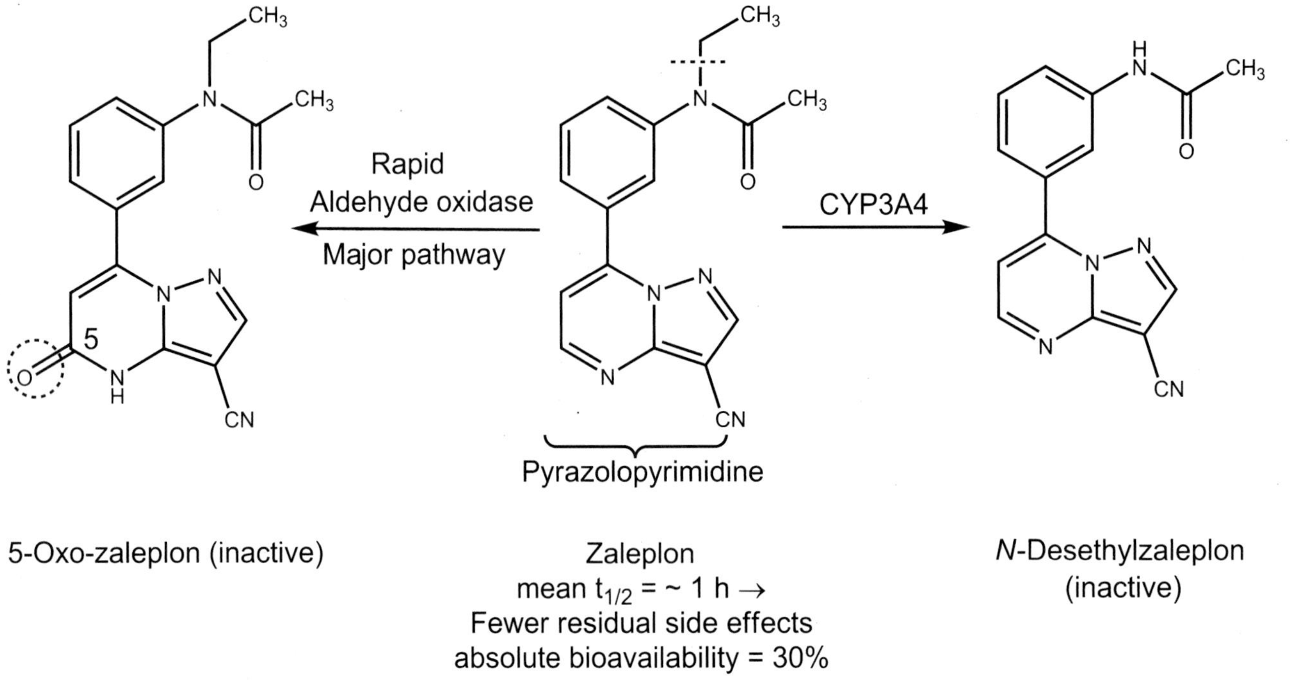
Rapid
Aldehyde oxidase
Major pathway
CYP3A4
Pyrazolopyrimidine
5-Oxo-zaleplon (inactive)
Zaleplon
mean $t_{1/2}$ = ~ 1 h →
Fewer residual side effects
absolute bioavailability = 30%
N-Desethylzaleplon
(inactive)

Ramelteon (Rozerem). The melatonin molecule was modified mainly by replacing the nitrogen of the indole ring with a carbon to give an indane ring and by incorporating 5-methoxyl group in the indole ring into a more rigid furan ring. The selectivity of the resulting ramelteon for MT_1 receptor is eight times more than that of MT_2 receptor. Unlike melatonin, it is more effective in initiating sleep (MT_1 activity) rather than to readjust the circadian rhythm (MT_2 activity). It appears to be distinctly more efficacious than melatonin but less efficacious than benzodiazepines as a hypnotic. Importantly, this drug has no addiction liability (it is not a controlled substance). As a result, it has recently been approved for the treatment of insomnia.

Barbiturates

The barbiturates were used extensively as sedative–hypnotic drugs. Except for a few specialized uses, they have been replaced largely by the much safer benzodiazepine. Barbiturates act throughout the CNS. However, they exert most of their characteristic CNS effects mainly by binding to an allosteric recognition site on $GABA_A$ receptors that positively modulates the effect of the $GABA_A$ receptor—GABA binding. Unlike benzodiazepines, they bind at different binding sites and appear to increase the *duration* of the GABA-gated chloride channel openings. In addition, by binding to the barbiturate modulatory site, barbiturates can also increase chloride ion flux without GABA attaching to its receptor site on $GABA_A$. This has been termed a *GABA mimetic effect.* It is thought to be related to the profound CNS depression that barbiturates can produce.

The barbiturates are 5,5-disubstituted barbituric acids. Consideration of the structure of 5,5-disubstituted barbituric acids reveals their acidic character. Those without methyl substituents on the nitrogen have pK_a's of about 7.6; those with a methyl substituent have pK_a's of about 8.4. The free acids have poor water solubility and good lipid solubility (the latter largely a function of the two hydrocarbon substituents on the 5-position, although in the 2-thiobarbiturates, the sulfur atom increases lipid solubility).

Sodium salts of the barbiturates are readily prepared and are water soluble. Their aqueous solutions generate an alkaline pH. A classic incompatibility is the addition of an agent with an acidic pH in solution, which results in

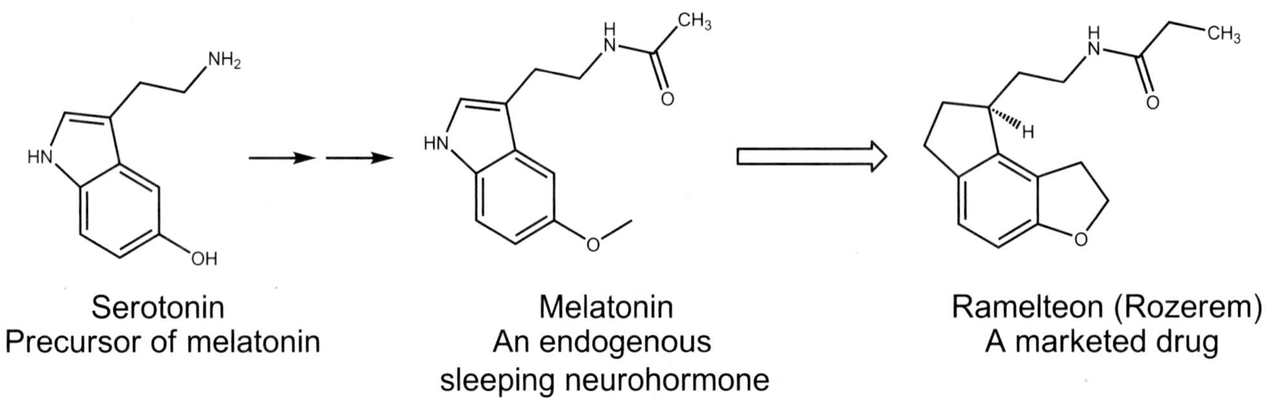
Serotonin
Precursor of melatonin
Melatonin
An endogenous
sleeping neurohormone
Ramelteon (Rozerem)
A marketed drug

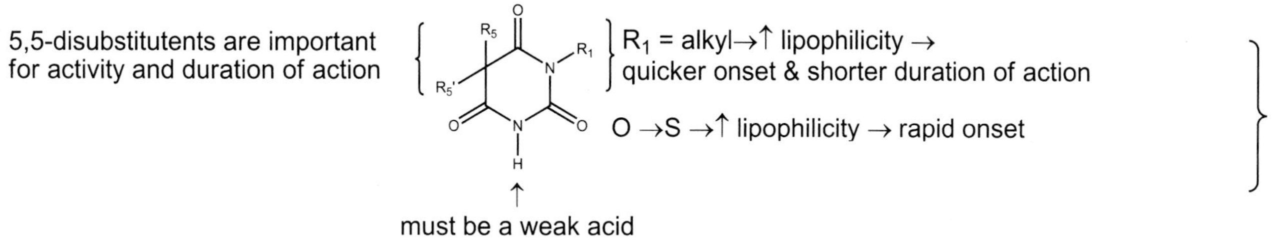

5,5-disubstitutents are important for activity and duration of action

R_1 = alkyl→↑ lipophilicity → quicker onset & shorter duration of action

O →S →↑ lipophilicity → rapid onset

must be a weak acid

Figure 12.3 ● Structure–activity relationship of barbiturates.

formation and precipitation of the free water-insoluble disubstituted barbituric acid. Sodium salts of barbiturates in aqueous solution decompose at varying rates by base-catalyzed hydrolysis, generating ring-opened salts of carboxylic acids.

Structure–Activity Relationships

Extensive synthesis and testing of the barbiturates over a long time span have produced well-defined SARs (see Fig. 12.3), which have been summarized.[18] The barbituric acid is 2,4,6-trioxohexahydropyrimidine, which lacks CNS depressant activity. However, the replacement of both hydrogens at position 5 with alkyl or aryl groups confers the activity. Both hydrogen atoms at the 5-position of barbituric acid must be replaced. This may be because if one hydrogen is available at position 5, tautomerization to a highly acidic trihydroxypyrimidine (pK_a ∼4) can occur. Consequently, the compound is largely in the anionic form at physiological pH, with little nonionic lipid-soluble compound available to cross the blood-brain barrier.

In general, increasing lipophilicity increases hypnotic potency and the onset of action and decreases the duration of action. Thus, beginning with lower alkyls, there is an increase in onset and a decrease in duration of action with increasing hydrocarbon content up to about seven to nine total carbon atoms substituted on the 5-position. It is because that lipophilicity and an ability to penetrate the brain in the first case and an ability to penetrate liver microsomes in the second may be involved. In addition for more lipophilic compounds, partitioning out of the brain to other sites can be involved in the second instance. There is an inverse correlation between the total number of carbon atoms substituted on the 5-position and the duration of action, which is even better when the character of these substituents is taken into account, for example, the relatively

polar character of a phenyl substituent (approximates a three- to four-carbon aliphatic chain), branching of alkyls, presence of an isolated double or triple bond, and so on. Additionally, these groups can influence the ease of oxidative metabolism by effects on bond strengths as well as by influencing partitioning.

Absorption from the GI tract is good. Binding to blood proteins is substantial. Compounds with low lipophilicity may be excreted intact in the urine, whereas highly lipophilic compounds are excreted after metabolism to polar metabolites. Increasing the lipophilicity generally increases the rate of metabolism, except for compounds with an extremely high lipophilicity (e.g., thiopental), which tend to depotize and are thus relatively unavailable for metabolism. Metabolism generally follows an ultimate (ω) or penultimate (ω-1) oxidation pattern. Ring-opening reactions are usually minor. *N*-methylation decreases duration of action, in large part, probably, by increasing the concentration of the lipid-soluble free barbituric acid. 2-Thiobarbiturates have a very short duration of action because its lipophilicity is extremely high, promoting depotization. Barbiturates find use as sedatives, as hypnotics, for induction of anesthesia, and as anticonvulsants.

Some of the more frequently used barbiturates are described briefly in the following sections. For the structures, the usual dosages required to produce sedation and hypnosis, the times of onset, and the duration of action, see Table 12.1.

BARBITURATES WITH A LONG DURATION OF ACTION (MORE THAN 6 HOURS)

Mephobarbital, USP. Mephobarbital, 3-methyl-5-ethyl-5-phenylbarbituric acid (metharbital), is metabolically *N*-demethylated to phenobarbital, which many consider to account for almost all of the activity. Its principal use is as an anticonvulsant.

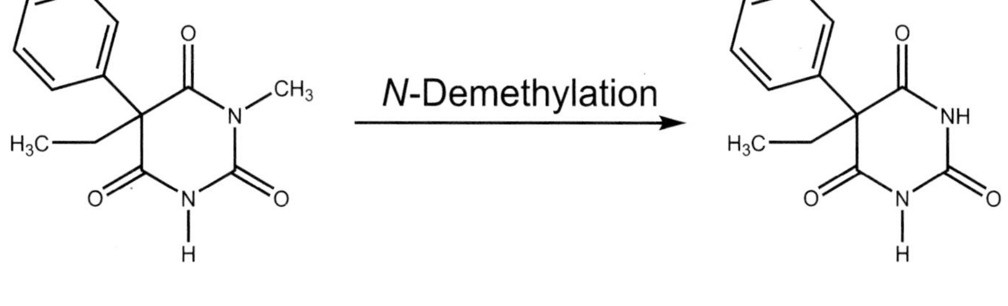

Mephobarbital (Mebaral)
Log P = 1.85

N-Demethylation

Phenobarbital (Luminal)
Log P = 1.71

TABLE 12.1 Barbiturates Used as Sedatives and Hypnotics

General Structure

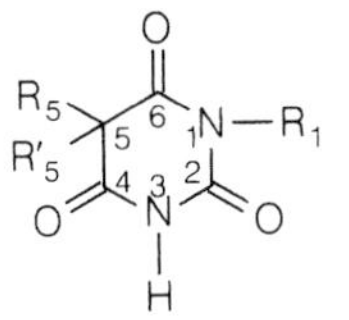

Generic Name *Proprietary Name*	Substituents			Sedative Dose (mg)	Hypnotic Dose (mg)	Usual Onset of Action (min)
	R_5	R'_5	R_1			
A. Long Duration of Action (more than 6 hours)						
Mephobarbital, *USP* *Mebaral*	C_2H_2	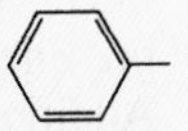 (phenyl)	CH_3	30–100[a]	100	30–60
Phenobarbital, *USP* *Luminal*	C_2H_2	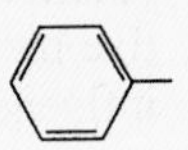 (phenyl)	H	15–30[a]	100	20–40
B. Intermediate Duration of Action (3–6 hours)						
Amobarbital, *USP* *Amytal*	CH_3CH_2-	$(CH_3)_2CHCH_2CH_2-$	H	20–40	100	20–30
Butabarbital sodium, *USP* *Butisol Sodium*	CH_3CH_2-	$CH_3CH_2\overset{CH_3}{\underset{\vert}{CH}}-$	H	15–30	100	20–30
C. Short Duration of Action (less than 3 hours)						
Pentobarbital sodium, *USP* *Nembutal Sodium*	CH_3CH_2-	$CH_3CH_2CH_2\overset{CH_3}{\underset{\vert}{CH}}-$	H	30	100	20–30
Secobarbital, *USP* *Seconal*	$CH_2{=}CHCH_2-$	$CH_3CH_2CH_2\overset{CH_3}{\underset{\vert}{CH}}-$	H	15–30	100	20–30

[a]Daytime sedative and anticonvulsant.

Phenobarbital, **USP.** Phenobarbital, 5-ethyl-5-phenyl-barbituric acid (Luminal), is a long-acting sedative and hypnotic. It is also a valuable anticonvulsant, especially in generalized tonic–clonic and partial seizures (see the discussion on anticonvulsants). Metabolism to the *p*-hydroxylphenyl compound followed by glucuronidation accounts for about 90% of a dose.

BARBITURATES WITH AN INTERMEDIATE DURATION OF ACTION (3–6 HOURS)

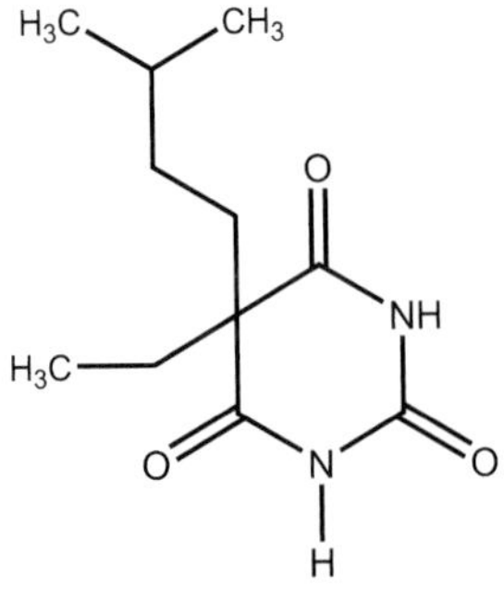

Amobarbital
Log P = 2.10

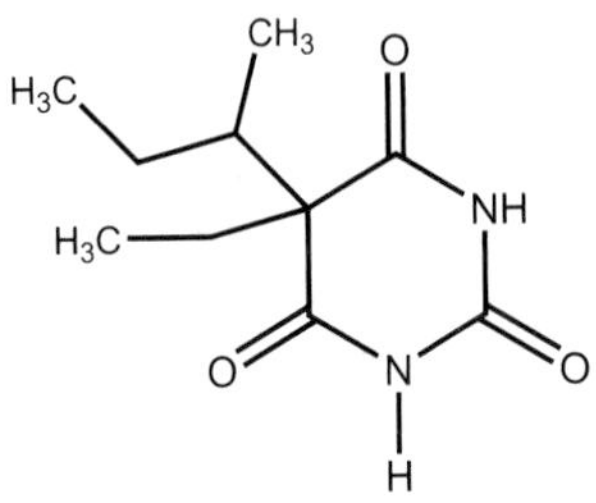

Butabarbital
Log P = 1.56

Barbiturates with an intermediate duration of action are used principally as sedative–hypnotics. They include amobarbital, *USP*, 5-ethyl-5-isopentylbarbituric acid (Amytal), and its water-soluble sodium salt, amobarbital sodium, *USP*, 5-allyl-5-isopropylbarbituric acid (aprobarbital [Alurate]); butabarbital sodium, *USP*, the water-soluble sodium salt of 5-*sec*-butyl-5-ethylbarbituric acid (Butisol Sodium).

BARBITURATES WITH A SHORT DURATION OF ACTION (LESS THAN 3 HOURS)

Barbiturates that have substituents in the 5-position promoting more rapid metabolism (e.g., by increasing the lipophilicity) than the intermediate group include pentobarbital-sodium, *USP*, sodium 5-ethyl-5-(1-methylbutyl)barbiturate (Nembutal); secobarbital, *USP*, 5-allyl-5-(1-methylbutyl)barbituric acid (Seconal); and the sodium salt sodium secobarbital. Barbiturates with an ultrashort duration of action are discussed under anesthetic agents.

Miscellaneous Sedative–Hypnotics

A wide range of chemical structures (e.g., imides, amides, alcohols) can produce sedation and hypnosis resembling those produced by the barbiturates. Despite this apparent structural diversity, the compounds have generally similar structural characteristics and chemical properties: a nonpolar portion and a semipolar portion that can participate in

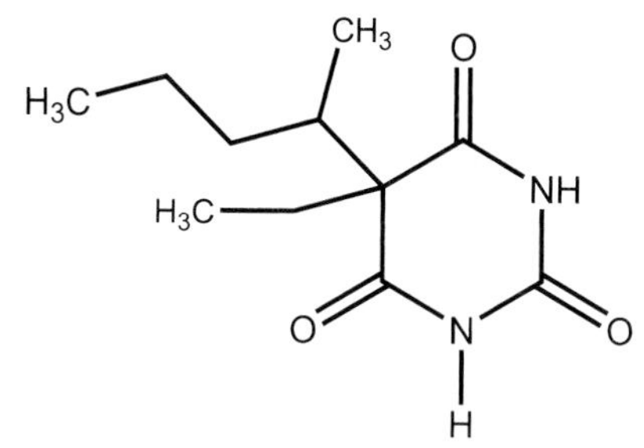

Pentobarbital
Log P = 2.10

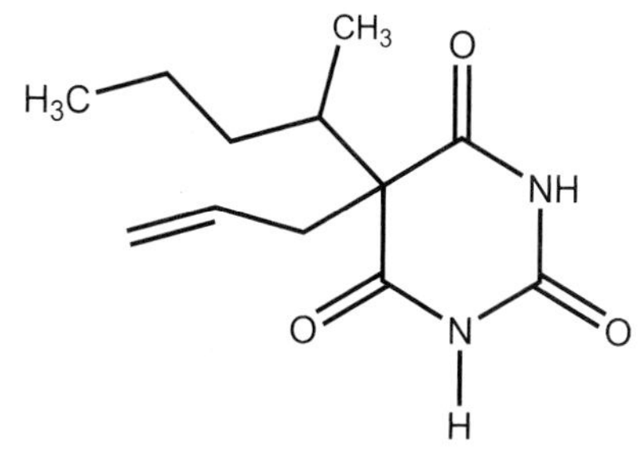

Secobarbital
Log P = 2.33

H-bonding. In some cases, modes of action are undetermined. As a working hypothesis, most of the agents can be envisioned to act by mechanisms similar to those proposed for barbiturates and alcohols.

AMIDES AND IMIDES

Glutethimide, **USP.** Glutethimide, 2-ethyl-2-phenyl-glutarimide (Doriden), is one of the most active nonbarbiturate hypnotics that is structurally similar to the barbiturates, especially phenobarbital. Because of glutethimide's low aqueous solubility, its dissolution and absorption from the GI track is somewhat erratic. Consistent with its high lipophilicity, it undergoes extensive oxidative metabolism in the liver with a half-life of approximately 10 hours. Glutethimide is used as a racemic mixture with the (+) enantiomer being primarily metabolized on the glutarimide ring and the (−) enantiomer on the phenyl ring. The product of metabolic detoxification is excreted after conjugation with glucuronic acid at the hydroxyl group. The drug is an enzyme inducer. In the therapeutic dosage range, adverse effects tend to be infrequent. Toxic effects in overdose are as severe as, and possibly more troublesome than, those of the barbiturates.

Alcohols and Their Carbamate Derivatives

The very simple alcohol ethanol has a long history of use as a sedative and hypnotic. Its modes of action were described under the anesthetic heading and are said to apply to other alcohols. It is widely used in self-medication as a sedative–hypnotic. Because this use has so many hazards, it is seldom a preferred agent medically.

As the homologous series of normal alcohols is ascended from ethanol, CNS depressant potency increases up to eight carbon atoms, with activity decreasing thereafter. Branching of the alkyl chain increases depressant activity and, in an isometric series, the order of potency is tertiary > secondary > primary. In part, this may be because tertiary and secondary alcohols are not metabolized by oxidation to the corresponding carboxylic acids. Replacement of a hydrogen atom in the alkyl group by a halogen increases the alkyl portion and, accordingly, for the lower–molecular weight compounds, increases potency. Carbamylation of alcohols generally increases depressant potency. Carbamate groups are generally much more resistant to metabolic inactivation than hydroxyl functions. Most of the alcohols and carbamates have been superseded as sedative–hypnotics. Several difunctional compounds (e.g., diol carbamates) have depressant action on the cord in addition to the brain and are retained principally for their skeletal muscle relaxant properties.

Ethchlorvynol, **USP.** Ethchlorvynol, 1-chloro-3-ethyl-1-penten-4-yn-3-ol (Placidyl), is a mild sedative–hypnotic with a quick onset and short duration of action ($t_{1/2} = 5.6$ hours). Because of its highly lipophilic character, it is extensively metabolized to its secondary alcohol ($\sim$90%) prior to its excretion. It reportedly induces microsomal hepatic enzymes. Acute overdose shares several features with barbiturate overdose.

Meprobamate, **USP.** Meprobamate, 2-methyl-2-propyltrimethylene dicarbamate, 2-methyl-2-propyl-1,3-propanediol dicarbamate (Equanil, Miltown), is officially indicated as an antianxiety agent. It is also a sedative–hypnotic agent. It has several overall pharmacological

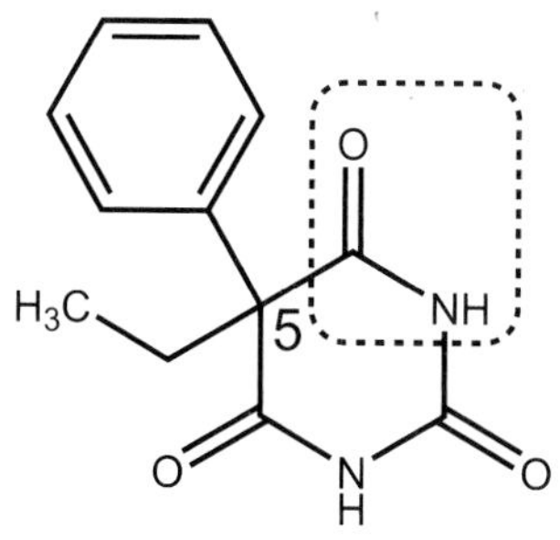

Phenobarbital, Log P = 1.71

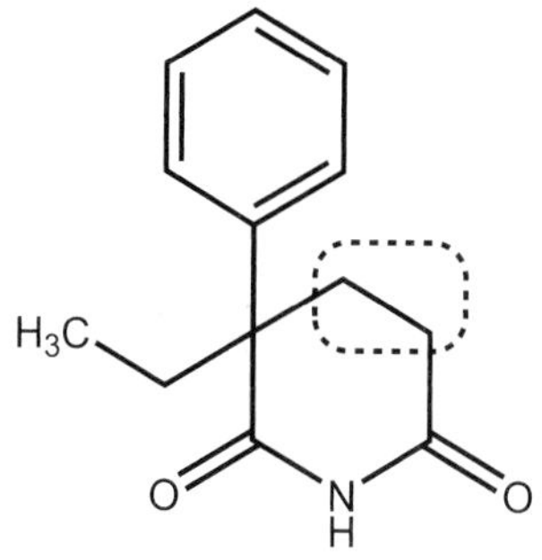

Glutethimide, Log P = 2.70

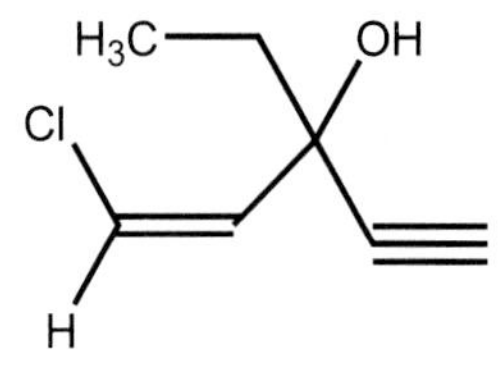

Ethchlorvynol

properties resembling those of benzodiazepines and barbiturates. The mechanism of action underlying anxiolytic effects is unknown but may involve effects on conductivity in specific brain areas.[19] It does not appear to act through effects on GABAergic systems. The drug is effective against absence seizures and may worsen generalized tonic–clonic seizures.

Meprobamate is also a centrally acting skeletal muscle relaxant. The agents in this group find use in several conditions, such as strains and sprains that may produce acute muscle spasm. They have interneuronal blocking properties at the level of the spinal cord, which are said to be partly responsible for skeletal muscle relaxation.[19] Also, the general CNS depressant properties they possess may contribute to, or be mainly responsible for, the skeletal muscle relaxant activity. Dihydric compounds and their carbamate (urethane) derivatives, as described previously in the discussion of meprobamate, are prominent members of the group.

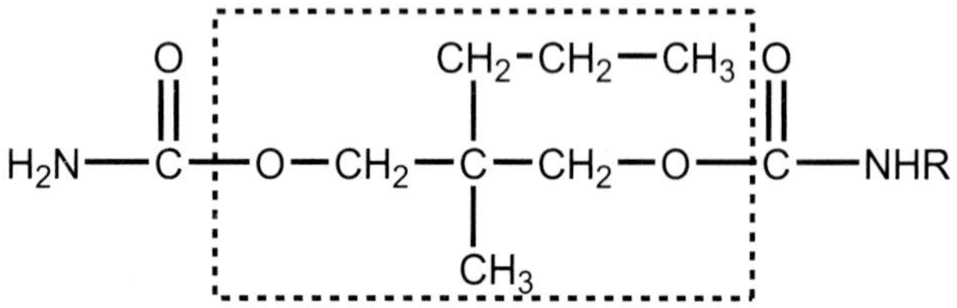

Meprobamate: R = H
Carisoprodol: R = CH (CH₃)₂

Carisoprodol, USP. Carisoprodol, *N*-isopropyl-2-methyl-2-propyl-1,3-propanediol dicarbamate, 2-methyl-2-propyl-1,3-propanediol carbamate isopropylcarbamate (Soma), is the mono-*N*-isopropyl–substituted relative of meprobamate. The structure is given in the discussion of meprobamate. It is indicated in acute skeletomuscular conditions characterized by pain, stiffness, and spasm. As can be expected, a major side effect of the drug is drowsiness.

Chlorphenesin Carbamate. Chlorphenesin carbamate, 3-(*p*-chlorophenoxy)-1,2-propanediol 1-carbamate (Maolate), is the *p*-chloro substituted and 1-carbamate derivative of the lead compound in the development of this group of agents, mephenesin. Mephenesin is weakly active and short-lived because of facile metabolism of the primary hydroxyl group. Carbamylation of this group increases activity. *p*-Chlorination increases the lipophilicity and seals off the *para* position from hydroxylation. Metabolism, still fairly rapid, involves glucuronidation of the secondary hydroxyl group. The biological half-life in humans is 3.5 hours.

Methocarbamol, USP. Methocarbamol, 3-(*o*-methoxyphenoxy)-1,2-propanediol 1-carbamate (Robaxin), is said to be more sustained in effect than mephenesin. Likely sites for metabolic attack include the secondary hydroxyl group and the two ring positions opposite the ether functions. The dihydric parent compound, guaifenesin, is used as an expectorant.

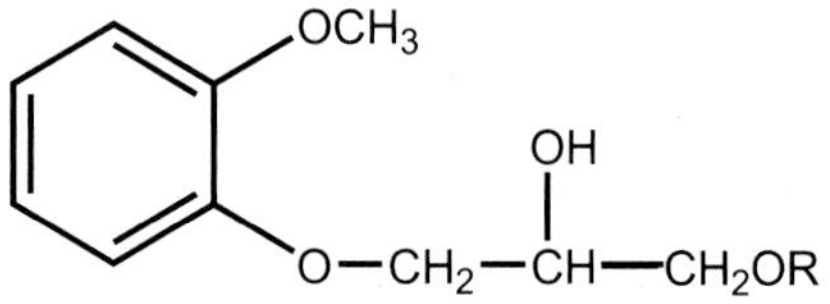

Guaifenesin: R = H
Methocarbamol: R = CONH₂

ALDEHYDES AND THEIR DERIVATIVES

For chemical reasons that are easily rationalized, few aldehydes are valuable hypnotic drugs. The aldehyde in use, chloral (as the hydrate), is thought to act principally through a metabolite, trichloroethanol. Acetaldehyde is used as the cyclic trimer derivative, paraldehyde, which could also be grouped as a cyclic polyether.

Chloral Hydrate, USP. Chloral hydrate, trichloroacetaldehyde monohydrate, $CCl_3CH(OH)_2$ (Noctec), is an aldehyde hydrate stable enough to be isolated. The relative stability of this *gem*-diol is largely a result of an unfavorable dipole–dipole repulsion between the trichloromethyl carbon and the carbonyl carbon present in the parent carbonyl compound.[20]

Chloral hydrate is unstable in alkaline solutions, undergoing the last step of the haloform reaction to yield chloroform and formate ion. In hydroalcoholic solutions, it forms the hemiacetal with ethanol. Whether or not this compound is the basis for the notorious and potentially lethal effect of

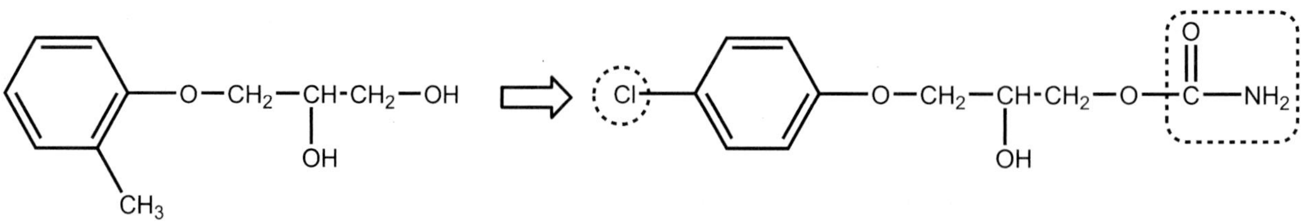

Mephenesin

Chlorphenesin Carbamate

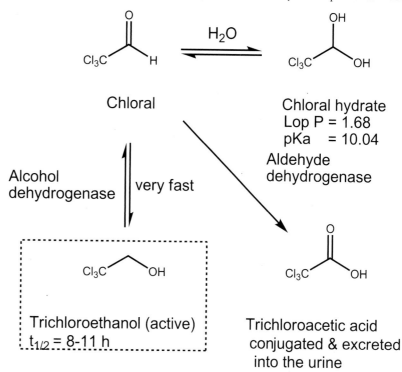

Figure 12.4 ● Reaction and metabolism of chloral.

the combination of ethanol and chloral hydrate (the "Mickey Finn") is controversial. Synergism between two different CNS depressants also could be involved. Additionally, ethanol, by increasing the concentration of nicotinamide adenine dinucleotide (NADH), enhances the reduction of chloral to the more active metabolite trichloroethanol, and chloral can inhibit the metabolism of alcohol because it inhibits alcohol dehydrogenase. Chloral hydrate is a weak acid because its CCl_3 group is very strong electron withdrawing. A 10% aqueous solution of chloral hydrate has pH 3.5 to 4.4, which makes it irritating to mucous membranes in the stomach. As a result, GI upset commonly occurs for the drug if undiluted or taken on an empty stomach. Chloral hydrate as a capsule, syrup, or suppository is currently available. Although it is suggested that chloral hydrate per se may act as a hypnotic,[21] chloral hydrate is very quickly converted to trichloroethanol, which is generally assumed to account for almost all of the hypnotic effect. The trichloroethanol is metabolized by oxidation to chloral and then to the inactive metabolite, trichloracetic acid (see Fig. 12.4), which is also extensively metabolized to acylglucuronides via conjugation with glucuronic acid. It appears to have potent barbiturate-like binding to GABA$_A$ receptors. Although an old drug, it still finds use as a sedative in nonoperating room procedures for the pediatric patient.

Paraldehyde, USP. Paraldehyde, 2,4,6-trimethyl-*s*-trioxane, paracetaldehyde, is recognizable as the cyclic trimer of acetaldehyde. It is a liquid with a strong characteristic odor detectable in the expired air and an unpleasant taste. These properties limit its use almost exclusively to an institutional setting (e.g., in the treatment of delirium tremens). In the past, when containers were opened and air admitted and then reclosed and allowed to stand, fatalities occurred because of oxidation of paraldehyde to glacial acetic acid.

Paraldehyde

ANTIPSYCHOTICS

The psychoses affect approximately 1% of the population in all cultures. They are psychogenic mental disorders involving a loss of contact with reality. The psychotic disorders include schizophrenia, the manic phase of bipolar (manic–depressive) illness, acute idiopathic psychotic illness, and other conditions marked by severe agitation. The most common is schizophrenia, in which perception, thinking, communication, social functioning, and attention are altered.

Schizophrenia is a particular kind of psychosis characterized mainly by a clear sensorium but a marked thinking disturbance. Symptoms are called *positive* (e.g., delusions, hallucinations) or *negative* (e.g., flat affect, apathy); cognitive dysfunction may occur. In the schizophrenias, which have an extremely complex and multifactored etiology,[22,23] the fundamental lesion appears to be a defect in the brain's informational gating mechanism. Basically, the gating system has difficulty discriminating between relevant and irrelevant stimuli. The etiology of psychosis remains unknown, although genetic, neurodevelopmental and environmental causative factors have all been proposed. Psychoses can be organic and related to a specific toxic chemical (e.g., delirium produced by central anticholinergic agents), an *N*-methyl D-aspartate (NMDA) receptor antagonist (e.g., phencyclidine [PCP]), a definite disease process (e.g., dementia), or they can be idiopathic.

Although the actual structural or anatomical lesions are not known, the basic defect appears to involve overactivity of dopaminergic neurons in the mesolimbic system. DA hypothesis for schizophrenia is the most fully developed of several hypotheses and is the basis for much of the rationale for drug therapy because (a) drugs that increase dopaminergic neurotransmission, such as levodopa (a DA precursor), amphetamines (a DA releaser), and apomorphine (a DA agonist), induce or exacerbate schizophrenia. Amphetamine-induced psychosis was determined to be caused by overactivation of mesolimbic D_2 receptors and judged to be the closest of the various chemically induced model psychoses to the schizophrenias; (b) DA receptor density is increased in certain brain regions of untreated schizophrenics; (c) many antipsychotic drugs strongly block postsynaptic D_2 receptors in CNS; and (d) successful treatment of schizophrenic patients has been reported to change the amount of homovanillic acid (HVA), a DA metabolite, in the cerebrospinal fluid, plasma, and urine. Consequently, the antipsychotic action is now thought to be produced (at least in part) by their ability to block DA receptors in the mesolimbic and mesofrontal systems. Moreover, extrapyramidal side effects of antipsychotic drugs correlate with their D_2 antagonism effect. The hyperprolactinemia that follows treatment with antipsychotics is caused by blockade of DA's tonic inhibitory effect on prolactin release from the pituitary. Nevertheless, the defects of DA hypothesis are significant, and it is now appreciated that schizophrenia is far more complex than originally supposed. Several classes of drugs are effective for symptomatic treatment.

Interest in DA, 5-HT, and Glu NTs led to most early drugs targeting the DA system, primarily as DA D_2 receptor. Typical antipsychotics (e.g., chlorpromazine, haloperidol) are better for treating positive signs than negative signs. For treating negative signs, the newer (atypical) antipsychotic drugs (e.g., clozapine, risperidone) target D_2 receptor and other receptors. The bases of the atypical group's activity against negative symptoms may be serotonin-2$_A$ receptor (5-HT$_{2A}$) block, block at receptors yet to be determined, and possibly decreased striatal D_2 block.[24] A classic competitive antagonism has been demonstrated at D_2 and D_3 receptors. Also, in recombinantly expressed receptors, inverse agonism has been demonstrated. Recent studies show that essentially all clinically used antipsychotic drugs are D_2 inverse agonists, suggesting that biochemical as well as clinical effects may not be explained by simple D_2 receptor blockade hypothesis.[25]

Typical antipsychotics began with the serendipitous discovery of the antipsychotic activity of chlorpromazine. A clear association between the ability to block DA at mesolimbic D_2 receptors was established. The conventional typical antipsychotics (neuroleptics) are characterized by the production of EPS, roughly approximating the symptoms of Parkinson disease. These are reversible on discontinuing or decreasing the dose of the drug and are associated with blockade of DA at D_2 striatal receptors. After sustained high-dose therapy with antipsychotics, a late-appearing EPS, tardive dyskinesia, may occur. The overall symptomatology resembles the symptoms of Huntington chorea. Atypical antipsychotics date from the discovery of clozapine, its antipsychotic properties, and its much lower production of EPS. Also contributing to the development of atypical antipsychotics was the introduction of risperidone. It has reduced EPS, has increased activity against negative symptoms, and, in addition to its DA-blocking ability, is a 5-HT$_{2A}$ antagonist. The view has been proposed that 5-HT$_{2A}$ receptors are involved in part (the negative symptoms) or wholly in schizophrenia. So far, the evidence appears to be that 5-HT$_{2A}$ blocking agents do not relieve positive effects of schizophrenia.[24] The view that 5-HT$_{2A}$ overactivity is the source of negative symptoms (part of the basis of psychosis) is not disproved at present, although some say it has been weakened.[24]

One result of the development of atypical antipsychotics has been a renewed interest in models of psychosis other than the amphetamine model. In line with possible dual involvement of 5-HT and DA, the lysergic acid diethylamide (LSD, a 5-HT agonist) model has been cited as better fitting schizophrenias than the amphetamine model. However, this has been disputed. Interest in serotoninergic involvement is still high and involves elucidating the roles of 5-HT$_6$ and 5-HT$_7$ receptors.

Interest remains in understanding the psychosis produced by several central anticholinergics. Muscarinic (M$_1$ and M$_4$) agonists appear to offer the best approach at this time.[26] The role of the M$_5$ receptor awaits synthesis of M$_5$-specific drugs.[27]

PCP (an NMDA antagonist)-induced psychosis has been proposed as a superior model for schizophrenia, because it presents both positive and negative symptoms.[24] It suggests that deficits in glutaminergic function occur in schizophrenia. Results of agonists of NMDA receptors, overall, have not been productive because of the excitatory and neurotoxic effects of the agents tested. Identification of susceptible receptor subtypes as targets, using glycine modulation or group II metabotropic receptor agonists to modulate NMDA receptors, has been proposed to circumvent the problems associated with the NMDA agonists.

The ionotropic glutamic acid α-amino-3-hydroxy-5-methyl-4-isoxazole propionic acid (AMPA) receptors are activated by brain-penetrating ampakines. There are suggestions that these agents exert some antipsychotic actions by increasing glutaminergic activity.

The individual antipsychotic agents are now considered. The substituted DA motif is useful as an organizational device. Antipsychotics can be classified into four groups (Table 12.2).

Phenothiazines

Several dozen phenothiazine antipsychotic drugs are chemically related agents used worldwide. Other phenothiazines are marketed primarily for their antiemetic, antihistaminic, or anticholinergic effect. The large body of information permits accurate statements about the structural features associated with activity (see Fig. 12.5). Many of the features were summarized and interpreted by Gordon et al.[28] Phenothiazines have a tricyclic structure (6-6-6 system) in which two benzene rings are linked by a sulfur and a nitrogen atom. The best position for substitution is the 2-position. Activity increases (with some exceptions) as

TABLE 12.2 Classification of Antipsychotics

Drug Groups	Structure Features	Examples	Comments
Phenothiazines	Aliphatic side chain Piperidine side chain Piperazine side chain	Chlorpromazine Thioridazine Fluphenazine	Least potent Least potent and ↓ EPS More potent and more EPS
Thioxanthenes	Double bond on C10	Thiothixene	Less potent than other phenothiazines
Butyrophenones	Aromatic butylpiperidines and diphenylbutylpiperidines	Haloperidol	More potent Fewer autonomic SEs Greater EPS
Newer drugs	Miscellaneous	Risperidone Clozapine Olanzapine	Less EPS Also good for negative symptoms

electron-withdrawing ability of the 2-substituent increases (e.g., chlorpromazine vs. promazine). Another possibly important structural feature in the more potent compounds is the presence of an unshared electron pair on an atom or atoms of the 2-substituent. Substitution at the 3-position can improve activity over nonsubstituted compounds but not as significantly as substitution at the 2-position. Substitution at position 1 has a deleterious effect on antipsychotic activity, as does (to a lesser extent) substitution at the 4-position.

The significance of these substituent effects could be that the hydrogen atom of the protonated amino group of the side chain H-bonds with an electron pair of an atom of the 2-substituent to develop a DA-like arrangement.

Horn and Snyder,[29] from x-ray crystallography, proposed that the chlorine-substituted ring of chlorpromazine base could be superimposed on the aromatic ring of DA base, with the sulfur atom aligned with the *p*-hydroxyl group of DA and the aliphatic amino groups of the two compounds also aligned. The model used here is based on the interpretation of the SARs by Gordon et al.[28] and on the Horn and Snyder[29] proposal but involves the protonated species rather than the free base. The effect of the substituent at the 1-position might be to interfere with the side chain's ability to bring the protonated amino group in proximity with the 2-substituent. In the Horn and Snyder[29] scheme, the sulfur atom at position 5 is in a position analogous to the *p*-hydroxyl group of DA, and it was also assigned a receptor-binding function by Gordon et al.[28] A substituent at position 4 might interfere with receptor binding by the sulfur atom.

The three-carbon chain between position 10 and the aliphatic amino nitrogen is critical for neuroleptic activity. Shortening or lengthening the chain at this position drastically decreases the activity. The three-atom chain length

may be necessary to bring the protonated amino nitrogen in proximity with the 2-substituent. Shortening the chain to two carbons has the effect of amplifying the antihistaminic and anticholinergic activities. For example, promethazine is effective antihistamine, whereas the amino ethyl derivatives diethazine (anticholinergic) and ethopropazine (antimuscarinic) have proved useful in the treatment of Parkinson disease. The amine is always tertiary. *N*-dealkylation of the side chain or increasing the size of amino *N*-alkyl substituents reduces antidopaminergic and antipsychotic activity.

As expected, branching with large groups (e.g., phenyl) decreases activity, as does branching with polar groups. Methyl branching on the *β*-position has a variable effect on activity. More importantly, the antipsychotic potency of *levo* (the more active) and *dextro* isomers differs greatly. This has long been taken to suggest that a precise fit (i.e., receptor site occupancy) is involved in the action of these compounds.

Decreases in size from a dimethylamino group (e.g., going to a monomethylamino) greatly decrease activity, as do effective size increases, such as the one that occurs with *N*,*N*-diethylamino group. Once the fundamental requirement of an *effective* size of about that equivalent to a dimethylamino is maintained, as in fusing *N*,*N*-diethyl substituents to generate a conformational restricted pyrrolidino group, activity can be enhanced with increasing chain length, as in *N*2-substituted piperizino compounds.

The critical size of groups on the amino atom suggests the importance of the amino group (here protonated) for receptor attachment. The effect of the added chain length, once the critical size requirement is met, could be increased affinity. It appears to have been reasonably proved that the

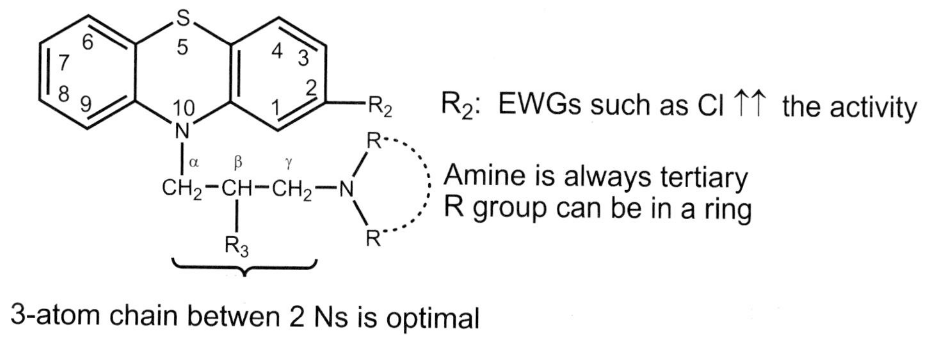

R2: EWGs such as Cl ↑↑ the activity

Amine is always tertiary
R group can be in a ring

3-atom chain betwen 2 Ns is optimal

Figure 12.5 ● SAR of phenothiazine antipsychotic agents.

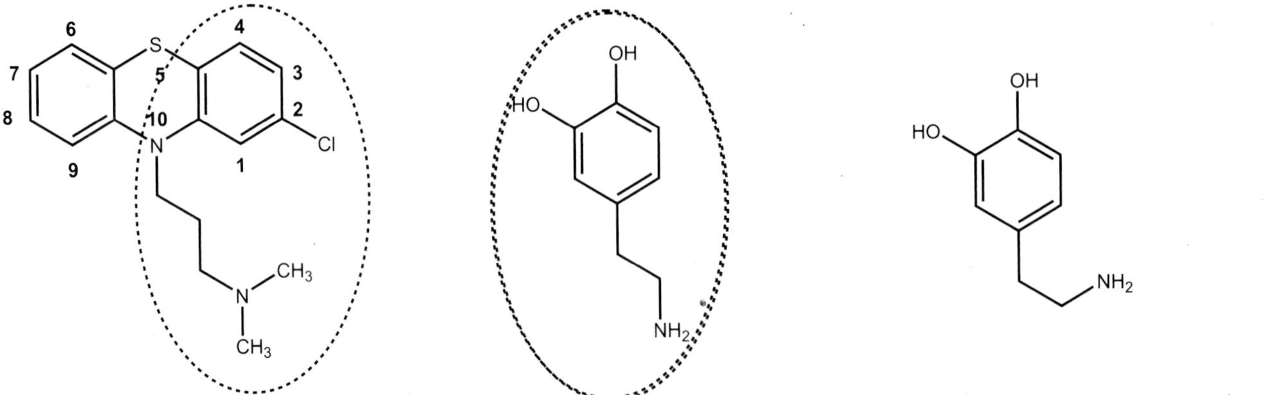

Phenothiazine

trans-α-Rotamer of dopamine (active)

cis-α-Rotamer of dopamine

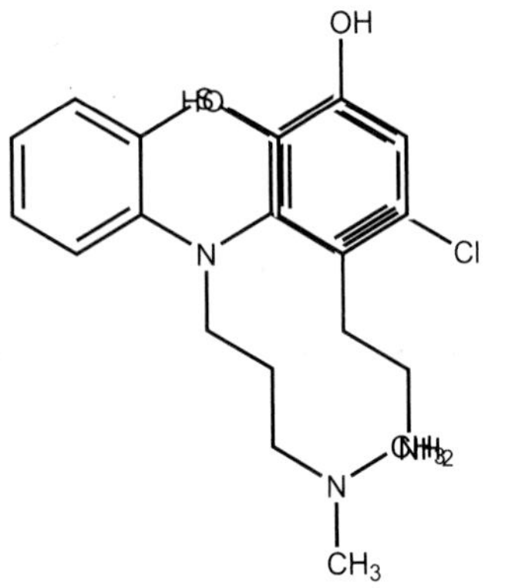

Superimposition of phenothiazine and active *trans*-α-rotamer of dopamine

protonated species of the phenothiazines can bind to DA receptors.[30]

Several piperazine phenothiazines are esterified at a free hydroxyl with long-chain fatty acids to produce highly lipophilic and long-acting prodrugs. They tend to have large volumes of distribution, probably because they are sequestered in lipid compartments of the body and have very high affinity for selected NT receptors in the CNS. They generally have a much longer clinical duration of action than would be estimated from their plasma half-lives. This is paralleled by prolonged occupancy of DA D_2 receptors in brain. The decanoates of fluphenazine and haloperidol are used commonly in the United States; several others (including esters of pipotiazine and perphenazine) are available elsewhere.

Because of the high lipophilicity of most antipsychotic drugs, they are highly membrane and protein bound (92%–99%) mostly to albumin. They accumulate in the brain, lung, and other tissues with a rich blood supply and also enter the fetal circulation and breast milk.

Most phenothiazines undergo significant first-pass metabolism. Chlorpromazine and other phenothiazines are metabolized extensively by CYP2D6. Thus, oral doses of chlorpromazine and thioridazine have systemic availability of 25% to 35%, whereas parenteral (intramuscular) administration increases the bioavailability of active drug fourfold to tenfold. In contrast, haloperidol, which is less likely to be metabolized, has an average systemic availability of about 65%. Metabolism of the phenothiazines is complex in detail.

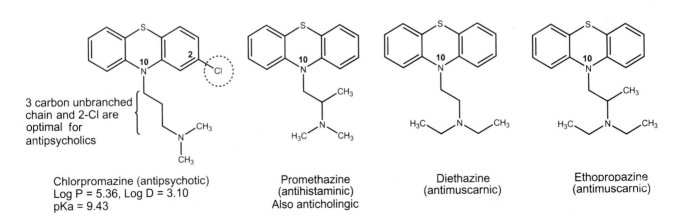

3 carbon unbranched chain and 2-Cl are optimal for antipsycholics

Chlorpromazine (antipsychotic)
Log P = 5.36, Log D = 3.10
pKa = 9.43

Promethazine
(antihistaminic)
Also anticholingic

Diethazine
(antimuscarnic)

Ethopropazine
(antimuscarnic)

A major route is 7-hydroxylation of the tricyclic system. Because electron-withdrawing 2-Cl substituent blocks the hydroxylation on chlorophenyl ring, the hydroxylation occurs at 7-position rather than 2-position. Thus, the major initial metabolite is frequently the 7-hydroxy compound (active metabolite). This compound is further metabolized by conjugation with glucuronic acid, and the conjugate is excreted. Metabolites of chlorpromazine may be excreted in the urine weeks after the last dose of chronically administered drug. Full relapse may not occur until 6 weeks or more after discontinuation of many antipsychotics. Detailed reviews of the metabolites of phenothiazines (as well as SARs and pharmacokinetic factors) are available.[31]

PRODUCTS

The structures of the phenothiazine derivatives described later are given in Table 12.3.

Chlorpromazine Hydrochloride, **USP.** Chlorpromazine hydrochloride, 2-chloro-10-[3-(dimethylamino)propyl]phenothiazine monohydrochloride (Thorazine), was the first phenothiazine compound introduced into therapy. It is still useful as an antipsychotic. Other uses are in nausea, vomiting, and hiccough. Oral doses of chlorpromazine and thioridazine have systemic availability of 25% to 35% because of significant first-pass metabolism. Chlorpromazine and other phenothiazines are metabolized extensively by CYP2D6 (Fig. 12.6). In contrast, bioavailability of chlorpromazine may be increased up to 10-fold with injections, but the clinical dose usually is decreased by only threefold to fourfold. Chlorpromazine may weakly induce its own hepatic metabolism, because its concentration in blood is lower after several weeks of treatment at the same dosage. Alterations of GI motility also may contribute. The drug has significant sedative and hypotensive properties, possibly reflecting central histaminergic and peripheral α_1-noradrenergic blocking activity, respectively. Effects of peripheral anticholinergic activity are common. As with the other phenothiazines, the effects of other CNS-depressant drugs, such as sedatives and anesthetics, can be potentiated.

TABLE 12.3 Phenothiazine Derivatives

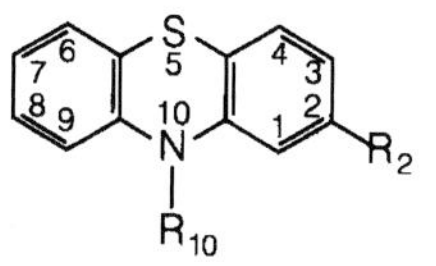

Generic Name *Proprietary Name*	R_{10}	R_2
Propyl Dialkylamino Side Chain		
Promazine hydrochloride, *USP* *Sparine*	—$(CH_2)_3N(CH_3)_2$ · HCl	H
Chlorpromazine hydrochloride, *USP* *Thorazine*	—$(CH_2)_3N(CH_3)_2$ · HCl	Cl
Triflupromazine hydrochloride, *USP* *Vesprin*	—$(CH_2)_3N(CH_3)_2$ · HCl	CF_3
Akyl Piperidyl Side Chain		
Thioridazine hydrochloride, *USP* *Mellaril*	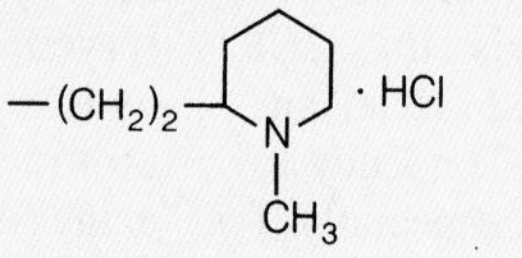 —$(CH_2)_2$— (N-CH₃ piperidyl) · HCl	SCH_3
Mesoridazine besylate, *USP* *Serentil*	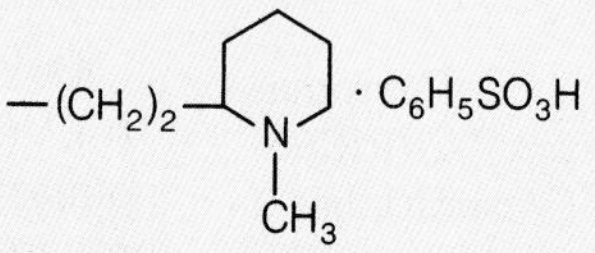 —$(CH_2)_2$— (N-CH₃ piperidyl) · $C_6H_5SO_3H$	O ↑ SCH_3
Propyl Piperazine Side Chain		
Prochlorperazine maleate, *USP* *Compazine*	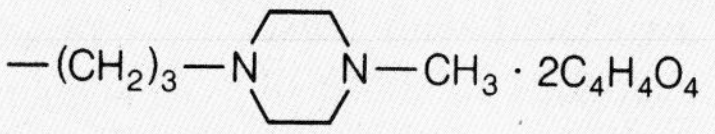 —$(CH_2)_3$—N(piperazine)N—CH_3 · $2C_4H_4O_4$	Cl
Trifluoperazine hydrochloride, *USP* *Stelazine*	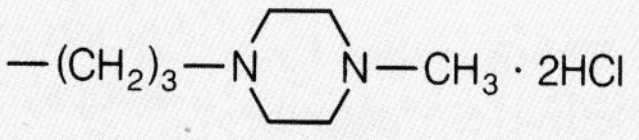 —$(CH_2)_3$—N(piperazine)N—CH_3 · 2HCl	CF_3
Perphenazine, *USP* *Trilafon*	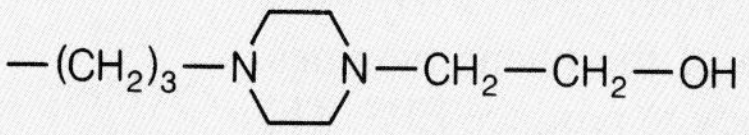 —$(CH_2)_3$—N(piperazine)N—CH_2—CH_2—OH	Cl
Fluphenazine hydrochloride, *USP* *Permitil, Prolixin*	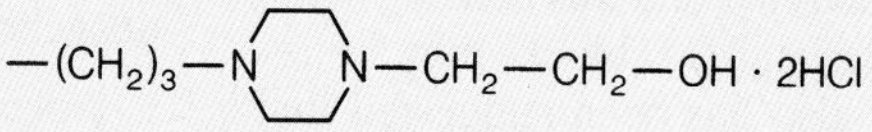 —$(CH_2)_3$—N(piperazine)N—CH_2—CH_2—OH · 2HCl	CF_3

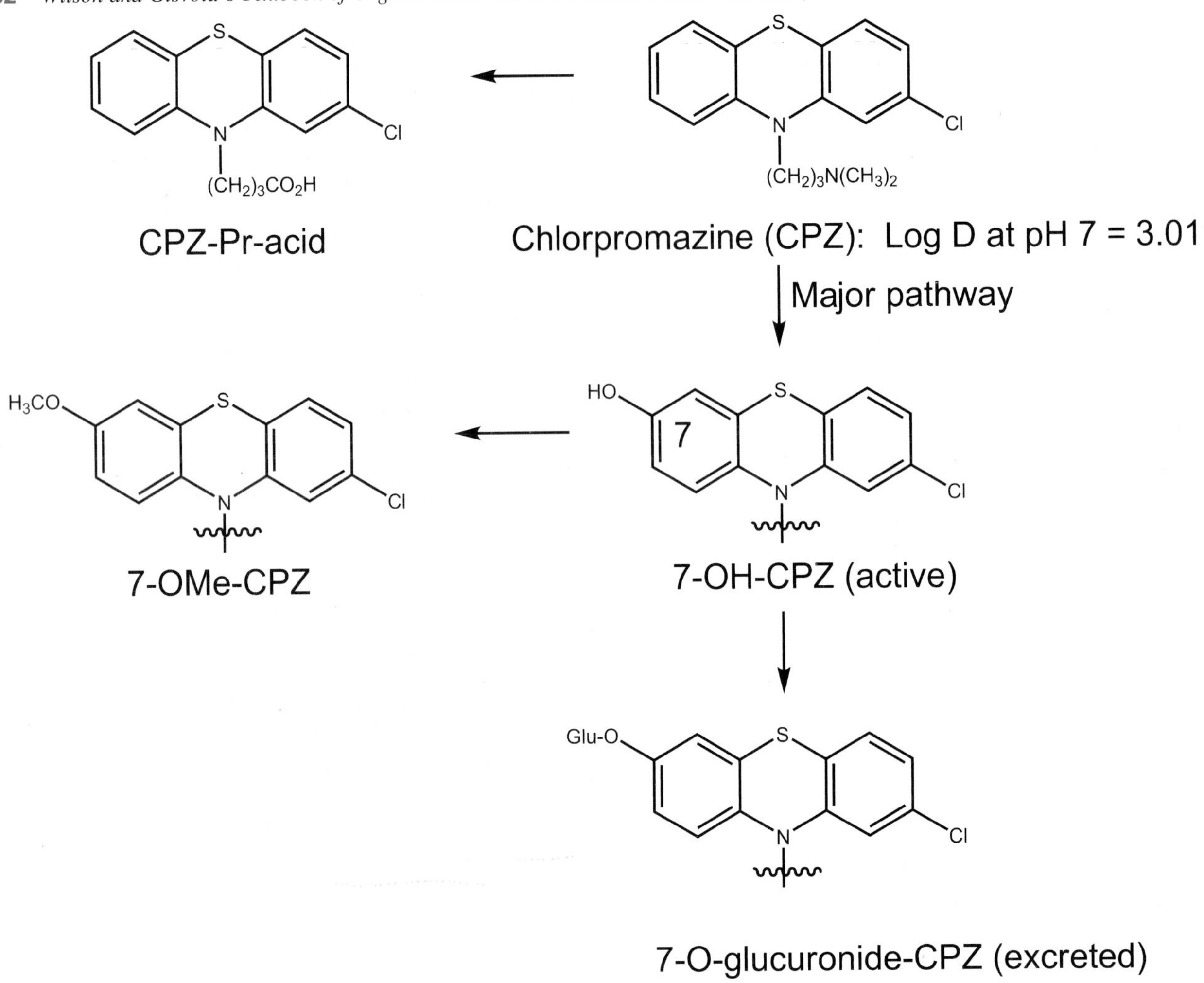

CPZ-Pr-acid

Chlorpromazine (CPZ): Log D at pH 7 = 3.01

Major pathway

7-OMe-CPZ

7-OH-CPZ (active)

7-O-glucuronide-CPZ (excreted)

Figure 12.6 ● Some metabolic pathways for chlorpromazine.

Promazine. Promazine, 10-[3-(dimethylamino) propyl-(phenothiazine monohydrochloride (Sparine), was introduced into antipsychotic therapy after its 2-chloro-substituted relative. The 2H-substituent vis-à-vis the 2Cl substituent gives a milligram potency decrease as an antipsychotic, as encompassed in Gordon's rule. Tendency to EPS is also lessened, which may be significant, especially if it is decreased less than antipsychotic potency.

Triflupromazine Hydrochloride, USP. Triflupromazine hydrochloride, 10-[3-(dimethylamino)propyl]-2-(trifluoromethyl)phenothiazine monohydrochloride (Vesprin), has a greater milligram potency as an antipsychotic, higher EPS, but lower sedative and hypotensive effects than chlorpromazine. The 2-CF$_3$ versus the 2-Cl is associated with these changes. Overall, the drug has uses analogous to those of chlorpromazine.

Thioridazine Hydrochloride, USP. Thioridazine hydrochloride, 10-[2-(1-methyl-2-piperidyl)ethyl]-2-(methylthio)phenothiazine monohydrochloride (Mellaril), is a member of the piperidine subgroup of the phenothiazines. The drug has a relatively low tendency to produce EPS. The drug has high anticholinergic activity, and this activity in the striatum, counterbalancing a striatal DA block, may be responsible for the low EPS. It also has been suggested that there may be increased DA receptor selectivity, which may

be responsible. The drug has sedative and hypotensive activity in common with chlorpromazine and less antiemetic activity. At high doses, pigmentary retinopathy has been observed. Its major metabolites include *N*-demethylated, ring-hydroxylated, and *S*-oxidized products. Thioridazine is prominently converted to the active metabolite mesoridazine (discussed next), which probably contributes to the antipsychotic activity of thioridazine.

Mesoridazine Besylate, USP. Mesoridazine besylate, 10-[2-(methyl-2-piperidyl)ethyl]-2-(methylsulfinyl)phenothiazine monobenzenesulfonate (Serentil), shares many properties with thioridazine. However, no pigmentary retinopathy has been reported.

Prochlorperazine Maleate, USP. Prochlorperazine maleate, 2-chloro-10-[3-(4-methyl-1-piperazinyl)propyl]phenothiazine maleate (Compazine), is in the piperazine subgroup of the phenothiazines, characterized by high-milligram antipsychotic potency, a high prevalence of EPS, and low sedative and autonomic effects. Prochlorperazine is more potent on a milligram basis than its alkylamino counterpart, chlorpromazine. Because of the high prevalence of EPS, however, it is used mainly for its antiemetic effect, not for its antipsychotic effect.

Perphenazine, USP. Perphenazine, 4-[3-(2-chlorophenothiazine-10-yl)propyl]piperazineethanol; 2-chloro-10-[3-

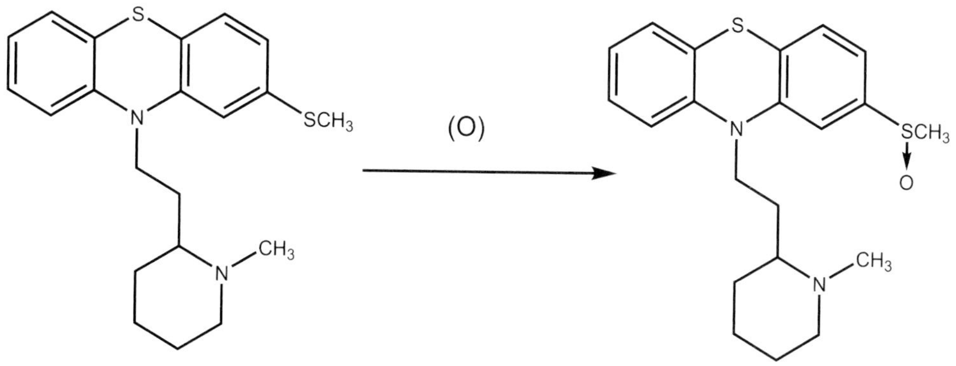

Thioridazine

(O)

Mesoridazine

[4-(2-hydroxyethyl)piperazinyl]propyl]phenothiazine (Trilafon), is an effective antipsychotic and antiemetic.

Fluphenazine Hydrochloride, USP. The member of the piperazine subgroup with a trifluoromethyl group at the 2-position of the phenothiazine system and the most potent antipsychotic phenothiazine on a milligram basis is fluphenazine hydrochloride, 4-[3-[2-(trifluoromethyl)phenazin-10-yl] propyl]-1-piperazineethanol dihydrochloride, 10[3-[4-(2-hydroxyethyl)piperazinyl]propyl]-2-trifluoromethylphenothiazine dihydrochloride (Permitil, Prolixin). It is also available as two lipid-soluble esters for depot intramuscular injection, the enanthate (heptanoic acid ester) and the decanoate ester. These long-acting preparations have use in treating psychotic patients who do not take their medication or are subject to frequent relapse.

Thiothixene, USP. The thioxanthene system differs from the phenothiazine system by replacement of the N-H moiety with a carbon atom doubly bonded to the propylidene side chain. With the substituent in the 2-position, Z- and E-isomers are produced. In accordance with the concept that the presently useful antipsychotics can be superimposed on DA, the Z-isomers are the more active antipsychotic isomers. The compounds of the group are very similar in pharmacological properties to the corresponding phenothiazines. Thus, thiothixene (Z-N-dimethyl-9-[3-(4-methyl-1-piperazinyl)propylidene]thioxanthene-2-sulfonamide (Navane), displays properties similar to those of the piperazine subgroup of the phenothiazines.

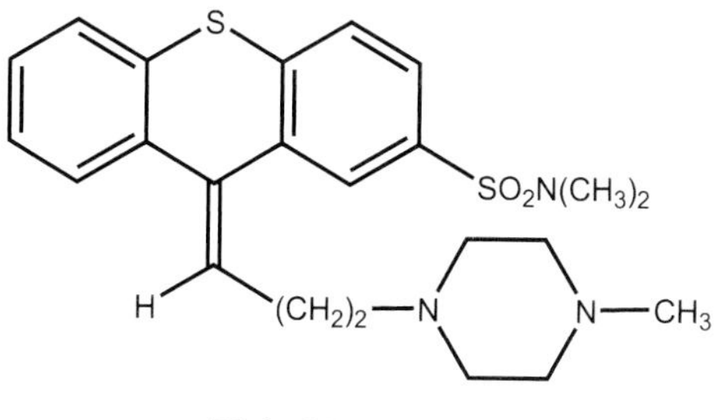

Thiothixene

Ring Analogs of Phenothiazines: Benzazepines, Dibenzoxazepines, and Dibenzodiazepines

Additional tricyclic antipsychotic agents are the benzazepines, containing a seven-membered central ring (6-7-6 system). These newer atypical antipsychotics include diben-

zodiazepines (clozapine with 2-Cl), dibenzoxazepines (loxapine with 2-Cl), thienobenzodiazepines (olanzapine without 2-substituent), and dibenzothiazepines (quetiapine without 2-substituent). These ring analogs of phenothiazines are structural relatives of the phenothiazine antipsychotics; therefore, most of them share many clinical properties with the phenothiazines. However, they have some important differences, *notably low production of EPS and reduction of negative symptoms*. These benzazepines and other atypical antipsychotics including risperidone, ziprasidone, and aripiprazole block both D_2 and $5-HT_{2A}$ receptor, other DA and serotonin receptor subtypes, adrenergic, histamine, and muscarinic receptors. The low D_2 receptor affinity and the high $5-HT_{2A}$ receptor affinity of atypical antipsychotics including clozapine and olanzapine led to the proposal that $5-HT_{2A}$ antagonism accounts for their lower EPS.

PRODUCTS

Loxapine. A dibenzoxazepine derivative in use is *loxapine succinate*, 2-chloro-11-(4-methyl-1-piperazinyl)dibenz[b, f][1,4]oxazepine succinate (Daxolin). The structural relationship to the phenothiazine antipsychotics is apparent. Examples in this group are clothiapine, metiapine, zotepine, and others. They have electron-withdrawing groups at position 2, relatively close to the side-chain nitrogen atoms. Loxapine, an effective antipsychotic, blocks D_2-type receptors and has side effects similar to those reported for the phenothiazines. Its metabolism involves aromatic hydroxylation to give several phenolic metabolites that have higher affinity for D_2 receptors than the parent. It is also N-demethylated to yield amoxapine (an antidepressant drug), which inhibits norepinephrine (NE) neurotransporter to block neuronal NE reuptake.

Clozapine. The dibenzodiazepine derivative is *clozapine* (Clozaril). It is not a potent antipsychotic on a milligram basis (note the orientation of the N-methyl piperazino group relative to the chlorine atom). In addition to their moderate potencies at DA receptors (mainly D_4), clozapine interact with varying affinities at several other classes of receptors (α_1 and α_2 adrenergic, $5-HT_{1A}$, $5-HT_{2A}$, $5-HT_{2C}$, muscarinic cholinergic, histamine H_1, and others). It is effective against both positive and negative symptoms of schizophrenia and has a low tendency to produce EPS. Clozapine has proved effective even in chronically ill patients who respond poorly to standard neuroleptics. However, there are legal restrictions on its use because of a relatively high frequency of agranulocytosis. As a rule, two other antipsychotics are tried before recourse to therapy with clozapine. Clozapine is metabolized

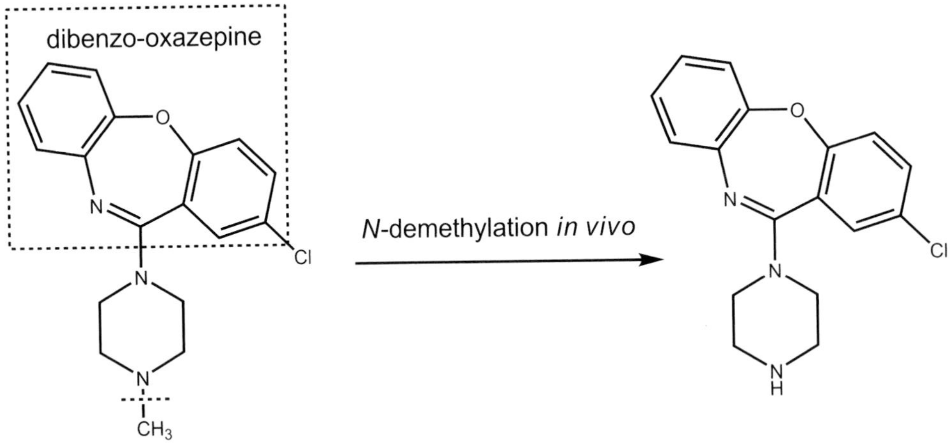

dibenzo-oxazepine

Loxapine
an antipsychotic

N-demethylation *in vivo*

Amoxapine
an antidepressant

preferentially by CYP3A4 into demethylated, hydroxylated, and *N*-oxide derivatives that are excreted in urine and feces. Elimination half-life averages about 12 hours. Other clozapine-like atypical antipsychotics may lack a 2-Cl substituent on the aromatic ring (e.g., olanzapine and quetiapine).

Olanzapine and Quetiapine. Clozapine analogs, olanzapine (Zyprexa) and quetiapine (Seroquel) possess tricyclic systems with greater electron density than chlorpromazine. The drugs are atypical antipsychotics. Olanzapine is a more potent antagonist at D_2 and 5-HT_{2A} receptors than clozapine and is well absorbed, but about 40% of an oral dose is metabolized before reaching the systemic circulation. Plasma concentrations of olanzapine peak at about 6 hours after oral administration, and its elimination half-life ranges from 20 to 54 hours. Major readily excreted metabolites of olanzapine are the inactive 10-*N*-glucuronide and 4'-nor derivatives, formed mainly by the action of CYP1A2, with CYP2D6 as a minor alternative pathway. It may have even lower risk than risperidone and has achieved widespread use.

Overall, these two compounds should bind less strongly to D_2 receptors and permit more receptor selectivity among receptor subtypes than typical antipsychotics. This could

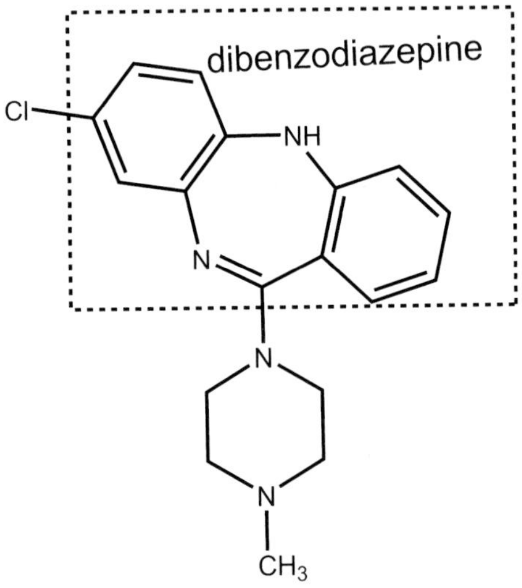

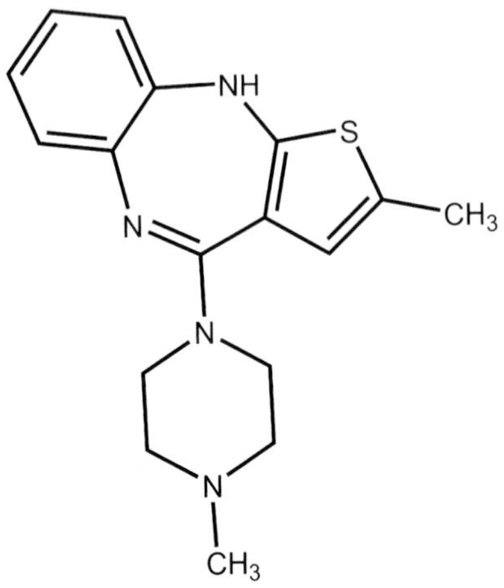

dibenzodiazepine

Clozapine

dibenzothiazepine

Olanzapine

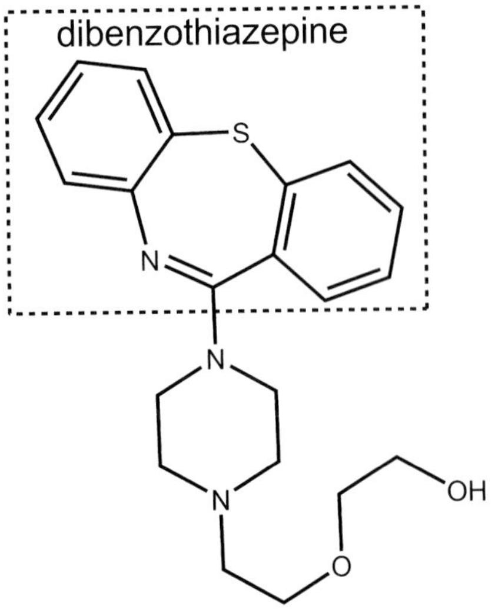

Quetiapine

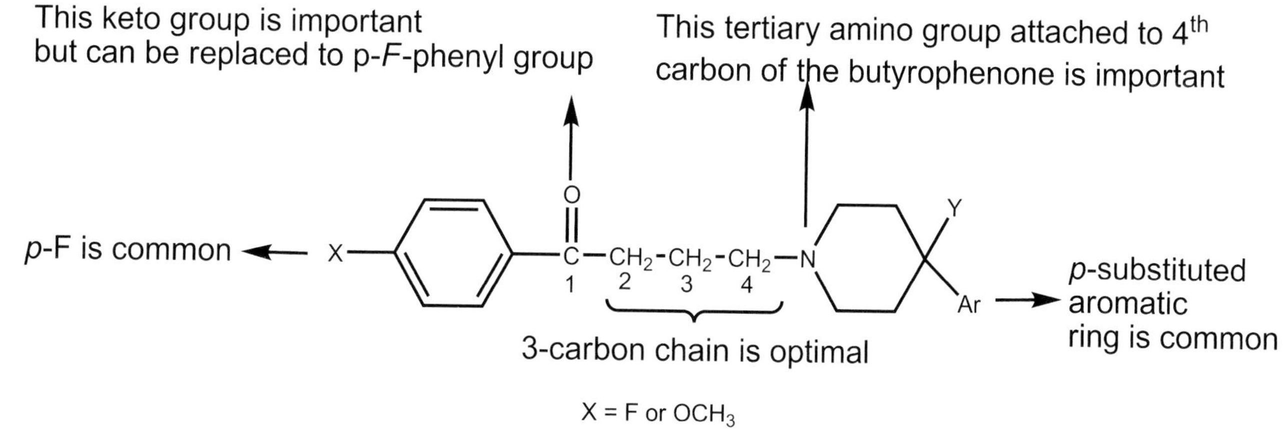

This keto group is important but can be replaced to p-*F*-phenyl group

This tertiary amino group attached to 4th carbon of the butyrophenone is important

p-F is common

p-substituted aromatic ring is common

3-carbon chain is optimal

X = F or OCH$_3$

Figure 12.7 ● General structure and SAR of fluorobutyrophenones.

account for decreased striatal D$_2$-blocking activity (EPS). Quetiapine is highly metabolized by hepatic CYP3A4 to inactive and readily excreted sulfoxide and acidic derivatives.

Fluorobutyrophenones

The fluorobutyrophenones belong to a much-studied group of compounds, many of which possess high antipsychotic activity. The structural requirements for antipsychotic activity in the group are well worked out.[32] General structure and SAR are expressed in the following structure (Fig. 12.7).

Attachment of a tertiary amino group to the fourth carbon of the butyrophenone skeleton is essential for neuroleptic activity; lengthening, shortening, or branching of the three-carbon propyl chain decreases neuroleptic potency. This aliphatic amino nitrogen is required, and highest activity is seen when it is incorporated into a cyclic form. A *p*-fluoro substituent aids activity. The C=O group gives optimal activity, although other groups, C(H)OH and C(H)aryl, also give good activity. The Y group can vary and assist activity, and an example is the hydroxyl group of haloperidol.

The empirical SARs could be construed to suggest that the 4-aryl piperidino moiety is superimposable on the 2-phenylethylamino moiety of DA and, accordingly, could promote affinity for D$_2$ and D$_3$ receptors. The long *N*-alkyl substituent could help promote receptor affinity and produce receptor antagonism activity and/or inverse agonism.

Some members of the class are D$_2$ and D$_3$ receptor antagonists and are extremely potent antipsychotic agents. EPS are extremely marked in some members of this class, which may, in part, be because of a potent DA block in the striatum and almost no compensatory striatal anticholinergic block. Most of the compounds do not have the structural features associated with effective anticholinergic activity.

Haloperidol, USP. Haloperidol, 4[4-(p-chlorophenyl)-4-hydroxypiperidone]-4′-*n*-fluorobutyrophenone (Haldol), the representative of several related classes of aromatic butylpiperidine derivatives, is a potent antipsychotic useful in schizophrenia and in psychoses associated with brain damage. It is frequently chosen as the agent to terminate mania and often used in therapy for Gilles de la Tourette syndrome. Haloperidol-induced dyskinesias may involve neurotoxicological metabolite similar to dopaminergic toxicant MPP$^+$ (Fig. 12.8).

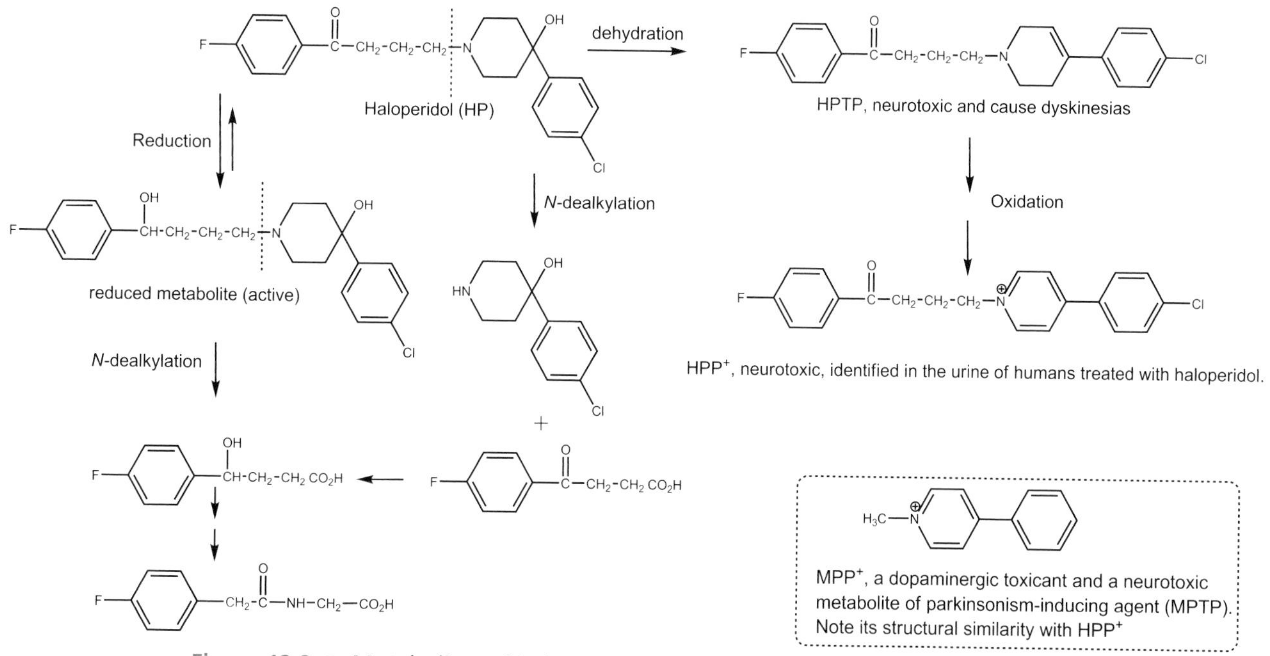

Figure 12.8 ● Metabolism of haloperidol and its possible neurotoxic metabolites.

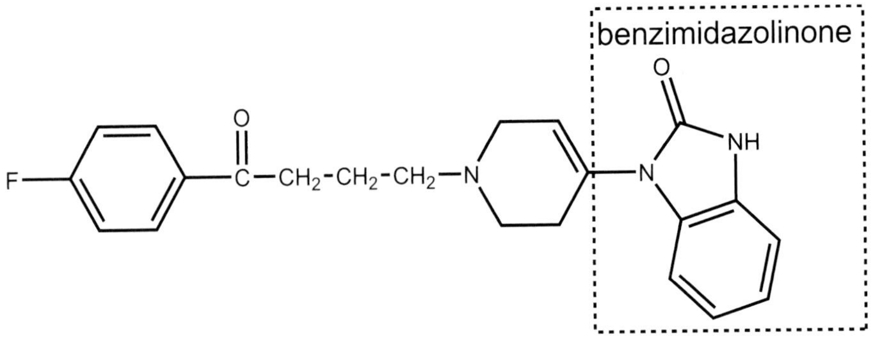

Droperidol

Droperidol, USP. Droperidol, 1-{1-[3-(*p*-fluorobenzoyl)propyl]-1,2, 3,6-tetrahydro-4-pyridyl}-2-benzimidazolinone (Inapsine), may be used alone as a preanesthetic neuroleptic or as an antiemetic. Because of its very short-acting and highly sedating properties, its most frequent use is in combination (Innovar) with the narcotic agent fentanyl (Sublimaze) preanesthetically.

Risperidone. Risperidone (Risperdal, a benzisoxazole) has the structural features of a hybrid molecule between a butyrophenone antipsychotic and a trazodone-like antidepressant. Its superior side effects profile (compared with haloperidol) at dosage of 6 mg/d or less and the lower risk of tardive dyskinesia have contributed to its very widespread use. It benefited refractory psychotic patients, with parkinsonism controlled at one tenth the dose of antiparkinsonian drugs used with haloperidol.[33] Coexisting anxiety and depressive syndromes were also lessened. It is reported to decrease the negative (e.g., withdrawal, apathy) as well as the positive (e.g., delusions, hallucinations) symptoms of schizophrenia. This is reportedly a consequence of the compound's combination 5-HT$_2$–D$_2$ receptor antagonistic properties.[34] Overall, the reasons for the decreased EPS and

effectiveness against negative symptom are still under investigation. It is an important atypical antipsychotic. Risperidone is metabolized in the liver by CYP2D6 to an active metabolite, 9-hydroxyrisperidone. Because this metabolite and risperidone are nearly equipotent, the clinical efficacy of the drug reflects both compounds.

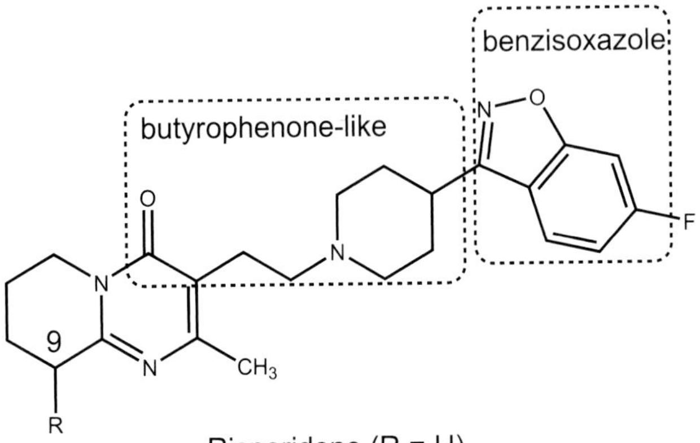

Risperidone (R = H)
Risperidone active metabolite (R = OH)

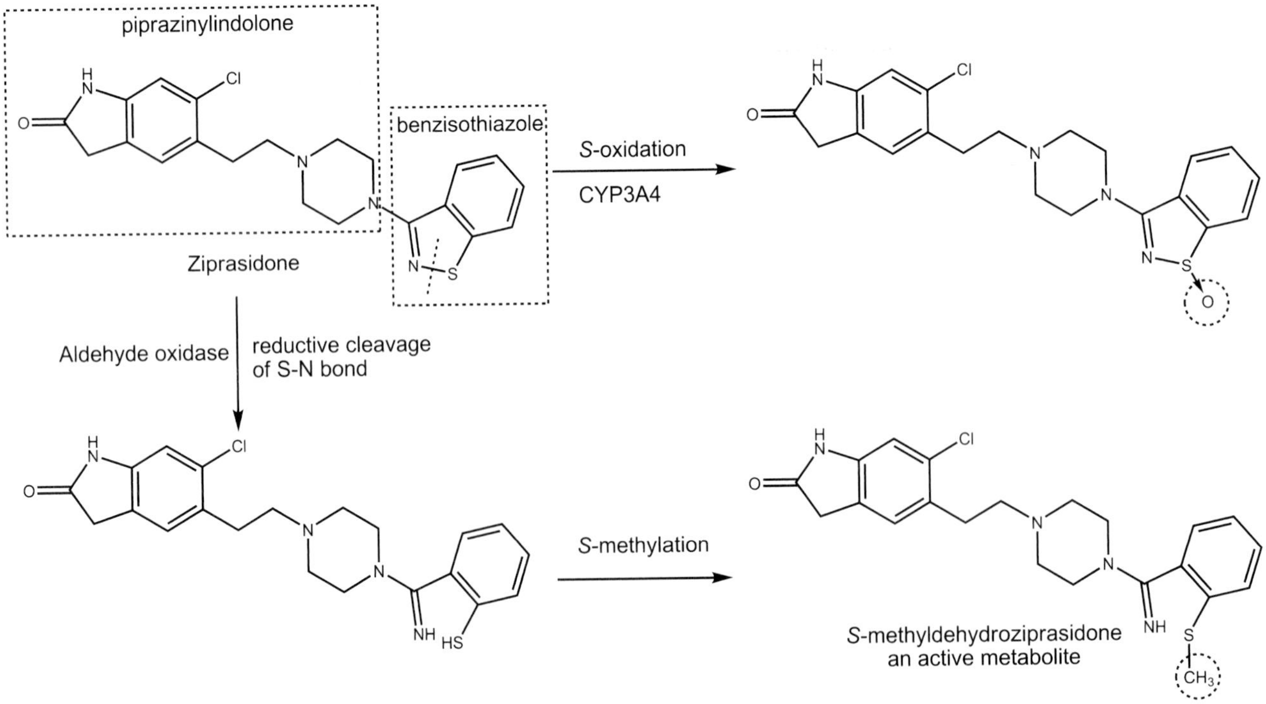

Figure 12.9 ● Major metabolic pathway of ziprasidone.

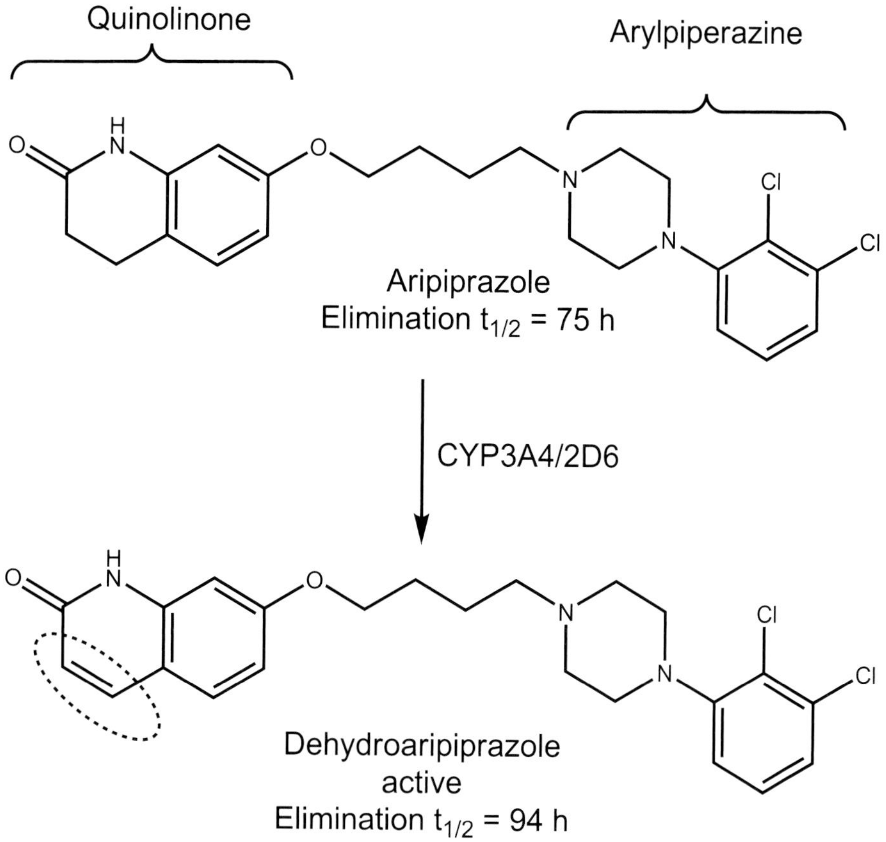

Quinolinone   Arylpiperazine

Aripiprazole
Elimination $t_{1/2}$ = 75 h

CYP3A4/2D6

Dehydroaripiprazole
active
Elimination $t_{1/2}$ = 94 h

Figure 12.10 ● Major metabolic pathway for aripiprazole.

Ziprasidone. Ziprasidone (Geodon, a benzisothiazolpiprazinylindolone derivative) also has the structural features of a hybrid molecule between a butyrophenone antipsychotic and a trazodone-like antidepressant. It is highly metabolized to four major metabolites, only one of which, *S*-methyldihydroziprasidone, likely contributes to its clinical activity (see Fig. 12.9). In humans, less than 5% of the dose is excreted unchanged. Reduction by aldehyde oxidase accounts for about 66% of ziprasidone metabolism; two oxidative pathways involving hepatic CYP3A4 account for the remainder.

Aripiprazole. Aripiprazole (Abilify). The newest, long-acting aripiprazole (an arylpiperazine quinolinone derivative), appears to be partial agonist of D_2 receptors (i.e., it stimulates certain D_2 receptors while blocking others depending on their locations in the brain and the concentration of drug). Bioavailability of aripiprazole is around 87%, with

peak plasma concentration attained at 3 to 5 hours after dosing. It is metabolized by dehydrogenation (see Fig. 12.10), oxidative hydroxylation, and *N*-dealkylation, largely mediated by hepatic CYPs 3A4 and 2D6.

The diphenylbutylpiperidine class can be considered a modification of the fluorobutyrophenone class. Because of their high lipophilicity, the compounds are inherently long acting. Pimozide has been approved for antipsychotic use, and penfluridol has undergone clinical trials in the United States. Overall, side effects for the two compounds resemble those produced by the fluorobutyrophenones.

β-AMINOKETONES

Several *β*-aminoketones have been examined as antipsychotics.[31] They evolved out of research on the alkaloid lobeline. The overall structural features associated with activity

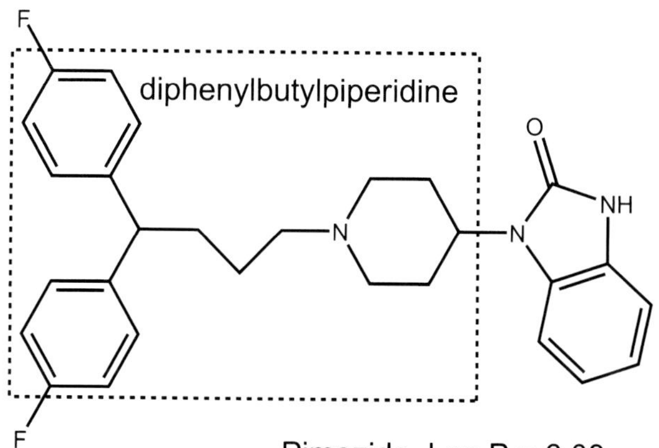

Pimozide, Log P = 6.08

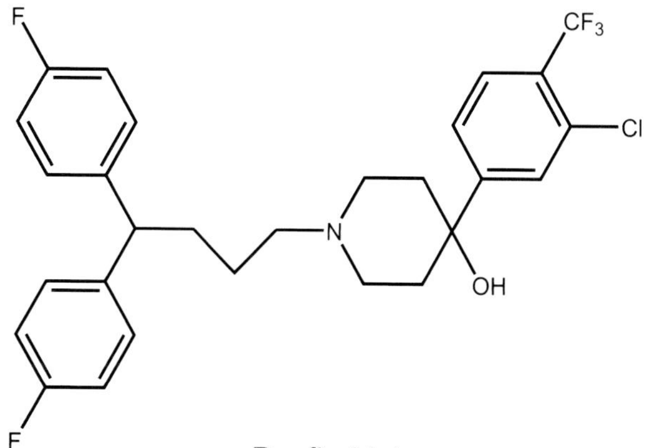

Penfluridol

can be seen in the structure of molindone. In addition to the β-aminoketone group, there must be an aryl group positioned as in molindone. It might be conjectured that the proton on the protonated amino group in these compounds H-bonds with the electrons of the carbonyl oxygen atom. This would produce a cationic center, two-atom distance, and an aryl group that could be superimposed on the analogous features of protonated DA.

Molindone Hydrochloride. Molindone hydrochloride, 3-ethyl-6,7-dihydro-2-methyl-5-morpholinomethyl)indole-4(5*H*)-one monohydrochloride (Moban), is about as potent an antipsychotic as trifluoperazine. Overall, side effects resemble those of the phenothiazines.

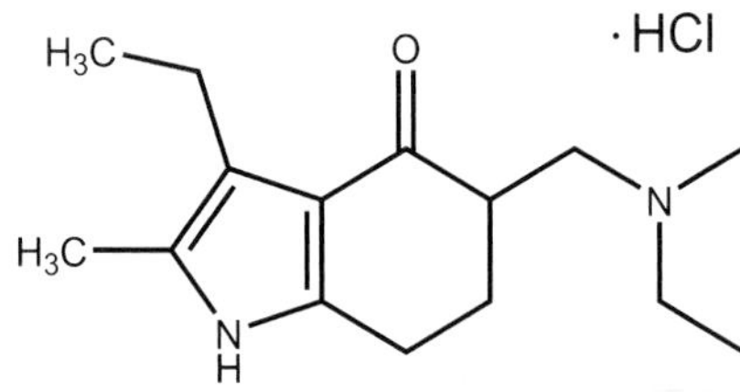

Molindone Hydrochloride

BENZAMIDES

The benzamides evolved from observations that the gastroprokinetic and antiemetic agent, metoclopramide, has antipsychotic activity related to D$_2$ receptor block. It was hoped that the group might yield compounds with diminished EPS liability. This expectation appears to have been met. An H-bond between the amido H and the unshared electrons of the methoxyl group to generate a pseudo ring is considered important for antipsychotic activity in these compounds. Presumably, when the protonated amine is superimposed on that of protonated DA, this pseudo ring would superimpose on DA's aromatic ring.[34] These features can be seen in sulpiride and remoxipride.

Remoxipride (Roxiam). Remoxipride is a D$_2$ receptor blocker.[35] It is as effective as haloperidol with fewer EPS and autonomic side effects. Negative symptoms of schizophrenia are diminished. The drug is classed as an atypical antipsychotic. Life-threatening aplastic anemia was reported with its use, which prompted its withdrawal from the market.

With respect to the atypical antipsychotics, two events long in the past may shed some light on the events of today.

The field of reuptake-inhibiting antidepressants arose when only a very small structural change was made in an antipsychotic drug, and the new activity noted. (The antipsychotic activity remained.) Therefore, small changes in structure can produce antipsychotics that are active against depressive symptoms. Likewise, small changes in structure could provide selectivity among D$_2$ receptors.

Almost 40 years ago, it was noted that thioridazine was far less unpleasant for patients than its relatives.[36] Its tricyclic system is far more nucleophilic than that of most other drugs. The emphasis at the time, however, was to increase milligram potency by increasing D$_2$ receptor affinity by lowering tricyclic electron density. The experience of clozapine, with increased electron density of the receptor-binding rings and thus lower affinity, appears to validate the observation about thioridazine and appears to allow more selectivity among D$_2$ receptors. Lessening blocks on, for example, striatal D$_2$ receptors, and possibly mesocortical D$_2$ receptors could produce drugs that are much less unpleasant for the patient. Additionally, a less intense D$_2$ block could allow the effects of other blocks to make up more of the drug's total action (e.g., 5-HT transporter block). Several atypical antipsychotics have rings with enhanced nucleophility. Of course, other structural features could be influencing receptor selectivity, for example, increasing steric hindrance to receptor binding by the protonated amino group or to the ring binding.

Antimanic Agents

LITHIUM SALTS

The lithium salts used in the United States are the carbonate (tetrahydrate) and the citrate. Lithium chloride is not used because of its hygroscopic nature and because it is more irritating than the carbonate or citrate to the GI tract.

The active species in these salts is the lithium ion. The classic explanation for its antimanic activity is that it resembles the sodium ion (as well as potassium, magnesium, and calcium ions) and can occupy the sodium pump. Unlike the sodium ion, it cannot maintain membrane potentials. Accordingly, it might prevent excessive release of NTs (e.g., DA) that characterize the manic state. Many of the actions of lithium ion have been reviewed.[37] Despite considerable investigation, the mode of action of lithium remains unclear. The major possibility is that lithium reduces signal transduction through the phosphatidylinositol signaling pathway by uncompetitive inhibition of inositol phosphatase. As a result, the pool of inositol available for the

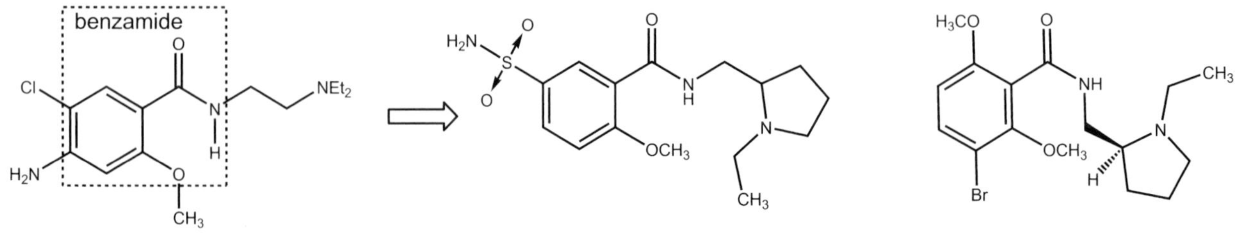

Metoclopramide
an gastroprokinetic & antiemetic agent
an 5-HT$_4$- partial agonists and D$_2$ antagonist

Sulpiride

Remoxipride

resynthesis of phosphatidylinositol-4,5-bisphosphate (PIP_2) is depleted, the cellular levels of PIP_2 is decreased, thereby, enzymatic formation of the second messengers is reduced.

The indications for lithium salts are acute mania (often with a potent neuroleptic agent for immediate control, because lithium is slow to take effect) and as a prophylactic to prevent occurrence of the mania of bipolar manic–depressive illness. Lithium salts are also used in severe recurrent unipolar depression. One effect of the drug that might be pertinent is an increase in the synthesis of presynaptic serotonin. Some have speculated that simply evening out transmission, preventing downward mood swing, for example, could be a basis for antidepressant action.

Because of its water solubility, the lithium ion is extensively distributed in body water. It tends to become involved in the many physiological processes involving sodium, potassium, calcium, and magnesium ions, hence, many side effects and potential drug interactions exist. The margin of safety is low; therefore, lithium should be used only when plasma levels can be monitored routinely. In the desired dose range, side effects can be adequately controlled.

Because of the toxicity of lithium, there is substantial interest in design of safer compounds. As more is learned about lithium's specific actions, the likelihood of successful design of compounds designed to act on specific targets is increased. Actually, carbamazepine and valproic acid, which target sodium channels, are proving to be effective.[38] These two drugs are discussed in the anticonvulsant section.

Lithium Carbonate, USP, and Lithium Citrate. Lithium carbonate (Eskalith, Lithane) and lithium citrate (Cibalith-S) are the salts commercially available in the United States.

⬡ ACKNOWLEDGMENT

Portions of this text were taken from Dr. Eugene I. Isaacson's chapter in the 11th edition of this book.

◆ R E V I E W   Q U E S T I O N S ◆

1. What is the mechanism of action of the benzodiazepines?

2. What is the mechanism by which antipsychotics work?

3. What pharmacokinetic properties are shared by most of the antipsychotic drugs?

4. Which benzodiazepines shown below is/are short acting?

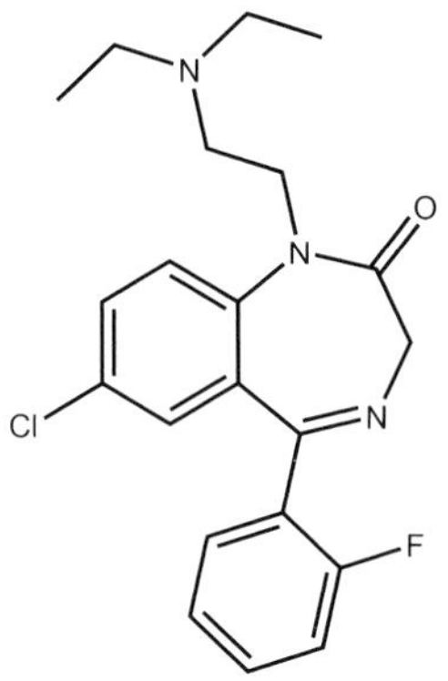

5. Which of the following drugs is/are metabolized to a compound that will continue to have significant sedative and hypnotic effect?

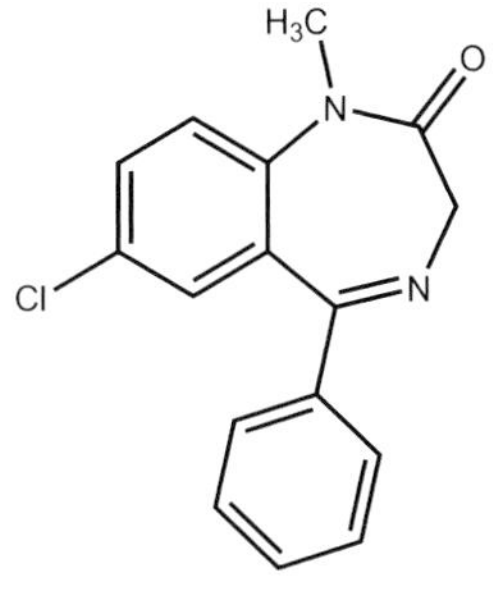

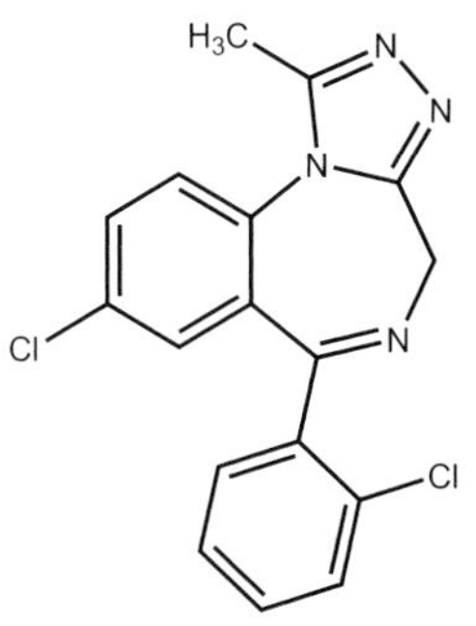

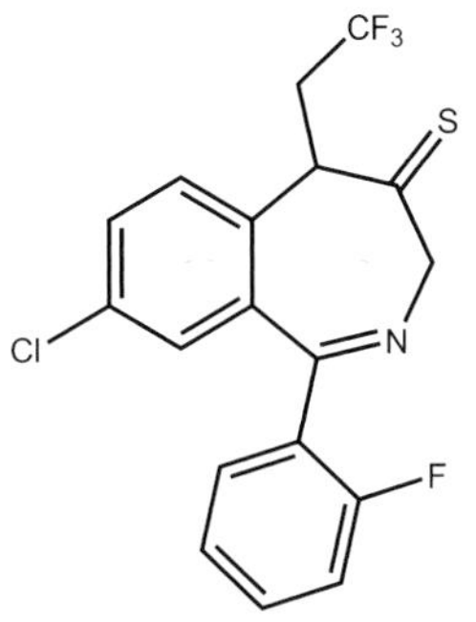

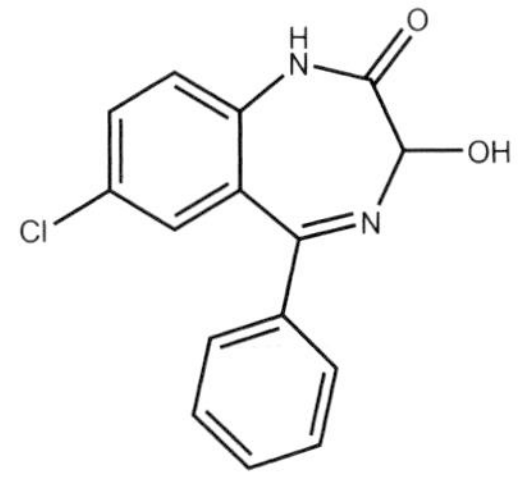

1

2

3

4

1. Oxazepam

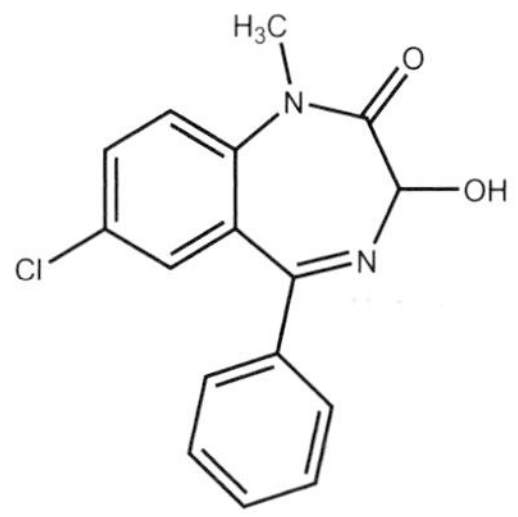

2. Temazepam

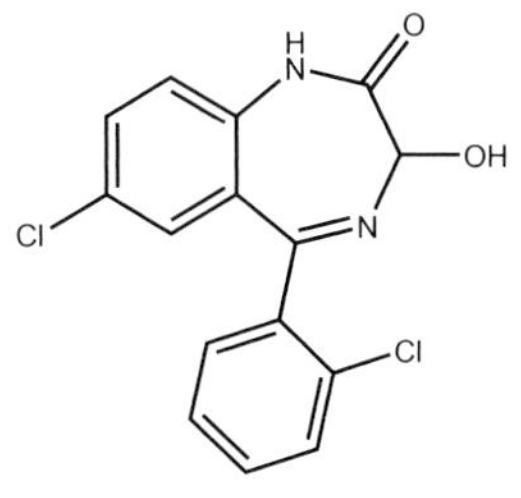

3. Lorazepam

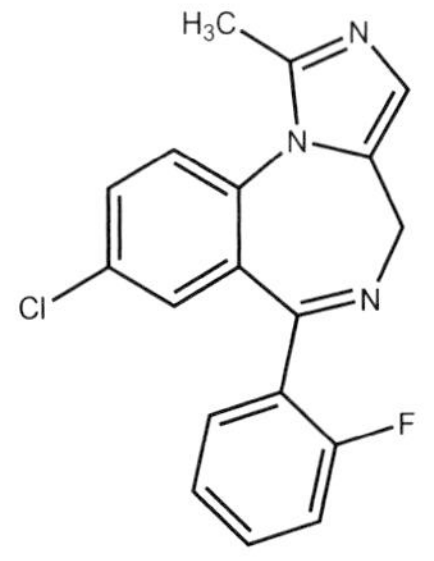

4. Midazolam

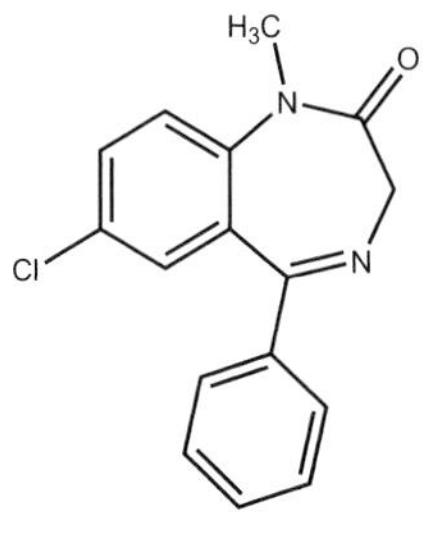

5. Diazepam

REFERENCES

1. Sateia, M. J., et al.: Sleep Med. Rev. 12:319, 2008.
2. Huang, J.-K., and Jan, C.-R.: Life Sci. 68:611, 2000.
3. Tariq, S. H., et al.: Clin. Geriatr. Med. 24:93, 2008.
4. Azabadi, E.: Br. J. Clin. Pharmacol. 61(6):761, 2006.
5. Weinberger, D. R.: N. Engl. J. Med. 344:1247, 2001.
6. Nemeroff, C. B.: Psychopharmacol. Bull. 37(4):113, 2003
7. Xue, H., et al.: J. Med. Chem. 44:1883, 2001.
8. Xue, H., et al.: J. Mol. Biol. 296:739, 2000.
9. Renard, S., et al.: J. Biol. Chem. 274:13370, 1999.
10. Buhr, A., et al.: Mol. Pharmacol. 49:1080, 1996.
11. Buhr, A., et al.: Mol. Pharmacol. 52:672, 1997.
12. Buhr, A., et al.: J. Neurochem. 74:1310, 2000.
13. Sternbach, L. H.: In Garattini, S., Mussini, E., and Randall, L. O. (eds.). The Benzodiazepines. New York, Raven Press, 1972, p. 1.
14. Currie, K. S.: Antianxiety agents. In Abraham, D. J. (ed.). Burger's Medicinal Chemistry, vol. 6, 6th ed. Hoboken, NJ, John Wiley and Sons, 2003, p. 525.
15. Hadjipavlou-Litina, D., et al.: Chem. Rev. 104:3751, 2004.
16. Greenblatt, D. J., and Shader, R. I.: Benzodiazepines in Clinical Practice. New York, Raven Press, 1974, p. 17 (and references therein).
17. Greenblatt, D. J., Shader, R. I., and Abernethy, D. R.: N. Engl. J. Med. 309:345, 410, 1983.
18. Daniels, T. C., and Jorgensen, E. C.: Central nervous system depressants. In Doerge, R. F. (ed.). Wilson and Gisvold's Textbook of Organic Medicinal and Pharmaceutical Chemistry, 8th ed. Philadelphia, J. B. Lippincott, 1982, p. 335.
19. Berger, F. M.: Meprobamate and other glycol derivatives. In Usdin, E., and Forrest, I. S. (eds.). Psychotherapeutic Drugs, part II. New York, Marcel Dekker, 1977, p. 1089.
20. Cram, D. J., and Hammond, G. S.: Organic Chemistry, 2nd ed. New York, McGraw-Hill, 1964, p. 295.
21. Mackay, F. J., and Cooper, J. R.: J. Pharmacol. Exp. Ther. 135:271, 1962.
22. Karlsson, H., et al.: Proc. Natl. Acad. Sci. U. S. A. 98:4634, 2001.
23. Lewis, D. A.: Proc. Natl. Acad. Sci. U. S. A. 98:4293, 2000.
24. Rowley, M., Bristow, L. J., and Hutson, P. H.: J. Med. Chem. 44:477, 2001.
25. Akam, E., and Strange P. G.: Biochem. Pharmacol. 6:2039, 2004.
26. Felder, C. C.: Life Sci. 68:2605, 2001.
27. Yeomans, J., et al.: Life Sci. 68:2449, 2001.
28. Gordon, M., Cook, L., Tedeschi, D. H., et al.: Arzneim. Forsch. 13:318, 1963.
29. Horn, A. S., and Snyder, S. H.: Proc. Natl. Acad. Sci. U. S. A. 68:2325, 1971.
30. Miller, D. D., et al.: J. Med. Chem. 30:163, 1987.
31. Altar, C. A., Martin, A. R., and Thurkauf, A.: Antipsychotic agents. In Abraham, D. J. (ed.). Burger's Medicinal Chemistry, vol. 6, 6th ed. Hoboken, NJ, John Wiley and Sons, 2003, p. 599.
32. Janssen, P. A. J., and Van Bever, W. F. M.: Butyrophenones and diphenylbutylamines. In Usdin, E., and Forrest, I. S. (eds.). Psychotherapeutic Drugs, part II. New York, Marcel Dekker, 1977, p. 869.
33. Chen, X.-M.: Annu. Rep. Med. Chem. 29:331, 1994.
34. van de Waterbeemd, H., and Testa, B.: J. Med. Chem. 26:203, 1983.
35. Howard, H. R., and Seeger, T. F.: Annu. Rep. Med. Chem. 28:39, 1993 (and references therein).
36. Potter, W. Z., and Hollister, L. E.: Antipsychotic agents and lithium. In Katzung, B. G. (ed.). Basic and Clinical Pharmacology, 10th ed. New York, Lange Medical Books/McGraw-Hill, Medical Publishing Division, 2007, p. 457.
37. Emrich, H. M., Aldenhoff, J. B., and Lux, H. D. (eds.): Basic Mechanisms in the Action of Lithium. Symposium Proceedings. Amsterdam, Excerpta Medica, 1981.
38. Leysen, D., and Pinder, R. M.: Annu. Rep. Med. Chem. 29:1, 1994.

SELECTED READING

Cooper, J. R., Bloom, F. E., and Roth, R. H.: The Biochemical Basis of Neuropharmacology, 8th ed. New York, Oxford University Press, 2003.
Timmermans, P. B. M. W. M., Chiu, A. T., and Thoolen, M. J. M. C.: α-Adrenergic receptors. In Hansch, C., Sammes, P. G., and Taylor, J. B. (eds.). Comprehensive Medicinal Chemistry, vol. 3, Membranes and Receptors. Oxford, Pergamon Press, 1990, p. 133.
Roweley, M., Bristow, L. J., and Hutson, P. H.: Current and novel approaches to the drug treatment of schizophrenia. J. Med. Chem. 44:477, 2001.
Strange, P. G.: Antipsychotic drugs: importance of dopamine receptors for mechanisms of therapeutic actions and side effects. Pharmacol. Rev. 53:119, 2001.
Weinberger, D. R.: Anxiety at the frontier of molecular medicine. N. Engl. J. Med. 344:1247, 2001.

CHAPTER 13

Central Dopaminergic Signaling Agents

A. MICHAEL CRIDER, MARCELO J. NIETO, AND KENNETH A. WITT

CHAPTER OVERVIEW

The understanding and development of dopamine (DA)-focused pharmacotherapy, with regard to central nervous system (CNS) disorders, requires the insight and integration of multiple disciplines. The structure–activity relationship (SAR) between drug and target, forming the foundation of medicinal chemistry, must be grounded by the ability to assess and discern the diseases under investigation. It is necessary to evaluate the drug with regard not only to the target, but also to the effects of the body on the drug, the nature of disease, subsequent actions of the target, and any potential "nontarget" actions. In this regard, DA-focused pharmacotherapy possesses numerous caveats owing to our lack of complete understanding of specific diseases and the overlapping action of the dopaminergic systems within the brain. Nevertheless, the respective drugs addressed in this chapter have proven to be effective in the symptomological management of Parkinson disease (PD) and schizophrenia, significantly enhancing the quality of life of individuals suffering from these disease states.

⬡ DOPAMINE

DA acts as a CNS neurotransmitter, controlling emotion, movement, and reward mechanisms, as well as serving as the metabolic precursor of norepinephrine and epinephrine. DA is classified as a catecholamine neurotransmitter based on its catechol nucleus and is derived from the amino acid tyrosine. Tyrosine is transported across the blood-brain barrier (BBB) into the brain, where it is then taken up by dopaminergic neurons. Conditions affecting tyrosine transport into the brain significantly impact DA formation. Once L-tyrosine enters the dopaminergic neuron, it is converted to L-dihydroxyphenylalanine (L-DOPA) by the enzyme tyrosine hydroxylase (TH), which is the rate-limiting step in DA synthesis. Subsequently, the enzyme L-aromatic amino acid decarboxylase (AADC) converts L-DOPA to DA (Fig. 13.1). The normally high levels of AADC in the brain will allow for the substantial increase in DA levels if levels of L-DOPA are increased. DA itself does not cross the BBB; however, L-DOPA crosses via the large neutral amino acid carrier.

Dopamine Storage and Release

DA is stored in neuronal presynaptic vesicles, with its release controlled by both nerve impulse and DA-autoreceptors present on presynaptic neurons (Fig. 13.2). The nerve impulse (i.e., action potential) results in rapid depolarization causing calcium ion channels to open. Calcium then stimulates the transport of vesicles to the synaptic membrane; the vesicle and cell membrane fuse, which leads to the release of the DA. In general, the degree of DA release is dependent on the rate and pattern of the nerve impulse. The greater the speed and number of impulses, the more DA is released into the synaptic cleft—at least until the DA vesicle concentrations are depleted. The release process can also be modulated via DA-autoreceptors, which are present on presynaptic neurons. DA-autoreceptors act as a negative-feedback control mechanism that modifies both the release and synthesis of DA. In this regard, agonists with selectivity for presynaptic DA-autoreceptors (D_2-subtype) act to reduce DA levels and antagonists act to enhance DA levels.

Dopamine Receptors

Dopaminergic-mediated physiological effects are dependent on affinity and selectivity of a ligand (agonist or antagonist) for DA receptors. DA receptors fall into the larger class of metabotropic G-protein–coupled receptors that are prominent in the vertebrate CNS. Endogenous DA is the primary ligand for DA receptors. Once DA is released from presynaptic neurons, it acts at presynaptic DA-autoreceptors and postsynaptic receptors (Fig. 13.2). DA receptors are divided into five subtypes, D_1 to D_5. These five subtypes are grouped into two principal categories based on structure and signaling transduction mechanisms. D_1 and D_5 receptors are members of the "D1-family" of DA receptors; whereas the D_2, D_3, and D_4 receptors are members of the "D2-family."[2] Activation of D1-family receptors stimulates the formation of cyclic adenosine monophosphate (cAMP) and phosphatidyl inositol hydrolysis. Increased cAMP in neurons is typically excitatory and can induce an action potential by modulating the activity of ion channels. Whereas, D2-family receptor activation inhibits cAMP synthesis, as well as suppresses Ca^{2+} currents and activates receptor-operated K^+ currents. Decreased cAMP in neurons is typically inhibitory and reduces DA release. DA-autoreceptors are of the D2-family.

Although D1- and D2-family receptors have opposite effects with regard to cAMP, the physiological significance of their interactions is much more complex. DA receptors are widespread throughout the brain, but each subtype has a unique distribution. Additionally, postsynaptic DA receptors exist on multiple neuronal subtypes (e.g., gamma-aminobutyric acid [GABA]ergic, glutamatergic,

L- Tyrosine → TH → Levodopa → AADC → Dopamine

Figure 13.1 ● Synthesis of DA.

and cholinergic neurons). Drugs that act as DA receptor agonists or antagonists often have differing affinity and selectivity for respective DA receptor subtypes. Thus, the net effect of any DA receptor agonist or antagonist on dopaminergic activity is dependent on both its presynaptic and postsynaptic effects. This complexity is further compounded by the receptor adaptations during disease states, such as PD and schizophrenia[3,4]; as some DA receptor subtypes will upregulate (increased number of receptors), whereas other subtypes will downregulate (decreased number of receptors) dependent on stage of disease and time profile of drug treatment.

Dopamine Transporter

The dopamine transporter (DAT) is the primary mechanism by which DA is removed from the synaptic cleft. The DAT plays a critical role in the inactivation and recycling of DA by actively pumping the extracellular DA back into presynaptic nerve terminals. Regional brain distribution of DAT is found in areas with established dopaminergic circuitry (e.g., mesostriatal, mesolimbic, and mesocortical pathways). Its cellular localization at presynaptic terminals provides an

excellent marker of dopaminergic neurons that are damaged in PD.[5] Additionally, the DAT has a well-established pharmacologic profile and is the principal target of psychostimulants (e.g., cocaine, amphetamine, and methylphenidate), which inhibit the reuptake of DA in the synaptic cleft resulting in locomotor stimulation.

Dopamine Metabolism

DA metabolism occurs through enzymatic action, via monoamine oxidase (MAO) or catechol-*O*-methyltransferase (COMT) (Fig. 13.3). There are two forms of MAO, MAO-A and MAO-B, both of which oxidize DA. DA is metabolized by intraneuronal MAO-A and by glial and astrocyte cells by MAO-A and MAO-B.[6] Depending on the pathway, DA can be converted to either dihydroxyphenylacetic acid (DOPAC) or homovanillic acid (HVA). In humans, the major brain metabolite is HVA, followed by DOPAC. Accumulation of HVA in the cerebrospinal fluid (CSF) and brain can be used as a measure of the functional activity of dopaminergic neurons in the brain. Drugs that increase the turnover of DA (e.g., antipsychotics) also increase the amount of HVA in the brain and CSF.[7]

Dopaminergic Pathways

To understand the actions of DA-focused pharmacotherapy and the associated adverse effects, it is necessary to identify the principal dopaminergic pathways in the brain.[3,4,7] The neurotransmission of DA can be divided into several major pathways: the nigrostriatal, mesocortical, mesolimbic, and tuberohypophyseal DA neuronal pathways (Fig. 13.4). The nigrostriatal pathway accounts for ~75% of the DA in the brain, consisting of cell bodies in the substantia nigra whose axons terminate in the striatum (principal connective nuclei of the basal ganglia). It is involved in the production of movement, as part of a system called the basal ganglia motor loop and is directly affected in PD. This system may also be involved in short-term side effects of antipsychotic medication (i.e., tremor and muscle rigidity), as well as long-term side effects of tardive dyskinesia. The mesocortical pathway originates in the ventral tegmental area and projects to the prefrontal cortex. It is essential to the normal cognitive function of the prefrontal cortex and is thought to be involved in motivation and emotional response. The mesolimbic pathway originates in cell bodies in the ventral tegmental area of the midbrain and project to the mesial components of the limbic system. Mesolimbic DA neurons are involved with pleasure and reward behavior and are heavily implicated in addiction. The tuberohypophyseal pathway emanates from the periventricular and arcuate nuclei of the hypothalamus, with projections to the pituitary gland and the median eminence of the hypothalamus (i.e., tuberoinfundibular DA tract). The tuberohypophyseal pathway is involved in the regulation of prolactin.

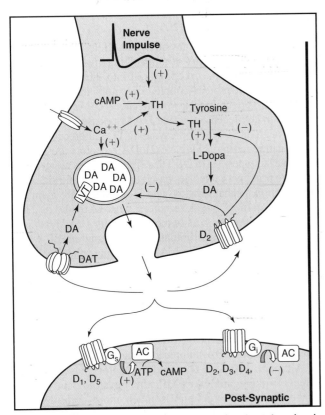

Figure 13.2 ● Schematic model of mechanisms involved in DA synthesis, release, storage, reuptake, and receptor activity in presynaptic and postsynaptic neurons. (AC, adenylate cyclase; cAMP, cyclic adenosine monophosphate; VT, vesicular monoamine transporter.)

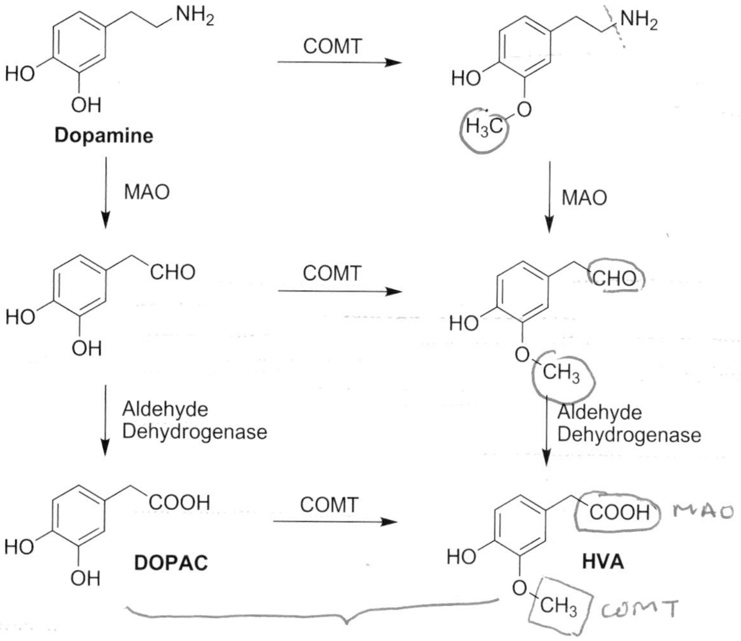

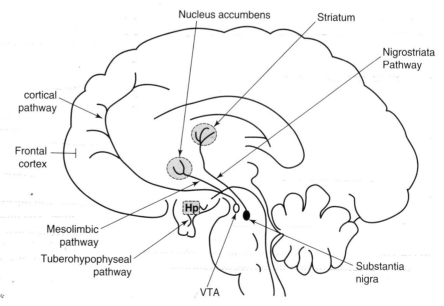

Figure 13.3 ● Metabolic pathway of DA.

PARKINSON DISEASE

PD is a progressive neurodegenerative illness characterized by tremor, muscular rigidity, bradykinesia (slowness of movement), and postural imbalance.[8] The incidence of PD is estimated to be about 1% in the general population older than 60 years of age.[9] Although characterized as a neuromuscular disorder, dementia also occurs at a much greater rate in PD patients over the normal age-matched population.[10] Although the etiology of PD remains unknown, several factors appear to play a role, including the aging process, environmental chemicals, oxidative stress, and genetic aspects.[9] The discovery that drug addicts exposed to the pyridine derivative 1-methyl-4-phenyl-1,2,3,6-tetrahydropyridine (MPTP), a byproduct of "synthetic heroin," developed a profound parkinsonian state led to intense study of the pathogenesis of PD.[11,12] On the basis of investigations in the treatment of MPTP-treated primates, a working

understanding of neurochemical basis of PD has developed. The primary motor control–related symptoms have shown to be the result of dysregulation of the motor cortex via the nigrostriatal pathway. The dysregulation is caused by the depletion of DA-producing neurons within the pars compacta region of the substantia nigra that project to the striatum. This is often accompanied by Lewy bodies, which are abnormal aggregates of protein that develop inside nerve cells. In healthy individuals, stimulation of D_1 receptors within the striatum results in an increased excitatory outflow from the thalamus to the motor cortex and is known as the "direct pathway"; whereas stimulation of the D_2 receptors within the striatum results in a decreased excitatory outflow from the thalamus to the motor cortex and is known as the "indirect pathway." However, under conditions of PD, the loss of dopaminergic input to the striatum leads to a decreased activity in the direct pathway and an increased activity in the indirect pathway (via D_1 and D_2 receptors, respectively). Both of these changes lead to

Figure 13.4 ● Dopamine pathways in the brain (*pathway projections not shown in their entirety*). (Hp, hypothalamus; VTA, ventral tegmental area.)

decreased excitatory input to the motor cortex and the hypokinetic symptomology associated with PD. Nevertheless, the symptoms of PD are not seen until about 80% of the dopaminergic neurons in the striatum have been destroyed. Thus, significant disease progression must occur before there is an observable reduction of motor movement and control.

Although DA loss within the striatum is the primary neurological factor associated with PD, other DA pathways and receptors have also been implicated. It has been postulated that dysregulation of mesolimbic and mesocortical dopaminergic pathways directly contributes to the depression states common with PD.[13] Dementia with PD has been shown to correlate with a loss of response to dopaminergic drugs, which has been correlated with reduced D_3 receptors.[14] DA D_3 receptors have also been postulated to play a role in motor control deficits associated with PD because they are often found colocalized with D_1 and D_2 and have shown to have a reduced expression in the basal ganglia of postmortem PD brains.[14–16] However, the recognition of dopaminergic pathway and receptor changes has not led to any more effective treatment than levodopa, which remains the gold standard. Clinical trials on the $D_1/D_2/D_3$ agonist rotigotine have shown promise in alleviating symptoms of early PD.[17] Yet, simply obtaining an optimal ratio of drug activity at these receptors will not slow the degeneration of dopamineric neurons. Nevertheless, current PD pharmacotherapy is centered on replacement of dopaminergic activity within the striatum. Whether this is to enhance DA release from remaining neurons, increase DA synthesis, provide exogenous DA agonists, or reduce DA metabolism, none of these approaches or combinations therein have shown to provide successful long-term treatment of symptoms.

Levodopa/Carbidopa

The first significant breakthrough in the treatment of PD came about with the introduction of high-dose levodopa. Fahn[18] referred to this as a revolutionary development in treating parkinsonian patients. The rationale for the use of levodopa for the treatment of PD was established in the early 1960s. Parkinsonian patients were shown to have decreased striatal levels of DA and reduced urinary excretion of DA. Since then, levodopa has shown to be remarkably effective for treating the symptoms of PD.[19] Because of enzymatic action of MAO-A in the gastrointestinal (GI) tract and AADC in the periphery, only a small percentage (1%–2%) of levodopa is delivered into the CNS. Coadministration of levodopa with the AADC inhibitor, carbidopa, prevents decarboxylation of levodopa outside of the CNS. The combination of levodopa and carbidopa results in a substantial increase in DA delivery to the CNS with a decrease in peripheral side effects. Long-term therapy with levodopa leads to predictable motor complications. These include loss of efficacy before the next dose ("wearing off"), motor response fluctuations ("on/off"), and unwanted movements (dyskinesias).[20,21] These effects are thought to be caused by the inability of levodopa therapy to restore normal DA levels in the CNS.[22] As a result, the use of longer-acting DA agonists may benefit parkinsonian patients.

Levodopa, **United States Pharmacopeia (USP).** Levodopa, (S)-2-amino-3-(3,4-dihydroxyphenyl) propanoic acid, is a white or almost white crystalline powder, slightly soluble in water, soluble in acidic and basic solutions, and practically insoluble in alcohol, chloroform, and ether. Aqueous solutions are neutral to slightly acidic (pK$_a$'s = 9.9 and 11.8).[23] Levodopa is rapidly absorbed from the small intestine by an active transport system for aromatic amino acids. It is widely distributed to most body tissues, but less to the CNS, and is bound to plasma proteins only to a minor extent (10%–30%). Levodopa is extensively decarboxylated by first-pass metabolism in the liver. A small amount is methylated to 3-O-methyldopa (3OMD), which accumulates in the CNS because of its long half-life. Most of levodopa is converted to DA, small amounts of which in turn are metabolized to norepinephrine and epinephrine. At least 30 metabolites of levodopa have been identified. Metabolites of DA are rapidly excreted in the urine. The principal metabolites DOPAC and HVA (Fig. 13.3) account for up to 50% of the administered dose. After prolonged therapy with levodopa, the ratio of DOPAC and HVA excreted may increase, probably reflecting a depletion of methyl donors necessary for metabolism by COMT. Antipsychotic drugs, such as phenothiazines, butyrophenones, and reserpine interfere with the therapeutic effects of levodopa, and nonspecific MAO inhibitors interfere with inactivation of DA. Anticholinergic drugs (e.g., trihexyphenidyl, benztropine, and procyclidine) act synergistically with levodopa to improve certain symptoms of PD, especially tremor. However, large doses of anticholinergic drugs can slow gastric emptying sufficiently to cause a delay in reabsorption of levodopa by the small intestine. Sympathomimetic agents such as epinephrine or isoproterenol may also enhance the cardiac side effects of levodopa. In some patients, the coadministration of antacids may enhance the GI absorption of levodopa. Levodopa is essentially a prodrug; that is itself inactive, but after penetrating the BBB is metabolized to DA. Levodopa is indicated for the treatment of idiopathic, postencephalitic, and symptomatic parkinsonism.

Carbidopa

Carbidopa, **USP.** Carbidopa, (S)-3-(3,4-dihydroxyphenyl)-2-hydrazinyl-2-methylpropanoic acid, is a white crystalline powder, slightly soluble in water (pK$_a$ = 7.8). Carbidopa is absorbed slower than levodopa and is 36% plasma protein bound.[23] Carbidopa is metabolized to two main metabolites (α-methyl-3-methoxy-4-hydroxyphenylpropionic acid and α-methyl-3,4-dihydroxyphenylpropionic acid). These two metabolites are primarily eliminated in the urine unchanged or as glucuronide conjugates. Unchanged carbidopa accounts for 30% of the total urinary excretion. No drug interactions have been described.

MAO B Inhibitors

MAO inhibitors are utilized to prolong the plasma half-life of levodopa or block the striatal metabolism of DA. Initially, the use of nonselective MAO inhibitors led to serious adverse effects caused by peripheral inhibition of monoamines. The use of selective MAO-B inhibitors decreases the risk of a hypertensive crisis that is associated with nonselective MAO inhibitors. The addition of a selective MAO-B inhibitor to levodopa therapy decreases both the metabolism of DA that is produced from levodopa and DA that is already present in the striatum.

Selegiline is an irreversible MAO-B inhibitor. Unlike compounds that inhibit MAO-A, selegiline does not produce the so-called cheese effect. This is a hypertensive crisis of the cardiovascular system caused by elevated levels of *p*-tyramine and other indirectly acting sympathomimetic amines that are found in certain foods (e.g., red wine, cheese, and herring).[24] Selegiline potentiates the effects of levodopa by blocking its metabolism by MAO. When administered with levodopa, selegiline allows for a reduction in the daily dosage and appears to improve the wearing-off effect of levodopa. However, whether selegiline is able to exert a neuroprotective effect in PD is inconclusive.[25] Selegiline is extensively first-pass metabolized to yield *N*-desmethylselegiline, l-methamphetamine, and l-amphetamine. These metabolites have been implicated in some of the psychomotor and cardiovascular adverse effects of selegiline.[26]

Rasagiline is a selective irreversible inhibitor of MAO-B that is approximately five times more potent than selegiline. The *R*-isomer is the active enantiomer whereas the *S*-isomer demonstrates only weak inhibition of MAO-B. Similar to selegiline, rasagiline does not produce the characteristic cheese effect that is observed for nonselective MAO inhibitors.[27] The neuroprotective effect of rasagiline is inferred by the propargyl group. This effect is observed at drug concentrations well below those necessary to cause MAO-B inhibition. Several mechanisms have been proposed for the neuroprotective effect of rasagiline including (a) a decrease in proapoptotic proteins (Bax and Bad), (b) an increase in antiapoptotic proteins (Bcl-2 and Bcl-xL), and (c) stabilization of mitochondrial membrane potential, thus preventing subsequent release of proapoptotic proteins.[28,29]

Selegiline   Rasagiline

Selegiline Hydrochloride, USP. Selegiline hydrochloride, (*R*)-*N*-methyl-*N*-(1-phenylpropan-2-yl)prop-2-yn-1-amine hydrochloride (Eldepryl), is an off-white powder, freely soluble in water and methanol (pK_a = 7.4).[30] Selegiline is readily absorbed from the GI tract. It is well distributed in the body and it penetrates the CNS. Selegiline has a high apparent volume of distribution, short half-life, and a very high oral clearance, indicating an extensive metabolism not only in the liver but also through extrahepatic biotransformation. Transdermal delivery reduces the first-pass metabolism and provides higher and more prolonged plasma levels of unchanged selegiline and lower levels of metabolites compared with the oral administration.[31] Selegiline transdermal system (EMSAM) has recently been approved for the treatment of depression.[23] Selegiline administered with fluoxetine may produce a "serotonin" syndrome (CNS irritability, increased

muscle tone, altered consciousness), and with meperidine could result in agitation, seizures, diaphoresis, and fever, which may progress to coma, apnea, and death. Drug reactions may occur several weeks following withdrawal of selegiline. The use of selegiline as monotherapy is limited to younger patients with early disease and without disabling symptoms.

Rasagiline Mesylate. Rasagiline mesylate, (*R*)-*N*-(prop-2-ynyl)-2,3-dihydro-1*H*-inden-1-amine methanesulfonate (Azilect), belongs to the propargylamine family and is a white to off-white powder, soluble in water or ethanol, slightly soluble in isopropanol. Rasagiline is rapidly absorbed. Plasma protein binding for rasagiline ranges from 88% to 94%, with specific binding to serum albumin being 61% to 63%. It undergoes complete biotransformation before excretion, mainly via *N*-dealkylation and hydroxylation, to yield three major metabolites: 1(*R*)-aminoindan, 3-hydroxy-*N*-propargyl-1-aminoindan, and 3-hydroxy-1-aminoindan. Both oxidative pathways are catalyzed by cytochrome P450 (CYP) enzymes, mainly the 1A2 isozyme. Rasagiline and its metabolites undergo glucuronide conjugation with subsequent urinary excretion.[29] Inhibitors of the CYP1A2 may increase plasma concentrations of rasagiline up to twofold.[32,33] Because rasagiline is a selective and irreversible inhibitor of MAO-B, its duration of action is independent of the drug's half-life and is instead determined by the regeneration rate of MAO-B. This characteristic is potentially beneficial in PD, where rasagiline's prolonged effect may be able to limit the fluctuating responses that are characteristic of long-term drug treatment with levodopa.[34]

Dopamine Agonists

The addition of DA agonists to levodopa therapy has gained widespread popularity in the treatment of PD.[35] DA agonists not only produce less dyskinesia, but also have been hypothesized to slow the progressive degeneration of DA neurons.[36] DA agonists are classified into ergot derivatives (pergolide, cabergoline, and bromocriptine) and nonergot derivatives (apomorphine, pramipexole, ropinirole, and rotigotine).

ERGOT DERIVATIVES

Pergolide binds with high affinity as an agonist at D_2-type and 5-HT$_{2B}$ receptors.[37] The compound also binds at D_1 receptors but with approximately 300-fold less affinity than at D_2 receptors. Pergolide is believed to induce valvular heart disease by acting on 5-HT$_{2B}$ receptors.[38] Because of the potential for cardiac valve damage, pergolide has been recently withdrawn from the market.[23] Cabergoline exhibits high affinity at D_2-like receptors with over 50-fold selectivity compared with D_1-like receptors.[39] Additionally, cabergoline binds with high affinity at 5-HT$_{2A}$ and 5-HT$_{2B}$ receptors.[37] The compound is approved in the United States only for hyperprolactinemia but is used in other countries for the treatment of PD. At the low dose used in the treatment of hyperprolactinemia, cabergoline does not appear to increase the risk of cardiac valve complications.[23] Bromocriptine acts as an agonist at D_2-like receptors and an antagonist at D_1-like receptors.[40] Additionally, it exhibits high affinity at 5-HT$_{2A}$ and 5-HT$_{2B}$ receptors. Although bromocriptine acts as an agonist at 5-HT$_{2A}$ receptors, it shows partial agonism at 5-HT$_{2B}$

receptors.[41] Compared with cabergoline, bromocriptine exhibits less dyskinesia, which may be related to its D_1-antagonist activity.[37]

Bromocriptine Mesylate, USP. Bromocriptine mesylate, (6a*R*,9*R*)-5-bromo-*N*-((2*R*,5*S*,10a*S*,10b*S*)-10b-hydroxy-5-isobutyl-2-isopropyl-3,6-dioxooctahydro-2*H*-oxazolo[3,2-a]pyrrolo[2,1c]pyrazin-2-yl)-7-methyl-4,6,6a,7,8,9-hexahydroindolo[4,3-fg]quinoline-9-carboxamide methanesulfonate (Parlodel), is a white solid soluble in ethanol and slightly soluble in water (pKₐ's = 6.6 and 15). Bromocriptine is rapidly absorbed after oral administration and it has low systemic bioavailability because of its extensive first-pass metabolism. Bromocriptine enters the brain quickly with a half-life for uptake into the brain of approximately 0.3 hours; 8% of the drug crosses the BBB.[23] The metabolites are excreted primarily in the bile and feces. The high first-pass hepatic metabolism implies an increased risk of drug interactions. Concomitant administration with the DA antagonists, metoclopramide, or domperidone may aggravate parkinsonian symptoms and induce extrapyramidal side effects (EPS). Other drugs that may interact with bromocriptine are highly plasma protein–bound drugs (e.g., warfarin, increased dyskinesia caused by bromocriptine); macrolides antibacterials (enhanced dopaminergic effects); and caffeine (elevation in plasma bromocriptine concentrations). The combination of levodopa/AADC inhibitors with bromocriptine permits a reduction of the dose of levodopa. Thus, the side effects of levodopa are decreased, resulting in a more continuous stimulation of DA receptors.

Cabergoline. Cabergoline, (6a*R*,9*R*,10a*R*)-7-allyl-*N*-(3-(dimethylamino)propyl)-*N*-(ethylcarbamoyl)-4,6,6a,7,8,9,10,10a-octahydroindolo[4,3-fg]quinoline-9-carboxamide (Dostinex), is a white powder soluble in alcohol, chloroform, and *N,N*-dimethylformamide; slightly soluble in acidic solutions and in *n*-hexane; and insoluble in water. Following oral administration, peak plasma concentrations are reached within 2 to 3 hours. Cabergoline is moderately bound to plasma proteins in a concentration-independent manner. The absolute bioavailability of cabergoline is unknown. Cabergoline is extensively metabolized by the liver, predominantly via hydrolysis of the acylurea bond of the urea moiety. CYP450 metabolism appears to be minimal. The major metabolites identified thus far do not contribute to the therapeutic effect of cabergoline. Less than 4% is excreted unchanged in the urine. Fecal excretion represents the main route of cabergoline elimination. There are no reports of interactions of cabergoline with other antiparkinsonian agents. Clarithromycin may elevate the plasma concentration of cabergoline by the inhibition of both CYP3A4 and P-glycoprotein.[42] Cabergoline is a potent D_2 receptor agonist and is indicated for the treatment of hyperprolactinemic disorders, either idiopathic or caused by pituitary adenomas.

NONERGOT DERIVATIVES

Pramipexole acts as an agonist at D_2 and D_3 receptors with greater affinity for D_3 than D_2 receptors. The compound has no appreciable affinity for D_1, D_5, 5-HT$_{2A}$, and 5-HT$_{2B}$ receptors.[37] The reduced dyskinesia associated with pramipexole compared with cabergoline may be related to its low affinity for the D_1 receptor. Ropinirole has about 20-fold selectivity for cloned human D_3 receptors compared with D_2 receptors. Additionally, ropinirole has low affinity for 5-HT$_{2A}$, 5-HT$_{2B}$, and D_1-like receptors.[37] A recent study suggests that D_3-agonists may be able to restore DA neurons and exert a neuroprotective effect.[43] These developments could offer exciting new therapeutic options for parkinsonian patients.

Apomorphine Hydrochloride, USP. Apomorphine hydrochloride, (6a*R*)-6-methyl-5,6,6a,7-tetrahydro-4*H*-dibenzo[de,g]quinolone-10,11-diol hydrochloride (Apokyn), is a white or off-white powder or crystal soluble in hot water (pKₐ = 8.92). Apormorphine is an aporphine alkaloid of the benzoquinoline class. Oral apomorphine is poorly absorbed and has a bioavailability of less than 4%. Upon subcutaneous administration, apomorphine is completely absorbed. Within 10 to 20 minutes, the maximum concentration of the drug is distributed from the blood plasma to the CSF. Other potential routes of administration include continuous subcutaneous infusion, intravenous infusion, intranasal spray application, sublingual, and rectal administration.[23] The agent is highly lipophilic in nature, allowing for rapid diffusion across the BBB after injection. Apomorphine has a short plasma half-life; however, clinical effects may last from 60 to 90 minutes. Apomorphine displays a significant degree of interpatient variability in its pharmacokinetic profile. Studies of both intravenous and subcutaneous injection routes found this

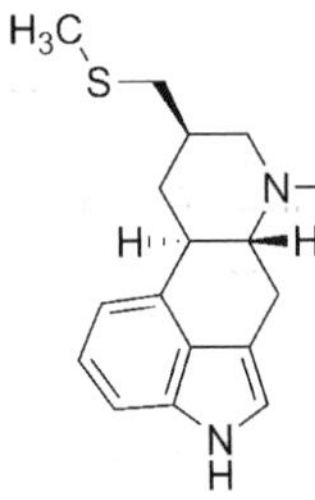

Pergolide (withdrawn)

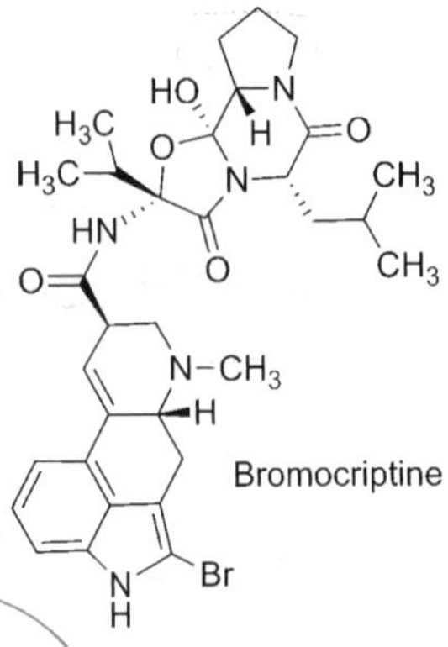

Bromocriptine

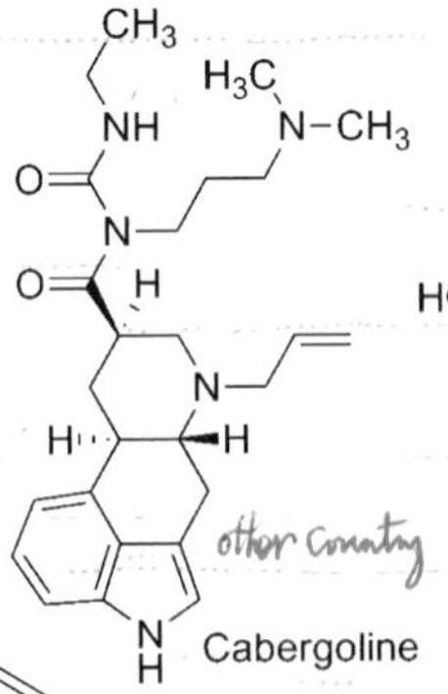

Ropinirole   *Indolin*

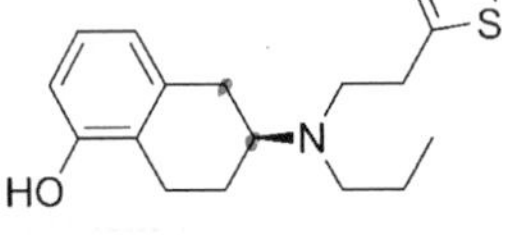

Rotigotine

Cabergoline   *other Country*

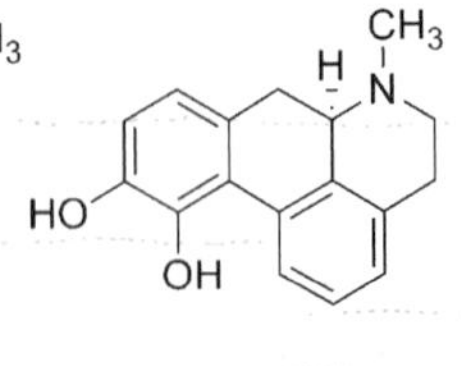

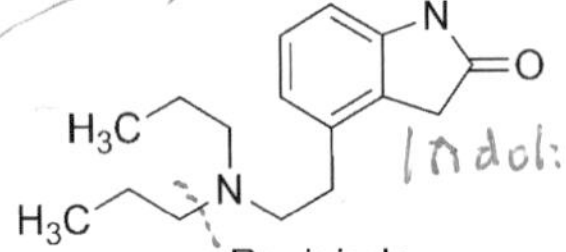

Apomorphine

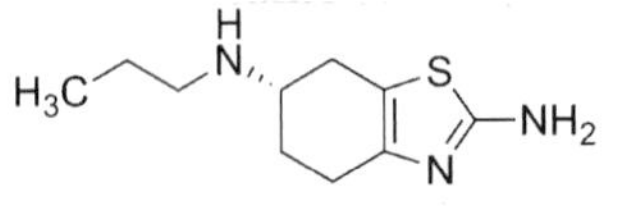

Pramipexole

variation was not attributable to body weight, age, gender, and duration of PD or L-DOPA dose/duration alone. Apomorphine is extensively metabolized. Hypothesized routes include sulfation, *N*-demethylation, glucuronidation, and oxidation. Subcutaneous injections of apomorphine are renally and hepatically cleared, with the majority appearing to be renally cleared. Dosage adjustments are needed in both liver and renal impairment. The activity of apomorphine is believed to be caused by stimulation of postsynaptic D_1- and D_2-type receptors within the caudate/putamen in the brain. Apomorphine is indicated for the acute, intermittent treatment of hypomobility, "off" episodes ("end-of-dose wearing off" and unpredictable on/off episodes) associated with advanced PD.[23]

more polar

Pramipexole Dihydrochloride. Pramipexole dihydrochloride, (*S*)-2-amino-6-propylamino-dihydrochloride (Mirapex), is a white to off-white powder soluble in water, slightly soluble in methanol and ethanol, and practically insoluble in dichloromethane. Following oral administration, pramipexole is readily absorbed. Pharmacokinetic properties differ between men and women, with area under the curve (AUC) for each dose level being 35% to 43% greater in women, mainly because of a 24% to 27% lower oral clearance. The drug undergoes minimal hepatic biotransformation and is excreted virtually unchanged in the urine by the renal tubular secretion. Pramipexole interacts with drugs excreted by renal tubular secretion (H_2-antagonists, diuretics, verapamil, quinidine, quinine), which leads to a decreased clearance of pramipexole.[44,45] Pramipexole is indicated for treatment of the signs and symptoms of idiopathic PD, alone or in combination with levodopa. It is also indicated for symptomatic treatment of moderate to severe idiopathic restless legs syndrome (RLS).

Less polar

Ropinirole Hydrochloride. Ropinirole hydrochloride, 4-(2-(dipropylamino)ethyl)indolin-2-one hydrochloride (Requip), is a white to pale greenish yellow powder that is very soluble in water. Ropinirole is rapidly absorbed after oral administration with maximal plasma concentrations generally reached after about 1.5 hours, and the elimination half-life appears to be approximately 3 hours. Ropinirole is also rapidly and extensively distributed from the vascular compartment and shows low plasma protein binding that is independent of its plasma concentration. This drug is cleared by metabolism in the liver, with only 10% being excreted unchanged. The main metabolite of ropinirole is the *N*-despropyl metabolite. The glucuronide of this metabolite and the carboxylic acid metabolite, 4-carboxymethylindolin-2-one, account only for 10% of the administered dose. None of the metabolites is pharmacologically active, and the excretion of ropinirole-derived products is mainly via the urine. The main CYP450 isozyme involved in the metabolism of ropinirole is CYP1A2. Inhibitors or inducers of this enzyme have been shown to alter the clearance of ropinirole.[46,47] Ropinirole is believed to act as an agonist at postsynaptic D_2 receptors. Ropinirole is indicated for the treatment of the signs and symptoms of idiopathic PD and moderate to severe primary RLS.

Rotigotine. Rotigotine, (6*S*)-6-{propyl[2-(2-thienyl) ethyl]amino}-5,6,7,8-tetrahydro-1-naphthalenol (Neupro), is a nonergoline that is available as a silicone-based, self-adhesive matrix, transdermal system for continuous delivery over a 24-hour period. Approximately 45% of the drug is released within 24 hours. The terminal half-life of rotigotine is 5 to 7 hours after removal of the patch. Rotigotine is 90% bound to plasma proteins. The compound undergoes extensive metabolism and has low bioavailability by the oral route. The major metabolites of rotigotine are the glucuronide and sulfate conjugates of rotigotine and sulfate conjugates of *N*-despropylrotigotine and *N*-desthienylethyl rotigotine. Rotigotine is excreted in the urine (71%) and feces (11%).[23] Studies using human liver microsomes did not find any interactions with CYP1A2, CYP2C9, CYP2C19, CYP2D6, and CYP3A4 substrates.[48] Rotigotine transdermal system contains sodium metabisulfite, and individuals sensitive to sulfite could be at risk for allergic reactions. Additionally, somnolence is a common adverse reaction with individuals on rotigotine, and patients should be closely monitored during therapy.[23] In transfected Chinese hamster ovary (CHO) cells, rotigotine binds with high affinity at D_3 and D_{2L} receptors (variants in the D_2 receptor subtype are caused by insertion of the 29 amino acids into the third loop to give D_{2S} and D_{2L}).[49] Using rat CHO cells, rotigotine shows over 30-fold selectivity at D_3 versus D_2 receptors.[48] Rotigotine was approved in May 2007 for the treatment of early-stage PD.

COMT Inhibitors

When administered with an AADC inhibitor, circulating levodopa is mainly metabolized by COMT. In the presence of a COMT inhibitor, the peripheral metabolism of levodopa is therefore decreased.

Tolcapone is a selective and reversible inhibitor of COMT in the CNS and periphery. Inhibition of COMT in the periphery reduces the formation of 3OMD in tissues that have significant COMT activity. It has been speculated that 3OMD may compete with the uptake of levodopa into the CNS and thereby contributes to the wearing-off effect of levodopa. Administration of levodopa in combination with a dopa decarboxylase inhibitor (carbidopa) and a COMT inhibitor (tolcapone) increases CNS delivery of levodopa. Therefore, more continuous levels of levodopa and DA are maintained.[50] Unlike tolcapone, entacapone does not penetrate the BBB to any extent. Thus, the compound only inhibits peripheral COMT. When combined with levodopa and carbidopa, entacapone provides less motor fluctuations in parkinsonian patients. Another advantage of entacapone over tolcapone is its lack of hepatotoxicity.[51]

polar

Tolcapone   Entacapone

Tolcapone. Tolcapone, 3,4-dihydroxy-4′-methyl-5-nitrobenzophenone (Tasmar), is a yellow, odorless, nonhygroscopic, crystalline compound ($pK_a = 4.78$). Tolcapone is rapidly absorbed after oral administration. Tolcapone is highly bound to plasma albumin (>98%), and its distribution is therefore restricted. Tolcapone has low first-pass metabolism. It is almost completely metabolized in the liver before excretion, and 60% is excreted by the kidney. The major metabolite of tolcapone is an inactive glucuronide conjugate. COMT inhibitors increase chronotropic and arrhythmogenic effects of epinephrine.[52,53] Tolcapone is indicated as an adjunct to levodopa/carbidopa for the management of signs and symptoms of PD.

Entacapone. Entacapone, (*E*)-2-cyano-3-(3,4-dihydroxy-5-nitrophenyl)-*N*,*N*-diethyl-2-propenamide (Comtan), is a nitrocatechol that is practically insoluble in water (pK_a = 4.50). Entacapone is rapidly absorbed after oral administration and does not cross the BBB. Entacapone does not distribute widely into tissues because of its high plasma protein binding and it is completely metabolized before excretion. The main metabolic pathway is by isomerization to the *cis*-isomer followed by direct glucuronidation of the parent and the *cis*-isomer. The glucuronide conjugates are inactive. Entacapone is eliminated in the feces (90%) and urine (10%). Entacapone is indicated as an adjunct to levodopa/carbidopa to treat patients with idiopathic PD who experience the signs and symptoms of end-of-dose wearing off.

Carbidopa/Levodopa/Entacapone. Levodopa, carbidopa, and entacapone (Stalevo) are formulated together to take advantage of each compound's mechanism of action. When entacapone is coadministered with levodopa and carbidopa, plasma levels of levodopa are greater and more sustained.[23] For absorption, distribution, metabolism, and excretion (ADME) properties and drug interactions, refer to the preceding monograph.

Other Antiparkinsonian Drugs

Anticholinergic agents have been used in the early stages of PD, frequently with amantadine and selegiline. The most commonly employed anticholinergics are benztropine, trihexyphenidyl, orphenadrine, and procyclidine. These compounds are most useful for treating the tremor aspect of PD. Because most individuals with PD are elderly, anticholinergics may impair cognitive function. Additionally, anticholinergics may produce various side effects through blockade of peripheral muscarinic receptors.[21,26]

Amantadine has demonstrated beneficial effects in the treatment of PD, especially in attenuating dyskinesias.[26] Although amantadine has DA-releasing properties, other pharmacological mechanisms appear to be involved in its antiparkinsonian effect. The compound is a weak noncompetitive *N*-methyl D-aspartate (NMDA) antagonist, yet it differs in its action from the NMDA antagonist MK-801 in a rodent model of PD.[54] Additionally, amantadine potently inhibits nicotinic acetylcholine function in the hippocampus.[55]

Trihexyphenidyl   Benztropine   Amantadine

◆ ANTIPSYCHOTIC DRUGS

Psychotic illness is a compilation of multiple disorders, including schizophrenia, the manic phase of bipolar syndrome, acute idiopathic psychosis, and other conditions marked by severe agitation,[56] yet the term "psychosis" is most often associated with schizophrenia. Schizophrenia affects approximately 1% of the U.S. population,[57] with both genetic[58] and neurodevelopmental[59] implications. Schizophrenia is characterized by delusions, abnormal behaviors, hallucinations, and thought disorders (i.e., positive symptoms), as well as loss of normal emotions, abilities, and motivation (i.e., negative symptoms). Although the etiology of schizophrenia is unknown, the principal neurochemical theories focus on DA[60] and, more recently, on glutamate and serotonin.[61,62] Much of our current knowledge of the mechanisms involved in schizophrenia has come from analyzing effects of antipsychotic drugs.

The DA hypothesis of schizophrenia (DHS) has been the principal neurochemical theory of schizophrenia for more than 30 years. The basis of the DHS lies in the capacity of antipsychotic drugs to block DA receptors (D_2 receptor subtype) positively correlated to their clinical potency in alleviating the symptoms of schizophrenia.[60,63] Nevertheless, the observed inactivity of D_2-antagonists in some individuals with schizophrenia and the pharmacological independence of positive and negative symptoms indicate further level of complexity. Other variants of the DHS suggest an imbalance between dopaminergic pathways, which may be phasic in nature.[64,65] With regard to symptomology, it is thought that a dysregulation in the mesocortical DA pathway contributes to negative symptoms.[66,67] Positron emission tomography (PET) studies suggest that individuals with schizophrenia may have decreased densities of D_1 receptors in the prefrontal cortex.[68] Presynaptic D_1 receptors within the prefrontal cortex are believed to modulate glutamatergic activity, directly effecting working memory in individuals with schizophrenia.[69] The positive symptoms are believed to be derived from D_2 receptor hyperactivity or upregulation within the in mesolimbic pathway.[66,70] Although it remains uncertain as to exactly how the different dopaminergic pathways and DA receptor subtype activities mediate the positive and negative symptoms of schizophrenia, it is clear that DA is a critical mediator. Yet, other transmitters have also been implicated. Glutamate NMDA receptor antagonists (e.g., phencyclidine, ketamine) produce psychotic symptoms in humans. A combined glutamate and DA dysregulation has also been implicated with schizophrenia.[71] Likewise, serotonin has modulatory effects on DA pathways in the brain and has been implicated in the reduction of side effects induced by D_2 receptor antagonists.

Typical Antipsychotic Agents

Typical antipsychotics (also known as first-generation or conventional antipsychotics, classical neuroleptics, or major tranquilizers) are a class of antipsychotic drugs first developed in the 1950s and used to treat psychosis (in particular, schizophrenia). Typical antipsychotics include phenothiazines, thioxanthenes, butyrophenones, diphenylbutylpiperidines, and the dihydroindolones (e.g., molindone, not commercially available in the United States). The conventional antipsychotic drugs can be classified as high (haloperidol and fluphenazine) or low potency (chlorpromazine) based on their affinity for DA D$_2$ receptors and the average therapeutic dose.[72] This group of antipsychotics is also associated with a significant degree of EPS. Some EPS are defined as acute dystonias (i.e., involuntary movements: muscle spasms, protruding tongue), which tend to occur within the first few weeks of treatment and decline over time. However, the EPS that is most widely associated with these drugs is tardive dyskinesia (i.e., impairment of voluntary movements, often in the face and tongue), which develops over months to years and is often irreversible. High-potency typical antipsychotics tend to be associated with more EPS and less histaminic (sedation), alpha adrenergic (orthostasis), and anticholinergic (dry mouth) side effects. Low-potency typical antipsychotics are associated with less EPS but more H1, α_1, and muscarinic side effects. Currently, the only patients in which the typical antipsychotic agents are preferred are those for whom there is a clear indication for short- or long-acting injectable preparations, and/or a tolerance to the side effects.

Phenothiazines and Thioxanthenes

The phenothiazine nucleus was first synthesized in 1876 (methylene blue) by Badische Anilin und Soda Fabrik (BASF) chemist H. Caro and elucidated by A. Bernstein in 1883 (thiodiphenylamine). It was not until 1950 that chlorpromazine (Table 13.1) was synthesized to explore its antihistaminic properties. The observations on the side effects of chlorpromazine prompted French psychiatrists Delay, Denicker, and Harl to use it in schizophrenic patients, publishing their seminal paper in 1952.[73] In 1958, Petersen et al.[74,75] synthesized the first thioxanthene. The structural difference with the phenothiazines is the bioisosteric replacement of the *N* at the 10-position for a carbon atom in the thioxanthenes. The side chain (R10) in the thioxanthenes is attached by a double bond to the tricyclic system. This portion of the molecule is not involved in the interaction with the receptor, but it serves to position correctly the other elements of the molecule. Thioxanthenes that have a double bond in the side chain can be either *cis*- or *trans*-isomers (Fig. 13.5).[76,77] The active form is the *cis*-isomer, which can be perfectly superimposed with the phenothiazine and the DA molecules, meaning that the Z-configuration is the preferred one for optimal receptor affinity. In general, thioxanthenes are more potent than the structurally related phenothiazines.

STRUCTURE–ACTIVITY RELATIONSHIPS

The SAR of phenothiazines is relatively simple because only position 2 (ring A) and the side chain afford active antipsychotic molecules. Conformational studies on chlorpromazine reveal that tilting of the side chain toward ring A allows favorable van der Waals interactions of the side chain with the chlorine substituent.[78] The resulting conformation permits the superimposition of DA. Substitution at the 1-position sterically hinders the ability of the side chain to approach ring A. On the other hand, a substituent at the 3-position will be too far from the side chain to provide van der Waals attractions. A trifluoromethyl group will give more van der Waals contacts with the side chain than a chloro substituent and, in fact, triflupromazine is more potent than chlorpromazine (Table 13.1). As a general rule, electron-withdrawing groups at the 2-position increase the antipsychotic efficacy (chlorpromazine vs. promazine).

In the thioxanthenes, the substituent at the 2-position does not govern the side chain in the same way as with the phenothiazines to assume a DA-like conformation.[79] The *cis* or *trans* conformation of unsubstituted thioxanthenes does not show any differential potency. For thioxanthenes, the 2-substituent of the *cis* form provides a closer approximation of the side chain toward ring A, enabling the substituent to enter into the van der Waals attractive forces with the side chain.[78,80,81]

A major requirement for the antipsychotic activity of phenothiazines is that the basic amino group be separated by three carbon atoms from the parent ring system. Molecular models indicate that a shorter or a branched side chain prohibits the assumption of the DA-like conformation caused by van der Waals repulsive forces between the side chain and the phenothiazine ring. The nature of the substituent on the side chain amine may also influence the conformation of the phenothiazine side chain. A piperazine ring affords more van der Waals contacts with the 2-substituent than does an alkylamino side chain. Piperazinyl phenothiazines are more potent in their antischizophrenic effects, their ability to elicit EPS, and their affinity for the DA-sensitive adenylate cyclase than alkylamino phenothiazines.[78,82]

PHARMACOKINETIC PROPERTIES

In general, these classes of drugs are rapidly absorbed from the GI tract (Table 13.1), but there is considerable individual patient variation in peak plasma concentrations.[83] Chlorpromazine has been the most widely studied phenothiazine, and it is believed that thioxanthenes and phenothiazines are metabolized following a very similar pathway. Compared with the phenothiazines, the thioxanthenes are less likely to form phenolic metabolites.[84] Chlorpromazine undergoes extensive first-pass metabolism yielding numerous metabolites. Numerous sites of attack by microsomal CYP450 system (especially CYP2D6) are possible, and most of these reactions happen to various degrees.[85,86] Several metabolites have been isolated and characterized. Phase I reactions include oxidative *N*-demethylation to give primary and secondary amines, aromatic hydroxylation that yields phenols, side chain tertiary amine oxidation that affords *N*-oxide metabolites, *S*-oxidation to give sulfoxide and sulfones, oxidative deamination that yields side chain carboxylic acids, and *N*-10 dealkylation to give chlorophenothiazine. Most of these metabolites are subject of further reactions similar to those already mentioned. From the 168 proposed metabolites, only 45 have been isolated, and the 7-hydroxy-chlorpromazine metabolite has been evaluated and found to be effective in schizophrenia. More recently, the sulfoxide metabolite was found to have a diminished therapeutic response.[87,88] Excretion is primarily via the kidneys with less than 1% of a dose excreted unchanged in the urine and 20% to 70% as conjugated or unconjugated metabolites. Approximately 5% of a dose is excreted in feces via biliary elimination. Some metabolites can still be detected up to 18 months after discontinuation of long-term therapy.

SPECIFIC AGENTS

Chlorpromazine Hydrochloride, USP. Chlorpromazine hydrochloride, 2-chloro-10-[3-(dimethylamino)propyl]phenothiazine (Thorazine), is a white to slightly creamy white, odorless, bitter tasting, crystalline powder (pK$_a$ = 9.43). The

TABLE 13.1 Structure and Pharmacokinetic Properties of Phenothiazines and Thioxanthenes

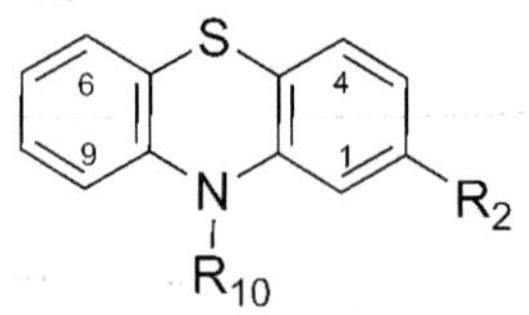

Name	R_2	R_{10}	log P	Absorption %[89]	PPB %[89]	Half-life (h)[89]
Promazine	H		5.37	Erratic*	94	
Chlorpromazine	Cl			40*	98	8–35
Thioridazine	SCH$_3$			60	95	21–25
Perphenazine	Cl			40		8–12
Prochlorperazine	Cl				91–99	6–8
Fluphenazine	CF$_3$			40–50	90	4–12
Trifluoperazine	CF$_3$			erratic	91–99	4–12
Chlorprothixene						17–24
Thiothixene			3.9	Erratic	91–99	3.5–34

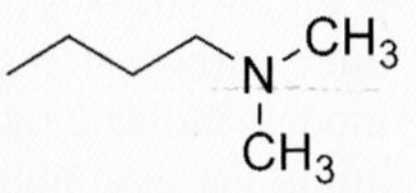

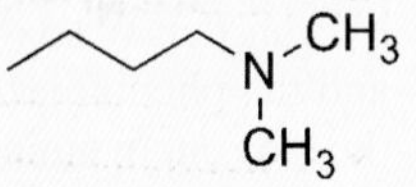

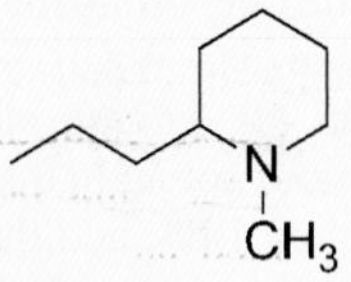

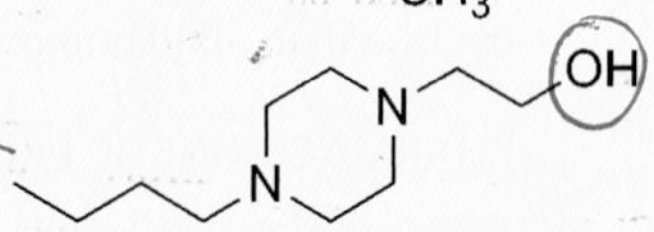

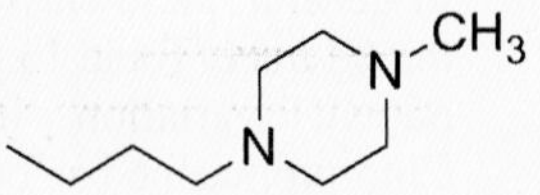

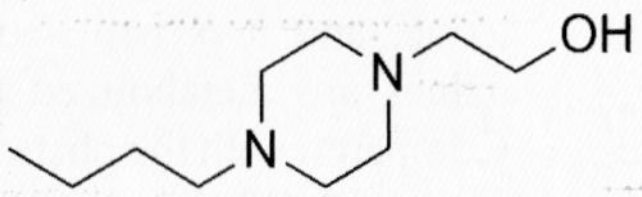

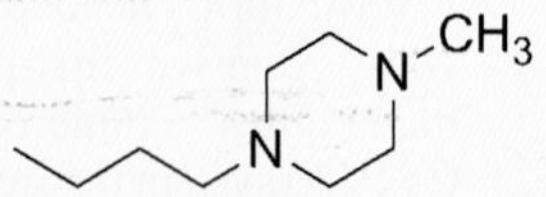

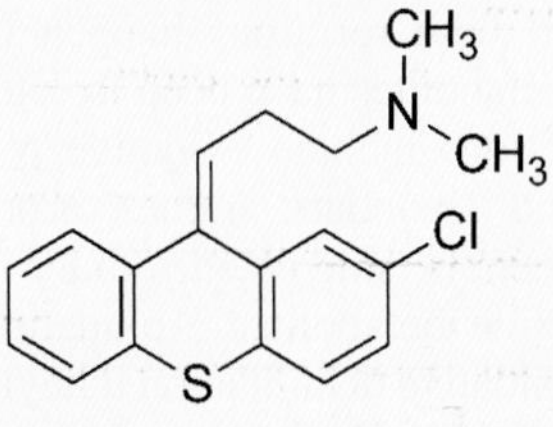

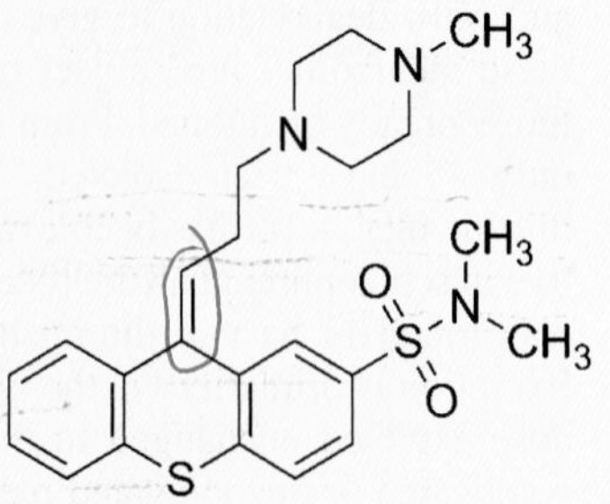

*Erratic because of variable metabolism in the intestinal wall and liver (marked first-pass effect).
PPB %, percentage of plasma protein binding.

drug has significant sedative and hypotensive properties, possibly reflecting central and peripheral α_1-adrenergic blocking activity, respectively. As with the other phenothiazines, the effects of the other CNS-depressant drugs, such as sedatives and anesthetics, can be potentiated.[90] Chlorpromazine is a minor substrate of CYP1A2 and 3A4 and a major substrate of CYP2D6.[91] Chlorpromazine also is a strong inhibitor of CYP2D6 and a weak inhibitor of CYP2E1. Inhibitors of the CYP2D6 enzyme may increase the levels/effects of chlorpromazine and chlorpromazine may increase the levels/effects of CYP2D6 substrates. Chlorpromazine may also decrease the bioactivation of CYP2D6 prodrug substrates.[91]

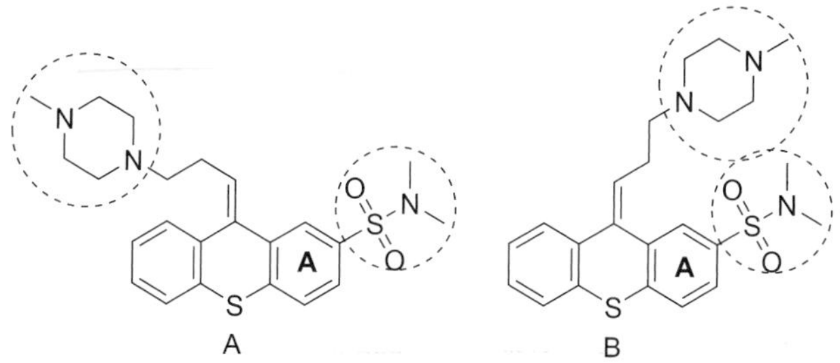

Figure 13.5 ◆ *Trans*-(A) versus *cis*-(B) isomers in the thiothixenes.

Chlorpromazine has strong anticholinergic and sedative effects and is a potent antiemetic. It is considered a low-potency neuroleptic agent and therefore the associated incidence of EPS is low. The incidence of sedative, anticholinergic, and cardiovascular side effects is high, however. It is indicated for the symptomatic relief of nausea, vomiting, hiccups, and porphyria; for preoperative sedation; and for the treatment of psychotic disorders.

Thioridazine Hydrochloride, USP. Thioridazine hydrochloride, 10-[2-(1-methyl-2-piperidyl)ethyl]-2-(methylthio)phenothiazine (Mellaril), is a member of the piperidine subgroup of the phenothiazines. Thioridazine occurs as a white or slightly yellow, crystalline or micronized powder, which is odorless or has a faint odor and is practically insoluble in water and freely soluble in dehydrated alcohol ($pK_a = 9.66$). Thioridazine has relatively low tendency to produce EPS. The drug has sedative and hypotensive activity in common with chlorpromazine and less antiemetic activity. At high doses, pigmentary retinopathy has been observed. Thioridazine has similar activity toward the CYP450 family of enzymes as chlorpromazine. Thioridazine is indicated for the treatment of schizophrenic patients who fail to respond adequately to treatment with other antipsychotic drugs.

Perphenazine, USP. Perphenazine, 2-[4-[3-(2-chloro-10H-phenothiazin-10-yl)propyl]piperazin-1-yl]ethanol. Perphenazine is a minor substrate of CYP1A2, 2C9, 2C19, and 3A4 and a major substrate for 2D6. Perphenazine is indicated for use in the management of the manifestations of psychotic disorders and for the control of severe nausea and vomiting in adults.

Trifluoperazine Hydrochloride, USP. Trifluoperazine hydrochloride, 10-[3-(4-Methyl-1-piperazinyl)propyl-[2-(trifluoromethyl)phenothiazine dihydrochloride (Stelazine). The absorption of trifluoperazine is erratic and variable and it is widely distributed into tissues. The excretion of trifluoperazine occurs 50% via kidneys and the other 50% is through enterohepatic circulation. The metabolism and drug interactions of trifluoperazine are the same as with the other phenothiazines. Trifluoperazine does not show any specific drug interactions. Trifluoperazine is indicated for the management of schizophrenia and short-term treatment of nonpsychotic anxiety.

Thiothixene, USP. Thiothixene, N,N-dimethyl-9-[3-(4-methyl-1-piperazinyl)propylidene]thioxanthene-2-sulfonamide (Navane). The absorption of thiothixene is erratic because of its high lipophilicity. Thiothixene is

$\log P \approx 3.9$

widely distributed into tissues and it is more than 90% bound to plasma proteins. Thiothixene has a similar metabolic pathway as the phenothiazines. Thiothixene is a major substrate of CYP1A2, and CYP1A2 inducers may decrease the levels/effects of thiothixene, whereas CYP1A2 inhibitors may increase the levels/effects of thiothixene. Thiothixene is also a weak inhibitor of CYP2D6. As with other antipsychotic agents, some patients who are resistant to previous medications have responded favorably to thiothixene. Thioxanthenes may also be of value in the management of withdrawn, apathetic schizophrenic patients.

BUTYROPHENONES AND RELATED STRUCTURES

Haloperidol was discovered by Janssen Laboratories (1958) as a byproduct while they were investigating analgesics structurally related to meperidine.[73] The behavioral profile of haloperidol was found to be very similar to that of chlorpromazine, but the required dose was about 50-fold less to exert the same behavioral effect. It was rapidly studied and pursued as a new drug. Soon after, Janssen Laboratories discovered and developed droperidol, another butyrophenone analog. Conformationally, the butyrophenones can assume a conformation resembling portions of the phenothiazine molecule. The three-carbon side chain of the phenothiazines may be analogous to the three-carbon bridge that separates the amino function from the carbonyl moiety of haloperidol. Moreover, the piperidine ring would correspond to the side chain amine or piperazine of the phenothiazines. After the introduction of haloperidol and droperidol, a great number of SAR studies were carried out.[92] As for the pharmacophore of the butyrophenones (Fig. 13.6), it is known that a tertiary amino group at the fourth carbon as well as the *para*-substituted (F is preferred) phenyl ring at the 1-position are required for D_2 affinity.[93,94] Possible variations on the butyrophenone group are at the piperidine moiety, in particular at the 4-position of the ring. Modifications by lengthening, shortening, or branching of the three-carbon propyl chain decrease neuroleptic activity. Replacement of the keto group also decreases D_2 affinity. The tertiary amino group is usually part of an N-containing heterocycles, preferably a piperidine ring. Replacement of the six-member basic ring by smaller or larger heterocyclic rings or by noncyclic amines decreases DA affinity.

Conformationally restricted butyrophenones also possess high D_2 affinity. Haloperidol and droperidol are the only butyrophenones currently commercially available in the United States. Replacement of the keto group for a di-4-fluorophenylmethane moiety produced diphenylbutylpiperidines, another class of neuroleptics. Pimozide, the prototype of this group of drugs, is structurally related to droperidol and is the only member commercially available within the diphenylbutylpiperidines class.

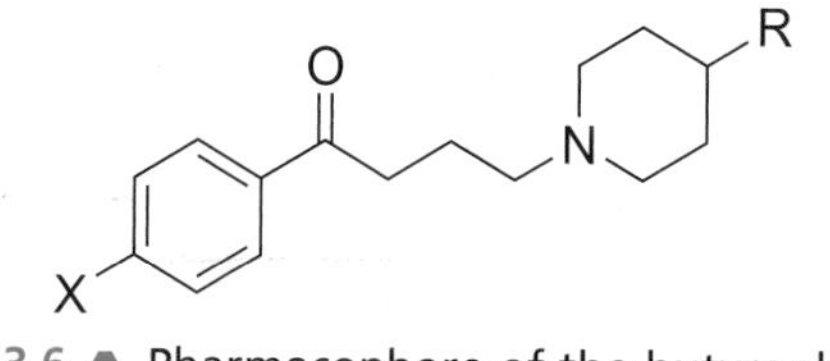

Figure 13.6 ◆ Pharmacophore of the butyrophenones.

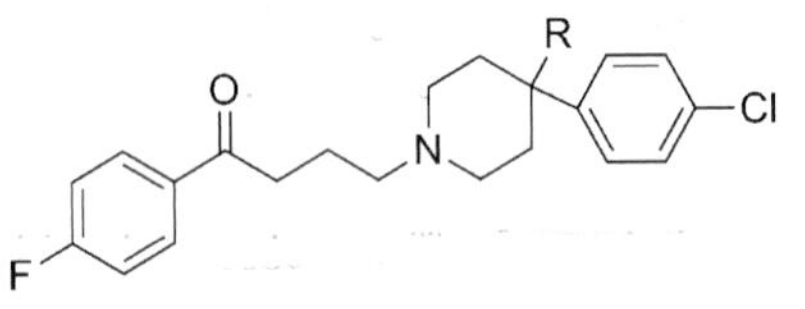

R = OH, Haloperidol
R = OCO(CH$_2$)$_8$CH$_3$, Haloperidol decanoate

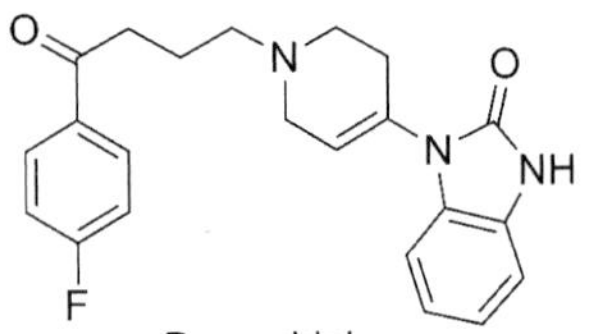

Droperidol

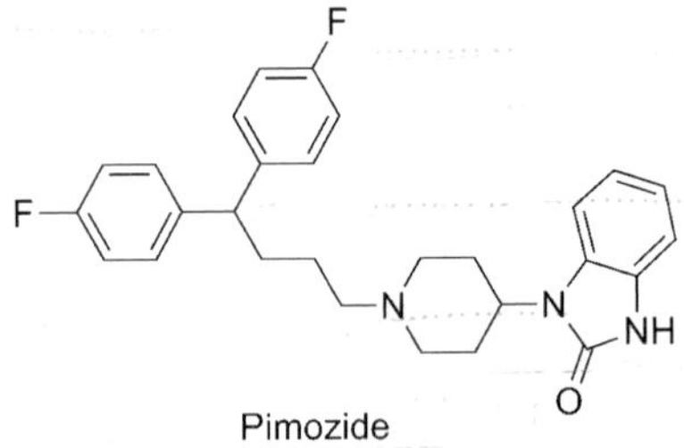

Pimozide

PHARMACOKINETIC PROPERTIES

Haloperidol is the prototype of the butyrophenones and the one that has been studied the most. Haloperidol and droperidol, the two butyrophenones available in the United States, are well absorbed from the GI tract.[83] First-pass metabolism in the liver reduces the bioavailability of haloperidol to approximately 60%. Haloperidol undergoes extensive metabolism including N-dealkylation, reduction, oxidation, and N-oxidation. Most of the metabolites of haloperidol are inactive. Hydroxyhaloperidol, the reduced (ketone) metabolite of haloperidol, is the only active metabolite and it is also subject to extensive hepatic metabolism (Fig. 13.7).[83,95]

SPECIFIC AGENTS

Haloperidol, USP. Haloperidol, 4-[4-(p-chlorophenyl)-4-hydroxypiperidino]-4-fluorobutyrophenone (Haldol), is an odorless white to yellow crystalline powder. Haloperidol is well and rapidly absorbed and has a high bioavailability. It is more than 90% bound to plasma proteins. Haloperidol is excreted slowly in the urine and feces. About 30% of a dose is excreted in urine and about 20% of a dose in feces via biliary elimination,[96] and only 1% of a dose is excreted as unchanged drug in the urine.[97] Haloperidol is a minor substrate of CYP1A2 and a major substrate of CYP2D6 and CYP3A4. CYP2D6 inhibitors may increase the levels/effects of haloperidol.[91] Haloperidol may increase the levels/effects of CYP2D6 substrates[98] and it may decrease the bioactivation of CYP2D6 prodrugs substrates. Haloperidol also is a moderate inhibitor of CYP2D6 and CYP3A4. CYP3A4 inducers may decrease the levels/effects of haloperidol, whereas CYP3A4 inhibitors may increase the levels/effects of haloperidol. Centrally acting acetylcholinesterase inhibitors may increase the risk of antipsychotic-related EPS. The precise mechanism of antipsychotic action is unclear but is considered to be associated with the potent DA D$_2$ receptor–blocking activity in the mesolimbic system and the resulting adaptive changes in the brain. Haloperidol is used primarily for the long-term treatment of psychosis and is especially useful in patients who are noncompliant with their drug treatment.

Haloperidol Decanoate. Haloperidol decanoate, 4-[4-(4-chlorophenyl)-4-hydroxypiperidino]-4-fluorobutyrophenone decanoate (Haldol Decanoate), is the decanoate ester (prodrug) of haloperidol. Peak plasma concentrations occur within 3 to 9 days and then decrease slowly. Haloperidol decanoate has no intrinsic activity. Haloperidol decanoate

4-(4-chlorophenyl)piperidin-4-ol

4-(4-chlorophenyl)-1-(4-(4-fluorophenyl)-4-oxobutyl)pyridinium

Haloperidol

Hydroxyhaloperidol

4-(4-chlorophenyl)-1-(4-(4-fluorophenyl)-4-hydroxybutyl)pyridinium

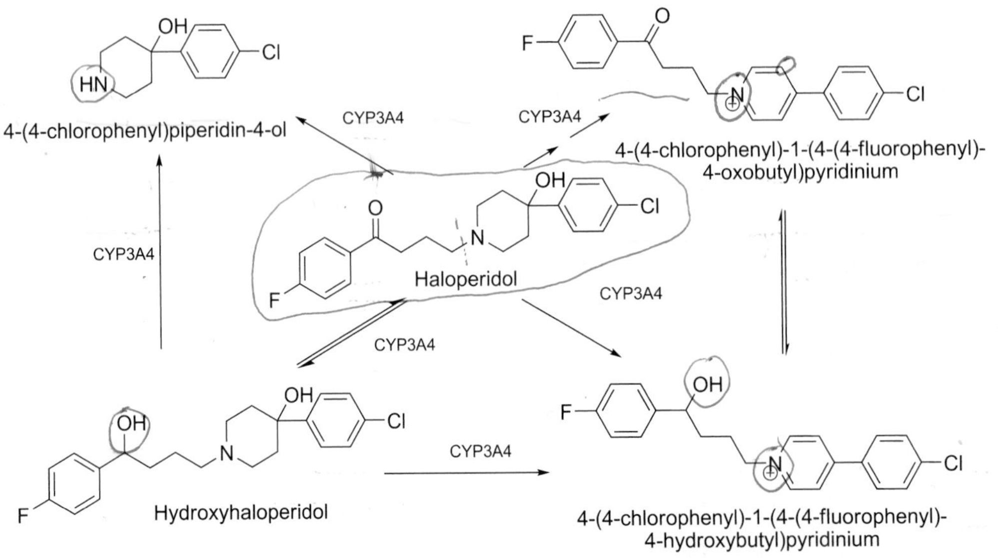

Figure 13.7 ● Metabolic pathway for haloperidol.

undergoes hydrolysis by plasma and/or tissue esterases to form haloperidol and decanoic acid, subsequently; haloperidol is metabolized in the liver. The pharmacological effects are those of haloperidol, which is released by bioconversion. Haloperidol decanoate is indicated for the treatment of long-term maintenance in schizophrenia, psychoses especially paranoid, and other mental and behavioral problems.

Droperidol, USP. Droperidol, 1-1-[3-(*p*-fluorobenzoyl)propyl]-1,2,[3,6-tetrahydro-4-pyridyl]-2-benzimidazolinone (Inapsine). Centrally acting acetylcholinesterase inhibitors may increase the risk of antipsychotic-related EPS. CNS depressants may produce additive sedative effects (benzodiazepines, barbiturates, antipsychotics, ethanol, opiates, and other sedative medications). Droperidol in combination with certain forms of inhalation anesthetics may produce peripheral vasodilatation and hypotension. Metoclopramide may increase the risk of EPS produced by droperidol.

Pimozide, USP. Pimozide, 1-[1-[4,4-*bis*(*p*-fluorophenyl)butyl]-4-piperidyl]-2-benzimidazolinone (Orap), is a white to creamy white solid ($pK_a = 9.42$). Pimozide is 50% absorbed after oral administration. It is metabolized by CYP450 enzymes, in particular the CYP3A4 and CYP1A2 isozymes, to inactive metabolites. Pimozide is excreted in the urine and to a lesser extent in the feces. Toxic effects may be produced with pimozide in the presence of inducers or inhibitors of CYP3A4 and CYP1A2. Pimozide is also a strong inhibitor of CYP2D6 without appearing to be an important substrate of this isoform.[99] The use of pimozide in the United States is small, but it is a critical drug for many patients with Gilles de la Tourette disorder who cannot tolerate haloperidol.

Atypical Antipsychotic Agents

Atypical antipsychotics (also known as second-generations) include drugs such as clozapine, olanzapine, quetiapine, risperidone, aripiprazole, and ziprasidone. With the development of the first atypical antipsychotic, clozapine, a clear division in treatment outcomes was observed. Atypical antipsychotics have generally shown to provide a greater reduction in both the positive and negative symptoms of schizophrenia, as well as an improvement in cognitive function. Thus, atypical antipsychotics are currently considered to be the first line of treatment for individuals with schizo-

phrenia. Affinity for 5-HT_{2A} receptors is a feature of several of the recently developed atypical antipsychotics. Many researchers believe that D_2 receptor antagonism, coupled with 5-HT_{2A} receptor antagonism, is responsible for the differentiation of effects observed with atypical antipsychotics. Inhibitory 5-HT neurons terminate on presynaptic DA neurons in the striatum. Thus, antagonism of presynaptic 5-HT_{2A} receptors leads to an increase in DA release. This increase in DA release is thought to attenuate D_2 blockade caused by antipsychotics. The decreased EPS associated with some of the atypical antipsychotics has also been suggested to be caused by 5-HT_{2A} receptor blockade.[100] Nevertheless, high 5-HT_{2A} receptor occupancy does not ensure that an antipsychotic will exhibit an atypical profile. Even at 80% to 90% 5-HT_{2A} receptor occupancy, no antipsychotic effect is observed unless D_2 receptor occupancy exceeds the 65% threshold.[101,102]

Other theories regarding the mechanisms of action of atypical antipsychotics have also been suggested. Kapur and Seeman[101] proposed that a low occupancy of D_2 receptors is sufficient to account for an atypical action. These investigators have suggested that a fast dissociation rate from D_2 receptors allows for DA neurotransmission that is more physiological. Yet, this theory has been questioned because several typical antipsychotics dissociate at similar rates as atypical agents.[103] The atypical profile of clozapine was initially suggested to be related to its high affinity for D_4 receptors; however, classical antipsychotics such as chlorpromazine and haloperidol also bind with high affinity at the D_4 receptor (Table 13.2). Additionally, the atypical antipsychotic, quetiapine, has no appreciable affinity for the D_4 receptor. Thus, it seems that antagonism at the D_4 receptor cannot explain the unique profile of atypical antipsychotics.[104,105] In the end, no single theory to date has been able to globally define and/or differentiate the actions of antipsychotics. This is as much caused by the complexity of the disease and interpretation of respective drug-mediated behavioral effects, as it is to determining the actual mechanism of action of any individual drug.

SPECIFIC AGENTS

Clozapine. Clozapine, 8-chloro-11-(4-methyl-1-piperazinyl) 5*H*-dibenzo[b,e] [1,4] diazepine (Clozaril), is a yellow crystalline powder that is only slightly soluble in water. With the introduction of clozapine, a different pharmacological

TABLE 13.2 Affinity Data for Antipsychotics

Compound	D2*	D3*	D4*	HT_{1A}#	HT_{2A}*
Chlorpromazine	4.80	1.8	9.5	3,100.0	2.8
Clozapine	180.00	270.0	22.0	105.0	5.2
Fluphenazine	1.20	0.2	30.00	145.0	5.8
Haloperidol	2.90	15.0	2.0	1,202.0	103.0
Olanzapine	21.0	23.0	14.0	2,063.0	4.9
Quetiapine	680.0	520.0	2,000.0	431.0	200.0
Risperidone	4.0	3.6	4.4	427.0	0.19
Trifluoperazine	3.8	0.95	39.0	950.0	12.0
Ziprasidone	2.6		>1,000.0	76.0	0.31
Aripiprazole				5.6	

Receptor binding profiles were generously provided by the National Institute of Mental Health's Psychoactive Drug Screening Program, Contract # NO1MH32004 (NIMH PDSP). The NIMH PDSP is directed by Bryan L. Roth MD, PhD at the University of North Carolina at Chapel Hill and Project Officer Jamie Driscol at NIMH, Bethesda MD, USA.

*Hot ligand: 3*H*-Spiperone.
#Hot ligand: 3*H*-8-OH-DPAT.

profile was observed compared with the classical antipsychotics.[106] Unlike typical antipsychotics, clozapine is largely devoid of EPS. The lack of EPS with this compound was postulated to be caused by its preferential binding to mesolimbic rather than striatal DA receptors.[107] Furthermore, clozapine was shown to exhibit potent affinity for 5-HT$_{2A}$ receptors.[108] When administered at a dose of 100 mg twice a day (bid [L. *bis in die*]), an average steady state plasma concentration of 319 ng/mL resulted at an average of 2.5 hours after administration. Because food does not apparently affect absorption, clozapine may be given with or without food. The compound is 97% bound to plasma proteins; however, interactions with other drugs have not been fully investigated.[23] Clozapine is extensively metabolized after absorption with 50% of an administered dose excreted in the urine and 30% in the feces. Clozapine is metabolized to two major metabolites by *N*-oxidation and *N*-demethylation. Clozapine *N*-oxide (CZNO) is thought to be formed by the action of CYP3A4 and flavin monooxygenase 3 (FMO3), whereas *N*-desmethyl-clozapine (DMCZ) appears to result by the action of CYP3A4 and CYP1A2 (Fig. 13.8).[109] Clozapine also binds with high affinity at M_1 and M_4 muscarinic receptors in the limbic area of the brain.[104] Whether affinity for muscarinic receptors contributes to the atypical profile for clozapine has not been established.[103]

DMCZ shows partial agonism at D_2 and D_3 receptors and exhibits a distinctly different pharmacological profile compared with clozapine and other atypical antipsychotics. Unlike clozapine, which is a potent M_1 muscarinic antagonist, DMCZ is a potent M_1 agonist. Agonism at muscarinic receptors has been proposed to be useful for impaired cognition in schizophrenia. Burnstein et al.[110] found that DMCZ acted as a partial agonist at DA D_2 and D_3 receptors. These investigators suggested that the low incidence of EPS associated with clozapine may be caused by the partial agonism of DMCZ at D_2 and D_3 receptors. Thus, DMCZ may be of interest as an atypical antipsychotic with an improved side effect profile compared with clozapine.

Although clozapine demonstrates a favorable pharmacological profile compared with typical antipsychotics, its use is restricted by a relatively high incidence of agranulocytosis. The exact mechanism for the cause of agranulocytosis has not been confirmed, but a highly reactive nitrenium ion that is formed by the action of hepatic enzymes appears to be involved.[111] The mean elimination half-life of clozapine

following a single 75-mg dose is 8 hours. Because of several adverse effects, clozapine is only used in refractory cases of schizophrenia. Individuals with a history of seizures or predisposed to seizures should be cautioned when taking clozapine. Similar to other atypical antipsychotic agents, clozapine causes an increased risk of mortality in elderly individuals with dementia-related psychoses.[23]

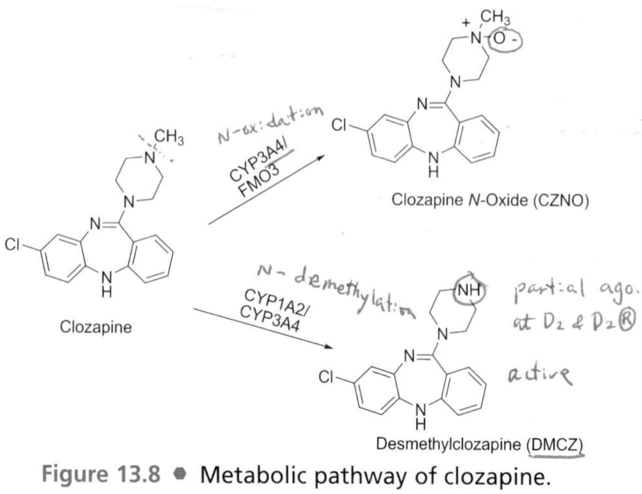

Olanzapine. Olanzapine, 2-methyl-4-(4-methyl-1-piperazinyl)-10*H*-thieno[2,3-b][1,5] benzodiazepine (Zyprexa), is a yellow crystalline solid that is essentially insoluble in water. Olanzapine orally disintegrating tablets (Zyprexa Zydis) is a solid dosage form that immediately disintegrates when exposed to saliva. This product is useful for elderly patients who have difficulty in swallowing. An injectable form, olanzapine for injection (Zyprexa IM), is indicated for agitation associated with schizophrenia or bipolar I mania. Olanzapine is combined with fluoxetine (Symbyax) for use in depression that is associated with bipolar I disorder. Peak concentrations of oral olanzapine are reached at 6 hours after oral administration, and absorption of the compound is not affected by food.[23] Olanzapine is 93% bound to plasma proteins, and its mean half-life is 27 hours.[112,113] Olanzapine undergoes extensive first-pass metabolism, and about 40% of an oral dose is metabolized prior to reaching the systemic circulation. The major metabolite of olanzapine in human subjects is the 10-*N*-glucuronide. Other human metabolites that have identified include the *N*-desmethyl, the *N*-oxide, and the 2-hydroxymethyl metabolites (Fig. 13.9). The *N*-desmethyl and the 2-hydroxymethyl metabolites are products of CYP1A2 and CYP2D6 action, respectively.[112,113]

Olanzapine binds with high affinity at DA D_2, 5-HT$_{2A}$, 5-HT$_{2C}$, 5-HT$_6$, α_1, and H_1 histamine receptors. The effects of olanzapine for the treatment of schizophrenia are presumably mediated through antagonism at D_2 and 5-HT$_{2A}$ receptors.[23,112,113] The use of olanzapine in acute mania that is associated with bipolar I disorder is thought to be mediated by antagonism at D_2 and other monamine receptors. Additionally, olanzapine is postulated to produce its mood stabilizing and antidepressant effects through 5-HT$_{2A}$ receptor blockade and increased cortical DA and NE concentrations.[114] Several studies have investigated the effect of olanzapine-induced weight gain and new-onset type 2 diabetes.[115,116] In a comparison study with risperidone, olanzapine was shown to have a greater risk of producing dyslipidemia and type 2 diabetes.[105,116]

Quetiapine. Quetiapine, 2-[2-(4-dibenzo[b,f][1,4]thiazepin-11-yl-1-piperazinyl)ethoxy]-ethanol fumarate (2:1, salt) (Seroquel), is a white to off-white crystalline powder that is moderately water soluble. Quetiapine is rapidly absorbed, and peak plasma levels occur 1 to 2 hours after administration. Food does not appreciably affect the absorption of quetiapine. The compound is 83% bound to plasma proteins and it has a mean elimination half-life of 7 hours. Administration of a single dose of ^{14}C-quetiapine showed that only 1% of the drug was excreted unchanged, with 73% excreted into the urine and approximately 30% excreted in the feces.[23] Numerous metabolites of quetiapine are known, and the sulfoxide metabolite represents the major metabolite present in plasma (Fig. 13.10). This metabolite is pharmacologically inactive. The remaining metabolites represent only 5% of the total radioactivity found in plasma. The 7-hydroxy and the 7-hydroxy-*N*-desalkyl are active metabolites, but

Figure 13.8 ● Metabolic pathway of clozapine.

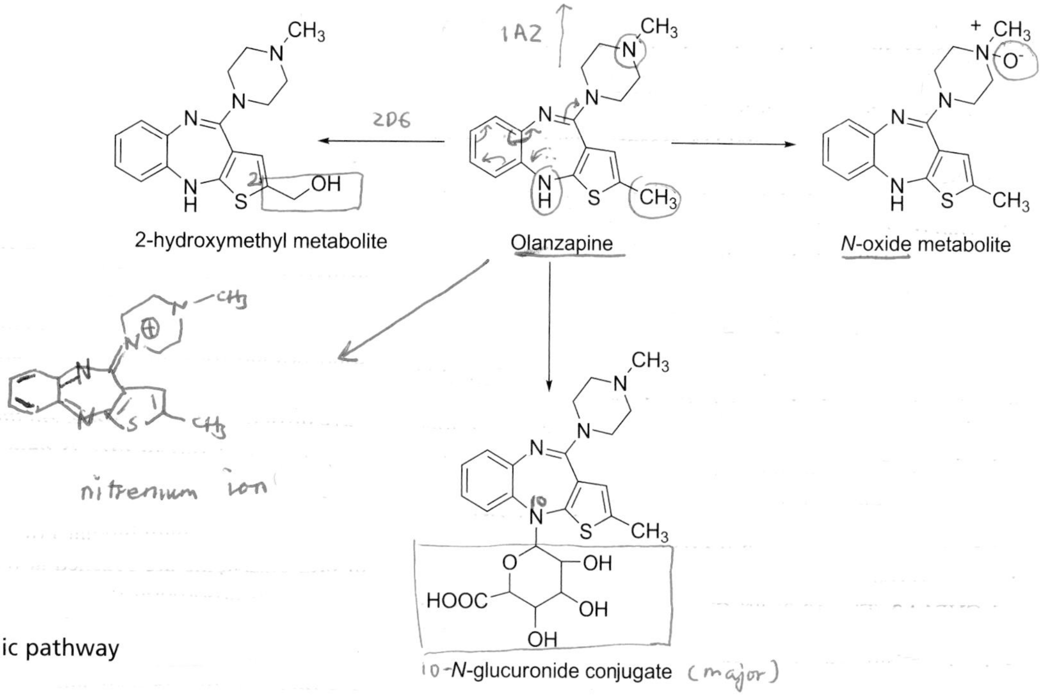

Figure 13.9 ● Metabolic pathway of olanzapine.

because of their low concentrations in plasma are not thought to contribute to the overall effects of quetiapine.[107,117]

In human liver microsomes, four primary metabolites of quetiapine are formed. These include quetiapine sulfoxide, 7-hydroxyquetiapine, and the *N*- and *O*-desalkylated metabolites (Fig. 13.10). This study showed that CYP3A4 is the major isoform of P450 responsible for quetiapine metabolism. CYP3A4 inducers (carbamazepine) or CYP3A4 inhibitors (ketoconazole) can either decrease or increase plasma levels of quetiapine.[118]

Common side effects associated with quetiapine therapy are orthostatic hypotension and somnolence. These effects are presumably caused by α-adrenergic and histamine H_1 receptor blockade, respectively. As with other atypical antipsychotics, patients treated with quetiapine should be monitored for hyperglycemic symptoms. Also, children and adolescents with major depressive disorder may experience an increase in their depression or suicidal tendencies.[23,107] Quetiapine binds with high affinity at α_1, α_2, H_1, and 5-HT$_{2A}$ receptors but has much lower affinity for D_2 and 5-HT$_{1A}$ receptors. The action of quetiapine at D_2 and 5-HT$_{2A}$ receptors is that of an antagonist, whereas it shows agonist effects at 5-HT$_{1A}$ receptors.[119,120] Quetiapine dissociates rapidly from D_2 receptors, and this leads to lower D_2 receptor occupancy compared with

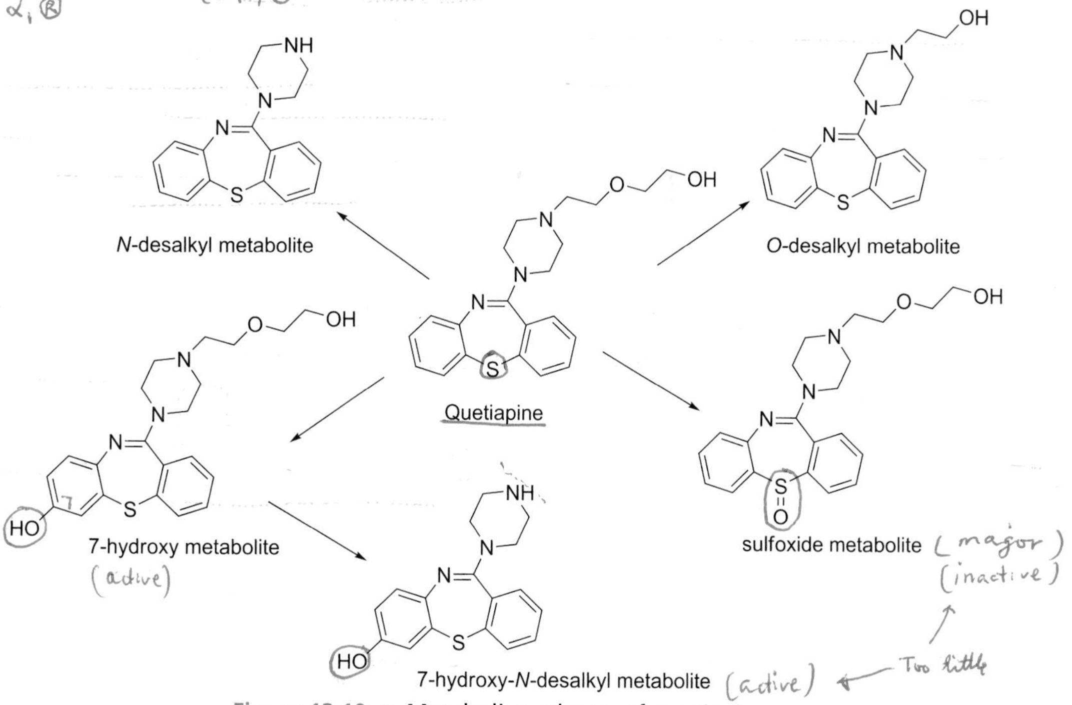

Figure 13.10 ● Metabolic pathway of quetiapine.

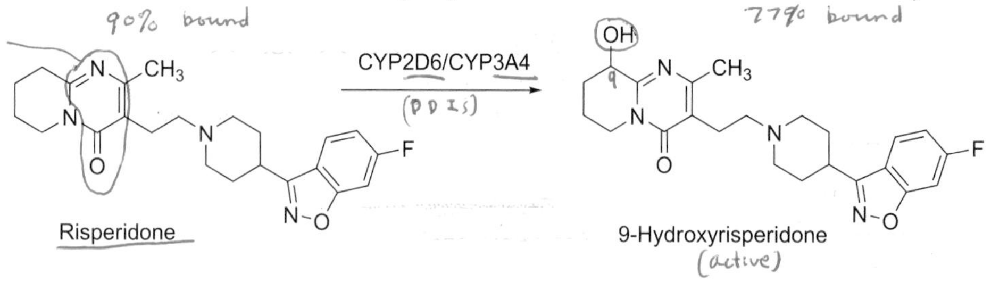

Figure 13.11 • Metabolic pathway of risperidone.

typical antipsychotics such as chlorpromazine.[121] This finding may explain the lack of EPS associated with quetiapine.[107]

Risperidone. Risperidone, 3-[2-[4-(6-fluoro-1,2-benzisoxazol-3-yl)-1-piperidinyl]ethyl-6,7,8,9-tetrahydro-2-methyl-4*H*-pyrido[1,2]pyrimidin-4-one (Risperdal), is a white to slightly beige powder that is essentially insoluble in water. Risperidone is also available as a 1-mg/mL oral solution and as orally disintegrating tablets (Risperdal M-Tab). Risperidone is well absorbed, and peak levels occur about 1 hour after administration. The absorption of risperidone is not affected by food. Risperidone is about 90% bound to albumin and α_1-acid glycoprotein, whereas its metabolite 9-hydroxyrisperidone is bound about 77%.[23] Risperidone is primarily metabolized in humans to the active metabolite 9-hydroxyrisperidone (Fig. 13.11). Although CYP2D6 was thought to be the major P450 isoform in the formation of the 9-hydroxy metabolite, a recent report suggests that CYP3A4 is involved.[121] The potent CYP3A4 inducer, rifampin, was shown to significantly reduce plasma concentrations of risperidone,[122] whereas ketoconazole, a CYP3A4 inhibitor, decreased the formation of the 9-hydroxy metabolite.[123] The metabolism of risperidone appears to be stereoselective. In human microsomes, the CYP2D6 inhibitor, quinidine, strongly inhibited the formation of (+)-9-hydroxyrisperidone, whereas the CYP3A4 inhibitor, ketoconazole, inhibited the formation of (−)-9-hydroxyrisperidone.[124] Individuals concurrently on risperidone and other medications should be carefully monitored because impaired CYP2D6 activity could increase the risk for drug interactions.[125,126] Renal excretion is the main route of elimination for risperidone and its metabolites. The mean half-life of risperidone is 3 hours in extensive metabolizers and 21 hours in poor metabolizers, respectively. The elimination half-life for the 9-hydroxy metabolite is similar to risperidone in extensive and poor metabolizers, with an overall elimination half-life of about 20 hours.[23] The major side effects associated with risperidone therapy are orthostatic hypotension, dose-related hyperprolactinemia, mild weight gain, EPS, and insomnia.[127] At higher doses (6 mg/day), risperidone is the atypical antipsychotic that most closely resembles conventional agents. A PET study in a group of individuals with schizophrenia showed that D_2 receptor occupancy was dose dependent. If the dose was increased such that D_2 receptor occupancy was 79% to 85%, the majority of patients developed EPS.[126] Risperidone is associated with increased mortality in elderly patients with dementia-related psychosis and is not recommended for these individuals.[23] Risperidone binds with high affinity at 5-HT$_{2A}$, 5-HT$_7$, D_2, α_1, α_2, and H_1 receptors. The antipsychotic action of risperidone has been proposed to be the result of D_2 and 5-HT$_{2A}$ antagonism.[23,107] Risperidone is effective in treating the positive and negative symptoms of schizophrenia and as adjunct therapy in bipolar mania.[127] The U.S. Food and Drug Administration (FDA) granted ap-

proval of risperidone orally disintegrating tablets in October 2006 for the treatment of irritability in autistic children and adolescents.[23]

Paliperidone. Paliperidone, (±)-3-[2-[4-(6-fluoro-1,2-benzisoxazol-3-yl)-1-piperidinyl]ethyl]-6,7,8,9-tetrahydro-9-hydroxy-2-methyl-4*H*-pyrido[1,2-*a*]pyrimidin-4-one (Invega), is essentially insoluble in water and is available as extended-release tablets. Paliperidone is delivered at a constant rate using an osmotic drug release device (Osmotic Release Oral Systems [OROS]). The absolute bioavailability of paliperidone is 28%, and studies in healthy subjects on a high-fat, high-calorie meal showed an increase in AUC. Paliperidone is 74% bound to plasma proteins. After a single, 1-mg dose of ^{14}C-paliperidone, 59% of the dose was excreted in the urine as unchanged drug, and 32% of the dose was recovered as metabolites. Most of the drug (80%) is excreted by the kidneys. Paliperidone is metabolized by dealkylation, hydroxylation, dehydrogenation, and scission of the benzoxazole ring. None of these metabolic pathways account for more than 10% of the dose. The terminal elimination half-life of paliperidone is 23 hours.[23]

Aripiprazole. Aripiprazole, (7-[4-[4-(2,3-dichlorophenyl)-1-piperazinyl]butoxy]-3,4-dihydro-2(1*H*)-quinolone, is an atypical antipsychotic that is available in tablets (Abilify), orally disintegrating tablets (Abilify Discmelt), and a 1-mg/mL oral solution. Unlike the other atypical antipsychotics, aripiprazole exhibits partial agonist activity at D_2, D_3, D_4, and 5-HT$_{1A}$ receptors, and antagonist action at 5-HT$_{2A}$ receptors. Although aripiprazole exhibits a low incidence of EPS, the compound occupies about 95% of striatal D_2 receptors at therapeutic doses. Additionally, aripiprazole does not have a fast rate of dissociation from D_2 receptors. Although the mechanism of action of this compound remains to be elucidated, the atypical profile for aripiprazole may be related to its action at other monoamine receptors.[105,128] The compound is well absorbed with peak plasma levels occurring 3 to 5 hours after oral administration. Food does not affect absorption of aripiprazole. Aripiprazole is extensively metabolized in the liver by the action of CYP2D6 and CYP3A4. The primary metabolite in humans is dehydroaripiprazole (Fig. 13.12). This metabolite represents about 40% of aripiprazole at steady state.[23] In the presence of CYP3A4 and CYP2D6 inhibitors or inducers, dosage adjustments of aripiprazole may be required. The mean elimination half-lives in extensive and poor metabolizers are 75 hours and 146 hours, respectively.[23] The major adverse effects of aripiprazole are headache, anxiety, and insomnia.[129] Similar to other atypical antipsychotics, aripiprazole shows an increased risk in mortality in elderly patients with dementia-related psychosis.[23] Aripiprazole demonstrates a different pharmacological profile from all other atypical antipsychotics. The compound exhibits partial agonist activity at 5-HT$_{1A}$ receptors and antagonist action at 5-HT$_{2A}$ receptors. The partial agonism at 5-HT$_{1A}$ may

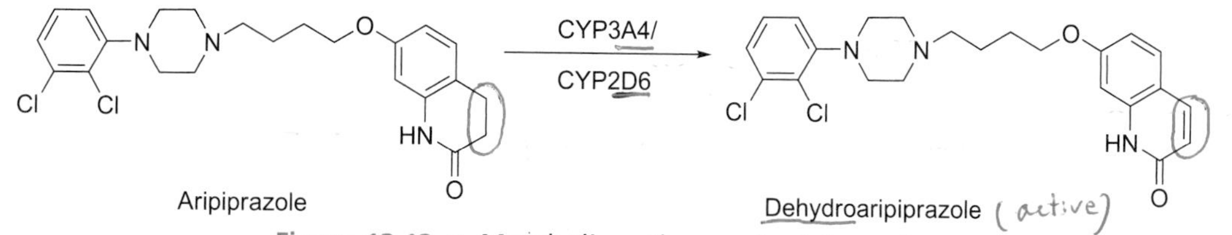

Figure 13.12 ● Metabolic pathway of aripiprazole.

contribute to the effects of aripiprazole against the negative symptoms of schizophrenia.[130] Unlike other antipsychotics, aripiprazole acts as a partial agonist at D_2 receptors. Additionally, the major metabolite, dehydroaripiprazole, shows similar pharmacological properties as aripiprazole, and it also acts as a partial agonist at D_2 receptors.[131] It has been suggested that a partial D_2 agonist will exhibit functional agonist activity in areas of the brain (mesocortical pathway) that have low DA levels, whereas a D_2 partial agonist can function as an antagonist in areas of the brain (mesolimbic pathway) where DA levels are high. Thus, positive symptoms of schizophrenia are reduced without significant EPS.[132] Aripiprazole is indicated for schizophrenia and for acute mania that is associated with bipolar I disorder.[23]

Ziprasidone. Ziprasidone, 5-[2-[4-(1,2-benzisothiazol-3-yl)-1-piperazinyl]ethyl]-6-chloro-1,3-dihydro-2*H*-indol-2-one, is available as the hydrochloride monohydrate for oral administration (Geodon) and as the mesylate trihydrate salt for intramuscular (IM) injection. The compound is well absorbed with peak plasma levels occurring at 6 to 8 hours after oral administration. The oral absorption is enhanced approximately twofold in the presence of food. Ziprasidone is bound about 99% to plasma proteins, primarily to albumin and α_1-acid glycoprotein. Ziprasidone is not displaced in the presence of two highly protein bound drugs, warfarin and propranolol. Ziprasidone is extensively metabolized with only about 5 % of the drug excreted unchanged.[23] In humans, two major pathways are responsible for the metabolism of ziprasidone: (a) oxidation by CYP3A4 (one third) and (b) reduction by aldehyde oxidase (two thirds).[133,134] The combined action of these metabolic pathways leads to four major circulating metabolites: benzisothiazole piperazine sulfoxide (BITP-sulfoxide), benzisothiazole piperazine sulfone (BITP-sulfone), ziprasidone sulfoxide, and *S*-methyldihydroziprasidone (Fig. 13.13).

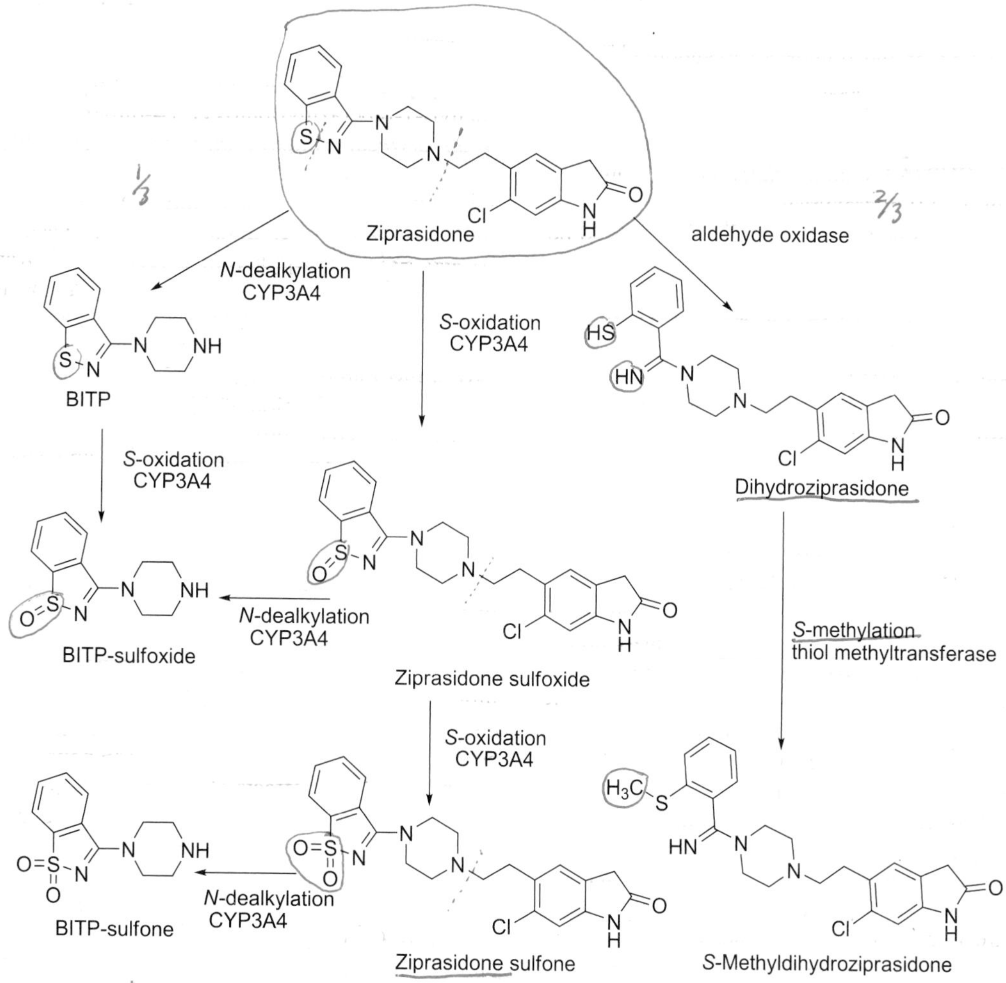

Figure 13.13 ● Metabolic pathway of ziprasidone.[133,134]

Multidrug therapy involving ziprasidone does not appear to be a serious concern, because the reductive activity of aldehyde oxidase is not affected by other drugs.[134] The elimination half-life of ziprasidone is 4 hours with about 20% of the drug excreted in urine and 66% eliminated in the feces.[23,107] Ziprasidone has a low incidence of sedation, EPS, and postural hypotension. Unlike other atypical antipsychotics, ziprasidone does not cause weight gain or elevated glucose levels. Ziprasidone has been shown to cause a mild-to-moderate increase in the QTc interval.[134] Prolongation of the QTc interval in some other drugs is associated with potentially life-threatening ventricular arrhythmias and sudden death. As with other atypical antipsychotic agents, ziprasidone can increase the risk of mortality in elderly patients with dementia-related psychosis and is not indicated in these individuals.[23] Ziprasidone binds with high affinity at D_2, D_3, 5-HT_{1A}, 5-HT_{1D}, 5-HT_{2A}, 5-HT_{2C}, and α_1-receptors. The compound acts as an agonist at 5-HT_{1A} receptors and as an antagonist at D_2 and 5-HT_{2A} receptors. Ziprasidone also inhibits synaptic uptake of serotonin and norepinephrine. Thus, it has been postulated that ziprasidone has potential use as an anxiolytic and an antidepressant.[107,135] Ziprasidone is indicated for schizophrenia and acute mania that is associated with bipolar disorder, whereas the injectable form of ziprasidone is indicated for the treatment of acute agitation in schizophrenic patients.[23]

⬡ FUTURE DIRECTIONS

DA has long been linked with PD and schizophrenia in a unique and multifaceted relationship. Although this close association ensures that DA and the dopaminergic systems will remain a primary focus for the treatment of both PD and schizophrenia, other avenues of therapy are on the horizon. A focus on neuroprotective agents for the treatment of PD may provide a more efficacious approach than DA symptomology-based therapies. Such treatments would target the mechanisms involved in the pathogenesis of the disease. A promising antioxidant, coenzyme Q_{10} (ubiquinone), has been proposed to slow down functional decline.[136] Based on findings that mitochondrial dysregulation and oxidative damage may play a role in the loss of nigral neurons, it is hypothesized that coenzyme Q_{10} could be an effective neuroprotectant.[136,137] Inhibitors of glutamate, anti-inflammatory, and antiapoptotic drugs have also been proposed as PD neuroprotectants,[138,139] although currently there is a lack of clinical verification. Yet, another approach is the use of gene therapy, using a glial cell line-derived neurotrophic factor to slow neurodegeneration in PD.[18,140,141] New approaches are also being explored in terms of schizophrenia treatment. Over the past decade, a dysfunction of glutaminergic neurons has been suggested to contribute to the pathophysiology of schizophrenia. This theory is supported by the fact that a noncompetitive inhibitor at NMDA receptors (a subtype of glutamate receptors) produces positive and negative symptoms of schizophrenia in normal subjects. Compounds that target the NMDA receptor may offer an alternative treatment for schizophrenia.[142] Ultimately, future strategies for the pharmacological treatment of PD and schizophrenia will likely evolve into a combination DA and non-DA approaches, appropriately tailored to each patients needs.

⬡ R E V I E W Q U E S T I O N S ⬡

1. Using chlorpromazine as the prototype, discuss the SAR of the phenothiazine antipsychotics.

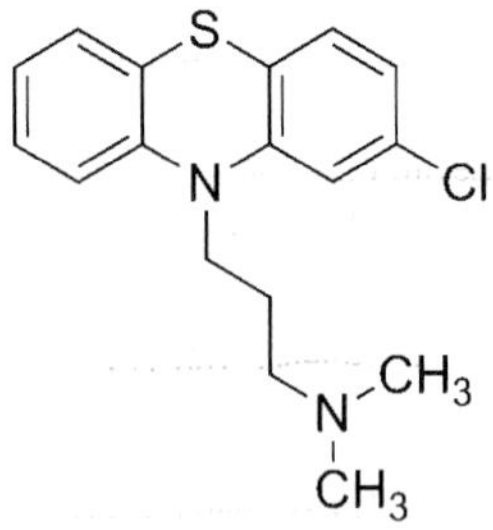

2. Ropinirole and rotigotine act as agonists at D_3 receptors. Compare the structures of these two compounds with that of DA. Clearly specify the pharmacophoric groups in ropinirole and rotigotine that impart D_3 agonist activity.

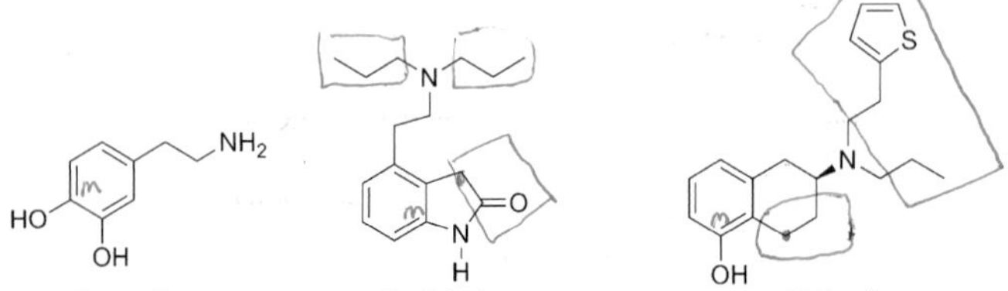

Dopamine   Ropinirole   Rotigotine

3. Shown below is the structure of the typical antipsychotic trifluoperazine. Give the structure of five likely metabolites for this compound.

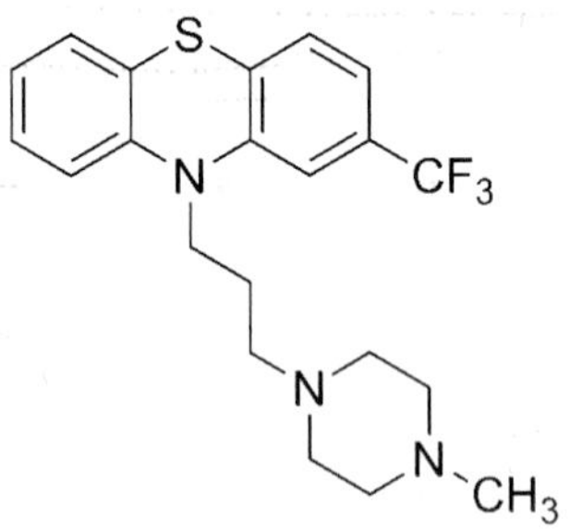

4. Explain the rationale for the combination product levodopa/carbidopa/entacapone in the treatment of PD.

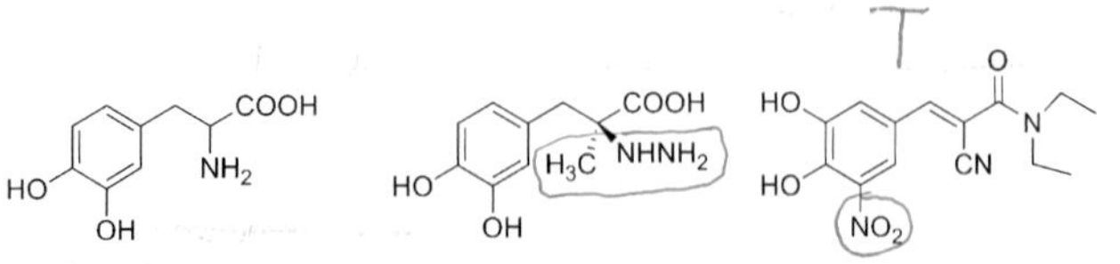

Levodopa   Carbidopa   Entacapone

5. Shown on the next column are the structures of the atypical antipsychotics olanzapine and clozapine. Describe the pharmacological action of these compounds at the D_2 and $5\text{-}HT_{2A}$ receptors. What is the relationship between the circled phenyl ring in clozapine and the 2-methylthiophene ring in olanzapine?

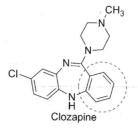

Clozapine

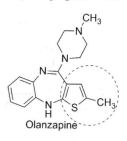

Olanzapine

REFERENCES

1. Wade, L. A., and Katzman, R.: J. Neurochem. 25:837–842, 1975.
2. Sokoloff, P., and Schwartz, J. C.: Trends Pharmacol. Sci. 16:270–275, 1995.
3. Hurley, M. J., and Jenner, P.: Pharmacol. Ther. 111:715–728, 2006.
4. Goto, Y., and Grace, A. A.: Int. Rev. Neurobiol. 78C:41–68, 2007.
5. Uhl, G. R.: Mov. Disord. 18 Suppl 7:S71–S80, 2003.
6. Youdim, M. B., Edmondson, D., and Tipton, K. F.: Nat. Rev. Neurosci. 7:295–309, 2006.
7. Cooper, J. R., Bloom, F. E., and Roth, R. H.: Dopamine. The Biochemical Basis of Neuropharmacology, 8th ed. New York, Oxford University Press, Inc., 2003, pp. 225–270.
8. Standaert, D. G., and Young, A. B.: Treatment of Central Nervous System Degenerative Disorders. In Brunton, L. L., Lazo, J. S., and Parker, K. L. (eds.). Goodman & Gillman's The Pharmacological Basis of Therapeutics, 11th ed. New York, McGraw Hill, 2006, pp. 527–546.
9. Samii, A., Nutt, J. G., and Ransom, B. R.: Lancet 363:1783–1793, 2004.
10. Lang, A. E., and Lozano, A. M.: N. Engl. J. Med. 339, 1044–1053, 1998.
11. Davis, G. C., Williams, A. C., Markey, S. P., et al.: Psychiatry Res. 1:249–254, 1979.
12. Langston, J. W., et al.: Science 219:979–980, 1983.
13. Lieberman, A.: Acta Neurol. Scand. 113:1–8, 2006.
14. Joyce, J. N., Ryoo, H. L., Beach, T. B., et al.: Brain Res. 955:138–152, 2002.
15. Piggott, M. A., Marshall, E. F., Thomas, N., et al.: Brain 122 (Pt 8):1449–1468, 1999.
16. Ryoo, H. L., Pierrotti, D., and Joyce, J. N.: Mov. Disord. 13:788–797, 1998.
17. Jenner, P.: Neurology 65:S3–S5, 2005.
18. Fahn, S.: Exp. Neurol. 144:21–23, 1997.
19. Pletscher, A., and DaPrada, M.: Acta Neurol. Scand. Suppl. 146:26–31, 1993.
20. Standaert, D. G., and Galanter J. M.: Pharmacology of Dopaminergic Neurotransmission. In Golan D. E., et al. (eds.). Principles of Pharmacology: the Pathologic Basis of Drug Therapy, 2nd ed. Lippincott, Williams & Wilkins, 2008, pp. 185–206.
21. Sweeney, P. J.: Parkinson's Disease: An Overview. In Carey, W. D. (ed.). The Cleveland Clinic Disease Management Project. The Cleveland Clinic, 2005.
22. Chase, T. N.: Drugs 55 Suppl 1:1–9, 1998.
23. US Food and Drug Administration, 2007, http://www.fda.gov.
24. Youdim, M. B. H., and Bakhle, Y. S.: Br. J. Pharmacol. 147:S287–S296, 2006.
25. Ebadi, M., et al.: J. Neurosci. Res. 67:285–289, 2002.
26. Lees, A.: Drugs Aging 22:731–740, 2005.
27. Chen, J. J., and Ly, A. V.: Am. J. Health Syst. Pharm. 63:915–928, 2006.
28. Mandel, S., et al.: Brain Res. Rev. 48:379–387, 2005.
29. Guay, D. R. P.: Am. J. Geriatr. Pharmacother. 4:330–346, 2006.
30. Chafetz, L., Desai, M. P., and Sukonik, L.: J. Pharm. Sci. 83:1250–1252, 1994.
31. Magyar, K., Pálfi, M., Tábi, T., et al.: Curr. Med. Chem. 11:2017–2031, 2004.
32. Siddiqui, M. A. A., and Plosker Greg, L.: Drugs Aging 22:83–91, 2005.
33. Med. Lett. Drugs Ther. 48:97–99, 2006.
34. Stocchi, F.: Int. J. Clin. Pract. 60:215–221, 2006.
35. Olanow, C. W., Watts, R. L., and Koller, W. C.: Neurology 56:S1–S88, 2001.
36. Clarke, C. E., and Guttman, M.: Lancet 360:1767–1769, 2002.

37. Kvernmo, T., Härtter, S., and Burger, E.: Clin. Ther. 28:1065–1078, 2006.
38. Waller, E. A., Kaplan, J., and Heckman, M. G.: Mayo Clin. Proc. 80:1016–1020, 2005.
39. Hagan, J. J., et al.: Trends Pharmacol. Sci. 18:156–163, 1997.
40. Tan, E. K., and Jankovic, J.: Clin. Neuropharmacol. 24:247–253, 2001.
41. Jähnichen, S., Horowski, R., and Pertz, H. H.: Eur. J. Pharmacol. 513:225–228, 2005.
42. Nakatsuka, A., Nagai, M., Yabe, H., et al.: J. Pharmacol. Sci. 100:59–64, 2006.
43. Joyce, J. N., and Millan, M. J.: Curr. Opin. Pharmacol. 7:100–105, 2007.
44. Dooley, M., and Markham, A.: Drugs Aging 12:495–514, 1998.
45. Deleu, D., Northway, M. G., and Hanssens, Y.: Clin. Pharmacokinet. 41:261–309, 2002.
46. Kaye, C. M., and Nicholls, B.: Clin. Pharmacokinet. 39:243–254, 2000.
47. Matheson, A. J., and Spencer, C. M.: Drugs 60:115–137, 2000.
48. Reynolds, N. A., Wellington, K., and Easthope, S. E.: CNS Drugs 19:973–981, 2005.
49. Kreiss, D. S., Bergstrom, D. A., Gonzalez, A. M., et al.: Eur. J. Pharmacol. 277:209–214, 1995.
50. Keating, G. M., and Lyseng-Williamson, K. A.: CNS Drugs 19:165–184, 2005.
51. Gordin, A., Kaakkola, S., and Teräväinen, H.: J. Neural Transm. 111:1343–1363, 2004.
52. Jorga, K., et al.: Br. J. Clin. Pharmacol. 49:39–48, 2000.
53. LeWitt, P. A.: Pharmacotherapy 20:26S–32S, 2000.
54. Allers, K. A., et al.: Exp. Neurol. 191:104–118, 2005.
55. Matsubayashi, H., Swanson, K. L., and Albuquerque, E. X.: J. Pharmacol. Exp. Ther. 281:834–844, 1997.
56. Baldessarini, R. J., and Tarazi, F. I.: Pharmacotherapy of Psychosis and Mania. In Brunton, L. L., Parker, K., and Lazo, J. S. (eds.). Goodman & Gilman's The Pharmacological Basis of Therapeutics, 11th ed. New York, McGraw-Hill, 2006, pp. 429–460.
57. Lewis, D. A., and Lieberman, J. A.: Neuron 28:325–334, 2000.
58. McDonald, C., and Murphy, K. C.: Psychiatr. Clin. North. Am. 26:41–63, 2003.
59. Lewis, D. A., and Levitt, P.: Annual Rev. Neurosci. 25:409–432, 2002.
60. Seeman, P.: Synapse 1:133–152, 1987.
61. Moghaddam, B.: Neuron 40:881–884, 2003.
62. Abi-Dargham, A.: Int. Rev. Neurobiol. 78:133–164, 2007.
63. Seeman, P., and Lee, T.: Science 188:1217–1219, 1975.
64. Grace, A. A.: Neuroscience 41:1–24, 1991.
65. Abi-Dargham, A., and Laruelle, M.: Eur. Psychiatry 20:15–27, 2005.
66. Davis, K. L., et al.: Am. J. Psychiatry 148:1474–1486, 1991.
67. Lieberman, J. A., Sheitman, B. B., and Kinon, B. J.: Neuropsychopharmacology 17:205–229, 1997.
68. Okubo, Y., Suhara, T., Suzuki, K., et al: Nature 385:634–636, 1997.
69. Frankle, W. G., Lerma, J., and Laruelle, M.: Neuron 39:205–216, 2003.
70. Weinberger, D. R., and Laruelle, M.: Neurochemical and Neuropharmacological Imaging in Schizophrenia. In Davis, K. L., et al. (eds.). Neuropsychopharmacology: Fifth Generation of Progress. Philadelphia, Lippincott, Williams and Wilkins, 2002, pp. 833–855.
71. Stone, J. M., Morrison, P., and Pilowsky, L. S.: J. Psychopharmacol. 21:440–452, 2007.
72. Miyamoto, S., et al.: Therapeutics of Schizophrenia. Neuropsychopharmacology: The Fifth Generation of Progress; Davis, K. L., et al., (eds.). Philadelphia, Lippincott, Williams and Wilkins, 2002, pp. 775–808.
73. Lehmann, H. E., and Ban, T. A.: Can. J. Psychiatry 42:152–162, 1997.

74. Petersen, P. V., et al.: Arzneimittelforschung 8:395–397, 1958.
75. Petersen, P. V., Lassen, N. O., and Holm, T. O.: 2-Chloro-9-(3-dimethylaminopropylidene) thiaxanthene and its amine exchange reactions; (Kefalas A/S). United States, 1964; US 3149103, 6 pp.
76. Wilhelm, M.: Pharm. J. 214:414–416, 1975.
77. Froimowitz, M., and Cody, V.: J. Med. Chem. 36:2219–2227, 1993.
78. Feinberg, A. P., and Snyder, S. H.: Proc. Natl. Acad. Sci. U. S. A. 72:1899–1903, 1975.
79. Kaiser, C., Pavloff, A. M. Garvey, E., et al.: J. Med. Chem. 15:665–673, 1972.
80. Horn, A. S., and Snyder, S. H.: Proc. Natl. Acad. Sci. U. S. A. 68:2325–2328, 1971.
81. Grol, C. J., et al.: J. Med. Chem. 25:5–9, 1982.
82. Kaiser, C., Tedeschi, D. H., Fowler, P. J., et al.: J. Med. Chem. 14:179–186, 1971.
83. Gareri, P., et al.: Clin. Drug Investig. 23:287–322, 2003.
84. Belal, F., Hefnawy, M. M., and Aly, F. A.: J. Pharm. Biomed. Anal. 16:369–376, 1997.
85. Shen, W. W.: Biol. Psychiatry 41:814–826, 1997.
86. Fang, J., and Gorrod, J. W.: Cell. Mol. Neurobiol. 19:491–510, 1999.
87. Chetty, M., et al.: Eur. Neuropsychopharmacol. 6:85–91, 1996.
88. Terry, A. V., Gearhart, D. A., Mahadik, S. P., et al.: Neuroscience 136:519–529, 2005.
89. Wishart, D. S., Knox, C., Guo, A. C., et al.: Nucleic Acids Res. 34:D668–D672, 2006.
90. IPCS Intox Databank, 2007, http://www.intox.org/databank/index.htm.
91. Mula, M., and Monaco, F.: Clin. Neuropharmacol. 25:280–289, 2002.
92. Janssen, P. A. J.: Haloperidol and related Butyrophenones. In Gordon, M. (ed.). Psychopharmacological Agents. Philadelphia, Academic Press, 1967, pp. 199–248.
93. Sikazwe, D. M. N., Li, S., Mardenborough, L., et al.: Bioorg. Med. Chem. Lett. 14:5739–5742, 2004.
94. Raviña, E., and Masaguer, C. F.: Curr. Med. Chem. 1:43–62, 2001.
95. Fang, J., McKay, G., Song, J., et al.: Drug Metab. Dispos. 29:1638–1643, 2001.
96. Beresford, R., and Ward, A.: Drugs 33:31–49, 1987.
97. Forsman, A., et al.: Curr. Ther. Res. 21:606–617, 1977.
98. Glue, P., and Banfield, C.: Human Psychopharmacol. 11:97–114, 1996.
99. Desta, Z., Kerbusch, T., Soukhova, N., et al.: J. Pharmacol. Exp. Ther. 285:428–437, 1998.
100. Matsui-Sakata, A., Ohtani, H., and Sawada, Y.: Drug Metab. Pharmacokinet. 20:368–378, 2005.
101. Kapur, S., and Seeman, P.: Am. J. Psychiatry 158:360–369, 2001.
102. Weiner, D. M., Burstein, E. S., Nash, N., et al.: J. Pharmacol. Exp. Ther. 299:268–276, 2001.
103. Roth, B. L., Sheffler, D., and Potkin, S. G.: Clin. Neurosci. Res. 3:108–117, 2003.
104. Dean, B., and Scarr, E.: Curr. Drug Targets CNS Neurol. Disord. 3: 217–225, 2004.
105. Horacek, J., Bubenikova-Valesova, V., Kopecek, M., et al.: CNS Drugs 20:389–409, 2006.
106. Kiss, B., and Bitter, I.: Structural Analogues of Clozapine. Analogue-Based Drug Discovery, 1st ed. In Fisher, J., and Ganellin, CR. (eds.). Research Triangle Park, Wiley-VCH, 2006, pp. 297–314.
107. Raggi, M. A., et al.: Curr. Med. Chem. 11:279–296, 2004.
108. Meltzer, H. Y.: Psychopharmacology 99:S18–S27, 1989. Psychopharmacology (Berl) 163:1–3, 2002.
109. Fang, J., et al.: Naunyn Schmiedebergs Arch. Pharmacol. 358:592–599, 1998.
110. Burstein, E. S., Ma, J., Wong, S., et al.: J. Pharmacol. Exp. Ther. 315:1278–1287, 2005.
111. Williams, D. P., et al.: J. Pharmacol. Exp. Ther. 283:1375–1382, 1997.
112. Kassahun, K., Mattiuz, E., Nyhart, E., Jr., et al.: Drug Metab. Dispos. 25:81–93, 1997.
113. Kassahun, K., et al.: Drug Metab. Dispos. 26:848–855, 1998.
114. Bymaster, F. P., and Felder, C. C.: Mol. Psychiatry 7:S57–S63, 2002.
115. Lambert, M. T., et al.: Prog. Neuropsychopharmacol. Biol. Psychiatry 30:919–923, 2006.
116. Moisan, J., et al.: Pharmacoepidemiol. Drug Saf. 14:427–436, 2005.
117. DeVane, C. L., and Nemeroff, C. B.: Clin. Pharmacokinet. 40:509–522, 2001.
118. Grimm, S. W., et al.: Br. J. Clin. Pharmacol. 61:58–69, 2006.
119. Nemeroff, C. B., Kinkead, B., and Goldstein, J.: J. Clin. Psychiatry 63:5–11, 2002.
120. Newman-Tancredi, et al.: Eur. J. Pharmacol. 428:177–184, 2001.
121. Berecz, R., Dorado, P., De La Rubia, A., et al.: Curr. Drug Targets 5:573–579, 2004.
122. Mahatthanatrakul, W., Dorado, P., De La Rubia, A., et al.: J. Clin. Pharm. Ther. 32:161–167, 2007.
123. Fang, J., Bourin, M., and Baker, G. B.: Naunyn Schmiedebergs Arch. Pharmacol. 359:147–151, 1999.
124. Yasui-Furukori, N., Hidestrand, M., Spiná, E., et al.: Drug Metab. Dispos. 29:1263–1268, 2001.
125. Bork, J. A., et al.: J. Clin. Psychiatry 60:469–476, 1999.
126. Nyberg, S., et al.: Am. J. Psychiatry 156:869–875, 1999.
127. Garver, D. L.: Curr. Drug Targets 7:1205–1215, 2006.
128. Harrison, T. S., and Perry, C. M.: Drugs 64:1715–1736, 2004.
129. Winans, E.: Am. J. Health Syst. Pharm. 60:2437–2445, 2003.
130. Jordan, S., Koprivica, V., Chen, R., et al.: Eur. J. Pharmacol. 441:137–140, 2002.
131. Wood, M. D., Scott, C., Clarke, K., et al.: Eur. J. Pharmacol. 546:88–94, 2006.
132. Potkin, S. G., Saha, A. R., Kujawa, M. J., et al.: Arch. Gen. Psychiatry 60:681–690, 2003.
133. Obach, R. S., and Walsky, R. L.: J. Clin. Psychopharmacol. 25:605–608, 2005.
134. Beedham, C., Miceli, J. J., and Obach, R. S.: J. Clin. Psychopharmacol. 23:229–232, 2003.
135. Stimmel, G. L., Gutierrez, M. A., and Lee, V.: Clin. Ther. 24:21–37, 2002.
136. Beal, M. F.: J. Bioenerg. Biomembr. 36:381–386, 2004.
137. Shults, C. W., Haas, R. H., and Beal, M. F.: Biofactors 9:267–272, 1999.
138. Bonuccelli, U., and Del Dotto, P.: Neurology 67(7 Suppl 2):S30–S38, 2006.
139. Djaldetti, R., and Melamed, E.: J. Neurol. 249 Suppl 2:II30–II35, 2002.
140. Bohn, M. C.: Mol. Ther. 1:494–496, 2000.
141. Gash, D. M., Zhang, Z., Ovadia, A., et al.: Nature 380:252–255, 1996.
142. Kristiansen, L. V., Huerta, I., Beneyto, M., et al.: NMDA receptors and schizophrenia. Curr. Opin. Pharmacol. 7:48–55, 2007.

CHAPTER 14

Anticonvulsants

MATTHIAS C. LU

The terms *anticonvulsant* and *antiepileptic* drug (AED) are used interchangeably in the literature to describe a diverse group of medications used clinically to provide seizure control in patients with epilepsies. However, because some anticonvulsants described in this chapter are used to treat neuropathic pains and/or to control severe mood changes in patients with mania and other mood disorders, the term AED will be used only when discussing the therapeutic usage of these drugs in the context of epilepsy treatment.

Epilepsy is the most prevalent neurological disorder affecting more than 0.5% of the world's population.[1] It is characterized by recurrent seizures, unprovoked by any identifiable causes. The etiology of epilepsy is largely unknown even though recent evidence suggests that it may have a genetic component associated with its disease development.[2,3] Seizures, on the other hand, are symptoms of disturbed electrical activity in the brain characterized by episodes of abnormal, excessive, and synchronous discharge of a group of neurons within the brain that cause involuntary movement, sensation, or thought.[4] It is generally agreed that seizures may result from primary or acquired neurological disturbances of brain function as a result of an imbalance between excitatory and inhibitory processes in the brain. There are many possible causes of seizures including brain tumors or infections, head trauma, neurological diseases, systemic or metabolic disorders, alcohol abuse, drug overdose, or toxicities.

In North America, the incidence of newly diagnosed epilepsy (~50–100 cases/100,000 per year) is highest among children younger than 5 years of age and the elderly older than 65 years of age.[1,5] Most of these newly diagnosed seizure disorders can be effectively controlled initially with the use of AEDs such as valproic acid (VPA), carbamazepine (CBZ), ethosuximide, and phenytoin to prevent recurrence of seizure activity.[6] However, the success of pharmacotherapy of epilepsy with these conventional AEDs is often hampered by the loss of effectiveness after prolonged drug exposure (~1/3 of the newly diagnosed patients become resistant to current pharmacotherapy).[7] The reason for this refractory to an AED may be a result of the coexistence of factors related to the epileptogenesis of the disease state or to the development of pharmacodynamic or pharmacokinetic tolerances.[8] In addition, the usage of these AEDs as first-line treatment options is associated with a wide range of clinical problems including drug interactions, idiosyncratic reactions, hepatotoxicity, and AED-induced teratogenesis.[6,9,10] These intolerable adverse events can negatively influence patient compliance and significantly diminish quality of life in patients with epilepsies.[6] Furthermore, even with recent market introduction of at least 10 newer AEDs with much improved side effects and toxicities profile, only less than 5% of patients with refractory epilepsy have their seizures effectively controlled with these newer AEDs.[11]

Thus, the goal of this chapter is to provide the readers with a basic understanding of how each of the drug molecules works, how they are metabolized, and the role these metabolite(s) might play in the development of idiosyncratic reactions or toxicities. Some of the basic concepts presented in this chapter will allow clinicians to assess potential drug–drug/food interactions and to provide optimal treatment plan for their patients. The inclusion of the structure–activity relationships (SARs) within each drug or structure type in this chapter should also provide readers with a much needed tool to evaluate future drug development in this area.

DISEASE STATES REQUIRING ANTICONVULSANT THERAPY

The diagnosis of a first epileptic seizure or epilepsy, at primary care facilities, is often subjective and prone to error because it is usually based on eyewitness accounts of the episodes.[6,12] An incorrect diagnosis, especially of the seizure type, however, can have far-reaching negative consequences for the patient, including loss of work and driving privileges, potential toxic or ineffective medication given, and other socioeconomic consequences.[13]

Classification of Epileptic Seizures and Recommended Initial Drug Therapy

The 1981 classification of the epileptic seizure types[14] and the 1989 classification of epileptic syndromes and epilepsies[15] are still widely accepted and workable because their accuracy facilitates diagnosis, drug selection, and precise discussion of seizure disorders.[6,16] Seizures are classified, based on their initial signs and symptoms and the pattern seen on the electroencephalogram (EEG), into two broad categories as generalized seizures or as partial seizures.[13]

Each of the epilepsy types is characterized by an abnormal pattern in the EEG. The EEG indicates sudden, excessive electrical activity in the brain. Most of the currently available AEDs work by preventing, stopping, or lessening this electrical activity. The precise causes of these abnormal changes is still unknown; however, it has been hypothesized that there is a site or focus of damaged or abnormal hyperexcitable neurons in the brain. These neurons can fire excessively and sometimes recruit adjacent neurons that in turn induce other neurons to fire. Thus, the location and the extent of the abnormal firing is essential for the determination of the epilepsy types.[16]

PRIMARY GENERALIZED SEIZURES

Two major types of generalized seizures are the primarily generalized tonic–clonic seizures (grand mal) and the absence (petit mal) seizures. The typical primarily generalized tonic–clonic seizure is often preceded by a series of bilateral muscular jerks followed by loss of consciousness, which in turn is followed by a series of tonic and then clonic spasms. The typical absence seizure (classic petit mal) consists of a sudden brief loss of consciousness (~10 seconds), sometimes with no motor activity, although often some minor clonic motor activity exists. Based on a recent evidence-based metaanalysis of AED efficacy and effectiveness, the recommended initial monotherapy for patients with generalized seizures are CBZ, oxcarbazepine (OXC), lamotrigine, VPA, phenytoin, and topiramate (TPM), whereas children with absence seizures are best treated with lamotrigine, VPA, or ethosuximide.[6,13]

PARTIAL SEIZURES

Major types of partial seizure are simple partial seizures (focal) and complex partial seizures (temporal lobe or psychomotor). Partial seizures are the most common seizure types experienced by approximately 60% to 70% of the adult patients. A prototypic simple partial seizure is Jacksonian motor epilepsy in which the Jacksonian march may be seen. As the abnormal discharge proceeds over the cortical site involved, the visible seizure progresses over the area of the body controlled by the cortical site. Partial seizures, if not controlled, may progress to another seizure type known as the secondarily generalized partial seizures (tonic–clonic or grand mal). The first-line treatment for patients with newly diagnosed or untreated simple partial seizures are CBZ or phenytoin for adults, lamotrigine or gabapentin for elderly adults, and OXC for children.[6,13]

The complex partial seizure is represented by the psychomotor or temporal lobe seizure. There is an aura, then a confused or bizarre but seemingly purposeful behavior lasting 2 to 3 minutes, often with no memory of the event. The seizure may be misdiagnosed as a psychotic episode. Although the initial treatment is the same, it is much harder to control complex partial seizures.

Anticonvulsants Used in Neuropathic Pain

Neuropathic pain, despite its heterogeneity in etiology and anatomical locations, is characterized by a neuronal hyperexcitability in damaged areas of the nerves. This neuronal hyperexcitability and many of the corresponding cellular changes is quite similar to that of epilepsy. Thus, it is not surprising that anticonvulsants such as CBZ, gabapentin, and more recently its close analog, pregabalin were approved for relieving pains associated with diabetic neuropathy, trigeminal neuralgia, and other neuropathic pains.[17] Both gabapentin and pregabalin have become an important treatment option in neuropathic pain because of their lack of potential drug interactions and minimal side effect profiles.

MECHANISMS OF ACTION OF ANTICONVULSANTS

At the cellular level, three basic mechanisms are believed to contribute to the antiepileptic action of the currently marketed anticonvulsants.[18,19] These are (a) modulation of voltage-gated ion channels (Na^+, Ca^{2+}, and K^+), (b) enhancement of γ-aminobutyric acid (GABA)-mediated inhibitory neurotransmission, and (c) attenuation of excitatory (particularly glutamate-mediated) neurotransmission in the brain. Many of AEDs, especially the newer drugs, work by more than one of the above mechanisms of actions, therefore possessing a broader spectrum of antiepileptic action.

Voltage-Gated Ion Channels as Targets for Anticonvulsants

VOLTAGE-GATED SODIUM CHANNELS

Voltage-gated sodium channels (VGSCs) in the presynaptic nerve terminal of the excitatory glutamate receptors are the molecular target for phenytoin, CBZ, and lamotrigine as well as some of the newer AEDs, such as OXC, felbamate (FBM), and zonisamide.[18] These aromatic AEDs inhibit excessive neuronal firing by binding to a site near the inactivation gate, thereby prolonging inactivation of VGSCs.[20] Figure 14.1 illustrates how phenytoin interacts with the hypothetical *inactivation gate* receptor according to a pharmacophore model suggested by Unverferth et al.[21] as a result of molecular simulations with these aromatic AEDs. This model includes an aromatic binding site and two separate hydrogen bonding sites for interacting with potent AEDs such as phenytoin and lamotrigine.

VOLTAGE-GATED CALCIUM CHANNELS

The voltage-gated calcium channels (VGCCs) are essential in regulating Ca^{2+} signaling, which is associated with many important cellular events such as the release of excitatory glutamate neurotransmitters, the plasticity changes

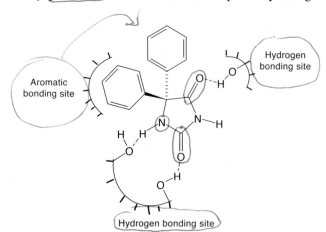

Figure 14.1 ● Binding of phenytoin to the hypothetical "inactivation gate" receptor on the voltage-gated sodium channels.

of long-term potentiation in learning and memory, and the maintenance of homeostasis of nerve cells. It has been suggested that excessive influx of Ca^{2+} plays a critical role in the induction and progression of epileptic seizures.[22,23] There are distinct classes of VGCCs. The high-threshold L-type Ca^{2+} channels in the presynaptic glutaminergic receptors require strong depolarization for activation and are the primary molecular targets of gabapentin and pregabalin, both of which are effective in refractory partial seizures.[22,24] On the other hand, the low-threshold T-type Ca^{2+} channels require only weak depolarization for activation and are the molecular targets of AEDs such as ethosuximide and zonisamide.[18,25]

VOLTAGE-GATED POTASSIUM CHANNELS

Potentiation of the voltage-gated K^+ channels is another attractive target for designing of newer AEDs, because they are intimately associated with the membrane repolarization processes.[20] Levetiracetam (LEV), a novel AED recently marketed for the adjunctive therapy of refractory partial seizures in adults, has been suggested to work by reducing the voltage-operated A-type potassium currents as one of its mechanism of actions.[26,27]

GABA_A Receptors as Targets for Anticonvulsants

It is now well recognized that cellular excitability leading to convulsive seizures can be attenuated by GABAergic stimulation in the brain.[19] The $GABA_A$ receptor is one of two ligand-gated ion channels responsible for mediating the effects of GABA, the major inhibitory neurotransmitter in the brain.[18,19] Activation of the $GABA_A$/benzodiazepine (BZD) receptors/chloride channel complex allows increased chloride conductance, thereby preventing the spread of neuronal excitations.[28,29]

The potential targets for AED's action on the GABAergic inhibitory synapses include (a) drugs that enhance the biosynthesis of GABA (gabapentin, pregabalin, and VPA), (b) drugs that inhibit GABA degradation (vigabatrin), (c) drugs that inhibit the reuptake of GABA (tiagabine), and (d) drugs that bind to an allosteric site on the postsynaptic $GABA_A$ receptor complex that increase chloride conductance (barbiturates, BZDs, neurosteroids, FBM, TPM).[19]

DRUGS THAT ENHANCE THE BIOSYNTHESIS OF GABA

GABA, the major inhibitory neurotransmitter in the brain, is biosynthesized at the GABAergic neurons by the decarboxylation of the amino acid, L-glutamic acid (itself an excitatory amino acid neurotransmitter in the brain). The rate-limiting enzyme that catalyzes this conversion is L-glutamic acid decarboxylase (GAD). The essential cofactor for this enzymatic reaction is pyridoxal phosphate (vitamin B_6) (see Fig. 14.2). GABA, after its release from the synaptic nerve terminal, is degraded by another pyridoxal-dependent enzyme, the GABA transaminase (GABA-T), which transfers an amino group from GABA to α-ketoglutarate producing L-glutamic acid and succinic acid semialdehyde (SSA). As shown in Figure 14.2, SSA is further oxidized by the action of the enzyme succinic semialdehyde dehydrogenase (SSADH, an aldehyde dehydrogenase) to succinic acid that can enter the TCA cycle for the production of additional α-ketoglutarate or be further reduced by SSA reductase (an alcohol dehydrogenase that catalyzes the interconversion of SSA and 4-hydroxybutyric acid).[30]

Being a 3-substituted GABA, gabapentin and especially pregabalin, may have the ability to activate GAD,[31] in addition to their major anticonvulsant action at the high-threshold L-type Ca^{2+} channels in the presynaptic glutaminergic receptors.[24] Both of these drugs are weak activators of GAD; however, their pharmacological actions on the GAD can not be discounted because gabapentin was able to elevate brain GABA levels ($\sim$75%–100%) in patients with epilepsy within hour after the first dosing.[32]

Similar to gabapentin and pregabalin, VPA, also elevates brain levels of GABA in patients with epilepsy.[30] It is generally agreed that VPA inhibits SSADH, the enzyme responsible for conversion of SSA to succinic acid. The exact mechanism of action of how this inhibition enhances GABA levels in the brain is still the subject of much debate (i.e., from an indirect stimulation of GAD to an inhibition of GABA-T). However, if we take into account that GABA also inhibits SSA reductase, an enzyme that reduces SSA to γ-hydroxybutyric acid, an epitogenic metabolite of GABA. Thus, it is reasonable to propose that VPA elevates GABA levels by reversing the transamination reaction mediated by GABA-T because of the accumulation of its product, SSA at the enzyme active site of GABA-T (Fig 14.2).

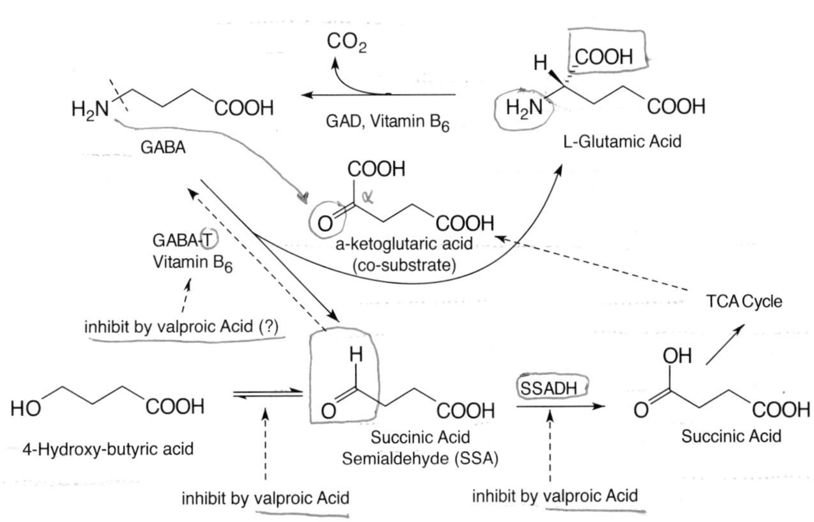

Figure 14.2 ● Biosynthesis and metabolism of GABA.

DRUGS THAT INHIBIT GABA DEGRADATION

Vigabatrin (γ-vinyl-GABA) is an irreversible inhibitor of GABA-T, rationally designed based on the biochemical mechanism of transamination reaction.[19,33] Briefly, vigabatrin, because of its structural similarity, competes with GABA for binding to GABA-T and forms a Schiff base intermediate with the cofactor, pyridoxal phosphate similar to GABA. However, unlike its substrate GABA, during the process of transferring the amino group to the pyridoxal phosphate, a reactive intermediate is formed with vigabatrin that immediately attaches itself to the active site of the enzyme, thereby irreversibly inhibiting GABA-T and increasing GABA levels in the brain.

DRUGS THAT INHIBIT REUPTAKE OF GABA

Released GABA is actively taken back into the GABAergic neurons or glial cells in the brain by GABA transporters (GATs).[28,34] Tiagabine, structurally related to nipecotic acid, is a selective inhibitor of the neuronal and glial GAT1 at the GABAergic neurons and an effective drug for the treatment of patients with refractory epilepsy.[34] Addition of two lipophilic heterocyclic rings to the nicopetic acid moiety did not interfere with its ability to bind GAT1 but actually allows tiagabine to cross into the brain freely and also more selectively than nicopetic acid toward GAT1.[34]

DRUGS THAT BIND TO THE GABA$_A$ RECEPTOR COMPLEX AND MODULATE CHLORIDE INFLUX

Many clinically useful anxiolytic hypnotic–sedatives and some AED drugs such as BZDs, and barbiturates (e.g., phenobarbital) exert their pharmacological actions by interacting with a discrete neuronal site on the GABA$_A$- BZD receptor-chloride channel complex.[35] The GABA$_A$-chloride ionophore is a glycoprotein pentamer that contains two α, two β, and one γ subunit and is present throughout the mammalian brain.[28,35] It has been hypothesized that binding of BZD agonists such as clonazepam to its receptor enhances GABA-mediated inhibitory neurotransmission by increasing the frequency of chloride channel openings. TPM, a broad-spectrum AED, also binds and increases the frequency of chloride channel opening but at a different site than the BZDs.[18] Barbiturates, on the other hand, bind to a third binding site on the GABA$_A$ receptor complex and increases the duration of chloride channel openings.[35] It has been hypothesized that the binding of these drugs to their respective binding sites induces conformational changes, thereby allowing GABA to work more efficiently to modulate chloride channel openings.

Excitatory Glutamate-Mediated Receptors as Target for Anticonvulsants

The acidic amino acids, L-glutamate and L-aspartate, are the most important excitatory neurotransmitters in the brain acting through two distinct families of glutamate receptors, the ligand-gated, ionotropic receptors and the G-protein–coupled metabotropic receptors.[36] The ligand-gated glutamate receptors such as N-methyl-D-aspartic acid (NMDA)/α-amino-3-hydroxyl-5-methyl-4-isoxazole propionic acid (AMPA) receptors modulate sodium and calcium influx and are involved in mediating excitatory synaptic transmission including the initiation and spread of seizure activity. Activation of these receptors is responsible for important functions in the brain including long-term potentiation in memory acquisition, learning, and some neurodegenerative disorders.[22,37] These receptors are potential therapeutic targets for epilepsy and other neurodegenerative disorders such as stroke and head injury, Alzheimer, and other chronic debilitating disorders. However, efforts in finding effective and safe NMDA antagonists have failed because of their toxicities and intolerable side effects.[38] Thus, with the exception of TPM, which deriving some of its antiepileptic action by modulating the AMPA receptor and FBM, which appears to bind to the glycine binding site on the NMDA receptor, none of the current AEDs has any direct action at the postsynaptic glutamate receptors.[19] Metabotropic glutamate receptors, on the other hand, modulate the release of glutamic acid, GABA, and other important neurotransmitters in the brain. Thus, these receptors are exciting new therapeutic targets for designing medications for pain, addiction, Parkinson disease, schizophrenia, and other neurodegenerative disorders.[28]

⬡ CLINICALLY IMPORTANT ANTICONVULSANTS

There is very little SAR among the clinically useful anticonvulsants except within each structure type, primarily effecting their side effects and toxicities. Thus, these aspects of medicinal chemistry will be covered under each structure type or under the individual drug monographs covered in this section.

Valproic Acid (Depakote, Depakene, Depacon)

VPA is an established AED with a simple chemical structure but an unusually broad spectrum of action. It is generally well tolerated, but its use is limited by two rare but significant toxic side effects (hepatotoxicity and teratogenicity) that can be dose-dependent or idiosyncratic in nature.[9,39,40] These drawbacks are apparently shared by its equipotent active metabolite, (E)-2-propyl-2-pentenoic acid (2-ene-VPA) (Fig. 14.3).

VPA is also an important inhibitor of the cytochrome P450 isozymes, mainly of CYP2C9 and also of uridine diphosphate (UDP)-glucuronyl transferase and epoxide hydrolase.[10] This inhibition is competitive and dose-dependent, and its effect is observed when sufficient concentrations of VPA is achieved (usually within 24 hours). Thus, an increase in the plasma concentrations of other AEDs such as lamotrigine is to be expected after dosing with VPA.

Metabolism of VPA is very complex and is the result of hepatic mitochondrial β-oxidation and microsomal oxidations, catalyzed by CYP2C9, CYP2C19, and CYP2E1 and possibly CYP3A4, and glucuronidations.[39,40] At least 10 metabolites have been identified. The major urinary inactive metabolite is 2-propyl-3-keto-pentanoic acid (3-keto-VPA) and an equipotent active metabolite, (E)-2-ene-VPA. Other minor metabolites identified are their hydroxylated or dehydrated products, and 2-propylglutaric acid (see Fig.14.3 for their structures). All of these metabolites are excreted as O-glucuronides.

The hepatotoxicity of VPA is most likely associated with 2, 4-diene-VPA and/or 4-epoxy-VPA rather than the 4-ene-VPA originally suggested because its closely related

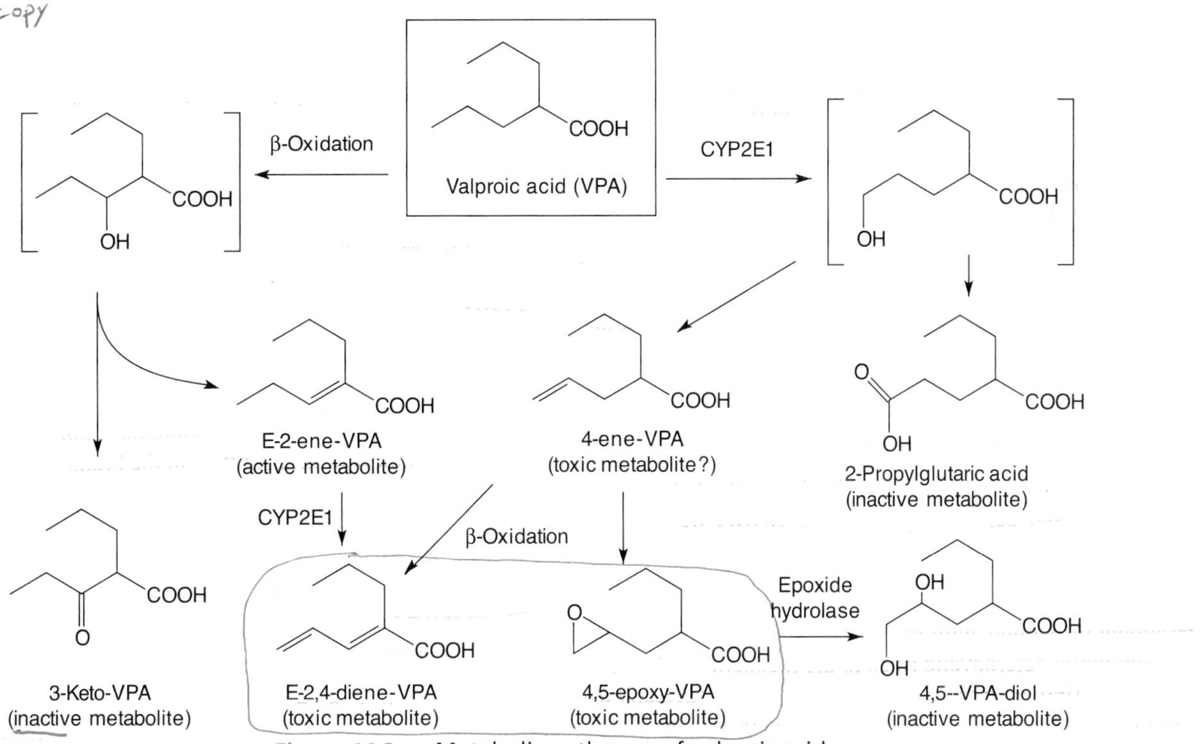

copy

Figure 14.3 ● Metabolic pathways of valproic acid.

analogs, α-fluoro-4-ene-VPA and α-fluoro-VPA, were not found to have any liver toxicity.[41] These toxic or reactive metabolites are normally detoxified as a cysteine conjugate via the GSH/glutathione transferase metabolic pathway.[41] Alternatively, the 4-epoxy-VPA can also be deactivated by epoxy hydrolase to form the corresponding inactive VPA-4, 5-diol (Fig. 14.3). It should be pointed out that these toxic metabolites may also react with the sulfhydryl group or other nucleophiles on the cellular proteins, thereby forming covalently bonded haptens. These drug-modified proteins then elicit and become the target of an immune response, thereby producing the observed idiosyncratic allergic reactions in clinically susceptible patients.

Valrocemide (valproyl glycinamide, VLR) and DP-VPA (SPD-421) are two novel VPA analogs currently in phase II clinical trials[42,43] (Fig. 14.4). The anticonvulsant properties of VLR were found to be a result of the parent molecule and not because of its metabolic biotransformation to VPA or glycine (i.e., itself an inhibitory neurotransmitter in the brain). The major in vivo inactive metabolite is valproyl glycine, which is formed via the normal metabolic inactivation of peptide drugs.[42] SPD-421, on the other

hand, is a phosphatidylcholine derivative of VPA. The phospholipid part of the molecule significantly increases its lipid solubility and facilitates its transport into the brain. Furthermore, SPD-421 was found to be minimally metabolized in the liver with most of the drug renally eliminated. However, upon entry into the brain, SPD-421 is specifically cleaved by the enzyme, phosplipase A_2 (PLA$_2$), at the site of seizure to release VPA (there is evidence that the activity of PLA$_2$ is significantly increased in neurons associated with epileptiform activity prior to seizure attack).[43] Thus, unlike VPA, both of these drugs are said to have low drug-interaction potentials.

Phenytoin (Dilantin, Kapseals, Phenytek) and Fosphenytoin (Cerebyx)

Phenytoin, 5,5-diphenylhydantoin (Dilantin), is a prime example of an effective anticonvulsant acting through its action at the VGSC.[18] Phenytoin is structurally very similar to phenobarbital but lacks the dependence liability (see the discussion of barbiturate-type anxiolytic hypnotic–sedative drugs under "CNS Depressants" in this

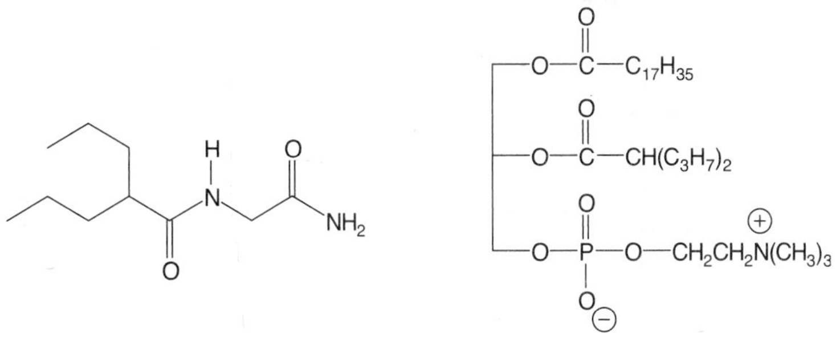

Figure 14.4 ● Novel valproic acid analogs in phase II trials.

Valrocemide

DP-VPA (SPD-421)

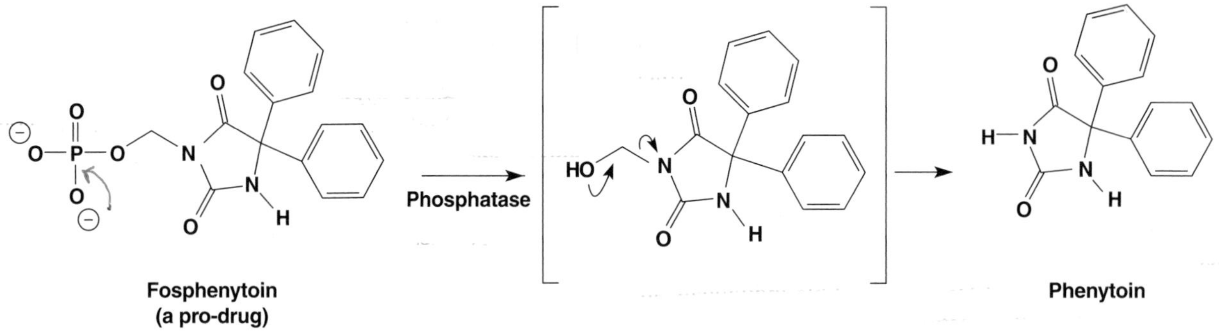

Figure 14.5 ● Biotransformation of fosphenytoin to phenytoin.

text). Phenytoin is very effective against all seizure types except absence; however, the drug may be incompletely or erratically absorbed from sites of administration because of its very low water solubility. For this reason, fosphenytoin, a prodrug of phenytoin, was developed and marketed to avoid complications such as vein irritation, tissue damage, and muscle necrosis associated with parenteral phenytoin administration. Fosphenytoin is rapidly absorbed either by intravenous or intramuscular administration.[43] It is converted into phenytoin through phosphatase

catalyzed hydrolysis of the phosphate ester as shown in Figure 14.5.

METABOLISM OF PHENYTOIN

The principal metabolic pathway of phenytoin in humans is aromatic hydroxylation, catalyzed by the cytochrome P450 isozymes (CYP2C9 and CYP2C19).[10,44] The metabolic biotransformations and its in vivo detoxification pathways are depicted in Figure 14.6. The major metabolites of phenytoin

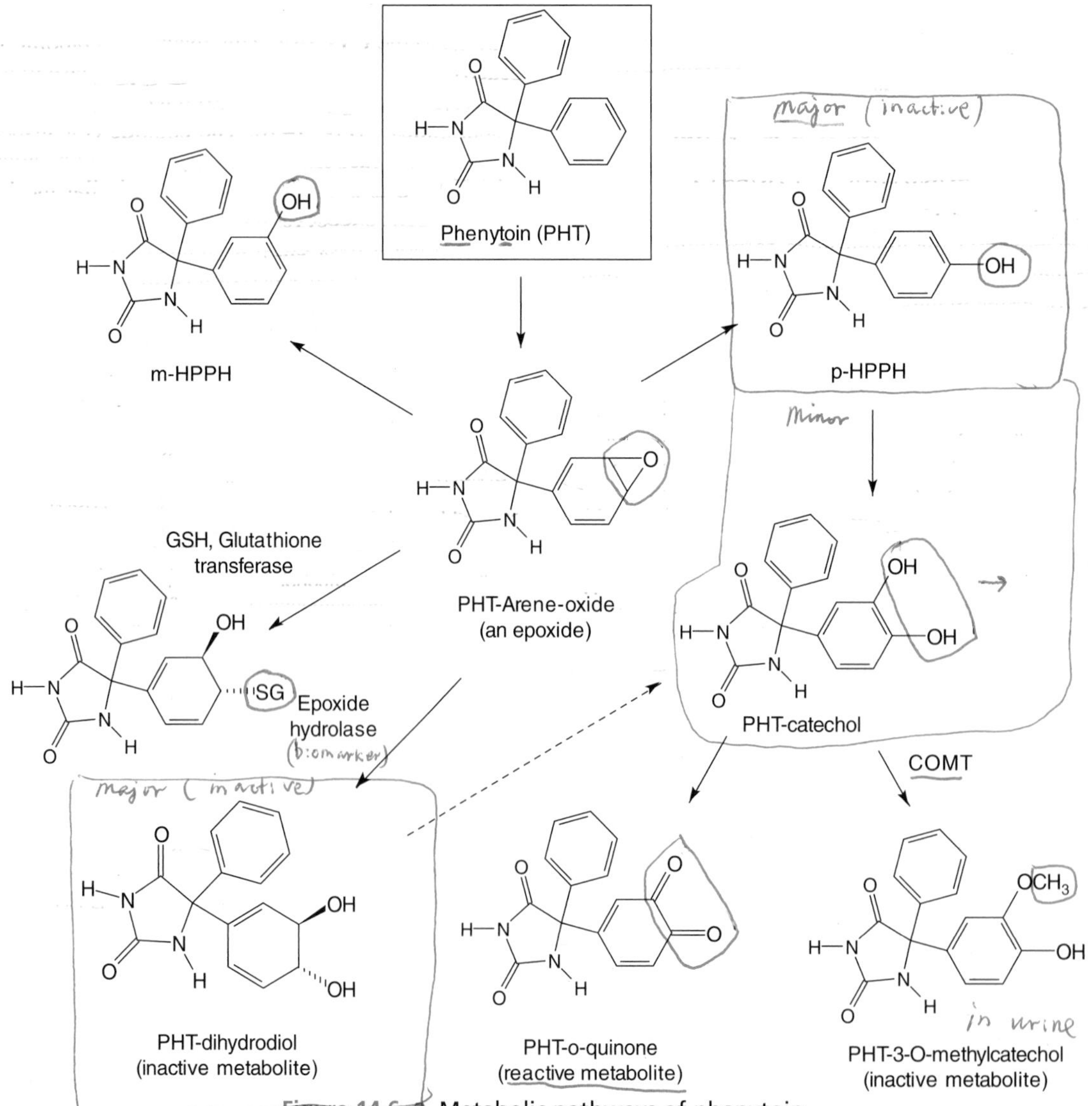

Figure 14.6 ● Metabolic pathways of phenytoin.

are the 5-(4-hydroxyphenyl)-5-phenyl hydantoins (*p*-HPPH) and dihydrodiol. Both of these inactive metabolites are excreted as the corresponding *O*-glucuronides. Further oxidation of *p*-HPPH leads to a catechol metabolite, which appears in the urine as a methyl conjugate by the action of catechol-*O*-methyltransferase (COMT).

HYPERSENSITIVITY REACTION OF PHENYTOIN

Hypersensitivity reactions (idiosyncratic toxicity) to phenytoin and other aromatic AEDs in susceptible individuals are believed to stem from the reactions of these reactive intermediates (i.e., arene oxide, catechol, or *o*-quinone) with hepatic enzymes or other cellular proteins forming covalently bonded haptens.[45] The reactive intermediate, arene oxide, is deactivated by either epoxide hydrolase to dihydrodiol (a major urinary metabolite) or by the action of GSH and glutathione transferase. It has also been suspected that these reactive arene oxides or epoxides mediate the teratogenicity of phenytoin and other AEDs. Recent studies indicate that epoxide hydrolase might be useful as a biomarker for prenatal determination of risk of fetal hydantoin syndrome.[46,47] Again, glutathione and epoxide hydrolase are important for detoxification of these reactive metabolites. Furthermore, a normal level of COMT in the liver or kidneys also greatly reduces the amount of catechol, which can be easily oxidized to the reactive *o*-quinone. Thus, COMT and the NADPH-dependent quinine oxidoreductase may play a protective role in phenytoin-induced toxicities.[48]

Both phenytoin and phenobarbital are potent liver enzyme inducers. Both of these drugs induce cytochrome P450 isozymes CYP1A2, CYP2C9/19, and CYP3A4, as well as epoxide hydrolase and UDP-glucuronyl transferase (phase II enzyme responsible for glucuronide formation).[10] Thus, for patients who are using multiple drugs, their plasma concentrations for drugs metabolized by these enzymes will be greatly affected.

Phenobarbital and Primidone (Mysoline)

Although sedative–hypnotic barbiturates commonly display anticonvulsant properties, only phenobarbital display enough anticonvulsant selectivity for use as antiepileptics. Primidone (Mysoline) is metabolized by CPY2C9/19 to phenobarbital and phenylethylmalonamide (PEMA) as shown in Figure 14.7. Both of these metabolites have anticonvulsant activities. However, it is generally believed that the pharmacological action of primidone is mainly a result of the minor metabolite, phenobarbital. Thus, primidone is much less potent/toxic than phenobarbital, because most of the drug is rapidly degraded to the less potent metabolite, PEMA.[49]

Carbamazepine (Tegretol) and Oxcarbazepine (Trileptal)

CBZ, 5H dibenz[b,f]lazepine 5 carboxamide is an iminostilbene derivative of tricyclic antidepressants.[50] The two phenyls substituted on the urea nitrogen fit the pharmacophore pattern suggested for binding to the VGSC[21] (Fig. 14.1). Like phenytoin, CBZ is useful in generalized tonic–clonic and partial seizures.

The major metabolic pathway of CBZ is the formation of a stable metabolite, 10,11-CBZ epoxide by cytochrome P450 isozyme CYP3A4. This reactive metabolite is further deactivated by the action of epoxide hydrolase to give inactive 10,11-CBZ-diol that is excreted as the corresponding glucuronides[50] (Fig. 14.8). The epoxide is a suspect in the idiosyncratic reactions CBZ may produce (e.g., aplastic anemia).[48] OXC is a newer AED with a similar mechanism of action to CBZ except for its metabolic inactivation pathway. It is also not a liver enzyme inducer like CBZ and phenytoin.[43,50] With the presence of a carbonyl function at the C-10 carbon, OXC is reduced to the corresponding CBZ-10-ol by the action of alcohol dehydrogenase that is excreted as its

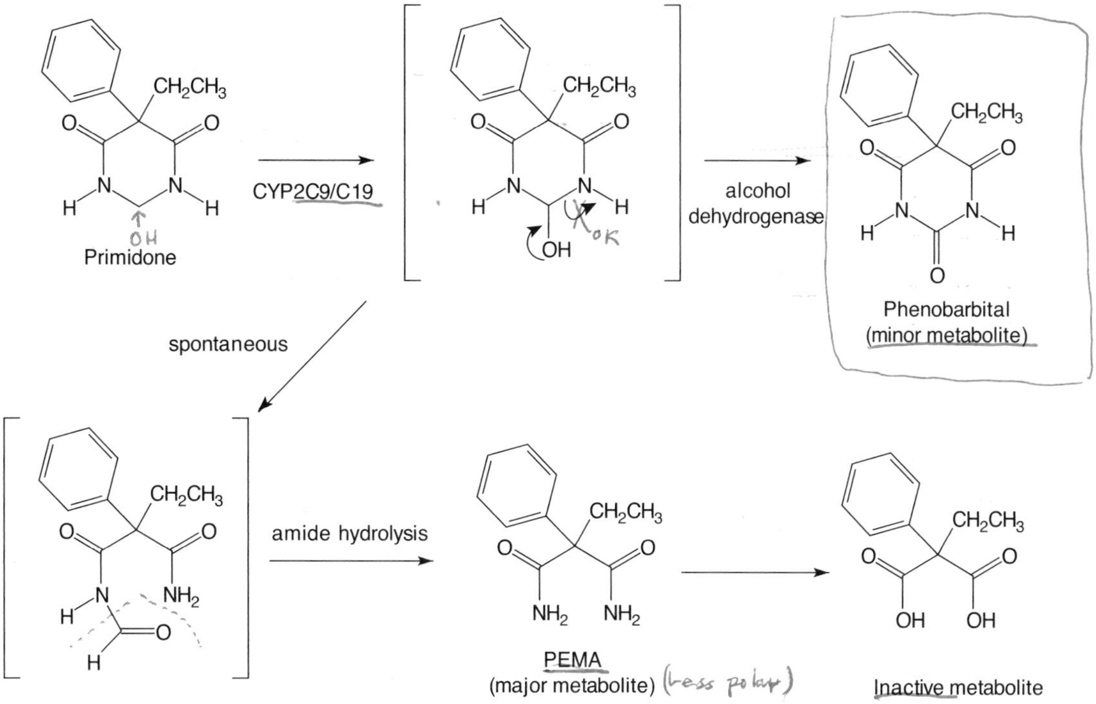

Figure 14.7 ● Metabolic biotransformation of primidone.

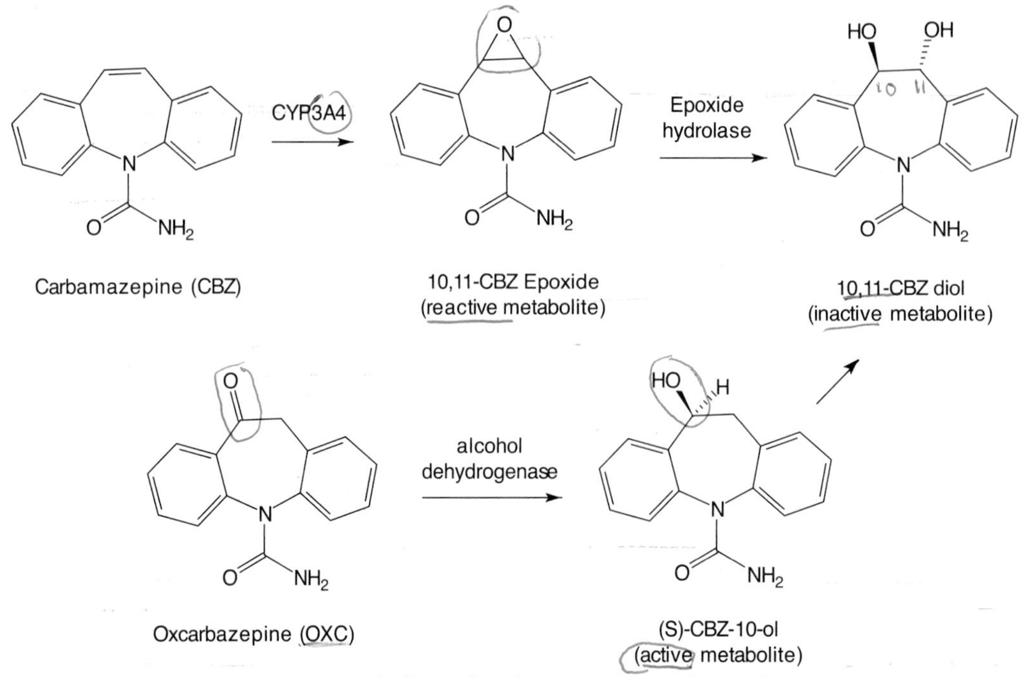

Figure 14.8 • Metabolism of carbamazepine and oxcarbazepine.

O-glucuronide or can be further oxidized to the 10,11-CBZ-diol as an inactive metabolite (Fig. 14.8). Thus, OXC is said to have much fewer hepatic and idiosyncratic side effects associated with CBZ.[23] Although OXC does not induce its own metabolism, it is a weak inducer of CYP3A4 and UDP-glucuronyl transferase and also inhibits CYP2C19. Thus, severe drug–drug interactions with medications metabolized by these enzymes are to be expected.[43]

Gabapentin (Neurontin) and Pregabalin (Lyrica)

Gabapentin and its closely related analog pregabalin, (S)-3-isobutyl-GABA (Fig. 14.9), are broad-spectrum anticonvulsants with multiple mechanisms of action.[24,51] In addition to modulating calcium influx and stimulate GABA biosynthesis as discussed earlier, they also compete for the biosynthesis of L-glutamic acid because of their structural similarity to L-leucine.[51] Gabapentin and pregabalin have very little liability for causing metabolic-based drug–drug interactions, particularly when used in combination with other AEDs because they are not metabolized in humans. More than 95% of the drug is excreted unchanged through the kidneys. However, there are some differences in their bioavailability. Unlike gabapentin, which exhibits 60% bioavailability when given in low doses because of intestinal uptake by a saturable small neutral L-amino acid transporter, the absorption of pregabalin is almost complete (98%) and exhibits an ideal linear

pharmacokinetic profile.[24] This high bioavailability of pregabalin can be attributed to its closer structure similarity to the essential amino acid, L-leucine.

FELBAMATE (FELBATOL) AND FLUROFELBAMATE

FBM, another potent and effective AED with a broad spectrum of action, is a carbamate ester of 2-phenyl-1, 3-propanediol, structurally similar to the anxiolytic drug meprobamate.[43] The carbamate ester is stable to esterases and therefore provides good oral bioavailability. However, the FBM therapy was found to be associated with rare but severe side effects such as aplastic anemia, idiosyncratic reactions, and hepatic failures within 6 months of its market introduction.[52,53] Extensive clinical metabolic studies with FBM have been able to link the formation of reactive metabolite(s) and the clinically observed toxicities.[52] FBM undergoes hepatic cytochrome P450-mediated hydroxylations (i.e., catalyzed by hepatic isozymes, CYP3A4, and CYP2E1) to give 2-hydroxyfelbamate (2-OH-FBM) and *p*-hydroxyfelbamate (pOH-FBM) that are excreted as their corresponding glucuronides (Fig. 14.10).

However, FBM also undergoes esterase-catalyzed hydrolysis to give two minor metabolites, 2-phenyl-1, 3-propandiol monocarbamate (MCF) and 3-carbamoyl-2-phenylpropionic acid (CPPA). It has been suggested that during the oxidative degradation of MCF to CPPA, the intermediate, 3-carbamoyl-2-phenylpropionaldehyde could be converted to a potentially toxic reactive metabolite, 2-

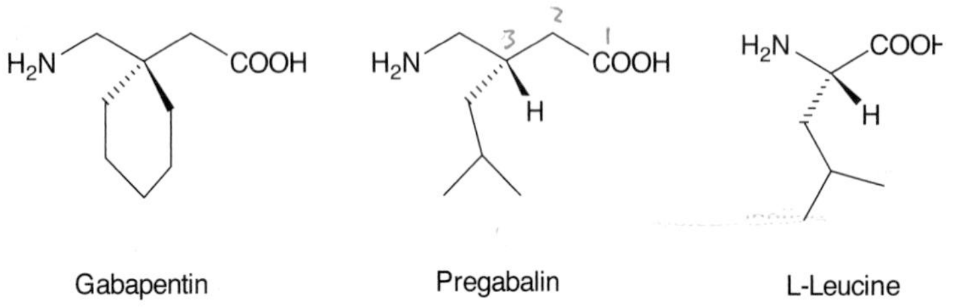

Figure 14.9 • Gabapentin, pregabalin, and L-leucine.

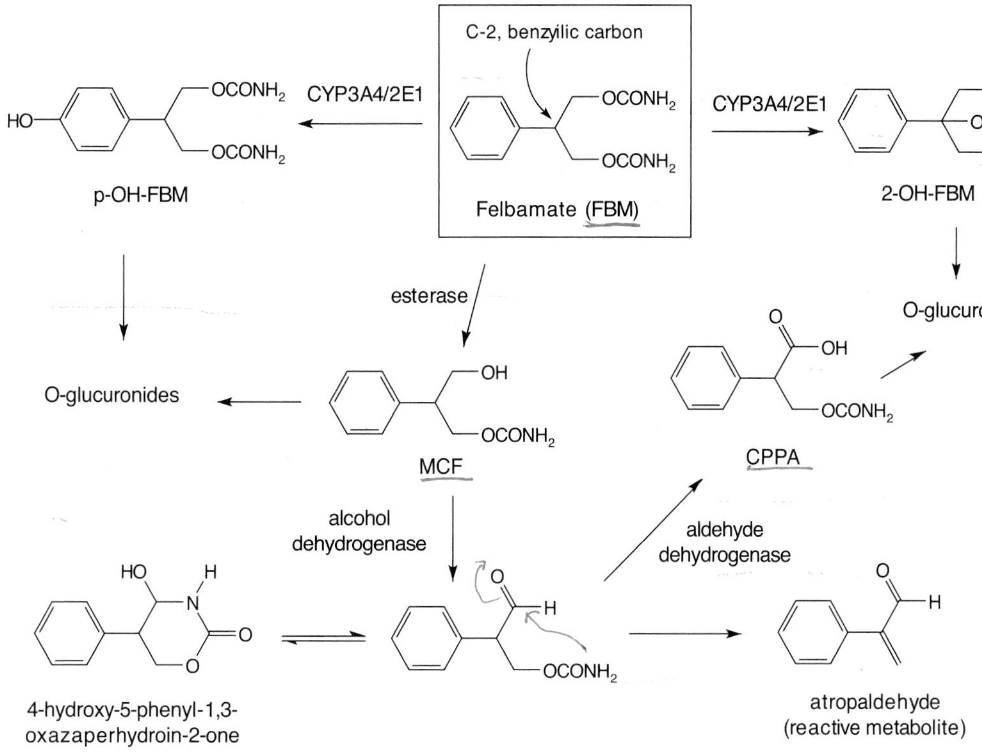

Figure 14.10 ● Metabolic biotransformation of felbamate.

phenylpropanal (atropaldehyde) that is normally deactivated as a cysteine conjugate via the GSH/glutathione transferase pathway discussed earlier under the metabolism of VPA.[39] Isolation of 4-hydroxy-5-phenyl-1, 3-oxazaperhydroin-2-one (i.e., a precursor for 2-phenylpropionaldehyde in human urine) provided further evidence linking this toxic metabolite to the observed clinical toxicities.[53] Similar to VPA discussed earlier, placement of a fluorine atom at the C-2 position of FBM resulted in a very potent anticonvulsant, 2-fluorofelbamate that lacks the idiosyncratic properties of FBM. Fluorofelbamate is currently under phase II clinical trials.[54]

It should be pointed out that although FBM has no effect on CYP2C9, it is an inhibitor of CYP2C19 and also inhibits the mitochondrial enzymes responsible for β-oxidation. Thus, drug interactions between FBM and VPA are to be expected.[55]

Novel Broad-Spectrum Anticonvulsants

Chemical structures of these newer broad-spectrum anticonvulsants are shown in Figure 14.11. All of these drugs have unique mechanisms of action and will be discussed in individual drug monographs.

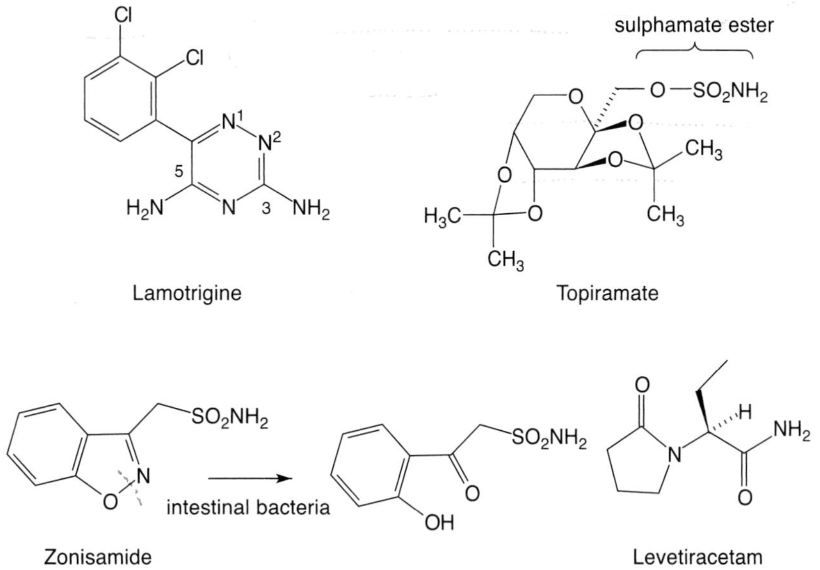

Figure 14.11 ● Newer broad-spectrum anticonvulsants.

LAMOTRIGINE (LAMICTAL)

Lamotrigine, an AED of the phenyltriazine class, has been found effective against refractory partial seizures. Like phenytoin and CBZ, its main mechanism of action appears to be blockade of sodium channels that is both voltage- and use-dependent. It also inhibits the high-threshold calcium channel, possibly through inhibition of presynaptic N-type calcium channels and also blocks glutamate release.[18,19] Lamotrigine is metabolized predominantly by glucuronidation. The major inactive urinary metabolites isolated are 2-N-glucuronide (76%) and 5-N-glucuronide (10%) because the aromatic ring is somewhat deactivated by the presence of chlorine atoms toward arene oxide formation.[56] Coadministration of lamotrigine with valproate, however, greatly increases the incidence of its idiosyncratic reactions.[56] It is conceivable that in the presence of VPA, an inhibitor of UDP-glucuronyl transferase, the concentration of the reactive arene oxide intermediate may be increased because of the reduced capacity of UDP-glucuronyl transferase to metabolize lamotrigine via normal glucuronidation pathways.

TOPIRAMATE (TOPAMAX)

TPM is a sulphamate-substituted monosaccharide, a derivative of the naturally occurring sugar D-fructose that exhibits broad and potent AED actions at both glutamate and GABA receptors.[19] It has good oral bioavailability of 85% to 95%, most likely resulting from its structural similarity to D-glucose. Thus, it may be actively transported into the brain by the D-glucose transporter. (Recall that D-fructose and D-glucose have identical stereochemistry at many of their chiral centers.) Only about 20% of the drug is eliminated by hepatic metabolism (CYP2C19), the remaining drug is excreted unchanged by the kidneys.[57] The sulphamate ester is hydrolyzed by sulfatases to the corresponding primary alcohol, which is further oxidized to the corresponding carboxylic acid. Even though there are no reports of significant interactions between TPM and other AEDs, TPM is said to have a weak carbonic anhydrase inhibitory activity because of the presence of the sulphamate moiety. Thus, concomitant use of TPM with other carbonic anhydrase inhibitors should be avoided.[57] The exact mechanism of actions are still unknown, but TPM appears to block glutamate release, antagonize glutamate kainic acid/AMPA receptors, and increase GABAergic transmission by binding to a site distinct from BZDs or barbiturates on the GABA$_A$ receptor complex.[19]

ZONISAMIDE (ZONEGRAN, EXCEGRAN)

Zonisamide, a sulfonamide-type anticonvulsant was recently approved for adjunctive therapy in the treatment of partial seizures in adults with epilepsy.[43] Zonisamide is primarily metabolized by reductive ring cleavage of the 1, 2-benzisoxazole ring to 2-sulfamoyl-acetyl-phenol (Fig. 14.11). This biotransformation is mainly carried out by the intestinal bacteria rather than the mammalian cytosolic aldehyde oxidase suggested earlier.[58] Again, because of the presence of a sulfonamide moiety in zonisamide molecule, precaution should be given to patients who have a history of hypersensitivity reactions toward sulfonamide drugs and concomitant use of zonisamide with other carbonic anhydrase inhibitors should also be avoided.[59]

LEVETIRACETAM (KEPPRA)

LEV is an analog of the nootropic agent, piracetam. Only the S-isomer shown in Figure 14.11 has any anticonvulsant activity. Unlike piracetam, LEV does not have any affinity for the AMPA receptor thereby has no nootropic activity for the treatment of Alzheimer disease. LEV also has no affinity for GABA receptors, BZD receptors, the various excitatory amino acid related receptors, or the voltage-gated ion channels.[43,60] For this reason, its mechanism of anticonvulsant action remains unclear, but it appears to exert its antiepileptic action by modulating kainite/AMPA-induced excitatory synaptic currents, thus decreasing membrane conductance.[60] Furthermore, the anticonvulsant activity of this drug appears to be mediated by the parent molecule rather than by its inactive metabolite, (S)-α-ethyl-2-oxo-1-pyrrolidineacetic acid (i.e., via the hydrolysis of amide group).[61] Like gabapentin, LEV has few drug interactions with other AEDs thereby can be used in combination to treat refractory epilepsy.[10,56]

Anticonvulsants Acts on a Selective Molecular Target

TIAGABINE (GABITRIL)

A glance at tiagabine's structure (Fig. 14.12) suggests an uptake inhibitor. Reportedly, it blocks GABA reuptake as a major mode of its anticonvulsant activity. Its use is against partial seizures. Inhibitors of GABA transporter-1 (GAT-1 inhibitors) increase extracellular GABA concentration in the hippocampus, striatum, and cortex, thereby prolonging the inhibitory action of GABA released synaptically. Nipecotic acid is a potent inhibitor of GABA reuptake into synaptosomal membranes, neurons, and glial cells. However, nipecotic acid fails to cross the blood-brain barrier following systemic administration because of its high degree of ionization. Tiagabine, marketed as the single R($-$)-enantiomer, a potent GAT-1 inhibitor structurally related to nipecotic acid, has an improved ability to cross the blood-brain barrier, and it has recently received Food and Drug Administration (FDA) approval as an AED.[43] It is well absorbed and readily metabolized by CYP3A4 to an inactive metabolite, 5-oxo-tiagabine (oxidation of the thiophen ring) or eliminated as glucuronide of the parent molecule.

Over 90% of tiagabine is metabolized by CYP3A4 isozymes.[62] The primary site of metabolic attack is the oxidation of the thiophen rings leading to 5-oxo-tiagabine that lacks anticonvulsant activity and the glucuronidation via the carboxylic function. Thus, the plasma concentrations of tiagabine would be greatly effected by any compound that induces or inhibits CYP3A4.

ETHOSUXIMIDE (ZARONTIN) AND METHSUXIMIDE (CELONTIN)

Ethosuximide is considered the prototypical anticonvulsant needed for treating patients with absence seizures.[6,19,25] Ethosuximide and the N-dealkylated active metabolite of methsuximide (Fig. 14.12) work by blocking the low-threshold T-type calcium channels, thereby reducing the hyperexcitability of thalamic neurons that is specifically associated with absence seizure.[20]

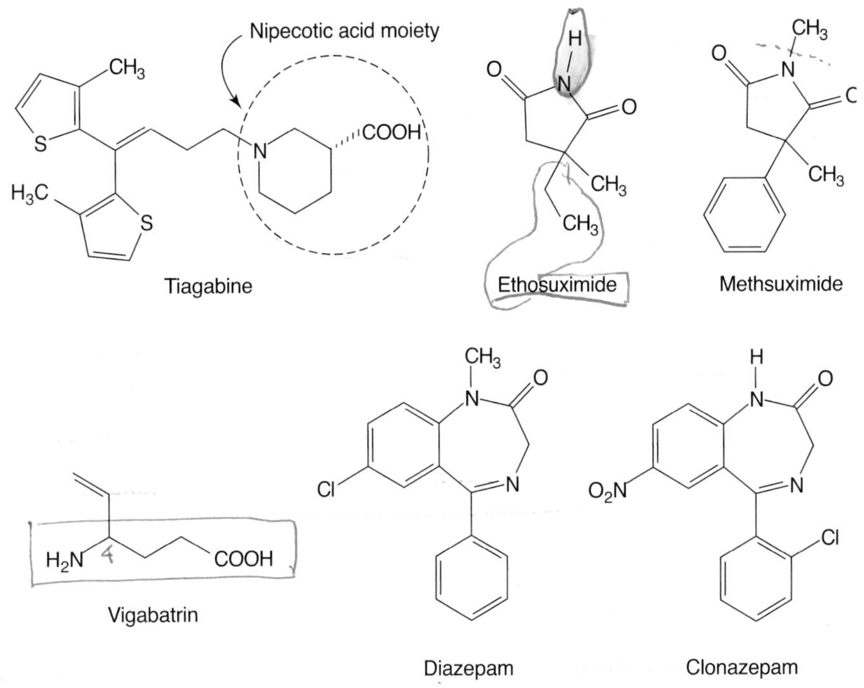

Nipecotic acid moiety

Tiagabine

Ethosuximide

Methsuximide

Vigabatrin

Diazepam

Clonazepam

Figure 14.12 ● Anticonvulsants acts on a selective molecular target.

VIGABATRIN (SABRIL)

Vigabatrin, a 4-vinyl analog of GABA, produces its pharmacological action by irreversibly blocking GABA catabolism catalyzed by GABA-T as discussed earlier. It is marketed in Europe and Canada as an adjunctive treatment of patients with partial seizures, but it has yet to gain FDA approval in the United States even after extensive clinical trials.[56] The main concern with this drug is its ability to cause a reversible visual field defect associated with retinal function in the eyes.[63]

BENZODIAZEPINES

For details of the chemistry and SARs of the BZDs, see the discussion of anxiolytic sedative–hypnotic drugs. Among the current clinically useful drugs, the structural features associated with anticonvulsant activity are identical with those associated with anxiolytic sedative–hypnotic activity.

Clonazepam (Klonopin)

Clonazepam is useful in absence seizures and in myoclonic seizures. Tolerance to the anticonvulsant effect of the clonazepam often developed rather quickly, and it is a common problem with the BZDs. Metabolism involves hydroxylation of the C-3 position, followed by glucuronidation and nitro group reduction, followed by acetylation.

Diazepam (Valium, Diastat)

Diazepam is given orally (Valium) or rectally (Diastat) as an adjunctive treatment in patients with generalized tonic–clonic status epilepticus (i.e., an acute and potentially fatal seizure) or in patients with refractory epilepsy in combination with other AEDs.[4] For details on diazepam (Valium), see its discussion under anxiolytics and sedative–hypnotic agents.

⬡ FUTURE DEVELOPMENT OF ANTIEPILEPTIC DRUGS

As stated earlier, even with the recent introduction of newer AEDs, greater than a third of newly diagnosed patients with epilepsy are still in need of an effective AED to control their seizures.[3,11,20] Furthermore, all current AEDs work only as prophylaxis against the symptoms of epilepsy, they do not prevent disease progression into refractory epilepsy. Future directions in the development of AEDs must come from either a better understanding of the epileptogenesis, especially the genetic mechanisms that underlie disease progression or the development of resistance after prolonged pharmacotherapy,[3] or from an innovative design strategy that produce new AEDs with unique mechanisms of action.[11] Several of these agents are currently undergoing different phases of clinical trials. The readers are to consult recent reviews for further details of these agents.[64–66]

● R E V I E W   Q U E S T I O N S ●

1. Provide a biochemical reason why pregabalin has better bioavailability than gabapentin.

2. SSADH deficiency, a rare inborn error of human metabolism, disrupts the normal metabolism of the inhibitory neurotransmitter GABA. Explain why these individuals are more susceptible to seizure activity.

3. Explain chemically/biochemically why 2-fluoro-VPA, a synthetic analog of VPA currently in clinical trials, may not possess similar hepatotoxic/teratogenic side effects as VPA.

4. Provide a biochemical rationale why valrocemide, a VPA analog, lacks epoxide hydrolase inhibitory activity and teratogenicity of VPA at clinically relevant concentrations.

5. Explain why coadministering valproate with phenytoin will increase its idiosyncratic toxicities. Identify at least two possible reactive metabolites of phenytoin that may be responsible for this observation.

6. Explain why there are cross-sensitivities among phenytoin, phenobarbital, fosphenytoin and primidone.

7. What will be the expected metabolic profile of CBZ if a specific inhibitor of CYP3A4 such as ketoconazole, an antifungal drug or the flavones present in grapefruit is taken concurrently?

8. Explain why lamotrigine is eliminated more rapidly in patients who have been taking CBZ or phenytoin.

9. Provide a possible rationale for why CYP3A4 inducers can increase the clearance of FBM, yet CYP3A4 inhibitors have little or no effect on its pharmacokinetic profile.

10. Explain why some dose adjustment of VPA may be required if FBM is added to a regimen of VPA.

REFERENCES

1. McAfee, A. T., Chilcott, K. E., Johannes, C. B., et al.: Epilepsia 48:1075–1082, 2007.
2. Tan, N. C. K., Mulley, J. C., and Berkovic, S. F.: Epilepsia 45:1429–1442, 2004.
3. Steinlein, O. K.: Nat. Rev. Neurosci. 5:400–408, 2004.
4. Pheops, S. J., Wheless, J. W., and Aldredge, B. K.: Seizure Disorders. In Helms, R.A., Quan, D. J., Herfindal, E. T., et al. (eds.). Textbook of Therapeutics—Drug and Disease Management, 8th ed. Philadelphia, Lippincott Williams & Wilkins, 2006, pp. 1608–1645.
5. Theodore, W. H., Spencer, S. S., Wiebe, S., et al.: Epilepsia 47:1700–1722, 2006.
6. Galuser, T., Ben-Menachem, E., Bourgeois, B., et al.: Epilepsia 47:1094–1120, 2006.
7. Avanzini, G.: Epilepsia 47:1285–1287, 2006.
8. Oby, E., and Janigro, D.: Epilepsia 47:1761–1774, 2006.
9. Lindhout, D.: Neurology 42(Suppl. 5):43–46, 1992.
10. Patsalos, P. N., and Perucca, E.: Lancet Neurol. 2:347–356, 2003.
11. Dichter, M. A.: Epilepsia 48(Suppl. 1):26–30, 2007.
12. Van Donselaar, C. A., and Stroink, H.: Epilepsia 47(Suppl. 1):9–13, 2006.
13. Browne, T. R., and Holmes, G. L.: N. Engl. J. Med. 344:1145–1151, 2001.
14. Commission on Classification and Terminology of the International League Against Epilepsy. Epilepsia 22:489–501, 1981.
15. Commission on Classification and Terminology of the International League Against Epilepsy. Epilepsia 30:389–399, 1989.
16. Engel, Jr.: J. Epilepsia 47:1558–1568, 2006.
17. Jensen, T. S.: Eur. J. Pain 6(Suppl. A):61–68, 2002.
18. Czapinski, P., Blaszczyk, B., and Czuczwar, S.: J. Curr. Top. Med. Chem. 5:3–14, 2005.
19. Rho, J. M., and Sankar, R.: Epilepsia 40:1471–1483, 1999.
20. Errington, A. C., Stöhr, T., and Lees G.: Curr. Top. Med. Chem. 5:15–30, 2005.
21. Unverferth, K., Engel, J., Höfgen, N., et al.: J. Med. Chem. 41:63–73, 1998.
22. DeLorenzo, R. J., Sun, D. A., and Deshpande, L. S.: Pharmacol. Ther. 105:229–266, 2005.
23. Cunningham, M. O., Woodhall, G. L., Thompson, S. E., et al.: Eur. J. Neurosci. 20:1566–1576, 2004.
24. Taylor, C. P., Angelotti, T., and Fauman, E.: Epilepsy Res. 73:137–150, 2007.
25. Gomora, J. C., Daud, A. N., Weiergräber, M., et al.: Mol. Pharmacol. 60:1121–1132, 2001.
26. Madeja, M., Margineanu, D. G., Gorji, A., et al.: Neuropharmacology 45:661–671, 2003.
27. De Smedt, T., Raedt, R., Vonck, K., et al.: CNS Drugs Rev. 13:43–56, 2007.
28. Foster, A. C., and Kemp, J. A.: Curr. Opin. Pharmacol. 6:7–17, 2006.
29. Costa, E.: Annu. Rev. Pharmacol. Toxicol. 38:321–350, 1998.
30. Johannessen, C. U.: Neurochem. Internat. 37:103–110, 2000.
31. Silverman, R. B., Andruszkiewicz, R., Nanavati, S. M., et al.: J. Med. Chem. 34:2295–2198, 1991.
32. Petroff, Q. A. C., Hyder, F., Rothman, D. L., et al.: Epilepsia 41:675–680, 2000.
33. Jung, M. J., Lippert, B., Metcalf, B. W., et al.: J. Neurochem. 29:797–802, 1977.
34. Schousboe, A., Sarup, A., Larsson, O. M., et al.: Biochem. Pharmacol. 68:1557–1563, 2004.
35. Chebib, M., and Johnston, G. A. R.: J. Med. Chem. 43:1427–1447, 2000.
36. Ozawa, S., Kamiya, H., and Tsuzuki, K.: Progress Neurobiol. 54:581–618, 1998.
37. Nakanishi, S.: Sciences 258:597–603, 1992.
38. Albensi, B. C., Igoechi, C., Janigro, D., et al.: Am. J. Alzheimers Dis. Other Demen. 19:269–274, 2004.
39. Jurima-Romet, M., Abbott, F. S., Tang, W., et al.: Toxicology 112:69–85, 1996.
40. Neuman, M. G., Shear, N. H., Jacobson-Brown, P. M., et al.: Clin. Biochem. 34:211–218, 2001.
41. Tang, W., Borel, A. G., Fujimiya, T., et al.: Chem. Res. Toxicol. 8:671–682, 1995.
42. Spiegelstein, O., Yagen, B., and Bialer, M.: Epilepsia 40:545–552, 1999.
43. Bialer, M., Johannessen, S. I., Kupferberg, H. J., et al.: Epilepsy Research 51:31–71, 2002.
44. Browne, T. R., and LeDuc, B.: Phenytoin—Chemistry and biotransformation. In Levy, R. H., Mattson, R. H., and Meldrum, B. S. (eds.). Antiepleptic Drugs, 4th ed. New York, Raven Oress, Ltd., 1995, pp. 283–300.
45. Yasumori, T., Chen, L. S., Li, Q. H., et al.: Biochem. Pharmacol. 57:1297–1303, 1999.
46. Buehler, B. A., Delimont, D., van Waes, M., et al.: New Engl. J. Med. 322:1567–1572, 1990.
47. Hartsfield, J. K., Benford, S.A., and Hilbelink, D. R.: Biochem. Mol. Med. 56:144–151, 1995.
48. Leeder, J. S.: Epilepsia 39(Suppl. 7):S8–S16, 1998.
49. Ferranti, V., Chabenat, C., Ménager, S., et al.: J. Chromatography B. 718:199–204, 1998.
50. Benes, J., Parada, A., Figueiredo, A. A., et al.: J. Med. Chem. 42:2582–2587, 1999.
51. Taylor, C. P., Gee, N. S., Su, T. Z., et al.: Epilepsy Res. 29:233–249, 1998.
52. Dieckhaus, C. M., Thompson, C. D., Roller, S. G., et al.: Chem. Biol. Interact. 142:99–117, 2002.
53. Dieckhaus, C. M., Santos, W. L., Sofia, R. D., et al.: Chem. Res. Toxicol. 14:958–964, 2001.
54. Hovinga, C. A.: Expert Opin. Investig. Drugs, 11:1387–1406, 2002.
55. Wagner, M. L., Graves, N. M., Leppik, I. E., et al.: Clin. Pharmacol. Ther. 56:494–502, 1994.
56. Walker, M. C., and Patsalos, P. N.: Pharmac. Ther. 67:351–384, 1995.
57. Mimrod, D., Specchio, L. M., Britzi, M., et al.: Epilepsia 46:1046–1054, 2005.
58. Kitamura, S., Sugihara, K., Kuwasako, M., et al.: J. Pharm. Pharmacol. 49:253–256, 1997.
59. Fukushima, Y., and Seino, M.: Epilepsia 47:1860–1864, 2006.
60. Carunchio, I., Pieri, M., Ciotti, M. T., et al.: Epilesia 48:654–662, 2007.
61. Patsalos, P. N., Ghattaura, S., Ratnaraj, N., et al.: Epilesia 47:1818–1821, 2006.
62. Ingwersen, S. H., Pedersen, P. C., Groes, L., et al.: Eur. J. Pharm. Sci. 11:247–254, 2000.
63. Banin, E., Shalev, R. S., Obolensky, A., et al.: Arch. Ophthalmol. 121:811–816, 2003.
64. Schmidt, B.: Amer. Soc. Exp. Neurotherapeutics 4:62–69, 2007.
65. Löscher, W., and Schmidt, D.: Epilepsy Res. 69:183–272, 2006.
66. Malawska, B.: Curr. Top. Med. Chem. 5:69–85, 2005.

SELECTED READING

Castilla-Guerra, L., Fernández-Moreno, M. del C., López-Chozas, J. M., et al.: Electrolytes Disturbances and Seizures. Epilepsia 47:1990–1998, 2006.

Gidal, B. E., and Garnett, W. R.: Epilepsy. In DiPiro, J. T., Talbert, R. L., Yee, G. C., et al. (eds.). Pharmacotherapy—A Pathophysiologic Approach, 6th ed. New York, NY, McGraw-Hill, 2005, pp. 1023–1048.

Johannessen, C. U., and Johannessen, S. I.: Valroate: past, present, and future. CNS Drug Rev. 9:199–216, 2003.

Kaneko, S., Okada, M., Iwasa, H., et al.: Genetics of epilepsy: current status and perspectives. Neurosci. Res. 44:11–30, 2002.

Kwan, P., Sills, G. J., and Brodie, M. J.: The mechanisms of action of commonly used antiepileptic drugs. Pharmacol. Ther. 90:21–34, 2001.

Patsalos, P. N., and Perucca, E.: Clinically important drug interactions in epilepsy: interactions between antiepileptic drugs and other drugs. Lancet Neurol. 2:473–481, 2003.

Trevor, A. J., and Way, W. L.: Sedative-hypnotic drugs. In Katzung, B. G. (ed.). Basic & Clinical Pharmacology, 9th ed. New York, NY, McGraw-Hill, 2004, pp. 351–366.

CHAPTER 15

Central Nervous System Stimulants

JOHN M. BEALE, JR.

CHAPTER OVERVIEW

This chapter discusses a broad range of agents that stimulate the central nervous system (CNS). The *analeptics* classically are a group of agents with a limited range of use because of the general nature of their effects. The *methylxanthines* have potent stimulatory properties, mainly cortical at low doses but with more general effects as the dose is increased. The *central sympathomimetic agents* amphetamine and close relatives have alerting and antidepressant properties but are medically used more often as anorexiants. The *antidepressant drugs* are used most frequently in depressive disorders and can be broadly grouped into the monoamine oxidase inhibitors (MAOIs), the monoamine reuptake inhibitors, and agents acting on autoreceptors. A small group of miscellaneously acting drugs, which includes several hallucinogens, cocaine, and cannabinoids, concludes the chapter.

ANALEPTICS

The traditional analeptics are a group of potent and relatively nonselective CNS stimulants. The convulsive dose lies near their analeptic dose. They can be illustrated by picrotoxinin and pentylenetetrazole. Both are obsolete as drugs but remain valuable research tools in determining how drugs act. Newer agents, modafinil and doxapram, are more selective and have use in narcolepsy and as respiratory stimulants.

Picrotoxin
Picrotoxinin, the active ingredient of picrotoxin, has the following structure:

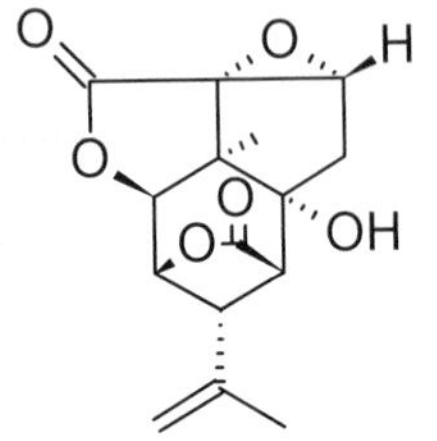

According to Jarboe et al.,[1] the hydroxylactonyl moiety is mandatory for activity, with the 2-propenyl group assisting. Picrotoxinin exerts its effects by interfering with the inhibitory effects of γ-aminobutyric acid (GABA) at the level of the GABA$_A$ receptor's chloride channel. The drug is obsolete medically. Pharmacologically, it has been useful in determining mechanisms of action of sedative–hypnotics and anticonvulsants. Butyrolactones bind to the picrotoxinin site.

Pentylenetetrazole
Pentylenetetrazole, 6,7,8,9-tetrahydro-5*H*-tetrazolo[*1,5-a*]azepine, 1,5-pentamethylenetetrazole (Metrazol), has been used in conjunction with the electroencephalograph to help locate epileptic foci. It is used as a laboratory tool in determining potencies of potential anticonvulsant drugs in experimental animals. The drug acts as a convulsant by interfering with chloride conductance.[2] It binds to an allosteric site on the GABA$_A$ receptor and acts as a negative modulator. Overall, it appears to share similar effects on chloride conductance with several other convulsive drugs, including picrotoxinin.

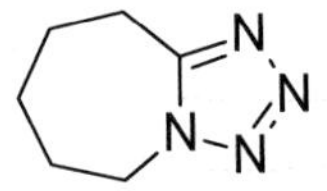

Modafinil
Modafinil (Provigil) has overall wakefulness-promoting properties similar to those of central sympathomimetics. It is considered an atypical α_1-norepinephrine (NE) receptor stimulant and is used to treat daytime sleepiness in narcolepsy patients. Adverse reactions at therapeutic doses are reportedly not severe and may include nervousness, anxiety, and insomnia. Modafinil is used by oral administration.

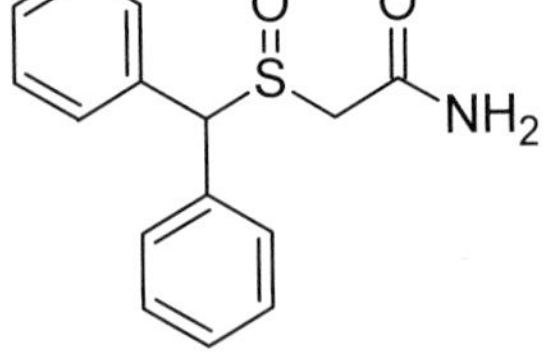

Doxapram Hydrochloride
Doxapram, 1-ethyl-4-(2-morpholinoethyl)-3,3-diphenyl-2-pyrrolidinone hydrochloride hydrate (Dopram), has an obscure molecular mechanism of action. Overall, it stimulates respiration by action on peripheral carotid chemoreceptors. It has use as a respiratory stimulant postanesthetically, after CNS depressant drug overdose, in chronic obstructive pulmonary diseases, and in the apneas. Dopram is administered exclusively by intravenous injection. Because of the benzyl alcohol content of the injectable formulation, Dopram must never be given to neonates.

METHYLXANTHINES

The naturally occurring methylxanthines are caffeine, theophylline, and theobromine. See Table 15.1 for their structures and occurrence and Table 15.2 for their relative potencies.

Caffeine is a widely used CNS stimulant. Theophylline has some medical use as a CNS stimulant, but its CNS-stimulant properties are encountered more often as sometimes severe, and potentially life-threatening, side effects of its use in bronchial asthma therapy. Theobromine has very little CNS activity (probably because of poor physicochemical properties for distribution to the CNS).

Caffeine is often used as it occurs in brewed coffee, brewed tea, and cola beverages. In most subjects, a dosage of 85 to 250 mg of caffeine acts as a cortical stimulant and facilitates clear thinking and wakefulness, promotes an ability to concentrate on the task at hand, and lessens fatigue. As the dose is increased, side effects indicating excessive stimulation (e.g., restlessness, anxiety, nervousness, tremulousness) become more marked. (They may be present in varying degrees at lower-dose levels.) With further increases in dosage, convulsions can occur. A review of the actions of caffeine in the brain with special reference to factors that contribute to its widespread use appears to be definitive.[3]

The CNS effects of theophylline at low-dose levels have been little studied. At high doses, the tendency to produce convulsions is greater for theophylline than for caffeine. In addition to being cortical stimulants, theophylline and caffeine are medullary stimulants, and both are used as such. Caffeine may be used in treating poisoning from CNS-depressant drugs, although it is not a preferred drug.

The important use of theophylline and its preparations in bronchial asthma is discussed elsewhere. Caffeine also is reported to have valuable bronchodilating properties in asthma. Finally, because of central vasoconstrictive effects, caffeine has value in treating migraine and tension headaches and may have actual analgesic properties in the latter use.

The CNS-stimulating effects of the methylxanthines were once attributed to their phosphodiesterase-inhibiting ability. This action is probably irrelevant at therapeutic doses. Evidence indicates that the overall CNS-stimulant ac-

tion is related more to the ability of these compounds to antagonize adenosine at A_1 and A_{2A} receptors.[3–6] All of the roles of these receptors are still under study. The adenosine receptor subtypes and their pharmacology have been reviewed.[3,7–9] Problems with the present compounds, such as caffeine and theophylline, are lack of receptor selectivity and the ubiquitous nature of the various receptor subtypes.

Caffeine and theophylline have pharmaceutically important chemical properties. Both are weak Brønsted-Lowry bases. The reported pK_a values are 0.8 and 0.6 for caffeine and 0.7 for theophylline. These values represent the basicity of the imino nitrogen at position 9. As acids, caffeine has a pK_a above 14, and theophylline, a pK_a of 8.8. In theophylline, a proton can be donated from position 7 (i.e., it can act as a Brønsted acid). Caffeine cannot donate a proton from position 7 and does not act as a Brønsted acid at pH values less than 14. Caffeine does have electrophilic sites at positions 1, 3, and 7. In addition to its Brønsted acid site at 7, theophylline has electrophilic sites at 1 and 3. In condensed terms, both compounds are electron-pair donors, but only theophylline is a proton donor in most pharmaceutical systems.

Although both compounds are quite soluble in hot water (e.g., caffeine 1:6 at 80°C), neither is very soluble in water at room temperature (caffeine about 1:40, theophylline about 1:120). Consequently, various mixtures or complexes designed to increase solubility are available (e.g., citrated caffeine, caffeine and sodium benzoate, theophylline–ethylenediamine compound [aminophylline]).

Caffeine in blood is not highly protein bound; theophylline is about 50% bound. Differences in the substituent at the 7-position may be involved. Additionally, caffeine is

TABLE 15.1 **Chemical Structures of the Xanthine Alkaloids**

Xanthine

(R, R', & R" = H)

Compound	R	R′	R″	Common Source
Caffeine	CH_3	CH_3	CH_3	Coffee, tea
Theophylline	CH_3	CH_3	H	Tea
Theobromine	H	CH_3	CH_3	Cocoa

TABLE 15.2 **Relative Pharmacological Potencies of the Xanthine Alkaloids**

Xanthine	CNS Stimulation	Respiratory Stimulation	Diuresis	Coronary Dilation	Cardiac Stimulation	Skeletal Muscle Stimulation
Caffeine	1[a]	1	3	3	3	1
Theophylline	2	2	1	1	1	2
Theobromine	3	3	2	2	2	3

[a]1, most potent

more lipophilic than theophylline and reputedly achieves higher brain concentrations. The half-life of caffeine is 5 to 8 hours, and that of theophylline, about 3.5 hours. About 1% of each compound is excreted unchanged. The compounds are metabolized in the liver. The major metabolite of caffeine is 1-methyluric acid, and that of theophylline, 1,3-dimethyluric acid.[10] Neither compound is metabolized to uric acid, and they are not contraindicated in gout.

CENTRAL SYMPATHOMIMETIC AGENTS (PSYCHOMOTOR STIMULANTS)

Sympathomimetic agents, whose effects are manifested mainly in the periphery, are discussed in Chapter 16. A few simple structural changes in these peripheral agents produce compounds that are more resistant to metabolism, more nonpolar, and better able to cross the blood-brain barrier. These effects increase the ratio of central to peripheral activity, and the agents are designated, somewhat arbitrarily, as *central sympathomimetic agents*.

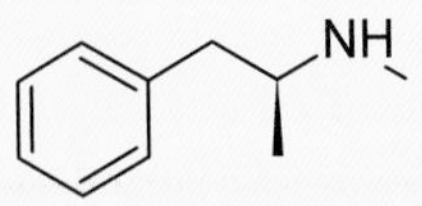

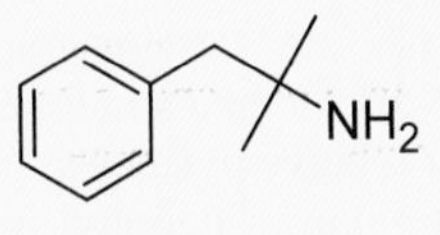

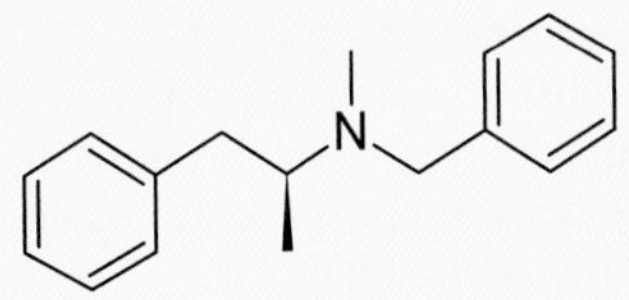

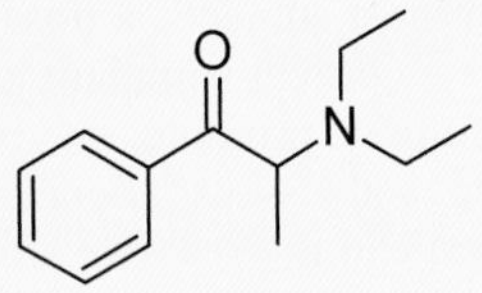

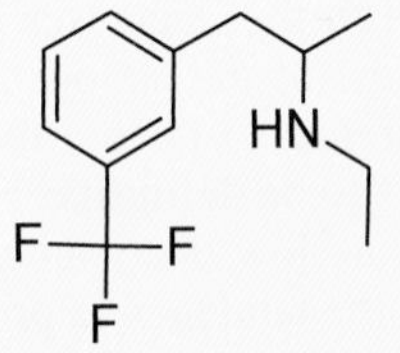

In addition to CNS-stimulating effects, manifested as excitation and increased wakefulness, many central sympathomimetics exert an anorexiant effect. Central sympathomimetic (noradrenergic) action is often the basis for these effects. Other central effects, notably dopaminergic and serotoninergic effects, can be operative, however.[11] In some agents, the ratio of excitation and increased wakefulness to anorexiant effects is decreased, and the agents are marketed as anorexiants. Representative structures of this group of compounds are given in Table 15.3. The structures of the anorexiants phendimetrazine and sibutramine and the alerting agents methylphenidate and pemoline, useful in attention-deficit disorders, are given in the text.

Structural features for many of the agents can be visualized easily by considering that within their structure, they contain a β-phenethylamine moiety, and this grouping can give some selectivity for presynaptic or postsynaptic noradrenergic systems. β-Phenethylamine, given peripherally, lacks central activity. Facile metabolic inactivation by monoamine oxidases (MAOs) is held responsible. Branching with lower alkyl groups on the carbon atom adjacent (α) to the amino nitrogen increases CNS rather than peripheral activity (e.g., amphetamine, presumably by retarding metabolism). The α branching generates a chiral center. The *dextro*(*S*)-isomer of amphetamine is up to 10 times as potent as the *levo*(*R*)-isomer for alerting activity and about twice as active as a psychotomimetic agent. Hydroxylation of the ring or hydroxylation on the β-carbon (to the nitrogen) decreases activity, largely by decreasing the ability to cross the blood-brain barrier. For example, phenylpropanolamine, with a β-hydroxyl (OH), has about 1/100th the ability to cross the blood-brain barrier of its deoxy congener, amphetamine.

Halogenation (F, Cl, Br) of the aromatic ring decreases sympathomimetic activity. Other activities may increase. *p*-Chloroamphetamine has strong central serotoninergic activity (and is a neurotoxin, destroying serotoninergic neurons in experimental animals).[12,13]

Methoxyl or methylenedioxy substitution on the ring tends to produce psychotomimetic agents, suggesting tropism for dopaminergic (D2) receptors.

N-methylation increases activity (e.g., compare methamphetamine with dextroamphetamine). Di-*N*-methylation de-

TABLE 15.3 Structures of Sympathomimetics with Significant Central Stimulant Activity

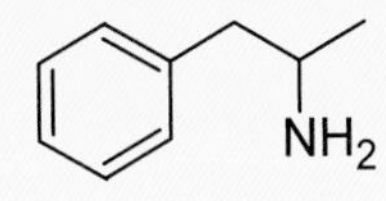

creases activity. Mono-*N* substituents larger than methyl decrease excitatory properties, but many compounds retain anorexiant properties. Consequently, some of these agents are used as anorexiants, reportedly with less abuse potential than amphetamine.

There can be some departure from the basic β-phenethylamine structure when compounds act by indirect noradrenergic mechanisms. A β-phenethylamine–like structure, however, can be visualized in such compounds.

The abuse potential of the more euphoriant and stimulatory of the amphetamines and amphetamine-like drugs is well documented. They produce an exceedingly destructive addiction. Apparently, both a euphoric "high" (possibly related to effects on hedonistic D2 receptors) and a posteuphoric depression (especially among amine-depleting drugs) contribute to compulsive use of these agents. Abuse of these drugs (especially methamphetamine) in recent years has reached disastrous proportions.

Recognized medical indications for dextroamphetamine and some very close congeners include narcolepsy, Parkinson disease, attention-deficit disorders, and, although not the preferred agents for obesity, appetite suppression. In some conditions, such as Parkinson disease, for which its main use is to decrease rigidity, the antidepressant effects of dextroamphetamine can be beneficial. It is also reportedly an effective antidepressant in terminal malignancies. In almost all cases of depression, and especially in major depressive disorders of the unipolar type, however, dextroamphetamine has long been superseded by other agents, notably the MAOIs and the monoamine reuptake-inhibiting antidepressants.

The compounds and their metabolites can have complex, multiple actions. In a fundamental sense, the structural basis for action is quite simple. The compounds and their metabolites resemble NE and can participate in the various neuronal and postsynaptic processes involving NE, such as synthesis, release, reuptake, and presynaptic and postsynaptic receptor activation. Also, because dopamine (DA) and, to a lesser extent, serotonin (5-hydroxytryptamine [5-HT]) bear a structural resemblance to NE, processes in DA- and 5-HT–activated systems can be affected. To illustrate the potential complexity, the receptor activations that can be associated with just one parameter, reduction in food intake, reportedly are α_1, β_1, β_2, 5-HT$_{1B}$, 5-HT$_{2A}$, 5-HT$_{2C}$, D$_1$, and D$_2$.

PRODUCTS

Amphetamine Sulfate

Amphetamine, ($\pm$)-1-phenyl-2-aminopropane (Benzedrine), as the racemic mixture has a higher proportion of cardiovascular effects than the *dextro* isomer. For most medical uses, the dextrorotatory isomer is preferred.

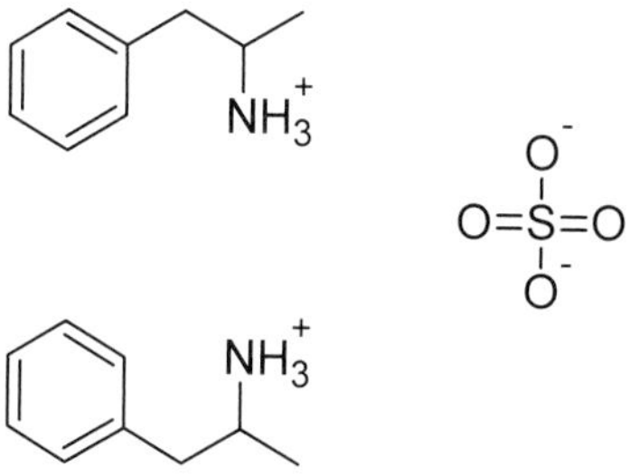

Dextroamphetamine Sulfate and Dextroamphetamine Phosphate

Dextroamphetamine, (+)-(S)-methylphenethylamine, forms salts with sulfuric acid (Dexedrine) and with phosphoric acids. The phosphate is the more water-soluble salt and is preferred if parenteral administration is required. The dextrorotatory isomer has the (S) configuration and fewer cardiovascular effects than the levorotatory (R)-isomer. Additionally, it may be up to 10 times as potent as the (R)-isomer as an alerting agent and about twice as potent a psychotomimetic agent. Although it is a more potent psychotomimetic agent than the (R)-isomer, it has a better ratio of alerting to psychotomimetic effects.

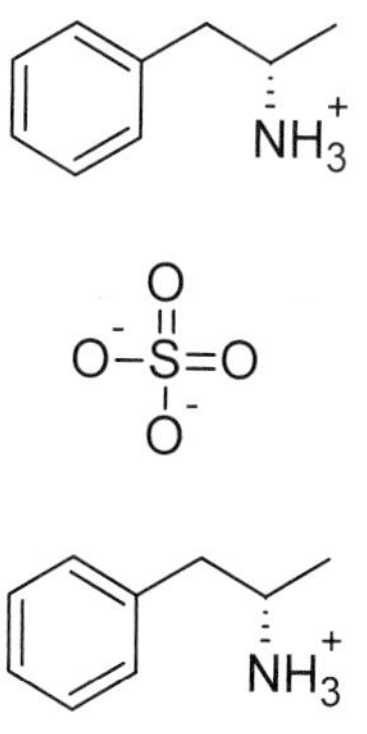

The major mode of action of dextroamphetamine is release of NE from the mobile pool of the nerve terminal. Other mechanisms, such as inhibition of uptake, may make a small contribution to the overall effects. The alerting actions relate to increased NE available to interact with postsynaptic receptors (α_1). Central β-receptor activation has classically been considered the basis for most of the anorexiant effect.

The psychotomimetic effects are linked to release of DA and activation of postsynaptic receptors. D$_2$ and mesolimbic D$_3$ receptors would be involved. Effects on 5-HT systems also have been linked to some behavioral effects of dextroamphetamine. Effects via 5-HT receptors would include 5-HT$_{1A}$ receptors and, theoretically, all additional receptors through 5-HT$_7$.

Dextroamphetamine is a strongly basic amine, with values from 9.77 to 9.94 reported. Absorption from the gastrointestinal tract occurs as the lipid-soluble amine. The drug is not extensively protein bound. Varying amounts of the drug are excreted intact under ordinary conditions. The amount is insignificant under conditions of alkaline urine. Under conditions producing systemic acidosis, 60% to 70% of the drug can be excreted unchanged. This fact can be used to advantage in treating drug overdose.

The α-methyl group retards, but does not terminate, metabolism by MAO. Under most conditions, the bulk of a dose of dextroamphetamine is metabolized by N-dealkylation to phenylacetone and ammonia. Phenylacetone is degraded further to benzoic acid.

In experimental animals, about 5% of a dose accumulates in the brain, especially the cerebral cortex, the thalamus, and the corpus callosum. It is first p-hydroxylated and then β-hydroxylated to produce p-hydroxynorephedrine, which has been reported to be the major active metabolite involved in NE and DA release.[14]

Methamphetamine Hydrochloride

Methamphetamine, (+)-1-phenyl-2-methylaminopropane hydrochloride desoxyephedrine hydrochloride (Desoxyn), is the N-methyl analog of dextroamphetamine. It has more marked central and less peripheral action than dextroamphetamine. It has a very high abuse potential, and by the intravenous route, its salts are known as "speed." The overall abuse problem presented by the drug is a national disaster. Medicinally acceptable uses of methamphetamine are analogous to those of dextroamphetamine.

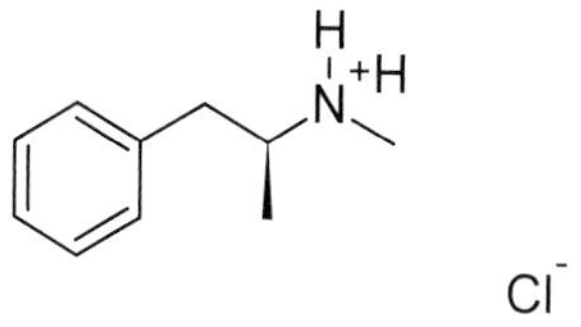

Phentermine Ion-Exchange Resin and Phentermine Hydrochloride

The free base is α,α-dimethylphenethylamine, 1-phenyl-2-methylaminopropane. In the resin preparation (Ionamin), the base is bound with an ion-exchange resin to yield a slow-release product; the hydrochloride (Wilpowr) is a water-soluble salt.

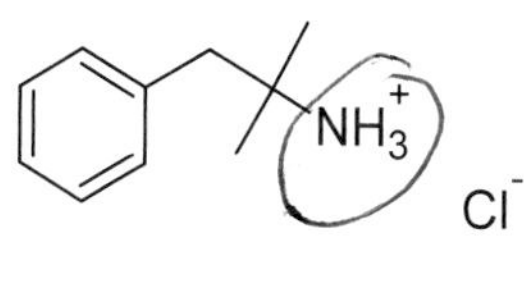

Phentermine has a quaternary carbon atom with one methyl oriented like the methyl of (S)-amphetamine and one methyl oriented like the methyl of (R)-amphetamine, and it reportedly has pharmacological properties of both the (R)- and (S)-isomers of amphetamine. The compound is used as an appetite suppressant and is a Schedule IV agent, indicating less abuse potential than dextroamphetamine.

Benzphetamine Hydrochloride

Benzphetamine hydrochloride, (+)-N-benzyl-N,α-dimethylphenethylamine hydrochloride, (+)-1-phenyl-2-(N-methyl-N-benzylamine)propane hydrochloride (Didrex), is N-benzyl–substituted methamphetamine. The large (benzyl) N-substituent decreases excitatory properties, in keeping with the general structure–activity relationship (SAR) for the group. Anorexiant properties are retained. Classically, amphetamine-like drugs with larger than N-methyl substituents are cited as anorexiant through central β-agonism. No claims for selectivity among β-receptor subtypes have been made in such citations. The compound shares mechanism-of-action characteristics with methylphenidate. Overall, it is said to reduce appetite with fewer CNS excitatory effects than dextroamphetamine.

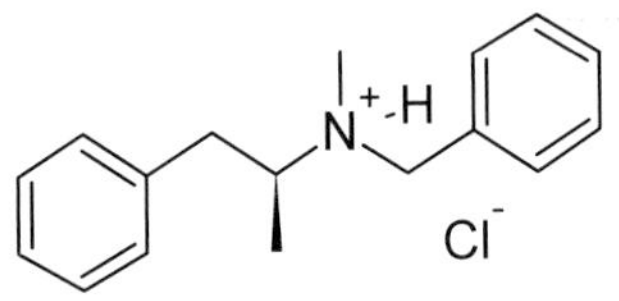

Diethylpropion Hydrochloride

Because it has two large (relative to H or methyl) N-alkyl substituents, diethylpropion hydrochloride, 1-phenyl-2-diethylaminopropan-1-one hydrochloride (Tenuate, Tepanil), has fewer sympathomimetic, cardiovascular, and CNS-stimulatory effects than amphetamine. It is reportedly an anorexiant agent that can be used for the treatment of obesity in patients with hypertension and cardiovascular disease. According to the generalization long used for this group of drugs, increasing N-alkyl size reduces central α_1 effects and increases β effects, even though the effects are likely mediated principally by indirect NE release.

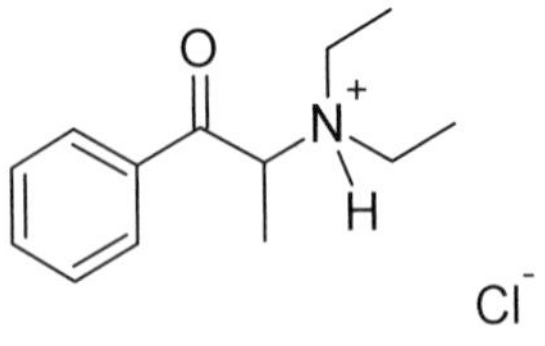

Fenfluramine Hydrochloride

Fenfluramine hydrochloride, (±)N-ethyl-α-methyl-m-(trifluoromethyl)phenethylamine hydrochloride (Pondimin), is unique in this group of drugs, in that it tends to produce sedation rather than excitation. Effects are said to be mediated principally by central serotoninergic, rather than central noradrenergic, mechanisms. In large doses in experimental animals, the drug is a serotonin neurotoxin.[15] It was withdrawn from human use after reports of heart valve damage and pulmonary hypertension. From its structure, more apolar or hydrophobic character than amphetamine, tropism for serotoninergic neurons would be expected. Likewise, the structure suggests an indirect mechanism. If an indirect mechanism were operative, then all postsynaptic 5-HT re-

ceptors could be activated. Evidence from several studies indicates that the 5-HT$_{1B}$ and the 5-HT$_{2C}$ receptors are most responsible for the satiety effects of 5-HT. 5-HT may also influence the type of food selected (e.g., lower-fat food intake).[11] The (+) isomer, dexfenfluramine (Redux), has a greater tropism for 5-HT systems than the racemic mixture. It, too, was withdrawn because of toxicity.

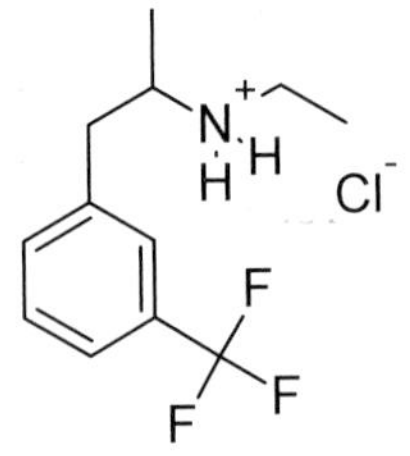

Phendimetrazine Tartrate

The optically pure compound phendimetrazine tartrate, (2S,3S)-3,4-dimethyl-2-phenylmorpholine-L-(+)-tartrate (Plegine), is considered an effective anorexiant that is less abuse prone than amphetamine. The stereochemistry of (+)phendimetrazine is as shown.[16]

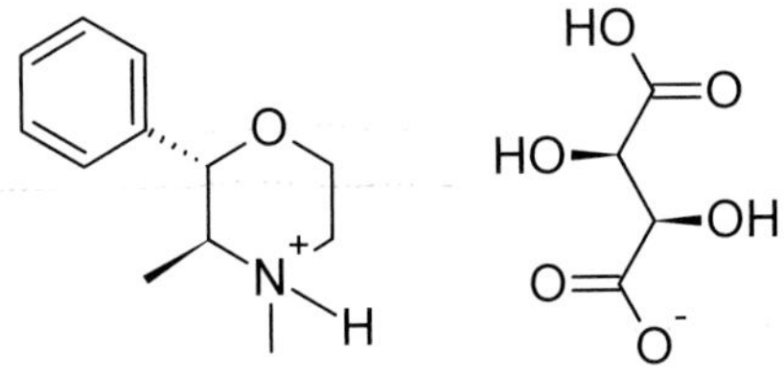

Sibutramine

Sibutramine (Meridia) is said to be an uptake inhibitor of NE and 5-HT. These mechanisms fit its structure. It is reportedly an antidepressant and an anorexiant drug. This mechanism implies that activation of all presynaptic and postsynaptic receptors in NE and 5-HT systems is possible. The data are not completely clear, but studies to date indicate that the receptors principally involved are α_1, β_1, and 5-HT$_{2C}$.[11]

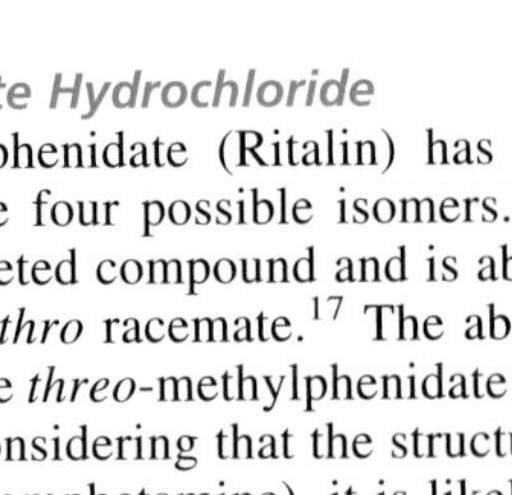

Methylphenidate Hydrochloride

Because methylphenidate (Ritalin) has two asymmetric centers, there are four possible isomers. The *threo* racemate is the marketed compound and is about 400 times as potent as the *erythro* racemate.[17] The absolute configuration of each of the *threo*-methylphenidate isomers has been determined.[18] Considering that the structure is fairly complex (relative to amphetamine), it is likely that one of the two components of the *threo* racemate contains most of the activity. Evidence indicates that the (+) -(2R,2'R)*threo* isomer is involved principally in the behavioral and pressor effects of the racemate.[19] As is likely with many central psychomotor stimulants, there are multiple modes of action.

Methylphenidate, probably largely via its *p*-hydroxy metabolite, blocks NE reuptake, acts as a postsynaptic agonist, depletes the same NE pools as reserpine, and has effects on dopaminergic systems, such as blocking DA reuptake.

Methylphenidate is an ester drug with interesting pharmacokinetic properties arising from its structure. The pK_a values are 8.5 and 8.8. The protonated form in the stomach reportedly resists ester hydrolysis. Absorption of the intact drug is very good. After absorption from the gastrointestinal tract, however, 80% to 90% of the drug is hydrolyzed rapidly to inactive ritalinic acid.[20] (The extent of hydrolysis may be about five times that for (+) versus (−).[21]) Another 2% to 5% of the racemate is oxidized by liver microsomes to the inactive cyclic amide. About 4% of a dose of the racemate reportedly reaches the brain in experimental animals and there is *p*-hydroxylated to yield the putative active metabolite.

Methylphenidate is a potent CNS stimulant. Indications include narcolepsy and attention-deficit disorder. The structure of the (2*R*,2′*R*) isomer of the *threo* racemic mixture is shown.

Pemoline

Pemoline, 2-amino-5-phenyl-4(5*H*)-oxazolone (Cylert), has a unique structure.

The compound is described as having an overall effect on the CNS like that of methylphenidate. Pemoline requires 3 to 4 weeks of administration, however, to take effect. A partial explanation for the delayed effect may be that one of the actions of the agent, as observed in rats, is to increase the rate of synthesis of DA.

◆ ANTIDEPRESSANTS

Monoamine Oxidase Inhibitors (MAOIs)

Antidepressant therapy usually implies therapy directed against major depressive disorders of the unipolar type and is centered on three groups of chemical agents: the MAOIs, the monoamine reuptake inhibitors, and autoreceptor desensitizers and antagonists. Electroshock therapy is another option. The highest cure or remission rate is achieved with electroshock therapy. In some patients, especially those who

are suicidal, this may be the preferred therapy. MAOIs and monoamine reuptake inhibitors have about the same response rate (60%–70%). In the United States, the latter group is usually chosen over MAOIs for antidepressant therapy. A key prescribing tenet is that if a member of the patient's family has been successfully treated with an antidepressant drug, then the patient will likely respond to that same drug.

A severe problem associated with the MAOIs that has been a major factor in relegating them to second-line drug status is that the original compounds inhibit liver MAOs irreversibly in addition to brain MAOs, thereby allowing dietary pressor amines that normally would be inactivated to exert their effects systemically. Several severe hypertensive responses, some fatal, have followed ingestion of foods high in pressor amines. It was hoped that the development of agents such as selegiline that presumably spare liver MAO might solve this problem. The approach of using MAO selectivity did solve the hypertensive problem, but the compound was not an antidepressant (it is useful in Parkinson disease). Another approach using a reversible MAOI has yielded antidepressants that lacked the hypertensive "cheese" effect. Another prominent side effect of MAOIs is orthostatic hypotension, said to arise from a block of NE released in the periphery. Actually, one MAOI, pargyline, was used clinically for its hypotensive action. Finally, some of the first compounds produced serious hepatotoxicity. Compounds available today reportedly are safer in this regard but suffer the stigma of association with the older compounds.

The history of MAOI development illustrates the role of serendipity. Isoniazid is an effective antitubercular agent but is a very polar compound. To gain better penetration into the *Mycobacterium tuberculosis* organism, a more hydrophobic compound, isoniazid substituted with an isopropyl group on the basic nitrogen (iproniazid), was designed and synthesized. It was introduced into clinical practice as an effective antitubercular agent. CNS stimulation was noted, however, and the drug was withdrawn. Later, it was determined in experimental animals and in vitro experiments with a purified MAO that MAO inhibition, resulting in higher synaptic levels of NE and 5-HT, could account for the CNS effects. The compound was then reintroduced into therapy as an antidepressant agent. It stimulated an intense interest in hydrazines and hydrazides as antidepressants and inaugurated effective drug treatment of depression.[22] It continued to be used in therapy for several years but eventually was withdrawn because of hepatotoxicity.

The present clinically useful irreversible inactivators can be considered mechanism-based inhibitors of MAO.[23] They are converted by MAO to agents that inhibit the enzyme. They can form reactants that bond covalently with the enzyme or its cofactor. A consequence of irreversible inactivation is that the action of the agents may continue for up to 2 weeks after administration is discontinued. The delay is caused by the necessity of synthesizing new, active MAO to replace the covalently inactivated enzyme. Consequently, many drugs degraded by MAO or drugs that elevate levels of MAO substrates cannot be administered during that time.

For a long time, because the agents that opened the field and then dominated it were irreversible inactivator, MAO inhibition was almost always regarded as irreversible. From the beginning, however, it was known that it was possible to have agents that act exclusively by competitive enzyme inhibition. For example, it has long been known that the harmala alkaloids harmine and harmaline act as CNS stimulants by competitive inhibition of MAO. Reversible (competitive) inhibitors selective for each of the two major MAO subtypes (A and B) are reportedly forthcoming.

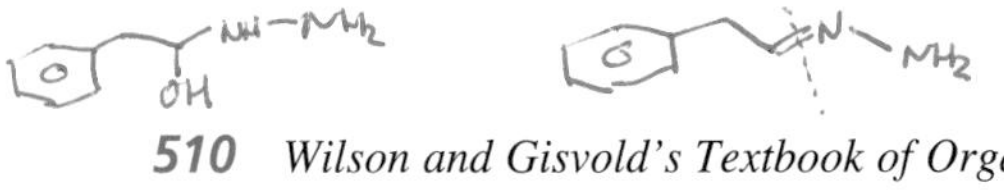

Moclobemide has received considerable attention abroad. A reversible inhibitor of MAO-A, it is considered an effective antidepressant and permits metabolism of dietary tyramine.[24] Metabolites of the drug are implicated in the activity. Reversible inhibitors of MAO-A (RIMAs) reportedly are antidepressant without producing hypertensive crises. Reversible inhibitors of MAO-B have also been studied. Presently, selective MAO-B inhibition has failed to correlate positively with antidepressant activity; selegiline, however, has value in treating Parkinson disease. A transdermal patch (Emsam) is useful in the treatment of depression.

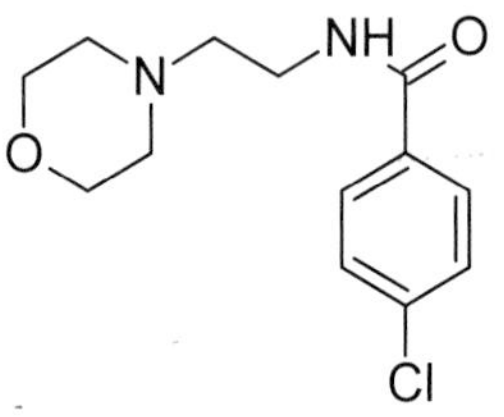

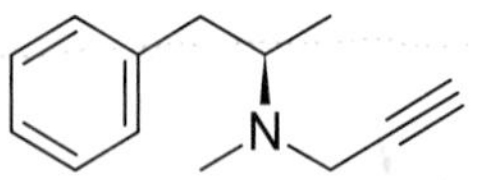

The clinically useful MAOI antidepressants are nonselective between inhibiting metabolism of NE and 5-HT. Agents selective for a MAO that degrades 5-HT have been under study for some time. The structures of phenelzine and tranylcypromine are given in Table 15.4.

Phenelzine Sulfate
Phenelzine sulfate, 2-(phenylethyl)hydrazine sulfate (Nardil), is an effective antidepressant agent. A mechanism-based inactivator, it irreversibly inactivates the enzyme or its cofactor, presumably after oxidation to the diazine, which can then break up into molecular nitrogen, a hydro-

gen atom, and a phenethyl free radical. The latter would be the active species in irreversible inhibition.[25]

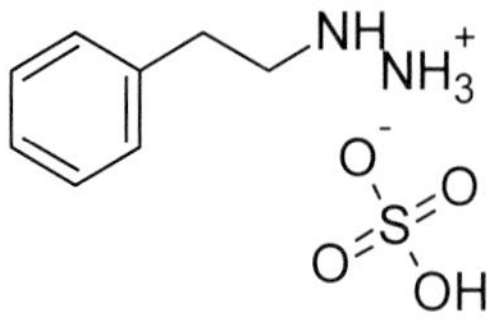

Tranylcypromine Sulfate
Tranylcypromine sulfate, (±)-*trans*-2-phenylcyclopropylamine sulfate (Parnate), was synthesized to be an amphetamine analog (visualize the α-methyl of amphetamine condensed onto the β-carbon atom).[26] It does have some amphetamine-like properties, which may be why it has more immediate CNS-stimulant effects than agents that act by MAO inhibition alone. For MAO inhibition, there may be two components to the action of this agent. One is thought to arise because tranylcypromine has structural features (the basic nitrogen and the quasi-π character of the α- and β-cyclopropane carbon atoms) that approximate the transition state in a route of metabolism of β-arylamines.[27,28] As α- and β-hydrogen atoms are removed from the normal substrate of the enzyme, the quasi-π character develops over the α,β-carbon system. Duplication of the transition state permits extremely strong, but reversible, attachment to the enzyme. Additionally, tranylcypromine is a mechanism-based inactivator. It is metabolized by MAO, with one electron of the nitrogen pair lost to flavin. This, in turn, produces homolytic fission of a carbon–carbon bond of cyclopropane, with one electron from the fission pairing with the remaining lone nitrogen electron to generate an imine (protonated) and with the other residing on a methylene carbon. Thus, a free radical is formed that reacts to form a covalent bond with the enzyme or with reduced flavin to inactivate the enzyme.[29]

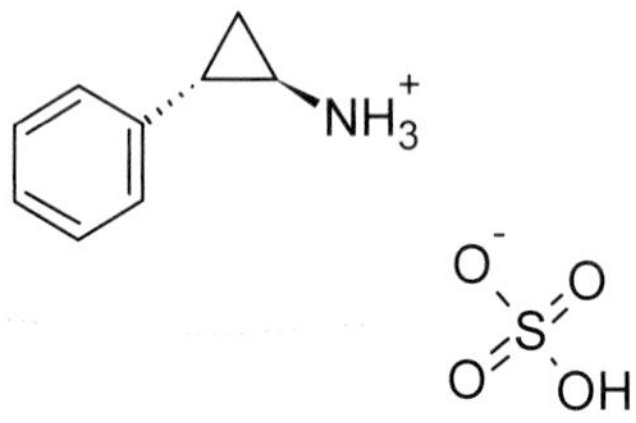

Monoamine Reuptake Inhibitors

Originally, the monoamine reuptake inhibitors were a group of closely related agents, the tricyclic antidepressants (TCAs), but now they are quite diverse chemically. Almost all of the agents block neuronal reuptake of NE or 5-HT or both (i.e., are selective).

Reuptake inhibition by these agents is at the level of the respective monoamine transporter via competitive inhibition of binding of the monoamine to the substrate-binding compartment. Probably the same site on the protein is involved for inhibitor and monoamine, but this has not yet been proved. The mechanism of reuptake by monoamine transporters has been reviewed.[30]

The net effect of the drug is to increase the level of the monoamine in the synapse. Sustained high synaptic levels of 5-HT, NE, or both appear to be the basis for the antidepressant effect of these agents. There is a time lag of 2 or more

TABLE 15.4 Structures of Monoamine Oxidase Inhibitors

Generic Name *Proprietary Name*	Structure
Phenelzine Sulfate *Nardil*	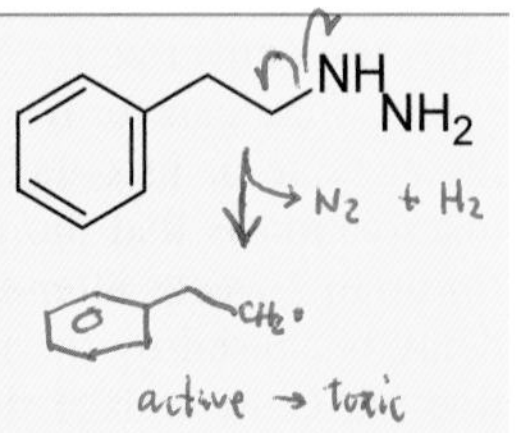
Tranylcypromine Sulfate *Parnate*	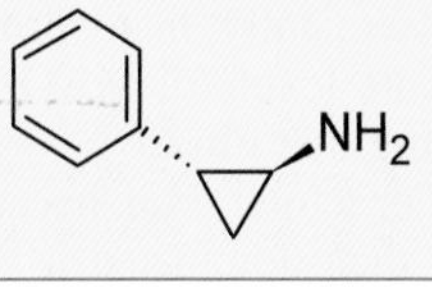

weeks before antidepressant action develops. It is considered that (in the case of 5-HT) 5-HT$_{1A}$ receptors and (in the case of NE) α_2 receptors undergo desensitization and transmitter release is maintained. Of course, activation of postsynaptic receptors and sustained transmission is the ultimate result of sustained synaptic levels of neurotransmitter.[31]

Tricyclic Antidepressants

The SARs for the TCAs are compiled in detail in the eighth edition of this text.[32] The interested reader is referred to this compilation. In summary, there is a large, bulky group encompassing two aromatic rings, preferably held in a skewed arrangement by a third central ring, and a three- or, sometimes, two-atom chain to an aliphatic amino group that is monomethyl or dimethyl substituted. The features can be visualized by consulting the structures of imipramine and desipramine as examples. The overall arrangement has features that approximate a fully extended *trans* conformation of the β-arylamines. To relate these features to the mechanism of action, reuptake block, visualize that the basic arrangement is the same as that found in the β-arylamines, plus an extra aryl bulky group that enhances affinity for the substrate-binding compartment of the transporter. The overall concept of a β-arylamine–like system with added structural bulk, usually an aryl group, appears to be applicable to many newer compounds—selective serotonin reuptake inhibitors (SSRIs), selective norepinephrine reuptake inhibitors (SNERIs)—that do not have a tricyclic grouping.

The TCAs are structurally related to each other and, consequently, possess related biological properties that can be summarized as characteristic of the group. The dimethylamino compounds tend to be sedative, whereas the monomethyl relatives tend to be stimulatory. The dimethyl compounds tend toward higher 5-HT to NE reuptake block ratios: in the monomethyl compounds, the proportion of NE uptake block tends to be higher and, in some cases, is considered selective NE reuptake. The compounds have anticholinergic properties, usually higher in the dimethylamino compounds. When treatment is begun with a dimethyl compound, a significant accumulation of the monomethyl compound develops as *N*-demethylation proceeds.

The TCAs are extremely lipophilic and, accordingly, very highly tissue bound outside the CNS. Because they have anticholinergic and noradrenergic effects, both central and peripheral side effects are often unpleasant and sometimes dangerous. In overdose, the combination of effects, as well as a quinidine-like cardiac depressant effect, can be lethal. Overdose is complicated because the agents are so highly protein bound that dialysis is ineffective.

PRODUCTS

Imipramine Hydrochloride

Imipramine hydrochloride, 5-[3-(dimethylamino)propyl]-10,11-dihydro-5*H*-dibenz[*b,f*]azepine monohydrochloride (Tofranil), is the lead compound of the TCAs. It is also a close relative of the antipsychotic phenothiazines (replace the 10–11 bridge with sulfur, and the compound is the antipsychotic agent promazine). It has weaker D$_2$ postsynaptic blocking activity than promazine and mainly affects amines (5-HT, NE, and DA) via the transporters. As is typical of dimethylamino compounds, anticholinergic and sedative (central H$_1$ block) effects tend to be marked. The compound per se has a

tendency toward a high 5-HT-to-NE uptake block ratio and probably can be called a *serotonin transport inhibitor* (SERTI). Metabolic inactivation proceeds mainly by oxidative hydroxylation in the 2-position, followed by conjugation with glucuronic acid of the conjugate. Urinary excretion predominates (about 75%), but some biliary excretion (up to 25%) can occur, probably because of the large nonpolar grouping. Oxidative hydroxylation is not as rapid or complete as that of the more nucleophilic ring phenothiazine antipsychotics; consequently, appreciable *N*-demethylation occurs, with a buildup of norimipramine (or desimipramine).

The demethylated metabolite is less anticholinergic, less sedative, and more stimulatory and is a SNERI.[31] Consequently, a patient treated with imipramine has two compounds that contribute to activity. Overall, the effect is nonselective 5-HT versus NE reuptake. The activity of desimipramine or norimipramine is terminated by 2-hydroxylation, followed by conjugation and excretion. A second *N*-demethylation can occur, which in turn is followed by 2-hydroxylation, conjugation, and excretion.

Desipramine Hydrochloride

The structure and salient properties of desipramine hydrochloride, 10,11-dihydro-*N*-methyl-5*H*-dibenz[*b,f*]azepine-5-propanamine monohydrochloride, 5-(3-methylaminopropyl)-10,11-dihydro-5*H*-dibenz[*b,f*]azepine hydrochloride (Norpramin, Pertofrane), are discussed under the heading, Imipramine. Among tricyclics, desipramine would be considered when few anticholinergic effects or a low level of sedation are important. It is a SNERI.[31]

Clomipramine Hydrochloride

Clomipramine (Anafranil) is up to 50 times as potent as imipramine in some bioassays. This does not imply clinical superiority, but it might be informative about tricyclic and, possibly, other reuptake inhibitors. The chloro replacing the H-substituent could increase potency by increasing distribution to the CNS, but it is unlikely that this would give the potency magnitude seen. It might be conjectured that an H-bond between the protonated amino group (as in vivo) and the unshared electrons of the chloro substituent might stabilize a β-arylamine–like shape and give more efficient competition for the transporter. The drug is an antidepressant. It is used in obsessive-compulsive disorder, an anxiety disorder that may have an element of depression.

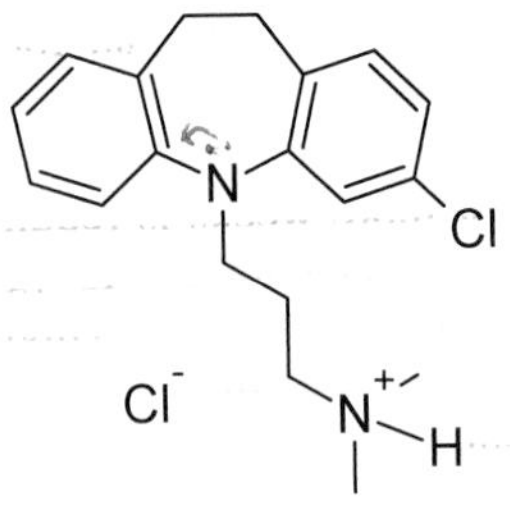

Amitriptyline Hydrochloride

Amitriptyline, 3-(10,11-dihydro-5H-dibenzo[a,d]cyclohepten-5-ylidene)-N,N-dimethyl-1-propanamine hydrochloride, 5-(3-dimethylaminopropylidene)-10,11-dihydro-5H-dibenzo[a,d]cycloheptene hydrochloride (Elavil), is one of the most anticholinergic and sedative of the TCAs. Because it lacks the ring-electron–enriching nitrogen atom of imipramine, metabolic inactivation mainly proceeds not at the analogous 2-position but at the benzylic 10-position (i.e., toluene-like metabolism predominates). Because of the 5-exocyclic double bond, E- and Z-hydroxy isomers are produced by oxidation metabolism. Conjugation produces excretable metabolites. As is typical of the dimethyl compounds, N-demethylation occurs, and nortriptyline is produced, which has a less anticholinergic, less sedative, and more stimulant action than amitriptyline. Nortriptyline is a SNERI[31]; the composite action of drug and metabolite is nonselective.

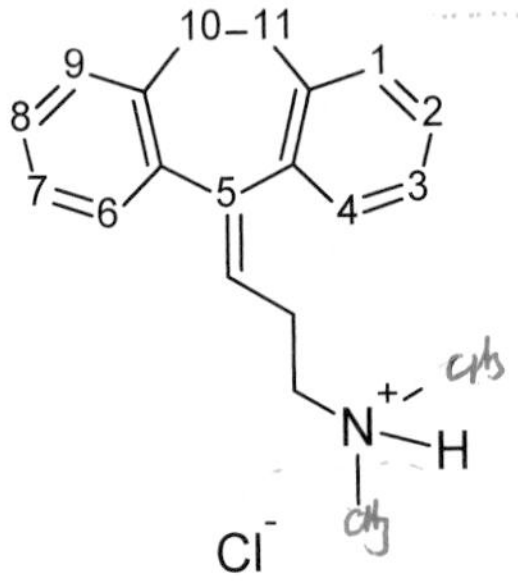

Nortriptyline Hydrochloride

Pertinent biological and chemical properties for nortriptyline, 3-(10,11-dihydro-5H-dibenzo[a,d]cyclohepten-5-ylidene)N-methyl-1-propanamine hydrochloride, 5-(3-methyl-amino-propylidene)-10,11-hydro-5H-dibenzo[a,d] cycloheptene hydrochloride (Aventyl, Pamelor), are given previously in the discussion of amitriptyline. Metabolic inactivation and elimination are like those of amitriptyline. Nortriptyline is a selective NE transporter (NET) inhibitor.[31]

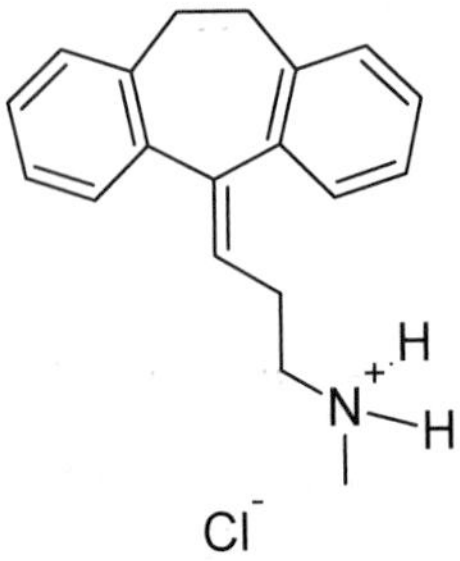

Protriptyline Hydrochloride

Protriptyline hydrochloride, N-methyl-5H-dibenzo[a,d]-cycloheptene-5-propylamine hydrochloride, 5-(3-methyl-aminopropyl)-5H-dibenzo[a,d]cycloheptene hydrochloride (Vivactil), like the other compounds under consideration, is an effective antidepressant. The basis for its chemical naming can be seen by consulting the naming and the structure of imipramine. Protriptyline is a structural isomer of nortriptyline. Inactivation can be expected to involve the relatively localized double bond. Because it is a monomethyl compound, its sedative potential is low.

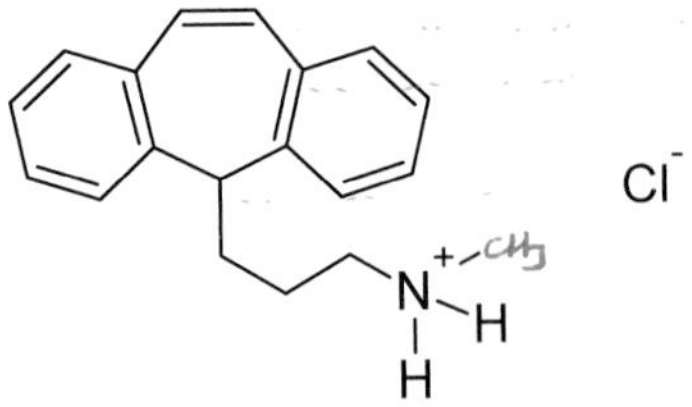

Trimipramine Maleate

For details of chemical nomenclature, consult the description of imipramine. Replacement of hydrogen with an α-methyl substituent produces a chiral carbon, and trimipramine (Surmontil) is used as the racemic mixture. Biological properties reportedly resemble those of imipramine.

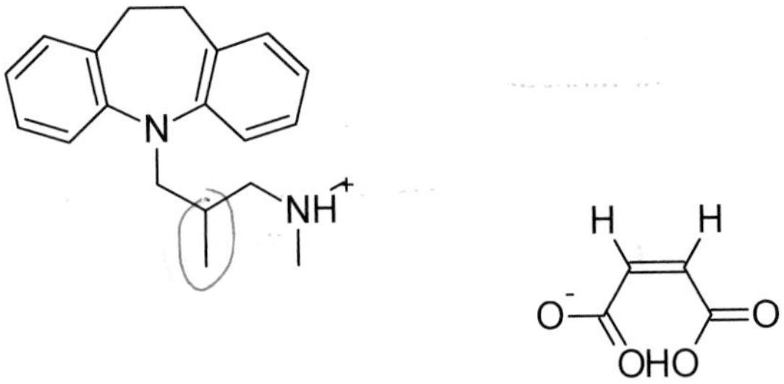

Doxepin Hydrochloride

Doxepin, 3-dibenz[b,e]-oxepin-11(6H)ylidine-N,N-dimethyl-1-propanamine hydrochloride, N,N-dimethyl-3-(dibenz[b,e] oxepin-11(6H)-ylidene)propylamine (Sinequan, Adapin), is an oxa congener of amitriptyline, as can be seen from its structure.

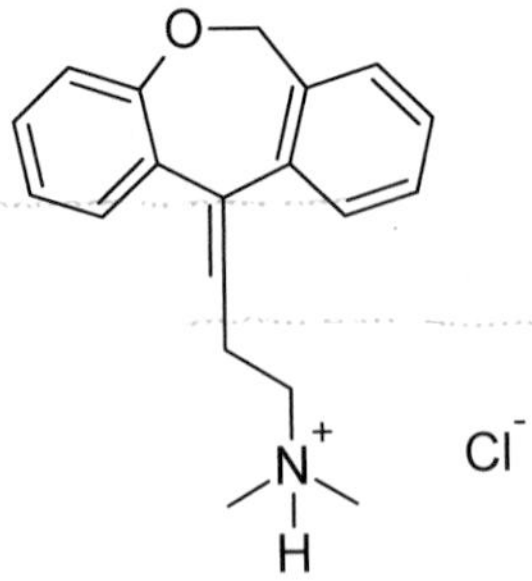

The oxygen is interestingly placed and should influence oxidative metabolism as well as postsynaptic and presynaptic binding affinities. The (Z)-isomer is the more active, although the drug is marketed as the mixture of isomers. The drug overall is a NE and 5-HT reuptake blocker with significant anticholinergic and sedative properties. It can be anticipated that the nor- or des- metabolite will contribute to the overall activity pattern.

Maprotiline Hydrochloride

Maprotiline hydrochloride, *N*-methyl-9,10-ethanoanthracene-9(10*H*)-propanamine hydrochloride (Ludiomil), is sometimes described as a tetracyclic rather than a tricyclic antidepressant. The description is chemically accurate, but the compound, nonetheless, conforms to the overall TCA pharmacophore. It is a dibenzobicyclooctadiene and can be viewed as a TCA with an ethylene-bridged central ring. The compound is not strongly anticholinergic and has stimulant properties. It can have effects on the cardiovascular system. It is a SNERI.[31]

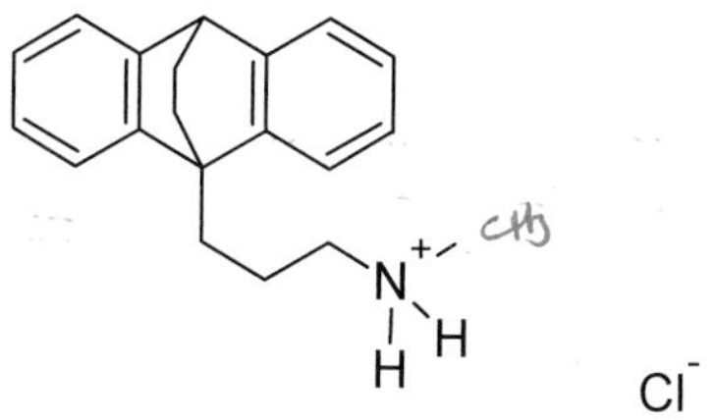

Amoxapine

Consideration of the structure of amoxapine, 2-chloro-11-(1-piperazinyl)dibenz-[*b,f*] [1,4]oxazepine (Asendin), reinforces the fact that many antidepressants are very closely related to antipsychotics. Indeed, some, including amoxapine, have significant effects at D_2 receptors. The *N*-methyl–substituted relative of amoxapine is the antipsychotic loxapine (Loxitane). The 8-hydroxy metabolite of amoxapine is reportedly active as an antidepressant and as a D_2 receptor blocker.

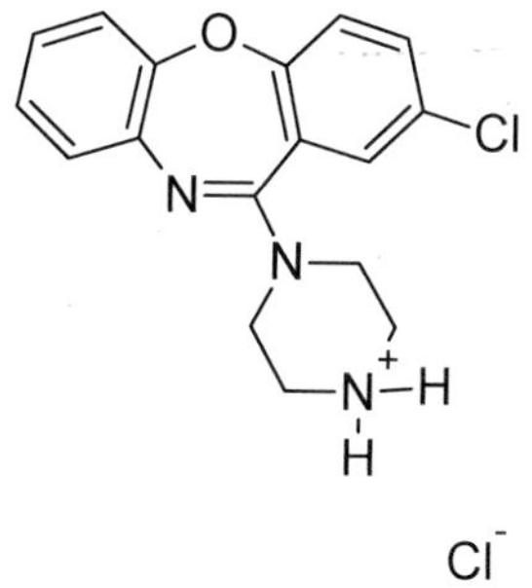

Selective Serotonin Reuptake (SSRI) Inhibitors

Structurally, the SSRIs differ from the tricyclics, in that the tricyclic system has been taken apart in the center. (This abolishes the center ring, and one ring is moved slightly forward from the tricyclic "all-in-a-row" arrangement.) The net effect is that the β-arylamine–like grouping is present, as in the tricyclics, and the compounds can compete for the substrate-binding site of the serotonin transporter protein (SERT). As in the tricyclics, the extra aryl group can add extra affinity and give favorable competition with the substrate, serotonin.

Many of the dimethylamino tricyclics are, in fact, SSRIs. Because they are extensively *N*-demethylated in vivo to nor-compounds, which are usually SNERIs, however, the overall effect is not selective. Breaking up the tricyclic system breaks up an anticholinergic pharmacophoric group and gives compounds with diminished anticholinergic effects. Overall, this diminishes unpleasant CNS effects and increases cardiovascular safety. Instead, side effects related to serotonin predominate.

Fluoxetine

In fluoxetine (Prozac), protonated in vivo, the protonated amino group can H-bond to the ether oxygen electrons, which can generate the β-arylamino–like group, with the other aryl serving as the characteristic "extra" aryl. The *S*-isomer is much more selective for SERT than for NET. The major metabolite is the *N*-demethyl compound, which is as potent as the parent and more selective (SERT versus NET).

Therapy for 2 or more weeks is required for the antidepressant effect. Somatodendritic 5-HT$_{1A}$ autoreceptor desensitization with chronic exposure to high levels of 5-HT is the accepted explanation for the delayed effect for this and other serotonin reuptake inhibitors.

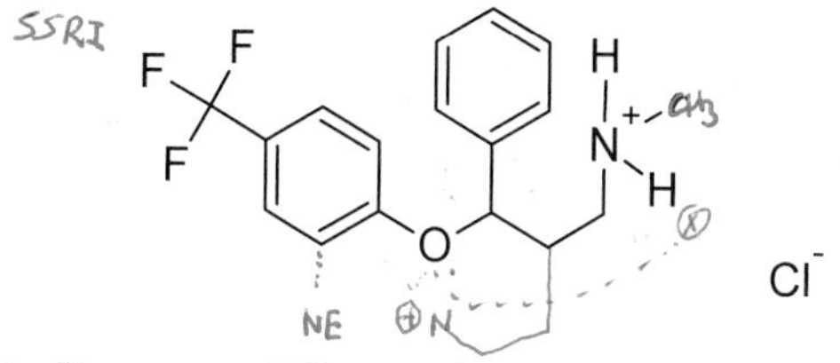

To illustrate a difference between selectivity for a SERT and a NET, if the *para* substituent is moved to the *ortho* position (and is less hydrophobic, typically), a NET is obtained. This and other SERTs have anxiolytic activity. One of several possible mechanisms would be agonism of 5-HT$_{1A}$ receptors, diminishing synaptic 5-HT. Presumably, synaptic levels of 5-HT might be high in an anxious state.

Paroxetine

In the structure of paroxetine (Paxil), an amino group, protonated in vivo could H-bond with the –CH$_2$–O– unshared electrons. A β-arylamine–like structure with an extra aryl group results. The compound is a very highly selective SERT. As expected, it is an effective antidepressant and anxiolytic.

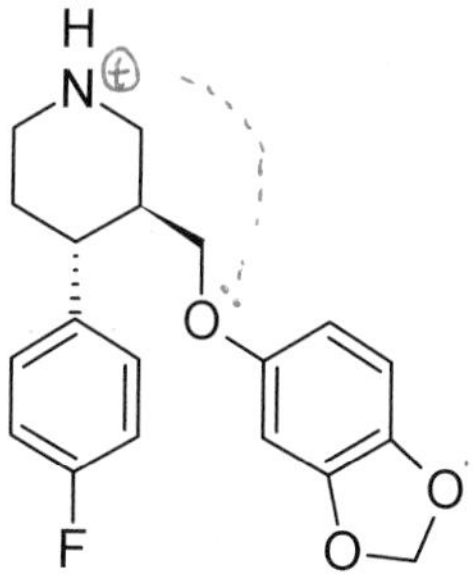

Sertraline

Inspection of sertraline (Zoloft) (1*S*,4*S*) reveals the pharmacophore for SERT inhibition. The Cl substituents also predict tropism for a 5-HT system. The depicted stereochemistry is important for activity.

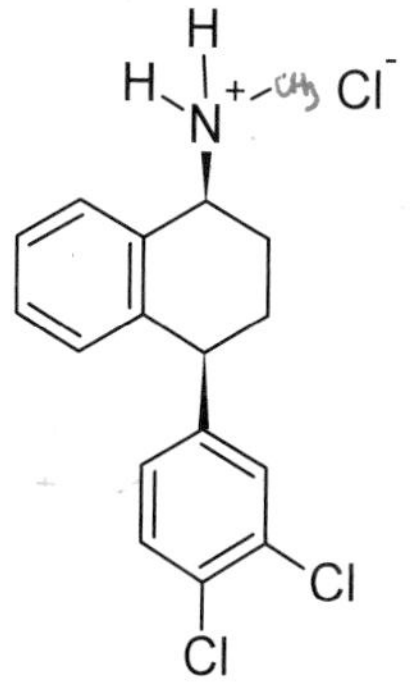

Fluvoxamine

The *E*-isomer of fluvoxamine (Luvox) (shown) can fold after protonation to the β-arylamine–like grouping. Here, the "extra" hydrophobic group is aliphatic.

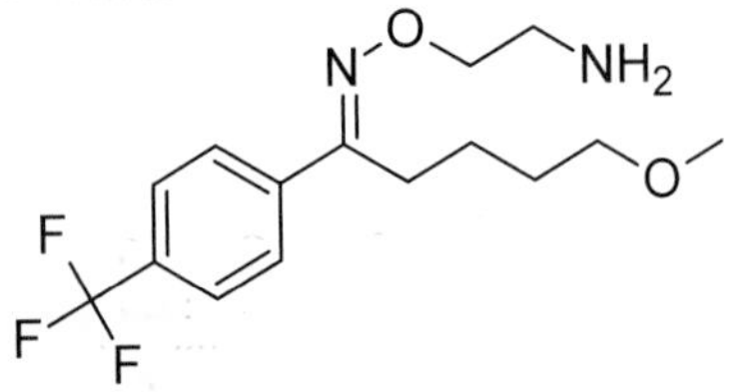

Citalopram

Citalopram (Celexa) is a racemic mixture and is very SERT selective. The *N*-monodemethylated compound is slightly less potent but is as selective. The aryl substituents are important for activity. The ether function is important and probably interacts with the protonated amino group to give a suitable shape for SERT binding.

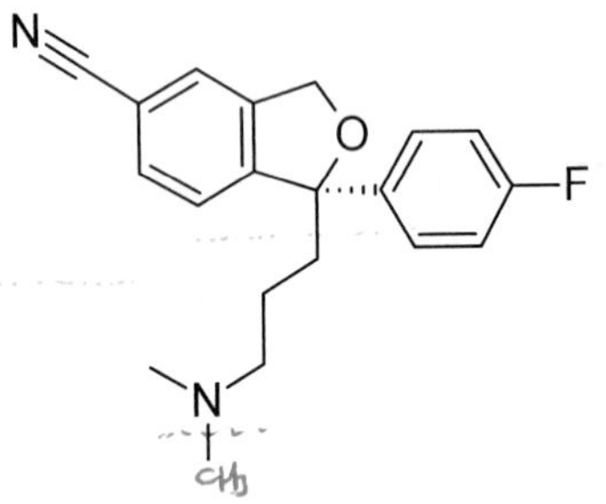

Selective Norepinephrine Reuptake Inhibitors

The discussion of fluoxetine opened the subject of SNERIs. That is, movement of a *para* substituent of fluoxetine (and relatives) to an *ortho* position produces a SNERI.

Nisoxetine

Nisoxetine is a SNERI and is an antidepressant. Most activity resides in the β-isomer.

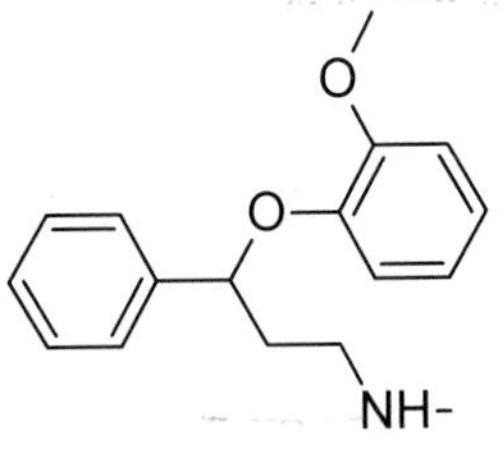

Reboxetine

Most of the activity of reboxetine resides in the *S,S*-isomer (The marketed compound is *RR* and *SS*.) It is claimed to be superior to fluoxetine in severe depression. It is marketed in Europe. At least three tricyclic compounds, desipramine, nortriptyline, and the technically tetracyclic maprotiline are SNERIs. They, of course, have typical characteristic TCA side effects but lower anticholinergic and H_1-antihistaminic (sedative) effects than dimethyl compounds. SNERIs are clinically effective antidepressants.

It would be expected that in the case of SNERIs, α_2 presynaptic receptors would be desensitized, after which sustained NE transmission would be via one or more post-synaptic receptors; α_1, β_1, and β_2 receptors are possibilities.

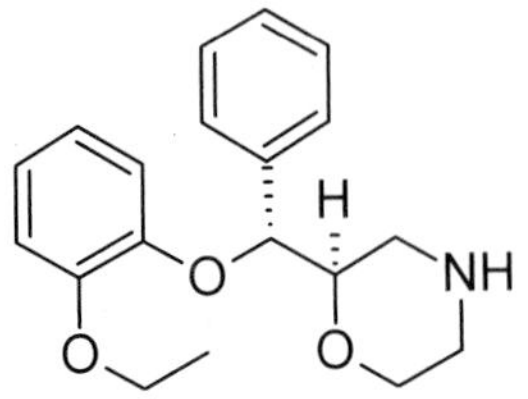

Newer (Nontricyclic) Nonselective 5-HT And NE Reuptake Inhibitors

Presently, one such compound is clinically used in the United States.

Venlafaxine

The structure and activity of venlafaxine (Effexor) are in accord with the general SARs for the group. As expected, it is an effective antidepressant. Venlafaxine is a serotonin–norepinephrine reuptake inhibitor (SNRI).

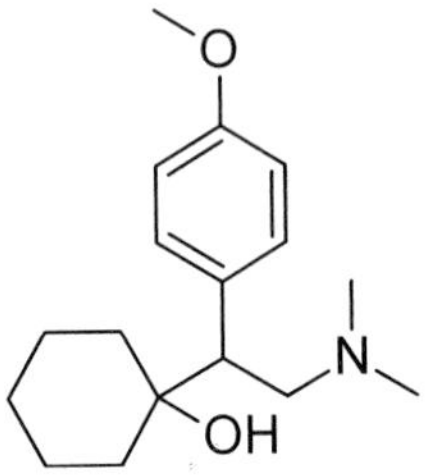

Selective Serotoninergic Reuptake Inhibitors and 5-HT$_{2A}$ Antagonists

The SSRIs and 5-HT$_{2A}$ antagonists are represented by trazodone (Desyrel) and nefazodone (Serzone).

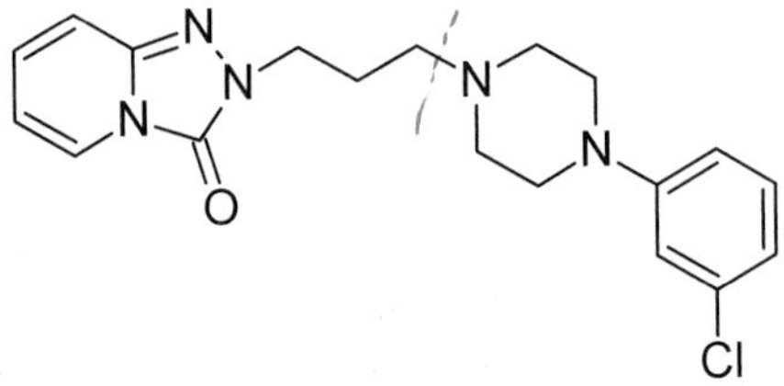

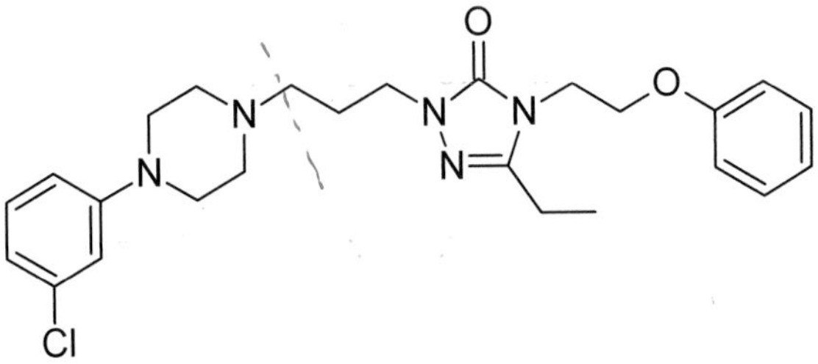

The structures of these two compounds derive from those of the fluorobutyrophenone antipsychotics. They have β-arylamine–like structures that permit binding to the SERT and inhibit 5-HT reuptake. In these compounds, the additional hydrophobic substituent can be viewed as being attached to the nitrogen of the β-arylamine–like group. Additionally, they are 5-HT$_{2A}$ antagonists. That antagonism may or may not afford antipsychotic effectiveness is discussed under antipsychotics. 5-HT$_{2A}$ antagonists appear to have antidepressant and anxiolytic activities. They may act, at least in part, by enhancing 5-HT$_{1A}$ activities.[33] Also, some of the effects may be mediated through 5-HT$_{2C}$ agonism (perhaps generally so for 5-HT–acting antidepressants). Some of the side effects of SSRIs are considered to be mediated through 5-HT$_{2A}$ receptors, so a 5-HT$_{2A}$ blocker would reduce them.[33] The two compounds yield the same compound on *N*-dealkylation. It is a serotonin reuptake inhibitor.

The most common use of trazodone is not as an antidepressant. A 100-mg dose can be used as a sedative–hypnotic. Despite this use, it has been shown that nefazodone produces better sleep hygiene than does trazodone, which is a rapid eye movement (REM)-suppressing compound.

5-HT$_{1A}$ Agonists and Partial Agonists

Buspirone

The initial compound in this series, buspirone (BuSpar), has anxiolytic and antidepressant activities and is a partial 5-HT$_{1A}$ agonist. Its anxiolytic activity is reportedly caused by its ability to diminish 5-HT release (via 5-HT$_{1A}$ agonism). High short-term synaptic levels of 5-HT are characteristic of anxiety. Also, because it is a partial agonist, it can stimulate postsynaptic receptors when 5-HT levels are low in the synapse, as is the case in depression. Several other spirones are in development as anxiolytics and antidepressants.[34]

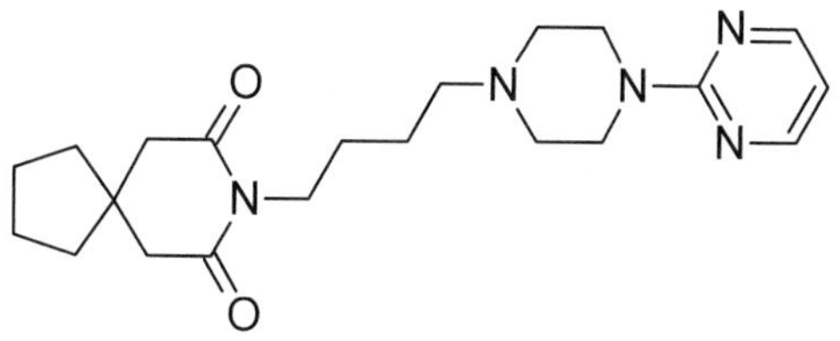

α$_2$ Antagonists

Mirtazapine

Mirtazapine (Remeron) was recently introduced for clinical use in the United States; its parent mianserin (pyridyl N replaced with C-H) was long known to be an antidepressant. It is reported to be faster acting and more potent than certain SSRIs. The mode of action gives increased NE release via α$_2$-NE receptor antagonism and increased 5-HT release via antagonism of NE α$_2$ heteroreceptors located on serotoninergic neurons.[33,34]

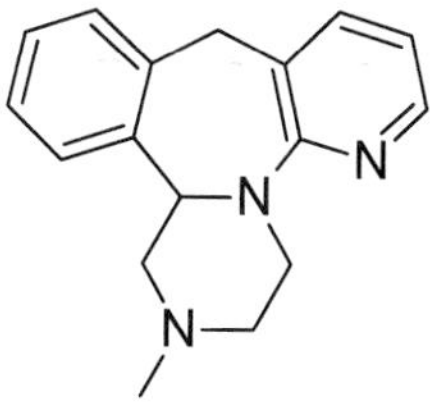

Miscellaneous Antidepressants

Bupropion

The mechanism of action of bupropion (Wellbutrin) is considered complex and reportedly involves a block of DA reuptake via the dopamine transporter (DAT), but the overall antidepressant action is noradrenergic. A metabolite that contributes to the overall action and its formation can be easily rationalized. Oxidation of one of the methyl groups on the *t*-butyl substituent yields hydroxybupropion, an active metabolite. Reduction of the keto group also occurs, yielding threohydrobupropion and erythrohydrobupropion. Both of these metabolites are also active.

Hydroxybupropion is half as potent as the parent bupropion, and the hydrobupropion isomers are five times less potent. The presence of these metabolites, especially hydroxybupropion which is formed by cytochrome P450 2D6 (CYP2D6), suggests that there will be a myriad of drug interactions with bupropion.

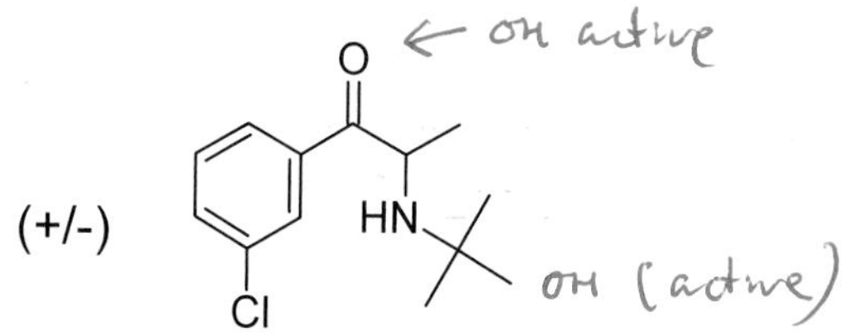

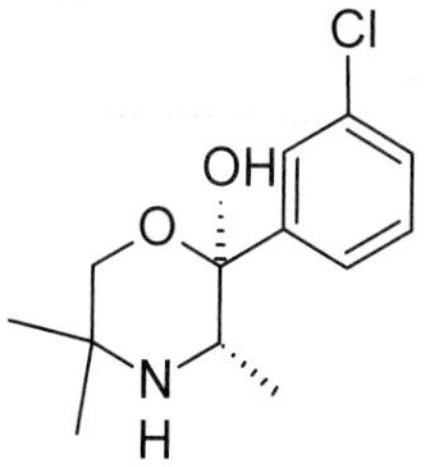

Bupropion Metabolite

Duloxetine (Cymbalta)

Duloxetine (Cymbalta) is a newer antidepressant. It is largely like venlafaxine, which is an SNERI (selective norepinephrine reuptake inhibitor).

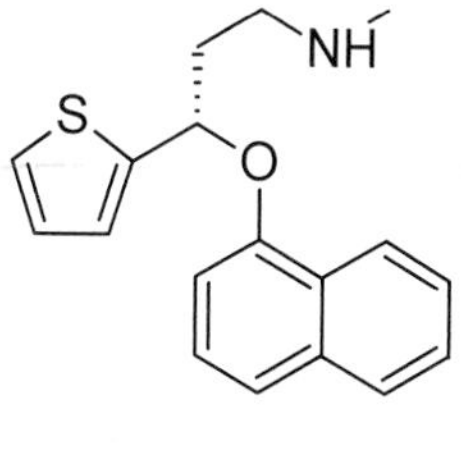

⬡ MISCELLANEOUS CNS-ACTING DRUGS

This section deals with a collection of drugs that do not fit easily under other topic headings in this chapter or the chapter on CNS depressants (Chapter 12). All of the drugs are drugs of abuse and could be organized under that heading.

The β-arylamino hallucinogens arose because of interest in the naturally occurring hallucinogens psilocin and mescaline and in modifying the amphetamines, which were popular drugs at the time. Lysergic acid diethylamide (LSD) was accidentally discovered during research on ergot alkaloids. It is of scientific interest because it serves as one model for clinical psychosis. Phencyclidine (PCP) is scientifically interesting because it gives information about the ionotropic *N*-methyl-D-aspartate glutamic acid receptor, and its CNS effects serve as a model for schizophrenia.

Cocaine as a CNS stimulant is a pernicious drug of abuse. Research on why it is so strongly addictive and on drug measures that might mitigate its effects has been intense in the past 2 decades.

Δ^1-Tetrahydrocannabinol and its relatives were studied for many years to determine the SARs. The field was given stimulus with the discovery of the endogenous cannabinoid receptors. Presently, the endogenous cannabinoid system is under investigation.

1β-Arylamino Hallucinogens

A property of the 1β-arylamino hallucinogens is alteration of the perception of stimuli. Reality is distorted, and the user may undergo depersonalization. Literally, the effects are those of a psychosis. Additionally, the drugs can produce anxiety, fear, panic, frank hallucinations, and additional symptoms that may be found in a psychosis. Accordingly, they are classed as hallucinogens and psychotomimetics.

This group can be subgrouped into those that possess an indolethylamine moiety, those that possess a phenylethylamine moiety, and those with both. In the first group, there is a structural resemblance to the central neurotransmitter 5-HT, and in the second, there is a structural resemblance to NE and DA. This resemblance is suggestive, and there may be some selectivity of effects on the respective transmitter systems. With structures of the complexity found in many of these agents, however, a given structure may possibly affect not just the closest structurally related neurotransmitter systems but other systems as well. Thus, a phenethylamine system could affect not only NE and DA systems but also 5-HT systems, and an indolethylamine system could affect not only 5-HT but also NE and DA systems.

INDOLETHYLAMINES

Dimethyltryptamine

Dimethyltryptamine is a very weak hallucinogen, active only by inhalation or injection, with a short duration of action. It possesses pronounced sympathomimetic (NE) side effects.

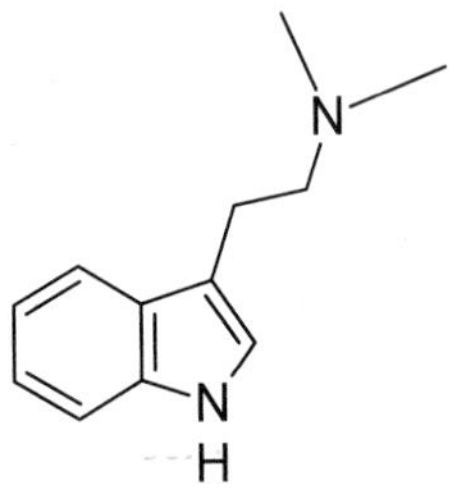

Psilocybin and Psilocin

Psilocybin is the phosphoric acid ester of psilocin and appears to be converted to psilocin as the active species in vivo. It occurs in a mushroom, *Psilocybe mexicana*. Both drugs are active orally, with a short duration of action.

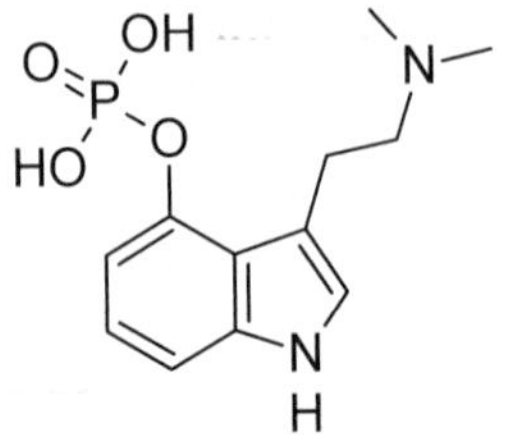

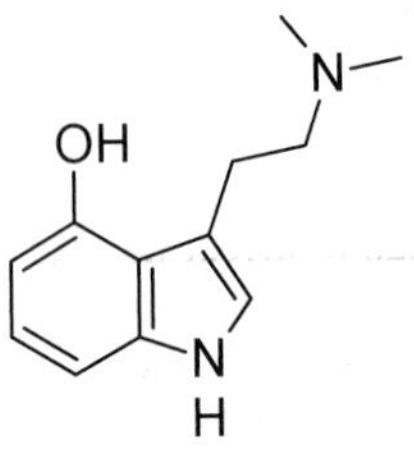

Synthetic α-methyl–substituted relatives have a much longer duration of action and enhanced oral potency.[35] This suggests that psilocin is metabolized by MAOs.

2-PHENYLETHYLAMINES

Mescaline

Mescaline, 3,4,5-trimethoxyphenethylamine, is a much-studied hallucinogen with many complex effects on the CNS. It occurs in the peyote cactus. The oral dose required for its hallucinogenic effects is very high, as much as 500 mg of the sulfate salt. The low oral potency probably results from facile metabolism by MAO. α-Methylation increases CNS activity. Synthetic α-methyl–substituted relatives are more potent.[35,36] The drugs 2,5-dimethoxy-4-methylamphetamine (DOM), 3,4-methylenedioxyamphetamine (MDA), and 2,5-dimethyl-dicyanoquinonediimine (DMDA; ecstasy) are extremely potent and are dangerous drugs of abuse.

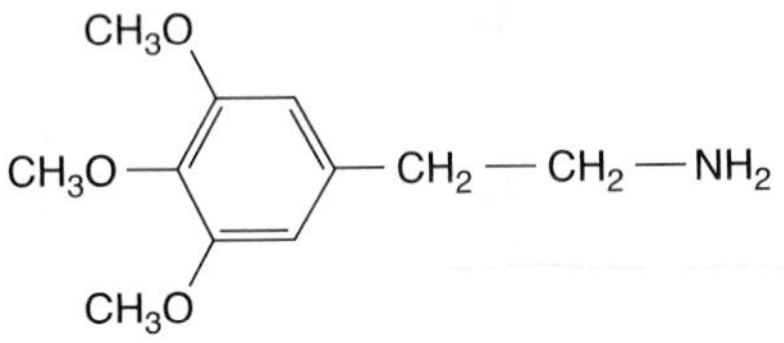

Mescaline

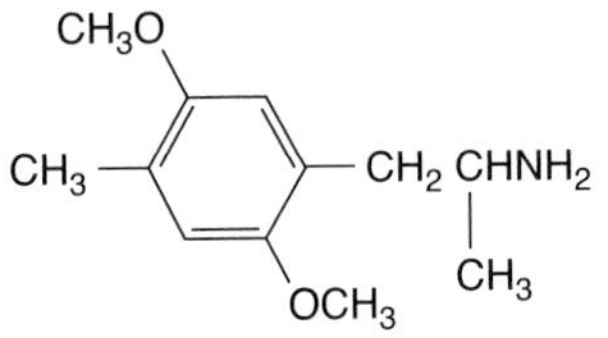

1-(2,5-Dimethoxy-4-methyphenyl)-2-aminopropane
(DOM, STP)

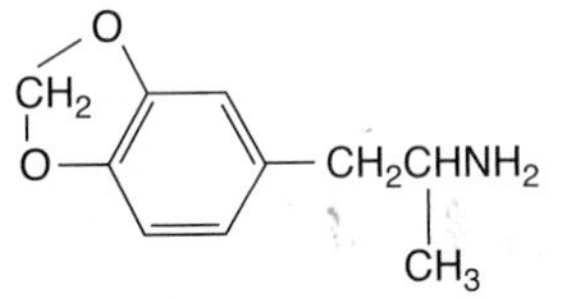

3,4-Methylenedioxyamphetamine
(MDA)

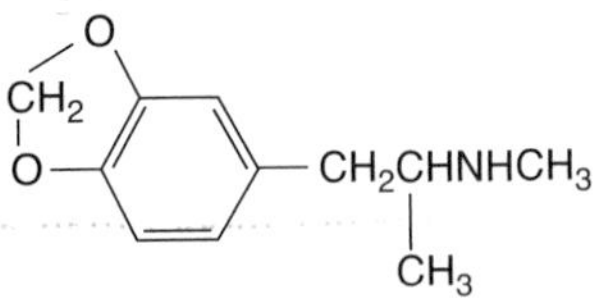

DMDA (ecstasy)

The presence of methoxyl or dioxymethylene (methylenedioxy) substituents on a 2-phenethylamine system is a characteristic of many psychotomimetic compounds and strongly suggests DA involvement.

AN AGENT POSSESSING BOTH AN INDOLETHYLAMINE AND A PHENYLETHYLAMINE MOIETY

(+)-Lysergic Acid Diethylamide

Both an indolethylamine group and a phenylethylamine group can be seen in the structure of the extraordinarily potent hallucinogen <u>LSD</u>. The stereochemistry is exceedingly important. Chirality, as shown, must be maintained or activity is lost; likewise, the location of the double bond, as shown, is required.[37] Experimentally, LSD has marked effects on <u>serotoninergic and dopaminergic neurons</u>. The bases for all of its complex CNS actions are not completely understood, however. Recently, its actions have been suggested as being <u>more typical of schizophrenic psychotic</u> reactions than the model based on amphetamine. For more on this, see the discussion of atypical antipsychotics (Chapter 12).

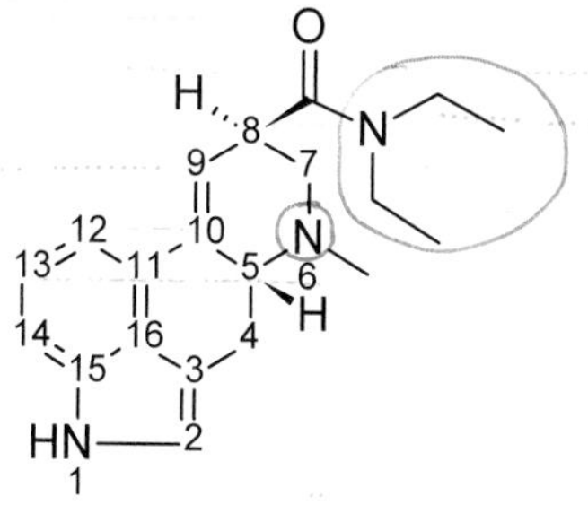

Dissociative Agents

Phencyclidine

Phencyclidine was introduced as a dissociative anesthetic for animals. Its close structural relative ketamine is still so used and may be used in humans (Chapter 22). In humans, PCP produces a sense of intoxication, hallucinogenic experiences not unlike those produced by the anticholinergic hallucinogens, and often, amnesia.

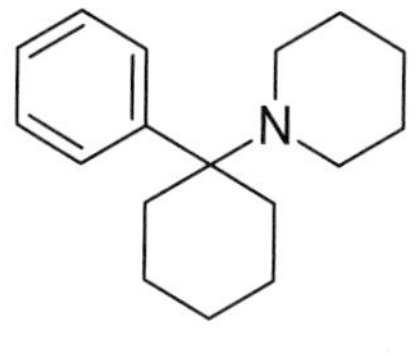

The drug affects many systems, including those of NE, DA, and 5-HT. It has been proposed that PCP (and certain other psychotomimetics) produces a unique pattern of activation of ventral tegumental area dopaminergic neurons.[38] It blocks glutaminergic *N*-methyl-D-aspartate receptors.[39] This action is the basis for many of its CNS effects. PCP itself appears to be the active agent. The psychotic state produced by this drug is also cited as a better model than amphetamine psychosis for the psychotic state of schizophrenia.[40]

Euphoriant–Stimulant

Cocaine

Cocaine as a euphoriant–stimulant, psychotomimetic, and drug of abuse could as well be discussed with amphetamine and methamphetamine, with which it shares many biological properties. At low doses, it produces feelings of well-being, decreased fatigue, and increased alertness. Cocaine tends to produce compulsive drug-seeking behavior, and a full-blown toxic psychosis may emerge. Many of these effects appear to be related to the effects of increased availability of DA for interaction with postsynaptic receptors (D_2 and D_3 receptors are pertinent). Cocaine is a potent DA reuptake blocker, acting by competitive inhibition of the DAT. A phenethylamine moiety

with added steric bulk may suffice for this action. An interaction between a hydrogen atom on the nitrogen of the protonated form of cocaine and an oxygen of the benzoyl ester group, or alternatively, an interaction between the unshared electron pair of the freebase nitrogen and the carbonyl of the benzoyl ester group, could approximate this moiety.

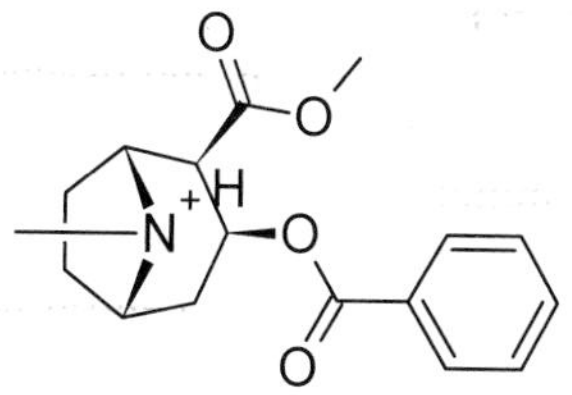

Considerable research on drugs affecting the DAT has been published in recent years. A review of pharmacotherapeutic agents for cocaine abuse is available.[41]

Depressant–Intoxicant

Δ^1-Tetrahydrocannabinol or Δ^9-THC

There are two conventions for numbering THC: that arising from terpenoid chemistry produces Δ^1-THC and that based on the dibenzopyran system results in a Δ^9-THC designation. The terpenoid convention is used here.

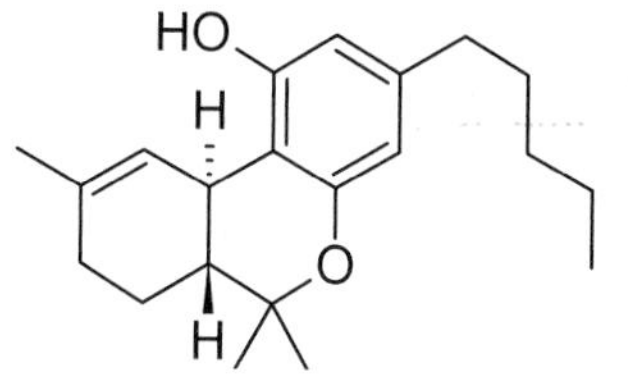

Tetrahydrocannabinoid is a depressant with apparent stimulant sensations arising from depression of higher centers. Many effects, reputedly subjectively construed as pleasant, are evident at low doses. The interested reader may consult a pharmacology text for a detailed account. At higher doses, psychotomimetic actions, including dysphoria, hallucinations, and paranoia, can be marked. Structural features associated with activity among cannabis-derived compounds have been reviewed.[42] Notably, the phenolic OH is required for activity. Certain SARs (especially separation of potency between enantiomers) for cannabinoids suggested action at receptors.[43] Two receptors for THC have been discovered. The relevant receptor for CNS actions is CB_1.[44] CB_2 occurs in immune tissues. The first natural ligand found for the receptor is the amide derivative of arachidonic acid, anandamide.[45] Other natural cannabinoids are arachidonic acid 2-glycerol ester and 2-arachidonyl glycerol ether.[46] The endogenous cannabinoid system appears to function as a retrograde messenger system at both stimulatory synapses and depressant synapses. The synaptic transmitter causes postsynaptic syntheses of endocannabinoids that are then transported to CB_1 receptors located presynaptically where they fine-tune both excitatory and inhibitory neurons.[47–51] Because CB_1 receptors appear to be present in all brain areas and affect both excitatory and inhibitory systems, the prospect of developing selective cannabinoid drugs acting at receptors is considered not good. Designing drugs to affect the transporter is considered the most promising research route.

Endocannabinoids, as regulated by leptin, are also involved in maintaining food intake and in other behaviors.[52,53]

● R E V I E W   Q U E S T I O N S ●

1. What is the definition of an analeptic?

2. How do the xanthine alkaloids produce their pharmacological effects?

3. Describe the SARs of the β-phenethylamine sympathomimetics.

4. What is fenfluramine? How does its effect differ from amphetamine?

5. Why is phentermine formulated with an ion-exchange resin?

6. Why is it necessary to wait for 2 to 3 weeks after an MAOI is discontinued and before another antidepressant is administered?

7. Why do we say that phenelzine is irreversible?

8. How does cocaine produce its effects?

9. What are the uses of methylphenidate (Ritalin)?

10. What is the evidence that psilocin is metabolized by monoamine oxidase?

11. MW is a 40-year-old WF who earns a living driving a taxicab. MW has just been diagnosed with major depressive disorder. Her mother has been depressed for about 15 years and has been successfully treated with phenelzine (Nardil). Consider the classes of antidepressants, their pharmacological effects and side effects. What would your selection be for treating MW?

REFERENCES

1. Jarboe, C. H., Porter, L. A., and Buckler, R. T.: J. Med. Chem. 11:729, 1968.
2. Pellmar, T. C., and Wilson, W. A.: Science 197:912, 1977.
3. Fredholm, B. B., et al.: Pharmacol. Rev. 51:83, 1999.
4. Daly, J. W.: J. Med. Chem. 25:197, 1982.
5. Williams, M., and Huff, J. R.: Annu. Rep. Med. Chem. 18:1, 1983.
6. Snyder, S. H., et al.: Proc. Natl. Acad. Sci. U. S. A. 78:3260, 1981.
7. Tucker, A. L., and Linden, J.: Cardiovasc. Res. 27:62, 1993.
8. Erion, M. D.: Annu. Rep. Med. Chem. 28:295, 1993.
9. DeNinno, M. P.: Annu. Rep. Med. Chem. 33:111, 1998.
10. Arnaud, M. J.: Products of metabolism of caffeine. In Dews, P. B. (ed.). Caffeine, Perspectives From Recent Research. New York, Springer-Verlag, 1984, p. 3.
11. Halford, J. C. G., and Blundell, J. E.: Prog. Drug Res. 54:25, 2000.
12. Fuller, R. W.: Ann. N. Y. Acad. Sci. 305:147, 1978.
13. Harvey, J. A.: Ann. N. Y. Acad. Sci. 305:289, 1978.
14. Groppetti, A., and Costa, E.: Life Sci. 8:635, 1969.
15. Clineschmidt, B. V., et al.: Ann. N. Y. Acad. Sci. 305:222, 1987.
16. Dvornik, D., and Schilling, G.: J. Med. Chem. 8:466, 1965.
17. Weisz, I., and Dudas, A.: Monatsh. Chem. 91:840, 1960.
18. Shaffi'ee, A., and Hite, G.: J. Med. Chem. 12:266, 1969.
19. Patrick, K. S., et al.: J. Pharmacol. Exp. Ther. 241:152, 1987.
20. Perel, J. M., and Dayton, P. G.: Methylphenidate. In Usdin, E., and Forrest, I. S. (eds.). Psychotherapeutic Drugs, part II. New York, Marcel Dekker, 1977, p. 1287.
21. Srinvas, N. R., et al.: J. Pharmacol. Exp. Ther. 241:300, 1987.
22. Whitelock, O. V. (ed.): Ann. N. Y. Acad. Sci., 80:000–000, 1959.
23. Richards, L. E., and Burger, A.: Prog. Drug Res. 30:205, 1986.
24. Strupczewski, J. D., Ellis, D. B., and Allen, R. C.: Annu. Rep. Med. Chem. 26:297, 1991.
25. Green, A. L.: Biochem. Pharmacol. 13:249, 1964.
26. Burger, A.: J. Med. Pharm. Chem. 4:571, 1961.
27. Belleau, B., and Moran, J. F.: J. Am. Chem. Soc. 82:5752, 1960.
28. Belleau, B., and Moran, J. F.: J. Med. Pharm. Chem. 5:215, 1962.
29. Silverman, R. B.: J. Biol. Chem. 258:14766, 1983.
30. Rudnick, G., and Clark, J.: Biochim. Biophys. Acta 1144:249, 1993.
31. Olivier, B.: Prog. Drug Res. 54:59, 2000.
32. Daniels, T. C., and Jorgensen, E. C.: Central nervous system stimulants. In Doerge, R. F. (ed.). Wilson and Gisvold's Textbook of Organic Medicinal and Pharmaceutical Chemistry, 8th ed. Philadelphia, J. B. Lippincott, 1982, p. 383.
33. Evrad, D. A., and Harrison, B. L.: Annu. Rep. Med. Chem. 34:1, 1999.
34. Olivier, B., et al.: Prog. Drug Res. 52:103, 1999.
35. Murphree, H. B., et al.: Clin. Pharmacol. Ther. 2:722, 1961.
36. Shulgin, A. T.: Nature 201:120, 1964.
37. Stoll, A., and Hofmann, A.: Helv. Chim. Acta 38:421, 1955.
38. Bowers, M. B., Bannon, M. J., and Hoffman, F. J., Jr.: Psychopharmacology 93:133, 1987.
39. Foster, A. C., and Fogg, G. E.: Nature 329:395, 1987.
40. Rowley, M., Bristow, L. J., and Hutson, P. H.: J. Med. Chem 44:477, 2001.
41. Carroll, F. I., Howell, L. L., and Kuhov, M. J.: J. Med. Chem. 42:2721, 2000.
42. Edery, H., et al.: Ann. N. Y. Acad. Sci. 191:40, 1971.
43. Hollister, L. E., Gillespie, H. K., and Srebnik, M.: Psychopharmacology 92:505, 1987.
44. Matsuda, L. A., et al.: Nature 346:561, 1990.
45. Davanne, W. A., et al.: Science 258:1946, 1992.
46. Mechoulam, R., et al.: Proc. Natl. Acad. Sci. U. S. A. 98:3602, 2001.
47. Egertova, M., et al.: Proc. R. Soc. London B 265:208, 1998.
48. Wilson, R. I., and Nicoll, R. A.: Nature 410:588, 2001.
49. Ohn-Shosaku, T., Maejqma, T., and Kano, N.: Neuron 29:729, 2001.
50. Kreitzer, A. C., and Regehr, W. G.: Neuron 29:717, 2001.
51. Christie, M. J., and Vaughn, C. W.: Nature 410:527, 2001.
52. DiMarzo, V., et al.: Nature 410:822, 2001.
53. Mechoulam, R., and Fride, E.: Nature 410:763, 2001.

SELECTED READING

Carroll, F. I., Howell, F. I., and Kuhar, M. J.: Pharmacotherapies for treatment of cocaine abuse: preclinical aspects. J. Med. Chem. 42:2721, 1999.

Fredholm, B. B., Bättig K., Holmén, J., et al.: Actions of caffeine in the brain with special reference to factors that contribute to its widespread use. Pharmacol. Rev. 51:83, 1999.

Halford, J. C. G., and Blundell, J. E.: Pharmacology of appetite suppression. Prog. Drug. Res. 54:25, 2000.

Olivier, B., Soudijn, W., and van Wijngaarden, I.: Serotonin, dopamine and norepinephrine transporters in the central nervous system and their inhibitors. Prog. Drug Res. 54:59, 2000.

Xiang, J.-N., and Lee, J. C.: Pharmacology of cannabinoid receptor agonists and antagonists. Annu. Rep. Med. Chem. 54:199, 2000.

CHAPTER 16

Adrenergic Agents

SHENGQUAN LIU

Adrenergic drugs exert their principal pharmacological and therapeutic effects by either enhancing or reducing the activity of the various components of the sympathetic division of the autonomic nervous system. In general, substances that produce effects similar to stimulation of sympathetic nervous activity are known as *sympathomimetics* or *adrenergic stimulants*. Those that decrease sympathetic activity are referred to as *sympatholytics*, *antiadrenergics*, or *adrenergic-blocking agents*.

Adrenergic agents act on adrenergic receptors (adrenoceptors, ARs) or affect the life cycle of adrenergic neurotransmitters (NTs), including norepinephrine (NE, noradrenaline), epinephrine (E, adrenaline), and dopamine (DA). These NTs modulate many vital functions, such as the rate and force of cardiac contraction, constriction, and dilation of blood vessels and bronchioles, the release of insulin, and the breakdown of fat. Therefore, adrenergic drugs constitute a broad class of agents, including albuterol (a bronchodilator), atenolol (an antihypertensive), and many common over-the-counter (OTC) cold remedies (Table 16.1). This chapter examines the biochemical basis for adrenergic action, adrenoceptors and then discusses the agents that affect the synthesis, storage, uptake, metabolism, or release of the adrenergic NTs and especially those that act directly on the various types of adrenoceptors.

ADRENERGIC NEUROTRANSMITTERS

Structure and Physicochemical Properties

NE, E, and DA are chemically catecholamines (CAs), which refer generally to all organic compounds that contain a catechol nucleus (ortho-dihydroxybenzene) and an ethylamine group (Fig. 16.1). In a physiological context, the term usually means DA and its metabolites NE and E. E contains one secondary amino group and three hydroxyl groups. Using the polyfunctional solubilizing potential and calculated log P (-0.63) of E, one would expect the molecule is polar and soluble in water, and, indeed, this turns out to be the case.

E is a weak base ($pK_a = 9.9$) because of its aliphatic amino group. It is also a weak acid ($pK_a = 8.7$) because of its phenolic hydroxyl group. It can be predicted that ionized species (the cation form) of E at physiological pH is predominant (log D at pH 7 = -2.75). This largely accounts for the high water solubility of this compound as well as other CAs. Because log P with a value of 0 to 3 is an optimal window

for absorption, we can predict that E has poor absorption and poor central nervous system (CNS) penetration.

Like most phenols, the catechol functional groups in CAs are highly susceptible to facile oxidation. E and NE undergo oxidation in the presence of oxygen (air) or other oxidizing agents to produce a quinone analog, which undergoes further reactions to give mixtures of colored products, one of which is adrenochrome (Fig. 16.2). Hence, solutions of these drugs often are stabilized by the addition of an antioxidant (reducing agent) such as ascorbic acid or sodium bisulfite.

E and NE each possess a chiral carbon atom; thus, each can exist as an enantiomeric pair of isomers. The enantiomer with the (R) configuration is biosynthesized by the body and possesses the biological activity. This (R) configuration of many other adrenergic agents also contributes to their high affinity to the corresponding adrenoceptors.

Biosynthesis

The CA biosynthesis and physiological regulation in neuroendocrine cells has been reviewed.[1] A summary view of the events and life cycle of NE are given in Figure 16.3.

CAs in neuroendocrine cells are in a state of constant flux. They are continuously being synthesized, released, and metabolized, yet they maintain a remarkable constant level in tissues. CAs are widely distributed in mammals, and their levels and physiological functions are regulated at many sites. The biosynthesis involves a sequence of enzymatic reactions.[2] The steps in the biosynthesis of CAs and related enzyme inhibitors are shown in Figure 16.4.

The first step in CA biosynthesis is the 3'-hydroxylation of the amino acid L-tyrosine to form L-dihydroxyphenylalanine (L-DOPA). L-Tyrosine is normally present in the circulation and transported actively into the adrenergic neuron, where it is 3'-hydroxylated by tyrosine hydroxylase (TH, tyrosine-3-monooxygenase). TH is stereospecific and requires molecular O_2, Fe^{2+}, and a tetrahydropteridine cofactor. As usual for the first enzyme in a biosynthetic pathway, TH hydroxylation is the rate-limiting step in the biosynthesis of NE. Further proof that this step is rate limiting in CA biosynthesis is that inhibitors of TH markedly reduce endogenous NE and DA in the brain and NE in the heart, spleen, and other sympathetically innervated tissues. This enzyme plays a key role in the regulation of CA biosynthesis and is, therefore, the logical biological target of some drugs.

Some effective TH inhibitors include α-methyl-*p*-tyrosine, α-methyl-3'-iodotyrosine, and α-methyl-5-hydroxytryptophan. In general, α-methyl analogs are more potent than the unmethylated analogs. Most of the agents in this category act

(text continues on page 522)

TABLE 16.1 Most Commonly Used Adrenergic Prescription Drugs

Mechanism of Action	Drug	Major Indications
α_1-Agonists	Naphazoline (Privine)	Nasal & ophthalmic congestion
α_2-Agonists	Clonidine (Catapres)*	Hypertension
	Methyldopa (Aldomet)	Hypertension
α_1-Blockers	Prazosin (Minipress)	Hypertension & benign prostatic hyperplasia (BPH)
	Terazosin (Hytrin)*	Hypertension & BPH
	Doxazosin (Cardura)*	Hypertension & BPH
	Tamsulosin (Flomax)	BPH & hypertension
β_2-Agonists	Albuterol (Ventolin)*	Asthma
α_1-, β_1-, & β_2-Blockers	Labetalol (Normodyne)*	Hypertension
	Carvedilol (Coreg)	Hypertension & heart failure
β_1- & β_2-Blockers	Propranolol (Inderal)*	Hypertension, arrhythmias, & angina
	Nadolol (Corgard)*	Hypertension, angina, & hyperthyroidism
	Timolol (Timoptic)*	Glaucoma & hypertension
	Sotalol (Betapace)*	Arrhythmias
	Levobunolol (Betagan)	Glaucoma
β_1-Blockers	Acebutolol (Sectral)	Hypertension, angina, & hyperthyroidism
	Atenolol (Tenormin)*	Hypertension, angina, & hyperthyroidism
	Metoprolol (Lopressor)*	Hypertension
	Bisoprolol (Zebeta)*	Hypertension

*Indicates adrenergic prescription drugs in the top 200 for 2005.

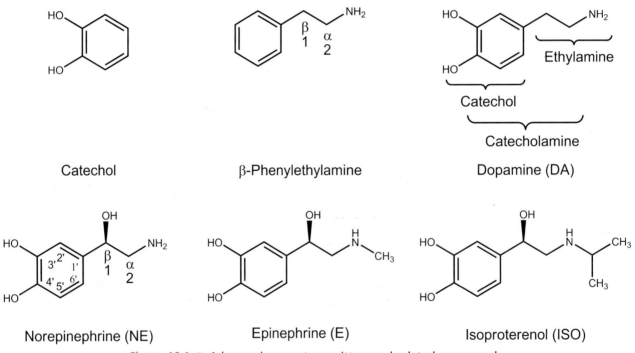

Catechol   β-Phenylethylamine   Dopamine (DA)

Norepinephrine (NE)   Epinephrine (E)   Isoproterenol (ISO)

Figure 16.1 ● Adrenergic neurotransmitters and related compounds.

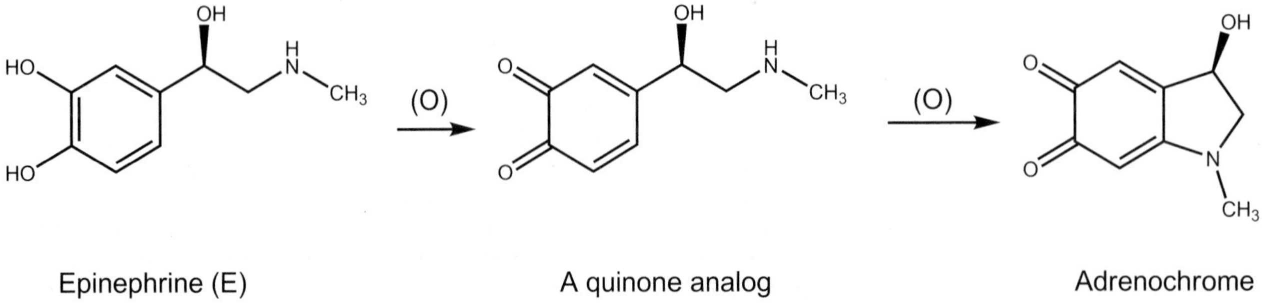

Epinephrine (E)   A quinone analog   Adrenochrome

Figure 16.2 ● Oxidation of Epinephrine (E).

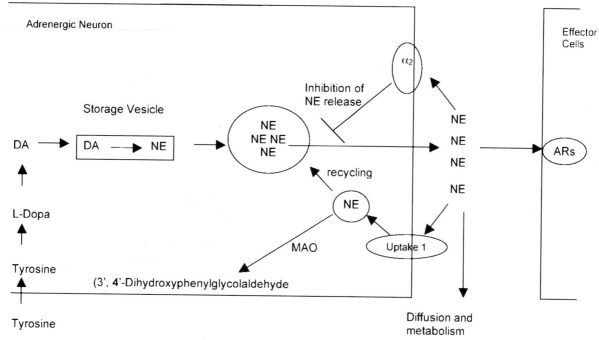

Adrenergic Neuron

Effector Cells

Storage Vesicle

Inhibition of NE release

DA → DA → NE → NE NE NE NE

recycling

NE

MAO

Uptake 1

L-Dopa

Tyrosine

(3', 4'-Dihydroxyphenylglycolaldehyde)

Tyrosine

Diffusion and metabolism

NE NE NE NE

ARs

Figure 16.3 ● Model of life cycle of NE.

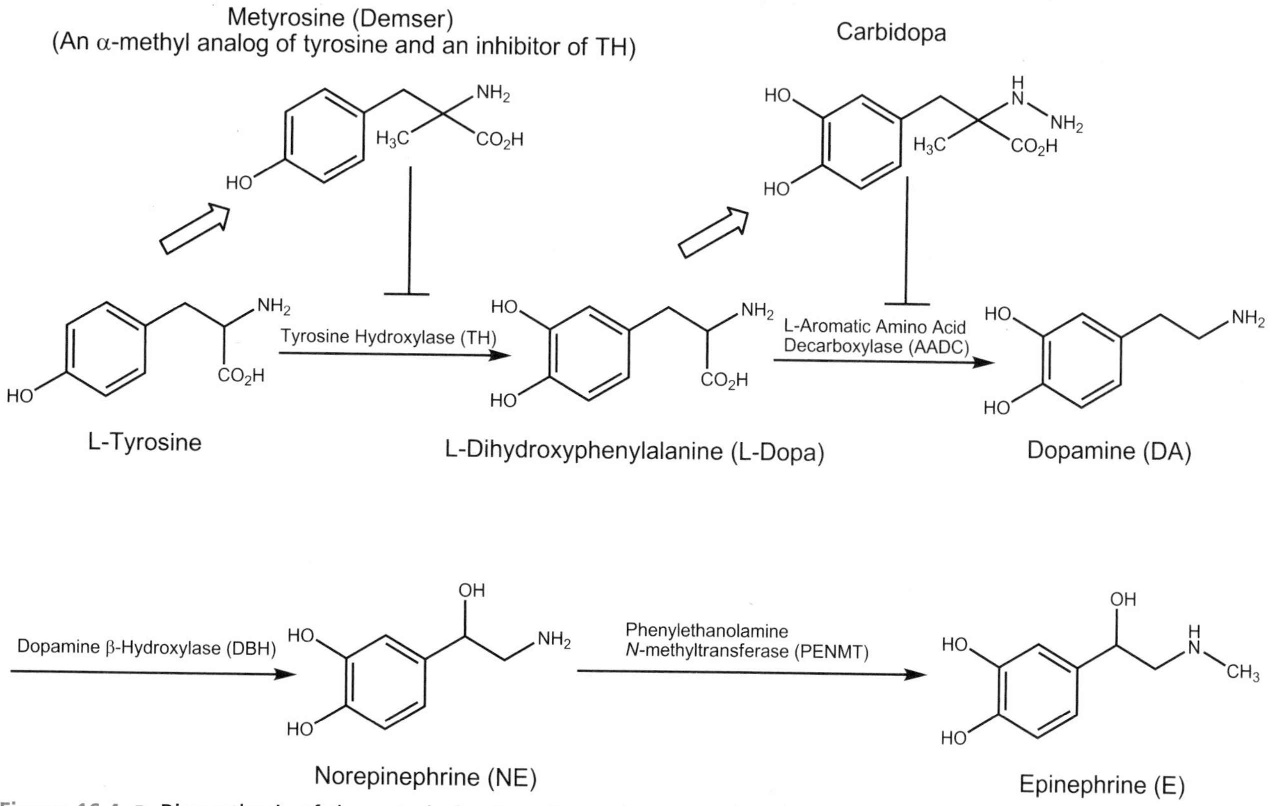

Metyrosine (Demser)
(An α-methyl analog of tyrosine and an inhibitor of TH)

Carbidopa

L-Tyrosine

Tyrosine Hydroxylase (TH)

L-Dihydroxyphenylalanine (L-Dopa)

L-Aromatic Amino Acid Decarboxylase (AADC)

Dopamine (DA)

Dopamine β-Hydroxylase (DBH)

Norepinephrine (NE)

Phenylethanolamine *N*-methyltransferase (PENMT)

Epinephrine (E)

Figure 16.4 ● Biosynthesis of the catecholamines dopamine, norepinephrine, and epinephrine.

as competitive inhibitors of TH. α-Methyl-*p*-tyrosine (metyrosine, Demser, Fig. 16.4) and its methyl ester have been the TH inhibitors most widely used to demonstrate the effects of exercise, stress, and various drugs on the turnover of CAs and to lower NE formation in patients with pheochromocytoma and malignant hypertension.

TH is a specific phenotypic marker of CA-producing cells in the CNS and peripheral nervous system (PNS). The activity of TH is carefully controlled. For example, adrenergic nerve stimulation leads to activation of a protein kinase that phosphorylates TH, thereby increasing its activity.[3] In addition, through end-product inhibition, NE markedly reduces TH activity. The basis of this feedback inhibition is believed to be a competition between the CA product and the pterin cofactor.

The second step in CA biosynthesis is the decarboxylation of L-DOPA to give DA, which is an important NT and a drug in its own right discussed in Chapter 13. The enzyme involved is DOPA decarboxylase. Although originally believed to remove carboxyl groups only from L-DOPA, a study of purified enzyme preparations and specific inhibitors demonstrated that DOPA decarboxylase acts on all naturally occurring aromatic L-amino acids, including L-histidine (precursor in the biosynthesis of histamine), L-tyrosine, L-tryptophan (precursor in the biosynthesis of 5-HT), and L-phenylalanine in addition to both L-DOPA and L-5-hydroxytryptophan. Therefore, this enzyme is more appropriately referred to as *L-aromatic amino acid decarboxylase* (AADC). In addition to being found in catecholaminergic neurons, AADC is found in high concentrations in many other tissues, including the liver and kidneys.

In simplest term, parkinsonism can be characterized as a DA deficiency in the brain. Thus, increasing brain levels of DA should ameliorate the symptoms. Unfortunately, direct parenteral DA administration is useless because the compound does not penetrate the blood-brain barrier (BBB). However, oral dosing with L-DOPA (levodopa, Dopar) could act as a prodrug because it entered the brain (on a specific carrier) and then was decarboxylated to DA there. L-DOPA is effective and decrease tremor and rigidity. Unfortunately, many adverse systemic effects were the result of the high doses needed to achieve the desired results. The main reason is the relatively higher concentration of AADC in peripheral system than in the brain. Inhibition of peripheral AADC activity by coadministration of at peripheral decarboxylase inhibitor such as carbidopa (charged at physiological pH), can markedly increase the proportion of levodopa that crosses the BBB. (see Chapter 13).

The third step in CA biosynthesis is side-chain β-hydroxylation of DA to give NE. DA formed in the cytoplasm of the neuron is actively transported into storage vesicles by a 12-helix membrane–spanning proton antiporter called the vesicular monoamine transporter (VMAT) and is then hydroxylated stereospecifically at the β-carbon to NE inside the vesicle by dopamine β-hydroxylase (DBH, dopamine β-monooxygenase). The NE formed is stored in the vesicles until depolarization of the neuron initiates the process of vesicle fusion with the plasma membrane and extrusion of NE into the synaptic cleft. DBH has rather low substrate specificity and acts in vitro on various substrates besides DA, hydroxylating almost any phenylethylamine to its corresponding phenylethanolamine (e.g., tyramine to octopamine, α-methyldopamine to α-methylnorepinephrine).

A number of the resultant structurally analogous metabolites can replace NE at the noradrenergic nerve endings and function as "false" NTs.

The last step in CA biosynthesis is the *N*-methylation of NE to give E in the adrenal medulla. The reaction is catalyzed by the enzyme phenylethanolamine-*N*-methyltransferase (PNMT). PNMT is a cytosolic enzyme and the methyl donor *S*-adenosyl methionine (SAM) is required for the *N*-methylation of NE. The adrenal medullary enzyme has rather low substrate specificity and transfers methyl groups to the nitrogen atom on various β-phenylethanolamines. The reaction occurs in the cell cytoplasm, and the E formed is transported into the storage granules of the chromaffin cells. Although PNMT is mostly found in the adrenal medulla, low levels of activity exist in heart and mammalian brain. Regulation of this enzyme in the brain has not been extensively studied, but glucocorticoids are known to regulate the activity of PNMT in the adrenal gland.

Storage, Release, Uptake, and Metabolism

Storage and Release. A large percentage of the NE present is located within highly specialized subcellular particles (later shown to be synaptic vesicles but colloquially referred to as *granules*) in sympathetic nerve endings and chromaffin cells. Much of the NE in CNS is also located within similar vesicles. The concentration in the vesicles is maintained also by the VMAT.

Following its biosynthesis and storage in granules, the entrance of Ca^{2+} into these cells results in the extrusion of NE by exocytosis of the granules. Ca^{2+}-triggered secretion involves interaction of highly conserved molecular scaffolding proteins leading to docking of granules at the plasma membrane and then NE is released from sympathetic nerve endings into the synaptic cleft, where it interacts with specific presynaptic and postsynaptic adrenoceptors, on the effector cell, triggering a biochemical cascade that results in a physiologic response by the effector cell. Indirectly acting and mixed sympathomimetics (e.g., tyramine, amphetamines, and ephedrine) are capable of releasing stored transmitter from noradrenergic nerve endings by a calcium-independent process. These drugs are poor agonists (some are inactive) at adrenoceptors, but they are excellent substrates for VMAT. They are avidly taken up into noradrenergic nerve endings by NE reuptake transporter (NET) responsible for NE reuptake into the nerve terminal. In the nerve ending, they are then transported by VMAT into the vesicles, displacing NE, which is subsequently expelled into the synaptic space by reverse transport via NET. Their action does not require vesicle exocytosis.

Uptake. Once NE has exerted its effect at adrenergic receptors, there must be mechanisms for removing the NE from the synapse and terminating its action at the receptors. These mechanisms include (a) reuptake of NE into the presynaptic neuron (recycling, major mechanism) by NET and into extraneuronal tissues, (b) conversion of NE to an inactive metabolite, and (c) diffusion of the NE away from the synapse. The first two of these mechanisms require specific transport proteins or enzymes, and therefore are targets for pharmacologic intervention. By far, the most important of these mechanisms is recycling the NE. This process is termed *uptake-1* and involves a Na^+/Cl^--dependent transmembrane (TM) NET that has a high affinity for NE.[4] This reuptake system also transports certain amines other than NE into the nerve terminal, and can be blocked by such drugs as cocaine and some of the tricyclic antidepressants (see Chapter 15). Similar transporters, dopamine transporter (DAT) and serotonin transporter (SERT) are responsible for the reuptake of DA and 5-HT (serotonin), respectively, into the neurons that release these transmitters. Some of the NE that reenters the sympathetic neuron is transported from the cytoplasm into the storage granules carried out by an H^+-dependent TM VMAT.[5] There, it is held in a stable complex with adenotriphosphate (ATP) and proteins until sympathetic nerve activity or some other stimulus causes it to be released into the synaptic cleft. Certain drugs, such as reserpine, block this transport, preventing the refilling of synaptic vesicles with NE and eventually cause nerve terminals to become depleted of their NE stores. By this mechanism, reserpine inhibits neurotransmission at adrenergic synapses.

In addition to the neuronal uptake of NE, there exists an extraneuronal uptake process, called *uptake-2* with relatively low affinity for NE. Although its physiological significance is unknown, it may play a role in the disposition of circulating CAs, because CAs that are taken up into extraneuronal tissues are metabolized quite rapidly.

Metabolism. The second mechanism of CA removal is metabolism. The major mammalian enzymes of importance in the CA metabolism are monoamine oxidase (MAO) and catechol-*O*-methyltransferase (COMT).[6,7] The comparison of the two enzymes is shown in Table 16.2.

Both E and NE are orally inactive and have short durations of action because of their high hydrophilicity, ionization, and extensive first-pass metabolic deactivation by COMT and MAO. The lack of substrate specificity of COMT and MAO is manifested in the metabolism of NE and E, shown in Figure 16.5. Not only do both MAO and COMT use NE and E as substrates, but each also acts on the metabolites produced by the other. Drugs that are catechols are subject to metabolism by COMT, whereas drugs with unsubstituted or secondary *N*-methyl-amino amino groups are often substrates for MAO.

The first enzyme of importance in the metabolism of CAs in the adrenergic neurons of human brain and peripheral tissues is MAO. MAOs oxidatively deaminate CAs to their corresponding aldehydes, which are rapidly oxidized to the corresponding acid by the enzyme aldehyde dehydrogenase (AD). In some circumstances, the aldehyde is reduced to the glycol by aldehyde reductase (AR). For example, NE is deaminated oxidatively by MAO to give 3′,4′-dihydroxyphenylglycolaldehyde (DOPGA), which then is reduced by AR to 3′,4′-dihydroxyphenylethylene glycol. It is primarily this glycol metabolite that is released into the circulation, where it undergoes methylation by the COMT that it encounters in nonneuronal tissues. The product of methylation, 3′-methoxy-4′-hydroxyphenylethylene glycol, is oxidized by alcohol dehydrogenase and AD to give 3′-methoxy-4′-hydroxymandelic acid. This metabolite commonly is referred to as *vanillylmandelic acid* (VMA), and is the major end product of several pathways of NE metabolism. An estimate of CA turnover can be obtained from laboratory analysis of total metabolites (sometimes referred to as *VMA and metanephrines*) in 24-hour urine sample. In the oxidative deamination of NE and E at extraneuronal sites such as the liver, the aldehyde formed is oxidized usually by AD to give 3,4-dihydroxymandelic acid (DOMA). MAO inhibitors (MAOIs) prevent MAO-catalyzed deamination of NE, DA, and 5-HT following their reuptake into the nerve terminal from the synaptic cleft. As a result, higher concentration of the NTs will be stored in the vesicles and become available for release from the presynaptic terminals on demand. Antidepressants such as phenelzine (Nardil), isocarboxazid (Marplan), and tranylcypromine (Parnate) are MAOIs.

There are two types of MAOs, and these exhibit different substrate selectivity.[8] MAO-B primarily metabolizes DA and thus MAO-B inhibitors would tend to preserve brain DA and be effective by themselves and/or potentiate levodopa. Selegiline (Eldepryl) is a specific type MAO-B inhibitor and does extend the duration and increase the efficacy of levodopa. The drug is promising, probably as an adjunct to levodopa or in levodopa refractory patients.

The understanding of CAs metabolism can be important in the management of certain drug therapies and may even aid in diagnosis. For example, changes resulting from drugs may indicate the success of a treatment. The cerebrospinal fluid (CSF) levels of methylhydroxyphenylglycoaldehyde (MOPEG) are indicative of NE levels. Just as they can be related to the intensity of depression, the degree of improvement expected with antidepressants can be monitored in the weeks it may take before the clinical symptoms improve. A CSF level of homovanillic acid (HVA, the major metabolite of brain DA, which is a counterpart of end metabolite of NE) is understandably low in parkinsonism.

The second enzyme of importance in the metabolism of CAs is COMT that *O*-methylates 3′-OH group of CAs and renders them inactive. Methylation by COMT occurs almost

TABLE 16.2 Comparison of MAO and COMT

	MAO	COMT
Location in Neurons	In neuronal mitochondria metabolism of intraneuronal CAs	Not in sympathetic neuron metabolism of extraneuronal CAs
Reaction	Deaminate CAs to aldehydes	*O*-methylate CAs to 3′-OMe-CAs
Substrates	Compounds with a terminal aliphatic amino group (primary or *N*-methyl-amino groups) preference:	Catechol-containing molecules
	MAO-A MOA-B	
	NE and 5-HT DA β-phenylethylamine benzylamine	DA, E, NE, ISO, etc.

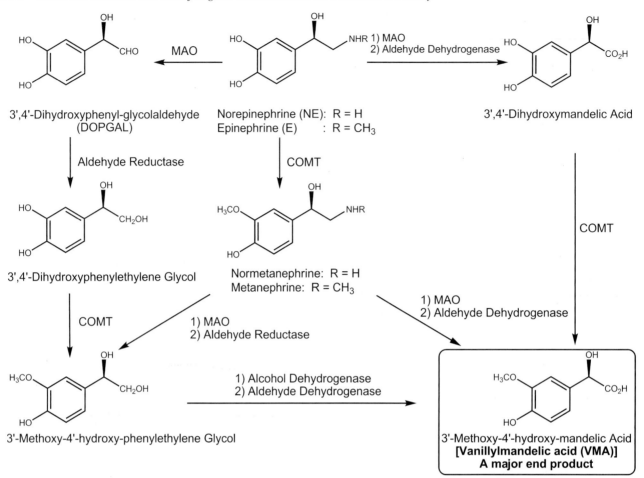

Figure 16.5 • Metabolism of norepinephrine and epinephrine by MAO and COMT.

exclusively on the *meta*-OH group of the catechol, regardless of whether the catechol is NE, E, or one of the metabolic products. For example, the action of COMT on NE and E gives normetanephrine and metanephrine, respectively. A converging pattern of the metabolism of NE and E in which 3′-methoxy-4′-hydroxymandelic acid (VMA) and 3′-methoxy-4′-hydroxyphenylethylene glycol are common end products thus occurs, regardless of whether the first metabolic step is oxidation by MAO or *O*-methylation by COMT. In patients with tumors of chromaffin tissue that secrete these amines (a rare cause of high blood pressure), the urinary excretion of VMA is markedly increased and is used as a diagnostic test for this condition.

Under normal circumstances, VMA is the principal urinary metabolite of NE, although substantial amounts of 3′-methoxy-4′-hydroxyphenylethylene glycol are excreted along with varying quantities of other metabolites, both in the free form and as sulfate or glucuronide conjugates (not shown in the schemes). Endogenous E is excreted primarily as metanephrine and VMA. These pathways of metabolism are also important to drugs that are structural analogs of NE. Tolcapone (Tasmar) and entacapone (Comtan) are COMT inhibitors presently available.

CAs released from either noradrenergic nerve terminals or the adrenal medulla are recognized by and bind to specific receptor molecules on the plasma membrane of the neuroeffector cells. These receptor ligand interactions produce a physiological response. Many cells possess these

receptors, and the binding of an agonist will generally cause the organism to respond in a fight-or-flight manner. For instance, the heart rate will increase and the pupils will dilate, energy will be mobilized, and blood flow will be diverted from other organs to skeletal muscle.

ADRENERGIC RECEPTORS

Adrenergic Receptor Subtypes

Membrane receptors transfer information from the environment to the cell's interior. A few nonpolar signal molecules such as estrogens and other steroid hormones are able to diffuse through the cell membranes and, hence, enter the cell. However, most signaling molecules such as CAs are too polar to pass through the membrane, and no appropriate transport systems are available. Thus, the information that they present must be transmitted across the cell membrane without the molecules themselves entering the cell. A membrane-associated receptor protein such as adrenergic receptors often performs the function of information transfer across the membrane.

In 1948, Ahlquist[9] proposed and designated α- and β-adrenoceptors based on their apparent drug sensitivity. The diverse physiological responses of CAs are mediated via α_1-, α_2-, and β-adrenoceptors, which are further divided into α_{1A}, α_{1B}, α_{1D}, α_{2A}, α_{2B}, α_{2C}, β_1, β_2, and β_3. They all belong

TABLE 16.3 Distribution and Effects of Adrenoceptors and Main Uses of the Adrenergic Drugs

Organ or Tissue	Predominant Adrenoceptors	Effect of Activation	Physiological Effect	Drugs	Therapeutic Uses
Blood vessels and skin	α_1	Vasoconstriction	↑ Blood pressure	α_1-Agonists	Shock, hypotension
Mucous membranes	α_1	Vasoconstriction		α_1-Agonists α_1-Antagonists	Nasal congestion Hypertension
Prostatic gland muscle	α_{1A}	Contraction	Prostatic hyperplasia	α_{1A}-Antagonists	BPH
CNS	α_2	↓ NE release	↓ Blood pressure	α_2-Agonists	Hypertension
Heart muscle	β_1 (minor β_2, β_3)	Muscle contraction	↑ Heart rate & force	β_1-Antagonists	Hypertension Arrhythmias
Bronchial smooth muscle	α_1	Smooth muscle contraction	Closes airways		
	β_2 (Bronchodilation)	Smooth muscle relaxation	Dilates & opens airways	β_2-Agonists	Asthma and COPD
Uterus (pregnant)	α_1	Muscle contraction			
	β_2	Smooth muscle relaxation	(−) Uterine contractions	β_2-Antagonists	Premature labor
Kidney	β_1	Increases rennin secretion	↑ Blood pressure		

to the superfamily of guanine nucleotide (G)-regulatory proteins (G-protein)–coupled receptors (GPCR), which have seven-transmembrane (7TM) helical regions. Elucidation of the characteristics of these receptors and the biochemical and physiological pathways they regulate has increased our understanding of the seemingly contradictory and variable effects of CAs on various organ systems. Although structurally related, different receptors regulate distinct physiological process by controlling the synthesis or release of various second messengers. An important factor in the response of any cell or organ to adrenergic drugs is the density and proportion of α- and β-adrenoceptors. For example, NE has relatively little capacity to increase bronchial airflow, because the receptors in bronchial smooth muscle are largely of the β_2-subtype. In contrast, isoproterenol (ISO) and E are potent bronchodilators.

The various adrenoceptor types and subtypes are not uniformly distributed with certain tissues containing more of one type than another. Table 16.3 describes various tissues they predominate, types of adrenoceptors, the result of activating these receptors, and the principal therapeutic uses of adrenergic agonists and antagonists. The clinical use of receptors-selective drugs becomes obvious when one considers the adrenoceptor subtypes and their locations.

α_1-Agonists as Vasoconstrictors and Nasal Decongestants. In blood vessels, the principal effect is vasoconstriction. Blood vessels with α_1-receptors are present in skin and during the fight-or-flight response, vasoconstriction results in the decreased blood flow to this organ. This accounts for an individual's skin appearing pale when frightened. Agonists acting selectively on α_1-receptors cause vasoconstriction and thus can be used alongside local anesthetics in dentistry to localize and prolong the effect on the anesthetic at the site of injection. They are also used as nasal decongestants (vasoconstriction of mucous membranes) and for raising blood pressure (vasoconstriction of blood vessels) in shock.

α_1-Antagonists for Treatment of Hypertension. Because α_1-agonists are vasoconstrictor and hypertensive, α_1-antagonists would be expected to be vasodilators and

hypotensive with clear implications of treating hypertension. Similarly, they should block α_{1A}-receptor in prostate smooth muscle and relax the muscle with implication of treating benign prostatic hyperplasia (BPH).

α_2-Agonists for Treatment of Hypertension. α_2-Agonists (e.g., clonidine) act at CNS sites to decrease sympathetic outflow to the periphery, resulting in decreased NE release at sympathetic nerve terminal and, therefore, relaxed vascular smooth muscle.

β_1-Blockers for Treatment of Hypertension, Angina, and Certain Cardiac Arrhythmias. Activation of the β_1-receptors in heart causes an increase in rate and force of contraction and β_1-blockers should be expected to slow the heart rate and decrease the force of contraction. They are used in treating hypertension, angina, and certain cardiac arrhythmias.

β_2-Agonists for Treatment of Asthma and Premature Labor. A major clinical use for adrenergic agonists is in treatment of asthma. Activation of β_2-receptors relaxes the smooth muscles in the bronchi, thus dilating and opening airways. Similarly, activation of β_2-receptors in the uterus relaxes the muscle, and some β_2-agonists are thus used to inhibit uterine contractions.

α-Adrenergic Receptors

The subtypes of adrenoceptor and their effector systems are summarized in Table 16.4. In the early 1970s, the discovery that certain adrenergic agonists and antagonists exhibited various degrees of selectivity for presynaptic and postsynaptic α-receptors led to the proposal that postsynaptic α-receptors be designated α_1 and that presynaptic α-receptors be referred to as α_2.[10] Later, a functional classification of the α-receptors was proposed wherein α_1-receptors were designated as those that were excitatory, while α_2-receptors purportedly mediated inhibitory responses.[11] Further developments revealed, however, that both α_1- and α_2-receptors could be either presynaptic or postsynaptic and either excitatory or inhibitory in their responses. However, the physiologic significance of postsynaptic α_2-receptors is less well understood.[12]

TABLE 16.4 Subtypes of Adrenoceptors and Their Effector Systems

Receptor	Agonists	Antagonists	G Protein	Main Biochemical Effectors
α_1	E ≥ NE >> ISO Phenylephrine Methoxamine	Prazosin Corynanthine	G_q	(+) PLC → ↑ IP$_3$ & DAG ↑ Ca^{2+}
α_2	E ≥ NE >> ISO Clonidine	Yohimbine	G_i G_i($\beta\gamma$ subunits)	(−) AC → ↓ cAMP ↑ K$^+$ channels
β-type	Isoproterenol	Propranolol	G_s	(+) AC → ↑ cAMP
β_1	ISO > E = NE Dobutamine	Metoprolol Betaxolol	G_s	(+) AC → ↑ cAMP ↑ L-type Ca^{2+} channels
β_2	ISO > E > NE Terbutaline	Butoxamine	G_s	(+) AC → ↑ cAMP

G_s, the *s* in subscript indicates the subunit's stimulatory role; G_i, the *i* in subscript indicates the subunit's inhibitory role; Gq, the *q* in subscript indicates the protein coupling receptors to phospholipase C.

Pharmacological and molecular biological methods have shown that it is possible to subdivide the α_1- and α_2-receptors into additional subtypes. The α_1- and α_2-receptors each have been divided into at least three subtypes, which have been designated α_{1A}, α_{1B}, α_{1D} and α_{2A}, α_{2B}, α_{2C}, respectively.[13–15]

Both receptor subtypes belong to a superfamily of membrane receptors whose general structure consists of 7TM α-helical segments. The interaction of adrenergic drugs and the receptors alters the tertiary or quaternary structure of the receptor, including the intracellular domain. These structural changes are not sufficient to yield an appropriate response, because they are restricted to a small number of receptor molecules in the cell membrane. The information embodied by CAs or drugs, which act as primary messengers, must be transduced into downstream activity that can alter the biochemistry of the cell. The signal–transduction mechanisms involve coupling to G proteins. Each G protein is a heterotrimer consisting of α-, β-, and γ-subunit and is classified based on their distinctive α subunits. G proteins of particular importance for adrenoceptor function include G_s, the stimulatory G protein of adenylyl cyclase (AC); G_i, the inhibitory G protein of AC; and G_q, the protein coupling receptors to phospholipase C (PLC).

The α- and β-receptors differ from each other in their structures, functions, and in the second-messenger system that is affected.[16,17] Stimulation of α_1-receptors results in the regulation of multiple effector systems. A primary mode of signal transduction involves (a) activation of the G_q-PLC-IP$_3$-Ca^{2+} pathway and (b) the activation of other Ca^{2+} and calmodulin-sensitive pathway such as CaM kinases. The α_1-receptor subtype is coupled to the enzyme PLC via a G_q. When stimulated by activation of the α_1-receptor, PLC hydrolyzes phosphatidylinositol-4,5-bisphosphate (PIP$_2$) to give the second messengers inositol-1,4,5-triphosphate (IP$_3$) and 1,2-diacylglycerol (DAG). In smooth muscle, IP$_3$ stimulates the release of Ca^{2+} from the sarcoplasmic reticulum, resulting in an increase in free intracellular calcium levels. Increased free intracellular calcium is correlated with smooth muscle contraction, whereas DAG activates protein kinase C (PKC), which phosphorylates proteins, and may induce slowly developing contractions of vascular smooth muscle (Fig. 16.6).

Vasoconstriction is commonly initiated by the opening of voltage-gated L-type Ca^{2+} channels in the sarcolemma during plasma membrane depolarization, which mediates Ca^{2+} flux into the cytoplasm. Ca^{2+} entry into the cell activates calmodulin (CaM). The Ca^{2+}-CaM complex activates myosin light chain kinase (MLCK) to phosphorylate myosin light chain (myosin-LC). The phosphorylated myosin-LC interacts with actin to form actin-myosin cross-bridges, a process that initiates vascular smooth muscle cell contraction. The vascular constriction thus causes an increase in blood pressure. In contrast, relaxation is a coordinated series of steps that act to dephosphorylate and hence inactivate myosin-LC.

Activation of α_2-receptors leads to a reduction in the catalytic activity of AC, which in turn results in a lowering of intracellular levels of cyclic adenosine monophosphate (cAMP) (Fig. 16.7). The α_2-receptor–mediated inhibition of AC is regulated by the G_i.

α-Receptors of the CNS and in peripheral tissues perform a number of important physiological functions.[16] In particular, α-receptors are involved in control of the cardiovascular system. For example, constriction of vascular smooth muscle is mediated by both postjunctional α_1- and α_2-receptors, though the predominant receptor mediating this effect is α_1.[18] In the heart, activation of α_1-receptors results in a selective inotropic response with little or no change in heart rate.[19] This is in contrast to the β_1-receptor, which is the predominant postjunctional receptor in the heart, mediating both inotropic and chronotropic effects. In the brain, activation of postjunctional α_2-receptors reduces sympathetic outflow from the CNS, which in turn causes a lowering of blood pressure.[20] The prototypical α_2-receptor is the presynaptic α-receptor found on the terminal sympathetic neuron.[10,11,21] Interaction of this receptor with agonists such as NE and E results in inhibition of NE release from the neuron. The α_2-receptors not only play a role in the regulation of NE release but also regulate the release of other NTs, such as acetylcholine and serotonin. Both α_1- and α_2-receptors also play an important role in the regulation of several metabolic processes, such as insulin secretion and glycogenolysis.[22]

β-Adrenergic Receptors

Three β-receptor subtypes have been cloned, including β_1, β_2, and β_3. In 1967, Lands et al.[23] suggested that β-receptors could be subdivided into β_1 and β_2 types. Seventeen years later, Arch et al.[24] identified a third subtype of β-receptor in brown adipose tissue designated as the β_3 subtype.[13] All clinically relevant α_1-, β_1-, β_2-, and β_3-receptors are postsynaptic

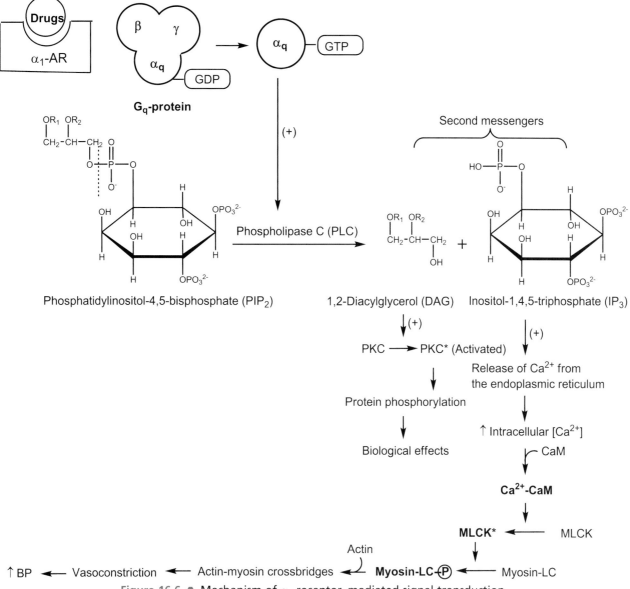

Figure 16.6 ● Mechanism of α_1-receptor–mediated signal transduction.

receptors that are linked to stimulation of biochemical processes in the postsynaptic cell. The function of presynaptic β-receptors is, however, unclear. The β-adrenoceptor subtypes also differ in terms of the rank order of potency of the adrenergic receptor agonists NE, E, and ISO (Table 16.4).

The use of β_2-agonists as bronchodilators and β_1- or β_1/β_2-blockers as antihypertensives is well established. The β_1-receptors are located mainly in the heart, where they mediate the positive inotropic and chronotropic effects of the CAs. They are also found on the juxtaglomerular cells of the kidney, where they are involved in increasing renin secretion. The β_2-receptors are located on smooth muscle throughout the body, where they are involved in relaxation of the smooth muscle, producing such effects as bronchodilation and vasodilation. They are also found in the liver, where they promote glycogenolysis. The β_3-receptor is located on brown adipose tissue and is involved in the stimulation of lipolysis.

All three β-receptors are coupled to AC, which catalyzes the conversion of ATP to cAMP (Fig. 16.7). This coupling is via the G-protein G_s.[25,26] In the absence of an agonist, guanosine diphosphate (GDP) is bound reversibly to the G_s protein. Interaction of the agonist with the receptor causes a conformational change in the receptor, which decreases the affinity of the G_s protein for GDP and a concomitantly increases the affinity for guanosine triphosphate (GTP). The α_s-subunit of G_s-protein complex dissociates from the receptor–G protein tertiary complex and then binds to and activates AC.

The intracellular function of the second-messenger cAMP is activation of protein kinases, which phosphorylate specific proteins, thereby altering their function.[27] The action of cAMP is terminated by a class of enzymes known as phosphodiesterase (PDE) that catalyzes the hydrolysis of cAMP to AMP (Fig. 16.7) and is related to the mechanism of action of caffeine and theophylline.

Cloning of the gene and complementary DNA (cDNA) for the mammalian β-receptor has made it possible to explore the structure–function relationships of the receptor.[28] Through such studies of single point mutations, it has

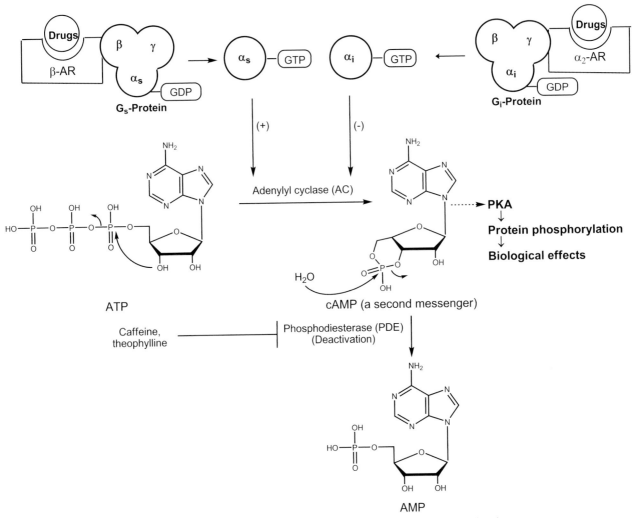

Figure 16.7 ● Mechanism of β_2-receptor–mediated signal transduction.

been proposed that the adrenergic agonist-binding site is within the TM-spanning regions, whereas the cytoplasmic regions of the receptor interact with the G_s protein. Specifically, aspartic acid residue 113 in transmembrane region III (TM-III) acts as the counterion to the cationic amino group of the adrenergic agonist. This aspartic acid residue is found not only in a comparable position in all the other adrenoceptors but also in other known GPCRs that bind substrates having positively charged nitrogens in their structure. Two serine residues, at positions 204 and 207 in TM-V, form H-bonds with the catechol OH groups of the adrenergic agonists. The β-OH group of adrenergic agonists is thought to form an H-bond with the side chain of asparagine 293 in TM-VI, whereas the phenylalanine residue at position 290 in the same TM-VI is believed to interact with the catechol ring (Fig. 16.8). Because the serine is in the fifth membrane-spanning region and the aspartic acid is in the third, it is likely that CAs bind parallel to the plane of the membrane, forming a bridge between the two TM-spanning regions.

Molecular biological techniques have shown the existence of adrenergic receptor polymorphism for both the α- and β-receptors. It is postulated that such polymorphisms may be an important factor behind individual differences in responses to drugs acting at these receptors. In addition, there

may be an association between the polymorphisms of adrenergic receptor genes and disease states.[29]

DRUGS AFFECTING ADRENERGIC NEUROTRANSMISSION

Drugs Affecting Catecholamine Biosynthesis

Metyrosine (α-Methyl-L-tyrosine, Demser). Although inhibition of any of the three enzymes involved in CA biosynthesis should decrease CAs, inhibitors of the first and the rate-limiting enzyme TH would be the most effective. As such, metyrosine is a much more effective competitive inhibitor of E and NE production than agents that inhibit any of the other enzymes involved in CA biosynthesis. It is often possible to "fool" the enzymes into accepting a structurally similar and unnatural substrate such as metyrosine. Metyrosine differs structurally from tyrosine only in the presence of an α-methyl group (Fig. 16.9). It is one example of a CA-biosynthesis inhibitor in clinical use.[30] Although metyrosine is used as a racemic mixture, it is the ($-$) isomer that possesses the inhibitory activity. Metyrosine, which is given orally in dosages ranging from

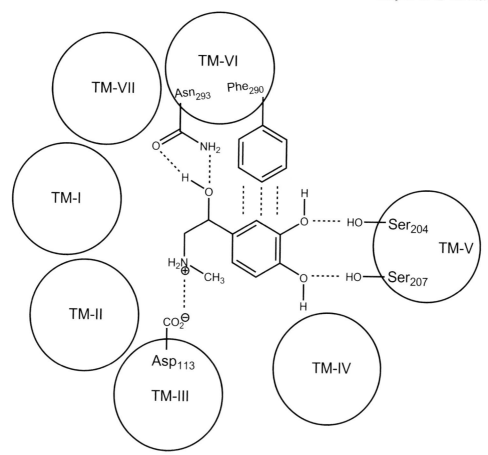

Figure 16.8 ● Model of β_2-AR binding sites: Illustration of the Easson-Stedman hypothesis representing the interaction of three critical pharmacophoric groups of norepinephrine with the complementary binding areas on the adrenergic receptor as suggested by site-directed mutagenesis studies.

Metyrosine (Methyl tyrosine, log P = 0.73, an inhibitor of TH): ↓ bp

Tyrosine Hydroxylase (TH)

L-Tyrosine (a precursor of NE and a substrate of TH)

Epinephrine (E): ↑ bp

Figure 16.9 ● Mechanism of action of metyrosine.

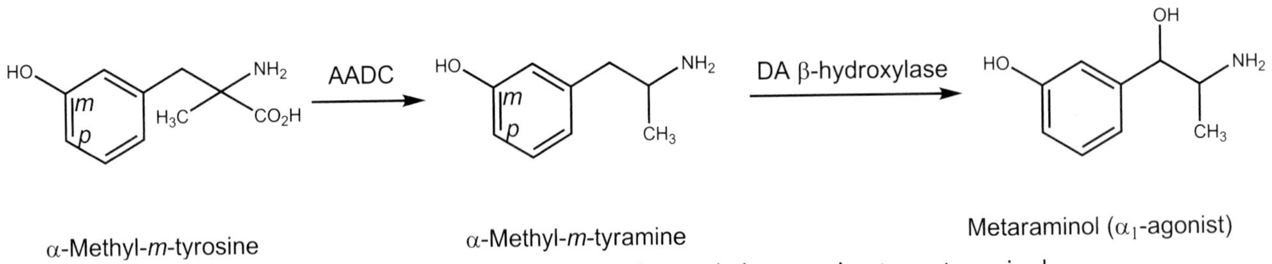

Figure 16.10 ● Metabolic activation of α-methyl-*m*-tyrosine to metaraminol.

1 to 4 g/day, is used principally for the preoperative management of pheochromocytoma, chromaffin cell tumors that produce large amounts of NE and E. Although these adrenal medullary tumors are often benign, patients frequently suffer hypertensive episodes. Metyrosine reduces the frequency and severity of these episodes by significantly lowering CA production (35%–80%). The drug is polar (log P = 0.73) and excreted mainly unchanged in the urine. Because of its limited solubility in water caused by intramolecular bonding of the zwitterions, crystalluria is a potential serious side effect. It can be minimized by maintaining a daily urine volume of more than 2 L. Inhibitors of CA synthesis have limited clinical utility because such agents nonspecifically inhibit the formation of all CAs and result in many side effects. Sedation is the most common side effect of this drug.

A similar example is the use of α-methyl-*m*-tyrosine in the treatment of shock. It differs structurally from metyrosine only in the presence of *m*-OH instead of *p*-OH in metyrosine. This unnatural amino acid is accepted by the enzymes of the biosynthetic pathway and converted to metaraminol (an α-agonist) as shown (Fig. 16.10).

Inhibitors of AADC (e.g., carbidopa) have proven to be clinically useful, but not as modulators of peripheral adrenergic transmission. Rather these agents are used to inhibit the metabolism of drug L-DOPA administered in the treatment of Parkinson disease (Chapter 13).

Drugs Affecting Catecholamine Storage and Release

Reserpine (an NT Depleter). Reserpine, a prototypical and historically important drug, is an indole alkaloid obtained from the root of *Rauwolfia serpentina* found in India.

As is typical of many indole alkaloids, reserpine is susceptible to decomposition by light and oxidation. Reserpine is extensively metabolized through hydrolysis of the ester function at position 18 and yields methyl reserpate and 3,4,5-trimethoxybenzoic acid. It not only depletes the vesicle storage of NE in sympathetic neurons in PNS, neurons of the CNS, and E in the adrenal medulla, but also depletes the storage of serotonin and DA in their respective neurons in the brain. Reserpine binds extremely tightly with and blocks VMAT that transports NE and other biogenic amines from the cytoplasm into the storage vesicles.[31] Thus in sympathetic neurons, NE, which normally is transported into the storage vesicles, is instead metabolized by mitochondrial MAO in the cytoplasm. In addition, there is a gradual loss of vesicle-stored NE as it is used up by release resulting from sympathetic nerve activity so that the storage vesicles eventually become dysfunctional. The end result is a depletion of NE in the sympathetic neuron. Analogous effects are seen in the adrenal medulla with E and with 5-HT in serotonergic neurons.

When reserpine is given orally, its maximum effect is seen after a couple of weeks. A sustained effect up to several weeks is seen after the last dose has been given. This is because the tight binding of reserpine to storage vesicles continues for a prolonged time, and recovery of sympathetic function requires synthesis of new vesicles over a period of days to weeks after discontinuation of the drug. Most adverse effects of reserpine (log P = 4.37) are caused by CNS effects because it readily enters the CNS. Sedation and inability to concentrate or perform complex tasks are the most common adverse effects. More serious is the occasional psychotic depression that can lead to suicide, which support monoamine theory of pathology of depression. Agents with fewer side effects have largely replaced reserpine in clinical use.

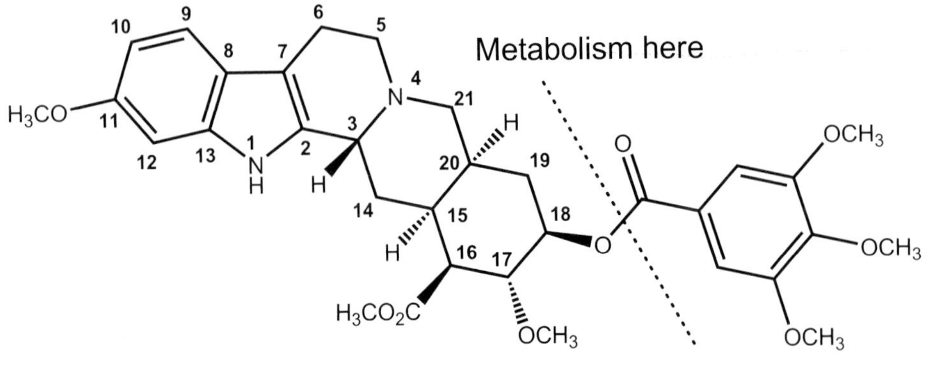

Reserpine (Log P = 4.37, Log D = 3.93)

guanidino moiety

Guanethidine
pKa = 13.43
No CNS activity

guanidino moiety

Guanadrel
pKa = 12.76
No CNS activity

Guanethidine (Ismelin) and guanadrel (Hylorel) are seldom used orally active antihypertensives. Drugs of this type enter the adrenergic neuron by way of the uptake-1 process and accumulate within the neuronal storage vesicles. There they bind to the storage vesicles and stabilize the neuronal storage vesicle membranes, making them less responsive to nerve impulses. The ability of the vesicles to fuse with the neuronal membrane is also diminished, resulting in inhibition of NE release into the synaptic cleft in response to a neuronal impulse and generalized decrease in sympathetic tone. Long-term administration of some of these agents also can produce a depletion of NE stores in sympathetic neurons.

Both neuronal blocking drugs possess a guanidino moiety [CNHC(=NH)NH$_2$], which is attached to either a hexahydroazocinyl ring linked by an ethyl group as in guanethidine, or a dioxaspirodecyl ring linked by a methyl group as in guanadrel. The presence of the more basic guanidino group (pK$_a$ >12) than the ordinary amino group in these drugs means that at physiological pH, they are essentially completely protonated. Thus, these agents do not get into the CNS. As a result, this drug has none of the central effects seen with many of the other antihypertensive agents described in this chapter. Guanethidine contains two basic nitrogen atoms with pK$_a$ values of 9.0 and 13.43, and can therefore form guanethidine monosulfate (C$_{10}$H$_{22}$N$_4$ · H$_2$SO$_4$) or guanethidine sulfate [(C$_{10}$H$_{22}$N$_4$)$_2$ · H$_2$SO$_4$].

Although guanethidine and guanadrel have virtually the same mechanism of action on sympathetic neurons, they differ in their pharmacokinetic properties. For example, although guanethidine is absorbed incompletely after oral administration (3%–50%), guanadrel is well absorbed, with a bioavailability of 85%.[32] These two agents also differ in terms of half-life: Guanethidine has a half-life of about 5 days, whereas guanadrel has a half-life of 12 hours. Both agents are partially metabolized (~50%) by the liver, and both are used to treat moderate-to-severe hypertension, either alone or in combination with another antihypertensive agent.

● SYMPATHOMIMETIC AGENTS

Sympathomimetic agents produce effects resembling those produced by stimulation of the sympathetic nervous system. They may be classified as agents that produce effects by a direct, indirect, or mixed mechanism of action. Direct-acting agents elicit a sympathomimetic response by interacting directly with adrenergic receptors. Indirect-acting agents produce effects primarily by causing the release of NE from adrenergic nerve terminals; the NE that is released by the indirect-acting agent activates the receptors to produce the response. Compounds with a mixed mechanism of action interact directly with adrenergic receptors and indirectly cause the release of NE. As described later, the mechanism by which an agent produces its sympathomimetic effect is related intimately to its chemical structure.

Direct-Acting Sympathomimetics

STRUCTURE–ACTIVITY RELATIONSHIPS

The structure–activity relationships (SARs) summary is shown in Figure 16.11. Comprehensive reviews of the SARs of α- and β-agonists and antagonists[33–35] covered their developments in the late 1980s. The parent structure with the features in common for many of the adrenergic drugs is β-phenylethylamine. The manner in which β-phenylethylamine is substituted on the *meta*- and *para*-positions of the aromatic ring, on the amino (R$_1$), and on α-, (R$_2$)-, and β-positions of the ethylamine side chain influences not only their mechanism of action, the receptor selectivity, but also their absorption, oral activity, metabolism, degradation, and thus duration of action (DOA). For the direct-acting sympathomimetic amines, maximal activity is seen in β-phenylethylamine derivatives containing (a) a catechol and (b) a (1R)-OH group on the ethylamine portion of the molecule. Such structural features are seen in the prototypical direct-acting compounds NE, E, and ISO. The SARs are supported by the model of β$_2$-AR binding studies (Fig. 16.8).

Optical Isomerism. A critical factor in the interaction of adrenergic agonists with their receptors is stereoselectivity. Substitution on either carbon-1 or carbon-2 yields optical isomers. (1R,2S) isomers seem correct configuration for direct-acting activity. For CAs, the more potent enantiomer has the (1R) configuration. This enantiomer is typically several 100-fold more potent than the enantiomer with the (1S) configuration. It appears that for all direct-acting, phenylethylamine-derived agonists that are structurally similar to NE, the more potent enantiomer is capable of assuming a conformation that results in the arrangement in space of the catechol group, the amino group, and the (1R)-OH group in a fashion resembling that of (1R)-NE. This explanation of stereoselectivity is based on the presumed interaction of these three critical pharmacophoric groups with three complementary binding areas on the receptor and is known as the Easson-Stedman hypothesis.[17,36] This three-point interaction is supported by site-directed mutagenesis studies[28] on the adrenergic receptor and is illustrated in Figure 16.8.

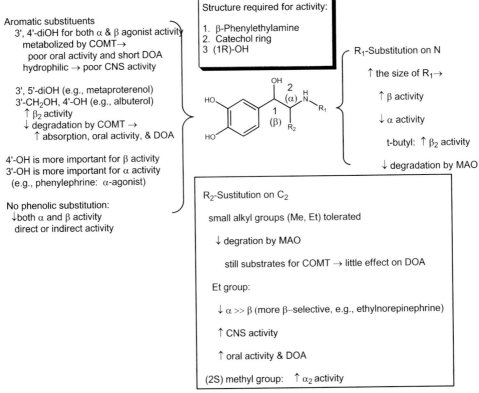

Figure 16.11 ● Structure–activity relationship of adrenergic phenylethylamine agonists.

Separation of Aromatic Ring and Amino Group. By far, the greatest adrenergic activity occurs when two carbon atoms separate the aromatic ring from the amino group. This rule applies with few exceptions to all types of activities.

R₁, Substitution on the Amino Nitrogen Determines α- or β-Receptor Selectivity. The amine is normally ionized at physiological pH. This is important for direct agonist activity, because replacing nitrogen with carbon results in a large decline in activity. The activity is also affected by the number of substituents on the nitrogen. Primary and secondary amines have good adrenergic activity, whereas tertiary amines and quaternary ammonium salts do not. The nature of the amino substituent also dramatically affects the receptor selectivity of the compound. As the size of the nitrogen substituent increases, α-receptor agonist activity generally decreases and β-receptor agonist activity increases. Thus, NE has more α-activity than β-activity and E is a potent agonist at α-, β₁-, and β₂-receptors. ISO, however, is a potent β₁- and β₂-agonist but has little affinity for α-receptors.

Norepinephrine (NE)
α > β agonist
α agonist

Epinephrine (E)
α, β₁ and β₂ agonist
nonselective α and β agonist

Isoproterenol (ISO)
β₁ and β₂ agonists
nonselective β agonist

N-t-Butylnorepinephrine (Colterol)
selective β₂ agonist

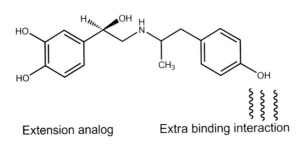

Extension analog   Extra binding interaction

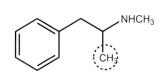

Ephedrine (Log P = 1.05)
more α and β activity
less lipophilic → less CNS activity

Methamphetamine (Log P = 1.97)
less α and β activity
more lipophilic → more CNS activity

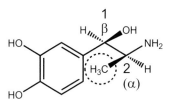

(1R, 2S)-α-Methylnorepinephrine
active isomer
selective α2 agonist

The nature of the substituents can also affect β_1- and β_2-receptor selectivity. In several instances, it has been shown that a β_2-directing *N-tert*-butyl group enhances β_2-selectivity. For example, *N-tert*-butylnorepinephrine (Colterol) is 9 to 10 times more potent as an agonist at tracheal β_2-receptors than at cardiac β_1-receptors. These results indicate that the β-receptor has a larger lipophilic binding pocket adjacent to the amine-binding aspartic acid residue than do the α-receptors. Increasing the length of the alkyl chain offers no advantage, but if a polar functional group is placed at the end of the alkyl group, the situation changes. In particular, adding a phenol group to the end of a C2 alkyl chain results in a dramatic rise in activity, indicating that an extra polar-binding region has been accessed, which can take part in H-bonding. Experiments have shown the activity of the extension analog is thereby increased by a factor of 800. As R_1 becomes larger than butyl group, it can provide compounds with α_1-blocking activity (e.g., tamsulosin and labetalol). Large substituents on the amino group also protect the amino group from undergoing oxidative deamination by MAO.

R_2, Substitution on the α-Carbon (Carbon-2). Substitution by small alkyl group (e.g., CH_3- or C_2H_5-) slows metabolism by MAO but has little overall effect on DOA of catechols because they remain substrates for COMT. However, the resistance to MAO activity is more important in noncatechol indirect-acting phenylethylamines. The DOA of drugs such as ephedrine or amphetamine is thus measured in hours rather than in minutes. Because addition of small alkyl group increases the resistance to metabolism and lipophilicity, such compounds often exhibit enhanced oral effectiveness and greater CNS activity than their counterparts that do not contain an α-alkyl group. In addition, compounds with an α-methyl substituent persist in the nerve terminals and are more likely to release NE from storage sites. For example, metaraminol is an α-agonist and also exhibits a greater degree of indirect sympathomimetic activity.

Methyl or ethyl substitution on the α-carbon of the ethylamine side chain reduces direct agonist activity at both α- and β-receptors. α-Substitution also significantly affects receptor selectivity. An ethyl group in this position diminishes α-activity far more than β-activity, affording compounds with β-selectivity (e.g., ethylnorepinephrine and isoetharine). In the case of β-receptors, for example, α-methyl or ethyl substitution results in compounds toward the β_2-selectivity, whereas in the case of α-receptors, α-methyl substitution gives compounds toward the α_2-selectivity. Another effect of α-substitution is the introduction of a chiral center, which has pronounced effects on the stereochemical requirements for activity. For example, with α-methylnorepinephrine, it is the *erythro* (1R,2S) isomer that possesses significant activity at α_2-receptors.

OH substitution on the β-carbon (carbon-1) generally decreases CNS activity largely because it lowers lipid solubility. However, such substitution greatly enhances agonist activity at both α- and β-receptors. For example, ephedrine is less potent than methamphetamine as a central stimulant, but it is more powerful in dilating bronchioles and increasing blood pressure and heart rate. Compounds lacking the β-OH group (e.g. DA) have a greatly reduced adrenergic receptor activity. Some of the activity is retained, indicating that the OH group is important but not essential. The R-enantiomer of NE is more active than the S-enantiomer, indicating that the secondary alcohol is involved in an H-bonding interaction.

Substitution on the Aromatic Ring. Maximal α- and β-activity also depends on the presence of 3′ and 4′ OH groups. Tyramine, which lacks two OH groups, has no affinity for adrenoceptors, indicating the importance of the OH groups. Studies of β-adrenoceptor structure suggest that the OH groups on serine residues 204 and 207 probably form H-bonds with the catechol OH groups at positions 3′ and 4′, respectively.

Phenylephrine
less α and β activity than NE
selective α1 agonist
almost no β activity

Metaproterenol
selective β2 agonist
not metabolized by COMT →
better absorption & longer DOA

Albuterol
selective β2 agonist
not metabolized by COMT →
better oral bioavailability

Resorcinal

Although the catechol moiety is an important structural feature in terms of yielding compounds with maximal agonist activity at adrenoceptors, it can be replaced with other substituted phenyl moieties to provide selective adrenergic agonists. This approach has been used in particular in the design of selective β_2-agonists. For example, replacement of the catechol function of ISO with the resorcinol structure gives a selective β_2-agonist, metaproterenol. Furthermore, because the resorcinol ring is not a substrate for COMT, β-agonists that contain this ring structure tend to have better absorption characteristics and a longer DOA than their catechol-containing counterparts. In another approach, replacement of the *meta*-OH of the catechol structure with a hydroxymethyl group gives agents, such as albuterol, which show selectivity to the β_2-receptor. Because they are not catechols, these agents are not metabolized by COMT and thus show improved oral bioavailability and longer DOA.

Modification of the catechol ring can also bring about selectivity at α-receptors as it appears that the catechol moiety is more important for α_2-activity than for α_1-activity. For example, removal of the *p*-OH group from E gives phenylephrine, which, in contrast to E, is selective for the α_1-receptor. Phenylephrine is less potent than E at both α- and β-receptors, with β_2-activity almost completely absent. However, the OH group can be replaced by other groups capable of interacting with the binding site by H-bonding. This is particularly true for the *meta*-OH group, which can be replaced by CH_2OH, NHMe, NHCOR, NMe_2, or $NHSO_2R$ group.

CAs without OH Groups. Phenylethylamines that lack OH groups on the ring and the β-OH group on the side chain act almost exclusively by causing the release of NE from sympathetic nerve terminals and thus results in a loss of direct sympathomimetic activity. Because substitution of OH groups on the phenylethylamine structure makes the resultant compounds less lipophilic, unsubstituted or alkyl-substituted compounds cross the BBB more readily and have more central activity. Thus, amphetamine and methamphetamine exhibit considerable CNS activity.

CAs per oral have only a brief DOA and are almost inactive, because they are rapidly inactivated in the intestinal mucosa and in the liver before reaching the systemic circulation. In contrast, compounds without one or both phenolic OH substituents are, however, not metabolized by COMT, and they are orally active and have longer DOA.

Imidazolines and α-Adrenergic Agonists. Although nearly all β-agonists are β-phenylethanolamine derivatives, it is α-adrenoceptors that exhibit a far more diverse assortment of structures. A second chemical class of α-agonists, the

X = usually CH_2 (α_1 agonists) or NH (α_2 agonists)

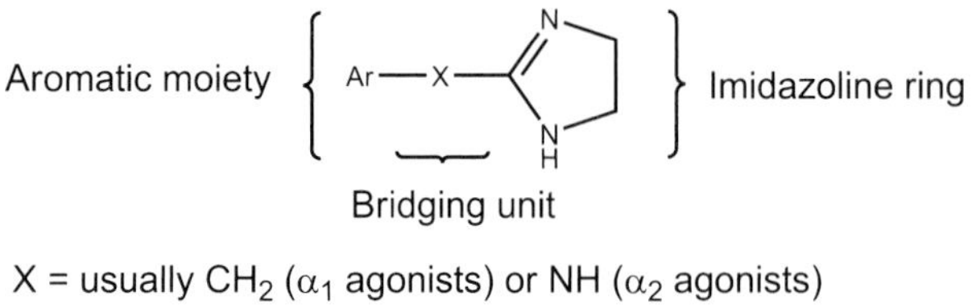

Figure 16.12 ● General structural features of the imidazoline α-adrenergic receptor agonists.

imidazolines, which give rise to α-agonists and are thus vasoconstrictors. These imidazolines can be nonselective, or they can be selective for either α_1- or α_2-receptors. Structurally, most imidazolines have their heterocyclic imidazoline nucleus linked to a substituted aromatic moiety via some type of bridging unit (Fig. 16.12).[34] The optimum bridging unit (X) is usually a single methylene group or amino group. Although modification of the imidazoline ring generally results in compounds with significantly reduced agonist activity, there are examples of so-called open-ring imidazolines that are highly active. The nature of the aromatic moiety, as well as how it is substituted, is quite flexible. However, agonist activity is enhanced when the aromatic ring is substituted with halogen substituents like chlorine (Cl) or small alkyl groups like methyl group, particularly when they are placed in the two *ortho* positions. Because the SARs of the imidazolines are quite different from those of the β-phenylethylamines, it has been postulated that the imidazolines interact with α-receptors differently from the way the β-phenylethylamines do, particularly with regard to the aromatic moiety.[37]

ENDOGENOUS CATECHOLAMINES

The three naturally occurring catecholamines DA, NE, and E are used as therapeutic agents.

Dopamine. (DA, 3′,4′-dihydroxyphenylethylamine) differs from NE in lacking of 1-OH group. It is the immediate precursor of NE and is a central NT particularly important in the regulation of movement (see Chapter 13). As a catechol and primary amine, DA is rapidly metabolized by COMT and MAO and has a short DOA with no oral activity. It is used intravenously in treatment of shock. In contrast with the NE and E, DA increases blood flow to the kidney in doses that have no chronotropic effect on the heart or that cause no increase in blood pressure. The increased blood flow to the kidneys enhances glomerular filtration rate, Na^+ excretion, and, in turn, urinary output. The dilation of renal blood vessels produced by DA is the result of its agonist action on the D_1-DA receptor.

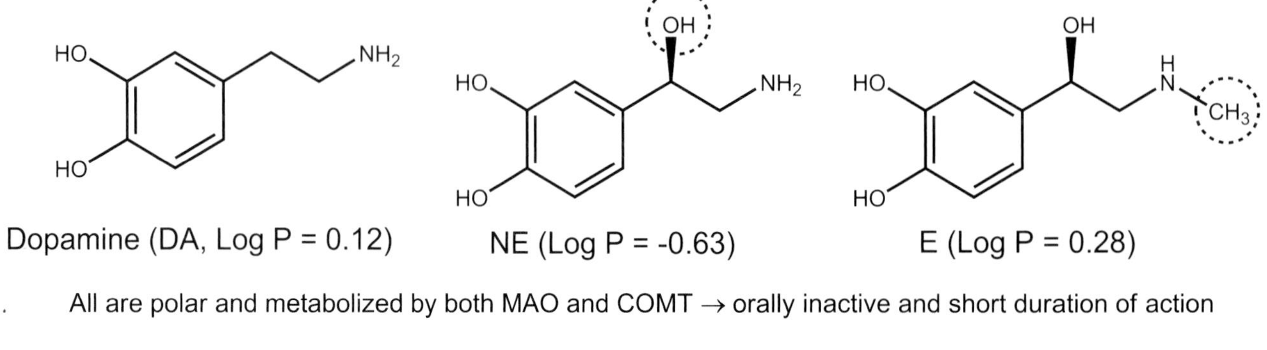

Dopamine (DA, Log P = 0.12)   NE (Log P = −0.63)   E (Log P = 0.28)

All are polar and metabolized by both MAO and COMT → orally inactive and short duration of action

In doses slightly higher than those required to increase renal blood flow, DA stimulates the β_1-receptors of the heart to increase cardiac output. Some of the effects of DA on the heart are also caused by NE release. Infusion at a rate greater than 10 μg/kg per minute results in stimulation of α_1-receptors, leading to vasoconstriction and an increase in arterial blood pressure. DA should be avoided or used at a much reduced dosage (one tenth or less) if the patient has received an MAO inhibitor. Careful adjustment of dosage also is necessary in patients who are taking tricyclic antidepressants.

Norepinephrine (NE, Levophed) differs from DA only by addition of a 1-OH substituent (β-OH-DA) and from E only by lacking the *N*-methyl group. Like DA, it is polar and rapidly metabolized by both COMT and MAO, resulting in poor oral bioavailability and short DOA (1 or 2 minutes even when given intravenously). It is a stimulant of α_1-, α_2-, and β_1-adrenoceptors (notice that lacking the *N*-methyl group results in lacking β_2- and β_3-activity). It is used to counteract various hypotensive crises, because its α-activity raises blood pressure and as an adjunct treatment in cardiac arrest because its β-activity stimulates the heart. It has limited clinical application caused by the nonselective nature of its activities.

Epinephrine (E, Adrenalin) differs from NE only by the addition of an *N*-methyl group. Like the other CAs, E is light sensitive and easily oxidized on exposure to air because of the catechol ring system. The development of a pink-to-brown color indicates oxidative breakdown. To minimize oxidation, solutions of the drug are stabilized by the addition of reducing agents such as sodium bisulfite. E is also destroyed readily in alkaline solutions and by metals (e.g., Cu, Fe, Zn) and weak oxidizing agents. It is used in aqueous solution for inhalation as the free amine. Like other amines, it forms salts with acids, hydrochloride, and the bitartrate being the most common.

Like NE, it lacks oral activity and has short DOA. However, it is much more widely used clinically than NE. E is a potent stimulant of all α_1-, α_2-, β_1-, β_2-, and β_3-adrenoceptors, and thus it switches on all possible adrenergic receptors, leading to a whole range of desired and side effects. Particularly prominent are the actions on the heart and on vascular and other smooth muscle. It is a very potent vasoconstrictor and cardiac stimulant. NE has, in general, greater β-activity caused by an additional *N*-methyl group. Therefore, E is used to stimulate the heart in cardiac arrest. Although intravenous infusion of E has pronounced effects on the cardiovascular system, its use in the treatment of

heart block or circulatory collapse is limited because of its tendency to induce cardiac arrhythmias.

The ability of epinephrine to stimulate β_2-receptors has led to its use by injection and by inhalation to relax bronchial smooth muscle in asthma and in anaphylactic reactions. Several OTC preparations (e.g., Primatene, Bronkaid) used for treating bronchial asthma use E. It is also used in inhibiting uterine contraction. Because of its α-activity, E is used to treat hypotensive crises and nasal congestion, to enhance the activity of local anesthetics, and as a constrictor in hemorrhage.

In addition, E is used in the treatment of open-angle glaucoma, where it apparently reduces intraocular pressure by increasing the rate of outflow of aqueous humor from the anterior chamber of the eye. The irritation often experienced on instillation of E into the eye has led to the development of other preparations of the drug that potentially are not as irritating. One such example is dipivefrin.

Dipivefrin (Propine, Dipivalyl Epinephrine). To overcome several of the pharmacokinetic and pharmaceutical shortcomings of E as an ophthalmic agent, the prodrug approach has been successfully applied. Dipivefrin is a prodrug of E that is formed by the esterification of the catechol OH groups of E with pivalic acid. Most of the advantages of this prodrug over E stem from improved bioavailability. The greatly increased lipophilicity allows much greater penetrability into the eye through the corneal epithelial and endothelial layer. The stroma in between requires hydrophilicity for penetration. Dipivefrin has that, too, due to the 1-OH group and cationic nitrogen (the eyedrops contain the hydrochloride [HCl] salt). This dual solubility permits much greater penetrability into the eye than the very hydrophilic E hydrochloride. Increased DOA is also achieved because the drug is resistant to the metabolism by COMT. In addition to its increased in vivo stability, it is also less easily oxidized by air due to the protection of the catechol OH groups. This high bioavailability and in vivo and in vitro stability translate into increased potency such that the 0.1% ophthalmic solution is approximately equivalent to a 2% E solution. After its absorption, it is converted to E by esterases slowly in the cornea and anterior chamber. Dipivefrin also offers the advantage of being less irritating to the eye than E.

α-ADRENERGIC RECEPTOR AGONISTS

All selective α_1-agonists have therapeutic activity as vasoconstrictors. Structurally, they include (a) phenylethanolamines

Epinephrine (E)
catechol: easily oxidized
             less lipophilic than dipivefrin
             poor absorption and poor penetration of the eye
             irritating to eyes when used in treatment of glaucoma

Dipivefrin: Ester and prodrug of E
Noncatechol: less easily oxidazied
                 more lipophilic than E
                 better absorption and penetration of the eye
                 less irritating to the eye than E

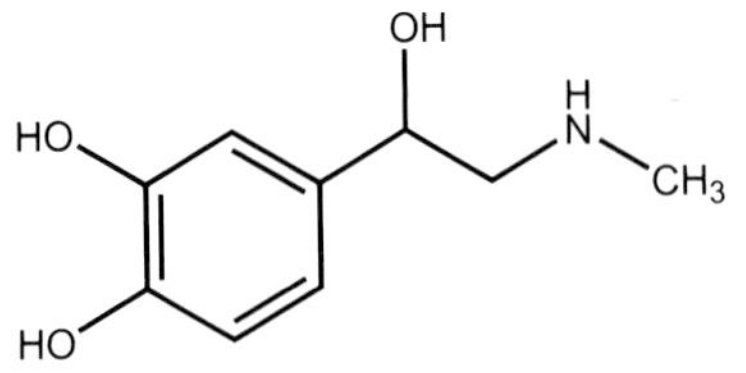

Epinephrine (E)

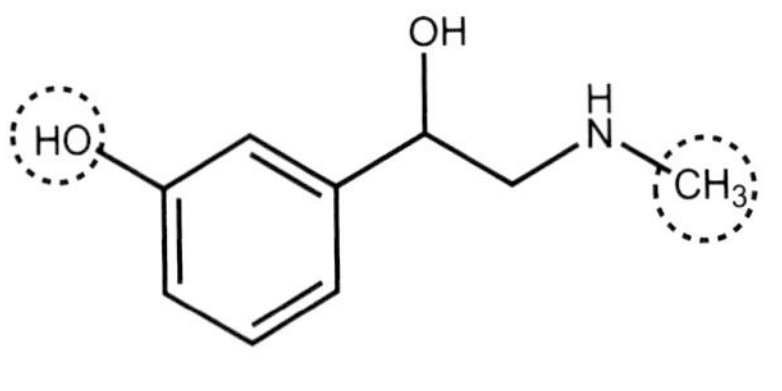

Phenylephrine

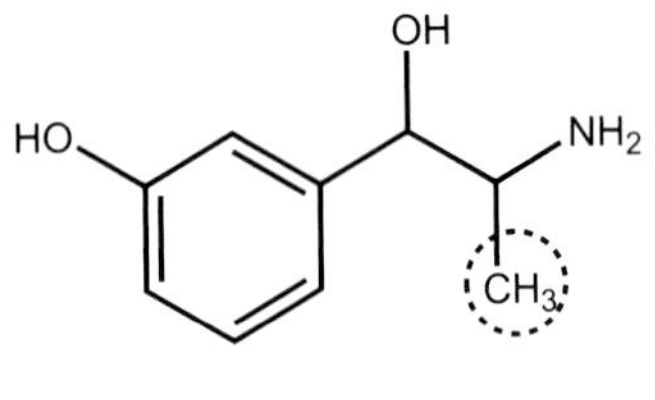

Metaraminol

such as phenylephrine, metaraminol, and methoxamine and (b) 2-arylimidazolines such as xylometazoline, oxymetazoline, tetrahydrozoline, and naphazoline.

Phenylephrine. (Neo-Synephrine, a prototypical selective direct-acting α_1-agonist) differs from E only in lacking a *p*-OH group. It is orally active, and its DOA is about twice that of E because it lacks the catechol moiety and thus is not metabolized by COMT. However, its oral bioavailability is less than 10% because of its hydrophilic properties (log P = −0.3), intestinal 3'-*O*-glucuronidation/sulfation and metabolism by MAO. Lacking the *p*-OH group, it is less potent than E and NE but it is a selective α_1-agonist and thus a potent vasoconstrictor. It is used similarly to metaraminol and methoxamine for hypotension. Another use is in the treatment of severe hypotension resulting from either shock or drug administration. It also has widespread use as a nonprescription nasal decongestant in both oral and topical preparations. When applied to mucous membranes, it reduces congestion and swelling by constricting the blood vessels of the membranes. In the eye, it is used to dilate the pupil and to treat open-angle glaucoma. In addition, it is used in spinal anesthesia to prolong the anesthesia and to prevent a drop in blood pressure during the procedure. It is relatively nontoxic and produces little CNS stimulation. Metaraminol is just another example.

Methoxamine (Vasoxyl) is another α_1-agonist and parenteral vasopressor used therapeutically and so have few cardiac stimulatory properties. It is bioactivated by *O*-demethylation to an active *m*-phenolic metabolite. In fact, it tends to slow the ventricular rate because of activation of the carotid sinus reflex. It is less potent than phenylephrine as a vasoconstrictor. Methoxamine is used primarily during surgery to maintain adequate arterial blood pressure, especially in conjunction with spinal anesthesia. It does not stimulate the CNS. Because it is not a substrate for COMT, its DOA is significantly longer than NE.

Midodrine (ProAmatine) is the *N*-glycyl prodrug of the selective α_1-agonist desglymidodrine. Removal of the *N*-glycyl moiety from midodrine occurs readily in the liver as well as throughout the body, presumably by amidases. Midodrine is orally active and represents another example of a dimethoxy-β-phenylethylamine derivative that is used therapeutically for its vasoconstrictor properties. Specifically, it is used in the treatment of symptomatic orthostatic hypotension.

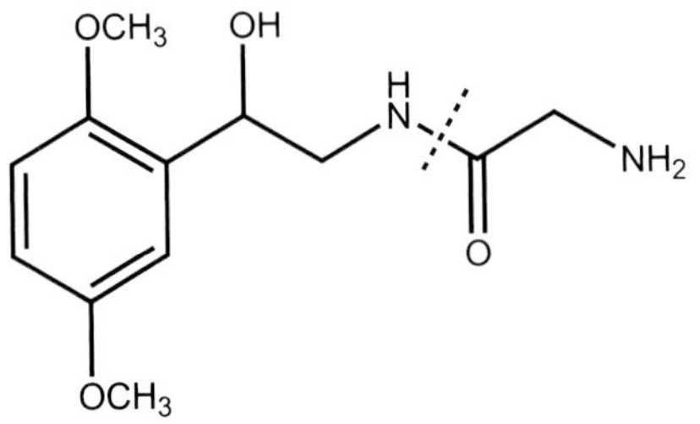

Midodrine: *N*-glycyl prodrug of desglymidodrine

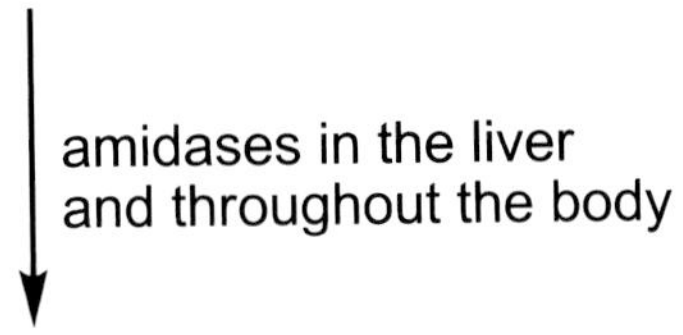

amidases in the liver
and throughout the body

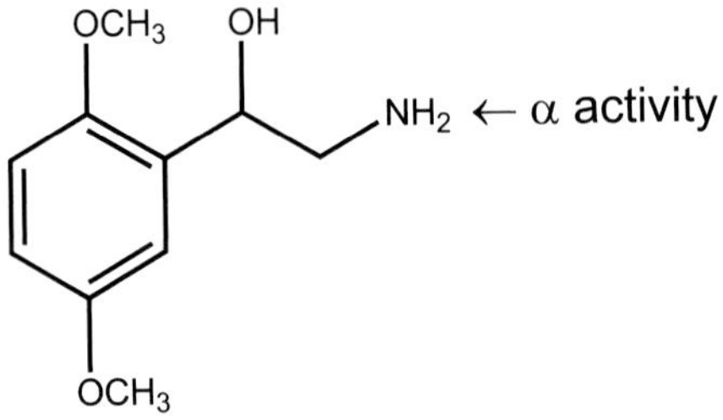

$NH_2 \leftarrow \alpha$ activity

Desglymidodrine
α_1 agonist and vasoconstrictor
differs from methoxamine in lacking α-CH$_3$

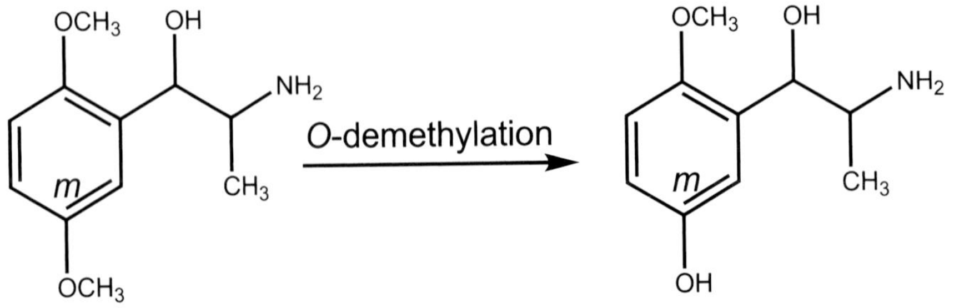

Methoxamine
Prodrug

O-demethylation

An active *m*-phenolic metabolite
α_1 agonist and vasoconstrictor

Naphazoline (Privine), tetrahydrozoline (Tyzine, Visine), xylometazoline (Otrivin), and oxymetazoline (Afrin) are 2-aralkylimidazolines α_1-agonists. These agents are used for their vasoconstrictive effects as nasal and ophthalmic decongestants. Although nearly all β-agonists are phenylethanolamine derivatives, α-receptors accommodate more diverse chemical structures. All 2-aralkylimidazoline α_1-agonists contain a one-carbon bridge between C-2 of the imidazoline ring and a phenyl ring, and thus a phenylethylamine structure feature is there. *Ortho*-lipophilic groups on the phenyl ring are important for α-activity. However, *meta*- or *para*-bulky lipophilic substituents on the phenyl ring may be important for the α_1-selectivity. They have limited access to the CNS, because they essentially exist in an ionized form at physiological pH caused by the very basic nature of the imidazoline ring (pK_a = 10–11). Xylometazoline and oxymetazoline have been used as topical nasal decongestants because of their ability to promote constriction of the nasal mucosa. When taken in large doses, oxymetazoline may cause hypotension, presumably because of a central clonidine-like effect. Oxymetazoline also has significant affinity for α_{2A}-receptors.

Clonidine (Catapres) differs from 2-arylimidazoline α_1-agonists mainly by the presence of *o*-chlorine groups and a NH bridge. The *o*-chlorine groups afford better activity than *o*-methyl groups at α_2 sites. Importantly, clonidine contains a NH bridge (aminoimidazolines) instead of CH_2 bridge in 2-arylimidazoline. The uncharged form of clonidine exists as a pair of tautomers as shown next. Clonidine is an example of a (phenylimino) imidazolidine derivative that possesses central α_2-selectivity. The α_1:α_2 ratio is 300:1. Under certain conditions, such as intravenous infusion, clonidine can briefly exhibit vasoconstrictive activity as a result of stimulation of peripheral α-receptors. However, this hypertensive effect, if it occurs, is followed by a much longer-lasting hypotensive effect as a result of the ability of clonidine to enter into the CNS and stimulate

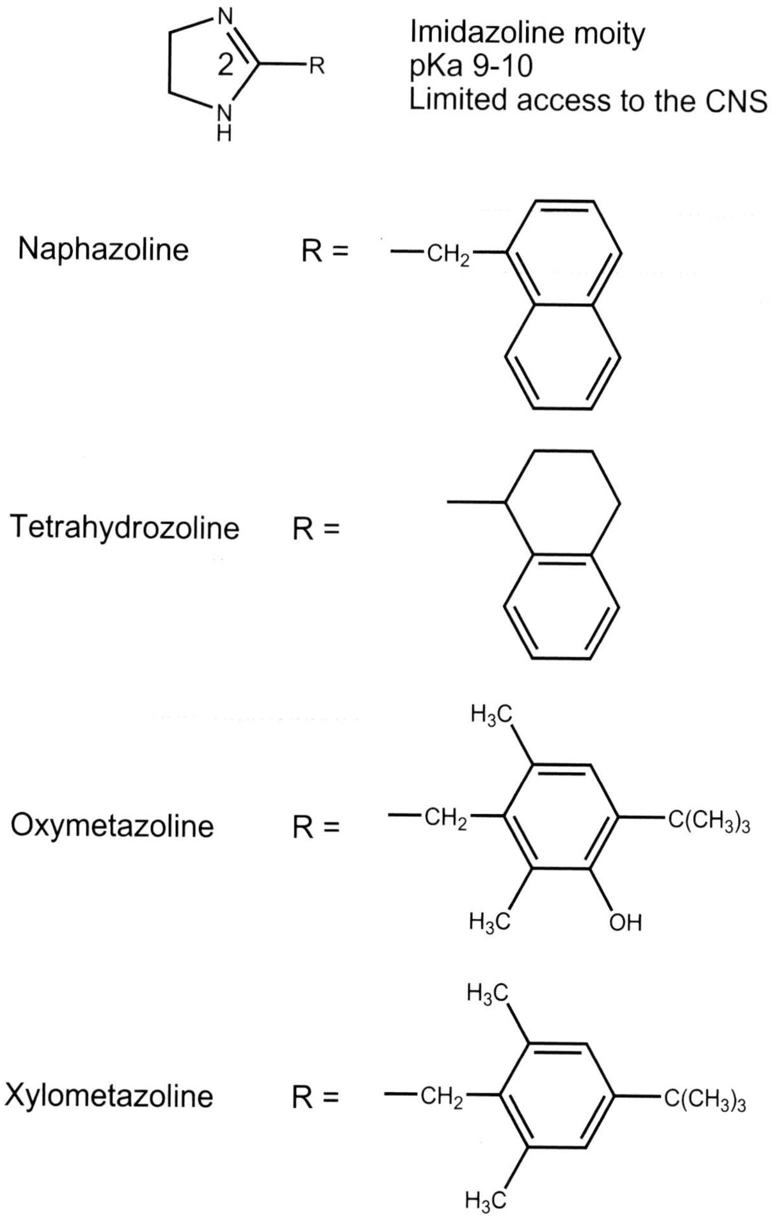

Imidazoline moity
pKa 9-10
Limited access to the CNS

Naphazoline   R =

Tetrahydrozoline   R =

Oxymetazoline   R =

Xylometazoline   R =

Clonidine (pKa = 8.0)   : R = H   some passage into the CNS

4-Hydroxyclonidine   : R = OH   no passage into the CNS
Apraclonidine (pKa = 9.22) : R = NH$_2$ no passage into the CNS

α_2-receptors located in regions of the brain such as the nucleus tractus solitarius. Stimulation of these α_2-receptors brings about a decrease in sympathetic outflow from the CNS, which in turn leads to decreases in peripheral vascular resistance and blood pressure.[20,38] Bradycardia is also produced by clonidine as a result of a centrally induced facilitation of the vagus nerve and stimulation of cardiac prejunctional α_2-receptors.[39] These pharmacological actions have made clonidine quite useful in the treatment of hypertension.

The ability of clonidine and its analogs to exert an antihypertensive effect depends on the ability of these compounds not only to interact with the α_2-receptor in the brain but also to gain entry into the CNS. For example, in the case of clonidine, the basicity of the guanidine group (typically $pK_a = 13.6$) is decreased to 8.0 (the pK_a of clonidine) because of the inductive and resonance effects of the dichlorophenyl ring. Thus, at physiological pH, clonidine will exist to a significant extent in the nonionized form required for passage into the CNS. It has an oral bioavailability of more than 90%.

Although various halogen and alkyl substitutions can be placed at the two ortho positions of the (phenylimino)imidazolidine nucleus without affecting the affinity of the derivatives for α_2-receptors, methyl analogs are much more readily metabolized to the corresponding acids (inactive) and thus have short DOA. Halogen substituents such as chlorine seem to provide the optimal characteristics in this regard.[40] One of the metabolites of clonidine, 4-hydroxyclonidine, has good affinity for α_2-receptors, but because it is too polar to get into the CNS, it is not an effective antihypertensive agent.

In addition to binding to the α_2-adrenergic receptor, clonidine, as well as some other imidazolines, shows high affinity for what has been termed the *imidazoline* receptor.[41,42] Through the use of imidazoline and α_2-antagonists, specific nonadrenergic imidazoline binding sites (I$_1$-IBS) have recently been characterized in CNS control of blood pressure, which are GPCR, with agmatine (decarboxylated arginine) being the endogenous ligand for IBS.[43,44] However, other studies involving both site-directed mutagenesis of the α_{2A}-receptor subtype and genetically engineered knockout mice deficient in either the α_{2A}- or α_{2B}-receptor subtypes provide evidence that the hypotensive response of the α_2-receptor agonists such as clonidine primarily involves the α_{2A}-receptor

subtype.[45,46] Thus, the central hypotensive activity for clonidine and other 2-aminoimidazolines need both α_2-receptors and I$_1$-IBS to produce their central sympatholytic response. Clonidine appears to be more selective for α_2-receptors than for I$_1$-IBS.

Apraclonidine (Iopidine) and Brimonidine (Alphagan). In addition to its therapeutic use as an antihypertensive agent, clonidine has been found to provide beneficial effects in several other situations,[47] including glaucoma, spasticity, migraine prophylaxis, opiate withdrawal syndrome, and anesthesia. This has prompted the development of analogs of clonidine for specific use in some of the mentioned areas. Two of such examples are apraclonidine and brimonidine. Apraclonidine does not cross the BBB. However, brimonidine can cross the BBB and hence can produce hypotension and sedation, although these CNS effects are slight compared with those of clonidine. CNS effects of these drugs are correlated well to their log P, pK_a, and thus log D value. Both apraclonidine and brimonidine are selective α_2-agonists with $\alpha_1:\alpha_2$ ratios of 30:1 and 1,000:1, respectively. Brimonidine is a much more selective α_2-agonist than clonidine or apraclonidine and is a first-line agent for treating glaucoma. Apraclonidine's primary mechanism of action may be related to a reduction of aqueous formation, whereas brimonidine lowers intraocular pressure by reducing aqueous humor production and increasing uveoscleral outflow. Apraclonidine is used specifically to control elevations in intraocular pressure that can occur during laser surgery on the eye. Another example is tizanidine (Zanaflex), which finds use in treating spasticity associated with multiple sclerosis or spinal cord injury. By stimulating α_2-adrenergic receptors, it is believed to decrease the release of excitatory amino acid NTs from spinal cord interneurons.[48]

Guanabenz (Wytensin) and Guanfacine (Tenex) (Open-Ring Imidazolidines). Studies on SAR of central α_2-agonists showed that the imidazoline ring was not necessary for α_2-activity. Two clonidine analogs, guanabenz ($pK_a = 8.1$) and guanfacine ($pK_a = 7$), which are closely related chemically and pharmacologically, are also used as antihypertensive drugs. In these compounds, the 2,6-dichlorophenyl moiety found in clonidine is connected to a guanidino group by a two-atom bridge. In the case of

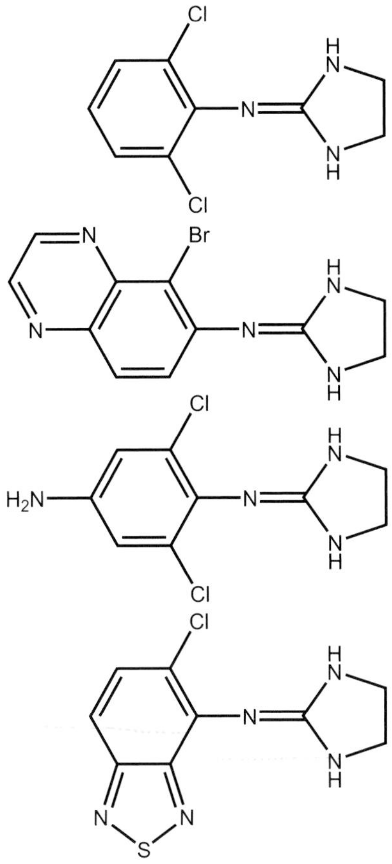

Drugs	Log P	pKa	Log D at pH 7	CNS activity
Clonidine	1.6	8.3	0.8	++
Brimonidine	0.9	9.63	-1.34	+
Apraclonidine	0.3	9.22	-1.91	--
Tizanidine	0.65	9.18	-1.47	+

guanabenz, this bridge is a —CH=N— group, whereas for guanfacine, it is a —CH$_2$CO— moiety. For both compounds, conjugation of the guanidino moiety with the bridging moiety helps to decrease the pK$_a$ of the basic group, so that at physiological pH a significant portion of each drug exists in its nonionized form. This accounts for their CNS penetration and high oral bioavailability (70%–80% for guanabenz and >80% for guanfacine).

Guanfacine is more selective for α_2-receptors than is clonidine. Their mechanism of action is the same as that of clonidine. Differences between clonidine and its two analogs are seen in their elimination half-life values and in their metabolism and urinary excretion patterns. The elimination half-life of clonidine ranges from 20 to 25 hours, whereas that for guanfacine is about 17 hours. Guanabenz has the shortest DOA of these three agents, with a half-life of about 6 hours. Clonidine and guanfacine are excreted unchanged in the urine to the extent of 60% and 50%, respectively. Very little of guanabenz is excreted unchanged in the urine.

Methyldopa (L-α-methyldopa, Aldomet) differs structurally from L-DOPA only in the presence of a α-methyl group. Originally synthesized as an AADC inhibitor, methyldopa ultimately decreases the concentration of DA, NE, E, and serotonin in the CNS and periphery. However, its mechanism of action is not caused by its inhibition of AADC but, rather, by its metabolism in the CNS to its active metabolite (α-methylnorepinephrine). Methyldopa is transported actively into CNS via an aromatic amino acid transporter, where it is decarboxylated by AADC in the brain to (1R,2S)-α-methyldopamine. This intermediate, in turn, is stereospecifically β-hydroxylated by DBH to give the (1R,2S)-α-methylnorepinephrine. This active metabolite is a selective α_2-agonist because it has correct (1R,2S) configuration (Fig. 16.13). It is currently postulated

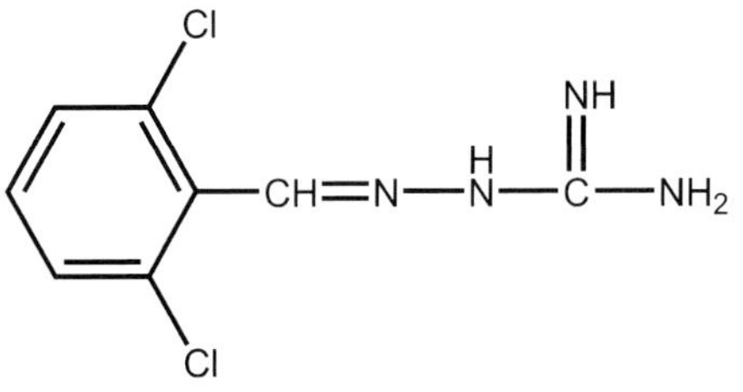

Guanabenz
pKa = 8.1 → mainly nonionized→
penetrate the CNS
oral bioavailability = 70-80%

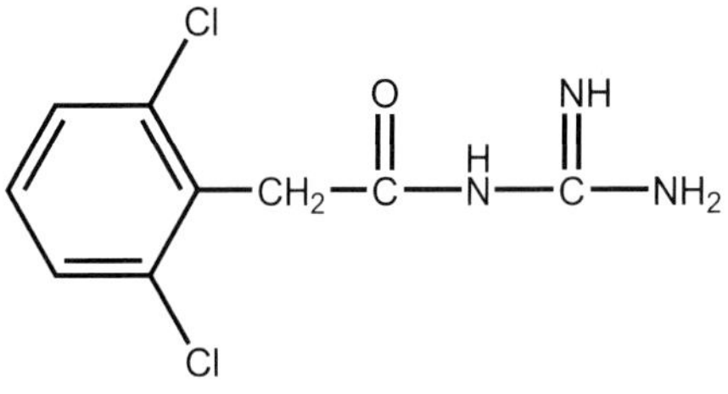

Guanfacine
pKa = 7 → mainly nonionized→
penetrate the CNS
oral bioavailability = >80%

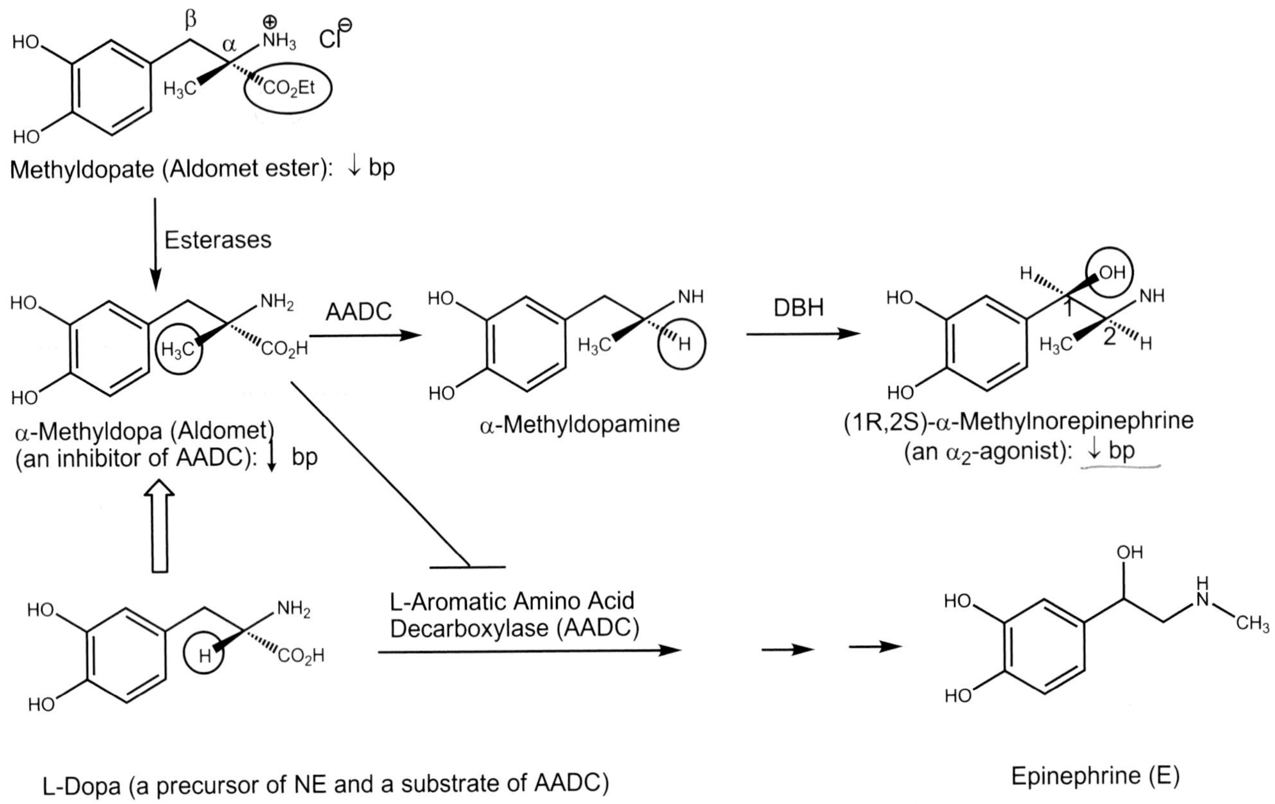

Figure 16.13 ● Metabolic conversion of methyldopate and methyldopa to α-methyl-norepinephrine.

that α-methylnorepinephrine acts on α_2-receptors in the CNS in the same manner as clonidine, to decrease sympathetic outflow and lower blood pressure.

Absorption can range from 8% to 62% and appears to involve an amino acid transporter. Absorption is thus affected by food, and about 40% of that absorbed is converted to methyldopa-*O*-sulfate by the intestinal mucosal cells. Methyldopa is used only by oral administration because its zwitterionic character limits its solubility. The ester hydrochloride salt of methyldopa, methyldopate (Aldomet ester), was developed as a highly water-soluble derivative that could be used to make parenteral preparations. It is converted to methyldopa in the body through the action of esterases (Fig. 16.13).

DUAL α- AND β-AGONISTS/ANTAGONISTS

Dobutamine (Dobutrex) is a positive inotropic agent administered intravenously for congestive heart failure. It resembles DA structurally but possesses a bulky 1-(methyl)-3-(4-hydroxyphenyl)propyl group on the amino group. It possesses a center of asymmetry, and both enantiomeric forms are present in the racemic mixture used clinically. The ($-$) isomer of dobutamine is a potent α_1-agonist, which is capable of causing marked pressor responses. In contrast, ($+$)-dobutamine is a potent α_1-antagonist, which can block the effects of ($-$)-dobutamine. Importantly, the effects of these two isomers are mediated via β_1-receptors. Both isomers appear to be full agonists, but the ($+$) isomer is a more potent β_1-agonist than the ($-$) isomer (approximately tenfold).[49,50]

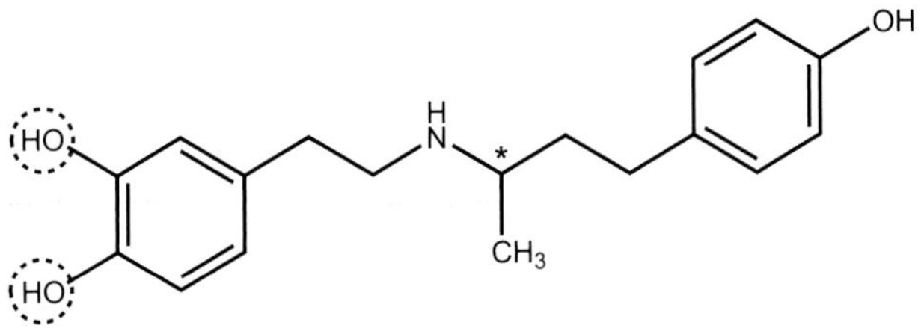

Dobutamine
oxidazed slightly by air
COMT metabolism and conjugation $\rightarrow$
orally inactive and short DOA

Dobutamine contains a catechol group and is orally inactive and thus is given by intravenous infusion. Solutions of the drug can exhibit a slight pink color because of oxidation of the catechol function. It has a plasma half-life of about 2 minutes because it is metabolized by COMT and by conjugation, although not by MAO.

β-ADRENERGIC RECEPTOR AGONISTS

Isoproterenol (Isuprel) is a nonselective and prototypical β-agonist ($\beta_2/\beta_1 = 1$). After oral administration, the absorption of ISO is rather erratic and undependable. The principal reason for its poor absorption characteristics and relatively short DOA is its facile metabolism by sulfate and glucuronide conjugation of the phenolic OH groups and *o*-methylation by COMT. Because it is a catechol, it is sensitive to light and air. Aqueous solutions become pink on standing. Unlike E and NE, ISO does not appear to

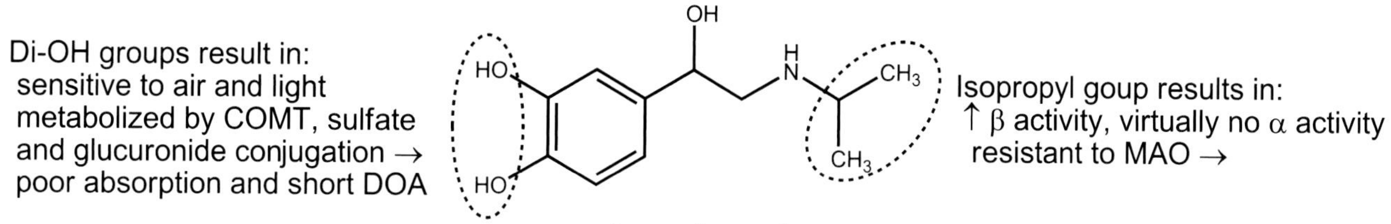

Di-OH groups result in:
sensitive to air and light
metabolized by COMT, sulfate
and glucuronide conjugation →
poor absorption and short DOA

Isopropyl goup results in:
↑ β activity, virtually no α activity
resistant to MAO →

Isoproterenol

undergo oxidative deamination by MAO. The drug has DOA of 1 to 3 hours after inhalation.

Because of an isopropyl substitution on the nitrogen atom, it has virtually no α-activity. However, it does act on both β_1- and β_2-receptors. It thus can produce an increase in cardiac output by stimulating cardiac β_1-receptors and can bring about bronchodilation through stimulation of β_2-receptors in the respiratory tract. In fact, it is one of the most potent bronchodilators available and is available for use by inhalation and injection. Cardiac stimulation is an occasionally dangerous adverse effect. This effect of ISO on the heart is sometimes used in the treatment of heart block.

The cardiac stimulation caused by its β_1-activity and its lack of oral activity have led to its diminished use in favor of more selective β-agonists. The problems have been overcome at least partially by the design and development of several noncatechol selective β_2-agonists. These agents relax smooth muscle of the bronchi, uterus, and skeletal muscle vascular supply. They find their primary use as bronchodilators in the treatment of acute and chronic bronchial asthma and other obstructive pulmonary diseases.

Metaproterenol (Alupent), terbutaline (Bricanyl, Brethine), and fenoterol (an investigational drugs) belong to the structural class of resorcinol bronchodilators that have 3',5'-diOH groups of the phenyl ring (rather than 3',4'-diOH groups as in catechols). 3',5'-diOH groups confer β_2-receptor selectivity on compounds with large amino substituents. For example, metaproterenol (a resorcinol analog of ISO), terbutaline (an *N-t*-butyl analog of metaproterenol), and other similar compounds are resorcinol β_2-selective agonists. They relax the bronchial musculature in patients with asthma but cause less direct cardiac stimulation than do the nonselective β-agonists. Because metaproterenol has a β-directing *N*-isopropyl group and it is less β_2 selective than either terbutaline or albuterol (both

have β_2-directing *t*-butyl groups), and hence is more prone to cause cardiac stimulation. Although these agents are more selective for β_2-receptors, they have a lower affinity for β_2-receptors than ISO. However, they are much more effective when given orally, and they have a longer DOA. This is because they are resistant to the metabolism by either COMT or MAO. Instead, their metabolism primarily involves glucuronide conjugation. Although both metaproterenol and terbutaline exhibit significant β_2-receptor selectivity, the common cardiovascular effects associated with other adrenergic agents can also be seen with these drugs when high doses are used.

Albuterol (Proventil, Ventolin), pirbuterol (Maxair), and salmeterol (Serevent) are examples of selective β_2-agonists whose selectivity results from replacement of the *meta*-OH group of the aromatic ring with a hydroxymethyl moiety. Pirbuterol is closely related structurally to albuterol ($\beta_2/\beta_1 = 60$); the only difference between the two is that pirbuterol contains a pyridine ring instead of a benzene ring. As in the case of metaproterenol and terbutaline, these drugs are not metabolized by either COMT or MAO. Instead, they are conjugated with sulfate. They are thus orally active, and exhibit a longer DOA than ISO. The DOA of terbutaline, albuterol, and pirbuterol is in the range of 3 to 6 hours. (*S*)-albuterol enhances bronchial muscle contraction, and this undesirable effect is completely avoided by using the pure (*R*)-albuterol, levalbuterol (Xopenex). Therefore, the efficacy is achieved at one-fourth dose of racemic albuterol with markedly reduced adverse effects.

Salmeterol has an *N*-phenylbutoxyhexyl substituent in combination with a β-OH group and a salicyl phenyl ring for optimal direct-acting β_2-receptor selectivity and potency. It has a potency similar to that of ISO. This drug associates with the β_2-receptor slowly resulting in slow onset of action and dissociates from the receptor at an even slower rate.[51] It

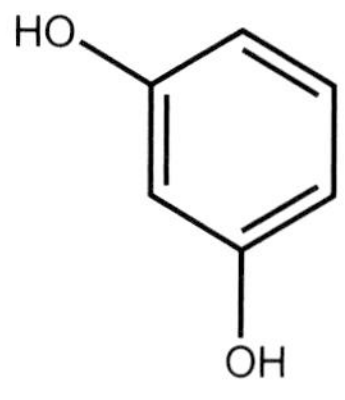

Resorcinal

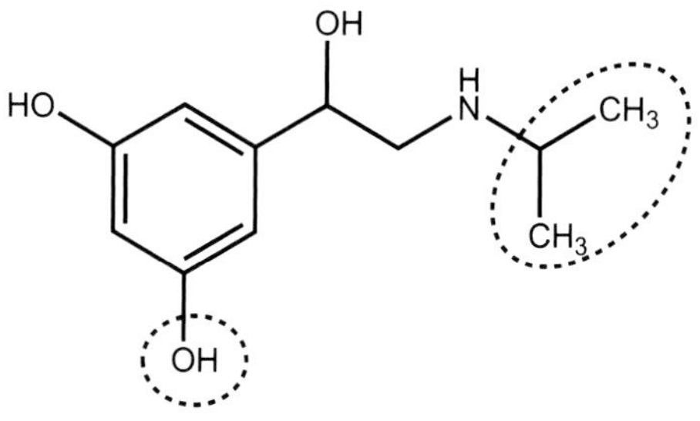

Metaproterenol
3, 5, Di-OH group result in:
↑ β_2 activity:
not metabolized by COMT
orally active and longer DOA

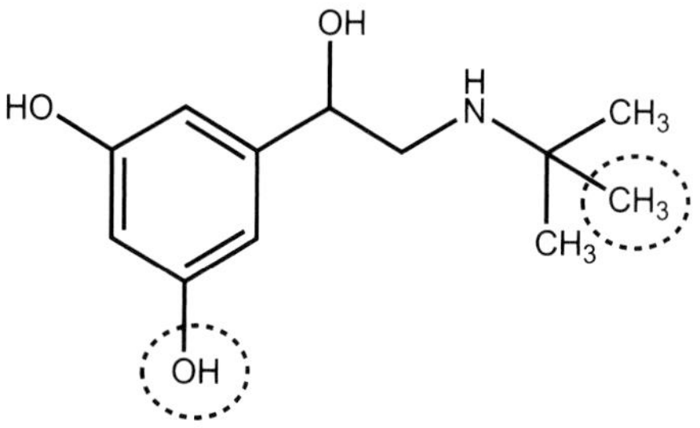

Terbutaline
Bulk *N-R* goup results in:
↑ β_2 activity & virtually no α activity
not metabolized by MAO
orally active and longer DOA

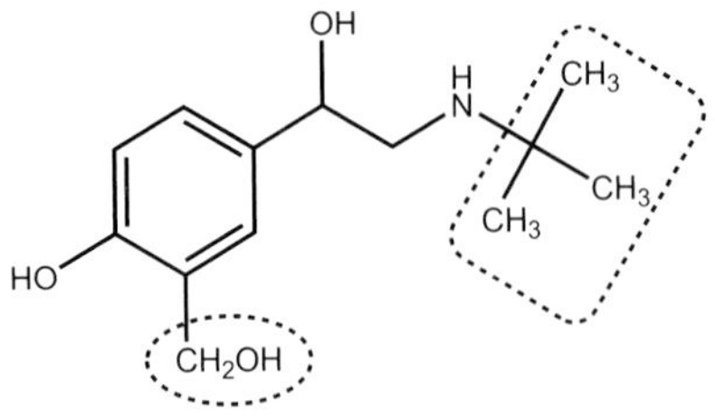

Albuterol

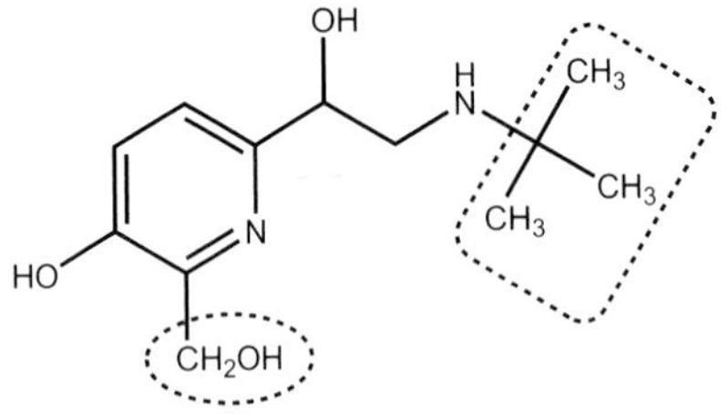

Pirbuterol

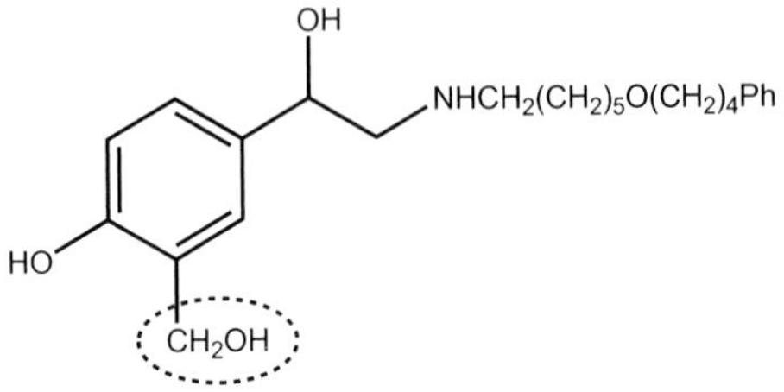

Salmeterol

is resistant to both MAO and COMT and highly lipophilic (log P = 3.88). It is thus very long acting (12 hours), an effect also attributed to the highly lipophilic phenylalkyl substituent on the nitrogen atom, which is believed to interact with a site outside but adjacent to the active site.

Formoterol and Levalbuterol. Formoterol (Foradil) is also a lipophilic (log P = 1.6) and long-acting β_2-agonist. It has 3'-formylamino (β-directing) and 4'OH groups on one phenyl ring and a lipophilic β-directing *N*-isopropyl-*p*-methoxyphenyl group on the nitrogen atom. Its long DOA (12 hours), which is comparable to that of salmeterol, has been suggested to result from its association with the membrane lipid bilayer,[52] from which it gradually diffuses to provide prolonged stimulation of β_2 receptors and its resistance to MAO and COMT. Formoterol has a much faster onset of action than does salmeterol as result of its lower lipophilicity. Both of these long-acting drugs are used by inhalation and are recommended for maintenance treatment of asthma, usually in conjunction with an inhaled corticosteroid.

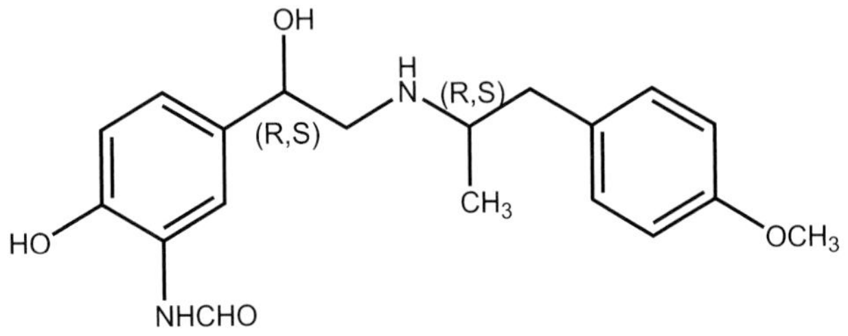

Formoterol (Log p = 1.6)

All of the previously mentioned β_2-agonists possess at least one chiral center and are used as racemic mixtures. Formoterol possesses two chiral centers and is used as the racemic mixture of the (R,R) and (S,S) enantiomers. As mentioned previously, it is the (R) isomer of the phenylethanolamines that possesses the pharmacological activity. There is no clinical advantage for using (R,R)-formoterol as bronchodilators compared with the racemic mixture because of its high potency and low dose. However, concerns have been raised about the use of racemic mixtures under the belief that the inactive isomer may be responsible for some of the adverse effects. Levalbuterol (Xopenex), the pure (R) isomer of racemic albuterol, represents the first attempt to address this issue as mentioned earlier.

Isoetharine. (α-ethyl ISO) was the first β_2-selective drug widely used for the treatment of airway obstruction. However, its degree of selectivity and activity for β_2-receptors may not approach that of some of the other agents such as terbutaline, albuterol, or even ISO. Because of the presence of the β_2-directing α-ethyl group and β-directing isopropyl group, isoetharine is a β_2-agonist and is resistant to MAO. However, because it contains the catechol ring system, it is metabolized by COMT and *O*-sulfated quite effectively. Consequently, it has a short DOA similar to that of ISO and is used only by inhalation for the treatment of acute episodes of bronchoconstriction.

Bitolterol (Tornalate, a Prodrug). Colterol (active metabolite of bitolterol) differs from ISO by replacing the β-directing *N*-isopropyl to β_2-directing *N-tert*-butyl group, which results in the increased β_2-selectivity. Bitolterol (Tornalate) is a prodrug of colterol (a β_2-selective agonist) in which the catechol OH groups have been converted to di-*p*-toluate esters, providing increased lipid solubility caused by the presence of the two lipophilic di-*p*-toluate esters in bitolterol. The presence of the bulky di-ester and bulky *N-tert*-butyl groups also prolong the DOA (8 hours) because it is resistant to COMT and MAO metabolism. Bitolterol is administered by inhalation for bronchial asthma and reversible bronchospasm. The highly bulky *p*-toluoyl groups apparently inhibit the efficiency of the esterases. After absorption, it is hydrolyzed by esterases slowly enough in the

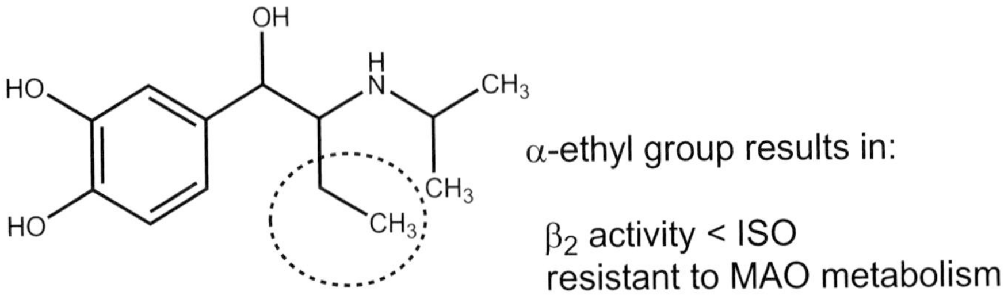

α-ethyl group results in:

β_2 activity < ISO
resistant to MAO metabolism

Isoetharine

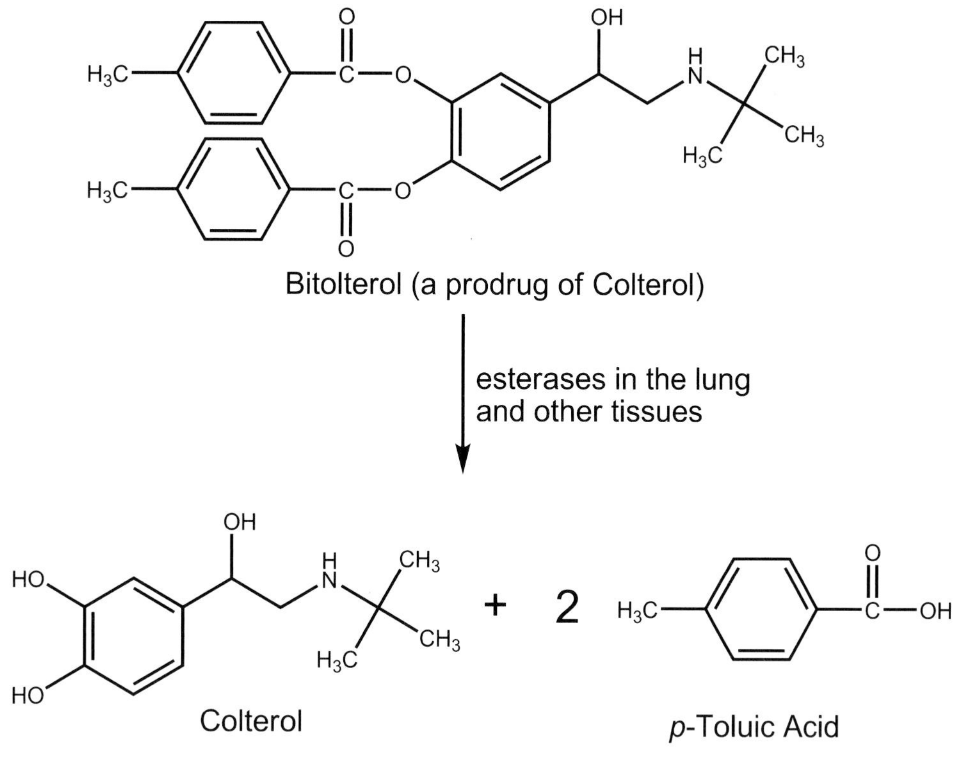

Bitolterol (a prodrug of Colterol)

esterases in the lung
and other tissues

Colterol

p-Toluic Acid

lung and other tissues to produce the active agent (colterol) affording sustained bronchodilation. The DOA of a single dose of the prodrug bitolterol is twice that of a single dose of colterol, permitting less frequent administration and greater convenience to the patient. Colterol is then metabolized after pharmacological action by COMT and conjugation.

Ritodrine (Yutopar) is a selective β_2-agonist that was developed specifically for use as a uterine relaxant. Its uterine inhibitory effects are more sustained than its effects on the cardiovascular system, which are minimal compared with those caused by nonselective β-agonists. The cardiovascular effects usually associated with its administration are mild tachycardia and slight diastolic pressure decrease. Usually, it is administered initially by intravenous infusion to stop premature labor and subsequently it may be given orally.

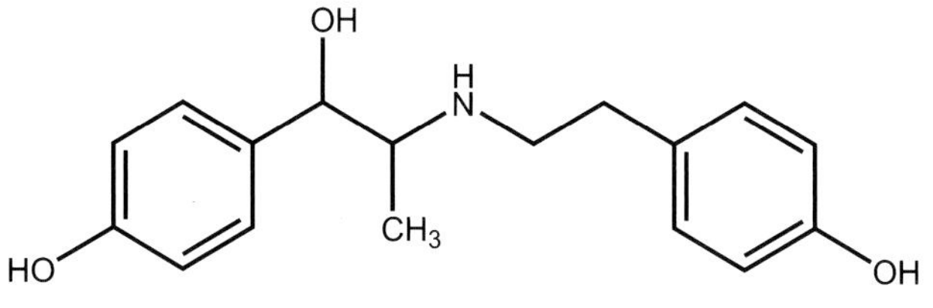

Ritodrine

β_3-Adrenergic Receptor Agonists. The β_3-receptor has been shown to mediate various pharmacological effects such as lipolysis, thermogenesis, and relaxation of the urinary bladder. Activation of the β_3-receptor is thought to be a possible approach for the treatment of obesity, type 2 diabetes mellitus, and frequent urination. Therefore, it is recognized as an attractive target for drug discovery. Selective β_3-agonists have been developed, but they have not been approved for therapeutic

use. Continuing clinical studies will clarify the physiologic effects mediated by β_3-receptors and elucidate the potential therapeutic uses of its agonists in humans.[53]

Indirect-Acting Sympathomimetics

Indirect-acting sympathomimetics act by releasing endogenous NE. They also enter the nerve ending by way of the active-uptake process and displace NE from its storage granules. As with the direct-acting agents, the presence of the catechol OH groups enhances the potency of indirect-acting phenylethylamines. However, the indirect-acting drugs that are used therapeutically are not catechol derivatives and, in most cases, do not even contain an OH moiety. In contrast with the direct-acting agents, the presence of a β-hydroxyl group decreases, and an α-methyl group increases, the effectiveness of indirect-acting agents. The presence of nitrogen substituents decreases indirect activity, with substituents larger than methyl groups rendering the compound virtually inactive. Phenylethylamines that contain a tertiary amino group are also ineffective as NE-releasing agents. Given the foregoing structure–activity considerations, it is easy to understand why amphetamine and *p*-tyramine are often cited as prototypical indirect-acting sympathomimetics. Because amphetamine-type drugs exert their primary effects on the CNS, they are discussed in more detail in Chapter 15. This chapter discusses those agents that exert their effects primarily on the periphery.

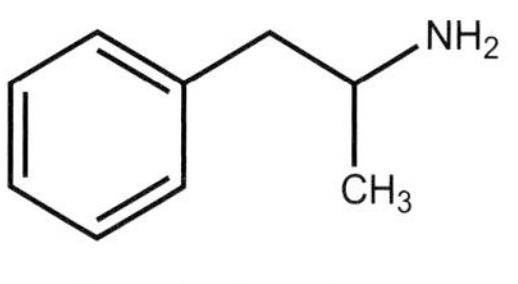

Amphetamine
Log P = 2.81

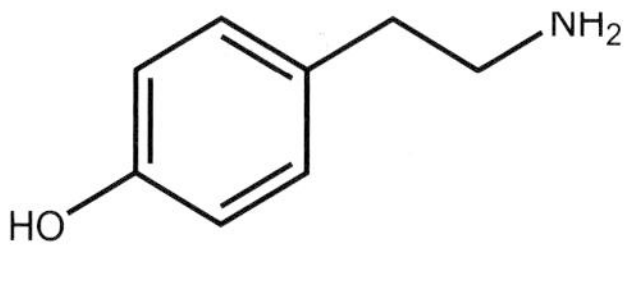

p-Tyramine

Hydroxyamphetamine (Paredrine) is an effective, indirect-acting sympathomimetic drug. It differs from amphetamine in the presence of *p*-OH group and so it has little or no CNS-stimulating action. It is used to dilate the pupil for diagnostic eye examinations and for surgical procedures on the eye. It is sometimes used with cholinergic blocking drugs like atropine to produce a mydriatic effect, which is more pronounced than that produced by either drug alone.

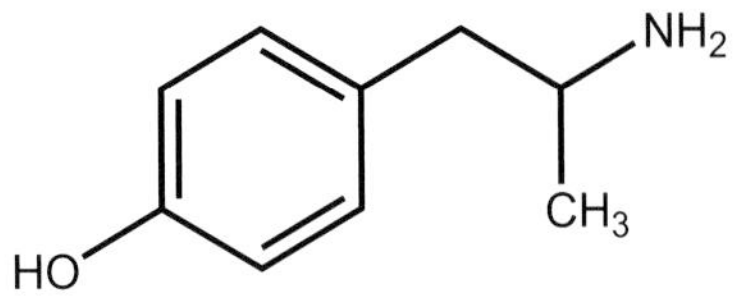

Hydroxyamphetamine
Log P = 1.07
pKa = 10.71

Propylhexedrine (Benzedrex) is another analog of amphetamine in which the aromatic ring has been replaced with a cyclohexane ring. This drug produces vasoconstriction and a decongestant effect on the nasal membranes, but it has only about one half the pressor effect of amphetamine and produces decidedly fewer effects on the CNS. Its major use is for a local vasoconstrictive effect on nasal mucosa in the symptomatic relief of nasal congestion caused by the common cold, allergic rhinitis, or sinusitis.

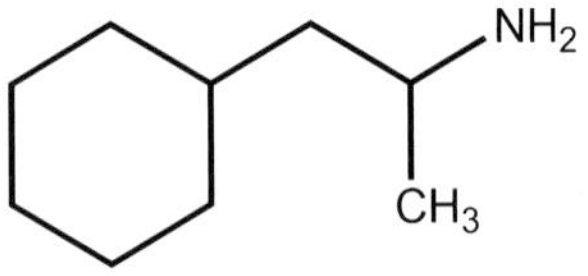

Propylhexedrine

L-(+)-Pseudoephedrine. (Sudafed, Afrinol, Drixoral) is the (*S,S*) diastereoisomer of ephedrine. Whereas ephedrine has a mixed mechanism of action, L-(+)-pseudoephedrine acts mostly by an indirect mechanism and has virtually no direct activity. The structural basis for this difference in mechanism is the stereochemistry of the carbon atom possessing the β-OH group. In pseudoephedrine, this carbon atom possesses the (*S*) configuration, the wrong stereochemistry at this center for a direct-acting effect at adrenoceptors. Although it crosses the BBB (log P = 1.05, pK_a = 9.38), L-(+)-pseudoephedrine's lack of direct activity affords fewer CNS effects than does ephedrine. It is a naturally occurring alkaloid from the *Ephedra* species. This agent is found in many OTC nasal decongestant and cold medications. Although it is less prone to increase blood pressure than ephedrine, it should be used with caution in hypertensive individuals, and it should not be used in combination with MAO inhibitors.

Sympathomimetics with a Mixed Mechanism of Action

Those phenylethylamines considered to have a mixed mechanism of action usually have no hydroxyls on the aromatic ring but do have a β-hydroxyl group.

D-(−)-Ephedrine. The pharmacological activity of (1*R*,2*S*)-D-(−)-ephedrine resembles that of E. The drug acts on both α- and β-receptors. Its ability to activate β-receptors probably accounted for its earlier use in asthma. It is the classic example of a sympathomimetic with a mixed mechanism of action.

Lacking H-bonding phenolic OH groups, ephedrine is less polar (log P = 1.05, pK_a = 9.6) and, thus, crosses the BBB far better than do other CAs. Therefore, ephedrine has been used as a CNS stimulant and exhibits side effects related to its action in the brain. It causes more pronounced stimulation of the CNS than E. The drug is not metabolized

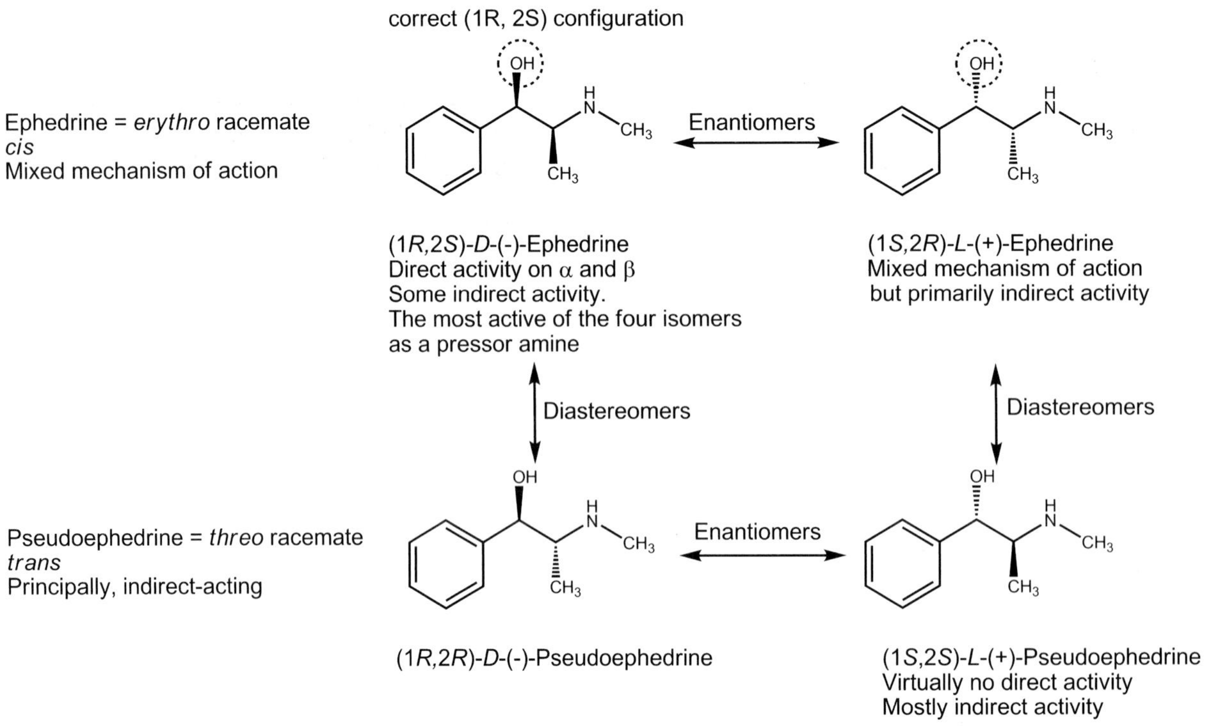

correct (1R, 2S) configuration

Ephedrine = *erythro* racemate
cis
Mixed mechanism of action

⟵ Enantiomers ⟶

(1*R*,2*S*)-D-(-)-Ephedrine
Direct activity on α and β
Some indirect activity.
The most active of the four isomers
as a pressor amine

(1*S*,2*R*)-L-(+)-Ephedrine
Mixed mechanism of action
but primarily indirect activity

↕ Diasteromers

↕ Diasteromers

Pseudoephedrine = *threo* racemate
trans
Principally, indirect-acting

⟵ Enantiomers ⟶

(1*R*,2*R*)-D-(-)-Pseudoephedrine

(1*S*,2*S*)-L-(+)-Pseudoephedrine
Virtually no direct activity
Mostly indirect activity

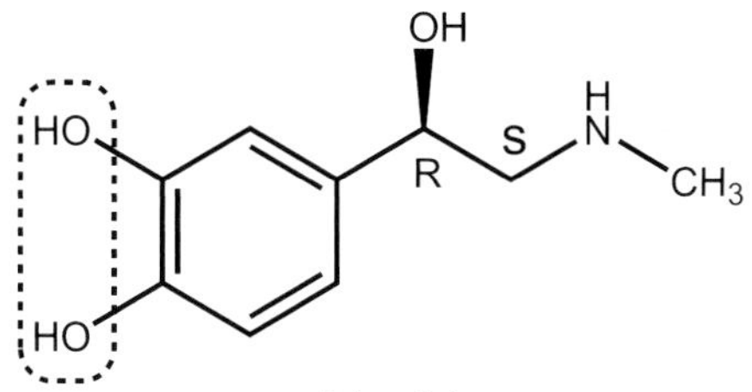

correct (1R) (2S) configuration

Epinephrine
Log P = -1.63

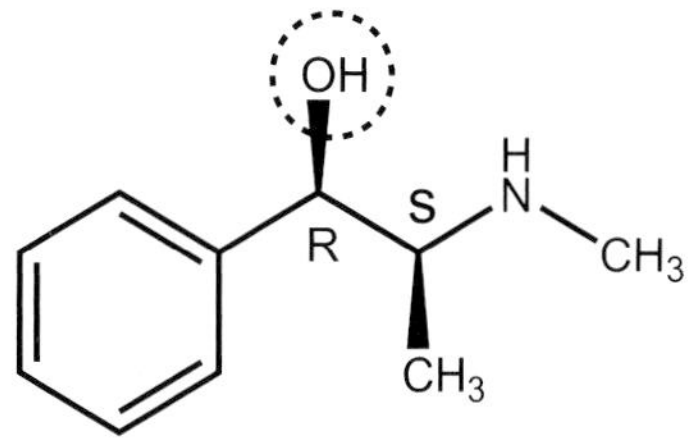

D-(-)-Ephedrine
Log P = 1.05

by either MAO or COMT and therefore has more oral activity and longer DOA than E. Like many other phenylisopropylamines, a significant fraction of the drug is excreted unchanged in the urine although it can be *p*-hydroxylated and *N*-demethylated by cytochrome P450 mixed-function oxidases. Because it is a weak base, its excretion can be accelerated by acidification of the urine.

Ephedrine has two asymmetric carbon atoms; thereby creating four optically active isomers. The *erythro* racemate is called *ephedrine*, and the *threo* racemate is known as *pseudoephedrine* (ψ-ephedrine). Natural ephedrine is the D (−) isomer, and it is the most active of the four isomers as a pressor amine. This is largely because of the fact that this isomer has the correct (1*R*,2*S*) configuration for optimal direct action at adrenergic receptors.

Ephedrine decomposes gradually and darkens when exposed to light. The free alkaloid is a base, and an aqueous solution of the free alkaloid has a pH above 10. The salt form has a pK$_a$ of 9.6. Ephedrine and its salts are used orally, intravenously, intramuscularly, and topically for various conditions, such as allergic disorders, colds, hypotensive conditions, and narcolepsy. It is used locally to constrict the nasal mucosa and cause decongestion and to dilate the pupil or the bronchi. Systemically, it is effective for asthma, hay fever, and urticaria.

This drug is an alkaloid that can be obtained from the stems of various species of *Ephedra*. Ma huang, the plant containing ephedrine, was known to the Chinese in 2000 BC, but the active principle, ephedrine, was not isolated until 1885. In recent years, various companies have begun marketing extracts of *Ephedra* shrubs for such purposes as weight loss and enhancement of athletic performance. Herbalists also market them as "alternative medicines" for cold and cough relief. It has been estimated that nearly one third of young, obese women have used a weight-loss supplement containing *Ephedra*.[54] Pharmacists must be aware that some patients may be taking such ma huang

containing herbal remedies or dietary supplements in addition to regulated drugs that could lead to serious adverse reactions.

Phenylpropanolamine (Propadrine) is the *N*-desmethyl analog of ephedrine and thus has many similar properties. Lacking the *N*-methyl group, phenylpropanolamine is slightly more polar, and therefore does not enter the CNS as well as ephedrine. This modification gives an agent that has slightly higher vasopressive action and lower central stimulatory action than ephedrine. Its action as a nasal decongestant is more prolonged than that of ephedrine. It is orally active. Phenylpropanolamine was a common active component in OTC appetite suppressants and cough and cold medications until 2001 when the Food and Drug Administration (FDA) recommended its removal from such medications, because studies showed an increased risk of hemorrhagic stroke in young women who took the drug.

Metaraminol (Aramine) is the *N*-desmethyl-α-methyl analog of phenylephrine. It possesses a mixed mechanism of action, with its direct-acting effects mainly on α_1-receptors. It is used parenterally as a vasopressor in the treatment and prevention of the acute hypotensive state occurring with spinal anesthesia. It also has been used to treat severe hypotension brought on by other traumas that induce shock.

⬡ ADRENERGIC RECEPTOR ANTAGONISTS (BLOCKERS)

α-Blockers

Because α-agonists cause vasoconstriction and raise blood pressure, α-blockers should be therapeutically used as antihypertensive agents. Unlike the β-blockers, which bear clear structural similarities to the adrenergic agonists NE,

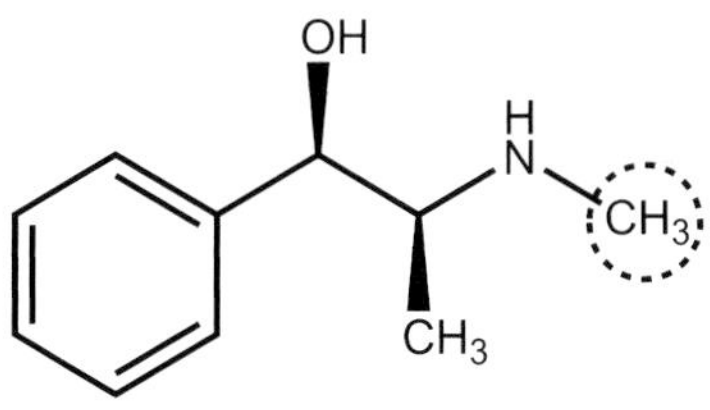

Ephedrine
Log P = 1.05

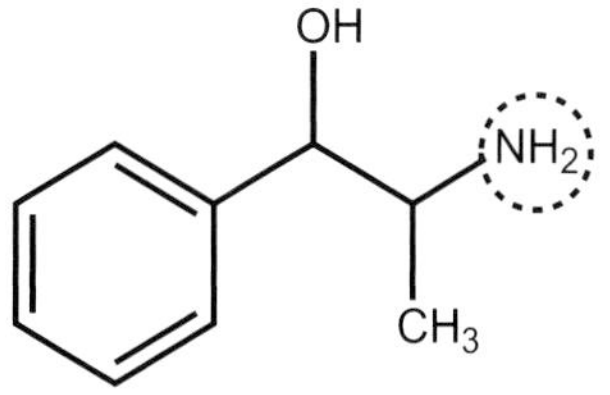

Phenylpropanolamine

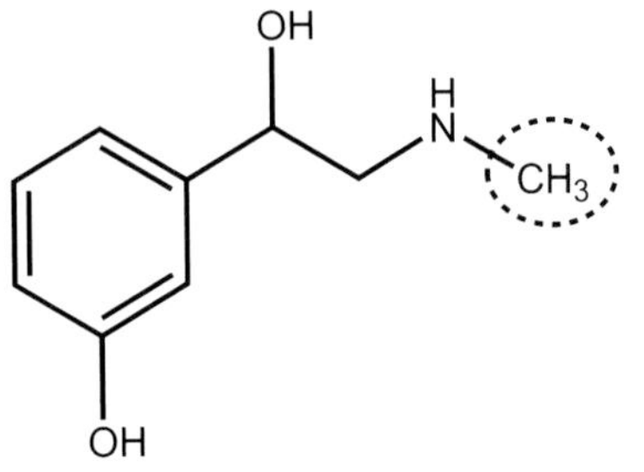

Phenylephrine

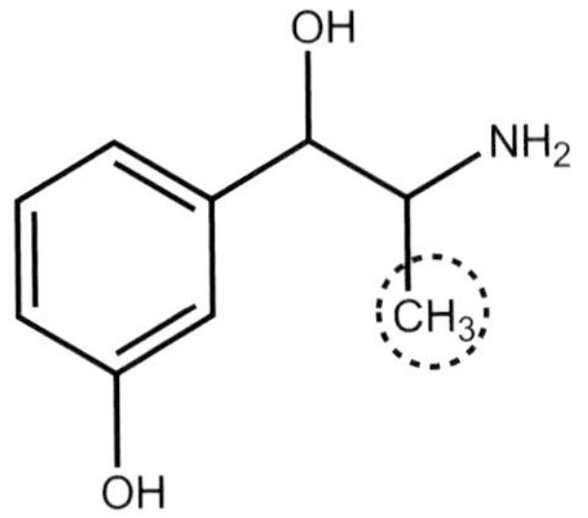

Metaraminol

E, and ISO, the α-blockers consist of several compounds of diverse chemical structure that bear little obvious resemblance to the α-agonists.[34]

NONSELECTIVE α-BLOCKERS

Tolazoline (Priscoline) and phentolamine (Regitine) are imidazoline competitive α-blockers, and primarily of historical interest. The structure of tolazoline are similar to the imidazoline α_1-agonists, but does not have the lipophilic substituents required for agonist activity. The type of group attached to the imidazoline ring thus dictates whether an imidazoline is an agonist or a blocker. Phentolamine is the more effective α-blocker, but neither drug is useful in treating essential hypertension for following reasons. (a) Tolazoline and phentolamine have both α_1- and α_2-blocking activity and produce tachycardia. Presumably, the blocking actions of these agents at presynaptic α_2-receptors contribute to their cardiac stimulatory effects by enhancing the release of NE. Both agents also have a direct vasodilatory action on vascular smooth muscle that may be more prominent than their α-blocking effects. (b) The blocking action of tolazoline is relatively weak, but its histamine-like and acetylcholine-like agonistic actions probably contribute to its vasodilatory activity. Its histamine-like effects include stimulation of gastric acid secretion, rendering it inappropriate for administration to patients who have gastric or peptic ulcers.

It has been used to treat Raynaud syndrome and other conditions involving peripheral vasospasm. Tolazoline is available in an injectable form and is indicated for use in persistent pulmonary hypertension of the newborn when supportive measures are not successful. Phentolamine is used to prevent or control hypertensive episodes that occur in patients with pheochromocytoma. It also has been used in combination with papaverine to treat impotence.

IRREVERSIBLE α-BLOCKERS

Agents in this class, when given in adequate doses, produce a slowly developing, prolonged adrenergic blockade that is not overcome by E. They are irreversible α-blockers, because β-haloalkylamines in the molecules alkylate α-receptors (recall that β-haloalkylamines are present in nitrogen mustard anticancer agents and are highly reactive alkylating agents). Although dibenamine is the prototypical agent in this class, it is phenoxybenzamine that is used therapeutically today.

The mechanism whereby β-haloalkylamines produce a long-lasting, irreversible α-receptor blockade is depicted in Figure 16.14. The initial step involves the formation of an intermediate aziridinium ion (ethylene iminium ion). The positively charged aziridinium ion electrophile then reacts with a nucleophilic group on the α-receptor (if this occurs in the vicinity of the α-receptor), resulting in the formation of a covalent bond between the drug and the receptor. Unfortunately, these nonselective drugs alkylate not only α-receptors but also other biomolecules, leading to their toxicity. It is thus used only to relieve the sympathetic effects of pheochromocytoma.

Phenoxybenzamine (Dibenzyline) an old but powerful α-blocker, is a haloalkylamine that blocks α_1- and α_2-receptors irreversibly. Phenoxybenzamine administration has been described as producing a "chemical sympathectomy" because of its selective blockade of the excitatory

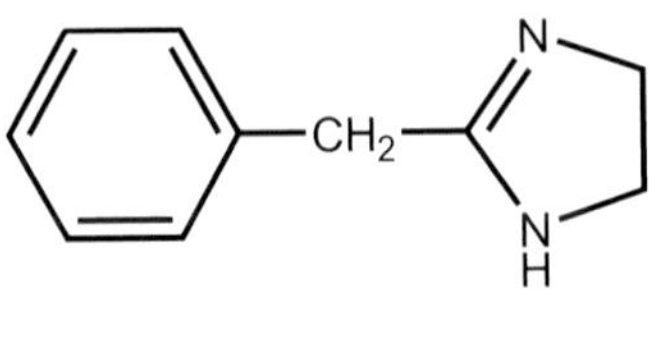

Tolazoline

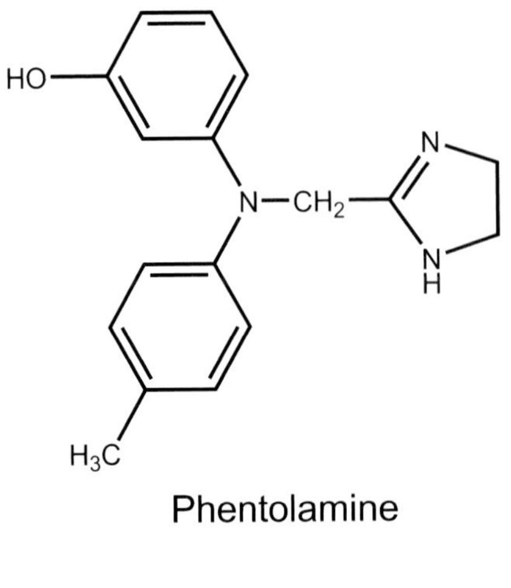

Phentolamine

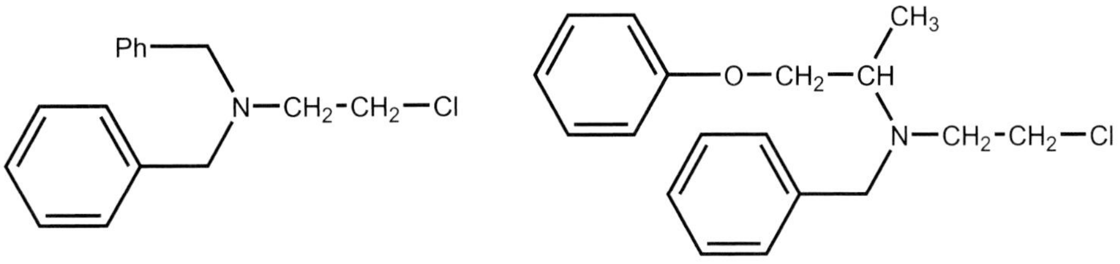

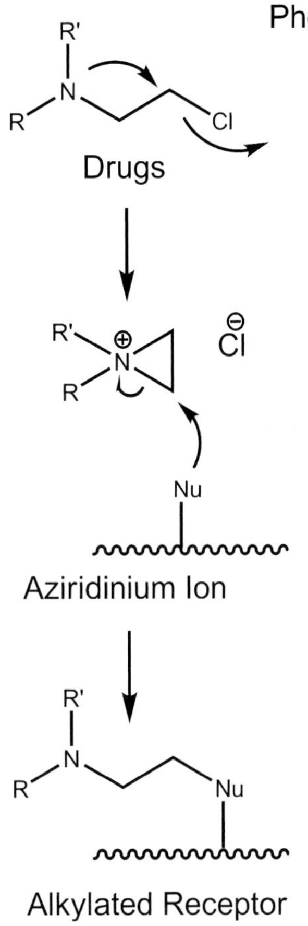

Figure 16.14 ● Mechanism of inactivation of α-adrenergic receptors by β-haloalkylamines.

responses of smooth muscle and of the heart muscle. Although phenoxybenzamine is capable of blocking acetylcholine, histamine, and serotonin receptors, its primary pharmacological effects, especially that of vasodilation, may be attributed to its α-adrenergic blocking capability. As would be expected of a drug that produces such a profound α-blockade, administration is frequently associated with reflex tachycardia, increased cardiac output, and postural hypotension. There is also evidence indicating that blockade of presynaptic α_2-receptors contribute to the increased heart rate produced by phenoxybenzamine.

The onset of action of phenoxybenzamine is slow, but the effects of a single dose of drug may last 3 to 4 days, because essentially new receptors must be made to replace those that have been inhibited irreversibly. The principal peripheral effects following its administration are an increase in systemic blood flow, an increase in skin temperature, and a lowering of blood pressure. It has no effect on the parasympathetic system and little effect on the gastrointestinal tract. The most common side effects are miosis, tachycardia, nasal stuffiness, and postural hypotension, all of which are related to the production of adrenergic blockade.

Oral phenoxybenzamine is used for the preoperative management of patients with pheochromocytoma and in the chronic management of patients whose tumors are not amenable to surgery. Only about 20% to 30% of an oral dose is absorbed.

SELECTIVE α_1-BLOCKERS

Prazosin (Minipress), terazosin (Hytrin), and doxazosin (Cardura) are quinazoline α_1-blockers. As a result, in part, of its greater α_1-receptor selectivity, the quinazoline class of α-blockers exhibits greater clinical utility and has largely replaced the nonselective haloalkylamine and imidazoline α-blockers. Structurally, these agents consist of three components: the quinazoline ring, the piperazine ring, and the acyl moiety. The 4-amino group on the quinazoline ring is very important for α_1-receptor affinity. Although they possess a piperazine moiety attached to the quinazoline ring, this group can be replaced with other heterocyclic moieties (e.g., piperidine moiety) without loss of affinity. The nature of the acyl group has a significant effect on the pharmacokinetic properties.[55]

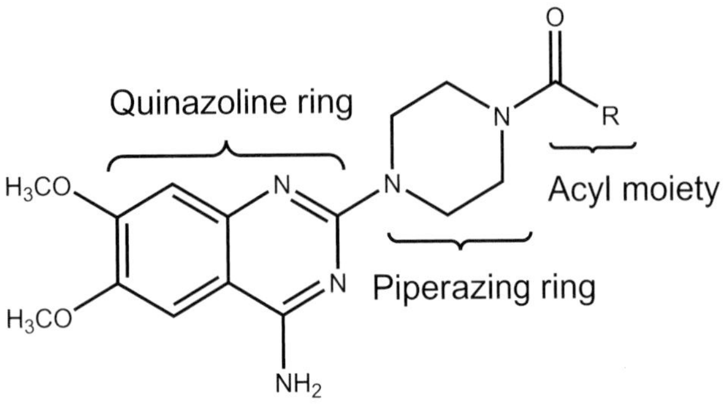

Prazosin: R =

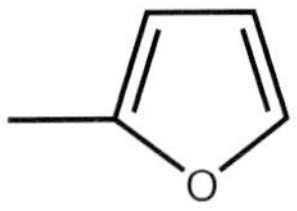

Terazosin: R =

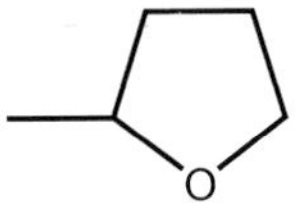

Doxazosin: R =

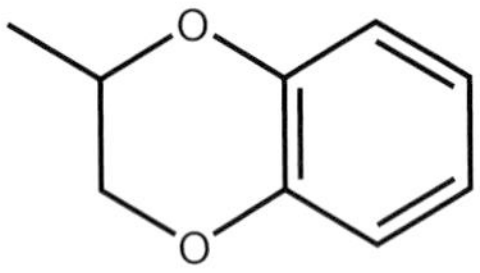

These drugs dilate both arterioles and veins and are thus used in the treatment of hypertension. They offer distinct advantages over the other α-blockers, because they produce peripheral vasodilation without an increase in heart rate or cardiac output. This advantage is attributed, at least in part, to the fact that prazosin blocks postjunctional α_1-receptors selectively without blocking presynaptic α_2-receptors. Contraction of the smooth muscle of prostate gland, prostatic urethra, and bladder neck is also mediated by α_1-adrenoceptors, with α_{1A} being predominant, and blockade of these receptors relaxes the tissue. For this reason, these agents are also used in the treatment of BPH, where they help improve urination flow rates.

Although the adverse effects of these drugs are usually minimal, the most frequent one, known as the *first-dose phenomenon*, is sometimes severe. This is a dose-dependent effect characterized by marked excessive postural hypotension and syncope, and can be minimized by giving an initial low dose at bedtime.

The main difference between prazosin, terazosin, and doxazosin lies in their pharmacokinetic properties. As mentioned previously, these differences are dictated by the nature of the acyl moiety attached to the piperazine ring. These drugs are metabolized extensively with the metabolites excreted in the bile. The fact that a single α_{1A}-adrenoceptor subtype is found in the prostatic and urethral smooth muscle cells led to the design of drugs with uroselectivity for this receptor subtype. Thus, alfuzosin and tamsulosin are uroselective α_1-blockers and first-line drugs for treatment of BPH without utility in treating hypertension.

Alfuzosin (Uroxatral) is also a quinazoline α_1-blocker but differs from terazosin in replacing the piperazine ring in terazosin with an open piperazine ring (a rotatable propylenediamine group). Alfuzosin is more selective for the subtype of α_{1A}-receptor in the prostate gland than those in vascular tissue. Thus, it has been used extensively in treating BPH as a first-line drug with fewer cardiovascular side effects than terazosin and doxazosin.

Tamsulosin (Flomax), a nonquinazoline benzensulfonamide, is the first in the class of subtype selective α_{1A}-blocker. It is many folds more selective for α_{1A}-receptors than for the other α_1-receptors. This selectivity may favor blockade of α_{1A}-receptors found in the prostate gland over those found in vascular tissue. Tamsulosin is efficacious in the treatment of BPH with little effect on blood pressure. Orthostatic hypotension is not as great with this agent as with the nonselective quinazolines.

SELECTIVE α_2-BLOCKERS

Yohimbine and Corynanthine. Yohimbine (Yocon) is a competitive and selective α_2-blocker. The compound is an indolealkylamine alkaloid and is found in the bark of the tree *Pausinystalia yohimbe* and in *Rauwolfia* root; its structure resembles that of reserpine. These isomeric indole alkaloids known as the yohimbanes exhibit different degrees of selectivity toward the α_1- and α_2-receptors, depending on their stereochemistry. For example, yohimbine is a

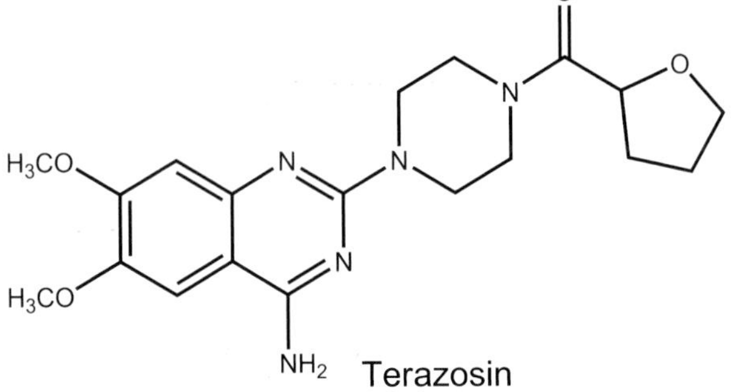

Terazosin

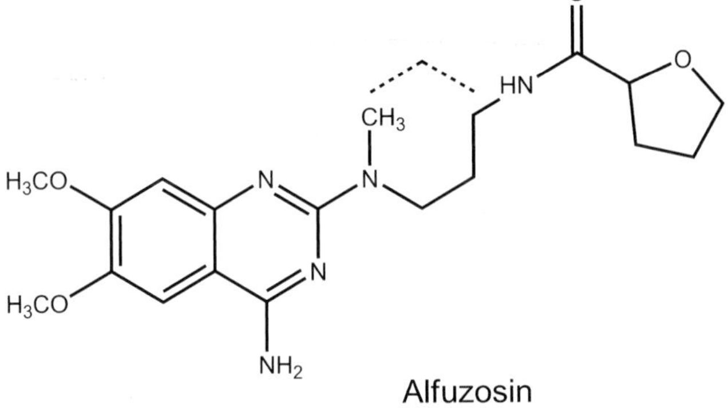

Alfuzosin

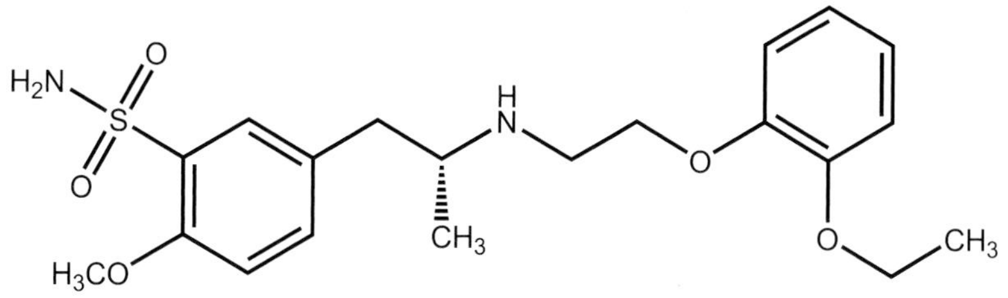

Tamsulosin

selective α_2-blocker, whereas corynanthine is a selective α_1-blocker. The only difference between these two compounds is the relative stereochemistry of the carbon containing the carbomethoxy substituent. In yohimbine, this group lies in the plane of the alkaloid ring system, whereas in corynanthine, it lies in an axial position and thus is out of the plane of the rings.[56]

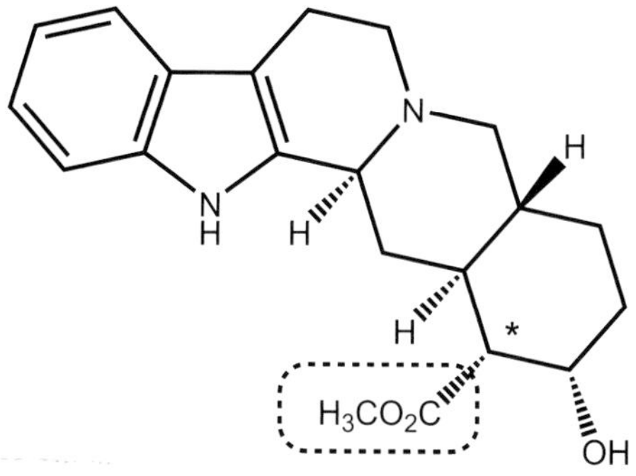

Yohimbine

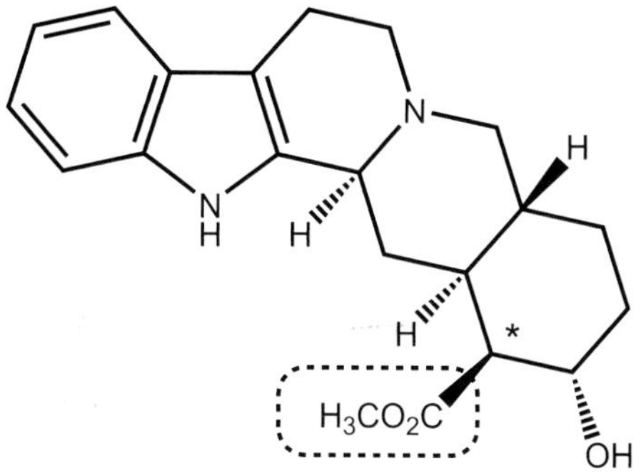

Corynanthine

Yohimbine increases heart rate and blood pressure as a result of its blockade of α_2-receptors in the CNS. It has been used experimentally to treat male erectile impotence.

Mirtazapine (Remeron) is another example of tetracyclic α_2-blockers that shows selectivity for α_2-receptors versus α_1-receptors.[57] Blockade of central α_2-receptors results in an increased release of NE and serotonin. This has prompted its use as an antidepressant. This agent also has activity at nonadrenergic receptors. It is a potent blocker of 5-HT$_2$ and 5-HT$_3$ serotonin receptors and at histamine H$_1$-receptors.

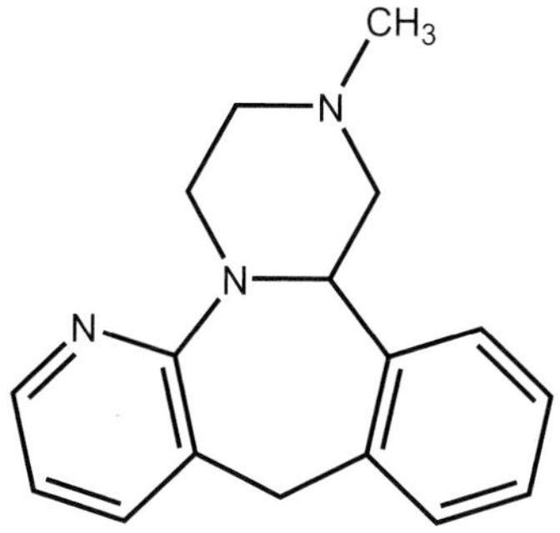

Mirtazapine (Log D = 1.38)

β-Blockers

STRUCTURE–ACTIVITY RELATIONSHIPS

β-Blockers are among the most widely employed antihypertensives and are also considered the first-line treatment for glaucoma. Most of β-blockers are in the chemical class of aryloxypropanolamines. The first β-blocker, dichloroisoproterenol (DCI), was reported in 1958 by Powell and Slater.[58] DCI differs structurally from ISO in that the agonist directing 3'4'-di-OH groups have been replaced by two chloro groups. This simple structural modification, involving the replacement of the aromatic OH groups, has provided the basis for nearly all of the approaches used in subsequent efforts to design and synthesize therapeutically useful β-blockers.[35] Unfortunately, DCI is not a pure antagonist but a partial agonist. The substantial direct sympathomimetic action of DCI precluded its development as a clinically useful drug.

Pronethalol was the next important β-blocker developed. Although it had much less intrinsic sympathomimetic activity (ISA) than DCI, it was withdrawn from clinical testing because of reports that it caused thymic tumors in mice. Within 2 years of this report, however, Black and Stephenson[59] described the β-blocking actions of propranolol, a close structural relative of pronethalol. Propranolol has become one of the most thoroughly studied and widely used drugs in the therapeutic armamentarium. It is the standard against which all other β-blockers are compared.

Propranolol belongs to the group of β-blockers known as *aryloxypropanolamines*. This term reflects the fact that an —OCH$_2$— group has been incorporated into the molecule between the aromatic ring and the ethylamino side chain. Because this structural feature is frequently found in β-blockers, the assumption is made that the —OCH$_2$— group is responsible for the antagonistic properties of the molecules. However, this is not true; in fact,

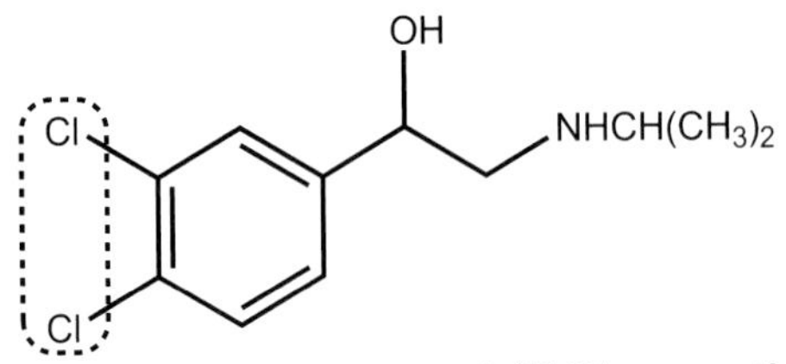

*Dichloro*isoproterenol (DCI, a partial β agonist)

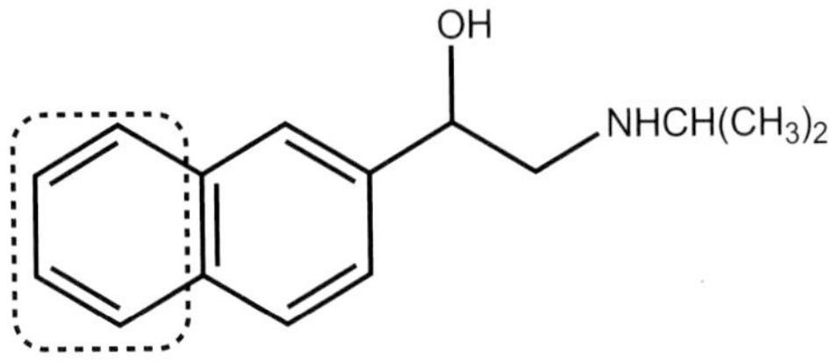

Pronethalol (a β blocker with toxicity)

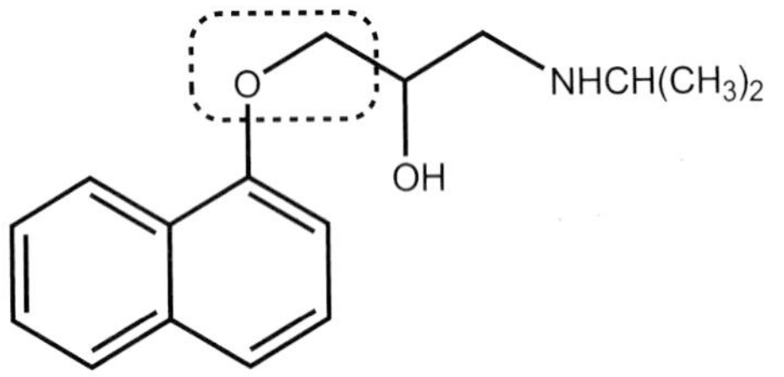

Propranolol (a prototype of β blockers)

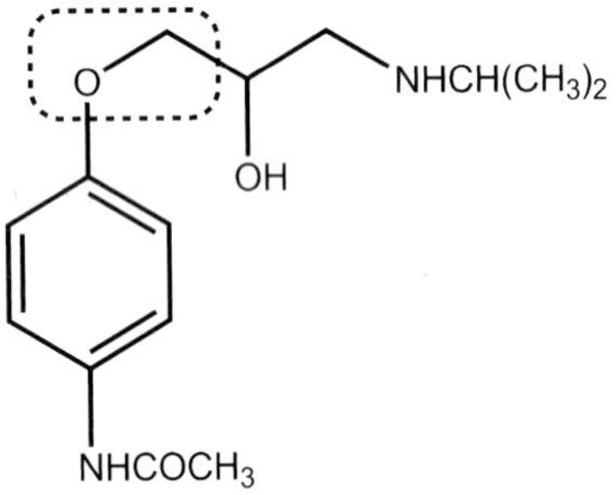

Practolol (a prototype of β₁ blockers)

the —OCH$_2$— group is present in several compounds that are potent β-agonists.[60] This latter fact again leads to the conclusion that it is the nature of the aromatic ring and its substituents that is the primary determinant of β-antagonistic activity. The aryl group also affects the absorption, excretion, and metabolism of the β-blockers.[61] Note that the side chain has been moved from C2′ to the C1′ position from the naphthyl ring.

The nature of the aromatic ring is also a determinant in their β₁-selectivity. One common structural feature of many cardioselective β-blockers is the presence of a *para*-substituent of sufficient size on the aromatic ring along with the absence of *meta*-substituents. Practolol is the prototypical example of a β₁-blocker of this structural type. It was the first cardioselective β₁-blocker to be used extensively in humans. Because it produced several toxic effects, however, it is no longer in general use in most countries.

Like β-agonists, β-directing *tert*-butyl and isopropyl groups, are normally found on the amino function of the aryl-oxypropanolamine β-blockers. It must be a secondary amine for optimal activity.

For arylethanolamine adrenergic agonists, the β-OH-substituted carbon must be in the *R* absolute configuration for maximal direct activity. However, for β-blockers, the β-OH-substituted carbon must be in the *S* absolute configuration for maximal β-blocking activity. Because of the insertion of an oxygen atom in the side chain of the aryl-oxypropanolamines, the Cahn-Ingold Prelog priority of the substituents around the asymmetric carbon differs from the agonists. This is effect of the nomenclature rules. The pharmacologically more active enantiomer of β-blockers interacts with the receptor recognition site in same manner as that of the agonists. In spite of the fact that nearly all of the β-blocking activity resides in one enantiomer, propranolol and most other β-blockers are used clinically as racemic mixtures. The only exceptions are levobunolol, timolol, and penbutolol, with which the (S) enantiomer is used.

Propranolol (log P = 3.10) is the most lipophilic drug among the available β-blockers, and thus it enters the CNS much better than the less lipophilic drug such as atenolol (log P = 0.10) or nadolol (log P = 1.29). The use of lipophilic β-blockers such as propranolol has been associated with more CNS side effects, such as dizziness, confusion, or depression. These side effects can be avoided, however, with the use of hydrophilic drugs, such as atenolol or nadolol. The more lipophilic drugs are primarily cleared by the liver, and so their doses need to be adjusted in patients with liver disease. In contrast, the less lipophilic drugs are cleared by the kidney and so their doses need to be adjusted in patients with impaired renal function.

NONSELECTIVE β-BLOCKERS (FIRST GENERATION)

Propranolol (Inderal, others) is the prototypical and nonselective β-blocker. It blocks the β₁- and β₂-receptors with equal affinity, lacks ISA, and does not block α-receptors. Propranolol, like the other β-blockers discussed, is a competitive blocker whose receptor-blocking actions can be reversed with sufficient concentrations of β-agonists. Currently, propranolol is approved for use in the United States for hypertension, cardiac arrhythmias, angina pectoris, postmyocardial infarction, hypertrophic cardiomyopathy, pheochromocytoma, migraine prophylaxis, and essential tremor. In addition, because of its high lipophilicity (log P = 3.10) and thus its ability to penetrate the CNS, propranolol has found use in treating anxiety and is under investigation for the treatment of a variety of other conditions, including schizophrenia, alcohol withdrawal syndrome, and aggressive behavior.

Some of the most prominent effects of propranolol are on the cardiovascular system. By blocking the β-receptors of the heart, propranolol slows the heart, reduces the force of contraction, and reduces cardiac output. Because of reflex sympathetic activity and blockade of vascular β₂-receptors, administration may result in increased peripheral resistance. The antihypertensive action, at least in part, may be attributed to its ability to reduce cardiac output, as well as to its suppression of renin release from the kidney. Because it exhibits no selectivity for β₁-receptors, it is contraindicated in the presence of conditions such as asthma and bronchitis.

A facet of the pharmacological action of propranolol is its so-called membrane-stabilizing activity. This is a nonspecific effect (i.e., not mediated by a specific receptor), which

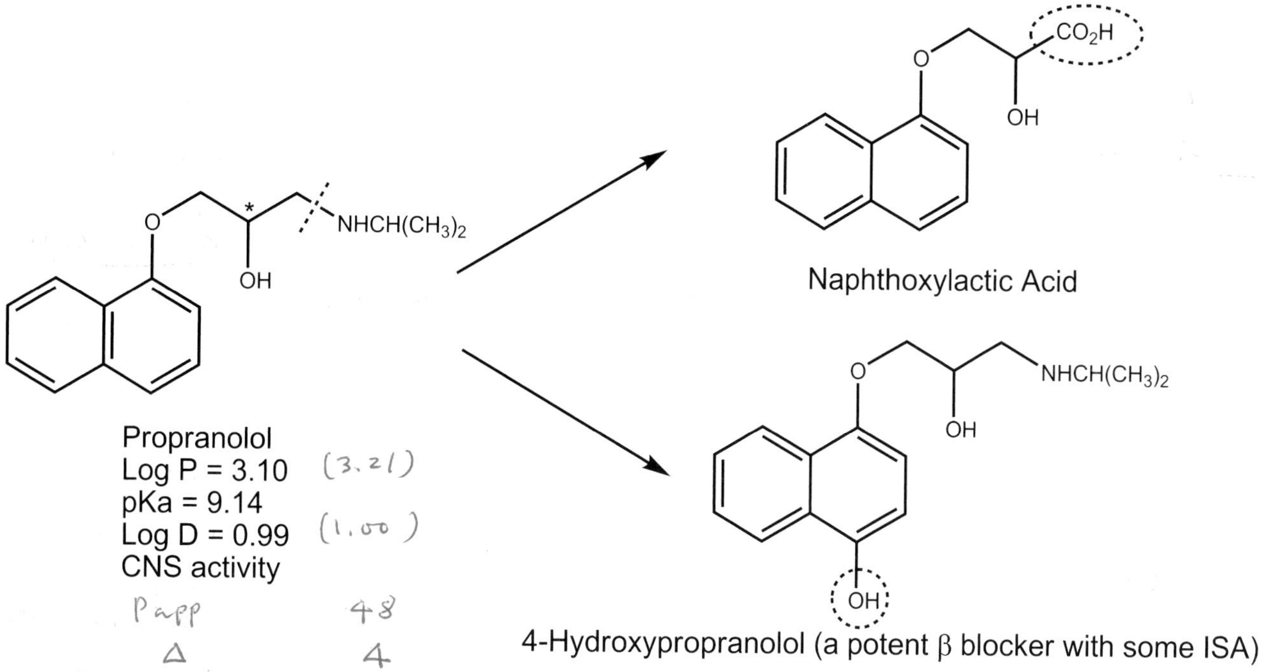

Naphthoxylactic Acid

Propranolol
Log P = 3.10 *(3.21)*
pKa = 9.14
Log D = 0.99 *(1.00)*
CNS activity

Papp   48
Δ   4

but Too lipophilic for Glaucoma.

4-Hydroxypropranolol (a potent β blocker with some ISA)

is also referred to as a *local anesthetic effect*. Both enantiomers possess membrane-stabilizing activity. Because the concentrations required to produce this effect far exceed those obtained with normal therapeutic doses of propranolol and related β-blockers, it is unlikely that the nonspecific membrane-stabilizing activity plays significant role in the clinical efficacy of β-blockers.

Propranolol is well absorbed after oral administration, but it undergoes extensive first-pass metabolism before it reaches the systemic circulation. Lower doses are extracted more efficiently than higher doses, indicating that the extraction process may become saturated at higher doses. In addition, the active enantiomer is cleared more slowly than the inactive enantiomer.[62]

One of the major metabolites after a single oral dose is naphthoxylactic acid. It is formed by a series of metabolic reactions involving *N*-dealkylation, deamination, and oxidation of the resultant aldehyde. Another metabolite of particular interest is 4-hydroxypropranolol, which is a potent β-blocker that has some ISA. It is not known what contribution, if any, 4-hydroxypropranolol makes to the pharmacological effects seen after administration of propranolol. The half-life of propranolol after a single oral dose is 3 to 4 hours, which increases to 4 to 6 hours after long-term therapy.

Other Nonselective β-Blockers. Several other clinically used nonselective β-blockers include *nadolol* (Corgard), *pindolol* (Visken), *penbutolol* (Levatol), *carteolol* (Cartrol, Ocupress), *timolol* (Blocadren, Timoptic), *levobunolol* (Betagan), *sotalol* (Betapace), and *metipranolol* (OptiPranolol). Structures of these compounds are shown in Figure 16.15. The first five of these blockers are used to treat hypertension. Nadolol is also used in the long-term management of angina pectoris, whereas timolol finds use in the prophylaxis of migraine headaches and in the therapy following myocardial infarction. Sotalol is used as an antiarrhythmic in treating ventricular arrhythmias and atrial fibrillation because in addition to its β-adrenergic

blocking activity, this agent blocks the inward K^+ current that delays cardiac repolarization.

Carteolol, timolol, levobunolol, and metipranolol are used topically to treat open-angle glaucoma. These agents lower intraocular pressure with virtually no effect on pupil size or accommodation. They thus offer an advantage over many of the other drugs used in the treatment of glaucoma. Although the precise mechanism whereby β-blockers lower intraocular pressure is not known with certainty, it is believed that they may reduce the production of aqueous humor. Even though these agents are administered into the eye, systemic absorption can occur, producing such adverse effects as bradycardia and acute bronchospasm in patients with bronchospastic disease.

Pindolol possesses modest membrane-stabilizing activity and significant intrinsic β-agonistic activity. Penbutolol and carteolol also have partial agonistic activity but not to the degree that pindolol does. The β-blockers with partial agonistic activity cause less slowing of the resting heart rate than do agents without this capability. The partial agonistic activity may be beneficial in patients who are likely to exhibit severe bradycardia or who have little cardiac reserve.

Timolol, pindolol, penbutolol, and carteolol have half-life values in the same range as propranolol. Nadolol undergoes very little hepatic metabolism and most of this drug is excreted unchanged in the urine. As a result, the half-life of nadolol is about 20 hours, making it one of the longest-acting β-blockers. Timolol undergoes first-pass metabolism but not to the same extent that propranolol does. Timolol and penbutolol are metabolized extensively such that little or no unchanged drug excreted in the urine. Pindolol is metabolized by the liver to the extent of 60%, with the remaining 40% being excreted in the urine unchanged.

β_1-SELECTIVE BLOCKERS (SECOND GENERATION)

The discovery that β-blockers are useful in the treatment of cardiovascular disease, such as hypertension, stimulated a search for cardioselective β-blockers. Cardioselective

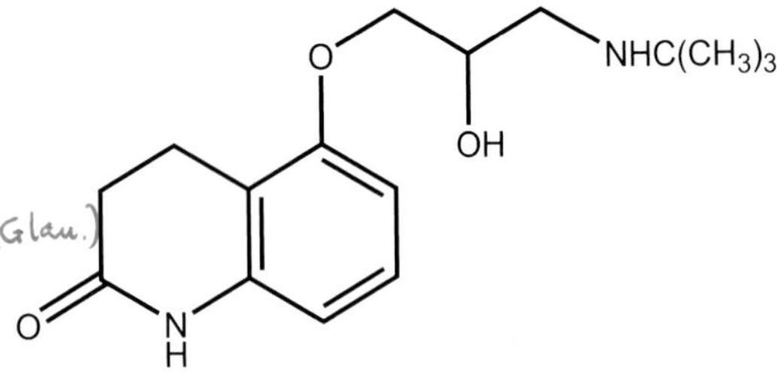

Log P 1.67
Log D -0.42
Δ   2.09 (Glau.)

Carteolol: antihypertensive Glucoma
& antiglaucoma

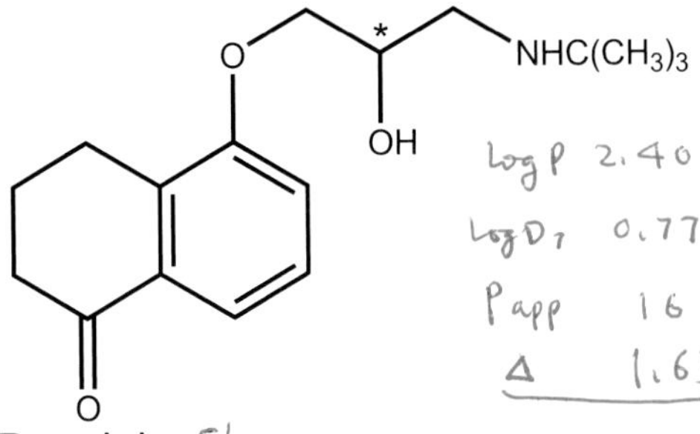

Log P 2.40
Log D7 0.77
Papp 16
Δ   1.63 (Glau)

Bunolol Glucoma
Levobunolol, S(-) isomer of bunolol
antiglaucoma

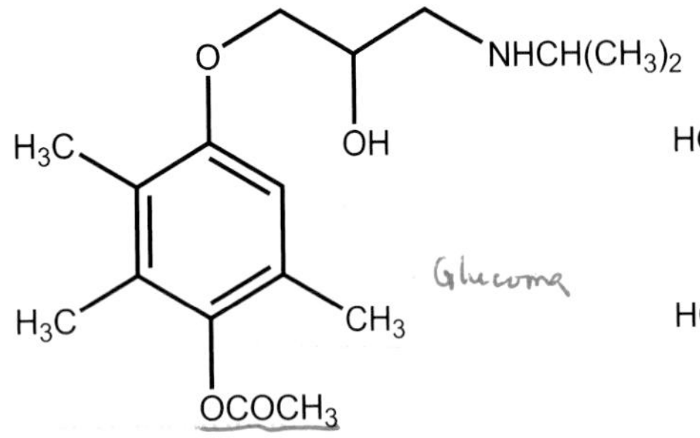

Log P 1.88
Log D7 -0.33
Papp 22
Δ   2.21 (Glau) Glucoma

Metipranolol: antiglaucoma

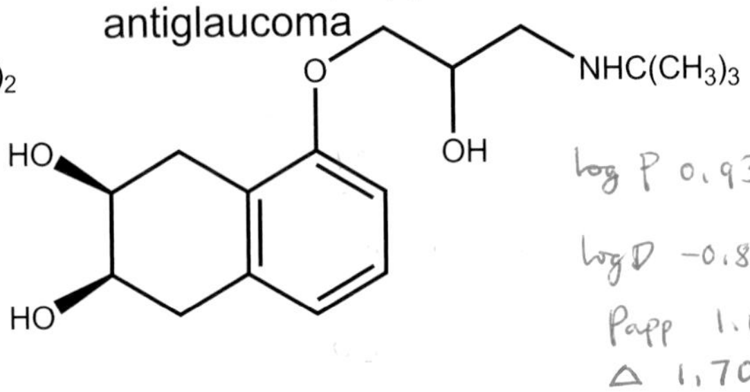

Log P 0.93
Log D -0.83
Papp 1.0
Δ 1.70 (HTN)

Nadolol: antihypertensive

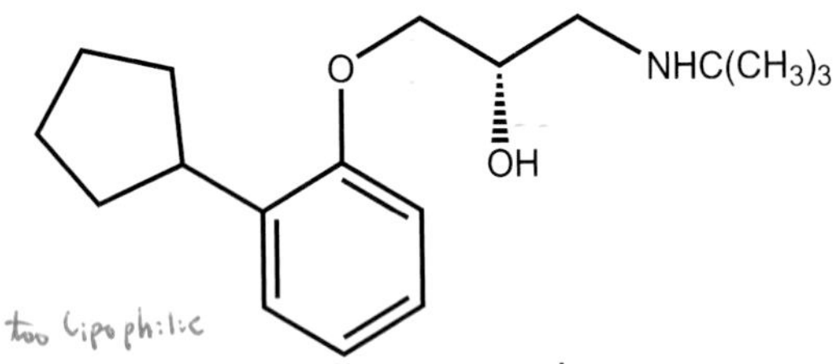

Log P 4.15
Log D7 2.05
Papp 45
Δ   2.1, but too lipophilic

Penbutolol: antihypertensive

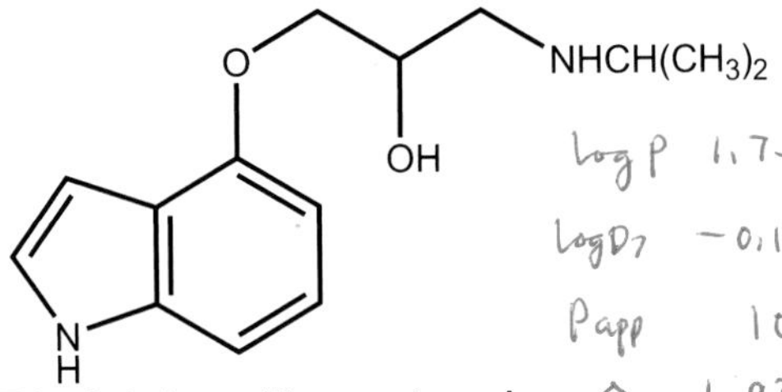

Log P 1.75
Log D7 -0.18
Papp 10
Δ 1.93 (HTN)

Pindolol: antihypertensive

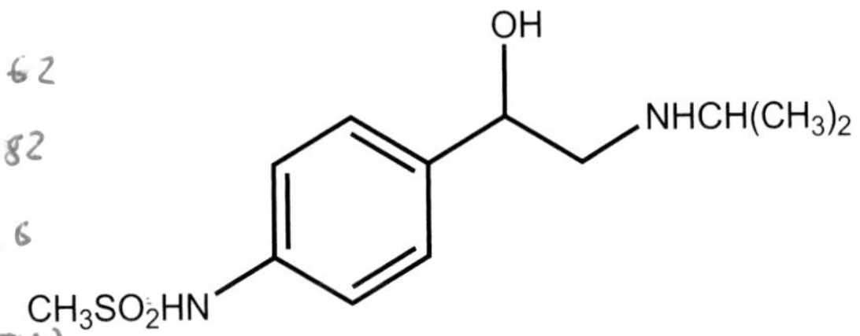

Log P -0.62
Log D7 -1.82
Papp 1.6
Δ 1.2 (HTN)

Sotalol: antiarrhythmias &
only phenylethylamine

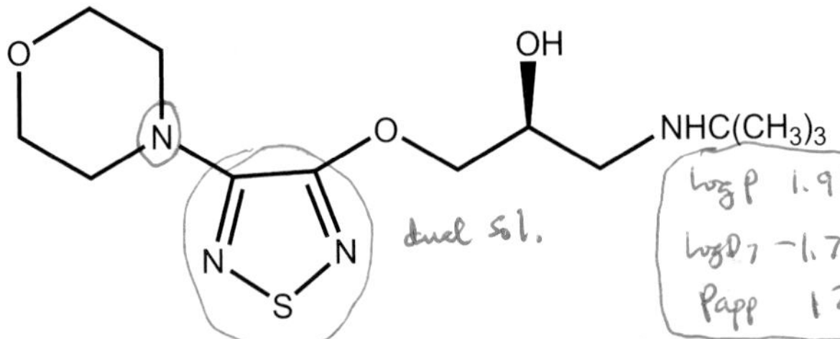

dual Sol.

Δ 3.68
Log P 1.91
Log D7 -1.77
Papp 12

Δ 3.68 .
Glaucoma

Timolol: antihypertensive &
antiglaucoma

Figure 16.15 • Nonselective β-blockers.

β_1-blockers are drugs that have a greater affinity for the β_1-receptors of the heart than for β_2-receptors in other tissues. Such cardioselective agents should provide two important therapeutic advantages. The first advantage should be the lack of a blocking effect on the β_2-receptors in the bronchi. Theoretically, this would make β_1-blockers safe for use in patients who have bronchitis or bronchial asthma. The second advantage should be the absence of blockade of the vascular β_2-receptors, which mediate vasodilation. This would be expected to reduce or eliminate the increase in peripheral resistance that sometimes occurs after the administration of nonselective β-blockers. Unfortunately, cardioselectivity is usually observed with β_1-blockers at only relatively low doses. At normal therapeutic doses, much of the selectivity is lost.

At present, the following β_1-selective blockers are used therapeutically: *acebutolol* (Sectral), *atenolol* (Tenormin), *betaxolol* (Kerlone, Betoptic), *bisoprolol* (Zebeta), *esmolol* (Brevibloc), and *metoprolol* (Lopressor). Structures of these agents are depicted in Figure 16.16. All of these agents except esmolol are indicated for the treatment of hypertension. Atenolol and metoprolol are also approved for use in treating angina pectoris and in therapy following myocardial infarction. Betaxolol is the only β_1-selective blocker indicated for the treatment of glaucoma.

Esmolol was designed specifically to possess a very short DOA; it has an elimination half-life of 9 minutes. Its effects disappear within 20 to 30 minutes after the infusion is discontinued. Esmolol must be diluted with an injection

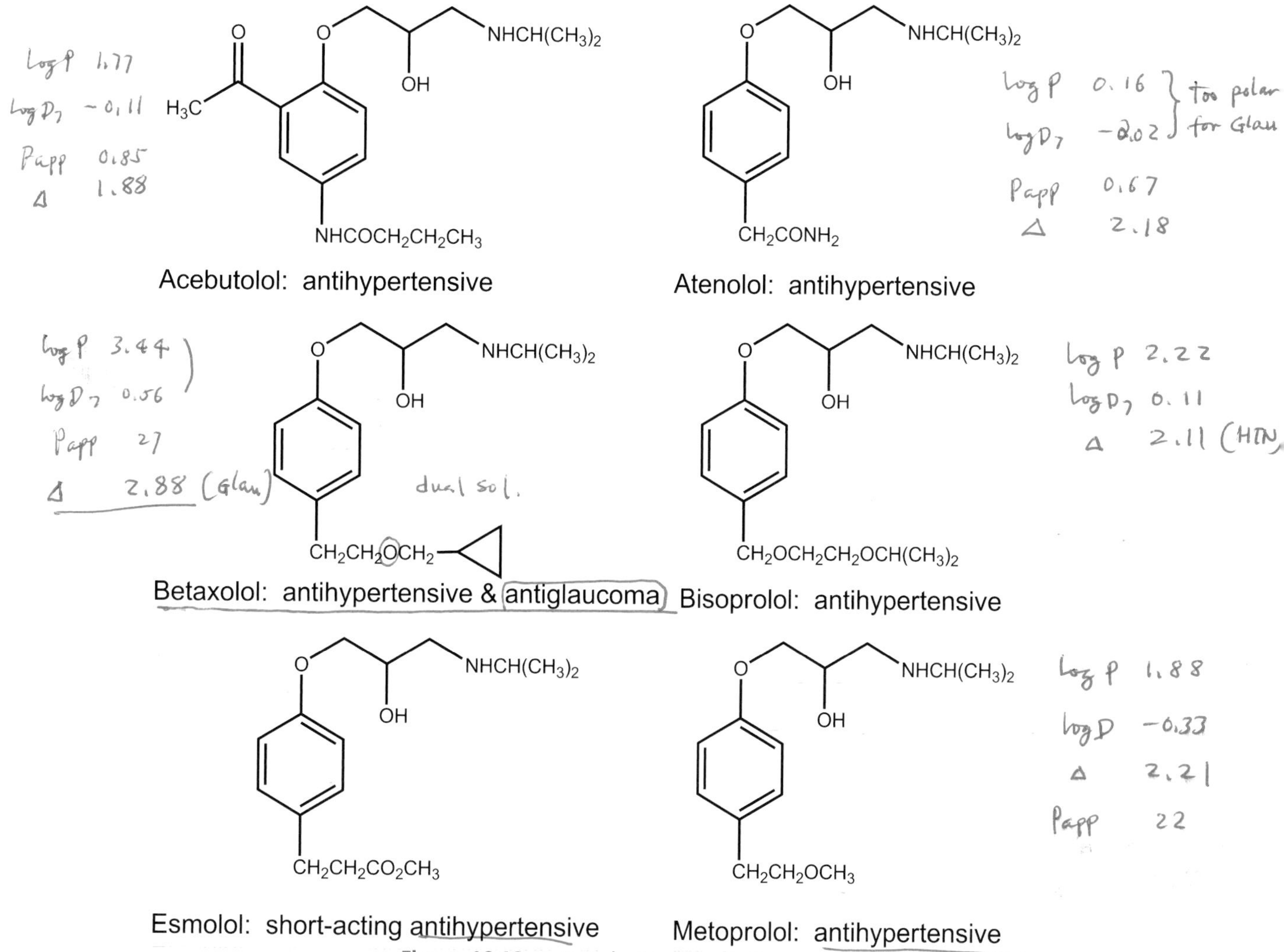

Log P 1.77
Log D₇ ~0.11
Papp 0.85
Δ 1.88

Acebutolol: antihypertensive

Log P 0.16 } too polar
Log D₇ −2.02 } for Glau
Papp 0.67
Δ 2.18

Atenolol: antihypertensive

Log P 3.44
Log D₇ 0.56
Papp 27
Δ 2.88 (Glau)

dual sol.

Betaxolol: antihypertensive & antiglaucoma

Log P 2.22
Log D₇ 0.11
Δ 2.11 (HTN)

Bisoprolol: antihypertensive

Esmolol: short-acting antihypertensive

Log P 1.88
Log D −0.33
Δ 2.21
Papp 22

Metoprolol: antihypertensive

Figure 16.16 ● β_1-Selective blockers.

solution before administration; it is incompatible with sodium bicarbonate. The short DOA of esmolol is the result of rapid hydrolysis of its ester functionality by esterases present in erythrocytes (Fig. 16.17). The resultant carboxylic acid is an extremely weak β-blocker that does not appear to exhibit clinically significant effects. The acid metabolite has an elimination half-life of 3 to 4 hours and is excreted primarily by the kidneys. This agent is administered by continuous intravenous infusion for control of ventricular rate in patients with atrial flutter, atrial fibrillation, or sinus tachycardia. Its rapid onset and short DOA render it useful during surgery, after an operation, or during emergencies for short-term control of heart rates. Esmolol and acebutolol are also indicated for treating certain cardiac arrhythmias.

In the class of β_1-selective blockers, only acebutolol possesses ISA. However, this activity is very weak. Acebutolol and betaxolol possess membrane-stabilizing activity, but the activity is much weaker than that seen with propranolol.

The half-life values of acebutolol and metoprolol are comparable to that seen with propranolol, and those of atenolol and bisoprolol are about twice that of propranolol. Betaxolol, with a half-life ranging between 14 and 22 hours, has the longest DOA of the β_1-selective blockers. Like pro-

pranolol, metoprolol has low bioavailability because of significant first-pass metabolism. Although the bioavailability of betaxolol is very high, it is metabolized extensively by the liver, with very little unchanged drug excreted in the urine. Atenolol (log P = 0.10), like nadolol (log P = 1.29), has low lipid solubility and does not readily cross the BBB. It is absorbed incompletely from the gastrointestinal tract, the oral bioavailability being approximately 50%. Little of the absorbed portion of the dose is metabolized; most of it is excreted unchanged in the urine. In the case of bisoprolol, about 50% of a dose undergoes hepatic metabolism, whereas the remaining 50% is excreted in the urine unchanged.

Acebutolol is one of the very few β-blockers whose metabolite plays a significant role in its pharmacological actions. This drug is absorbed well from the gastrointestinal tract, but it undergoes extensive first-pass metabolic conversion to diacetolol by hydrolytic conversion of the amide group to the amine, followed by acetylation of the amine (Fig. 16.18). After oral administration, plasma levels of diacetolol are higher than those of acebutolol. Diacetolol is also a selective β_1-blocker with partial agonistic activity; it has little membrane-stabilizing activity. It has a longer half-life (8–12 hours) than the parent drug and is excreted by the kidneys.

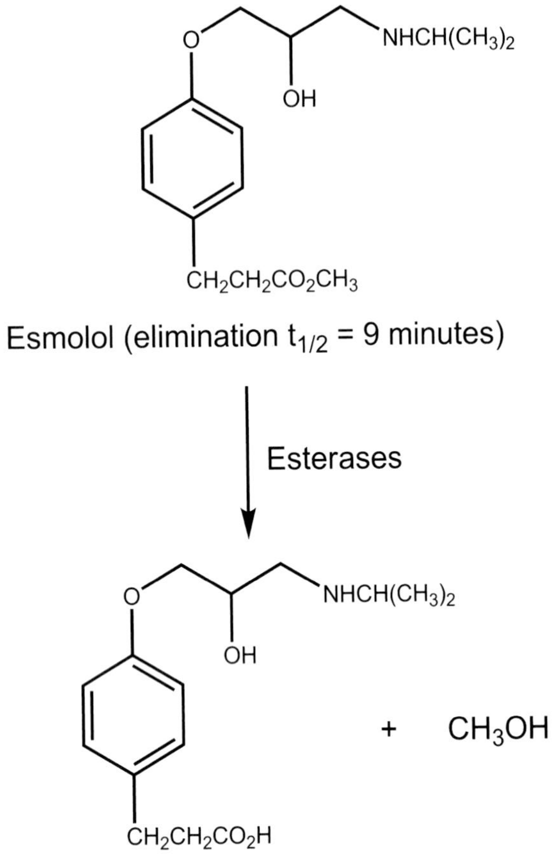

Esmolol (elimination $t_{1/2}$ = 9 minutes)

Esterases

+ CH_3OH

Figure 16.17 ● Metabolism of esmolol.

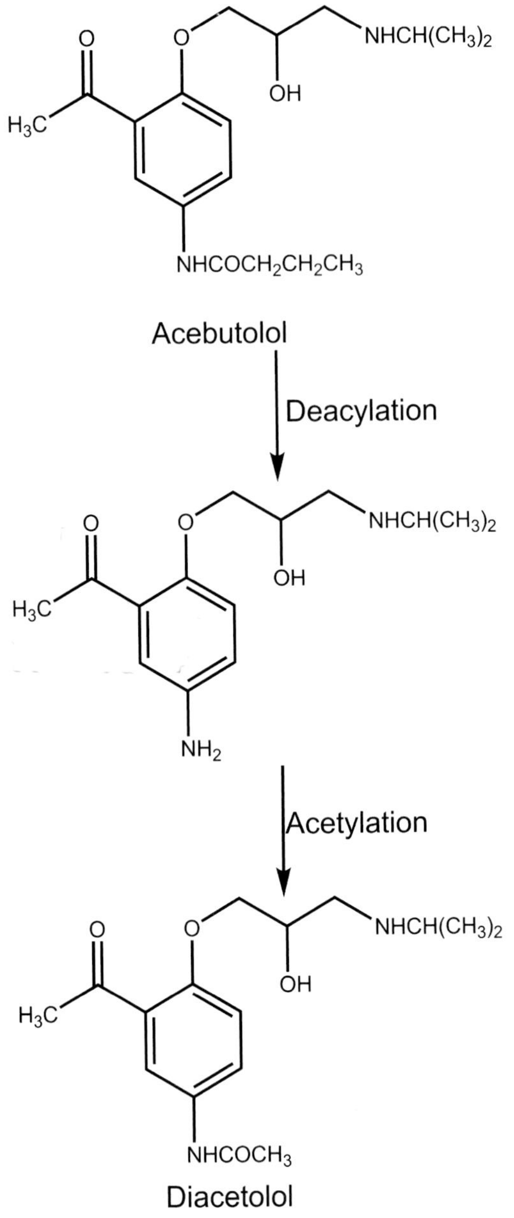

Acebutolol

Deacylation

Acetylation

Diacetolol

Figure 16.18 ● Metabolism of acebutolol.

β-BLOCKERS WITH α_1-ANTAGONIST ACTIVITY (THIRD GENERATION)

Several drugs have been developed that possess both β- and α-receptor–blocking activities within the same molecule. Two examples of such molecules are labetalol (Normodyne) and carvedilol (Coreg). As in the case of dobutamine, the arylalkyl group with nearby methyl group in these molecules is responsible for its α_1-blocking activity. The bulky *N*-substituents and another substituted aromatic ring are responsible for its β-blocking activity.

Labetalol (Normodyne, Trandate, others), a phenylethanolamine derivative, is representative of a class of drugs that act as competitive blockers at α_1-, β_1-, and β_2-receptors. It is a more potent β-blocker than α-blocker. Because it has two asymmetric carbon atoms (1 and 1'), it exists as a mixture of four isomers. It is this mixture that is used clinically in treating hypertension. The different isomers, however, possess different α- and β-blocking activities. The β-blocking activity resides solely in the (1R,1'R) isomer, whereas the α_1-blocking activity is seen in the (1S,1'R) and (1S,1'S) isomers, with the (1S,1'R) isomer possessing the greater therapeutic activity.[63] Labetalol is a clinically useful antihypertensive agent. The rationale for its use in the management of hypertension is that its α-receptor–blocking effects produce vasodilation and its β-receptor–blocking effects prevent the reflex tachycardia usually associated with vasodilation. Although labetalol is very well absorbed, it undergoes extensive first-pass metabolism.

Carvedilol. Carvedilol (Coreg) is a β-blocker that has a unique pharmacological profile. Like labetalol, it is a β-blocker that possesses α_1-blocking activity. Only the (S) enantiomer possesses the β-blocking activity, although both enantiomers are blockers of the α_1-receptor.[64] Overall, its β-blocking activity is 10- to 100-fold of its α-blocking activity. This drug is also unique in that it possesses antioxidant activity and an antiproliferative effect on vascular smooth muscle cells. It thus has a neuroprotective effect and the ability to provide major cardiovascular organ protection.[65] It is used in treating hypertension and congestive heart failure.

⬡ ACKNOWLEDGMENT

The author wishes to express his gratitude to Dr. Paul Goldsmith for proofreading. Portions of this text were taken from Dr. Rodney L. Johnson's chapter in the 11th edition of this book.

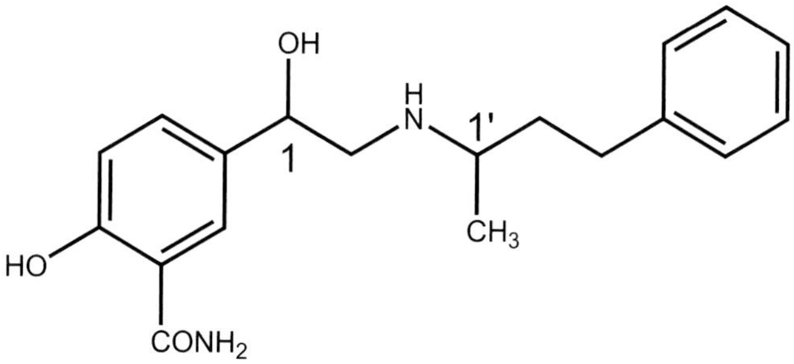

Labetalol

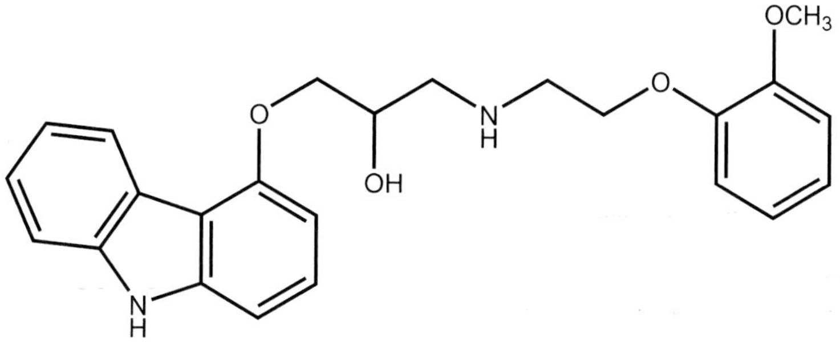

Carvedilol

● R E V I E W   Q U E S T I O N S ●

1. What functional group interactions between the cate-cholamines and adrenoceptors are most likely? Which functional groups are considered pharmacophores of catecholamines?

2. Which of the following drugs would be resistant to metabolism by COMT and why?

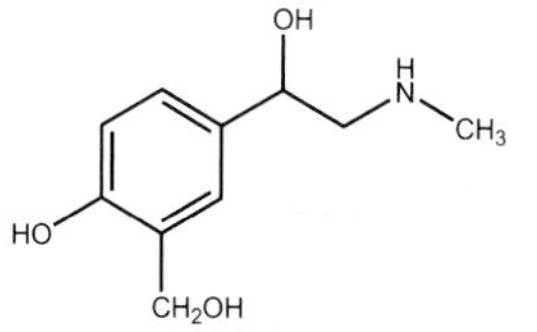

Drug A

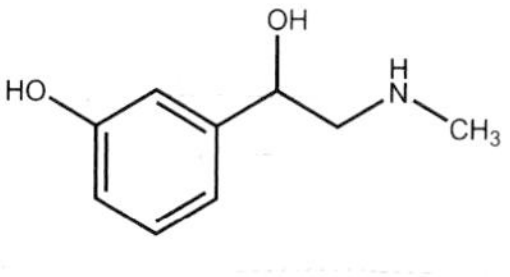

Drug B

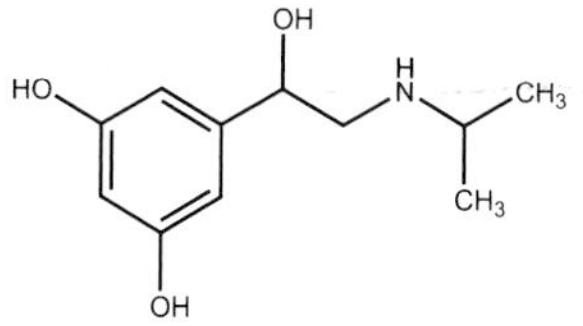

Drug C

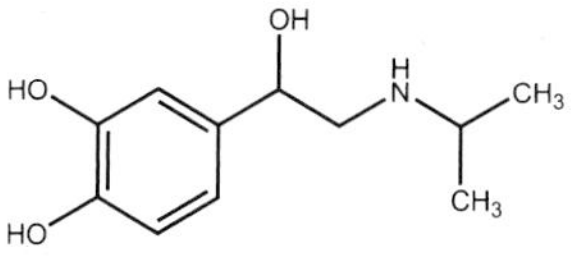

Drug D

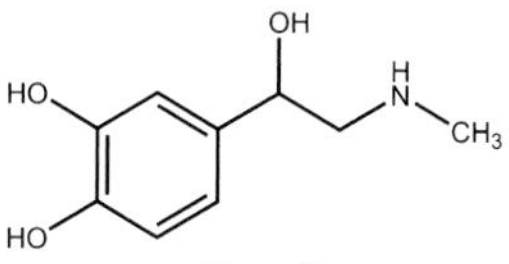

Drug E

3. Which of the drug(s) shown would be the least orally active and have the shortest duration of action and why?

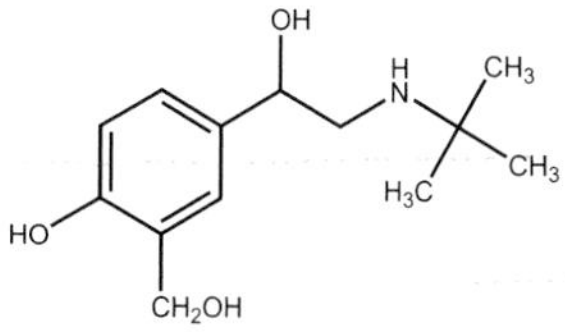

Drug A

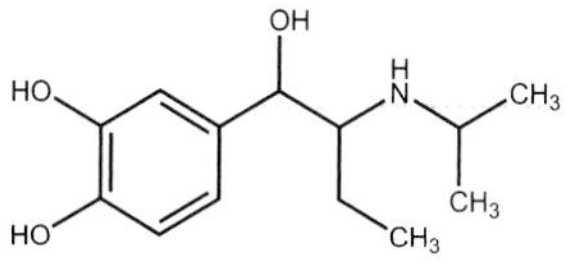

Drug B

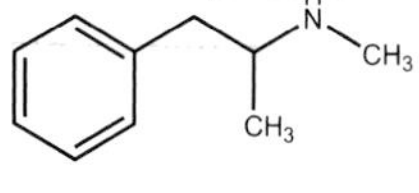

Drug C

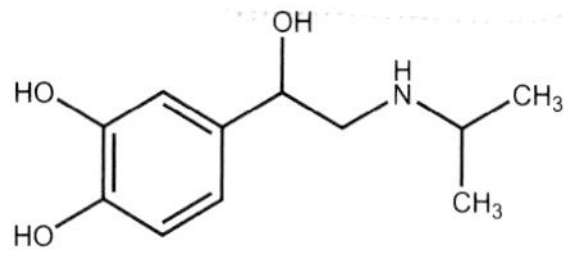

Drug D

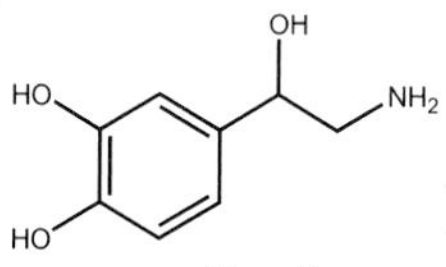

Drug E

4. Which of the following drugs is the most likely to be selective β_2-agonist?

Drug A

Drug B

Drug C

Drug D

Drug E

5. Which of the following drugs is considered to be a prodrug?

Drug A

Drug B

Drug C

Drug D

Drug E

REFERENCES

1. Flatmark, T.: Acta. Physiol. Scand. 168:1, 2000.
2. Musacchio, J. M.: Enzymes involved in the biosynthesis and degradation of catecholamines. In Iversen, L. L., Iversen, S. D., and Snyder, S. H. (eds.). Handbook of Psychopharmacology, vol. 3, Biochemistry of Biogenic Amines. New York, Plenum Press, 1975.
3. Masserano, J. M., et al.: The role of tyrosine hydroxylase in the regulation of catecholamine synthesis. In Trendelenburg, U., and Weiner, N. (eds.). Handbook of Experimental Pharmacology, vol. 90/II, Catecholamines II. Berlin, Springer-Verlag, 1989.
4. Borowsky, B., and Hoffman, B. J.: Int. Rev. Neurobiol. 38:139, 1995.
5. Schuldiner, S.: J. Neurochem. 62:2067, 1994.
6. Kopin, I. J.: Pharmacol. Rev. 37:333, 1985.
7. Dostert, P. L., Benedetti, M. S., and Tipton, K. F.: Med. Res. Rev. 9:45, 1989.
8. Boulton, A. A., and Eisenhofer, G.: Adv. Pharmacol. 42:273, 1998.
9. Ahlquist, R. P.: Am. J. Physiol. 153:586, 1948.
10. Langer, S. Z.: Biochem. Pharmacol. 23:1793, 1974.
11. Berthelsen, S., and Pettinger, W. A.: Life Sci. 21:595, 1977.
12. McGrath, J. C.: Biochem. Pharmacol. 31:467, 1982.
13. Hein, P., and Michel, M. C.: Biochem. Pharmacol. 73:1097, 2007.
14. Perez, D. M.: Biochem. Pharmacol. 73:1051, 2007
15. Carrieri, A., and Fano, A.: Curr. Top. Med. Chem. 7:195, 2007.
16. Ruffolo, R. R., Jr., and Hieble, J. P.: Pharmacol. Ther. 61:1, 1994.
17. Koshimizu, T., et al.: Pharmacol. Ther. 98:235, 2003.
18. Ruffolo, R. R., Jr., Nichols, A. J., and Hieble, J. P.: Functions mediated by alpha-2 adrenergic receptors. In Limbird, L. E. (ed.). The Alpha-2 Adrenergic Receptor. Clifton, NJ, Humana Press, 1988, p. 187.
19. Broadley, K. J.: J. Auton. Pharmacol. 2:119, 1982.
20. Timmermans, P. B. M. W. M.: Centrally acting hypotensive drugs. In van Zwieten, P. A. (ed.). Handbook of Hypertension, Vol 3. Pharmacology of Antihypertensive Drugs. Amsterdam, Elsevier, 1984, p. 102.
21. Langer, S. Z., and Hicks, P. E.: J. Cardiovasc. Pharmacol. 6(Suppl. 4):S547, 1984.
22. Ruffolo, R. R., Jr., Nichols, A. J., and Hieble, J. P.: Life Sci. 49:171, 1991.
23. Lands, A. M., et al.: Nature 214:597, 1967.
24. Arch, J. R., et al.: Nature 309:163, 1984.
25. Gilman, A. G.: Annu. Rev. Biochem. 56:615, 1987.
26. Lefkowitz, R. J., et al.: Trends Pharmacol. Sci. 7:444, 1986.
27. Nestor, E. J., Walaas, S. I., and Greengard, P.: Science 225:1357, 1984.
28. Ostrowski, J., et al.: Annu. Rev. Pharmacol. Toxicol. 32:167, 1992.
29. Buscher, R., Herrmann, V., and Insel, P. A.: Trends Pharmacol. Sci. 20:94, 1999.
30. Brogden, R. N., et al.: Drugs 21:81, 1981.
31. Rudnick, G., et al.: Biochemistry 29:603, 1990.
32. Palmer, J. D., and Nugent, C. A.: Pharmacotherapy 3:220, 1983.
33. Triggle, D. J.: Adrenergics: catecholamines and related agents. In Wolff, M. E. (ed.). Burger's Medicinal Chemistry, 4th ed., part III. New York, John Wiley & Sons, 1981.
34. Nichols, A. J., and Ruffolo, R. R., Jr.: Structure–activity relationships for α-adrenoceptor agonists and antagonists. In Ruffolo, R. R., Jr. (ed.). α-Adrenoceptors: Molecular Biology, Biochemistry, and Pharmacology. Progress in Basic Clinical Pharmacology, vol. 8. Basel, Karger, 1991, p. 75.
35. Hieble, J. P.: Structure–activity relationships for activation and blockade of β-adrenoceptors. In Ruffolo, R. R., Jr. (ed.). β-Adrenoceptors: Molecular Biology, Biochemistry, and Pharmacology. Progress in Basic Clinical Pharmacology, vol. 7. Basel, Karger, 1991, p. 105.
36. Easson, L. H., and Stedman, E.: Biochem. J. 27:1257, 1933.
37. Ruffolo, R. R., Jr., and Waddel, J. E.: J. Pharmacol. Exp. Ther. 224:559, 1983.
38. Langer, S. Z., Cavero, I., and Massingham, R.: Hypertension 2:372, 1980.
39. de Jonge, A., Timmermans, P. B., and van Zwieten, P. A.: Naunyn Schmiedebergs Arch. Pharmacol. 317:8, 1981.
40. Comer, W. T., and Matier, W. L.: Antihypertensive agents. In Wolff, M. E., and Matier, W. L.: Antihypertensive agents. In Wolff, M. E. (ed.). Burger's Medicinal Chemistry, 4th ed., part III. New York, John Wiley & Sons, 1981, p. 285.
41. Bousquet, P., et al.: Ann. N. Y. Acad. Sci. 881:272, 1999.
42. Head, G. A.: Ann. N. Y. Acad. Sci. 881:279, 1999.
43. Piletz, J. E., et al.: Ann. N. Y. Acad. Sci. 1009–1043, 2003.
44. Dardonville, C., and Rozas, I.: Med. Res. Rev. 24:639, 2004.
45. MacMillan, L. B., et al.: Science 273:801, 1996.
46. Link, R. E., et al.: Science 273:803, 1996.
47. Ruffolo, R. R., Jr., et al.: Annu. Rev. Pharmacol. Toxicol. 33:243, 1993.
48. Davies, J., and Quinlan, J. E.: Neuroscience 16:673, 1985.
49. Ruffolo, R. R., Jr., et al.: J. Pharmacol. Exp. Ther. 219:447, 1981.
50. Majerus, T. C., et al.: Pharmacotherapy 9:245, 1989.
51. Clark, R. B., et al.: Mol. Pharmacol. 49:182, 1996.
52. Anderson, G. P., Linden, A., and Rabe, K. F.: Eur. Respir. J. 7:569, 1994.
53. Sawa, M., and Harada, H.: Curr. Med. Chem. 13:25, 2006.
54. Andraws, R., et al.: Prog. Cardiovasc. Dis. 47:271, 2005.
55. Honkanen, E., et al.: J. Med. Chem. 26:1433, 1983.
56. Ferry, N., et al.: Br. J. Pharmacol. 78:359, 1983.

57. Holm, K. J., and Markham, A.: Drugs 57:607, 1999.
58. Powell, C. E., and Slater, I. H.: J. Pharmacol. Exp. Ther. 122:480, 1958.
59. Black, J. W., and Stephenson, J. S.: Lancet 2:311, 1962.
60. Kaiser, C., et al.: J. Med. Chem. 20:687, 1977.
61. Riddell, J. G., Harron, D. W. G., and Shank, R. G.: Clin. Pharmacokinet. 12:305, 1987.
62. Walle, T., et al.: Biochem. Pharmacol. 37:115, 1988.
63. Gold, E. H., et al.: J. Med. Chem. 25:1363, 1982.
64. Nichols, A. J., et al.: Chirality 1:265, 1989.
65. Lysko, P. G., Feuerstein, G. Z., and Ruffolo, R. R., Jr.: Pharm. News 2:12, 1995.

SELECTED READING

Abraham, D. J. (ed): Adrenergics and adrenergic-blocking agents. In Burgers' medicinal chemistry and drug discovery, 6th ed., vol. 6. Hoboken, NJ, John Wiley and Sons, 2003.

Burnham, T. H., and Schwalm, A. (eds.). Drug Facts and Comparisons. St. Louis, Wolters-Kluwer, 2007.
Cooper, J. R., Bloom, F. E., and Roth, R. H.: The Biochemical Basis of Neuropharmacology, 8th ed. New York, Oxford University Press, 2003.
Westfall, T. C., and Westfall, D. P.: Adrenergic agonists and antagonists. In Brunton, L. L., Lazo, J. S., and Parker, K. L. (eds.). Goodman and Gilman's The Pharmacological Basis of Therapeutics, 11th ed. New York, McGraw-Hill, 2006, p. 237.
Westfall, T. C., and Westfall, D. P.: Neurotransmission: The autonomic and somatic motor nervous systems. In Brunton, L. L., Lazo, J. S., and Parker, K. L. (eds.). The Pharmacological Basis of Therapeutics, 11th ed. New York, McGraw-Hill, 2006, p. 137.

CHAPTER 17

Cholinergic Drugs and Related Agents (Prof. in Micsio)

STEPHEN J. CUTLER

ANS

This chapter describes the role that the autonomic nervous system plays in regulating the mammalian system. This chapter supports the fact that acetylcholine (ACh) plays a critical role in the mechanisms of regulation of human physiology. This, in turn, not only serves in the development of agents that mimic the effect of ACh, but also those that block its effects as therapeutic agents. Through these developments, scientists are gaining a better understanding of how to treat diseases such as Alzheimer disease, Parkinson disease, and, most recently, overactive bladder. For pharmacists to be good practitioners, it is necessary that they understand how the autonomic nervous system influences normal physiological function as well as to how they can be used in manipulating diseases.

Few systems, if any, have been studied as extensively as those innervated by neurons that release ACh at their endings. Since the classic studies of Dale,[1] who described the actions of the esters and ethers of choline on isolated organs and their relationship to muscarine, pharmacologists, physiologists, chemists, and biochemists have applied their knowledge to understand the actions of the cholinergic nerve and its neurotransmitter. Advances in the applications of biotechnology and chemistry have developed probes that have uncovered the complexity of the action of ACh on cholinergic neurons and receptors, unknown when ACh was first demonstrated in the frog heart in 1921 by Loewi as the substance released by vagus nerve stimulation.[2]

This chapter includes the drugs and chemicals that act on cholinergic nerves or the tissues they innervate to either mimic or block the action of ACh. Drugs that mimic the action of ACh do so either by acting directly on the cholinergic receptors in the tissue or by inhibiting acetylcholinesterase (AChE), the enzyme that inactivates ACh at the nerve terminal. Chemicals that bind or compete with ACh for binding to the receptor may block cholinergic neurotransmission.

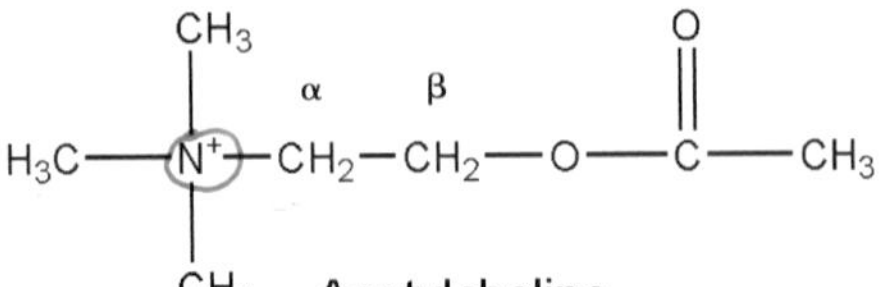

Acetylcholine

Cholinergic nerves are found in the peripheral nervous system and central nervous system (CNS) of humans. Its presence in the CNS is currently receiving the most attention, as researchers are beginning to unlock the mysteries surrounding cognitive impairment and, most particularly, Alzheimer disease. Synaptic terminals in the cerebral cortex, corpus striatum, hippocampus, and several other regions in the CNS are rich in ACh and in the enzymes that synthesize and hydrolyze this neurotransmitter. Many experiments show that agonists and antagonists of cholinergic receptors can modify the output of neurotransmitters, including ACh, from brain preparations. Although the function of ACh in the brain and brainstem is not clear, it has been implicated in memory and behavioral activity in humans.[3] The *peripheral nervous system* consists of those nerves outside the cerebrospinal axis and includes the somatic nerves and the autonomic nervous system. The *somatic nerves* are made up of a sensory (afferent) nerve and a motor (efferent) nerve. The *motor nerves* arise from the spinal cord and project uninterrupted throughout the body to all skeletal muscle. ACh mediates transmission of impulses from the motor nerve to skeletal muscle (i.e., neuromuscular junction).

(PNS)

The *autonomic nervous system* is composed of two divisions: *sympathetic* and *parasympathetic*. ACh serves as a neurotransmitter at both sympathetic and parasympathetic preganglionic nerve endings, postganglionic nerve fibers in the parasympathetic division, and some postganglionic fibers (e.g., salivary and sweat glands) in the sympathetic division of the autonomic nervous system. The autonomic nervous system regulates the activities of smooth muscle and glandular secretions. These, as a rule, function below the level of consciousness (e.g., respiration, circulation, digestion, body temperature, metabolism). The two divisions have contrasting effects on the internal environment of the body. The sympathetic division frequently discharges as a unit, especially during conditions of rage or fright, and expends energy. The parasympathetic division is organized for discrete and localized discharge and stores and conserves energy.

Drugs and chemicals that cause the parasympathetic division to react are termed *parasympathomimetic*, whereas those blocking the actions are called *parasympatholytic*. Agents that mimic the sympathetic division are *sympathomimetic*, and those that block the actions are *sympatholytic*. Another classification used to describe drugs and chemicals acting on the nervous system or the structures that the fibers innervate are based on the neurotransmitter released at the nerve ending. Drugs acting on the autonomic nervous system are divided into *adrenergic*, for those postganglionic sympathetic fibers that release norepinephrine and epinephrine, and *cholinergic*, for the remaining fibers in the autonomic nervous system and the motor fibers of the somatic nerves that release ACh.

CHOLINERGIC RECEPTORS

There are two distinct receptor types for ACh that differ in composition, location, and pharmacological function and have specific agonists and antagonists. Cholinergic receptors have been characterized as *nicotinic* and *muscarinic* on the basis of their ability to be bound by the naturally occurring alkaloids nicotine and muscarine, respectively. Receptor subtypes that differ in location and specificity to agonists and antagonists have been identified for both the nicotinic and muscarinic receptors.

Nicotinic Receptors

Nicotinic receptors are coupled directly to ion channels and, when activated by Ach, mediate very rapid responses. Ion channels are responsible for the electrical excitability of nerve and muscle cells and for the sensitivity of sensory cells. The channels are pores that open or close in an all-or-nothing fashion on time scales ranging from 0.1 to 10 milliseconds to provide aqueous pathways through the plasma membrane that ions can transverse. Factors affecting selectivity of ion pores include both the charge and size of the ion. Ions in aqueous solution are hydrated. The water around the ion is characterized by the presence of two distinct water structures: a tightly bound, highly ordered layer immediately surrounding the ion and a second, less structured layer[4] (Fig. 17.1). Ion transport through a channel requires some denuding of the surrounding water shell. The degree of organization of the water structure determines the energy required to remove the hydration

TABLE 17.1 Radii of Alkali and Alkali Earth Cations

Ion	Ionic Radius (Å)	Effective Hydrated Radius (Å)
Li^+	0.60	4.5
Na^+	0.95	3.4
K^+	1.33	2.2
Rb^+	1.48	1.9
Cs^+	1.69	1.9
Mg^{2+}	0.65	5.9
Ca^{2+}	0.99	4.5
Sr^{2+}	1.13	3.7
Ba^{2+}	1.35	3.7

From Triggle, D. J.: Neurotransmitter-Receptor Interactions. San Diego, Academic Press, 1971.

shell and is a factor in the selectivity of that ion channel.[5] Table 17.1 lists the effective radii of alkali and alkaline earth cations.

The nicotinic ACh receptor was the first neurotransmitter isolated and purified in an active form.[6] It is a glycoprotein embedded into the polysynaptic membrane that can be obtained from the electric organs of the marine ray, *Torpedo californica* and the electric eel, *Electrophorus electricus*. The receptor is pictured as a cylindrical protein of about 250,000 Da and consists of five-subunit polypeptide chains, of which two appear to be identical.[7,8] The subunit stoichiometry of the polypeptide units from the *Torpedo* receptor is $\alpha_2,\beta,\gamma,\delta$.[9] The peptide chains of the receptor are arranged to form an opening in the center, which is the ion channel. Each α chain contains a negatively charged binding site for the quaternary ammonium group of ACh. The receptor appears to exist as a dimer of the two five-subunit polypeptide chain monomers linked through a disulfide bond between δ chains. A structural protein of molecular weight 43,000 binds the nicotinic receptor to the membrane (Fig. 17.2). With so many variables in the subunits, many combinations of nicotinic subtype receptors are available.

When the neurotransmitter ACh binds to the nicotinic receptor, it causes a change in the permeability of the membrane to allow passage of small cations Ca^{2+}, Na^+, and K^+. The physiological effect is to temporarily depolarize the end plate. This depolarization results in muscular contraction at a neuromuscular junction or, as occurs in autonomic ganglia, continuation of the nerve impulse. Neuromuscular nicotinic ACh receptors are of interest as targets for autoimmune antibodies in myasthenia gravis and for muscle relaxants used during the course of surgical procedures. Nicotinic receptors in autonomic ganglia, when blocked by drugs, can play a role in the control of hypertension.

NICOTINIC RECEPTOR SUBTYPES

Nicotinic receptors located in the neuromuscular junction differ from those on neurons, such as those in the CNS and autonomic ganglia, in that they have different ligand specificities. Nicotinic receptors at the neuromuscular junction (N_1) are blocked by succinylcholine, *d*-tubocurarine, and decamethonium and stimulated by phenyltrimethylammonium. N_2-nicotinic receptors are found in autonomic ganglia. They are blocked by hexamethonium and trimethaphan but stimulated by tetramethylammonium and dimethyl-4-phenylpiperazinium (DMPP). Nicotinic receptor subtypes

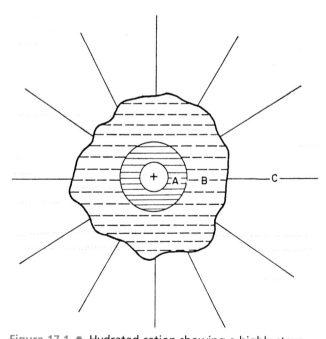

Figure 17.1 ● Hydrated cation showing a highly structured shell of water around the cation (**A**), a less structured layer surrounding the inner water shell (**B**), and water in a "normal" state (**C**). (With permission from the author and the Royal Society of Chemistry.)

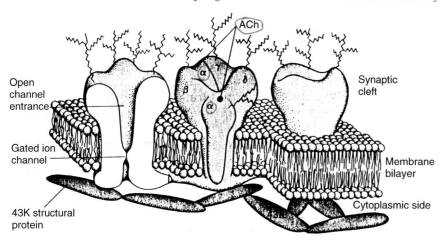

Figure 17.2 ● Model of the nicotinic receptor consisting of five protein subunits embedded in a cell membrane, based on electron microscopy and neutron scattering data. *Jagged lines* represent oligosaccharide chains on the upper part of the receptor. A 43K protein is bound to the receptor on the cytosolic side of the cell membrane. The ACh-binding sites are shown on the two-subunit proteins. (Reprinted with permission from Lindstrom, J. M., et al.: Cold Spring Harbor Symp. Quant. Biol. 48:93, 1983.)

have also been identified in many regions of the CNS; however, their pharmacological function is not yet fully understood.[10] Even so, great attempts are being made to understand the role of so many receptor subtypes, particularly those found in the CNS.[11,12]

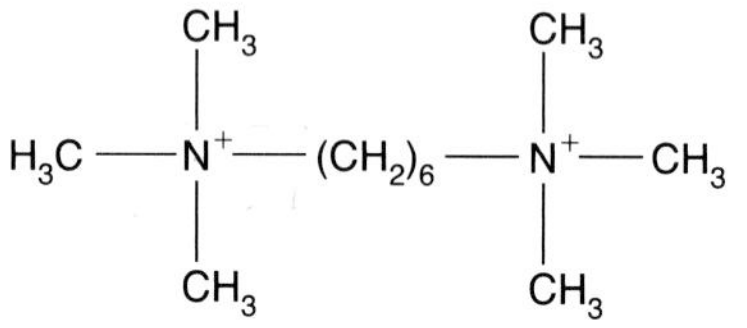

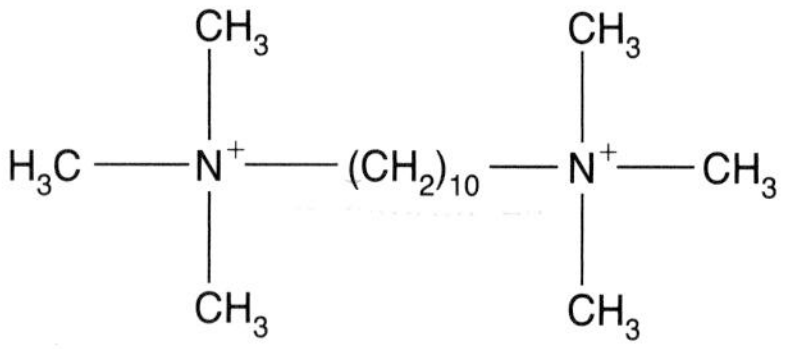

Decamethonium

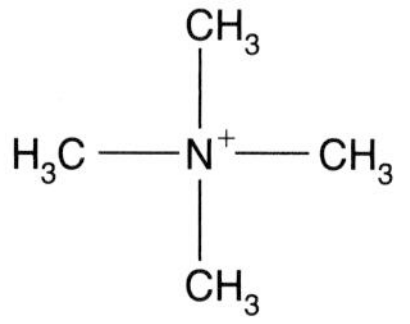

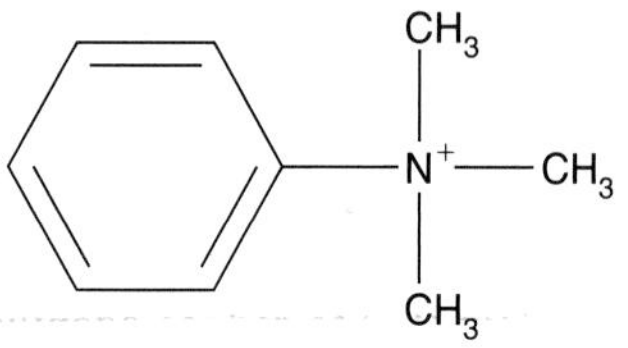

Phenyltrimethylammonium

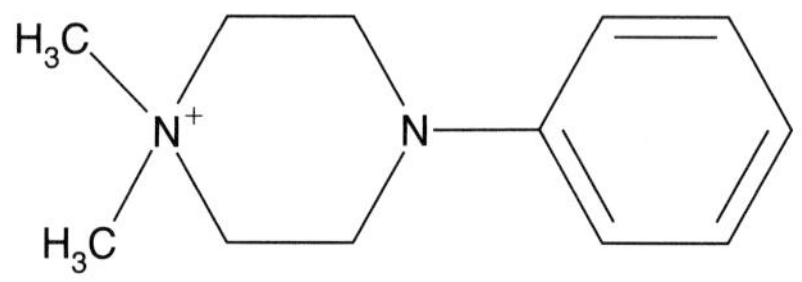

Hexamethonium

Tetramethylammonium

DMPP

Muscarinic Receptors

Muscarinic receptors play an essential role in regulating the functions of organs innervated by the autonomic nervous system to maintain homeostasis of the organism. The action of ACh on muscarinic receptors can result in stimulation or inhibition of the organ system affected. ACh stimulates secretions from salivary and sweat glands, secretions and contraction of the gut, and constriction of the airways of the respiratory tract. It inhibits contraction of the heart and relaxes smooth muscle of blood vessels.

As early as 1980, it became apparent that a single muscarinic receptor type could not mediate the actions of ACh. Research on cholinergic receptors has increased since the 1980s, as these receptors represent potential targets for useful drugs for disease states that are becoming more prevalent because of our increasing population of aged persons. The outcome of these studies has been the discovery of several muscarinic receptor subtypes.

Muscarinic receptors mediate their effects by activating guanosine triphosphate (GTP)-binding proteins (G proteins). These receptors have seven protein helixes that transcend the plasma membrane, creating four extracellular domains and four intracellular domains (Fig. 17.3). The extracellular domain of the receptor contains the binding site for ACh. The intracellular domain couples with G proteins to initiate biochemical changes that result in pharmacological action from receptor activation.

MUSCARINIC RECEPTOR SUBTYPES

Evidence from both pharmacological and biochemical studies shows that subtypes of muscarinic receptors are located in the CNS and peripheral nervous system.[13,14] Molecular cloning studies have revealed the existence of five different molecular mammalian muscarinic receptor proteins. The cloned receptors have been identified as m_1 to m_5. In another

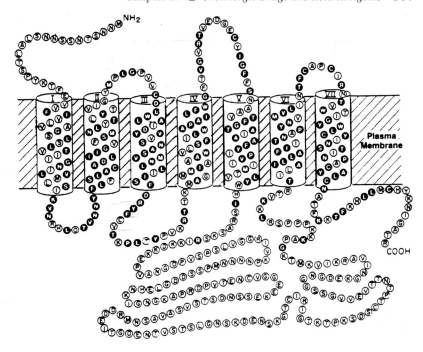

Figure 17.3 ● Hypothetical model of a muscarinic receptor showing the location of the transmembrane helical protein domains and the extracellular and intracellular domains connecting the seven α-helical proteins in the membrane. (Reprinted from Goyal, R. K.: N. Engl. J. Med. 321:1024, 1989, with permission from the author and the Massachusetts Medical Society.)

method of identification, muscarinic receptor subtypes have been defined on the basis of their affinity for selective agonists and antagonists and the pharmacological effects they cause. These receptors are designated with capital letters and subscript numbers as M_1 to M_5. The nomenclature convention adopted for these receptors is that the pharmacologically defined subtypes M_1, M_2, and M_3 correspond to the genetically defined subtypes m_1, m_2, and m_3. The m_4 gene-derived protein is referred to as the M_4 subtype and has many pharmacological properties similar to those of the M_2 subtype. The m_5 receptor gene product does not have an equivalent pharmacological profile.

M_1 Receptors. Even though molecules do not have exclusive selectivity on muscarinic receptor subtypes, M_1 receptors have been defined as those with high affinity for pirenzepine and low affinity for compounds such as AF-DX 116. They have been termed *neural* because of their distribution within particular brain structures. In addition to the CNS, M_1 receptors are located in exocrine glands and autonomic ganglia. In humans, these receptors seem to affect arousal attention, rapid eye movement (REM) sleep, emotional responses, affective disorders including depression, and modulation of stress. They are believed to participate in higher brain functions, such as memory and learning. Alzheimer disease research has implicated cholinergic neurons and receptors, but evidence does not show conclusively that these are the primary causes of the disease. M_1 receptors have been identified in submucosal glands and some smooth muscle. They are located in parietal cells in the gastrointestinal (GI) tract and in peripheral autonomic ganglia,

such as the intramural ganglia of the stomach wall. When stimulated, M_1 receptors cause gastric secretion.[15] Although McN-A-343 is a selective agonist, pirenzepine hydrochloride (HCl) acts as an antagonist and has been used outside the United States for the treatment of peptic ulcer disease.

M_2 Receptors. M_2 receptors are identified by their high affinity for methoctramine, a polyamine, and by their low affinity for pirenzepine. M_2 receptors are also called *cardiac* muscarinic receptors because they are located in the atria and conducting tissue of the heart. Their stimulation causes a decrease in the strength and rate of cardiac muscle contraction. These effects may be produced by affecting intracellular K^+ and Ca^{2+} levels in heart tissue. M_2 receptors activate K^+ channels to cause hyperpolarization of cardiac cells, resulting in bradycardia. These receptors may also act through an inhibitory G protein (G_i) to reduce adenylate cyclase activity and lower cyclic 3′,5′-adenosine monophosphate (cAMP) levels in cardiac cells. Lower cAMP levels decrease the amount of free Ca^{2+} in cardiac cells and slow down the heart rate.[16] M_2 receptors can also serve as autoreceptors on presynaptic terminals of postganglionic cholinergic nerves to inhibit ACh release. The balance of the effects of multiple muscarinic receptor subtypes determines the size of the airway of the smooth muscle in the bronchioles. Contraction is primarily the result of the action of ACh on M_3 receptors (see on next page) following stimulation of the vagus. At the same time, ACh stimulates inhibitor M_2 autoreceptors located on nerve endings to limit release of ACh. In asthmatics, neuronal M_2 receptors in the lungs do not function normally.[17]

[handwritten: negative feedback]

$H_3C - \overset{\overset{\displaystyle CH_3}{|}}{\underset{\underset{\displaystyle CH_3}{|}}{N^+}} - CH_2 - C \equiv C - CH_2 - O - \overset{\overset{\displaystyle O}{\|}}{C} - \overset{\overset{\displaystyle H}{|}}{N} -$ (phenyl ring with Cl)

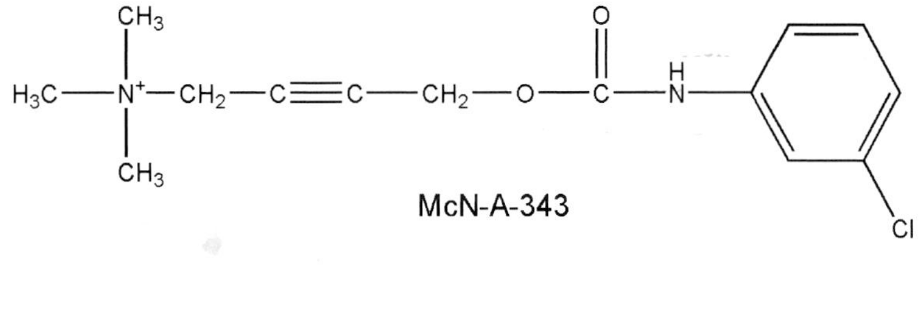

McN-A-343

M3 Receptors. M_3 receptors, referred to as *glandular* muscarinic receptors, are located in exocrine glands and smooth muscle. Their effect on these organ systems is mostly stimulatory. Glandular secretions from lacrimal, salivary, bronchial, pancreatic, and mucosal cells in the GI tract are characteristic of M_3 receptor activation. Contraction of visceral smooth muscle is also a result of M_3 receptor stimulation. These stimulant effects are mediated through G protein activation of phospholipase C (PLC) to form the second-messenger inositol triphosphate (IP_3) and diacylglycerol (DAG). Discoveries in the past decade have revealed that the endothelium can control the tone of vascular smooth muscle by the synthesis of a potent relaxant, endothelium-derived relaxing factor (EDRF), now identified as nitric oxide (NO), and a vasoconstrictor substance, endothelium-derived contracting factor (EDCF). The synthesis and release of these substances contribute to the tone of the vascular epithelium. M_3 receptors, when activated in endothelial cells, cause the release of EDRF and contribute to vasodilation.[18]

M4 Receptors. M_4 receptors, like M_2 receptors, act through G_i protein to inhibit adenylate cyclase. They also function by a direct regulatory action on K^+ and Ca^{2+} ion channels. M_4 receptors in tracheal smooth muscle, when stimulated, inhibit the release of ACh[19] in the same manner that M_2 receptors do.

M5 Receptors. A great deal of research remains to be performed on the M_5 subclass of receptors. Because the M_5 receptor messenger RNA (mRNA) is found in the substantia nigra, it has been suggested that M_5 receptors may regulate dopamine release at terminals within the striatum.

BIOCHEMICAL EFFECTS OF MUSCARINIC RECEPTOR STIMULATION

Transmission at the synapse involving second messengers is much slower, about 100 ms, compared with the few milliseconds at synapses where ion channels are activated directly. The delayed reaction to receptor stimulation is caused by a cascade of biochemical events that must occur to cause the pharmacological response (Fig. 17.4). The sequence of events in these second-messenger systems begins with activation of the receptors by an agonist and involves the activation of G proteins that are bound to a portion of the intracellular domain of the muscarinic receptor.[20] G proteins are so called because of their interaction with the guanine nucleotides GTP and guanosine diphosphate (GDP). They translate drug–receptor interactions at the surface of the cell to components inside the cell to create the biological response. G proteins consist of three subunits, α, β, and γ. When the receptor is occupied, the α subunit, which has enzymatic activity, catalyzes the conversion of GTP to GDP. The α subunit bound with GTP is the active form of the G protein that can associate with various enzymes (i.e., PLC and adenylate cyclase) and ion channels (K^+ and Ca^{2+}). G proteins are varied, and the α subunit may cause activation (G_s) or inactivation (G_i) of the enzymes or channels. Recent studies suggest that β and γ subunits also contribute to pharmacological effects.[21]

A single drug–receptor complex can activate several G protein molecules, and each in turn can remain associated with a target molecule (e.g., an enzyme) and cause the production of many molecules, amplifying the result of the

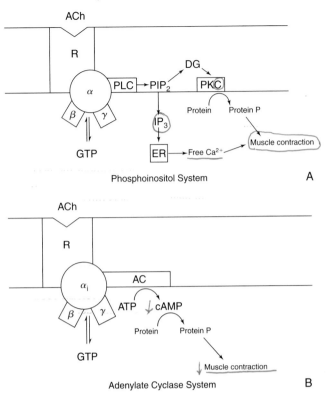

Figure 17.4 ● Proposed biochemical mechanisms of cholinergic receptor action. **A.** ACh activates a G protein (α, β, γ) in the phospholipase system to activate the membrane enzyme phospholipase C (PLC), enhancing muscle contraction. **B.** Inhibition of adenylate cyclase system through an inhibitory G protein (α_1) to cause muscle relaxation.

initial drug–receptor combination. M_1, M_3, and M_5 receptors activate PLC, causing the release of IP_3 and DAG, which in turn release intracellular Ca^{2+} and activate protein kinases, respectively. M_2 and M_4 receptors produce inhibition of adenylate cyclase.

Phosphoinositol System. The phosphoinositol system requires the breakdown of membrane-bound phosphatidylinositol 4,5-diphosphate (PIP_2) by PLC to IP_3 and DAG, which serve as second messengers in the cell. IP_3 mobilizes Ca^{2+} from intracellular stores in the endoplasmic reticulum to elevate cytosolic free Ca^{2+}. The Ca^{2+} activates Ca^{2+}-dependent kinases (e.g., troponin C in muscle) directly or binds to the Ca^{2+}-binding protein calmodulin, which activates calmodulin-dependent kinases. These kinases phosphorylate cell-specific enzymes to cause muscle contraction. DAG is lipidlike and acts in the plane of the membrane through activation of protein kinase C to cause the phosphorylation of cellular proteins, also leading to muscle contraction (Fig. 17.4).[22,23]

Adenylate Cyclase. Adenylate cyclase, a membrane enzyme, is another target of muscarinic receptor activation. The second-messenger cAMP is synthesized within the cell from adenosine triphosphate (ATP) by the action of adenylate cyclase. The regulatory effects of cAMP are many, as it can activate various protein kinases. Protein kinases catalyze the phosphorylation of enzymes and ion channels, altering the amount of calcium entering the cell and thus affecting muscle contraction. Muscarinic receptor activation causes lower levels of cAMP, reducing cAMP protein-dependent kinase activity, and a relaxation of muscle contraction. Some have suggested that a GTP-inhibitory protein (G_i) reduces the activity of adenylate cyclase, causing smooth muscle relaxation (Fig. 17.4).[20,24]

Ion Channels. In addition to the action of protein kinases that phosphorylate ion channels and modify ion conductance, G proteins are coupled directly to ion channels to regulate their action.[24] The Ca^{2+} channel on the cell membrane is activated by G proteins without the need of a second messenger to allow Ca^{2+} to enter the cell. The α subunit of the G protein in heart tissue acts directly to open the K^+ channel, producing hyperpolarization of the membrane and slowing the heart rate.

CHOLINERGIC NEUROCHEMISTRY

Cholinergic neurons synthesize, store, and release ACh (Fig. 17.5). The neurons also form choline acetyltransferase (ChAT) and AChE. These enzymes are synthesized in the soma of the neuron and distributed throughout the neuron by axoplasmic flow. AChE is also located outside the neuron and is associated with the neuroglial cells in the synaptic cleft. ACh is prepared in the nerve ending by the transfer of an acetyl group from acetyl-coenzyme A (CoA) to choline. The reaction is catalyzed by ChAT. Cell fractionation studies show that much of the ACh is contained in synaptic vesicles in the nerve ending but that some is also free in the cytosol. Choline is the limiting substrate for the synthesis of ACh. Most choline for ACh synthesis comes from the hydrolysis of ACh in the synapse. Choline is recaptured by the presynaptic terminal as part of a high-affinity uptake system under the influence of sodium ions[25] to synthesize ACh.

Several quaternary ammonium bases act as competitive inhibitors of choline uptake. Hemicholinium (HC-3), a bisquaternary cyclic hemiacetal, and the triethyl analog of choline, 2-hydroxyethyltriethylammonium, act at the presynaptic membrane to inhibit the high-affinity uptake of choline into the neuron. These compounds cause a delayed paralysis at repetitively activated cholinergic synapses and can produce respiratory paralysis in test animals. The delayed block is caused by the depletion of stored ACh, which may be

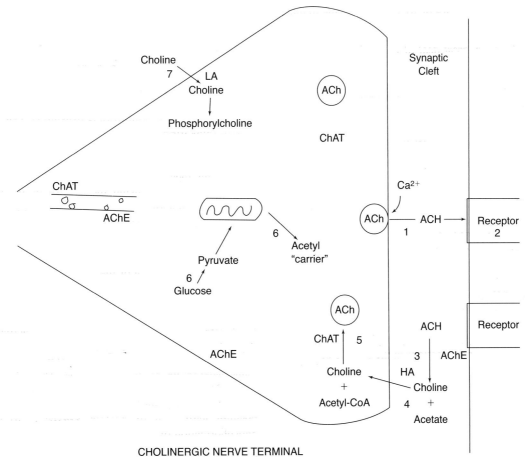

CHOLINERGIC NERVE TERMINAL

Figure 17.5 ● Hypothetical model of synthesis, storage, and release of ACh. **1.** ACh is released from storage granules under the influence of the nerve action potential and Ca^{2+}. **2.** ACh acts on postsynaptic cholinergic receptors. **3.** Hydrolysis of ACh by AChE occurs in the synaptic cleft. **4.** A high-affinity uptake system returns choline to the cytosol. **5.** ChAT synthesizes ACh in the cytosol, and the ACh is stored in granules. **6.** Glucose is converted to pyruvate, which is converted to acetyl-CoA in the mitochondria. Acetyl-CoA is released from the mitochondria by an acetyl carrier. **7.** Choline is also taken up into the neuron by a low-affinity uptake system and converted partly to phosphorylcholine.

Hemicholinium (HC-3)

2-Hydroxethyltriethylammonium

reversed by choline. The acetyl group used for the synthesis of ACh is obtained by conversion of glucose to pyruvate in the cytosol of the neuron and eventual formation of acetyl-CoA. Because of the impermeability of the mitochondrial membrane to acetyl-CoA, this substrate is brought into the cytosol by the aid of an acetyl "carrier."

The synthesis of ACh from choline and acetyl-CoA is catalyzed by ChAT. Transfer of the acetyl group from acetyl-CoA to choline may be by a random or an ordered reaction of the Theorell-Chance type. In the ordered sequence, acetyl-CoA first binds to the enzyme, forming a complex (EA) that then binds to choline. The acetyl group is transferred, and the ACh formed dissociates from the enzyme active site. The CoA is then released from the enzyme complex, EQ, to regenerate the free enzyme. The scheme is diagrammed in Figure 17.6. ChAT is inhibited in vitro by *trans-N-*methyl-4-(1-naphthylvinyl)pyridinium iodide[26]; however, its inhibitory activity in whole animals is unreliable.[27]

Newly formed ACh is released from the presynaptic membrane when a nerve action potential invades a presynaptic nerve terminal.[28] The release of ACh results from depolarization of the nerve terminal by the action potential, which alters membrane permeability to Ca^{2+}. Calcium enters the nerve terminal and causes release of the contents of several synaptic vesicles containing ACh into the synaptic cleft. This burst, or quantal release, of ACh causes depolarization of the postsynaptic membrane. The number of quanta of ACh released may be as high as several hundred at a neuromuscular junction, with each quantum containing between 12,000 and 60,000 molecules. ACh is also released spontaneously in small amounts from presynaptic membranes. This small amount of neurotransmitter maintains

muscle tone by acting on the cholinergic receptors on the postsynaptic membrane.

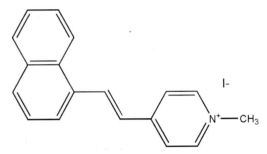

*trans-N-*Methyl-4-(1-napthylvinyl)pyridinium iodide

After ACh has been released into the synaptic cleft, its concentration decreases rapidly. It is generally accepted that there is enough AChE at nerve endings to hydrolyze into choline and acetate any ACh that has been liberated. For example, there is sufficient AChE in the nerve junction of rat intercostal muscle to hydrolyze about 2.7×10^8 ACh molecules in 1 ms; this far exceeds the 3×10^6 molecules released by one nerve impulse.[29]

◆ CHOLINERGIC AGONISTS

Cholinergic Stereochemistry

Three techniques have been used to study the conformational properties of ACh and other cholinergic chemicals: x-ray crystallography, nuclear magnetic resonance (NMR), and molecular modeling by computation. Each of these methods may report the spatial distribution of atoms in a molecule in terms of torsion angles. A *torsion angle* is defined as the angle formed between two planes, for example, by the O1—C5—C4—N atoms in ACh. The angle between the oxygen and nitrogen atoms is best depicted by means of Newman projections (Fig. 17.7). A torsion angle has a positive sign when the bond of the front atom is rotated to the right to eclipse the bond of the rear atom. The spatial orientation of ACh is described by four torsion angles (Fig. 17.8).

The conformation of the choline moiety of ACh has drawn the most attention in studies relating structure and

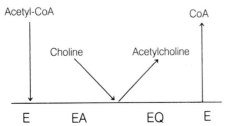

Figure 17.6 ● Ordered synthesis of acetylcholine (ACh) by choline acetyltransferase (ChAT).

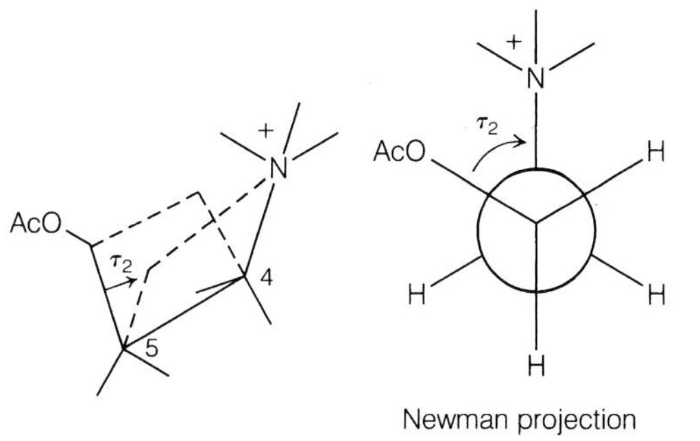

Figure 17.7 ● Spatial orientation of O1—C5—C4—N atoms in ACh.

TABLE 17.2 Conformational Properties of Some Cholinergic Agents

Compound	O1-C5-C4-N Torsion Angle
Acetylcholine bromide	+77
Acetylcholine chloride	+85
(+)-2S,3R,5S-Muscarine iodide	+73
Methylfurmethide iodide	+83
(+)-Acetyl-(S)-β-methylcholine iodide	+85
(−)-Acetyl-(R)-α-methylcholine iodide	
Crystal form A	+89
Crystal form B	−150
(+)-*cis*(2S)-Methyl-(4R)-trimethylammonium-1,3-dioxolane iodide	+68
(+)-*trans*(1S, 2S)-Acetoxycyclopropyltrimethyl ammonium iodide	+137
Carbamoylcholine bromide	+178
Acetylthiocholine bromide	+171
Acetyl-(Rα, Sβ)-dimethylcholine iodide (*erythro*)	+76

From Shefter, E.: Structural variations in cholinergic legends. In Triggle, D. J., Moran, J. F., and Barnard, E. A. (eds.). Cholinergic Ligand Interactions. New York, Academic Press, 1971, pp. 87–89.

pharmacological activity. The torsion angle (τ_2) determines the spatial orientation of the cationic head of ACh to the ester group. X-ray diffraction studies have shown that the torsion angle (τ_2) on ACh has a value of +77°. Many compounds that are muscarinic receptor agonists containing a choline component (e.g., O—C—C—N$^+$[CH$_3$]$_3$) have a preferred synclinal (gauche) conformation, with τ_2 values ranging from 68° to 89° (Table 17.2). Intermolecular packing forces in the crystal as well as electrostatic interactions between the charged nitrogen group and the ether oxygen of the ester group are probably the two dominant factors that lead to a preference for the synclinal conformation in the crystal state. Some choline esters display an antiperiplanar (*trans*) conformation between the onium and ester groups. For example, carbamoyl choline chloride (τ_2, +178°) is stabilized in this *trans* conformation by several hydrogen bonds. Acetylthiocholine iodide (τ_2, +171°) is in this conformation because of the presence of the bulkier and less electronegative sulfur atom, and (+) *trans*-(1S,2S)-acetoxycyclopropyltrimethylammonium iodide (τ_2, +137°) is fixed in this conformation by the rigidity of the cyclopropyl ring.

NMR spectroscopy of cholinergic molecules in solution is more limited than crystallography in delineating the conformation of compounds and is restricted to determining the torsion angle O1—C5—C4—N. Most NMR data are in agreement with the results of x-ray diffraction studies. NMR studies indicate that ACh and methacholine apparently are not in their most stable *trans* conformation but exist in one of two gauche conformers[30] (Fig. 17.9). This may result from strong intramolecular interactions that stabilize the conformation of these molecules in solution.[31]

Molecular orbital calculations based on the principles of quantum mechanics may be used to determine energy minima of rotating bonds and to predict preferred conformations for the molecule. By means of molecular mechanics, theoretical conformational analysis has found that ACh has an energy minimum for the τ_2 torsion angle at about 84° and that the preferred conformation of ACh corresponds closely in aqueous solution to that found in the crystal state.

The study of interactions between bimolecules and small molecules is of great interest and importance toward the understanding of drug action. These studies are challenging because of the large size of at least one molecule. For the first time, the conformation of a neurotransmitter has been determined for a molecule in the bound state. ACh is transformed from the gauche conformation in the free state to a nearly *trans* conformation when bound to the nicotinic receptor.[32] The active conformation of muscarinic agonists on their receptor has a dihedral angle of τ_2 between 110° and 117°.[33]

The parasympathomimetic effects of muscarine were first reported in 1869,[34] but its structure was not elucidated until 1957.[35] Muscarine has four geometric isomers: muscarine, epimuscarine, allomuscarine, and epiallomuscarine (Fig. 17.10). None has a center or plane of symmetry. Each geometric isomer can exist as an enantiomeric pair. The activity of muscarine, a nonselective muscarinic receptor agonist, resides primarily in the naturally occurring (+)-muscarine enantiomer.

It is essentially free of nicotinic activity and apparently has the optimal stereochemistry to act on the muscarinic receptor subtypes. Synthetic molecules with a substituent on the carbon atom that corresponds to the β carbon of ACh also show great differences in muscarinic activity between their isomers. Acetyl-(+)-(S)-β-methylcholine, (+)-*cis*-(2S)-methyl-(4R)-trimethylammonium-1,3-dioxolane, (+)-*trans*-(1S,2S)-acetoxycyclopropyltrimethylammonium, and naturally occurring (+)-(2S,3R,5S)-muscarine are more potent than their enantiomers and have very high ratios of activity between the (S)- and (R)-isomer (Table 17.3). A similar observation may be made of (+)-acetyl-(S)-β-methylcholine, (+)-*cis*-(2S)-methyl-(4R)-trimethylammonium-1,3-dioxolane, and (+)-*trans*-(1S,2S)-acetoxycyclopropyltrimethylammonium, all of

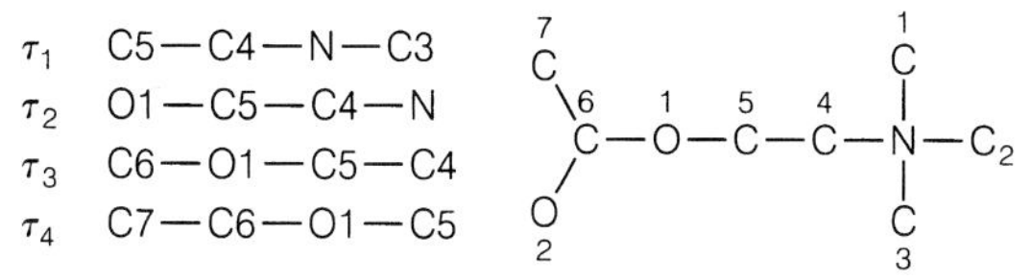

τ_1 C5—C4—N—C3
τ_2 O1—C5—C4—N
τ_3 C6—O1—C5—C4
τ_4 C7—C6—O1—C5

Figure 17.8 ● ACh torsion angles.

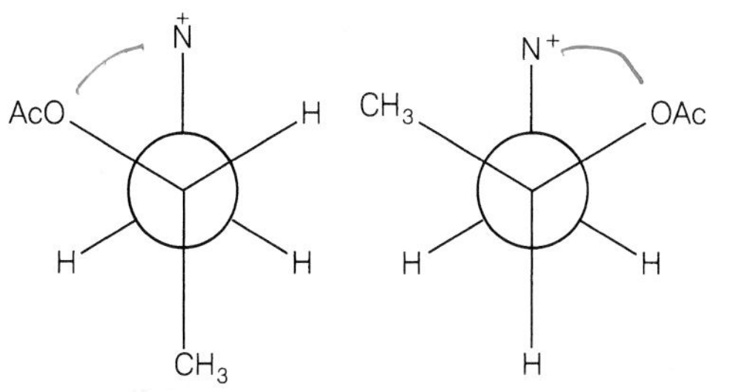

Figure 17.9 ● Gauche conformers of methacholine.

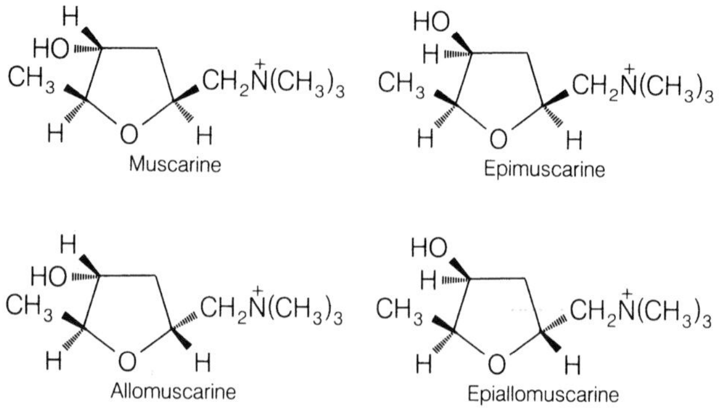

Muscarine

Epimuscarine

Allomuscarine

Epiallomuscarine

Figure 17.10 • Geometric isomers of muscarine.

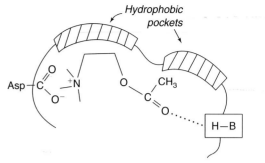

Figure 17.11 • Hypothetical structure of the muscarinic receptor.

which have an (*S*) configuration at the carbon atom that corresponds to the β carbon of ACh. Each of these active muscarinic molecules may be deployed on the receptor in the same manner as ACh and (+)-muscarine. Their (*S*)/(*R*) ratios (Table 17.3) show the greatest stereoselectivity of the muscarinic receptor in guinea pig ileum for the configuration at the carbon adjacent to the ester group. In contrast, the nicotinic receptors are not considered as highly stereoselective as their muscarinic counterparts.

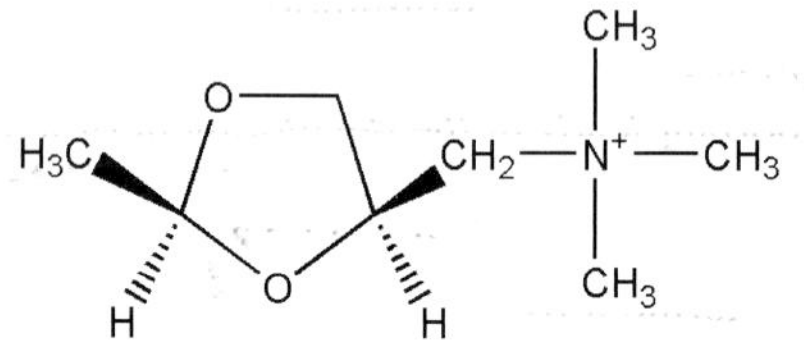

cis-2-Methyl-4-trimethylammonium-1,3-dioxolane

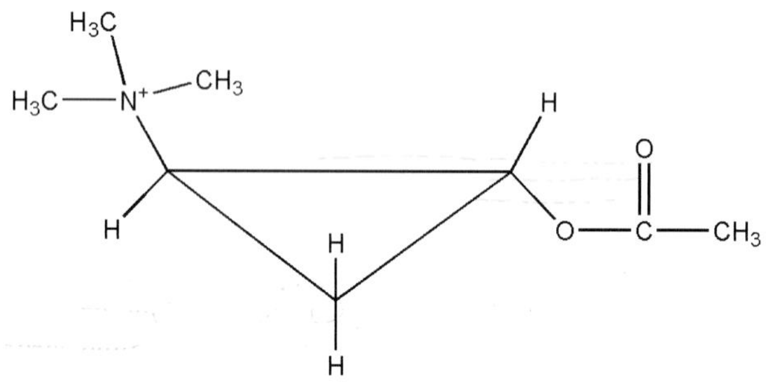

trans-2-Acetoxycyclopropyltrimethylammonium

Structure–Activity Relationships

Although muscarinic receptors have been cloned and the amino acid sequences are known, their three-dimensional structures remain unresolved. Thus, it is not possible to use this information alone to design specific drug molecules. Scientists still use pharmacological and biochemical tests to determine optimal structural requirements for activity. ACh is a relatively simple molecule. The chemistry and ease of testing for ACh biological activity have allowed numerous chemical derivatives to be made and studied. Alterations on the molecule may be divided into three categories: the onium group, the ester function, and the choline moiety.

The onium group is essential for intrinsic activity and contributes to the affinity of the molecule for the receptors, partially through the binding energy and partially because of its action as a detecting and directing group. Molecular modeling data show the binding site to be a negatively charged aspartic acid residue in the third of the seven transmembrane helixes of the muscarinic receptor.[36] Hydrophobic pockets are located in helices 4, 5, 6, and 7 of the muscarinic receptor (Fig. 17.11).[37] The trimethylammonium group is the optimal functional moiety for activity, although some significant exceptions are known (e.g., pilocarpine, arecoline, nicotine, and oxotremorine). Phosphonium, sulfonium, arsenonium isosteres, or substituents larger than methyl on the nitrogen increase the size of the onium moiety, produce diffusion of the positive charge, and interfere sterically with proper drug–receptor interaction, resulting in decreased activity (Table 17.4).

The ester group in ACh contributes to the binding of the compound to the muscarinic receptor because of hydrogen bond formation with threonine and asparagine residues at

TABLE 17.3 Equipotent Molar Ratios of Isomers on Guinea Pig Ileum: Ratios Relative to Acetylcholine

Compound	Guinea Pig Ileum	(*S*)/(*R*) Ratio
(+)-Acetyl-(*S*)-β-methylcholine chloride	1.0[a]	24
(−)-Acetyl-(*R*)-β-methylcholine chloride	24.0[a]	
(+)-(2*S*,3*R*,5*S*)-Muscarine iodide	0.33[b]	394
(−)-(2*R*,3*S*,5*R*)-Muscarine iodide	130[b]	
(+)-*cis*(2*S*)-Methyl-(4*R*)-trimethylammonium-1,3-dioxolane iodide	6.00[c]	100
(−)-*cis*(2*R*)-Methyl-(4*S*)-trimethylammonium-1,3-dioxolane iodide	0.06[c]	
(+)-*trans*(1*S*,2*S*)-Acetoxycyclopropyltrimethylammonium iodide	00.88[d]	517
(−)-*trans*(1*R*,2*R*)-Acetoxycyclopropyltrimethylammonium iodide	455[d]	

[a]Beckett, A. H., et al.: Nature 189:671, 1961.
[b]Waser, P. I.: Pharmacol. Rev. 13:465, 1961.
[c]Belleau, B., and Puranen, J.: J. Med. Chem. 6:235–328, 1963.
[d]Armstrong, P. D., Cannon, J. G., and Long, J. P.: Nature 220:65–66, 1968.

TABLE 17.4 Activity of Acetoxyethyl Onium Salts: Equipotent Molar Ratios Relative to Acetylcholine

$CH_3COOCH_2CH_2$	Cat Blood Pressure	Intestine	Frog Heart
N_+Me_3	1	1 (Rabbit)	1
N^+Me_2H	50	40	50
N^+MeH_2	500	1,000	500
N^+H_3	2,000	20,000	40,000
N^+Me_2Et	3	2.5 (Guinea pig)	2
N^+MeEt_2	400	700	1,500
N^+Et_3	2,000	1,700	10,000[a]
N^+PMe_3	13	12 (Rabbit)	12
As^+Me_3	66	90	83
S^+Me_2	50	30 (Guinea pig)	96
N	d = 1.47 Å	d' = 2.4 Å	
P	1.87	3.05	
S	1.82	—	
As	1.98	3.23	

Data are from Barlow, R. B.: Introduction to Chemical Pharmacology. London, Methuen and Co., 1964; Welsh, A. D., and Roepke, M. H.: J. Pharmacol. Exp. Ther. 55:118, 1935; Stehle, K. L., Melville, K. J., and Oldham, F. K.: J. Pharmacol. Exp. Ther. 56:473, 1936; Holton, P., and Ing, H. R.: Br. J. Pharmacol. 4:190, 1949; Ing, H. R., Kordik, P., and Tudor Williams, D. P. H.: Br. J. Pharmacol. 7:103, 1952.
[a]Reduces effect of acetylcholine.

the receptor site. A comparison of the cholinergic activity of a series of alkyltrimethylammonium compounds [R-$N^+(CH_3)$, R = C_1–C_9] shows *n*-amyltrimethylammonium,[38] which may be considered to have a size and mass similar to those of ACh and to be one magnitude weaker as a muscarinic agonist. The presence of the acetyl group in ACh is not as critical as the size of the molecule. Studying a series of *n*-alkyltrimethylammonium salts revealed[39] that for maximal muscarinic activity, the quaternary ammonium group should be followed by a chain of five atoms; this has been referred to as the *five-atom rule*.

Shortening or lengthening the chain of atoms that separates the ester group from the onium moiety reduces muscarinic activity. An α substitution on the choline moiety decreases both nicotinic and muscarinic activity, but muscarinic activity is decreased to a greater extent. Nicotinic activity is decreased to a greater degree by substitution on the β carbon. Therefore, acetyl α-methylcholine, although less potent than ACh, has more nicotinic than muscarinic activity, whereas acetyl-β-methylcholine (methacholine) exhibits more muscarinic than nicotinic activity. Hydrolysis by AChE is more affected by substitutions on the β than the α carbon. The hydrolysis rate of racemic acetyl β-methylacetylcholine is about 50% of that of ACh; racemic acetyl α-ACh is hydrolyzed about 90% as fast.

Oxotremorine. Oxotremorine [1-(-pyrrolidono)-4-pyrrolidino-2-butyne] has been regarded as a CNS muscarinic stimulant. Its action on the brain produces tremors in experimental animals. It increases ACh brain levels in rats up to 40% and has been studied as a drug in the treatment of Alzheimer disease. Although earlier studies suggested that this approach of elevating levels of ACh to treat Alzheimer disease is useful, this belief was highly disputed by many researchers. Nevertheless, oxotremorine, as a cholinergic agonist, facilitates memory storage.[40] These findings have served as important leads in the development of agents useful in treating Alzheimer disease. Although it possesses groups that do not occur in other highly active muscarinic agents, oxotremorine's *trans* conformation shows that distances between possible active centers correspond with (+)-muscarine (Fig. 17.12).[41]

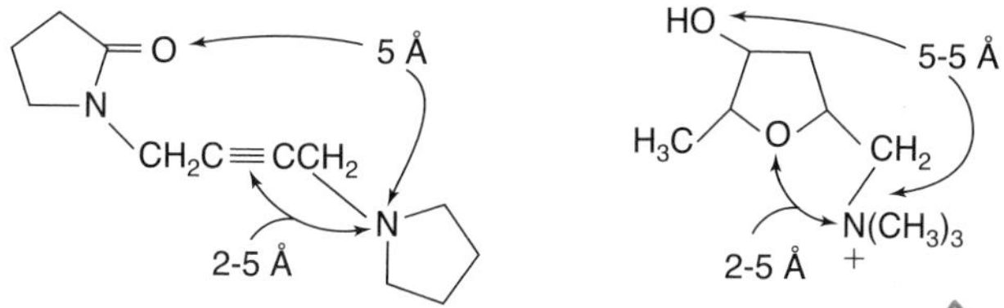

Arecoline. Arecoline is an alkaloid obtained from the seeds of the betel nut (*Areca catechu*). For many years, natives of the East Indies have consumed the betel nut as a source of a euphoria-creating substance.

CHOLINERGIC RECEPTOR ANTAGONISTS

Characterization of muscarinic receptors can now be extended beyond the pharmacological observations on organ systems (e.g., smooth muscle, heart) to determine structure–activity relationships. Dissociation constants of antagonists from radioligand-binding experiments on the various muscarinic receptors have played a major role in identifying these receptors and the selectivity of antagonists to the five muscarinic receptor subtypes. Antagonists with high affinity for one receptor and a low affinity for the other four receptor types are very few, however, and many antagonists bind to several subtypes with equal affinity. M_1 receptors have been identified as those with high affinity for pirenzepine and low affinity for a compound such as AF-DX 116. Pirenzepine can distinguish between M_1 and M_2, M_3, or M_5 but has significant affinity for M_4 receptors. Himbacine can distinguish between M_1 and M_4 receptors. Methoctramine, a polymethylenetetramine, not only discriminates between M_1 and M_2 receptors but also has good selectivity for M_2 muscarinic receptors. M_2 receptors bind to AF-DX 116 and gallamine, a neuromuscular blocking agent. M_3 receptors have a high affinity for 4-diphenylacetoxy-*N*-methylpiperidine (4-DAMP) and hexahydrosiladifenidol (HHSiD) but

Figure 17.12 ● Comparison of the geometries of oxotremorine and muscarine.

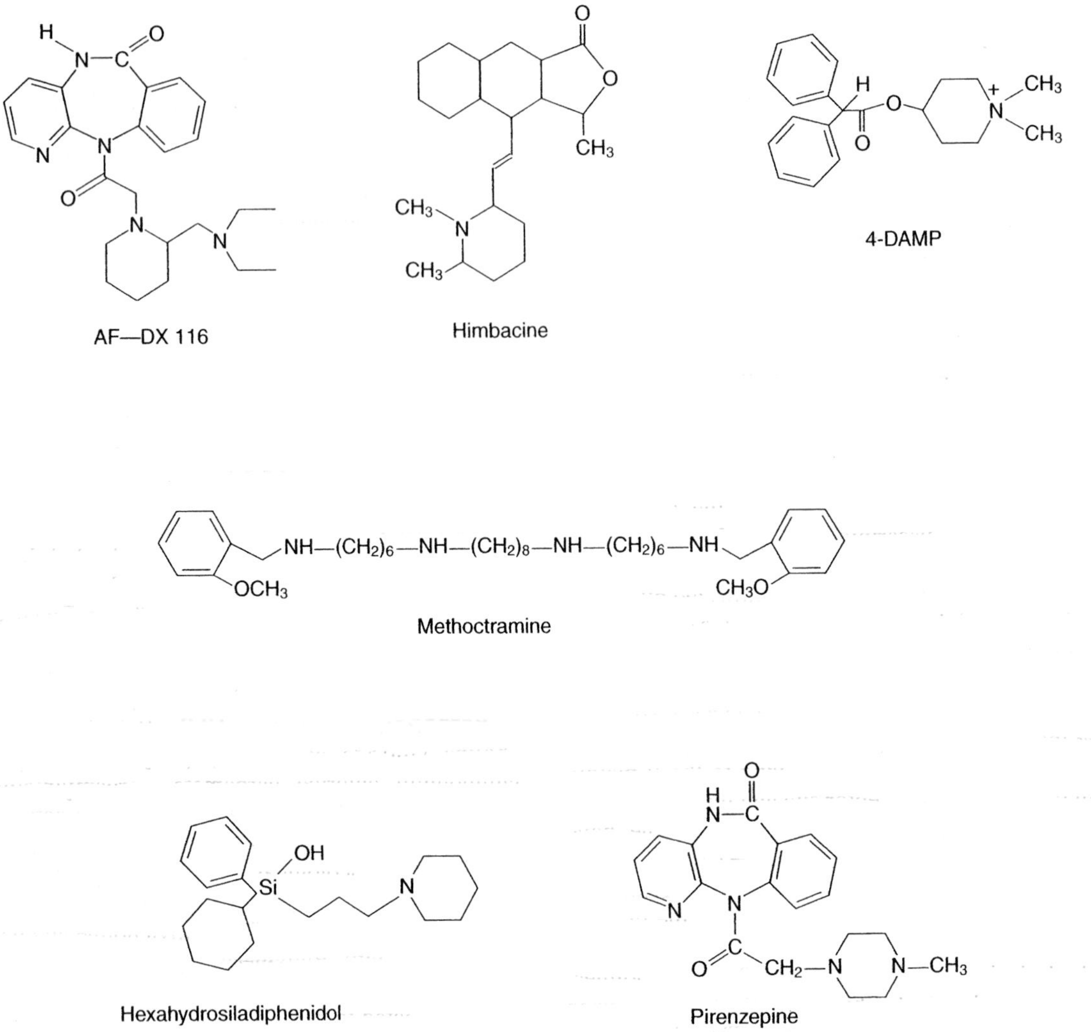

AF—DX 116

Himbacine

4-DAMP

Methoctramine

Hexahydrosiladiphenidol

Pirenzepine

Figure 17.13 ● Chemical structures of partially selective muscarinic antagonists.

also exhibit affinity for M_1 and M_2 receptors.[21] Tropicamide has been reported to be a putative M_4 receptor antagonist. Figure 17.13 includes structures of some receptor subtype antagonists.

① ↓ DOA ← hydrolysis
② non selective

Products

Acetylcholine Chloride. ACh chloride exerts a powerful stimulant effect on the parasympathetic nervous system. Attempts have been made to use it as a cholinergic agent, but its duration of action is too short for sustained effects, because of rapid hydrolysis by esterases and lack of specificity when administered for systemic effects. It is a cardiac depressant and an effective vasodilator. Stimulation of the vagus and the parasympathetic nervous system produces a tonic action on smooth muscle and induces a flow from the salivary and lacrimal glands. Its cardiac-depressant effect results from (a) a negative chronotropic effect that causes a decrease in heart rate and (b) a negative inotropic action on heart muscle that produces a decrease in the force of myocardial contractions. The vasodilatory action of ACh is primarily on the arteries and the arterioles, with distinct effect on the peripheral vascular system. Bronchial constriction is a characteristic side effect when the drug is given systemically.

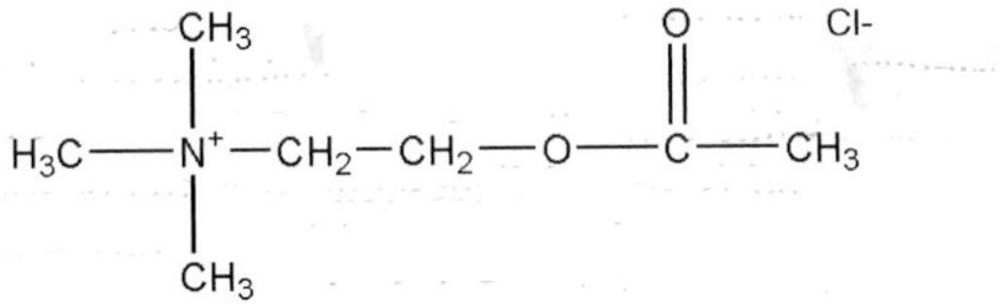

Acetylcholine Chloride

One of the most effective antagonists to the action of ACh is atropine, a nonselective muscarinic antagonist. Atropine blocks the depressant effect of ACh on cardiac muscle and its production of peripheral vasodilation (i.e., muscarinic effects) but does not affect the skeletal muscle contraction (i.e., nicotinic effect) produced.

ACh chloride is a hygroscopic powder that is available in an admixture with mannitol to be dissolved in sterile water for injection shortly before use. It is a short-acting miotic when introduced into the anterior chamber of the eye and is especially useful after cataract surgery during the placement of sutures. When applied topically to the eye, it has little therapeutic value because of poor corneal penetration and rapid hydrolysis by AChE.

Methacholine Chloride, United States Pharmacopeia (USP). Methacholine chloride, acetyl-β-methylcholine chloride or (2-hydroxypropyl)trimethylammonium chloride acetate, is the acetyl ester of β-methylcholine. Unlike ACh, methacholine has sufficient stability in the body to give sustained parasympathetic stimulation. This action is accompanied by little (1/1,000 that of ACh) or no nicotinic effect.

Methacholine Chloride

Methacholine can exist as (S) and (R) enantiomers. Although the chemical is used as the racemic mixture, its muscarinic activity resides principally in the (S)-isomer. The (S)/(R) ratio of muscarinic potency for these enantiomers is 240:1.

(+)-Acetyl-(S)-β-methylcholine is hydrolyzed by AChE, whereas the (R)(−)-isomer is not. (−)-Acetyl-(R)-β-methylcholine is a weak competitive inhibitor (K_i, 4×10^{-4} M) of AChE obtained from the electric organ of the eel (*E. electricus*). The hydrolysis rate of the (S)(+)-isomer is about 54% that of ACh. This rate probably compensates for any decreased association (affinity) owing to the β-methyl group with the muscarinic receptor site and may account for the fact that ACh and (+)-acetyl-β-methylcholine have equimolar muscarinic potencies in vivo. (−)-Acetyl-(R)-β-methylcholine weakly inhibits AChE and slightly reinforces the muscarinic activity of the (S)(+)-isomer in the racemic mixture of acetyl-β-methylcholine.

In the hydrolysis of the acetyl α- and β-methylcholines, the greatest stereochemical inhibitory effects occur when the choline is substituted in the β-position. This also appears to be true of organophosphorous inhibitors. The (R)(−)- and (S)(+)-isomers of acetyl-α-methylcholine are hydrolyzed at 78% and 97% of the rate of ACh, respectively.

Methacholine chloride occurs as colorless or white crystals or as a white crystalline powder. It is odorless or has a slight odor and is very deliquescent. It is freely soluble in water, alcohol, or chloroform, and its aqueous solution is neutral to litmus and bitter. It is hydrolyzed rapidly in alkaline solutions. Solutions are relatively stable to heat and will keep for at least 2 or 3 weeks when refrigerated to delay growth of molds.

Carbachol. Choline chloride carbamate is nonspecific in its action on muscarinic receptor subtypes. The pharmacological activity of carbachol is similar to that of ACh. It is an ester of choline and thus possesses both muscarinic and nicotinic properties by cholinergic receptor stimulation. It can also act indirectly by promoting release of ACh and by its weak anticholinesterase activity. Carbachol forms a carbamyl ester in the active site of AChE, which is hydrolyzed more slowly than an acetyl ester. This slower hydrolysis rate reduces the amount of free enzyme and prolongs the duration of ACh in the synapse. Carbachol also stimulates the autonomic ganglia and causes contraction of skeletal muscle but differs from a true muscarinic agent in that it does not have cardiovascular activity despite the fact that it seems to affect M_2 receptors.[42]

Carbachol is a miotic and has been used to reduce the intraocular tension of glaucoma when a response cannot be obtained with pilocarpine or neostigmine. Penetration of the cornea is poor but can be enhanced by the use of a wetting agent in the ophthalmic solution. In addition to its topical use for glaucoma, carbachol is used during ocular surgery, when a more prolonged miosis is required than can be obtained with ACh chloride.

Carbachol Chloride

Carbachol differs chemically from ACh in its stability to hydrolysis. The carbamyl group of carbachol decreases the electrophilicity of the carbonyl and, thus, can form resonance structures more easily than ACh can. The result is that carbachol is less susceptible to hydrolysis and, therefore, more stable in aqueous solutions.

Bethanechol Chloride, USP. Bethanechol, β-methylcholine chloride carbamate, (2-hydroxypropyl)trimethylammonium chloride carbamate, carbamylmethylcholine chloride (Urecholine), is nonspecific in its action on muscarinic receptor subtypes but appears to be more effective at eliciting pharmacological action of M_3 receptors.[43] It has pharmacological properties similar to those of methacholine. Both are esters of β-methylcholine and have feeble nicotinic activity. Bethanechol is inactivated more slowly by AChE in vivo than is methacholine. It is a carbamyl ester and is expected to have stability in aqueous solutions similar to that of carbachol.

The main use of bethanechol chloride is in the relief of urinary retention and abdominal distention after surgery. The drug is used orally and by subcutaneous injection. It must never be administered by intramuscular or intravenous injection because of the danger from cholinergic overstimulation and loss of selective action. Proper administration of the drug is associated with low toxicity and no serious side effects. Bethanechol chloride should be used with caution in asthmatic patients; when used for glaucoma, it produces frontal headaches from the constriction of the sphincter muscle in the eye and from ciliary muscle spasms. Its duration of action is 1 hour.

Bethanechol Chloride

Pilocarpine Hydrochloride, USP. Pilocarpine monohydrochloride is the hydrochloride of an alkaloid obtained from the dried leaflets of *Pilocarpus jaborandi* or *P. microphyllus*, in which it occurs to the extent of about 0.5% together with other alkaloids.

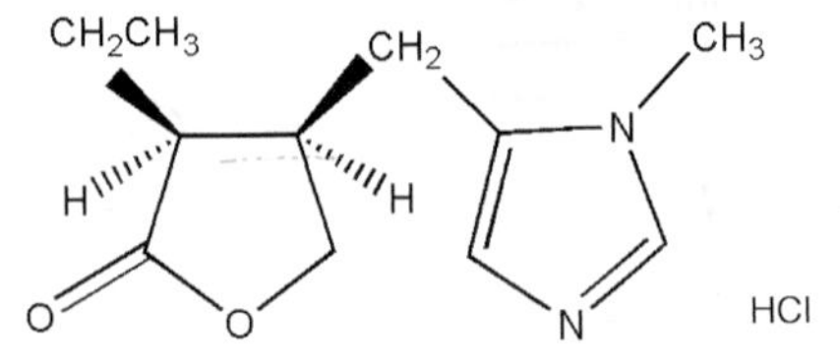

Pilocarpine Hydrochloride

It occurs as colorless, translucent, odorless, faintly bitter crystals that are soluble in water (1:0.3), alcohol (1:3), and chloroform (1:360). (In this chapter, a solubility expressed as 1:360 indicates that 1 g is soluble in 360 mL of the solvent at 25°C. Solubilities at other temperatures are so indicated.) It is hygroscopic and affected by light; its solutions are acid to litmus and may be sterilized by autoclaving. Alkalies saponify the lactone group to give the pharmacologically inactive hydroxy acid (pilocarpic acid). Base-catalyzed epimerization at the ethyl group position occurs to an appreciable extent and is another major pathway of degradation.[44] Both routes result in loss of pharmacological activity.

Pilocarpine is a nonselective agonist on the muscarinic receptors. Despite this, it reportedly acts on M_3 receptors in smooth muscle to cause contractions in the gut, trachea, and eye.[45,46] In the eye, it produces pupillary constriction (miosis) and a spasm of accommodation. These effects are valuable in the treatment of glaucoma. The pupil constriction and spasm of the ciliary muscle reduce intraocular tension by establishing better drainage of ocular fluid through the canal of Schlemm, located near the corner of the iris and cornea. Pilocarpine is used as a 0.5% to 0.6% solution (i.e., of the salts) in treating glaucoma. Systemic effects include copious sweating, salivation, and gastric secretion.

Pilocarpine Nitrate, USP. Pilocarpine mononitrate occurs as shining white crystals that are not hygroscopic but are light sensitive. It is soluble in water (1:4) and alcohol (1:75) but insoluble in chloroform and ether. Aqueous solutions are slightly acid to litmus and may be sterilized in the autoclave. The alkaloid is incompatible with alkalies, iodides, silver nitrate, and reagents that precipitate alkaloids.

Cevimeline Hydrochloride. Cevimeline (Evoxac) is *cis*-2'-methylspiro {1-azabicyclo [2.2.2] octane-3, 5' -[1,3] oxathiolane} hydrochloride, hydrate (2:1). Cevimeline has a molecular weight of 244.79 and is a white to off white crystalline powder. It is freely soluble in alcohol, chloroform, and water. Cevimeline is a cholinergic agonist which binds to the M_3 muscarinic receptor subtype, which results in an increase secretion of exocrine glands, such as salivary and sweat glands. Because of these effects, it was approved for use in the treatment of dry mouth associated with Sjögren syndrome. By stimulating the salivary muscarinic receptors cevimeline promotes secretion thereby alleviating dry-mouth in these patients. Cevimeline is metabolized by the isozymes CYP2D6 and CYP3A3 and CYP3A4. It has a half-life of 5 hours.[47]

Cholinesterase Inhibitors

There are two types of cholinesterases in humans, AChE and butyrylcholinesterase (BuChE). The cholinesterases differ in their location in the body and their substrate specificity. AChE is associated with the outside surface of glial cells in the synapse and catalyzes the hydrolysis of ACh to choline and acetic acid. Inhibition of AChE prolongs the duration of the neurotransmitter in the junction and produces pharmacological effects similar to those observed when ACh is administered. These inhibitors are indirect-acting cholinergic agonists. AChE inhibitors have been used in the treatment of myasthenia gravis, atony in the GI tract, and glaucoma. They have also been used as agricultural insecticides and nerve gases. More recently, they have received attention as symptomatic drug treatments in patients suffering from Alzheimer disease.[48]

BuChE (pseudocholinesterase) is located in human plasma. Although its biological function is not clear, it has catalytic properties similar to those of AChE. The substrate specificity is broader (Table 17.5), and it may hydrolyze dietary esters and drug molecules in the blood.

Three different chemical groupings, acetyl, carbamyl, and phosphoryl, may react with the esteratic site of AChE. Although the chemical reactions are similar, the kinetic parameters for each type of substrate differ and result in differences between toxicity and usefulness.

The initial step in the hydrolysis of ACh by AChE is a reversible enzyme–substrate complex formation. The association rate (k_{+1}) and dissociation rate (k_{-1}) are relatively large. The enzyme–substrate complex, E_A–ACh, may also

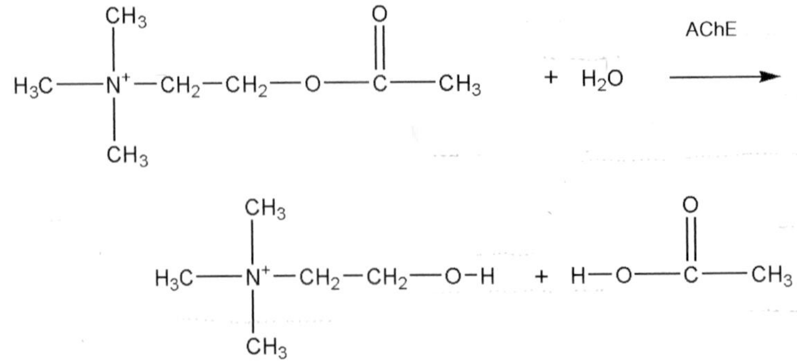

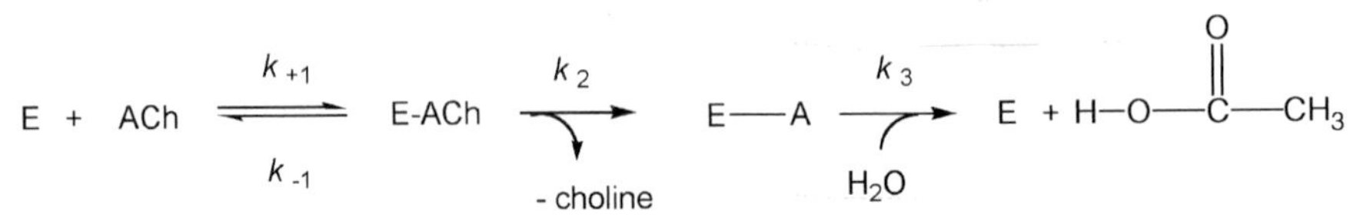

TABLE 17.5 **Hydrolysis of Various Substrates by AChE and BuChE**

	AChE		BuChE	
Enzyme Substrate	Source	Relative Rate[a]	Source	Relative Rate[a]
Acetylcholine	Human or bovine RBC	100	Human or horse plasma	100
Acetylthiocholine	Bovine RBC	149	Horse plasma	407
Acetyl-β-methylcholine	Bovine RBC	18	Horse plasma	0
Propionylcholine	Human RBC	80	Horse plasma	170
Butyrylcholine	Human RBC	2.5	Horse plasma	250
Butyrylthiocholine	Bovine RBC	0	Horse plasma	590
Benzoylcholine	Bovine RBC	0	Horse plasma	67
Ethyl acetate	Human RBC	2	Human plasma	1
3,3-Dimethylbutyl acetate	Human RBC	60	Human plasma	35
2-Chloroethyl acetate	Human RBC	37	Human plasma	10
Isoamyl acetate	Human RBC	24	Horse plasma	7
Isoamyl propionate	Human RBC	10	Horse plasma	13
Isoamyl butyrate	Human RBC	1	Horse plasma	14

Adapted from Heath, D. F.: Organophosphorus Poisons—Anticholinesterases and Related Compounds. New York, Pergamon Press, 1961.
[a]Relative rates at approximately optimal substrate concentration; rate with acetylcholine = 100.

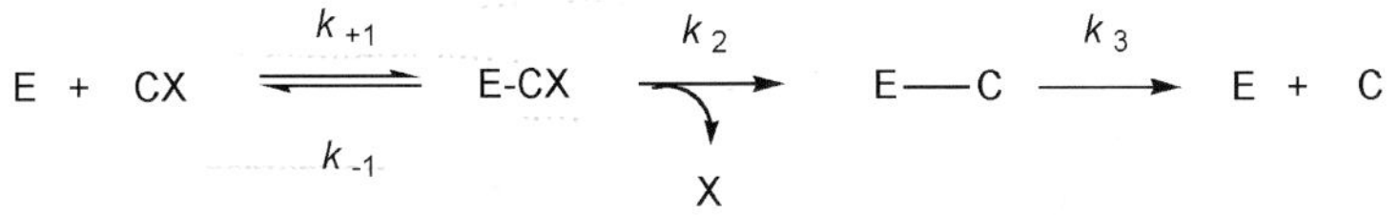

$$E \; + \; CX \; \underset{k_{-1}}{\overset{k_{+1}}{\rightleftharpoons}} \; E\text{-}CX \; \overset{k_2}{\underset{X}{\searrow}} \; E\text{---}C \; \overset{k_3}{\longrightarrow} \; E \; + \; C$$

where CX = carbamylating substrate

form an acetyl-enzyme intermediate at a rate (k_2) that is slower than either the association or dissociation rates. Choline is released from this complex with the formation of the acetyl-enzyme intermediate, EA. This intermediate is then hydrolyzed to regenerate the free enzyme and acetic acid. The acetylation rate, k_2, is the slowest step in this sequence and is rate-limiting (see discussion that follow).

Kinetic studies with different substrates and inhibitors suggest that the active center of AChE consists of several major domains: an anionic site, to which the trimethylammonium group binds; an esteratic site, which causes hydrolysis of the ester portion of ACh; and hydrophobic sites, which bind aryl substrates, other uncharged ligands, and the alkyl portion of the acyl moiety of ACh. There is also a peripheral anionic site, removed by at least 20 Å from this active center, which allosterically regulates activity at the esteratic site.[49] The anionic site was believed to have been formed by the γ-carboxylate group of a glutamic acid residue,[50] but more recent studies suggest that the aromatic moieties of tryptophan and phenylalanine residues bind the quaternary ammonium group of ACh in the anionic site through cation$-\pi$ interactions.[51] The location and spatial organization in the esteratic site by serine, histidine, and glutamic acid residues constitute the esteratic site. The triad of these amino acid residues contributes to the high catalytic efficiency of AChE (Fig. 17.14).[52]

AChE attacks the ester substrate through a serine hydroxyl, forming a covalent acyl-enzyme complex. The serine is activated as a nucleophile by the glutamic acid and histidine residues that serve as the proton sink to attack the carbonyl carbon of ACh. Choline is released, leaving the acetylated serine residue on the enzyme. The acetyl-enzyme

intermediate is cleaved by a general base catalysis mechanism to regenerate the free enzyme. The rate of the deacetylation step is indicated by k_3.

Carbamates such as carbachol are also able to serve as substrates for AChE, forming a carbamylated enzyme intermediate (E–C). The rate of carbamylation (k_2) is slower than the rate of acetylation. Hydrolysis (k_3, decarbamylation) of the carbamyl-enzyme intermediate is 10^7 times slower than that of its acetyl counterpart. The slower hydrolysis rate limits the optimal functional capacity of AChE, allowing carbamate substrates to be semireversible inhibitors of AChE.

In the mechanism above, k_3 is rate-limiting. The rate k_2 depends not only on the nature of the

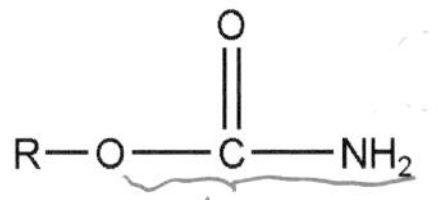

$$R\text{---}O\text{---}\overset{\displaystyle O}{\overset{\|}{C}}\text{---}NH_2$$

alcohol moiety of the ester but also on the type of carbamyl ester. Esters of carbamic acid are better

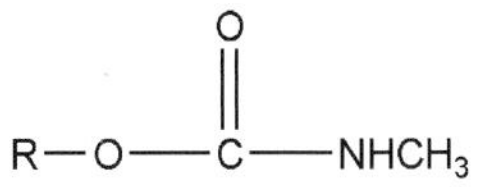

$$R\text{---}O\text{---}\overset{\displaystyle O}{\overset{\|}{C}}\text{---}NHCH_3$$

carbamylating agents of AChE than the methylcarbamyl

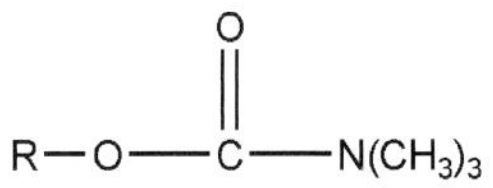

$$R\text{---}O\text{---}\overset{\displaystyle O}{\overset{\|}{C}}\text{---}N(CH_3)_3$$

and dimethylcarbamyl analogs.[53]

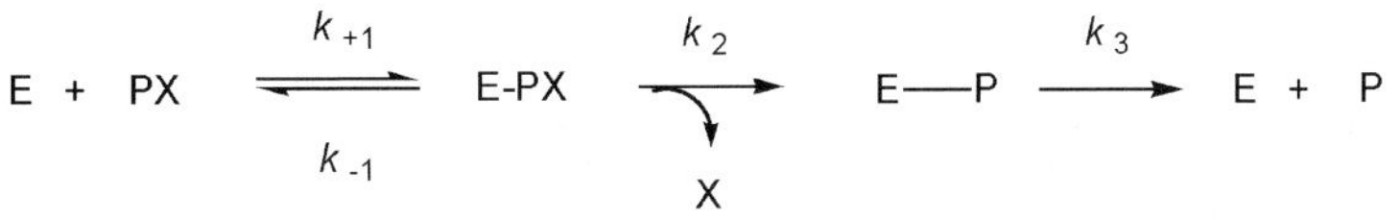

$$E \; + \; PX \; \underset{k_{-1}}{\overset{k_{+1}}{\rightleftharpoons}} \; E\text{-}PX \; \overset{k_2}{\underset{X}{\searrow}} \; E\text{---}P \; \overset{k_3}{\longrightarrow} \; E \; + \; P$$

where PX = phosphorylating substrate

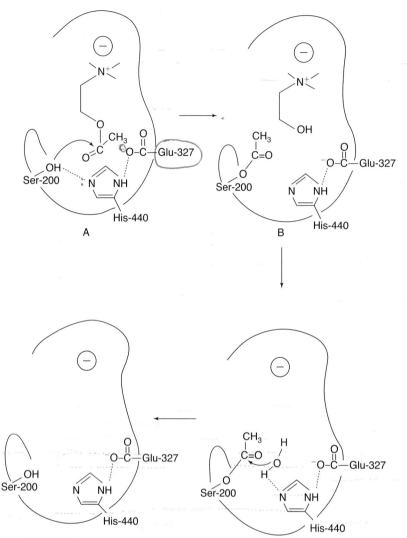

Figure 17.14 ● Mechanism of hydrolysis of ACh by AChE. **A.** ACh–AChE reversible complex. **B.** Acetylation of esteratic site. **C.** General base-catalyzed hydrolysis of acetylated enzyme. **D.** Free enzyme.

Organophosphate esters of selected compounds can also esterify the serine residue in the active site of AChE. The hydrolysis rate (k_3) of the phosphorylated serine is extremely slow, and hydrolysis to the free enzyme and phosphoric acid derivative is so limited that the inhibition is considered irreversible. These organophosphorous compounds are used in the treatment of glaucoma as agricultural insecticides, and, at times, as nerve gases in warfare and bioterrorism. Finally, some have either been or are currently being evaluated for use against Alzheimer disease. Table 17.6 shows the relative potencies of several AChE inhibitors.

Reversible Inhibitors

Physostigmine, USP. Physostigmine is an alkaloid obtained from the dried ripe seed of *Physostigma venenosum.* It occurs as a white, odorless, microcrystalline powder that is slightly soluble in water and freely soluble in alcohol, chloroform, and the fixed oils. The alkaloid, as the free base, is quite sensitive to heat, light, moisture, and bases, undergoing rapid decomposition. In solution, it is hydrolyzed to methyl carbamic acid and eseroline, neither of which inhibits AChE. Eseroline is oxidized to a red compound, rubreserine,[54] and then further decomposed to eserine blue and eserine brown. Addition of sulfite or ascorbic acid prevents oxidation of the phenol, eseroline, to rubreserine. Hydrolysis does take place, however, and the physostigmine is inactivated. Solutions are most stable at pH 6 and should never be sterilized by heat.

TABLE 17.6 **Inhibition Constants for Anticholinesterase Potency of Acetylcholinesterase Inhibitors**

Reversible and Semireversible Inhibitors	K_1 (M)
Ambenonium	4.0×10^{-8}
Carbachol	1.0×10^{-4}
Demecarium	1.0×10^{-10}
Edrophonium	3.0×10^{-7}
Neostigmine	1.0×10^{-7}
Physostigmine	1.0×10^{-8}
Pyridostigmine	4.0×10^{-7}

Irreversible Inhibitors	K_2 (mol/min)
Isoflurophate	1.9×10^{4}
Echothiophate	1.2×10^{5}
Paraoxon	1.1×10^{6}
Sarin	6.3×10^{7}
Tetraethylpyrophosphate	2.1×10^{8}

Physostigmine

Eseroline

Red

Rubreserine

Physostigmine is a relatively poor carbamylating agent of AChE and is often considered a reversible inhibitor of the enzyme. Its cholinesterase-inhibiting properties vary with the pH of the medium (Fig. 17.15). The conjugate acid of physostigmine has a pKa of about 8, and as the pH of the solution is lowered, more is present in the protonated form. Inhibition of cholinesterase is greater in acid media, suggesting that the protonated form makes a contribution to the inhibitory activity well as its carbamylation of the enzyme.

Physostigmine Salicylate *(for Glaucoma)*

Physostigmine was used first as a topical application in the treatment of glaucoma. Its lipid solubility properties permit adequate absorption from ointment bases. It is used systemically as an antidote for atropine poisoning and other anticholinergic drugs by increasing the duration of action of ACh at cholinergic sites through inhibition of AChE. Physostigmine, along with other cholinomimetic drugs acting in the CNS, has been studied for use in the treatment of Alzheimer disease.[55] Cholinomimetics that are currently used or which have been recently evaluated in the treatment of Alzheimer disease include donepezil, galantamine, metrifonate, rivastigmine, and tacrine.[48] It is anticipated that this list will continue to grow as the etiology of this disease becomes better understood.

Physostigmine Salicylate, USP. The salicylate of physostigmine (eserine salicylate) may be prepared by neutralizing an ethereal solution of the alkaloid with an ethereal solution of salicylic acid. Excess salicylic acid is removed from the precipitated product by washing it with ether. The salicylate is less deliquescent than the sulfate.

Physostigmine salicylate occurs as a white, shining, odorless crystal or white powder that is soluble in water (1:75), alcohol (1:16), or chloroform (1:6) but much less soluble in ether (1:250). On prolonged exposure to air and light, the crystals turn red. The red may be removed by washing the crystals with alcohol, although this causes loss of the compound as well. Aqueous solutions are neutral or slightly acidic and take on a red coloration after a period. The coloration may be taken as an index of the loss of activity of physostigmine solutions.

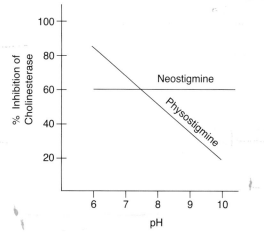

Figure 17.15 ● *Effect of pH on inhibition of cholinesterase by physostigmine and neostigmine.*

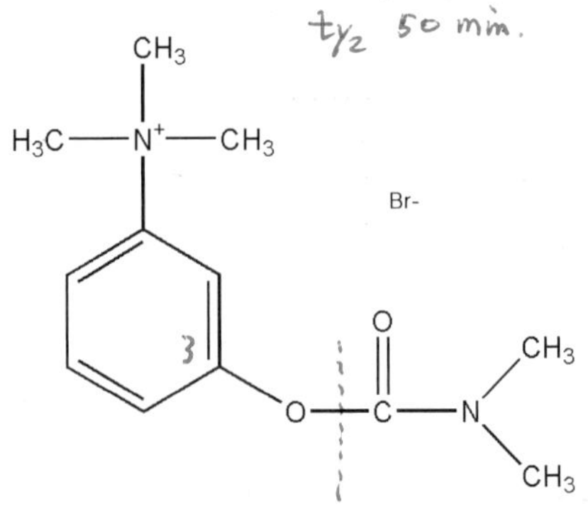

Neostigmine Bromide

Solutions of physostigmine salicylate are incompatible with the usual reagents that precipitate alkaloids (alkalies) and with iron salts. Incompatibility also occurs with benzalkonium chloride and related wetting agents because of the salicylate ion.

Physostigmine Sulfate, USP. Physostigmine sulfate occurs as a white, odorless, microcrystalline powder that is deliquescent in moist air. It is soluble in water (1:4), alcohol (1:0.4), and ether (1:1,200). It has the advantage over the salicylate salt of being compatible in solution with benzalkonium chloride and related compounds.

Neostigmine Bromide. Neostigmine bromide, (*m*-hydroxyphenyl)trimethylammonium bromide dimethylcarbamate or the dimethylcarbamic ester of 3-hydroxyphenyltrimethylammonium bromide (Prostigmin bromide), is used as an antidote to nondepolarizing neuromuscular blocking drugs and in the treatment of myasthenia gravis. It occurs as a bitter, odorless, white, crystalline powder. It is soluble in water and alcohol. The crystals are much less hygroscopic than those of neostigmine methylsulfate and thus may be used in tablets. Solutions are stable and may be sterilized by boiling. Aqueous solutions are neutral to litmus.

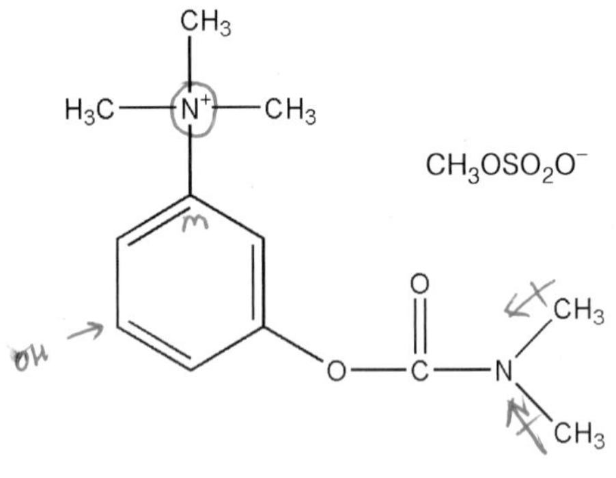

Neostigmine Methylsulfate

Use of physostigmine, as a prototype of an indirect-acting parasympathomimetic drug, facilitated the development of stigmine, in which a trimethylamine group was placed *para* to a dimethylcarbamate group in benzene. Better inhibition of cholinesterase was observed when these groups were placed *meta* to each other as in neostigmine, a more active and useful agent. Although physostigmine contains a methylcarbamate functional group, greater chemical stability toward hydrolysis was obtained with the dimethylcarbamyl group in neostigmine.[56]

Neostigmine has a half-life of about 50 minutes after oral or intravenous administration. About 80% of a single intramuscular dose is excreted in the urine within 24 hours; approximately 40% is excreted unchanged, and the remainder is excreted as metabolites. Of the neostigmine that reaches the liver, 98% is metabolized in 10 minutes to 3-hydroxyphenyltrimethyl ammonium, which has activity similar to, but weaker than, neostigmine. Its transfer from plasma to liver cells and then to bile is probably passive. Because cellular membranes permit the passage of plasma proteins synthesized in the liver into the bloodstream through capillary walls or lymphatic vessels, they may not present a barrier to the diffusion of quaternary amines such as neostigmine. The rapid hepatic metabolism of neostigmine may provide a downhill gradient for the continual diffusion of this compound.[57] A certain amount is hydrolyzed slowly by plasma cholinesterase.

Neostigmine has a mechanism of action quite similar to that of physostigmine. It effectively inhibits cholinesterase at about 10^{-6} M concentration. Its activity does not vary with pH, and at all ranges it exhibits similar cationic properties (Fig. 17.15). Skeletal muscle is also stimulated by neostigmine, a property that physostigmine does not have.

The uses of neostigmine are similar to those of physostigmine but differ in exhibiting greater miotic activity, fewer and less unpleasant local and systemic manifestations, and greater chemical stability. The most frequent application of neostigmine is to prevent atony of the intestinal, skeletal, and bladder musculature. An important use is in the treatment of myasthenia gravis, a condition caused by an autoimmune mechanism that requires an increase in ACh concentration in the neuromuscular junction to sustain normal muscular activity.

Neostigmine Methylsulfate. Neostigmine methylsulfate, (*m*-hydroxyphenyl)trimethylammonium methylsulfate dimethylcarbamate or the dimethylcarbamic ester of 3-hydroxyphenyltrimethylammonium methylsulfate (Prostigmin methylsulfate), is a bitter, odorless, white, crystalline powder. It is very soluble in water and soluble in alcohol. Solutions are stable and can be sterilized by boiling. The compound is too hygroscopic for use in a solid form and thus is always used as an injection. Aqueous solutions are neutral to litmus.

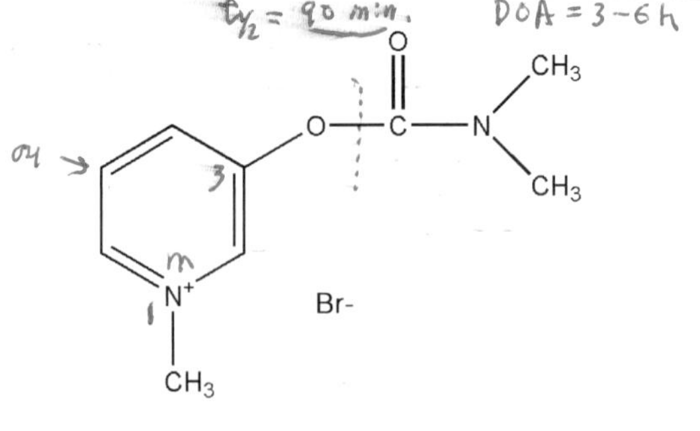

Pyridostigmine Bromide

The methylsulfate salt is used postoperatively as a urinary stimulant and in the diagnosis and treatment of myasthenia gravis.

Pyridostigmine Bromide, USP. Pyridostigmine bromide, 3-hydroxy-1-methylpyridinium bromide dimethylcarbamate or pyridostigmine bromide (Mestinon), occurs as a white, hygroscopic, crystalline powder with an agreeable, characteristic odor. It is freely soluble in water, alcohol, and chloroform.

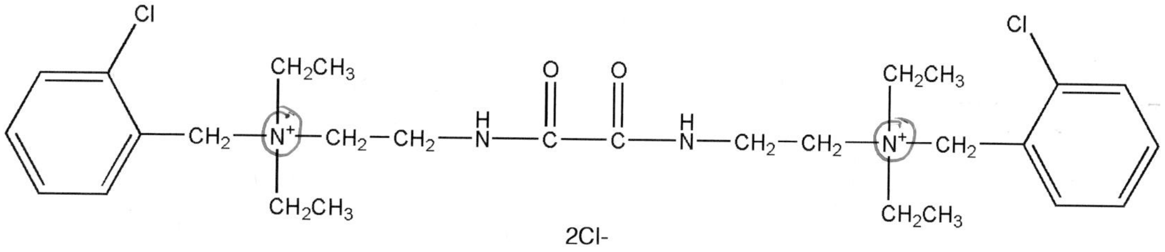

Ambenonium Chloride

Pyridostigmine bromide is about one fifth as toxic as neostigmine. It appears to function in a manner similar to that of neostigmine and is the most widely used anticholinesterase agent for treating myasthenia gravis. The liver enzymes and plasma cholinesterase metabolize the drug. The principal metabolite is 3-hydroxy-*N*-methylpyridinium. Orally administered pyridostigmine has a half-life of 90 minutes and a duration of action of between 3 and 6 hours.

Ambenonium Chloride. Ambenonium chloride, [oxalylbis(iminoethylene)]bis[(*o*-chlorobenzyl)diethylammonium] dichloride (Mytelase chloride), is a white, odorless powder, soluble in water and alcohol, slightly soluble in chloroform, and practically insoluble in ether and acetone. Ambenonium chloride is used for the treatment of myasthenia gravis in patients who do not respond satisfactorily to neostigmine or pyridostigmine.

This drug acts by suppressing the activity of AChE. It possesses a relatively prolonged duration of action and causes fewer side effects in the GI tract than the other anticholinesterase agents. The dosage requirements vary considerably, and the dosage must be individualized according to the response and tolerance of the patient. Because of its quaternary ammonium structure, ambenonium chloride is absorbed poorly from the GI tract. In moderate doses, the drug does not cross the blood-brain barrier. Ambenonium chloride is not hydrolyzed by cholinesterases.

Demecarium Bromide, USP. Demecarium bromide, (*m*-hydroxyphenyl)trimethylammonium bromide, decamethylenebis[methylcarbamate] (Humorsol), is the diester of (*m*-hydroxyphenyl)trimethylammonium bromide with decamethylene-bis-(methylcarbamic acid) and thus is comparable to a bis-prostigmine molecule.

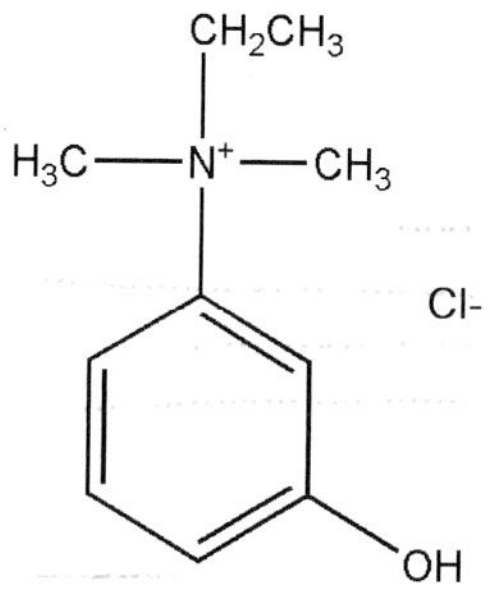

Edrophonium Chloride

It occurs as a slightly hygroscopic powder that is freely soluble in water or alcohol. Ophthalmic solutions of the drug have a pH of 5 to 7.5. Aqueous solutions are stable and may be sterilized by heat. Its efficacy and toxicity are comparable to those of other potent anticholinesterase inhibitor drugs. It is a long-acting miotic used to treat wide-angle glaucoma and accommodative esotropia. Maximal effect occurs hours after administration, and the effect may persist for days.

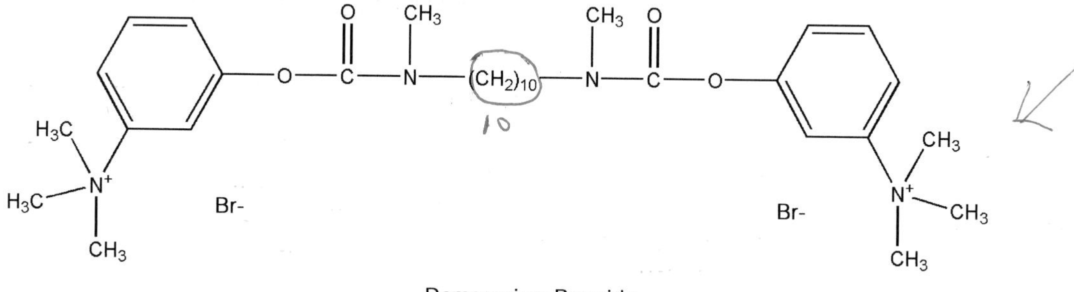

Demecarium Bromide

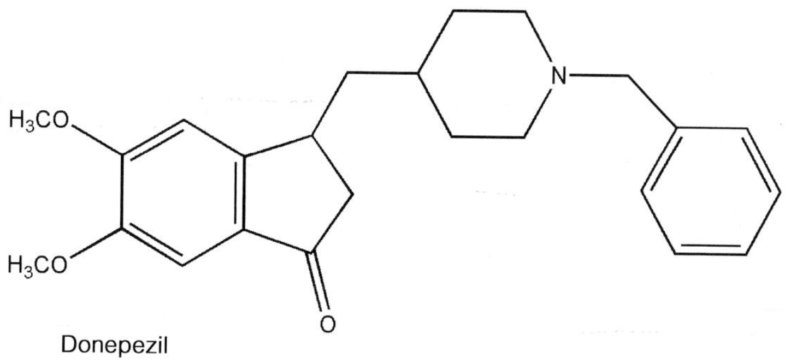

Donepezil

Donepezil. Donepezil, (±)-2,3-dihydro-5,6-dimethoxy-2-[[1-(phenylmethyl)-4-piperidinyl]methyl]-1*H*-inden-1-one (Aricept), commonly referred to in the literature as E2020, is a reversible inhibitor of AChE. It is indicated for the treatment of symptoms of mild-to-moderate Alzheimer disease. Donepezil is approximately 96% bound to plasma proteins, with an elimination half-life of 70 hours. It is metabolized principally by the 2D6 and 3A4 isozymes of the P450 system. *96% protein binding → DₒA = 70 h*

Edrophonium Chloride, USP. Edrophonium chloride, ethyl(*m*-hydroxyphenyl)dimethylammonium chloride (Tensilon), is a reversible anticholinesterase agent. It is bitter and very soluble in water and alcohol. Edrophonium chloride injection has a pH of 5.2 to 5.5. On parenteral administration, edrophonium has a more rapid onset and shorter duration of action than neostigmine, pyridostigmine, or ambenonium. It is a specific anticurare agent and acts within 1 minute to alleviate overdose of *d*-tubocurarine, dimethyl *d*-tubocurarine, or gallamine triethiodide. The drug is also used to terminate the action of any one of these drugs when the physician so desires. It is of no value, however, in terminating the action of the depolarizing (i.e., noncompetitive) blocking agents, such as decamethonium and succinylcholine. In addition to inhibiting AChE, edrophonium chloride has a direct cholinomimetic effect on skeletal muscle, which is greater than that of most other anticholinesterase drugs.

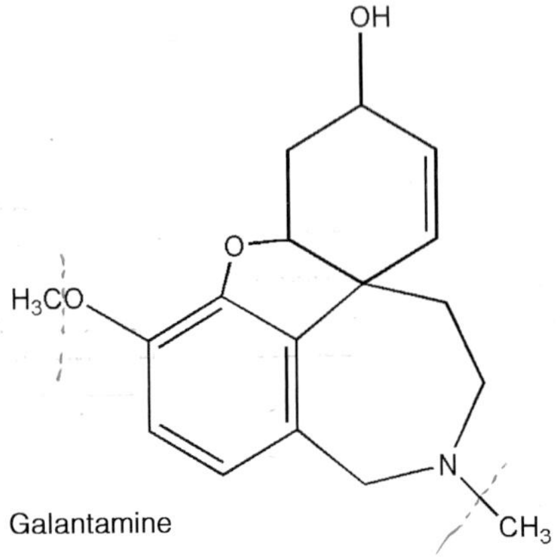

Galantamine

Edrophonium chloride is structurally related to neostigmine methylsulfate and has been used as a potential diagnostic agent for myasthenia gravis. This is the only degenerative neuromuscular disease that can be temporarily improved by administration of an anticholinesterase agent. Edrophonium chloride brings about a rapid increase in muscle strength without significant side effects.

Galantamine. Galantamine, 4a,5,9,10,11,12-hexahydro-3-methoxy-11-methyl-6*H*-benzofuro-[3a,3,2,ef][2]-benzazepin-6-ol (Nivalin, Reminyl), is an alkaloid extracted from the tuberous plant *Leucojum aestivum* (L.) belonging to the Amaryllidaceae family and from the bulbs of the daffodil, *Narcissus pseudonarcissus*. It is a reversible cholinesterase inhibitor that appears to have no effect on butyrylcholinesterase. In addition, it acts at allosteric nicotinic sites, further enhancing its cholinergic activity. Galantamine undergoes slow and minor biotransformation with approximately 5% to 6% undergoing demethylation. It is primarily excreted in the urine.

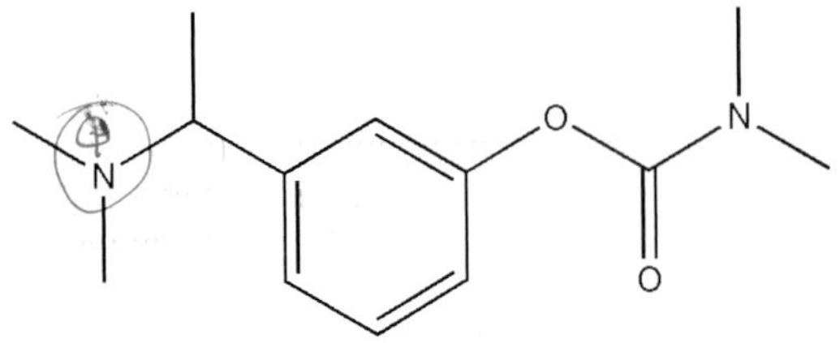

Rivastigmine

Metrifonate. Metrifonate is an organophosphate that was originally developed to treat schistosomiasis under the trade name Bilarcil. It is an irreversible cholinesterase inhibitor with some selectivity for BuChE over AChE. It achieves sustained cholinesterase inhibition by its nonenzymatic metabolite dichlorvos (DDVP), a long-acting organophosphate. Its use in mild-to-moderate Alzheimer disease was suspended recently because of adverse effects experienced by several patients during the clinical evaluation of this product. Toxicity at the neuromuscular junction is probably attributable to the inhibition by the drug of neurotoxic esterase, a common feature of organophosphates.

Rivastigmine. Rivastigmine (Exelon, EA 713) is a pseudoirreversible noncompetitive carbamate inhibitor of AChE. Although the half-life is approximately 2 hours, the inhibitory properties of this agent last for 10 hours because of the slow dissociation of the drug from the enzyme. The Food and Drug Administration (FDA) approved its use in mild-to-moderate Alzheimer disease in April 2000. In July 2007, rivastigmine was granted approval for use in managing mild-to-moderate dementia associated with Parkinson disease.

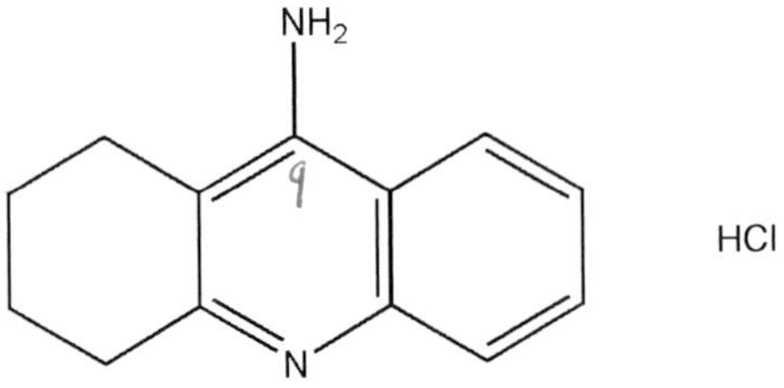

Tacrine Hydrochloride

Tacrine Hydrochloride. Tacrine hydrochloride, 1,2,3,4-tetrahydro-9-aminoacridine hydrochloride (THA, Cognex), is a reversible cholinesterase inhibitor that has been used in the treatment of Alzheimer disease for several years. The drug has been used to increase the levels of ACh in these patients on the basis of observations from autopsies that concentrations of ChAT and AChE are markedly reduced in the brain, whereas the number of muscarinic receptors is almost normal. The use of the drug is not without controversy, as conflicting results on efficacy have been reported.[58,59] The drug has been used in mild-to-moderate Alzheimer dementia.

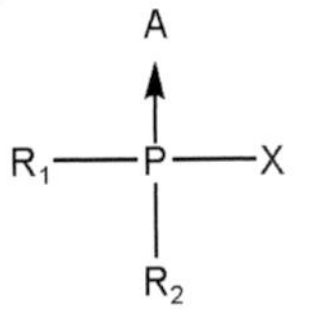

where R₁ = alkoxy
R₂ = alkoxyl, alkyl, or tertiary amine
X = a good leaving group
(e.g., F, CN, thiomalate, *p*-nitrophenyl)

Irreversible Inhibitors

Both AChE and BuChE are inhibited irreversibly by a group of phosphate esters that are highly toxic (LD_{50} for humans is 0.1–0.001 mg/kg). These chemicals are nerve poisons and have been used in warfare, in bioterrorism, and as agricultural insecticides. They permit ACh to accumulate at nerve endings and exacerbate ACh-like actions. The compounds belong to a class of organophosphorous esters. A general formula for such compounds follows:

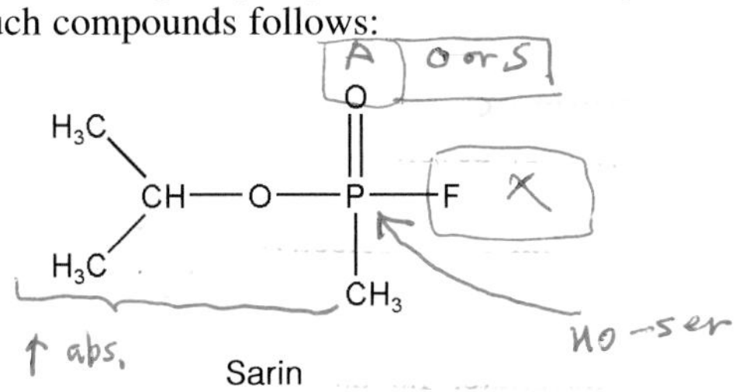

[handwritten: A | O or S]

H₃C—CH—O—P(=O)—F [handwritten box: X]
H₃C

CH₃ [handwritten: HO–ser]

[handwritten: ↑ abs.]

Sarin

A is usually oxygen or sulfur but may also be selenium. When *A* is other than oxygen, biological activation is required before the compound becomes effective as an inhibitor of cholinesterases. Phosphorothionates [$R_1R_2P(S)X$] have much poorer electrophilic character than their oxygen analogs and are much weaker hydrogen bond-forming molecules because of the sulfur atom.[60] Their anticholinesterase activity is 10^5-fold weaker than their oxygen analogs. *X* is the leaving group when the molecule reacts with the enzyme. Typical leaving groups include fluoride, nitrile, and *p*-nitrophenoxy. The *R* groups may be alkyl, alkoxy, aryl, aryloxy, or amino. The *R* moiety imparts lipophilicity to the molecule and contributes to its absorption through the skin. Inhibition of AChE by organophosphorous compounds takes place in two steps, association of enzyme and inhibitor and the phosphorylation step, completely analogous to acylation by the substrate (Fig. 17.16). Stereospecificity is mainly caused by interactions of enzyme and inhibitor at the esteratic site.

The serine residue at the esteratic site forms a stable phosphoryl ester with the organophosphorous inhibitors. This stability permits labeling studies[61] to be carried out on this and other enzymes (e.g., trypsin, chymotrypsin) that have the serine hydroxyl as part of their active site.

Although insecticides and nerve gases are irreversible inhibitors of cholinesterases by forming a phosphorylated serine at the esteratic site of the enzyme, it is possible to reactivate the enzyme if action is taken soon after exposure to

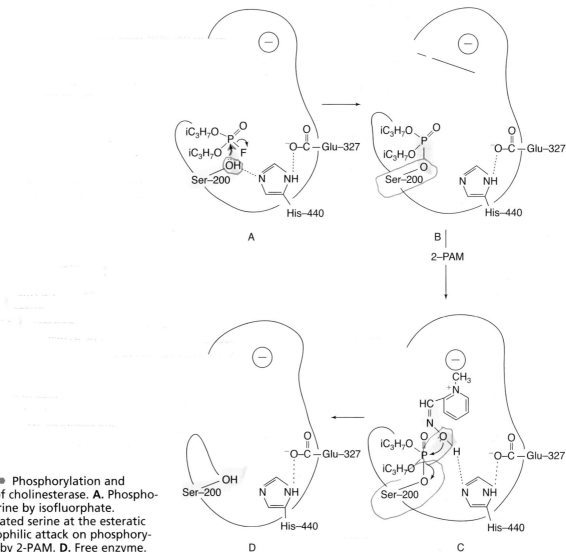

Figure 17.16 ● Phosphorylation and reactivation of cholinesterase. **A.** Phosphorylation of serine by isofluorphate. **B.** Phosphorylated serine at the esteratic site. **C.** Nucleophilic attack on phosphorylated residue by 2-PAM. **D.** Free enzyme.

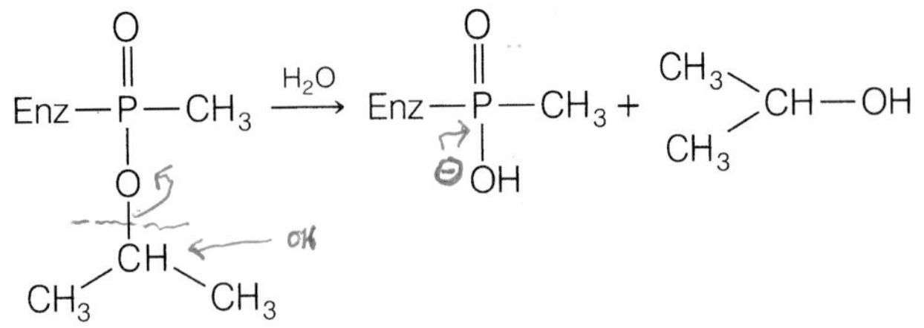

Figure 17.17 ● Aging of phosphorylated enzyme.

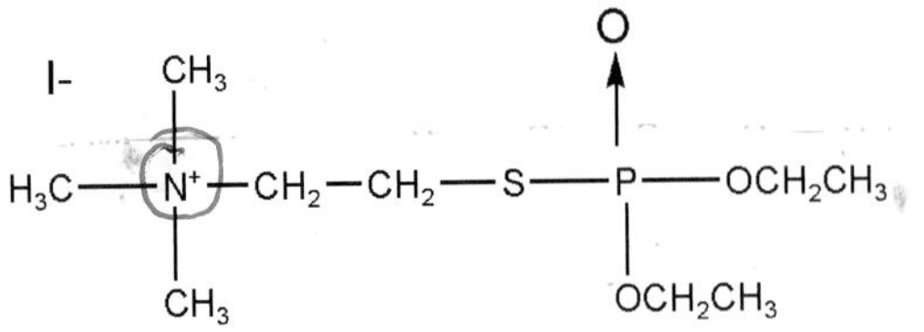

these poisons. Several compounds can provide a nucleophilic attack on the phosphorylated enzyme and cause regeneration of the free enzyme. Substances such as choline, hydroxylamine, and hydroxamic acid have led to the development of more effective cholinesterase reactivators, such as nicotinic hydroxamic acid and pyridine-2-aldoxime methiodide (2-PAM). A proposed mode of action for the reactivation of cholinesterase that has been inactivated by isoflurophate by 2-PAM is shown in Figure 17.16.

Cholinesterases that have been exposed to phosphorylating agents (e.g., sarin) become refractory to reactivation by cholinesterase reactivators. The process is called *aging* and occurs both in vivo and in vitro with AChE and BuChE. Aging occurs by partial hydrolysis of the phosphorylated moiety that is attached to the serine residue at the esteratic site of the enzyme (Fig. 17.17).

Phosphate esters used as insecticidal agents are toxic and must be handled with extreme caution. Symptoms of toxicity are nausea, vomiting, excessive sweating, salivation, miosis, bradycardia, low blood pressure, and respiratory difficulty, which is the usual cause of death.

The organophosphate insecticides of low toxicity, such as malathion, generally cause poisoning only by ingestion of relatively large doses. Parathion or methylparathion, however, cause poisoning by inhalation or dermal absorption. Because these compounds are so long acting, cumulative and serious toxic manifestations may result after several small exposures.

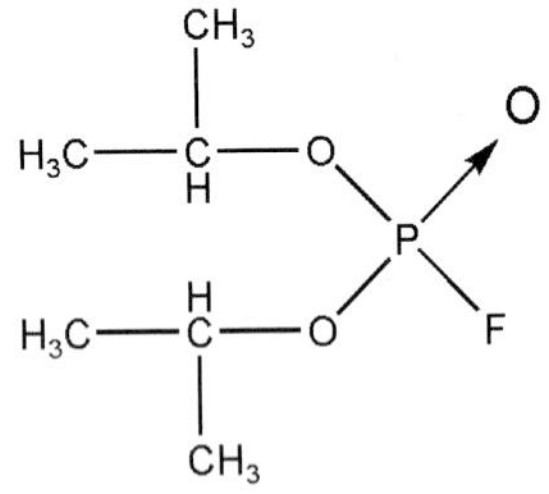

Isofluorphate

Products

Isofluorphate, USP. Isofluorphate, diisopropylphosphorofluoridate (Floropryl), is a colorless liquid soluble in water to the extent of 1.54% at 25°C, which decomposes to give a pH of 2.5. It is soluble in alcohol and to some extent in peanut oil. It is stable in peanut oil for a period of 1 year but decomposes in water in a few days. Solutions in peanut oil can be sterilized by autoclaving. The compound should be stored in hard glass containers. Continued contact with soft glass is said to hasten decomposition, as evidenced by discoloration.

Echothiophate Iodide

Isofluorphate must be handled with extreme caution. Contact with eyes, nose, mouth, and even skin should be avoided because it can be absorbed readily through intact epidermis and more so through mucous tissues.

Because isofluorphate irreversibly[62] inhibits cholinesterase, its activity lasts for days or even weeks. During this period, new cholinesterase may be synthesized in plasma, erythrocytes, and other cells.

A combination of atropine sulfate and magnesium sulfate protects rabbits against the toxic effects of isofluorphate. Atropine sulfate counteracts the muscarinic effect, and magnesium sulfate counteracts the nicotinic effect of the drug.[63] Isofluorphate has been used in the treatment of glaucoma.

Echothiophate Iodide, USP. Echothiophate iodide, (2-mercaptoethyl)trimethylammonium iodide, S-ester with O,O-diethylphosphorothioate (Phospholine Iodide), occurs as a white, crystalline, hygroscopic solid that has a slight mercaptan-like odor. It is soluble in water (1:1) and dehydrated alcohol (1:25); aqueous solutions have a pH of about 4 and are stable at room temperature for about 1 month.

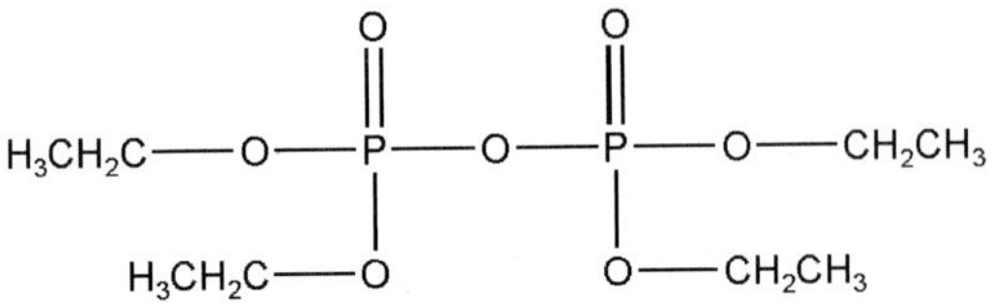

Tetraethylpyrophosphate

Echothiophate iodide is a long-lasting cholinesterase inhibitor of the irreversible type, as is isofluorphate. Unlike the latter, however, it is a quaternary salt, and when applied locally, its distribution in tissues is limited, which can be very desirable. It is used as a long-acting anticholinesterase agent in the treatment of glaucoma.

Hexaethyltetraphosphate (HETP) and Tetraethyl pyrophosphate (TEPP). HETP and TEPP are compounds that also show anticholinesterase activity. HETP was developed by the Germans during World War II and is used as an insecticide against aphids. When used as insecticides, these compounds have the advantage of being hydrolyzed rapidly to the relatively nontoxic, water-soluble compounds phosphoric acid and ethyl alcohol. Fruit trees or vegetables sprayed with this type of compound retain no harmful residue after a period of a few days or weeks, depending on the weather conditions. Workers spraying with these agents should use extreme caution so that the vapors are not breathed and none of the vapor or liquid comes in contact with the eyes or skin.

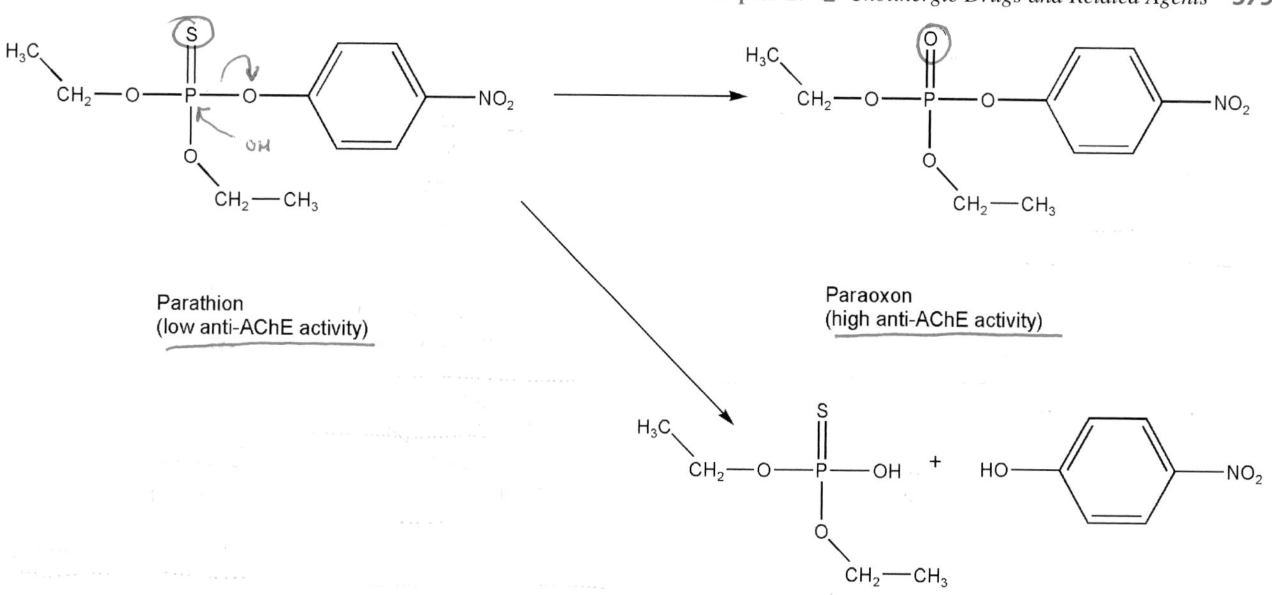

Parathion
(low anti-AChE activity)

Paraoxon
(high anti-AChE activity)

Malathion. Malathion, 2-[(dimethoxyphosphinothioyl) thio]butanedioic acid diethyl ester, is a water-insoluble phosphodithioate ester that has been used as an agricultural insecticide. Malathion is a poor inhibitor of cholinesterases. Its effectiveness as a safe insecticide is a result of the different rates at which humans and insects metabolize the chemical. Microsomal oxidation, which causes desulfuration, occurs slowly to form the phosphothioate (malaoxon), which is 10,000 times more active than the phosphodithioate (malathion) as a cholinesterase inhibitor. Insects detoxify the phosphothioate by a phosphatase, forming dimethyl phosphorothioate, which is inactive as an inhibitor. Humans, however, can rapidly hydrolyze malathion by a carboxyesterase enzyme, yielding malathion acid, a still poorer inhibitor of AChE. Phosphatases and carboxyesterases further metabolize malathion acid to dimethylphosphothioate. The metabolic reactions are shown in Figure 17.18.

Parathion. Parathion, *O,O*-diethyl *O-p*-nitrophenyl phosphorothioate (Thiophos), is a yellow liquid that is freely soluble in aromatic hydrocarbons, ethers, ketones, esters, and alcohols but practically insoluble in water, petroleum ether, kerosene, and the usual spray oils. It is decomposed at a pH above 7.5. Parathion is used as an agricultural insecticide. It is a relatively weak inhibitor of cholinesterase;

OMPA
(weak cholinesterase inhibitor)

liver microsomes

(O)

Hydroxymethyl OMPA
(strong cholinesterase inhibitor)

OMPA-*N*-methoxide
(strong cholinesterase inhibitor)

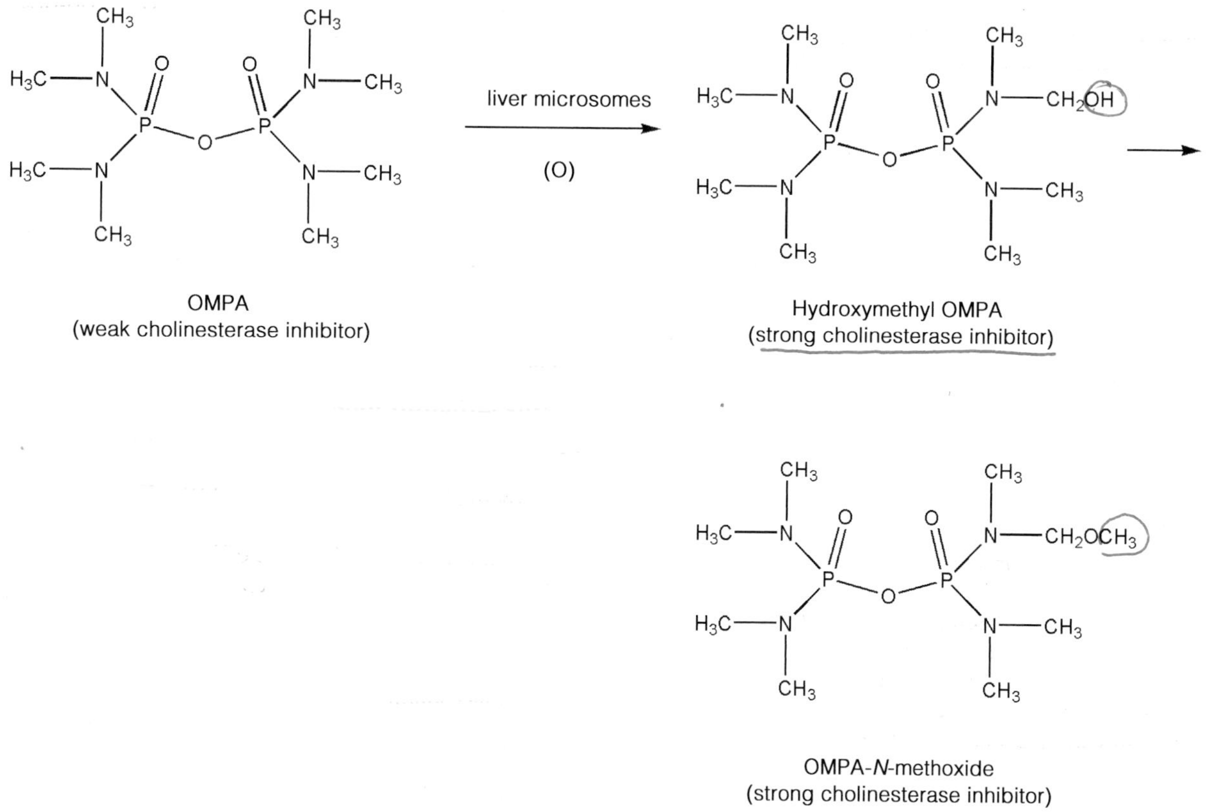

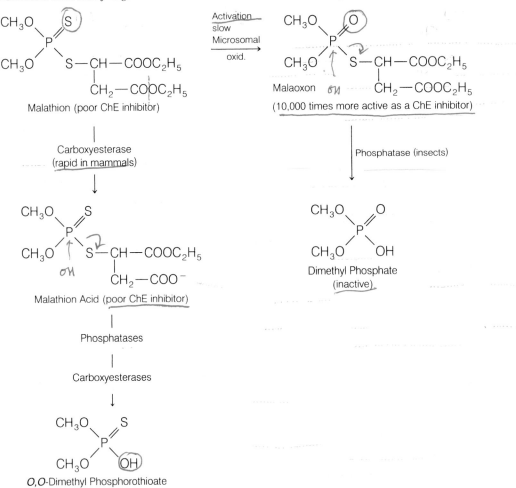

Figure 17.18 ● Comparison of metabolism of malathion by mammals and insects.

however, enzymes present in liver microsomes and insect tissues convert parathion (pI_{50} <4) to paraoxon, a more potent inhibitor of cholinesterase (pI_{50} >8).[64] Parathion is also metabolized by liver microsomes to yield *p*-nitrophenol and diethylphosphate; the latter is inactive as an irreversible cholinesterase inhibitor.[65]

Schradan. Schradan, octamethyl pyrophosphoramide (OMPA), *bis*[bisdimethylaminophosphonous] anhydride (Pestox III), is a viscous liquid that is miscible with water and soluble in most organic solvents. It is not hydrolyzed by alkalies or water but is hydrolyzed by acids. Schradan is used as a systemic insecticide for plants, being absorbed by the plants without appreciable injury. Insects feeding on the plant are incapacitated.

Schradan is a weak inhibitor of cholinesterases in vitro. In vivo, it is metabolized to the very strong inhibitor hydroxymethyl OMPA. Hydroxymethyl OMPA is not stable and is metabolized further to the *N*-methoxide, which is a weak inhibitor of cholinesterase.[66]

Pralidoxime Chloride, USP. Pralidoxime chloride, 2-formyl-1-methylpyridinium chloride oxime, 2-PAM chloride, or 2-pyridine aldoxime methyl chloride (Protopam chloride), is a white, nonhygroscopic, crystalline powder that is soluble in water, 1 g in less than 1 mL.

Pralidoxime chloride is used as an antidote for poisoning by parathion and related pesticides. It may be effective

against some phosphates that have a quaternary nitrogen. It is also an effective antagonist for some carbamates, such as neostigmine methylsulfate and pyridostigmine bromide. The mode of action of pralidoxime chloride is described in Figure 17.16.

Pralidoxime Chloride

A, B = bulky groups,
e.g., cycloalkyl,
aromatic

C = H, OH
carboxamide

The biological half-life of pralidoxime chloride in humans is about 2 hours, and its effectiveness is a function of its concentration in plasma, which reaches a maximum 2 to 3 hours after oral administration.

Pralidoxime chloride, a quaternary ammonium compound, is most effective by intramuscular, subcutaneous, or intravenous administration. Treatment of poisoning by an anticholinesterase will be most effective if given within a few hours. Little will be accomplished if the drug is used more than 36 hours after parathion poisoning has occurred.

⬡ CHOLINERGIC BLOCKING AGENTS

A wide variety of tissues respond to ACh released by the neuron or exogenously administered chemicals to mimic this neurotransmitter's action. Peripheral cholinergic receptors are located at parasympathetic postganglionic nerve endings in smooth muscle, sympathetic and parasympathetic ganglia, and neuromuscular junctions in skeletal muscle. Although ACh activates these receptors, there are antagonists that are selective for each. Atropine is an effective blocking agent at parasympathetic postganglionic terminals. Like most classic blocking agents, it acts on all muscarinic receptor subtypes. *d*-Tubocurarine blocks the effect of ACh on skeletal muscle, which is activated by N_1 nicotinic receptors. Hexamethonium blocks transition at N_2 nicotinic receptors located in autonomic ganglia.

Anticholinergic action by drugs and chemicals apparently depends on their ability to reduce the number of free receptors that can interact with ACh. The theories of Stephenson[67] and Ariens[68] have explained the relationship between drug–receptor interactions and the observed biological response (see Chapter 2). These theories indicate that the amount of drug–receptor complex formed at a given time depends on the affinity of the drug for the receptor and that a drug that acts as an agonist must also possess another property, called *efficacy* or *intrinsic activity*. Another explanation of drug–receptor interactions, the Paton rate theory,[69] defines a biological stimulus as proportional to the rate of drug–receptor interactions (see Chapter 2). Both of these theories are compatible with the concept that a blocking agent that has high affinity for the receptor may decrease the number of available free receptors and the efficiency of the endogenous neurotransmitter.

Structure–Activity Relationships

A wide variety of compounds possess anticholinergic activity. The development of such compounds has been largely empiric and based principally on atropine as the prototype. Nevertheless, structural permutations have resulted in compounds that do not have obvious relationships to the parent molecule. The following classification delineates the major chemical types encountered:

- Solanaceous alkaloids and synthetic analogs
- Synthetic aminoalcohol esters
- Aminoalcohol ethers
- Aminoalcohols
- Aminoamides
- Miscellaneous
- Papaveraceous

The chemical classification of anticholinergics acting on parasympathetic postganglionic nerve endings is complicated somewhat because some agents, especially the quaternary ammonium derivatives, act on the ganglia that have a muscarinic component to their stimulation pattern and, at high doses, at the neuromuscular junction in skeletal muscle.

There are several ways in which the structure–activity relationship could be considered, but in this discussion we follow, in general, the considerations of Long et al.,[70] who based their postulations on the 1-hyoscyamine molecule being one of the most active anticholinergics and, therefore, having an optimal arrangement of groups.

Anticholinergic compounds may be considered chemicals that have some similarity to ACh but contain additional substituents that enhance their binding to the cholinergic receptor.

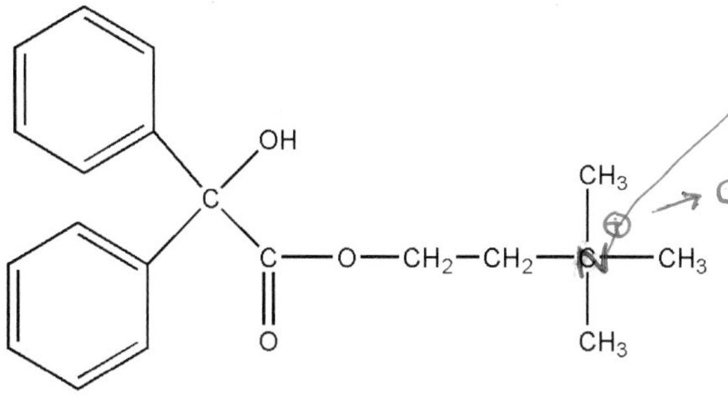

Benzilylcarbocholine

As depicted above, an anticholinergic agent may contain a quaternary ammonium function or a tertiary amine that is protonated in the biophase to form a cationic species. The nitrogen is separated from a pivotal carbon atom by a chain that may include an ester, ether, or hydrocarbon moiety. The substituent groups *A* and *B* contain at least one aromatic moiety capable of van der Waals interactions to the receptor surface and one cycloaliphatic or other hydrocarbon moiety for hydrophobic bonding interactions. *C* may be hydroxyl or carboxamide to undergo hydrogen bonding with the receptor.

THE CATIONIC HEAD

It is generally considered that the anticholinergic molecules have a primary point of attachment to cholinergic sites through the *cationic head* (i.e., the positively charged nitrogen). For quaternary ammonium compounds, there is no question of what is implied, but for tertiary amines, one assumes, with good reason, that the cationic head is achieved by protonation of the amine at physiological pH. The nature of the substituents on this cationic head is critical insofar as a parasympathomimetic response is concerned. Steric factors that cause diffusion of the onium charge or produce a less-than-optimal drug–receptor interaction result in a decrease of parasympathomimetic properties and allow the drug to act as an antagonist because of other bonding interactions. Ariens[68] has shown that carbocholines (e.g., benzilylcarbocholine) engage in a typical competitive action with ACh, although they are less effective than the corresponding compounds possessing a cationic head, suggesting

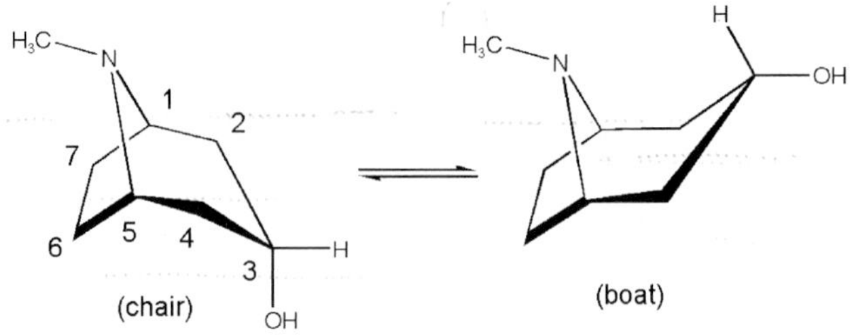

TROPINE
(3α-Hydroxytropane or
3α-Tropanol)

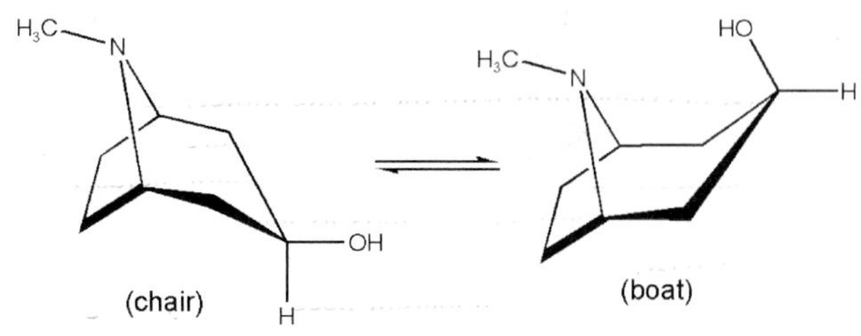

PSEUDOTROPINE
(3β-Hydroxytropane or
3β-Tropanol)

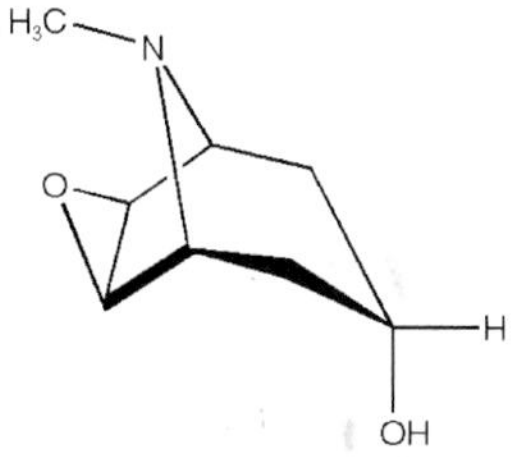

SCOPINE
(6:7 β-Epoxy-3-α-hydroxytropane
or 6:7 β-Epoxy-3-α-tropanol

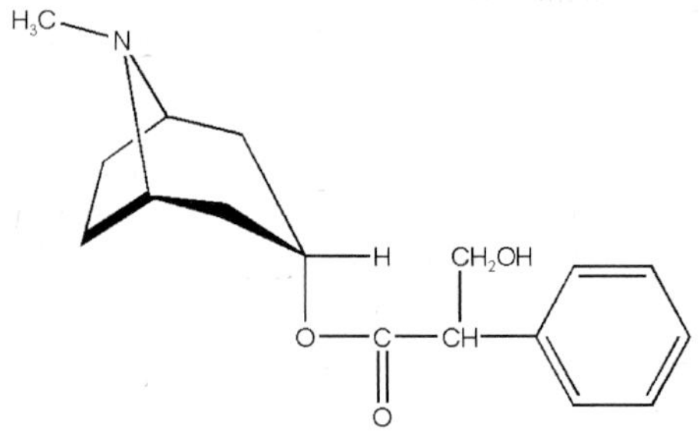

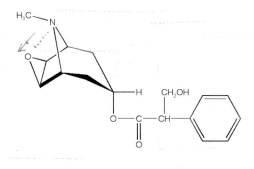

ATROPINE
(or hyoscyamine)

SCOPOLAMINE
(or hyoscine)

that hydrophobic bonding may play an important role in these drug–receptor interactions.

THE HYDROXYL GROUP

Although not requisite for activity, a suitably placed alcoholic hydroxyl group enhances antimuscarinic activity over that of a similar compound without the hydroxyl group. The position of the hydroxyl group relative to the nitrogen appears to be fairly critical, with the diameter of the receptive area estimated to be about 2 to 3 Å. It is assumed that the hydroxyl group contributes to the strength of binding, probably by hydrogen bonding to an electron-rich portion of the receptor surface.

THE ESTERATIC GROUP

Many of the highly potent antimuscarinic compounds possess an ester grouping, and this may be a contributing feature for effective binding. This is reasonable because the agonist (i.e., ACh) possesses a similar function for binding to the same site. An esteratic function is not necessary for activity, because several types of compounds do not possess such a group (e.g., ethers, aminoalcohols).

CYCLIC SUBSTITUTION

Examination of the active compounds discussed in the following sections reveals that at least one cyclic substituent (phenyl, thienyl, or other) is a common feature in almost all anticholinergic molecules. Aromatic substitution is often used in connection with the acidic moiety of the ester function. Virtually all acids used, however, are of the aryl-substituted acetic acid variety. Use of aromatic acids leads to low activity of these compounds as anticholinergics but potential activity as local anesthetics.

In connection with the apparent need for a cyclic group, Ariens[68] points out that the "mimetic" molecules, richly endowed with polar groups, undoubtedly require a complementary polar receptor area for effective binding. As a consequence, it is implied that a relatively nonpolar area surrounds such sites. Thus, increasing the binding of the molecule in this peripheral area by introducing flat, nonpolar groups (e.g., aromatic rings) should achieve compounds with excellent affinity but without intrinsic activity. This postulate is consistent with most antimuscarinic drugs, whether they possess an ester group or not.

PARASYMPATHETIC POSTGANGLIONIC BLOCKING AGENTS

Parasympathetic postganglionic blocking agents are also known as antimuscarinic, anticholinergic, parasympatholytic, or cholinolytic drugs. Antimuscarinic drugs act by competitive antagonism of ACh binding to muscarinic receptors. Endogenous neurotransmitters, including ACh, are relatively small molecules. Ariens[68] noted that competitive reversible antagonists generally are larger molecules capable of additional binding to the receptor surface. The most potent anticholinergic drugs are derived from muscarinic agonists that contain one or sometimes two large or bulky groups. Ariens[68] suggested that molecules that act as competitive reversible antagonists generally are capable of binding to the active site of the receptor but have an additional binding interaction that increases receptor affinity but does not contribute to the intrinsic activity (efficacy) of the drug. Several three-dimensional models of G-protein–coupled receptors, including the muscarinic receptor, have been reported. Despite knowledge of their amino acid sequences, it is not yet possible to provide an unambiguous description of the docking of molecules to these receptors. The concepts of Ariens[68] and others, however, appear consistent with the binding site models proposed. Bebbington and Brimblecombe[41] proposed in 1965 that there is a relatively large area lying outside the agonist–receptor binding site, where van der Waals interactions can take place between the agonist and the receptor area. This, too, is not inconsistent with contemporary theories on cholinergic receptor interaction with small molecules.

Therapeutic Actions

Organs controlled by the autonomic nervous system usually are innervated by both the sympathetic and the parasympathetic systems. There is a continual state of dynamic balance between the two systems. Theoretically, one should achieve the same end result by either stimulation of one of the systems or blockade of the other. Unfortunately, there is usually a limitation to this type of generalization. There are, however, three predictable and clinically useful results from blocking the muscarinic effects of ACh.

1. *Mydriatic effect*: dilation of the pupil of the eye; and *cycloplegia*, a paralysis of the ciliary structure of the eye, resulting in a paralysis of accommodation for near vision
2. *Antispasmodic effect*: lowered tone and motility of the GI tract and the genitourinary tract
3. *Antisecretory effect*: reduced salivation (*antisialagogue*), reduced perspiration (*anhidrotic*), and reduced acid and gastric secretion

These three general effects of parasympatholytics can be expected in some degree from any of the known drugs, although, occasionally, one must administer rather heroic doses to demonstrate the effect. The mydriatic and cycloplegic effects, when produced by topical application, are not subject to any greatly undesirable side effects because of limited systemic absorption. This is not true for the systemic antispasmodic effects obtained by oral or parenteral administration. Drugs with effective blocking action on the GI tract are seldom free of adverse effects on the other organs. The same is probably true of drugs used for their antisecretory effects. Perhaps the most common side effects experienced from the oral use of these drugs, under ordinary conditions, are dryness of the mouth, mydriasis, and urinary retention. The latter effects have been exploited in the development of agents used to manage overactive bladder with symptoms of the urge of urinary incontinence, urgency, and frequency.

Mydriatic and cycloplegic drugs are generally prescribed or used in the office by ophthalmologists. Their principal use is for refraction studies in the process of fitting lenses. This permits the physician to examine the eye retina for possible abnormalities and diseases and provides controlled conditions for the proper fitting of glasses. Because of the inability of the iris to contract under the influence of these drugs, there is a definite danger to the patient's eyes during the period of drug activity unless they are protected from strong light by the use of dark glasses. These drugs also are used to treat inflammation of the cornea (keratitis), inflammation of the iris and the ciliary organs (iritis and iridocyclitis), and inflammation of the choroid (choroiditis). A dark-colored iris appears to be more difficult to dilate than a light-colored one and may require more concentrated solutions. Caution in the use of mydriatics is advisable because of their demonstrated effect in raising the intraocular pressure. Pupil dilation tends to cause the iris to restrict drainage of fluid through the canal of Schlemm by crowding the angular space, thereby leading to increased intraocular pressure. This is particularly true for patients with glaucomatous conditions.

Atropine is used widely as an antispasmodic because of its marked depressant effect on parasympathetically innervated smooth muscle. It appears to block all muscarinic receptor subtypes. Atropine is, however, the standard by which other similar drugs are measured. Also, atropine has a blocking action on the transmission of the nerve impulse, rather than a depressant effect directly on the musculature. This action is termed *neurotropic*, in contrast with the action of an antispasmodic such as papaverine, which appears to act by depression of the muscle cells and is termed *musculotropic*.

Papaverine is the standard for comparison of musculotropic antispasmodics and, although not strictly a parasympatholytic, is treated together with its synthetic analogs later in this chapter. The synthetic antispasmodics appear to combine neurotropic and musculotropic effects in greater or lesser measure, together with a certain amount of ganglion-blocking activity for the quaternary derivatives.

Anticholinergic drugs have a minor role in the management of peptic ulcer disease.[71] For the present, the most rational therapy involving anticholinergic drugs seems to be a combination of a nonirritating diet to reduce acid secretion, antacid therapy, and reduction of emotional stress. Most of the anticholinergic drugs are offered either as the chemical alone, or in combination with a CNS depressant such as phenobarbital, or with a neuroleptic drug to reduce the CNS contribution to parasympathetic hyperactivity. In addition to the antisecretory effects of anticholinergics on hydrochloric acid and gastric acid secretion, there have been some efforts to use them as antisialagogues and anhidrotics.

Paralysis agitans or parkinsonism (Parkinson disease), first described by the English physician James Parkinson in 1817, is another condition that is often treated with anticholinergic drugs. It is characterized by tremor, "pill rolling," cogwheel rigidity, festinating gait, sialorrhea, and masklike facies. Fundamentally, it represents a malfunction of the extrapyramidal system. Parkinsonism is characterized by progressive and selective degeneration of dopaminergic neurons, which originate in the substantia nigra of the midbrain and terminate in the basal ganglia (i.e., caudate nucleus, putamen, and pallidum). Skeletal muscle movement is controlled to a great degree by patterns of excitation and inhibition resulting from the feedback of information to the cortex and mediated through the pyramidal and extrapyramidal pathways. The basal ganglia structures, such as the pallidum, corpus striatum, and substantia nigra, serve as data processors for the pyramidal pathways and the structures through which the extrapyramidal pathways pass on their way from the spinal cord to the cortex. Lesions of the pyramidal pathways lead to a persistent increase in muscle tone, resulting in an excess of spontaneous involuntary movements, along with changes in the reflexes. Thus, the basal ganglia are functional in maintaining normal motor control. In parkinsonism, there is degeneration of the substantia nigra and corpus striatum, which are involved with controlled integration of muscle movement. The neurons in the substantia nigra and basal ganglia use the neurotransmitter dopamine and interact with short cholinergic interneurons. When dopamine neurons degenerate, the balance between them is altered. The inhibitory influence of dopamine is reduced, and the activity of cholinergic neurons is increased. The principal goal of anticholinergic drugs in the treatment of parkinsonism is to decrease the activity of cholinergic neurons in the basal ganglia.

The usefulness of the belladonna group of alkaloids for the treatment of parkinsonism was an empiric discovery. Since then, chemists have prepared many synthetic analogs of atropine in an effort to retain the useful antitremor and antirigidity effects of the belladonna alkaloid while reducing the adverse effects. In this process, it was discovered that antihistamine drugs (e.g., diphenhydramine) reduced tremor and rigidity. The antiparkinsonian-like activity of

antihistamines has been attributed to their anticholinergic properties. The activity of these drugs is confined to those that can pass through the blood-brain barrier.

SOLANACEOUS ALKALOIDS AND ANALOGS

The solanaceous alkaloids, represented by (−)-hyoscyamine, atropine [(−)-hyoscyamine], and scopolamine (hyoscine), are the forerunners of the class of antimuscarinic drugs. These alkaloids are found principally in henbane (*Hyoscyamus niger*), deadly nightshade (*Atropa belladonna*), and jimson weed (*Datura stramonium*). There are other alkaloids that are members of the solanaceous group (e.g., apoatropine, noratropine, belladonnine, tigloidine, meteloidine) but lack sufficient therapeutic value to be considered in this text.

Crude drugs containing these alkaloids have been used since early times for their marked medicinal properties, which largely depend on inhibition of the parasympathetic nervous system and stimulation of the higher nervous centers. Belladonna, probably as a consequence of the weak local anesthetic activity of atropine, has been used topically for its analgesic effect on hemorrhoids, certain skin infections, and various itching dermatoses. Application of sufficient amounts of belladonna or its alkaloids results in mydriasis. Internally, the drug causes diminution of secretions, increases the heart rate (by depression of the vagus nerve), depresses the motility of the GI tract, and acts as an antispasmodic on various smooth muscles (ureter, bladder, and biliary tract). In addition, it directly stimulates the respiratory center. The multiplicity of actions exerted by the drug is looked on with some disfavor, because the physician seeking one type of response unavoidably also obtains the others. The action of scopolamine-containing drugs differs from those containing hyoscyamine and atropine in having no CNS stimulation; rather, a narcotic or sedative effect predominates. The use of this group of drugs is accompanied by a fairly high incidence of reactions because of individual idiosyncrasies; death from overdosage usually results from respiratory failure. A complete treatment of the pharmacology and uses of these drugs is not within the scope of this text. The introductory pages of this chapter briefly review some of the more pertinent points in connection with the major activities of these drug types.

Structural Considerations

All of the solanaceous alkaloids are esters of the bicyclic aminoalcohol 3-hydroxytropane or of related aminoalcohols. The structural formulas that follow show the piperidine ring system in the commonly accepted chair conformation because this form has the lowest energy requirement. The alternate boat form can exist under certain conditions, however, because the energy barrier is not great. Inspection of the 3-hydroxytropane formula also indicates that even though there is no optical activity because of the plane of symmetry, two stereoisomeric forms (tropine and pseudotropine) can exist because of the rigidity imparted to the molecule through the ethylene chain across the 1,5 positions.

In tropine, the axially oriented hydroxyl group, *trans* to the nitrogen bridge, is designated α, and the alternate *cis* equatorially oriented hydroxyl group is designated β.

The aminoalcohol derived from scopolamine, namely scopine, has the axial orientation of the 3-hydroxyl group but, in addition, a β-oriented epoxy group bridged across the 6,7 positions, as shown. Of the several different solanaceous alkaloids known, it has been indicated that (−)-hyoscyamine, atropine, and scopolamine are the most important. Their structures are shown, but antimuscarinic activity is associated with all of the solanaceous alkaloids that possess the tropinelike axial orientation of the esterified hydroxyl group. Studying the formulas reveals that in each case tropic acid is the esterifying acid. Tropic acid contains an easily racemized asymmetric carbon atom, the moiety accounting for optical activity in these compounds in the absence of racemization. The proper enantiomorph is necessary for high-antimuscarinic activity, as illustrated by the potent (−)-hyoscyamine in comparison with the weakly active (+)-hyoscyamine. The racemate, atropine, has intermediate activity. The marked difference in antimuscarinic potency of the optical enantiomorphs apparently does not extend to the action on the CNS, inasmuch as both seem to have the same degree of activity.[72]

The solanaceous alkaloids have been modified by preparing other esters of 3-α-tropanol or making a quaternary of the nitrogen in tropanol or scopine with a methyl halide. These compounds represent some of the initial attempts to separate the varied actions of atropine and scopolamine. Few aminoalcohols have been found that impart the same degree of neurotropic activity as that exhibited by the ester formed by combination of tropine with tropic acid. Similarly, the tropic acid portion is highly specific for the anticholinergic action, and substitution by other acids decreases neurotropic potency, although the musculotropic action may increase. The earliest attempts to modify the atropine molecule retained the tropine portion and substituted various acids for tropic acid.

Besides changing the acid residue, other changes have been directed toward the quaternization of the nitrogen. Examples of this type of compound are methscopolamine bromide, homatropine methylbromide, and anisotropine methylbromide. Quaternization of the tertiary amine produces variable effects in terms of increasing potency. Decreases in activity are apparent in comparing atropine with methylatropine (no longer used) and scopolamine with methscopolamine. Ariens et al.[73] ascribed decreased activity, especially when the groups attached to nitrogen are larger than methyl, to a possible decrease in affinity for the anionic site on the cholinergic receptor. They attributed this decreased affinity to a combination of greater electron repulsion by such groups and greater steric interference to the approach of the cationic head to the anionic site. In general, quaternization reduces parasympathomimetic action much more than parasympatholytic action. This may be partially a result of the additional blocking at the parasympathetic ganglion induced by quaternization, which could offset the decreased affinity at the postganglionic site. However, quaternization increases the curariform activity of these alkaloids and aminoesters, a usual consequence of quaternizing alkaloids. Another disadvantage in converting an alkaloidal base to the quaternary form is that the quaternized base is absorbed more poorly through the intestinal wall, so that the activity becomes erratic and, in some instances, unpredictable. Bases (such as alkaloids) are absorbed through the lipoidal gut wall only in the dissociated form, which can be expected to exist for a tertiary base, in the small intestine. Quaternary nitrogen bases cannot revert to an undissociated form, even in basic media and, presumably, may have difficulty passing through the gut wall. Since quaternary compounds can be absorbed, other less efficient mechanisms for absorption probably prevail. Quaternary ammonium compounds combine reversibly with endogenous substances in the gut, such as mucin, to form neutral ion-pair complexes. These complexes penetrate the lipid membrane by passive diffusion.

Products

Atropine, USP. Atropine is the tropine ester of racemic tropic acid and is optically inactive. It possibly occurs naturally in various Solanaceae, although some claim, with justification, that whatever atropine is isolated from natural sources results from racemization of (−)-hyoscyamine during the isolation process. Conventional methods of alkaloid isolation are used to obtain a crude mixture of atropine and hyoscyamine from the plant material. This crude mixture is racemized to atropine by refluxing in chloroform or by treatment with cold dilute alkali. Because the racemization process makes atropine, an official limit is set on the hyoscyamine content by restricting atropine to a maximum levorotation under specified conditions.

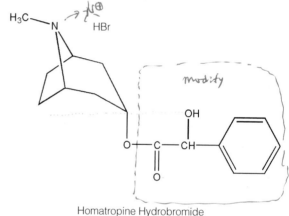

Homatropine Hydrobromide

Atropine occurs in the form of optically inactive, white, odorless crystals possessing a bitter taste. It is not very soluble in water (1:460, 1:90 at 80°C) but is more soluble in alcohol (1:2, 1:1.2 at 60°C). It is soluble in glycerin (1:27), in chloroform (1:1), and in ether (1:25). Saturated aqueous solutions are alkaline in reaction (pH ~9.5). The free base is useful when nonaqueous solutions are to be made, such as in oily vehicles and ointment bases. Atropine has a plasma half-life of about 2 to 3 hours. It is metabolized in the liver to several products, including tropic acid and tropine.

Atropine Sulfate, USP. Atropine sulfate (Atropisol) is prepared by neutralizing atropine in acetone or ether solution with an alcoholic solution of sulfuric acid, with care used to prevent hydrolysis. The salt occurs as colorless crystals or as a white, crystalline powder. It is efflorescent in dry air and should be protected from light to prevent decomposition.

Atropine sulfate is freely soluble in water (1:0.5), in alcohol (1:5, 1:2.5 at boiling point), and in glycerin (1:2.5). Aqueous solutions are not very stable, although solutions may be sterilized at 120°C (15 lb pressure) in an autoclave if the pH is kept below 6. Sterilization probably is best effected by the use of aseptic techniques and a bacteriological filter. It has been suggested that no more than a 30-day supply of an aqueous solution should be made and that for small quantities the best procedure is to use hypodermic tablets and sterile distilled water.[73] Kondritzer and Zvirblis[74] have studied the kinetics of alkaline and proton-catalyzed hydrolyses of atropine in aqueous solution. The region of maximal stability lies between pH 3 and approximately 5. They have also proposed an equation to predict the half-life of atropine undergoing hydrolysis at constant pH and temperature.

The action of atropine or its salts is the same. It produces a mydriatic effect by paralyzing the iris and the ciliary muscles and, for this reason, is used by the oculist in iritis and corneal inflammations and lesions. Its use is rational in these conditions because one of the first rules in the treatment of inflammation is rest, which, of course, is accomplished by the paralysis of muscular motion. Its use in the eye (0.5%–1% solutions or gelatin disks) for fitting glasses is widespread. Atropine is administered in small doses before general anesthesia to lessen oral and air passage secretions and, when administered with morphine, to lessen the respiratory depression induced by morphine.

Atropine causes restlessness, prolonged pupillary dilation, and loss of visual accommodation and, furthermore, gives rise to arrhythmias such as atrioventricular dissociation, ventricular extrasystoles, and even ventricular fibrillation. Even though ether has been gradually replaced by other anesthetics, thereby eliminating problems with respiratory secretions caused by ether and thus requiring atropine, surgeons and anesthesiologists today continue to use it as an anesthetic premedicant to reduce excessive salivary and airway secretions and to prevent vagal reflexes.

Its ability to dry secretions has also been used in the so-called rhinitis tablets for symptomatic relief in colds. In cathartic preparations, atropine or belladonna has been used as an antispasmodic to lessen the smooth muscle spasm (griping) often associated with catharsis.

Atropine may be used to treat some types of arrhythmias. It increases the heart rate by blocking the effects of ACh on the vagus. In this context, it is used to treat certain reversible bradyarrhythmias that may accompany acute myocardial infarction. It is also used as an adjunct to anesthesia to protect against bradycardia, hypotension, and even cardiac arrest induced by the skeletal muscle relaxant succinylcholine chloride.

Another use for atropine sulfate emerged following the development of the organophosphates, which are potent inhibitors of AChE. Atropine is a specific antidote to prevent the muscarinic effects of ACh accumulation, such as vomiting, abdominal cramps, diarrhea, salivation, sweating, bronchoconstriction, and excessive bronchial secretions. It is used intravenously but does not protect against respiratory failure caused by depression of the respiratory center and the muscles of respiration.

Hyoscyamine, USP. Hyoscyamine is a levorotatory alkaloid obtained from various solanaceous species. One of the commercial sources is Egyptian henbane (*Hyoscyamus muticus*), in which it occurs to the extent of about 0.5%. Usually, it is prepared from the crude drug in a manner similar to that used for atropine and is purified as the oxalate. The free base is obtained easily from this salt.

It occurs as white needles that are sparingly soluble in water (1:281), more soluble in ether (1:69) or benzene (1:150), very soluble in chloroform (1:1), and freely soluble in alcohol. It is used as the sulfate and hydrobromide. The principal reason for the popularity of the hydrobromide has been its nondeliquescent nature. The salts have the advantage over the free base in being quite water soluble.

Hyoscyamine is the *levo* form of the racemic mixture known as atropine. The *dextro* form does not exist naturally but has been synthesized. Cushny[75] compared the activities of (−)-hyoscyamine, (+)-hyoscyamine, and the racemate (atropine) in 1904 and found greater peripheral potency for the (−) isomer and twice the potency of the racemate. All later studies have essentially confirmed that the (+) isomer is only weakly active and that the (−) isomer is, in effect, the active portion of atropine. Inspection of the relative doses of atropine sulfate and hyoscyamine sulfate illustrates the differences very nicely. The principal criticism offered against the use of hyoscyamine sulfate exclusively is that it tends to racemize to atropine sulfate rather easily in solution, so that atropine sulfate then becomes the more stable of the two. All of the isomers behave very much the same in the CNS.

Hyoscyamine is used to treat disorders of the urinary tract more so than any other antispasmodic, although there is no evidence that it has any advantages over the other belladonna preparations and the synthetic anticholinergics. It is used to treat spasms of the bladder and, in this manner, serves as a urinary stimulant. It is used together with a narcotic to counteract the spasm produced by the narcotic when the latter is used to relieve the pain of urethral colic. Hyoscyamine preparations are also used as antispasmodics in the therapy of peptic ulcers.

Hyoscyamine Sulfate, USP. Hyoscyamine sulfate (Levsin sulfate) is a white, odorless, crystalline compound of a deliquescent nature that also is affected by light. It is soluble in water (1:0.5) and alcohol (1:5) but almost insoluble in ether. Solutions of hyoscyamine sulfate are acidic to litmus.

This drug is used as an anticholinergic in the same manner and for the same indications as atropine and hyoscyamine, but it possesses the disadvantage of being deliquescent.

Scopolamine. Scopolamine (hyoscine) is found in various members of the Solanaceae (e.g., *H. niger*, *Duboisia myoporoides*, *Scopolia* spp., and *Datura metel*). Scopolamine usually is isolated from the mother liquor remaining from the isolation of hyoscyamine.

Hyoscine is the older name for this alkaloid, although *scopolamine* is the accepted name in the United States. Scopolamine is the *levo* component of the racemic mixture that is known as *atroscine*. The alkaloid is racemized readily in the presence of dilute alkali.

The alkaloid occurs in the form of a levorotatory, viscous liquid that is only slightly soluble in water but very soluble in alcohol, chloroform, or ether. It forms crystalline salts with most acids, with the hydrobromide being the most stable and the most popularly accepted. An aqueous solution of the hydrobromide containing 10% mannitol is said to be less prone to decomposition than unprotected solutions. The commercially available transdermal system of scopolamine comprises an outer layer of polymer film and a drug reservoir containing scopolamine, polyisobutylene, and mineral oil, which is interfaced with a microporous membrane to control diffusion of the drug. In this dosage form, scopolamine is effective in preventing motion sickness. The action is believed to be on the cortex or the vestibular apparatus. Whereas atropine stimulates the CNS, causing restlessness and talkativeness, scopolamine usually acts as a CNS depressant.

Scopolamine Hydrobromide, USP. Scopolamine hydrobromide (hyoscine hydrobromide) occurs as white or colorless crystals or as a white, granular powder. It is odorless and tends to effloresce in dry air. It is freely soluble in water (1:1.5), soluble in alcohol (1:20), only slightly soluble in chloroform, and insoluble in ether.

Scopolamine is a competitive blocking agent of the parasympathetic nervous system as is atropine, but it differs markedly from atropine in its action on the higher nerve centers. Both drugs readily cross the blood-brain barrier and, even at therapeutic doses, cause confusion, particularly in the elderly.

A sufficiently large dose of scopolamine will cause an individual to sink into a restful, dreamless sleep for about 8 hours, followed by a period of approximately the same length in which the patient is in a semiconscious state. During this time, the patient does not remember events that take place. When scopolamine is administered with morphine, this temporary amnesia is termed *twilight sleep.*

Homatropine Hydrobromide, USP. Homatropine hydrobromide, $1\alpha H,5\alpha H$-tropan-3α-ol mandelate (ester) hydrobromide (Homatrocel), occurs as white crystals or as a white, crystalline powder that is affected by light. It is soluble in water (1:6) and alcohol (1:40), less soluble in chloroform (1:420), and insoluble in ether.

Solutions are incompatible with alkaline substances, which precipitate the free base, and with the common reagents that precipitate alkaloids. As with atropine, solutions are sterilized best by filtration through a bacteriological filter.

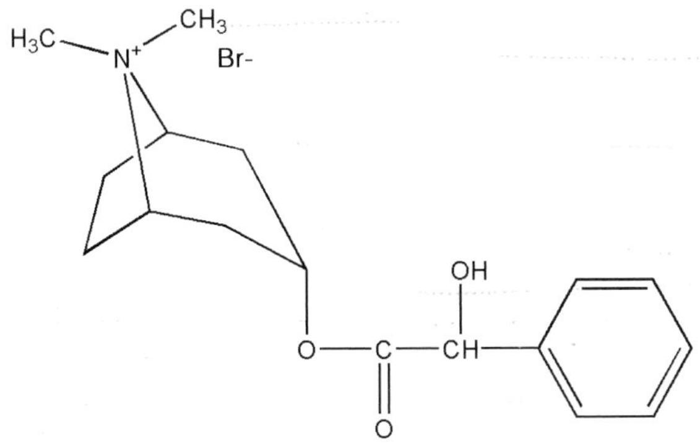

Homatropine Methylbromide

Homatropine hydrobromide is used topically to paralyze the ciliary structure of the eye (cycloplegia) and to effect mydriasis. It behaves very much like atropine but is weaker and less toxic. In the eye, it acts more rapidly but less persistently than atropine. Dilation of the pupil takes place in about 15 to 20 minutes, and the action subsides in about 24 hours. By using a miotic, such as physostigmine, it is possible to restore the pupil to normality in a few hours.

Homatropine Methylbromide, USP. Homatropine methylbromide, 3α-hydroxy-8-methyl-$1\alpha H,5\alpha H$-tropanium bromide mandelate (Novatropine, Mesopin), occurs as a bitter, white, odorless powder and is affected by light. The compound is readily soluble in water and alcohol but insoluble in ether. The pH of a 1% solution is 5.9 and that of a 10% solution is 4.5. Although a solution of the compound yields a precipitate with alkaloidal reagents, such as mercuric potassium iodide test solution, addition of alkali hydroxides or carbonates does not cause the precipitate that occurs with nonquaternary nitrogen salts (e.g., atropine, homatropine).

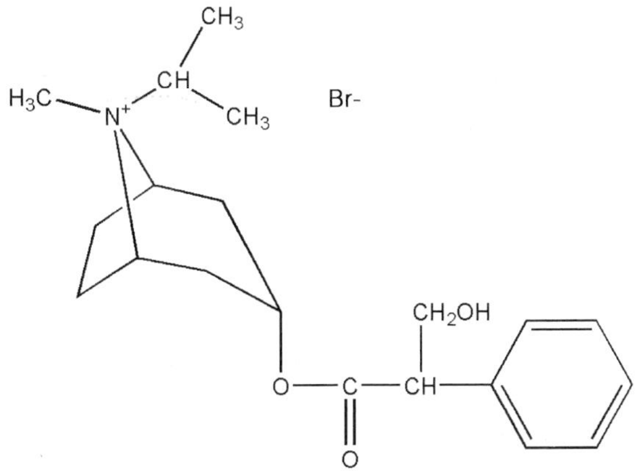

Ipratropium Bromide

Homatropine methylbromide is transported poorly across the blood-brain barrier because of its quaternary ammonium group and, therefore, has far fewer stimulant properties than atropine. It does have all the characteristic peripheral parasympathetic depressant properties of atropine and is used to reduce oversecretion and to relieve GI spasms.

Ipratropium Bromide. Ipratropium bromide, 3-(3-hydroxy-1-oxo-2-phenylpropoxy)-8-methyl-8-(1-methylethyl)-8-azoniabicyclo[3.2.1]octane bromide (Atrovent), is a quaternary ammonium derivative of atropine. It is freely soluble in water and ethanol but insoluble in chloroform and ether. The salt is stable in neutral and acidic solutions but rapidly hydrolyzed in alkaline solutions.

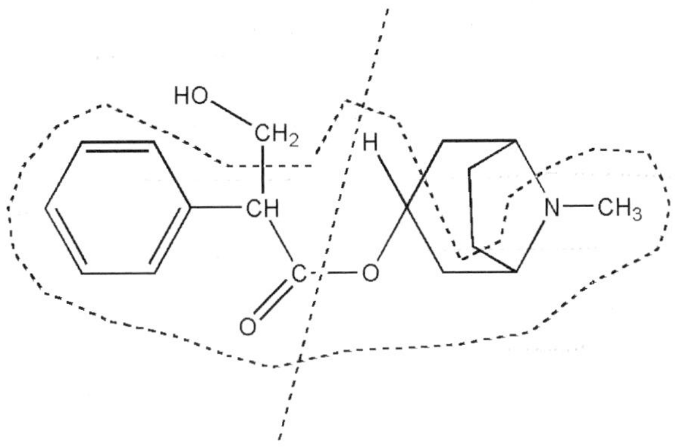

Tropic Acid   Tropine

Ipratropium bromide is used in inhalation therapy to produce dilation of bronchial smooth muscle for acute asthmatic attacks. The drug produces bronchodilation by competitive inhibition of cholinergic receptors bound to smooth muscle of the bronchioles. Ipratropium may also act on the surface of mast cells to inhibit ACh-enhanced release of chemical mediators. The drug has a slow onset of action, within 5 to 15 minutes after being administered by inhalation, and should not be used alone for acute asthmatic attacks. The peak therapeutic effect from one dose is observed between 1 and 2 hours. The effects of the drug last for about 6 hours. It has a half-life of 3.5 hours.

Tiotropium Bromide. Tiotropium bromide, $(1\alpha,2\beta,4\beta,7\beta)$-7-[(hydroxidi-2-thienylacetyl)oxy]-9,9-dimethyl-3-oxa-9-azoniatricyclo[3.3.1.0^{2,4}]nonane, (Spiriva) is an antimuscarinic agent that is used in an inhalation device to deliver the drug into the lungs. It is indicated in the treatment of chronic obstructive pulmonary disease (COPD), including chronic bronchitis and emphysema. The standard once-daily dose is 18 μg of tiotropium.

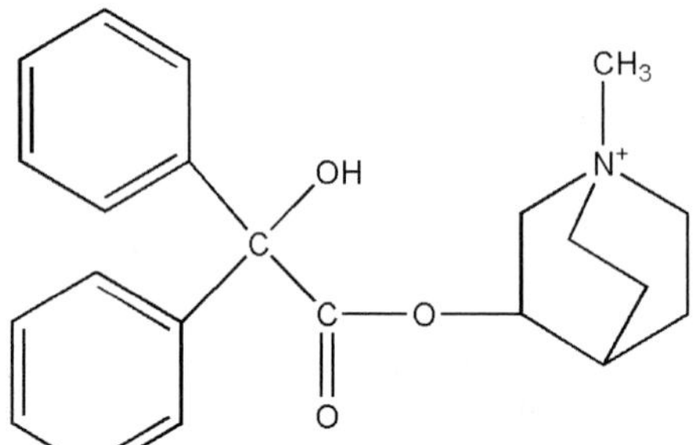

Clidinium Bromide

SYNTHETIC CHOLINERGIC BLOCKING AGENTS

Aminoalcohol Esters

The solanaceous alkaloids are generally agreed to be potent parasympatholytics, but they have the undesirable property of producing a wide range of effects through their nonspecific blockade of autonomic functions. Efforts to use the antispasmodic effect of the alkaloids most often result in side effects such as dryness of the mouth and fluctuations in pulse rate. Therefore, synthesis of compounds possessing specific cholinolytic actions has been a very desirable field of study. Few prototypical drugs were as avidly dissected in the minds of researchers as atropine in attempts to modify its structure to separate the numerous useful activities (i.e., antispasmodic, antisecretory, mydriatic, and cycloplegic). Most early research was carried out in the pre– and post–World War II era before muscarinic receptor subtypes were known.

Efforts at synthesis started with rather minor deviations from the atropine molecule, but a review of the commonly used drugs today indicates a marked departure from the rigid tropane aminoalcohols and tropic acid residues. Examination of the structures of antispasmodics shows that the acid portion has been designed to provide a large hydrophobic moiety rather than the stereospecific requirement of (*S*)-tropic acid in (−)-hyoscyamine that was once considered important. One of the major developments in the field of aminoalcohol esters was the successful introduction of the quaternary ammonium derivatives as contrasted with

the tertiary amine-type esters synthesized originally. Although some effective tertiary amine esters are in use today, the quaternaries, as a group, represent the more popular type and appear to be slightly more potent than their tertiary amine counterparts.

The accompanying formula shows the portion of the atropine molecule (enclosed in the curved dotted line) believed to be responsible for its major activity. This is sometimes called the *spasmophoric* group and compares with the *anesthesiophoric* group obtained by similar dissection of the cocaine molecule. The validity of this conclusion has been amply borne out by the many active compounds having only a simple diethylaminoethyl residue replacing the tropine portion.

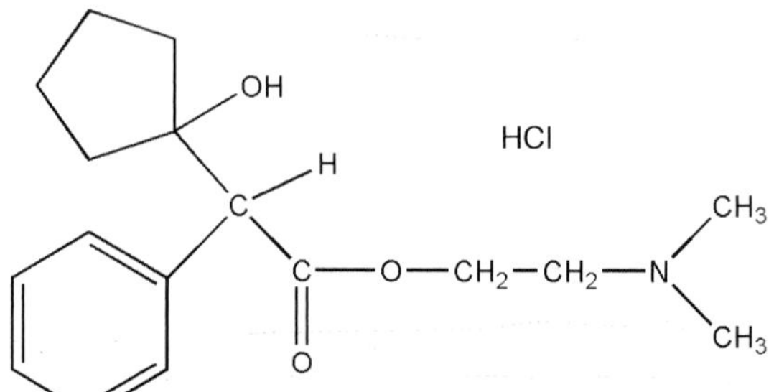

Cyclopentolate Hydrochloride

The aminoalcohol portion of eucatropine may be considered a simplification of the atropine molecule. In eucatropine, the bicyclic tropine has been replaced by a monocyclic aminoalcohol and mandelic acid replaces tropic acid (see under "Products").

Although simplification of the aminoalcohol portion of the atropine prototype has been a guiding principle in most research, many of the anticholinergics now used still include a cyclic aminoalcohol moiety. The aminoalcohol ester anticholinergics are used primarily as antispasmodics or mydriatics, and cholinolytic compounds classed as aminoalcohol or aminoalcohol ether analogs of atropine are, with few exceptions, used as antiparkinsonian drugs.

Another important feature in many of the synthetic anticholinergics used as antispasmodics is that they contain a quaternary nitrogen, presumably to enhance activity. The initial synthetic quaternary compound methantheline bromide has served as a forerunner for many others. These compounds combine anticholinergic activity of the antimuscarinic type with some ganglionic blockade to reinforce the parasympathetic blockade. Formation of a quaternary ammonium moiety, however, introduces the possibility of blockade of voluntary synapses (curariform activity); this can become evident with sufficiently high doses.

Products

The antimuscarinic compounds now in use are described in the following monographs.

Clidinium Bromide, USP. Clidinium bromide, 3-hydroxy-1-methylquinuclidinium bromide benzilate (Quarzan), is a white or nearly white, almost odorless, crystalline powder that is optically inactive. It is soluble in water and alcohol but only very slightly soluble in ether and benzene.

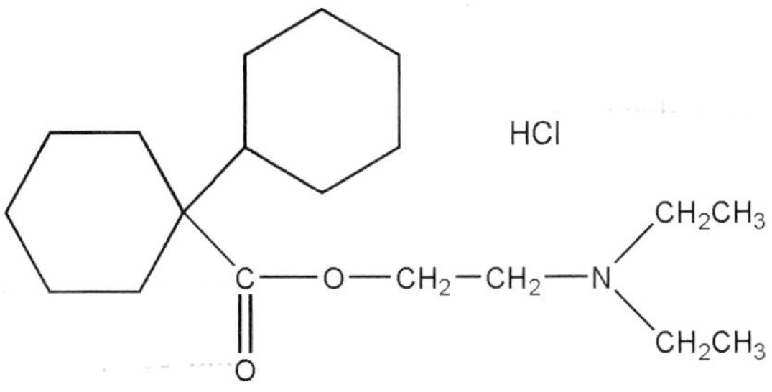

Dicyclomine Hydrochloride

This anticholinergic agent is marketed alone and in combination with the minor tranquilizer chlordiazepoxide (Librium) in a product known as Librax. The rationale of the combination for the treatment of GI complaints is the use of an anxiety-reducing agent together with an anticholinergic agent, based on the recognized contribution of anxiety to the development of the diseased condition. It is suggested for peptic ulcer, hyperchlorhydria, ulcerative or spastic colon, anxiety states with GI manifestations, nervous stomach, irritable or spastic colon, and others. Clidinium bromide is contraindicated in glaucoma and other conditions that may be aggravated by the parasympatholytic action, such as prostatic hypertrophy in elderly men, which could lead to urinary retention.

Cyclopentolate Hydrochloride, **USP.** Cyclopentolate hydrochloride, 2-dimethylaminoethyl 1-hydroxy-α-phenylcyclopentaneacetate hydrochloride (Cyclogyl), is a crystalline, white, odorless solid that is very soluble in water, easily soluble in alcohol, and only slightly soluble in ether. A 1% solution has a pH of 5.0 to 5.4.

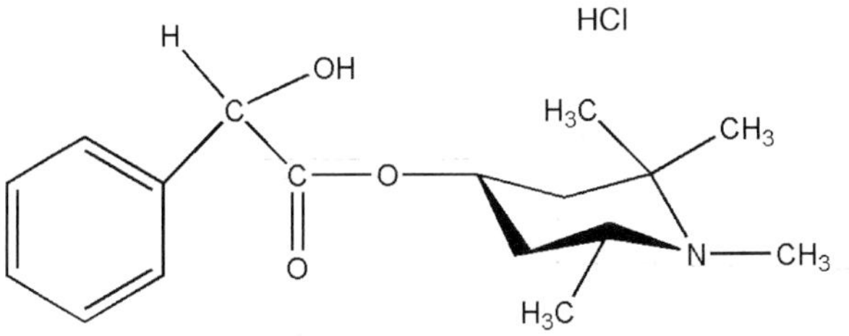

Eucatropine Hydrochloride

It is used only for its effects on the eye, where it acts as a parasympatholytic. When placed in the eye, it quickly produces cycloplegia and mydriasis. Its primary field of usefulness is in refraction studies. Cyclopentolate hydrochloride can be used, however, as a mydriatic in the management of iritis, iridocyclitis, keratitis, and choroiditis. Although it does not seem to affect intraocular tension significantly, it is best to be very cautious with patients with high intraocular pressure and with elderly patients with possible unrecognized glaucomatous changes.

Cyclopentolate hydrochloride has one half of the antispasmodic activity of atropine and is nonirritating when instilled repeatedly into the eye. If not neutralized after the refraction studies, its effect dissipates within 24 hours. Neutralization with a few drops of pilocarpine nitrate solution, 1% to 2%, often results in complete recovery in 6 hours. It is supplied as a ready-made ophthalmic solution in concentrations of either 0.5% or 2%.

Dicyclomine Hydrochloride, **USP.** Dicyclomine hydrochloride, 2-(diethylamino)ethyl bicyclohexyl-1-carboxyl-

ate hydrochloride (Bentyl), has some muscarinic receptor subtype selectivity. It binds more firmly to M_1 and M_3 than to M_2 and M_4 receptors.[76]

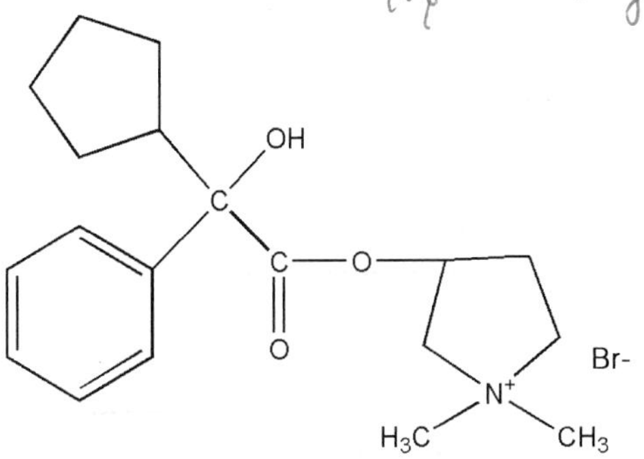

Trp 200 drugs

Glycopyrrolate   *⅛*

Dicyclomine hydrochloride has one eighth of the neurotropic activity of atropine and approximately twice the musculotropic activity of papaverine. This preparation, first introduced in 1950, has minimized the adverse effects associated with the atropine-type compounds. It is used for its spasmolytic effect on various smooth muscle spasms, particularly those associated with the GI tract. It is also useful in dysmenorrhea, pylorospasm, and biliary dysfunction.

Eucatropine Hydrochloride, **USP.** Eucatropine hydrochloride, euphthalmine hydrochloride or 1,2,2,6-tetramethyl-4-piperidyl mandelate hydrochloride, possesses the aminoalcohol moiety characteristic of one of the early local anesthetics (e.g., β-eucaine) but differs in the acidic portion of the ester by being a mandelate instead of a benzoate. The salt is an odorless, white, granular powder, providing solutions that are neutral to litmus. It is very soluble in water, freely soluble in alcohol and chloroform, but almost insoluble in ether.

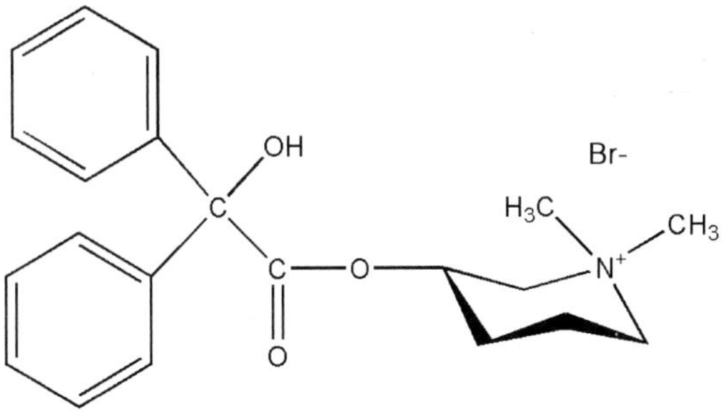

Mepenzolate Bromide

The action of eucatropine hydrochloride closely parallels that of atropine, although it is much less potent than the latter. It is used topically in a 0.1 mL dose as a mydriatic in 2% solution or in the form of small tablets. Use of concentrations from 5% to 10% is, however, not uncommon. Dilation, with little impairment of accommodation, takes place in about 30 minutes, and the eye returns to normal in 2 to 3 hours.

Glycopyrrolate, **USP.** Glycopyrrolate, 3-hydroxy-1, 1-dimethylpyrrolidinium bromide α-cyclopentylmandelate (Robinul), occurs as a white, crystalline powder that is soluble in water or alcohol but practically insoluble in chloroform or ether.

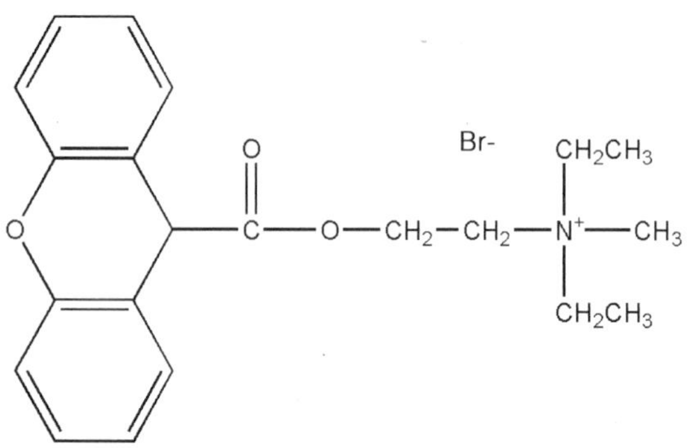

Methantheline Bromide

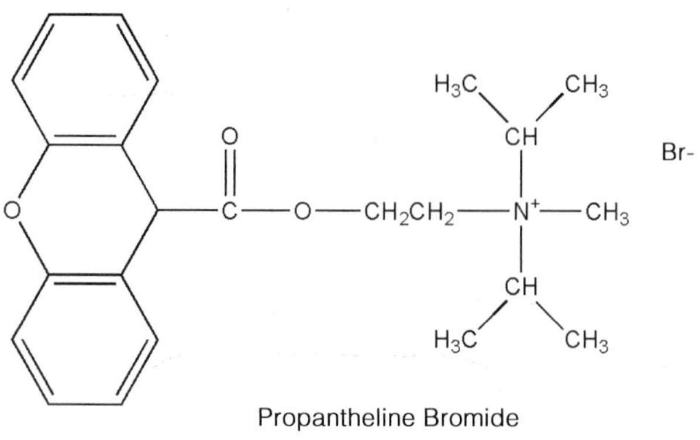

Propantheline Bromide

Glycopyrrolate is a typical anticholinergic and possesses, at adequate dosage levels, the atropine-like effects characteristic of this class of drugs. It has a spasmolytic effect on the musculature of the GI tract as well as the genitourinary tract. It diminishes gastric and pancreatic secretions and the quantity of perspiration and saliva. Its side effects are also typically atropine-like (i.e., dryness of the mouth, urinary retention, blurred vision, constipation). Glycopyrrolate is a more potent antagonist on M_1 than on M_2 and M_3 receptors. The low affinity of M_2 receptors may, in part, explain the low incidence of tachycardia during use of this drug as an antispasmodic.[77] Because of its quaternary ammonium character, glycopyrrolate rarely causes CNS disturbances, although in sufficiently high dosage, it can bring about ganglionic and myoneural junction block.

The drug is used as an adjunct in the management of peptic ulcer and other GI ailments associated with hyperacidity, hypermotility, and spasm. In common with other anticholinergics, its use does not preclude dietary restrictions or use of antacids and sedatives if these are indicated.

Mepenzolate Bromide. Mepenzolate bromide, 3-hydroxy-1,1-dimethylpiperidinium bromide benzilate (Cantil), has an activity about one half that of atropine in reducing ACh-induced spasms of the guinea pig ileum. The selective action on colonic hypermotility is said to relieve pain, cramps, and bloating and to help curb diarrhea.

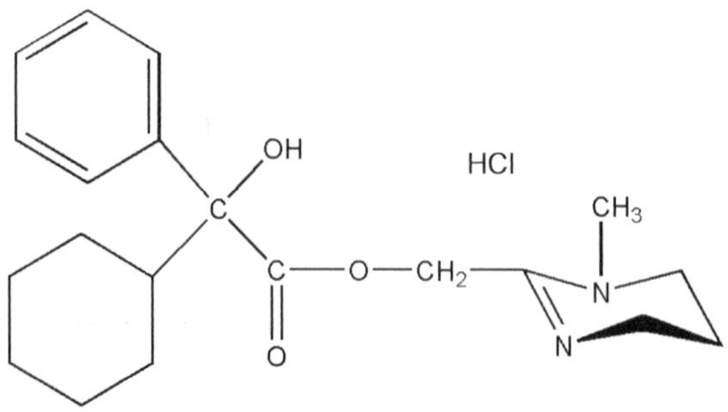

Oxyphencyclimine Hydrochloride

Methantheline Bromide, USP. Methantheline bromide, diethyl(2-hydroxyethyl)methylammonium bromide xanthene-9-carboxylate (Banthine Bromide), is a white, slightly hygroscopic, crystalline salt that is soluble in water to produce solutions with a pH of about 5. Aqueous solutions are not stable and hydrolyze in a few days. The bromide form is preferable to the very hygroscopic chloride.

This drug, introduced in 1950, is a potent anticholinergic agent and acts at the nicotinic cholinergic receptors of the sympathetic and parasympathetic systems, as well as at the myoneural junction of the postganglionic cholinergic fibers. Like other quaternary ammonium drugs, methantheline bromide is absorbed incompletely from the GI tract.

Among the conditions for which methantheline bromide is indicated are gastritis, intestinal hypermotility, bladder irritability, cholinergic spasm, pancreatitis, hyperhidrosis, and peptic ulcer, all of which are manifestations of parasympathotonia.

Side reactions are atropine-like (mydriasis, cycloplegia, dryness of mouth). The drug is contraindicated in glaucoma. Toxic doses may bring about a curare-like action, a not too surprising fact when it is considered that ACh is the mediating factor for neural transmission at the somatic myoneural junction. This side effect can be counteracted with neostigmine methylsulfate.

Oxyphencyclimine Hydrochloride. Oxyphencyclimine hydrochloride, 1,4,5,6-tetrahydro-1-methyl-2-pyrimidinyl) methyl α-phenylcyclohexaneglycolate monohydrochloride (Daricon, Vistrax), was introduced in 1958 and promoted as a peripheral anticholinergic–antisecretory agent, with little or no curare-like activity and little or no ganglionic blocking activity. These activities are probably absent because of the tertiary character of the molecule. This activity is in contrast with that of compounds that couple antimuscarinic action with ganglionic blocking action. The tertiary character of the nitrogen promotes intestinal absorption of the molecule. Perhaps the most significant activity of this compound is its marked ability to reduce both the volume and the acid content of the gastric juices, a desirable action in view of the more recent hypotheses pertaining to peptic ulcer therapy. Another important feature of this compound is its low toxicity in comparison with many of the other available anticholinergics. Oxyphencyclimine hydrochloride is hydrolyzed in the presence of excessive moisture and heat. It is absorbed from the GI tract and has a duration of action of up to 12 hours.

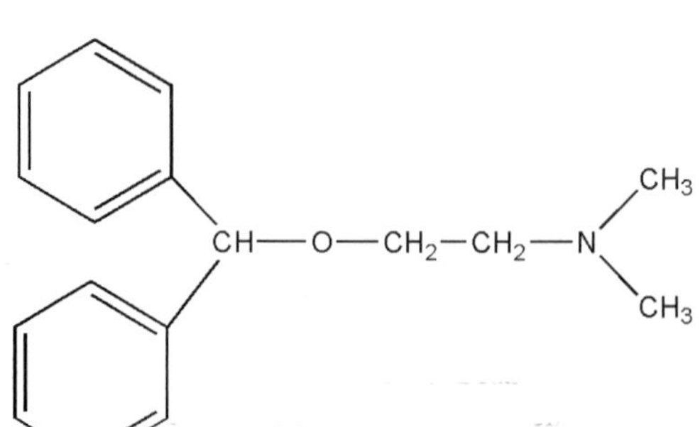

Diphenhydramine

Oxyphencyclimine hydrochloride is suggested for use in peptic ulcer, pylorospasm, and functional bowel syndrome. It is contraindicated, as are other anticholinergics, in patients with prostatic hypertrophy and glaucoma.

Propantheline Bromide, USP. Propantheline bromide, 2-hydroxy-ethyl)diisopropylmethylammonium bromide xanthene-9-carboxylate (Pro-Banthine), is prepared in a manner exactly analogous to that used for methantheline bromide. It is a white, water-soluble, crystalline substance, with properties quite similar to those of methantheline bromide. Its chief difference from methantheline bromide is in its potency, which has been estimated variously to be 2 to 5 times as great.

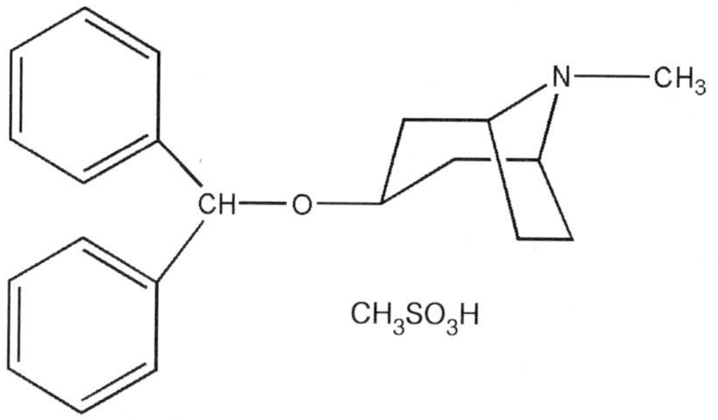

Benztropine Mesylate

Oxybutynin. Oxybutynin, 4-Diethylaminobut- 2-ynyl2-cyclohexyl-2- hydroxy-2-phenyl-ethanoate, (Oxytrol) was one of the first agents specifically developed to exploit the effects that cholinergic blocking agents have on the bladder. By competitively blocking the muscarinic receptors, it has direct spasmolytic effects on bladder smooth muscle. This reduction in smooth muscle tone allows for greater volumes of urine to be stored in the bladder, which results in less urinary incontinence, urgency, and frequency. Oxybutynin acts as a competitive antagonist on M_1, M_2, and M_3 receptor subtypes.[78]

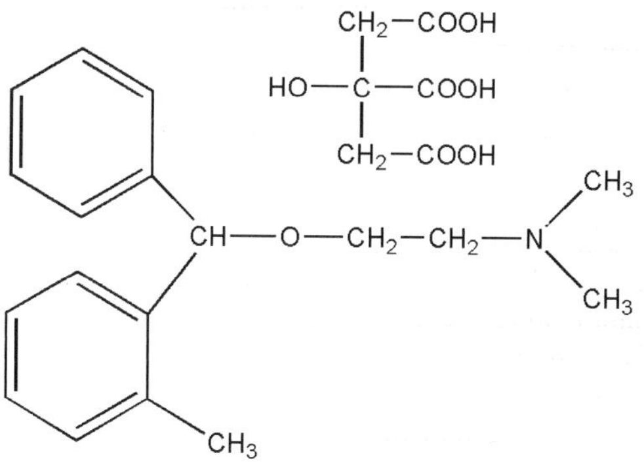

Orphenadrine Citrate

Trospium Chloride. Trosoium chloride, 3α-benziloy-loxynortropane-8-spiro-1′-pyrrolidinium chloride, (Sanctura) was available in Europe for almost 20 years before gaining approval in the United States in May 2004. Much like oxybutynin, it too is a competitive antagonist for muscarinic receptors and is used to manage overactive bladder. The quaternary amine reduces the likelihood that this agent will cross the blood-brain barrier. In addition, it has a limited

metabolic profile, largely a result of its highly water-soluble characteristics.[79]

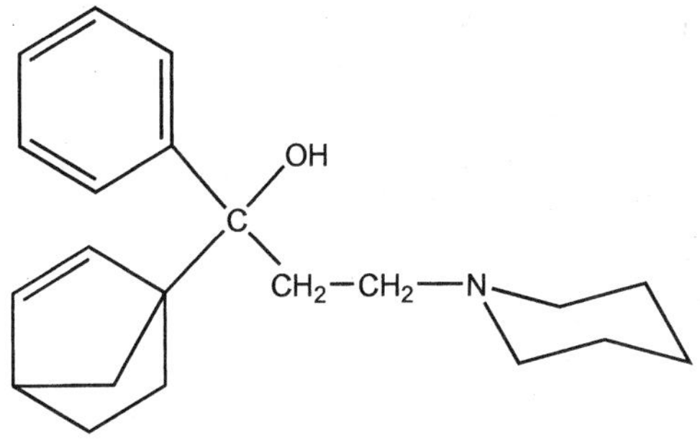

Biperiden

Solifenacin Succinate. Solifenacin succinate (Vesicare), (+)-(1S, 3′R)-quinuclidin-3′-yl 1-phenyl-1,2,3,4-tetrahy-droisoquinoline-2-carboxylate, is a competative antagonist for M_1, M_2, and M_3 receptor subtypes. One of the issues surrounding the use of such antagonists is the selectivity for the bladder over other tissue such as the salivary glands. It is reported that the selectivity of solifenacin for bladder muscarinic receptors over salivary receptors is superior to the effects observed with oxybutynin.[80]

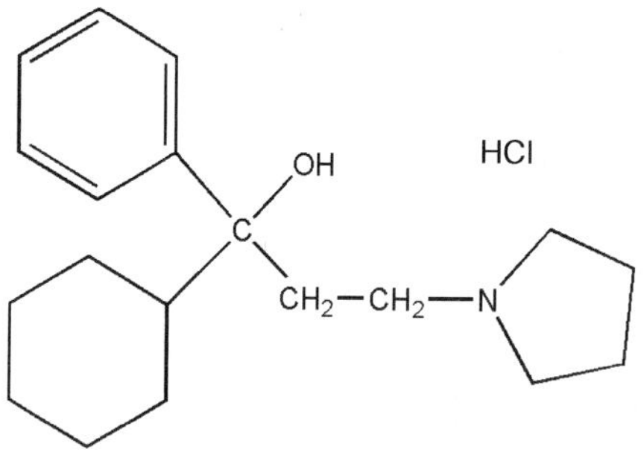

Procyclidine Hydrochloride

Aminoalcohol Ethers

The aminoalcohol ethers thus far introduced have been used as antiparkinsonian drugs rather than as conventional anticholinergics (i.e., as spasmolytics or mydriatics). In general, they may be considered closely related to the antihistaminics and, indeed, do possess substantial antihistaminic properties. In turn, the antihistamines possess anticholinergic activity and have been used as antiparkinsonian agents. Comparison of chlorphenoxamine and orphenadrine with the antihistaminic diphenhydramine illustrates the close similarity of structure. The use of diphenhydramine in parkinsonism has been cited previously. Benztropine may also be considered a structural relative of diphenhydramine, although the aminoalcohol portion is tropine and, therefore, more distantly related than chlorphenoxamine and orphenadrine. In the structure of benztropine, a three-carbon chain intervenes between the nitrogen and oxygen functions, whereas the others evince a two-carbon chain. However, the rigid ring structure possibly orients the nitrogen and oxygen functions into more nearly the two-carbon chain interprosthetic distance than is apparent at first glance. This, combined with the flexibility of the alicyclic chain, would help to minimize the distance discrepancy.

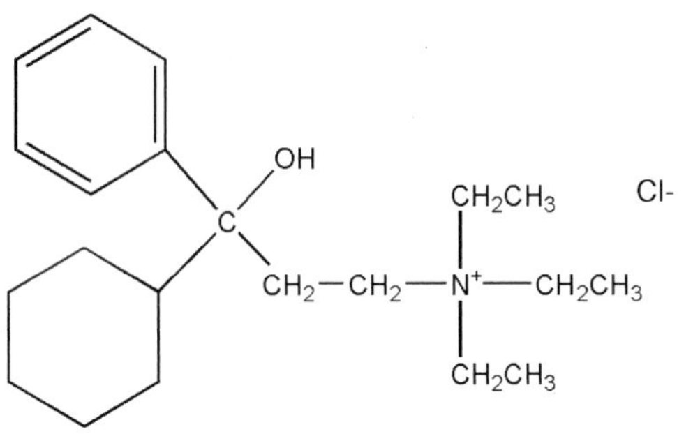

Tridihexethyl Chloride

Benztropine Mesylate, USP. Benztropine mesylate, 3α-(diphenylmethoxy)-1αH,5αH-tropane methanesulfonate (Cogentin), has anticholinergic, antihistaminic, and local anesthetic properties. Its anticholinergic effect makes it applicable as an antiparkinsonian agent. It is about as potent an anticholinergic as atropine and shares some of the side effects of this drug, such as mydriasis and dryness of mouth. Importantly, however, it does not produce central stimulation but instead exerts the characteristic sedative effect of the antihistamines.

The tremor and rigidity characteristic of parkinsonism are relieved by benztropine mesylate, and it is particularly valuable for those patients who cannot tolerate central excitation (e.g., aged patients). It may also have a useful effect in minimizing drooling, sialorrhea, masklike facies, oculogyric crises, and muscular cramps.

The usual caution exercised with any anticholinergic in glaucoma and prostatic hypertrophy is observed with this drug.

Orphenadrine Citrate. Orphenadrine citrate, *N,N*-dimethyl-2-(*o*-methyl-α-phenylbenzyloxy)ethylamine citrate (1:1) (Norflex), introduced in 1957, is closely related to diphenhydramine structurally but has much lower antihistaminic activity and much higher anticholinergic action. Likewise, it lacks the sedative effects characteristic of diphenhydramine. Pharmacological testing indicates that it is not primarily a peripherally acting anticholinergic because it has only weak effects on smooth muscle, on the eye, and on secretory glands. It does reduce voluntary muscle spasm, however, by a central inhibitory action on cerebral motor areas, a central effect similar to that of atropine.

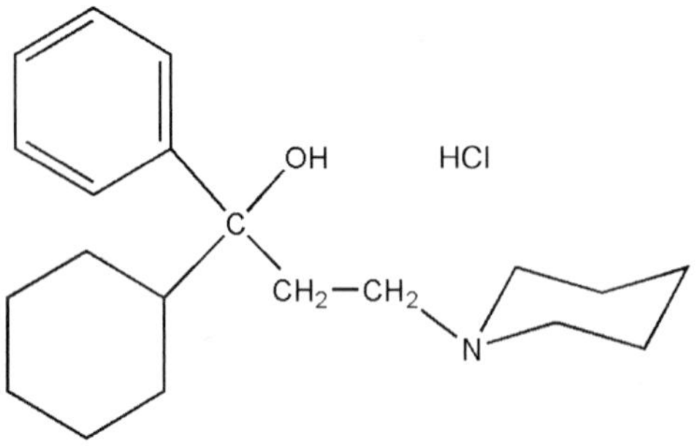

Trihexyphenidyl Hydrochloride

This drug is used for the symptomatic treatment of Parkinson disease. It relieves rigidity better than it does tremor, and in certain cases, it may accentuate the latter. The drug combats mental sluggishness, akinesia, adynamia, and lack of mobility, but this effect seems to diminish rather rapidly with prolonged use. It is best used as an adjunct to the other agents, such as benztropine, procyclidine, cycrimine, and trihexyphenidyl, in the treatment of paralysis agitans. Orphenadrine citrate is also used as an adjunct to rest, physiotherapy, and other measures to relieve pain of local muscle spasm (e.g., nocturnal leg cramps).

The drug has a low incidence of the usual side effects for this group, namely, dryness of mouth, nausea, and mild excitation.

Aminoalcohols

The development of aminoalcohols as parasympatholytics took place in the 1940s. It was soon established, however, that these antispasmodics were equally efficacious in parkinsonism.

Several of the drugs in this class of antimuscarinic agents possess bulky groups in the vicinity of hydroxyl and cyclic amino functional groups. These compounds are similar to the classic aminoester anticholinergic compounds derived from atropine. The presence of the alcohol group seems to substitute adequately as a prosthetic group for the carboxyl function in creating an effective parasympathetic blocking agent. The aminoester group, per se, is not a necessary adjunct to cholinolytic activity, provided that other polar groupings, such as the hydroxyl, can substitute as a prosthetic group for the carboxyl function. Another structural feature common to all aminoalcohol anticholinergics is the γ-aminopropanol arrangement, with three carbons intervening between the hydroxyl and amino functions. All of the aminoalcohols used for paralysis agitans are tertiary amines. Because the desired locus of action is central, formation of a quaternary ammonium moiety destroys the antiparkinsonian properties. These aminoalcohols have been quaternized, however, to enhance the anticholinergic activity to produce an antispasmodic and antisecretory compound, such as tridihexethyl chloride.

Biperiden, USP. Biperiden, α-5-norbornen-2-yl-α-phenyl-1-piperidinepropanol (Akineton), introduced in 1959, has a relatively weak visceral anticholinergic, but a strong nicotinolytic, action in terms of its ability to block nicotine-induced convulsions. Therefore, its neurotropic action is rather low on intestinal musculature and blood vessels. It has a relatively strong musculotropic action, which is about equal to that of papaverine, in comparison with most synthetic anticholinergic drugs. Its action on the eye, although mydriatic, is much lower than that of atropine. These weak anticholinergic effects add to its usefulness in Parkinson syndrome by minimizing side effects.

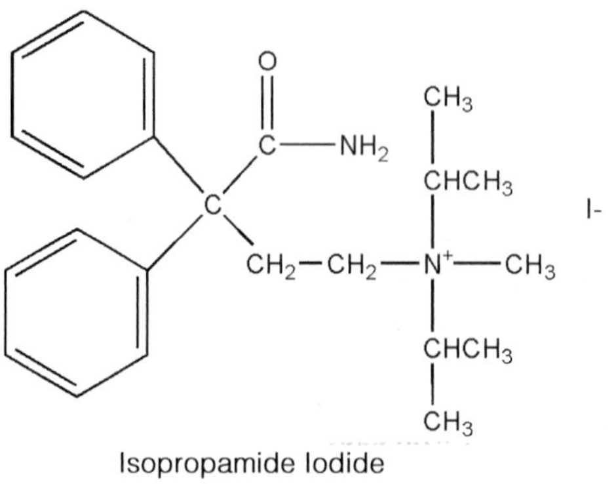

Isopropamide Iodide

The drug is used in all types of Parkinson disease (postencephalitic, idiopathic, arteriosclerotic) and helps to eliminate akinesia, rigidity, and tremor. It is also used in drug-induced extrapyramidal disorders to eliminate symptoms and permit continued use of tranquilizers. Biperiden is also of value in spastic disorders not related to parkinsonism, such as multiple sclerosis, spinal cord injury, and cerebral palsy. It is contraindicated in all forms of epilepsy.

Biperiden Hydrochloride, USP. Biperiden hydrochloride, α-5-norbornen-2-yl-α-phenyl-1-piperidinepropanol hydrochloride (Akineton hydrochloride), is a white, optically inactive, crystalline, odorless powder that is slightly soluble in water, ether, alcohol, and chloroform and sparingly soluble in methanol.

Biperiden hydrochloride has all of the actions described for biperiden. The hydrochloride is used for tablets because it is better suited to this dosage form than is the lactate salt. As with the free base and the lactate salt, xerostomia (dryness of the mouth) and blurred vision may occur.

Procyclidine Hydrochloride, USP. Procyclidine hydrochloride, α-cyclohexyl-α-phenyl-1-pyrrolidinepropanol hydrochloride (Kemadrin), was introduced in 1956. Although it is an effective peripheral anticholinergic and, indeed, has been used for peripheral effects similar to its methochloride (i.e., tricyclamol chloride), its clinical usefulness lies in its ability to relieve voluntary muscle spasticity by its central action. Therefore, it has been used with success in the treatment of Parkinson syndrome. It is said to be as effective as trihexyphenidyl and is used to reduce muscle rigidity in postencephalitic, arteriosclerotic, and idiopathic types of the disease. Its effect on tremor is not predictable and probably should be supplemented by combination with other similar drugs.

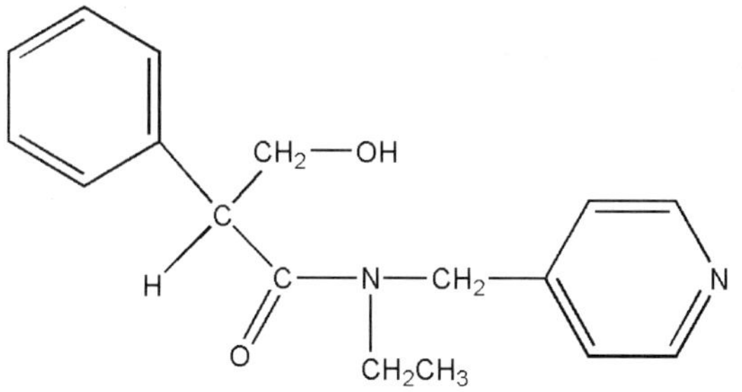

Tropicamide

The toxicity of the drug is low, but when the dosage of the drug is high, side effects are noticeable. At therapeutic dosage levels, dry mouth is the most common side effect. The same care should be exercised with this drug as with all other anticholinergics when it is administered to patients with glaucoma, tachycardia, or prostatic hypertrophy.

Tridihexethyl Chloride, USP. Tridihexethyl chloride, 3-cyclohexyl-3-hydroxy-3-phenylpropyl)triethylammonium chloride (Pathilon), is a white, bitter, crystalline powder with a characteristic odor. The compound is freely soluble in water and alcohol, with aqueous solutions being nearly neutral in reaction.

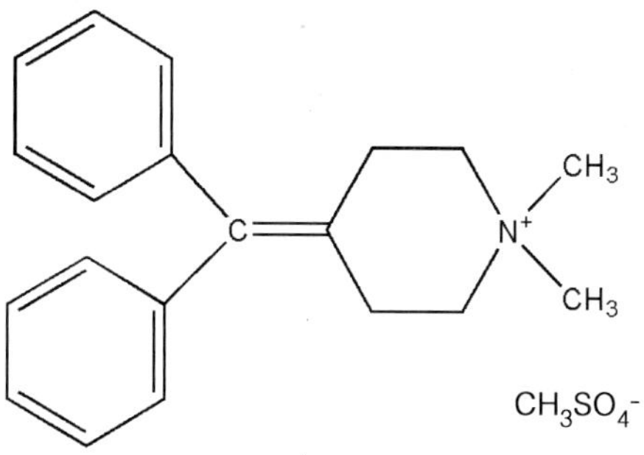

Diphemanil Methylsulfate

Although this drug, introduced in 1958, has ganglion-blocking activity, its peripheral atropine-like activity predominates; therefore, its therapeutic application has been based on the latter activity. It possesses the antispasmodic and the antisecretory activities characteristic of this group, but because of its quaternary character, it is valueless in relieving Parkinson syndrome.

The drug is useful for adjunctive therapy in a wide variety of GI diseases, such as peptic ulcer, gastric hyperacidity, and hypermotility and spastic conditions, such as spastic colon, functional diarrhea, pylorospasm, and other related conditions. Because its action is predominantly antisecretory, it is more effective in gastric hypersecretion than in hypermotility and spasm. It is best administered intravenously for the latter conditions.

The side effects usually found with effective anticholinergic therapy occur with the use of this drug. These are dryness of mouth, mydriasis, and such. As with other anticholinergics, care should be exercised when administering the drug to patients with glaucomatous conditions, cardiac decompensation, and coronary insufficiency. It is contraindicated in patients with obstruction at the bladder neck, prostatic hypertrophy, stenosing gastric and duodenal ulcers, or pyloric or duodenal obstruction.

Trihexyphenidyl Hydrochloride, USP. Trihexyphenidyl hydrochloride, α-cyclohexyl-α-phenyl-1-piperidinepropanol hydrochloride (Artane, Tremin, Pipanol), introduced in 1949, is approximately half as active as atropine as an antispasmodic but is claimed to have milder side effects, such as mydriasis, drying of secretions, and cardioacceleration. It has a good margin of safety, although it is about as toxic as atropine. It has found a place in the treatment of parkinsonism and is claimed to provide some measure of relief from the mental depression often associated with this condition. It

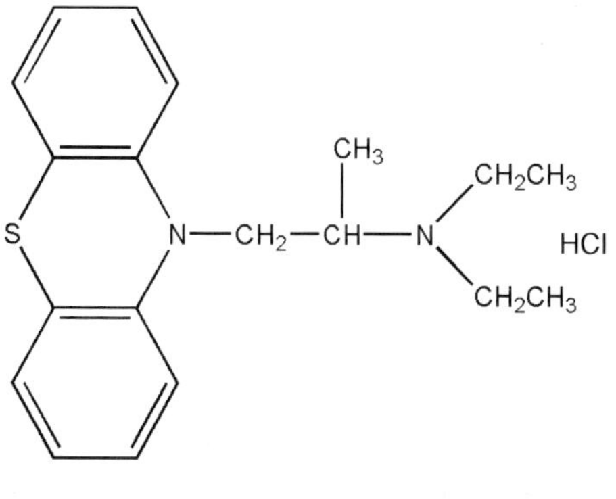

Ethopropazine Hydrochloride

does, however, exhibit some of the side effects typical of the parasympatholytic-type preparation, although adjusting the dose carefully may often eliminate these.

Tolterodine. Tolterodine (Detrol), 2-[3-[bis(1-methylethyl)amino]-1-phenyl-propyl]-4-methyl-phenol, is an antimuscarinic agent that acts on M_2 and M_3 muscarinic subtype receptors. By competitively blocking of the muscarinic receptors results in a reduction of the smooth muscle tone, allowing for greater volume of urine to be stored in the bladder. This results in less urinary incontinence, urgency, and frequency.[81]

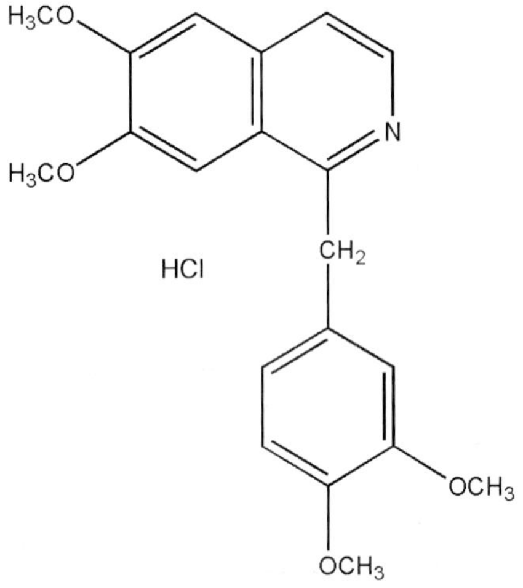

Papaverine Hydrochloride

Aminoamides

From a structural standpoint, the aminoamide type of anticholinergic represents the same type of molecule as the aminoalcohol group, with the important exception that the polar amide group replaces the corresponding polar hydroxyl group. Aminoamides retain the same bulky structural features found at one end of the molecule or the other in all of the active anticholinergics. Isopropamide iodide is the only drug of this class currently in use.

Another amide-type structure is that of tropicamide, formerly known as bis-tropamide, a compound with some of the atropine features.

Isopropamide Iodide, USP. Isopropamide iodide, 3-carbamoyl-3,3-diphenylpropyl)diisopropylmethylammonium iodide (Darbid), occurs as a bitter, white to pale yellow, crystalline powder that is only sparingly soluble in water but freely soluble in chloroform and alcohol.

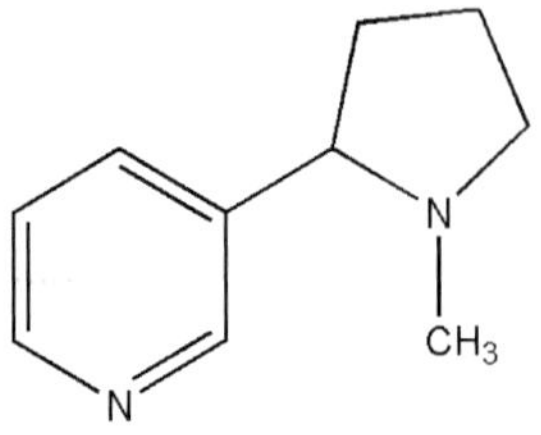

Nicotine

This drug, introduced in 1957, is a potent anticholinergic, producing atropine-like effects peripherally. Even with its quaternary nature, it does not cause sympathetic blockade at the ganglionic level except at high dosages. Its principal distinguishing feature is its long duration of action. A single dose can provide antispasmodic and antisecretory effects for as long as 12 hours.

It is used as adjunctive therapy in the treatment of peptic ulcer and other conditions of the GI tract associated with hypermotility and hyperacidity. It has the usual side effects of anticholinergics (dryness of mouth, mydriasis, difficult urination) and is contraindicated in glaucoma, prostatic hypertrophy, etc.

Tropicamide, USP. Tropicamide, *N*-ethyl-2-phenyl-*N*-(4-pyridylmethyl)hydracrylamide (Mydriacyl), is an effective anticholinergic for ophthalmic use when mydriasis is produced by relaxation of the sphincter muscle of the iris, allowing adrenergic innervation of the radial muscle to dilate the pupil. Its maximum effect is achieved in about 20 to 25 minutes and lasts for about 20 minutes, with complete recovery in about 6 hours. Its action is more rapid in onset and wears off more rapidly than that of most other mydriatics. To achieve mydriasis, either 0.5% or 1.0% concentration may be used, although cycloplegia is achieved only with the stronger solution. Its uses are much the same as those described above for mydriatics in general, but opinions differ on whether the drug is as effective as homatropine, for example, in achieving cycloplegia. For mydriatic use, however, in examination of the fundus and treatment of acute iritis, iridocyclitis, and keratitis, it is quite adequate; and because of its shorter duration of action, it is less prone to initiate a rise in intraocular pressure than the more potent, longer-lasting drugs. As with other mydriatics, however, pupil dilation can lead to increased intraocular pressure. In common with other mydriatics, it is contraindicated in patients with glaucoma, either known or suspected, and should not be used in the presence of a shallow anterior chamber. Thus far, no allergic reactions or ocular damage has been observed with this drug. The ability to clone the various muscarinic receptor subtypes has allowed the observation that tropicamide has modest selectivity for the M_4 receptor.[82]

n = 5 or 6, active as ganglionic blockers (feeble curariform activity)

n = 9 to 12, weak ganglionic blockers (strong curariform activity)

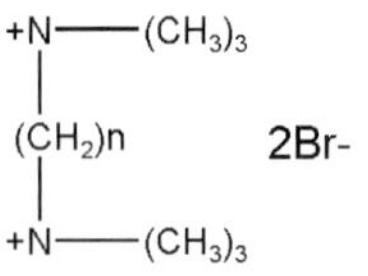

Darifenacin Hydrobromide. Darfenacin (Enablex), (s)-2-{1-[2-(2,3-dihydrobenzofuran-5-yl)ethyl]-3-pyrrolidinyl}-2,2-diphen-ylacetamide, is an antimuscarinic agent that has selectivity for the M_3 muscarinic subtype receptor. By competitively blocking of the muscarinic receptors results in a reduction of the smooth muscle tone, allowing for greater volume of urine to be stored in the bladder. This results in less urinary incontinence, urgency, and frequency. It is a white to almost white, crystalline powder, with a molecular weight of 507.5. Darifenacin is metabolized by the isozymes CYP2D6 and CYP3A4 with the primary metabolic routes being monohydroxylation of the dihydrobenzofuran ring, opening of the dihydrobenzofuran ring, and *N*-dealkylation of the pyrrolidine nitrogen.[83]

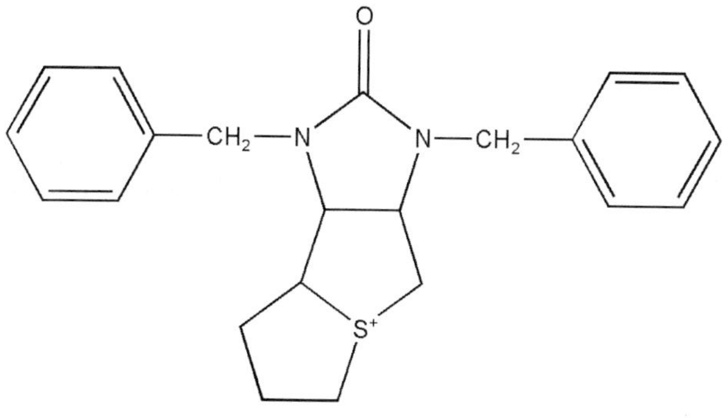

Trimethaphan Camsylate

Miscellaneous

Further structural modification of classic antimuscarinic agents can be found in the drugs described next. Each of them has the typical bulky group characteristic of the usual anticholinergic molecule. One modification is represented by the diphenylmethylene moiety (e.g., diphemanil); a second, by a phenothiazine (e.g., ethopropazine); and a third, by a thioxanthene structure (e.g., methixene).

Diphemanil Methylsulfate, USP. Diphemanil methylsulfate, 4-(diphenylmethylene)-1,1-dimethylpiperidinium methylsulfate (Prantal), or diphemanil methylsulfate is a potent cholinergic blocking agent. In the usual dosage range, it acts as an effective parasympatholytic by blocking nerve impulses at the parasympathetic ganglia, but it does not invoke a sympathetic ganglionic blockade. It is claimed to be highly specific in its action on those innervations that activate gastric secretion and GI motility. Although this drug can produce atropine-like side effects, they rarely occur at recommended doses. The highly specific nature of its action on gastric functions makes the drug useful in the treatment of peptic ulcer, and its lack of atropine-like effects makes its use much less distressing than other antispasmodic drugs. In addition to its action in decreasing gastric hypermotility, diphemanil methylsulfate is valuable in hyperhidrosis in low doses (50 mg twice daily) or topically. The drug is not well absorbed from the GI tract, particularly in the presence of food, and should be administered between meals. The methylsulfate salt was chosen as the best, because the chloride is hygroscopic and the bromide and iodide ions have exhibited toxic manifestations in clinical use.

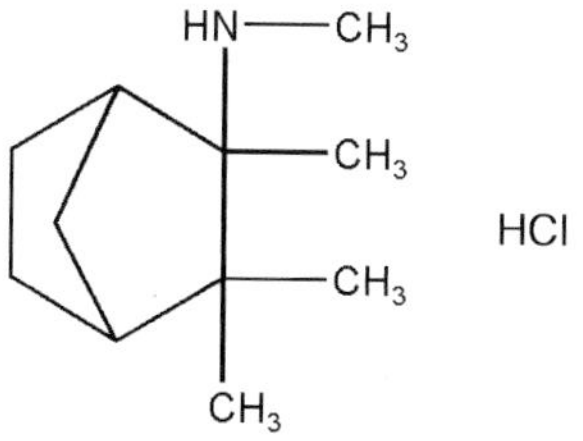

Mecamylamine Hydrochloride

Ethopropazine Hydrochloride, USP. Ethopropazine hydrochloride, 10-[2-(diethylamino)propyl]phenothiazine monohydrochloride (Parsidol), introduced to therapy in 1954, has antimuscarinic activity and is especially useful in the symptomatic treatment of parkinsonism. In this capacity, it has value in controlling rigidity, and it also has a favorable effect on tremor, sialorrhea, and oculogyric crises. It is often used in conjunction with other antiparkinsonian drugs for complementary activity.

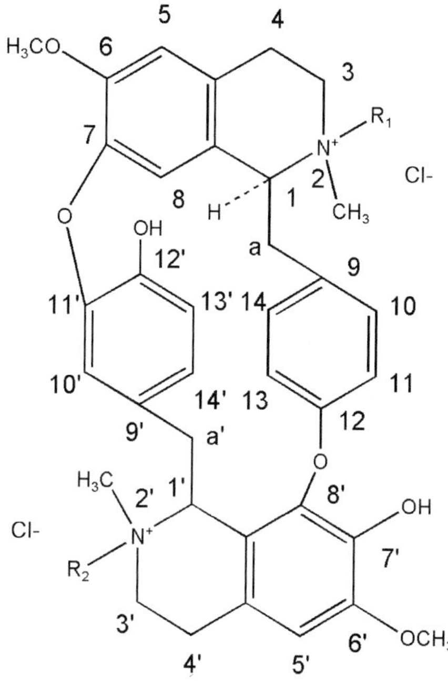

(Ia) R₁=R₂=CH₃
(Ib) R₁=H; R₂=CH₃
(Ic) R₁=CH₃; R₂=H

Side effects are common with this drug but are usually not severe. Drowsiness and dizziness are the most common side effects at ordinary dosage levels, and as the dose increases, xerostomia, mydriasis, and others become evident. It is contraindicated in conditions such as glaucoma because of its mydriatic effect.

Papaverine Hydrochloride, USP. Papaverine hydrochloride, 6,7-dimethoxy-1-veratrylisoquinoline hydrochloride, was isolated by Merck in 1848 from opium, in which it occurs to the extent of about 1%. Although its natural origin is closely related to morphine, the pharmacological actions of papaverine hydrochloride are unlike those of morphine. Its main effect is as a spasmolytic on smooth muscle, acting as a direct, nonspecific relaxant on vascular, cardiac, and other smooth muscle. Because of its broad antispasmodic action on ACh muscarinic receptors, it is often called a *nonspecific antagonist*. Papaverine hydrochloride has been used in the treatment of peripheral vascular disorders, but its use is limited by lack of potency.

Papaverine hydrochloride interferes with the mechanism of muscle contraction by inhibiting the cyclic nucleotide phosphodiesterases in smooth muscle cells responsible for converting cAMP and cyclic guanosine monophosphate (cGMP) to 5′-AMP and 5′-GMP, respectively. The increased levels of cAMP and cGMP are associated with

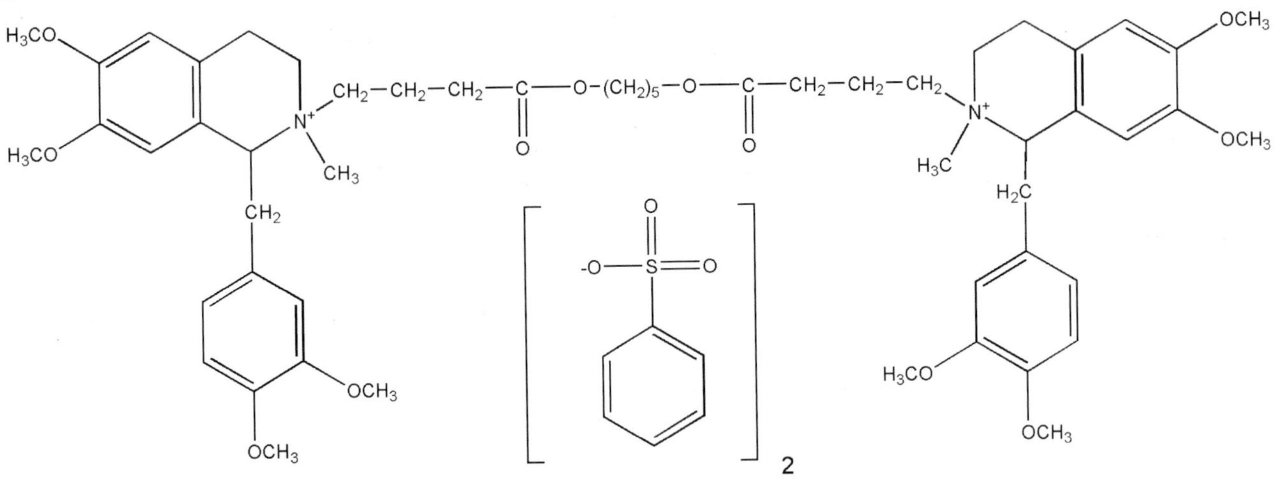

Atracurium Besylate

muscle relaxation through their phosphorylation of myosin light-chain kinase.

GANGLIONIC BLOCKING AGENTS

Autonomic ganglia have been the subject of interest for many years in the study of interactions between drugs and nervous tissues. The first important account[84] was given by Langley and described the stimulating and blocking actions of nicotine on sympathetic ganglia. It was found that small amounts of nicotine stimulated ganglia and then produced a blockade of ganglionic transmission because of persistent depolarization. From these experiments, Langley was able to outline the general pattern of innervation of organs by the autonomic nervous system. *Parasympathetic* ganglia usually are located near the organ they innervate and have preganglionic fibers that stem from the cervical and thoracic regions of the spinal cord. *Sympathetic* ganglia consist of 22 pairs that lie on either side of the vertebral column to form lateral chains. These ganglia are connected both to each other by nerve trunks and to the lumbar or sacral regions of the spinal cord.

Using the sympathetic cervical ganglion as a model revealed that transmission in the autonomic ganglion is more complex than formerly believed. Traditionally, stimulation of autonomic ganglia by ACh was considered to be the nicotinic action of the neurotransmitter. It is now understood that stimulation by ACh produces a triphasic response in sympathetic ganglia. Impulse transmission through the ganglion occurs when ACh is released from preganglionic fibers and activates the N_2 nicotinic receptors of the neuronal membrane. This triggers an increase in sodium and potassium conductances of a subsynaptic membrane, resulting in an initial excitatory postsynaptic potential (EPSP) with a latency of 1 ms, followed by an inhibitory postsynaptic potential (IPSP) with a latency of 35 ms, and, finally, a slowly generating EPSP with a latency of several hundred milliseconds. The ACh released by preganglionic fibers also activates M_1 muscarinic receptors of the ganglion and probably of the small-intensity fluorescent (SIF) cell. This results in the appearance of a slow IPSP and a slow EPSP in the neurons of the ganglion.[85] The initial EPSP is blocked by conventional competitive nondepolarizing ganglionic blocking agents, such as hexamethonium, and is considered the primary

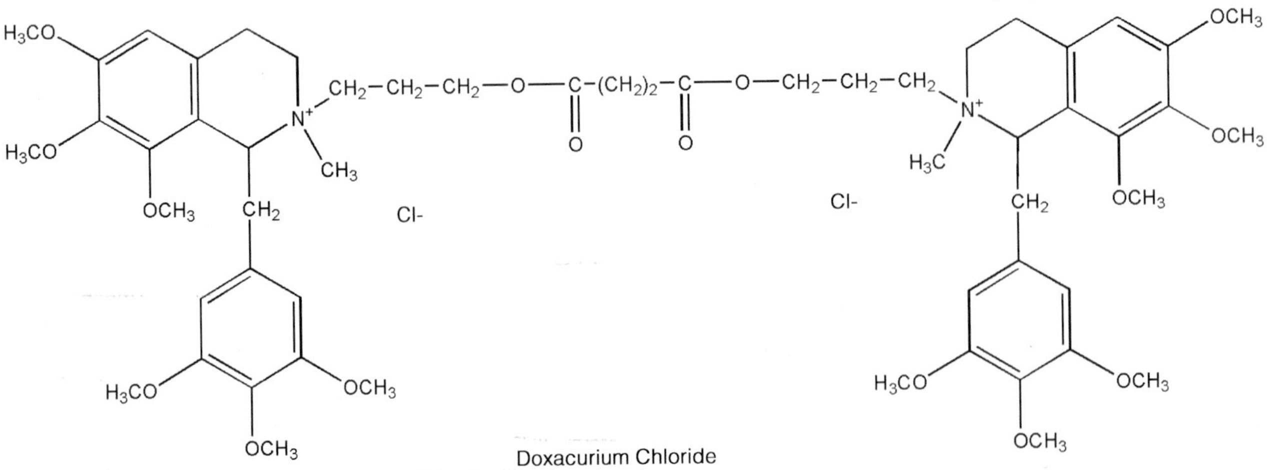

Doxacurium Chloride

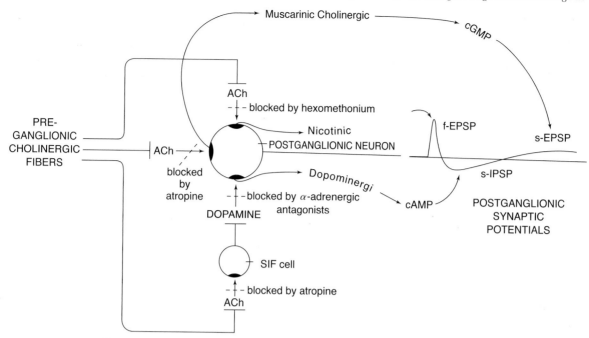

Figure 17.19 ● Neurotransmission at the sympathetic cervical ganglion.

pathway for ganglionic transmission.[86] The slowly generating or late EPSP is blocked by atropine but not by the traditional ganglionic blocking agents. This receptor has muscarinic properties because methacholine causes generation of the late EPSP without causing the initial spike characteristic of ACh. Atropine also blocks the late EPSP produced by methacholine. There may be more than one type of muscarinic receptor in sympathetic ganglia. Atropine blocks both high-affinity (M_1) and low-affinity (M_2) muscarinic receptors in the ganglion.[87] In addition to the cholinergic pathways, the cervical sympathetic ganglion has a neuron that contains a catecholamine.[88] These neuronal cells, identified initially by fluorescence histochemical studies and shown to be smaller than the postganglionic neurons, are now referred to as SIF cells. Dopamine has been identified as the fluorescent catecholamine in the SIF cells that are common to many other sympathetic ganglia. Dopamine apparently mediates an increase in cAMP, which causes hyperpolarization of postganglionic neurons (Fig. 17.19). The IPSP phase of the transmission of sympathetic ganglia following ACh administration can be blocked by both atropine and α-adrenergic blocking agents.[85]

If a similar nontraditional type of ganglionic transmission occurs in the parasympathetic ganglia, it has not yet become evident. With the anatomical and physiological differences between sympathetic and parasympathetic ganglia, it should be no surprise that ganglionic agents may show some selectivity between the two types of ganglia. Although we do not have drug classifications such as "parasympathetic ganglionic blockers" and "sympathetic ganglionic blockers," we do find that certain ganglia have a predominant effect over certain organs and tissues and that a nondiscriminant blockade of autonomic ganglia results in a change in the effect of the autonomic nervous system on that organ (Table 17.7).

None of the commonly known ganglionic blockers has yet been identified as a selective blocker of parasympathetic ganglia.

Van Rossum[89,90] has reviewed the mechanisms of ganglionic synaptic transmission, the mode of action of ganglionic stimulants, and the mode of action of ganglionic blocking agents. They have been classified as blocking agents in the following manner.

Depolarizing Ganglionic Blocking Agents

Depolarizing blocking agents are actually ganglionic stimulants. Thus, for nicotine, small doses give an action similar to that of the natural neuroeffector ACh, an action

TABLE 17.7 Results of Ganglionic Blockers on Organs

Organ	Predominant System	Results of Ganglionic Blockade
Cardiovascular system		
Heart	Parasympathetic	Tachycardia
Arterioles	Sympathetic	Vasodilation
Veins	Sympathetic	Dilation
Eye		
Iris	Parasympathetic	Mydriasis
Ciliary muscle	Parasympathetic	Cycloplegia
GI tract	Parasympathetic	Relaxation
Urinary bladder	Parasympathetic	Urinary retention
Salivary glands	Parasympathetic	Dry mouth
Sweat glands	Sympathetic[a]	Anhidrosis

Adapted from Goth, A.: Medical Pharmacology, 9th ed. St. Louis, C. V. Mosby, 1978.
[a]Neurotransmitter is ACh.

known as the "nicotinic effect of ACh." Larger amounts of nicotine, however, bring about a ganglionic block characterized initially by depolarization, followed by a typical competitive antagonism. To conduct nerve impulses, the cell must be able to carry out a polarization and depolarization process, and if the depolarized condition is maintained without repolarization, obviously no conduction occurs. ACh itself, in high concentration, will bring about an autoinhibition. Chemicals that cause this type of ganglionic block are not of therapeutic significance. The classes of ganglionic blocking agents that are described are therapeutically useful.

Nondepolarizing Competitive Ganglionic Blocking Agents

Compounds in the class of nondepolarizing competitive ganglionic blocking agents possess the necessary affinity to attach to the nicotinic receptor sites that are specific for ACh, but they lack the intrinsic activity necessary for impulse transmission (i.e., they cannot effect depolarization of the cell). Under experimental conditions, in the presence of a fixed concentration of blocking agent of this type, a large enough concentration of ACh can offset the blocking action by competing successfully for the specific receptors. When such a concentration of ACh is administered to a ganglion preparation, it appears that the intrinsic activity of the ACh is as great as it was when no antagonist was present, the only difference being in the larger concentration of ACh required. It is evident, then, that such blocking agents are "competitive" with ACh for the specific receptors involved and that either the agonist or the antagonist, if present in sufficient concentration, can displace the other. Drugs falling into this class are tetraethylammonium salts, hexamethonium, and trimethaphan. Mecamylamine possesses a competitive component in its action but is also noncompetitive, a so-called dual antagonist.

Nondepolarizing Noncompetitive Ganglionic Blocking Agents

Nondepolarizing noncompetitive ganglionic blocking agents produce their effect not at the specific ACh receptor site but at some point farther along the chain of events that is necessary for transmission of the nerve impulse. When the block has been imposed, increasing the concentration of ACh has no effect; thus, apparently, ACh does not act competitively with the blocking agent at the same receptors. Theoretically, a pure noncompetitive blocker should have a high-specific affinity for the noncompetitive receptors in the ganglia and a very low affinity for other cholinergic synapses, together with no intrinsic activity. Mecamylamine, as mentioned above, has a noncompetitive component but is also a competitive blocking agent.

The first ganglionic blocking agents used in therapy were tetraethylammonium chloride and bromide. Although one might assume that curariform activity would be a deterrent to their use, the curariform activity of the tetraethyl compound is less than 1% of that of the corresponding tetramethylammonium compound. A few years after the introduction of the tetraethylammonium compounds, Paton and Zaimis[91]

investigated the usefulness of the bis-trimethylammonium polymethylene salts:

Gallamine Triethiodide

As shown, their findings indicate that there is a critical distance of about five to six carbon atoms between the onium centers for good ganglionic blocking action. Interestingly, the pentamethylene and hexamethylene compounds are effective antidotes against the curare effect of the decamethylene compound. Hexamethonium bromide and hexamethonium chloride emerged from this research as clinically useful products.

Trimethaphan camphorsulfonate, a monosulfonium compound, bears some similarity to the quaternary ammonium types because it, too, is a completely ionic compound. Although it produces a prompt ganglion-blocking action on parenteral injection, its action is short, and it is used only for controlled hypotension during surgery. Almost simultaneously with the introduction of chlorisondamine (now long removed from the market), announcement was made of the powerful ganglionic blocking action of mecamylamine, a secondary amine *without* quaternary ammonium character. As expected, the latter compound showed uniform and predictable absorption from the GI tract as well as a longer duration of action. Its action was similar to that of hexamethonium.

Drugs of this class have limited usefulness as diagnostic and therapeutic agents in the management of peripheral vascular diseases (e.g., thromboangiitis obliterans, Raynaud disease, diabetic gangrene). The principal therapeutic application has been in the treatment of hypertension through blockade of the sympathetic pathways. Unfortunately, the action is nonspecific, and the parasympathetic ganglia, unavoidably, are blocked simultaneously to a greater or lesser extent, causing visual disturbances, dryness of the mouth, impotence, urinary retention, and constipation. Constipation, in particular, probably caused by unabsorbed drug in the intestine (poor absorption), has been a drawback because the condition can proceed to a paralytic ileus if extreme care is not exercised. For this reason, cathartics or a parasympathomimetic (e.g., pilocarpine nitrate) is frequently administered simultaneously. Another adverse effect is the production of orthostatic (postural) hypotension (i.e., dizziness when the patient stands up in an erect position). Prolonged administration of the ganglionic blocking agents results in diminished effectiveness because of a buildup of tolerance, although some are more prone to this than others. Because of the many serious side effects, more effective hypotensive agents have replaced this group of drugs.

In addition to these adverse effects, there are several limitations to the use of these drugs. For instance, they are contraindicated in disorders characterized by severe reduction of blood flow to a vital organ (e.g., severe coronary insufficiency, recent myocardial infarction, retinal and cerebral

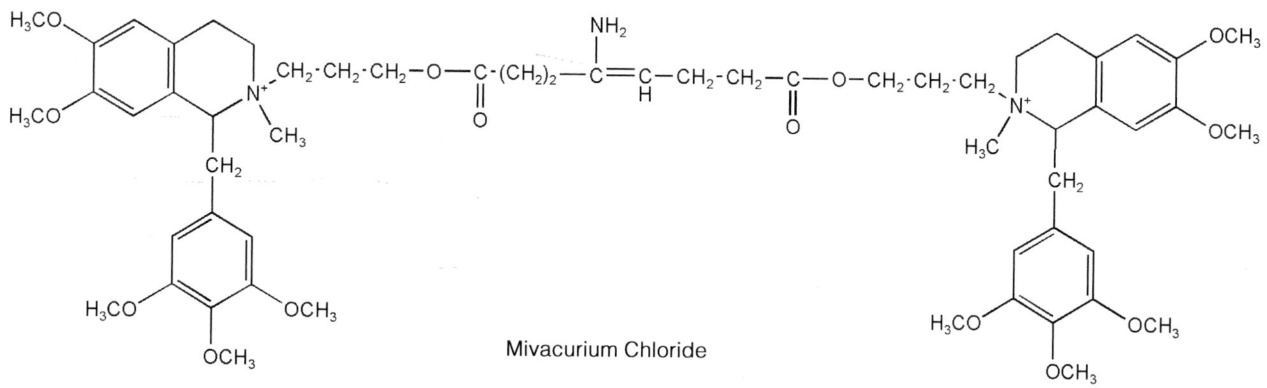

Mivacurium Chloride

thrombosis) as well as situations in which there have been large reductions in blood volume. In the latter, the contraindication exists because the drugs block the normal vasoconstrictor compensatory mechanisms necessary for homeostasis. A potentially serious complication, especially in older men with prostatic hypertrophy, is urinary retention. These drugs should be used with care or not at all in the presence of renal insufficiency, glaucoma, uremia, and organic pyloric stenosis.

Trimethaphan Camsylate, USP. Trimethaphan camsylate, (+)-1,3-dibenzyldecahydro2-oxoimidazo[4,5-*c*] thieno[1,2- *α*]-thiolium 2-oxo-10-bornanesulfonate (1:1) (Arfonad), consists of white crystals or a crystalline powder with a bitter taste and a slight odor. It is soluble in water and alcohol but only slightly soluble in acetone and ether. The pH of a 1% aqueous solution is 5.0 to 6.0.

This ganglionic blocking agent is short acting and is used for certain neurosurgical procedures in which excessive bleeding obscures the operative field. Certain craniotomies are included among these operations. The action of the drug is direct vasodilation, and because of its transient action, it is subject to minute-by-minute control. This fleeting action, however, makes it useless for hypertensive control. The drug is ineffective when given orally. The usual route of administration is intravenous. Trimethaphan camsylate is indicated in the treatment of hypertensive emergencies to reduce blood pressure rapidly. These emergencies may include pulmonary hypertension associated with systemic hypertension and acute dissecting aneurysm.

Mecamylamine Hydrochloride. The secondary amine mecamylamine hydrochloride, *N*,2,3,3-tetramethyl-2-norbornanamine hydrochloride (Inversine), has a powerful ganglionic blocking effect that is almost identical to that of hexamethonium. It has an advantage over most of the ganglionic blocking agents in being absorbed readily and smoothly from the GI tract. It is rarely used, however, for the treatment of moderate-to-severe hypertension because severe orthostatic hypotension occurs when the drug blocks sympathetic ganglia.

◉ NEUROMUSCULAR BLOCKING AGENTS

Agents that block the transmission of ACh at the motor end plate are called *neuromuscular blocking agents*. The therapeutic use of these compounds is primarily as adjuvants in surgical anesthesia to obtain relaxation of skeletal muscle. They also are used in various orthopedic procedures, such as alignment of fractures and correction of dislocations.

The therapeutically useful compounds in this group sometimes are referred to as possessing *curariform* or *curarimimetic* activity in reference to the original representatives of the class, which were obtained from curare. Since then, synthetic compounds have been prepared with similar activity. Although all of the compounds falling into this category, natural and synthetic alike, bring about substantially the same end result (i.e., voluntary-muscle relaxation), there are some significant differences in mechanisms.

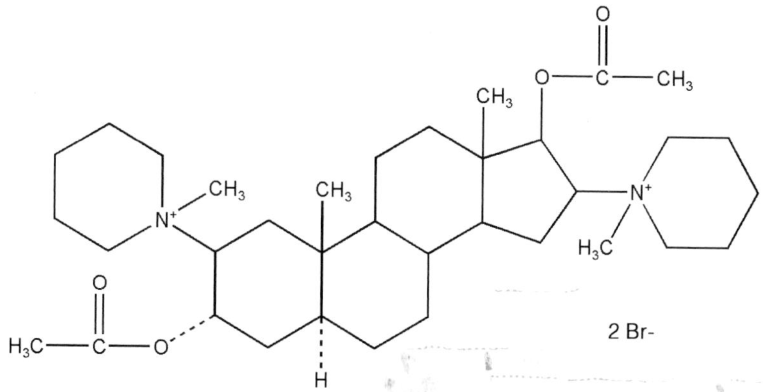

2 Br-

Pancuronium Bromide

The possible existence of a junction between muscle and nerve was suggested as early as 1856, when Claude Bernard observed that the site of action of curare was neither the nerve nor the muscle. Since that time, it has been agreed that ACh mediates transmission at the neuromuscular junction by a sequence of events described previously in this chapter. The neuromuscular junction consists of the axon impinging onto a specialized area of the muscle known as the muscle end plate. The axon is covered with a myelin sheath, containing the nodes of Ranvier, but is bare at the ending. The nerve terminal is separated from the end plate by a gap of 200 Å. The subsynaptic membrane of the end plate contains the cholinergic receptor, the ion-conducting channels (which are opened under the influence of ACh), and AChE.

One of the anatomical differences between the neuromuscular junction and other ACh-responsive sites is the absence in the former of a membrane barrier or sheath that envelopes the ganglia or constitutes the blood-brain barrier. This is important in the accessibility of the site of action to drugs, particularly quaternary ammonium compounds, because they pass through living membranes with considerably greater difficulty and selectivity than do compounds that can exist in a nonionized species. The essentially bare nature (i.e., lack of lipophilic barriers) of the myoneural junction permits ready access by quaternary ammonium compounds. In addition, compounds with considerable molecular dimensions are accessible to the receptors in the myoneural junction. As a result of this property, variations in the chemical structure of quaternaries have little influence on the potential ability of the molecule to reach the cholinergic receptor in the neuromuscular junction. Thus, the following types of neuromuscular junction blockers have been noted.

Nondepolarizing Blocking Agents

Traditionally, *nondepolarizing blocking agents* is a term applied to categorize drugs that compete with ACh for the recognition site on the nicotinic receptor by preventing depolarization of the end plate by the neurotransmitter. Thus, by decreasing the effective ACh–receptor combinations, the end plate potential becomes too small to initiate the propagated action potential. This results in paralysis of neuromuscular transmission. The action of these drugs is quite analogous to that of atropine at the muscarinic receptor sites of ACh. Many experiments suggest that the agonist (ACh) and the antagonist compete on a one-to-one basis for the end plate receptors. Drugs in this class are tubocurarine, dimethyltubocurarine, pancuronium, and gallamine.

Depolarizing Blocking Agents

Drugs in the category of depolarizing blocking agents depolarize the membrane of the muscle end plate. This depolarization is quite similar to that produced by ACh itself at ganglia and neuromuscular junctions (i.e., its so-called nicotinic effect), with the result that the drug, if in sufficient concentration, eventually will produce a block. Either smooth or voluntary muscle, when challenged repeatedly with a depolarizing agent, eventually becomes insensitive.

This phenomenon is known as *tachyphylaxis*, or *desensitization*, and is demonstrated convincingly under suitable experimental conditions with repeated applications of ACh itself, the results indicating that within a few minutes the end plate becomes insensitive to ACh. These statements may imply that a blocking action of this type is clear-cut, but under experimental conditions, it is not quite so unambiguous, because a block that begins with depolarization may regain the polarized state even before the block. Furthermore, depolarization induced by increasing the potassium ion concentration does not prevent impulse transmission. For these and other reasons, it is probably best to consider the blocking action a desensitization until a clearer picture emerges. Drugs falling in this class are decamethonium and succinylcholine.

Curare and Curare Alkaloids

Originally *curare* was a term used to describe collectively the very potent arrow poisons used since early times by the South American Indians. The arrow poisons were prepared from numerous botanic sources and often were mixtures of several different plant extracts. Some were poisonous by virtue of a convulsant action and others by a paralyzant action. Only the latter type is of value in therapeutics and is spoken of ordinarily as curare.

Chemical investigations of the curares were not especially successful because of difficulties in obtaining authentic samples with definite botanic origin. Not until 1935 was a pure crystalline alkaloid, *d*-tubocurarine chloride, possessing in great measure the paralyzing action of the original curare, isolated from a plant. Wintersteiner and Dutcher,[92] in 1943, isolated the same alkaloid. They showed, however, that the botanic source was *Chondodendron tomentosum* (Menispermaceae) and, thus, provided a known source of the drug.

Following the development of quantitative bioassay methods for determining the potency of curare extracts, a purified and standardized curare was developed and marketed under the trade name Intocostrin (purified *C. tomentosum* extract), the solid content of which consisted of almost one-half (+)-tubocurarine solids. Following these essentially pioneering developments, (+)-tubocurarine chloride and dimethyltubocurarine iodide appeared on the market as pure entities.

Tubocurarine Chloride, USP. Tubocurarine chloride, (+)-tubocurarine chloride hydrochloride pentahydrate, is prepared from crude curare by a process of purification and crystallization. Tubocurarine chloride occurs as a white or yellowish white to grayish white, odorless, crystalline powder that is soluble in water. Aqueous solutions of it are stable to heat sterilization.

The structural formula for (+)-tubocurarine was long thought to be that of Ia (see structure diagram). Through the work of Everett et al.,[93] the structure is now known to be that of Ib. The monoquaternary nature of Ib thus revealed has caused some reassessment of thinking concerning the theoretical basis for the blocking action, because all had previously assumed a diquaternary structure (i.e., Ia). Nevertheless, this does not negate the earlier conclusions that a diquaternary nature of the molecule

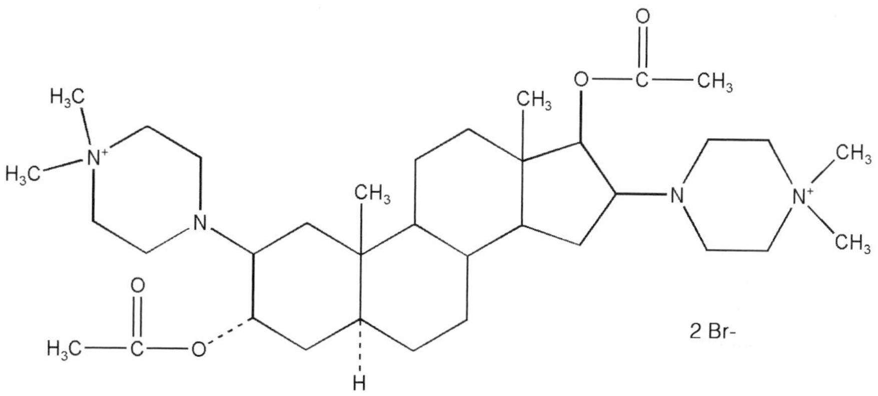

Pipecurium Bromide

provides better blocking action than does a monoquaternary nature (e.g., Ib is approximately fourfold less potent than dimethyl tubocurarine iodide). Further, (+)-isotubocurarine chloride (Ic) has twice the activity of Ib in the particular test used.

Tubocurarine is a nondepolarizing blocking agent used for its paralyzing action on voluntary muscles, the site of action being the neuromuscular junction. Its action is inhibited or reversed by the administration of AChE inhibitors, such as neostigmine, or by edrophonium chloride (Tensilon). Such inhibition of its action is necessitated in respiratory embarrassment caused by overdosage. Additionally, in somewhat higher concentrations, *d*-tubocurarine may enter the open ion channel and add a noncompetitive blockade. Cholinesterase inhibitors do not restore this latter action easily or fully. Often, adjunctive artificial respiration is needed until the maximal curare action has passed. The drug is inactive orally because of inadequate absorption through lipoidal membranes in the GI tract, and when used therapeutically, it usually is injected intravenously.

d-Tubocurarine binds for only 1 ms to the receptor, yet its pharmacological effect of muscle paralysis, produced by administration of the drug intravenously during surgery, lasts for up to 2 hours. The basis of this action is the pharmacokinetics of the drug. *d*-Tubocurarine is given intravenously, and although 30% to 77% is bound to plasma proteins, the drug is distributed rapidly to central body compartments, including neuromuscular junctions. About 45% of *d*-tubocurarine is eliminated unchanged by the kidneys. Its half-life is 89 minutes.

Tubocurarine, in the form of a purified extract, was used first in 1943 as a muscle relaxant in shock therapy for mental disorders. Its use markedly reduced the incidence of bone and spine fractures and dislocations from convulsions because of shock. Following this, it was used as an adjunct in general anesthesia to obtain complete muscle relaxation, a use that persists to this day. Before its use began, satisfactory muscle relaxation in various surgical procedures (e.g., abdominal operations) was obtainable only with "deep" anesthesia with the ordinary general anesthetics. Tubocurarine permits a lighter plane of anesthesia, with no sacrifice in the muscle relaxation so important to the surgeon. A reduced dose of tubocurarine is administered with ether because ether itself has curare-like action.

Metocurine Iodide, USP. Metocurine iodide, (+)-*O,O'*-dimethylchondrocurarine diiodide (Metubine iodide), is prepared from natural crude curare by extracting the curare with methanolic potassium hydroxide. When the extract is treated with an excess of methyl iodide, the (+)-tubocurarine is converted to the diquaternary dimethyl ether and crystallizes out as the iodide (see "Tubocurarine Chloride"). Other ethers besides the dimethyl ether have been made and tested. For example, the dibenzyl ether was one third as active as tubocurarine chloride, and the diisopropyl compound had only one half the activity. For comparison, the dimethyl ether has approximately 4 times the activity of tubocurarine chloride.

The pharmacological action of this compound is the same as that of tubocurarine chloride, namely, a nondepolarizing competitive blocking effect on the motor end plate of skeletal muscles. It is considerably more potent than *d*-tubocurarine, however, and has the added advantage of exerting much less effect on respiration. The effect on respiration is not a significant factor in therapeutic doses. Accidental overdosage is counteracted best by forced respiration.

Synthetic Compounds with Curariform Activity

Curare, until relatively recent times, remained the only useful curarizing agent; and it, too, suffered from a lack of standardization. The original pronouncement in 1935 of the structure of (+)-tubocurarine chloride, unchallenged for 35 years, led other workers to hope for activity in synthetic substances of less complexity. The quaternary ammonium character of the curare alkaloids coupled with the known activity of the various simple onium compounds hardly seemed to be coincidental, and it was natural for research to follow along these lines. One of the synthetic compounds discovered was marketed in 1951 as Flaxedil (gallamine triethiodide). Other various neuromuscular blocking agents have followed.

Atracurium Besylate. Atracurium besylate, 2-(2-carboxyethyl)-1,2,3,4-tetrahydro-6,7-dimethoxy-2-methyl-1-veratrylisoquinolinium benzenesulfonate pentamethylene ester (Tracrium), is a nondepolarizing neuromuscular blocking agent that is approximately 2.5 times more potent than *d*-tubocurarine. Its duration of action (half-life, 0.33 hours) is much shorter than that of *d*-tubocurarine. The drug is

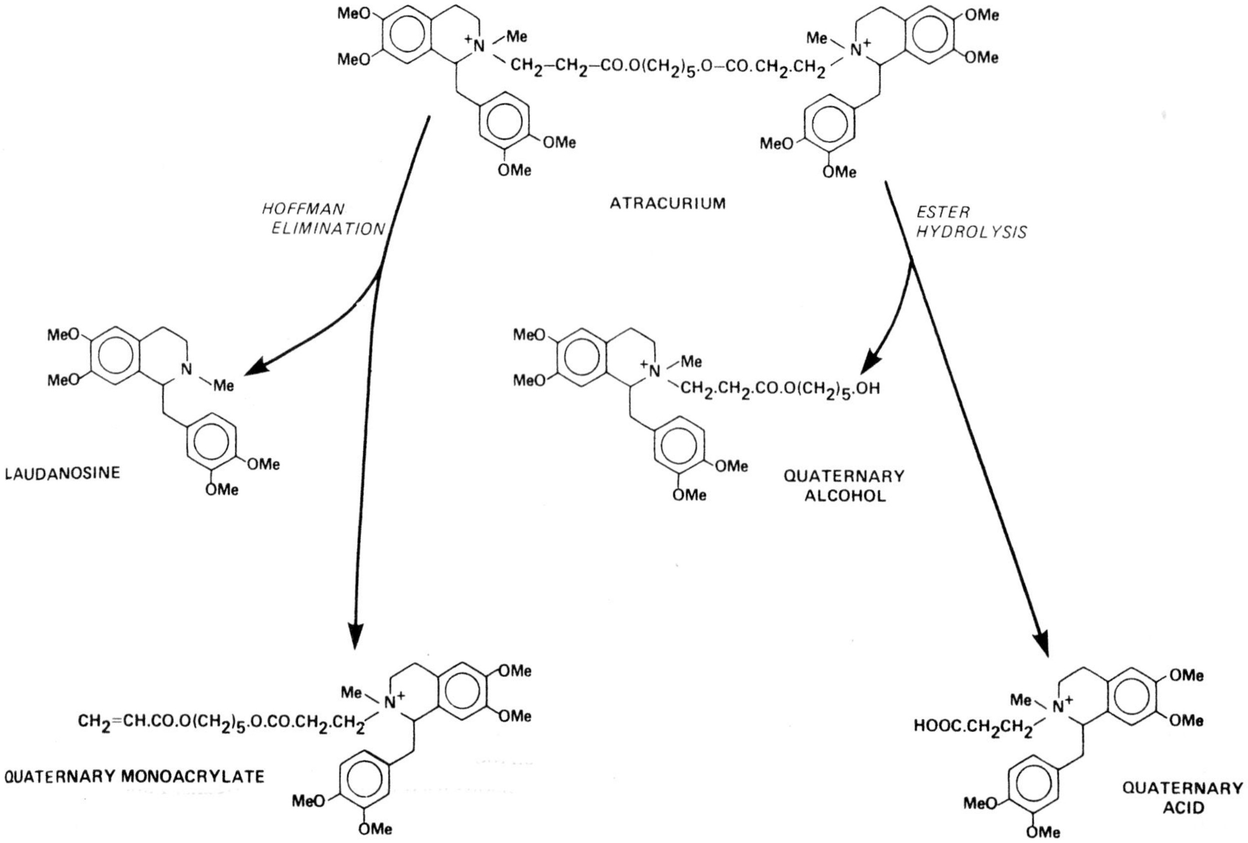

Figure 17.20 • Hoffman elimination and hydrolysis reactions of atracurium.

metabolized rapidly and nonenzymatically to yield laudanosine and a smaller quaternary compound (Fig. 17.20), which do not have neuromuscular blocking activity. In vitro experiments show that atracurium besylate breaks down at pH 7.4 and 37°C by a Hoffman elimination reaction.[94] Atracurium besylate undergoes enzymatic decomposition of its ester function to yield an inactive quaternary alcohol and quaternary acid. AChE inhibitors such as neostigmine, edrophonium, and pyridostigmine antagonize paralysis by atracurium besylate.

Doxacurium Chloride. The molecular structure of doxacurium chloride, 1,2,3,4-tetrahydro-2-(3-hydroxypropyl)-6,7,8-trimethoxy2-methyl-1-(3,4,5-trimethoxybenzyl) isoquinolinium chloride succinate (Nuromax), provides the possibility for 10 stereoisomers: 4 *d,l* pairs and two *meso*

forms. Of the 10 stereoisomers, 3 are all-*trans* configuration, and these are the only active ones.[95] Doxacurium chloride is a long-acting nondepolarizing blocking agent. The drug differs from drugs such as gallium and pancuronium in that it has no vagolytic activity. It is used as a skeletal muscle relaxant in surgical procedures expected to last longer than 90 minutes.

Gallamine Triethiodide, USP. Gallamine triethiodide, [*v*-phenenyl-tris(oxyethylene)]tris[triethylammonium] triiodide (Flaxedil), is a skeletal muscle relaxant that works by blocking neuromuscular transmission in a manner similar to that of *d*-tubocurarine (i.e., a nondepolarizing blocking agent). It does have some differences, however. It has a strong vagolytic effect and a persistent decrease in neuromuscular function after successive doses that cannot be

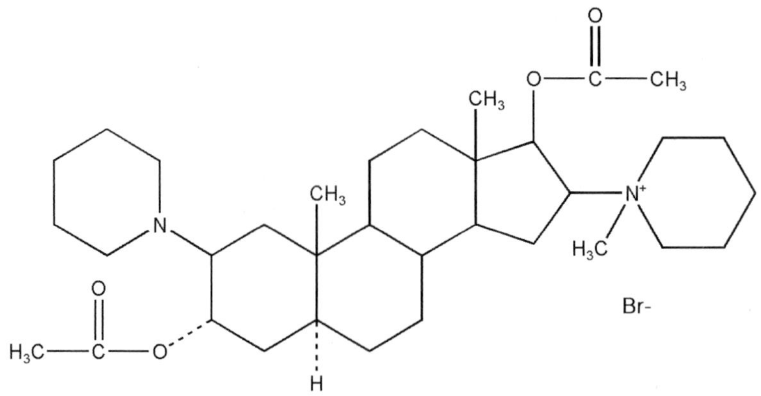

Vecoronium Bromide

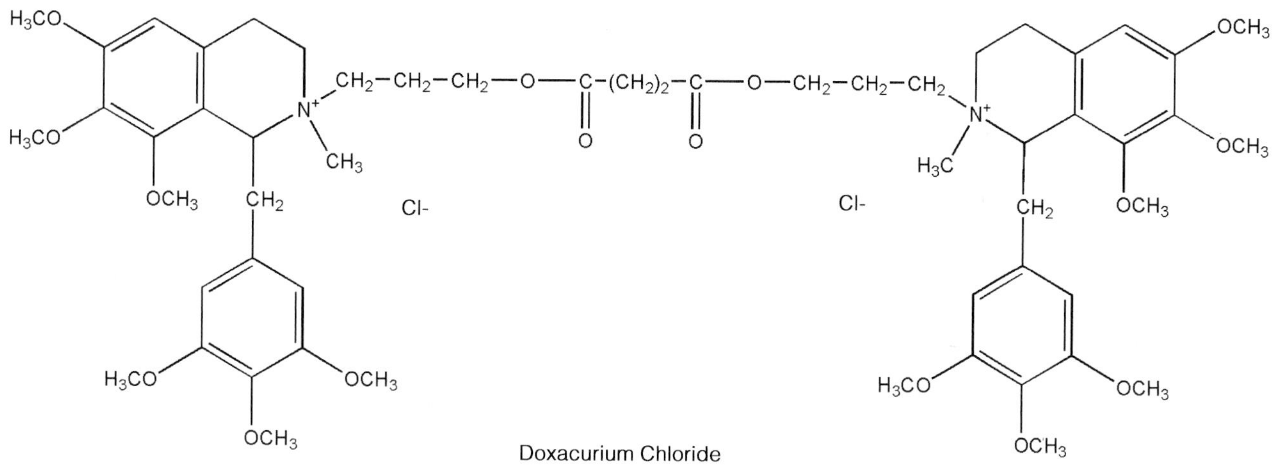

Doxacurium Chloride

overcome by cholinesterase inhibitors. Gallamine triethiodide also has muscarinic antagonistic properties and binds with greater affinity to the M_2 receptors than to the M_1 receptor. This latter characteristic may cause its strong vagolytic action.[95, 96]

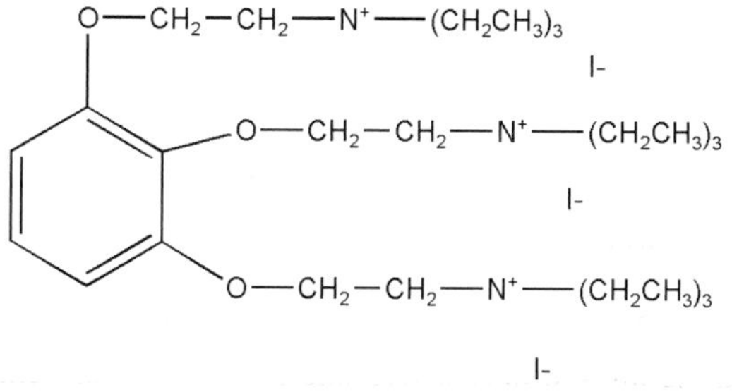

Gallamine Triethiodide

The drug is contraindicated in patients with myasthenia gravis, and one should remember that its action is cumulative, as with curare. The antidote for gallamine triethiodide is neostigmine.

Mivacurium Chloride. Mivacurium chloride, 1,2,3,4-tetrahydro-2-(3-hydroxypropyl)-6,7-dimethoxy-2-methyl-1-(3,4,5-trimethoxybenzyl)isoquinolinium chloride, (E)-4-octandioate (Mivacron), is a mixture of three stereoisomers, the *trans-trans*, *cis-trans*, and *cis-cis* diesters, each of which has neuromuscular blocking properties. The *cis-cis* isomer is about one tenth as potent as the other isomers. Mivacurium chloride is a short-acting nondepolarizing drug

used as an adjunct to anesthesia to relax skeletal muscle. The drug is hydrolyzed by plasma esterases, and it is likely that anticholinesterase agents used as antidotes could prolong rather than reverse the effects of the drug.

Pancuronium Bromide. Although pancuronium bromide, $2\beta,16\beta$-dipiperidino-5α-androstane-$3\alpha,17\beta$-diol diacetate dimethobromide (Pavulon), is a synthetic product, it is based on the naturally occurring alkaloid malouetine, found in arrow poisons used by primitive Africans. Pancuronium bromide acts on the nicotinic receptor and in the ion channel, inhibiting normal ion fluxes.

This blocking agent is soluble in water and is marketed in concentrations of 1 or 2 mg/mL for intravenous administration. It is a typical nondepolarizing blocker, with a potency approximately 5 times that of (+)-tubocurarine chloride and a duration of action approximately equal to the latter. Studies indicate that it has little or no histamine-releasing potential or ganglion-blocking activity and that it has little effect on the circulatory system, except for causing a slight rise in the pulse rate. As one might expect, ACh, anticholinesterases, and potassium ion competitively antagonize it, whereas its action is increased by inhalation anesthetics such as ether, halothane, enflurane, and methoxyflurane. The latter enhancement in activity is especially important to the anesthetist because the drug is frequently administered as an adjunct to the anesthetic procedure to relax the skeletal muscle. Perhaps the most frequent adverse reaction to this agent is occasional prolongation of the neuromuscular block beyond the usual time course, a situation that can usually be controlled with neostigmine or by manual or mechanical

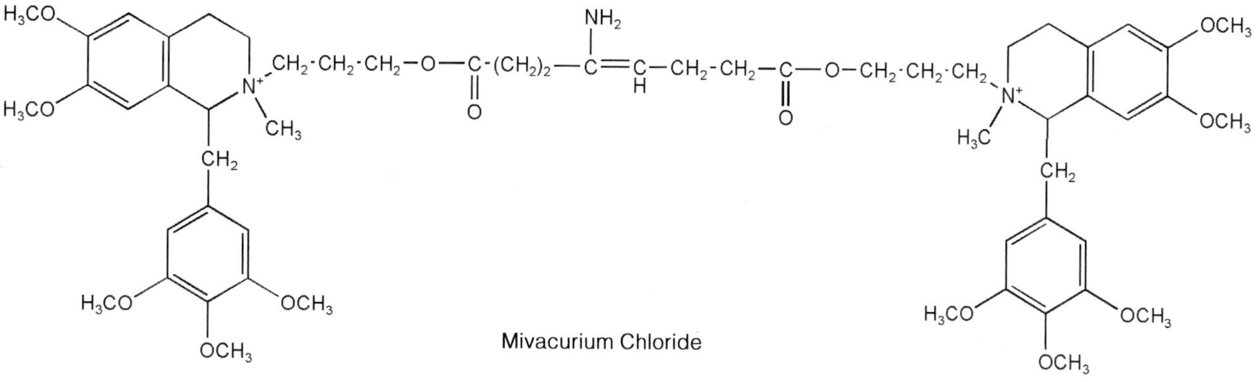

Mivacurium Chloride

ventilation, since respiratory difficulty is a prominent manifestation of the prolonged blocking action.

As indicated, the principal use of pancuronium bromide is as an adjunct to anesthesia, to induce relaxation of skeletal muscle, but it is also used to facilitate the management of patients undergoing mechanical ventilation. Only experienced clinicians equipped with facilities for applying artificial respiration should administer it, and the dosage should be adjusted and controlled carefully.

Pipecurium Bromide. Pipecurium bromide, 4,4′-(3α, 17β-dihydroxy-5α-androstan-2β,16β-ylene)bis(1,1-dimeth-ylpiperazinium)dibromide diacetate (Arduan), is a nondepolarizing muscle relaxant similar, both chemically and clinically, to pancuronium bromide. It is a long-acting

drug indicated as an adjunct to anesthesia and in patients undergoing mechanical ventilation.

Vecuronium Bromide. Vecuronium bromide, 1-(3α, 17β-dihydroxy-2β-piperidino-5α-androstan-16β-yl)-1-methylpiperidinium bromide diacetate (Norcuron), is the monoquaternary analog of pancuronium bromide. It belongs to the class of nondepolarizing neuromuscular blocking agents and produces effects similar to those of drugs in this class. It is unstable in the presence of acids and undergoes gradual hydrolysis of its ester functions in aqueous solution. Aqueous solutions have a pH of about 4.0. This drug is used mainly to produce skeletal muscle relaxation during surgery and to assist in controlled respiration after general anesthesia has been induced.

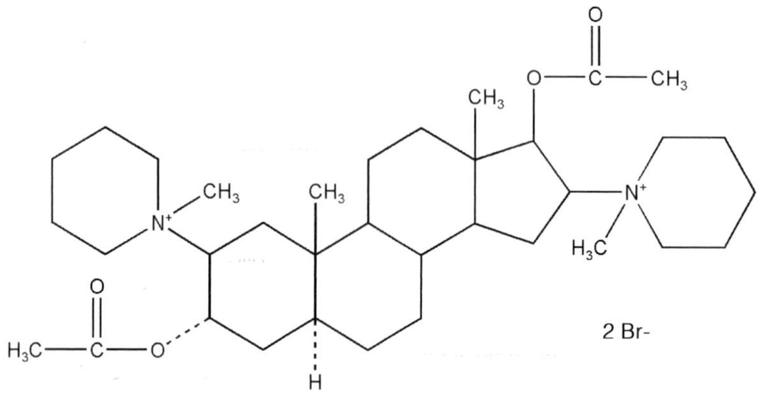

Pancuronium Bromide

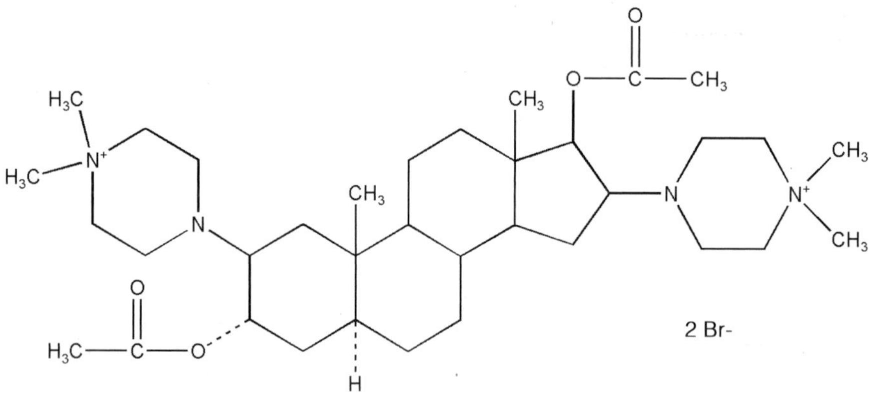

Pipecurium Bromide

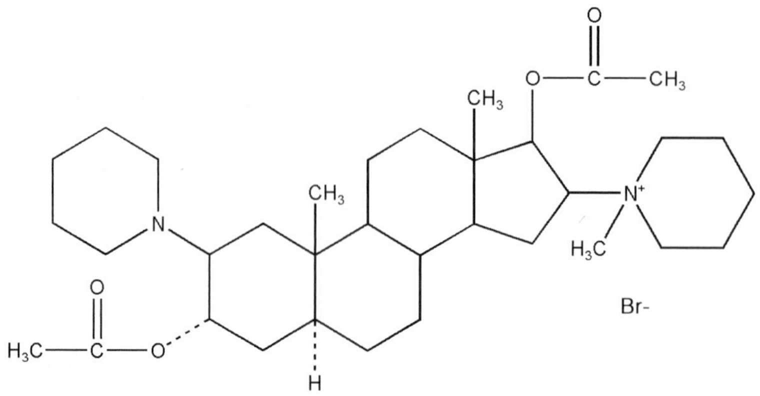

Vecoronium Bromide

Succinylcholine Chloride, USP. Succinylcholine chloride, choline chloride succinate (2:1) (Anectine, Sucostrin), is a white, odorless, crystalline substance that is freely soluble in water to give solutions with a pH of about 4. It is stable in acidic solutions but unstable in alkali. Aqueous solutions should be refrigerated to ensure stability.

Succinylcholine chloride is characterized by a very short duration of action and a quick recovery because of its rapid hydrolysis after injection. It brings about the typical muscular paralysis caused by blocking nervous transmission at the myoneural junction. Large doses may cause temporary respiratory depression, as with similar agents. Its action, in contrast with that of (1)-tubocurarine, is not antagonized by neostigmine, physostigmine, or edrophonium chloride. These anticholinesterase drugs actually prolong the action of succinylcholine chloride, which suggests that the drug is probably hydrolyzed by cholinesterases. The brief duration of action of this curare-like agent is said to render an antidote unnecessary if the proper supportive measures are available. Succinylcholine chloride has a disadvantage, however, in that the usual antidotes cannot terminate its action promptly.

It is used as a muscle relaxant for the same indications as other curare agents. It may be used for either short or long periods of relaxation, depending on whether one or several injections are given. In addition, it is suitable for continuous intravenous drip administration.

Succinylcholine chloride should not be used with thiopental sodium because of the high alkalinity of the latter. If used together, they should be administered immediately after mixing; however, separate injection is preferable.

● R E V I E W   Q U E S T I O N S ●

1. When discussing the structure–activity relationship of acetylcholine what will alkyl substitutions on the beta carbon cause to the molecule?
   a. decrease rate of hydrolysis by esterases ✓
   b. decrease nicotinic action ✓
   c. increase muscarinic action
   d. All of the above are correct.
   e. Only a and c are correct.

2. The therapeutic usefulness of the agent represented below is:

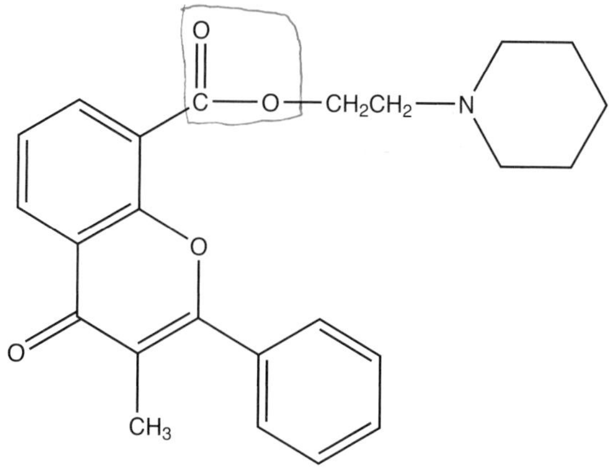

   a. incontinence
   b. glaucoma
   c. myasthenia gravis
   d. insecticidal agent
   e. irritable bowel syndrome

3. The therapeutic usefulness of the agent represented below is in treating Alzheimer disease. Please describe why this agent has usefulness in treating this disease.

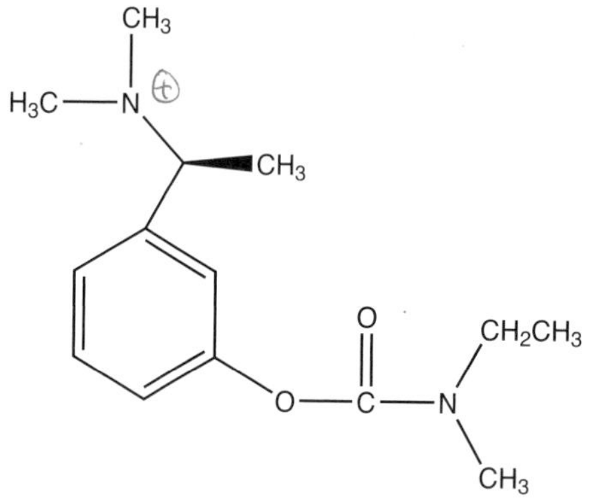

4. Describe the reason cholinergics can be used in myasthenia gravis.

REFERENCES

1. Dale, H. H.: J. Pharmacol. Exp. Ther. 6:147, 1914.
2. Loewi, O.: Arch. Gesamte. Physiol. (Pfluegers) 189:239, 1921.
3. Zola-Morgan, S., and Squire, L. R.: Annu. Rev. Neurosci. 16:547, 1994.
4. Frank, H. S., and Wen, W.-Y.: Discuss. Faraday Soc. 24:133, 1957.
5. Hille, B.: Annu. Rev. Physiol. 38:139, 1976.
6. Karlin, A.: In Cotman, C. U., Poste, G., and Nicolson, G. L. (eds.). Cell Surface and Neuronal Function. Amsterdam, Elsevier Biomedical, 1980, p. 191.
7. Changeaux, J. P., Devillers-Thiery, A., and Chermoulli, P.: Science 225:1335, 1984.
8. Anholt, R., et al.: In Martonosi, A. N. (ed.). The Enzymes of Biological Membranes, vol. 3. New York, Plenum Press, 1985.
9. Raftery, M. A., et al.: Science 208:1445, 1980.
10. Sargent, P. B.: Neuroscience 16:403, 1994.
11. Dani, J. A.: Biol. Psychiatry 49:166, 2001.
12. Rattray, M.: Biol. Psychiatry 49:185, 2001.
13. Goyal, R. K.: N. Engl. J. Med. 321:1022, 1989.
14. Birdsall, N. J. M., et al.: Pharmacology 37(Suppl.):22, 1988.
15. Mutschlur, E., et al.: Prog. Pharmacol. Clin. Pharmacol. 7:13, 1989.
16. Doods, H. N., et al.: Prog. Pharmacol. Clin. Pharmacol. 7:47, 1989.
17. Barnes, P. J.: Life Sci. 52:521, 1993.
18. Rubanyi, G. M.: J. Cell Biol. 46:27, 1991.

19. Kilbinger, H., Dietricht, C., and von Bardeleben, R. S.: J. Physiol. Paris 87:77, 1993.
20. Linder, M. E., and Gilman, A. E.: Sci. Am. 27:56, 1992.
21. Caufield, M. P.: Pharmacol. Ther. 58:319, 1993.
22. Berridge, M. J., and Irvine, R. F.: Nature 312:315, 1984.
23. Berridge, M. J.: Annu. Rev. Biochem. 56:159, 1987.
24. Clapham, D. E.: Annu. Rev. Neurosci. 17:441, 1994.
25. Haga, T., and Nada, H.: Biochim. Biophys. Acta. 291:564, 1973.
26. Cavallito, C. J., et al.: J. Med. Chem. 12:134, 1969.
27. Aquilonius, S. M., et al.: Acta Pharmacol. Toxicol. 30:129, 1979.
28. Whittaker, V. P.: Trends Pharmacol. Sci. 7:312, 1986.
29. Namba, T., and Grob, D.: J. Neurochem. 15:1445, 1968.
30. Partington, P., Feeney, J., and Burgen, A. S. V.: Mol. Pharmacol. 8:269, 1972.
31. Casey, A. F.: Prog. Med. Chem. 11:1, 1975.
32. Behling, R. W., et al.: Proc. Natl. Acad. Sci. U. S. A. 85:6721, 1988.
33. Nordvall, G., and Hacksell, U.: J. Med. Chem. 36:967, 1993.
34. Schmeideberg, O., and Koppe, R.: Das Muscarine, das Giftege Alka id des Fiielgenpiltzes. Leipzig, Vogel, 1869.
35. Hardegger, E., and Lohse, F.: Helv. Chim. Acta 40:2383, 1957.
36. Trumpp-Kallmeyer, S., et al.: J. Med. Chem. 35:3448, 1992.
37. Triggle, D. J., et al.: J. Med. Chem. 34:3164, 1991.
38. Ariens, E. J., and Simonis, A. M.: In deJong, H. (ed.). Quantitative Methods in Pharmacology. Amsterdam, Elsevier, 1969.
39. Ing, H. R.: Science 109:264, 1949.
40. Hernandez, M., et al.: Br. J. Pharmacol. 110:1413, 1993.
41. Bebbington, A., and Brimblecombe, R. W.: Adv. Drug Res. 2:143, 1965.
42. Ren, L. N., Nakane, T., and Chiba, S.: J. Cardiovasc. Pharmacol. 22:841, 1993.
43. Morrison, K. J., and Vanhoutte, P. M.: Br. J. Pharmacol. 106:672, 1992.
44. Nunes, M. A., and Brochmann-Hanssen, E. J.: J. Pharm. Sci. 63:716, 1974.
45. Williams, P. D., et al.: Pharmacology 23:177, 1992.
46. Gabelt, B. T., and Kaufman, P. L.: J. Pharmacol. Exp. Ther. 263:1133, 1992.
47. Ramos-Casals, M., and Brito-Zeron, P.: Expert Rev. Clin. Immun. 3:195, 2007.
48. Mallarkey, G.: Cholinesterase Inhibitors in Alzheimer's Disease. Auckland, Adis International, 1999.
49. Berman, A. H., Yguerabide, J., and Taylor, P.: Biochemistry 19:2226, 1980.
50. Englehard, N., Prchal, K., and Nenner, M.: Angew. Chem. Int. Ed. 6:615, 1967.
51. Ordentlich, A., et al.: J. Biol. Chem. 268:17083, 1993.
52. Shafferman, A., et al.: J. Biol. Chem. 267:17040, 1992.
53. Wilson, I. B., Harrison, M. A., and Ginsberg, S.: J. Biol. Chem. 236:1498, 1961.
54. Ellis, S., Krayer, O., and Plachte, F. L.: J. Pharmacol. Exp. Ther. 79:309, 1943.
55. Enz, A., et al.: Prog. Brain Res. 98:431, 1993.
56. O'Brien, R. D.: Mol. Pharmacol. 4:121, 1968.
57. Calvey, H. T.: Biochem. Pharmacol. 16:1989, 1967.
58. Summers, W. K., et al.: N. Engl. J. Med. 315:1241, 1986.
59. Molloy, D. W., et al.: Can. Med. Assoc. J. 144:29, 1991.
60. Heath, D. F.: Organophosphorus Poisons. Oxford, Pergamon Press, 1961.
61. Oosterban, R. A., and Cohen, J. A.: The active site of esterases. In Goodwin, T. W., Harris, I. J., and Hartley, B. S. (eds.). Structure and Activity of Enzymes. New York, Academic Press, 1964.
62. Linn, J. G., and Tomarelli, R. C.: Am. J. Ophthalmol. 35:46, 1952.
63. Comroe, J. H., et al.: J. Pharmacol. Exp. Ther. 87:281, 1946.
64. Gage, J. C.: Biochem. J. 54:426, 1953.
65. Nakatsugawa, T., Tolman, N. M., and Dahm, P. A.: Biochem. Pharmacol. 17:1517, 1968.
66. Mountner, L. A., and Cheatam, R. M.: Enzymologia 25:215, 1963.
67. Stephenson, R. P.: Br. J. Pharmacol. Chemother. 11:379, 1956.
68. Ariens, E. J.: Adv. Drug Res. 3:235, 1966.
69. Paton, W. D. M.: Proc. R. Soc. Lond. B 154:21, 1961.
70. Long, J. P., et al.: J. Pharmacol. Exp. Ther. 117:29, 1956.
71. AMA Drug Evaluations Annual 1994. Chicago, American Medical Association, 1994, p. 894.
72. Gyermek, L., and Nador, K.: J. Pharm. Pharmacol. 9:209, 1957.
73. Ariens, E. J., Simonis, A. M., and Van Rossum, J. M.: In Ariens, E. J. (ed.). Molecular Pharmacology. New York, Academic Press, 1964, p. 205.
74. Kondritzer, A. A., and Zvirblis, P.: J. Am. Pharm. Assoc. Sci. Ed. 46:531, 1957.
75. Cushny, A. R.: J. Physiol. 30:176, 1904.
76. Doods, H. N., et al.: Eur. J. Pharmacol. 250:223, 1993.
77. Fuder, M., and Meincke, M.: Naunyn Schmiedebergs Arch. Pharmakol. 347:591, 1993.
78. Abramov, Y., and Sand, P. K.: Expert Opinion Pharmaco. 5:2351, 2004.
79. Madersbacher, H., and Rovner, E.: Expert Opinion Pharmaco. 7:1373, 2006.
80. Ohtake, A., Ukai, M., Hatanaka, T., et al.: Eur. J. Pharmacol. 492:243, 2004.
81. Clemett, D., and Jarvis, B.: Drugs & Aging 18:277, 2001.
82. Lazareno, S., and Birdsall, N. J.: Br. J. Pharmacol. 109:1120, 1993.
83. Blok, B. F. M., and Corcos, J.: Aging Health 3:143, 2007.
84. Karczmar, A. G. (ed.): International Encyclopedia of Pharmacology and Therapeutics, Sect. 12, Ganglionic Blocking and Stimulating Agents, vol. 1. Berlin, Springer-Verlag, 1980.
85. Skok, V. I.: In Karkevich, D. A. (ed.). Pharmacology of Ganglionic Transmission. Berlin, Springer-Verlag, 1980, p. 7.
86. Greengard, P., and Kebabian, J. W.: Fed. Proc. 33:1059, 1974.
87. Hammer, R., and Giachetti, A.: Life Sci. 31:2291, 1982.
88. Volle, R. L., and Hancock, J. C.: Fed. Proc. 29:1913, 1970.
89. Van Rossum, J. M.: Int. J. Neuropharmacol. 1:97, 1962.
90. Van Rossum, J. M.: Int. J. Neuropharmacol. 1:403, 1962.
91. Paton, W. D. M., and Zaimis, E. J.: Br. J. Pharmacol. 4:381, 1949.
92. Wintersteiner, O., and Dutcher, J. D.: Science 97:467, 1943.
93. Everett, A. J., Lowe, L. A., and Wilkinson, S.: Chem. Commun. 1020, 1970.
94. Stenlake, J. B., et al.: Br. J. Anaesth. 55:3S, 1983.
95. USAN and the USP Dictionary of Drug Names. Rockville, MD, United States Pharmacopeial Convention, 1994, p. 231.
96. Burke, R. E.: Mol. Pharmacol. 30:58, 1986.

CHAPTER 18

Drugs Acting on the Renal System

STEPHEN J. CUTLER

CHAPTER OVERVIEW

Drugs acting on the renal system describes the role renin–angiotensin system plays in regulating the cardiovascular system. This chapter supports the fact that this system plays a critical role in the mechanisms of hypertension and heart failure (formally recognized as congestive heart failure [CHF]). This, in turn, serves in the development of therapeutic agents that act on the various enzymes and receptors associated with the renin–angiotensin system. For pharmacists to be good practitioners, it is necessary that they understand how the renin–angiotensin system influences normal physiological functions as well as how components of the system, such as renin, angiotensin I and II, and angiotensin-converting enzyme, can be used in manipulating specific cardiovascular diseases.

The Renin–Angiotensin System and Hypertension

The renin–angiotensin system is a hormonal system that plays a central role in the control of sodium excretion and body fluid volume. It interacts closely with the sympathetic nervous system and aldosterone secretion in the regulation of blood pressure. Figure 18.1 shows the relationship of the component parts of the renin–angiotensin system and their main physiological effects.

The relationship between the renin–angiotensin system and blood pressure in humans has been known since before the beginning of the 20th century. Tigerstedt and Bergman[1] demonstrated in 1898 that, when injected in a host, kidney extract produced a potent vasopressor response. The substance was named *renin*. Many years later, this substance was shown to require a cofactor to produce vasoconstriction.[2] Eventually, in 1939, this hypertensive substance was isolated, identified as a decapeptide, and later called *angiotensin*. This cofactor existed as an inactive precursor, angiotensinogen. Later studies revealed that angiotensin existed in two forms, the biologically inactive decapeptide angiotensin I and the active octapeptide angiotensin II.[3]

The precursor of angiotensin, angiotensinogen, is a glycoprotein of molecular weight (MW) 58,000 to 61,000, synthesized primarily in the liver and brought into the circulatory system. Renin, an aspartyl protease (MW 35,000–40,000), whose primary source is the kidney, cleaves the Leu-Val bond from the aspartic acid end of the angiotensinogen polypeptide molecule to release the decapeptide angiotensin I (Fig. 18.2). The biochemical conversion continues with the cleavage of a dipeptide (His-Leu) from the carboxyl terminal of angiotensin I by angiotensin-converting enzyme (ACE) to form the octapeptide angiotensin II, a potent vasoconstrictor. Angiotensin III is formed by removal of the *N*-terminal aspartate residue of angiotensin II, a reaction catalyzed by glutamyl aminopeptidase. In contrast to angiotensin II, angiotensin III has a less potent but significant regulatory effect on sodium excretion by the renal tubules. This is primarily resulting from the effect angiotensin III has in stimulating aldosterone secretion, a potent mineralcorticoid.

The vasoconstrictive effects of angiotensin II are a result of many factors. In the kidneys, it constricts glomerular arterioles. The effects are greater on efferent arterioles than afferent ones. Constriction of afferent arterioles results in increased arteriolar resistance, which raises systemic arterial blood pressure. In addition, angiotensin II stimulates the release of vasopressin from the hypothalamus. Vasopressin is also known as the *antidiuretic hormone* (ADH), because this peptidic hormone is typically released to conserve water when the body is dehydrated. In the kidneys, it increases the permeability to water of the distal convoluted tubules and collecting tubules in the nephrons. This, in turn, results in concentrating the urine and reducing urine volume. By inducing moderate vasoconstriction, this peptide results in an increase in blood pressure. Additionally, angiotensin II has been shown to stimulate the production of endothelin, a 21 amino acid peptide that is produced in the vascular endothelium and which plays a role in the regulation of smooth muscle contraction and which contributes to blood pressure regulation (see Chapter 19).[4] Lastly, angiotensin II plays a primary role in regulating aldosterone secretion. Upon stimulation by the renin–angiotensin system, aldosterone is secreted by the adrenal cortex and elicits its effects at various sites, including the nephrons. It is responsible for the reabsorption of sodium into the bloodstream. This results in increased levels of sodium in the plasma, which in turn result in increased blood volume and vascular resistance.[5] If aldosterone levels in the body become too high, then symptoms such as elevated blood pressure or heart failure (formally classified as CHF) can occur.

The regulatory action of the renin–angiotensin system in controlling sodium and potassium balance and arterial blood pressure is modified by vasodilators called kinins. Proteolytic enzymes that circulate in the plasma form *kinins*. Kallikrein is activated in plasma by noxious influences to act on a kinin, callidin, which is converted to bradykinin by tissue enzymes. Bradykinin enhances release of the prostaglandins PGE2 and PGI2 within certain tissues to produce a vasodilatory effect (Fig. 18.3). Bradykinin is converted to inactive products by

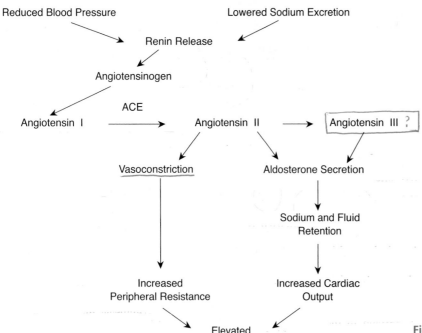

↓BP
⋮
↑BP

Figure 18.1 ● Renin–angiotensin system of blood pressure control.

ACE and other carboxypeptidases.[6] Although ACE causes activation of angiotensin and inactivation of bradykinin, actions that appear to be opposite, the balance of the system seems to favor vasoconstriction.

ACE is a membrane-bound enzyme anchored to the cell membrane through a single transmembrane domain located near the carboxy-terminal extremity. The enzyme is a zinc-containing glycoprotein with an MW about 130,000. It is a nonspecific peptidyldipeptide hydrolase, widely distributed in mammalian tissues, that cleaves dipeptides from the car-boxy terminus of several endogenous peptides. The minimum structural requirement for binding and cleavage of a substrate by ACE is that it is a tripeptide with a free carboxylate group. A general exception is that this enzyme does not cleave peptides with a penultimate prolyl residue. This accounts for the biological stability of angiotensin II.[7] The important binding points at the active site of ACE are a cationic site to attract a carboxylate ion and a zinc ion that can polarize a carbonyl group of an amide function to make it more susceptible to hydrolysis. In the active site, there is

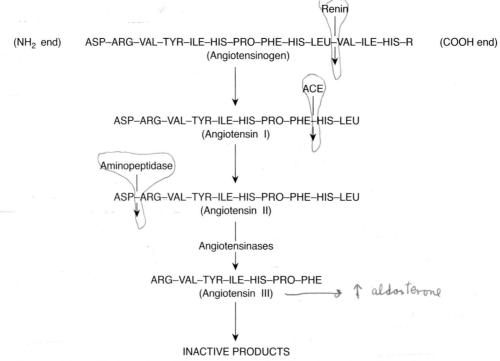

Figure 18.2 ● Biochemistry of the renin–angiotensin system: formation of angiotensins from angiotensinogen.

Rallikrein

Calladin ———————→ Bradykinin ———————→ Prostaglandin Release

|ACE

Inactive Products   Vasodilatation

Figure 18.3 ● Bradykinin formation and action.

a nucleophilic attack of the amide carbonyl by the γ-carbonyl group of a glutamic acid residue to cause hydrolysis of the peptide. Figure 18.4 shows a hypothetical model of the hydrolysis of angiotensin I by the active site of ACE. ACE exists in more than one form. Somatic ACE that regulates blood pressure, found in most tissues, differs from the isoenzyme ACE found in the testis. Somatic ACE, in contrast to testicular ACE, contains two binding domains. The principal active site for hydrolysis is the domain located in the C-terminal half of somatic ACE.[8]

Because the renin–angiotensin system plays such an important role in regulating kidney function,[9] aldosterone release,[10] electrolyte balance, and blood volume, it is easy to recognize why targeting this pathway is beneficial in the management of high blood pressure and heart failure. Inhibitors of angiotensin-converting enzyme (ACE in-

hibitors) are often used to reduce the formation of the more potent angiotensin II. In addition, angiotensin receptor blockers (ARBs) can be used to prevent angiotensin II from acting on angiotensin receptors.[11]

Recently, there have been several agents investigated for their ability to inhibit renin, which in turn results in less angiotensin II being produced.[12]

◗ RENIN–ANGIOTENSIN SYSTEM INHIBITORS

Angiotensin-Converting Enzyme Inhibitors

PRODUCTS

Captopril. Captopril, 1-[(2*S*)-3-mercapto-2-methyl-1-oxopropionyl]proline (Capoten), blocks the conversion of angiotensin I to angiotensin II by inhibiting the converting enzyme. The rational development of captopril as an inhibitor of ACE was based on the hypothesis that ACE and carboxypeptidase A functioned by similar mechanisms. It was noted that *d*-2-benzylsuccinic acid[7] was a potent inhibitor of carboxypeptidase A, but not ACE. By use of this small

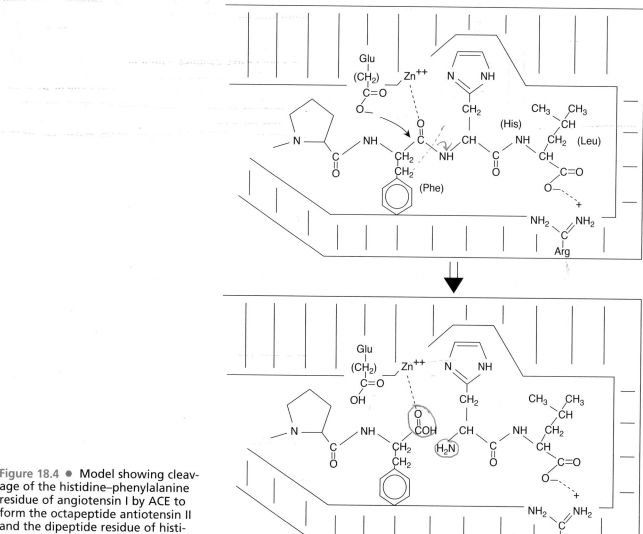

Figure 18.4 ● Model showing cleavage of the histidine–phenylalanine residue of angiotensin I by ACE to form the octapeptide antiotensin II and the dipeptide residue of histidine and leucine.

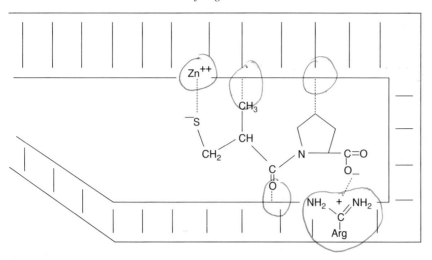

Figure 18.5 ● Accommodation of captopril to the active site of ACE.

molecule as a prototype, captopril was designed with a carboxyl group on a proline and a thiol group was introduced to enhance the binding to the zinc ion of ACE. The important binding points at the active site of ACE are thought to be an arginine residue, which provides a cationic site that attracts a carboxylate ion, and a zinc ion, which can polarize a carbonyl group of an amide function to make it more susceptible to hydrolysis. Hydrophobic pockets lie between these groups in the active site, as does a functional group that forms a hydrogen bond with an amide carbonyl. Figure 18.5 shows the hypothetical binding of captopril in the active site of ACE.

Captopril
(Capoten)

Lisinopril. Lisinopril, 1-[N^2-[S-1-carboxy-3-phenyl-propyl]-L-lysyl]-L-proline dihydrate (Prinivil, Zestril), is a lysine derivative of enalaprilat, the active metabolite of enalapril. Like all ACE inhibitors, it is an active site-directed inhibitor of the enzyme, with the zinc ion used in an effective binding interaction at a stoichiometric ratio of 1:1. The pharmacological effects of lisinopril are similar to those of captopril and enalapril.

Lisinopril
(Prinivil)
(Zestril)

ACE-INHIBITOR PRODRUGS

Many new ACE inhibitors became available for the treatment of hypertension following the clinical effectiveness of enalapril. Enalapril is a non–thiol-containing ACE inhibitor devoid of the side effects of rash and loss of the sense of taste characteristic of the thiol-containing compound captopril. With the exception of the phosphorus-containing fosinopril, these antihypertensive agents have a 2-(S)-aminophenylbutyric acid ethyl ester moiety differing only in the substituents on the amino group. They have the common property of acting as prodrugs, being converted to the active enzyme inhibitor following absorption and metabolism by liver and intestinal enzymes. These drugs (Fig. 18.6), like the prototypical drug captopril, are used in the treatment of mild-to-moderate hypertension, either alone or in conjunction with diuretics or calcium channel blockers. Table 18.1 compares some of their properties.

PRODUCTS

Enalapril Maleate. Enalapril maleate, 1-[N[(S)-1-carboxy-3-phenylpropyl]-L-alanyl]-L-proline 1′-ethyl ester maleate (Vasotec), is a long-acting ACE inhibitor. It requires activation by hydrolysis of its ethyl ester to form the diacid enalaprilat. Enalapril is devoid of the side effects of rash and loss of taste seen with captopril. These side effects are similar to those of the mercapto-containing drug penicillamine. The absence of the thiol group in enalapril maleate may free it from these side effects. The half-life is 11 hours.

Enalapril
(Vasotec)

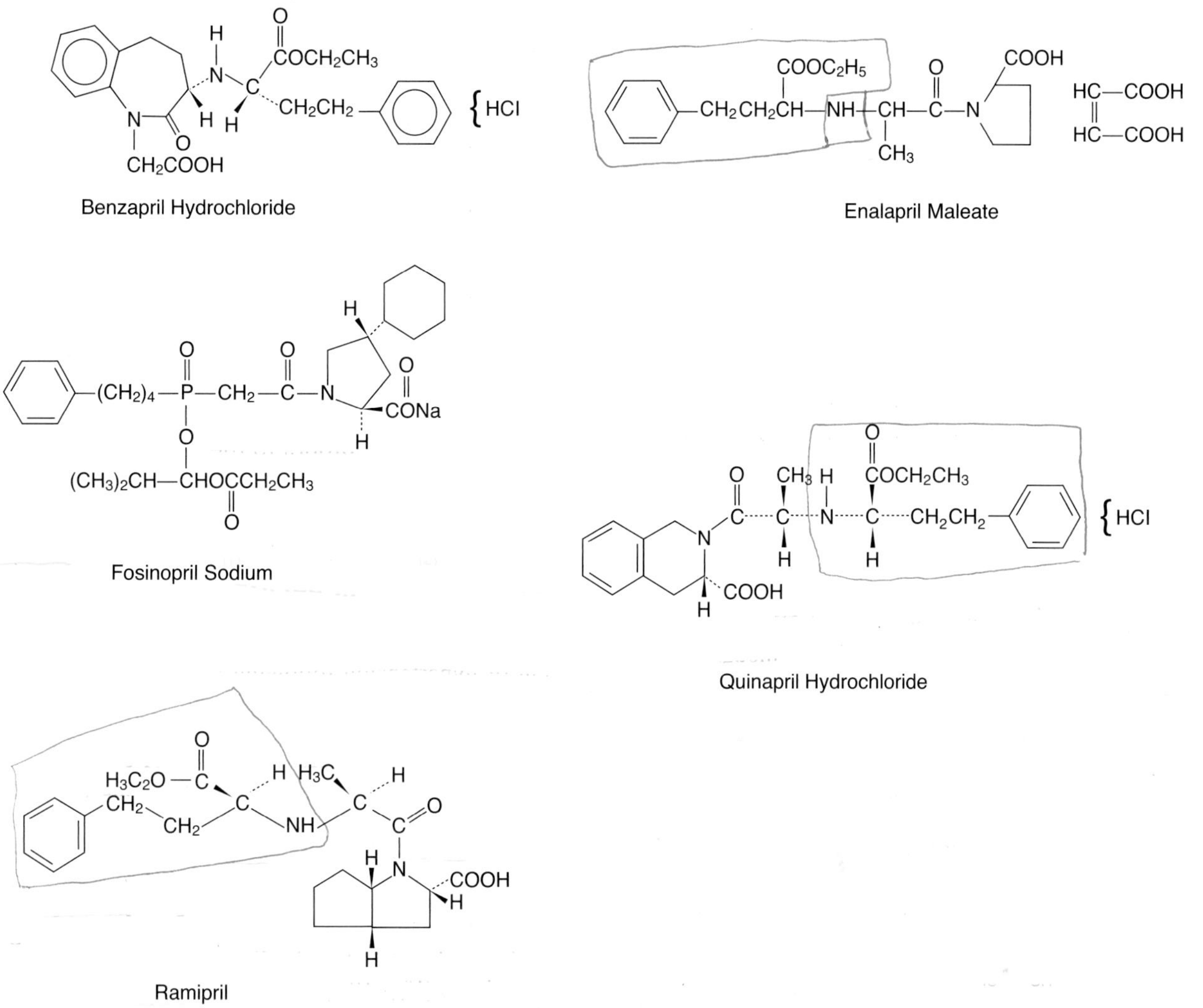

Figure 18.6 ● ACE-inhibitor prodrugs.

Benazepril Hydrochloride. Benazepril hydrochloride, (3S)-3-[[(1S)-1-carbethoxy-3-phenylpropyl]amino]-2,3,4,5-tetrahydro-2-oxo-1H-1-benzazepine-1-acetic acid 3-ethyl ester hydrochloride (Lotensin), is metabolized rapidly to the active diacid benazaprilat. As with the ACE prodrugs, no mutagenicity has been found, even though these drugs cross the placenta.

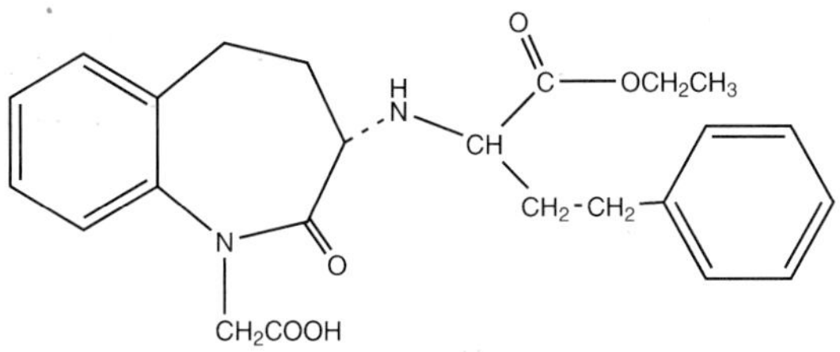

Benazepril
(Lotensin)

Quinapril Hydrochloride. Quinapril hydrochloride, (S)-[(S)-N-[(S)21-carboxy3-phenylpropyl]alanyl]-1,2,3,4-tetrahydro-3-isoquinolinecarboxylic acid 1-ethyl ester hydrochloride (Acuretic), forms the diacid quinaprilate in the

body. It is more potent than captopril and equipotent to the active form of enalapril.

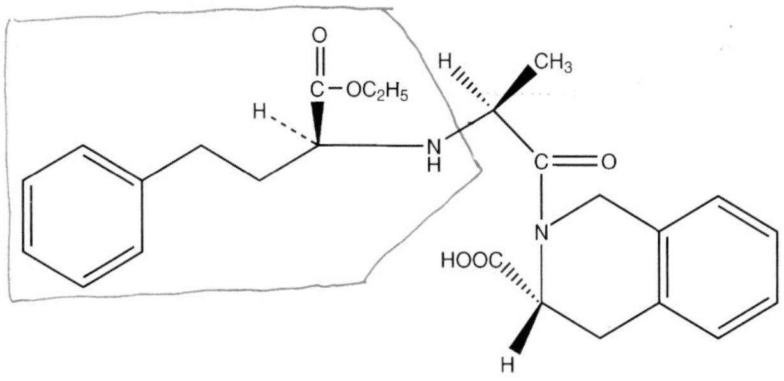

Quinapril
(Accupril)

Ramipril. Ramipril, (2S, 3aS, 6aS)-1-[(S)-N-[(S)-1-carboxy-3-phenylpropyl]alanyl]octahydrocyclopenta[b]-pyrrole-2-carboxylic acid 1-ethyl ester (Altace), is hydrolyzed to ramiprilat, its active diacid form, faster than enalapril is hydrolyzed to its active diacid form. Peak serum concentrations from a single oral dose are achieved between 1.5 and 3 hours. The ramiprilate formed completely

TABLE 18.1 Comparison of Properties of ACE-Inhibitor Prodrugs

Prodrug	Metabolite	Metabolite Protein Binding (%)	Metabolite Plasma $t_{1/2}$ (hours)	Mode of Excretion
Benazepril	Benazeprilat	95	10–11	Renal
Enalapril	Enalaprilat	50–60	11.0	Renal
Fosinopril	Fosinoprilat	97	11.5	Renal/fecal
Quinapril	Quinaprilat	97	3.0	Renal/fecal
Ramipril	Ramiprilat	56	13–17	Renal/fecal

suppresses ACE activity for up to 12 hours, with 80% inhibition of the enzyme still observed after 24 hours.

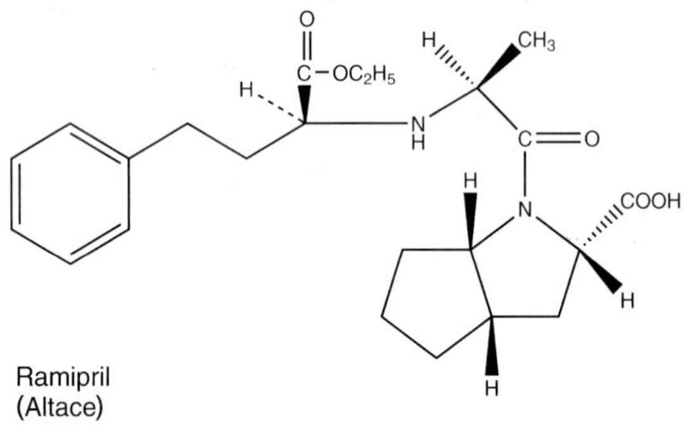

Ramipril
(Altace)

Fosinopril Sodium. Fosinopril sodium, (4S)-4-cyclohexyl-1-[[[(RS)-1-hydroxy-2-methylpropoxy](4-phenylbutyl)phosphinyl]acetyl]-L-proline sodium salt (Monopril), is a phosphorus-containing ACE inhibitor. It is inactive but serves as a prodrug, being completely hydrolyzed by intestinal and liver enzymes to the active diacid fosinoprilat.

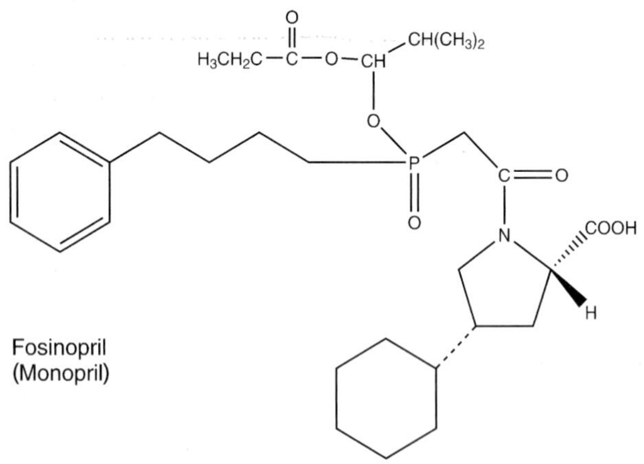

Fosinopril
(Monopril)

Trandolapril. Trandolapril, 1-[2-(1-ethoxycarbonyl-3-phenylpropylamino)propionyl]octahydroindole-2-carboxylic acid (Mavik), is an indole-containing ACE inhibitor that is structurally related to most of the preceding agents discussed. Enalapril is very similar to trandolapril, with the primary difference occurring in the heterocyclic systems. The pyrrolidine of enalapril has been replaced with an octahydroindole system. Much like enalaprilate, trandolapril must be hydrolyzed to tranolaprilate, which is the bioactive species.

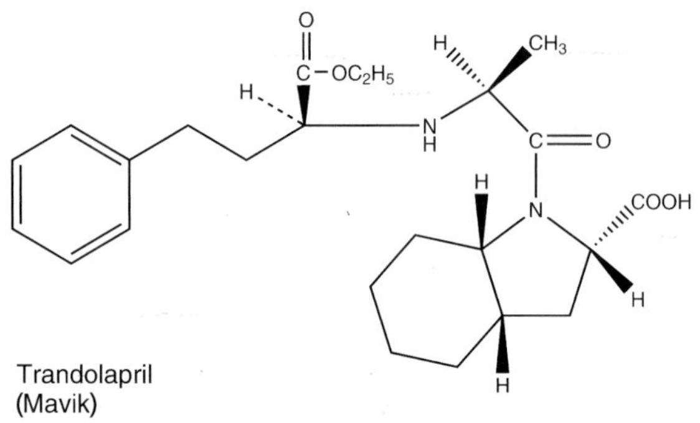

Trandolapril
(Mavik)

◉ ANGIOTENSIN ANTAGONISTS

There are four different subtypes of angiotensin II receptor subclasses identified to date and include AT_1, AT_2, AT_3, and AT_4. These belong to the class of G-protein–coupled receptors and are responsible for the signal transduction of the hormone. Although there is some understanding of the role AT_2 plays in development of a fetus or neonate, there is very little known about the role of AT_2 and AT_3 in the human body. However, it is the AT_1 receptors that are of particular interest in managing specific cardiovascular diseases. Studies have demonstrated that stimulation of AT_1 receptors by angiotensin II result in vasoconstriction, aldosterone synthesis and secretion, increased vasopressin secretion, decreased renal blood flow, renal tubular sodium reuptake, and several other physiological events.

Administration of a competitive antagonist that inhibits angiotensin II at the AT_1 receptor will produce a vasodilatory effect. Because the substrate for this receptor is an octapeptide, much of the earlier work was performed by using various peptide systems. One such agent, saralasin, is an octapeptide that differs from angiotensin by two amino acids. This agent's use was limited because it had some partial agonistic properties. Nevertheless, it served as a lead in the development of other agents that are useful in antagonizing the angiotensin II receptor. The most significant lead in the development of this class came from a series of imidazole-5-acetic acid derivatives that attenuated pressor response to angiotensin II in test animals. Molecular modeling revealed that the imidazole-5-acetic acid could be exploited to mimic more closely the pharmacophore of angiotensin II. The first successful agent to be developed through this method is losartan. Later, four other agents were introduced into the U.S. market. These tend to be biphenylmethyl derivatives that possess certain acidic moieties, which can interact with various positions on the receptor, much like the substrate, angiotensin II.

● ANGIOTENSIN II BLOCKERS

PRODUCTS

Losartan. Losartan, 2-butyl-4-chloro-1-[*p*-(*o*-1*H*-tetra-zol-5-yl-phenyl)benzyl]imidazole-5-methanol monopotassium salt (Cozarr), was the first nonpeptide imidazole to be introduced as an orally active angiotensin II antagonist with high specificity for AT$_1$. When administered to patients, it undergoes extensive first-pass metabolism, with the 5-methanol being oxidized to a carboxylic acid. This metabolism is mediated by CYP 2C9 and 3A4 isozymes. The 5-methanol metabolite is approximately 15 times more potent than the parent hydroxyl compound. Because the parent hydroxyl compound has affinity for the AT$_1$ receptor, strictly speaking, it is not a prodrug.[13]

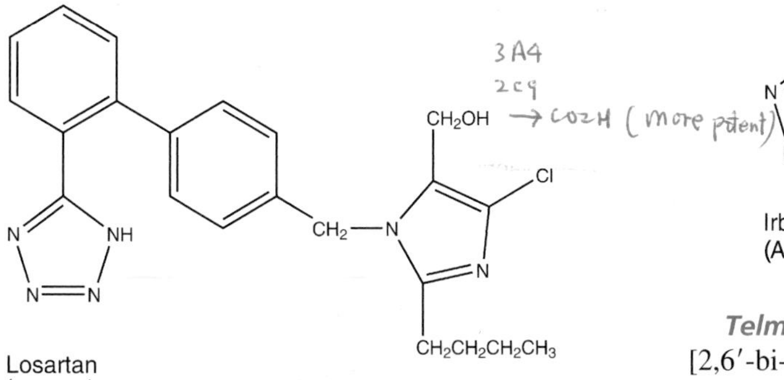

Losartan
(Cozaar)

Candesartan. Candesartan, (+)-1-[[(cyclohexyloxy)carbonyl]-oxy]ethyl 2- ethoxy-1-[[2′-(1*H*-tetrazol-5-yl)[1,1′-biphenyl]-4-yl]methyl]-1*H*-benzimidazole-7-carboxylate (Atacand), like losartan, possesses the acidic tetrazole system, which most likely plays a role in binding to the angiotensin II receptor similarly to the acidic groups of angiotensin II. Also, the imidazole system has been replaced with a benzimidazole possessing an ester at position 7. This ester must be hydrolyzed to the free acid. Fortunately, this conversion takes place fairly easily because of the carbonate in the ester side chain. This facilitates hydrolysis of the ester so much that conversion to the free acid takes place during absorption from the gastrointestinal tract.

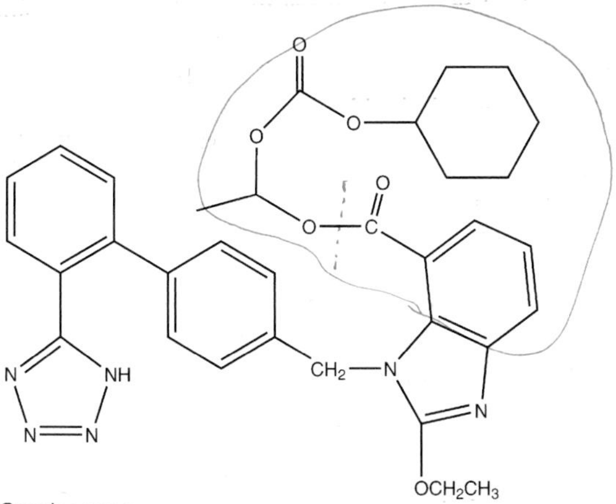

Candesartan
(Atacand)

Irbesartan. Irbesartan, 2-butyl-3-[[29-(1*H*-tetrazol-5-yl)[1,19-biphenyl]-4-yl]methyl]1,3-diazaspiro[4,4]non-1en-4-one (Avapro), like losartan, possesses the acidic tetrazole system, which most likely plays a role, similar to the acidic groups of angiotensin II, in binding to the angiotensin II receptor. In addition, the biphenyl system that serves to separate the tetrazole from the aliphatic nitrogen is still present. A major difference in this agent is that it does not possess the acidic side chain. Even so, irbesartan has good affinity for the angiotensin II receptor because of hydrogen bonding with the carbonyl moiety of the amide system. Also, this particular agent does not require metabolic activation as candesartan does.

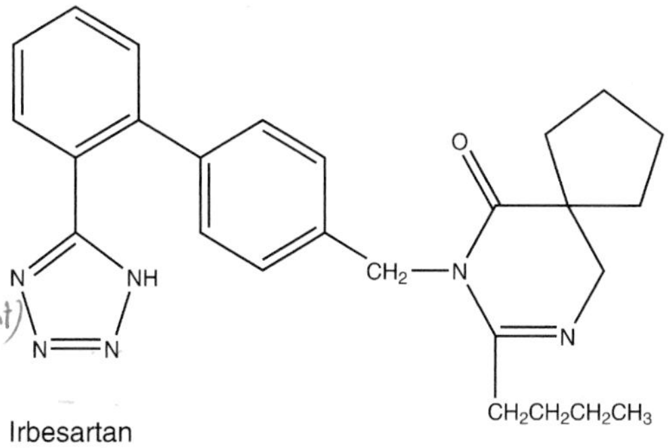

Irbesartan
(Avapro)

Telmisartan. Telmisartan, 4′-[(1,4′-dimethyl-2′-propyl [2,6′-bi-1*H*-benzimidazol]-1′-yl)methyl]-[1,1′-biphenyl]-2-carboxylic acid (Micardis), does not appear to bear any structural relationship to this class, but there is actually a great deal of overlap in the chemical architecture with other agents. The first, and most significant, difference is the replacement of the acidic tetrazole system with a simple carboxylic acid. This acid, like the tetrazole, plays a role in receptor binding. The second difference is the lack of a carboxylic acid near the imidazole nitrogen that also contributes to receptor binding.[14] As with irbesartan, however, there is not a need for this group to be acidic but, rather, to be one that participates in receptor binding. The second imidazole ring, much like a purine base in deoxyribonucleic acid (DNA), can hydrogen bond with the angiotensin II receptor.

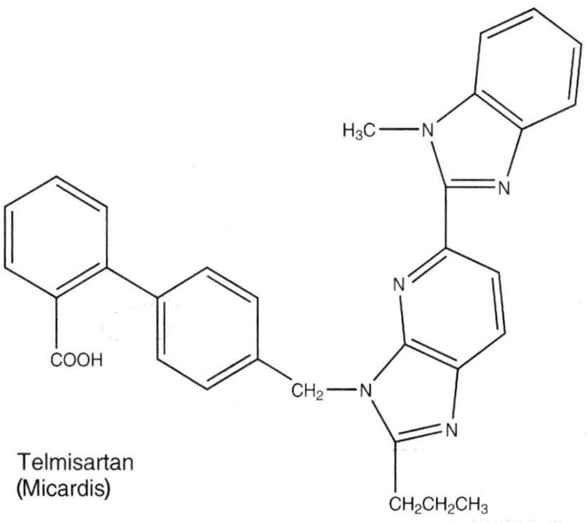

Telmisartan
(Micardis)

Olmesartan. Olmesartan medoxomil, (5-methyl-2-oxo-1,3-dioxol-4-yl)methyl-5-(2-hydroxypropan-2-yl)-2-

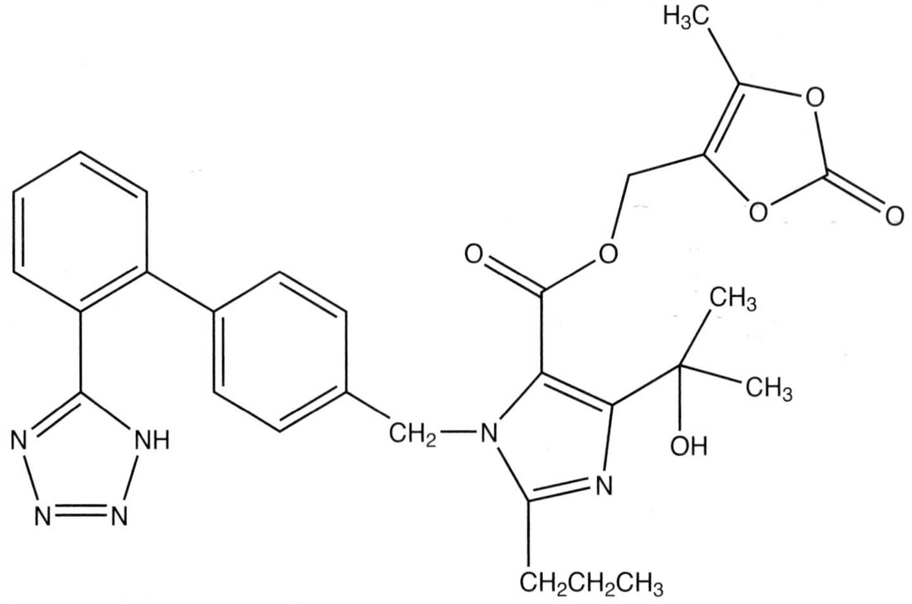

Olmesartan medoxomil

propyl-3-[[4-[2-(2H-tetrazol-5-yl)phenyl]phenyl]methyl] imidazole-4-carboxylate (Benicar, Olmetec) uses the tetrazole ring system as its acidic system, which participates in receptor binding.[14] When administered to a patient, the drug is rapidly and completely bioactivated by ester hydrolysis of the medoxomil during absorption from the gastrointestinal tract. Once the prodrug is converted to the active form, virtually no further metabolism occurs. In September 2007, the Food and Drug Administration (FDA) approved its use as a combination product with the calcium channel blocker amlodipine for the management of hypertension. This combination product is sold under the tradename of Azor.

Valsartan. Valsartan, *N*-(1-oxopentyl)-*N*-[[2′-(1*H*-tetrazol-5-yl)[1,1′-biphenyl]-4-yl]methyl]-L-valine (Diovan), like losartan, possesses the acidic tetrazole system, which most likely plays a role, similar to that of the acidic groups of angiotensin II, in binding to the angiotensin II receptor. In addition, the biphenyl system that serves to separate the tetrazole from the aliphatic nitrogen is still present. In addition, there is a carboxylic acid side chain in the valine moiety that also serves to bind to the angiotensin II receptor.[15]

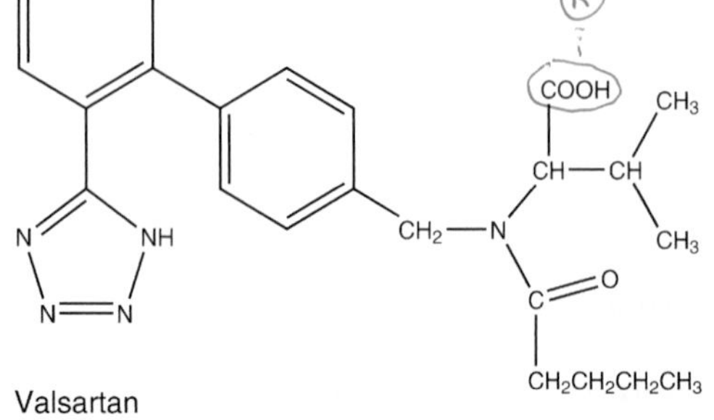

Valsartan
(Diovan)

RENIN INHIBITORS

Renin is a circulating enzyme that is secreted by the kidneys in response to decreases in glomerular filtration rate, which is typically a result of low blood volume. It is a 340-amino acid protein that participates in the renin–angiotensin system. It is responsible for cleaving angiotensinogen, which is produced in the liver, to angiotensin I. As indicated previously in this chapter, angiontensin I is converted to angiotensin II, which plays an important role in regulating blood pressure, among other physiological events. Inhibitors of renin have usefulness in managing cardiovascular diseases such as hypertension and heart failure because of their ability in reducing the influence on the renin–angiotensin system through reduced biosynthesis of angiotensin II and other bioactive intermediates.[16]

Although this drug target has been investigated for more than 30 years, it represents the first new class of orally active antihypertensive agents and joins at least seven other classes of antihypertensive drugs. The other classes, as described in Chapter 19, include diuretics, α-blockers, β-blockers, calcium channel blockers, as well as those discussed in this chapter and include ACE inhibitors, ARBs, and aldosterone receptor antagonists.

PRODUCTS

Aliskiren. Aliskiren, (2*S*,4*S*,5*S*,7*S*)-5-amino-*N*-(2-carbamoyl-2-methyl-propyl)-4-hydroxy-7-{[4-methoxy-3-(3-methoxypropoxy)phenyl]methyl}-8-methyl-2-propan-2-yl-nonanamide (Tekturna), is the first renin inhibitor introduced into the U. S. market.[17] It was approved by the FDA in 2007 for the management of hypertension. The trade name for aliskiren in the United Kingdom is Rasilez.

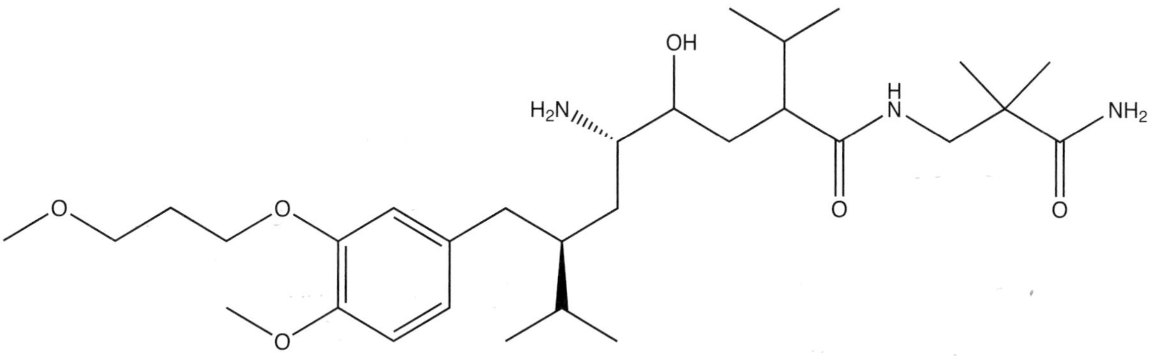

Aliskiren

⬡ ALDOSTERONE ANTAGONISTS

Aldosterone antagonists are, as the name implies, receptor antagonists at the mineralcorticoid receptor. Antagonism of these receptors inhibits sodium resorption in the distal tubule of the nephron, which in turn, interferes with sodium/potassium exchange, reducing urinary potassium excretion. Overall, this results in a weak diuretic effect and decreases cardiac workload. Agents that block aldosterone may be used in the management of hypertension or heart failure. The two agents approved for use in the United States are spironolactone (Aldactone) and eplerenone (Inspra) and are discussed in greater detail in the diuretic chapter of this textbook.

◆ R E V I E W   Q U E S T I O N S ◆

1. The renin–angiotensin system plays an important role in regulation of blood pressure. For that reason, this pathway encompasses the conversion of an approximately 400 amino acid sequence to a decapeptide, then to the biologically active octapeptide, and is an excellent target for drug therapy to manage hypertension. Describe the starting protein and its conversion to the biologically active metabolite. Be sure to include the enzymes involved in the conversion of the protein and peptides.

2. The therapeutic usefulness of the agent represented below (candesartan [Atacand]) is:

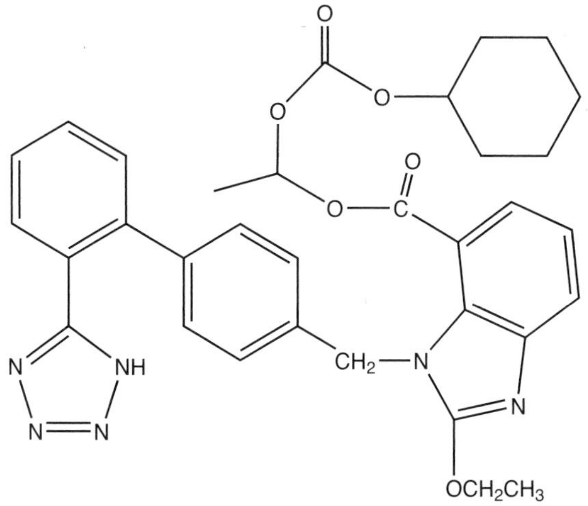

a. angiotensin-converting enzyme inhibitor
b. angiotensin II receptor blocker
c. renin inhibitor
d. aldosterone antagonist
e. More than one answer is correct.

3. Although the agent represented below (losartan [Cozaar]) has some pharmacological effects, one of its metabolites is reported to be more potent. Identify the metabolite and describe its production.

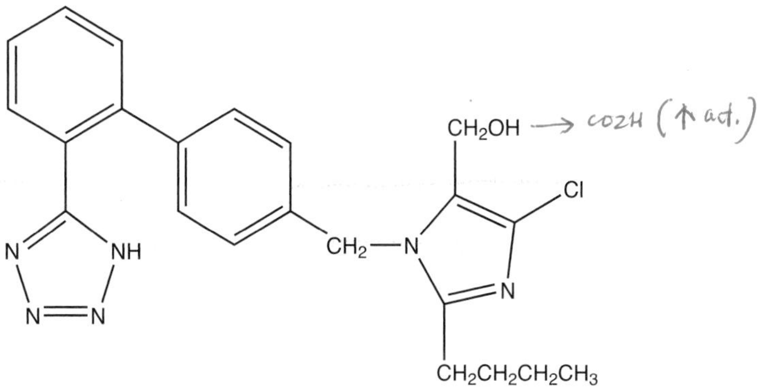

REFERENCES

1. Tigerstedt, R., and Bergman, P. G.: Scand. Arch. Physiol. 8:223, 1898.
2. Page, F., and Helmer, O. A.: J. Exp. Med. 71:29, 1940.
3. Skeggs, L., Marsh, W. H., Kahn, J. R., et al.: J. Exp. Med. 99:275, 1954.
4. Moreau, P., Laplante, M.-A., Beaucage, P., et al.: HHandb. Exp. Pharmacol. 163:149, 2004.
5. Jackson, E. K.: In Hardman, J. G., and Limbird, L. E. (eds.). Goodman and Gilman's The Pharmacological Basis of Therapeutics, 10th ed. New York, Macmillan, 2001, pp. 809–841.
6. Ceconi, C., Francolini, G., Olivares, A., et al.: Eur. J. Pharmacol. 577:1, 2007.
7. Shapiro, R., and Riordan, J. F.: Biochemistry 23:5225, 1984.
8. Ehlers, M. R., and Riordan, J. F.: Biochemistry 30:7118, 1991.
9. Levens, N. R., Peach, M. J., and Carey, R. M.: Circ. Res. 48:157, 1981.
10. Jordan, J., Tank, J., Diedrich, A., et al.: Hypertension 36:e3, 2000.
11. Aulakh, G. K., Sodhi, R. K., and Singh, M.: Life Sci. 81:615, 2007.
12. Li, Y. C.: Current Opinion in Investigational Drugs 8:750, 2007.
13. Schmidt, B., Drexler H., and Schieffer B.: Am. J. Cardiovasc. Drugs 4:361, 2004.
14. Le, M. T., Pugsley, M. K., Vauquelin, G., et al.: Br. J. Pharmacol. 151:952, 2007.
15. de Gasparo, M., and Whitebread, S.: Regul. Pept. 59:303, 1995.
16. Venkata, C., and Ram, S.: J. Clin. Hypertens. 9:615, 2007.
17. Sealey, J. E., and Laragh, J. H.: Am. J. Hypertens. 20(5):587, 2007.

C H A P T E R 19

Cardiovascular Agents

STEPHEN J. CUTLER

CHAPTER OVERVIEW

Proteins, cardiovascular agents, describe the role various chemical entities play in controlling cardiovascular diseases. This chapter describes the agents used in the treatment of angina, cardiac arrhythmias, hypertension, erectile dysfunction, hyperlipidemias, and disorders of blood coagulation. For pharmacists to be good practitioners, it is necessary that they understand the pathophysiology of cardiovascular diseases and the agents used to treat these syndromes.

The treatment and therapy of cardiovascular disease have undergone dramatic changes since the 1950s. Data show that since 1968 and continuing through the 1990s, there has been a noticeable decline in mortality from cardiovascular disease. The bases for advances in the control of heart disease have been (a) a better understanding of the disease state, (b) the development of effective therapeutic agents, and (c) innovative medical intervention techniques to treat problems of the cardiovascular system.

The drugs discussed in this chapter are used for their action on the heart or other parts of the vascular system, to modify the total output of the heart or the distribution of blood to the circulatory system. These drugs are used in the treatment of angina, cardiac arrhythmias, hypertension, hyperlipidemias, and disorders of blood coagulation. This chapter also includes a discussion of hypoglycemic agents, thyroid hormones, and antithyroid drugs.

ANTIANGINAL AGENTS AND VASODILATORS

Most coronary artery disease conditions are caused by deposits of atheromas in the intima of large and medium-sized arteries serving the heart. The process is characterized by an insidious onset of episodes of cardiac discomfort caused by ischemia from inadequate blood supply to the tissues. Angina pectoris (angina), the principal symptom of ischemic heart disease, is characterized by a severe constricting pain in the chest, often radiating from the precordium to the left shoulder and down the arm. The syndrome has been described since 1772, but not until 1867 was amyl nitrite introduced for the symptomatic relief of angina pectoris.[1] It was believed at that time that anginal pain was precipitated by an increase in blood pressure and that the use of amyl nitrite reduced both blood pressure and, concomitantly, the work required of the heart. Later, it was generally accepted that nitrites relieved angina pectoris by dilating the coronary arteries and that changes in the work of the heart were of only secondary importance. We now know that the coronary blood vessels in the atherosclerotic heart already are dilated, and that ordinary doses of dilator drugs do not significantly increase blood supply to the heart; instead, anginal pain is relieved by a reduction of cardiac consumption of oxygen.[2]

Although vasodilators are used in the treatment of angina, a more sophisticated understanding of the hemodynamic response to these agents has broadened their clinical usefulness to other cardiovascular conditions. Because of their ability to reduce peripheral vascular resistance, vasodilators, including organonitrates, angiotensin-converting enzyme (ACE) inhibitors, and angiotensin receptor–blocking agents, are used to improve cardiac output in some patients with congestive heart failure (CHF).

The coronary circulation supplies blood to the myocardial tissues to maintain cardiac function. It can react to the changing demands of the heart by dilating its blood vessels to provide sufficient oxygen and other nutrients and to remove metabolites. Myocardial metabolism is almost exclusively aerobic, which makes blood flow critical to the support of metabolic processes of the heart. This demand is met effectively by the normal heart, because it extracts a relatively large proportion of the oxygen delivered to it by the coronary circulation. The coronary blood flow depends strongly on myocardial metabolism, which in turn is affected by work done by the heart and the efficiency of the heart. The coronary system normally has a reserve capacity that allows it to respond by vasodilation to satisfy the needs of the heart during strenuous activity by the body.

Coronary atherosclerosis, one of the more prevalent cardiovascular diseases, develops with increasing age and may lead to a reduction of the reserve capacity of the coronary system. It most often results in multiple stenosis and makes it difficult for the coronary system to meet adequately the oxygen needs of the heart that occur during physical exercise or emotional duress. Insufficient coronary blood flow (*myocardial ischemia*) in the face of increased oxygen demand produces angina pectoris.

The principal goal in the prevention and relief of angina is to limit the oxygen requirement of the heart, so that the amount of blood supplied by the stenosed arteries is adequate. Nitrate esters, such as nitroglycerin, lower arterial blood pressure and, in turn, reduce the work of the left ventricle. This action is produced by the powerful vasodilating effect of the nitrates on the arterial system and, to an even greater extent, on the venous system. The result is reduced cardiac filling pressure and ventricular size. This reduces the work required of the ventricle and decreases the oxygen requirements, allowing the coronary system to satisfy the oxygen demands of myocardial tissue and relieve anginal pain.

Intermediary Myocardial Metabolism

Energy metabolism by heart tissue provides an adequate supply of high-energy phosphate compounds to replace the adenosine triphosphate (ATP) that is continually being consumed in contraction, ion exchange across membranes, and other energy-demanding processes. Because of the high turnover rate of ATP in heart muscle, a correspondingly high rate of ATP production in the mitochondria is required.

Normal myocardial metabolism is aerobic, and the rate of oxygen use parallels the amount of ATP synthesized by the cells.[3] Free fatty acids (FFAs) are the principal fuel for myocardial tissue, but lactate, acetate, acetoacetate, and glucose are also oxidized to carbon dioxide and water. A large volume of the myocardial cell consists of mitochondria in which two-carbon fragments from FFA breakdown are metabolized through the Krebs cycle. The reduced flavin and nicotinamide dinucleotides formed by this metabolism are reoxidized by the electron-transport chain because of the presence of oxygen (Fig. 19.1). In the hypoxic or ischemic heart, the lack of oxygen inhibits the electron-transport chain function and causes an accumulation of reduced flavin and nicotinamide coenzymes. As a result, fatty acids are converted to lipids rather than being oxidized. To compensate for this, glucose use and glycogenolysis increase, but the resulting pyruvate cannot be oxidized; instead, it is converted to lactate. A great loss of efficiency occurs as a result of the change of myocardial metabolism from aerobic to anaerobic pathways. Normally, 36 mol of ATP are formed from the oxidation of 1 mol of glucose, but only 2 mol are formed from its glycolysis. This great loss of high-energy stores during hypoxia thus limits the functional capacity of the heart during stressful conditions and is reflected by the production of anginal pain.

Nitrovasodilators

SMOOTH MUSCLE RELAXATION

The contractile activity of all types of muscle (smooth, skeletal) is regulated primarily by the reversible phosphorylation of myosin. Myosin of smooth muscle consists of two heavy chains (molecular weight [MW] 200,000 each) that are coiled to produce a filamentous tail. Each heavy chain is associated with two pairs of light chains (MW 20,000 and 16,000) that serve as substrates for calcium- and calmodulin-dependent protein kinases in the contraction process. Together with actin (MW 43,000), they participate in a cascade of biochemical events that are part of the processes of muscle contraction and relaxation (Fig. 19.2).

Cyclic nucleotides, cyclic adenosine monophosphate (cAMP), and, especially, cyclic guanosine monophosphate (cGMP) play important roles in the regulation of smooth muscle tension. cAMP is the mediator associated with the smooth muscle relaxant properties of drugs such as β-adrenergic agonists. It activates the protein kinases that phosphorylate myosin light-chain kinase (MLCK). Phosphorylation of MLCK inactivates this kinase and prevents its action with Ca^{2+} and calmodulin to phosphorylate myosin, which interacts with actin to cause contraction of smooth muscle (Fig. 19.2).

The activity of cGMP in smooth muscle relaxation is affected by exogenous and endogenous agents. It is suggested[4] that nitrovasodilators undergo metabolic transformation in

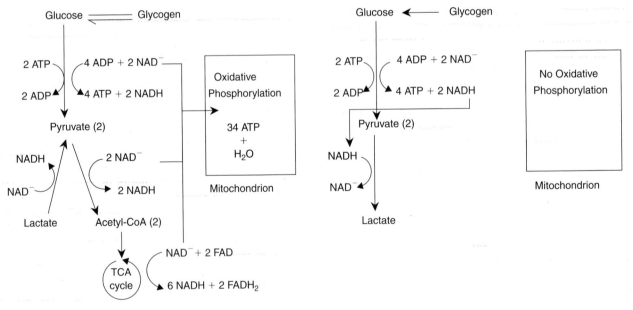

NORMAL GLUCOSE METABOLISM   ISCHEMIC GLUCOSE METABOLISM

Figure 19.1 ● Normal and ischemic myocardial metabolism of glucose. A total production of 36 mol of ATP results from the aerobic catabolism of 1 mol of glucose and use of NADH and $FADH_2$ in the oxidative phosphorylation process in mitochondria. When oxygen is not available, NADH and $FADH_2$ levels rise and shut off the tricarboxylic acid (TCA) cycle. Pyruvate is converted to lactate. Only 2 mol of ATP are formed from anaerobic catabolism of 1 mol of glucose. (Adapted from Giuliani, E. R., et al.: Cardiology: Fundamentals and Practice, 2nd ed. By permission of the Mayo Foundation, Rochester, MN.)

Figure 19.2 ● Regulation of smooth muscle contraction. Contraction is triggered by an influx of Ca^{2+}. The increase of free Ca^{2+} causes binding to calmodulin (CM). The Ca^{2+}—CM complex binds to myosin light-chain kinase (MLCK) and causes its activation (MLCK*). MLCK* phosphorylates myosin, which combines with actin to produce contraction of smooth muscle. Myosin is dephosphorylated in the presence of myosin phosphatase to cause muscle relaxation. The β-agonists activate adenylate cyclase (AC) to raise levels of cAMP, which in turn activates kinases that phosphorylate MLCK, inactivating it to prevent muscle contraction.

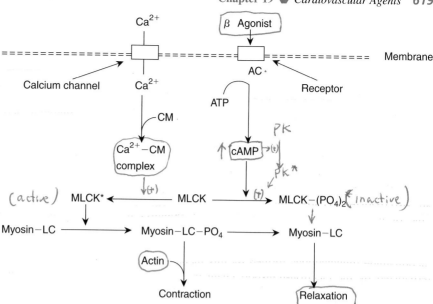

vascular smooth muscle cells to form nitric oxide (NO). NO mediates smooth muscle relaxation by activating guanylate cyclase to increase intracellular concentrations of cGMP. cGMP activates protein kinases that can regulate free Ca^{2+} levels in the muscle cell and cause relaxation of smooth muscle by phosphorylating MLCK.

A short-lived free radical gas, NO is widely distributed in the body and plays an important role by its effect through cGMP on the smooth muscle vasculature. It is synthesized in the vascular endothelial cell from the semiessential amino acid L-arginine by NO synthase. After production in the cell, it diffuses to the smooth muscle cell, where it activates the enzyme guanylate cyclase, which leads to an increase in cGMP and then muscle relaxation (Fig. 19.3). Endothelium-derived relaxing factor (EDRF), released from the endothelial cell to mediate its smooth muscle–relaxing properties through cGMP, is identical with NO.

Inhibitors of phosphodiesterases of cAMP and cGMP also cause smooth muscle relaxation. These inhibitors increase cellular levels of cAMP and cGMP by preventing their hydrolysis to AMP and GMP, respectively. Drugs such as papaverine (see Chapter 17), theophylline (see chapter on

Diuretics), and sildenafil (this chapter), which relax smooth muscle, do so in part by inhibiting phosphodiesterases.

METABOLISM OF NITROVASODILATORS

After oral administration, organic nitrates are metabolized rapidly by the liver, kidney, lungs, intestinal mucosa, and vascular tissue. Buccal absorption reduces the immediate hepatic destruction of the organic nitrates because only 15% of the cardiac output is delivered to the liver; this allows a transient but effective circulating level of the intact organic nitrate before it is inactivated.[5]

Organic nitrates, nitrites, nitroso compounds, and a variety of other nitrogen-containing substances, such as sodium nitroprusside, for the most part cause their pharmacological effects by generating or releasing NO in situ. In some ways, these drugs are viewed as "replacement agents" for the endogenous NO generated by the NO synthase pathway from arginine. The mechanisms by which vasodilatory drugs release NO have become better understood recently. Table 19.1 shows the oxidation state of various nitrosyl compounds that are common in nitrovasodilatory drugs. A common feature of these drugs is that they release nitrogen in the form of NO and contain nitrogen in an oxidation state higher than +3 (as would occur in ammonia, amines, amides, and most biological nitrogen compounds). The nitrogen in NO has an oxidation state of +2. Compounds such as nitroprusside, nitrosoamines, and nitrothiols with oxidation states of +3 release NO nonenzymatically. Although their spontaneous liberation of NO is by an unknown mechanism, it involves only a one-electron reduction, which may occur on exposure of these chemicals to various reducing agents in the tissue of vascular smooth muscle membranes. Organic nitrites such as amyl nitrite react with available thiol groups to form unstable S-nitrosothiols, which rapidly decompose to NO by homolytic cleavage of their S—N bond. In mammalian smooth muscle, this will occur almost exclusively with glutathione as the most abundant thiol compound.[6]

The pharmacodynamic action of nitroglycerin is preceded by metabolic changes that follow various paths. Biotransformation of nitroglycerin to the dinitrates and the

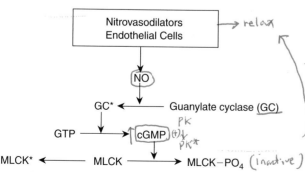

Figure 19.3 ● Mechanism of nitrovasodilators. Nitric oxide (NO) formed in smooth muscle from nitrovasodilators or from endothelial cells (EDRF) activates guanylate cyclase (GC*). GC* activates cGMP-dependent protein kinases that phosphorylate myosin light-chain kinase (MLCK), causing its inactivation and subsequent muscle relaxation (see also Fig. 19.2).

TABLE 19.1 Nitrosyl Vasodilatory Substances and Their Oxidation State

Nitrosyl Compound	Structure	Nitrogen Oxidation State
Nitric oxide	N═O	+2
Nitrite	—ONO	+3
Nitrate	—ONO$_2$	+5
Organic nitrite	R—O—N═O	+3
Nitrosothiol	R—S—N═O	+3
Organic nitrate	R—O—NO$_2$	+5
Thionitrate	R—S—NO$_2$	+5
Nitroprusside	[(CN)$_5$Fe—N═O]^2	+3

Reprinted from Harrison, D. G., and Bates, J. M.: Circulation 87:1462, 1993, with permission from the American Heart Association.

increase of intracellular cGMP precede vascular relaxation. Sulfhydryl-containing compounds, such as cysteine, react chemically with organic nitrates to form inorganic nitrite ions. The release of NO from an organic nitrate, such as nitroglycerin, appears to occur in a stepwise fashion involving nonenzymatic and enzymatic steps. Because nitroglycerin requires a three-electron reduction to release NO, thiols may be involved in the process. Nitroglycerin may decompose nonenzymatically by interaction with various thiols, such as cysteine or *N*-acetylcysteine, which may be present in tissue, to form a nitrosothiol intermediate before undergoing enzymatic transformation to release NO. Nitroglycerin also readily releases NO by acting on an enzyme system attached to the cellular surface membrane of smooth muscle. The process may include glutathione-*S*-transferases, which convert nitroglycerin to a vasoinactive nitrite, which then may release NO nonenzymatically.[7]

ESTERS OF NITROUS AND NITRIC ACIDS

Inorganic acids, like organic acids, will form esters with an alcohol. Pharmaceutically, the important ones are sulfate, nitrite, and nitrate. Sulfuric acid forms organic sulfates, of which methyl sulfate and ethyl sulfate are examples.

Nitrous acid (HNO$_2$) esters may be formed readily from an alcohol and HNO$_2$. The usual procedure is to mix sodium nitrite, sulfuric acid, and the alcohol. Organic nitrites are generally very volatile liquids that are only slightly soluble in water but soluble in alcohol. Preparations containing water are very unstable because of hydrolysis.

The organic nitrates and nitrites and the inorganic nitrites have their primary utility in the prophylaxis and treatment of angina pectoris. They have a more limited application in treating asthma, gastrointestinal spasm, and certain cases of migraine headache. Their application may be regarded as causal therapy, because they act by substituting an endogenous factor, the production or release of NO, which may be impaired under pathophysiological circumstances associated with dysfunction of the endothelial tissue. Nitroglycerin (glyceryl trinitrate) was one of the first members of this group to be introduced in medicine and remains an important member of the group. Varying the chemical structure of the organic nitrates yields differences in speed of onset, duration of action, and potency (Table 19.2). Although the number of nitrate ester groups may vary from two to six or more, depending on the compound, there is no direct relationship between the number of nitrate groups and the level of activity.

It appears that the higher the oil/water partition coefficient of the drug, the greater the potency. The orientation of the groups within the molecule also may affect potency. Lipophilicity of the nitrogen oxide–containing compound produces a much longer response of vasodilatory action. The highly lipophilic ester nitroglycerin permeates the cell membrane, allowing continual formation of NO within the cell. The same effect appears to occur for sodium nitroprusside, nitroso compounds, and other organic nitrate and nitrite esters.[4]

ANTIANGINAL ACTION OF NITROVASODILATORS

The action of short-acting sublingual nitrates in the relief of angina pectoris is complex. Although the sublingual nitrates relax vascular smooth muscle and dilate the coronary arteries of normal humans, there is little improvement of coronary blood flow when these chemicals are administered to individuals with coronary artery disease. Nitroglycerin is an effective antianginal agent because it causes redistribution of coronary blood flow to the ischemic regions of the heart and reduces myocardial oxygen demand. This latter effect is produced by a reduction of venous tone resulting from the nitrate vasodilating effect and a pooling of blood in the peripheral veins, which results in a reduction in ventricular volume, stroke volume, and cardiac output. It also causes reduction of peripheral resistance during myocardial contractions. The combined vasodilatory effects cause a decrease in cardiac work and reduce oxygen demand.

PRODUCTS

Amyl Nitrite, United States Pharmacopeia (USP). Amyl nitrite, isopentyl nitrite [(CH$_3$)$_2$CHCH$_2$CH$_2$ONO], is a mixture of isomeric amyl nitrites but is principally isoamyl nitrite. It may be prepared from amyl alcohol and HNO$_2$ by several procedures. Usually, amyl nitrite is dispensed in

TABLE 19.2 Relationship between Speed and Duration of Action of Sodium Nitrite and Certain Inorganic Esters

Compound	Action Begins (minutes)	Maximum Effect (minutes)	Duration of Action (minutes)
Amyl nitrite	0.25	0.5	1
Nitroglycerin	2	8	30
Isosorbide dinitrate	3	15	60
Sodium nitrite	10	25	60
Erythrityl tetranitrate	15	32	180
Pentaerythritol tetranitrate	20	70	330

ampul form and used by inhalation or orally in alcohol solution. Currently, it is recommended for treating cyanide poisoning; although not the best antidote, it does not require intravenous injections.

Amyl nitrite is a yellowish liquid with an ethereal odor and a pungent taste. It is volatile and inflammable at room temperature. Amyl nitrite vapor forms an explosive mixture in air or oxygen. Inhalation of the vapor may involve definite explosion hazards if a source of ignition is present, as both room and body temperatures are within the flammability range of amyl nitrite mixtures with either air or oxygen. It is nearly insoluble in water but is miscible with organic solvents. The nitrite also will decompose in valeric acid and nitric acid.

Nitroglycerin. Glyceryl trinitrate is the trinitrate ester of glycerol and is listed as available in tablet form in the *USP*. It is prepared by carefully adding glycerin to a mixture of nitric and fuming sulfuric acids. This reaction is exothermic, and the reaction mixture must be cooled to between 10°C and 20°C.

The ester is a colorless oil, with a sweet, burning taste. It is only slightly soluble in water, but it is soluble in organic solvents.

$$H_2C-ONO_2$$
$$HC-ONO_2$$
$$H_2C-ONO_2$$

Nitroglycerin	
Transmucosal	Nitrogard
Translingual	Nitrolingual
Oral	Nitrobid
	Nitroglyn
Ointment	Nitroglyn
Injection	Nitrobid IV
	Tridil
Transdermal	Nitrodur
	Nitrodisc
	Minitran
	Deponit
	Transderm-Nitro

Nitroglycerin is used extensively as an explosive in dynamite. A solution of the ester, if spilled or allowed to evaporate, will leave a residue of nitroglycerin. To prevent an explosion of the residue, the ester must be decomposed by adding alkali. Even so, the material dispensed is so dilute that the risk of explosions does not exist. It has a strong vasodilating action and, because it is absorbed through the skin, is prone to cause headaches among workers associated with its manufacture. This transdermal penetration is why nitroglycerin is useful in a patch formulation. In medicine, it has the action typical of nitrites, but its action develops more slowly and is of longer duration. Of all the known coronary vasodilatory drugs, nitroglycerin is the only one capable of stimulating the production of coronary collateral circulation and the only one able to prevent experimental myocardial infarction by coronary occlusion.

Previously, the nitrates were thought to be hydrolyzed and reduced in the body to nitrites, which then lowered the blood pressure. This is not true, however. The mechanism of vasodilation of nitroglycerin through its formation of NO is described previously.

Nitroglycerin tablet instability was reported in molded sublingual tablets.[8] The tablets, although uniform when manufactured, lost potency both because of volatilization of nitroglycerin into the surrounding materials in the container and intertablet migration of the active ingredient. Nitroglycerin may be stabilized in molded tablets by incorporating a "fixing" agent such as polyethylene glycol 400 or polyethylene glycol 4000.[9] In addition to sublingual tablets, the drug has been formulated into an equally effective lingual aerosol for patients who have problems with dissolution of sublingual preparations because of dry mucous membranes. Transdermal nitroglycerin preparations appear to be less effective than other long-acting nitrates, as absorption from the skin is variable.

Diluted Erythrityl Tetranitrate, **USP.** Erythritol tetranitrate, 1,2,3,4-butanetetrol, tetranitrate (*R**, *S**)-(Cardilate), is the tetranitrate ester of erythritol and nitric acid. It is prepared in a manner analogous to that used for nitroglycerin. The result is a solid, crystalline material. This ester is also very explosive and is diluted with lactose or other suitable inert diluents to permit safe handling; it is slightly soluble in water and soluble in organic solvents.

$$H_2C-ONO_2$$
$$HC-ONO_2$$
$$HC-ONO_2$$
$$H_2C-ONO_2$$

Erythrityl Tetranitrate
(Cardilate)

Erythrityl tetranitrate requires slightly more time than nitroglycerin to produce its effect, which is of longer duration. It is useful when mild, gradual, and prolonged vascular dilation is warranted. The drug is used in the treatment of, and as prophylaxis against, attacks of angina pectoris and to reduce blood pressure in arterial hypertonia.

Erythrityl tetranitrate produces a reduction of cardiac preload as a result of pooling blood on the venous side of the circulatory system by its vasodilating action. This action results in a reduction of blood pressure on the arterial side during stressful situations and is an important factor in preventing the precipitation of anginal attacks.

Diluted Pentaerythritol Tetranitrate, **USP.** Pentaerythritol tetranitrate, 2,2-bis (hydroxymethyl)-1,3-propanediol tetranitrate (Peritrate, Pentritol), is a white, crystalline material with a melting point of 140°C. It is insoluble in water, slightly soluble in alcohol, and readily soluble in acetone. The drug is a nitric acid ester of the tetrahydric alcohol pentaerythritol and is a powerful explosive. Accordingly, it is diluted with lactose, mannitol, or other suitable inert diluents to permit safe handling.

$$O_2NOH_2C-\overset{\overset{\displaystyle H_2C-ONO_2}{|}}{\underset{\underset{\displaystyle H_2C-ONO_2}{|}}{C}}-CH_2ONO_2$$

Pentaerythritol Tetranitrate
(Peritrate)
(Pentritol)

It relaxes smooth muscle of smaller vessels in the coronary vascular tree. Pentaerythritol tetranitrate is used prophylactically to reduce the severity and frequency of anginal attacks and is usually administered in sustained-release preparations to increase its duration of action.

Diluted Isosorbide Dinitrate, USP. Isosorbide dinitrate, 1,4:3,6-dianhydro-D-glucitol dinitrate (Isordil, Sorbitrate), occurs as a white, crystalline powder. Its water solubility is about 1 mg/mL.

Isosorbide Dinitrate
(Isordil)

Isosorbide Mononitrate
(ISMO Imdur)
This molecule is lacking one of the nitro substitutions

Isosorbide dinitrate, as a sublingual or chewable tablet, is effective in the treatment or prophylaxis of acute anginal attacks. When it is given sublingually, the effect begins in about 2 minutes, with a shorter duration of action than when it is given orally. Oral tablets are not effective in acute anginal episodes; the onset of action ranges from 15 to 30 minutes. The major route of metabolism involves denitration to isosorbide 5-mononitrate. This metabolite has a much longer half-life than the parent isosorbide dinitrate. As such, this particular metabolite is marketed in a tablet form that has excellent bioavailability with much less first-pass metabolism than isosorbide dinitrate. Isosorbide is marketed as a combination therapy with hydralazine under the tradename BiDil specifically for African Americans with CHF.

Calcium Antagonists

EXCITATION–CONTRACTION COUPLING MUSCLE

Stimulation of the cardiac cell initiates the process of excitation, which has been related to ion fluxes through the cell membrane. Depolarization of the tissue in the atria of the heart is mediated by two inwardly directed ionic currents. When the cardiac cell potential reaches its threshold, ion channels in the membrane are opened, and Na^+ enters the cell through ion channels. These channels give rise to the fast sodium current that is responsible for the rapidly rising phase, phase 0, of the ventricular action potential (Fig. 19.4). The second current is caused by the slow activation of an L-type Ca^{2+} ion channel that allows the movement of Ca^{2+} into the cell. This "slow channel" contributes to the maintenance of the plateau phase (phase 2) of the cardiac action potential. We now understand that the Ca^{2+} that enters with the action potential initiates a second and larger release of Ca^{2+} from the sarcoplasmic reticulum in the cell. This secondary release of Ca^{2+} is sufficient to initiate the contractile process of cardiac muscle.

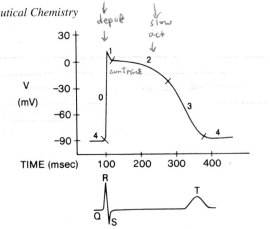

Figure 19.4 • Diagrammatic representation of the membrane action potential, as recorded from a Purkinje fiber, and an electrogram recorded from an isolated ventricular fiber. The membrane resting potential is 90 mV relative to the exterior of the fiber. At the point of depolarization, there is a rapid change (phase 0) to a more positive value. Phases 0 to 4 indicate the phases of depolarization and repolarization. Note that phases 0 and 3 of the membrane action potential correspond in time to the inscription of the QRS and T waves, respectively, of the local electrogram.

Contraction of cardiac and other muscle occurs from a reaction between actin and myosin. In contrast to smooth vascular muscle, the contractile process in cardiac muscle involves a complex of proteins (troponins I, C, and T and tropomyosin) attached to myosin, which modulates the interaction between actin and myosin. Free Ca^{2+} ions bind to troponin C, uncovering binding sites on the actin molecule and allowing interaction with myosin, causing contraction of the muscle. The schematic diagram in Figure 19.5 shows the sequence of events.[10] Contraction of vascular smooth muscle, like that of cardiac muscle, is regulated by the concentration of cytoplasmic Ca^{2+} ions. The mechanism by which the contraction is effected, however, includes a calcium- and calmodulin-dependent kinase as opposed to a Ca^{2+}-sensitive troponin–tropomyosin complex (Fig. 19.2). The activating effect depends on a different type of reaction. The elevated free cytosolic Ca^{2+} in vascular smooth muscle cells binds to a high-affinity binding protein, calmodulin.

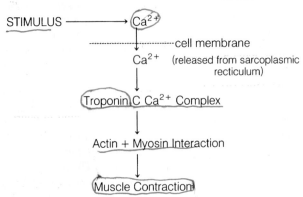

Figure 19.5 • Sequence of events showing excitation–contraction coupling in cardiac muscle.

ION CHANNELS AND CALCIUM

Calcium ions play an important role in the regulation of many cellular processes, such as synaptic transmission and muscle contraction. The role of calcium in these cellular functions is as a second messenger, for example, regulating enzymes and ion channels. The entry of extracellular Ca^{2+} in the cytosol of myocardial cells and the release of Ca^{2+} from intracellular storage sites is important for initiating contractions of the myocardium. Normally, the concentration of Ca^{2+} in the extracellular fluid is in the millimolar range, whereas the intracellular concentration of free Ca^{2+} is less than 10^{-7} M, even though the total cellular concentration may be 10^{-3} M or higher. Most of the Ca^{2+} is stored within intracellular organelles or tightly bound to intracellular proteins. The free Ca^{2+} needed to satisfy the requirements of a contraction resulting from a stimulus may result from activation of calcium channels on the cell membrane and/or the release of calcium from bound internal stores. Each of these methods of increasing free cytosolic Ca^{2+} involves channels that are selective for the calcium ion. Calcium channel blockers reduce or prevent the increase of free cytosolic calcium ions by interfering with the transport of calcium ions through these pores.

Calcium is one of the most common elements on earth. Most calcium involved in biological systems occurs as hydroxyapatite, a static, stabilizing structure like that found in bone. The remaining calcium is ionic (Ca^{2+}). Ionic calcium functions as a biochemical regulator, more often within the cell. The importance of calcium ions to physiological functions was realized first by Ringer, who observed in 1883 the role of Ca^{2+} in cardiac contractility.

The ionic composition of the cytosol in excitable cells, including cardiac and smooth muscle cells, is controlled to a large extent by the plasma membrane, which prevents the free movement of ions across this barrier. Present in the membranes are ion-carrying channels that open in response to either a change in membrane potential or binding of a ligand. Calcium-sensitive channels include (a) Na^+ to Ca^{2+} exchanger, which transports three Na^+ ions in return for one Ca^{2+}; (b) a voltage-dependent Ca^{2+} channel, which provides the route for entry of Ca^{2+} for excitation and contraction in cardiac and smooth muscle cells and is the focus of the channel-blocking agents used in medicine; and (c) receptor-operated Ca^{2+} channels mediated by ligand binding to membrane receptors such as in the action of epinephrine on the α-adrenergic receptor. The membrane of the sarcolemma within the cell also has ion-conducting channels that facilitate movement of Ca^{2+} ions from storage loci in the sarcoplasmic reticulum.

Four types of calcium channels, differing in location and function, have been identified: (a) L type, located in skeletal, cardiac, and smooth muscles, causing contraction of muscle cells; (b) T type, found in pacemaker cells, causing Ca^{2+} entry, inactivated at more negative potentials and more rapidly than the L type; (c) N type, found in neurons and acting in transmitter release; and (d) P type, located in Purkinje cells but whose function is unknown at this time.

Calcium antagonists act only on the L-type channel to produce their pharmacological effects. The L channels are so called because once the membrane has been depolarized, their action is long lasting. Once the membrane has been depolarized, L channels must be phosphorylated to open.

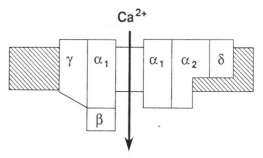

Ca^{2+}

Figure 19.6 ● Schematic representation of an L-type Ca^{2+} channel.

Although there are similarities between L-type calcium channels that exist in cardiac and smooth muscle, there are distinct differences between the two. Cardiac L channels are activated through β-adrenergic stimulation via a cAMP-dependent phosphorylation process,[11] whereas L channels in smooth muscle may be regulated by the inositol phosphate system linked to G-protein–coupled, receptor-linked phospholipase C activation.[12]

CALCIUM CHANNEL BLOCKERS

The L-type calcium channel, acted on by calcium channel blockers, consists of five different subunits, designated α_1, α_2, β, γ, and δ. The α_1 subunit provides the central pore of the channel (Fig. 19.6). Calcium channel blockers can be divided conveniently into the three different chemical classes of the prototype drugs that have been used: phenylalkylamines (verapamil), 1,4-dihydropyridines (nifedipine), and benzothiazepines (diltiazem). These prototype compounds sometimes are termed the "first generation" of calcium channel blockers because two of the groups of drug classes have been expanded by the introduction of a "second generation" of more potent analogs (Table 19.3).

The specific Ca^{2+} channel antagonists verapamil, nifedipine, and diltiazem interact at specific sites on the calcium channel protein. These blockers do not occlude the channel physically but bind to sites in the channel, because they can promote both channel activation and antagonism. Affinity for binding sites on the channel varies, depending on the status of the channel. The channel can exist in either an open (O), resting (R), or inactivated (I) state, and the equilibrium between them is determined by stimulus frequency and membrane potential (Fig. 19.7). Verapamil

TABLE 19.3 First- and Second-Generation Calcium Channel Blockers

Chemical Classification	First Generation	Second Generation
Phenylalkylamines	Verapamil	Anipamil
		Bepridil
1,4-Dihydropyridine	Nifedipine	Amlodipine
		Felodipine
		Isradipine
		Nicardipine
		Nimodipine
Benzothiazepine	Diltiazem	—

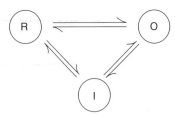

Figure 19.7 • Schematic representation of an ion channel existing in an equilibrium of resting (*R*), open (*O*), and inactivated (*I*) states.

and diltiazem do not bind to a channel in the resting state, only after the channel has been opened. They are ionized, water-soluble Ca^{2+}-entry blockers that reach their binding sites by the hydrophilic pathway when the channel is open. Verapamil and diltiazem are use dependent (i.e., their Ca^{2+}-blocking activity is a function of the frequency of contractions). An increase in contraction frequency causes a reduction, rather than an augmentation, of contractions. Nifedipine is a neutral molecule at physiological pH and can cause interference with the Ca^{2+} in the open or closed state. In the closed state, nifedipine can traverse the phospholipid bilayer to reach its binding site because of its lipid solubility.

CARDIOVASCULAR EFFECTS OF CALCIUM ION CHANNEL BLOCKERS

All Ca^{2+} antagonists yet developed are vasodilators. Vasodilation is a result of the uncoupling of the contractile mechanism of vascular smooth muscle, which requires Ca^{2+}. Coronary artery muscle tone is reduced in healthy humans but is particularly pronounced in a condition of coronary spasm. Peripheral arteriole resistance is reduced more than venous beds. The vasodilatory effect of these drugs is the basis for their use in the control of angina and hypertension.[13]

Although verapamil, nifedipine, and diltiazem can cause vasodilation, they are not equally effective at blocking the Ca^{2+} channels found in various tissues. The phenylalkylamine verapamil and the benzothiazepine diltiazem have both cardiac and vascular actions. These drugs have antiarrhythmic, antianginal, and antihypertensive activity. They depress the cardiac neural network, and so slow sinus node automaticity, prolong atrioventricular (AV) nodal conductance, and depress myocardial contractility, as well as reduce peripheral vascular resistance to prevent a coronary vascular spasm. Nifedipine and other 1,4-dihydropyridines are more effective at causing vasodilation than affecting pacemaker and tension responses in the heart. This is especially important because selectivity occurs as a consequence of disease states. Hypertensive smooth muscle is more sensitive to Ca^{2+} channel blockers than is normotensive tissue.[14] This makes verapamil and diltiazem more useful in ischemic conditions, because they have a more profound effect on cardiac muscle calcium channels.[15]

The inhibition of Ca^{2+} influx into cardiac tissue by Ca^{2+} antagonists is also the basis for the use of these drugs as antiarrhythmic agents. The Ca^{2+} channel blockers dampen Ca^{2+}-dependent automaticity in the regular pacemaker cells in the sinoatrial (SA) node and depress the

origination of ectopic foci. Calcium antagonists can block reentry pathways in myocardial tissue, an integral component of arrhythmias. Numerous side effects in the heart, such as bradycardia, decreased cardiac contractility, and reduced AV conductance, are traced to Ca^{2+} channel–blocking activity.

PRODUCTS

Verapamil. Verapamil, 5-[(3,4-dimethoxyphenethyl) methylamino]-2-(3,4-dimethoxyphenyl)-2-isopropylvaleronitrile (Calan, Isoptin), was introduced in 1962 as a coronary vasodilator and is the prototype of the Ca^{2+} antagonists used in cardiovascular diseases. It is used in the treatment of angina pectoris, arrhythmias from ischemic myocardial syndromes, and supraventricular arrhythmias.

Verapamil's major effect is on the slow Ca^{2+} channel. The result is a slowing of AV conduction and the sinus rate. This inhibition of the action potential inhibits one limb of the reentry circuit believed to underlie most paroxysmal supraventricular tachycardias that use the AV node as a reentry point. It is categorized as a class IV antiarrhythmic drug (see "Classes of Antiarrhythmic Drugs" later in this chapter). Hemodynamically, verapamil causes a change in the preload, afterload, contractility, heart rate, and coronary blood flow. The drug reduces systemic vascular resistance and mean blood pressure, with minor effects on cardiac output.

Verapamil is a synthetic compound possessing slight structural similarity to papaverine. It can be separated into its optically active isomers, of which the levorotatory enantiomer is the most potent. It is absorbed rapidly after oral administration. The drug is metabolized quickly and, as a result, has low bioavailability. The liver is the main site of first-pass metabolism, forming several products. The preferential metabolic step involves *N*-dealkylation, followed by *O*-demethylation, and subsequent conjugation of the product before elimination. The metabolites have no significant biological activity. Verapamil has an elimination half-life of approximately 5 hours.

Verapamil
(Isoptin)
(Calan)

The route traveled by a Ca^{2+} channel blocker, such as verapamil, to its receptor site parallels that observed with many local anesthetic-like antiarrhythmic agents. It is believed that verapamil, like most of the Ca^{2+} channel blockers, crosses the cell membrane in an uncharged form to gain access to its site of action on the intracellular side of the membrane. Data show a greater affinity of verapamil and other Ca^{2+} channel blockers to the inactivated state of the channel.[16]

Diltiazem Hydrochloride. Diltiazem hydrochloride, (+)-*cis*-3-(acetoxy)-5-[2(dimethylamino)ethyl]-2,3-dihydro-2-(4-methoxyphenyl)1,5-benzothiazepin-4(5*H*)one hydrochloride (Cardizem), was developed and introduced in Japan as a cardiovascular agent to treat angina pectoris. It was observed to dilate peripheral arteries and arterioles. The drug increases myocardial oxygen supply by relieving coronary artery spasm and reduces myocardial oxygen demand by decreasing heart rate and reducing overload. Diltiazem hydrochloride is used in patients with variant angina. The drug has electrophysiological properties similar to those of verapamil and is used in clinically similar treatment conditions as an antiarrhythmic agent, but it is less potent.

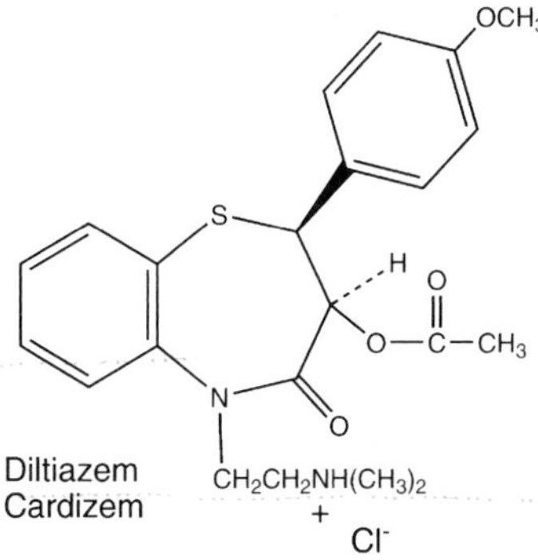

Diltiazem
Cardizem

The drug is absorbed rapidly and almost completely from the digestive tract. It reaches peak plasma levels within 1 hour after administration in gelatin capsules. Oral formulations on the market are sustained-release preparations providing peak plasma levels 3 to 4 hours after administration.

Diltiazem hydrochloride is metabolized extensively after oral dosing, by first-pass metabolism. As a result, the bioavailability is about 40% of the administered dose. The drug undergoes several biotransformations, including deacetylation, oxidative *O*- and *N*-demethylations, and conjugation of the phenolic metabolites. Of the various metabolites (Fig. 19.8), only the primary metabolite, deacetyldiltiazem, is pharmacologically active. Deacetyldiltiazem has about 40% to 50% of the potency of the parent compound.

Nifedipine. Nifedipine, 1,4-dihydro-2, 6-dimethyl-4-(2-nitrophenyl)-3,5-pyridinedicarboxylate dimethyl ester

(Adalat, Procardia), is a dihydropyridine derivative that bears no structural resemblance to the other calcium antagonists. It is not a nitrate, but its nitro group is essential for its antianginal effect.[17] As a class, the dihydropyridines possess a central pyridine ring that is partially saturated. To this, positions 2 and 6 are substituted with an alkyl group that may play a role in the agent's duration of action. In addition, positions 3 and 5 are carboxylic groups that must be protected with an ester functional group. Depending on the type of ester used at these sites, the agent can be distributed to various parts of the body. Finally, position 4 requires an aromatic substitution possessing an electron-withdrawing group (i.e., Cl or NO$_2$) in the *ortho* and/or *meta* position.

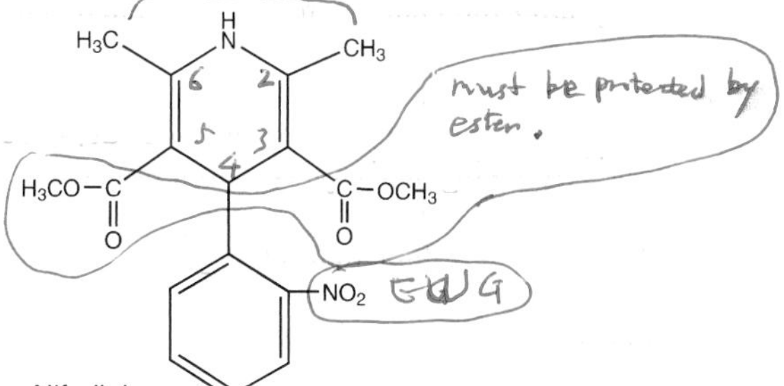

Nifedipine
(Procardia)
(Adalat)

The prototype of this class, nifedipine, has potent peripheral vasodilatory properties. It inhibits the voltage-dependent calcium channel in the vascular smooth muscle but has little or no direct depressant effect on the SA or AV nodes, even though it inhibits calcium current in normal and isolated cardiac tissues. Nifedipine is more effective in patients whose anginal episodes are caused by coronary vasospasm and is used in the treatment of vasospastic angina as well as classic angina pectoris. Because of its strong vasodilatory properties, it is used in selected patients to treat hypertension.

Nifedipine is absorbed efficiently on oral or buccal administration. A substantial amount (90%) is protein bound. Systemic availability of an oral dose of the drug may be approximately 65%. Two inactive metabolites are the major products of nifedipine metabolism and are found in equilibrium with each other (Fig. 19.9). Only a trace of unchanged nifedipine is found in the urine.[18]

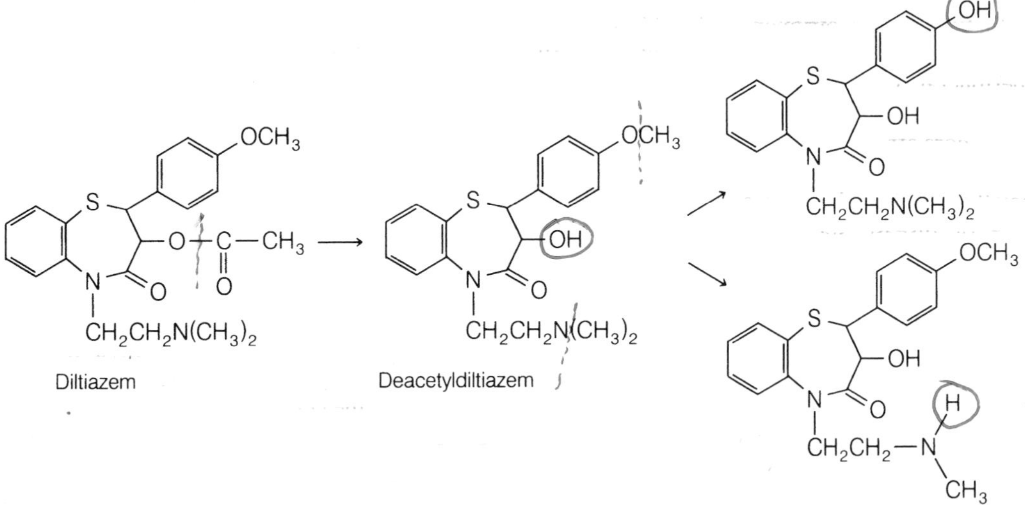

Diltiazem   Deacetyldiltiazem

Figure 19.8 ● Biotransformations of diltiazem.

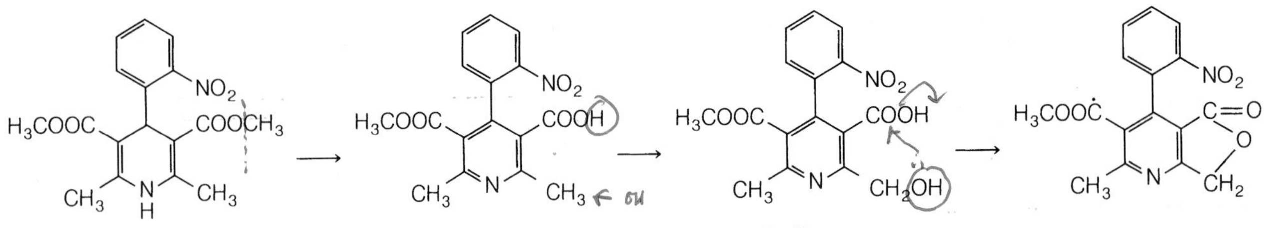

Figure 19.9 ● Nifedipine metabolism.

Amlodipine. Amlodipine, 2-[(2-aminoethoxy)methyl]4-(2-chlorophenyl)-1,4-dihydro-6-methyl-3,5-pyridinedicarboxylic acid 3-ethyl 5-methyl ester (Norvasc), is a second-generation 1,4-dihyropyridine derivative of the prototypical molecule nifedipine. Like most of the second-generation dihydropyridine derivatives, it has greater selectivity for the vascular smooth muscle than myocardial tissue, a longer half-life (34 hours), and less negative inotropy than the prototypical nifedipine. Amlodipine is used in the treatment of chronic stable angina and in the management of mild-to-moderate essential hypertension. It is marketed as the benzene sulfonic acid salt (besylate). Amlodipine was approved in September 2007 as a combination product with olmesartan (Azor), an angiotensin II receptor antagonist (Chapter 18), for the treatment of hypertension. Amlodipine is also marketed as a combination therapy with atorvastatin under the tradename Norvasc for the management of high cholesterol and high blood pressure.

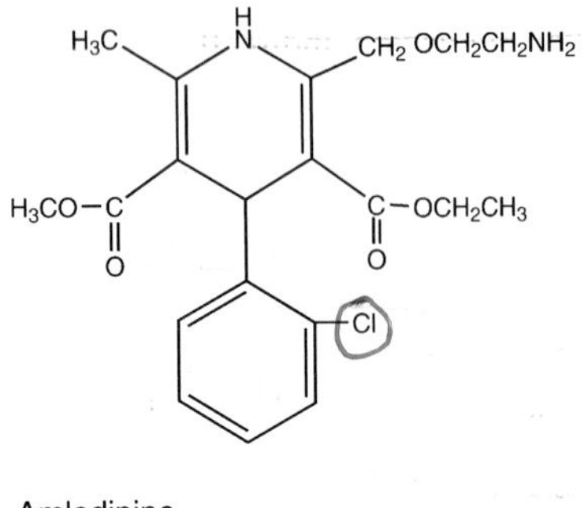

more vaso-selective
↑DOA

Amlodipine
(Norvasc)

Felodipine. Felodipine, 4-(2,3-dichlorophenyl)-1,4-dihydro-2,6-dimethyl-3,5-pyridinedicarboxylic acid ethyl methyl ester (Plendil), is a second-generation dihydropyridine channel blocker of the nifedipine type. It is more selective for vascular smooth muscle than for myocardial tissue and serves as an effective vasodilator. The drug is used in the treatment of angina and mild-to-moderate essential hypertension. Felodipine, like most of the dihydropyridines, exhibits a high degree of protein binding and has a half-life ranging from 10 to 18 hours.

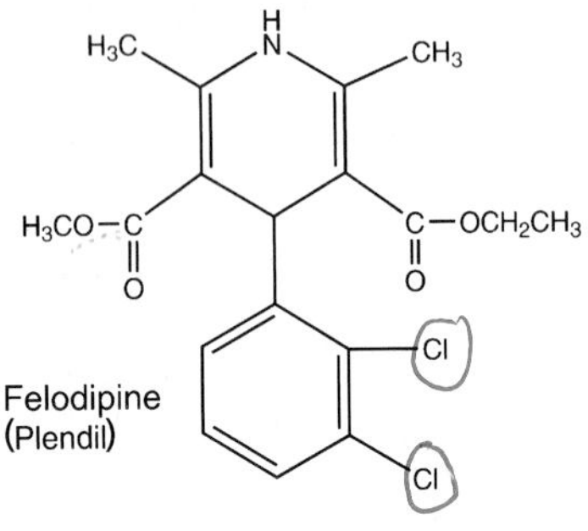

Felodipine
(Plendil)

Isradipine. Isradipine, 4-(4-benzofuranazyl)-1,4-dihydro-2,6-dimethyl-3,5-pyridinecarboxylic acid methyl 1-methylethyl ester (DynaCirc), is another second-generation dihydropyridine-type channel blocker. This drug, like the other second-generation analogs, is more selective for vascular smooth muscle than for myocardial tissue. It is effective in the treatment of stable angina, reducing the frequency of anginal attacks and the need to use nitroglycerin.

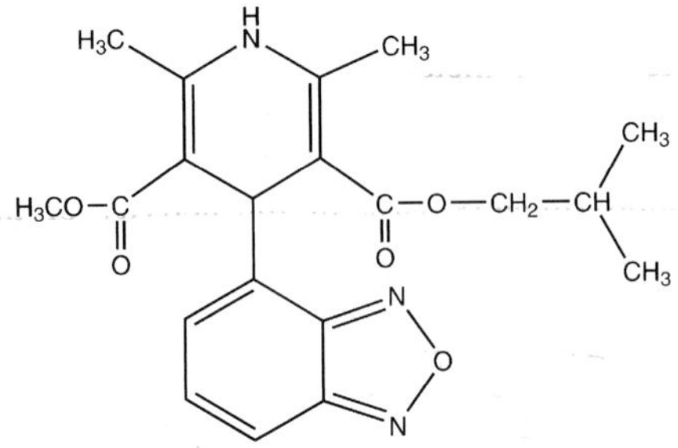

Isradipine
(DynaCirc)

Nicardipine Hydrochloride. Nicardipine hydrochloride, 1,4-dihydro-2,6-dimethyl-4-(3-nitrophenyl)-3,5-pyridinedicarboxylic acid methyl 2-[methyl(phenylmethyl)amino]ethyl ester hydrochloride (Cardene), is a more potent vasodilator of the systemic, coronary, cerebral, and renal vasculature and has been used in the treatment of mild, moderate, and severe hypertension. The drug is also used in the management of stable angina.

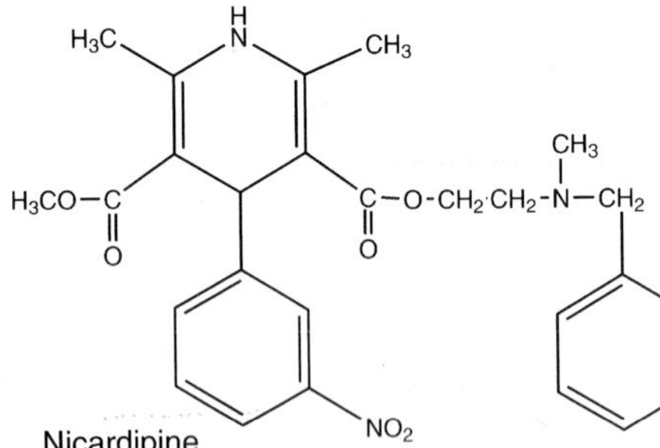

Nicardipine
(Cardene)

Nimodipine. Nimodipine, 1,4-dihydro-2,6-dimethyl-4-(3-nitrophenyl)- 3,5-pyridinedicarboxylic acid 2-methoxyethyl 1-methylethyl ester (Nimotop), is another dihydropyridine calcium channel blocker but differs in that it dilates the cerebral blood vessels more effectively than do the other dihydropyridine derivatives. This drug is indicated for treatment of subarachnoid hemorrhage-associated neurological deficits.

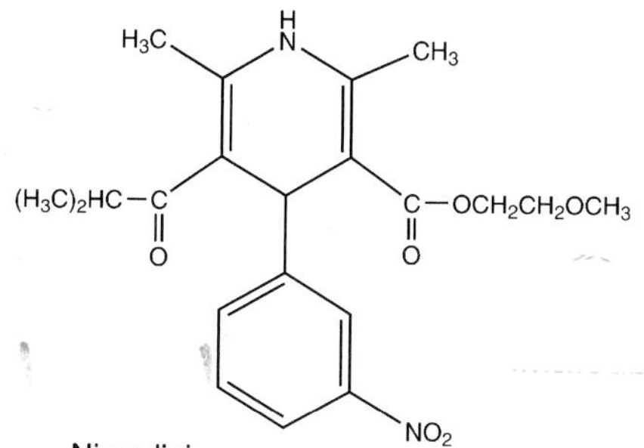

Nimodipine
(Nimotop)

Nisoldipine. In vitro studies show that the effects of nisoldipine, 1,4-dihydro-2, 6-dimethyl-4-(2-nitrophenyl)-3,5-pyridinecarboxylic acid methyl 2-methylpropyl ester (Sular), on contractile processes are selective, with greater potency on vascular smooth muscle than on cardiac muscle.

Nisoldipine is highly metabolized, with five major metabolites identified. As with most of the dihydropyridines, the cytochrome P450 (CYP) 3A4 isozyme is mainly responsible for the metabolism of nisoldipine. The major biotransformation pathway appears to involve the hydroxylation of the isobutyl ester side chain. This particular metabolite has approximately 10% of the activity of the parent compound.

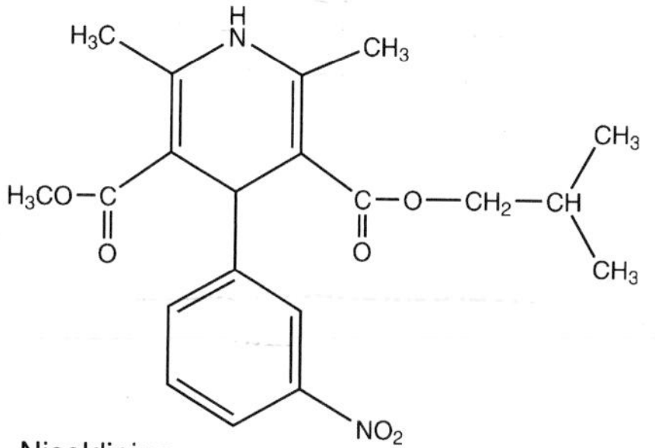

Nisoldipine
(Sular)

Nitrendipine. Nitrendipine, 1,4-dihydro-2,6-dimethyl-4-(3-nitrophenyl)-3,5-pyridinecarboxylic acid methyl ethyl ester (Baypress), is a second-generation dihydropyridine channel blocker of the nifedipine type. It is more selective for vascular smooth muscle than for myocardial tissue and serves as an effective vasodilator. The drug is used in the treatment of mild-to-moderate essential hypertension.

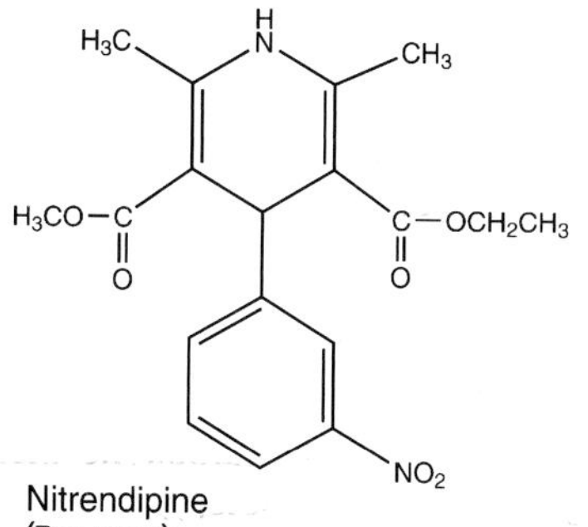

Nitrendipine
(Baypress)

Bepridil Hydrochloride. Bepridil hydrochloride, β-[(2-methylpropoxy)methyl]-*N*-phenyl-*N*-(phenylmethyl)-1-pyrrolidineethylamine hydrochloride (Vascor), is a second-

generation alkylamine-type channel blocker, structurally unrelated to the dihydropyridines. Its actions are less specific than those of the three prototypical channel blockers, verapamil, diltiazem, and nifedipine. In addition to being a Ca^{2+} channel blocker, it inhibits sodium flow into the heart tissue and lengthens cardiac repolarization, causing bradycardia. Caution should be used if it is given to a patient with hypokalemia. Bepridil hydrochloride is used for stable angina. The drug has a half-life of 33 hours and is highly bound to protein (99%).

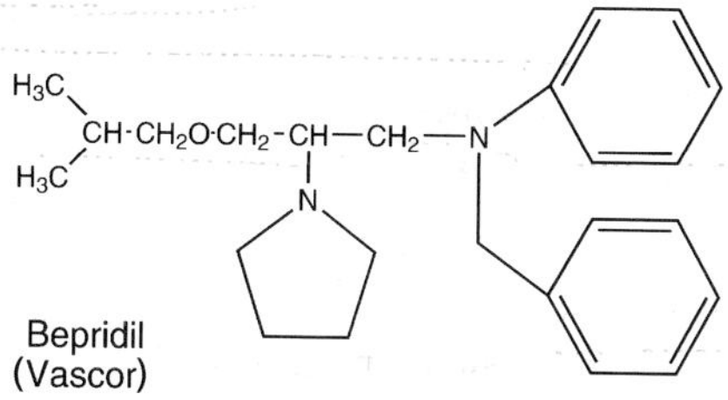

Bepridil
(Vascor)

Sodium Channel Blocker

Ranolazine. Ranolazine, *N*-(2,6-dimethylphenyl)-2-[4-[2-hydroxy-3-(2-methoxyphenoxy)propyl]piperazin-1-yl]acetamide (Ranexa), is an antianginal medication that was approved by the Food and Drug Administration (FDA) in January 2006 for the treatment of chronic angina. Ranolazine is believed to elicit its effects by altering the transcellular late sodium current. This, in turn, alters the sodium-dependent calcium channels during myocardial ischemia. Thus, ranolazine indirectly prevents the calcium overload that is associated with cardiac ischemia. Ranolazine is metabolized by the cytochrome CYP3A enzymes in the liver.[19]

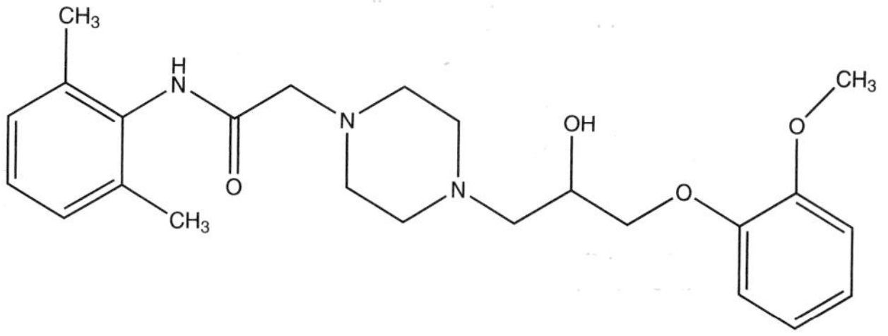

Ranolazine

From P658

Antithrombotic Agents

Platelet activation and platelet aggregation play an important role in the pathogenesis of thromboses. These, in turn, play an important role in unstable angina, myocardial infarction, stroke, and peripheral vascular thromboses. Because many cardiovascular diseases are associated with platelet activation, many agents possessing antiplatelet or antithrombotic effects have been investigated. This has revolutionized cardiovascular medicine, in which vascular stenting or angioplasty can be used without compromising normal hemostasis or wound healing. Although most of these agents act by different mechanisms, many of the newer agents are being developed to antagonize the GPIIb/IIIa receptors of platelets.

Aspirin. Aspirin, acetylsalicylic acid, has an inhibitory effect on platelet aggregation not only because of its ability to inhibit cyclooxygenase (COX) but also because of its ability to acetylate the enzyme. Aspirin irreversibly inhibits COX (prostaglandin H synthase), which is the enzyme involved in converting arachidonate to prostaglandin G_2 and ultimately thromboxane 2, an inducer of platelet aggregation. Aspirin's mechanism of action includes not only the inhibition in the biosynthesis of thromboxane 2, but also its ability to acetylate the serine residue (529) in the polypeptide chain of platelet prostaglandin H synthetase-1. This explains why other nonsteroidal anti-inflammatory agents that are capable of inhibiting the COX enzyme do not act as antithrombotics—they are not capable of acetylating this enzyme. Because platelets cannot synthesize new enzymes, aspirin's ability to acetylate COX lasts for the life of the platelet (7–10 days) and is, thus, irreversible.

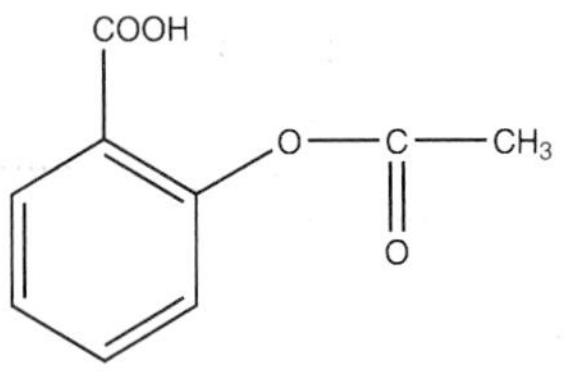

Aspirin

Dipyridamole. Dipyridamole, 2,2',2'',2'''-[(4,8-di-1piperidinylpyrimido[5,4-*d*]pyrimidine-2,6-diyl)dinitrilo]-tetrakisethanol (Persantine), may be used for coronary and myocardial insufficiency. Its biggest use today, however, is as an antithrombotic in patients with prosthetic heart valves. It is a bitter, yellow, crystalline powder, soluble in dilute acids, methanol, or chloroform. A formulation containing dipyridamole and aspirin (Aggrenox) is currently being marketed as an antithromobotic.

Dipyridamole is a long-acting vasodilator. Its vasodilating action is selective for the coronary system; it is indicated for long-term therapy of chronic angina pectoris. The drug also inhibits adenosine deaminase in erythrocytes and interferes with the uptake of the vasodilator adenosine by erythrocytes. These actions potentiate the effect of prostacyclin (PGI_2), which acts as an inhibitor to platelet aggregation.

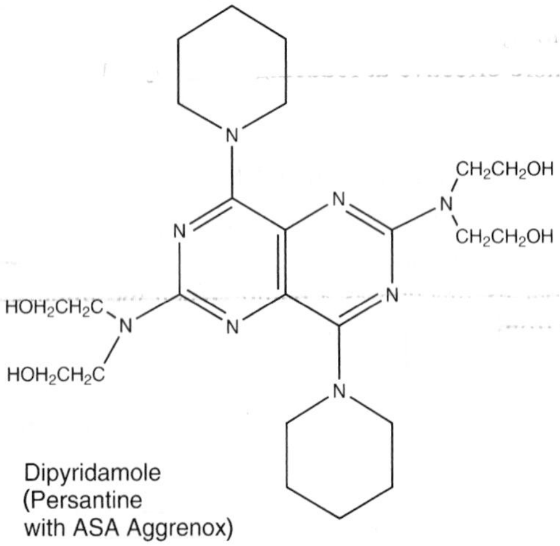

Dipyridamole
(Persantine
with ASA Aggrenox)

⚘ ***Clopidogrel.*** Clopidogrel, methyl (+)-(*S*)-α-(2-chlorophenyl)-6,7-dihydrothieno[3,2-c]pyridine-5(4H)-acetate sulfate (Plavix), is useful for the preventative

management of secondary ischemic events, including myocardial infarction, stroke, and vascular deaths. It may be classified as a thienopyridine because of its heterocyclic system. Several agents possessing this system have been evaluated as potential antithrombotic agents. These agents have a unique mechanism, in that they inhibit the purinergic receptor located on platelets. Normally, nucleotides act as agonists on these receptors, which include the P2Y type. Two P2Y receptor subtypes (P2Y1 and P2Y2) found on platelets, when stimulated by adenosine diphosphate (ADP), cause platelet aggregation. Clopidogrel acts as an antagonist to the P2Y2 receptor. It is probably a prodrug that requires metabolic activation, because in vitro studies do not interfere with platelet aggregation. Although platelet aggregation is not normally seen in the first 8 to 11 days after administration to a patient, the effect lasts for several days after the drug therapy is discontinued. Unlike other thienopyridines currently used, clopidogrel does not seriously reduce the number of white cells in the blood, and therefore, routine monitoring of the white blood cell count is not necessary during treatment.

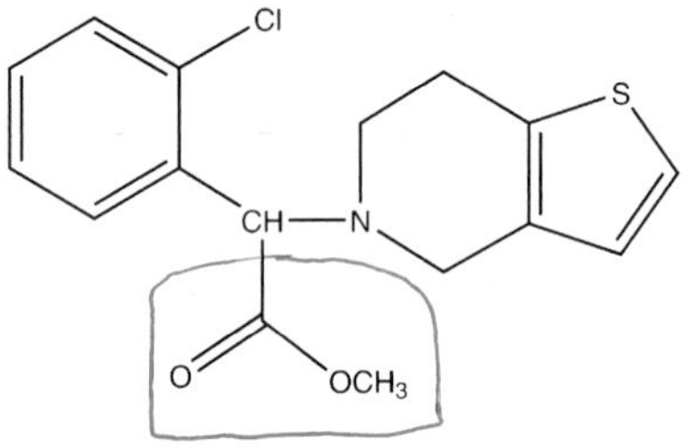

Clopidrogel
(Plavix)

Ticlopidine. Ticlopidine, 5-[(2-chlorophenyl)methyl]-4,5,6,7-tetrahydrothieno [3,2-c]pyridine hydrochloride (Ticlid), is useful in reducing cardiac events in patients with unstable angina and cerebrovascular events in secondary prevention of stroke. It belongs to the thienopyridine class and facilitated the development of clopidogrel. One of the drawbacks to this agent is its side effect profile, which includes neutropenia, and patients receiving this antithrombotic should have their blood levels monitored. Its mechanism of action is similar to that of clopidogrel, in that it inhibits the purinergic receptors on platelets.

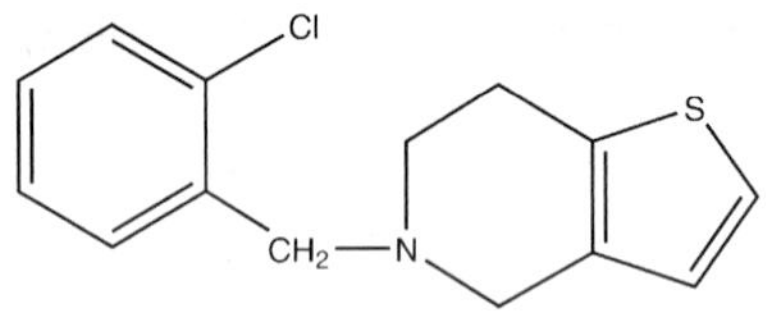

Ticlopidine
(Ticlid)

GPIIB/IIIA RECEPTORS

Located on platelets is a site that serves to recognize and bind fibrinogen. This site is a dimeric glycoprotein that allows fibrinogen to bind, leading to the final step of platelet aggregation. The receptor must be activated before it will associate with fibrinogen, and this may be accomplished by thrombin, collagen, or thromboxane A_2 (TXA_2). Once the receptor is activated, fibrinogen most likely binds to the platelet through the arginine-glycine-aspartic acid (RGD) sequences at residues 95-96-97 and 572-573-574 of the α-chain of fibrinogen. This particular feature has been used in the design of nonpeptide antagonists that mimic the RGD system in which a distance of 15 to 17Å (16–18 atoms) separates the amine group of arginine and the carbonyl oxygen of aspartic acid.

Eptifibatide. Eptifibatide (Integrilin) is a synthetic cyclic heptapeptide that acts as a GPIIb/IIIa receptor antagonist, thus causing inhibition of platelet aggregation. Its structure is based on the natural product barbourin, a peptide isolated from the venom of a pygmy rattlesnake (*Sistrurus milarud barbouri*). As part of the structure, there is a sequence RGD that can bind to the RGD receptor found on platelets and block its ability to bind with fibrinogen. This agent is used in the treatment of unstable angina and for angioplastic coronary interventions.

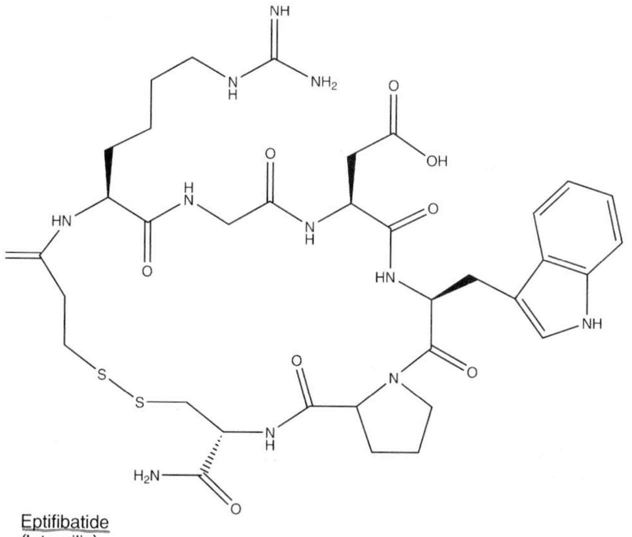

Eptifibatide
(Integrilin)

Tirofiban. Tirofiban is a nonpeptide that appears unrelated chemically to eptifibatide, but actually has many similarities. The chemical architecture incorporates a system that is mimicking the RGD moiety that is present in eptifibatide. This can be seen in the distance between the nitrogen of the piperidine ring, which mimics the basic nitrogen of arginine in the RGD sequence, and the carboxylic acid, which mimics the acid of aspartate in the RGD sequence. The basic nitrogen and the carboxylic acid of tirofiban are separated by approximately 15 to 17Å (16–18 atoms). This is the optimum distance seen in the RGD sequence of the platelet receptor. Tirofiban is useful in treating non–Q wave myocardial infarction and unstable angina.

Abciximab. Abciximab (ReoPro) is a chimeric Fab fragment monoclonal antibody that can bind to the GPIIa/IIIb receptor of platelets and block the ability of fibrinogen to associate with the platelet. This results in less platelet aggregation. Abciximab is useful in treating unstable angina and as an adjunct to percutaneous coronary intervention (PCI). The half-life of abciximab is about 30 minutes, whereas its effects when bound to the GPIIa/IIIb may last up to 24 hours. A significant drawback to using abciximab lies in its cost, which is approximately $1,500 for a single dose.

ANTIARRHYTHMIC DRUGS

Cardiac arrhythmias are caused by a disturbance in the conduction of the impulse through the myocardial tissue, by disorders of impulse formation, or by a combination of these factors. The antiarrhythmic agents used most commonly affect impulse conduction by altering conduction velocity and the duration of the refractory period of heart muscle tissue. They also depress spontaneous diastolic depolarization, causing a reduction of automaticity by ectopic foci.

Many pharmacological agents are available for the treatment of cardiac arrhythmias. Agents such as oxygen, potassium, and sodium bicarbonate relieve the underlying cause of some arrhythmias. Other agents, such as digitalis, propranolol, phenylephrine, edrophonium, and neostigmine, act on the cardiovascular system by affecting heart muscle or on the autonomic nerves to the heart. Finally, there are drugs that alter the electrophysiological mechanisms causing arrhythmias. The latter group of drugs is discussed in this chapter.

Within the past 5 decades, research on normal cardiac tissues and, in the clinical setting, on patients with disturbances of rhythm and conduction has brought to light information on the genesis of cardiac arrhythmias and the mode of action of antiarrhythmic agents. In addition, laboratory tests have been developed to measure blood levels of antiarrhythmic drugs such as phenytoin, disopyramide, lidocaine, procainamide, and quinidine, to help evaluate the pharmacokinetics of these agents. As a result, it is possible to maintain steady-state plasma levels of these drugs, which allows the clinician to use these and other agents more effectively and with greater safety. No other clinical intervention has been more effective at reducing mortality and morbidity in coronary care units.

Cardiac Electrophysiology

The heart depends on the synchronous integration of electrical impulse transmission and myocardial tissue response to carry out its function as a pump. When the impulse is released from the SA node, excitation of the heart tissue takes

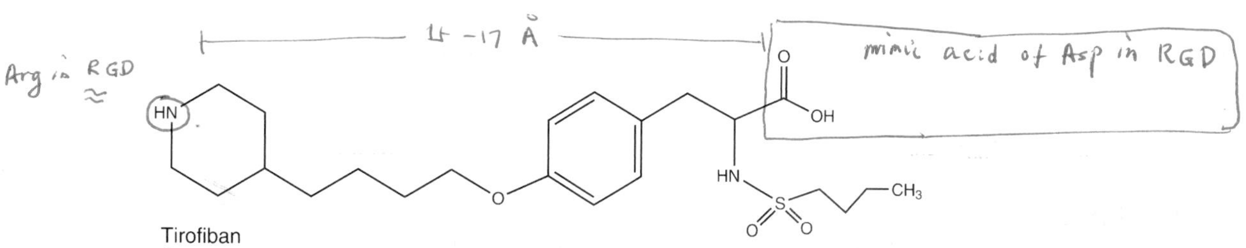

Tirofiban
(Aggrastat)

place in an orderly manner by a spread of the impulse throughout the specialized automatic fibers in the atria, the AV node, and the Purkinje fiber network in the ventricles. This spreading of impulses produces a characteristic electrocardiographic pattern that can be equated to predictable myocardial cell membrane potentials and Na^+ and K^+ fluxes in and out of the cell.

A single fiber in the ventricle of an intact heart, during the diastolic phase (see phase 4, Fig. 19.4), has a membrane potential (resting potential) of 90 mV. This potential is created by differential concentrations of K^+ and Na^+ in the intracellular and extracellular fluid. An active transport system (pump) on the membrane is responsible for concentrating the K^+ inside the cell and maintaining higher concentrations of Na^+ in the extracellular fluid. Diastolic depolarization is caused by a decreased K^+ ionic current into the extracellular tissue and a slow inward leakage of Na^+ until the threshold potential (60–55 mV) is reached. At this time, the inward sodium current suddenly increases, and a self-propagated wave occurs to complete the membrane depolarization process. Pacemaker cells possess this property, which is termed *automaticity*. This maximal rate of depolarization (MRD) is represented by phase 0 or the spike action potential (Fig. 19.4).

The form, duration, resting potential level, and amplitude of the action potential are characteristic for different types of myocardial cells. The rate of rise of the response (phase 0) is related to the level of the membrane potential at the time of stimulation and has been termed *membrane responsiveness*. Less negative potentials produce smaller slopes of phase 0 and are characterized by slower conduction times. The phase 0 spike of the SA node corresponds to the inscription of the P wave on the electrocardiogram (Fig. 19.10). Repolarization is divided into three phases. The greatest amount of repolarization is represented by phase 3, in which there is a passive flux of K^+ ions out of the cell. Phase 1 repolarization is caused by an influx of Cl^- ions. During phase 2, a small inward movement of Ca^{2+} ions occurs through a slow channel mechanism that is believed to be important in the process of coupling excitation with contraction. The process of repolarization determines the duration of the action potential and is represented by the QT interval. The action potential duration is directly related to the refractory period of cardiac muscle.

Mechanisms of Arrhythmias

The current understanding of the electrophysiological mechanisms responsible for the origin and perpetuation of cardiac arrhythmias is caused by altered impulse formation (i.e., change in automaticity), altered conduction, or both, acting simultaneously from different locations of the heart. The generation of cardiac impulses in the normal heart is usually confined to specialized tissues that spontaneously depolarize and initiate the action potential. These cells are located in the right atrium and are referred to as the *SA node* or the *pacemaker cells*. Although the spontaneous electrical depolarization of the SA pacemaker cells is independent of the nervous system, these cells are innervated by both sympathetic and parasympathetic fibers, which may cause an increase or decrease of the heart rate, respectively. Other special cells in the normal heart that possess the property of automaticity may influence cardiac rhythm when the normal pacemaker is suppressed or when pathological changes occur in the myocardium to make these cells the dominant source of cardiac rhythm (i.e., ectopic pacemakers). Automaticity of subsidiary pacemakers may develop when myocardial cell damage occurs because of infarction or from digitalis toxicity, excessive vagal tone, excessive catecholamine release from sympathomimetic nerve fibers to the heart, or even high catecholamine levels in plasma. The development of automaticity in specialized cells, such as that found in special atrial cells, certain AV node cells, bundle of His, and Purkinje fibers, may lead to cardiac arrhythmias. Because production of ectopic impulses is often caused by a defect in the spontaneous phase 4 diastolic depolarization ("T wave"), drugs that can suppress this portion of the cardiac stimulation cycle are effective agents for these types of arrhythmia.

Arrhythmias are also caused by disorders in the conduction of impulses and changes in the refractory period of the myocardial tissue. Pharmacological intervention is based on these two properties. The Purkinje fibers branch into a network of interlacing fibers, particularly at their most distant positions. This creates several pathways in which a unidirectional block in a localized area may establish circular (circus) microcellular or macrocellular impulse movements that reenter the myocardial fibers and create an arrhythmia (Fig. 19.11). Unidirectional block results from localized

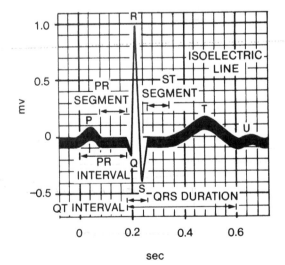

Figure 19.10 ● Normal electrocardiogram. (From Ganong, W. F.: Review of Medical Physiology, 9th ed. San Francisco, Lange Medical Publications, 1985.)

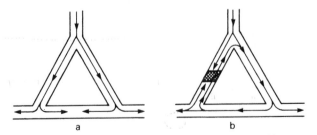

Figure 19.11 ● Reentry mechanism of Purkinje fibers. **A.** Normal conduction of impulses through triangular arrangement of cardiac fibers. **B.** Unidirectional block on left arm of triangular section allows impulse to reenter the regional conducting system and recycle.

TABLE 19.4 Classes of Antiarrhythmic Drugs

Class	Drugs	Mechanism of Action
IA	Quinidine, procainamide, disopyramide	Lengthens refractory period
IB	Lidocaine, phenytoin, tocainide, mexiletine	Shortens duration of action potential
IC	Encainide, flecainide, lorcainide, moricizine, propafenone	Slows conduction
II	β-Adrenergic blockers (e.g., propranolol)	Slows AV conduction time, suppresses automaticity
III	Amiodarone, bretylium, sotalol	Prolongs refractoriness
IV	Calcium channel blockers (e.g., verapamil, diltiazem)	Blocks slow inward Ca^{2+} channel

myocardial disease (*infarcts*) or from a change in dependence of the tissue to Na^+ fluxes that causes a longer conduction time and allows the tissue to repolarize to propagate the retrograde impulse.

Classes of Antiarrhythmic Drugs

Antiarrhythmic drugs can be placed into four separate classes, based on their mechanism of action or pattern of electrophysiological effects produced on heart tissue. Table 19.4 summarizes the four-part classification of antiarrhythmic drugs as first proposed by Vaughan Williams[20] in 1970 and expanded in 1984.[21] Note that drugs within the same category are placed there because they demonstrate similar clinical actions. That patients do not respond to a drug in this class, however, should not rule out use of other drugs in the same class.[22] Despite the well-intentioned use of these agents, most antiarrhythmic drugs have the potential to aggravate the arrhythmia they treat (*proarrhythmia*). Proarrhythmia develops from an increase in the density of single ectopic beats and is more likely to occur in patients who have a dysfunction in the left ventricle or sustained ventricular tachycardia. Class I antiarrhythmic agents (discussed under "Class I. Membrane-Depressant Drugs") are especially proarrhythmic in myocardial infarction patients.

CLASS I. MEMBRANE-DEPRESSANT DRUGS

Class I antiarrhythmic agents are drugs that have membrane-stabilizing properties (i.e., they shift membranes to more negative potentials). Drugs in this class act on the fast Na^+ channels and interfere with the process by which the depolarizing charge is transferred across the membrane. It is assumed that these drugs bind to the Na^+ channel and block its function, preventing Na^+ conductance as long as the drug is bound. The prototypical drugs in this class are quinidine and procainamide. During the 1970s, several drugs were studied for their antiarrhythmic effects. Most of them were local anesthetics that affected Na^+ membrane channels, and they were grouped in a single class (class I). Studies on the antiarrhythmic properties of these chemicals have shown that there are sufficient differences to place them into separate subgroups.[22]

Class I antiarrhythmic drugs can be subdivided based on the relative ease with which they dissociate from the Na^+ ion channel. Drugs in class IC, such as encainide,

lorcainide, and moricizine, are the most potent sodium channel–blocking agents of the class I antiarrhythmic drugs. They slowly dissociate from the Na^+ channel, causing a slowing of the conduction time of the impulse through the heart. Class IB drugs, which include lidocaine, tocainide, and mexiletine, dissociate rapidly from the Na^+ channels and thus have the lowest potency as sodium channel blockers. They produce little, if any, change in action potential duration. Quinidine, procainamide, and disopyramide are drugs that have an intermediate rate of dissociation from Na^+ channels. These are categorized as class IA antiarrhythmic agents, and they lengthen the refractory period of cardiac tissue to cause cessation of arrhythmias.[23]

Studies have shown that Na^+ channels on the membranes of Purkinje fiber cells normally exist in at least three states: *R*, rested, closed near the resting potential but able to be opened by stimulation and depolarization; *A*, activated, allowing Na^+ ions to pass selectively through the membrane; and *I*, inactivated and unable to be opened (i.e., inactive).[24] The affinity of the antiarrhythmic drug for the receptor on the ion channel varies with the state of the channel or with the membrane potential. Because of this, *R*, *A*, and *I* ion channels can have different kinetics of interaction with antiarrhythmic drugs. A review of the recent literature shows that the antiarrhythmic drugs have low affinity for *R* channels but relatively high affinity for the *A* or *I* channels or both. Regardless of which channel state is blocked by class I antiarrhythmic drugs, the unblocking rate directly determines the amount of depression present at normal heart rates.

CLASS II. β-ADRENERGIC BLOCKING AGENTS

β-Adrenergic blocking drugs cause membrane-stabilizing or depressant effects on myocardial tissue. Their antiarrhythmic properties, however, are considered to be principally the result of inhibition of adrenergic stimulation to the heart. The principal electrophysiological property of these β-blocking agents is reduction of the phase 4 slope of potential sinus or ectopic pacemaker cells, such that the heart rate decreases and ectopic tachycardias are either slowed or converted to sinus rhythm.

CLASS III. REPOLARIZATION PROLONGATORS

Drugs in this class (e.g., amiodarone, bretylium, sotalol, ibutilide, dofetilide) cause several different electrophysiological changes on myocardial tissue but share one common effect, prolonging the action potential, which increases the effective refractory period of the membrane action potential without altering the phase of depolarization or the resting membrane potential. Drugs in this class produce their effects by more than one mechanism. Sotalol is a K^+ channel blocker and has some β-adrenergic blocking properties.[2] Amiodarone and bretylium, drugs that also prolong the action potential by means that are unclear, also have Na^+ channel–blocking properties.

CLASS IV. CALCIUM CHANNEL BLOCKERS

Although not all Ca^{2+} channel blockers possess antiarrhythmic activity, some members of this class of antiarrhythmic drugs (verapamil, diltiazem) block the slow inward current of Ca^{2+} ions during phase 2 of the membrane action potential in cardiac cells. For example, the prototypical drug in this group, verapamil, selectively blocks entry of Ca^{2+} into the myocardial cell. It acts on the slow-response fibers found in the sinus node and the AV node, slowing conduction velocity and increasing refractoriness in the AV node.

pH and Activity

The action of class I local anesthetic-type antiarrhythmic drugs is pH dependent and may vary with each drug.[25] Antiarrhythmic drugs are weak bases, with most having pK_a values ranging from 7.5 to 9.5. At physiological pH of 7.40, these bases exist in an equilibrium mixture consisting of both the free base and the cationic form. Ionizable drugs, such as lidocaine (pK_a 7.86), have stronger electrophysiological effects in ischemic rather than normal myocardial cells. This potentiation has been attributed in part to the increase in H^+ concentration within the ischemic areas of the heart. Acidosis increases the proportion of Na^+ ion channels occupied by the protonated form of the antiarrhythmic agent. Nevertheless, the effect of pH on the antiarrhythmic activity of drugs can be complex, as both the free base and cationic species have been proposed as the active form of some drugs. The uncharged form of the Na^+ channel blocker can penetrate directly from the lipid phase of the surrounding cell membrane to block the channel.

Small changes in pH can alter these drugs' effectiveness by changing the charged-to-uncharged molecular ratio in the myocardial cells. Acidosis external to the myocardial cell promotes the cationic form. Because this species does not partition in the membrane as readily, onset of these drugs' action would be delayed. Furthermore, concentration of these drugs in the membrane would be reduced. Therefore, drugs that act on the channel only in the inactivated (closed) state would have a reduced effect in acidotic conditions. Acidosis may also prolong the effect of these drugs. External acidosis facilitates protonation of receptor-bound drugs. Because only neutral drugs can dissociate from closed channels, recovery is prolonged by acidosis.

Alkalosis tends to hyperpolarize the cell membrane and, thereby, reduces the effect of antiarrhythmic drugs. Because of this, alkalosis promotes the formation of more of the free-base antiarrhythmic agent, increasing the rate of recovery from the block. Alkalosis-inducing salts such as sodium lactate have been used to counteract toxicity caused by the antiarrhythmic quinidine.

CLASS I ANTIARRHYTHMICS

Quinidine Sulfate, USP. Quinidine sulfate is the sulfate of an alkaloid obtained from various species of *Cinchona* and their hybrids. It is a dextrorotatory diastereoisomer of quinine. The salt crystallizes from water as the dihydrate, in the form of fine, needlelike, white crystals. Quinidine sulfate contains a hydroxymethyl group that serves as a link between a quinoline ring and a quinuclidine moiety. The structure contains two basic nitrogens, of which the quinuclidine nitrogen is the stronger base (pK_a 10). Quinidine sulfate is bitter and light sensitive. Aqueous solutions are nearly neutral or slightly alkaline. It is soluble to the extent of 1% in water and more highly soluble in alcohol or chloroform.

Quinidine
(Cardioquin)
(Quinora)
(Auinidex)

Quinidine sulfate is the prototype of antiarrhythmic drugs and a class IA antiarrhythmic agent according to the Vaughan Williams classification. It reduces Na^+ current by binding the open ion channels (i.e., state A). The decreased Na^+ entry into the myocardial cell depresses phase 4 diastolic depolarization and shifts the intracellular threshold potential toward zero. These combined actions diminish the spontaneous frequency of pacemaker tissues, depress the automaticity of ectopic foci, and, to a lesser extent, reduce impulse formation in the SA node. This last action results in bradycardia. During the spike action potential, quinidine sulfate decreases transmembrane permeability to passive influx of Na^+, thus slowing the process of phase 0 depolarization, which decreases conduction velocity. This is shown as a prolongation of the QRS complex of electrocardiograms. Quinidine sulfate also prolongs action potential duration, which results in a proportionate increase in the QT interval. It is used to treat supraventricular and ventricular ectopic arrhythmias, such as atrial and ventricular premature beats, atrial and ventricular tachycardia, atrial flutter, and atrial fibrillation.

Quinidine sulfate is used most frequently as an oral preparation and is occasionally given intramuscularly. Quinidine sulfate that has been absorbed from the gastrointestinal tract or from the site of intramuscular injection is bound 80% to serum albumin.[18] The drug is taken up quickly from the bloodstream by body tissues; consequently, a substantial concentration gradient is established within a few minutes. Onset of action begins within 30 minutes, with the peak effect attained in 1 to 3 hours. Quinidine is metabolized primarily in the liver by hydroxylation, and a small amount is excreted by the liver.[26] Because of serious side effects and the advent of more effective oral antiarrhythmic agents, quinidine is now used less, except in selected patients for long-term oral antiarrhythmic therapy.

Quinidine Gluconate, USP. Quinidinium gluconate (Duraquin, Quinaglute) occurs as an odorless, very bitter, white powder. In contrast with the sulfate salt, it is freely soluble in water. This is important because there are emergencies when the condition of the patient and the need for a rapid response make the oral route of administration inappropriate. The high water solubility of the gluconate salt along with a low irritant potential makes it valuable when an injectable form is needed in these emergencies. Quinidine gluconate forms a stable aqueous solution. When used for injection, it usually contains 80 mg/mL, equivalent to 50 mg of quinidine or 60 mg of quinidine sulfate.

Quinidine Polygalacturonate. Quinidine polygalacturonate (Cardioquin) is formed by reacting quinidine and polygalacturonic acid in a hydroalcoholic medium. It contains the equivalent of approximately 60% quinidine. This salt is only slightly ionized and slightly soluble in water, but studies have shown that although equivalent doses of quinidine sulfate give higher peak blood levels earlier, a more uniform and sustained blood level is achieved with the polygalacturonate salt.

In many patients, the local irritant action of quinidine sulfate in the gastrointestinal tract causes pain, nausea, vomiting, and especially diarrhea, often precluding oral use in adequate doses. Studies with the polygalacturonate salt yielded no evidence of gastrointestinal distress. It is available as 275-mg tablets. Each tablet is the equivalent of 200 mg of quinidine sulfate or 166 mg of free alkaloid.

Procainamide Hydrochloride, USP. Procainamide hydrochloride, *p*-amino-*N*-[2-(diethylamino)ethyl]benzamide monohydrochloride, procainamidium chloride (Pronestyl, Procan SR), has emerged as a major antiarrhythmic drug. It was developed in the course of research for compounds structurally similar to procaine, which had limited effect as an antiarrhythmic agent because of its central nervous system (CNS) side effects and short-lived action caused by rapid hydrolysis of its ester linkage by plasma esterases. Because of its amide structure, procainamide hydrochloride is also more stable in water than is procaine. Aqueous solutions of procainamide hydrochloride have a pH of about 5.5. A kinetic study of the acid-catalyzed hydrolysis of procainamide hydrochloride showed it to be unusually stable to hydrolysis in the pH range 2 to 7, even at elevated temperatures.[27]

Procainamide
(Pronestyl)
(Procan SR)

Procainamide hydrochloride is metabolized through the action of *N*-acetyltransferase. The product of enzymatic metabolism of procainamide hydrochloride is *N*-acetylprocainamide (NAPA), which possesses only 25% of the activity of the parent compound.[26] A study of the disposition of procainamide hydrochloride showed that 50% of the drug was excreted unchanged in the urine, with 7% to 24% recovered as NAPA.[28,29] Unlike quinidine, procainamide hydrochloride is bound only minimally to plasma proteins. Between 75% and 95% of the drug is absorbed from the gastrointestinal tract. Plasma levels appear 20 to 30 minutes after administration and peak in about 1 hour.[30]

Procainamide hydrochloride appears to have all of the electrophysiological effects of quinidine. It diminishes automaticity, decreases conduction velocity, and increases action potential duration and, thereby, the refractory period of myocardial tissue. Clinicians have favored the use of procainamide hydrochloride for ventricular tachycardias and

quinidine for atrial arrhythmias, even though the two drugs are effective in either type of disorder.

Disopyramide Phosphate, USP. Disopyramide phosphate, α-[2(diisopropylamino)ethyl]-α-phenyl-2-pyridineacetamide phosphate (Norpace), is an oral and intravenous class IA antiarrhythmic agent. It is quite similar to quinidine and procainamide in its electrophysiological properties, in that it decreases phase 4 diastolic depolarization, decreases conduction velocity, and has vagolytic properties.[31] It is used clinically in the treatment of refractory, life-threatening ventricular tachyarrhythmias. Oral administration of the drug produces peak plasma levels within 2 hours. The drug is bound approximately 50% to plasma protein and has a half-life of 6.7 hours in humans. More than 50% is excreted unchanged in the urine. Therefore, patients with renal insufficiency should be monitored carefully for evidence of overdose. Disopyramide phosphate commonly exhibits side effects of dry mouth, constipation, urinary retention, and other cholinergic blocking actions because of its structural similarity to anticholinergic drugs.

Disopyramide
(Norpace)

Lidocaine Hydrochloride, USP. Lidocaine hydrochloride, 2-(diethylamino)-2′,6′-acetoxylidide monohydrochloride (Xylocaine), was conceived as a derivative of gramine (3-dimethylaminomethylindole) and introduced as a local anesthetic. It is now being used intravenously as a standard parenteral agent for suppression of arrhythmias associated with acute myocardial infarction and cardiac surgery. It is the drug of choice for the parenteral treatment of premature ventricular contractions.

Lidocaine
(Xylocaine)

Lidocaine hydrochloride is a class IB antiarrhythmic agent with a different effect on the electrophysiological properties of myocardial cells from that of procainamide and quinidine. It binds with equal affinity to the active (A) and inactive (I) Na^+ ion channels. It depresses diastolic depolarization and automaticity in the Purkinje fiber network and increases the functional refractory period relative to action potential duration, as do procainamide and quinidine. It differs from the latter two drugs, however, in that it does not decrease, and may even enhance, conduction velocity

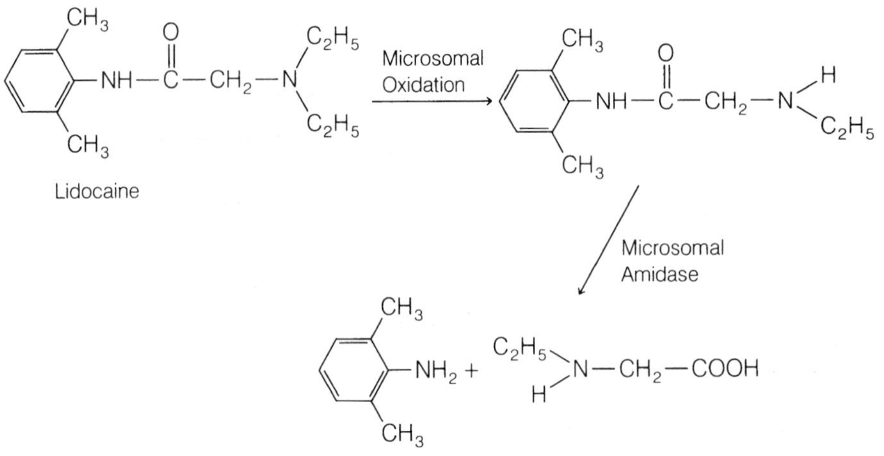

Figure 19.12 ● Metabolism of lidocaine.

and increase membrane responsiveness to stimulation. There are fewer data available on the subcellular mechanisms responsible for the antiarrhythmic actions of lidocaine than on the more established drug quinidine. It has been proposed that lidocaine has little effect on membrane cation exchange of the atria. Sodium ion entrance into ventricular cells during excitation is not influenced by lidocaine because it does not alter conduction velocity in this area. Lidocaine hydrochloride does depress Na^+ influx during diastole, as do all other antiarrhythmic drugs, to diminish automaticity in myocardial tissue. It also alters membrane responsiveness in Purkinje fibers, allowing increased conduction velocity and ample membrane potential at the time of excitation.[32]

Lidocaine hydrochloride administration is limited to the parenteral route and is usually given intravenously, although adequate plasma levels are achieved after intramuscular injections. Lidocaine hydrochloride is not bound to any extent to plasma proteins and is concentrated in the tissues. It is metabolized rapidly by the liver (Fig. 19.12). The first step is deethylation with the formation of monoethylglycinexylidide, followed by hydrolysis of the amide.[33] Metabolism is rapid, the half-life of a single injection ranging from 15 to 30 minutes. Lidocaine hydrochloride is a popular drug because of its rapid action and its relative freedom from toxic effects on the heart, especially in the absence of hepatic disease. Monoethylglycinexylidide, the initial metabolite of lidocaine, is an effective antiarrhythmic agent; its rapid hydrolysis by microsomal amidases, however, prevents its use in humans.

Precautions must be taken so that lidocaine hydrochloride solutions containing epinephrine salts are not used as cardiac depressants. Such solutions are intended only for local anesthesia and are not used intravenously. The aqueous solutions without epinephrine may be autoclaved several times, if necessary.

Phenytoin Sodium, USP. Phenytoin sodium, 5,5-diphenyl-2,4-imidazolidinedione, 5,5-diphenylhydantoin, diphenyl-hydantoin sodium (Dilantin), has been used for decades in the control of grand mal types of epileptic seizure. It is structurally analogous to the barbiturates but does not possess their extensive sedative properties. The compound is available as the sodium salt. Solutions for parenteral administration contain 40% propylene glycol and 10% alcohol to dissolve the sodium salt.

Phenytoin sodium's cardiovascular effects were uncovered during observation of toxic manifestations of the drug in patients being treated for seizure disorders. Phenytoin sodium was found to cause bradycardia, prolong the PR interval, and produce T-wave abnormalities on electrocardiograms. It is a class IB antiarrhythmic agent. Today, phenytoin sodium's greatest clinical use as an antiarrhythmic drug is in the treatment of digitalis-induced arrhythmias.[34] Its action is similar to that of lidocaine. It depresses ventricular automaticity produced by digitalis, without adverse intraventricular conduction. Because it also reverses the prolongation of AV conduction by digitalis, phenytoin sodium is useful in supraventricular tachycardias caused by digitalis intoxication.

Phenytoin sodium is located in high amounts in the body tissues, especially fat and liver, leading to large gradients between the drug in tissues and the plasma concentrations. It is metabolized in the liver.

Mexiletine Hydrochloride. Mexiletine hydrochloride, 1-methyl-2-(2,6-xylyloxy)ethylamine hydrochloride (Mexitil) (pK$_a$ 8.4), is a class IB antiarrhythmic agent that is effective when given either intravenously or orally. It resembles lidocaine in possessing a xylyl moiety but otherwise is different chemically. Mexiletine hydrochloride is an ether and is not subject to the hydrolysis common to the amides lidocaine and tocainide. Its mean half-life on oral administration is approximately 10 hours.

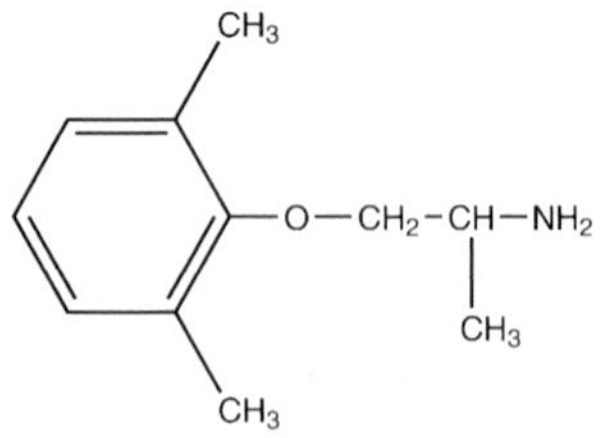

Mexiletine
(Mexitil)

Although not subject to hydrolysis, mexiletine hydrochloride is metabolized by oxidative and reductive processes in the liver. Its metabolites, *p*-hydroxymexiletine and hydroxymethylmexiletine, are not pharmacologically active as antiarrhythmic agents.[35]

Mexiletine hydrochloride, like class I antiarrhythmic agents, blocks the fast Na^+ channel in cardiac cells. It is especially effective on the Purkinje fibers in the heart. The drug increases the threshold of excitability of myocardial cells by reducing the rate of rise and amplitude of the action potential and decreases automaticity.

Mexiletine hydrochloride is used for long-term oral prophylaxis of ventricular tachycardia. The drug is given in 200- to 400-mg doses every 8 hours.

Tocainide Hydrochloride. Tocainide hydrochloride, 2-amino-2′,6′-propionoxyxylidide hydrochloride (Tonocard) (pK_a 7.7), is an analog of lidocaine. It is orally active and has electrophysiological properties like those of lidocaine.[36] Total body clearance of tocainide hydrochloride is only 166 mL/min, suggesting that hepatic clearance is not large. Because of low hepatic clearance, the hepatic extraction ratio must be small; therefore, tocainide hydrochloride is unlikely to be subject to a substantial first-pass effect. The drug differs from lidocaine, in that it lacks two ethyl groups, which provides tocainide hydrochloride some protection from first-pass hepatic elimination after oral ingestion. Tocainide hydrochloride is hydrolyzed in a manner similar to that of lidocaine. None of its metabolites is active.

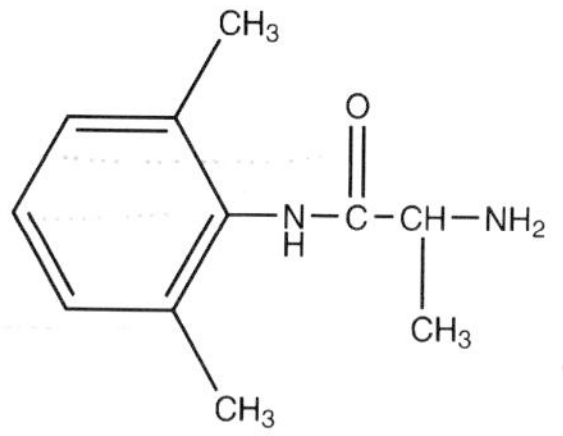

Tocainide
(Tonocard)

Tocainide hydrochloride is classed as a IB antiarrhythmic agent and used orally to prevent or treat ventricular ectopy and tachycardia. The drug is given in 400- to 600-mg doses every 8 hours.

Flecainide Acetate. Flecainide acetate, N-(2-piperidinylmethyl)-2,5-bis (2,2,2-trifluoroethoxy)benzamide monoacetate (Tambocor), is a class IC antiarrhythmic drug with local anesthetic activity; it is a chemical derivative of benzamide. The drug undergoes biotransformation, forming a meta-O-dealkylated compound, whose antiarrhythmic properties are half as potent as those of the parent drug, and a meta-O-dealkylated lactam of flecainide with little pharmacological activity.[37] Flecainide acetate is given orally to suppress chronic ventricular ectopy and ventricular tachycardia. It has some limitations because of CNS side effects.

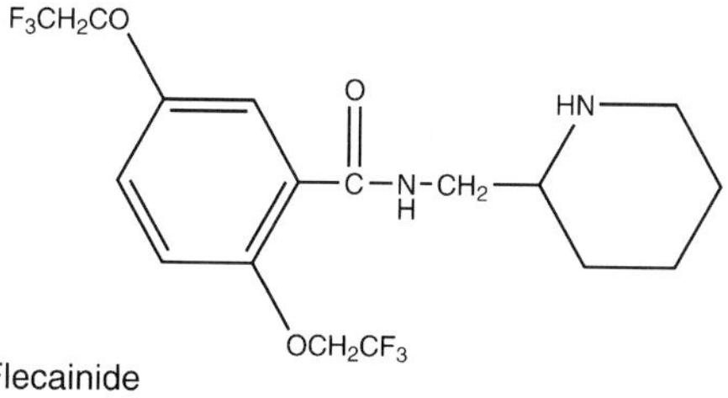

Flecainide
(Tambocor)

Moricizine. Moricizine, ethyl 10-(3-morpholinopropionyl)phenothiazine-2-carbamate (Ethmozine), is a phenothiazine derivative used for the treatment of malignant ventricular arrhythmias. It is categorized as a class IC antiarrhythmic agent, blocking the Na^+ channel with 1:1 stochiometry. The drug has higher affinity for the inactivated state than the activated or resting states. It appears to bind to a site on the external side of the Na^+ channel membrane.[38] It has been used to suppress life-threatening ventricular arrhythmias.

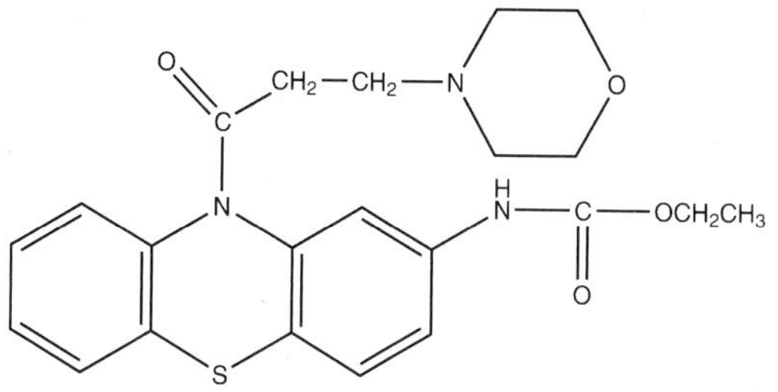

Moricizine
(Ethmozine)

Propafenone. Propafenone, 2-[2′-hydroxy-3-(propylamino)propoxy]-3-phenylpropiophenone (Rythmol), a class IC antiarrhythmic drug, contains a chiral center and is marketed as the racemic mixture. Therapy with the racemic mixture of propafenone produces effects that can be attributed to both (S) and (R) enantiomers. Although (R) and (S) enantiomers exert similar Na^+ channel–blocking effects, the (S) enantiomer also produces a β-adrenergic blockade. As a result, the (S) enantiomer is reported to be 40-fold more potent than the (R) enantiomer as an antiarrhythmic agent.[39] The enantiomers also display stereoselective disposition characteristics. The (R) enantiomer is cleared more quickly. Hepatic metabolism is polymorphic and determined genetically. Ten percent of Caucasians have a reduced capacity to hydroxylate the drug to form 5-hydroxypropafenone. This polymorphic metabolism accounts for the interindividual variability in the relationships between dose and concentration and, thus, variability in the pharmacodynamic effects of the drug. The 5-hydroxy metabolites of both enantiomers are as potent as the parent compound in blocking Na^+ channels. Propafenone also depresses the slow inward current of Ca^{2+} ions. This drug has been used for acute termination or long-term suppression of ventricular arrhythmias. It is bound in excess of 95% to α_1-acid glycoprotein in the plasma. It is absorbed effectively, but bioavailability is estimated to be less than 20% because of first-pass metabolism. Less than 1% is eliminated as unchanged drug. Therapy with propafenone may produce effects that can be attributed to both (S) and (R) enantiomers. Thus, the effects may be modulated because of an enantiomer–enantiomer interaction when patients are treated with the racemate.[40]

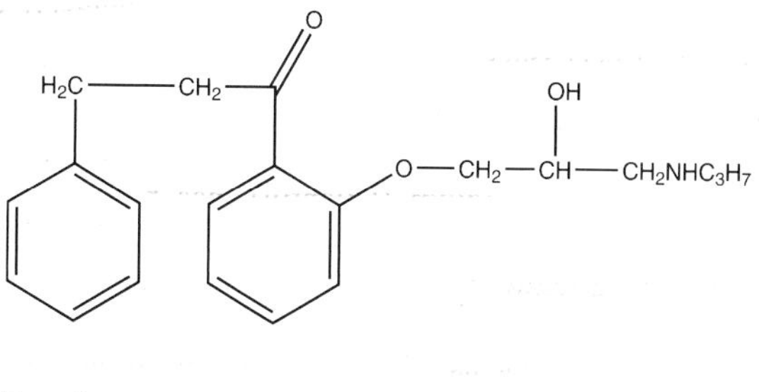

Propafenone
(Rythmol)

CLASS II ANTIARRHYTHMICS

Class II antiarrhythmics are discussed under the heading, "Adrenergic System Inhibitors."

CLASS III ANTIARRHYTHMICS

Amiodarone. Amiodarone, 2-butyl-3-benzofuranyl-4-[2-(diethylamino)ethoxy]-3,5-diiodophenyl ketone (Cordarone), was introduced as an antianginal agent. It has very pronounced class III action and is especially effective in maintaining sinus rhythm in patients who have been treated by direct current shock for atrial fibrillation.[41] Like class III antiarrhythmic drugs, amiodarone lengthens the effective refractory period by prolonging the action potential duration in all myocardial tissues. Amiodarone is eliminated very slowly from the body, with a half-life of about 25 to 30 days after oral doses.[42] Although the drug has a broad spectrum of antiarrhythmic activity, its main limitation is a slow onset of action. Drug action may not be initiated for several days, and the peak effect may not be obtained for several weeks.

Amiodarone has adverse effects involving many different organ systems. It also inhibits metabolism of drugs cleared by oxidative microsomal enzymes. It contains iodine in its molecular structure and, as a result, has an effect on thyroid hormones. Hypothyroidism occurs in up to 11% of patients receiving amiodarone.[43] The principal effect is the inhibition of peripheral conversion of T_4 to T_3. Serum reverse T_3 (rT_3) is increased as a function of the dose as well as the length of amiodarone therapy. As a result, rT_3 levels have been used as a guide for judging adequacy of amiodarone therapy and predicting toxicity.[44]

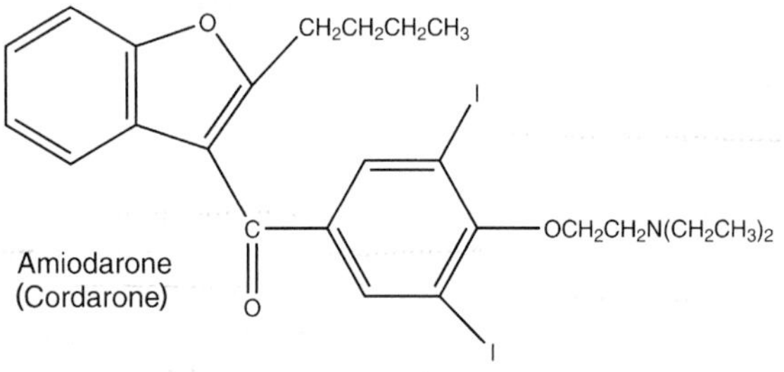

Amiodarone
(Cordarone)

Bretylium Tosylate. Bretylium tosylate, (*o*-bromobenzyl)ethyl dimethylammonium *p*-toluenesulfonate (Bretylol), is an extremely bitter, white, crystalline powder. The chemical is freely soluble in water and alcohol. Bretylium tosylate is an adrenergic neuronal-blocking agent that accumulates selectively in the neurons and displaces norepinephrine. Because of this property, bretylium was used initially, under the trade name of Darenthin, as an antihypertensive agent. It caused postural

decrease in arterial pressure.[44] This use was discontinued because of the rapid development of tolerance, erratic oral absorption of the quaternary ammonium compound, and persistent pain in the parotid gland on prolonged therapy. Currently, bretylium is reserved for use in ventricular arrhythmias that are resistant to other therapy. Bretylium does not suppress phase 4 depolarization, a common action of other antiarrhythmic agents. It prolongs the effective refractory period relative to the action potential duration but does not affect conduction time and is categorized as a class III antiarrhythmic agent. Because bretylium does not have properties similar to those of the other antiarrhythmic agents, it has been suggested that its action is a result of its adrenergic neuronal-blocking properties; the antiarrhythmic properties of the drug, however, are not affected by administration of reserpine. Bretylium is also a local anesthetic, but it has not been possible to demonstrate such an effect on atria of experimental animals, except at very high concentrations.[45] Therefore, the precise mechanism of the antiarrhythmic action of bretylium remains to be resolved.

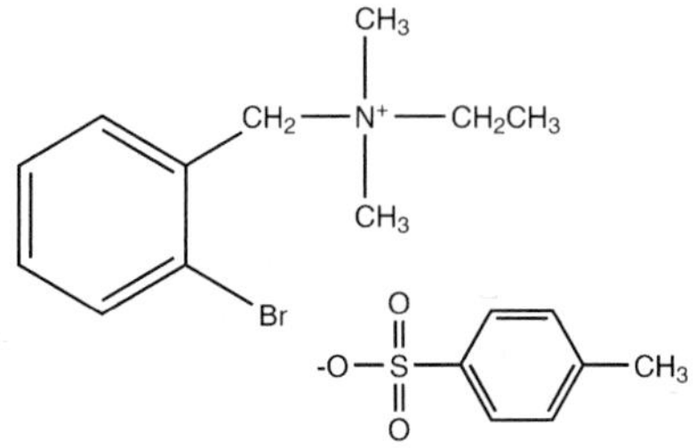

Bretylium
(Bretylol)

Dofetilide. Dofetilide, *N*-[4-(3-{[2-(4-methanesulfonylaminophenyl)ethyl]methylamino}propoxy)phenyl]methane-sulfonamide (Tikosyn), acts by blocking the cardiac ion channel carrying the rapid component of the delayed rectifier potassium currents (Ikr) and is used to terminate supraventricular arrhythmias, prevent the recurrence of atrial fibrillation, and treat life-threatening ventricular arrhythmias. Unlike sotalol and ibutilide, which are also methanesulfonanilides, it has no effect on adrenergic receptors or sodium channels, respectively. Dofetilide has high specificity for the delayed rectifier potassium currents.[46]

Ibutilide. Ibutilide, *N*-{4-[4-(ethylheptylamino)-1-hydroxybutyl]phenyl}methanesulfonamide (Corvert), a class III antiarrhythmic belonging to the methanesulfonanilide class of agents, is indicated for rapid conversion of atrial fibrillation or atrial flutter to normal sinus rhythm.

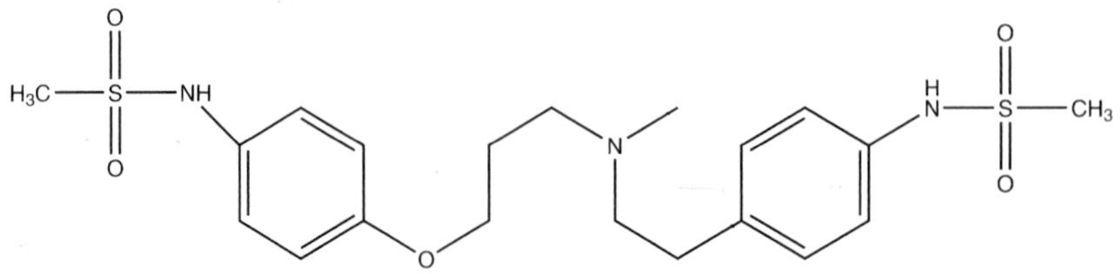

Dofetilide
(Tikosyn)

Unlike dofetilide, it is not highly specific for the delayed rectifier potassium currents (Ikr) and does have some affinity for sodium channels.

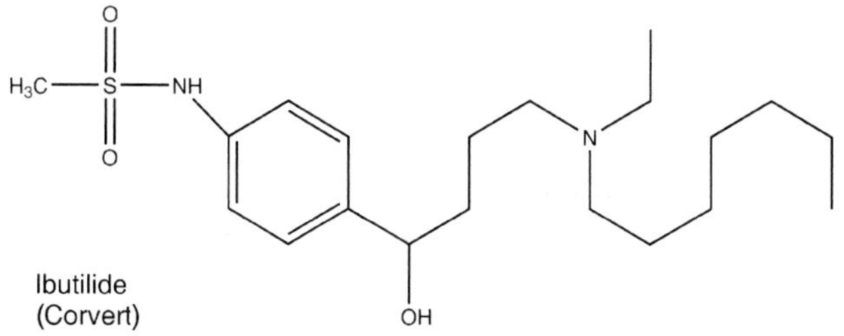

Ibutilide
(Corvert)

Sotalol. Sotalol, 4'[1-hydroxy-2-(isopropylamino) ethyl]methylsulfonanilide (Betapace), is a relatively new antiarrhythmic drug, characterized most often as a class III agent, and although it has effects that are related to the class II agents, it is not therapeutically considered a class II antiarrhythmic. It contains a chiral center and is marketed as the racemic mixture. Because of its enantiomers, its mechanism of action spans two of the antiarrhythmic drug classes. The *l*(−) enantiomer has both β-blocking (class II) and potassium channel-blocking (class III) activities. The d(+) enantiomer has class III properties similar to those of the (−) isomer, but its affinity for the β-adrenergic receptor is 30 to 60 times lower. The sotalol enantiomers produce different effects on the heart. Class III action of *d*-sotalol in the sinus node is associated with slowing of sinus heart rate, whereas β-adrenergic blockade contributes to the decrease in heart rate observed with *1*- or *d,1*-sotalol. Sotalol is not metabolized, nor is it bound significantly to proteins. Elimination occurs by renal excretion, with more than 80% of the drug eliminated unchanged. Sotalol is characteristic of class III antiarrhythmic drugs, in that it prolongs the duration of the action potential and, thus, increases the effective refractory period of myocardial tissue. It is distinguished from the other class III drugs (amiodarone and bretylium) because of its β-adrenergic receptor–blocking action.

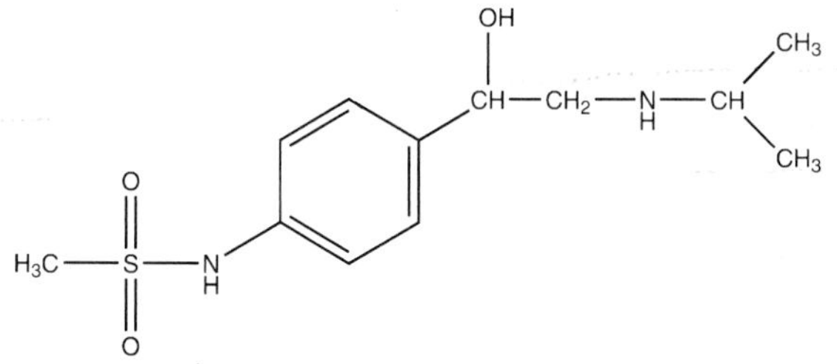

Sotalol
(Betapace)

Azimilide. Azimilide, *E*-1-[[[5-(4-chlorophenyl)-2-furanyl]methylene]amino]-3-[4-(4-methyl-1-piperazinyl) butyl]-2,4-imidazolidinedione, is a class III agent that sig-

nificantly blocks the delayed rectifier potassium current, Iks, including the Ikr component. Its ability to block multichannels may be caused by a lack of the methane sulfonamide group that is common to other class III agents, which selectively block the Ikr potassium current. It is believed that blocking both Ikr and Iks potassium currents yields consistent class III antiarrhythmic effects at any heart rate.[47]

CLASS IV ANTIARRHYTHMICS

Verapamil and Diltiazem. Both verapamil and diltiazem block the slow inward Ca^{2+} currents (voltage-sensitive channel) in cardiac fibers. This slows down AV conduction and the sinus rate. These drugs are used in controlling atrial and paroxysmal tachycardias and are categorized as class IV antiarrhythmic agents according to the Vaughan Williams classification.[21] (A more detailed description of calcium channel blockers is given previously.)

● ANTIHYPERTENSIVE AGENTS

Hypertension is a consequence of many diseases. Hemodynamically, blood pressure is a function of the amount of blood pumped by the heart and the ease with which the blood flows through the peripheral vasculature (i.e., resistance to blood flow by peripheral blood vessels). Diseases of components of the central and peripheral nervous systems, which regulate blood pressure and abnormalities of the hormonal system, and diseases of the kidney and peripheral vascular network, which affect blood volume, can create a hypertensive state in humans. Hypertension is generally defined as mild when the diastolic pressure is between 90 and 104 mm Hg, moderate when it is 105 to 114 mm Hg, and severe when it is above 115 mm Hg. It is estimated that about 15% of the adult population in the United States (about 40 million) are hypertensive.

Primary (essential) hypertension is the most common form of hypertension. Although advances have been made in the identification and control of primary hypertension, the etiology of this form of hypertension has not yet been resolved. *Renal hypertension* can be created by experimentally causing renal artery stenosis in animals. Renal artery stenosis also may occur in pathological conditions of the kidney, such as nephritis, renal artery thrombosis, renal artery infarctions, or other conditions that restrict blood flow through the renal artery. Hypertension also may originate from pathological states in the CNS, such as malignancies. Tumors in the adrenal medulla that cause release of large amounts of catecholamines create a hypertensive condition known as *pheochromocytoma.* Excessive secretion of aldosterone by the adrenal cortex, often because of adenomas, also produces hypertensive disorders.

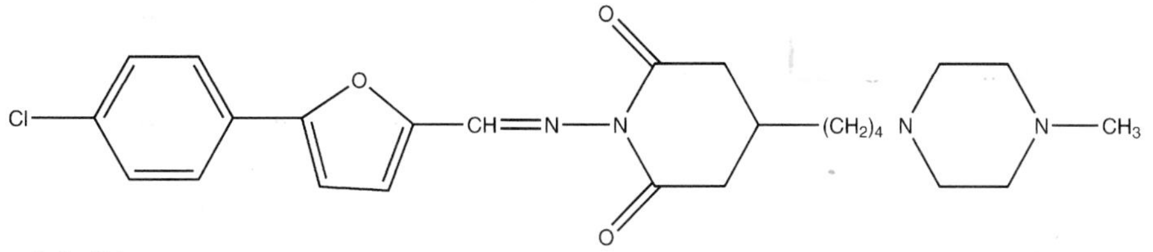

Azimilide

Arterial blood pressure is regulated by several physiological factors, such as heart rate, stroke volume, peripheral vascular network resistance, blood vessel elasticity, blood volume, and viscosity of blood. Endogenous chemicals also play an important part in the regulation of arterial blood pressure. The peripheral vascular system is influenced greatly by the sympathetic–parasympathetic balance of the autonomic nervous system, the control of which originates in the CNS. Enhanced adrenergic activity is a principal contributor to primary (essential) hypertension.

Therapy using antihypertensive agents evolved rapidly between 1950 and 1960. During that time, several drugs for the treatment and control of hypertensive disease were discovered. Despite the many years of experience, treatment remains empiric because the etiology of the principal form of hypertension, primary hypertension, is unknown. The first drugs used to produce symptomatic relief of hypertension were α-adrenergic blocking agents. These drugs had limitations because their duration of action was far too short and side effects precluded long-term therapy. Contemporary therapy of primary hypertension uses one of several drug classes as the first course. These drugs may be diuretics to reduce blood volume, inhibitors of the renin–angiotensin system (ACE inhibitors, Chapter 18), and agents that reduce peripheral vascular resistance (e.g., calcium channel blockers, vasodilators, and sympathetic nervous system depressants). The antihypertensive drug classes discussed in this section include endothelin receptor antagonists, sympathetic nervous system depressants, and vasodilators acting on smooth muscle. Calcium channel blockers and other vasodilators are included in previous discussions in this chapter. Diuretics and renin angiotensin system are discussed in Chapter 18.

ENDOTHELIN RECEPTOR ANTAGONISTS

Endothelin-1 is a 21-amino acid peptide that is produced in the vascular endothelium, which plays a role in the regulation of smooth muscle contraction. Two types of endothelin receptors, ET_A and ET_B, have been identified on smooth muscle. The physiological role these play varies depending on the location of the receptor. Overall, the receptors are linked to a Gq-protein and when activated, results in the formation of IP_3. This, in turn, results in the release of calcium by the sacroplasmic reticulum that results in increased smooth muscle contraction and vasoconstriction. It is of interest to note that ET_B receptors located on the endothelium have a slightly different role than those found on the vascular smooth muscle. When the endothelium ET_B receptors are stimulated, NO is formed from L-arginine. The NO that is released produces vasodilation in much the same fashion as nitroglycerin. This effect is generally transient, whereas the overall effects of stimulation of the vascular endothelin receptors is prolong. Agents that antagonize these receptors (edothelin receptor antagonists [ETRAs]) have usefulness in treating hypertension, heart failure, and coronary vasospasm. Currently, the approved agents are only indicated for pulmonary hypertension.[48]

PRODUCTS

Ambrisentan. Ambrisentan, (+)-(2S)-2-[(4,6-dimethyl-pyrimidin-2-yl)oxy]-3-methoxy-3,3-diphenylpropanoic acid (Letairis), is a potent ET_A selective endothelin antagonist that, is indicated, in the treatment of pulmonary arterial hypertension (PAH). PAH is a rare disease that if left untreated has a high mortality rate. In June of 2007, the FDA granted approval of ambrisentan for once-daily treatment of PAH. Studies have shown that it improves a 6-minute walk by about 30 to 60 m for patients receiving placebo.[49]

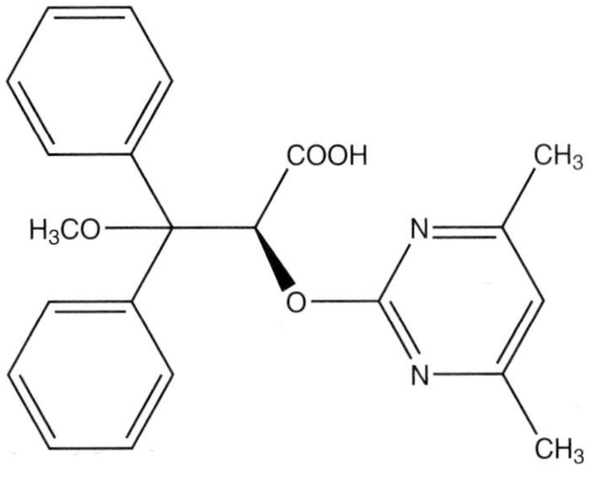

Ambrisentan

Bosentan. Bosentan, N-[6-(2-hydroxyethoxy)-5-(2-methoxyphenoxy)-2-pyrimidin-2-yl-pyrimidin-4-yl]-4-tert-butyl-benzenesulfonamide (Tracleer, Bozentan), was the first endothelin receptor antagonist marketed in the United States. Bosentan works by competitively blocking the endothelin receptor subtypes ET_A and ET_B. In binding to the receptors, it blocks the effects of endothelin, which include constriction of the vascular smooth muscle, which leads to narrowing of the blood vessels and hypertension. Although it is not selective for the ET_A receptors, it does have a higher affinity for that subtype over ET_B. However, the clinical significance of selectivity over preferential receptor binding has not been demonstrated. Bosentan is an inducer of CYP2C9 and CYP3A4, and patients using bosentan must be monitored for liver toxicity.[50]

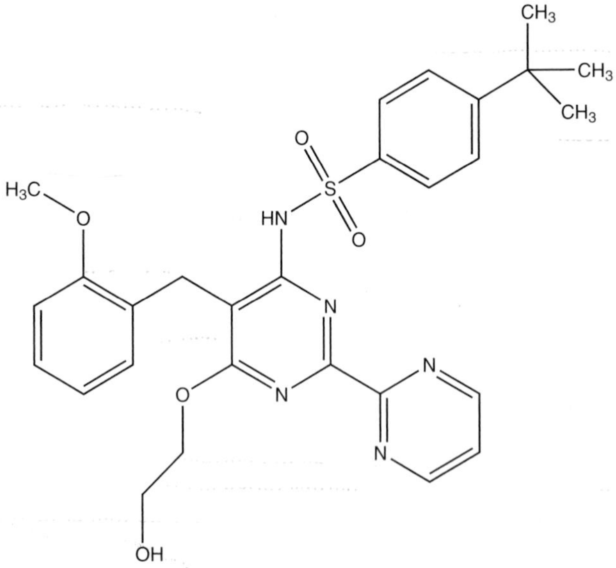

Bosentan

Sitaxsentan Sodium. Sitaxsentan, N-(4-chloro-3-methyl-oxazol-5-yl)-2-[2-(6-methylbenzo[1,3]dioxol-5-yl)acetyl]thiophene-3-sulfonamide (Thelin), belongs to the sulfonamide class of endothelin receptor antagonists.

Although it has 6,000-fold selectivity for the ET$_A$ receptor, clinical trials have not demonstrated a greater efficacy over bosentan. However, it has much lower liver toxicity than bosentan. The manufacturer is attempting to meet efficacy outcomes set by the FDA, which must be met before approval of sitaxsentan as a therapeutic agent will be granted.

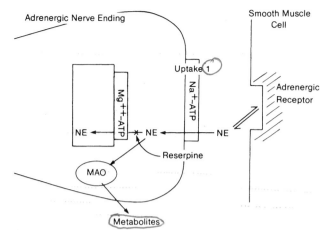

Figure 19.13 ● Action of reserpine at adrenergic nerve ending.

Sitaxsentan

ADRENERGIC SYSTEM INHIBITORS

Drugs that reduce blood pressure by depressing the activity of the sympathetic nervous system have been used as effective agents in the treatment of hypertension. This can be accomplished in several ways: (a) depleting the stores of neurotransmitter, (b) reducing the number of impulses traveling in sympathetic nerves, (c) antagonizing the actions of the neurotransmitter on the effector cells, and (d) inhibiting neurotransmitter release.

AGENTS DEPLETING NEUROTRANSMITTER STORES

Folk remedies prepared from species of *Rauwolfia*, a plant genus belonging to the Apocynaceae family, were reported as early as 1563. The root of the species *Rauwolfia serpentina* has been used for centuries as an antidote to stings and bites of insects, to reduce fever, as a stimulant to uterine contractions, for insomnia, and particularly for the treatment of insanity. Its use in hypertension was recorded in the Indian literature in 1918, but not until 1949 did hypotensive properties of *Rauwolfia* spp. appear in the Western literature.[51] *Rauwolfia* preparations were introduced in psychiatry for the treatment of schizophrenia in the early 1950s, following confirmation of the folk remedy reports on their use in mentally deranged patients. By the end of the 1960s, however, the drug had been replaced by more efficacious neurotropic agents. Reserpine and its preparations remain useful in the control of mild essential hypertension.

The effects of reserpine do not correlate well with tissue levels of the drug. The pharmacological effects of reserpine were still present in animals when it could no longer be detected in the brain.[52] Reserpine depletes catecholamines and serotonin from central and peripheral neurons by interfering with the uptake of these amines from the cytosol into the vesicles and granules.[53,54] As a consequence, norepinephrine cannot be stored intraneuronally in adrenergic neurons, and much of the norepinephrine in the cytosol is metabolized by monoamine oxidase (MAO) (Fig. 19.13). The binding of reserpine to the storage vesicle membrane is

firm, and as a result, the storage granule is destroyed, reducing the ability of the nerve to concentrate and store norepinephrine. Because reserpine acts on both central and peripheral adrenergic neurons, its antihypertensive effects may result from neurotransmitter depletion from both of these sites.

Chemical investigations of the active components of *R. serpentina* roots have yielded several alkaloids (e.g., ajmaline, ajmalicine, ajmalinine, serpentine, and serpentinine). Reserpine, which is the major active constituent of *Rauwolfia*,[55] was isolated in 1952 and is a much weaker base than the alkaloids just mentioned. Reserpinoid alkaloids are yohimbine-like bases that have an additional functional group on C-18. Only three naturally occurring alkaloids possess reserpine-like activity strong enough for use in treating hypertension: reserpine, deserpidine, and rescinnamine.

Reserpine is absorbed rapidly after oral administration. Fat tissue accumulates reserpine slowly, with a maximal level reached between 4 and 6 hours. After 24 hours, small amounts of reserpine are found in the liver and fat, but none is found in the brain or other tissues. Reserpine is metabolized by the liver and intestine to methyl reserpate and 3,4,5-trimethoxybenzoic acid.

Powdered Rauwolfia Serpentina, USP. Rauwolfia (Raudixin, Rauserpal, Rauval) is the powdered whole root of *R. serpentina* (Benth). It is a light tan to light brown powder, sparingly soluble in alcohol and only slightly soluble in water. It contains the total alkaloids, of which reserpine accounts for about 50% of the total activity. Orally, a dosage of 200 to 300 mg is roughly equivalent to 500 μg of reserpine. It is used in the treatment of mild or moderate hypertension or in combination with other hypotensive agents in severe hypertension.

Reserpine, USP. Reserpine (Serpasil, Reserpoid, Rau-Sed, Sandril) is a white to light yellow, crystalline alkaloid, practically insoluble in water, obtained from various species of *Rauwolfia*. In common with other compounds with an indole nucleus, it is susceptible to decomposition by light and oxidation, especially when in solution. In the dry state, discoloration occurs rapidly when reserpine is exposed to light, but the loss in potency is usually small. In solution,

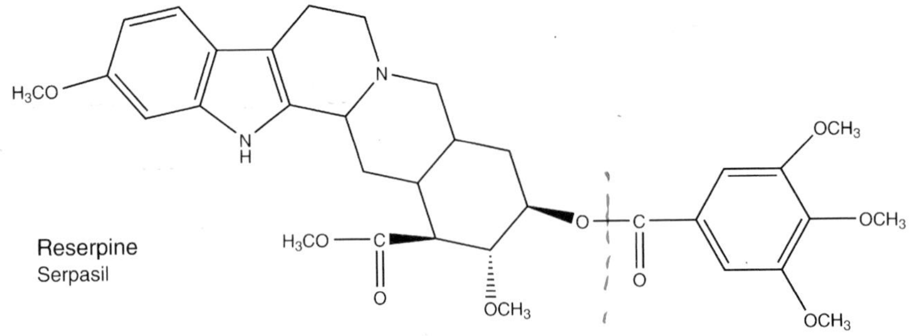

Reserpine
Serpasil

reserpine may break down with no appreciable color change when exposed to light, especially in clear glass containers; thus, color change cannot be used as an index of the amount of decomposition.

Reserpine is effective orally and parenterally for the treatment of hypertension. After a single intravenous dose, the onset of antihypertensive action usually begins in about 1 hour. After intramuscular injection, the maximum effect occurs within approximately 4 hours and lasts about 10 hours. When it is given orally, the maximum effect occurs within about 2 weeks and may persist up to 4 weeks after the final dose. When used in conjunction with other hypotensive drugs in the treatment of severe hypertension, the daily dose varies from 100 to 250 μg.

Guanethidine and Related Compounds. Guanethidine has been classified traditionally as an adrenergic blocking agent because it can prevent the release of norepinephrine from postganglionic neurons in response to adrenergic stimulation. Guanethidine and other compounds discussed in this section have other actions on catecholamine metabolism and can cause significant depletion of these amines in adrenergic neurons. They do not interfere with release of epinephrine from the adrenal medulla.

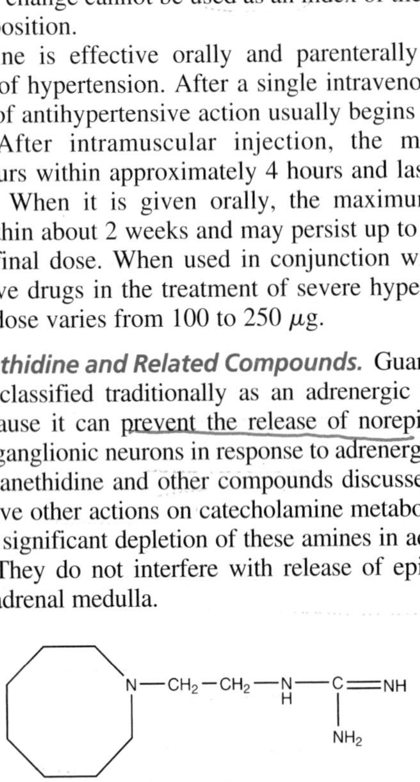

Guanethidine
(Ismelin)

Guanethidine Monosulfate, USP. Guanethidine monosulfate, [2-(hexahydro-1 (2*H*)-azocinyl)ethyl]guanidine sulfate (Ismelin sulfate), is a white, crystalline material that is very soluble in water. It was one of a series of guanidine compounds prepared in the search for potent antitrypanosomal agents. There is an absence of CNS effects, such as depression, because the drug is highly polar and does not easily cross the blood-brain barrier. Guanethidine monosulfate produces a gradual, prolonged fall in blood pressure. Usually, 2 to 7 days of therapy are required before the peak effect is reached, and usually, this peak effect is maintained for 3 or 4 days. Then, if the drug is discontinued, the blood pressure returns to pretreatment levels over a period of 1 to 3 weeks. Because of this slow onset and prolonged duration of action, only a single daily dose is needed.

Guanethidine monosulfate is metabolized by microsomal enzymes to 2-(6-carboxyhexylamino)ethylguanidine and guanethidine *N*-oxide (Fig. 19.14). Both metabolites have very weak antihypertensive properties. Guanethidine monosulfate is taken up by the amine pump located on the neuronal membrane and retained in the nerve, displacing norepinephrine from its storage sites in the neuronal granules. The displaced norepinephrine is metabolized to homovanillic acid by mitochondrial MAO, depleting the nerve ending of the neurotransmitter. The usefulness of guanethidine monosulfate also resides in the fact that once it is taken up by the nerve, it produces a sympathetic blockade by inhibiting release of nonepinephrine that would occur on neuronal membrane response to stimulation[29] by the nerve action potential. Guanethidine monosulfate stored in the granules is released by the nerve action potential but has very low intrinsic activity for the adrenergic receptors on the postjunctional membrane. Moderate doses for a prolonged period or large doses may produce undesirable side effects by causing neuromuscular blockade and adrenergic nerve conduction blockade.

Guanadrel Sulfate. Guanadrel sulfate, (1,4-dioxaspiro[4.5]dec-2-ylmethyl)guanadine sulfate (Hylorel), is similar to guanethidine monosulfate in the manner in which it reduces elevated blood pressure. It acts as a postganglionic adrenergic blocking agent by displacing norepinephrine in adrenergic neuron storage granules, thereby preventing release of the endogenous neurotransmitter on nerve stimulation. Guanadrel sulfate has a much shorter half-life (10 hours) than guanethidine monosulfate, whose

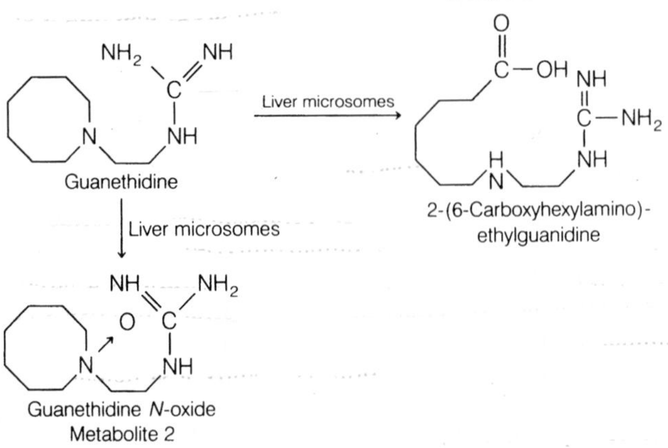

Figure 19.14 ● Metabolism of guanethidine monosulfate.

half-life is measured in days. In the stepped-care approach to hypertension, guanadrel sulfate is usually a step 2 agent.

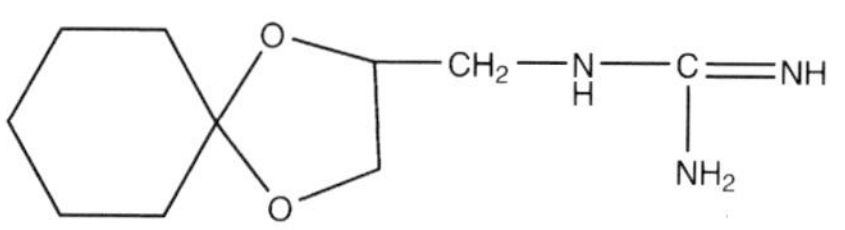

Guanadrel
(Hylorel)

SELECTIVE α-ADRENERGIC ANTAGONISTS

The principal clinical use of α-adrenergic antagonists is in the treatment of catecholamine-dependent hypertension. Classic drugs such as phentolamine and phenoxybenzamine are non-specific-blocking agents of both α_1- and α_2-receptors on the presynaptic membrane of the adrenergic neuron. Specific antagonists of α_1-receptors are effective antihypertensive agents by blocking the vasocontricting effect on smooth muscle and not interfering with the activation of α_2-receptors on the adrenergic neuron, which when activated inhibit further release of norepinephrine.

Prazosin Hydrochloride. The antihypertensive effects of prazosin hydrochloride, 1-(4-amino-6,7-dimethoxy-2-quinazolinyl)-4-(2-furoyl)piperazine monohydrochloride (Minipress), are caused by peripheral vasodilation as a result of its blockade of α_1-adrenergic receptors. In ligand-binding studies, prazosin hydrochloride has 5,000-fold greater affinity for α_1-receptors than for some α_2-adrenergic receptors.[56]

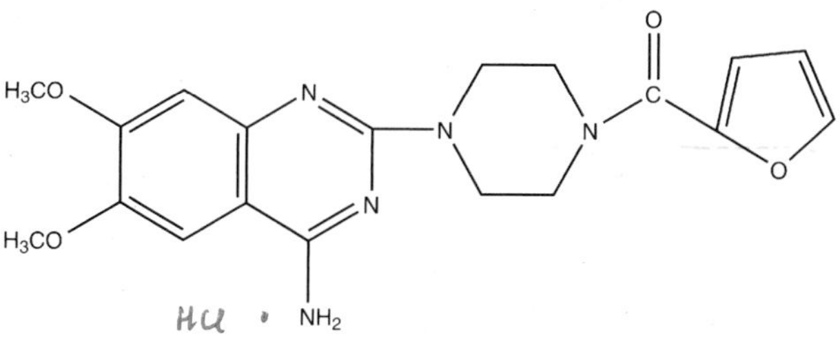

Prazosin
(Minipress)

Prazosin hydrochloride is readily absorbed, and plasma concentrations reach a peak about 3 hours after administration. Plasma half-life is between 2 and 3 hours. Prazosin hydrochloride is highly bound to plasma protein; it does not cause adverse reactions, however, with drugs that might be displaced from their protein-binding sites (e.g., cardiac glycosides). It may cause severe orthostatic hypertension because of its α-adrenergic blocking action, which prevents the reflex venous constriction that is activated when an individual sits up from a prone position.

Terazosin Hydrochloride. Terazosin hydrochloride, 1-(4-amino-6,7-dimethoxy-2-quinazolinyl)-4-(tetrahydro-2-furoyl)piperazine monohydrochloride (Hytrin), is a structural congener of prazosin hydrochloride. It possesses similar selective properties of specifically inhibiting α_1-adrenergic receptors. The drug is slightly less potent than prazosin hydrochloride. Terazosin hydrochloride has a half-life of approximately 12 hours, which is much longer than that of prazosin. This lends itself to a once-daily dose to control hypertension in many patients.

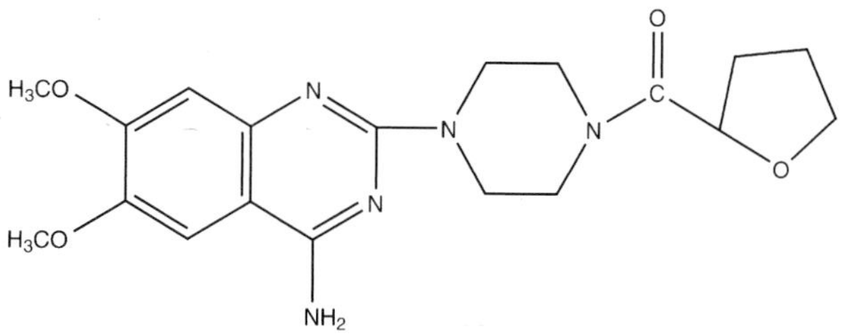

Terazosin
(Hytrin)

Doxazosin. Doxazosin, 1-(4-amino-6,7-dimethoxy-2-quinazolinyl)-4-(1,4-benzodioxan-2-ylcarbonyl)piperazine (Cardura), is a quinazoline compound that selectively inhibits the α_1-subtype of α-adrenergic receptors. This agent is very useful in the management of hypertension associated with pheochromocytoma.

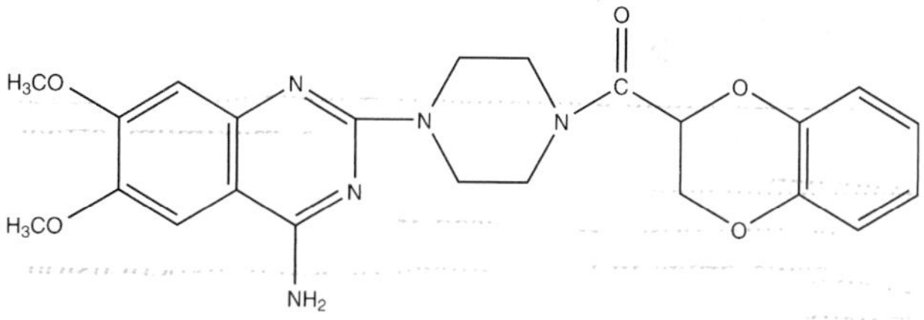

Doxazosin
(Cardura)

CENTRALLY ACTING ADRENERGIC DRUGS

The use of agents that directly affect the peripheral component of the sympathetic nervous system represents an important approach to the treatment of hypertension. A second approach to modifying sympathetic influence on the cardiovascular system is through inhibition or reduction of CNS control of blood pressure. Several widely used medications act by stimulating α_2-receptors, which in the CNS reduces sympathetic outflow to the cardiovascular system and produces a hypotensive effect.

Methyldopate Hydrochloride, USP. Methyldopate hydrochloride, L-3-(3,4-dihydroxyphenyl)-2-methylalanine ethyl ester hydrochloride (Aldomet ester hydrochloride), α-methyldopa, lowers blood pressure by inhibiting the outflow of sympathetic vasoconstrictor impulses from the brain. Early studies had suggested that the hypotensive action of α-methyldopa was a result of the peripheral properties of the drug as a decarboxylase inhibitor or a false transmitter.

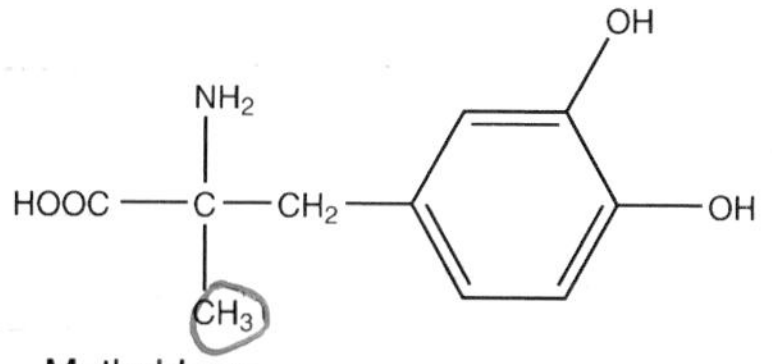

Methyldopa
(Aldomet)

The current hypothesis concerning the hypotensive activity of methyldopa involves the CNS as the site of action.[57] Methyldopa, on conversion to α-methylnorepinephrine, acts on α_2-adrenergic receptors to inhibit the release of norepinephrine, resulting in decreased sympathetic outflow from the CNS and activation of parasympathetic outflow.

Methyldopa is used as a step 2 agent and is recommended for patients with high blood pressure who are not responsive to diuretic therapy alone. Methyldopa, suitable for oral use, is a zwitterion and is not soluble enough for parenteral use. The problem was solved by making the ester, leaving the amine free to form the water-soluble hydrochloride salt. It is supplied as a stable, buffered solution, protected with antioxidants and chelating agents.

Clonidine Hydrochloride. Clonidine hydrochloride, 2-[(2,6-dichlorophenyl)imino]imidazolidine monohydrochloride (Catapres), was the first antihypertensive known to act on the CNS. It was synthesized in 1962 as a derivative of the known α-sympathomimetic drugs naphazoline and tolazoline, potential nasal vasoconstrictors, but instead it proved to be effective in the treatment of mild-to-severe hypertension.

Clonidine hydrochloride acts by both peripheral and central mechanisms in the body to affect blood pressure. It stimulates the peripheral α-adrenergic receptors to produce vasoconstriction, resulting in a brief period of hypertension. Clonidine hydrochloride acts centrally to inhibit the sympathetic tone and cause hypotension that is of much longer duration than the initial hypertensive effect. Administration of clonidine hydrochloride thus produces a biphasic change in blood pressure, beginning with a brief hypertensive effect and followed by a hypotensive effect that persists for about 4 hours. This biphasic response is altered by dose only. Larger doses produce a greater hypertensive effect and delay the onset of the hypotensive properties of the drug. Clonidine hydrochloride acts on α_2-adrenoreceptors located in the hindbrain to produce its hypotensive action. Clonidine hydrochloride also acts centrally to cause bradycardia and to reduce plasma levels of renin. Sensitization of baroreceptor pathways in the CNS appears to be responsible for the bradycardia transmitted by way of the vagus nerve. The central mechanism that results in decreased plasma renin is not known, however. The hypotensive properties of clonidine in animals can be blocked by applying α-adrenergic blocking agents directly to the brain.[58]

Clonidine hydrochloride has advantages over antihypertensive drugs such as guanethidine monosulfate and prazosin hydrochloride, in that it seldom produces orthostatic hypotensive side effects. It does, however, have some sedative properties that are undesirable; it also may cause constipation and dryness of the mouth.

Clonidine hydrochloride is distributed throughout the body, with the highest concentrations found in the organs of elimination: kidney, gut, and liver. Brain concentrations are low but higher than plasma concentrations. The high concentration in the gut is caused by an enterohepatic cycle in which clonidine hydrochloride is secreted into the bile in rather high concentrations. The half-life in humans is about 20 hours. Clonidine hydrochloride is metabolized by the body to form two major metabolites, *p*-hydroxyclonidine and its glucuronide. *p*-Hydroxyclonidine does not cross the blood-brain barrier and has no hypotensive effect in humans.

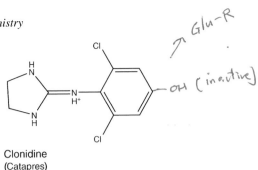

Clonidine
(Catapres)

Guanabenz Acetate. Guanabenz acetate, [(2,6-dichlorobenzylidene)amino]guanidine monoacetate (Wytensin), is a central α_2-adrenergic agonist that reduces the release of norepinephrine from the neuron when stimulated. The effect of the drug results in decreased sympathetic tone in the heart, kidneys, and peripheral blood vessels. The drug does not produce orthostatic hypotension.

Guanabenz
(Wytensin)

Guanfacine Hydrochloride. Guanfacine hydrochloride, N-(aminoiminomethyl)-2,6-dichlorobenzeneacetamide (Tenex), is structurally related to clonidine hydrochloride and guanabenz acetate and shares many of their pharmacological properties. The drug has a longer duration of action than either clonidine hydrochloride or guanabenz acetate. It lasts up to 24 hours. It also requires much longer (8–12 hours) for a peak effect to occur after the drug is administered.

Guanfacine
(Tenex)

VASODILATORY DRUGS ACTING ON SMOOTH MUSCLE

Reduction of arterial smooth muscle tone may occur by many mechanisms, such as reduction in sympathetic tone, stimulation of β-adrenergic receptors, or even direct action on the vasculature without interference from the autonomic innervation. Drugs acting on the arteriolar smooth muscle also increase sympathetic reflex activity, causing an increase in heart rate and cardiac output and stimulating renin release, which increases sodium retention and plasma volume. As a result, it is common to coadminister saluretics and β-adrenergic blocking drugs with these agents.

Antihypertensive agents that produce vasodilation of smooth muscle can be divided into two categories: direct-acting and indirect-acting vasodilators. Indirect-acting vasodilators may be distinguished from direct-acting vasodilators, in that they produce their effect by interfering with the vasoconstrictor stimuli, and their primary site of action is not necessarily the vascular smooth muscle itself. Indirect-acting vasodilators include sympatholytic drugs, such as reserpine; α-adrenergic antagonists, such as prazosin hydrochloride; ACE inhibitors; and angiotensin II receptor antagonists, such as saralysin. Direct-acting vasodilators include hydralazine hydrochloride, sodium nitroprusside, potassium channel openers, and calcium channel-blocking agents.[58]

Hydralazine Hydrochloride, USP. Hydralazine hydrochloride, 1-hydrazinophthalazine monohydrochloride (Apresoline hydrochloride), originated from the work of a chemist[59] attempting to produce some unusual chemical compounds and from the observation[60] that this compound had antihypertensive properties. It occurs as yellow crystals and is soluble in water to the extent of about 3%. A 2% aqueous solution has a pH of 3.5 to 4.5.

Hydralazine hydrochloride is useful in the treatment of moderate-to-severe hypertension. It is often used in conjunction with less potent antihypertensive agents, because side effects occur frequently when it is used alone in adequate doses. In combinations, it can be used in lower and safer doses. Its action appears to be centered on the smooth muscle of the vascular walls, with a decrease in peripheral resistance to blood flow. This results in increased blood flow through the peripheral blood vessels. It also has the unique property of increasing renal blood flow, an important consideration in patients with renal insufficiency.

Hydralazine hydrochloride acts on vascular smooth muscle to cause relaxation. Its mechanism of action is unclear. It interferes with Ca^{2+} entry and Ca^{2+} release from intracellular stores and reportedly causes activation of guanylate cyclase, resulting in increased levels of cGMP. All of these biochemical events can cause vasodilation.

Absorption of hydralazine hydrochloride taken orally is rapid and nearly complete. The maximal hypotensive effect is demonstrable within 1 hour. The drug is excreted rapidly by the kidneys, and within 24 hours, 75% of the total amount administered appears in the urine as metabolites or unchanged drug. Hydralazine hydrochloride undergoes benzylic oxidation, glucuronide formation, and *N*-acetylation by the microsomal enzymes in the tissues (Fig. 19.15). Acetylation appears to be a major determinant of the rate of hepatic removal of the drug from the blood and, therefore, of systemic availability.[61] Rapid acetylation results in a highly hepatic extraction ratio from blood and greater first-pass elimination.

Hydralazine hydrochloride is more effective clinically when coadministered with drugs that antagonize adrenergic transmission (e.g., β-adrenergic antagonists, reserpine, guanethidine monosulfate, methyldopa, and clonidine hydrochloride). When given with diuretics, it is useful in the treatment of CHF.

Hydralazine hydrochloride is marketed as a combination therapy with isosorbide under the trade name BiDil specifically for African Americans with CHF.

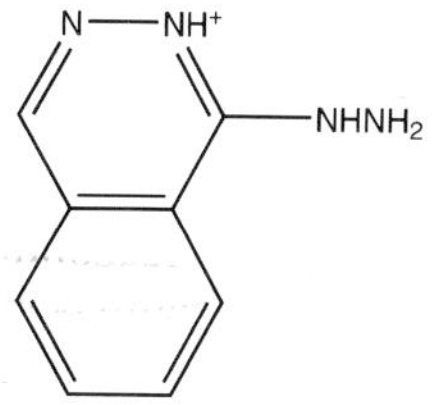

Hydralazine
(Apresoline)

Sodium Nitroprusside, USP. Sodium nitroprusside, sodium nitroferricyanide, disodium pentacyanonitrosylferrate(2) $Na_2[Fe(CN)_5NO]$ (Nipride, Nitropress), is one of the most potent blood pressure–lowering drugs. Its use is limited to hypertensive emergencies because of its short duration of action. The effectiveness of sodium nitroprusside as an antihypertensive has been known since 1928, but not until 1955 was its efficacy as a drug established.[62] The drug differs from other vasodilators, in that vasodilation occurs in both venous and arterial vascular beds. Sodium nitroprusside is a reddish brown water-soluble powder that is decomposed by light when in solution. The hypotensive effect of the chemical is a result of the formation of NO in situ (discussed under the heading, "Nitrovasodilators"), elevating cellular levels of cGMP. Sodium nitroprusside is metabolized by the liver, yielding thiocyanate. Because thiocyanate is excreted by the kidneys, patients with impaired renal function may suffer thiocyanate toxicity.

$$Na_2[Fe(CN)_5NO] \cdot 2H_2O$$

Sodium Nitroprusside
(Nipride)
(Nitropress)

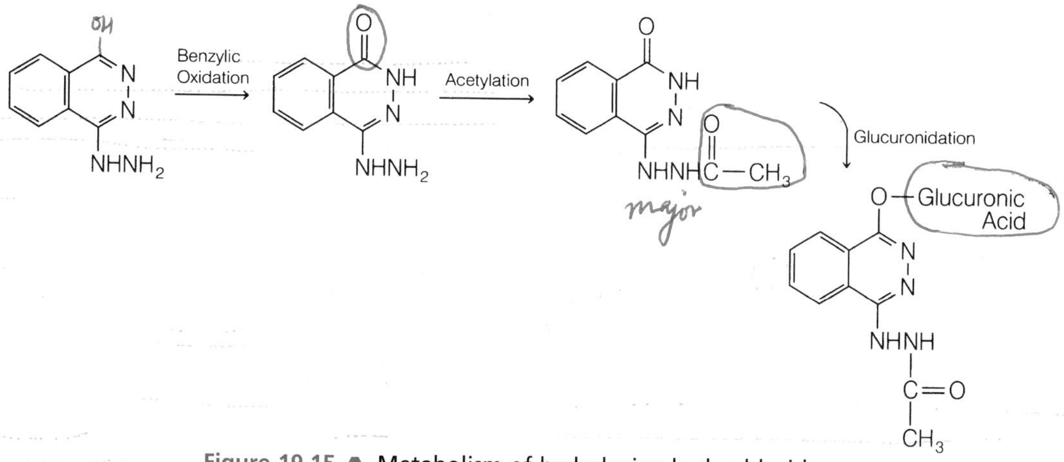

Figure 19.15 ● Metabolism of hydralazine hydrochloride.

PHOSPHODIESTERASE TYPE 5 INHIBITORS

As discussed throughout this chapter, the cyclic nucleotide phosphodiesterases constitute a group of enzymes that catalyze the hydrolysis of various cyclic nucleotides including cAMP and cGMP. The contractility of all muscle types is regulated primarily by reversible phosphorylation of the protein myosin. The phosphorylation of myosin allows it to interact with actin, which results in muscle contraction. Through different mechanisms, cAMP and cGMP interfere with the ability of myosin to be phosporylated and/or interact with actin. This, in turn, results in muscle relaxation. Agents that interfere with the degradation of the cyclic nucleotide have usefulness in treating hypertension, erectile dysfunction, etc. Phosphodiesterase type 5 (PDE5) is responsible for the catalytic hydrolysis of cGMP in the smooth muscle of the arteries in the penis and lungs. Inhibitors of this particular phosphodiesterase have been shown to relax arteries in the penis, thus allowing the corpus cavernosum to fill with blood and aiding in an erection.[63]

PRODUCTS

Silenafil Citrate. Sildenafil, 1-[4-ethoxy-3-(6,7-dihydro-1-methyl-7-oxo-3-propyl-1H-pyrazolo[4,3-d]pyrimidin-5-yl)-phenylsulfonyl]-4-methylpiperazine citrate (Viagra), is a potent inhibitor of PDE5. It was initially studied for use in hypertension and angina pectoris because of its ability to increase intracellular levels of cyclic nucleotides. However, during phase I clinical trials, it was noted that the drug had little effect on angina and was unpredictable in managing hypertension. However, patients noted that there were improved effects in their sexual dysfunction. Therefore, the manufacturer decided to develop the investigational compound for treating erectile dysfunction, rather than for angina or hypertension. In March 1998, the FDA approved the drug for use in erectile dysfunction, becoming the first oral agent approved to treat erectile dysfunction in the United States. Within a year, it soon had annual sales exceeding $1 billion per year. The chemical structure of sildenafil is similar to that of cGMP and acts as a competitive binding agent of PDE5.

Sildenafil is also effective in the rare disease, PAH (presented earlier in this chapter under "Endothelin Receptor Antagonist"). By increasing cycli nucleotide levels, it relaxes the arterial wall, leading to decreased pulmonary arterial resistance and pressure. As a result of the selective distribution of PDE-5 within the arterial smooth muscle of the lungs and penis, sildenafil acts selectively in these areas. In June 2005, the FDA approved sildenafil (Revatio) for the management of PAH. To avoid confusion with its use in either PAH or erectile dysfunction, the product used for erectile dysfunction is a blue oval tablet, whereas the product used for management of PAH is a round white tablet.[63]

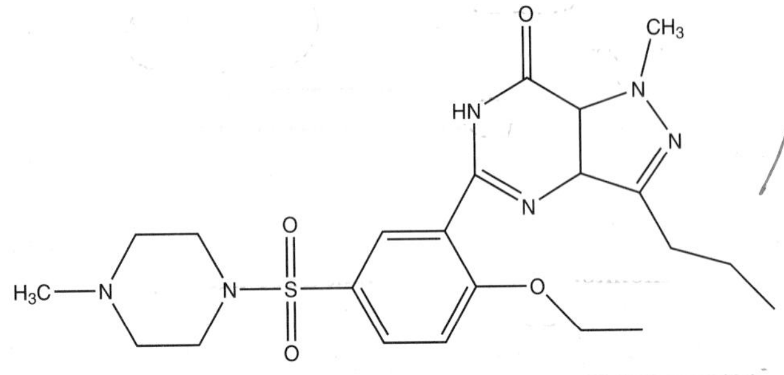

Sildenafil

Vardenafil Hydrochloride. Vardenafil, 4-[2-ethoxy-5-(4-ethylpiperazin-1-yl)sulfonyl-phenyl]-9-methyl-7-propyl-3,5,6,8-tetrazabicyclo[4.3.0]nona-3,7,9-trien-2-one (Levitra), was the second PDE5 introduced in the U.S. market. The metabolism of vardenafil is primarily by CYP3A4. As such, concomitant use of CYP3A4 inhibitors such as ritonavir, indinavir, ketoconazole, as well as moderate CYP3A inhibitors such as erythromycin typically results in significant increases of plasma levels of vardenafil.

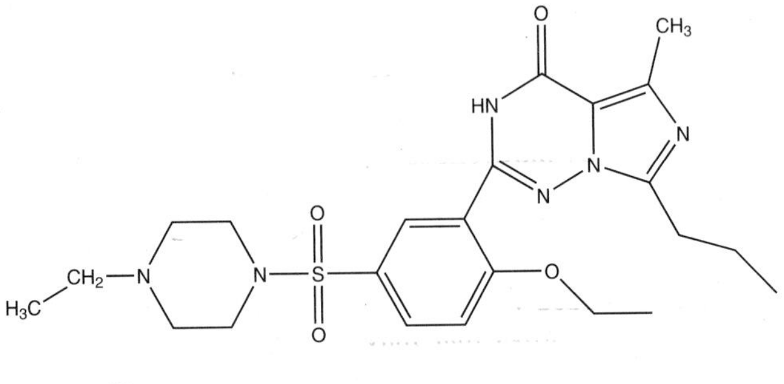

Vardenafil

Tadalafil. Tadalafil, (6R-trans)-6-(1,3-benzodioxol-5-yl)-2,3,6,7,12,12a-hexahydro-2-methyl-pyrazino[1′, 2′:1,6]pyrido[3,4-b]indole-1,4-dione (Cialis), is a potent PDE5 inhibitor. It received FDA approval for the treatment of erectile dysfunction in December 2003. Because of its half-life of 17.5 hours, it is marketed as a 36-hour treatment. Tadalafil is predominantly metabolized by hepatic enzymes, including CYP3A4. The concomitant use of CYP3A4 inhibitors such as ritonavir, indinavir, ketoconazole, as well as moderate CYP3A inhibitors such as erythromycin have been shown to result in significant increases in tadalafil plasma levels. Much like sildenafil, tadalafil is under clinical investigation for managing PAH.[64]

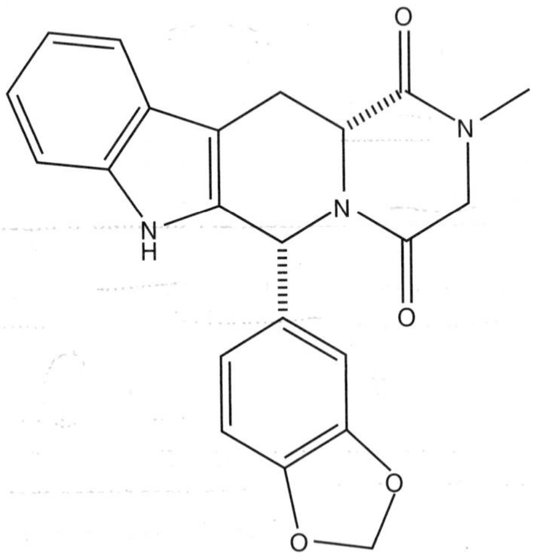

Tadalafil

POTASSIUM CHANNEL AGONISTS

The two agents that can be classified in this category are diazoxide and minoxidil. These drugs are also called *potassium channel openers*. These agents activate ATP-sensitive potassium channels, which leads to a decrease of intracellular Ca^{2+} and reduces the excitability of smooth muscle. The primary action of these drugs is to open potassium channels in the plasma membrane of vascular smooth muscle. An efflux of potassium from the cell follows, resulting in hyperpolarization of the membrane, which produces an inhibitory influence on membrane excitation and subsequent vasodilation.

***Diazoxide*, USP.** Diazoxide is used as the sodium salt of 7-chloro-3-methyl-2*H*-1,2,4-benzothiadiazine 1,1-dioxide (Hyperstat IV). Diazoxide lowers peripheral vascular resistance, increases cardiac output, and does not compromise renal blood flow.

This is a des-sulfamoyl analog of the benzothiazine diuretics and has a close structural similarity to chlorothiazide. It was developed intentionally to increase the antihypertensive action of the thiazides and to minimize the diuretic effect.

It is used by intravenous injection as a rapidly acting antihypertensive agent for emergency reduction of blood pressure in hospitalized patients with accelerated or malignant hypertension. More than 90% is bound to serum protein, and caution is needed when it is used in conjunction with other protein-bound drugs that may be displaced by diazoxide. The injection is given rapidly by the intravenous route to ensure maximal effect. The initial dose is usually 1 mg/kg of body weight, with a second dose given if the first injection does not lower blood pressure satisfactorily within 30 minutes. Further doses may be given at 4- to 24-hour intervals if needed. Oral antihypertensive therapy is begun as soon as possible.

The injection has a pH of about 11.5, which is necessary to convert the drug to its soluble sodium salt. There is no significant chemical decomposition after storage at room temperature for 2 years. When the solution is exposed to light, it darkens.

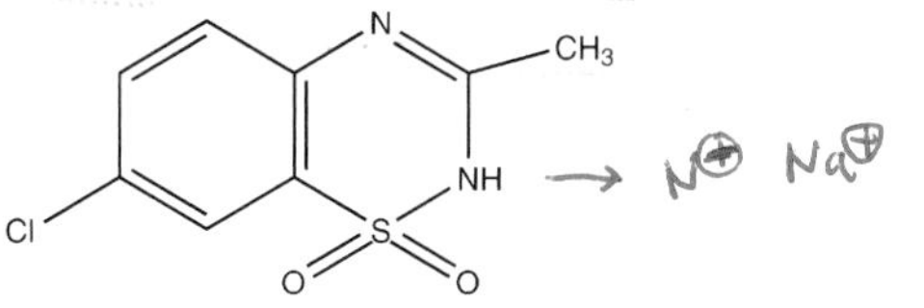

Diazoxide
(Hyperstat)

***Minoxidil*, USP.** Minoxidil, 2,4-diamino-6-piperidinopyrimidine-3-oxide (Loniten), was developed as a result of isosteric replacement of a triaminotriazine moiety by triaminopyrimidine. The triaminotriazines were initially observed to be potent vasodilators in cats and dogs, following their formation of *N*-oxides in these animals. The triazines were inactive in humans because of their inability to form *N*-oxide metabolites; this led to the discovery of minoxidil. Minoxidil is the only direct-acting vasodilator that requires metabolic activation to produce its antihypertensive effect (Fig. 19.16). It is converted to minoxidil sulfate in the liver by a sulfotransferase enzyme.[65]

The antihypertensive properties of minoxidil are similar to those of hydralazine hydrochloride, in that minoxidil can decrease arteriolar vascular resistance. Minoxidil exerts its vasodilatory action by a direct effect on arteriolar smooth muscle and appears to have no effect on the CNS or on the adrenergic nervous system in animals.[66] The serum half-life is 4.5 hours, and the antihypertensive effect may last up to 24 hours.

Minoxidil is used for severe hypertension that is difficult to control with other antihypertensive agents. The drug has

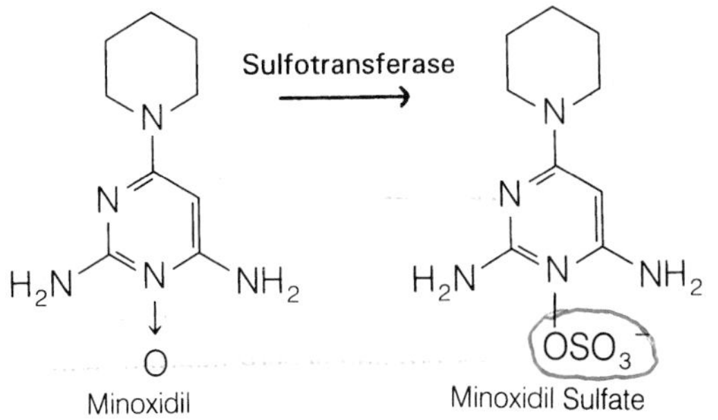

Figure 19.16 ● Activation of minoxidil.

some of the characteristic side effects of direct vasodilatory drugs. It causes sodium and water retention and may require coadministration of a diuretic. Minoxidil also causes reflex tachycardia, which can be controlled by use of a β-adrenergic blocking agent.

Minoxidil topical solution is used to treat alopecia androgenitica (male-pattern baldness). Although the mechanism is not clearly understood, topical minoxidil is believed to increase cutaneous blood flow, which may stimulate hair growth. The stimulation of hair growth is attributed to vasodilation in the vicinity of application of the drug, resulting in better nourishment of the local hair follicles.

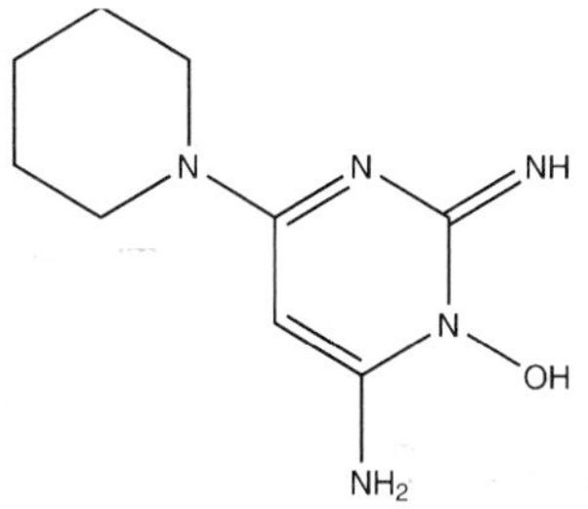

Minoxidil
(Loniten)

POSITIVE INOTROPIC AGENTS

Agents that successfully increase the force of contraction of the heart may be particularly useful in the treatment of CHF. In CHF, the heart cannot maintain sufficient blood flow to various organs to provide oxygen-rich blood. Agents that increase the force of contraction allow greater amounts of blood to be distributed throughout the body and, in turn, reduce the symptoms associated with CHF. Most of the positive inotropic agents exhibit their effects on the force of contraction by modifying the coupling mechanism involved in the myocardial contractile process.

Digitalis glycosides, a mixture of products isolated from foxglove, *Digitalis* spp., were first used as a heart medication as early as 1500 BC when in the *Ebers Papyrus*, the ancient Egyptians reported their success in using these products. Throughout history, these plant extracts have also been used as arrow poisons, emetics, and diuretics. The dichotomy of the poisonous effects and the beneficial heart properties is still evident today. Cardiac glycosides are still used today in the treatment of CHF and atrial fibrillation, with careful attention paid in monitoring the toxicity that these agents possess.

The cardiac glycosides include two distinct classes of compounds—the cardenolides and the bufadienolides. These differ in the substitutions at the C-17 position, where the cardenolides possess an unsaturated butyrolactone ring, whereas the bufadienolides have an α-pyrone ring. Pharmacologically, both have similar properties and are found in many of the same natural sources, including plant and toad species. By far, the most important sources include *Digitalis purpurea* and *Digitalis lanata*. In 1785, William Withering published *An Account of the Foxglove and Its Medical Uses: With Practical Remarks on Dropsy and Other Diseases*, in which he describes the beneficial use of foxglove in dropsy (edema), which often exists in CHF.

Even with recent advances in synthetic organic chemistry coupled with the use of combinatorial chemistry, no new therapeutics have displaced the cardiac glycosides. Furthermore, the perennial use of these agents over many centuries is even more remarkable when one considers the useful life of a "blockbuster" drug in today's marketplace. This remarkable fact is based, quite simply, on the unique ability of nature to produce extraordinarily bioactive substances, which characteristically possess both a lipophilic portion in the steroidal ring and a hydrophilic moiety in the glycosidic rings. The therapeutic use of these agents depends largely on a balance between the different solubility characteristics of the steroid structure, and the type and number of sugar units attached to it. Although the fundamental pharmacological properties reside with the steroidal nucleus, the sugars play a critical role in the biological effects elicited, because they increase the water solubility of the lipid system, making them more available for translocation in an aqueous environment and, at the same time, allowing transportation across fatty sites. These properties uniquely balance each other and allow successful translocation to the receptive sites in the body. Ultimately, the lipophilic steroid also plays a specific role in the agent's onset and duration of action. As the steroidal rings are modified with polar groups (e.g., hydroxyls), the onset increases, and the duration of action decreases. The sugar residues are substituted on C-3 of the steroid and generally are digitoxose, glucose, rhamnose, or cymarose.

The cardiac glycosides elicit their effects through inhibition of the Na^+/K^+-ATPase pump. Inhibition of this pump increases the intracellular Na^+ concentration, which affects Na^+/Ca^{2+} exchange. This increases intracellular concentrations of Ca^{2+}, which is available to activate the contractile proteins actin and myosin, thereby enhancing the force of contraction. Also, it is suggested that these agents have other compensatory mechanisms including baroreceptor sensitivity, which result in improved conditions for patients suffering from CHF.

Digoxin. Digoxin (Lanoxin) is a purified digitalis preparation from *D. lanata* and represents the most widely used digitalis glycoside. This wide use is primarily a result of its fast onset and short half-life. Position 3 of the steroid is substituted with three digitoxose residues that, when removed, provide a genin or aglycone steroid that is still capable of receptor binding but with altered pharmacokinetics.

Digitalis. Digitalis (Crystodigin) is isolated from *D. lanata* and *D. purpurea* among other *Digitalis* spp., and is the chief active glycoside in digitalis leaf, with 1 mg digitoxin equal to 1 g of digitalis leaf therapy. In patients who miss doses, digitalis is very useful for maintenance therapy because of the longer half-life it provides. The longer duration and increased half-life are a result of the lack of the C-12 hydroxy that is present in digoxin. In digoxin, this hydroxy plays two roles: (a) it serves as a site for metabolism, which

reduces the compound's half-life; and (b) it gives more hydrophilic character, which results in greater water solubility and ease in renal elimination.

Amrinone. During normal heart function, cAMP performs important roles in regulating intracellular calcium levels. That is, certain calcium channels and storage sites for calcium must be activated by cAMP-dependant protein kinases. Because cAMP plays an indirect role in the contractility process, agents that inhibit its degradation will provide more calcium for cardiac contraction. One phosphodiesterase enzyme that is involved in the hydrolysis of myocardium cAMP is F-III. Amrinone, 5-amino (3,4'-dipyridin)-6 1

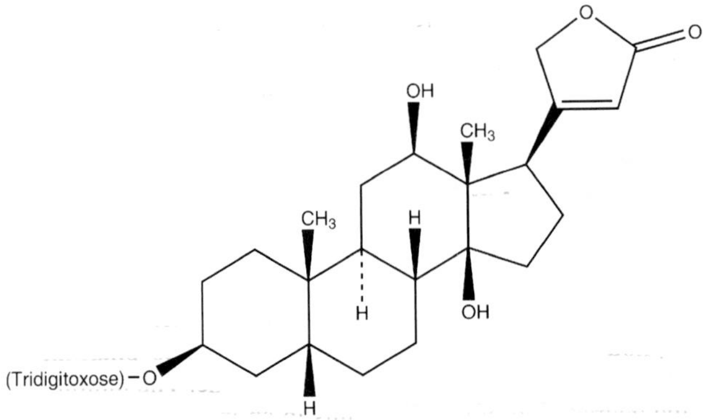

Digoxin
(Lanoxin)

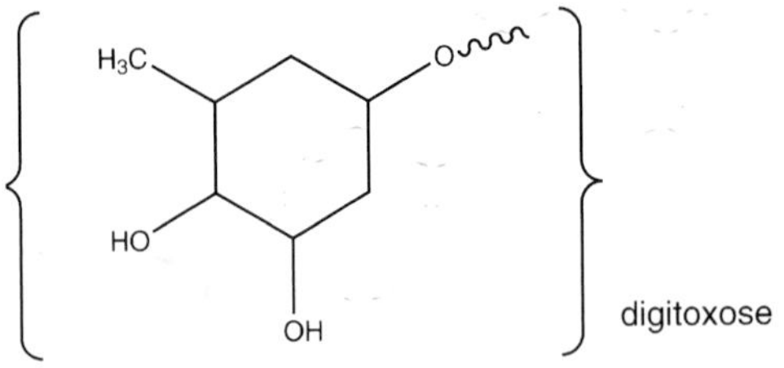

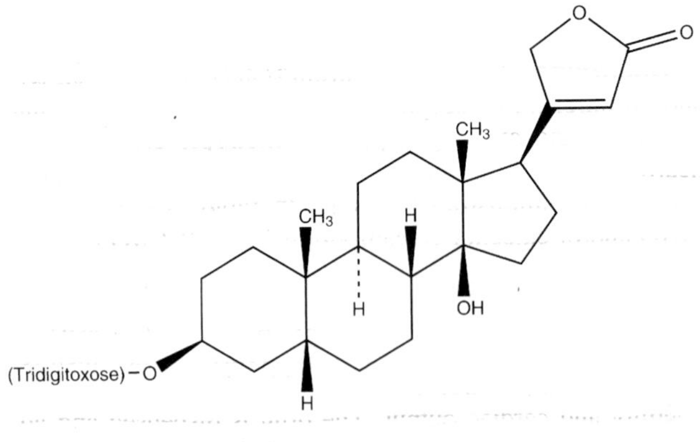

Digitalis
(Crystodigin)

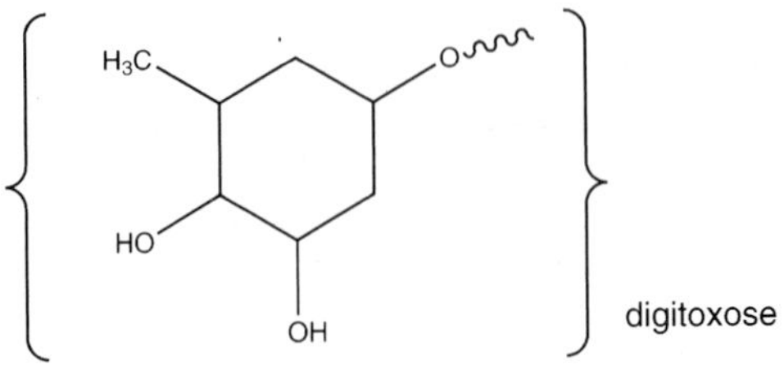

(*H*)-one (Inocor), possesses positive isotropic effects as a result of its ability to inhibit this phosphodiesterase. In 1999, the *USP* Nomenclature Committee and the United States Adopted Names (USAN) Council approved changing the nonproprietary name and the current official monograph title of amrinone to inamrinone. This change in nomenclature was a result of amrinone being confused with amiodarone because of the similarity of the names. This was reported to cause confusion between the products that led to medication errors, some of which resulted in serious injury or death.

Amrinone
(Inocor)

Milrinone. Milrinone, 1,6-dihydro-2-methyl-6-oxo-3,4′-bipyridine-5-carbonitrile (Primacor), is another dipyridine phosphodiesterase F-III inhibitor that possesses pharmacological properties similar to those of amrinone. The inhibition of the degradation of cAMP results in an increase in the cardiac muscle's force of contraction.

Milrinone
(Primacor)

Dopamine. Dopamine (Intropin) acts primarily on α_1- and β_1-adrenergic receptors, increasing systemic vascular resistance and exerting a positive inotropic effect on the heart. It must be administered by an intravenous route, because oral administration results in rapid metabolism by MAO and/or catechol-*O*-methyltransferase (COMT).

Dobutamine. Dobutamine (Dobutex) is a sympathomimetic drug that is a β_1-adrenergic agonist with α_1-activity. It is primarily used in cases of cardiogenic shock, which result from its β_1-inotropic effects, which increase heart contractility and cardiac output. The drug is dispensed and administered as a racemic mixture consisting of both (+) and (−) isomers. The (+) isomer is a potent β_1-agonist, whereas the (−) isomer is an α_1-agonist.

P647 - 654

ANTIHYPERLIPIDEMIC AGENTS

The major cause of death in the Western world today is vascular disease, of which the most prevalent form is atherosclerotic heart disease. Although many causative factors of this disease are recognized (e.g., smoking, stress, diet),

atherosclerotic disease can be treated through medication or surgery.

Hyperlipidemia is the most prevalent indicator for susceptibility to atherosclerotic heart disease; it is a term used to describe elevated plasma levels of lipids that are usually in the form of lipoproteins. Hyperlipidemia may be caused by an underlying disease involving the liver, kidney, pancreas, or thyroid, or it may not be attributed to any recognizable disease. In recent years, lipids have been implicated in the development of atherosclerosis in humans. *Atherosclerosis* may be defined as degenerative changes in the intima of medium and large arteries. This degeneration includes the accumulation of lipids, complex carbohydrates, blood, and blood products and is accompanied by the formation of fibrous tissue and calcium deposition on the intima of the blood vessels. These deposits or *plaques* decrease the lumen of the artery, reduce its elasticity, and may create foci for thrombi and subsequent occlusion of the blood vessel.

Lipoprotein Classes

Lipoproteins are macromolecules consisting of lipid substances (cholesterol, triglycerides) noncovalently bound with protein and carbohydrate. These combinations solubilize the lipids and prevent them from forming insoluble aggregates in the plasma. They have a spherical shape and consist of a nonpolar core surrounded by a monolayer of phospholipids whose polar groups are oriented toward the lipid phase of the plasma. Included in the phospholipid monolayer are a small number of cholesterol molecules and proteins termed *apolipoproteins*. The apolipoproteins appear to be able to solubilize lipids for transport in an aqueous surrounding such as plasma (Fig. 19.17).

The various lipoproteins found in plasma can be separated by ultracentrifugal techniques into chylomicrons, very–low-density lipoprotein (VLDL), intermediate-density lipoprotein (IDL), low-density lipoprotein (LDL), and high-density lipoprotein (HDL). These correlate with the electrophoretic separations of the lipoproteins as follows: chylomicrons, pre–β-lipoprotein (VLDL), broad

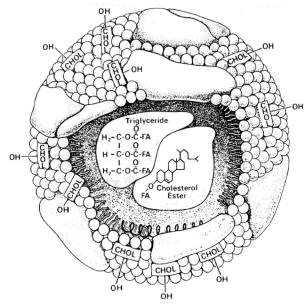

Figure 19.17 ● **Hypothetical model of lipoprotein particle.**

β-lipoprotein (IDL), β-lipoprotein (LDL), and α-lipoprotein (HDL).

Chylomicrons contain 90% triglycerides by weight and originate from exogenous fat from the diet. They are the least dense of the lipoproteins and migrate the least under the influence of an electric current. Chylomicrons are normally absent in plasma after 12 to 24 hours of fasting. The VLDL is composed of about 60% triglycerides, 12% cholesterol, and 18% phospholipids. It originates in the liver from FFAs. Although VLDL can be isolated from plasma, it is catabolized rapidly into IDL, which is degraded further into LDL. Normally, IDL also is catabolized rapidly to LDL, but it is usually not isolated from plasma. The LDL consists of 50% cholesterol and 10% triglycerides. This is the major cholesterol-carrying protein. In normal persons, this lipoprotein accounts for about 65% of the plasma cholesterol and is of major concern in hyperlipidemic disease states. The LDL is formed from the intravascular catabolism of VLDL. The HDL is composed of 25% cholesterol and 50% protein and accounts for about 17% of the total cholesterol in plasma.

Lipoprotein Metabolism

The rate at which cholesterol and triglycerides enter the circulation from the liver and small intestine depends on the supply of the lipid and proteins necessary to form the lipoprotein complexes. Although the protein component must be synthesized, the lipids can be obtained either from de novo biosynthesis in the tissues or from the diet. Reduction of plasma lipids by diet can delay the development of atherosclerosis. Furthermore, the use of drugs that decrease assimilation of lipids into the body plus diet decreases mortality from cardiovascular disease.[67]

The lipid transport mechanisms that exists shuttle cholesterol and triglycerides among the liver, intestine, and other tissues. Normally, plasma lipids, including lipoprotein cholesterol, are cycled in and out of plasma and do not cause extensive accumulation of deposits in the walls of arteries. Genetic factors and changes in hormone levels affect lipid transport by altering enzyme concentrations and apoprotein content, as well as the number and activity of lipoprotein receptors. This complex relationship makes the treatment of all hyperlipoproteinemias by a singular approach difficult, if not impractical.

Lipids are transported by both *exogenous* and *endogenous* pathways. In the exogenous pathway, dietary fat (triglycerides and cholesterol) is incorporated into large lipoprotein particles (chylomicrons), which enter the lymphatic system and are then passed into the plasma. The chylomicrons are acted on by lipoprotein lipase in the adipose tissue capillaries, forming triglycerides and monoglycerides. The FFAs cross the endothelial membrane of the capillary and are incorporated into triglycerides in the tissue for storage as fat or are used for energy by oxidative metabolism. The chylomicron remnant in the capillary reaches the liver and is cleared from the circulation by binding to a receptor that recognizes the apoprotein E and B-48 protein components of the chylomicron remnant.

In the endogenous pathway of lipid transport, lipids are secreted from the liver. These are triglycerides and cholesterol combined with apoprotein B-100 and apoprotein E to form VLDL. The VLDL is acted on by lipoprotein lipase in the capillaries of adipose tissue to generate FFAs and an IDL.

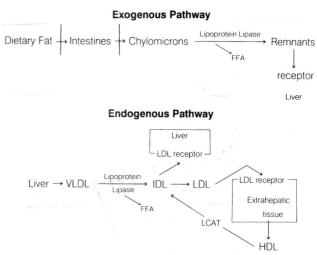

Figure 19.18 ● Exogenous and endogenous pathways of lipoprotein metabolism.

Some IDL binds to LDL receptors in the liver and is cleared from plasma by endocytosis. Approximately half of the circulating IDL is converted to LDL in the plasma by additional loss of triglycerides. This LDL has a half-life in plasma of about 1.5 days and represents 60% to 70% of the cholesterol in plasma. These LDL particles bind to LDL receptors in extrahepatic tissues and are removed from the plasma. Levels of LDL receptors vary depending on the need of extrahepatic tissues to bind LDL to use cholesterol. The extrahepatic tissue subsequently releases HDL. Free plasma cholesterol can be adsorbed onto HDL and the cholesterol esters formed by the enzyme lecithin–cholesterol acyltransferase (LCAT). These esters are transferred from HDL to VLDL or LDL in plasma to complete the cycle. The pathways for plasma lipoprotein metabolism by the exogenous and endogenous routes are shown in Figure 19.18.

Hyperlipoproteinemias

Lipid disorders are related to problems of lipoprotein metabolism[68] that create conditions of hyperlipoproteinemia. The hyperlipoproteinemias have been classified into six types, each of which is treated differently (Table 19.5).

The abnormal lipoprotein pattern characteristic of type I is caused by a decrease in the activity of lipoprotein lipase, an enzyme that normally hydrolyzes the triglycerides present in chylomicrons and clears the plasma of this lipoprotein fraction. Because the triglycerides found in chylomicrons come primarily from exogenous sources, this type of hyperlipoproteinemia may be treated by decreasing the intake of dietary fat. There are no drugs at present that can be used to counteract type I hyperlipidemia effectively.

Type II hyperlipoproteinemia has been divided into types IIa and IIb. Type IIa is characterized by elevated levels of LDL (β-lipoproteins) and normal levels of triglycerides. This subtype disorder is very common and may be caused by disturbed catabolism of LDL. Type IIb differs from type IIa, in that this hyperlipidemia has elevated VLDL levels in addition to LDL levels. Type II hyperlipoproteinemia is often clearly familial and frequently inherited as an autosomal dominant abnormality with complete penetrance and expression in infancy. Patients have been treated by use of dietary restrictions on cholesterol and saturated fats. This

TABLE 19.5   Characterization of Hyperlipoproteinemia Types

| Hyperlipo-proteinemia | Abnormality | | Appearance of Plasma[a] | Total Triglycerides | Cholesterol |
	Electrophoresis	Ultracentrifuge			
I	Massive chylomicronemia	Clear; creamy layer of chylomicronemia on top	Massively elevated	Slightly to moderately elevated	
IIa	β-Lipoproteins elevated	LDL increased	Clear	Normal	Heavily elevated
IIb	Pre–β-lipoproteins elevated	LDL + VLDL increased	Slightly turbid	Slightly elevated	Heavily elevated
III	Broad β-lipoprotein band	VLDL/LDL of abnormal composition	Slightly turbid to turbid	Elevated	Elevated
IV	Pre–β-lipoproteins elevated	VLDL increased	Turbid	Moderately to heavily elevated	Normal to elevated
V	Pre–β-lipoproteins elevated; chylomicronemia	VLDL increased; chylomicronemia	Turbid; on top, chylomicronemia	Massively elevated	Slightly elevated

Adapted from Witte, E. C.: Prog. Med. Chem. 11:199, 1975.
[a]After having been kept standing at 4°C for 25 hours.

type of hyperlipoproteinemia responds to some form of chemotherapy. The combined therapy may bring LDL levels back to normal.

Type III is a rare disorder characterized by a broad band of β-lipoprotein. Like type II, it is also familial. Patients respond favorably to diet and drug therapy.

In type IV hyperlipoproteinemia, levels of VLDL are elevated. Because this type of lipoprotein is rich in triglycerides, plasma triglyceride levels are elevated. The metabolic defect that causes type IV is still unknown; this form of hyperlipidemia, however, responds to diet and drug therapy.

Type V hyperlipoproteinemia has high levels of chylomicrons and VLDL, resulting in high levels of plasma triglycerides. The biochemical defect of type V hyperlipoproteinemia is not understood. Clearance of dietary fat is impaired, and reduction of dietary fat is indicated along with drug therapy.

Clofibrate, USP. Clofibrate, ethyl 2-(p-chlorophenoxy)-2-methylpropionate (Atromid-S), is a stable, colorless to pale yellow liquid with a faint odor and a characteristic taste. It is soluble in organic solvents but insoluble in water.

Clofibrate is prepared by a Williamson synthesis, condensing p-chlorophenol with ethyl α-bromoisobutyrate, or by the interaction of a mixture of acetone, p-chlorophenol, and chloroform in the presence of excess potassium hydroxide. The acid obtained by either of these methods is esterified to give clofibrate. Both acid and ester are active; the latter, however, is preferred for medicinal use. Clofibrate is hydrolyzed rapidly to 2-p-chlorophenoxy-2-methylpropionic acid by esterases in vivo and, bound to serum albumin, circulates in blood. The acid has been investigated as a hypolipidemic agent. It is absorbed more slowly and to a smaller extent than is the ester. The aluminum salt of the acid gives even lower blood levels than p-chlorophenoxy-2-methylpropionic acid.[69]

Clofibrate is the drug of choice in the treatment of type III hyperlipoproteinemias and may also be useful, to a lesser extent, in types IIb and IV hyperlipoproteinemias. The drug is not effective in types I and IIa.

Clofibrate can lower plasma concentrations of both triglycerides and cholesterol, but it has a more consistent clinical effect on triglycerides. It also affects lipoprotein plasma levels by enhancing removal of triglycerides from the circulation and causes reduction of VLDL by stimulating lipoprotein lipase to increase the catabolism of this lipoprotein to LDL.[70] Clofibrate lowers triglyceride levels in the serum much more than cholesterol levels and decreases levels of FFAs and phospholipids. The lowering of cholesterol levels may result from more than one mechanism. Clofibrate inhibits the incorporation of acetate into the synthesis of cholesterol, between the acetate and mevalonate step, by inhibiting sn-glyceryl-3-phosphate acyltransferase. Clofibrate also regulates cholesterol synthesis in the liver by inhibiting microsomal reduction of 3-hydroxy-3-methylglutaryl-CoA (HMG-CoA), catalyzed by HMG-CoA reductase. Clofibrate may lower plasma lipids by means other than impairment of cholesterol biosynthesis, such as increasing excretion through the biliary tract.

Clofibrate is tolerated well by most patients; the most common side effects are nausea and, to a smaller extent, other gastrointestinal distress. The dosage of anticoagulants, if used in conjunction with this drug, should be reduced by one third to one half, depending on the individual response, so that the prothrombin time may be kept within the desired limits.

Clofibrate
(Atromid)

Gemfibrozil. Gemfibrozil, 5-(2,5-dimethylphenoxy)-2,2-dimethylpentanoic acid (Lopid), is a congener of clofibrate that was used first in the treatment of hyperlipoproteinemia in the mid-1970s. Its mechanism of action and use are similar to those of clofibrate. Gemfibrozil reduces plasma levels of VLDL triglycerides and stimulates clearance of VLDL from plasma. The drug has little effect on cholesterol plasma levels but does cause an increase of HDL.

Gemfibrozil is absorbed quickly from the gut and excreted unchanged in the urine. The drug has a plasma half-life of 1.5 hours, but reduction of plasma VLDL concentration takes between 2 and 5 days to become evident. The peak effect of its hypolipidemic action may take up to 4 weeks to become manifest.

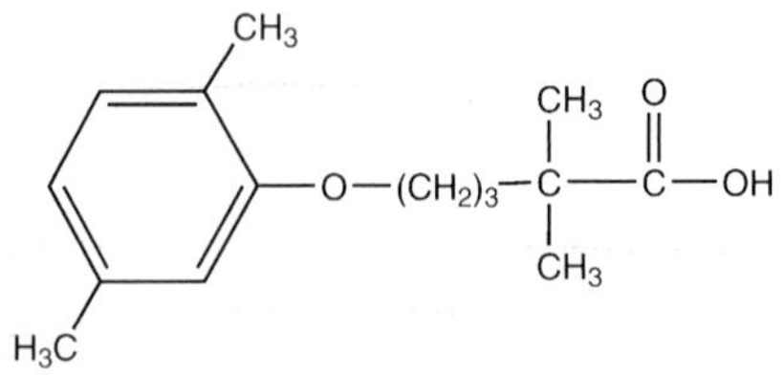

Gemfibrozil
(Lopid)

Fenofibrate. Fenofibrate, 2-[4-(4-chlorobenzoyl)phenoxy]-2-methylpropanoic acid 1-methylethyl ester (Tricor), has structural features represented in clofibrate. The primary difference involves the second aromatic ring. This imparts a greater lipophilic character than exists in clofibrate, resulting in a much more potent hypocholesterolemic and triglyceride-lowering agent. Also, this structural modification results in a lower dose requirement than with clofibrate or gemfibrozil.

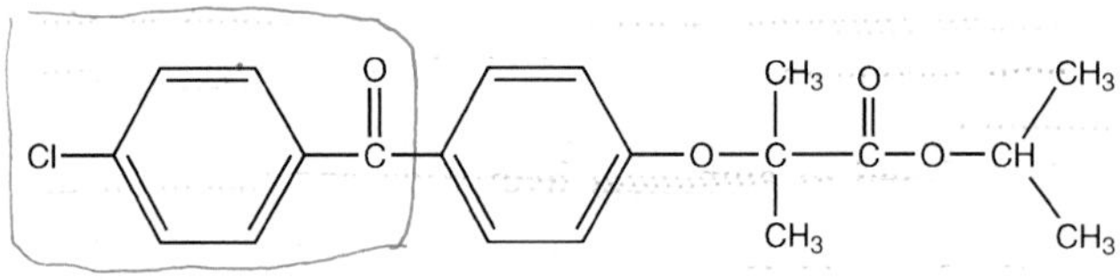

Fenofibrate
(Tricor)

Dextrothyroxine Sodium, USP. Dextrothyroxine sodium, *O*-(4-hydroxy-3,5-diiodophenyl)-3,5-diiodo-D-tyrosine monosodium salt hydrate, sodium D-3,3′,5,5′-tetraiodothyronine (Choloxin), occurs as a light yellow to buff powder. It is stable in dry air but discolors on exposure to light; hence, it should be stored in light-resistant containers. It is very slightly soluble in water, slightly soluble in alcohol, and insoluble in acetone, chloroform, and ether.

The hormones secreted by the thyroid gland have marked hypocholesterolemic activity along with their other well-known actions. The finding that not all active thyroid principles possessed the same degree of physiological actions led to a search for congeners that would cause a decrease in serum cholesterol levels without other effects such as angina pectoris, palpitation, and congestive failure. D-Thyroxine resulted from this search. At the dosage required, however, L-thyroxine contamination must be minimal; otherwise, it will exert its characteristic actions. One route to optically pure (at least 99% pure) D-thyroxine is the use of an L-amino acid oxidase from snake venom, which acts only on the L-isomer and makes separation possible.

The mechanism of action of D-thyroxine appears to be stimulation of oxidative catabolism of cholesterol in the liver through stimulation of 7-α-cholesterol hydroxylase, the rate-limiting enzyme in the conversion of cholesterol to bile acids. The bile acids are conjugated with glycine or taurine and excreted by the biliary route into the feces. Although thyroxine does not inhibit cholesterol biosynthesis, it increases the number of LDL receptors, enhancing removal of LDL from plasma.

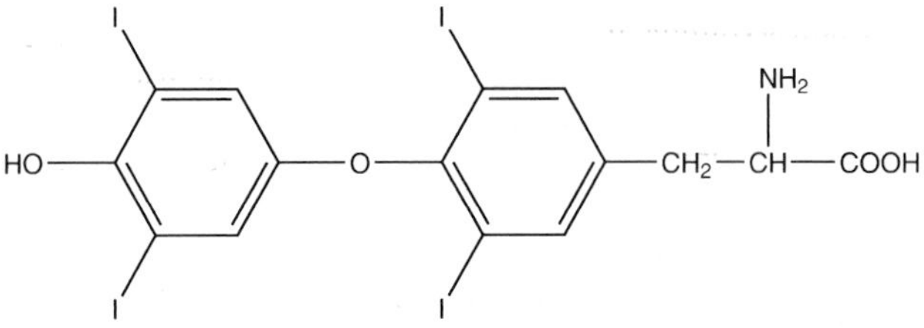

Dextrothyroxine
(Choloxin)

Use of thyroxine in the treatment of hyperlipidemias is not without adverse effects. The drug increases the frequency and severity of anginal attacks and may cause cardiac arrhythmias.

D-Thyroxine potentiates the action of anticoagulants such as warfarin or dicumarol; thus, the dosage of the anticoagulants used concurrently should be reduced by one third and then, if necessary, further modified to maintain the prothrombin time within the desired limits. Also, it may increase the dosage requirements for insulin or oral hypoglycemic agents if used concurrently with them.

Cholestyramine Resin, USP. Cholestyramine (Cuemid, Questran) is the chloride form of a strongly basic anion-exchange resin. It is a styrene copolymer with divinylbenzene with quaternary ammonium functional groups. After oral ingestion, cholestyramine resin remains in the gastrointestinal tract, where it readily exchanges chloride ions for bile acids in the small intestine, to be excreted as bile salts in the feces. Cholestyramine resin is also useful in lowering plasma lipids. The reduction in the amounts of reabsorbed bile acids results in increased catabolism of cholesterol in bile acids in the liver. The decreased concentration of bile acids returning to the liver lowers the feedback inhibition by bile acids of 7-α-hydroxylase, the rate-limiting enzyme in the conversion of cholesterol to bile acids, increasing the breakdown of hepatic cholesterol. Although biosynthesis of cholesterol is increased, it appears that the rate of catabolism is greater, resulting in a net decrease in plasma cholesterol levels by affecting LDL clearance. The increase of LDL receptors in the liver that occurs when its content of cholesterol is lowered augments this biochemical event.

Cholestyramine resin does not bind with drugs that are neutral or with amine salts; acidic drugs (in the anion form) could be bound, however. For example, in animal tests, absorption of aspirin given concurrently with the resin was depressed only moderately during the first 30 minutes.

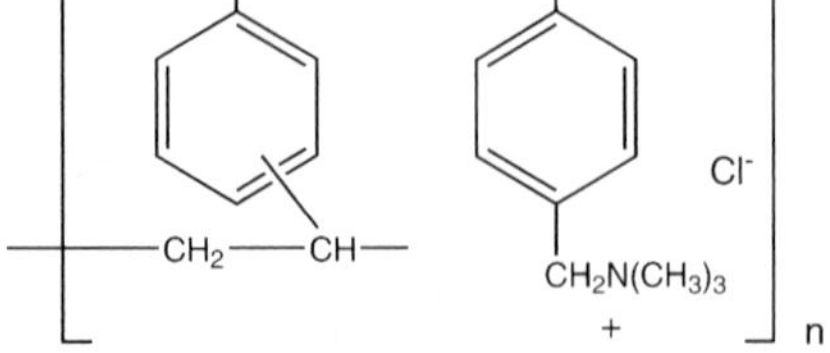

Cholestyramine Resin
(Cholybar)
(Questran)

Cholestyramine resin is the drug of choice for type IIa hyperlipoproteinemia. When used in conjunction with a controlled diet, it reduces β-lipoproteins. The drug is an insoluble polymer and, thus, probably one of the safest because it is not absorbed from the gastrointestinal tract to cause systemic toxic effects.

Colestipol Hydrochloride. Colestipol (Colestid) is a high–molecular-weight, insoluble, granular copolymer of tetraethylenepentamine and epichlorohydrin. It functions as an anion-exchange, resin-sequestering agent in a manner similar to that of cholestyramine resin. Colestipol hydrochloride reduces cholesterol levels without affecting triglycerides and seems to be especially effective in the treatment of type II hyperlipoproteinemias.

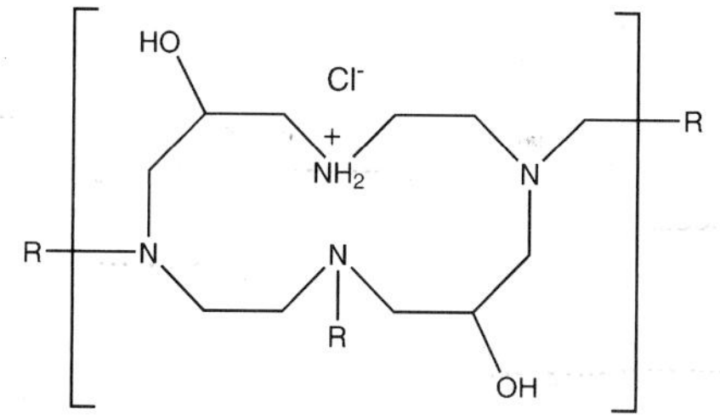

Colestipol
(Colestid)

Colesevelam. Colesevelam (Welchol) is one of the more recent additions to the class of bile acid-sequestering agents. Its structure is rather novel, and at first glance, it appears to look like the previous examples of cholestyramine and colestipol. It does not possess the chloride ions, however, and, strictly speaking, is not an anion-exchange resin. This compound has good selectivity for both the trihydroxy and dihydroxy bile acids. The selectivity for these hydroxylated derivatives lends some insight into the reduced side effects colesevelam possesses, compared with cholestyramine and colestipol. Unlike the older agents, colesevelam does not have a high incidence of causing constipation. This results from the compound's ability to "pick up" water as a result of its affinity for hydroxyl system (i.e., hydrogen bonding with either the bile acid or water). In turn, this yields softer, gel-like materials that are easier to excrete.

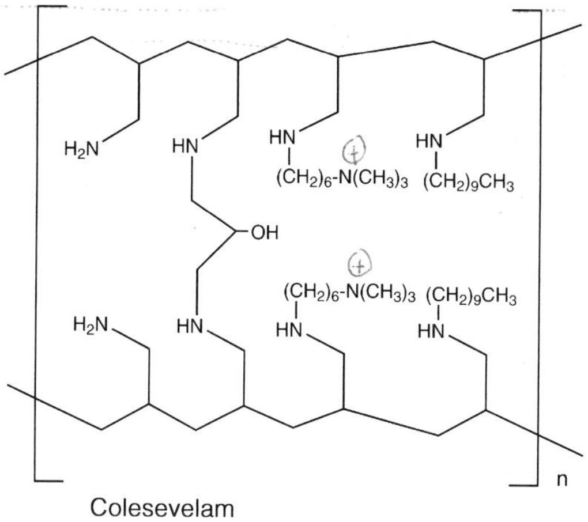

Colesevelam
(Welchol)

Nicotinic Acid. Nicotinic acid, 3-pyridinecarboxylic acid (Niacin), is effective in the treatment of all types of hyperlipoproteinemia except type I, at doses above those given as a vitamin supplement. The drug reduces VLDL synthesis and, subsequently, its plasma products, IDL and LDL. Plasma triglyceride levels are reduced because of the decreased VLDL production. Cholesterol levels are lowered, in turn, because of the decreased rate of LDL formation from VLDL. Although niacin is the drug of choice for type II hyperlipoproteinemias, its use is limited because of the vasodilating side effects. Flushing occurs in practically all patients but generally subsides when the drug is discontinued.

The hypolipidemic effects of niacin may be caused by its ability to inhibit lipolysis (i.e., prevent the release of FFAs and glycerol from fatty tissues). Therefore, there is a reduced reserve of FFA in the liver and diminution of lipoprotein biosynthesis, which reduces the production of VLDL. The decreased formation of lipoproteins leads to a pool of unused cholesterol normally incorporated in VLDL. This excess cholesterol is then excreted through the biliary tract.

Niacin (nicotinic acid) may be administered as aluminum nicotinate (Nicalex). This is a complex of aluminum hydroxy nicotinate and niacin. The aluminum salt is hydrolyzed to aluminum hydroxide and niacin in the stomach. The aluminum salt seems to have no advantage over the free acid. Hepatic reaction appears more prevalent than with niacin.

Nicotinic acid has been esterified to prolong its hypolipidemic effect. Pentaerythritol tetranicotinate has been more effective experimentally than niacin in reducing cholesterol levels in rabbits. Sorbitol and *myo*-inositol hexanicotinate polyesters have been used in the treatment of patients with atherosclerosis obliterans.

The usual maintenance dose of niacin is 3 to 6 g/day given in three divided doses. The drug is usually given at mealtimes to reduce the gastric irritation that often accompanies large doses.

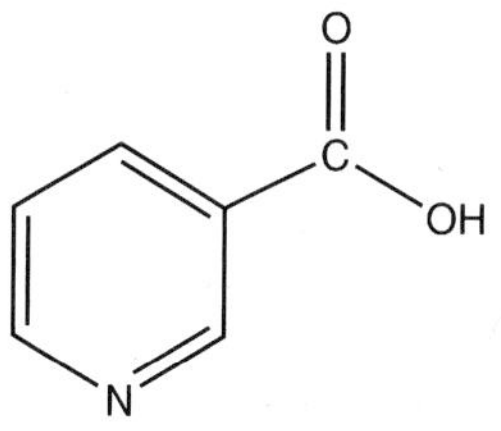

Nicotinic Acid
(Niacin)

β-Sitosterol. Sitosterol is a plant sterol, whose structure is identical with that of cholesterol, except for the substituted ethyl group on C-24 of its side chain. Although the mechanism of its hypolipidemic effect is not clearly understood, it is suspected that the drug inhibits the absorption of dietary cholesterol from the gastrointestinal tract. Sitosterols are absorbed poorly from the mucosal lining and appear to compete with cholesterol for absorption sites in the intestine.

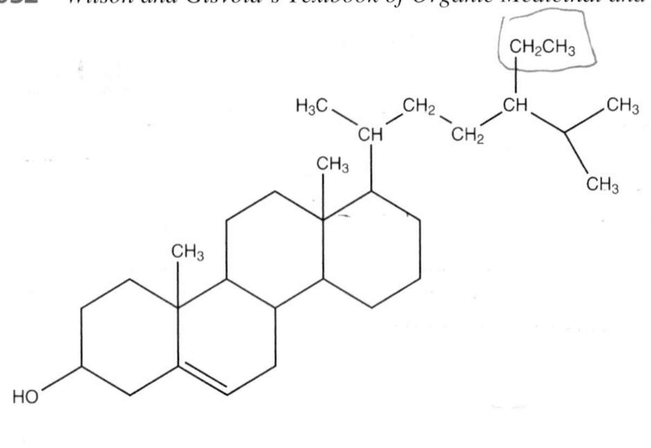

β-Sitosterol

responsible for cholesterol absorption. Although it may be used alone, it is marketed as a combination product with simvastatin under the trade name Vytorin.[72]

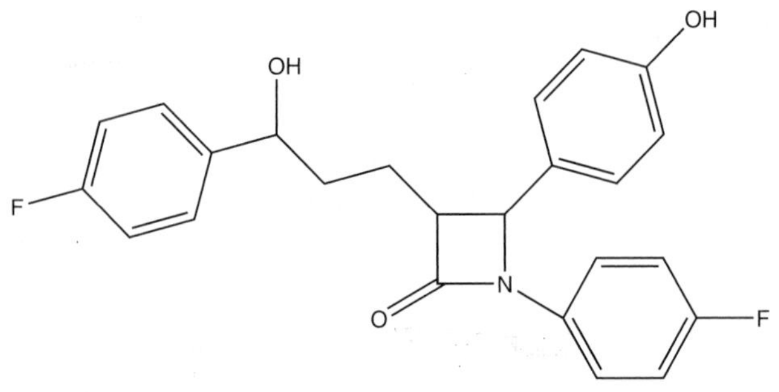

Ezetimibe

Probucol, USP. Probucol, 4,4'-[(1-methylethylidene) bis(thio)]bis[2,6-bis(1,1-dimethylethyl)phenol], DH-581 (Lorelco), is a chemical agent that was developed for the plastics and rubber industry in the 1960s. The probucol molecule has two tertiary butylphenol groups linked by a dithiopropylidene bridge, giving it a high lipophilic character with strong antioxidant properties. In humans, it causes reduction of both liver and serum cholesterol levels, but it does not alter plasma triglycerides. It reduces LDL and (to a lesser extent) HDL levels by a unique mechanism that is still not clearly delineated. The reduction of HDL may be caused by the ability of probucol to inhibit the synthesis of apoprotein A-1, a major protein component of HDL.[71] It is effective at reducing levels of LDL and is used in hyperlipoproteinemias characterized by elevated LDL levels.

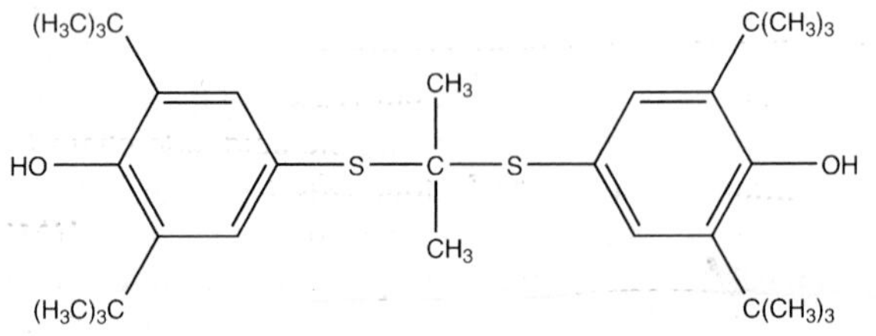

Probucol
(Lorelco)

Ezetimibe. Ezetimibe, (3R,4S)-1-(4-fluorophenyl)-3-((3S)-3-(4-fluorophenyl)-3-hydroxypropyl)-4-(4-hydroxyphenyl)-2-azetidinone (Zetia), is an antihyperlipidemic agent that has usefulness in lowering cholesterol levels. It acts by decreasing cholesterol absorption in the intestine by blocking the absorption of the sterol at the Brush boarder. Specifically, the β-lactam binds to the Niemann-Pick C1-Like 1 (NPC1L1) protein on the gastrointestinal tract that is

HMG-CoA Reductase Inhibitors

Drugs in this class of hypolipidemic agents inhibit the enzyme HMG-CoA reductase, responsible for the conversion of HMG-CoA to mevalonate in the synthetic pathway for the synthesis of cholesterol (Fig. 19.19). HMG-CoA reductase is the rate-limiting catalyst for the irreversible conversion of HMG-CoA to mevalonic acid in the synthesis of cholesterol. The activity of HMG-CoA reductase is also under feedback regulation. When cholesterol is available in sufficient amounts for body needs, the enzyme activity of HMG-CoA reductase is suppressed.

Elevated plasma cholesterol levels have been correlated with an increase in cardiovascular disease. Of the plasma lipoproteins, the LDL fraction contains the most cholesterol. The source of cholesterol in humans is either the diet or the de novo synthesis with the reduction of HMG-CoA by HMG-CoA reductase as the rate-limiting step. Ingested cholesterol as the free alcohol or ester is taken up after intestinal absorption and transported to the liver and other body organs through the exogenous pathway (Fig. 19.19). The LDL delivers cholesterol to peripheral cells. This process occurs after binding of LDL to specific LDL receptors located on the surface of cell membranes. After binding and endocytosis of the receptor and LDL, lysosomal degradation of this complex in the cell makes cholesterol available for use in cellular membrane synthesis. It is generally accepted that total plasma cholesterol is lowered most effectively by reducing LDL levels. Therefore, the population of LDL receptors is an important component of clearing the plasma of cholesterol. HMG-CoA reductase inhibitors contribute to this by directly blocking the active site of the enzyme. This action has a twofold effect on cholesterol plasma levels; it causes a decrease in de novo cholesterol synthesis and an increase in hepatic LDL receptors. These HMG-CoA reduc-

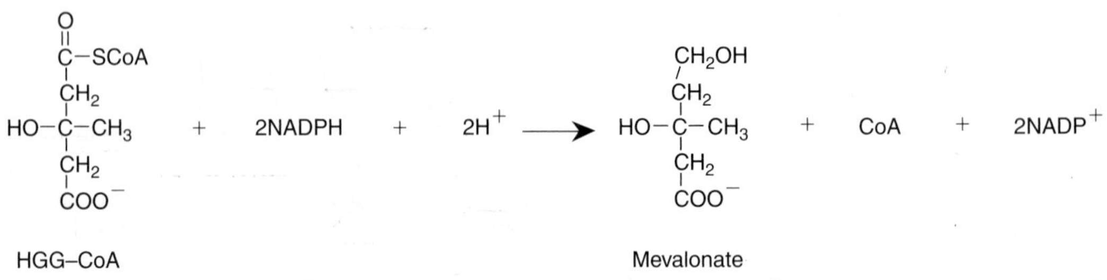

HGG–CoA   Mevalonate

Figure 19.19 ● HMG-CoA reductase reaction.

tase inhibitors are effective hypocholesteremic agents in patients with familial hypercholesteremia.

Three drugs, lovastatin, simvastatin, and pravastatin, compose the list of approved HMG-CoA reductase inhibitors for the treatment of hyperlipidemia in patients. The three drugs have structures similar to the substrate, HMG-CoA, of the enzyme HMG-CoA reductase. Lovastatin and simvastatin are lactones and prodrugs, activated by hydrolysis in the liver to their respective β-hydroxy acids. Pravastatin, in contrast, is administered as the sodium salt of the β-hydroxy acid.

Lovastatin. Lovastatin, 2-methylbutanoic acid 1,2,3,7, 8,8a-hexahydro-3,7-dimethyl-8-[2-(tetrahydro-4-hydroxy6-oxo-2H-pyran-2-yl)ethyl]-1-naphthalenyl ester, mevinolin, MK-803 (Mevacor) (formerly called mevinolin), is a potent inhibitor of HMG-CoA. The drug was obtained originally from the fermentation products of the fungi *Aspergillus terreus* and *Monascus ruber*. Lovastatin was one of two original HMG-CoA reductase inhibitors. The other drug, mevastatin (formerly called compactin), was isolated from cultures of *Penicillium cillium citrum*. Mevastatin was withdrawn from clinical trials because it altered intestinal morphology in dogs. This effect was not observed with lovastatin. For inhibitory effects on HMG-CoA reductase, the lactone ring must be hydrolyzed to the open-ring heptanoic acid.

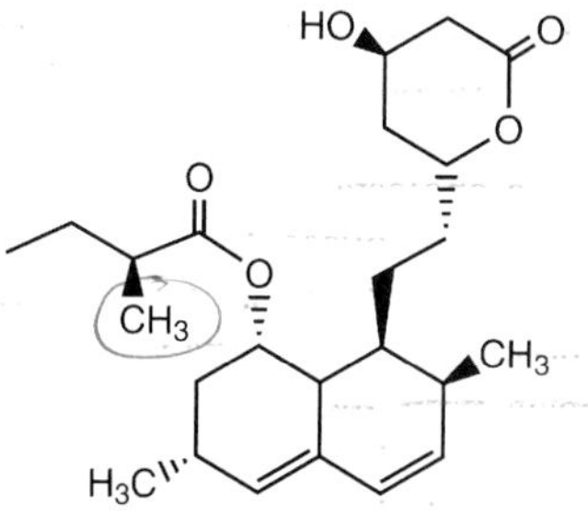

↓F (F≈5%)

Lovastatin
(Mevacor)

Simvastatin. Simvastatin, 2,2-dimethyl butanoic acid, 1,2,3,7,8,8a-hexahydro-3,7-dimethyl-8-[2-(tetrahydro-4-hydroxy-6-oxo-2-pyran-2-yl)ethyl]-1-naphthalenyl ester (Zocor), is an analog of lovastatin. These two drugs have many similar properties. Both drugs, in the prodrug form, reach the liver unchanged after oral administration, where they undergo extensive metabolism to several open-ring hydroxy acids, including the active β-hydroxy acids. They are also highly bound to plasma proteins. These actions make the bioavailability of simvastatin rather poor but better than that of lovastatin, which has been estimated to be 5%.

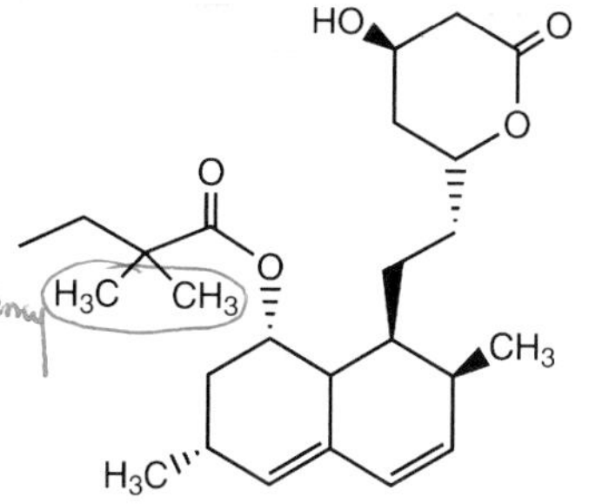

↑ poteny 2X · ↑F

Simvastatin
(Zocor)

Pravastatin. Pravastatin, sodium 1,2,6,7,8,8a-hexahydro-β,δ,6-trihydroxy-2-methyl-8-(2-methyl-1-oxobutoxy)-1-naphthaleneheptanoate (Pravachol), is the most rapid acting of the three HMG-CoA reductase inhibitor drugs, reaching a peak concentration in about 1 hour. The sodium salt of the β-hydroxy acid is more hydrophilic than the lactone forms of the other two agents, which may explain this property. In addition, the open form of the lactone ring contributes to a more hydrophilic agent, which, in turn, results in less CNS penetration. This explains, in part, why pravastatin has fewer CNS side effects than the more lipophilic lactone ester of this class of agents. Absorption of pravastatin following oral administration can be inhibited by resins such as cholestyramine because of the presence of the carboxylic acid function on the drug. The lactone forms of lovastatin and simvastatin are less affected by cholestyramine.

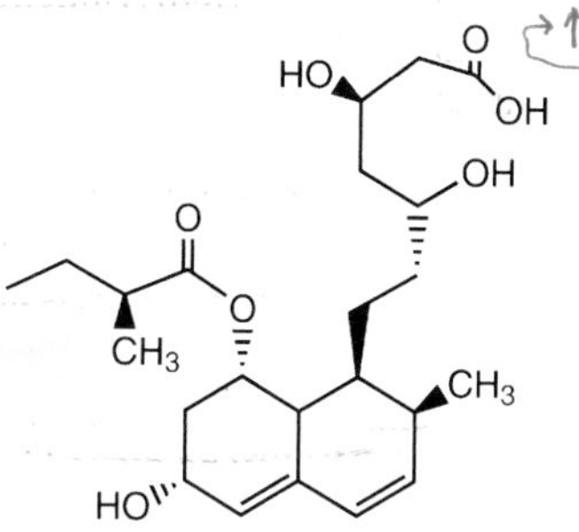

→↑ rapid-acting · ↑ polar than Lactone

Pravastatin
(Pravachol)

Fluvastatin. Fluvastatin, [R*,S*-(E)]-(±)-7-[3-(4-fluorophenyl)-1-(1-methylethyl)-1H-indol-2-yl]-3,5-dihydroxy-6-heptenoic acid monosodium salt (Lescol), is very similar to pravastatin. It possesses a heptanoic acid side chain that is superimposable over the lactone ring found in lovastatin and simvastatin. This side chain is recognized by HMG-CoA reductase. Also, much like pravastatin, the CNS side effects of this lipid-lowering agent are much lower than those of the agents that possess a lactone ring as part of their architectural design.

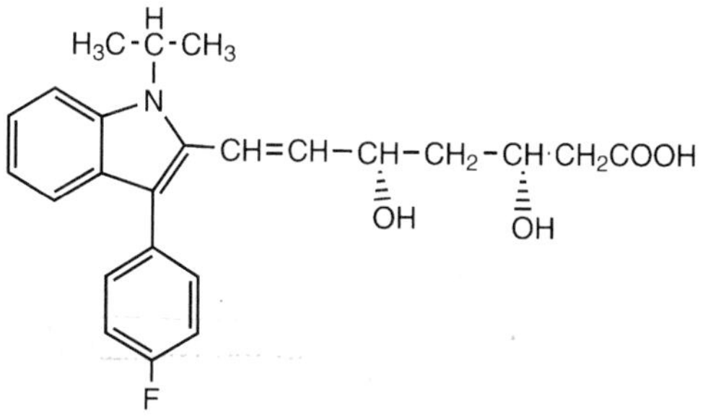

Fluvastatin
(Lescol)

Atorvastatin. Atorvastatin, [R-(R*,R*)]-2-(4-fluorophenyl)-b,d-dihydroxy-5-(1-methylethyl)-3-phenyl-4-[(phenylamino)carbonyl]-1H-pyrrole-1-heptanoic acid (Lipitor), also possesses the heptanoic acid side chain, which is critical for inhibition of HMG-CoA reductase. Although the side chain is less lipophilic than the lactone form, the high amount of lipophilic substitution causes this agent to have a slightly higher level of CNS penetration than pravastatin, resulting in a slight increase in CNS side effects. Even so, its CNS profile is much lower than that of lovastatin. Atorvastatin is marketed as a combination therapy with amlodipine under the trade name Norvasc for management of high cholesterol and high blood pressure.

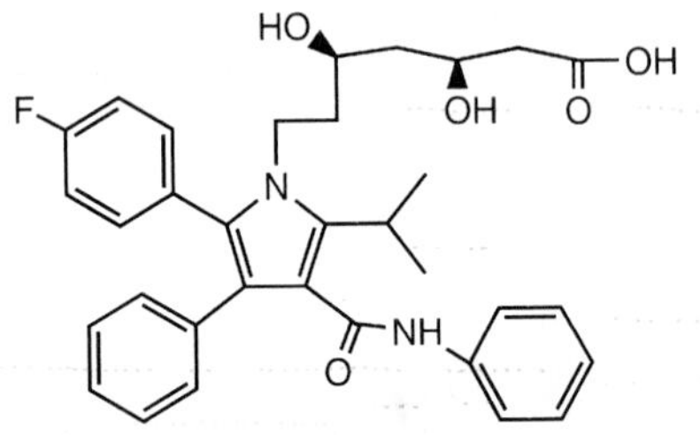

Atorvastatin
(Lipitor)

Rosuvastatin. Rosuvastatin, 7-[4-(4-fluorophenyl)-6-(1-methylethyl)-2-(methyl-methylsulfonyl-amino)-pyrimidin-5-yl]-3,5-dihydroxy-hept-6-enoic acid (Crestor), is one of the more recently introduced statins in the United States. As with all statins, there is a concern of rhabdomyolysis and as such, the FDA has mandated that a warning about this side effect, as well as a kidney toxicity warning, be added to the product label (http://www.fda.gov/CDER/Drug/advisory/crestor_3_2005.htm). This should not come as a surprise because of the relationship in the chemical architecture to cerivastatin, which was withdrawn from the market as a result of its adverse side effects.

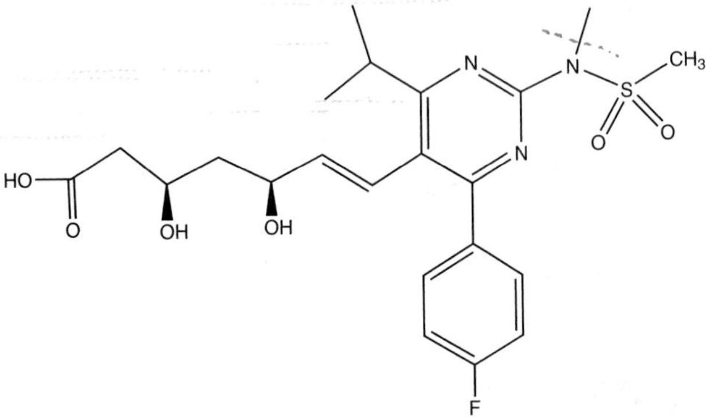

Rosuvastatin

Cerivastatin. Cerivastatin (Baycol) is one of the newer agents in this class of cholesterol-lowering agents. However, it carries a higher incidence of rhabdomyolysis and, as a result, was voluntarily withdrawn from the market by its manufacturer in 2001.

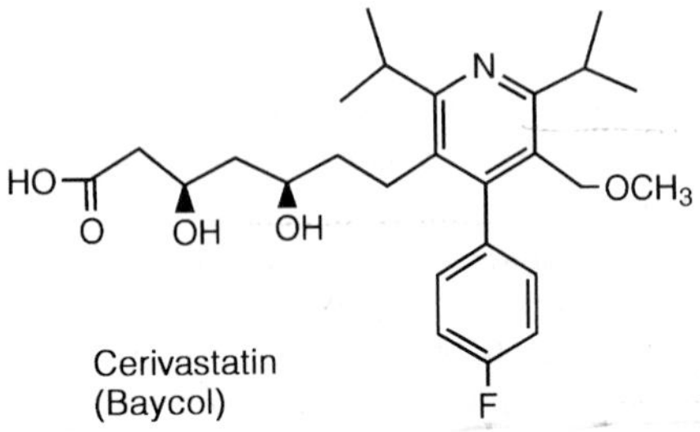

Cerivastatin
(Baycol)

ANTICOAGULANTS

A theory of blood clotting introduced in 1905 was based on the existence of four factors: thromboplastin (thrombokinase), prothrombin, fibrinogen, and ionized calcium. The clotting sequence proposed was that when tissue damage occurred, thromboplastin entered the blood from the platelets and reacted with prothrombin in the presence of calcium to form thrombin. Thrombin then reacted with fibrinogen to form insoluble fibrin, which enmeshed red blood cells (RBCs) to create a clot. The concept remained unchallenged for almost 50 years, but it has now been modified to accommodate the discovery of numerous additional factors that enter into the clotting mechanism (Table 19.6).

Mechanism of Blood Coagulation

The fluid nature of blood can be attributed to the flat cells (endothelial) that maintain a nonthrombogenic environment in the blood vessels. This is a result of at least four phenomena: (a) the maintenance of a transmural negative electric charge that prevents adhesion between platelets; (b) the release of a plasmalogen activator, which activates the fibrinolytic pathway; (c) the release of thrombomodulin, a cofactor that activates protein C, a coagulation factor inhibitor; and (d) the release of PGI$_2$, a potent inhibitor of platelet aggregation.

The process of blood coagulation (Fig. 19.20) involves a series of steps that occur in a cascade and terminate in the formation of a fibrin clot. Blood coagulation occurs by activation of either an intrinsic pathway, a relatively slow process of clot formation, or an extrinsic pathway, which has a much faster rate of fibrin formation. Both pathways merge into a common pathway for the conversion of prothrombin to thrombin and subsequent transformation of fibrinogen to the insoluble strands of fibrin. Lysis of intravascular clots occurs through a plasminogen–plasmin system, which consists of plasminogen, plasmin, urokinase, kallikrein, plasminogen activators, and some undefined inhibitors.

The *intrinsic* pathway refers to the system for coagulation that occurs from the interaction of factors circulating in the

TABLE 19.6 Roman Numerical Nomenclature of Blood-Clotting Factors and Some Common Synonyms

Factor	Synonyms
I	Fibrinogen
II	Prothrombin
III	Thromboplastin, tissue factor
IV	Calcium
V	Proaccelerin, accelerator globulin, labile factor
VI	(This number is not used now)
VII	Proconvertin, stable factor, autoprothrombin I, SPCA
VIII	Antihemophilic factor, antihemophilic globulin, platelet cofactor I, antihemophilic factor A
IX	Plasma thromboplastin component (PTC), Christmas factor, platelet cofactor II, autoprothrombin II, antihemophilic factor B
X	Stuart-Power factor, Stuart factor, autoprothrombin III
XI	Plasma thromboplastin antecedent (PTA), antihemophilic factor C
XII	Hageman factor
XIII	Fibrin-stabilizing factor, fibrinase, Laki-Lorand factor

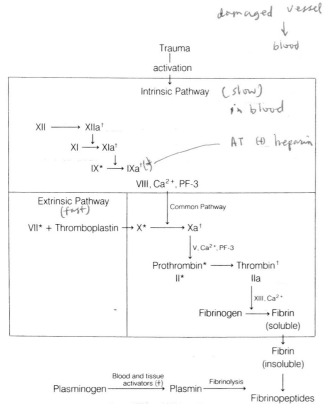

handwritten annotations:
damaged vessel wall
↓
blood

(slow)
in blood

AT ⊕ heparin

Intrinsic Pathway

Extrinsic Pathway (fast)

Figure 19.20 ● Scheme of blood coagulation and fibrinolysis. (*, a vitamin K–dependent factor; †, inhibition by heparin and antithrombin III.)

blood. It is activated when blood comes into contact with a damaged vessel wall or a foreign substance. Each of the plasma coagulation factors (Table 19.6), with the exception of factor III (tissue thromboplastin), circulates as an inactive proenzyme. Except for fibrinogen, which precipitates as fibrin, these factors are usually activated by enzymatic removal of a small peptide in the cascade of reactions that make up the clotting sequence (Fig. 19.20). The *extrinsic* clotting system refers to the mechanism by which thrombin is generated in plasma after the addition of tissue extracts. When various tissues, such as brain or lung (containing thromboplastin), are added to blood, a complex between thromboplastin and factor VII in the presence of calcium ions activates factor X, bypassing the time-consuming steps of the intrinsic pathway that form factor X.

The intrinsic and extrinsic pathways interact in vivo. Small amounts of thrombin formed early after stimulation of the extrinsic pathway accelerate clotting by the intrinsic pathway by activating factor VIII. Thrombin also speeds up the clotting rate by activating factor V, located in the common pathway. Thrombin then converts the soluble protein fibrinogen into a soluble fibrin gel by acting on Gly–Arg bonds to remove small fibrinopeptides from the N-terminus, enabling the remaining fibrinogen molecule to polymerize. It also activates factor XIII, which stabilizes the fibrin gel in the presence of calcium by cross-linking between the chains of the fibrin monomer through intermolecular γ-glutamyl–lysine bridges to form an insoluble mass.

Anticoagulant Mechanisms

In the milieu of biochemicals being formed to facilitate the clotting of blood, the coagulation cascade in vivo is controlled by a balance of inhibitors in the plasma to prevent all of the

blood in the body from solidifying. Thrombin plays a pivotal role in blood coagulation. It cleaves fibrinogen, a reaction that initiates formation of the fibrin gel, which constitutes the framework of the blood clot. As mentioned previously, it activates the cofactors factor V and factor VIII to accelerate the coagulation process. Intact endothelial cells express a receptor, thrombomodulin, for thrombin. When thrombin is bound to thrombomodulin, it does not have coagulant activity, which thus prevents clot formation beyond damaged areas and onto intact endothelium. In this bound state, however, thrombin does activate protein C, which then inactivates two cofactors and impedes blood clotting. Thrombin also activates factor XIII, leading to cross-linking of the fibrin gel. The activity of thrombin is regulated by its inactivation by plasma protein inhibitors: α_1-proteinase inhibitor, α_2-macroglobulin, antithrombin (antithrombin III), and heparin cofactor II. These belong to a family of proteins called *serpins*, an acronym for *serine protease inhibitors*.

Antithrombin III, an α_2-globin, neutralizes thrombin and the serine proteases in the coagulation cascade—Xa, IXa, XIa, and XIIa. Although antithrombin III is a slow-acting inhibitor, it becomes a rapid-acting inhibitor of thrombin in the presence of heparin. Heparin is a naturally occurring anticoagulant that requires antithrombin III (discussed previously) for its biological property of preventing blood clot formation. It binds at the lysine site of the antithrombin III molecule, causing a change in the conformation of antithrombin III and increasing its anticoagulant properties. Heparin can then dissociate from antithrombin III to bind to another antithrombin III molecule. An additional system, which controls unwanted coagulation, involves protein C, a vitamin K–dependent zymogen in the plasma. Protein C is converted to a serine protease when thrombin and factor Xa, formed in the blood in the coagulation cascade, interact with thrombomodulin. The now-activated protein C inhibits factors V and VIII and, in so doing, blocks further production of thrombin. Protein C also enhances fibrinolysis by causing release of the tissue plasminogen activator.

The biosynthesis of prothrombin (factor II) depends on an adequate supply of vitamin K. A deficiency of vitamin K results in the formation of a defective prothrombin molecule. The defective prothrombin is antigenically similar to normal prothrombin but has reduced calcium-binding ability and no biological activity. In the presence of calcium ions, normal prothrombin adheres to the surface of phospholipid vesicles and greatly increases the activity of the clotting mechanism. The defect in the abnormal prothrombin is in the NH_2-terminal portion, in which the second carboxyl residue has not been added to the γ-carbon atom of some glutamic acid residues on the prothrombin molecule to form γ-carboxyglutamic acid.[73] Administration of vitamin K antagonists decreases synthesis of a biologically active prothrombin molecule and increases the clotting time of blood in humans.[74] *e.g warfarin*

Vitamin K is critical to the formation of clotting factors VII, IX, and X. These factors are glycoproteins that have γ-carboxyglutamic acid residues at the N-terminal end of the peptide chain. The enzyme involved in forming an active prothrombin is a vitamin K–dependent carboxylase located in the microsomal fraction of liver cells. It has been suggested that vitamin K drives the carboxylase reaction by abstracting a proton from the relatively unreactive methylene carbon of the glutamyl residue, forming a 2,3-epoxide. Oral

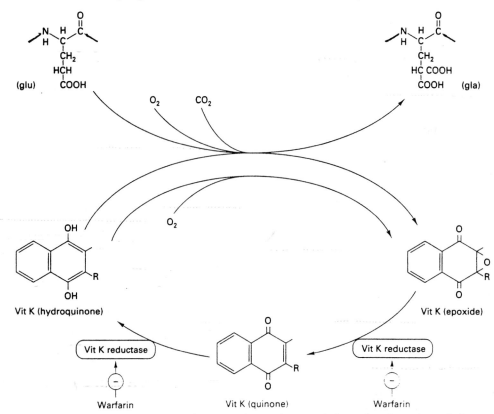

Figure 19.21 • Mechanism of action of vitamin K and sites of action of warfarin.

anticoagulants interfere with the γ-carboxylation of glutamic acid residues by preventing the reduction of vitamin K to its hydroquinone form (Fig. 19.21).

Hemophilia A, a blood disease characterized by a deficiency of coagulation factor VIII, is the most common inherited blood coagulation disorder. Treatment of this disease over the past 25 years has depended on the concentration of the antihemophilic factor (factor VIII) by cryoprecipitation and immunoaffinity chromatography separation technology. The impact of this therapy has been diminished by the presence of viruses that cause the acquired immunodeficiency syndrome (AIDS) and other less tragic viral diseases in humans. Recombinant antihemophilic factor preparations have been produced since 1989 with use of mammalian cells genetically altered to secrete human factor VIII. Kogenate and Helixate are recombinant preparations, obtained from genetically altering baby hamster kidney cells that contain high concentrations of factor VIII. Recombinant factor VIIa, an active factor in the extrinsic pathway, now in phase III clinical trials (Novo Seven), has been used to treat patients with hemophilia A factor VII deficiency. Hemophilia B, another genetic blood disorder, which constitutes about 20% of hemophilia cases, is caused by a deficiency of factor IX and has been treated from cryoprecipitated fractions obtained from plasma. Monoclonal antibody technology has produced an essentially pure, carrier-free preparation of native factor IX (Mononine). Recombinant technology has solved the problem of limited supply and viral contamination of these critical blood factors.

Blood Degredation

Some patients suffer from a rare, potentially life-threatening disease of the blood characterized by hemolytic anemia and thrombosis, which is known as paroxysmal nocturnal hemoglobinuria (PNH). One symptom of the disease includes red urine, which results from the breakdown of RBC products (hemoglobin and hemosiderin) in the urine. An inconsistent, but potentially life-threatening, complication of PNH is the development of venous thrombosis.

Platelet Aggregation and Inhibitors

Blood platelets play a pivotal role in hemostasis and thrombus formation. Actually, they have two roles in the cessation of bleeding: a hemostatic function, in which platelets, through their mass, cause physical occlusion of openings in blood vessels, and a thromboplastic function, in which the chemical constituents of the platelets take part in the blood coagulation mechanism. The circulatory system is self-sealing because of the clotting properties of blood. The pathological formation of clots within the circulatory system, however, creates a potentially serious clinical situation that must be dealt with through the use of anticoagulants.

Platelets do not adhere to intact endothelial cells. They do become affixed to subendothelial tissues, which have been exposed by injury, to cause hemostasis. Platelets bind to collagen in the vessel wall and trigger other platelets to adhere to them. This adhesiveness is accompanied by a change in shape of the platelets and may be caused by mobilization of calcium bound to the platelet membrane. The growth of the platelet mass depends on the ADP released by the first few adhering cells and enhances the aggregation process. A secondary phase (phase II) immediately follows, with additional platelet aggregation. In this secondary phase, the platelets undergo a secretory process during which enzymes such as cathepsin and acid hydrolases, along with fibrinogen, are

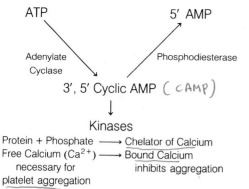

Figure 19.22 ● Role of adenosine 3′,5′-cyclic monophosphate (cAMP) in inhibition of platelet aggregation.

released from α-granules in the platelets and ADP, ATP, serotonin, and calcium are released from dense bodies in the platelets. The dense bodies are likened to the storage granules associated with adrenergic neurons. Increased levels of cAMP inhibit platelet aggregation. cAMP activates specific dependent kinases, which form protein–phosphate complexes that chelate calcium ions. The reduced levels of calcium inhibit aggregation (Fig. 19.22). Inhibitors of platelet aggregation can increase cAMP levels by either stimulating adenylate cyclase or inhibiting phosphodiesterase.[74] Substances such as glucagon, adenosine, and isoproterenol increase cAMP levels and inhibit platelet aggregation. Drugs such as theophylline, aminophylline, dipyramidole, papaverine, and adenosine inhibit phosphodiesterase and aggregation of platelets. Epinephrine, collagen, and serotonin inhibit adenylate cyclase and stimulate platelet aggregation.[75] The role of platelets in arterial thrombosis is similar to that in hemostasis. The factors contributing to venous thrombosis are circulatory stasis, excessive generation of thrombin formation of fibrin and, to a lesser extent than in the artery, platelet aggregation.

Aspirin, sulfinpyrazone, and indomethacin have an inhibitory effect on platelet aggregation. They inhibit COX, the enzyme that controls the formation of prostaglandin endoperoxides and increases the tendency for platelets to aggregate.[76] Aspirin also inhibits the platelet-release reaction. Dipyridamole inhibits adenosine deaminase and adenosine uptake by platelets. As a result, the increased plasma concentrations of adenosine inhibit ADP-induced aggregation of platelets.

Among the many pharmacological actions of prostaglandins is the ability of some to stimulate or inhibit the aggregation of platelets and alter the clotting time of blood. Prostaglandins are synthesized from 20-carbon polyunsaturated fatty acids containing from three to five double bonds. These fatty acids are present in the phospholipids of cell membranes of all mammalian tissues. The main precursor of prostaglandins is arachidonic acid. Arachidonic acid is released from membrane phospholipids by the enzyme phospholipase A_2. Once released, arachidonic acid is metabolized by COX synthetase to form unstable cyclic endoperoxides, PGG_2 and PGH_2, which subsequently are transformed into PGI_2 and TXA_2. The conversion to TXA_2 is aided by the enzyme thromboxane synthetase. The formation of PGI_2 can occur nonenzymatically. Blood platelets convert arachidonic acid to TXA_2, whereas PGI_2 is formed mainly by the vascular endothelium. Both PGI_2 and TXA_2

are unstable at physiological pH and temperatures. Their half-lives are 2 to 3 minutes.

PGI_2 inhibits platelet aggregation by stimulating adenylate cyclase to increase cAMP levels in the platelets. PGI_2 is also a vasodilator and, as a result, has potent hypotensive properties when given intravenously or by intra-arterial administration. TXA_2 induces platelet aggregation. Together with PGI_2, TXA_2 plays a role in the maintenance of vascular homeostasis. In addition to being a platelet aggregator, TXA_2 is a potent vasoconstrictor.

Retardation of clotting is important in blood transfusions, to avoid thrombosis after surgery or from other causes, to prevent recurrent thrombosis in phlebitis and pulmonary embolism, and to lessen the propagation of clots in the coronary arteries. This retardation may be accomplished by agents that inactivate thrombin (heparin) or substances that prevent the formation of prothrombin in the liver (the coumarin derivatives and the phenylindanedione derivatives).

Although heparin is a useful anticoagulant, it has limited applications. Many of the anticoagulants in use today were developed following the discovery of dicumarol, an anticoagulant present in spoiled sweet clover. These compounds are orally effective, but there is a lag period of 18 to 36 hours before they increase the clotting time significantly. Heparin, in contrast, produces an immediate anticoagulant effect after intravenous injection. A major disadvantage of heparin is that the only effective therapeutic route is parenteral.

Dicumarol and related compounds are not vitamin K antagonists in the classic sense. They appear to act by interfering with the function of vitamin K in the liver cells, which are the sites of synthesis of the clotting factors, including prothrombin. This lengthens the clotting time by decreasing the amount of biologically active prothrombin in the blood.

The discovery that dicumarol and related compounds were potent reversible competitors of vitamin K coagulant-promoting properties (although at high levels, dicumarol is not reversed by vitamin K) led to the development of antivitamin K compounds such as phenindione, which was designed in part according to metabolite–antimetabolite concepts. The active compounds of the phenylindanedione series are characterized by a phenyl, a substituted phenyl, or a diphenylacetyl group in the 2-position. Another requirement for activity is a keto group in the 1- and 3-position, one of which may form the enol tautomer. A second substituent, other than hydrogen, at the 2-position prevents this keto–enol tautomerism, and the resulting compounds are ineffective as anticoagulants.

PRODUCTS   (-) Heparin

Protamine Sulfate, USP. Protamine sulfate has an anticoagulant effect, but if used in the proper amount, it counteracts the action of heparin and is used as an antidote for the latter in cases of overdosage. It is administered intravenously in a dose that depends on the circumstances.

Dicumarol, USP. Dicumarol, 3,3′-methylenebis[4-hydroxycoumarin], is a white or creamy white crystalline powder with a faint, pleasant odor and a slightly bitter taste. It is practically insoluble in water or alcohol, slightly soluble in chloroform, and dissolved readily by solutions of fixed alkalies. The effects after administration require 12 to 72 hours to develop and persist for 24 to 96 hours after discontinuance.

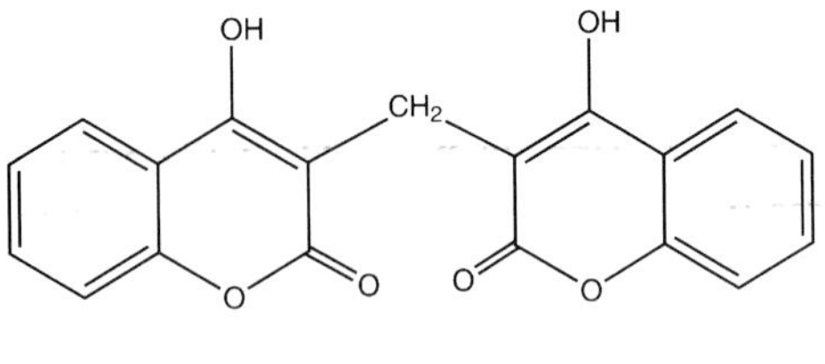

Dicumarol

Dicumarol is used alone or as an adjunct to heparin in the prophylaxis and treatment of intravascular clotting. It is used in postoperative thrombophlebitis, pulmonary embolus, acute embolic and thrombotic occlusion of peripheral arteries, and recurrent idiopathic thrombophlebitis. It has no effect on an already-formed embolus but may prevent further intravascular clotting. Because the outcome of acute coronary thrombosis depends largely on extension of the clot and formation of mural thrombi in the heart chambers, with subsequent embolization, dicumarol has been used in this condition. It has also been administered to arrest impending gangrene after frostbite. The dose, after determination of the prothrombin clotting time, is 25 to 200 mg, depending on the size and the condition of the patient. The drug is given orally in the form of capsules or tablets. On the second day and thereafter, it may be given in amounts sufficient to maintain the prothrombin clotting time at about 30 seconds. If hemorrhages should occur, a dosage of 50 to 100 mg of menadione sodium bisulfite is injected, supplemented by a blood transfusion.

Warfarin Sodium, USP. Warfarin sodium, 3-(α-acetonylbenzyl)-4-hydroxycoumarin sodium salt (Coumadin, Panwarfin), is a white, odorless, crystalline powder, with a slightly bitter taste; it is slightly soluble in chloroform and soluble in alcohol or water. A 1% solution has a pH of 7.2 to 8.5.

By virtue of its great potency, warfarin sodium at first was considered unsafe for use in humans and was used very effectively as a rodenticide, especially against rats. At the proper dosage level, however, it can be used in humans, especially through the intravenous route.

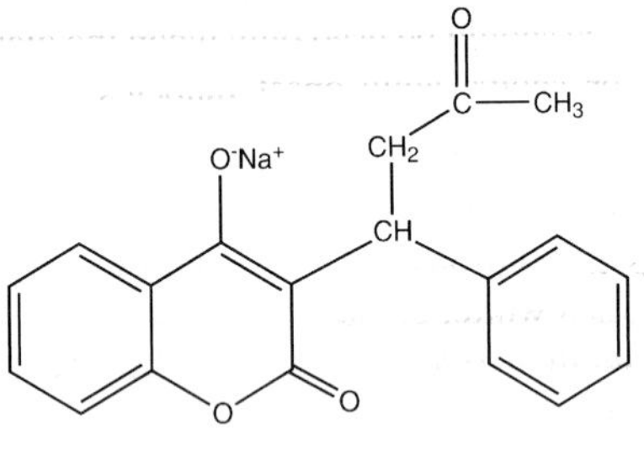

Wafarin Sodium
(Coumadin)

Warfarin Potassium, USP. Warfarin potassium, 3-(α-acetonylbenzyl)-4-hydroxycoumarin potassium salt (Athrombin-K), is readily absorbed after oral administration, and a therapeutic hypoprothrombinemia is produced within 12 to 24 hours after administration of 40 to 60 mg. This salt is therapeutically interchangeable with warfarin sodium.

Anisindione, USP. Anisindione, 2-(p-methoxyphenyl)-1,3-indandione, 2-(p-anisyl)-1,3-indandione (Miradon), is a p-methoxy congener of phenindione. It is a white, crystalline powder, slightly soluble in water, tasteless, and absorbed well after oral administration.

In instances when the urine may be alkaline, an orange color may be detected. This is caused by metabolic products of anisindione and is not hematuria.

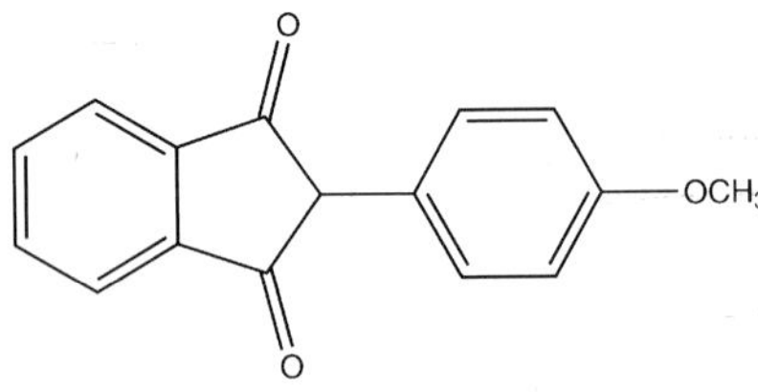

Anisindione
(Miradon)

Eculizumab. Eculizumab (Soliris) is a monoclonal antibody that binds to the terminal complement protein C5 in RBCs. This blocks the cleavage of C5 and halts the process of complement-mediated cell destruction of the RBCs. Eculizumab has been shown to be effective in treating PNH and in March 2007 was approved by the FDA for treating PNH.[77]

To P627

⬡ SYNTHETIC HYPOGLYCEMIC AGENTS

The discovery that certain organic compounds will lower the blood sugar level is not recent. In 1918, guanidine was shown to lower the blood sugar level. The discovery that certain trypanosomes need much glucose and will die in its absence was followed by the discovery that galegine lowered the blood sugar level and was weakly trypanocidal. This led to the development of several very active trypanocidal agents, such as the bisamidines, diisothioureas, bisguanidines, and others. Synthalin (trypanocidal at 1:250 million) and pentamidine are outstanding examples of very active trypanocidal agents. Synthalin lowers the blood sugar level in normal, depancreatized, and completely alloxanized animals. This may be caused by reduced oxidative activity of mitochondria, resulting from inhibition of the mechanisms that simultaneously promote phosphorylation of ADP and stimulate oxidation by nicotinamide adenine dinucleotide (NAD) in the citric acid cycle. Hydroxystilbamidine isethionate, *USP*, is used as an antiprotozoan agent.

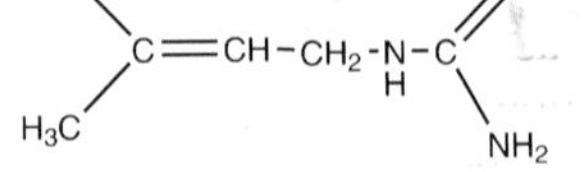

Galegine

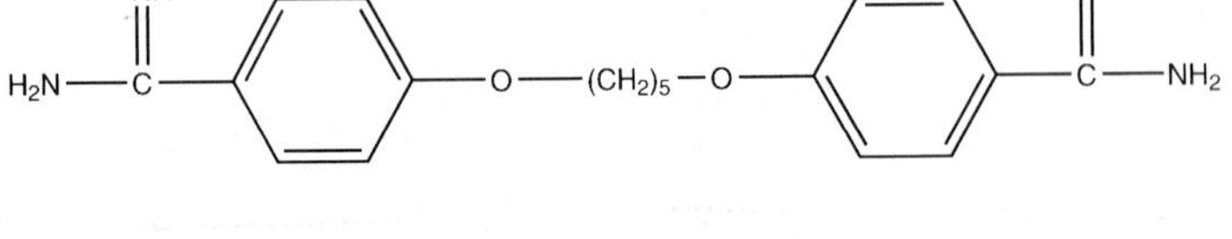

Pentamidine

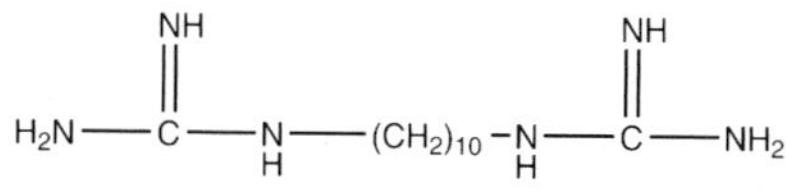

Synthalin

In 1942, *p*-aminobenzenesulfonamidoisopropylthiadiazole (an antibacterial sulfonamide) was found to produce hypoglycemia. This result stimulated research for the development of synthetic hypoglycemic agents, several of which are in use today.

Sulfonylureas became widely available in 1955 for the treatment of non–ketosis-prone mild diabetes and are still the drugs of choice. A second class of compounds, the biguanides, in the form of a single drug, phenformin, has been used since 1957. Phenformin was withdrawn from the U.S. market, however, because it causes lactic acidosis, from which fatalities have been reported.

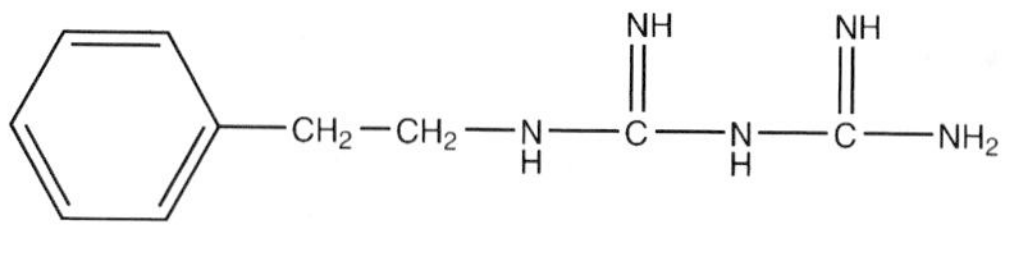

Phenformin

Sulfonylureas

The sulfonylureas may be represented by the following general structure:

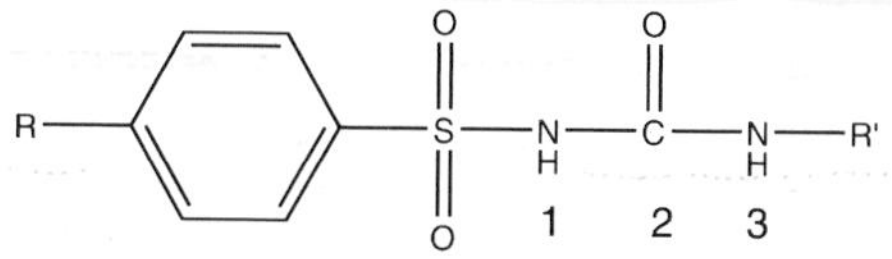

These are urea derivatives with an arylsulfonyl group in the 1-position and an aliphatic group at the 3-position. The aliphatic group, R′, confers lipophilic properties to the molecule. Maximal activity results when R′ consists of three to six carbon atoms, as in chlorpropamide, tolbutamide, and acetohexamide. Aryl groups at R′ generally give toxic compounds. The R group on the aromatic ring primarily influences the duration of action of the compound. Tolbutamide disappears quite rapidly from the bloodstream by being metabolized to the inactive carboxy compound, which is excreted rapidly. Chlorpropamide, however, is metabolized more slowly and persists in the blood much longer.

The mechanism of action of the sulfonylureas is to stimulate the release of insulin from the functioning β-cells of the intact pancreas. In the absence of the pancreas, they have no significant effect on blood glucose. The sulfonylureas may have other actions, such as inhibition of secretion of glucagon and action at postreceptor intracellular sites to increase insulin activity.

For a time, tolbutamide, chlorpropamide, and acetohexamide were the only oral hypoglycemic agents. Subsequently, a second generation of these drugs became available. Although they did not present a new method of lowering blood glucose levels, they were more potent than the existing drugs. Glipizide and glyburide are the second-generation oral hypoglycemic agents.

Whether they are first- or second-generation oral hypoglycemic drugs, this group of agents remains a valuable adjunct to therapy in adult-onset diabetes patients. Accordingly, the sulfonylureas are not indicated in juvenile-onset diabetes.

Tolbutamide, USP. Tolbutamide, 1-butyl-3-(*p*-tolylsulfonyl)urea (Orinase), occurs as a white, crystalline powder that is insoluble in water and soluble in alcohol or aqueous alkali. It is stable in air.

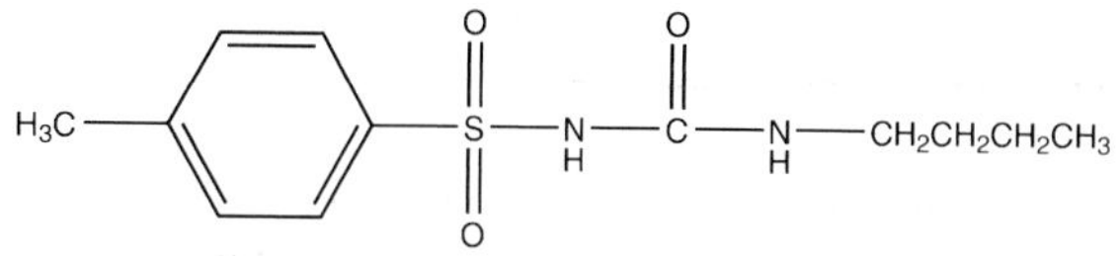

Tolbutamide
(Orinase)

Tolbutamide is absorbed rapidly in responsive diabetic patients. The blood sugar level reaches a minimum after 5 to 8 hours. It is oxidized rapidly in vivo to 1-butyl-3-(*p*-carboxyphenyl)sulfonylurea, which is inactive. The metabolite is freely soluble at urinary pH; if the urine is strongly acidified, however, as in the use of sulfosalicylic acid as a protein precipitant, a white precipitate of the free acid may be formed.

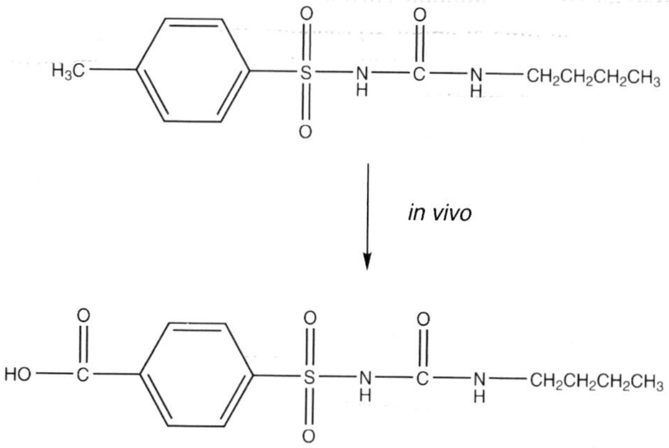

Tolbutamide should be used only when the diabetic patient is an adult or shows adult-onset diabetes, and the patient should adhere to dietary restrictions.

Tolbutamide Sodium, USP. Tolbutamide sodium, 1-butyl-3-(*p*-tolylsulfonyl)urea monosodium salt (Orinase Diagnostic), is a white, crystalline powder, freely soluble in water, soluble in alcohol and chloroform, and very slightly soluble in ether.

This water-soluble salt of tolbutamide is used intravenously for the diagnosis of mild diabetes mellitus and of functioning pancreatic islet cell adenomas. The sterile dry powder is dissolved in sterile water for injection to make a clear solution, which then should be administered within 1 hour. The main route of breakdown is to butylamine and sodium *p*-toluene sulfonamide.

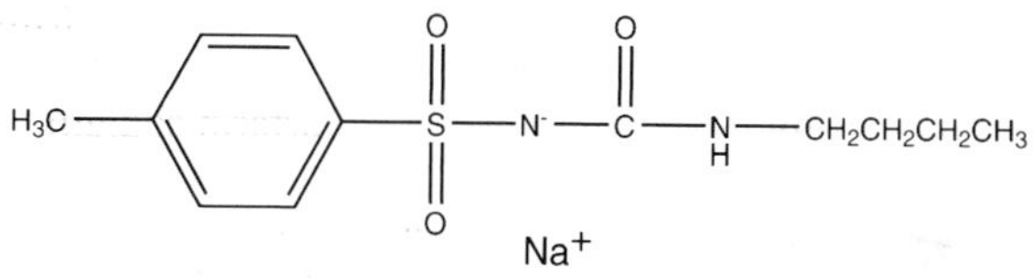

Tolbutamide Sodium

Chlorpropamide, USP. Chlorpropamide, 1-[(*p*-chlorophenyl)-sulfonyl]-3-propylurea (Diabinese), is a white, crystalline powder, practically insoluble in water, soluble in alcohol, and sparingly soluble in chloroform. It will form water-soluble salts in basic solutions. This drug is more resistant to conversion to inactive metabolites than is tolbutamide and, as a result, has a much longer duration of action. One study showed that about half of the drug is excreted as metabolites, with the principal one being hydroxylated in the 2-position of the propyl side chain.[78] After control of the blood sugar level, the maintenance dose is usually on a once-a-day schedule.

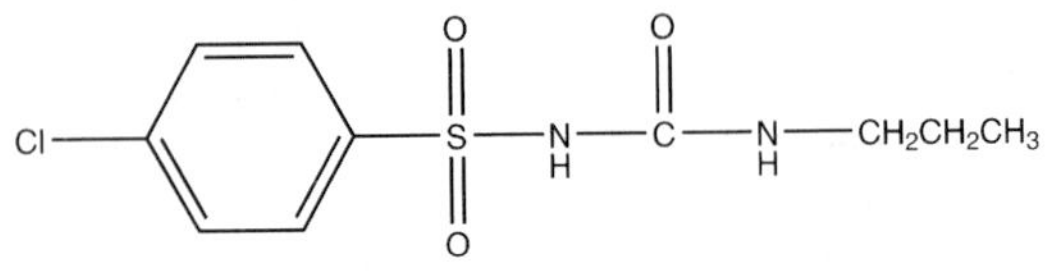

Chlorpropamide
(Diabinese)

Tolazamide, USP. Tolazamide, 1-(hexahydro-1*H*-azepin-1-yl)-3-(*p*-tolylsulfonyl)urea (Tolinase), is an analog of tolbutamide and is reported to be effective, in general, under the same circumstances in which tolbutamide is useful. Tolazamide, however, appears to be more potent than tolbutamide and is nearly equal in potency to chlorpropamide. In studies with radioactive tolazamide, investigators found that 85% of an oral dose appeared in the urine as metabolites that were more soluble than tolazamide itself.

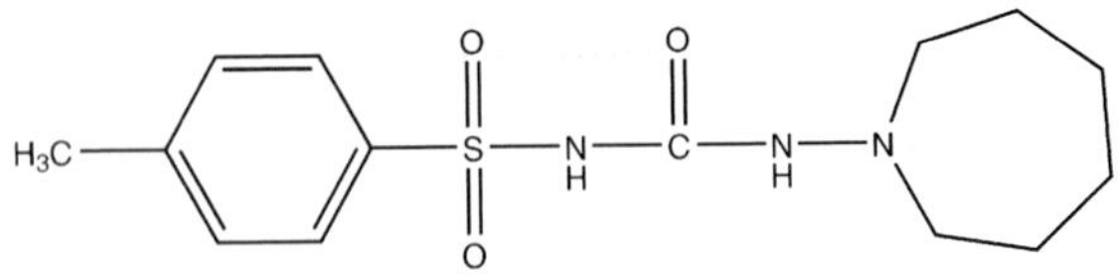

Tolazamide
(Tolinase)

Acetohexamide, USP. Acetohexamide, 1-[(*p*-acetyl-phenyl)sulfonyl]-3-cyclohexylurea (Dymelor), is related chemically and pharmacologically to tolbutamide and chlorpropamide. Like the other sulfonylureas, acetohexamide lowers the blood sugar level, primarily by stimulating the release of endogenous insulin.

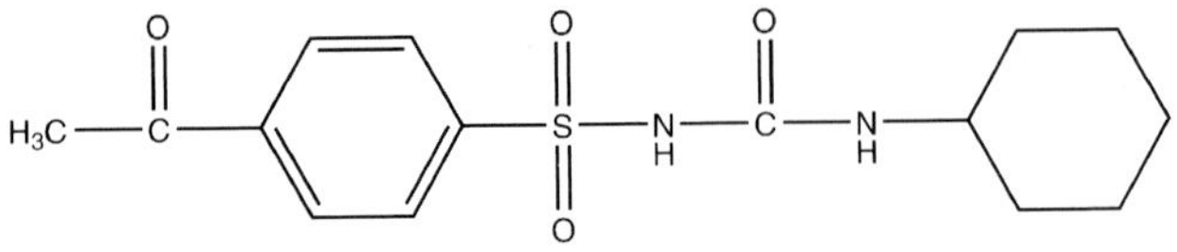

Acetohexamide
(Dymelor)

Acetohexamide is metabolized in the liver to a reduced form, the α-hydroxyethyl derivative. This metabolite, the main one in humans, possesses hypoglycemic activity. Acetohexamide is intermediate between tolbutamide and chlorpropamide in potency and duration of effect on blood sugar levels.

Glipizide. Structurally, glipizide, 1-cyclohexyl-3-[[*p*-[2(methylpyrazinecarboxamido)ethyl]phenyl]sulfonyl]urea (Glucotrol), is a cyclohexylsulfonylurea analog similar to acetohexamide and glyburide. The drug is absorbed rapidly on oral administration. Its serum half-life is 2 to 4 hours, and it has a hypoglycemic effect that ranges from 12 to 24 hours.

Glyburide. Similar to glipizide, glyburide, 1-[[*p*-[2-(5-chloro-*o*-anisamido)ethyl]-phenyl]sulfonyl]-3-cyclohexyl-urea (DiaBeta, Micronase, Glynase), is a second-generation oral hypoglycemic agent. The drug has a half-life elimination of 10 hours, but its hypoglycemic effect remains for up to 24 hours.

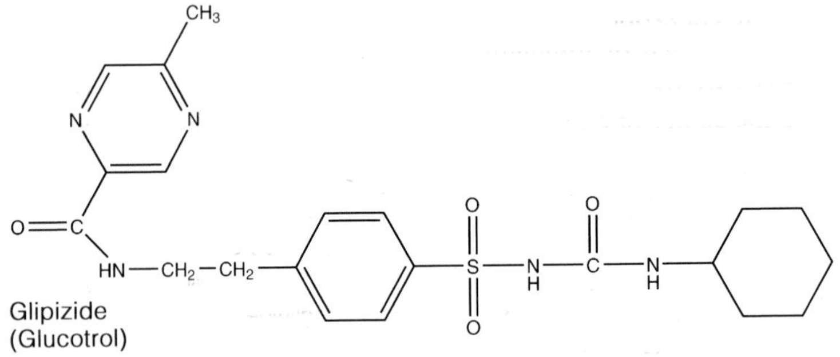

Glipizide
(Glucotrol)

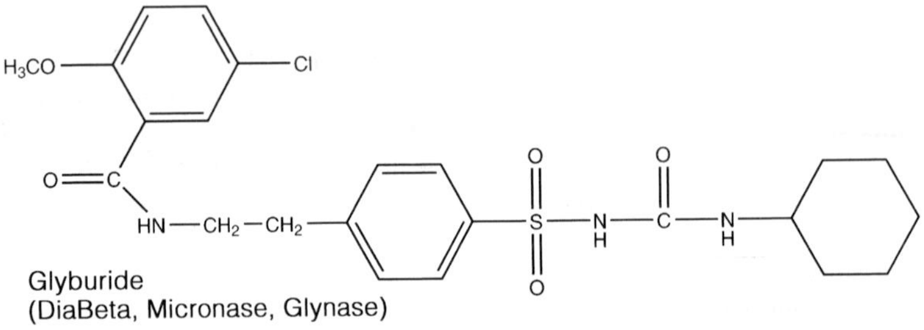

Glyburide
(DiaBeta, Micronase, Glynase)

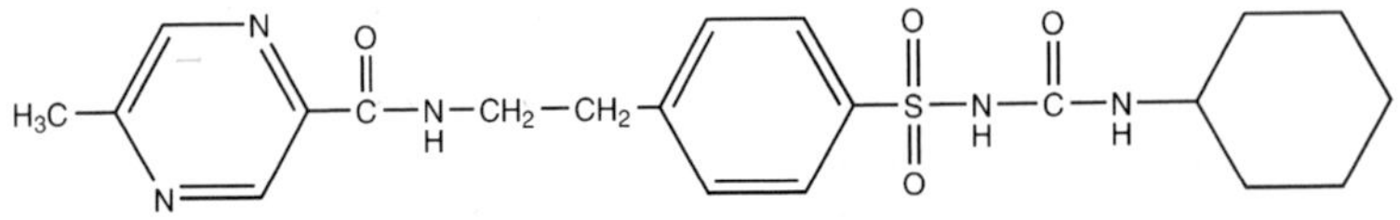

Glipizide
(Glucotrol)

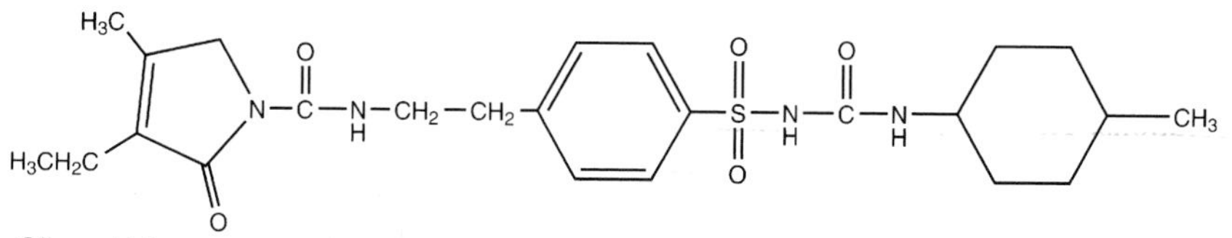

Glimepiride
(Amaryl)

Glipizide. Glipizide, 1-cyclohexyl-3-[[*p*-(2-(5-methyl-pyrazinecarboxamido)ethyl]phenyl]sulfonyl]urea (Glucotrol), is an off-white, odorless powder with a pK$_a$ of 5.9. It is insoluble in water and alcohols, but soluble in 0.1 N NaOH. Even though on a weight basis, it is approximately 100 times more potent than tolbutamide, the maximal hypoglycemic effects of these two agents are similar. It is rapidly absorbed on oral administration, with a serum half-life of 2 to 4 hours, whereas the hypoglycemic effects range from 12 to 24 hours. Metabolism of glipizide is generally through oxidation of the cyclohexane ring to the *p*-hydroxy and *m*-hydroxy metabolites. A minor metabolite that occurs involves the *N*-acetyl derivative, which results from the acetylation of the primary amine following hydrolysis of the amide system by amidase enzymes.

Glimepiride. Glimepiride, 1-[[*p*-[2-(3-ethyl-4-methyl-2-oxo-3-pyrroline-1-carboxamido)ethyl]phenyl]sulfonyl]-3-(*trans*-4-methylcyclohexyl)urea (Amaryl), is very similar to glipizide with the exception of their heterocyclic rings. Instead of the pyrazine ring found in glipizide, glimepiride contains a pyrrolidine system. It is metabolized primarily through oxidation of the alkyl side chain of the pyrrolidine, with a minor metabolic route involving acetylation of the amine.

Gliclazide. Chemically, gliclazide, 1-(3-azabicy-clo[3.3.0]oct-3-yl)-3-*p*-tolylsulphonylurea (Diamicron), is very similar to tolbutamide, with the exception of the bicyclic heterocyclic ring found in gliclazide. The pyrrolidine increases its lipophilicity over that of tolbutamide, which increases its half-life. Even so, the *p*-methyl is susceptible to the same oxidative metabolic fate as observed for tolbutamide, namely, it will be metabolized to a carboxylic acid.

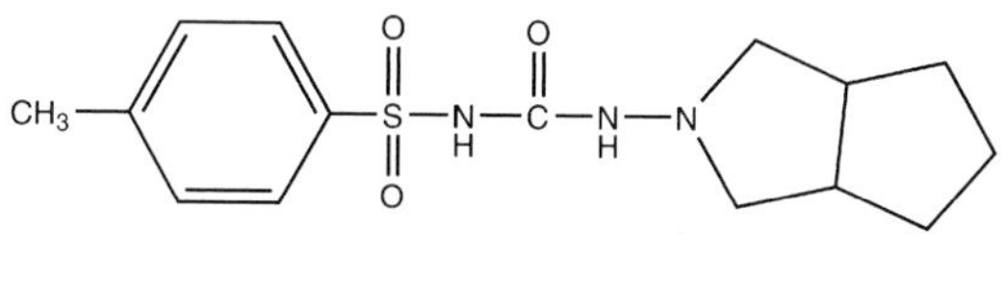

Gliclazide
(Diamicron)

Nonsulfonylureas—Metaglinides

The metaglinides are nonsulfonylurea oral hypoglycemic agents used in the management of type 2 diabetes (non–insulin-dependent diabetes mellitus, NIDDM). These agents tend to have a rapid onset and a short duration of action. Much like the sulfonylureas, these induce insulin release from functioning pancreatic β cells. The mechanism of action for the metaglinides, however, differs from that of the sulfonylureas. The mechanism of action is through binding to specific receptors in the β-cell membrane, leading to the closure of ATP-dependent K$^+$ channels. The K$^+$ channel blockade depolarizes the β-cell membrane, which in turn

leads to Ca^{2+} influx, increased intracellular Ca^{2+}, and stimulation of insulin secretion. Because of this different mechanism of action from the sulfonylureas, there are two major differences between these seemingly similar classes of agents. The first is that the metaglinides cause much faster insulin production than the sulfonylureas. As a result, the metaglinides should be taken during meals, as the pancreas will produce insulin in a much shorter period. The second difference is that the effects of the metaglinides do not last as long as the effects of the sulfonylureas. The effects of this class appear to last less than 1 hour, whereas sulfonylureas continue to stimulate insulin production for several hours. One advantage of a short duration of action is that there is less risk of hypoglycemia.

Repaglinide. Repaglinide, (+)-2-ethoxy-4-[*N*-[3-methyl-1-(*S*)-[2-(1-piperidinyl) phenyl]butyl]carbamoyl-methyl]benzoic acid (Prandin), represents a new class of nonsulfonylurea oral hypoglycemic agents. With a fast onset and a short duration of action, the medication should be taken with meals. It is oxidized by CYP 3A4, and the carboxylic acid may be conjugated to inactive compounds. Less than 0.2% is excreted unchanged by the kidney, which may be an advantage for elderly patients who are renally impaired. The most common side effect involves hypoglycemia, resulting in shakiness, headache, cold sweats, anxiety, and changes in mental state.

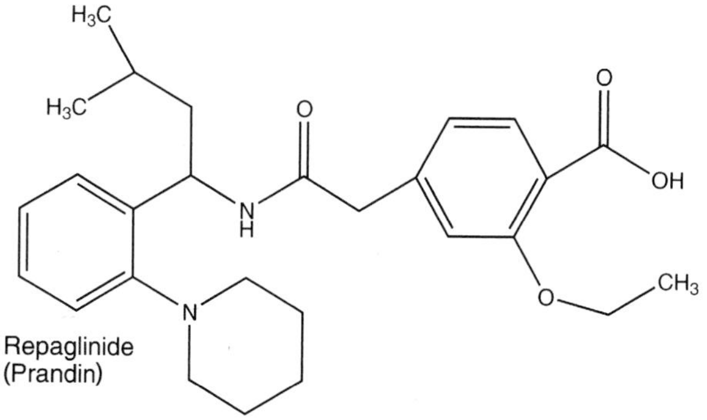

Repaglinide
(Prandin)

Nateglinide. Although nateglinide, *N*-(4-isopropylcyclohexanecarbonyl)-D-phenylalanine (Starlix), belongs to the metaglinides, it is a phenylalanine derivative and represents a novel drug in the management of type 2 diabetes.

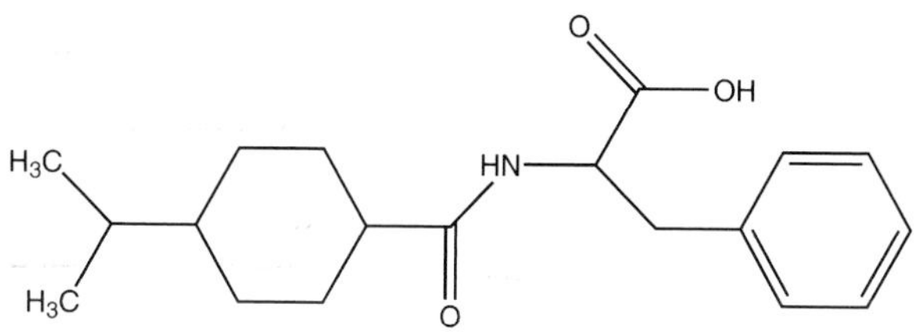

Nateglinide
(Starlix)

Thiazolindiones

The thiazolindiones represent a novel nonsulfonylurea class of hypoglycemic agents for the treatment of NIDDM. Much like the sulfonylureas, the use of these agents requires a functioning pancreas that can successfully secrete insulin from β cells. Although insulin may be released in normal levels from the cells, peripheral sensitivity to this hormone may be reduced or lacking. The thiazolidinediones are highly selective agonists for the peroxisome proliferator-activated receptor-γ (PPARγ), which is responsible for improving glycemic control, primarily through the improvement of insulin sensitivity in muscles and adipose tissue. In addition, they inhibit hepatic gluconeogenesis. These agents normalize glucose metabolism and reduce the amount of insulin needed to achieve glycemic control. They are only effective in the presence of insulin.

Rosiglitazone. Rosiglitazone, (±)-5-[[4-[2-(methyl-2-pyridinylamino)ethoxy]phenyl]methyl]-2,4-thiazolidine-dione (Avandia), is a white to off-white solid with pK$_a$ values of 6.8 and 6.1. Rosiglitazone is readily soluble in ethanol and a buffered aqueous solution with pH of 2.3; solubility decreases with increasing pH in the physiological range. The molecule has a single chiral center and is present as a racemate. Even so, the enantiomers are functionally indistinguishable because of rapid interconversion.

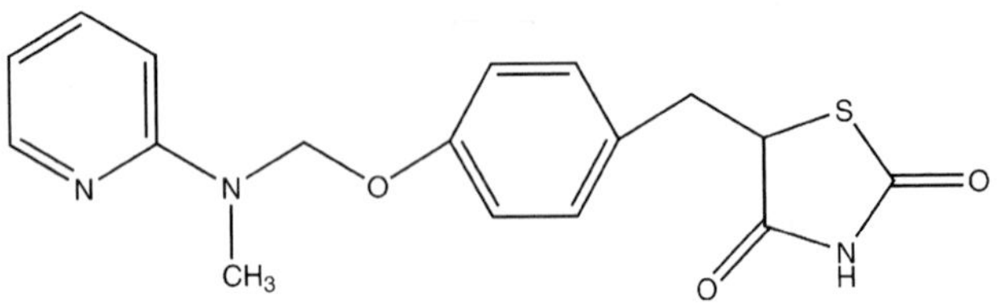

Rosiglitazone
(Avandia)

Pioglitazone. Pioglitazone, (±)-5-[[4-[2-(5-ethyl-2-pyri-dinyl)ethoxy]phenyl]methyl]-2,4-thiazolidinedione (Actos), is an odorless, white, crystalline powder that must be converted to a salt such as its hydrochloride before it will have any water solubility. Although the molecule contains one chiral center, the compound is used as the racemic mixture. This is primarily a result of the in vivo interconversion of the two enantiomers. Thus, there are no differences in the pharmacological activity of the two enantiomers.

Bisguanidines

Metformin. Metformin, *N,N*-dimethylimidodicarboni-midic diamide hydrochloride (Glucophage), is a bisguanidine. This class of agents is capable of reducing sugar absorption from the gastrointestinal tract. Also, they can decrease gluconeogenesis while increasing glucose uptake by muscles and fat cells. These effects, in turn, lead to lower blood glucose levels. Unlike the sulfonylureas, these are not hypoglycemic agents but rather can act as antihyperglycemics. This difference in nomenclature is caused by the inability of these agents to stimulate the release of insulin from the pancreas. Often, metformin is coadministered with the nonsulfonylureas to improve the efficacy of those agents.

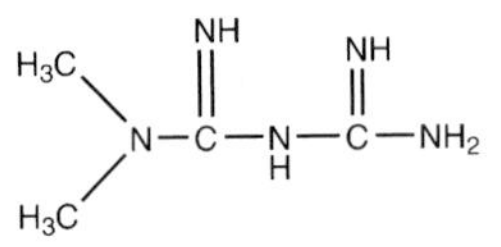

Metformin
(Glucophage)

α-Glucosidase Inhibitors

The enzyme α-glucosidase is present in the brush border of the small intestine and is responsible for cleaving dietary carbohydrates and facilitating their absorption into the body. Inhibition of this enzyme allows less dietary carbohydrate to be available for absorption and, in turn, less available in the blood following a meal. The inhibitory properties of these agents are greatest for glycoamylase, followed by sucrose, maltase, and dextranase, respectively. Because these do not enhance insulin secretion when used as monotherapy, hypoglycemia is generally not a concern when using these agents.

Acarbose. Acarbose, *O*-4,6-dideoxy-4-[[(1*S*,4*R*,5*S*,6*S*) 4,5,6-trihydroxy-3-(hydroxymethyl)-2-cyclohexen-1-yl]amino]α-D-glucopyranosyl-(1,4)-*O*-α-D-glucopyranosyl-(1,4)-D-glucose (Precose), is a naturally occurring oligosaccharide, which is obtained from the microorganism *Actinoplanes utahensis*. It is a white to off-white powder

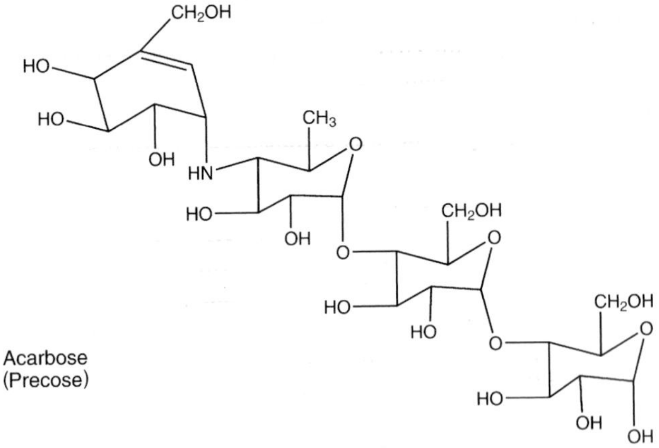

Acarbose
(Precose)

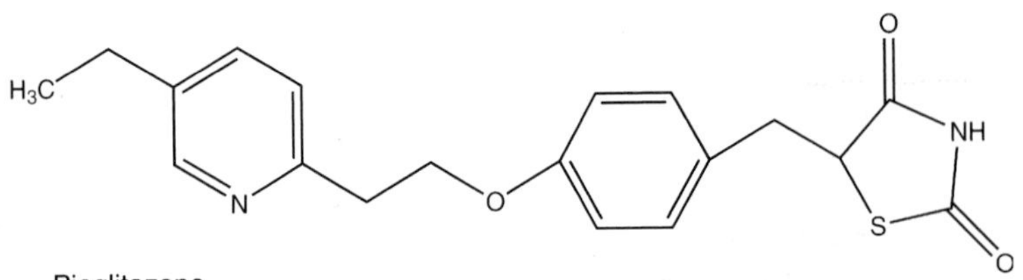

Pioglitazone
(Actos)

that is soluble in water and has a pK_a of 5.1. As one might expect, its affinity for α-glucosidase is based on it being a polysaccharide that the enzyme attempts to hydrolyze. This allows acarbose to act as a competitive inhibitor, which in turn reduces the intestinal absorption of starch, dextrin, and dissacharides.

Miglitol.   Miglitol, 1-(2-hydroxyethyl)-2-(hydroxymethyl)-[2R-(2α,3β,4α,5β)]-piperidine (Glyset), a desoxynojirimycin derivative, is chemically known as 3,4,5-piperidinetriol. It is a white to pale yellow powder that is soluble in water, with a pK_a of 5.9. In chemical structure, this agent is very similar to a sugar, with the heterocyclic nitrogen serving as an isosteric replacement of the sugar oxygen. This feature allows recognition by the α-glucosidase as a substrate. This results in competitive inhibition of the enzyme and delays complex carbohydrate absorption from the gastrointestinal tract.

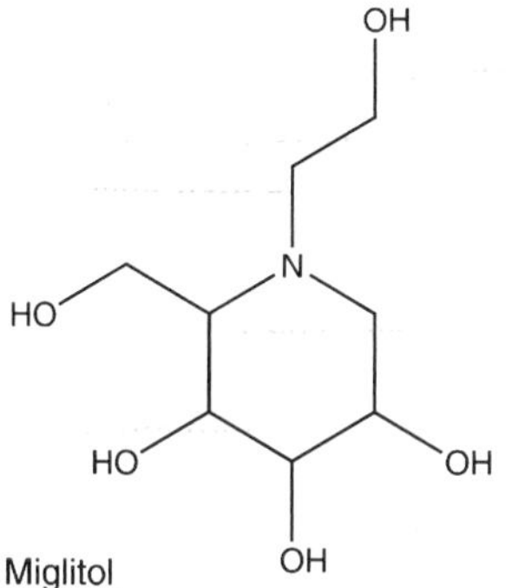

Miglitol
(Glyset)

THYROID HORMONES

Desiccated, defatted thyroid substance has been used for many years as replacement therapy in thyroid gland deficiencies. The efficacy of the whole gland is now known to depend on its thyroglobulin content. This is an iodine-containing globulin. Thyroxine was obtained as a crystalline derivative by Kendall[79] of the Mayo Clinic in 1915. It showed much the same action as the whole thyroid substance. Later, thyroxine was synthesized by Harington and Barger[80] in England. Later studies showed that an even more potent iodine-containing hormone existed, which is now known as triiodothyronine. Evidence now indicates that thyroxine may be the storage form of the hormone, whereas triiodothyronine is the circulating form. Another point of view is that in the blood, thyroxine is bound more firmly to the globulin fraction than is triiodothyronine, which can then enter the tissue cells.

Levothyroxine Sodium, USP.   Levothyroxine sodium, O-(4-hydroxy-3,5-diiodophenyl)-3,5-diiodo-2-tyrosine monosodium salt, hydrate (Synthroid, Letter, Levoxine, Levoid), is the sodium salt of the *levo* isomer of thyroxine, which is an active physiological principle obtained from the thyroid gland of domesticated animals used for food by humans. It is also prepared synthetically. The salt is a light yellow, tasteless, odorless powder. It is hygroscopic but stable in dry air at room temperature. It is soluble in alkali hydroxides, 1:275 in alcohol, and 1:500 in water, to give a pH of about 8.9.

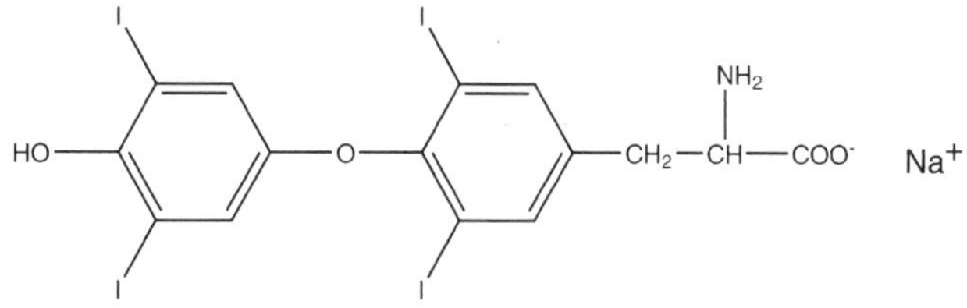

Levothyroxine Sodium
(Synthroid, Letter, Levoxine, Levoid)

Levothyroxine sodium is used in replacement therapy of decreased thyroid function (hypothyroidism). In general, a dosage of 100 μg of levothyroxine sodium is clinically equivalent to 30 to 60 mg of thyroid *USP*.

Liothyronine Sodium, USP.   Liothyronine sodium, O-(4-hydroxy-3-iodophenyl)-3,5-diiodo-L-thyroxine monosodium salt (Cytomel), is the sodium salt of L-3,3′,5-triiodothyronine. It occurs as a light tan, odorless, crystalline powder, which is slightly soluble in water or alcohol and has a specific rotation of +18 to 22 degrees in a mixture of diluted HCl and alcohol.

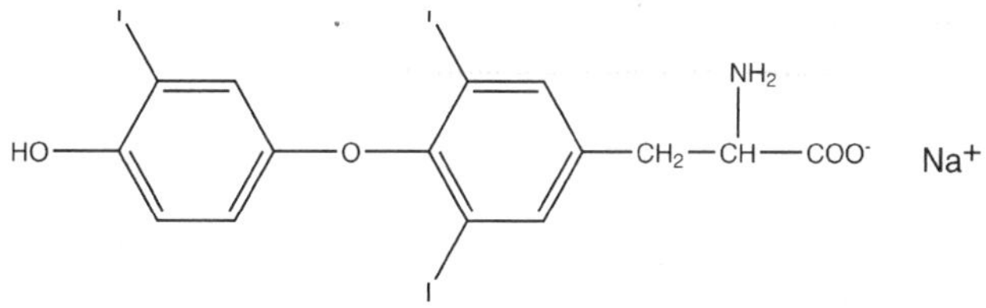

Liothyronine Sodium
(Cytomel)

Liothyronine sodium occurs in vivo together with levothyroxine sodium; it has the same qualitative activities as thyroxine but is more active. It is absorbed readily from the gastrointestinal tract, is cleared rapidly from the bloodstream, and is bound more loosely to plasma proteins than is thyroxine, probably because of the less acidic phenolic hydroxyl group.

Its uses are the same as those of levothyroxine sodium, including treatment of metabolic insufficiency, male infertility, and certain gynecological disorders.

ANTITHYROID DRUGS

Hyperthyroidism (excessive production of thyroid hormones) usually requires surgery, but before surgery the patient must be prepared by preliminary abolition of the hyperthyroidism through the use of antithyroid drugs. Thiourea and related compounds show an antithyroid activity, but they are too

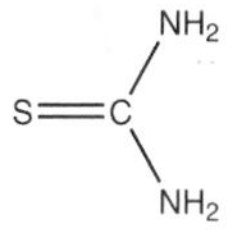

Thiourea

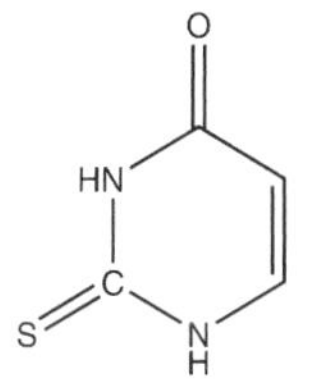

2-Thiouracil

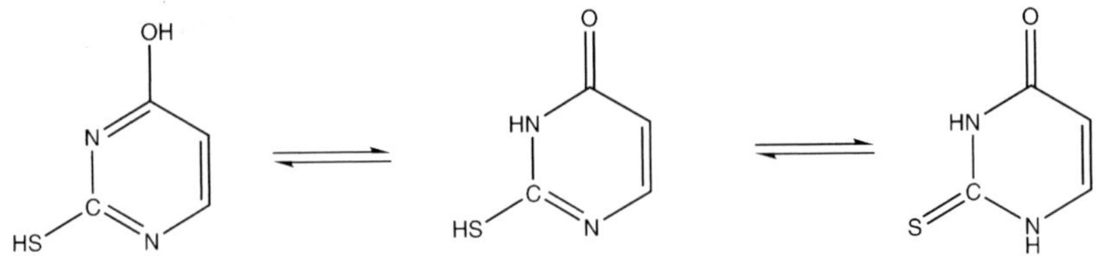

toxic for clinical use. The more useful drugs are 2-thiouracil derivatives and a closely related 2-thioimidazole derivative. All of these appear to have a similar mechanism of action (i.e., prevention of the iodination of the precursors of thyroxine and triiodothyronine). The main difference in the compounds lies in their relative toxicities.

These compounds are absorbed well after oral administration and excreted in the urine.

The 2-thiouracils, 4-keto-2-thiopyrimidines, are undoubtedly tautomeric compounds and can be represented as follows:

Some 300 related structures have been evaluated for antithyroid activity, but of these, only the 6-alkyl-2-thiouracils and closely related structures possess useful clinical activity. The most serious adverse effect of thiouracil therapy is agranulocytosis.

Propylthiouracil, USP. Propylthiouracil, 6-propyl-2-thiouracil (Propacil), is a stable, white, crystalline powder with a bitter taste. It is slightly soluble in water but readily soluble in alkaline solutions (salt formation).

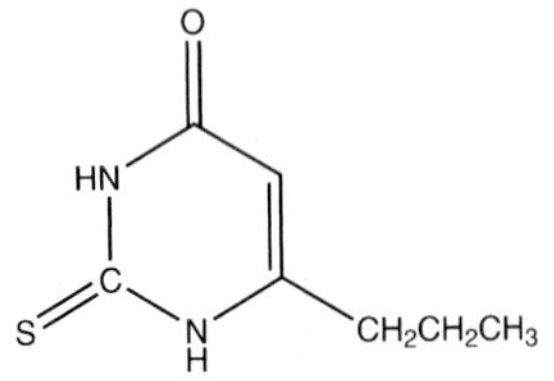

Propylthiouracil
(Propacil)

This drug is useful in the treatment of hyperthyroidism. There is a delay in appearance of its effects because propylthiouracil does not interfere with the activity of thyroid hormones already formed and stored in the thyroid gland. This lag period may vary from several days to weeks, depending on the condition of the patient. The need for three equally spaced doses during a 24-hour period is often stressed, but evidence now indicates that a single daily dose is as effective as multiple daily doses in the treatment of most hyperthyroid patients.[81]

Methimazole, USP. Methimazole, 1-methylimidazole-2-thiol (Tapazole), occurs as a white to off-white, crystalline powder with a characteristic odor and is freely soluble in water. A 2% aqueous solution has a pH of 6.7 to 6.9. It should be packaged in well-closed, light-resistant containers.

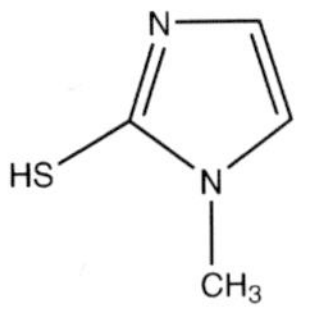

Methimazole
(Tapazole)

Methimazole is indicated in the treatment of hyperthyroidism. It is more potent than propylthiouracil. The side effects are similar to those of propylthiouracil. As with other antithyroid drugs, patients using this drug should be under medical supervision. Also, like the other antithyroid drugs, methimazole is most effective if the total daily dose is subdivided and given at 8-hour intervals.

◆ REVIEW QUESTIONS ◆

1. Nitroglycerin can be used as an antianginal agent because of its vasodilator effects. Also, nitroglycerin is a liquid used in dynamite; why does not Mrs. Smith blow up when using this drug as a vasodilator?

   a. It is not really the same nitroglycerin as the one used to make dynamite.
   b. Nitroglycerin must be used while it is fresh so it will not detonate.
   c. There are stabilizers added to nitroglycerin that prevent its detonation.
   d. Nitroglycerin is very dilute when used as an antianginal agent so it will not detonate.

2. Although the agent shown here (Losartan [Cozaar]) has some pharmacological effects, one of its metabolites is reported to be more potent. Identify this metabolite.

   a. *N*-dealkylation that releases the imidazole ring (*N*-deimidazole metabolite)

   b. oxidation of the 5-methanol to a carboxylic acid
   c. oxidation of the aromatic (benzene) ring to a phenol
   d. oxidation of the omega-1 carbon on the 2-position alkyl side chain
   e. None of the above is true because only the parent compound is active.

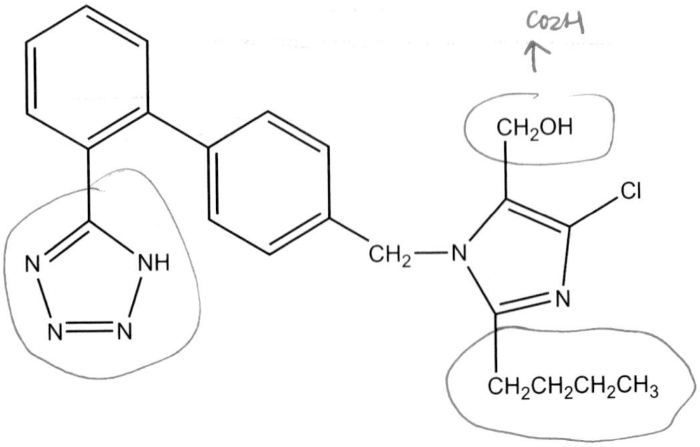

3. After a patient is administered an <u>organic nitrate,</u> these are then metabolized to nitric oxide (NO) by first reacting with _____ to form _____.

   a. sulfhydryls: *S*-nitrosothiols
   b. amidase; carboxylic acids and amines
   c. esterases; carboxylic acids and alcohols
   d. hydroxyl residues; *O*-nitrosoalcohols

4. Highlight the difference between digoxin and digitoxin and point out the two primary reasons why one is more toxic than the other.

REFERENCES

1. Robinson, B. F.: Adv. Drug. Res. 10:93, 1975.
2. Aronow, W. S.: Am. Heart J. 84:273, 1972.
3. Sonnenblick, E., Ross, J., Jr., and Braunwald, E.: Am. J. Cardiol. 22:328, 1968.
4. Ignarro, L. J., et al.: J. Pharmacol. Exp. Ther. 218:739, 1981.
5. Feelisch, M.: Eur. Heart J. 14(Suppl. I):123, 1993.
6. Needleman, P.: Annu. Rev. Pharmacol. Toxicol. 16:81, 1976.
7. Chung, S. J., and Fung, H. L.: J. Pharmacol. Exp. Ther. 253:614, 1990.
8. Fusari, S. A.: J. Pharm. Sci. 62:123, 1973.
9. Fusari, S. A.: J. Pharm. Sci. 62:2012, 1973.
10. McCall, D., et al.: Curr. Probl. Cardiol. 10:1, 1985.
11. Heschler, J., et al.: Eur. J. Biochem. 165:261, 1987.
12. Beridge, M. J.: Annu. Rev. Biochem. 56:159, 1987.
13. van Zweiten, P. A., and van Meel, J. C.: Prog. Pharmacol. 5:1, 1982.
14. Atkinson, J., et al.: Naunyn Schmeidbergs Arch. Pharmacol. 337:471, 1988.
15. Smith, H. J., and Briscoe, M. G.: J. Mol. Cell Cardiol. 17:709, 1985.
16. Sanguinetti, M. C., and Kass, R. S.: Circ. Res. 55:336, 1984.
17. Rosenkirchen, R., et al.: Naunyn Schmiedebergs Arch. Pharmacol. 310:69, 1979.
18. Triggle, D. J.: Calcium antagonists. In: Antonoccio, P. N. (ed.). Cardiovascular Pharmacology, 3rd ed. New York, Raven Press, 1990.
19. Dobesh, P. P., and Trujillo, T. C.: Pharmacotherapy 27:1659, 2007.
20. Vaughan Williams, E. M.: In Sandoe, E., Flensted-Jansen, E., and Olesen, K. H. (eds.). Symposium on Cardiac Arrhythmias. Sodertalje, Sweden, B. Astra, 1970, pp. 449–472.
21. Vaughan Williams, E. M.: J. Clin. Pharmacol. 24:129, 1984.
22. CAPS Investigators: Am. J. Cardiol. 61:501, 1988.
23. Woosley, R. L.: Annu. Rev. Pharmacol. Toxicol. 31:427, 1991.
24. Campbell, T. J.: Cardiovasc. Res. 17:344, 1983.
25. Yool, A. J.: Mol. Pharmacol. 46:970, 1994.
26. Hondeghem, L. M., and Katzung, B. G.: Annu. Rev. Pharmacol. Toxicol. 24:387, 1984.
27. Nies, A. S., and Shang, D. G.: Clin. Pharmacol. Exp. Ther. 14:823, 1973.
28. Koch-Wester, J.: Ann. N. Y. Acad. Sci. 179:370, 1971.
29. Giardinia, E. V., et al.: Clin. Pharmacol. Ther. 19:339, 1976.
30. Elson, J., et al.: Clin. Pharmacol. Ther. 17:134, 1975.
31. Belfer, B., et al.: Am. J. Cardiol. 35:282, 1975.
32. Bigger, T. J., and Jaffe, C. C.: Am. J. Cardiol. 27:82, 1971.
33. Hollunger, G.: Acta Pharmacol. Toxicol. 17:356, 1960.
34. Helfant, R. H., et al.: Am. Heart J. 77:315, 1969.
35. Beckett, A. H., and Chiodomere, E. C.: Postgrad. Med. J. 53(Suppl. 1):60, 1977.
36. Anderson, J. L., Mason, J. W., and Roger, M. D.: Circulation 57:685, 1978.
37. Guehler, J., et al.: Am. J. Cardiol. 55:807, 1985.
38. Saeki, T., et al.: Eur. J. Pharmacol. 261:249, 1994.
39. Groshner, K., et al.: Br. J. Pharmacol. 102:669, 1991.
40. Hii, J. T., Duff, H. J., and Burgess, E. D.: Clin. Pharmacokinet. 21:1, 1991.
41. Olsson, S. B., Brorson, L., and Varnauskas, E.: Br. Heart J. 35:1255, 1973.
42. Kannan, R., et al.: Clin. Pharmacol. 31:438, 1982.
43. Witt, D. M., Ellsworth, A. J., and Leversee, J. H.: Ann. Pharmacother. 27:1463, 1993.
44. Nadermanee, K., et al.: Circulation 66:202, 1982.
45. Papp, J. G., and Vaughan Williams, E. M.: Br. J. Pharmacol. 37:380, 1969.
46. Boyer, E. W., Stork, C., and Wang, R. Y.: Int. J. Med. Toxicol. 2001;4:16.
47. Salata, J. J., and Brooks, R. R.: Cardiol. Drug Rev. 15:137–156, 1997.
48. D'Orleans-Juste, P., Labonte, J., Bkaily, G., et al.: Pharmacol. Ther. 95:221, 2002.
49. Newman, J. H., Kar, S., and Kirkpatrick, P.: Nat. Rev. Drug Discov. 6:697, 2007
50. Oldfield, V., and Lyseng-Williamson, K. A.: Am. J. Cardiovasc. Drugs, 6:189, 2006.
51. Vakil, R.: Br. Heart J. 11:350, 1949.
52. Hess, S. M., Shore, P. A., and Brodie, P. P.: Br. J. Pharmacol. Exp. Ther. 118:84, 1956.
53. Kirshner, N.: J. Biol. Chem. 237:2311, 1962.
54. von Euler, U. S., and Lishajko, F.: Int. J. Neuropharmacol. 2:127, 1963.
55. Muller, J. M., Schlittler, E., and Brin, H. J.: Experientia 8:338, 1952.
56. U'Prichard, D., et al.: Eur. J. Pharmacol. 50:87, 1978.
57. Langer, S. Z., and Cavero, I.: Hypertension 2:372, 1980.
58. Starke, K., and Montel, H.: Neuropharmacology 12:1073, 1973.
59. Meisheri, K. D.: Direct-acting vasodilators. In Singh, B. J., et al. (eds.). Cardiovascular Pharmacology. New York, Churchill Livingstone, 1994, p. 173.
60. Gross, F., Druey, J., and Meier, R.: Experientia 6:19, 1950.
61. Zacest, R., and Koch-Wesesr, J.: Clin. Pharmacol. 13:4420, 1972.
62. Page, I. H., et al.: Circulation 11:188, 1955.
63. Corbin, J. D., Francis, S. H., and Webb, D. J.: Urology 60(2):4, 2002.
64. Ring, B. J., Patterson, B. E., Mitchell, M. I., et al.: Clin. Pharmacol. Ther. 77(1):63, 2005.
65. Cook, N. S.: Potassium Channels: Structure, Classification, Function and Therapeutic Potential. New York, John Wiley & Sons, 1990, p. 181.
66. DuCharme, D. W., et al.: Pharmacol. Exp. Ther. 184:662, 1973.
67. Levy, R. I., et al.: Circulation 69:325, 1984.
68. Levy, R. I.: Annu. Rev. Pharmacol. Toxicol. 47:499, 1977.
69. Mannisto, P. T., et al.: Acta Pharmacol. Toxicol. 36:353, 1975.
70. Kesaniemi, Y. A., and Grundy, S. M.: JAMA 251:2241, 1984.
71. Atmeh, R. F., et al.: J. Lipid Res. 24:588, 1983.
72. Sweeney, M. E., and Johnson, R. R.: Exp. Opin. Drug Metab. Toxicol. 3(3):441, 2007.
73. Stenflo, J., et al.: Proc. Natl. Acad. Sci. U. S. A. 71:2730, 1974.
74. Jackson, C. M., and Suttie, J. W.: Prog. Hematol. 10:333, 1978.
75. Triplett, D. A. (ed.): Platelet Function. Chicago, American Society of Clinical Pathology, 1978.
76. Hamberg, M., et al.: Proc. Natl. Acad. Sci. U. S. A. 71:345, 1974.
77. Kaplan, M.: Curr. Opin. Investig. Drugs 3(7):1017, 2002.
78. Thomas, R. C., and Ruby, R. W.: J. Med. Chem. 15:964, 1972.
79. Kendall, E. C.: JAMA 64:2042, 1915.
80. Harrington, C. R., and Barger, C.: Biochem. J. 21:169, 1927.
81. Greer, M. A., and Meihoff, W. C.: N. Engl. J. Med. 272:888, 1965.

CHAPTER 20

Hormone-Related Disorders: Nonsteroidal Therapies

RONALD A. HILL

A large and growing number of medicinal substances act on endocrine systems. Many are steroid analogs (i.e., ligands for estrogen, progestin, and androgen receptors), and, as suggested by the title of this chapter, will not be considered herein, but instead in Chapter 25. Neither will all nonsteroidal endocrine modulators be considered in the present chapter, however. Medicinals acting to modulate calcium deposition and resorption, particularly within bone, are discussed in Chapter 21 (including ligands for vitamin D receptors, parathyroid hormone receptors, and calcitonin receptors). Coverage of thyroid hormones, and of agents for treating hyperthyroid states, has been retained in Chapter 19 for this edition of the text. Numerous other endocrine system interventions are, at present, solely accomplished by administering a naturally occurring human protein produced by artificial means. For now, agents of this nature receive primary consideration within a chapter dedicated to "biologics" (Chapter 27); examples include human growth hormone, somatostatin, and the follitropins.

For more than 6 decades, a collection of disorders of primary metabolism, chiefly type 1 and type 2 diabetes, have, for obvious reasons, received great attention from the drug discovery community. These efforts have intensified over the past several decades, evolving to include a significant fraction of the biotechnology enterprise. Insulin remains central to the treatment of type 1 diabetes, and various details of insulin chemistry, biochemistry, and pharmacology are provided in Chapter 27. Within the past decade or so, however, various modified insulins have reached the market, and the molecular bases of their diverse characteristics are considered in the present chapter, along with a brief introduction to insulin itself. Two general classes of drugs that act primarily—but not necessarily exclusively—as insulin secretagogues for treating type 2 diabetes, namely the sulfonylureas and the glinides, are then considered in detail. It has long been realized that defective responsiveness to insulin plays a major role in the etiology and progression of type 2 diabetes. On this basis, biguanides that act, at least in part, as "insulin sensitizers" have been in clinical use for many years, and more recently the thiazolidinediones appeared on the market.

Hormones other than insulin and glucagon also play important roles in regulating the body's glucose handling and associated aspects of food consumption and primary metabolism. The identification of two of these, and subsequent characterization of their physiological actions and biochemistry, led to the creation of amylin and glucagon-like peptide type 1 (GLP-1) receptor agonists, which to date are represented in the market by analogs of the endogenous proteins. Enzymes catalyzing the degradation of these hormones were also identified as potential molecular targets for therapeutic intervention; thus, the first inhibitor of dipeptidyl peptidase type 4 (DPP-4 or DPP-IV), sitagliptin, recently reached the U.S. market, with others expected in the near future.

Given the fact that endocrine signals of a suitable nature are requisite to the survival and proliferation of many cancerous cells, various therapeutics used in oncology (Chapter 10) fall within the potential scope of this chapter. Among these, the gonadotropin-releasing hormone receptor (GnRH-R) agonists and antagonists receive consideration herein. These drugs represent treatment options for various gonadal hormone–dependent cancers, but also see such clinical uses as fertility modulation, mitigation of various uterine disorders, and in treating precocious puberty. The GnRH-R agonists and antagonists currently on the market are modified peptides, and examining how the molecular features of each of these drugs endow them with their particular pharmacological and biopharmaceutical properties offers the medicinal chemistry student some excellent lessons within a realm that is often lightly emphasized. Entry points to the literature in this area have been selected and provided to facilitate further explorations by students who may be motivated to expand the breadth and depth of these lessons.

DISORDERS OF GLUCOSE METABOLISM: DIABETES AND THE METABOLIC SYNDROME

Various forms of diabetes afflict a large and increasing proportion of the population of much of the developed world, and (somewhat surprisingly) rapidly increasing numbers of individuals in the developing world. Diabetes causes impairments, and eventually often kills, in large measure, because of the secondary effects of excessively elevated circulating and tissue glucose levels. Perhaps more insidiously, tolerance to hypoglycemic excursions as a result of progressively impaired counterregulatory responses to the administration of insulin and drugs that elicit insulin release can cause individuals to suffer severe hypoglycemic episodes, involving shock and, in more extreme cases, coma or death.

Diabetes can be broadly classified as "type 1" or "type 2." Type 1 diabetes is also often referred to as insulin-dependent diabetes mellitus (IDDM), or sometimes as juvenile-onset diabetes mellitus, although onset can in fact occur in adults. The hallmark of type 1 diabetes is absent or insufficient insulin secretion by the insulin-secreting cells of the pancreas, namely the beta cells (β cells) of the islets of Langerhans. In some individuals, this arises because of a genetic defect, whereas in other individuals, the disease is "idiopathic" (i.e., the cause is indeterminate), but in most cases, the β-islet cells are partially or completely destroyed as a result of an erroneous autoimmune response. Regardless of cause, type 1 diabetes must, at present, be treated with one or more types of insulin. Type 2 diabetes is often referred to as non–insulin-dependent diabetes mellitus (NIDDM). In type 2 diabetes, the insulin secretory response is impaired—increasingly so as the disease progresses with time, but in most cases, a comorbid defect is the failure of many cells of the body to properly respond to circulating insulin, particularly certain cells in the liver and skeletal muscles having a primary glucose storage role, and certain cells in adipose tissue. Another way of stating this is that the "insulin sensitivity" of these cells becomes impaired. This impairment often occurs secondary to obesity, although this contributor is apparently not obligatory, and the "obesity" may be so mild as to hardly be recognizable as such. In recent years, states of health have been characterized that, without intervention, often lead to type 2 diabetes. Such prediabetic states are now often broadly referred to as "the metabolic syndrome,"[1,2] and various medical organizations are establishing criteria and treatment guidelines intended to avert further development into full-blown type 2 diabetes— that is, preventive medicine tactics. Although historically type 2 diabetes has most often been treated with insulin secretagogues (such as one of the sulfonylurea drugs, vide infra) or, in some cases, insulin, the recognition that this disorder— which is really an array of related disorders—is most often one of defective cellular insulin responsiveness has, in recent years, guided basic and drug discovery research onto paths culminating with the testing and marketing of therapeutic agents, having completely new mechanisms of action. Clinical results in some cases provide the hope not only that the damaging out-of-safe-range excursions of blood and tissue glucose levels might be prevented, but also that individuals with type 2 diabetes might be cured, and individuals with prediabetic syndromes be saved from developing the full-blown disease. For type 1 diabetics or those type 2 patients requiring insulin supplementation, devices allowing for continuous monitoring of blood glucose and microprocessor-controlled on-demand insulin delivery seem likely to soon revolutionize treatment. Until very recently, though, alternatives to lifelong insulin therapy for such patients seemed no more than hopeful dreams. Yet, scientific advances now suggest that, before many more years pass, it should be possible to implant alternative glucose-responsive, insulin-secreting cells in the pancreas or liver. Even more excitingly, it appears that it will be possible to stimulate regeneration of β-cell populations within the pancreatic islets while simultaneously arresting the autoimmune attack that would otherwise destroy them; therefore, type 1 diabetes could, for all practical purposes, be cured.

Insulins and Modified Insulins

Type 1 diabetes must, for now, be treated with insulin replacement therapy. After the demonstration c. 1900 that this disorder, which was invariably fatal within a short time, was one of pancreatic β-cell failure, more than 20 years passed before insulin was isolated and purified from fetal calf pancreases, and its clinical relevance demonstrated. Commercially viable production was achieved by Eli Lilly and Co., with initial marketing in 1923 (Iletin). The primary structure of human insulin was not reported until 1958 (Nobel Prize in Chemistry to Frederick Sanger, 1964), and the tertiary structure was not available until reported by Dorothy Crowfoot Hodgkin in 1969, a triumph of x-ray crystallography. Prior to the 1980s, treatment of type 1 diabetes was achieved via injections of porcine or bovine insulin, or combinations thereof. Although preparations containing porcine or bovine insulin may remain in use around the globe, the availability of human insulin produced artificially via methods of "biotechnology" has widely supplanted insulin from animal sources, and, undoubtedly, will soon completely replace them as cost barriers are conquered. No animal-sourced preparations are now available in the United States. Moreover, several modified insulin preparations have come on the market in recent years, and the development of technology for alternative routes of administration besides injection is also rapidly changing the therapeutic landscape.

Human insulin is a heterodimer (Fig. 20.1), consisting of two different peptide subunits linked covalently by two disulfide bridges. This heterodimer is produced from a single, continuous, and substantially larger (110-amino-acid) protein, namely preproinsulin. Among other reasons, production in this manner ensures proper three-dimensional (3D) folding and cross-linking of insulin. Preproinsulin is converted to proinsulin (86-amino-acid residues), from which insulin is produced by removal of a 35-amino-acid segment joining the two subunits. Chapter 27 includes a more detailed treatment of the biosynthesis and structural attributes of human insulin, as well as further information regarding its storage within, and release from, pancreatic β cells.

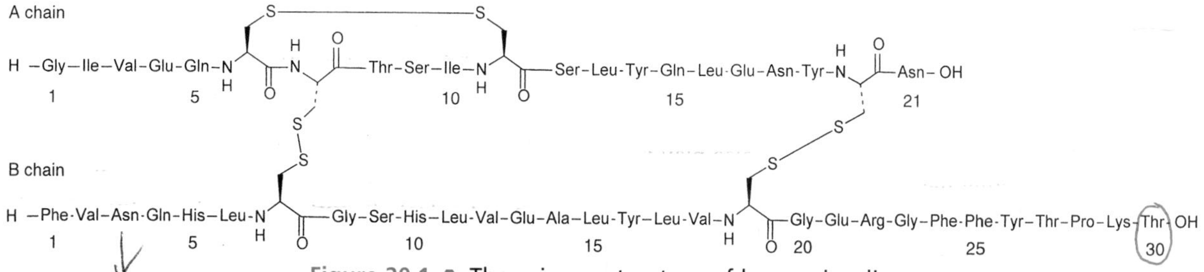

Figure 20.1 ● The primary structure of human insulin.

TABLE 20.1 Modified Insulins[a]

	Trade Name	Structural Differences vs. Human Insulin	Characteristics Achieved
Bovine insulin		$Thr^{A8} \to Ala$, $Ile^{A10} \to Val$ $Thr^{B30} \to Ala$	
Porcine insulin		A chain same as hIns $Thr^{B30} \to Ala$	
Insulin aspart	NovoLog	A chain same as hIns $Pro^{B28} \to Asp$	Rapidity of onset increased, duration substantially decreased vs. regular human insulin[b]
Insulin lispro	Humalog	A chain same as hIns $Pro^{B28} \to Lys$, $Lys^{B29} \to Pro$	Rapidity of onset increased, duration substantially decreased vs. regular human insulin[b]
Insulin glulisine	Apidra	A chain same as hIns $Asn^{B3} \to Lys$, $Lys^{B29} \to Glu$	Rapidity of onset increased, duration substantially decreased vs. regular human insulin[b]
Insulin glargine	Lantus	$Asn^{A21} \to Gly$ Arg^{B31} and Arg^{B32} added to B chain C terminus	Extended action
Insulin detemir	Levemir	A chain same as hIns Lys^{B29} derivatized: $N^{\epsilon}\text{-}CO(CH_2)_{12}CH_3$ Thr^{B30} removed	Soluble *and* long-acting

[a]See also Table 20.2 for other details and information pertaining to modified insulins.
[b]Solution dimerization is reduced or abolished, the onset rate is thus substantially increased because the monomer remains in solution; completion of release into the systemic circulation occurs substantially sooner because the molecules mostly stay in solution at the injection site.

Porcine insulin differs from human insulin by only a single amino acid: The carboxyl terminus residue of the B chain in human insulin is threonine, whereas in porcine insulin, it is alanine (Fig. 20.1 and Table 20.1). Bovine insulin differs in this same manner, but also at two additional positions in the A chain ($Thr^{A8}Ala$ and $Ile^{A10}Val$; again see Table 20.1). Even though these differences are quite modest, and allow either bovine or porcine insulin to bind to and activate human insulin receptors comparably to human insulin, immunogenicity to the animal insulins can and does occur. (Although it is now realized that, historically, more incidences of immune intolerance were likely traceable to minor impurities in the insulin preparations than to the animal insulin itself.) Human recombinant insulin is produced commercially in *Escherichia coli* or yeast. Because proper folding of the final product must be achieved, and purification is nontrivial, the production processes for human recombinant insulin are highly complex and demanding (see Chapter 27, and references therein, for further details). Human insulin had also been produced commercially by conversion of porcine insulin, which requires only the B^{30} Ala→Thr replacement, and can be done in such a way as to preserve 3D structure.

Insulin is monomeric in solution only at very low concentrations, less than about 0.1 μm. In many pharmaceutical preparations, it is dimeric; that is, it exists in a form in which one molecule of A-B covalently linked heterodimer associates noncovalently with another A-B heterodimer. In solutions of pH near neutral, the addition of suitable amounts of Zn^{2+} to such dimeric preparations results in the formation of hexamers (i.e., 6 × A-B heterodimer). Hexamer formation also occurs without Zn^{2+} in solutions having of concentrations higher than ~0.2 μm. Pharmaceutical advantage has been taken of the formation of such noncovalent multimers, because solubilities of the various insulin species differ and, thus, release rates from the injection site can be considerably altered, and reliably so. Consequently, products such as protamine zinc insulin suspension, semilente insulin, and ultralente insulin were created (see Chapter 27). The B21→B30 sequence was found to play a crucial role in this noncovalent insulin dimerization, and a more detailed understanding of this fact has allowed, yet additional pharmaceutical manipulations, resulting in such products as neutral protein Hagedorn (NPH) insulin, also known as isophane insulin. Amino acid substitutions in the B21→B30 region, in some cases in conjunction with a further single amino acid substitution elsewhere in the A-B heterodimer, have, over the past decade, provided several therapeutically valuable "modified insulins," including lispro insulin, insulin aspart, insulin glargine, insulin glulisine, and insulin detemir (see Table 20.2). In these products, enhanced solution stabilities, modified solubilities, increased rapidity of onset, and varied (shortened or extended) durations of action are achieved.

Sulfonylureas and Glinides

Sulfonylureas act at the molecular level primarily as "insulin secretagogues," that is, these compounds elicit insulin secretion from pancreatic β-islet cells. Glinides (also known as meglitinides) exert their action mainly by this means as well. A sufficient complement of functioning β cells must, therefore, be present in a patient in order for any one of these compounds to exert at least this component of its intended action, thus only patients with type 2 (not type 1) diabetes are candidates for pharmacotherapy with such compounds. In recent years, it has become apparent that for insulin secretagogues, homeostatic (biochemical) adjustments cause a progressive loss of at least some effectiveness over the course of several months after initiation of therapy.[3] The entirety of the consequent implications in clinical practice has not yet been established.

The insulin-secreting response that a sulfonylurea or glinide elicits from β cells is brought about at the macromolecular target level by interaction of these drug molecules with adenosine triphosphate (ATP)-sensitive K^+ channels. (Secondary pharmacological targets leading to significant differences between and among sulfonylureas and glinides will be briefly discussed later in the chapter.) More specifically, a sulfonylurea or glinide molecule binds to an sulfonylurea receptor (SUR) subunit

TABLE 20.2 Marketed Insulin Products[a]

	Trade Name	Formulation and Administration	Onset Characteristics	Peak (hr)	Duration	Other Information
Regular human insulin, recombinant[b]	Humulin R Humulin R Pen Novolin R	100 U/mL (OTC)	Rapid 0.5–1 hr	Varies by formulation	8–12 hr	
Regular human insulin, recombinant	Exubera (Pfizer)	Powder, 1 mg or 3 mg per inhalation	10–20 min	2 hr	~6 hr	Restricted availability
Regular human insulin, recombinant, concentrated	Humulin R (Lilly)	500 U/mL (R$_x$)	Rapid	Extended	up to 24 hr	Zinc-insulin preparation; clear solution but precipitates upon injection
Recombinant human insulin isophane suspension	Humulin N Novolin N	100 U/mL (OTC)	1–1.5 hr	4–12 hr	24 hr	NPH (neutral protein Hagedorn): a crystalline protamine zinc insulin suspension
Insulin suspension isophane human recombinant;	Humulin 70/30, Humulin 70/30 Pen (Lilly)	70 U/mL	Rapid	Mixed	24 hr	
insulin human recombinant	Novolin 70/30 (Novo Nordisk)	30 U/mL sc				
Insulin glulisine recombinant	Apidra, Apidra Solostar (Sanofi-Aventis)	100 U/mL sc 15 min before meal, or infusion sc or iv	Rapid	0.5–1.5 hr	1–2.5 hr	Produced in a nonpathogenic laboratory strain of *E. coli* (K12)
Insulin as part recombinant	NovoLog (Novo Nordisk)	100 U/mL sc	Rapid 0.25 hr	1–3 hr	3–5 hr	Produced in *Saccharomyces cerevisiae* (baker's yeast)
Insulin lispro recombinant	Humalog, Humalog Pen, Humalog Kwikpen (Lilly)	100 U/mL sc	Rapid 0.25 hr	0.5–1.5 hr	2–5 hr	Consists of zinc-insulin lispro crystals dissolved in clear aqueous fluid
Insulin glargine recombinant	Lantus (Sanofi-Aventis)	100 U/mL sc	1.1 hr	Extended release— no distinct peak	24+ hr	Formulated upon as a solution at pH 4; injection, hexameric insulin microcrystals precipitate, from which insulin in biologically active form is slowly released
Insulin detemir recombinant	Levemir (Novo Nordisk)	100 U/mL sc or iv infusion	0.8–2 hr	Extended release— no distinct peak	24 hr	
Insulin lispro protamine recombinant; insulin lispro recombinant	Humalog Mix, Humalog Mix Kwikpen (Lilly)	50 U/mL/50 U/mL or 75 U/mL/75 U/mL sc	Rapid	Mixed	up to 24 hr	
Insulin as part protamine recombinant; insulin aspart recombinant	NovoLog Mix 70/30 (Novo Nordisk)	70 U/mL	Rapid	Mixed	12–16 hr	
		30 U/mL sc				

[a]See Table 20.1 for structural details of modified insulins.
[b]Ultralente (U) and Lente (L) insulins have been discontinued in the United States, supplanted by newer modified insulins and insulin mixtures.
iv, intravenous; OTC, over-the-counter; rDNA, recombinant DNA; sc, subcutaneous; U, international activity units.

of an octameric protein complex (Fig. 20.2), which includes four channel-forming $K_{ir}6$ protein subunits, and four SUR1 protein subunits. SUR proteins are so named for their ability to bind various sulfonylureas with high affinity. Sulfonylurea (or glinide) binding favors channel closure, intracellular K^+ concentrations ($[K^+]_{in}$) consequently increase, which in turn increases the propensity of β cells to depolarize (Fig. 20.3). Sufficient β-cell depolarizations bring about insulin release from membrane-associated vesicular stores, which, under normal conditions, are continuously replenished from intracellular insulin storage vesicles. Normally functioning β-islet cells similarly release insulin in response to sufficiently elevated blood glucose concentrations: glucose catabolism (glycolysis) within the cells increases the intracellular ATP:adenosine diphosphate (ADP) concentration ratio (i.e., [ATP]/[ADP] increases), thereby increasing the chances that ATP rather than ADP will be bound to specific adenosine nucleotide–binding sites on the SUR subunits of ATP-sensitive K^+ channels, which in turn favors channel closure. Thus, sufficient tissue-level concentrations of sulfonylureas or glinides in effect mimic the high (ATP)/(ADP) situation that would normally result from elevated blood glucose concentrations, and can,

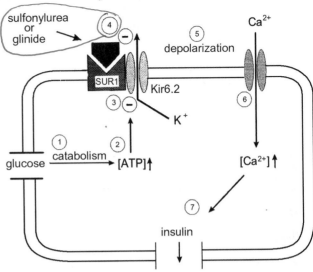

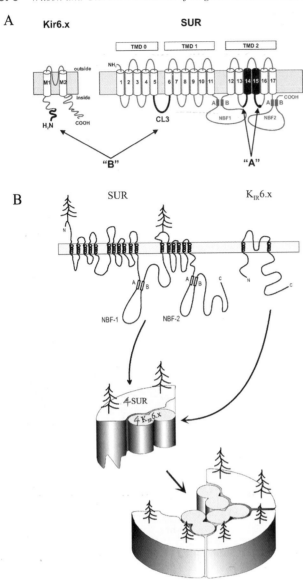

Figure 20.2 • Structure of SUR1/K$_{ir}$6.2 assemblies as pertains to sulfonylurea and glinide binding. **A.** Schematic of the 17-transmembrane SUR subunits,[4] indicating the two nucleotide binding folds NBF1 and NBF2; the two-transmembrane Kir6.X subunits; and the general locations of the "A" ligand-binding domains and the "B" ligand-binding domains (Fig. 20.7); **B.** Schematic of the octameric (4+4) channel assemblages illustrating the central pore created by four K$_{ir}$6.2 subunits, and the four surrounding SUR1 subunits.[5,6] A sulfonylurea or glinide ligand simultaneously engages the portions of the SUR1 and K$_{ir}$6.2 subunits comprising the "B" ligand-binding domain.

Figure 20.3 • Simplified diagram of sulfonylurea action on pancreatic β cells leading to insulin release (adapted from Bounds et al.,[7] with permission). Glucose entering the cell via a membrane transporter (*1*) results in ATP synthesis (*2*), and sufficiently elevated ATP/ADP ratios favor ATP binding (*3*) over ADP binding at the nucleotide binding sites on the channel assemblage, in turn favoring K$^+$ channel closure. Sulfonylureas or glinides also bind to the channel assemblage (*4*), also favoring channel closure. Increased K$^+$ channel closure traps a greater portion of K$^+$ ions within the cell, rendering the intracellular milieu less negative versus extracellular fluids (i.e., depolarization [*5*]). Sufficient depolarization favors calcium channel opening (*6*), allowing Ca^{2+} to flow into the cell. Sufficient increases in cytoplasmic [Ca^{2+}] cause insulin exocytosis (*7*), and also increase trafficking of insulin granules to the cell membrane.

Sulfonylureas were fortuitously discovered because of the hypoglycemic side effects of various sulfonamide antibiotics ("sulfa drugs"), including the isopropylthiadiazole derivative of sulfanilamide and, during its clinical testing, carbutamide (see Fig. 20.6). In the subsequent process of creating such first-generation insulin secretagogues as tolbutamide and chlorpropamide, and thereafter second-generation compounds such as glyburide and gliquidone, many thousands of analogs were synthesized and evaluated pharmacologically. The structure–activity results are somewhat self-evident from the information in Table 20.3, to the extent that molecular-level potency (insulin-releasing action) correlates with dose. In fact, upon accounting for the consequences of relatively modest oral bioavailability and pharmacokinetic differences, observed hypoglycemic potencies correlate very well with molecular-level affinities of the SUR1 binding of these compounds, and with functional potencies obtained from in vitro physiological assays. Invariably, optimized alkyl, cycloalkyl, or cycloazalkyl *N3* (*N'*) substituents provide the highest affinities and potencies. Substitution of *N1* with a benzenesulfonyl moiety (or a comparable arylsulfonyl moiety) is necessary, with *para* substituents generally increasing the potency. Further elaboration at the *para* position with a β-(acylamino)ethyl moiety (as in, for example, the structure of glyburide) was found to greatly enhance the activities among compounds of this general structural class, based on which finding all of the marketed second-generation hypoglycemic sulfonylureas were created.

in this way, compensate for a loss of proper intracellular responsiveness to food-associated hyperglycemic excursions.

Insulin secretagogue sulfonylureas are more specifically referred to as *N*-(phenylsulfonyl)-*N'*-alkylureas. Sulfonylureas commonly referred to as "first-generation" (Fig. 20.4) and "second-generation" (Fig. 20.5) molecules differ mainly with respect to elaboration on the benzene ring at the *para* position of the phenylsulfonyl moiety. Glimepiride is sometimes classified as a third-generation molecule, but structurally, there is no real basis for this distinction.

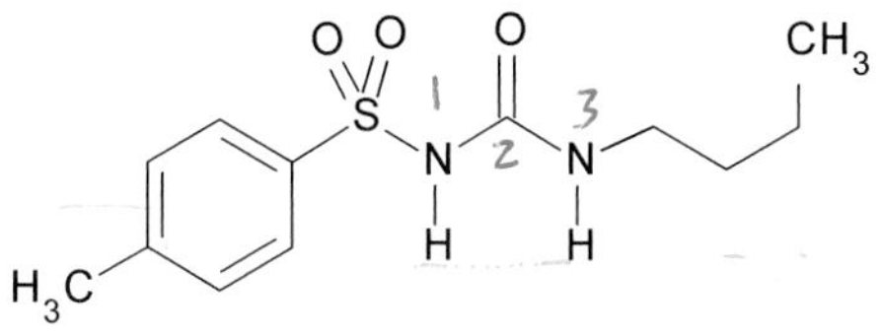

tolbutamide

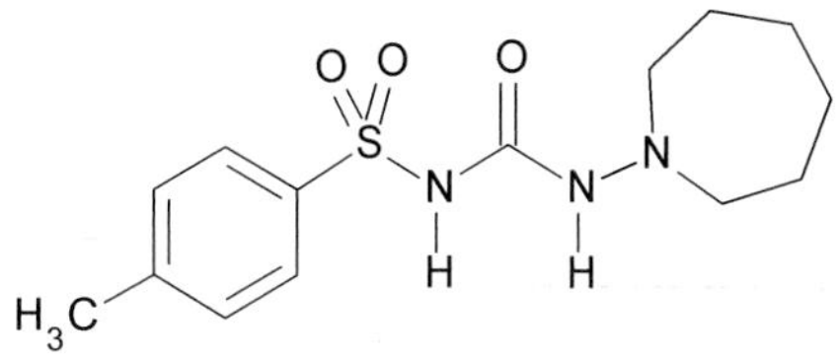

tolazamide

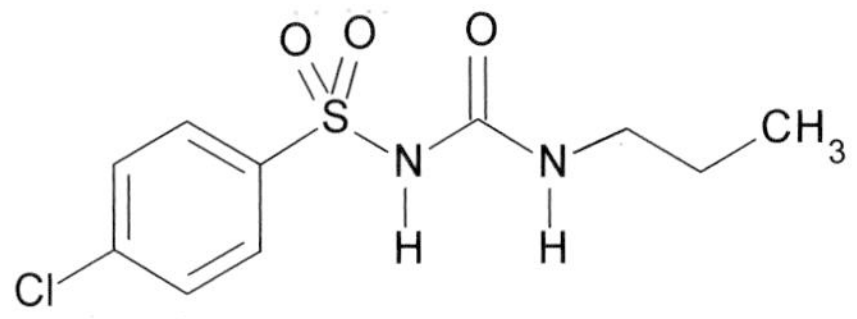

chlorpropamide

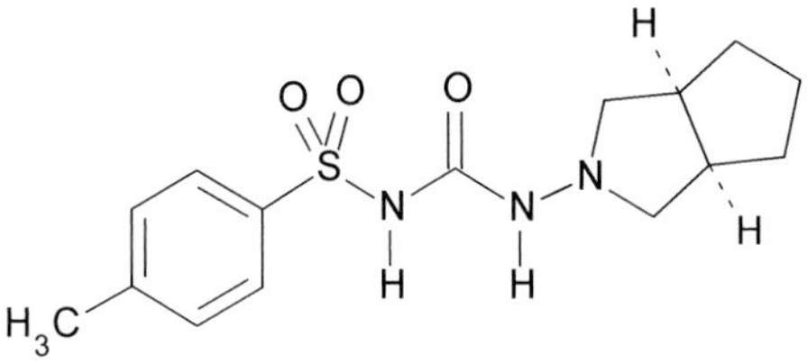

gliclazide

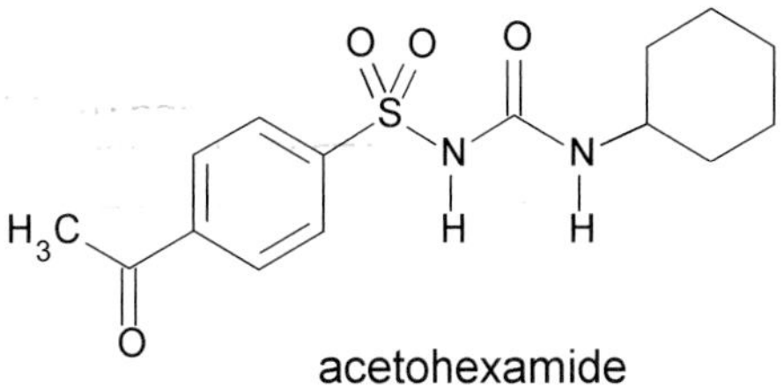

acetohexamide

Figure 20.4 ● First-generation sulfonylurea structures.

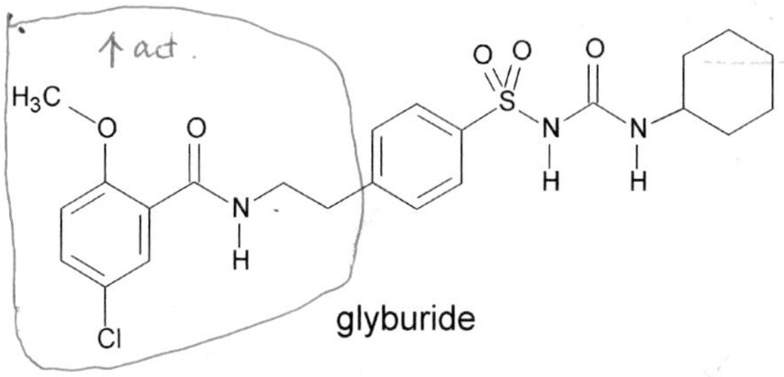

glyburide

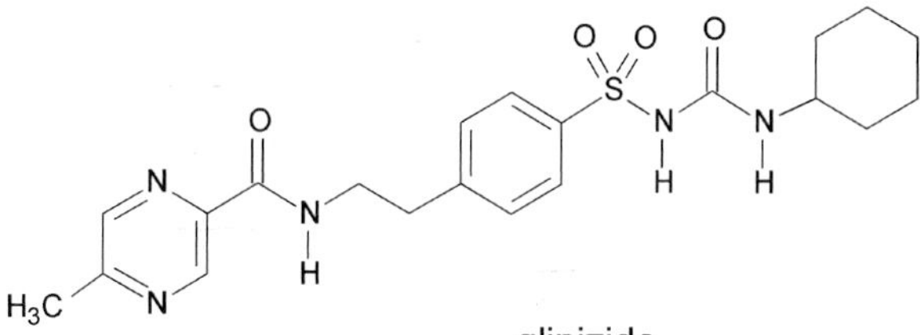

glipizide

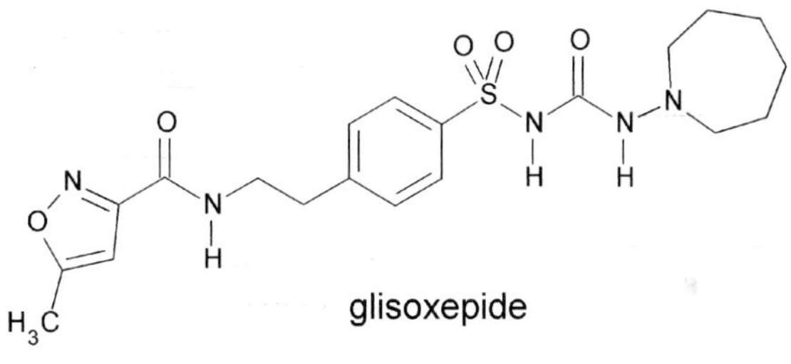

glisoxepide

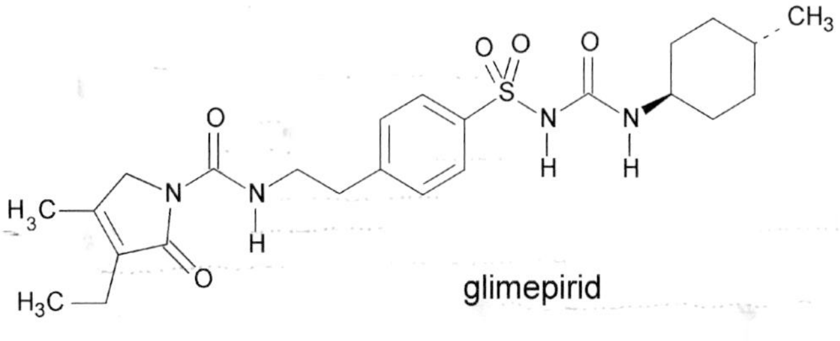

glimepirid

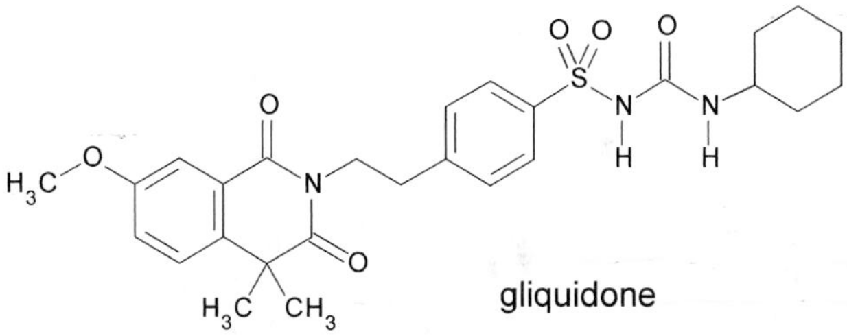

gliquidone

Figure 20.5 ● Second-generation sulfonylurea structures.

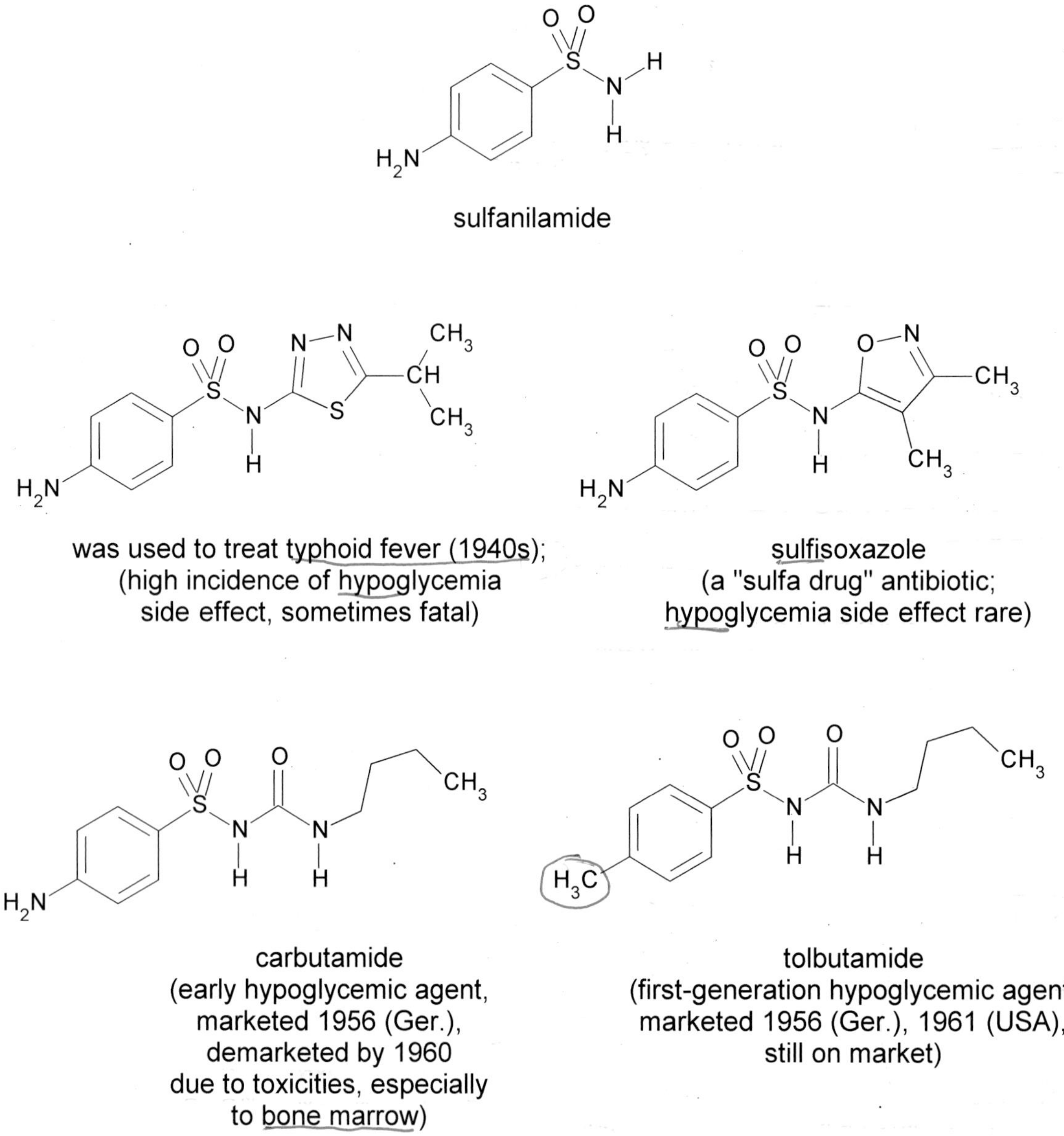

sulfanilamide

was used to treat typhoid fever (1940s); (high incidence of hypoglycemia side effect, sometimes fatal)

sulfisoxazole (a "sulfa drug" antibiotic; hypoglycemia side effect rare)

carbutamide (early hypoglycemic agent, marketed 1956 (Ger.), demarketed by 1960 due to toxicities, especially to bone marrow)

tolbutamide (first-generation hypoglycemic agent, marketed 1956 (Ger.), 1961 (USA), still on market)

Figure 20.6 • Structural genesis of hypoglycemic sulfonylureas.

The sulfonylureas behave as weak acids within the physiological pH range, with pK_a values typically 5 to 6 (Table 20.3); thus, at the pH of blood, the negatively charged conjugate base predominates to the extent of >95%. In addition to the presence of the anionic moiety, portions of these ionized molecules are also relatively lipophilic; such structural combinations often lend themselves to extensive binding to serum and tissue proteins, and this is found to be the case with all of these drugs. In their free acid states, all of the marketed sulfonylureas are quite lipophilic (see log P values, Table 20.3). This characteristic facilitates absorption from the gut lumen, especially in initial portions of the small intestine where the pH remains below or near the pK_a of the drug. Despite the lipophilicity of these molecules in their free-acid form, diffusion through the blood-brain barrier (BBB) is reported to be minimal for drugs of this class, presumably attributable to the combination of high serum protein binding and low percentage of free acid species in blood. Efflux transporters are known to be involved in some cases.[8] For some of these drugs, however, the high potency coupled with

the presence of ATP-sensitive K^+ channels within the brain might possibly account for certain undesirable side effects (notably, weight gain).

Glinides (Figs. 20.7 and 20.8) contain a carboxylic acid moiety that, in its carboxylate form, interacts with the same anion recognition site on ATP-sensitive K^+ channels as does the ionized (conjugate base) form of the sulfonylurea moiety.[10] The pK_a's for the carboxylic acid moieties of repaglinide and nateglinide fall within the expected range. Repaglinide includes a tertiary amine moiety, incorporated within a piperidine ring. The effective pK_a of this structural moiety (6.0–6.2),[12] which gives account of two dissociation microconstants (see Fig. 20.9), is well above the pK_a of aniline (4.6), owing to the sterically demanded twist of the piperidine nitrogen's lone-pair out of optimal conjugation with the benzene ring. Because of the presence of two ionizable moieties, at no solution pH does an uncharged form predominate. Even so, the carboxylate anion (with the piperidine moiety as uncharged free base), which is the predominant molecular species at plasma pH, is relatively

TABLE 20.3 Sulfonylureas

Drug	Protein Binding	Volume of Distribution	Acid–Base and Lipid Partitioning Character	Biotransformation	Elimination[a]	Forms and Dose Range
Tolbutamide	91%–96% hsa[b]	0.12 L/kg[#] / 10 L[h]	pKa 5.2,[c] 5.3[d] Log P 2.3[d] (free acid) Log $D_{7.4}$ = −0.98[c] Log $D_{7.4}$ = 0.81[e]	Extensive, CYP2C9[f]	No unchanged drug in urine[f] ~60% as carboxy metabolite, 30% as hydroxy metabolite in urine (48 hr)[h] Cl_{ss} = 0.9 L/hr[f] $t_{1/2}$ ~7 hr (4–25 hr)[f]	Tablets: 500 mg 250–3,000 mg/day
Acetohexamide	65%–88%[h] hsa	15 L[h]	pKa 4.3* Log P 2.44 (free acid)* Log $D_{7.0}$ 0.52*	Extensive	~85% of dose in urine, ~15% in feces[i] acetohexamide: $t_{1/2}$ ~ 1.5 hr (0.8–2.4 hr)[g] α-OH metabolite: $t_{1/2}$ ~ 5 hr (2–12)[g]	Tablets: 250 mg, 500 mg 250–1,500 mg/day
Chlorpropamide	96%[h] hsa	10 L[j]	pKa 4.7,[j] 5.1[k] Log P 2.3 (free acid)[j] Log $D_{7.0}$ 0.45*	~80%–82% biotransformed CYP2C9(?)[f]	18% of dose as unchanged drug, 75% as metabolites ([ω−1]-OH, 55%) in urine[m] $t_{1/2}$ ~33–43 hr[h]	Tablets: 100 mg, 250 mg 100–750 mg/day
Tolazamide	94%, hsa[n] 65%[e]	NA	pKa 3 (HB+)[d] pKa 5.7 (HA)[d] Log P 1.5,[d] 1.7* (uncharged) Log $D_{7.0}$ 0.02*	Extensive[o] Enzymes not reported	85% excreted in urine, <7% unchanged[o] $t_{1/2}$ ~7 hr (4–25 hr)[g]	Tablets: 100 mg, 200 mg, 500 mg 100–1,000 mg/day
Glipizide	98.4%[p] hsa[h]	0.17 L/kg[p] 15 L[h]; 12–14 L[p]	pKa 5.1,[j] 5.9[j] (HA) Log P 1.9 (free acid)[j] Log $D_{7.0}$ 0.29*	~90% biotransformed[f] ~95% biotransformed[h] CYP2C9[f]	61%–75% of total dose in urine, 3%–20% in feces,[s] <5% unchanged urine[p] Cl_{ss} = 2.1 L/hr[f] $t_{1/2}$ ~3.4 ± 0.7 h[p]	Tablets: 5 mg, 10 mg ER tablets: 2.5 mg, 5 mg, 10 mg 2.5–40 mg/day
Glyburide (glibenclamide)	>99% hsa[b]	0.20 L/kg[#] 15 L[h]	pKa 6.2–6.4[t] Log P 3.4 (free acid)[t] Log P 0.7 (conj base)[t]	Extensive CYP2C8, CYP2C9, CYP3A4[u]	60% urine (as metabolites), 40% feces (minimal excretion of unchanged drug)[v] Cl_{ss} = 7.8 L/hr[f] $t_{1/2}$ ~ 5–7 hr[w]	Tablets: 1.25 mg, 1.5 mg, 2.5 mg, 3 mg, 4.5 mg, 5 mg, 6 mg 0.75–20 mg/day
Glimepiride	>99.5%[x]	0.18 L/kg[#]	pKa 5.0* Log P 2.9 (free acid)[x] Log $D_{7.0}$ 1.3*	CYP2C9[y,z]	<0.5% unchanged drug in urine 37%–52% in urine as metabolites[x] Cl_{ss} = 4.3 L/hr[f] $t_{1/2}$ ~3.4 ± 2 hr[x]	Tablets: 1 mg, 2 mg, 3 mg, 4 mg, 6 mg, 8 mg 1–8 mg/day

[a]Half-lives ($t_{1/2}$) refer to terminal-phase elimination, unless otherwise noted.
[b]Brown, K. F., and Crooks, M. J.: Biochem. Pharmacol. 25(10):1175–1178, 1976.
[c]Jansson, R., Bredberg, U., and Ashton, M.: J. Pharm. Sci. 97(6):2324–2339, 2008.
[d]Hanai, T., et al.: Internet Electro. J. Mol. Des. 2(10):702–711, 2003.
[e]Plumb, R. S., Potts, W. B. III, and Rainville. P. D.: Rapid Commun. Mass Spectrom. 22(14):2139–2152, 2008.
[f]Kirchheiner, J., Roots, I., and Goldammer, M.: Clin. Pharmacokinet. 44(12):1209–1225, and references therein, 2005.
[g]Jackson J. E., and Bressler, R.: Drugs 22(3):211–245, 1981.
[h]Balant, L.: Clin. Pharmacokinet. 6(3):215–241, 1981.
[i]Galloway, J. A., McMahon, R. E., Culp, H. W., et al: Diabetes 16(2):118–127, 1967.
[j]Llinas, A., Glen, R. C., and Goodman, J. M.: J. Chem. Inf. Model. 48(7):1289–1303, 2008.
[k]Lipinski, C. A., Fiese, E. F., and Korst, R. J.: QSAR 10(2):109–117, 1991.
[l]Hughes, L. D., Palmer, D. S., and Nigsch, F., et al: J. Chem. Inf. Model. 48(1):220–232, 2008.
[m]Taylor, J. A.: Clin. Pharmacol. Ther. 13(5)(Pt. 1):710–718, 1972.
[n]Crooks, M. J., and Brown, K. F.: J. Pharm. Pharmacol. 26(5):304–311, 1974.
[o]Thomas, R. C., et al.: J. Med. Chem. 21(8):725–732, 1978.
[p]Kobayashi, K. A., Bauer, L.A., Horn, JR, et al.: Clin. Pharm. 7(3):224–228, 1988.
[q]Panten, U., Burgfeld, J., Goerke, F., et al.: Biochem. Pharmacol. 38(8):1217–1229, 1989.
[r]Fuccella, L. M., Tamassia, V., and Valzelli, G.: J. Clin. Pharmacol. New Drugs 13(2):68–75, 1973.
[s]Balant, L., Fabre, J., and Zahnd, G.R.: Eur. J. Clin. Pharmacol. 8:63–69, 1975.
[t]Uihlein, M., and Sistovaris, N.: J. Chromatogr. 227:93–101, 1982.
[u]Zharikova, O. L., Ravindran, S., Nanovskaya, T. N., et al.: Biochem. Pharmacol. 73:2012–2019, 2007. See also references therein.
[v]Rydberg, T., Wåhlin-Boll, E., Melander, A.: J. Chromatogr. 564(1):223–233, 1991.
[w]Balant, L., Fabre, J., Loutan, L., et al.: Arzneim. Forsch. 29:162–163, 1979.
[x]Langtry, H. D., and Balfour, J. A.: Drugs 55(4):563–584, 1998.
[y]Niemi, M., Neuvonen, P. J., and Kivistö, K. T.: Clin. Pharmacol. Ther. 70(5):439–445, 2001.
[z]Wang, R., Chen, K., Wen, S. Y., et al.: Clin. Pharmacol. Ther. 78(1):90–92, 2005.
*Calculated (Accelrys Software, ACD Labs), as reported via SciFinder (Chemical Abstracts Service) accessed Spring 2009.
[#]From data compiled in Table A-II-1: Goodman and Gilman's The Pharmacological Basis of Therapeutics, 11th Edition (McGraw-Hill, 2006).
α1GP, alpha 1 acid glycoprotein; ER, extended release; hsa, human serum albumin; NA, not available.

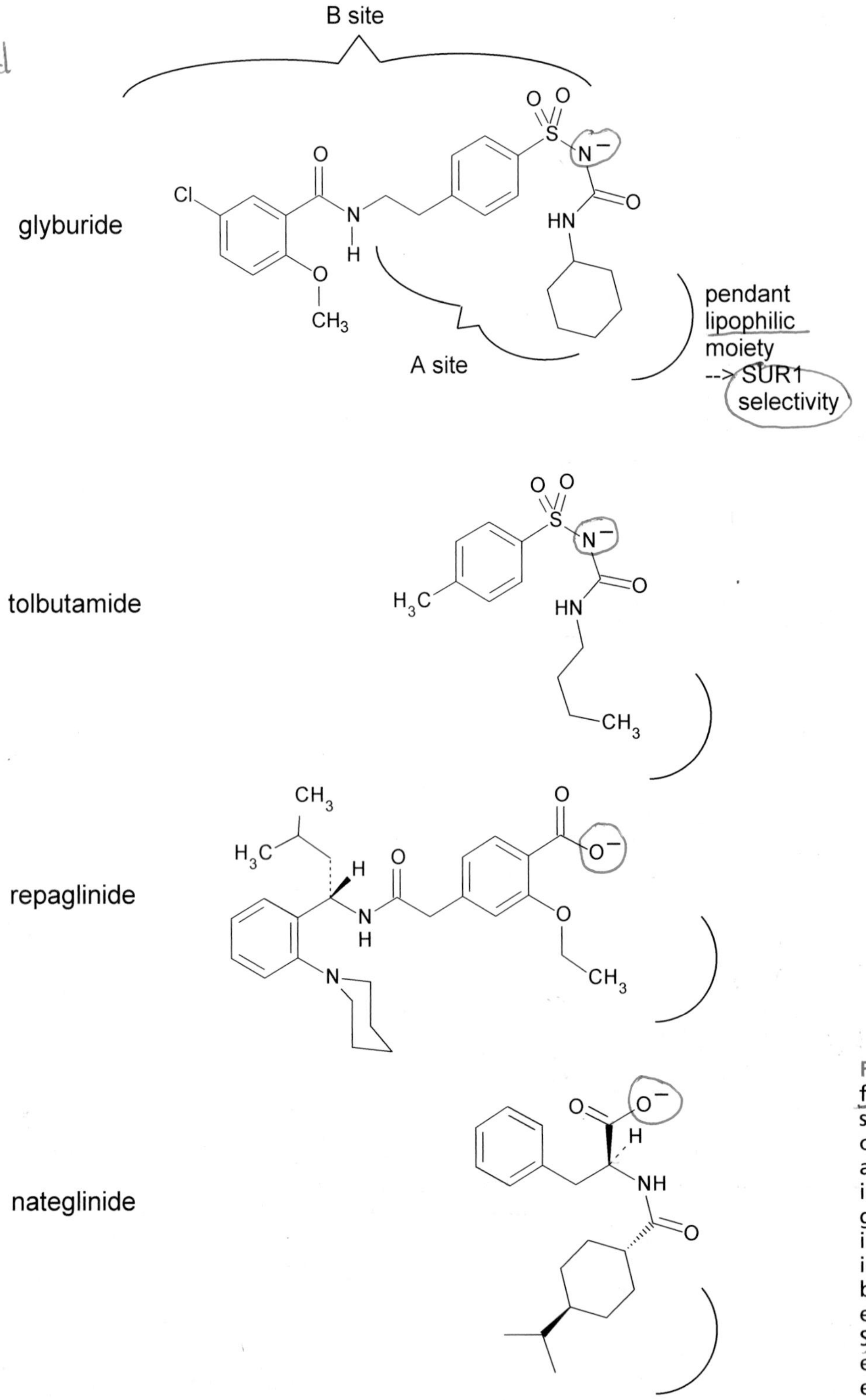

Good

glyburide

tolbutamide

repaglinide

nateglinide

Figure 20.7 ● Relationship of first- and second-generation sulfonylurea structures to those of repaglinide and nateglinide, and structural segments engaging the "A" and "B" binding regions at one of the four binding sites (at each SUR1:K$_{ir}$6.2 interface) of the channel assemblage. Ability to appropriately engage the "A" site confers SUR1 selectivity; after Winkler et al.,[4] Vila-Carriles et al.,[9] Grell et al.,[10] and Sleevi.[11]

lipophilic (log P ~1.8). Moreover, log D peaks near 4.0 between pH 5 and pH 6, even though the amphoteric (doubly charged) form predominates 76:1 over the uncharged species at the pH of log D maximum. Thus, absorption from the gut occurs readily, although there is significant loss caused by first-pass biotransformation (CYP3A4 and CYP2C8; see Table 20.4).

The "structural heritage" of repaglinide is made more obvious by comparison of the structure of meglitinide, a long-known molecule that has not been commercially marketed

as a hypoglycemic agent, to that of glyburide (Fig. 20.10). Moreover, structure–activity relationships reported by Grell et al.[10] in conjunction with the molecular biology studies of the receptor by several groups[4,9,13] clarify the interactions of these molecules at the interface of the SUR1 protein subunit and the K$_{ir}$6.2 protein subunits, and provide a basis for selectivity of hypoglycemic sulfonylureas and glinides for SUR$_1$ over the SUR$_{2A}$-containing channels found in heart and skeletal muscle or the SUR$_{2B}$-containing channels found in smooth muscle (Figs. 20.2 and 20.7).

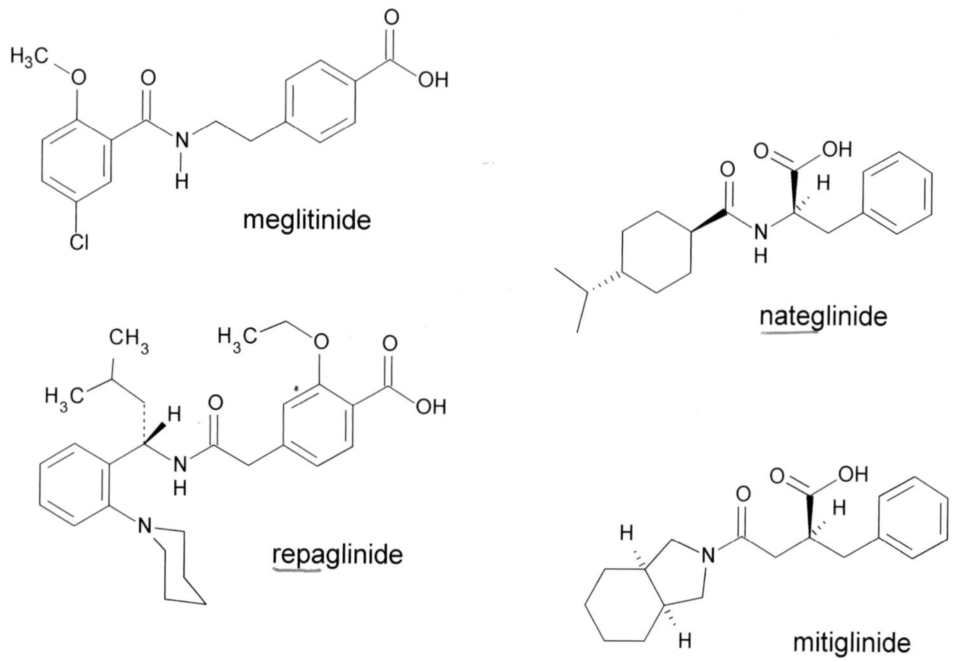

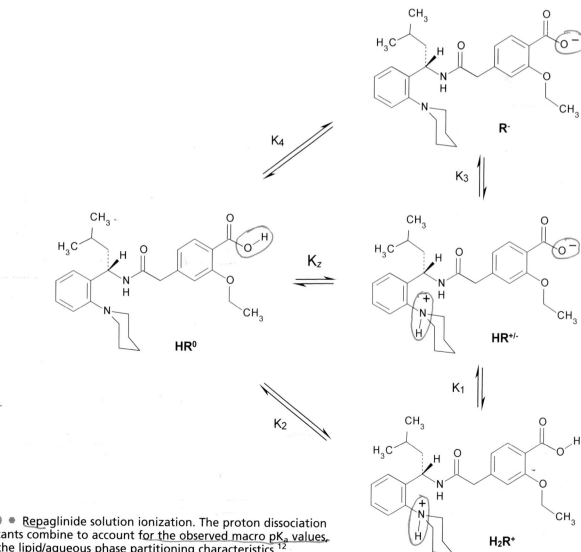

Figure 20.8 ● Glinide structures, including the prototypical compound meglitinide (see Fig. 20.10).

Figure 20.9 ● Repaglinide solution ionization. The proton dissociation microconstants combine to account for the observed macro pK_a values, as well as the lipid/aqueous phase partitioning characteristics.[12]

TABLE 20.4 Glinides Marketed in the United States[a]

Drug	Protein Binding	Volume of Distribution	Lipid Partitioning Character	Biotransformation	Oral Bioavailability	Elimination	Dosage Forms and Dose Range
Repaglinide	98%, hsa[b]	$V_{ss} = 31$ L	Log $D_{7.4}$ ~2.6[c]	Extensive → CYP3A4, CYP2C8	56%[d]	8% urine as metabolites, 90% feces (~2% unchanged)[e]	Tablets Low end: 0.5 mg b.i.d. (1 mg/day) High end: 4 mg q.i.d. (16 mg/day)
Nateglinide	98%, hsa, (α_1GP)[b]	10 L	Log D 0.76 (pH 7)[c] Log P 4.20[c] (free acid)	≥70% biotransformed[f] CYP2C9 (70%), CYP3A4 (30%)[f,g]	73%[b]	83%–87% urine (16% unchanged), 8%–10% feces[a,f]	Tablets Low end: 60 mg once a day; High end: 120 mg t.i.d. (360 mg/day)

[a]Information comes from manufacturer's product information unless otherwise indicated.
[b]Scheen, A. J.: Clin. Pharmacokinet. 46(2):93–108, 2007.
[c]Mandič, Z., and Gabelica, V.: J. Pharm. Biomed. Anal. 41(3):866–871, 2006.
[d]Hatorp, V.: Clin. Pharmacokinet. 41(7):471–483, 2002.
[e]van Heiningen, P. N., Hatorp, V., Kramer Nielsen, K., et al.: Eur. J. Clin. Pharmacol. 55(7):521–525, 1999.
[f]Weaver, M. L., Orwig, B. A., Rodriguez, L. C., et al.: Drug. Metab. Dispos. 29:415–421, 2001.
[g]Sabia, H., Sunkara, G., Ligueros-Saylan, M., et al.: Eur. J. Clin. Pharmacol. 60(6):407–412, 2004.
α_1GP, alpha glycoprotein; b.i.d., bis in die (twice a day); hsa, human serum albumin; q.i.d.,quater in die (4 times a day); t.i.d., ter in die (3 times a day).

Recently, evidence indicates that ATP-sensitive K$^+$ channels involved in mediating insulin secretion are found not only on the cell surface, but also at insulin-storage granules,[14] and various drugs may differ at least with respect to access to these two sites of action. Also, additional pharmacological targets probably have considerable clinical relevance. For example, gliquidone, glipizide, and nateglinide exhibit peroxisome proliferator–activated receptor–type gamma (PPARγ) activity at concentrations reached in tissues under standard pharmacotherapy regimens of these drugs.[15] The noteworthiness of this finding will be more apparent to the reader upon completing the section on thiazolidinediones further on in this chapter. Nateglinide and mitiglinide, but not sulfonylureas, evidently elicit insulin secretion in part via a ryanodine–receptor-mediated pathway.[16] Still, other molecular targets have been identified for various of these drugs, and these may partly account for the significant pharmacodynamic variations among the sulfonylureas and glinides that have yet to be fully explained. Active metabolites (see succeeding discussion), tissue and serum protein binding, and transporters also undoubtedly play important roles in these variations, some of which are already characterized, and in each such case, the possibility of pharmacogenomic variations among individuals accordingly arises. As an example, repaglinide and nateglinide are substrates of the *SLCO1B1*-encoded hepatic organic anion uptake transporter (i.e., OATP1B1), and at least one single-nucleotide polymorphism significantly alters repaglinide pharmacokinetics (PK)[17] and nateglinide PK.[18]

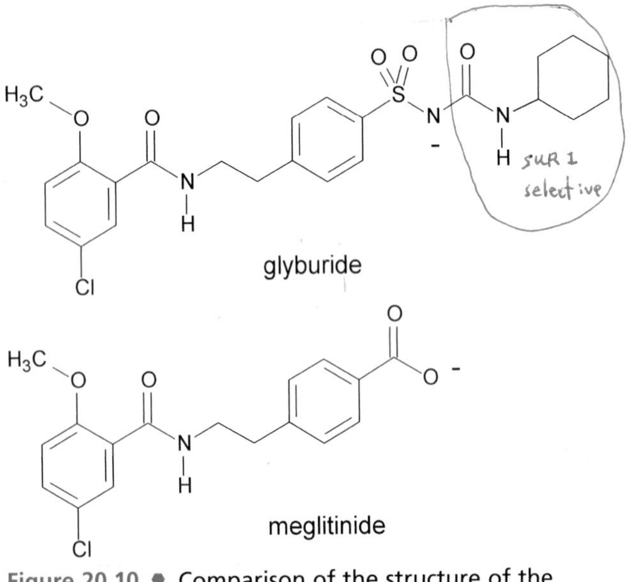

Regarding biotransformation ("drug metabolism") of the various hypoglycemic sulfonylureas in clinical use, although each drug exhibits a unique fate, common themes are, as is to be expected, associated with structural commonalities among the molecules (Fig. 20.11). Those that include a cyclohexyl ring are hydroxylated on that ring. Just within the past decade, it became clear that for glyburide, not only does hydroxylation occur in humans at each of the possible positions (2, 3, and 4), but with each of the possible stereochemical orientations (*cis* and *trans* in relative disposition to the attached urea nitrogen); see Figure 20.12.[19] Moreover, an ethylene-bridge–hydroxylated metabolite of glyburide (Fig. 20.13), presumably the benzylic hydroxylation product, was identified only within the past decade, and is now known to be a major metabolite in humans.[20] Some of these metabolites are known to confer a significant portion of the hypoglycemic effects of this drug, and may account for certain significant pharmacodynamic characteristics of this drug as well as for side effects, especially hypoglycemic episodes. Pharmacologically active metabolites are also known to be important for other sulfonylureas. Notably, the ketone moiety of the *p*-acetyl substituent on the phenyl ring of acetohexamide is reduced to the corresponding benzylic alcohol (Fig. 20.11), which exhibits a longer pharmacokinetic half-life than the parent drug, and is approximately

Figure 20.10 • Comparison of the structure of the prototypical glinide, meglitinide, with that of its "ancestor," glyburide. Comparison to Figure 20.7 will reveal that meglitinide lacks the SUR1 selectivity–bestowing pendant lipophilic group that engages the "A" binding site of the receptor (see Fig. 20.2).

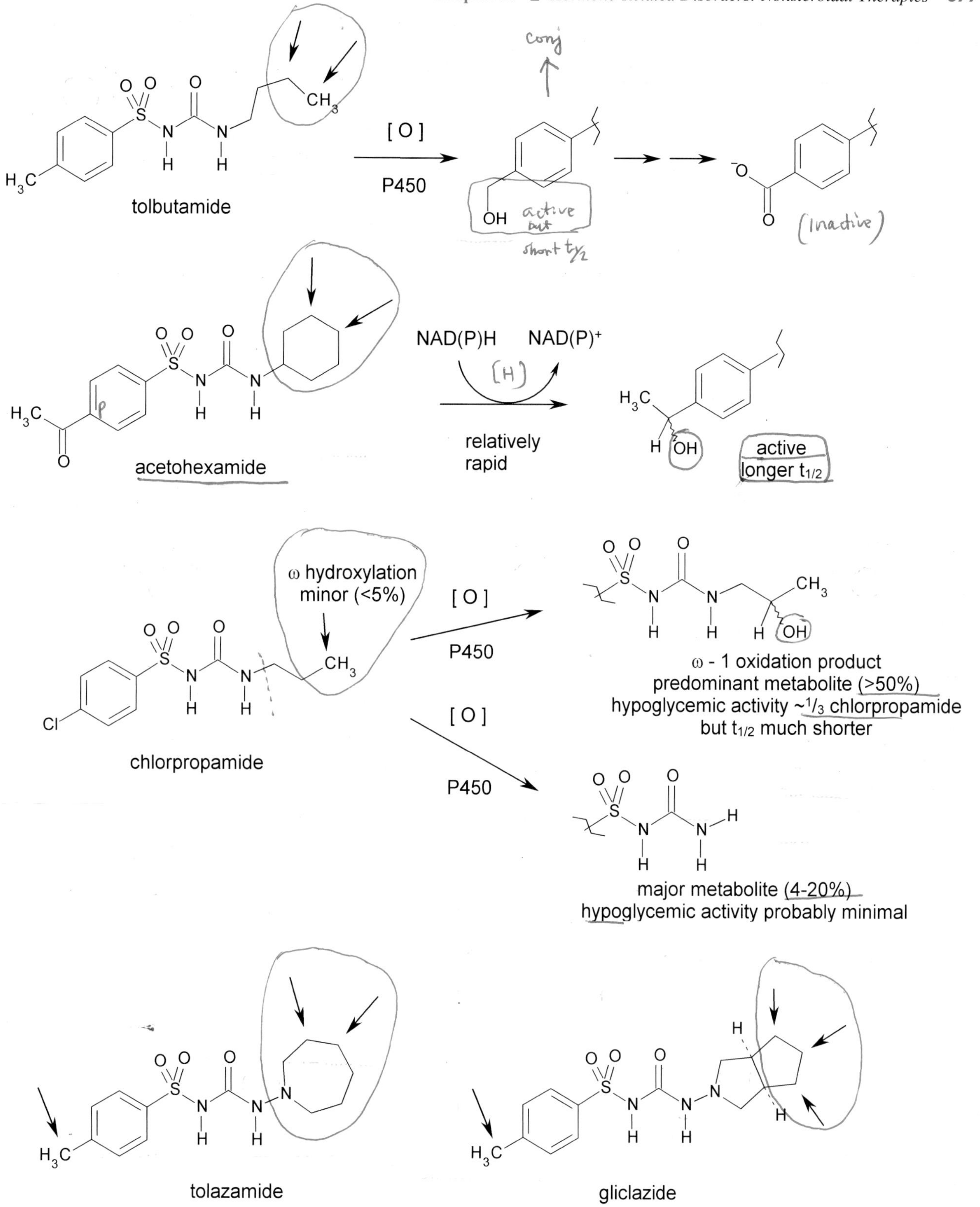

Figure 20.11 ● Biotransformations of first-generation sulfonylureas (see also Fig. 20.12).

equiactive with respect to hypoglycemic effect. ω-Hydroxylated or (ω–1)-hydroxylated metabolites of alkyl chain–containing sulfonylureas are formed and are either known or suspected to contribute to hypoglycemic activity. Those molecules having a *p*-methylphenyl moiety undergo benzylic hydroxylation. Because this transformation is

effected, at least in part, by CYP2C9, pharmacogenomic variations in PK are to be expected.[21] For gliclazide, CYP2C19 genetic polymorphism rather than CYP2C9 genetic polymorphism accounts for pharmacogenomic variations in PK.[22,23] In each case, though the resulting hydroxymethyl metabolite, which is either known to be able to

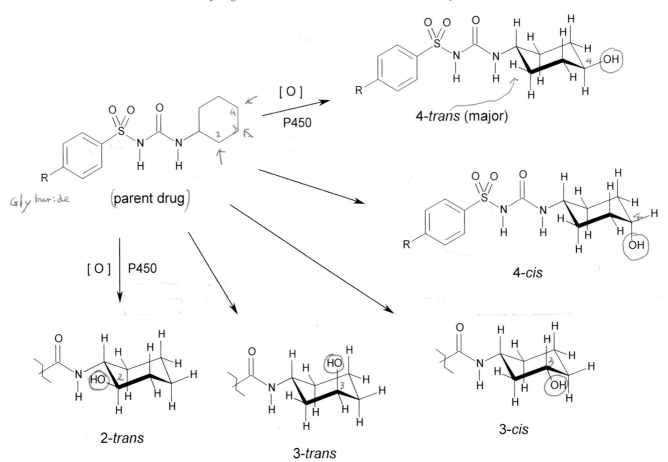

Figure 20.12 ● P450-catalyzed cyclohexane ring hydroxylations of glyburide. Evidence suggests that the 2-*cis*-hydroxy metabolite (not shown) is also formed, but definitive proof has not been obtained. Also note that some of these metabolites can exist as a pair of enantiomers, concerning which nothing is known.

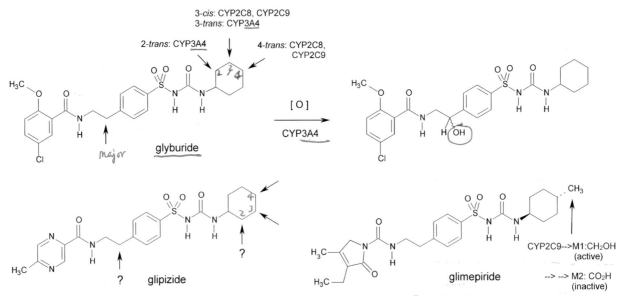

Figure 20.13 ● Major biotransformations of second-generation sulfonylureas.

exert significant target-level hypoglycemic activity (e.g., tolbutamide) or undoubtedly can, probably plays a relatively insignificant role with respect to in vivo pharmacological activity: because of relatively rapid oxidation to aldehyde and thence to inactive carboxylic acid, as well as conjugation to inactive β-D-glucuronide, blood and tissue concentrations do not build to sufficient levels. Similarly, because of rapid conversion to glucuronide or sulfate conjugates, which are eliminated mainly in bile, the *O*-demethylated metabolite of gliquidone (Fig. 20.13) does not contribute substantively to the hypoglycemic activity of this drug.

Repaglinide undergoes extensive biotransformation in humans,[24] and this fact primarily accounts for the modest 56% average oral bioavailability of this drug.[25] Oxidative biotransformation catalyzed predominantly by CYP3A4 and CYP2C8[26,27] produces a dicarboxylic acid (M2, see Fig. 20.14) as the major metabolite, reported to account for >65% of an administered dose of [^{14}C]-repaglinide, and to have no hypoglycemic effect.[24,28] Subsequent *N*-dealkylation to the aniline M1 also occurs, and M1 was found at a slightly higher concentration than M2 in urine,[24] but most (~90%) of an administered dose is excreted in feces, of which some 72% is M2. On the other hand, the major circulating fraction of an administered dose is repaglinide,

which is rapidly cleared from plasma. Direct phase II conjugation to the acyl glucuronide has been reported.

Biotransformation plays the predominant role in the clearance of nateglinide, with isopropyl side chain–centered phase I biotransformation and direct phase II conjugation as key components (Fig. 20.15). Although the *p*-hydroxyphenyl metabolite has been identified, with respect to phase I biotransformations, only products resulting from the actions of P450s on the isopropyl moiety are reported to be formed in significant quantities in humans. Monohydroxylation of the terminal isopropyl methyls produces two diastereomeric primary alcohols (M2 and M3), both of which are reportedly about a third as pharmacologically active as nateglinide.[29] Urinary excretion accounts for about 85% of the elimination of an administered dose, about half of which is M1 and unchanged nateglinide (2:1).[30] Following nateglinide administration, M1 is prominent in plasma but reportedly exerts about fivefold or sixfold less potent hypoglycemic activity (intravenous [iv]) than nateglinide. M7 is either formed via direct dehydrogenation of repaglinide, or by elimination of water from M1, M2, or M3. M7 is also interesting because it exhibits hypoglycemic activity of comparable potency and nature to nateglinide's, although circulating concentrations are almost 10-fold lower than that of nateglinide. Two

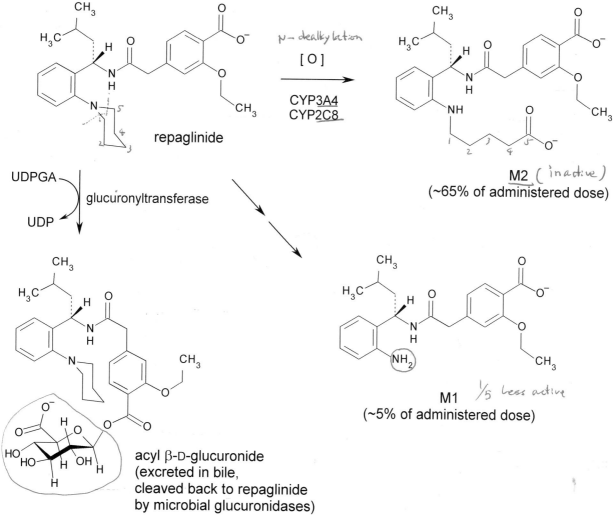

Figure 20.14 ● Important biotransformations of repaglinide. (UDP, uridine-3′,5′-diphosphate; UDPGA, 3′-phosphouridine-5′-phospho-β-D-glucuronic acid.)

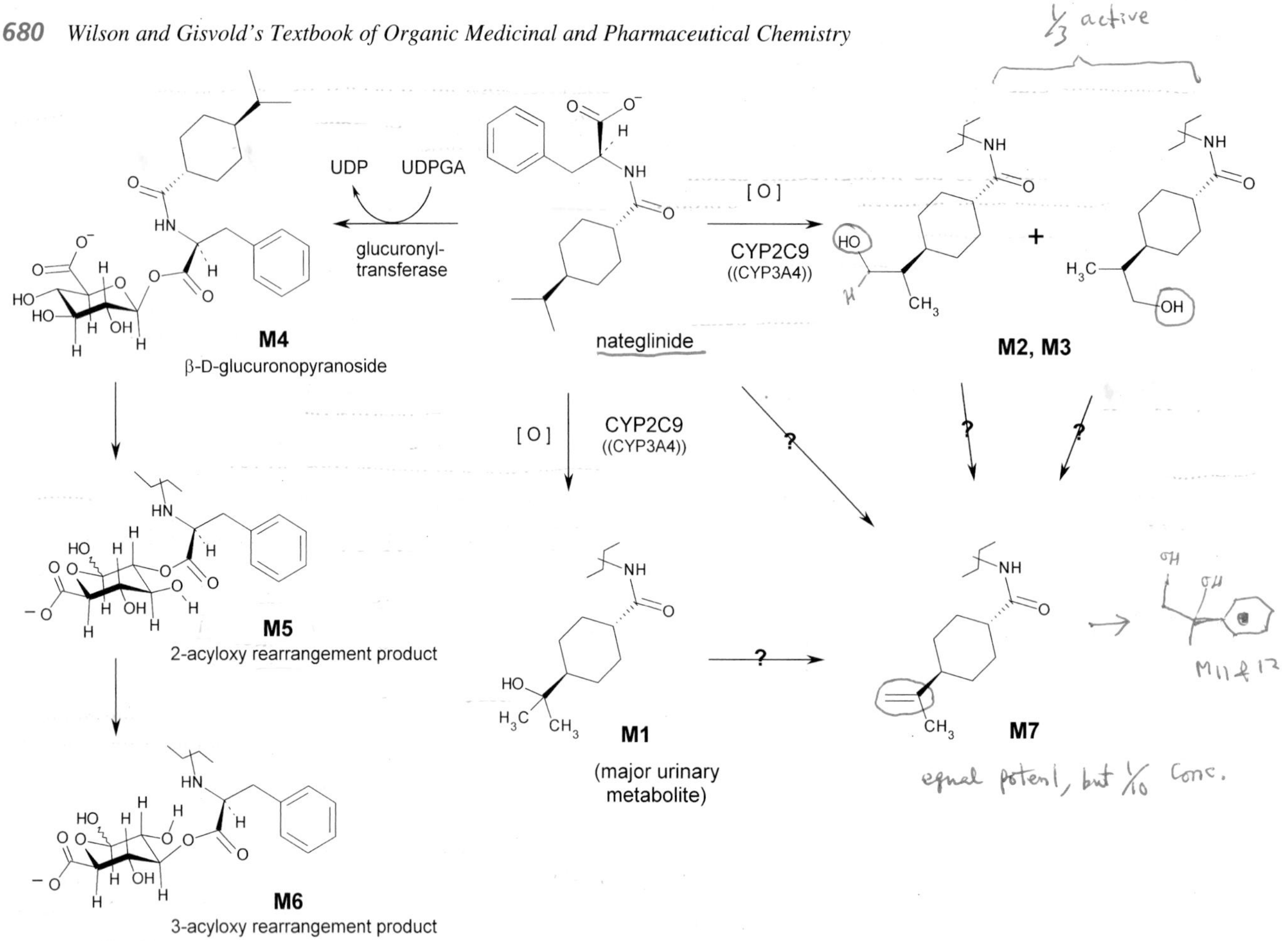

Figure 20.15 ● Important biotransformations of nateglinide. The abbreviations UDPGA and UDP are defined in the caption to Figure 20.14.

diastereomeric dihydroxylated metabolites (M11, M12, not pictured), together representing ~8% of administered dose, may be formed from M7 via epoxidation and spontaneous or epoxide hydrolase–mediated hydrolysis, but detection of the epoxide has yet to be reported, so direct ω–1 hydroxylation of M2 and M3, cannot be ruled out as pathways to M11 and M12. Although, apparently, no glucuronides of any of the isopropyl-hydroxylated species have been detected in humans, an acyl β-D-glucuronopyranoside is produced from the carboxylic acid moiety. Two apparent rearrangement products have also been characterized, in which the acyl group is shifted to the 2'-hydroxyl or 3'-hydroxyl of the sugar (Fig. 20.15), and the three glucuronides in aggregate appear in urine and account for 5% (oral) or 8% (iv) of an administered dose. Because CYP2C9 plays a major role in nateglinide biotransformation, pharmacogenomic variations in PK have been characterized.[21,31]

PRODUCTS (SEE ALSO TABLES 20.3 AND 20.4)

Tolbutamide is *N*-[(butylamino)carbonyl]-4-methylbenzenesulfonamide; or 1-butyl-3-(*p*-tolylsulfonyl)urea (Orinase, generic). Orinase Diagnostic was the sodium salt, which is freely soluble in water for injection, but this product was discontinued c. 2000.

Acetohexamide is 4-acetyl-*N*-[(cyclohexylamino)carbonyl]-benzenesulfonamide; or 1-[(*p*-acetylphenyl)sulfonyl]-3-cyclohexylurea; or 1-(*p*-acetylbenzenesulfonyl)-3-cyclohexylurea (generic). Acetohexamide incorporates the nearly op-

timal (for potency) cyclohexyl moiety in the "right-hand" side of its molecular structure, but a *p*-acetyl substituent on the "left-side" benzene ring that decreases lipophilicity and is rapidly biotransformed by reduction to an active metabolite that is cleared relatively rapidly (see preceding discussion) independently of any P450s.

Tolazamide is *N*-[[(hexahydro-1*H*-azepin-1-yl)amino]carbonyl]-4-methylbenzenesulfonamide; or 1-(hexahydro-1*H*-azepin-1-yl)-3-(*p*-tolylsulfonyl)urea; or 1-(4-methylphenylsulfonyl)-3-(hexahydro-1*H*-azepin-1-yl)urea (generic). Tolazamide incorporates a fully saturated azepine moiety that is but weakly basic, with a pKa of ~3.[32] The pKa of the sulfonylurea group lies within the typical range; thus, in areas of the duodenum wherein the pH falls within the range of 4 to 5, the uncharged form of the drug is the predominant species, and its lipophilicity lends to rapid absorption by passive diffusion.

Chlorpropamide is 4-chloro-*N*-[(propylamino)carbonyl]benzenesulfonamide; or 1-[(*p*-chlorophenyl)sulfonyl]-3-propylurea; or 1-(*p*-chlorobenzenesulfonyl)-3-propylurea (Diabinese, generic). The *p*-chlorophenyl moiety is quite resistant to P450-mediated hydroxylations; hence, blood levels of the drug are sustained for a markedly long length of time, as aliphatic hydroxylation constitutes most of the clearance, and this happens relatively slowly. Although the ω-hydroxyl and (ω–1)-hydroxyl metabolites (the latter formed in much greater portion) exert hypoglycemic potencies not much less than does the parent drug, elimination of these by conversion to the corresponding glucuronides occurs more rapidly than hydroxylation of chlorpropamide,[33] so blood levels of these metabolites remain low, and thus they probably do not make an appreciable contribution to the hypoglycemic action of this drug in clinical application. Removal of the entire propyl side chain (oxidative *N*-dealkylation) also occurs to a significant extent (up to 20% of an orally administered dose), creating the inactive metabolite *p*-chlorobenzenesulfonylurea, about 10% of which degrades to the corresponding benzenesulfonamide.[34]

Glipizide is *N*-[2-[4-[[[(cyclohexylamino)carbonyl]amino]sulfonyl]phenyl]ethyl]-5-methyl-2-pyrazinecarboxamide; this compound can also be named as the urea—see preceding discussion (Glucotrol, generic). In the United States, combinations are available with metformin (Metaglip, generic; tablets, mg glipizide/mg metformin as hydrochloride: 2.5/250, 2.5/500, 5/500). Extended-release tablets are available (Glucotrol XL, generic). The pyrazine moiety within this structure renders the molecule significantly more hydrophilic than the similar molecule glyburide, albeit also moderately less potent on a dosage as well as target-level basis.

Glyburide (glibenclamide) is 5-chloro-*N*-[2-[4-[[[(cyclohexylamino)carbonyl]amino]sulfonyl]phenyl]ethyl]-2-methoxybenzamide; this compound can also be named as the urea—see preceding discussion (Diabeta, Glynase, generic). Some tablet formulations contain micronized drug (formerly Micronase, now only generic). Combinations are available with metformin in the United States (Glucovance, generic; tablets, mg glipizide/mg metformin as hydrochloride: 1.25/250, 2.5/500, 5/500).

Glimepiride is 3-ethyl-2,5-dihydro-4-methyl-*N*-[2-[4-[[[[(*trans*-4-methylcyclohexyl)amino]-carbonyl]amino]sulfonyl]phenyl]ethyl]-2-oxo-1*H*-pyrrole-1-carboxamide; this compound can also be named as the urea—see preceding discussion (Amaryl, generic). Combinations are available with rosiglitazone in the United States (Avandaryl tablets; mg glimepiride/mg rosiglitazone as maleate salt: 1/4, 2/4, 4/4, 2/8, 4/8); and with pioglitazone (Duetact tablets; mg glimepiride/ mg pioglitazone as hydrochloride salt: 2/30, 4/30).

Repaglinide is 2-ethoxy-4-[2-[[(1*S*)-3-methyl-1-[2-(1-piperidinyl)phenyl]butyl]amino]-2-oxoethyl]benzoic acid (Prandin); approvals for generics are pending. Combinations are available with metformin in the United States (Prandimet), and the drug may also be coprescribed with one of the thiazolidinediones (typically pioglitazone or rosiglitazone; see previous discussion). To establish the most clinically valuable dose, the patient is titrated while monitoring blood glucose levels and hemoglobin glycosylation (HbA$_{1c}$) as an index of longer-term overall control.

Nateglinide (Starlix) is D-Phenylalanine, *N*-[[*trans*-4-(1-methylethyl)cyclohexyl]carbonyl]-; or (−)-*N*-[(*trans*-4-isopropylcyclohexyl)carbonyl]-D-phenylalanine. In addition to the information given previously and in Table 20.4, it is noteworthy that, although nateglinide is much less potent on a dosage basis than is repaglinide and most of the sulfonylureas, this drug seems to exhibit unique molecular pharmacodynamics. Nateglinide closes ATP-sensitive K$^+$ channels some threefold more rapidly than repaglinide, and exhibits an off-rate twice as fast as that of glyburide or glimepiride and five times faster than repaglinide.[35] These

characteristics are reflected by the systemic pharmacodynamics of this drug, translating clinically to improved safety, among other apparent benefits.

Thiazolidinediones (Glitazones)

The thiazolidinedione class of hypoglycemic agents, which are also commonly called glitazones, are represented on the U.S. market by rosiglitazone and pioglitazone (Fig. 20.16). The 2,4-thiazolidinedione (or thiazolidine-2,4-dione) moiety is acidic (Fig. 20.17), with the glitazones exhibiting pK$_a$ values near 6.5 to 6.8, and this characteristic is crucial to the target-level pharmacological activity: the negatively charged conjugate base mimics the carboxylate anion of the natural fatty acid ligands (Fig. 20.18).

On the molecular level, the glitazones are thought to mainly exert their hypoglycemic action via binding to the PPARγ. The endogenous ligands for PPARs are free fatty acids and eicosanoids (prostaglandins and leukotrienes). The PPARs are nuclear, wherein the glitazone-PPARγ complex binds with a retinoid X receptor (RXR). This interaction in turn causes release of corepressor protein by the RXR:HRE complex (HRE, hormone response elements), and upon recruitment of coactivator protein, interaction of the resulting multiprotein complex with DNA promotes transcription. Several biological effects result from the activation of PPARγ, but the action of main interest here is sensitization to insulin within key tissues, including the liver, skeletal muscle, and adipose tissue.[36,37] Induction of adiponectin synthesis may be a crucial component of this beneficial effect.[38,39] Expression levels of PPARγ (both subtypes—PPARγ1 and PPARγ2) are particularly high in adipose tissue, where thiazolidinediones can upregulate adipose triglyceride lipase,[40] and exert effects on the expression of several genes suggestive of significant adipose tissue remodeling.[37] Allowing for tissue access differences, the potency of the beneficial effects of these compounds on carbohydrate metabolism for type 2 diabetics parallels potency of agonist effect on PPARγ. A relatively recent body of evidence indicates that pancreatic β-cell function is improved as a result of chronic treatment with PPARγ agonists.[41]

Ciglitazone (see Fig. 20.16), a Takeda compound, was the first molecule of this series brought to clinical testing, from which it was withdrawn because of an elevated incidence of cataracts among patients enrolled in longer-term chronic studies. Takeda replaced ciglitazone with pioglitazone, which received Food and Drug Administration (FDA) approval (Actos) in 1999. During the same period, troglitazone was developed by Dai-ichi Sankyo and received FDA approval in January 1997. The trimethylchromanol moiety in troglitazone is the same as in the α-tocopherol form of vitamin E, and troglitazone thereby exhibits significant antioxidant activity. Unfortunately, incidence of hepatotoxicity was substantially higher for troglitazone than either rosiglitazone or pioglitazone, both of which came on the U.S. market in the summer of 1999. By this time, demarketing of troglitazone worldwide was already occurring, and the FDA issued a formal recall in the following year. A probable basis for troglitazone's hepatotoxicity, involving one or more reactive metabolites, has recently been elucidated (see succeeding discussion).

Selectivity for PPARγ over PPARα or PPARδ constitutes a necessary characteristic of molecules intended to therapeutically exploit this mechanism of obtaining insulin-sensitization (although there is rationale for PPARα activity,

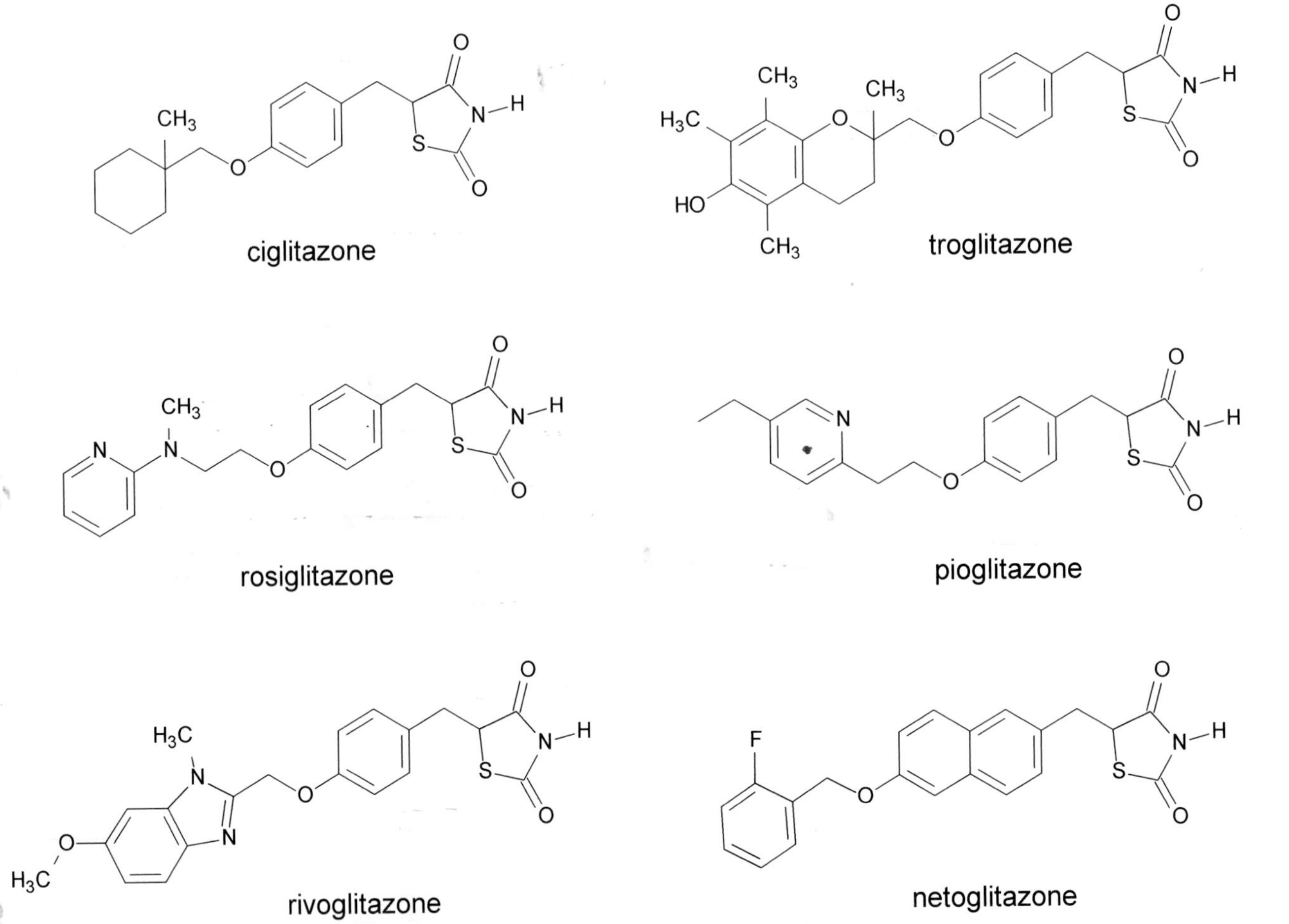

Figure 20.16 • Structures of thiazolidinediones used currently or historically, or in late-stage development for treating type 2 diabetes.

and aleglitazar—see structure Fig. 20.18—is a dual PPARγ/PPARα agonist currently in clinical trials). Extensive x-ray crystallographic, nuclear magnetic resonance (NMR), and computational chemistry studies provided an understanding that the thiazolidinedione ring not only constitutes a carboxylate anion isostere in receptor binding, but also that a network of hydrogen bonds to complementary side chain moieties of Ser-289, His-323, Tyr-473, and His-449 accounts for the PPARγ selectivity. Moreover, NMR studies suggest that agonist binding selects among a set of interchanging ligand-binding domain (LBD) conformations (i.e., the LBD region is mobile in the aporeceptor), bestowing a conformation that enables the coactivator recruitment necessary for promoting transcription, over conformations that are not enabling.[42–44] In PPARα, the residue corresponding to His-323 is instead a prohibitively positioned tyrosine, and in PPARδ the binding pocket is too narrow to accommodate the thiazolidinedione ring or substituents α to the acidic moiety, such as occurs in aleglitazar (structure Fig. 20.18). Structure–activity relationships for PPARγ ligands have been extensively investigated,[11] and many originally empirical observations can now be readily explained based on the knowledge of the binding-pocket structure as discussed previously.

Rosiglitazone and pioglitazone are formulated as their salts (maleate and hydrochloride, respectively). The salts are much more water soluble than the parent acids, conferring rapid dissolution of the drug upon disintegration of a tablet in the stomach. Although the monosubstitution at C5 of the thiazolidinedione ring allows for stereoisomers, interconversion is rapid under physiological conditions, caused by the acidity of the hydrogen at this position, and drugs of this class are therefore sold as racemates. Besides the two products in the list that follows, agents of the thiazolidine class in later stages of clinical development include netoglitazone (RWJ 241947, also known as isaglitazone, MCC 555) and rivoglitazone.[45]

PRODUCTS (SEE ALSO TABLE 20.5)

Rosiglitazone is 5-[4-[2-(N-methyl-N-(2-pyridyl)amino)ethoxy]benzyl]thiazolidine-2,4-dione, and is available as the maleate salt in tablets containing the drug alone (Avandia) or in combination products with metformin (Avandamet) or with glimepiride (Avandaryl). The 2-aminopyridine moiety allows for salt formation; the marketed formulations contain the 1:1 salt with maleic acid, in which the pyridine nitrogen accepts a proton, forming the 2-aminopyridinium species.

Although rosiglitazone is extensively biotransformed—essentially no unchanged drug appears in urine or feces—in humans, only ~35% of the administered radioactivity was recovered within 48 hours, and more than a week was required to reach 90% recovery.[46] The major routes of biotransformation (Fig. 20.19) are N-demethylation and hydroxylation of the pyridine ring *para* to the amino nitrogen, with CYP2C8

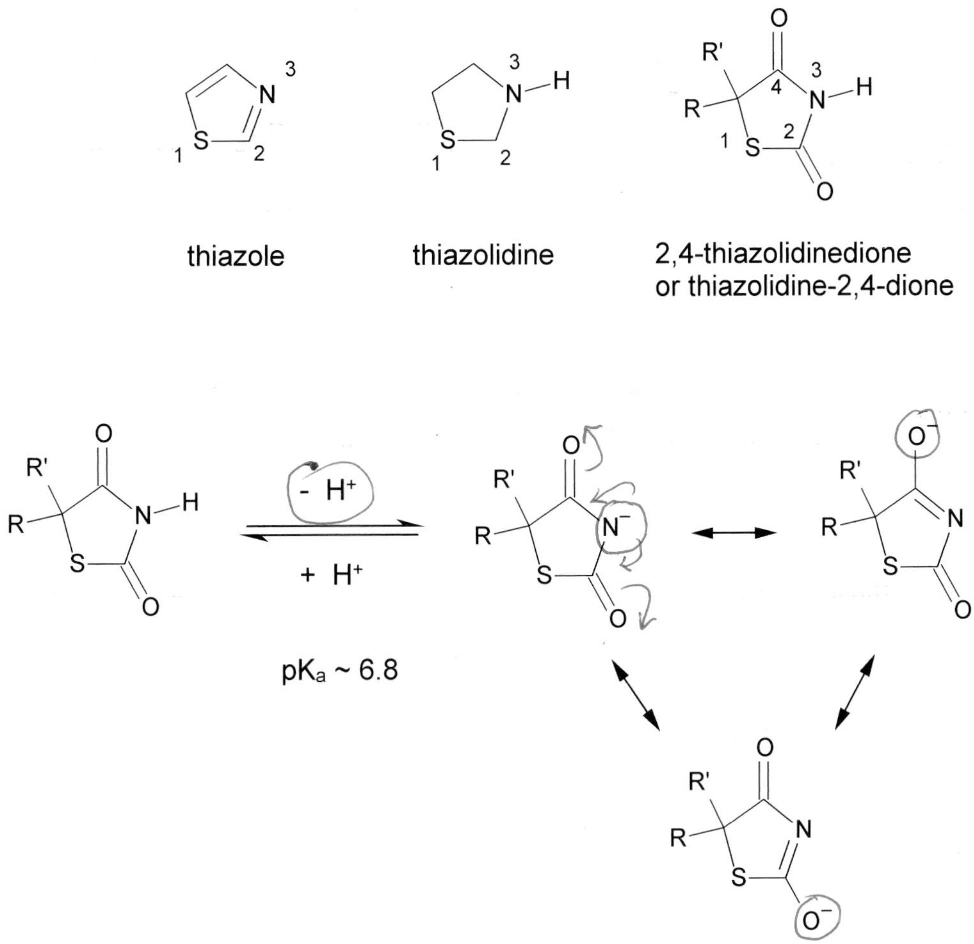

Figure 20.17 ● Thiazolidinedione nomenclature and numbering, and canonical (resonance) structures representing delocalization of the negative charge in the anionic conjugate base.

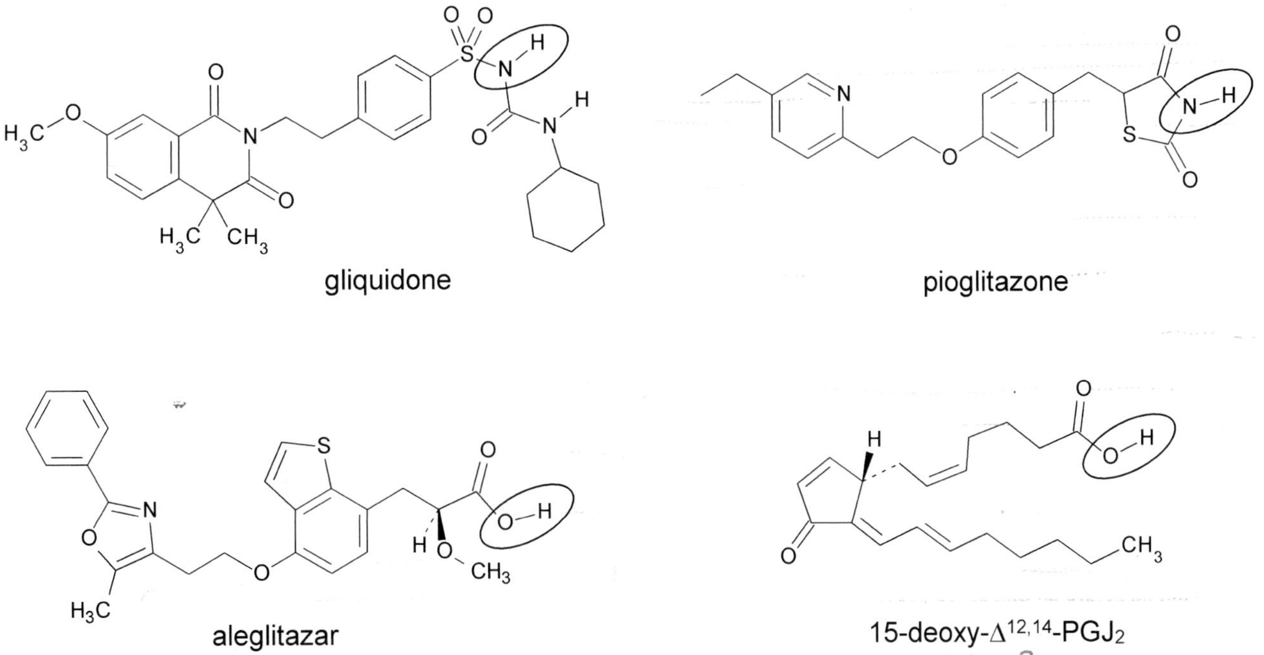

Figure 20.18 ● PPARγ ligands of diverse structure, including a natural prostanoid ligand, 15-deoxy-Δ^{12,14}-PGJ₂.

TABLE 20.5 Glitazones Marketed in the United States

Drug	Protein Binding	Volume of Distribution	Acid–Base and Lipid Partitioning Character	Biotransformation	Oral Bioavailability	Elimination	Dosage Forms and Dose Range
Rosiglitazone	99.8% (hsa)[a]	V_{ss} = 17.6 L[a]	pK$_a$ 6.5 (HB$^+$)[b] pK$_a$ 6.4 (HA)[b] Log P = 2.8 (uncharged form)[c] Log D$_{7.4}$ = 2.6[c]	extensive[d] CYP2C8 (major) CYP2C9 (minor)[a,e]	99%[a,d]	t$_{1/2}$ ~4 hr 64% urine (~0.1% unchanged); 23% feces (~no unchanged drug)[a,d]	Tablets: 2 mg, 4 mg, 8 mg (base eq.) 4–8 mg/day Combinations with metformin or glimepiride
Pioglitazone	99%, hsa[f]	0.63 L/kg[f]	pK$_a$ 5.5 (HB$^+$)[b] pK$_a$ 6.4 (HA)[b] Log P = 3.3 (uncharged form)[c] Log D$_{7.4}$ = 3.1[c]	CYP3A4 CYP2C8[f,g]	>80%[g]	t$_{1/2}$ 3–7 hr 15%–30% urine (metabolites and their conjugates); fate of remaining drug uncharacterized[f]	Tablets: 15 mg, 30 mg, 45 mg (base eq.) 15–45 mg/day combinations with metformin or glimepiride

[a]Avandia product information (20-Oct-2008 labeling).
[b]Calculated (Accelrys Software, ACD Labs), as reported via SciFinder (Chemical Abstracts Service) accessed Spring 2009. The proximity of the two pK$_a$ values renders experimental determination difficult, as noted by Giaginis et al.[c] NMR spectroscopic determination, with deconvolution, would be necessary, but such determinations were not discovered in the literature.
[c]Giaginis, C., Theocharis, S., and Tsantili-Kakoulidou, A.: J. Chromatogr. B. Analyt. Technol. Biomed. Life Sci. 857(2):181–187, 2007.
[d]Cox, P. J., Ryan, D. A., Hollis, F. J., et al.: Drug. Metab. Dispos. 28(7):772–780, 2000.
[e]Baldwin, S. J., Clarke, S. E., and Chenery, R. J.: Br. J. Clin. Pharmacol. 48(3):424–432, 1999.
[f]Actos product information (11-Dec-2008 labeling).
[g]Jaakkola, T., Backman, J. T., Neuvonen, M., et al.: Br. J. Clin. Pharmacol. 61(1):70–78, 2006, and references therein.
hsa, human serum albumin.

playing the major role in both transformations, and some involvement of CYP2C9.[21,47] The sulfate conjugate M10 is the predominant circulating metabolite by 4-hour postdose. The extraordinarily high plasma protein binding of this metabolite (and the N-demethylated sulfate conjugate M4) in humans accounts for the lengthy residence time of the radioactivity in the body, despite the relatively short pharmacokinetic half-life (4–4.5 hours) of rosiglitazone itself.

Pioglitazone is 5-(4-[2-(5-ethylpyridin-2-yl)ethoxy]benzyl)thiazolidine-2,4-dione, and is available in tablets containing the hydrochloride salt alone (Actos in the United

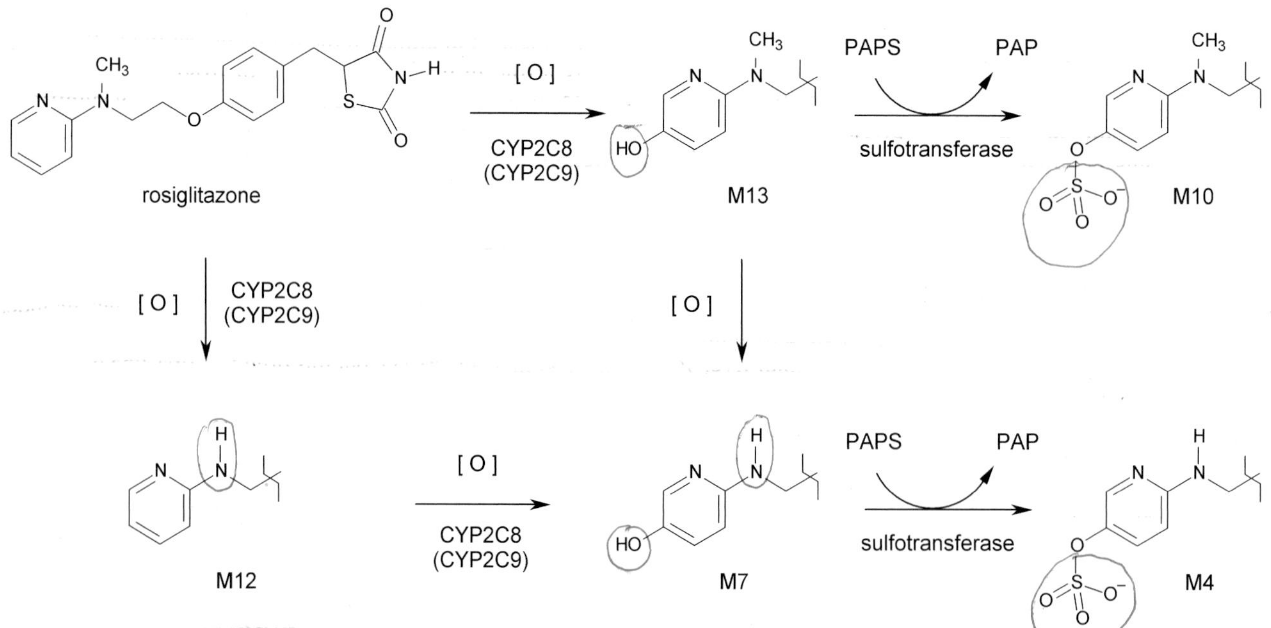

Figure 20.19 ● Important biotransformations of rosiglitazone. (PAP, 3'-phosphoadenosine-5'-phosphate; PAPS, 3'-phosphoadenosine-5'-phosphosulfate.)

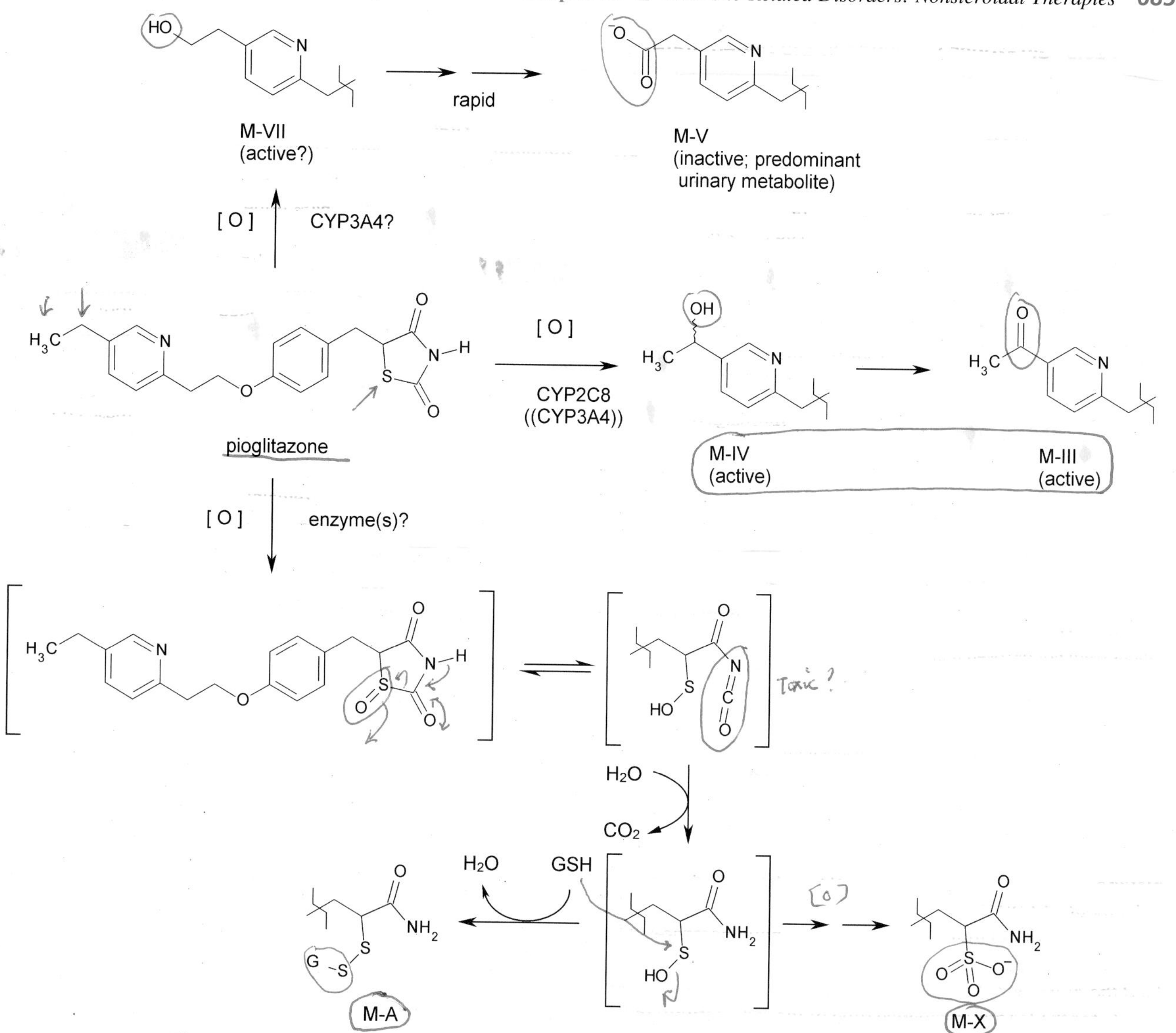

Figure 20.20 ● Important biotransformations of pioglitazone. (GSH, glutathione.)

States, Glustin in Europe and Zactos in Mexico), or in combination with glimepiride (Duetact, see "Glimepiride" previously in this chapter) or metformin (Actoplus Met; see under "Metformin" later in this chapter).

Pioglitazone is extensively biotransformed,[48–50] and at least three metabolites are known to be pharmacologically active, although only two of these (M-IV and M-III, see Fig. 20.20) are thought to significantly contribute to the therapeutic effects.[51] CYP2C8 and CYP3A4 predominantly account for the observed biotransformations, with the former playing a greater role. Ring-opened metabolites (M-X, M-A) have also been identified in human liver mi-

crosomes,[48] but although the pathway leading to these may play a role in the hepatotoxicity of troglitazone, pioglitazone seems not to have the same liability to any significant extent, most likely because the pioglitazone doses are sufficiently lower (by about 10-fold) than those that had been needed with troglitazone.

Biguanides

The biguanide class of insulin-sensitizing agents includes only one marketed medicinal in the United States, namely metformin (Fig. 20.21), but this drug is a first-line drug in the

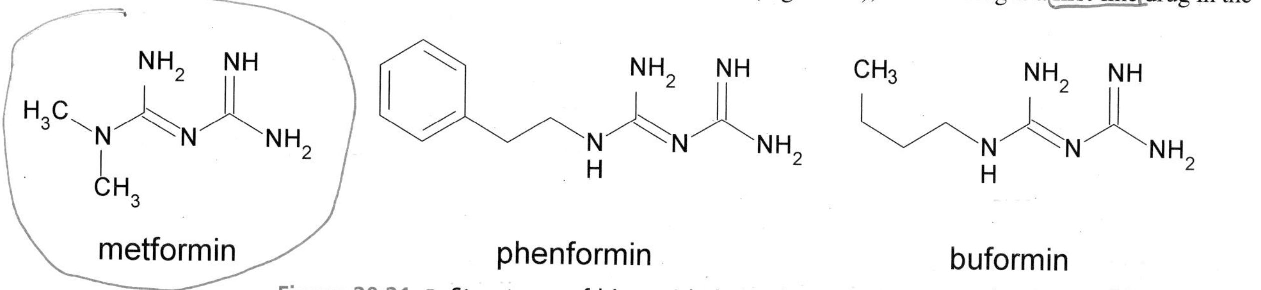

Figure 20.21 ● Structures of biguanide hypoglycemic agents.

treatment of type 2 diabetes, for which it is prescribed heavily, alone and in combinations. Having been brought to market in France in 1979 (though not until 1995 in the United States), metformin has a long history of use, despite which fact the mechanisms underlying its effects remain uncertain.[52–56] Activation by metformin of adenosine monophosphate-activated protein kinase (AMPK) has commonly been stated as the molecular mechanism in recent years; however, the as-yet-to-be-identified primary target(s) must either be upstream of AMPK, or trigger downstream mechanisms that deliver stimulatory feedback upstream of AMPK, or cause changes in crosstalk mechanisms (such as those involving insulin receptor substrate 1) to indirectly enhance AMPK action, or some combination thereof. A month of chronic metformin therapy increases basal levels of protein kinase C type zeta (PKC$_\zeta$) in the muscle tissue of type 2 diabetics, in turn restoring glucose handling to a more normal state,[57,58] and PKC$_\zeta$ acts through serine-threonine kinase 11 (STK11/LKB1) to modulate AMPK activity;[55] however, PKC$_\zeta$ is clearly not the direct macromolecular target of metformin, either. Some evidence suggests that subtle

metformin-caused changes in mitochondrial membrane potential may circuitously bring about the beneficial collateral changes in other pathways, including the aforementioned PKC$_\zeta$→STK11→AMPK signaling chain; metformin inhibits complex I (NADH:ubiquinone dehydrogenase) of the electron transport chain.[59,60] In any case, over a period of weeks, metformin enhances the sensitivity of various cells of the body to insulin. Recently, much activity has centered on fully characterizing the roles of the organic cation transporter 1 (OCT1), the functioning of which is clearly essential to metformin's action.[61] Presumably, this transporter allows the drug to reach its intracellular target(s), and pharmacogenomic variations with respect to the OCT1 complex that decrease or abolish the effectiveness of metformin have been identified.[61,62] OCT1 is richly expressed in those hepatocytes participating most directly in the regulation of glucose levels.

The bioavailability of metformin at normal clinical doses ranges from 40% to 60%, which is quite high for such an extensively ionized and hydrophilic drug (calculated log D ~ −6 at pH 7)[63]; the biguanide moiety is extremely basic (Fig. 20.22), thus, metformin exists almost

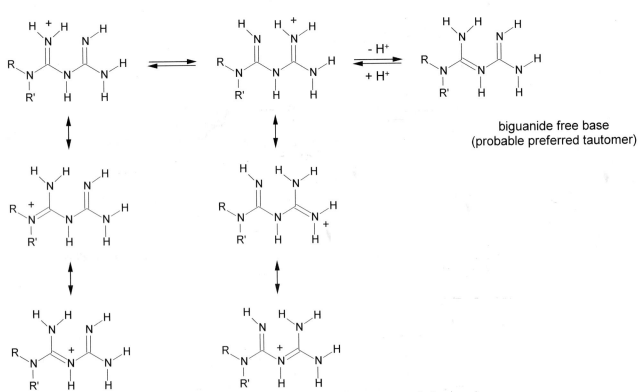

Figure 20.22 ● Biguanides: basis of the "biguanide" designation, tautomeric forms of the protonated species, and canonical (resonance) structures representing delocalization of the positive charge in the conjugate acid.

exclusively as protonated, positively charged molecular species throughout the entire physiological pH range. Absorption from the gut was recently shown to occur by a paracellular route, which, surprisingly, was found to be saturable;[64] the exact molecular basis for this observation, if yet known, has not been reported. Renal elimination is also transporter mediated (active tubular secretion). Elimination of absorbed metformin is essentially 100% by the kidneys, at a rate about 3.5-fold creatinine clearance, thus renal insufficiency precludes metformin pharmacotherapy because of the resultant risk of lactic acidosis that otherwise essentially never occurs with this drug. Other drugs of this class (phenformin, buformin, structures Fig. 20.21) were abandoned because of lactic acidosis-linked fatalities, even though the incidence with phenformin was actually quite rare. Little metformin binding to plasma proteins occurs, but partitioning into erythrocytes is considerable, significantly impacting the PK of this drug.

Metformin is *N,N*-dimethylimidodicarbonimidic diamide, but can accurately and much more simply be named as 1,1-dimethylbiguanide. Metformin is available, as its hydrochloride salt, in tablets ranging in strengths from 500-mg to 1-g (Glucophage, numerous generics), extended-release tablets (Fortamet, Glumetza), and an oral solution (Riomet); and in combinations with rosiglitazone (Avandamet), pioglitazone (Actoplus Met), glipizide (Metaglip, generics), glyburide (Glucovance), repaglinide (Prandimet), and most recently, sitagliptin (Janumet).

α-Glucosidase Inhibitors

Medicinals acting as α-glucosidase inhibitors slow the breakdown of disaccharides (notably sucrose) and starch-derived polysaccharides into monosaccharides in the gastrointestinal (GI) tract, delaying production and thereby absorption of glucose following consumption of meals. This approach to reducing peak postprandial serum glucose levels is highly effective, with the caveat that these drugs cause very uncomfortable GI side effects in a high percentage of patients; fortunately, artful inception of therapy, with monitoring, can greatly reduce the impact of this liability. The α-glucosidase inhibitors marketed in the United States include acarbose and miglitol; an additional α-glucosidase inhibitor, voglibose, is marketed in Japan and several other countries including Brazil (structures Fig. 20.23).

Digestion of amylose and amylopectin forms of starch begins with reactions catalyzed by a pair of related α-amylases, which are endoglucosidase enzymes contained in pancreatic secretions. Complete digestion also requires debranching for amylopectin, and further cleavage of various disaccharides and small oligosaccharides. These reactions are catalyzed by α-glucosidases, which are a highly similar set of enzymes that cleave the glycoside linkage between particular sugar moieties; more specifically, hydrolysis occurs at the acetal oxygen bridging the C1 of a glucose residue and either C4 or C6 of another glucose in α-(1→4) or α-(1→6) linkage (maltose or isomaltose, respectively; see Fig. 20.24), but not β-(1→4) glucose–glucose linkages (as in cellobiose) or the β-(1→4) galactose–glucose linkage in lactose. α-Glucosidases are exoglycosidases, cleaving terminal glucose residues from the nonreducing end of an oligosaccharide. Four separate maltase enzymes found in the luminal membrane of enterocytes (more specifically, the brush-border epithelial cells) actually constitute these activities: two associated with "sucrase-isomaltase" (SI)

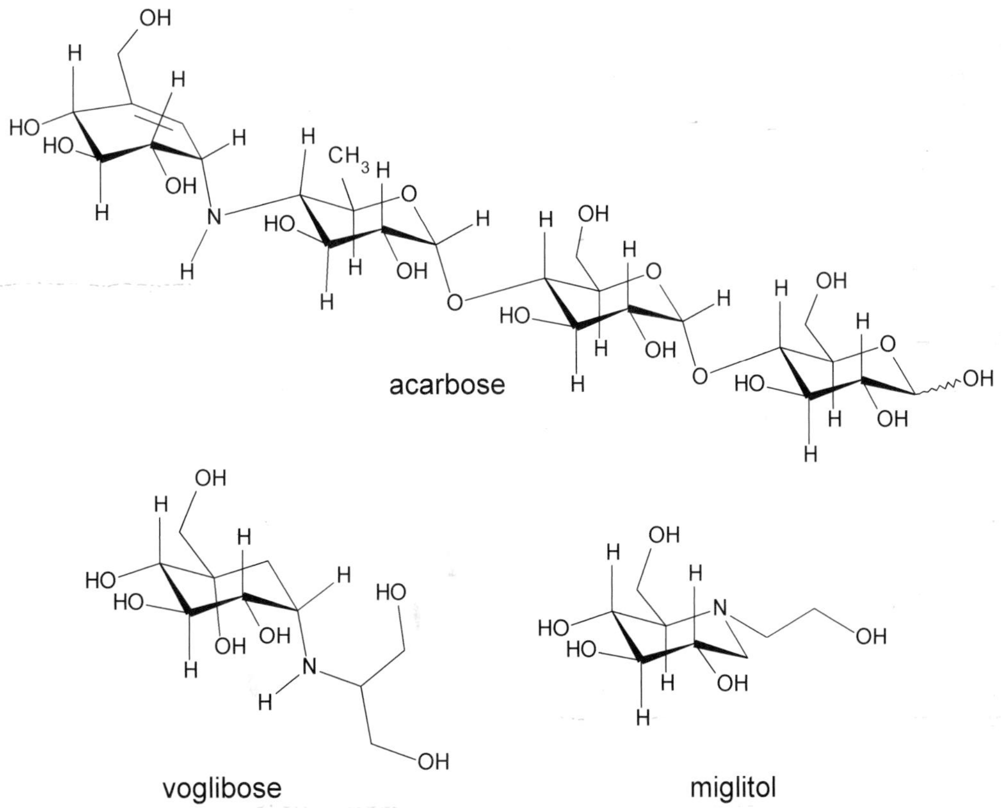

acarbose

voglibose

miglitol

Figure 20.23 ● Structures of antihyperglycemic α-glucosidase inhibitors on the market worldwide.

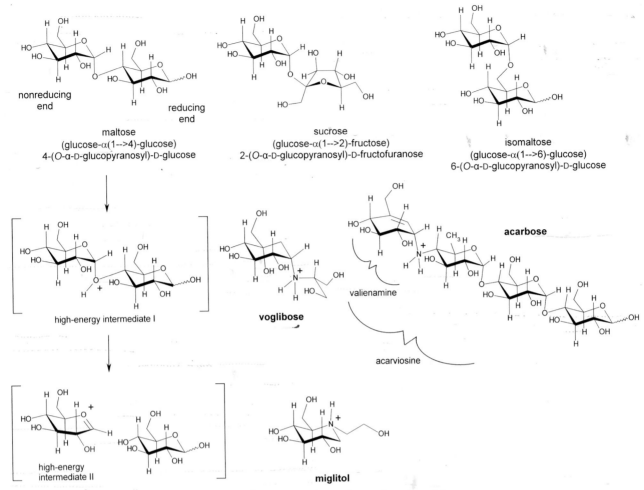

Figure 20.24 • Polysaccharide linkages of relevance to the actions of α-glucosidase inhibitors, and the relationship of inhibitor structures to postulated high-energy intermediates in the hydrolysis of the disaccharide bonds.

activity and two with "maltase–glucoamylase" (MGAM) activity.[65,66] The sucrase activity represents catalytic hydrolysis of the α-(1→2) linkage between glucose C1 and fructose C2 in sucrose.

Acarbose potently and competitively inhibits the MGAM activity,[66] and more specifically, the glucoamylase—but not the maltase—activity.[67] The former activity was recently shown to reside within the C-terminal subunit of the enzyme, which extends into the intestinal lumen, and to which acarbose binds with considerably higher affinity than it does to the N-terminal subunit.[68] The latter subunit is mostly membrane-imbedded, although both subunits are catalytically active and are closely related members of the glycosyl hydrolase family 31. Miglitol potently inhibits glucoamylase and sucrase activities, but not isomaltase activity.[69] Voglibose inhibits sucrase and maltase activities[70] with such potency that clinically effective doses of voglibose are more than 100-fold lesser than the doses required for acarbose or miglitol.

Structure–activity relationships for molecules inhibiting α-glucosidases were extensively reviewed in 1996 by Junge et al.[71]; however, interpretations are complicated by substrate-dependent inhibitor binding and inhibition kinetics for these enzymes. These complexities are now understood to arise, in part, as manifestations of allosteric crosstalk between binding sites in these multisubunit enzymes.[68,72]

PRODUCTS

Acarbose is *O*-4,6-dideoxy-4-[[(1*S*,4*R*,5*S*,6*S*)-4,5,6-trihydroxy-3-(hydroxymethyl)-2-cyclohexen-1-yl]amino]-α-D-glucopyranosyl-(1→4)-*O*-α-D-glucopyranosyl-(1→4)-D-glucose. It is sold as 25-, 50-, and 100-mg tablets (Precose, generics) dosed with the first bite of each meal, up to t.i.d. Acarbose potently inhibits the glucoamylase activity of MGAM α-glucosidases and the sucrase activity of SI α-glucosidases, whereas isomaltase activity is at most moderately inhibited at concentrations in the range of those in the intestinal lumen upon oral dosing, and trehalase and lactase are not significantly inhibited.[73] Some inhibition of pancreatic α-amylases may also contribute to the clinical effects.

Based on the structure of acarbose, it should come as no surprise that little intact acarbose reaches the systemic circulation; instead, acarbose is extensively biotransformed by the action of microbes and digestive enzymes in the gut. Only about 35% of the radioactivity in a dose of ^{14}C-labeled acarbose administered orally to men was excreted in the urine, appearing as several metabolites, some of which are phase II conversion products of 4-methylpyrogallol (*O*-methyl, *O*-sulfate, or *O*-glucuronide conjugates)[74]; the methylpyrogallol fragment arises from the terminal valienamine pseudosugar. That these biotransformation products are mostly formed in the gut is shown by the fact that nearly 90% of an intravenously administered dose of acarbose is excreted intact in urine.

Miglitol is (2R,3R,4R,5S)-1-(2-hydroxyethyl)-2-(hydroxymethyl)-3,4,5-piperidinetriol, or *N*-hydroxyethyl-1-deoxynorjirimycin. The drug is available as 25-, 50-, and 100-mg tablets (Glyset), for administration 25 to 100 mg t.i.d. with meals. In contrast to acarbose, miglitol is highly absorbed from a 25-mg oral dose, although absorption is reported to be saturable, and accordingly less complete at higher doses.[69] Binding to plasma proteins is minimal, and the volume of distribution (0.18 L/kg, corresponding to 12–13 L in a 70-kg adult) is characteristic of compounds distributed only to blood and extracellular fluids. Practically no systemic biotransformation of miglitol occurs in humans; essentially 100% of an orally administered dose is excreted intact in urine.

Amylin Analogs

Amylin is a circulating hormone released along with insulin from normally functioning pancreatic β cells. This 37-amino-acid polypeptide (Fig. 20.25) incorporates one intramolecular disulfide bridge between cysteine residues at positions 2 and 7. The physiological and biochemical roles of amylin are at present only rather vaguely understood, but some of these are discussed here. Amylin, in excess, causes amyloidogenesis. The ramifications of this fact, in terms of β cell loss in pancreatic islets or progressive amyloid tangle formation associated with Alzheimer disease, is an active area of investigation. The observation, though, that this property is not shared by rat amylin[75–77] was exploited in the design of pramlintide, which differs from human amylin at only three positions toward the *C*-terminal end, namely substitution in each case with proline (Fig. 20.25).

Pramlintide is the 25-L-proline-28-L-proline-29-L-proline trisubstitution product of human amylin. The marketed formulation (Symlin) is an acetate salt, the exact composition of which may not be public-domain knowledge, although salts containing up to four acetic acid molecules per pramlintide molecule would be possible by virtue of the free amino terminus and Lys[1], Arg[11], and His[18] residues. The carboxyl terminus of pramlintide, as in amylin, is amidated, and there are no appreciably acidic moities in the structure; thus, in solution at the pH of blood and tissues pramlintide would be present almost entirely as one or the other of two significant molecular species, one having a +3 charge (histidine imidazole deprotonated and uncharged) predominating modestly over the quadruply protonated (+4) species.

Pramlintide's labeled pharmacotherapeutic uses are (a) as an adjunct in type 1 diabetics who require mealtime insulin injections and yet fail to achieve desired glucose control (15 μg initially, titrated to 30 or 60 μg as tolerated); and (b) as an adjunct in type 2 diabetics who require mealtime insulin injections and yet fail to achieve desired glucose control (60 μg initially, increased after 3–7 days to 120 μg if tolerated), with or without ongoing management with metformin or a sulfonylurea. Pramlintide functions as an amylinomimetic; its administration slows gastric emptying, suppresses glucagon secretion (in turn inhibiting liver glucose output), and reduces the amount of food consumed via centrally mediated appetite suppression or satiety enhancement. Abnormal postprandial glucagon secretion occurs in diabetics, exacerbating hyperglycemic excursions, and pramlintide's glucagon-suppressing action serves to normalize this response. The multiple effects of pramlintide (and by analogy, endogenous amylin) are mediated directly or indirectly, or by some combination thereof, mechanistic understanding of which remains modest or even poor in many aspects.

Amylin receptors consist of short-form calcitonin receptors (CT[a]) in hetero-oligomeric complex with receptor activity–modifying proteins (RAMP1, RAMP2, RAMP3), thereby generating three subtypes of receptor complexes (AMY$_{1(a)}$, AMY$_{2(a)}$, and AMY$_{3(a)}$, or simply AMY1, AMY2, and AMY3).[78,79] CT receptors are G-protein–coupled receptors (GPCRs), and the short-form CTr is a splice variant lacking a 16-amino-acid insert in the first intracellular loop (thus, it is also known as "insert negative"). Compared with many other GPCRs, particularly those that are targets of currently marketed or late-stage investigational pharmacotherapeutic agents, characterization of anatomical distributions and tissue- and system-level functions of amylin receptors remain but lightly addressed in open literature reports.

Pramlintide's effects upon administration to patients almost certainly arise in significant measure from direct AMY-mediated actions within the brainstem.[80] Amylin receptors are abundant in the circumventricular organs, including the subfornical organ (where AMY$_{1(a)}$ receptors are known to be expressed in relative abundance), the organum vasculosum lateralis terminalis, and the area postrema (AMY$_{3(a)}$), where the action of pramlintide (or of β-cell–secreted amylin) is not precluded by a diffusional BBB. Amylin receptors are also expressed in various other brain areas, in particular the nucleus accumbens, but neither amylin or pramlintide circulating in the bloodstream are likely to exert any action at these BBB-shielded locations. Direct amylin receptor–mediated actions of pramlintide in

```
               +  +000000000+000000=000000000000000000000
Pramlintide:   KCNTATCATQRLANFLVHSSNNFGPILPPTNVGSNTY-(NH2)
Human Amylin:  KCNTATCATQRLANFLVHSSNNFGAILSSTNVGSNTY-(NH2)
Rat amylin:    KCNTATCATQRLANFLVRSSNNFGPVLPPTNVGSNTY-(NH2)
               1234567890123456789012345678901234567
                        1         2         3
```

Figure 20.25 ● Primary amino acid sequences of human amylin, rat amylin, and pramlintide. Charge symbols above the set of sequences indicate charges of the predominant molecular form of the side chain (the free N-terminal amino group is also indicated) at physiological pH (7.4): positive (+), neutral (0), or near-equal (=). Underlines indicate sites of amylin hydrolysis by insulin-degrading enzyme (IDE).

the periphery, if any, remain poorly characterized.[81] Unsurprisingly, though, the appetite-suppressing actions, and benefits of pramlintide and amylin agonists in general, are receiving significant clinical and scientific attention.

Pramlintide has a relatively short pharmacokinetic half-life of about 50 minutes. One conversion product, *des*-Lys[1]-pramlintide, retains full agonist activity and exhibits an elimination time-course similar to that of pramlintide itself. Amylin is degraded by IDE at three sites (as indicated in Fig. 20.25); in vivo administration of IDE inhibitors increases toxicities of the same nature as those associated with excessive endogenous or exogenously administered amylin.[82] Pramlintide possesses amino acid residue pairs identical with those of amylin at each of the IDE cleavage sites, thus this enzyme probably governs the elimination rates of pramlintide and *des*-Lys[1]-pramlintide.

Despite the fact that pramlintide is a relatively large and clearly nonnative polypeptide, systemic immunosensitivity has not proven to be an issue of clinical concern, even upon long-term pramlintide pharmacotherapy.

Incretin System Modulating Agents: Incretin Mimetics and Dipeptidyl Peptidase Type 4 Inhibitors

Several polypeptide hormones have been identified that are synthesized in the cells of the upper intestines and act to modulate carbohydrate metabolism. Among these are the *incretins*, a term first coined by La Barre in 1932.[83] The "incretin effect" refers to insulin secretion stimulated by orally administered glucose independent of any increase in blood glucose. Eventually, two incretins were identified, in 1971 and 1985, respectively: glucose-dependent insulinotropic peptide (GIP) and GLP-1.[84] GIP was originally named gastric inhibitory peptide by its discoverers,[85] but it was later renamed in such a way as to retain the acronym while better reflecting its physiological roles.

The gene encoding proglucagon (PG), besides being expressed in pancreatic islet α cells (and in some neurons in the hypothalamus and brainstem, and certain taste cells of the tongue), is also expressed in endocrine cells of the lower intestinal mucosa. From PG, gut L cells produce the peptides glicentin, oxyntomodulin, intervening peptide-2, and GLP-1. PG(72–108) is equivalent to GLP-1(1–37), and is derived from PG via the action of the convertase PC1/3. GLP-1(1–37) is further shortened, apparently also by PC1/3, to GLP-1(7–37) or GLP-1(7–36)amide (Fig. 20.26); at least 80% of "GLP-1" released into the bloodstream is the latter. Secretion occurs upon ingestion of lipid- or carbohydrate-containing foodstuffs.[86–88] Following their release, both bioactive forms of GLP-1 are very short-lived (plasma $t_{1/2}$ ~1–2 min): DPP-4 or DPP-IV rapidly cleaves two residues from the amino terminus, generating GLP-1(9–37) and GLP-1(9–36)amide, respectively.[88] Release of

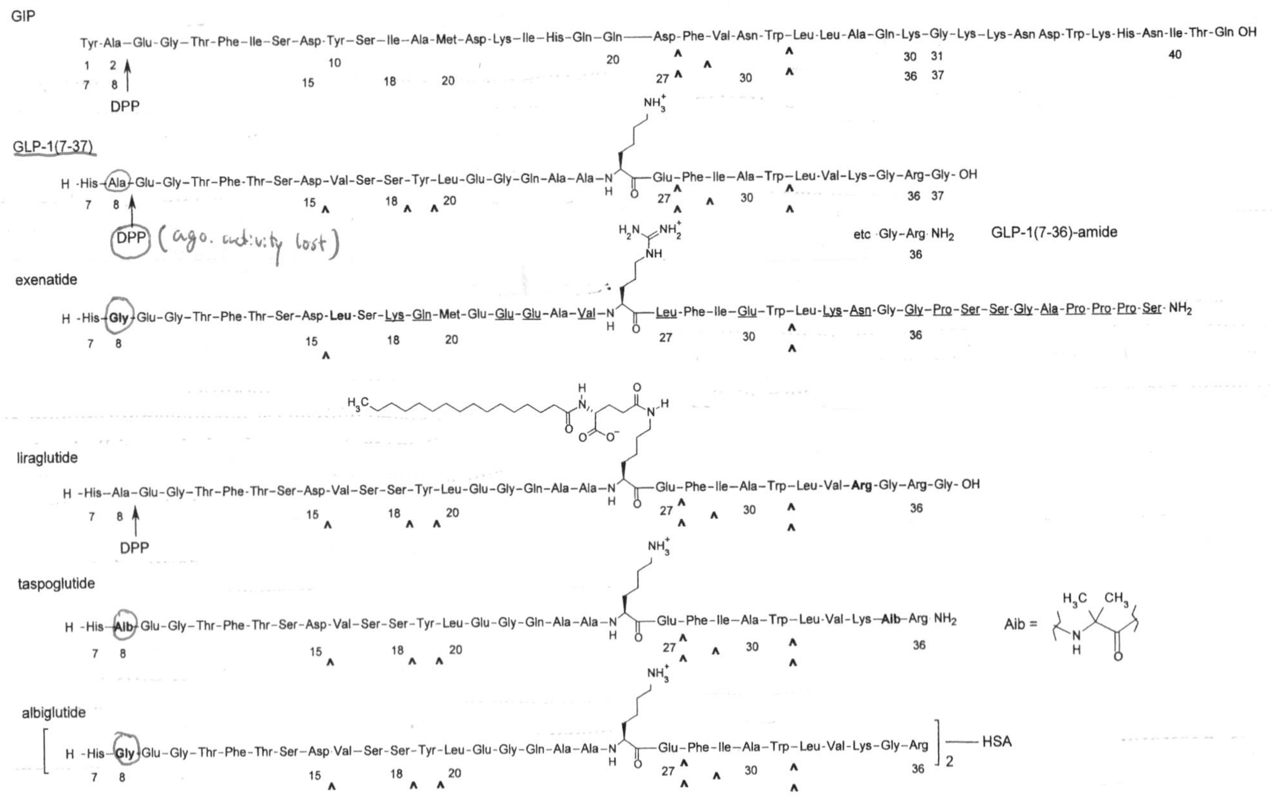

Figure 20.26 ● Primary sequences of endogenous human incretins and incretin mimetic pharmacotherapeutic agents. *Arrows* indicate a peptide bond cleaved by DPP-4 catalysis, carets (^) indicate sites of cleavage by neutral endopeptidase 24.11 (neprilysin) catalysis (double-caret–marked bonds are likely more prominently cleaved). Underscored residues in the structure of exenatide indicate nonconservative substitutions versus GLP-1 or GIP. The numbering for GLP-1 is "slipped" by six residues; the corresponding numberings are given below the GIP structure for reference. (HSA, human serum albumin.)

the bioactive forms of GLP occurs within minutes of food intake, even though L cells are found predominantly in the ileum and caecum, and considerable evidence indicates that some combination of neural or endocrine signaling mediates this response. GLP-1 acts via specific GPCRs in the portal vein to trigger vagal afferents that, mediated by neuronal pathways within the brain, generate efferent signals stimulating pancreatic insulin release and inhibiting glucagon release.[89] GPCRs for GLP-1 (GLP-1Rs) are also expressed in pancreatic islet β cells, as well as in the GI tract, kidney, vagus nerve, and neurons in areas of the brain, including the hypothalamus and hindbrain; in β-islet cells, agonist binding to GLP-1Rs increases the biosynthesis of insulin, as well as of glucokinase and the GLUT2 glucose transporter.[90]

Structure–activity studies indicate that the C-terminal portions of the GLP-1 peptides provide an important component of receptor binding, whereas the N-terminal segment is necessary for receptor activation.[91] Accordingly, once DPP-4 removes the N-terminal dipeptide from either GLP-1(7–37) or GLP-1(7–36)NH$_2$, agonist activity is lost. GLP-1(9–36)NH$_2$ finds some use as a pharmacological tool for its antagonist activity at GLP-1Rs.

GIP is synthesized via the action of a prohormone convertase on a 153-amino-acid proprotein coded by a specific gene in gut K cells, which are found mainly in the mucosa of the duodenum and jejunum.[84] In contrast to the mostly indirect stimulation of GLP-1 release, GIP secretion is mainly triggered directly by the enteral presence of glucose and lipids, providing what amounts to an early warning system for the pancreas. The bioactive GIP(1–42) is rapidly converted (plasma t_h ~5–7 min) to inactive GIP(3–42). Like the two GLP-1 hormones, this inactivation is also effected via DPP-4 catalyzed cleavage of a dipeptide from the amino terminus.[92] GIP activates insulin secretion via binding to seven-transmembrane–segment GPCRs on islet β cells, distinct receptors from those activated by GLP-1(7–37) and GLP-1(7–36)NH$_2$.[88] GIP-stimulated insulin secretion only occurs when blood glucose is substantively elevated, and receptor knockout studies in mice indicate that GIP receptors (GIPRs, which are also present in brain, pituitary, adipocytes, upper GI tract, adrenal cortex, and bone) are required for a proper gluconormative response to hyperglycemia. Notably, in type 2 diabetics, exogenously administered (iv) GIP cannot facilitate glucose-stimulated insulin secretion as it does in healthy patients.

Relatively recently, compelling direct evidence from rodent and in vitro experimentation and some indirect but inconclusive evidence from human clinical studies of incretin mimetics (see discussion that follows) and DPP-4 inhibitors suggests that incretins may exert preservative, proliferative, and even neogenerative effects on β-cell mass and β-cell populations, thereby arresting—and potentially even reversing—the progressive declines that have, heretofore, been inevitable in type 2 diabetes.[90,93] If so, a truly new age in the treatment of this common and insidious disorder has begun, particularly when technology allows reliable detection of prediabetic states amenable to prophylactic treatment.

Exenatide, at the time of this writing, is currently the only incretin mimetic approved (2005) for the U.S. market (Byetta, Amylin Pharmaceuticals). Exenatide must be administered parenterally (subcutaneous [sc]); injection is typically made in the abdomen about an hour before the first and last meals of the day. Exenatide is synthetically produced exendin-4, a 39-residue hormone (see Fig. 20.26) present in the venom of the Gila monster. Exenatide's actions mimic those of GLP-1; exenatide differs from GLP-1 in 14 of its first 30 amino acids (the length of GLP-1(7–36)NH$_2$), although at least four of these substitutions may be regarded as conservative. Exenatide is not, however, a DPP-4 substrate, by virtue of the presence of a glycine rather than an alanine in the second position, and partly for this reason has a greatly increased serum half-life of 2 to 3 hours[94]; some of the other amino acid changes almost certainly also render exenatide less susceptible to neutral endopeptidase 24.11 (NEP-24.11),[95] which is a membrane-bound zinc metallopeptidase also known as neprilysin, and which may account for as much as half of the elimination of GLP-1(7–37) and GLP-1(7–36)NH$_2$. Although approved as adjunctive therapy (with metformin, or with a sulfonylurea, or with metformin + a sulfonylurea, or with metformin + a thiazolidinedione), in fact none of these other medicinals are necessary for exenatide to produce its clinically beneficial effects. Exenatide administration alone in pharmacological doses restores the early stage insulin release, loss of which is a hallmark of type 2 diabetes, and increases the robustness of the second-stage insulin release. Premeal exenatide injections (5 or 10 μg) also suppress glucagon release following a meal (but do not affect normal hypoglycemia-stimulated glucagon release), slow gastric emptying, induce satiety, and promote normalcy of postprandial glucose uptake while suppressing hepatic glucose release. Moreover, the glucose dependency of exenatide-stimulated insulin secretion means that this drug cannot cause abnormal hypoglycemic episodes, although this can, of course, happen when the drug is adjunctive to a sulfonylurea. Although there are GLP-1 receptors expressed in hindbrain and hypothalamus that are probably involved in mediating exenatide-induced satiety effects, evidence suggests that direct agonist action on these receptors by circulating exenatide is likely not involved.[96]

Liraglutide is GLP-1(1–37) modified at Lys[26]: the ε-amino group is acylated with an (N-hexadecanoyl)glutam-γ-yl moiety (Fig. 20.26) that noncovalently but avidly binds to human serum albumin. (Also, Lys[34] is conservatively replaced with Arg.) These changes provide for a greatly extended serum t_h of ~10 to 15 hours after sc administration (0.6–1.8 mg), allowing for once-daily dosing.[97–99] Liraglutide (Victoza, Novo Nordisk) is awaiting approval by the FDA, EMEA, and the Kōrō-shō (Japan).

Albiglutide (also known as naliglutide, GSK 716155) is a sequential dimer of GLP-1(7–36)(Ala[8]→Gly) covalently linked to modified human serum albumin (i.e., it is a "fusion protein" with modified HSA). This molecule is currently well into phase III clinical trials. Although albiglutide, if marketed (Syncria, GlaxoSmithKline), will—like exenatide—be administered by injection, the half-life and duration of 6 to 7 days[100] would allow for weekly administration.

Taspoglutide (R1583, Roche) is GLP-1 modified at residues 8 and 35 (see Fig. 20.26) with α-methylalanine in place of the Ala and Gly, respectively. These modifications greatly retard degradation by DPP-IV and neutral endopeptidase 24.11, respectively (see preceding discussion for exenatide). The phase III trials, which commenced in 2008, are being conducted with a zinc-based preparation, prolonging the duration in a manner similar to zinc-containing insulin preparations, so that once-weekly injections of 20 to 30 mg will be possible.

Besides the aforementioned list of products, a number of other incretin mimetics are being created and developed. A long-acting version of exenatide ("exenatide LAR") consisting of microspheres of a poly(lactide-coglycolide) polymeric matrix has been devised, from which exenatide is slowly released from the injection site through diffusion and erosion.[101] An adenoviral vector has also been created for exenatide ("gene therapy," and was reported to successfully generate exenatide and modulate glucose control and other GLP-1-mediated responses in mice for at least 15 weeks following treatment[102]; other gene therapy approaches for delivering GLP-1 itself are also being explored. Boc5,[103] a cyclobutanedicarboxylic acid (CAS Reg. No. 917569-14-3, structure still undisclosed), is reported to be a nonpeptide GLP-1 agonist exerting incretin effects in C57BL/6J and *db/db* mice. The variety of the developments described above provide some sense of the current level of interest in incretin mimetics among researchers and clinicians, interest undoubtedly based on perceived strength of promise. The relative merits of incretin receptor agonists as compared to the indirect incretin-enhancing approach achieved with inhibitors of DPP-IV (discussed next) or neutral endopeptidase 24.11 largely remain to be discerned, which will likely happen during the coming decade or so.

DPP-4 or DPP-IV is a serine protease that selectively binds and hydrolyzes substrates that incorporate alanine (as in GLP(7–36)NH$_2$, see earlier discussion and Fig. 20.26) or proline (as in neuropeptide Y and peptide YY) at the second position. Because there are many serine proteases, excellent selectivity is an essential design feature requisite to bestowing pharmacotherapeutic usefulness.[104] In particular, minimizing inhibition of the closely related enzymes DPP-2, fibroblast activation protein (FAP), DPP-7 (also known as quiescent cell proline peptidase, QPP), DPP-8, and DPP-9 has proved to be crucial.[105,106] These serine proteases are among a relatively few peptidases that can cleave at proline, and they do so on the carboxyl side. Human DPP-4 is a 766-amino-acid transmembrane glycoprotein and a member of peptidase clan SC, and more specifically a member of family S9, subfamily S9B. Clan SC serine proteases include a catalytic triad in the specific order Ser, Asp, His—different from the classical serine proteases such as trypsin (class SA: His, Asp, Ser) or subtilisin (class SB: Asp, His, Ser).

DPP-4 was first identified in 1967, and early inhibitors were created by relatively simple modifications of proline-based structures. After the later realization that this enzyme might likely be an important pharmacotherapeutic target, compound library screening provided inhibitors with a variety of new base structures, including the lead compound from which sitagliptin was created (Fig. 20.27). In due course, a significant number of x-ray crystal structures were generated, for complexes in which the catalytic pocket is occupied with various inhibitors, the first two reports occurring in

2003.[107,108] This body of structural information very quickly grew to be sufficient to enable true de novo structure-based drug design; an excellent overview is provided by Kuhn et al.[109] The catalytic site of DPP-4 is extracellular, and includes an α/β-hydrolase fold containing the Ser^{630}-Asp^{708}-His^{740} catalytic triad, and an eight-bladed β-propeller domain[108] that participates in the binding of various known inhibitors, including sitagliptin.[109] The S1 pocket within the protein, which accommodates proline (or, less favorably, alanine, as is found in the GLP-1 peptides and in GIP), is enclosed by the largely hydrophobic residues Tyr^{631}, Val^{656}, Trp^{662}, Tyr^{666}, and Val^{711}, and among the reported x-ray structures of enzyme:inhibitor complexes the shape of this pocket changes very little, even for structurally very disparate inhibitors.

The discovery of sitagliptin at Merck preceded the availability of x-ray structures, and was accomplished by more classical (albeit highly refined) screening and lead-optimization approaches. Thornberry and Weber[106] provide an informative account of this process. Although initially commencing with preclinical development of in-licensed compounds, extensive screening of a very large compound collection was also conducted c. 2001, from which effort these authors report that relatively few hits—and only three suitable leads—were gleaned. Sitagliptin was ultimately created (Fig. 20.27) from one of these leads, which was a β-amino acid derivative and thus unlike the α-amino-acid–based compounds divulged prior to this discovery. The in-licensed compounds were abandoned at about the same time because of toxicities that were found to be traceable to DPP-8 or DPP-9 inhibition; the existence of these enzymes, as well as of QPP (see previous discussion), were first reported circa this same time frame. Some characteristics of a few of the "way-station" compounds created during the lead optimization process that led to sitagliptin provide a sense of the process, particularly the large changes in target-level activity, biopharmaceutics characteristics, and deleterious effects profile, which can result from seemingly very subtle changes to the molecular structure. The necessity to monitor and optimize multiple characteristics simultaneously (such as target affinity and oral bioavailability) during the process of creating a marketable drug should also be readily apparent from this outline. Sufficient preclinical studies were completed for sitagliptin by January 2002 that it was moved to first priority for development. (Marketing approval was obtained from the FDA in late 2006, representing an impressively and exceptionally compressed timeline from screening hit identification to marketing.)

An x-ray structure of DPP-4 with bound sitagliptin later provided an understanding of the structure–affinity observations.[110] The trifluorophenyl moiety occupies the S1 pocket. The triazolopyrazine-ring-attached trifluoromethyl substituent—where a buildup of electron density occurs—situates near the positively charged side chain of Arg^{358}; the protonated (cationic) form of the primary amino group forms a hydrogen bond with Tyr^{662}, and salt bridges to the γ-carboxylates of Glu^{205} and Glu^{206}; the triazolopiperazine group engages the phenyl group of residue Phe^{357}.

Other DPP-4 inhibitors are either on the market elsewhere (vildagliptin in the EU, Novartis [Galvus]), or are under regulatory review (alogliptin, Takeda; saxagliptin,

1

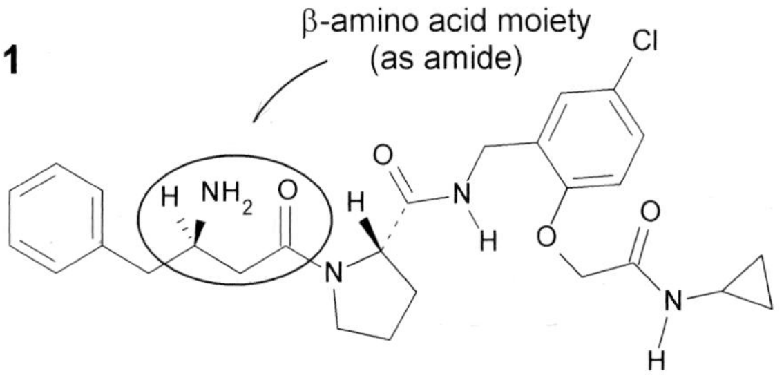

β-amino acid moiety
(as amide)

Merck β-amino acid lead from screening
DPP-4 IC$_{50}$ = 1900 nM

2

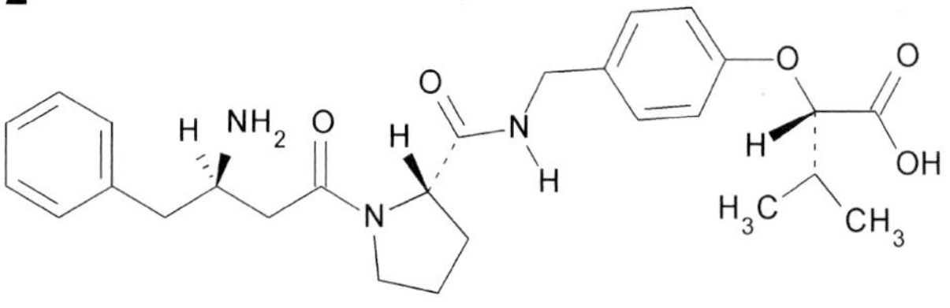

DPP-4 IC$_{50}$ = 0.4 nM
>100,000-fold selectivity vs. DPP-8, DPP-9
extremely poor oral absorption

3

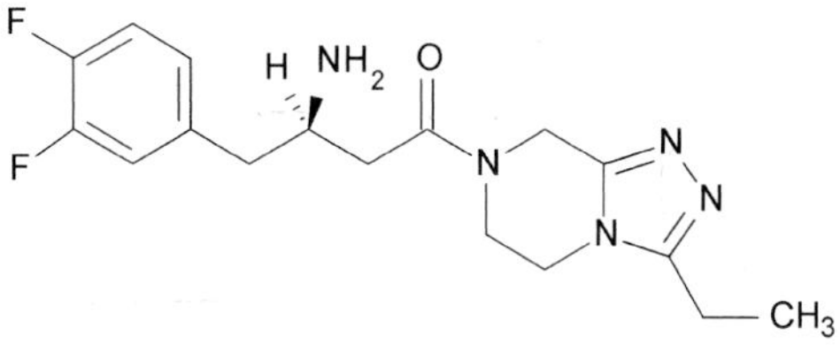

DPP-4 IC$_{50}$ = 230 nM
oral bioavailability (rat) poor: *F* = 2%

4

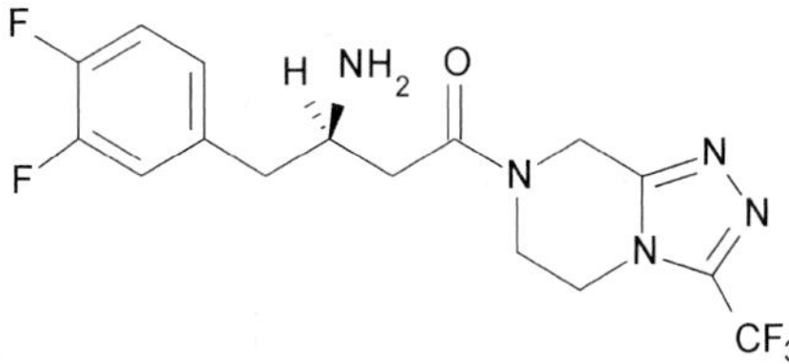

DPP-4 IC$_{50}$ = 130 nM
oral bioavailability (rat) much improved: *F* = 44%

5

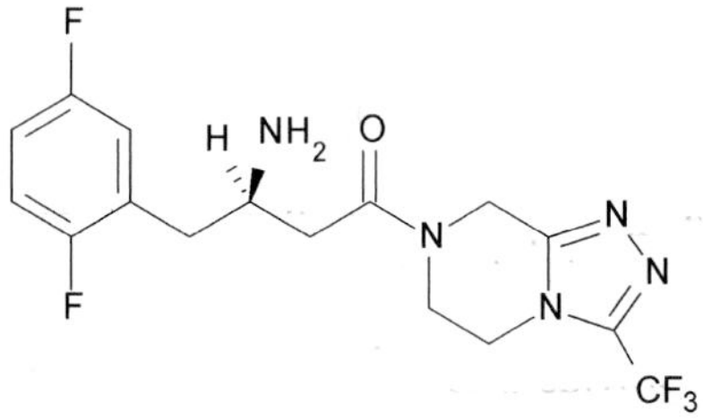

DPP-4 IC$_{50}$ = 27 nM
acute cardiovascular side-effects
(dogs, mild but concerning)

6

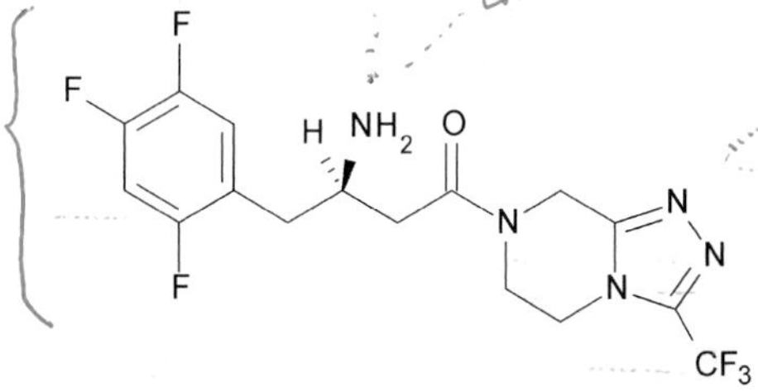

sitagliptin
DPP-4 IC$_{50}$ = 18 nM
>2500-fold selectivity vs. DPP-8, DPP-9

Figure 20.27 ● Sitagliptin creation outline. The β-amino acid–lead compound (**1**) was discovered by screening of a large library of compounds. Compound **2** bound with very high affinity to the enzyme but was not endowed with useful oral bioavailability. Changing the metabolically labile ethyl substituent in compound **3** to trifluoromethyl gave a compound (**4**) with acceptable bioavailability, albeit binding with considerably lower affinity than molecule **2**. Relocating the fluorines on the phenyl ring improved the binding affinity but a cardiovascular side effect appeared in preclinical studies of **5** in dogs. Adding one additional fluorine increased the affinity and eliminated the worrisome preclinical side effect; molecule **6** was ultimately marketed as sitagliptin phosphate.

Bristol Myers Squibb [Onglyza]),[111] or are well along in phase III studies (linagliptin, Boehringer Ingelheim). Three of these (Fig. 20.28) incorporate a nitrile (cyano) moiety: vildagliptin and saxagliptin a 2-cyanopyrrolidine, alogliptin a 2-cyanophenyl. In each case, the nitrile engages the enzyme at the same position as does the scissile[1] bond in peptide substrates such as GLP-1 or GIP. The nitrile group is attacked by the hydroxyl of the catalytic serine (Ser[630]), forming a covalent imidate species (Fig. 20.29). Hydrolysis of this imidate occurs slowly; thus, these inhibitors may be described as slowly reversible or pseudoirreversible.

Sitagliptin phosphate is the 1:1 phosphoric acid salt of sitagliptin free base (i.e., (2*R*)-4-oxo-4-[3-(trifluoromethyl)-5,6-dihydro[1,2,4]triazolo[4,3-*a*]pyrazin-7(8*H*)-yl]-1-(2,4,5-trifluorophenyl)-2-butanamine), see Figure 20.30, and is marketed (Junuvia, 2006) in 25-, 50-, and 100-mg tablets. A combination product with metformin (Janumet, 2007) in two strengths (50 mg/500 mg and 50 mg/1,000 mg sitagliptin/metformin) is also available, and sitagliptin may also be prescribed with a thiazolidinedione, or possibly a sulfonylurea. The phosphate salt provides very high water solubility.[112] The bioavailability of orally administered sitagliptin is ~87%.[113] The drug exhibits relatively low plasma protein

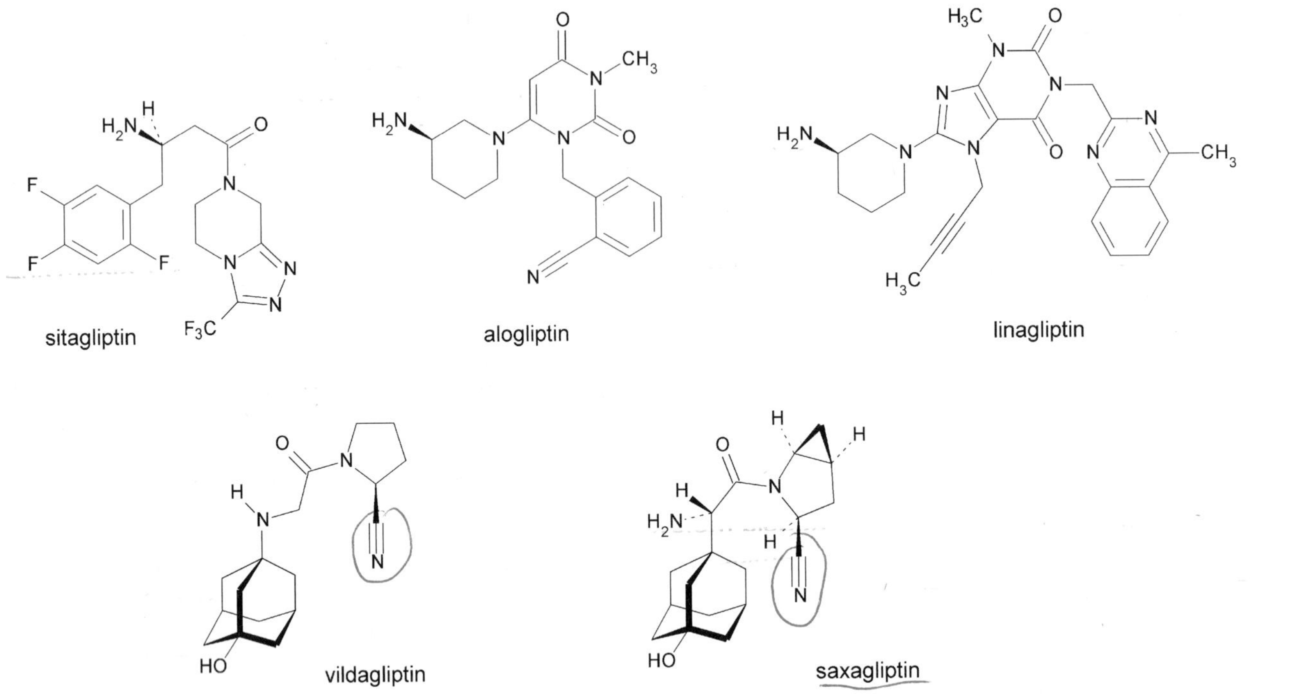

Figure 20.28 • Structures of DPP-4 inhibitors on the global market or in advanced stages of clinical development.

binding (~38%), a relatively large volume of distribution (198 L), and a terminal elimination half-life of ~12 hours. About 79% of a 100-mg oral dose is excreted unchanged in urine, the balance as trace-level metabolites (CYP3A4, lesser contribution by CYP2C8) in urine or feces: 87% of administered radioactivity is excreted in urine, and 13% in feces. Active tubular excretion is reported to play a key role in renal clearance of unchanged drug, and may be mediated at least in part via the organic anion transporter hOAT-3.

Glucose Elevating Agents

Apart from administration of glucose, either glucagon (rDNA origin) or diazoxide represent therapeutic options for pharmacotherapy of hypoglycemia. Applications are limited and specialized, as will be discussed here.

Glucagon produced by recombinant DNA technology is marketed by Novo Nordisk (glucagon [recombinant] hydrochloride, GlucaGen HypoKit, GlucaGen Diagnostic Kit) and by Eli Lilly (glucagon [recombinant] Emergency Kit). Details regarding the structure and chemistry of this 29-amino-acid peptide are available in Chapter 27. As discussed earlier in this chapter, endogenous glucagon is produced from the gene-derived protein PG in the α cells of the islets of Langerhans in the pancreas. The core function of this hormone is to renormalize blood glucose levels when they fall too low, by stimulating production from glycogen

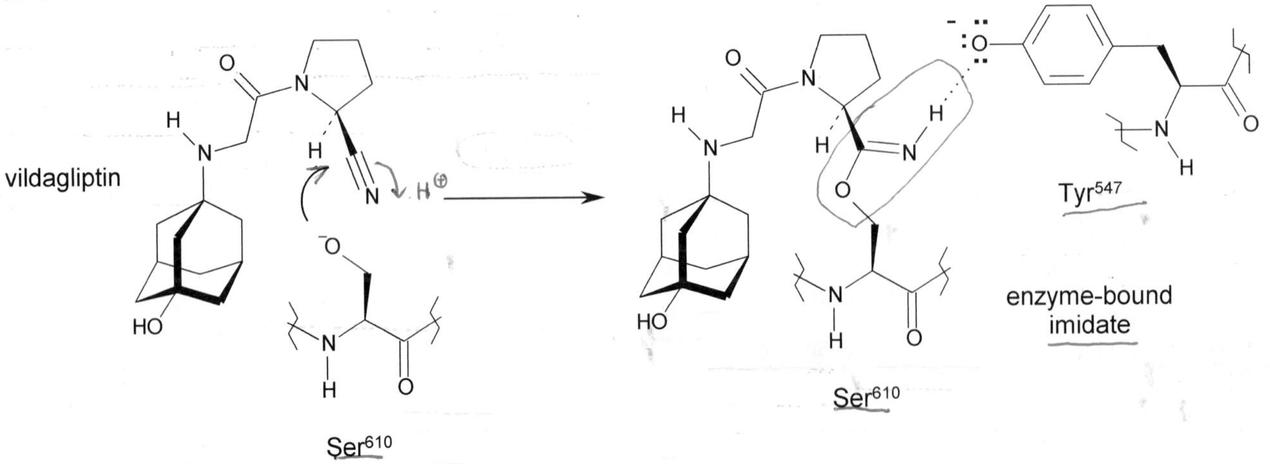

Figure 20.29 • Covalently bound imidate intermediate formed with nitrilo-containing DPP-4 inhibitors.

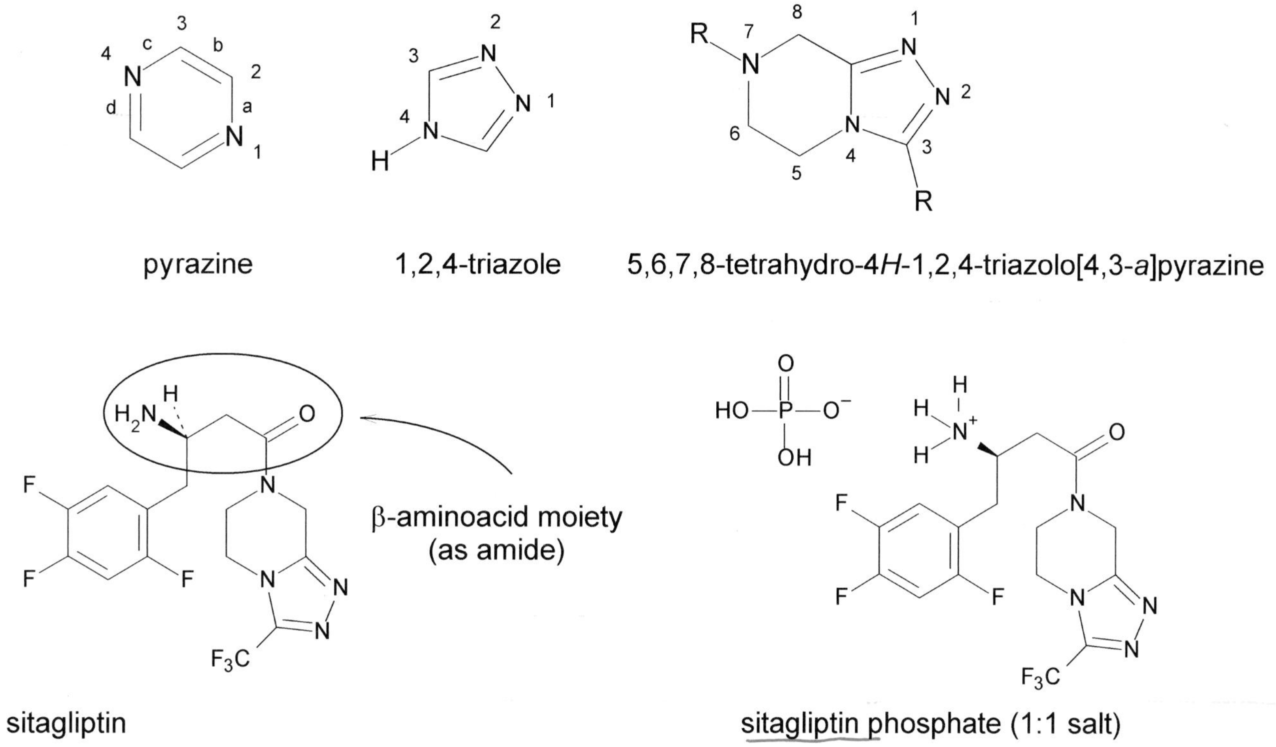

pyrazine   1,2,4-triazole   5,6,7,8-tetrahydro-4*H*-1,2,4-triazolo[4,3-*a*]pyrazine

β-aminoacid moiety
(as amide)

sitagliptin   sitagliptin phosphate (1:1 salt)

Figure 20.30 ● Basis of sitagliptin fused ring system nomenclature, and explicit structure of 1:1 phosphate salt.

Glucogon → ↑ hepatic Glu prodn.

stores in liver and muscle, and stimulating hepatic gluconeogenesis. Glucagon also elicits biochemical processes (such as fatty acid oxidation) that supply the needed precursors for gluconeogenesis. Glucagon supplied exogenously (i.e., injected) in response to emergency hypoglycemia acts rapidly to elicit these same responses. Clinically, glucagon also provides an alternative to cholinergic antagonists for reducing GI motility and secretory activity during radiologic imaging procedures.

Diazoxide is 7-chloro-3-methyl-4*H*-benzo[*e*][1,2,4] thiadiazine-1,1-dioxide (structure Fig. 20.31), and is currently available in the United States only as a 50-mg/mL oral suspension (Proglycem); discontinued formulations included capsules for oral administration, and injectable forms that typically found use for indications other than hypoglycemic conditions. Diazoxide is a cyclic benzenesulfonamide, although the free acid in solution can exist in three tautomeric forms, and the 4*H* tautomer most likely predominates to a very high proportion.[114] Partly because of the additional nitrogen in the quinazoline ring structure, the molecule is somewhat more acidic (pKa ~8.4,[115] 8.6[116]) than benzenesulfonamide (pKa ~10).

Diazoxide acts as an ATP-sensitive potassium channel opener, thus inhibiting basal insulin secretion. This action may be viewed as the reverse of the insulin secretagogue actions of the sulfonylureas discussed earlier in this chapter; however, diazoxide is much less selective for SUR$_1$ over SUR$_{2A}$, SUR$_{2B}$, or SUR$_{2C}$ receptor types,[117] acts on mitochondrial ATP-sensitive potassium channels,[118] and exerts various extrapancreatic effects that will not be discussed here.[119] The action of diazoxide on β-islet cells may trigger glucagon release from α-islet cells via paracrine pathways.[120]

Structurally, diazoxide closely resembles (Fig. 20.31) hydrochlorthiazide, a diuretic that inhibits the sodium chloride symporter in the distal convoluted tubule. Diazoxide does not act as a diuretic, however, instead exerting an antidiuretic effect. The discovery/creation/development of pancreas-selective ATP-sensitive potassium channel openers continues to be an area of ongoing investigation.[121–123]

Diazoxide binds extensively (>90%) to serum proteins, which greatly retards its renal excretion, by which route this drug is almost exclusively eliminated, with a terminal elimination half-life about 28 ± 8 hours. Lacking this serum binding (or active tubular reuptake), the hydrophilicity of this molecule would otherwise confer a much more rapid rate of renal excretion.

In contrast to the acute clinical uses of glucagon, diazoxide finds use in chronic hypoglycemic conditions: inoperable islet cell adenoma or carcinomas, extrapancreatic malignancies of insulin-secreting cells, or islet cell hyperplasias. In children, additional indications include congenital hyperinsulinemia[124] and leucine sensitivity. Experimentally, diazoxide is among an array of ATP-sensitive potassium channel openers being studied for intermittently bringing about β-cell rest (see discussion of β-cell "fatigue" earlier in this chapter).[125]

● GONADOTROPINS, GONADOTROPIN-RELEASING HORMONE, AND GNRH RECEPTOR AGONISTS AND ANTAGONISTS

As discussed elsewhere in this book (Chapters 25 and 27), the term *gonadotropin* encompasses three large-peptide

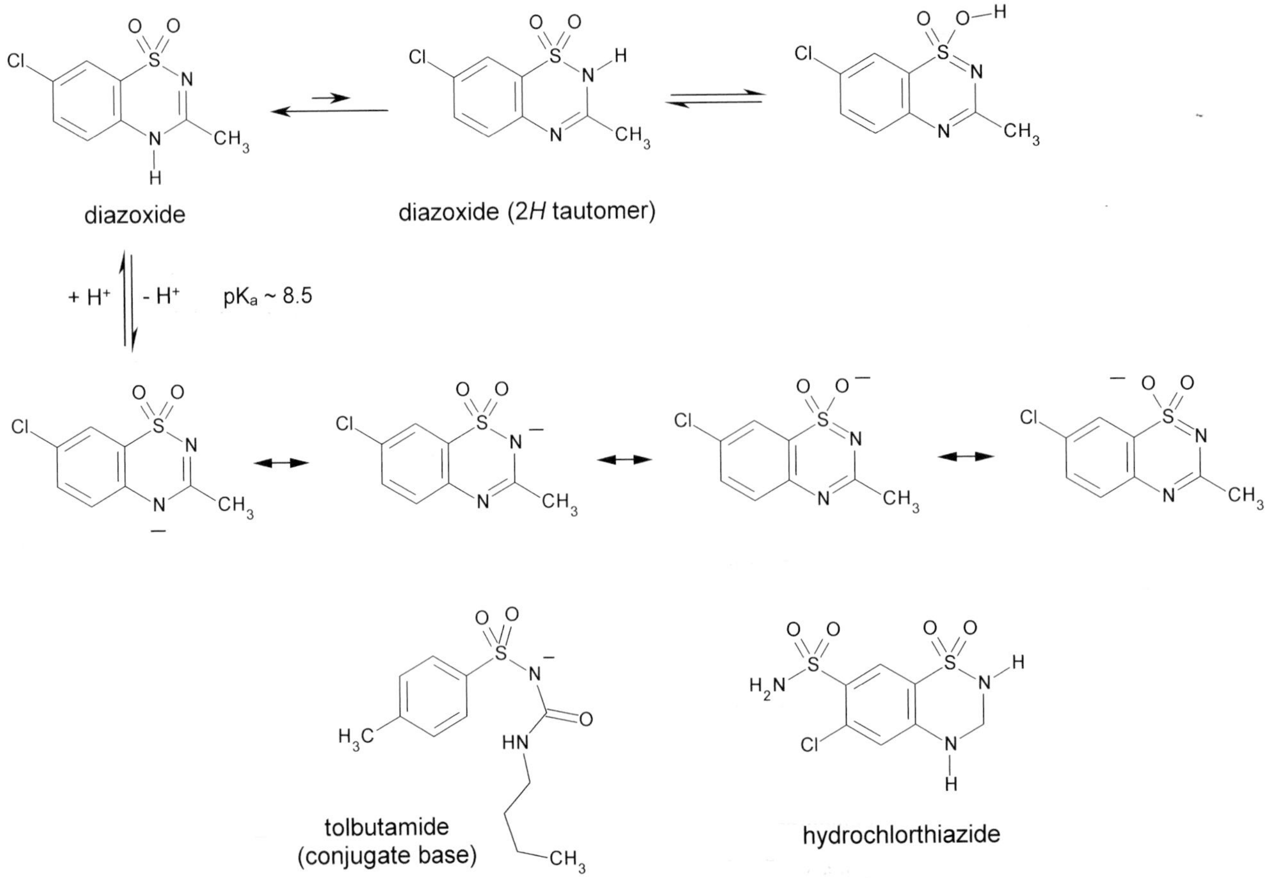

Figure 20.31 ● Diazoxide structure. The *4H* structure shown predominates in dimethylsulfoxide and is thought to predominate in aqueous solutions (although the solubility of the free acid is very low). Canonical (resonance) structures represent delocalization of the negative charge in the anionic conjugate base. Structures of the conjugate base of the sulfonylurea tolbutamide, and of the diuretic hydrochlorthiazide, are provided for comparison.

hormones: luteinizing hormone (LH), follicle-stimulating hormone (FSH), and chorionic gonadotropin (CG). LH and FSH are produced by the anterior pituitary, CG by the placenta during pregnancy; human CG is more commonly denoted as hCG. In broad brushstrokes sufficient for the needs of the information that follows, the major actions of LH and FSH in women are encapsulated by Figure 25.9 (Chapter 25). Release of LH and FSH by the pituitary is stimulated by gonadotropin-releasing hormone (GnRH, also known as luteinizing hormone–releasing hormone (LHRH), or simply—but less commonly—gonadoliberin). GnRH is produced in the arcuate nucleus and preoptic areas of the hypothalamus, and upon its release, is carried to the pituitary via the portal circulation. Although LH and FSH are named for their actions on the ovaries during the estrus cycle of women (see Chapter 25, Fig. 25.11), these hormones similarly regulate spermatogenesis in the testes of men (see Fig. 25.10). GnRH acts in the pituitary on cells known as gonadotropes, binding to seven-transmembrane–segment GPCRs (GnRH-Rs)[126] and activating them, thereby triggering signaling pathways involving phospholipase C, ultimately bringing about an increase in cytoplasmic calcium concentrations, which in turn prompts LH or FSH release.[127] The control of pituitary release of either LH or FSH or both, in disparate amounts and timings (as

depicted in Fig. 25.11) with only one hypothalamic releasing hormone, is made possible via variations in magnitude and frequency of the pulsatile release of GnRH, in conjunction with feedback regulation by circulating estrogens, progestins, and androgens. (For further details, the reader is referred to other information sources, as the focus herein is intended to be the medicinal chemistry rather than the intricacies of physiology; see, e.g., Knobil,[128] and references given in Chapter 25.) A relatively thorough understanding of these pathways and systems, gained over nearly a century at least, now allows for their therapeutic exploitation despite their complexities, although new findings regularly alter clinical practice as well as drug discovery directions.

Inadequate production by the pituitary of gonadotropins causes hypogonadism, the consequences of which include infertility. Exogenously administered gonadotropins thus provide one means of fertility enhancement (see Chapter 27). Functional deficits in the gonads diminish production of estrogen, progestin, and testosterone (depending on gender and cycle stage), which otherwise inhibit release of LH or FSH from the pituitary, and also of GnRH from the hypothalamus (negative feedback loops). Gonadotropin (LH, FSH) levels rise, so that in the hypothalamus, the net impacts on GnRH release are relatively complex.

Gonadotropin-Releasing Hormone Agonists

Upon acute administration, GnRH agonists produce an initial stimulation of either LH release (called the "flare" response) or FSH release (in this case to stimulate ovulation), but upon chronic administration, the effect is to downregulate pituitary release of gonadotropins. In turn, during the initial flare response there is an increase in gonadal steroidogenesis (testosterone and dihydrotestosterone in men, estrone and estradiol in premenopausal women). Following the flare response, steroidogenesis decreases over the next 2 to 4 weeks. Examples of therapeutic applications (see Table 20.6) include controlling timing of estrus cycle events in women and—in veterinary medicine—female animals to allow for artificial insemination or in vitro fertilization; suppression of precocious puberty; inducing ovarian suppression and a hypoestrogenic state in women when beneficial (e.g., menorrhagia, endometriosis, adenomyosis, or uterine fibroids); induction of hypogonadal states in oncology (notably, prostate cancer); and fertility suppression in male dogs. For chronic administration, long-lasting depot injections enable monthly or quarterly administration, and implantable devices allow release for as long as a year.

TABLE 20.6 GnRH Agonists

Drug	Indications	Dosing	Volume of Distribution	Serum Protein Binding	Serum Time-course	Elimination
Leuprolide acetate (Lupron, Eligard, Lupron Depot, Viadur, generic)	A, B, C, D off-label: E, F, G	Injection, implant, or depot; amount varies from 1–45 mg for adult indications, depending on indication and type of administration (i.e., immediate-release vs. depot).	27 L[a]	43%–49%[b]	(Bolus dose) terminal $t_{1/2} \approx 3$ hr (two-compartment model)[a] $Cl_{ss} = 140$ mL/min[a]	Not fully characterized
Histrelin acetate (Vantas) (Supprelin LA)	A B	50-mg sc implant once every 12 months → 50–60 μg/day release rate for Vantas → ca. 65 μg/day release rate for Supprelin LA	58 ± 8 L[c]	30 ± 9%[c]	(Bolus dose) terminal $t_{1/2}$ =3.9 ± 1.0 hr[c] (50-mg implant) Cl_{ss} = 174 ± 56.5 mL/min[c]	Not studied
Triptorelin pamoate (Trelstar LA, Trelstar Depot)	A, C, D off-label: F, H, I, J, K	Depot: im, 3.75 mg monthly LA: im, 11.25 mg every 84 days	30–33 L[d]	Minimal[d]	(Bolus dose) $t_{1/2}$ = 2.8 ± 1.2 hr[d]	~42% as intact drug in urine following iv bolus[d]; Cl_T ~210 mL/min, Cl_H ~80 mL/min, Cl_R ~91 mL/min[d]
Toserelin acetate (Zoladex)	A, C, E, N	3.6 mg (base equiv) implant 10.8 mg (base equiv) implant	(0.25 mg sc bolus): 44 ± 14 L men, 20 ± 4 L women[e]	27%[e]	(0.25-mg sc bolus): $t_{1/2}$ = 4.2 ± 1.1 hr in men, $t_{1/2}$ = 2.3 ± 0.6 hr in women[e]	>90% in urine (20% as unchanged drug)[e]
Nafarelin acetate (Synarel)	B, C	2 mg/mL intranasal, 200 μg/spray B: 1,600 mg/day C: starting dose: 200 μg b.i.d., increase to 800 μg/day if needed	NA	~80%[f]	Bioavailability 2%–6% (200 μg intranasal)[f] Peak plasma concentration 10–45 min $t_{1/2}$ = 2.5 hr (400 μg intranasal)[f]	44%–55% urine (3% of dose as unchanged drug)[f]

Indications: A, palliative treatment of advanced prostate cancer; B, treatment of children with central precocious puberty; C, endometriosis; D, uterine leiomyomata (fibroids); E, palliative treatment of advanced breast cancer; F, ovarian carcinoma; G, paraphilia; H, pancreatic carcinoma; I, hypergonadism; J, growth hormone deficiency; K, in vitro fertilization assistance; M, assisted reproduction (LH surge suppression for timing control); N, to bring about presurgical endometrial thinning.
[a]Sennello, L. T., Finley, R. A., Chu, S. Y., et al.: J. Pharm. Sci. 75(2):158–160, 1986.
[b]Eligard product information (8-Nov-2007 labeling).
[c]Vantas product information (8-Nov-2004 labeling).
[d]Trelstar product information (29-Jun-2001 labeling).
[e]Zoladex product information (27-Jul-1998 labeling), or Facts and Comparisons' Web site, accessed April 2009.
[f]Synarel product information (12-Apr-2006 labeling).
b.i.d., bis in die (twice a day); im, intramuscular; iv, intravenous; NA, not available; sc, subcutaneous.

```
GnRH        pyro-Glu-His-Trp-Ser-Tyr---Gly---------Leu-Arg-Pro-Gly-NH₂
leuprolide  pyro-Glu-His-Trp-Ser-Tyr-D-Leu---------Leu-Arg-Pro-NHEt
buserelin   pyro-Glu-His-Trp-Ser-Tyr-D-Ser(O-tBu)--Leu-Arg-Pro-NHEt
nafarelin   pyro-Glu-His-Trp-Ser-Tyr-D-Nal---------Leu-Arg-Pro-Gly-NH₂
histrelin   pyro-Glu-His-Trp-Ser-Tyr-D-His(Nτ-Bz)--Leu-Arg-Pro-NHEt
goserelin   pyro-Glu-His-Trp-Ser-Tyr-D-Ser(O-tBu)--Leu-Arg-Pro-NHNHC(=O)NH₂
triptorelin pyro-Glu-His-Trp-Ser-Tyr-D-Trp---------Leu-Arg-Pro-Gly-NH₂
deslorelin  pyro-Glu-His-Trp-Ser-Tyr-D-Trp---------Leu-Arg-Pro-NHEt
```

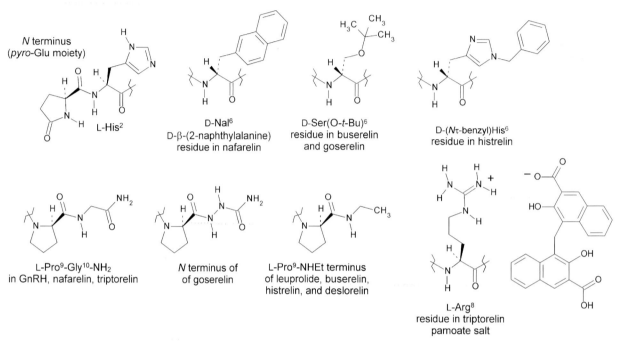

Figure 20.32 ● Primary sequences and selected substructures for endogenous human GnRH, and marketed GnRH agonists.

Nafarelin acetate is formulated for intranasal administration, the only nonparenteral formulation among the currently available GnRH agonists. Deslorelin acetate currently finds use only in veterinary medicine, such as for stimulating ovulation in mares (acute administration → flare effect) or helping to stabilize and maintain high-risk pregnancies in livestock, although clinical trials in humans for certain breast cancers, precocious puberty, and congenital adrenal hyperplasia are in progress or completed.

The marketed GnRH agonists are all close structural analogs of GnRH itself (Fig. 20.32). They are often called "superagonists" because they have increased potency and increased duration of action versus the endogenous agonist (GnRH), which is rapidly cleaved in the pituitary by endopeptidases (24.11 and 24.15)[129] and has a very short half-life (2–4 minutes) in the systemic circulation. The reported agonist potencies relative to GnRH for some of these molecules are leuprolide (15-fold), buserelin (20-fold), deslorelin (144-fold), and histrelin (210-fold).[130] All of the marketed synthetic agonists incorporate, like GnRH, *pyro*-glutamic acid at the amino terminus, in which the N-terminal α-amino group has undergone cyclocondensation with the γ-carboxyl moiety of the same glutamate residue, forming a five-membered amide-containing ring—that is, a lactam moiety (more specifically, this constitutes a 5-oxopyrrolidine-2-carboxylic acid residue). The

following four amino acids (positions 2–5) are also the same in all. Position 6 is the main point of structural variation among these GnRH-analog agonists; substitution is consistently with a D amino acid to confer peptidase resistance (see discussion that follows). Leuprolide (leuprorelin), buserelin, histrelin, and deslorelin are nonapeptides rather than decapeptides: They lack the amidated C-terminal glycine, instead terminating at Pro9, which is amidated with ethylamine, thus forming an *N*-ethylprolinamide terminus. This terminal N-ethyl moiety can be viewed as an abbreviated stand-in for the terminal glycinamide moiety of GnRH. Goserelin terminates in an unusual (among medicinal substances) aminocarbonylhydrazide moiety, whereas nafarelin and triptorelin maintain the same structure at the C-terminus as GnRH. The goserelin N-terminus can be seen as a bioisosteric substitution: It is identical to that of the natural hormone except that an −NH− is substituted for the methylene (−CH₂−) of the terminal glycine. All of the marketed agonists include the strongly basic Arg8 residue, so that, with no appreciably acidic groups elsewhere within the structure to provide an internal counterion, a salt form is obligatory; acetate is the counterion for most. Triptorelin is marketed in the United States as its pamoate salt (see Fig. 20.32), which provides for long duration of action by virtue of depot creation upon intramuscular injection.

The elimination processes and fates of these peptides are not fully characterized. For leuprolide, available information suggests that elimination is mostly via peptidase-catalyzed cleavage, and subsequent urinary excretion of peptide fragments.[131] In healthy men, a pentapeptide is the prominent metabolite, and formation is relatively rapid, with levels of this metabolite peaking between 2- and 6-hour postdose. Following administration of the 3.75-mg depot suspension formulation, less than 5% of an administered dose was recovered as leuprolide and the pentapeptide metabolite. Such extensive fragmentation does not occur with all of these analogous compounds; however, more than 40% of an iv bolus dose of triptorelin, for example, is recovered intact in urine.[132] Although the overall elimination of histrelin has reportedly not been studied following insertion of 50-mg implants, biotransformation in human hepatic microsomes showed the presence of a single prominent metabolite resulting from *N*-deethylation of the C-terminal amide moiety.[133] Peptidase-generated histrelin fragments are also likely, but the molecule is designed to be resistant to hydrolysis by endopeptidases 24.11 and 24.15. Nafarelin is extensively biotransformed. Following administration of (^{14}C)nafarelin subcutaneously to men, at least six metabolites appeared in urine, collectively accounting for about half of the dose, with ~3% of the dose appearing in urine as unchanged nafarelin.

Hexapeptide Tyr^5–$Gly^{10}(NH_2)$ was the most prominent metabolite.[134] The metabolites collectively persist in serum for much longer than the parent drug.

Gonadotropin-Releasing Hormone Antagonists

To some extent, the clinical uses of GnRH antagonists (Table 20.7) parallel those of the agonists discussed previously; however, antagonists do not, of course, generate the flare response.[135] Instead, GnRH receptors in the gonadotrope cells of the pituitary are blocked, so that pituitary output of FSH and LH is reduced or abolished. This response occurs rapidly, unlike the desensitization that develops over several weeks when GnRH agonists are used for gonadotropin suppression. Return to a pretreatment state also occurs relatively quickly, within 2 days after stopping lower doses of GnRH antagonists (except, of course, with depot injections).

The marketed GnRH antagonists (Fig. 20.33) were designed based on the GnRH structure,[136] but contain many more alterations as compared with agonists, including more D amino acids, and numerous unnatural or derivatized side chains (the full structure of ganirelix, Fig. 20.34, provides an exemplary illustration). His^2 was identified early on as important to receptor activation,[137] and this residue is re-

TABLE 20.7 GnRH Antagonists

Drug	Indications	Dosing	Volume of Distribution	Serum Protein Binding	Serum Time-course	Elimination
Cetrorelix (Cetrotide)	A (C, D, E)	0.25 mg daily, sc or 3 mg once, sc	~1.2 L/kg[a]	86%[a]	t_{max} ~1 hr (0.25 mg sc) t_{max} ~1.5 hr (3 mg sc) highly nonlinear pharmacokinetics (dose-dependent)[a]	Urine (unchanged, slow) bile (unchanged + metabolites, slow)
Ganirelix diacetate	A	0.25 mg daily, sc	43.7 L (single 0.25-mg iv dose), 76.5 L (daily dosing)[b]	82%[b]	$t_{1/2}$ = 13 hr (single 0.25-mg dose), $t_{1/2}$ = 16 hr (daily dosing)[b]	Feces (75%), urine (22%)
Degarelix acetate	C	sc 240 mg initial 80 mg once/ 28 days	>1 L/kg upon iv admin[c]	~90%[c]	Depot formed upon injection; serum concentration profile highly dependant on injection site conc[c]	~9 L/hr Cl$_{ss}$ in patients; peptide hydrolysis in hepatobiliary system, mainly biliary excretion (20%–30% renal excretion following depot injection)[c]
Abarelix acetate (Plenaxis) [Germany]	B	Depot	0.42 L/kg[d]	NA	t_{max} ~1 hr, $t_{1/2}$ ~ 5 ± 2 hr (single 15 μg/kg im dose)[d]	13% of a 15 μg/kg im dose excreted unchanged in urine[d]

Indications: A, assisted reproduction (LH surge suppression for timing control); B, in oncology, to reduce the amount of testosterone made in patients with advanced symptomatic prostate cancer for which no other treatment options are available; said to overcome the need for anti-androgen coprescribing; C, hormone-sensitive cancers of the prostate; D, hormone-sensitive cancers of the breast (in premenopausal/perimenopausal women); E, certain benign gynecological disorders (endometriosis, uterine fibroids and endometrial thinning).
[a]Cetrotide product information (FDA labeling approved 4-Apr-2008).
[b]Ganirelix Acetate (Organon) product information (30-June-2008 FDA labeling).
[c]Degarelix Acetate (Ferring) product information (24-Dec-2008 FDA labeling).
[d]Wong, S. L., Lau, D. T., Baughman, S. A., et al.: J. Clin. Pharmacol. 44(5):495–502, 2004.
iv, intravenous; im, intramuscular; NA, not available; sc, subcutaneous.

GnRH	*pyro*-Glu--His--Trp--Ser---Tyr------Gly-------Leu---Arg------Pro---Gly-NH₂
abarelix	Ac-D-Nal-D-Cpa-D-Pal-Ser-(*N*-Me)Tyr--D-Asn------Leu--ILys-----Pro-D-Ala-NH₂
cetrorelix	Ac-D-Nal-D-Cpa-D-Pal-Ser---Tyr------D-Cit-----Leu---Arg-----Pro-D-Ala-NH₂
degarelix	Ac-D-Nal-D-Cpa-D-Pal-Ser-4-Aph(hor)D-Aph(ur)---Leu--ILys-----Pro-D-Ala-NH₂
ganirelix	Ac-D-Nal-D-Cpa-D-Pal-Ser---Tyr------D-Lys(bem)-Leu-L-Lys(bem)-Pro-D-Ala-NH₂
	1 2 3 4 5 6 7 8 9 10

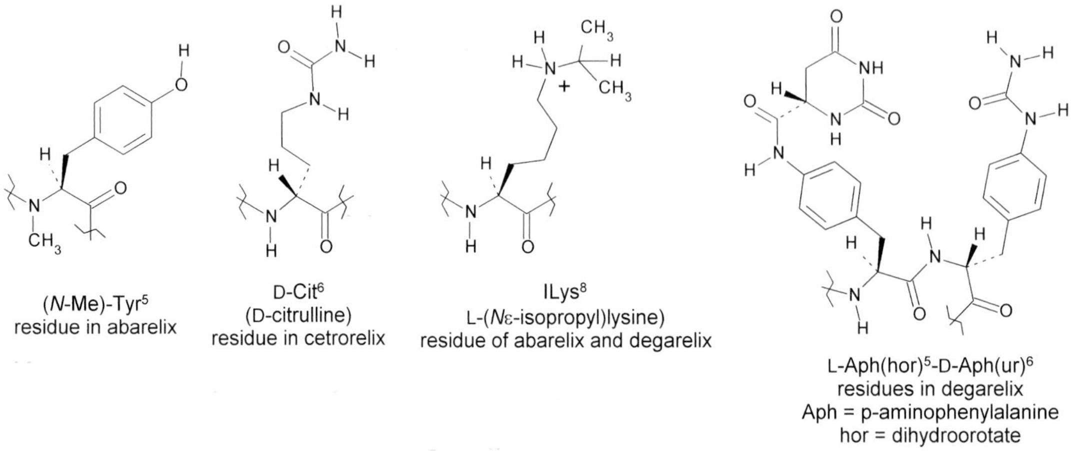

Figure 20.33 • Primary sequences and selected substructures for marketed GnRH antagonists.

placed in the antagonists with structural moieties that engage the receptor but do not allow receptor activation. Additional structure–activity information came from studies of cyclic peptides,[138,139] which, together with information from protein structure modeling (see discussion that follows), indicated a relatively large binding pocket formed within the bundle of the transmembrane helices I to VII of the GnRH-R. (Although there are genes corresponding to GnRH-R₁ and GnRH-R₂ subtypes, the latter is apparently not expressed in humans.) Abarelix incorporates backbone *N*-methylation at Tyr⁵. All are decapeptides like GnRH itself, but unlike GnRH, incorporate alaninamide rather than glycinamide at the *C*-terminus. Rather than having a *pyro*-Glu at the N-terminus as in the native hormone, all are instead *N*-acetylated. Each has at least one strongly basic amino acid in its sequence, at residue 8, thus these peptides are formulated as salts. The counterion is acetate in all cases. Ganirelix is a diacetate, having an additional basic

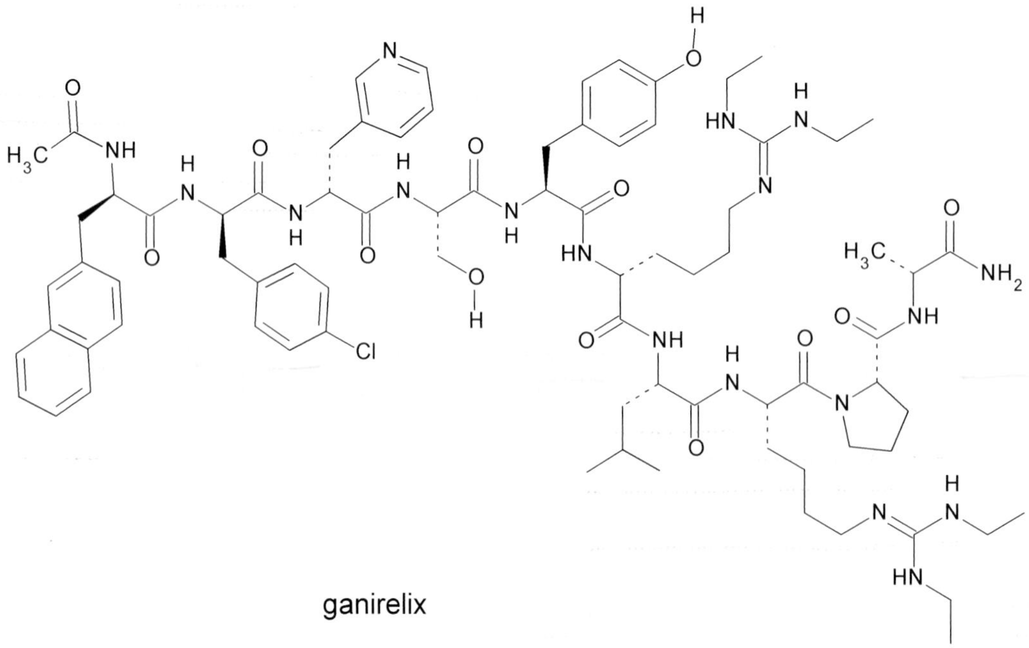

ganirelix

Figure 20.34 • Full structure of ganirelix.

residue—a derivatized lysine—at position 6; the diacetate salt endows the drug with excellent water solubility for preparation of an aqueous solution (0.5 mg/mL, pH 5.0) for parenteral administration (sc injection); the solution stability at pH 5.0 is such that ganirelix can be marketed as a sterile solution rather than a powder requiring reconstitution.

An overview of key structure–activity aspects for peptidic GnRH antagonists was provided within a pair of papers by Rivier et al.[140,141] Although structural determinants of GnRH-R affinity and efficacy are now rather well understood, structural bases for alterations in duration of action remain much less so. Changes in peptide structure alter solubility characteristics, resistance to degrading enzymes, and plasma and tissue protein binding, all of which affect duration, and none of which can readily and reliably be predicted at present. The need for parenteral administration, especially for chronic applications, represents a liability among all of the marketed GnRH antagonists. Also, there is a modest but significant incidence of severe generalized hypersensitivity reactions; this problem with the Plenaxis product of abarelix acetate undoubtedly played a part in the decision by Praecis Pharmaceuticals to voluntarily discontinue sales in 2005, although components of the formulation other than the drug may have accounted for many of these reactions. (Defined structure–activity relationships for stimulation of histamine release from mast cells by peptides of this class have been reported, however—notably for variation at position 8.[142]) In any case, nonpeptide, orally bioavailable GnRH antagonists have been sought, and several compounds have advanced through phase II trials. Developments in this area were reviewed in detail by Betz et al. in mid-2008[143]; the interested reader is particularly encouraged to study this review, as the authors provide a highly instructive exposition of the structural determinants for agonist and antagonist actions at GnRH-Rs, and for receptor selectivity among GPCR ligands in general, based on the picture that emerged from a large collection of elegant reports. This review also offers up important lessons with regard to molecular pharmacodynamics—notably, the significances of ligand-binding kinetics with regard to efficacy and affinity variations, and to the origins of insurmountable versus surmountable antagonism. As yet, no crystal structures have become available for either unliganded or ligand-bound GnRH-R, but the aggregate work in this area makes abundantly clear the power of advanced protein modeling in conjunction with analysis of the effects of site-directed mutagenesis on the binding and action of ligands from various structural classes. Readily apparent also is the great worth of time- and resource-demanding efforts to discover/create such a variety of ligands, and conduct artfully designed and executed biological experiments with them.

The biological fates of the peptidic GnRH antagonists are partly characterized. Cetrorelix elimination occurs by renal and biliary routes.[144–146] Following a 10-mg sc dose given to men and women, only unchanged cetrorelix was detected in urine, whereas chain-shortened fragments produced by the actions of peptidases were found in bile, with fragment (1–4) predominating and fragments (1–9), (1–7), and (1–6) present in significant quantities. Dose dependencies of elimination clearly show that these elimination pathways are saturable, and other than peptide hydrolysis, no other phase I biotransformations, nor any phase II transformations, occur significantly for cetrorelix. For ganirelix, cumulative elimination over 288 hours for a single 1-mg dose (iv) resulted in recovery of 75% of the dose in feces and 22% in urine.[147,148] Any excretion in urine was reported to be complete within the first 24 hours, whereas fecal elimination did not approach completion until nearly 200-hour postdose. Elimination was found to be dose-proportional within the range of 0.125 to 0.5 mg. Fragment peptides (1–4 and 1–6) were the major components of fecal radioactivity, whereas no unchanged drug was detected in feces. Following depot injection, degarelix undergoes peptide hydrolysis primarily in the hepatobiliary system, whereupon the majority of the cleavage products are excreted in bile.[149]

⬡ CONCLUDING REMARKS

Rapid advances in endocrinology on many scientific fronts (and similarly, with respect to autocrine, paracrine, and juxtacrine systems) have brought about the identification of numerous new potential molecular targets for therapeutic intervention in a wide range of maladies. Among the new medicinals that have been created as a result, enzyme inhibitors or ligands for GPCRs are prominently represented, and will undoubtedly continue to be; however, as intimated in a few instances in this chapter, we should anticipate that an ever-increasing fraction of emerging therapeutic agents will be of a less-traditional nature. Accordingly, gaining a solid understanding of the molecular-level attributes underlying the actions and limitations of medicinals will be of ever-greater importance to clinicians who seek the best choices for their patients.

⬢ R E V I E W   Q U E S T I O N S ⬢

1. Drugs of the hypoglycemic sulfonylurea class have the general molecular structure shown at right. The potencies of these molecules as oral hypoglycemic agents parallel to a very great extent the affinity with which they bind to ATP-sensitive potassium channels, as discussed in an early section of this chapter. Using the information from Table 20.3, and the structures shown in Figures 20.4 and 20.5, fill in the following table, listing the drugs from top to bottom according to daily dose range, with the least potent at the top. As an example, a row has been completed for gliclazide, which is not included in Table 20.3.

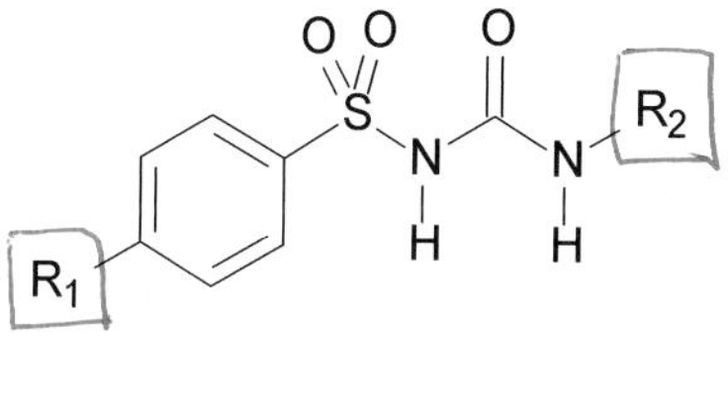

Drug	Daily Dose Range	R_1	R_2
gliclazide	80–240 mg	H_3C-	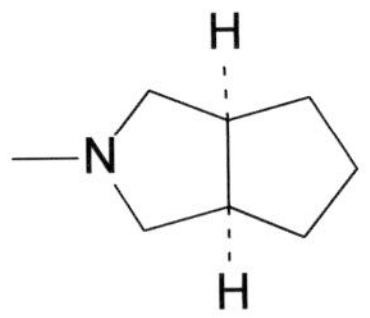 *(bicyclic N-containing ring structure)*

(handwritten note) ↑ Hₐₒ sol ⟶ salt → ↑ dissolution

2. The sulfonylureas are weak acids, and all drugs of this class are poorly water soluble, though some more so than others. One possible strategy for increasing the dissolution rate for a sulfonylurea to be formulated in an oral solid dosage form would be to make a salt, which would be expected to have a considerably greater water solubility (although none of the marketed sulfonylureas are currently formulated as their salts). Draw, explicitly, the structure of the potassium salt of glipizide.

3. (a) Draw the structure of *N1*-(*trans*-4-hydroxycyclohexyl)-*N3*-[*p*-(1-hydroxyethyl)phenyl-sulfonyl]urea.
   (b) Your structure, if correctly drawn, represents that of a metabolite of which hypoglycemic drug discussed in this chapter?
   (c) How many biotransformative steps are required to produce this metabolite from the parent drug you (hopefully) named in part b?
   (d) What enzymes are required to catalyze the biotransformations that can produce this metabolite from its parent drug?
   (e) Would you expect this metabolite to be a prominent one, or a minor one for this drug, and why?

4. Glipizide undergoes a pair of biotransformations that were not discussed in this chapter (a less-prominent route of biotransformation than those that were mentioned). A glipizide molecule is acted on by a liver amidase, and one of the two products thereby produced is then *N*-acetylated, a reaction catalyzed by an *N*-acetyltransferase.

   (a) Draw the structure of the product of these two steps of biotransformation, and also the structure of the other product (a carboxylic acid) produced in the first step.
   (b) Would you expect the *N*-acetylated metabolite to (1) have significant pharmacological activity at the molecular level of the same nature as that of the glipizide, or (2) to exert hypoglycemic activity of clinical importance following oral administration? In each case, provide a justification for your answer.

5. In each of the following blanks, list a drug discussed in this chapter that acts at the molecular level in a way meeting the given description.

   _____ an enzyme inhibitor

   _____ a ligand for a protein complex that activates gene transcription

   _____ an inhibitor of ion channel opening

   _____ an agonist for a G-protein–coupled receptor

6. Diazoxide increases the propensity of ATP-sensitive potassium channels in β-islet cells of the pancreas to open, whereas glyburide exerts essentially the opposite effect. Yet, diazoxide is being studied clinically as a prospective aid in the treatment of type 2 diabetes, and significant drug discovery activity currently focuses on finding molecules that exert the same action as diazoxide, but with greater target selectivity, for the same therapeutic purpose. What is the basis for these efforts?

7. Why, based on its molecular nature and physicochemical properties, must exenatide be administered only via a parenteral route?

8. Within the structure of ganirelix (Fig. 20.34), how many amino acid residues come from the set of 20 amino acids abundant in proteins (including stereochemistry)? List them.

REFERENCES

1. Arenillas, J. F., Moro, M. A., and Dávalos, A.: Stroke 38:2196–2203, 2007.
2. Blaha, M. J., Bansal, S., Rouf, R., et al.: Mayo Clin. Proc. 83(8): 932–943, 2008.
3. Remedi, M. S., and Nichols, C. G.: PLoS Med. 5(10):e206, 2008.
4. Winkler, M., Stephan, D., Bieger, S., et al.: J. Pharmacol. Exp. Ther. 322(2):701–708, 2007.
5. Babenko, A. P., Aguilar-Bryan, L., and Bryan, J: Annu. Rev. Physiol. 60:667–687, 1998.
6. Tusnády, G. E., Bakos E., Váradi A., et al.: FEBS Lett. 402(1):1–3, 1997.
7. Roane, D. S., and Bounds, J. K.: Nutr. Neurosci. 2(4):209–225, 1999.
8. Takanaga, H., Murakami, H., Koyabu, N., et al.: J. Pharmacy Pharmacol. 50:1027–1033, 1998.
9. Vila-Carriles, W. H., Zhao, G., and Bryan, J.: FASEB. J. 21(1): 18–25, 2007.
10. Grell, W., Hurnaus, R., Griss, G., et al.: J. Med. Chem. 41(26): 5219–5246, 1998.
11. Sleevi, M.: Insulin and hypoglycemic agents: In Abraham, D. J. (ed.). Burger's Medicinal Chemistry and Drug Discovery, 6th ed., vol. 4: Autocoids, Diagnostics, and Drugs from New Biology. New York, John Wiley, 2003, pp. 24–31.
12. Mandič, Z., and Gabelica, V: J. Pharm. Biomed. Anal. 41(3): 866–871, 2006.
13. Ashfield R., Gribble, F. M., Ashcroft S. J., et al.: Diabetes 8(6):1341–1347, 1999.
14. Geng, X., Li, L., Bottino, R., et al.: Am. J. Physiol. 293(1 Pt. 1): E293–E301, 2007.
15. Scarsi, M., Podvinec, M., and Roth, A.: Mol. Pharmacol. 71(2): 398–406, 2007.
16. Shigeto, M., Katsura, M., Matsuda, M., et al.: J. Pharmacol. Exp. Ther. 322(1):1–7, 2007.
17. Kalliokoski, A., Neuvonen, M., Neuvonen, P., et al.: J. Clin. Pharmacol. 48(3):311–321, 2008.
18. Zhang, W., He, Y. J., Han, C. T., et al.: Br. J. Clin. Pharmacol. 62(5):567–572, 2006.
19. Ravindran, S., Zharikova, O. L., Hill, R. A., et al.: Biochem. Pharmacol. 72(12):1730–1737, 2006. See also references therein.
20. Zharikova, O. L., Ravindran, S., and Nanovskaya, T. N.: Biochem. Pharmacol. 73:2012–2019, 2007. See also references therein.
21. Kirchheiner, J., Roots, I., Goldammer, M., et al.: Clin. Pharmacokinet. 44(12):1209–1225, 2005. See also references therein.
22. Zhang, Y., Si, D., Chen, X., et al.: Br. J. Clin. Pharmacol. 64(1):67–74, 2007.
23. Xu, H., Williams, K. M., Liauw, W. S., et al.: Br. J. Pharmacol. 153(7):1579–1586, 2008.
24. van Heiningen, P. N., Hatorp, V., Kramer Nielsen, K., et al.: Eur. J. Clin. Pharmacol. 55(7):521–525, 1999.
25. Tornio, A., Niemi, M., Neuvonen, M., et al.: Clin. Pharmacol. Ther. 84(3):403–411, 1998.
26. Bidstrup, T. B., Bjornsdottir, I., Sidelmann, U. G., et al.: Br. J. Clin. Pharmacol. 56(3):305–314, 2003.
27. Niemi, M., Backman, J. T., Kajosaari, L. I., et al.: Clin. Pharmacol. Ther. 77(6):468–478, 2005.
28. Niemi, M., Kajosaari, L., Neuvonen, L., et al.: Br. J. Clin. Pharmacol. 57(4):441–447, 2004.
29. Takesada, H., Matsuda, K., Ohtake, R., et al.: Bioorg. Med. Chem. 4(10):1771–1781, 1996.
30. Weaver, M. L., Orwig, B. A., Rodriguez, L. C., et al.: Drug Metab. Dispos. 29:415–421, 2001.
31. Sabia, H., Sunkara, G., Ligueros-Saylan, M., et al.: Eur. J. Clin. Pharmacol. 60(6):407–412, 2004.
32. Hanai, T., Miyazaki, R., Kamijima, E., et al.: Internet Electro. J. Mol. Des. 2(10):702–711, 2003.
33. Balant, L.: Clin. Pharmacokinet. 6(3):215–241, 1981.
34. Taylor, J. A.: Clin. Pharmacol. Ther. 13(5)(Pt. 1):710–718, 1972.
35. Hu, S., Boettcher, B. R., and Dunning, B. E.: Diabetologia 46 Suppl 1:M37–M43, 2003.
36. Yki-Järvinen, H.: N. Engl. J. Med. 351(11):1106–1118, 2004.
37. Kolak, M., Hannele, Y.-J., Katja K., et al.: J. Clin. Endocrinol. Metab. 92:720–724, 2007.
38. Ikeda, Y., Takata, H., Inoue, K., et al.: Diabetes Care 30:e48; doi:10. 2337/dc07-0308, 2007.
39. Kanatani, Y., Usui, Y., Ishizuka, K., et al.: Diabetes 56:795–803, 2007.
40. Kershaw, E. E., Schupp, M., Guan, H. P., et al.: Am. J. Physiol. Endocrinol. Metab. 293:E1736–E1745, 2007.
41. Evans-Molina, C., Robbins, R. D., Kono, T., et al.: Mol. Cell. Biol. 29:2053–2067, 2009.
42. Xu, H. E., Lambert, M. H., Montana, V. G., et al.: Proc. Natl. Acad. Sci. U. S. A., 98(24):13919–13924, 2001.
43. Cronet, P., Petersen, J. F. W., Folmer, R., et al.: Structure 9(8): 699–706, 2001.
44. Johnson, B. A., Wilson E. M., Li, Y., et al.: J. Mol. Biol. 298: 187–194, 2000.
45. Schimke, K., and Davis, T. M.: Curr. Opin. Investig. Drugs 8(4): 338–344, 2007.
46. Cox, P. J., Ryan, D. A., Hollis, F. J., et al.: Drug Metab. Dispos. 28(7):772–780, 2000.
47. Baldwin, S. J., Clarke, S. E., and Chenery, R. J.: Br. J. Clin. Pharmacol. 48(3):424–432, 1999.
48. Baughman, T. M., Graham, R. A., Wells-Knecht, K., et al.: Drug Metab. Dispos. 33(6):733–738, 2005.
49. Eckland, D. A., Danhof, M.: Exp. Clin. Endocrinol. Diabetes 108(Suppl 2):S234–S242, 2000.
50. Shen, Z., Reed, J. R., Creighton, M., et al.: Xenobiotica 33(5): 499–509, 2003.
51. Jaakkola, T., Backman, J. T., Neuvonen, M., et al.: Br. J. Clin. Pharmacol. 61(1):70–78, 2006.
52. Basu, R., Shah, P., Basu, A., et al.: Diabetes 57(1):24–31, 2008.
53. Mukhtar, M. H., Payne, V. A., Arden, C., et al.: Am. J. Physiol. Regul. Integr. Comp. Physiol. 294:R766-R774, 2008.
54. Saeedi, R., Parsons, H. L., Wambolt, R. B., et al.: Am. J. Physiol. Heart Circ. Physiol. 294(6):H2497–H2506, 2008.
55. Xie, Z., Dong, Y., Scholz, R., et al.: Circulation 117:952–962, 2008.
56. Correia, S., Carvalho, C., Santos, M. S., et al.: Mini Rev. Med. Chem. 8(13):1343–1354, 2008.
57. Luna, V., Casauban, L., Sajan, M. P., et al.: Diabetologia 49(2): 375–382, 2006.
58. Temofonte, N., Sajan, M. P., Nimal, S., et al.: Diabetologia 52(1): 60–64, 2009.
59. El-Mir, M. Y., Nogueira, V., Fontaine, E., et al.: J. Biol. Chem. 275 (1):223–228, 2000.
60. Mooney, M. H., Fogarty, S., Stevenson, C., et al.: Br. J. Pharmacol. 153(8):1669–1677, 2008.
61. Shu, Y., Sheardown, S. A., Brown, C., et al.: J. Clin. Invest. 117(5): 1422–1431, 2007.
62. Takane, H., Shikata, E., Otsubo, K., et al.: Pharmacogenomics 9(4): 415–422, 2008.
63. Saitoh, R., Sugano, K., Takata, N., et al.: Pharm. Res. 21(5):749–755, 2004.
64. Proctor, W. R., Bourdet, D. L., and Thakker, D. R.: Drug Metab. Dispos. 36(8):1650–1658, 2008.
65. Nichols, B. L., Eldering, J., Avery, S., et al.: J. Biol. Chem. 273(5): 3076–3081, 1998.
66. Quezada-Calvillo, R., Robayo-Torres, C. C., Opekun, A. R. et al.: J. Nutr. 137(7):1725–1733, 2007.

67. Quezada-Calvillo, R., Sim, L., Ao, Z., et al.: J. Nutr. 138(4):685–692, 2008.
68. Sim, L., Quezada-Calvillo, R., Sterchi, E. E., et al.: J. Mol. Biol. 375(3):782–792, 2008.
69. Scott, L. J., and Spencer, C. M.: Drugs 59(3):521–549, 2000.
70. Horii, S., Fukase, H., Matsuo, T., et al.: J. Med. Chem. 29(6): 1038–1046, 1986.
71. Junge, B., Matzke, M., and Stoltefuss, J.: Chemistry and structure-activity relationships of glucosidase inhibitors. Handbook of Experimental Pharmacology, vol. 119 (Oral Antidiabetics), 411–482, 2006.
72. Breitmeier, D., Gunther, S., and Heymann, H.: Arch. Biochem. Biophys. 346(1):7–14, 1997.
73. Caspary, W. F., and Graf, S.: Res. Exp. Med. (Berl) 175(1):1–6, 1979.
74. Boberg, M., Kurz, J., Ploschke, H. J., et al.: Arzneimittelforschung 40(5):555–563, 1990.
75. Konarkowska, B., Aitken, J. F., Kistler, J., et al.: FEBS J. 273(15): 3614–3624, 2006. See also references therein.
76. Götz, J., Ittner, L. M., and Lim, Y. A.: Cell Mol. Life Sci. 66(8): 1321–1325, 2009. Review.
77. Lim, Y. A., Ittner, L. M., and Lim, Y. L.: FEBS Lett. 582(15): 2188–2194, 2008.
78. Hay, D. L., Christopoulos, G., Christopoulos, A., et al.: Biochem. Soc. Trans. 32(5):865–867, 2004.
79. Qi, T., Christopoulos, G., Bailey, R. J., et al.: Mol. Pharmacol. 74(4):1059–1071, 2008.
80. Young, A.: Adv. Pharmacol. 52:47–65, 2005.
81. Roth, J. D., Maier, H., Chen, S., et al.: Arch. Neurol. 66(3):306–310, 2009.
82. Bennett, R. G., Hamel, F. G., and Duckworth, W. C.: Diabetes 52(9):2315–2320, 2003.
83. La Barre, J.: Bull. Acad. R. Med. Belg. 12:620–634, 1932.
84. Kim, W., and Egan, J. M.: Pharmacol. Rev. 60: 470–512, 2008.
85. Brown, J. C., and Dryburgh, J. R.: Can. J. Biochem. 49:867–872, 1971.
86. Holst, J. J.: Annu. Rev. Physiol. 59:257–271, 1997.
87. Drucker, D. J.: Cell Metab. 3(3):153–165, 2006.
88. Drucker, D. J., Nauck, M. A.: Lancet 368:1696–1705, 2006.
89. Vahl, T. P., Tauchi, M., Durler, T. S.: Endocrinology 148:4965–4973, 2007.
90. Salehi, M., Aulinger, B. A., and D'Alessio, D. A.: Endocr. Rev. 29: 367–379, 2008.
91. Adelhorst, K., Hedegaard, B. B., Knudsen, L. B., et al.: J. Biol. Chem. 4;269(9):6275–6278, 1994.
92. Kieffer, T. J., McIntosh, C. H., and Pederson R. A.: Endocrinology 136:3585–3596, 1995.
93. Nicolucci, A., and Rossi, M. C.: Acta. Biomed. 79(3):184–191, 2008.
94. Kolterman, O. G., Kim, D. D., Shen, L., et al.: Am. J. Health Syst. Pharm. 62(2):173, 2005.
95. Plamboeck, A., Holst, J. J., Carr, R. D., et al.: Diabetologia 48: 1882–1890, 2005.
96. Williams, D. L., Baskin, D. G., and Schwartz, M. W.: Endocrinology 150:1680–1687, 2009.
97. Elbrond, B., Jakobsen, G., Larsen, S., et al.: Diabetes Care 25(8): 1398–1404, 2002.
98. Madsen, K., Knudsen, L. B., Agersoe, H., et al.: J. Med. Chem. 50(24), 6126–6132, 2007.
99. Russell-Jones, D.: Mol. Cell Endocrinol. 297:137–140, 2009.
100. Matthews, J. E., Stewart, M. W., De Boever, E. H., et al.: J. Clin. Endocrinol. Metab. 93(12):4810–4817, 2008.
101. Kim, D., MacConell, L., Zhuang, D., et al.: Diabetes Care 30(6): 1487–1493, 2007.
102. Samson, S. L., Gonzalez, E. V., Yechoor, V., et al.: Mol. Ther. 16(11):1805–1812, 2008.
103. Su, H., He, M., Li, H., et al.: PLoS ONE 3(8):e2892, 2008. doi:10.1371/journal.pone.0002892.
104. Pei, Z.: Curr. Opin. Drug Discov. Devel. 11(4):515–532, 2008.
105. Van der Veken, P., Van der Haemers, A., and Augustyns, K.: Curr. Top. Med. Chem. 7:621–635, 2007.
106. Thornberry, N. A., and Weber, A. E.: Curr. Top. Med Chem 7(6): 557–568, 2007.
107. Rasmussen, H. B., Branner, S., Wiberg, F. C., et al.: Nat. Struct. Biol. 10:19–25, 2003.
108. Thoma, R., Löffler, B., Stihle, M., et al.: Structure 11(8):947–959, 2003.
109. Kuhn, B., Hennig, M., and Mattei, P.: Curr. Top. Med. Chem 7: 609–619, 2007.
110. Kim, D., Wang, L., Beconi, M., et al.: J. Med. Chem. 48(1):141–151, 2005.
111. Augeri, D. J., Robl, J. A., Betebenner, D. A., et al.: J. Med. Chem. 48(15):5025–5037, 2005.
112. Fitzpatrick, S., Taylor, S., Booth, S. W., et al.: Pharm. Dev. Technol. 11(4):521–528, 2006.
113. Januvia product information (22-July-2008): obtained via http://www.accessdata.fda.gov/drugsatfda_docs/label/2008/021995s007lbl.pdf
114. Jakobsen, P., and Treppendahl, S.: Tetrahedron 35(18):2151–2153, 1979.
115. Hennig, U. G. G., Chatten, L. G., Moskalyk, R. E., et al.: Analyst (Cambridge, United Kingdom) 106(1262):557–564, 1981.
116. Llinas, A., Glen, R. C., and Goodman, J. M.: J. Chem. Inf. Model. 48(7):1289–1303, 2008.
117. Wheeler, A., Wang, C., Yang, K., et al.: Mol. Pharmacol. 74(5), 1333–1344, 2008.
118. Riess, M. L., Camara, A. K., Heinen, A., et al.: J. Cardiovasc. Pharmacol. 51(5):483–491, 2008.
119. Adebiyi, A., McNally, E. M., and Jaggar, J. H.: Mol. Pharmacol. 74(3):736–743, 2008.
120. Jacobson, D. A., Wicksteed, B. L., and Philipson, L. H.: Diabetes 58:304–306, 2009.
121. Sebille, S., de Tullio, P., Florence, X., et al.: Bioorg. Med. Chem. 16(10):5704–5719, 2008.
122. de Tullio, P., Boverie, S., Becker, B., et al.: J. Med. Chem. 48:4990–5000, 2005.
123. Sharma, B. K., Sharma, S. K., Singh, P., et al.: J. Enzyme Inhib. Med. Chem. 23(1):1–6, 2008.
124. Mohnike, K., Blankenstein, O., Pfuetzner, A., et al.: Horm. Res. 70(1):59–64, 2008.
125. Grill, V., and Bjoerklund, A.: Mol. Cell Endocrinol. 297(1–2):86–92, 2009.
126. Millar, R. P., Lu, Z. L., Pawson, A. J., et al.: Endocr. Rev. 25(2):235–275, 2004.
127. Hsieh, K. P., and Martin, T. F.: Mol. Endocrinol. 6(10):1673–1681, 1992.
128. Knobil, E.: Recent Prog. Horm. Res. 36:53–88, 1980.
129. Molineaux, C. J., Lasdun, A., Michaud, C., et al.: J. Neurochem. 51(2):624–633, 1988.
130. Dineen, M. K., Tierney, D. S., Kuzma, P., et al.: J. Clin. Pharmacol. 45(11):1245–1249, 2005.
131. Sennello, L. T., Finley, R. A., Chu, S. Y., et al.: J. Pharm. Sci. 75(2):158–160, 1986.
132. Trelstar product information, as per 29-June-2001 FDA labeling.
133. Vantas product information, as per 8-Nov-2004 FDA labeling.
134. Synarel product information (12-Apr-2006 labeling).
135. Felberbaum, R. E., Ludwig, M., and Diedrich, K.: Mol. Cell Endocrinol. 166(1):9–14, 2000.
136. Karten, M. J., and Rivier, J. E.: Endocr. Rev. 7(1):44–66, 1986.
137. Vale, W., Grant, G., Rivier, J., et al.: Science 176(37):933–934, 1972.
138. Beckers, T., Bernd, M., Kutscher, B., et al.: Biochem. Biophys. Res. Commun. 289(3):653–663, 2001.
139. Koerber, S. C., Rizo, J., Struthers, R. S., et al.: J. Med. Chem. 43(5): 819–828, 2000.
140. Samant, M. P., Hong, D. J., Croston, G., et al.: J. Med. Chem. 49 (12):3536–3543, 2006.
141. Samant, M. P., Gulyas, J., Hong, D. J., et al.: J. Med. Chem. 48(15): 4851–4860, 2005.
142. Ljungqvist, A., Feng, D. M., Tang, P. F., et al.: Biochem. Biophys. Res. Commun. 148(2):849–856, 1987.
143. Betz, S. F., Zhu, Y. F., Chen, C., et al.: J. Med. Chem. 51(12): 3331–3348, 2008.
144. Norman, P.: Curr. Opin. Oncol. Endoc. Metab. Invest. Drugs 2(2):227–248, 2000.
145. Schwahn, M., Schupke, H., Gasparic, A., et al.: Drug Metab. Dispos. 28(1):10–20, 2000.
146. Cetrotide product information (4-Apr-2008 labeling); Cetrorelix: Facts and Comparisions 4.0, Wolters-Kluwer Health, accessed May 2009.
147. Rabasseda, X., Leeson, P., and Castaner, J.: Drugs Future 24(4):393–403, 1999.
148. Ganirelix Acetate (Organon) FDA Labeling approved 30-June-2008: http://www.accessdata.fda.gov/drugsatfda_docs/label/2008/021057s007lbl.pdf
149. Degarelix Acetate product information (labeling approved 24-Dec-2008).

CHAPTER 21

Agents Treating Bone Disorders

JOHN H. BLOCK

CHAPTER OVERVIEW

Bone is a dynamic tissue. Ninety-nine percent of the body's calcium is found in bone as a complex mixed salt called *hydroxyapetite* [($Ca_5(PO_4)_3(OH)$]. Because the crystal unit cell has two molecules of hydroxyapatite, it is also written as $Ca_{10}(PO_4)_6(OH)_2$. Bone is the body's calcium reservoir with calcium constantly being removed by osteoclast cells (bone resorption) and laid down by osteoblast cells (calcium deposition). The former are derived from monocyte–macrophage cell lines. Together, bone resorption and calcium deposition are known as *bone remodeling*. The large bones such as the femur and hip harbor the body's marrow containing stem cells that produce a wide variety of cells including erythrocytes, platelets, B cells, T cells, neutrophils, basophils, eosinophils, monocytes, and mast cells.

It should not be surprising that bone, being a dynamic tissue, is subject to several diseases, and there are pharmacological treatments for these diseases. These diseases range from deterioration of bone structure, defects in bone remodeling, and malignancies. Some of these pathological conditions have a genetic basis, others can be ascribed to lifestyle, and some attributed to an aging population. This chapter will be restricted to those bone diseases for which there are approved drug treatments. Antineoplastic agents used to treat malignancies of the bone are discussed in Chapter 10.

DISEASES OF BONE TISSUE UTILIZING APPROVED DRUG THERAPIES

Paget Disease of Bone (*Osteo Deformans*)

Paget disease can be thought of as improper resorption of bone. Essentially, bones grow larger leading to deformation of the affected bones and become weaker than normal with increasing risk of fracture. It can occur on several bones or be isolated to one bone. It most likely occurs in the pelvis, skull, spine, or leg bones. The bones may become misshapen and break more easily. There may or may not be pain. Manifestations of Paget disease tend to appear in the patient's late 40s. Although there is some evidence of hereditary factors, slow viruses also have been considered a cause. Diagnosis begins with a determination of the patient's alkaline phosphatase levels followed by bone scans and x-rays. Drug therapy includes bisphosphonates and calcitonin.[1]

Heterotopic Ossification

This diagnosis consists of various diseases resulting in abnormal formation of true bone within extraskeletal soft tissues. The latter include fascia, tendons, and other mesenchymal soft tissues. Many times the cause is related to traumatic injury. Treatment includes surgery, radiation, nonsteroidal anti-inflammatory drugs (NSAIDS, Chapter 24) and bisphosphonates.

Hypercalcemia of Malignancy

A malignancy is the most common cause of hypercalcemia and can be an indication of a malignancy, the most common being multiple myeloma, breast, or lung cancer. It is caused by increased osteoclastic activity within the bone. Primary hyperparathyroidism is the second most common cause of hypercalcemia. In addition to treating the cause, approved drug treatments for hypercalcemia of malignancy include bisphosphonates, calcitonin, gallium nitrate, and cinacalcet.

Osteoporosis

Osteoporosis is the most common of the bone diseases. It is a pathological condition characterized by decreased bone mass and structural deterioration of bone tissue.[2] The result is bone fragility leading to increased risk of fractures of the hip, spine, and wrist. Many times the broken hip is considered the result of the patient falling when, in actuality, the broken hip was the initial event causing the fall. The economic impact of this disease is tremendous. Osteoporosis is responsible for more than 1.5 million fractures annually distributed among 300,000 hips, 700,000 vertebrae, 250,000 wrists, and 300,000 other sites. It is more common in women than men because women, on average, have a smaller bone mass than men. Diagnosis, prior to an actual fracture, is done by bone density measurements.

Osteoporosis has been considered a disease of aging, but inflammation may be an important variable. Calcium flux favors bone mineralization through adolescence. Bone resorption and deposition are in balance in adults and become negative beginning in the late 50s. Loss of calcium from bone increases relative to calcium deposition onto bone increases with menopause. The importance of estrogen is shown by it acting directly on osteoblasts and possibly inhibiting osteoclasts. The loss of estrogen production results in a significant alteration of the osteoblast–osteoclast ratio because of increased osteoclastogenesis and decreased osteoclast apoptosis. The role of estrogen on osteoblast function has led to the development of selective estrogen receptor modifiers (SERM) for the prevention and treatment of osteoporosis. These are discussed in more detail in Chapter 25.

Associated with menopause and the loss of estrogen is an increase in the production of proinflammatory cytokines including interleukin-1 (IL-1), tumor necrosis factor-α (TNF-α), and interleukin-6 (IL-6). Paralleling this increased production of proinflammatory cytokines is increased osteoclastic bone resorption. Of particular importance for osteoclast differentiation and activation and, therefore, progression of osteoporosis, is the receptor activator of nuclear factor-κB (RANK), a membrane-bound receptor on osteoblast precursor cells and the receptor's functional ligand, RANK ligand (RANKL), also a cytokine. When RANKL binds to RANK, there is increased osteoclastic activity and increased osteoclast numbers because of decreased osteoclast apoptosis. Opposing RANKL is osteoprotegerin, an endogenous inhibitor of RANKL, specifically binding it and blocking its interaction with RANK. Osteoprotegerin, by inhibiting RANKL, normalizes the osteoblast–osteoclast ratio decreasing bone resorption and loss of calcium from bone.[3]

There are medical conditions that can increase the risk of osteoporosis (secondary osteoporosis) or exacerbate an existing osteoporotic condition. Chronic use of glucocorticoids can accelerate calcium loss. In addition, some anticonvulsants (i.e., phenobarbital and phenytoin) can negatively affect calcium flux involving bone. Medical conditions that immobilize individuals for extensive time periods can also lead to calcium loss.

There are controllable risk factors that reduce the risk and severity of the disease. These include anorexia in the age span when humans are accumulating dietary calcium, a diet low in calcium and vitamin D (cholecalciferol), inactive lifestyle, cigarette smoking, and excessive use of alcohol. Staying as physically active as possible throughout one's life span is important, particularly focusing on activities that include working against gravity (walking, hiking, jogging, stair climbing, and dancing). It is important for all age groups to consume calcium, but because calcium deposition onto bone is at its greatest through adolescence, it is important to consume quantities of calcium equal to the daily adequate intake (AI) of, depending on age, 500 to 1,300 mg/day. Younger people can obtain their calcium from diet, primarily dairy. Older individuals may need to take calcium supplements. Paralleling adequate calcium intake is vitamin D consumption. The current adult AI is 5 to 10 μg (200–400 IU). This has been considered too conservative with recommendations that it be increased to 20 to 25 μg (800–1,000 IU). A person's vitamin D status can be checked by measuring 25-hydroxycholecalciferol blood levels.

Osteoporosis is a greater problem in women mainly because women live longer and have less bone mass than men. Nevertheless, osteoporosis is a disease of older men. A 60-year-old white man has a 25% lifetime risk for an osteoporotic fracture, with consequences more severe than in women.[4] The 1-year mortality rate in men after hip fracture is twice than in women.[5] The factors that increase the risk of osteoporotic fracture in men are the same as those found in women.[6]

Osteomalacia

Osteomalacia is caused by a vitamin deficiency and can be thought of as the adult version of rickets. Whereas osteo-porosis is caused by loss of both calcium and cartilage from bone, the cartilage matrix of bone remains with osteomalacia. Because of the vitamin D deficiency, dietary calcium is not transported across the intestinal mucosa to be deposited onto adult bone. The latter process is referred to as mineralization of the bone. The result is "soft" bone that becomes misshapen, because the bones cannot support the body. Inward curvature of the vertebral column and collapsed pelvis are two common results from osteomalacia. Treatment is increased vitamin D intake, but it may not be possible to correct the misshapen bone.

DRUGS USED TO TREAT DISEASES OF THE BONE

Bisphosphonates

The general bisphosphonate structure is illustrated in Figure 21.1. Bisphosphonates should not be confused with bisphosphates. Bisphosphonates have covalent carbon–phosphorous bonds, and bisphosphates carbon-oxygen-phosphorous bonds. In other words, the latter are phosphate esters very similar in chemistry to biochemical phosphate esters. Most in vivo bisphosphates are substrates for phosphatase enzymes, whereas bisphosphonates are stable in the presence of hydrolytic phosphatases. The phosphonate groups are required both for binding to bone hydroxyapatite and cell-mediated antiresorptive activity.

Bisphosphonates were first reported in 1897. The discovery for treating and preventing osteoporosis began in the early 1960s with Procter & Gamble's detergent division searching for better additives for use in hard water areas. Bisphosphonates have excellent affinity for Ca^{2+} and Mg^{2+}. The research moved to the company's dental division where it was discovered that bisphosphonates prevent tartar buildup by forming a thin film on the surface of teeth because it is strongly chemisorbed onto hydroxyapetite.[7]

Bisphosphonates approved for treating bone diseases can be divided into two groups: non–N-containing and N-containing (Table 21.1). The rank order of bisphosphonates binding to hydroxyapatite, from weaker to stronger binding is clodronate (lowest) < etidronate < risedronate < ibandronate

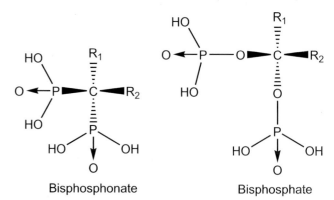

Figure 21.1 ● Bisphosphonate and bisphosphate chemistry. Bisphosphonates have carbon–phosphorous bonds, whereas bisphosphates are phosphate esters with carbon-oxygen-phosphorous bonds. The therapeutic bisphosphonates (Table 21.1) differ by the substituents at positions R_1 and R_2.

TABLE 21.1 Bisphosphonates

Generic Name	Brand Name	R₁	R₂	Approved Indications	Nonapproved Indications	Contraindications	Dosing
Non-*N*-containing Bisphosphonates							
Etidronate disodium	Didronel	$-OH$	$-CH_3$	Heterotopic ossification; Hypercalcemia of malignancy; Paget disease		Clinically overt osteomalacia	Daily
Tiludronate disodium	Skelid	$-OH$	(—S—phenyl—Cl)	Paget disease			Daily
N-Containing Bisphosphonates			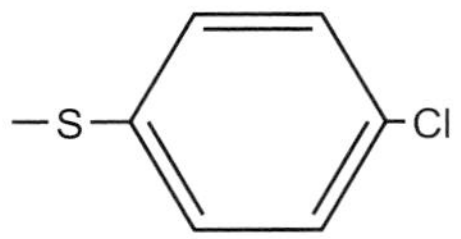				
Alendronate sodium	Fosamax	$-OH$	$-(CH_2)_3NH_2$	Male osteoporosis; Corticosteroid-induced osteoporosis; postmenopausal osteoporosis; prophylaxis of postmenopausal osteoporosis	Osteoporosis from Crohn disease; hypercalcemia of pregnancy	Esophageal abnormalities that delay esophageal emptying; Inability to stand or sit upright for 30 minutes; patients at increased risk of aspiration should not receive oral solution	Weekly or daily
Pamidronate disodium	Aredia	$-OH$	$-(CH_2)_2NH_2$	Osteolytic bone metastasis; hypercalcemia of pregnancy; Paget disease			Daily to monthly, depending on the condition
Risedronate sodium	Actonel	$-OH$	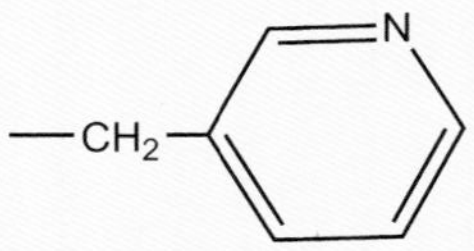 (—CH₂— pyridine)	Male osteoporosis; Corticosteroid-induced osteoporosis; prophylaxis of corticosteroids induced osteoporosis; postmenopausal osteoporosis; prophylaxis of postmenopausal osteoporosis; Paget disease		Hypocalcemia; Inability to sit or stand upright for at least 30 minutes	Daily to monthly
Zoledronic acid	Zometa	$-OH$	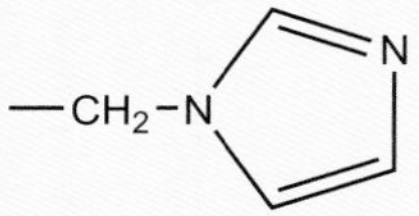 (—CH₂—N imidazole)	Bone metastasis; Hypercalcemia of malignancy; multiple myeloma; Paget disease; postmenopausal osteoporosis		Hypocalcemia	IV; spacing depends on the indication

< alendronate < pamidronate < zoledronate (highest). As noted in later discussion, this order does not completely parallel antiresorptive potency. A key difference between the non–N-containing and N-containing bisphosphonates is the ability of the latter to form positive charges on their nitrogens at physiological pH. In general, the more positively charged bisphosphonates (zoledronate, ibandronate, and alendronate) produce a positive surface on the bone, attracting additional bisphosphonates to bone.

The non–N-containing and N-containing bisphosphonates differ in their mechanism of action. The former's (etidronate, tiludronate) site of action is the osteoclast's aminoacyl-transverse ribonucleic acid (tRNA) synthetase reversing the reactions normally involved in activating amino acids during protein synthesis. These two bisphosphonates replace the terminal pyrophosphate moiety of adenosine triphosphate (ATP). This initiates apoptosis in the osteoclast leading to a decrease in bone resorption. There is some evidence that the bisphosphonate-modified ATP may affect mitochondrial function that also would lead to apoptosis. The two non–N-containing bisphosphonates are indicated for Paget disease and, in the case of etidronate disodium, also heterotopic ossification and hypercalcemia of malignancy.

The N-containing bisphosphonates have a different site of action. They interfere with the mevalonate pathway required for biosynthesis of cholesterol and subsequent sterols. The specific sites appear to be that portion of the pathway utilizing isoprenoid diphosphates as substrates for farnesyl diphosphate synthase (FPPS) as the primary target. The bisphosphonates may be false substrates for the isoprenoid diphosphates. The impact of FPPS inhibition may be more than inhibiting sterol synthesis. FPPS is required for the synthesis of farnesyl pyrophosphate, which is the precursor for geranylgeranyl diphosphate. Both farnesyl pyrophosphate and geranylgeranyl pyrophosphate are required for lipid modification (prenylation) of subcellular membranes where signaling proteins are located. This causes loss of osteoclast function and may be more important than apoptosis of the cells necessary for bone resorption to occur.

X-ray crystallography indicates the bisphosphonate nitrogen binds to the FPPS threonine (T201) or the backbone carbonyl of lysine (K200). The optimal distance between the drug's nitrogen and the amino acid oxygen is approximately 3 Å. From lowest to highest, binding to FPPS is pamidronate < alendronate < ibandronate < risedronate < zoledronate, which closely matches antiresorptive potency. The latter two with their heterocyclic nitrogens are significantly better inhibitors of FPPS than the other three.[8]

No drug is without adverse reactions, and this is true of bisphosphonates. They can be very irritating to the gastrointestinal mucous linings. The recommended procedure for oral administration directs the patient to sit upright, consume a full glass of water with the tablet, and remain in the upright position for at least 30 minutes. Oral bisphosphonates should be taken an hour before food. They are poorly absorbed.

A rare but serious adverse reaction is osteonecrosis of jaws. A suggested mechanism is oversuppression of bone turnover.[9] In the majority of reported cases, there had been a previous dental surgical procedure. In this model, bisphosphonates, by disrupting the osteoblast–osteoclast balance, impair proper healing of the jaw following surgery. Unfortunately, there are no definitive guidelines that help the clinician decide if the patient has medical condition that increase his or her risk of osteonecrosis when using bisphosphonates.[10]

The bisphosphonates also may cause severe and sometimes incapacitating pain in bone, joint, and/or muscle (musculoskeletal). This adverse reaction is difficult to define because it can appear within days, months, or years after starting treatment. Some patients report that the pain disappears after discontinuing the bisphosphonate, whereas others have reported slow or incomplete resolution after stopping the drug.[11]

It is difficult to describe any type of rank ordering of efficacy for bisphosphonates. There have been no head-to-head comparisons of several of the drugs in a single trial using the same diagnostic criteria. Measurements of efficacy include incidence of vertebral fracture, nonvertebral fracture, and bone mineral density. Comparisons are more likely focusing on convenience of dosing. Because bisphosphonates adhere strongly to the bone surface, dosing has moved from daily to weekly or monthly for oral administration. Depot injections permit annual administration.

⬡ HORMONE THERAPY

It is important to keep in mind that calcium's biochemical functions include much more than being the main mineral component of bones and teeth. All cells have calcium channels that strictly control calcium flux into and out of cells. Therefore, it is important that blood calcium levels be tightly regulated. This is done with three hormones: parathyroid, calcitonin, and 1,25-dihydroxycholecalciferol (1,25-diOH-D_3). Parathyroid hormone (PTH) is produced by the parathyroid gland located behind the thyroid gland. The parathyroid gland has calcium receptors that sense blood calcium levels. If there is hypocalcemia, PTH is released increasing osteoclastic activity on bone, resulting in increased bone resorption.[12] PTH also acts on the kidney, maximizing tubular reabsorption of calcium and activating the cytochrome P450 mixed function oxidase hydroxylation of 25-hydroxycholecalciferol to 1,25-diOH-D_3. The latter travels to the intestinal mucosa where it is a ligand for the vitamin D receptor (VDR). The result is active transport of dietary calcium into systemic circulation. 1,25-diOH-D_3 can be thought of as a kidney hormone. A patient with kidney failure is prescribed 1,25-diOH-D_3 because of the inability to carry out the final hydroxylation. In addition to regulating the uptake of dietary calcium from the intestinal tract, 1,25-diOH-D_3, along with PTH, enhances calcium flux from bone.

Calcitonin is produced in the thyroid gland and sometimes is called thyrocalcitonin. It is released when there is hypercalcemia. This hormone reduces blood calcium levels by suppressing tubular reabsorption of calcium, thereby enhancing calcium urinary excretion and inhibiting bone resorption minimizing calcium flux from bone.

Calcitonin-Salmon (sCT; Miacalcin, Calcimar)

Human and salmon calcitonins differ from each other by 16 of the total 32 amino acids. Although each calcitonin has a

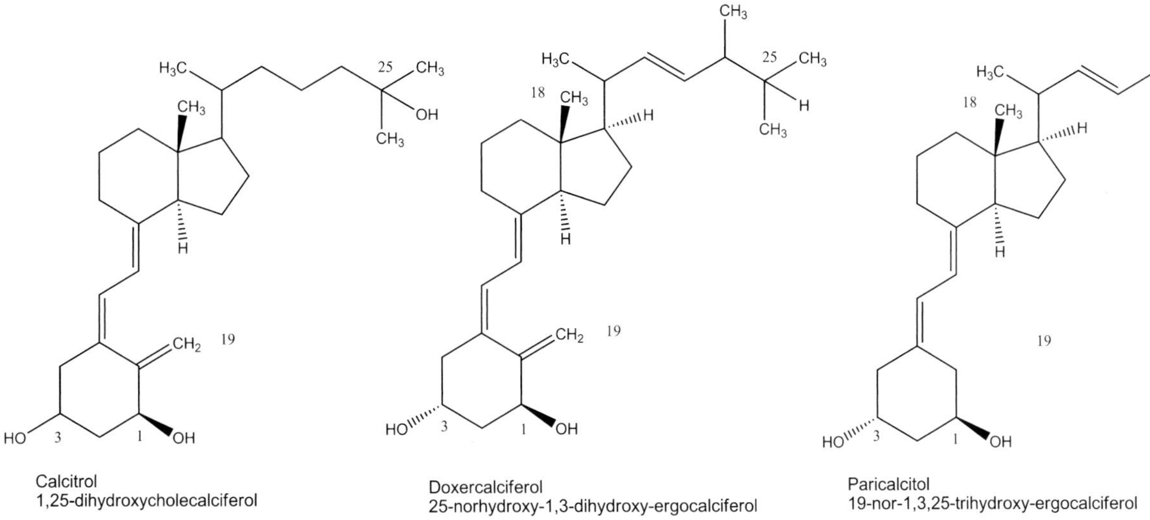

Figure 21.2 ● Drugs based on the ergocalciferol indicated for hyperparathyroidism.

cys-S-S-cys disulfide bridge between cysteines 1 and 7 at the amino terminal end, and each ends at the carboxyl end with a prolinamide, the differences in the other amino acids between the two differ in their tertiary structures. These differences cause calcitonin-salmon to be one order of magnitude greater than human calcitonin in reducing calcium concentration in the blood stream of mammals.[13,14] Nevertheless, these significant differences in amino acid sequence increase the risk of adverse reactions caused by the patient's immune system.

There are two dosage forms: intramuscular and nasal. Because of the adverse effects, there can be inflammation at the injection site plus flushing, nausea, and vomiting following an injection. Use of the nasal dosage form can cause backache and rhinitis. The approved indications for calcitonin-salmon are hypercalcemia, Paget disease, and postmenopausal osteoporosis.

Teriparatide Injection [hPTH(1–34); Forteo]

Teriparatide contains the first 34 amino acids of the 84 amino acid human parathyroid hormone and is produced by recombinant DNA technology. The N-terminal region of endogenous PTH contains most of the biological activity. Timing the administration of PTH determines the response. Teriparatide is administered once daily because once-daily administration stimulates new bone formation by stimulation of osteoblastic activity over osteoclastic activity. In contrast, continuous infusion leads to greater bone resorption than formation.

Teriparatide is indicated for primary postmenopausal osteoporosis in women who are at high risk of fracture and for increasing bone mass in men with primary or hypogonadal osteoporosis who are at high risk for fracture. It is not indicated for pseudohypoparathyroidism or secondary hypoparathyroidism. "True" hypoparathyroidism is caused by a PTH deficiency, and teriparatide acts as a PTH replacement. Pseudohypoparathyroidism usually is caused by a PTH receptor defect. Treatment for the latter includes calcium supplements and vitamin D with the goal to maintain blood calcium levels.

There is a boxed warning regarding a potential risk of developing osteosarcoma. It is based on studies in male and female rats. The effect was observed at systemic exposures to teriparatide ranging from 3 to 60 times the exposure in humans given a 20-μg dose. The boxed warning also warns against administering teriparatide to patients with Paget disease because of the active osteoblastic activity associated with this disease.

Hyperparathyroidism

The focus on this chapter has been on diseases that interfere with bone remodeling. A key gland is the parathyroid, particularly when there is hypoparathyroidism. The opposite can occur with an overactive gland or hyperparathyroidism. There are two vitamin D analogs that are indicated for renal failure when patients are on dialysis. These patients cannot carry out the final cytochrome P450–catalyzed hydroxylation of 25-hydroxycholecalciferol (25-OH-D$_3$) to 1,25-diOH-D$_3$ (calcitriol). It is common to prescribe calcitriol to prevent vitamin D–resistant rickets or osteomalacia. Because of the defective kidney, or lack of kidney, there is inactive feedback to the parathyroid, and the patient's parathyroid can over secrete parathyroid hormone to maintain blood calcium levels. There are two drugs (Fig. 21.2) based on the ergocalciferol structure that better regulate the parathyroid gland with less transport of dietary calcium and phosphorous. These are paricalcitol (19-nor-1,3,25-trihydroxyergocalciferol) and doxercalciferol (25-norhydroxy-1,3-dihydroxyergocalciferol). A third drug, cinacalcet (Fig. 21.3), either mimics calcium because it is a ligand for the calcium-sensing receptor on the parathyroid

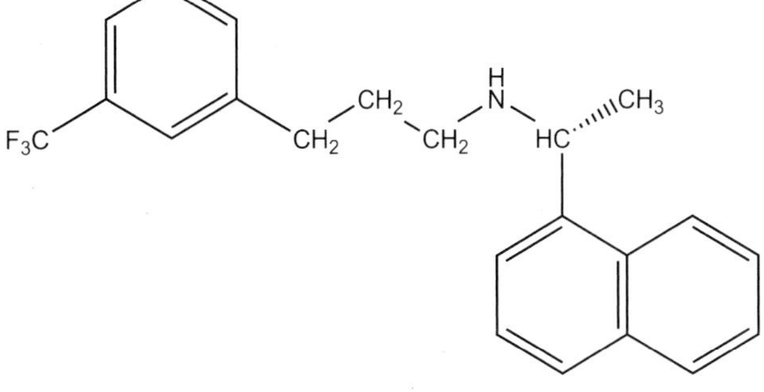

Figure 21.3 ● Cinacalcet (Sensipar).

gland or sensitize the receptor's sensitivity to extracellular calcium. The end result is that the parathyroid gland secretes less hormone. Cinacalcet is indicated for secondary hyperparathyroidism in patients undergoing renal dialysis and hypercalcemia caused by parathyroid carcinoma.

FUTURE DIRECTIONS

Serotonin Regulation of Bone Formation

The low-density lipoprotein (LDL)-receptor–related protein 5 (Lrp5) is a regulator of bone remodeling (balanced osteoblast and osteoclast activity). Among its functions is limiting biosynthesis of serotonin in the gut. Using knockout mice models that are deficient in Lrp5, increased serotonin levels results in decreased bone formation. The site of approximately 95% of the body's serotonin production is the gut, and this serotonin cannot cross the blood-brain barrier. Most of the gut-produced serotonin is taken up by platelets with much of the remainder possibly affecting bone formation by controlling osteoblast proliferation.[15] Consistent with this model is the observation that patients taking selective serotonin reuptake inhibitors (SSRIs), where there is increased peripheral serotonin, can have reduced bone mass.[16]

Monoclonal Antibodies

A monoclonal antibody target for the treatment of osteoporosis is the RANKL, which is the essential mediator of osteoclasts. As pointed out in the osteoporosis discussion, the loss of calcium by increased osteoclastic activity and decreased osteoclast apoptosis is opposed by a RANKL inhibitor, osteoprotegerin a 401-amino acid glycoprotein, and a member of the TNF superfamily. Rather than develop a pharmaceutically acceptable osteoprotegerin, a fully human monoclonal antibody, denosumab, that binds to the RANKL preventing its binding to RANK is being evaluated for the treatment of osteoporosis. The reported result is inhibition of all stages of osteoclast activity.[17] It is important to keep a perspective when administering drugs that interfere with the immune system over long periods of time. RANKL is part of the normal bone remodeling process as well as with pathological bone loss. The key is balance, and this will require long-term studies in patients with postmenopausal osteoporosis.

● R E V I E W   Q U E S T I O N S ●

1. Name the two cell lines responsible for bone remodeling and function of each.

2. What is found in the large bones and what is its function?

3. How does osteoporosis differ from osteomalacia?

4. How does the site of action of the non–*N*-bisphosphonates differ from the *N*-containing bisphosphonates?

5. What is the basis for the adverse reactions seen with administration of calcitonin-salmon?

6. What is teriparatide?

REFERENCES

1. The Paget Foundation www.page.org, accessed February 2009.
2. National Institutes of Health Osteoporosis and Related Bone Diseases—National Resources Center.
3. Mundy, G. R.: Nut. Rev. 65:S147–S151, 2007.
4. Nguyen, T. V., Eisman, J. A., and Kelly, P. J.: Am. J. Epidemiol. 144:255–263, 1966.
5. Kiebzak, G. M., Beinart, G. A., Perser, K., et al.: Arch. Intern. Med. 162:2217–2222, 2002.
6. Liu, H., Paige, N. M., Goldzweig, C. L., et al.: Ann. Intern. Med. 148:685–701, 2008.
7. Francis, M. D., and Centner, R. L.: J. Chem. Edu. 55:760–766, 1978.
8. Russell, R. G. G., Watts, N. B., Ebetino, F. H., et al.: Osteoporos. International 19:733–759, 2008.
9. Woo, S.-B., Hellstein, J. W., and Kalmar, J. R.: Ann. Intern. Med. 144:753–761, 2006.
10. Edwards, B. J., Hellstein, J. W., Jacobsen, P. L., et al.: J. Am. Dental. Assoc. 139:1674–1677, 2008.
11. Information on bisphosphonates. www.fda.gov/cder/drug/infopage/bisphosphonates/default.htm, accessed February 2009.
12. Shoback, D.: N. Eng. J. Med. 359:301–403, 2008.
13. Findlay, D. M., Michelangeli, V. P., Orlowski, R. C., et al.: Endocrinology 112:1288–1291, 1983.
14. Arvinte, T., and Drake, A. F.: J. Biol. Chem. 268:6408–6414, 1993.
15. Yadav, V. K., Ryu, J. H., and Suda, N.: Cell 135:825–837, 2008.
16. Richards, J. B., Papaioannou, A., Adachi, J. D., et al.: Arch. Intern. Med. 167:188–194, 2007.
17. McClung, M. R., Lewiecki, E. M., Cohen, S. B., et al.: N. Eng. J. Med. 354:821–831, 2006.

C H A P T E R 22

Anesthetics

CAROLYN J. FRIEL

CHAPTER OVERVIEW

This chapter focuses on the general and local anesthetic drugs used to block the transmission of pain. The general anesthetic section covers both the inhaled and the intravenous drugs. The local anesthetic section includes the topical and parenteral drugs. This chapter includes the mechanism of action, structure–activity relationships (SAR), and individual drug monographs for the general and the local anesthetic agents.

⬡ THE INHALED GENERAL ANESTHETICS

In 1846, a Boston dentist, William Morton, demonstrated the use of ether as a general anesthetic in a public demonstration. The publication of the successful operation led to the use of general anesthetics by surgeons and ushered in the "age of anesthesia." The first paper that described the use of the general anesthetic ended with the warning that "Its action is not yet thoroughly understood, and its use should be restricted to responsible persons."[1] Although it has been 160 years since that statement was written, the sentiment remains today.

The pharmacological mechanism of action of the anesthetic drugs is not clear. The idea that we can understand the mechanism of action for a general anesthetic supposes that we understand what the term anesthesia means. A clinical definition of general anesthesia is a state where no movement occurs in response to what should be painful. Although this gives us a working definition of the drug's action, it does not explain the physiology behind the action. Much research remains to be done on the physiological mechanism of action of the drugs discussed in this chapter. The general anesthetic section will begin by reviewing the stages of general anesthesia, followed by a summary of the SAR of the inhaled anesthetics and their proposed mechanism of action and will conclude with individual drug monographs.

Stages of General Anesthesia[2]

Analgesia (Stage I): The stage of analgesia lasts from onset of drowsiness to loss of eyelash reflex (blinking when the eyelash is stroked). Variable levels of amnesia and analgesia are seen in this stage. The patient is considered unconscious at the end of stage I.
Excitement (Stage II): The stage of excitement is characterized by agitation and delirium. During this stage, salivation may be copious. Heart rate and respiration

may be irregular. Induction agents are designed to move the patient through this undesirable stage quickly.
Surgical Anesthesia (Stage III): This stage is divided into four planes but for the purpose of this chapter, it is sufficient to understand that this stage of anesthesia is the target depth for the procedure. During this stage, a painful stimuli will not elicit a somatic reflex or deleterious autonomic response.
Impending Death (Stage IV): This stage lasts from onset of apnea to failure of circulation and respiration and ends in death.

The ideal anesthetic combination will allow the patient to proceed quickly from stage I to stage III and avoid stage IV. Inhaled anesthetics are used in combination with other drugs to induce anesthesia. The drug combinations used to achieve this are complex and will not be addressed here; the reader is referred to a general anesthesia textbook for a more detailed description.

The Ideal Inhaled Anesthetic

The ideal inhaled anesthetic will be inexpensive, potent, pleasant to inhale, minimally soluble in the blood and tissues, stable on the shelf and during administration, and lack undesirable side effects such as cardiotoxicity, hepatotoxicity, renal toxicity, and neurotoxicity. The ideal inhaled anesthetic has not been developed yet and all of these factors must be kept in mind when choosing an anesthetic for a particular patient.

POTENCY

The most common way to measure inhaled anesthetic potency is by recording the minimum alveolar concentration (MAC) needed to prevent movement to a painful stimulus. The MAC concentrations are recorded at 1 atmosphere and reported as the mean concentration needed to abolish movement in 50% of subjects. The MACs for the inhaled anesthetics are listed in Table 22.1. Potency of the inhaled anesthetics is extremely important as the anesthetic gas is displacing oxygen in the inspired gas. Inhaled agents with low potencies (high MACs) such as nitrous oxide require administration at increased pressure or are used only in combination with more potent inhaled agents.

SOLUBILITY

The ideal general anesthetic will have low solubility in blood conveyed by the blood:gas partition coefficient listed

TABLE 22.1 Properties of the Inhaled Anesthetics

Anesthetic	MAC (%)	Blood:Gas	Oil:Gas
Nitrous oxide	104	0.46	1.1
Halothane	0.75	2.4	137
Enflurane	1.68	1.8	98
Methoxyflurane	0.16	16.0	970
Isoflurane	1.15	1.43	90.8
Sevoflurane	2.10	0.65	50
Desflurane	7.3	0.42	18.7
Xenon	71	0.12	1.9

in Table 22.1. The blood:gas partition coefficient is defined as the ratio of the concentration of the drug in the blood to the concentration of the drug in the gas phase (in the lung), at equilibrium. The volatile anesthetic is inhaled into the lungs, diffuses into the blood, and when equilibrium is reached, it diffuses into tissues. For the drug to have a quick onset, the solubility in the blood should be low, thus saturation will occur quickly, and the drug can then move into the tissue compartment. Recovery is also expected to be faster for those drugs with a low blood:gas partition coefficient as the drug will be eliminated quicker if it has a low solubility in the blood and quickly passes into the lungs for exhalation.

When a patient is exposed to the volatile gas for prolonged procedures, greater than 5 hours, the solubility of the drug in the tissues will also effect the recovery period. In these cases, it is necessary to consider the solubility of the drug in fat and lean organs as well as the body mass of the individual patient to determine how recovery could be affected by drug solubility. Most inhaled anesthetics have similar solubilities in lean organs, but their solubilities in fat vary as predicted by their oil:gas partition coefficients listed in Table 22.1.[3] Obese patients may have increased recovery times if an inhaled anesthetics with high-fat solubility is used for a prolonged period.

STABILITY

The early inhaled anesthetics suffered from stability problems, leading to explosions and operating room fires. By halogenating the ether and hydrocarbon anesthetics, the explosiveness and flammability of the drugs were diminished, and the number of operating room fires decreased. Halogenation clearly stabilizes the inhaled agent and all inhaled anesthetics used today contain halogens.

Sporadic reports of fires involving sevoflurane can be found in the literature.[4–6] The operating room fires involving sevoflurane all involved the recapture process and recirculating equipment. In an attempt to decrease operating room personnel exposure to the volatile anesthetics being exhaled by the patient, as well as to reduce the acquisition costs of the drug, recirculating breathing apparatus were developed. These breathing apparatus are designed to capture the expired gas, remove the carbon dioxide, and then allow the patient to inhale the anesthetic gas again. Different carbon dioxide absorbents are used such as calcium hydroxide, barium hydroxide, and sodium hydroxide. When the absorbent inadvertently dries out, as a result of the continuous flow of fresh gas, sevoflurane can break down and produce hydrogen in an exothermic reaction. The generation of hydrogen and heat may have been responsible for the reported fires that began in the anesthetic equipment.[6] Other anesthetics have not had this same problem but all are monitored for their degradation products when exposed to carbon dioxide absorbents. Toxic metabolites of the inhaled anesthetics, such as the fluoride anion, are also a concern and discussed in the individual drug monographs.

Structure–Activity Relationships of the Volatile General Anesthetics

The inhalation anesthetics in use today are nitrous oxide, halothane, isoflurane, desflurane, and sevoflurane. The chemical structures for these compounds and some of historical interest can be seen in Figure 22.1. While it is true that there is no single pharmacophore for the inhaled anesthetics, the chemical structure is related to the activity of the drug molecule.

ALKANE/CYCLOALKANE

alkane series   cycloalkane series

The first SAR studies conducted independently by Meyer and Overton in the 1880s showed a distinct positive correlation between anesthetic potency and solubility in olive oil. Many series of compounds confirm this simple relationship but exceptions to the model exist. The potency of alkanes, cycloalkanes, and aromatic hydrocarbons increases in direct proportion to the number of carbon atoms in the structure up to a cutoff point.[7] Within the n-alkane series, the cutoff number is 10, with n-decane showing minimal anesthetic potency. In the cycloalkane series, the cutoff number in most studies is eight with cyclooctane showing no anesthetic activity in the rat. The reduced activity of the compounds beyond their cutoff number could be a result of problems getting to the site of action (reduced vapor pressure or high blood solubility) or inability to bind to the site of action and induce the conformational change required for anesthetic action.[8]

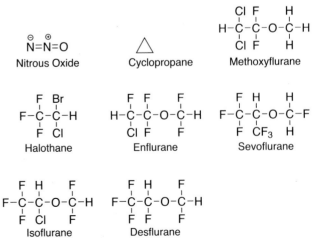

Figure 22.1 ● The chemical structures of the inhaled anesthetic agents.

The cycloalkanes are more potent anesthetics than the straight chain analog with the same number of carbons. For example, the MAC of cyclopropane in rats is about one fifth of the MAC of n-propane.[8]

ALKANOL SERIES

alkane series   alkanol series

A similar increase in potency with increase in carbon length was seen in the n-alkanol series. In addition, the n-alkanol with a given number of carbons is more potent than the n-alkane with the same chain length.[9]

EFFECT OF HALOGENATION/ETHER HALOGENATION

The first inhaled anesthetics used in the late 1800s, diethyl ether and cyclopropane caused laryngospasms. These compounds were also explosive and flammable requiring careful handling. Early studies found that halogenating the ethers decreased the flammability of the compounds, enhanced their stability and increased their potency. Higher atomic mass halogens increased potency compared to lower atomic mass halogens. For example, replacing the fluorine in desflurane ($CF_2HOCFHCF_3$) with a chlorine to form isoflurane ($CF_2HOCClHCF_3$) increased potency more than fourfold.[10] Replacing the chlorine with bromine in the investigational agent I-537 ($CF_2HOCBrHCF_3$) increased potency threefold further. In general, halogenated ether compounds also caused less laryngospasms than unhalogenated compounds. Unfortunately, halogenation also increased the propensity of the drugs to cause cardiac arrhythmias and/or convulsions.[11] Halogenated methyl ethyl ethers were found to be more stable and potent than halogenated diethyl ethers. The commonly used inhaled anesthetics are ethers or aliphatic hydrocarbons with 2 to 5 carbon atoms.

The effect of halogenating the alkane, cycloalkane, and alkanol compounds has been extensively studied in animal models. For the n-alkane series, fully saturating the alkane with fluorine abolished activity except when n equaled one.[7] When n was 2 to 4 carbons the highest potency was seen when the terminal carbon contained one hydrogen ($CHF_2(CF_2)_nCHF_2$). When n was greater than 5 carbons the potency decreased in this series. The potency of the dihydrogen compounds ($CH_2F(CF)_nCH_2F$) (n = 2–4) was greater than the equivalent nonfluorinated alkane compound. Similar findings for the n-alkanol series were found. The most potent fluorinated n-alkanols were the $CHF_2(CF_2)_nCH_2OH$ series, when n was between 2 and 5.[7] The decrease in activity for the completely fluorinated compounds would not be predicted by the Meyer-Overton hypothesis. Another interesting phenomenon that does not follow the Meyer-Overton hypothesis can be found using the structural isomers isoflurane and enflurane. (Fig. 22.1) The compounds have similar solubility in oil, yet the MAC for enflurane is greater than the MAC for isoflurane (Table 22.1). The stereoisomers of isoflurane (+) and (−) have also been isolated and tested for anesthetic potency in rats. The (+) isomer was found to be 53% more potent than the (−) isomer. This observation would not be predicted based on the Meyer-Overton hypothesis.

EFFECT OF SATURATION

Molecular flexibility of the inhaled anesthetics is not required. The addition of double and/or triple bonds to small anesthetic molecules having 6 carbon atoms or less increases potency.[12]

Mechanism of Action of the Inhaled Anesthetics

The mechanism of action of the inhaled anesthetics is not known. Most theories of the inhaled anesthetics leave room for the possibility of multiple mechanisms, receptors, and regions of the nervous system (spinal cord and brain) to explain their action. It seems likely that the individual anesthetic molecules act with different potencies on multiple receptors that lead to similar clinical states of anesthesia. Some of theories of anesthetic action are briefly covered below.

MEYER-OVERTON THEORY

As discussed, work of Meyer and Overton in the 1880s showed that there was strong correlation between the potency of the anesthetic and its solubility in olive oil. This correlation holds true for a surprising number of inhaled anesthetics but it does not explain the drugs mechanism of action. When biological membranes were found to be composed mainly of lipids, the work of Meyer and Overton was extended to offer a proposed mechanism of action of the inhaled anesthetics. Namely, that the lipid-soluble drug somehow disrupted the biological membrane and produced anesthesia. This "unitary hypothesis" has led to research focused on the effect of the anesthetics on the lipid membrane. The inhaled anesthetics do disrupt the lipid bilayer but it is unclear if they make enough changes to effect cell signaling.[13] If lipid solubility were the only factor for anesthetic potency, then chiral enantiomers would have the same potencies as their log P's are identical. This is not the case. The stereoisomers of isoflurane do not have the same in vivo potency (~20%) despite having the same effect on the lipid membrane.[13] It is also clear that all lipophilic chemicals are not anesthetics and thus the unitary theory of anesthesia cannot adequately explain the mechanism of action of the inhaled anesthetic drugs.

INTERACTION WITH ION CHANNELS[14]

Inhaled anesthetics interact with various ion channels to influence the electrical activity of cells and their physiological response. The most studied receptor that inhaled anesthetics act on is the $GABA_A$ receptor. Inhaled anesthetics enhance chloride ion conductance into the cell and thus hyperpolarize the cell membrane and prevent impulse transmission. They act at the $GABA_A$ receptor in a manner similar to the benzodiazepines but not identical. Molecular modeling studies based on mutagenesis data and structurally homologous proteins predict the existence of an inhaled anesthetic binding site on the $GABA_A$ receptor. The binding site is postulated to be between the second and third transmembrane segments of the $GABA_A$ α_1-receptor subunits.[15] Chloride channel blockers and benzodiazepine antagonists show only a small effect on the potency of the anesthetics, thus $GABA_A$ potentiation cannot universally explain their mechanism of action.[13] Inhaled anesthetics are also known to enhance the major inhibitory receptors in the spinal cord, the glycine receptors.

Inhaled anesthetics are also proposed to inhibit the excitatory synaptic channel activity of neuronal nicotinic acetylcholine receptors, glutamate receptors (*N*-methyl-D-aspartate [NMDA] and α-amino-3-hydroxy-5-methyl-4-isoxazole propionic acid [AMPA]), sodium channels, potassium channels, calcium channels (voltage-gated cardiac and neuronal), and ryanodine receptors. The multitude of receptor channels that are affected to various degrees by specific inhaled anesthetics leads to the current theory that multiple receptors are targets of the volatile anesthetics and no single receptor–drug interaction can fully explain their mechanism of action.

General Anesthetic Monographs, Individual Products Including Adverse Reactions

The chemical structures of the inhaled anesthetic agents are shown in Figure 22.1.

NITROUS OXIDE

Nitrous oxide is a gas at room temperature and is supplied as a liquid under pressure in metal cylinders. Nitrous oxide is a "dissociative anesthetic" and causes slight euphoria and hallucinations. The low potency of nitrous oxide (MAC = 104%) precludes it from being used alone for surgical anesthesia. To use it as the sole anesthetic agent the patient would have to breathe in pure N_2O to the exclusion of oxygen. This situation would obviously cause hypoxia and potentially lead to death. Nitrous oxide can inactivate methionine synthase, a B_{12}-dependent enzyme necessary for the synthesis of DNA and therefore should be used with caution in pregnant and B_{12}-deficient patients. Nitrous oxide is also soluble in closed gas containing body spaces and can cause these spaces to enlarge when administered possibly leading to adverse occurrences (occluded middle ear, bowel distension, pneumothorax). Nitrous oxide is a popular anesthetic in dentistry were it is commonly referred to as "laughing gas." It is used in combination with more potent anesthetics for surgical anesthesia and remains a drug of recreational abuse.[16] Nitrous oxide undergoes little or no metabolism.[3]

HALOTHANE

Halothane is a nonflammable, nonpungent, volatile, liquid, halogenated (F, Cl, and Br) ethane (bp = 50°C), introduced in 1956. Halothane may increase heart rate, cause cardiac arrhythmias, increase cerebral blood flow, and increase intracranial pressure.[17] It can undergo spontaneous oxidation when exposed to ultraviolet light to yield HCl, HBr, Cl^-, Br^-, and phosgene ($COCl_2$). To prevent oxidation it is packaged in amber bottles with a low concentration of thymol (0.01%) as a stabilizer. The drug has a high potency (MAC = 0.75%), a blood:gas partition coefficient of 2.4, and high adipose solubility. Halothane undergoes both reductive and oxidative processes with up to 20% of the dose undergoing metabolism (Fig. 22.2).[18] The trifluoroacetyl chloride metabolite is electrophilic and can form covalent bonds with proteins leading to immune responses and halothane hepatitis upon subsequent halothane exposure. Halothane hepatitis is rare with 1 case reported for every 6,000 to 35,000 patients exposed.[17,18]

The use of inhaled anesthetics and halothane in particular can produce malignant hyperthermia (MH) in genetically susceptible individuals. This results in an increase in body temperature, tachycardia, tachypnea, acidosis, and rhabdomyolysis. MH is a result of the excessive release of calcium from the sarcoplasmic reticulum (SR). Patients with an inherited mutation in the ryanodine receptor (RYR1), which is located in the SR, are at an increased risk of developing MH when exposed to an inhaled anesthetic triggering agent. Treatment entails discontinuing the anesthetic agent, rapid cooling, intravenous dantrolene sodium, and supportive measures. MH has been reported to occur with all anesthetics agents and with succinylcholine, a depolarizing neuromuscular blocker. The combination of halothane and succinylcholine appears to trigger a great extent of the MH episodes. Patients with a family history of MH can be genetically screened for MH susceptibility via the caffeine–halothane contracture test. This test is invasive requiring a piece of skeletal muscle to conduct and it is expensive costing approximately $5,000 (cost in 2008). Noninvasive molecular genetic screening is currently being developed.[19]

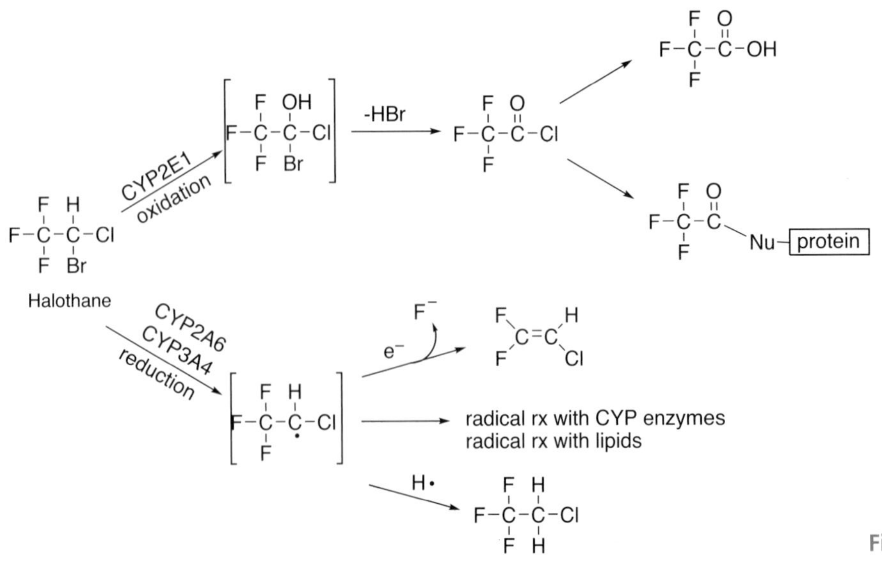

Figure 22.2 • Halothane metabolism.

METHOXYFLURANE

Methoxyflurane is a volatile liquid (bp = 105°C) with a high blood:gas partition coefficient and thus a slow induction and prolonged recovery.[20] Approximately 75% of the drug undergoes metabolism yielding dichloroacetate, difluoromethoxyacetate, oxalate, and fluoride ions. The intrarenal inorganic fluoride concentration, as a result of renal defluorination, may be responsible for the nephrotoxicity seen with methoxyflurane. Both the concentration of F^- generated and the duration for which it remained elevated were factors in the development of methoxyflurane nephrotoxicity.[21] Methoxyflurane was removed from the U.S. market in 2000 because of safer alternatives. Both isoflurane and enflurane produce less fluoride ion upon metabolism than methoxyflurane.

ENFLURANE

Enflurane is a volatile liquid (bp = 56.5°C) with a blood: gas partition coefficient of 1.8 and an MAC of 1.68%. Approximately 2% to 8% of the drug is metabolized primarily at the chlorofluoromethyl carbon. Little chlorofluoroacetic acid is produced suggesting minor metabolism at the difluoromethyl carbon. Difluoromethoxydifluoroacetate and fluoride ion have been reported as metabolites. Enflurane may increase heart rate, cause cardiac arrhythmias, increase cerebral blood flow, and increase intracranial pressure but all to a smaller degree than halothane.[17] Enflurane also causes electroencephalographic (EEG) patterns consistent with electrical seizure activity. It has caused tonic–clonic convulsive activity in patients when used at high concentrations or during profound hypocarbic periods. Enflurane is therefore not recommended in patients with seizure disorders.[22]

ISOFLURANE

Isoflurane is a volatile liquid (bp = 48.5°C) with an MAC of 1.15, a blood:gas partition coefficient of 1.43 and high solubility in fat. Isoflurane is a structural isomer of enflurane. It is a known respiratory irritant, but less so than desflurane. Approximately 0.2% of the administered drug undergoes metabolism, the rest is exhaled unchanged. The metabolism of isoflurane yields low levels of the nephrotoxic fluoride ion as well as a potentially hepatotoxic trifluoroacetylating compound (Fig. 22.3).[23] The relatively low concentrations of these compounds have resulted in very low risks of hepatotoxicity and nephrotoxicity. There have been no reports of

seizures caused by isoflurane and only transient increases in heart rate have been reported.

DESFLURANE

Desflurane is a nonflammable, colorless, very volatile liquid packaged in amber-colored vials. The boiling point is 22.8°C, and it requires a vaporizer specifically designed for desflurane. The manufacturer states that the vials can be stored at room temperature. Desflurane has a blood:gas partition coefficient of 0.42, an MAC of 7.3% and an oil:gas partition coefficient of 18.7. The low blood:gas partition coefficient leads to fast induction times and short recovery times. Desflurane is not recommended for induction anesthesia in children because of the high incidence of laryngospasms (50%), coughing (72%), breath holding (68%), and increase in secretions (21%).[24] Desflurane can produce a dose-dependent decrease in blood pressure and concentrations exceeding 1 MAC may cause transient increases in heart rate. Desflurane can react with desiccated carbon dioxide absorbents to produce carbon monoxide that may result in elevated levels of carboxyhemoglobin.[24]

Desflurane is metabolized minimally with less than 0.02% of the administered dose recovered as urinary metabolites. Desflurane produces minimal free fluoride ion and very little trifluoroacetic acid and has not been reported to cause either kidney or liver damage.

SEVOFLURANE

Sevoflurane is a volatile, nonpungent, nonflammable, and nonexplosive liquid with a boiling point of 58.6°C. The blood:gas partition coefficient is 0.65, the oil:gas partition coefficient is 50, and the MAC is 2.1%. Sevoflurane reacts with desiccated carbon dioxide adsorbents, to produce compounds (A and B) with known toxicity (Fig. 22.4). The type of CO_2 absorbent used, the temperature of the absorbent, and the duration of exposure can influence the degree to which sevoflurane breaks down.[25] The major breakdown product, compound A, pentafluoroisopropenyl fluoromethyl ether, (PIFE, $C_4H_2F_6O$) has been studied extensively.[25] Compound A is nephrotoxic in rats and nonhuman primates and remains a theoretical risk to humans.[26–28] As discussed previously under the stability of inhaled anesthetics, sevoflurane breakdown by CO_2 absorbents generates heat and has resulted in sporadic operating room fires.[5,29]

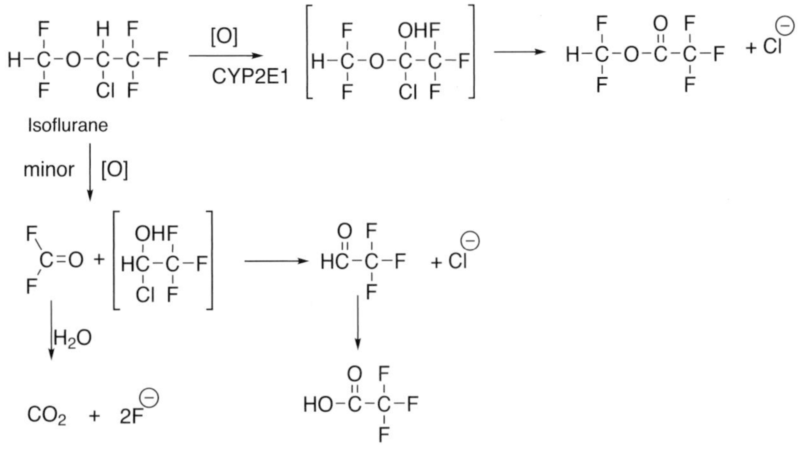

Figure 22.3 ● Isoflurane metabolism.

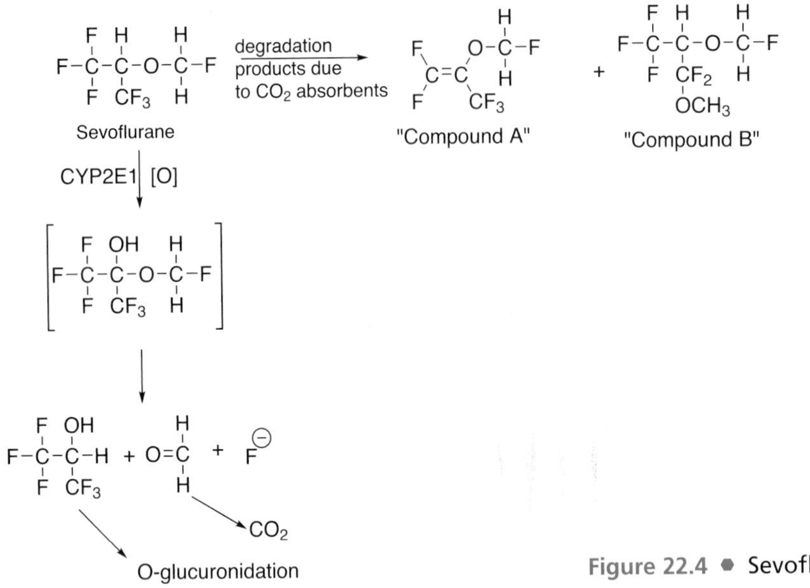

Figure 22.4 • Sevoflurane metabolism and chemical instability.

Approximately 5% to 8% of the administered dose of sevoflurane is metabolized in man by CYP2E1 to hexafluoroisopropanol, CO_2 and the potentially nephrotoxic fluoride ion. (Fig. 22.4).[27,30,31] Patients should be monitored for increases in blood urea nitrogen (BUN) and creatine levels as high fluoride ion levels, and concerns about Compound A exposure, may induce renal toxicity. Sevoflurane has been studied in a small number of patients with preexisting renal insufficiency (creatine >1.5 mg/dL). Creatinine levels increased in 7% of renally impaired patients and the manufacturer recommends that it be used with caution in this patient population.[32] To reduce the potential toxicity in humans the use of sevoflurane should be limited to less than 2 MAC hours.[17]

Sevoflurane has been shown to cause epileptic changes on EEGs and case reports of seizures during surgery, especially in children, have been reported.[33]

XENON

Xenon is an inert gas that is nonflammable and nonexplosive. The outer shell of xenon is complete thus it is not a highly reactive compound neither seeking, nor donating electrons to biological molecules. Despite its "inert" status, xenon has been shown to interact with biological molecules by forming an induced dipole in the presence of a cationic site.[34] An induced dipole could also result from an interaction with another fleeting dipole formed at the proposed binding site to form an induced dipole-induced dipole or London dispersion force.[35] The mechanism of xenon anesthesia and the site of action are still unknown.

The low blood:gas partition coefficient (0.12) leads to quick onset and recovery, but the potency is low with an MAC of 71%. Xenon gas is produced in low quantities and presently is expensive to obtain. The low incidence of reported side effects, lack of environmental concerns (it will not contribute to the destruction of the ozone layer), and absence of metabolites makes xenon an interesting anesthetic for development.[36,37] Xenon is being tested in Japan and Europe presently and if a closed system anesthetic circulator is developed that can recapture the exhaled xenon the fiscal concerns may lesson. Patents have been awarded in the United States for xenon anesthetic equipment.

THE INJECTABLE GENERAL ANESTHETICS

General anesthesia includes the use of the inhalation anesthetics covered previously in this chapter and many intravenous drugs used during surgical procedures. The reader is referred to other chapters in this textbook for information on the benzodiazepines (Chapter 12), the barbiturates (Chapter 12), and the neuromuscular blockers (Chapter 17). Three additional drugs will be covered here that are solely used for their anesthetic effects: propofol, etomidate, and ketamine.

Propofol

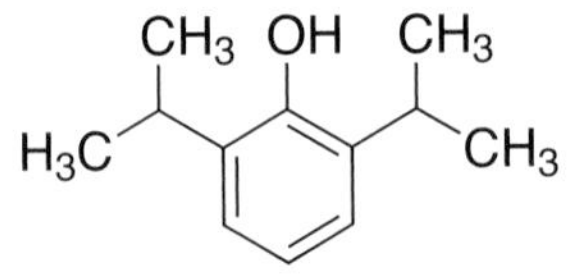

Propofol

Propofol is an injectable sedative–hypnotic used for the induction and maintenance of anesthesia or sedation. Propofol is only slightly soluble in water with an octanol/water partition coefficient of 6,761:1; thus, it is formulated as an oil-in-water emulsion. The fat component of the emulsion consists of soybean oil, glycerol, and egg lecithin. The pK_a of the propanol hydroxyl is 11 and the injectable emulsion has a pH of 7 to 8.5. Formulations contain either disodium ethylenediaminetetraacetic acid (EDTA) (0.005%) or sodium metabisulfite to retard the growth of microorganisms. EDTA is a metal chelator and patients on propofol containing EDTA for extended periods of time excrete more zinc and iron in their urine.[38] The clinical consequence of this is not known but the manufacturer recommends that a drug holiday or zinc supplementation be considered after 5 days of therapy.[39] Generic formulations of propofol may contain sodium metabisulfite as the antimicrobial agent, and patients allergic to sulfites, especially asthmatic patients, should avoid this formulation.[40] Aseptic technique must be followed and unused portions of the drug must be discarded according to the

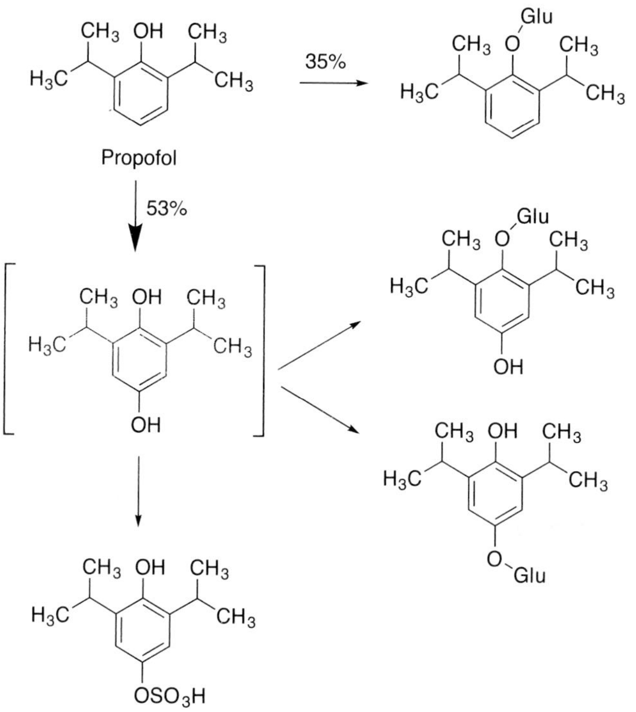

Figure 22.5 ● Metabolism of propofol.

manufacturer's instructions to prevent microbial contamination and possible sepsis.

Although unrelated chemically to the inhaled anesthetics, propofol has been shown to be a positive modulator of the $GABA_A$ receptor. The binding site on $GABA_A$ is distinct from the benzodiazepine binding site, and propofol binding is not inhibited by the benzodiazepine antagonist flumazenil.[41] The propofol binding site is believed to be on the β subunit. Propofol also directly activates Cl currents at glycine receptors, the predominant spinal inhibitory receptor. Unlike many volatile general anesthetics, propofol does not enhance the function of serotonin 5-HT_3 receptors and this may explain its low incidence of postoperative nausea and vomiting.[42] Propofol shows no analgesic properties, but it does not increase sensitivity to pain like some barbiturates.[43] Propofol causes a dose-dependent decrease in blood pressure and heart rate and a threefold to fourfold increase in serum triglyceride concentrations after 7 days of administration.[40]

Propofol is quickly and extensively metabolized with 88% of a ^{14}C-labelled intravenous administered dose appearing in the urine as conjugates. Less than 2% of the dose is found unchanged in the feces and less than 0.3% found unchanged in the urine (Fig 22.5). Thirty minutes after the ^{14}C-labelled dose was administered, 81% of the radioactivity was in the form of metabolites.[43] Propofol has a quick onset of action (arm-to-brain circulation time) and a quick recovery time.

Etomidate

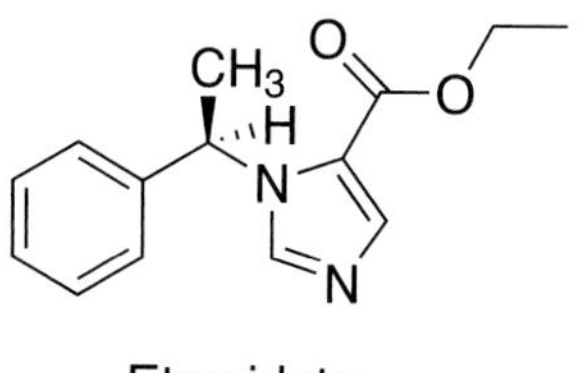

Etomidate

Etomidate is a carboxylated imidazole intended for the induction of general anesthesia. It is marketed as the more potent R (+) isomer. It is believed to exert its anesthetic effect via positive modulation of the $GABA_A$ receptor.[44] It is not water soluble and is available in the United States as a 2-mg/mL solution containing 35% v/v propylene glycol and in Europe as a soybean oil and medium-chain triglycerides formulation.[45,46] The propylene glycol has been associated with moderate-to-severe pain on injection and irritation of the vascular tissue.[46] A high incidence of skeletal muscle movements were noted in about 32% of patients following etomidate injection. Case reports of seizures are also found in the literature.[47] Administration of etomidate has little effect on cardiac output, peripheral, or pulmonary circulation. Studies have found that etomidate, even after a single dose, reduces plasma cortisol and aldosterone levels. Etomidate should not be used in patients with severe sepsis as the adrenal insufficiency has been shown to increase the risk of death in these patients.[48] This is probably a result of the inhibition of the 11 β-hydroxylase enzyme. Etomidate should only be used for induction of anesthesia when the cardiac benefits outweigh the risks associated with adrenal insufficiency.

Etomidate is quickly distributed throughout most organs in the body after intravenous administration and the tissue concentrations equal and sometimes exceed the plasma concentrations. The lipid solubility of the drug allows it to rapidly penetrate into the brain with peak concentrations occurring within 1 minute of administration. Etomidate is rapidly metabolized in the plasma and liver via esterases. About 75% of the drug is eliminated in the urine as the inactive ester hydrolyzed carboxylic acid.[49]

Ketamine

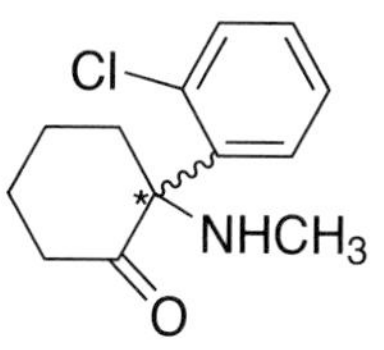

Ketamine

Ketamine is formulated as an acidic solution, pH 3.5 to 5.5, available with or without 0.1 mg/mL benzethonium chloride preservative. Ketamine is marketed as the racemic mixt⁻ and some properties of the individual isomers have elucidated.[50] Ketamine is a rapid-acting agent that ca. used for induction, used as the sole agent for general anesthesia or combined with other agents. Unlike the proposed mechanism of action for most anesthetics, ketamine does not act at the $GABA_A$ receptor. Ketamine acts as a noncompetitive antagonist at the glutamate, NMDA receptor, a nonspecific ion channel receptor. The NMDA receptor is located throughout the brain and contains four well-studied binding sites. The primary binding site binds L-glutamate, NMDA, and aspartate. The allosteric site binds glycine, which facilitates primary ligand binding. There is also a magnesium binding site that blocks ion flow through the channel and a phencyclidine (PCP) binding site that blocks the ion channel when occupied. Ketamine is believed to bind to the PCP site in a stereoselective manner and block the ion flow in the channel.[51] By blocking the flow of calcium ions into the cell, ketamine prevents the calcium

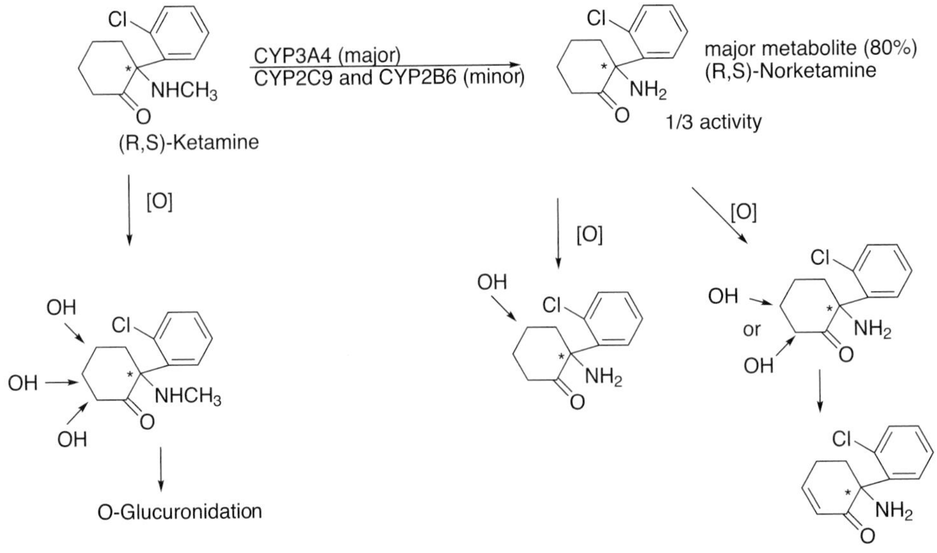

Figure 22.6 ● Metabolism of ketamine.

concentration from building and triggering excitatory synaptic transmissions in the brain and spinal cord.

Ketamine causes a transient increase in blood pressure after administration and is contraindicated in patients whom a significant elevation of blood pressure would constitute a serious hazard. Ketamine has also been found to bind to mu, delta, and kappa opioid receptors as well as the sigma receptors. The S(+) ketamine is two to three times more potent than the R(−) ketamine as an analgesic.[51] Ketamine has different effects at different doses on the opioid receptors and the use of ketamine as a postoperative analgesic or for chronic pain requires more study.[52,53]

Ketamine is classified as a "dissociative anesthetic," and psychological manifestations during emergence of anesthesia occur in 12% of patients. These vary from pleasant dreamlike states to vivid hallucinations and delirium. The duration is usually for only a few hours but patients have reported recurrences taking place up to 24 hours postoperatively. The incidence of this appears to be less in children younger than 16 years of age and in patients older than 65 years of age. Like other dissociative anesthetics, ketamine is abused for its hallucinatory effects. Most of the illegally used ketamine comes from stolen legitimate sources, particularly from veterinary clinics or smuggled in from Mexico.[54]

Ketamine is metabolized via *N*-demethylation to form the main metabolite norketamine. Norketamine has about one third the potency of the parent compound. Minor meta-bolic pathways include hydroxylation of the cyclohexanone ring; hydroxylation followed by glucuronide conjugation, and hydroxylation followed by dehydration to the cyclohexenone derivative (Fig. 22.6).[55,56]

THE LOCAL ANESTHETICS

Drugs classified as local anesthetics inhibit the conduction of action potentials in all afferent and efferent nerve fibers. Thus, pain and other sensations are not transmitted effectively to the brain, and motor impulses are not transmitted effectively to muscles. Local anesthetics have various clinical uses to treat acute or chronic pain or to prevent the sensation of pain during procedures. To understand the mechanism of action of the local anesthetics, an introduction to the physiology of nerve fibers and the transmission of pain sensation is briefly discussed below.

Physiology of Nerve Fibers and Neurotransmission

The nervous system functions to receive stimulation and transmit stimulus via the nerve cells or neurons. A neuron is a single cell typically composed of a cell body connected via an axon to the axon terminal (Fig. 22.7). The axon terminal is the presynaptic component of the nerve synapse and may contain neurotransmitters ready to be released upon receiving an action potential "message". The axon

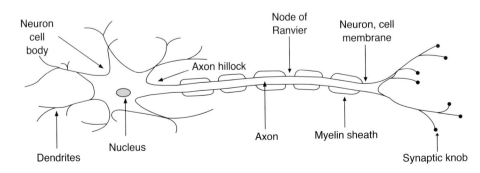

Figure 22.7 ● Schematic diagram of a neuron. Representation of the various branching found in dendrites.

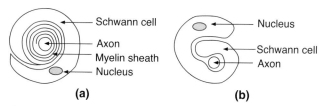

Figure 22.8 ● Representations of myelinated **(A)** and unmyelinated **(B)** axons.

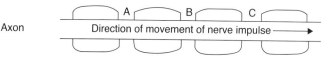

Figure 22.9 ● Representation of the transmission of a nerve impulse along a neuron fiber by saltatory conduction.

varies in length from a few millimeters to a meter or longer. Most axons are too long to transmit the signal to the terminal ending by simple chemical diffusion. Thus, the message received by the neuron cell body is transmitted as an electrical impulse to the axon terminal. The electrical impulse is most often generated at the axon hillock, the region of the cell body where the axon emerges. The electrical impulse is conducted by changes in the electrical potential across the neural membrane. The rate at which the message is transmitted down the axon depends on the thickness of the axon and the presence or absence of myelin. The axon may be bare or it may be surrounded by the membrane of a glial cell that forms a myelin sheath (Fig. 22.8). Between the myelin sheaths are areas of the axonal membrane that are unmyelinated, these bare areas are called the nodes of Ranvier. The nodes of Ranvier allow the nerve impulse to skip from node to node down the length of the axon to increase the speed of the action potential conduction (Fig. 22.9). In unmyelinated neurons, the change in the electrical potential of one part of the membrane causes a change in electrical potential of the adjacent membrane, thus the impulse moves along the axon slower. Nerve impulses travel at speeds of up to 120 m/s in myelinated axons and 10 m/s in unmyelinated axons.

The electrical potential difference between the inner and outer surfaces of the cell membrane is a result of the movement of ions across the membrane. At rest, most neurons have a resting potential of about −70 mV. This means that the inside of the neuron contains more anionic charges than the external side. The ions that move across the nerve membrane and contribute to most of the electrochemical potential are Ca^{2+}, Na^+, K^+, and Cl^-. For a nerve cell to transmit an impulse, the internal charge must increase about 20 mV to −50 mV, the firing threshold for a nerve cell. If this initial depolarization reaches the firing threshold, an action potential will be generated. During an action potential the internal charge will quickly increase to about +35 mV and the membrane is now *depolarized*. This spike is quickly followed by the *hyperpolarization* of the membrane, to

below −70 mV, followed by the return of the membrane to the resting potential (Fig. 22.10). The generation of the action potential from the axon hillock to the terminal end of the nerve may result in the release of neurotransmitters that cross the synaptic cleft to deliver the "message" to the adjacent neuron or target organ.

Neuronal Membrane Ion Permeability During an Action Potential

By definition, the membrane potential is the difference in the polarity of the inside of the cell compared to the outside of the cell, with the outside of the cell conventionally set at 0 mV. During an action potential, the membrane potential changes from a −70 to a +35 mV. Exactly how does a membrane change its electrical potential? It changes its potential by the movement of ions. For an ion to move from one side of the lipophilic membrane to the other, it must go through a channel. There are many specialized protein channels that can change their three-dimensional configuration to allow ions to flow through. If the ion is moving with its concentration gradient, it can simply diffuse through an open channel, no energy would be required. For an ion to move against the electrical gradient, energy is required and the channels are therefore coupled to ATP pumps.

The axolemma is more permeable to K^+ ions than to Na^+ ions. These ions diffuse out of the neuron through the so-called *potassium leak channels*, whose opening does not appear to require a specific membrane change. The movement of K^+ ions is concentration driven; K^+ ions move from inside the neuron, where the concentration is high, to the extracellular fluid, where the concentration is lower. This tendency of K^+ ions to leak out of the neuron (*driven by the concentration gradient*) is balanced to some extent by a limited movement of K^+ ions back into the neuron, both by diffusion through K^+ channels and by active transport mechanisms such as the sodium/potassium ATPase pump. These movements of K^+ result in a potential difference across the membrane, which is a major contributor to the *equilibrium potential* that exists between the opposite faces

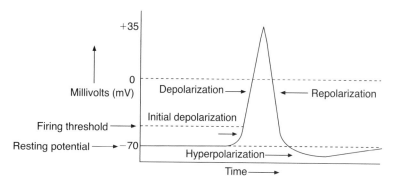

Figure 22.10 ● Changes in electrical potential observed during a nerve impulse.

of a biological membrane in a normal cell at rest with a switched-on sodium pump.

The initial depolarization of the neuron (Fig. 22.10) was shown by Hodgkin and Huxley in 1953 to be a result of increased movement of Na^+ into the neuron, which is followed almost immediately by increased movement of K^+ ions out of the neuron. It is thought that the action potential is triggered by a stimulation that causes a momentary shift of the membrane potential of a small section of the membrane to a less negative value (*depolarization of the membrane*). This causes the gated Na^+ channels in this section of the membrane to open, which allows Na^+ to enter the cell. This process depolarizes the membrane still further, until the action potential reaches a critical value (the *firing threshold*), when it triggers the opening of large numbers of adjacent Na^+ channels so that Na^+ ions flood into the axon. This process continues until the membrane potential of this section of membrane reaches the equilibrium potential for Na^+ ions when the cell is at rest. At this point, all the Na^+ channels of the membrane should be permanently open. This situation is not reached, however, because each channel has an automatic closing mechanism that operates even though the cell membrane is still depolarized. Once closed, the ion channel cannot open again until the membrane potential in its vicinity returns to its original negative value, which is brought about by the leakage of K^+ ions out of the neuron through K^+ channels. Hodgkin and Huxley showed that a membrane becomes more permeable to K^+ ions, a fraction of a millisecond after the Na^+ channels have started to open. As a result, K^+ ions flow out of the neuron, which reduces the electrical potential of the membrane, and so at the peak of the action potential, the membrane potential has a value of about $+40$ mV. The movement of the K^+ ions out of the axon, coupled with the automatic closing of the sodium channel gates and the slower action of the sodium/potassium ATPase pump that transports 3 Na^+ ions out of the neuron for every 2 K^+ ions into the neuron, results in a net flow of positive ions out of the neuron. This briefly *hyperpolarizes* the membrane and causes the membrane potential to drop below its resting potential. As the sodium channels close and K^+ ions flow back into the axon, the membrane potential returns to its resting value. The entire process of depolarization and repolarization is normally accomplished within 1 millisecond.

Ligand-Gated Sodium Channel Structure and Function

Based on mutation studies and electrophysiology studies, a three-dimensional picture relating the structure of the sodium channel to its function is emerging. The sodium channel is a complicated protein with multiple polypeptide sections that are responsible for specific functions of the channel. The channel must (a) be selective for sodium ions, (b) be able to detect and then open when the membrane is slightly depolarized, (c) be able to detect and then close when the membrane becomes hyperpolarized, and (d) convert to a resting state ready to depolarize again. There is much work currently being conducted on all of these functions of the sodium channel.

The mammalian brain sodium channel is comprised of an α subunit and one or more auxiliary β subunits (Figs.

22.11–22.12). The α subunit is composed of four domains (DI–DIV) that fold to make the pore that the sodium ions pass through. Each of the four domains is composed of six transmembrane α-helical segments (S1–S6). The β subunits are involved in the kinetics and voltage dependence of sodium channel opening and closing. The β subunits have large extracellular domains with many sites of glycosylation and only one transmembrane segment.[57]

The sodium channel contains specific amino acids that act as a *selectivity filter*, only allowing sodium ions to pass through the channel. The amino acids that make up the selectivity filter of an ion channel are referred to as the P region. Sodium channels have a P region that gives specificity to sodium ions, whereas potassium and calcium channels have their own P regions that confer selectivity for their respective ions. The selectivity filter of the sodium channel is composed of two rings made up of amino acids from the four homologous domains (DI–DIV). The first ring is composed entirely of negatively charged amino acids. Approximately two to three amino acids deeper into the pore, the second ring is found. The second ring of the P region of the sodium channel is composed of the amino acid sequence DEKA (Asp Glu Lys Ala), whereas the P region of a calcium channel is EEEE (Glu Glu Glu Glu).[58] By selectively mutating the four amino acids from DEKA to EEEE, selectivity for calcium could be conferred to the sodium channels.[59] Other studies also showed that when external solutions where made highly acidic the negative charges of the selectivity filter amino acids could be neutralized ($COO^- \rightarrow COOH$) and ion conductivity decreased.[58]

The sodium channel must also be able to change conformations in response to small changes in the membrane potential. How do sodium channels detect voltage changes and then change shape in response to them? The voltage sensing units of the sodium channels are the S4 segments of the α subunit. These segments contain positively charged amino acids at every third residue. It is postulated that the S4 segments move in response to the change in the local membrane potential and cause a further conformational change that opens the gate of the sodium channel, thus allowing sodium to flow in.[60] The S4 voltage sensors are also responsible for causing conformational changes in the receptor that close the channel to sodium conductance. Exactly how the conformational changes occur is being studied (Fig. 22.12).

Further down the pore of the sodium channel, beyond the selectivity filter lays the putative *local anesthetic binding site* (Fig. 22.13). Site directed mutagenesis studies and molecular modeling studies suggest that local anesthetic binding involves multiple interactions. The positively charged nitrogen of the local anesthetic molecule may form a cation $-\pi$ electron interaction with a phenylalanine residue from the DIVS6 domain.[61,62] The aromatic ring of the anesthetic may also interact with a tyrosine amino acid in the DIVS6 domain. The putative local anesthetic binding site is believed to involve the S6 subunits of the α DI, DIII, and DIV domains. The exact amino acids involved depend on the source and the state of the sodium channel being studied. These studies also suggest that the positively charged nitrogen of the local anesthetic may lie in the center of the pore to create an electrostatic repulsive force that, in addition to the steric block, would prevent sodium ion passage through the pore (Fig. 22.13).[57]

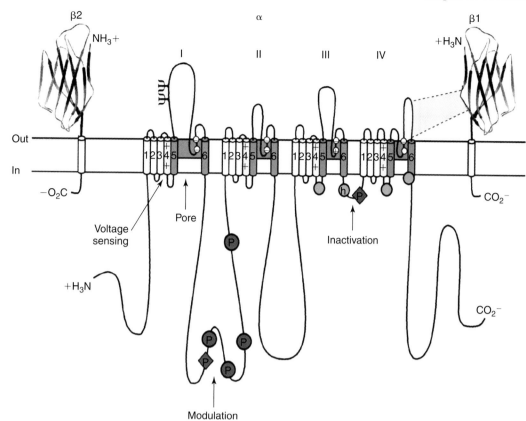

Figure 22.11 ● Structure of voltage-gated sodium channels. Schematic representation of the sodium-channel subunits. The α subunit of the Na$_v$1.2 channel is illustrated together with the β1 and β2 subunits; the extracellular domains of the β subunits are shown as immunoglobulin-like folds, which interact with the loops in the α subunits as shown. Roman numerals indicate the domains of the α subunit; segments 5 and 6 (*dark gray*) are the pore-lining segments and the S4 helices (*light gray*) make up the voltage sensors. Light gray circles in the intracellular loops of domains III and IV indicate the inactivation gate IFM motif and its receptor (h, inactivation gate); P, phosphorylation sites, in dark gray circles, sites for protein kinase A; in dark gray diamonds, sites for protein kinase C; ψ, probable *N*-linked glycosylation site. The circles in the re-entrant loops in each domain represent the amino acids that form the ion selectivity filter (the outer rings have the sequence EEDD and inner rings DEKA). (Reprinted from Catterall, W. A.: Ionic currents to molecular mechanisms: the structure and function of voltage-gated sodium channels. Neuron 26:13–25, 2000, with permission from Elsevier.)

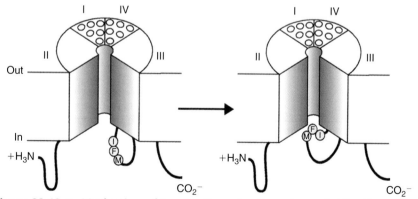

Figure 22.12 ● Mechanism of inactivation of sodium channels. The hinged-lid mechanism. The intracellular loop connecting domains III and IV of the sodium channel is depicted as forming a hinged lid with the critical phenylalanine (F1489) within the IFM motif shown occluding the mouth of the pore during the inactivation process. The circles represent the transmembrane helices. (Reprinted from Catterall, W. A.: Ionic currents to molecular mechanisms: the structure and function of voltage-gated sodium channels. Neuron, 26:13–25, 2000, with permission from Elsevier.)

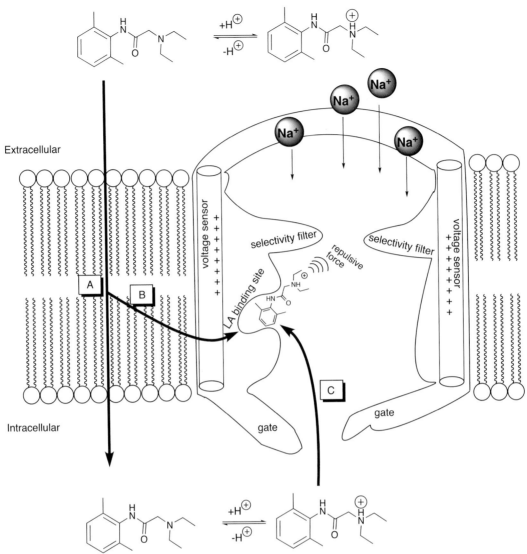

Figure 22.13 • Proposed mechanism of action of the local anesthetics:
(A) Hydrophobic pathway into the nerve cell, **(B)** Hydrophobic pathway to the binding site, **(C)** Hydrophilic pathway from the inside of the nerve cell to the binding site. (Adapted with permission from Hille, B.: Local anesthetics: hydrophilic and hydrophobic pathways for the drug-receptor reaction. J. Gen. Physiol. 69:497–515, 1977 and Strichartz, G., et al.: Fundamental properties of local anesthetics. II. Measured octanol: buffer partition coefficients and pK$_a$ values of clinically used drugs. Anesth. Analg. 71:158–170, 1990.)

Mechanism of Action of Local Anesthetics

The mechanism of action of the local anesthetics is believed to be via their sodium channel blocking effects. The local anesthetic drug binds to the channel in an area just beyond the selectivity filter or P region (Fig. 22.13). When the local anesthetic binds, it blocks sodium ion passage into the cell and thus blocks the formation and propagation of the action potential. This blocks the transmittance of the message of "pain" or even "touch" from getting to the brain. The ability of a local anesthetic to block action potentials depends on the ability of the drug to penetrate the tissue surrounding the targeted nerve as well as the ability of the drug to access the binding site on the sodium channel.

Local anesthetics do not access the binding site by entering into the sodium channel from the exterior of the neuron. The molecules are too big to pass by the selectivity filter. When local anesthetics are synthesized with a permanent charge, such as compound QX-314 below, they are unable to access the binding site unless they are applied directly to the interior of the neuron.[63] (For more information on QX-314 see "Future Directions," at the end of this chapter.)

QX-314

If local anesthetics do not access the binding site via the external side, how do they get to their site of action? There is much experimental evidence to show that local anesthetics must access the binding site via a hydrophobic or via a hydrophilic pathway (Fig. 22.13).[64,65] The anesthetics pass through the membrane in their uncharged form (Fig. 22.13 hydrophobic pathway A). In the axoplasm, they reequilibrate with their cationic species. It is postulated that the anesthetic molecule may access the binding site via a hydrophilic pathway by entering into the sodium channel from the interior of the pore, when the channel is open (Fig. 22.13 hydrophilic pathway C). The local anesthetic molecule is believed to bind to the binding site in its ionized form. Another possibility is that before passing all the way through the lipid membrane, the anesthetic may be able to directly access the local anesthetic binding site (Fig. 22.13 hydrophobic pathway B).

Studies using local anesthetics containing a tertiary nitrogen also confirm that the local anesthetic is accessing the binding site from either the hydrophobic or hydrophilic pathways described previously. When this type of anesthetic is applied externally, and the pH of the external media is increased, and thus the local anesthetic is predominantly in the unionized form, the onset of block is more rapid. The neutral form of the drug molecule penetrates the membrane and then accesses the binding site through pathway B or C described in Figure 22.13. The pH of the solution had no effect on sodium conduction block when the local anesthetic used was the neutral molecule benzocaine, suggesting that the change in pH affects the drug charge and not the receptor.[63,66]

The sodium channel has been shown to have a great deal of flexibility and can change shape when the electrical environment around the channel changes. There are at least three conformations that the sodium channel can form. (a) An open state, such as that depicted in Figure 22.12 (drawing on the left) where the sodium ion has a clear pathway from the external side of the membrane to the internal side of the membrane. (b) A "closed/inactive" state shown in Figure 22.12 (drawing on the right), where the sodium channel undergoes a conformational change to prevent sodium ion passage into the cell. The sodium channel undergoes this conformational change in response to the huge influx of sodium causing depolarization of the cell membrane. The sodium channel is now closed and inactive, it cannot open again until the membrane has reached its resting potential. (c) The third conformation of the sodium channel is formed when the membrane potential returns to the resting potential. The sodium channel is now closed but able to open when a stimulus reaches the threshold potential. At this point, the sodium channel is in a "closed/resting" state that is different from the "closed/inactive" state.

The affinity of the local anesthetics for the binding site has complex voltage and frequency dependant relationships. Affinity depends on what state the sodium channel is in as well as the specific drug being tested. In general, at resting states, when the membrane is hyperpolarized, the local anesthetics bind with low affinity. When the membrane has been depolarized and the channel is open, local anesthetics bind with high affinity. Local anesthetics also bind with high affinities when the sodium channel is in the "closed/inactive" conformation, perhaps stabilizing the inactive form of the receptor.

The ability of the local anesthetic to block conduction also depends on the targeted neuron. In general, autonomic fibers, small unmyelinated C fibers (mediating pain sensations), and small myelinated Aγ fibers (mediating pain and temperature sensations) are blocked before the larger myelinated Aγ, Aβ, and Aα fibers (mediating postural, touch, pressure, and motor information).[67]

SARs of Local Anesthetics

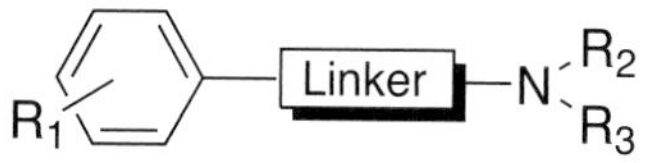

The structure of most local anesthetic agents consists of three parts as shown above. They contain (a) a lipophilic ring that may be substituted, (b) a linker of various lengths that usually contains either an ester or an amide, and (c) an amine group that is usually a tertiary amine with a pK_a between 7.5 and 9.0.

1. *The Aromatic Ring*
   The aromatic ring adds lipophilicity to the anesthetic and helps the molecule penetrate through biological membranes. It is also thought to have direct contact with the local anesthetic binding site on the sodium channel. The exact amino acids involved in binding depend on the sodium channel being studied as well as the state (open, closed/inactive, closed/active) of the sodium channel. The aromatic ring is believed to interact with the local anesthetic binding site in a π–π interaction or a π-cation interaction with the S6 domain of the α component of the sodium channel. Substituents on the aromatic ring may increase the lipophilic nature of the aromatic ring. An SAR study of para substituted ester type local anesthetics showed that lipophilic substituents and electron-donating substituents in the para position increased anesthetic activity.[68] The lipophilic substituents are thought to both increase the ability of the molecule to penetrate the nerve membrane and increase their affinity at the receptor site. Buchi and Perlia suggested that the electron-donating groups on the aromatic ring created a resonance effect between the carbonyl group and the ring, resulting in the shift of electrons from the ring to the carbonyl oxygen. As the electronic cloud around the oxygen increased, so did the affinity of the molecule with the receptor (Fig. 22.14).[69] When the aromatic ring was substituted with an electron-withdrawing group, the electron cloud around the carbonyl oxygen decreased and the anesthetic activity decreased as well.

2. *The Linker*
   The linker is usually an ester or an amide group along with a hydrophobic chain of various lengths. In general, when the number of carbon atoms in the linker is increased, the lipid solubility, protein binding, duration of action, and toxicity increases.[70] Esters and amides are bioisosteres having similar sizes, shapes, and electronic structures. The similarity in their structures means that esters and amides have similar binding properties and usually differ only in their stability in vivo and in vitro. For molecules that only differ at the linker functional groups, amides are more stable than esters and thus have longer half-lives than esters. Plasma protein binding may

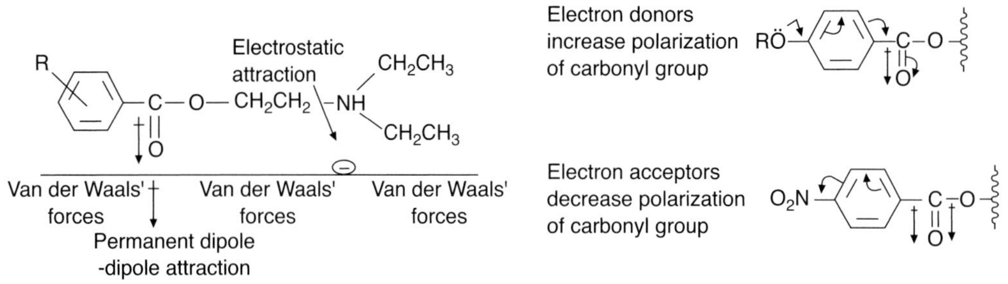

Figure 22.14 ● Schematic representation of the binding of an ester-type local anesthetic agent to a receptor site. (Reprinted with permission from Buchi, J., Perlia, X.: Design of local anesthetics. In Ariens, E. J. [ed.] Drug Design. New York, Academic Press, 1972, Vol. 3, p. 243.)

be more prevalent for the amide anesthetics as well, contributing to the increased half-life.[71] Individual drugs are discussed in the drug monograph section.

As described previously, the nature of the substituents on the aromatic ring can affect the electronic nature of the linker and can contribute to the drug's potency and stability. Substituents on the aromatic ring may also confer a steric block to protect the linker from metabolism. Thus, the binding affinity and stability of the anesthetic molecule is affected by the linker as well as the functional groups on the aromatic ring. In general, ester groups are more susceptible to hydrolysis than amide functional groups because of the prevalence of esterases in the blood and the liver. The first ester type local anesthetic synthesized was procaine (Novocain) in 1905. Procaine metabolism can be seen in Figure 22.15. The para-aminobenzoic acid (PABA) metabolite, common to the ester class of drugs, is believed to be responsible for the allergic reactions some patients have experienced with local anesthetics.[72]

3. *The Nitrogen*

Most local anesthetics contain a tertiary nitrogen with a pK_a between 7.5 and 9.5. Therefore, at physiological pH, both the cationic and neutral form of the molecule exists. At physiological pH, the ionized to unionized form of the anesthetic can be calculated using the Henderson-Hasselbalch equation:

$$pH = pK_a + \log ([B]/[BH^+])$$

Extensive work using both internally and externally applied compounds, changing the pH of the solution, and using permanently charged anesthetic analogs has led to the present theory of anesthetic SARs. Namely, that the anesthetic compounds bind to the anesthetic receptor site on the sodium channel in the ionized form. From Figure 22.13, it can be seen that the molecule can penetrate the nerve membrane in its neutral form and then reequilibrate with its cationic form on the internal side of the membrane. Permanently charged, quaternary anesthetics applied to the

external side of the nerve membrane do not penetrate and cannot access the local anesthetic binding site.

To keep the anesthetic soluble in commercial solutions, most preparations are acidified. In an attempt to decrease pain on injection and to increase the onset of action, some practitioners advocate adding sodium bicarbonate to the commercial preparation. By adding sodium bicarbonate, the solution will become less acidic and more of the drug will be found in the neutral form. The neutral form will thus cross the nerve membrane quicker and have a quicker onset of action. Although this theoretically makes sense, many studies have found no difference in the onset of action between alkalinized and nonadjusted anesthetics. Manufacturers formulate solutions at a pH that gives them adequate shelf life. When the pH is increased, the stability of the preparation decreases and outright precipitation can occur if too much of the water-soluble cationic form is converted to the anesthetic base. If this practice is followed, very careful titration of the added base is required. The solution should be observed for precipitation and the solution must be used immediately.

Vasoconstrictors Used in Combination with Local Anesthetics

Many anesthetic preparations are commercially available combined with the vasoconstrictor epinephrine. Some anesthetics are also combined with other agents such as norepinephrine, phenylephrine, oxymetolazone, or clonidine to achieve a desired formulation. The epinephrine in the anesthetic solution has multiple purposes. As a vasoconstrictor, the injected epinephrine will constrict capillaries at the injection site and thus limit blood flow to the area. The local anesthetic will thus stay in the immediate area of injection longer and not be carried away to the general circulation. This will help keep the drug where it is needed and allow minimal drug to be absorbed systemically. Thus, anesthetics with epinephrine used for infiltration anesthesia consistently result in lower plasma levels of the anesthetic. This will reduce the systemic toxicity from the anesthetic and increase

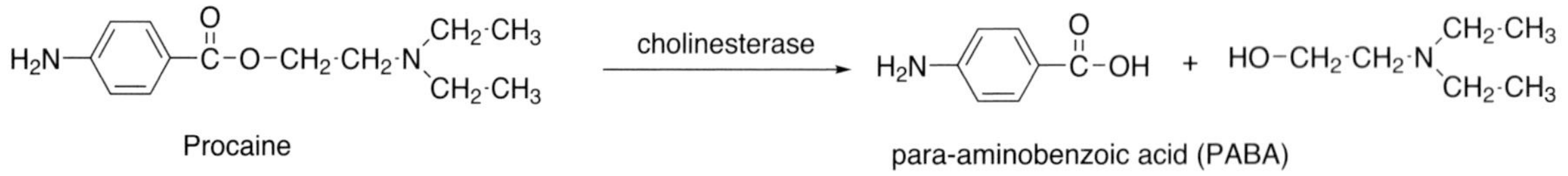

Figure 22.15 ● Metabolism of procaine.

the duration of anesthetic activity at the site of injection. The lack of blood flow in the immediate area will also decrease the presence of metabolizing enzymes and this also increase the duration of action of the anesthetic locally. The characteristic blanching that follows epinephrine infiltration anesthesia also makes suturing or manipulating the area easier because of the lack of blood flow in the area. It is not recommended that anesthetics with a vasoconstrictor be used in tissue served by end-arterial blood supply (fingers, toes, earlobes, etc.). This is to prevent ischemic injury or necrosis of the tissue. Epinephrine has also been shown to counteract the myocardial depressant effects of bupivacaine when added to a bupivacaine epidural solution.[73]

Allergic Reactions to Local Anesthetics

True allergic reactions to local anesthetics are very rare. Patients may be allergic to the anesthetic, a metabolite of the anesthetic or a preservative in the anesthetic. Allergies to the ester anesthetics are more common than allergies to the amide anesthetics. As discussed, the ester anesthetics may be metabolized to PABA, which is believed to be responsible for the allergic reactions (Fig. 22.15).

Although the amide type local anesthetics are not metabolized to PABA they may contain a paraben preservative that can be metabolized to PABA like compounds. Parabens are methyl, ethyl, propyl, and butyl aliphatic esters of PABA. In addition to parabens, anesthetics may be preserved with metabisulfites that are also known to cause allergic reactions in sensitive patients, especially patients with asthma.[74] Thus, patients that are allergic to ester type local anesthetics should receive a preservative free amide type anesthetic.

PABA also blocks the mechanism of action of the sulfonamide antibiotics. Sulfonamide antibiotics bind to and inhibit the action of the dihydropteroate synthetase enzyme, the enzyme bacteria used to convert PABA to folate. The inhibition of this enzyme is competitive, therefore if enough PABA is present it will compete with the antibiotic for the binding site on the enzyme and bacterial folate would be synthesized. Thus, there is at least a theoretical reason not to use a PABA forming anesthetic in a patient being treated with a sulfonamide antibiotic.

Methemoglobinemia

Cyanosis as a result of the formation of methemoglobinemia may occur after the administration of the local anesthetics lidocaine,[75] prilocaine,[76,77] and benzocaine.[78] When normal hemoglobin is oxidized by a drug or drug metabolite, it forms methemoglobin. Methemoglobin contains the oxidized form of iron, ferric iron (Fe^{3+}) rather than the reduced ferrous iron (Fe^{2+}) that hemoglobin contains. The oxidized iron cannot bind to oxygen, and methemoglobinemia results when the methemoglobin concentration in the blood reaches 10 to 20 g/L (6%–12% of the normal hemoglobin concentration). Cyanosis results and does not respond to treatment with 100% oxygen. Patients with increased risk factors for developing drug-induced methemoglobinemia include children younger than 2 years, anemic patients, those with a genetic deficiency of glucose-6-phosphate dehydrogenase or nicotinamide adenine dinucleotide methemoglobin reductase or those exposed to excessive doses of the causative local anesthetic. If clinical symptoms of methemoglobinemia occur, treatment is an intravenous infusion of a 1% methylene blue solution, 1 mg/kg body weight, over 5 minutes.

● LOCAL ANESTHETIC MONOGRAPHS, INDIVIDUAL PRODUCTS INCLUDING ADVERSE REACTIONS

The Ester Local Anesthetics

COCAINE

Cocaine

Cocaine was the first agent used for topical anesthesia. It was isolated from the coca leaves that native peoples of the Andes Mountains chew for multiple effects including local anesthesia and stimulant properties to ward off fatigue. Chemists working with the coca alkaloids noticed that the crystals could numb their tongues. In 1884, a German surgeon demonstrated the successful use of cocaine to anesthetize the cornea during eye surgery. One of the most prominent surgeons at Johns Hopkins University, Dr. William Halsted, read about this account and began investigations with cocaine for general surgery. They successfully used cocaine during surgery, but unfortunately Dr. Halsted and several colleagues became addicted.[79] Today, cocaine is used for topical anesthesia of mucous membranes using a 4% to 10% solution. If the solution remains on the membrane for 5 minutes, anesthesia and vasoconstriction of the area will occur. Cocaine has inherent vasoconstrictor properties thus requires no additional epinephrine. The toxicity of cocaine is a result of its vasoconstrictor properties and ability to inhibit catecholamine, including norepinephrine reuptake. Toxic manifestations include excitation, dysphoria, tremor, seizure activity, hypertension, tachycardia, myocardial ischemia, and infarction. Cocaine is used primarily for nasal surgeries, although its abuse potential has resulted in a decrease in use and a search for alternate anesthetics. When cocaine was compared with lidocaine/phenylephrine for nasal intubations, the results were the same with less toxicity in the lidocaine/phenylephrine group.[80]

PROCAINE

Procaine

Procaine was synthesized in 1904 to address the chemical instability of cocaine and the local irritation it produced. The

pK_a of procaine is 8.9; it has low lipid solubility and the ester group is unstable in basic solutions. Procaine is available in concentrations ranging from 0.25% to 10% with pHs adjusted to 5.5 to 6.0 for chemical stability. Procaine is also included in some formulations of penicillin G to decrease the pain of intramuscular injection. Procaine is very quickly metabolized in the plasma by cholinesterases and in the liver via ester hydrolysis by a pseudocholinesterase (Fig. 22.15). The in vitro elimination half-life is approximately 60 seconds. Any condition that decreases the cholinesterase concentration may increase exposure to procaine and potential toxicity. Decreased enzyme activity can be found with genetic deficiency, liver disease, malignancy, malnutrition, renal failure, burns, third trimester of pregnancy, and following cardiopulmonary bypass surgery. Ester hydrolysis produces PABA, the compound responsible for the allergic reactions common to the ester anesthetics. Procaine is not used topically because of its inability to pass through lipid membranes and finds use as an infiltration agent for cutaneous or mucous membranes, for short procedures. Procaine is also used for peripheral nerve block and as an epidural agent to diagnose pain syndromes.[73]

CHLOROPROCAINE

2-Chloroprocaine

The 2 chloride substitution on the aromatic ring of chloroprocaine is an electron-withdrawing functional group. Thus, it pulls the electron density from the carbonyl carbon into the ring. The carbonyl carbon is now a stronger electrophile and more susceptible to ester hydrolysis. Therefore, chloroprocaine has a more rapid metabolism than procaine. The in vitro plasma half-life is approximately 25 seconds. The 2-chloro-4-aminobenzoic acid metabolite precludes this from being used in patients allergic to PABA. The very short duration of action means that this drug can be used in large doses for conduction block (with rapid onset and short duration of action.) As with procaine, a decrease in the plasma cholinesterase activity will prolong the half-life. The pK_a of the chloroprocaine alkyl amine is 9.0 and thus chloroprocaine is almost exclusively ionized at physiological pH. Chloroprocaine is formulated with a pH between 2.5 and 4.0 using hydrochloric acid. The acidic pH of the formulation is responsible for considerable irritation and pain on injection.

Chloroprocaine is used for cutaneous or mucous membrane infiltration for surgical procedures, epidural anesthesia (without preservatives) and for peripheral conduction block.

TETRACAINE

Tetracaine

Tetracaine was developed to address the low potency and short duration of action of procaine and chloroprocaine. The addition of the butyl side chain on the para nitrogen increases the lipid solubility of the drug and enhances the topical potency of tetracaine. The plasma half-life is 120 to 150 seconds. Topically applied tetracaine to unbroken skin requires 30 to 45 minutes to confer topical anesthesia. Tetracaine 4% gel is superior than eutectic mixture with lidocaine (EMLA) (an emulsion of lidocaine and prilocaine) in preventing pain associated with needle procedures in children.[81] Tetracaine metabolism is similar to procaine ester metabolism yielding parabutylaminobenzoic acid and dimethylaminoethanol and conjugates excreted in the urine. The pK_a of the dimethylated nitrogen is 8.4 and tetracaine is formulated as a hydrochloride salt with a pH of 3.5 to 6.0. The increased absorption from topical sites has resulted in reported toxicity. Overdoses of tetracaine may produce central nervous system (CNS) toxicity and seizure activity with fatalities from circulatory depression reported.[82] No selective cardiac toxicity is seen with tetracaine although hypotension has been reported. Tetracaine is employed for infiltration anesthesia, spinal anesthesia, or topical use.

BENZOCAINE

Benzocaine

Benzocaine is a unique local anesthetic because it does not contain a tertiary amine. The pK_a of the aromatic amine is 3.5 ensuring that benzocaine is uncharged at physiological pH. Because it is uncharged, it is not water soluble but is ideal for topical applications. The onset of action is within 30 seconds and the duration of drug action is 10 to 15 minutes. Benzocaine is used for endoscopy, bronchoscopy, and topical anesthesia. Benzocaine is available as a 20% solution topical spray, in a 1% gel for mucous membrane application, and a 14% glycerin suspension for topical use in the outer ear.

Toxicity to benzocaine can occur when the topical dose exceeds 200 to 300 mg resulting in methemoglobinemia. Infants and children are more susceptible to this and methemoglobinemia has been reported after benzocaine lubrication of endotracheal tubes and after topical administration to treat a painful diaper rash.[83,84]

The Amino Amide Local Anesthetics

LIDOCAINE

Lidocaine

Lidocaine was the first amino amide synthesized in 1948 and has become the most widely used local anesthetic. The tertiary amine has a pK_a of 7.8 and it is formulated as the hydrochloride salt with a pH between 5.0 and 5.5. When lidocaine is formulated premixed with epinephrine the pH of the solution is adjusted to between 2.0 and 2.5 to prevent

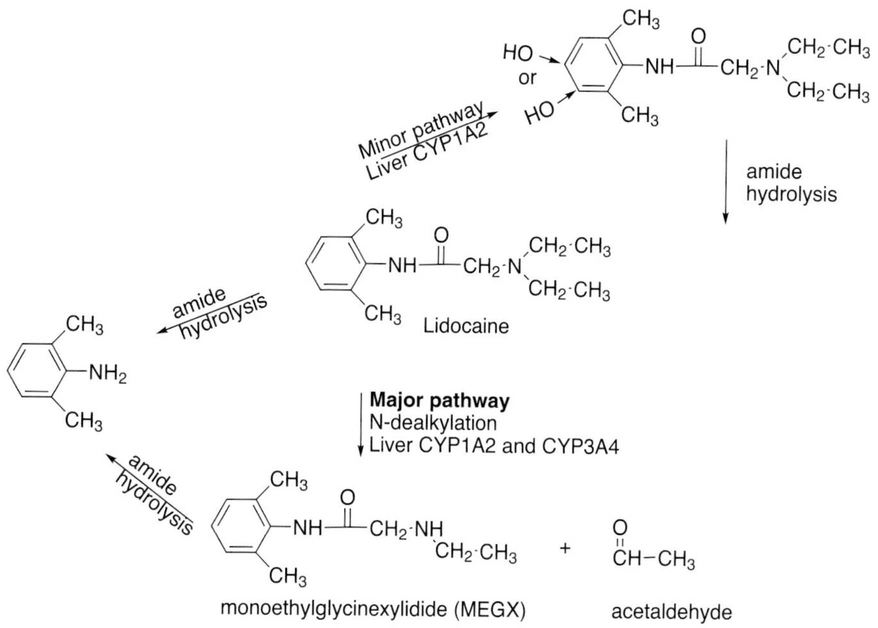

Figure 22.16 ● Metabolism of lidocaine.

the hydrolysis of the epinephrine. Lidocaine is also available with or without preservatives. Some formulations of lidocaine contain a methylparaben preservative that may cause allergic reactions in PABA-sensitive individuals. The low pK$_a$ and medium water solubility provide intermediate duration of topical anesthesia of mucous membranes. Lidocaine can also be used for infiltration, peripheral nerve and plexus blockade, and epidural anesthesia.

The metabolism of lidocaine is typical of the amino amide anesthetics and is shown in Figure 22.16. The liver is responsible for most of the metabolism of lidocaine and any decrease in liver function will decrease metabolism. Lidocaine is primarily metabolized by de-ethylation of the tertiary nitrogen to form monoethylglycinexylidide (MEGX). At low lidocaine concentrations, CYP1A2 is the enzyme responsible for most MEGX formation. At high lidocaine concentrations, both CYP1A2 and CYP3A4 are responsible for the formation of MEGX. The amide functional group is fairly stable because of the steric block provided by the ortho methyl groups although amide hydrolysis products are reported.[85–87]

The toxicity associated with lidocaine local anesthesia is low when used at appropriate doses. Absorption of lidocaine will be decreased with the addition of epinephrine to the local anesthetic. Toxicity increases in patients with liver disease and those with acidosis, which decreases plasma protein binding of lidocaine. CNS toxicity is low with seizure activity reported with high doses. The cardiac toxicity of lidocaine is manifested by bradycardia, hypotension, and cardiovascular collapse, which may lead to cardiac arrest and death.

MEPIVACAINE

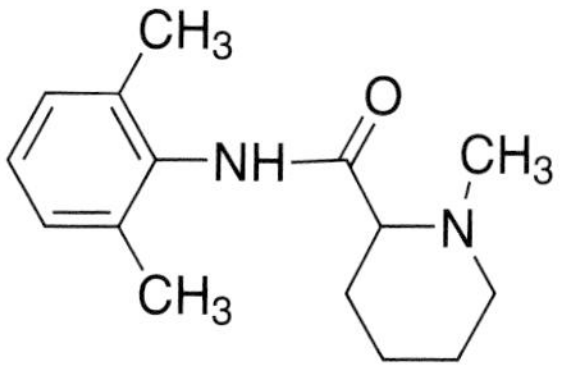

Mepivacaine

Mepivacaine hydrochloride is available in 1% to 3% solutions and is indicated for infiltration anesthesia, dental procedures, peripheral nerve block, or epidural block. The onset of anesthesia is rapid, ranging from about 3 to 20 minutes for sensory block. Mepivacaine is rapidly metabolized in the liver with 50% of the administered dose excreted into the bile as metabolites. The metabolites are reabsorbed in the intestine and excreted in the kidney with only a small percentage found in the feces. Less than 5% to 10% of the administered dose is found unchanged in the urine. The primary metabolic products are the *N*-demethylated metabolite and the 3 and 4 phenolic metabolites excreted as their glucuronide conjugates.

PRILOCAINE

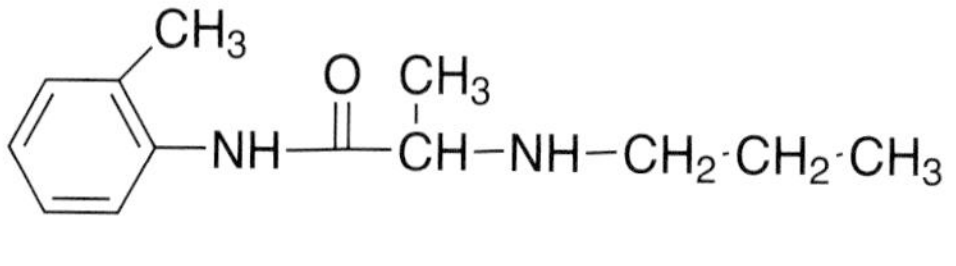

Prilocaine

Prilocaine hydrochloride is a water-soluble salt available as a solution for nerve block or infiltration in dental procedures. Prilocaine is used for intravenous regional anesthesia as the risk of CNS toxicity is low because of the quick metabolism. Prilocaine prepared in the crystal form is used in EMLA for topical administration to decrease painful needle sticks in children. Prilocaine 4% solution should be protected from light and the manufacturer recommends discarding if the solution turns pinkish or slightly darker than light yellow. Solutions are available in various concentrations up to 4%, with or without epinephrine and with or without preservatives.

The pK$_a$ of the secondary amine is 7.9 and commercial preparations have a pH of 5.0 to 5.6. Prilocaine has only one ortho substitution on the aromatic ring, making it more susceptible to amide hydrolysis and giving it a shorter duration

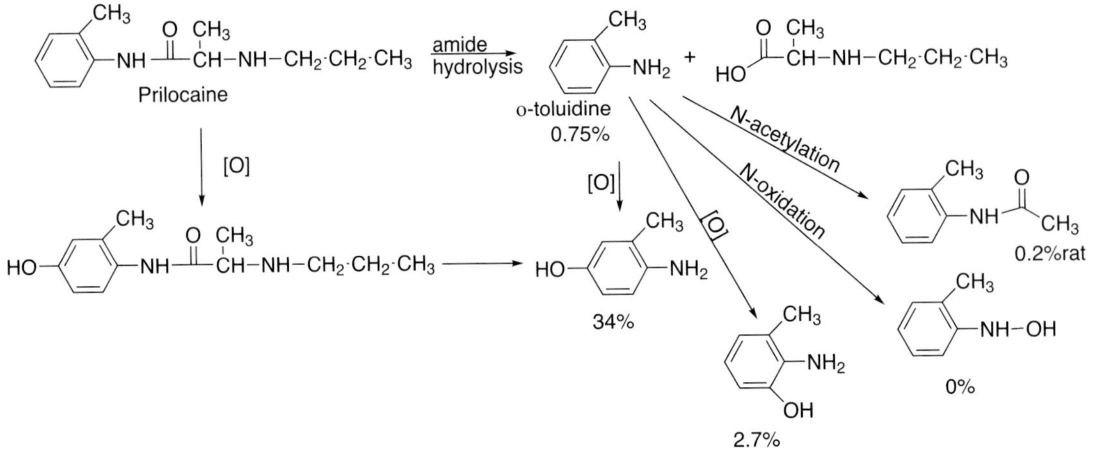

Figure 22.17 ● Metabolism of prilocaine.

of action than lidocaine. Prilocaine metabolism has been studied extensively in animal models, less is known about the human metabolites or the human CYP enzymes involved in their formation (Fig. 22.17).[88,89] The metabolism of prilocaine in the liver yields *o*-toluidine, which is a possible carcinogen. Many aromatic amines, including *o*-toluidine have been shown to be mutagenic, and metabolites of *o*-toluidine have been shown to form DNA adducts. Metabolites of *o*-toluidine are also believed to be responsible for the methemoglobinemia observed with prilocaine use. To decrease the potential for methemoglobinemia, strict adherence to the maximum recommended dose should be followed. Metabolism of prilocaine is extensive with less than 5% of a dose excreted unchanged in the urine.

ETIDOCAINE

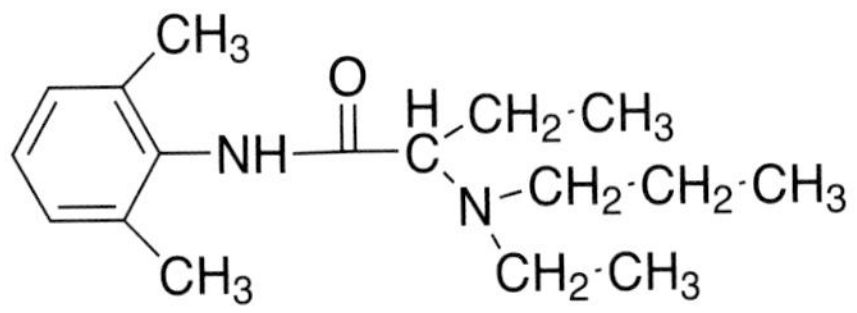

Etidocaine

Etidocaine differs from lidocaine by the addition of an alkyl chain and the extension of one ethyl group on the tertiary amine to a butyl group. The additional lipophilicity gives etidocaine a quicker onset, longer half-life, and an increased potency compared with lidocaine. This may make etidocaine desirable for use when A and C nerve fibers are being anesthetized for long surgical procedures (>2 hours).[90] The tertiary nitrogen pK$_a$ is 7.74, which is similar to lidocaine's pK$_a$ (7.8).

Etidocaine is the most potent amino amide local anesthetic and is used for epidural anesthesia, topical anesthesia, and for peripheral nerve or plexus block. Etidocaine blocks large fast-conducting neurons quicker than the sensory neurons and may leave epidural patients unable to move yet sensitive to painful procedures.[73] Etidocaine has the same potential for cardiac toxicity as bupivacaine and the decreased reports probably are results of the decreased use of etidocaine.

BUPIVACAINE AND LEVOBUVACAINE

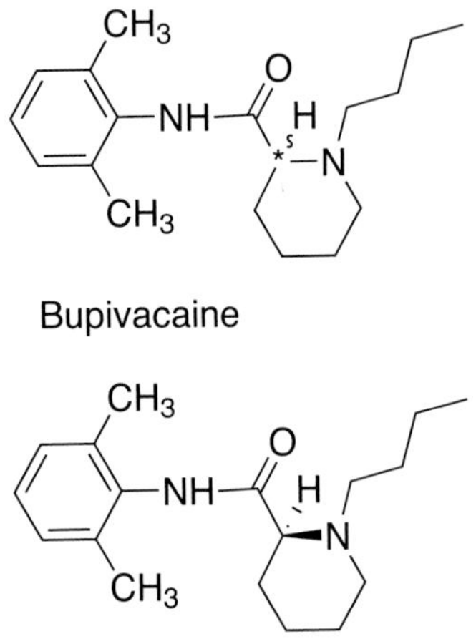

Bupivacaine

Levobupivacaine S (-)

Bupivacaine was synthesized simultaneously with mepivacaine in 1957 but was at first overlooked because of the increased toxicity compared with mepivacaine. When the methyl on the cyclic amine of mepivacaine is exchanged for a butyl group the lipophilicity, potency and the duration of action all increase. Literature reports of cardiovascular toxicity, including severe hypotension and bradycardia, are abundant in the literature.[91] Bupivacaine is highly bound to plasma proteins (95%), and thus the free concentration may remain low until all of the protein binding sites are occupied. After that point, the plasma levels of bupivacaine rise rapidly and patients may progress to overt cardiac toxicity without ever showing signs of CNS toxicity.[92] The cardiotoxicity of bupivacaine is a result of its affinity to cardiac tissues and its ability to depress electrical conduction and predispose the heart to reentry types of arrhythmias. The cardiotoxicity of bupivacaine was found to be significantly more prominent with the "R" isomer, or the racemic mixture, thus the "S" stereoisomer is now on the market as levobupivacaine.[93]

Levobupivacaine is the pure "S" enantiomer of bupivacaine and in vivo and in vitro studies confirm that it does not undergo metabolic inversion to R(+) bupivacaine. The pK$_a$ of the tertiary nitrogen is 8.09, the same as bupivacaine's pK$_a$. Levobupivacaine is available in solution for epidural administration, peripheral nerve block administration, and infiltration anesthesia. Clinical trials have shown that levobupivacaine and bupivacaine have similar anesthetic effects.[94] Levobupivacaine has lower CNS and cardiotoxicity than bupivacaine although unintended intravenous injection when performing nerve blocks may result in toxicity. Racemic bupivacaine is metabolized extensively with no unchanged drug found in the urine or feces. Liver enzymes including the CYP3A4 and CYP1A2 isoforms are responsible for *N*-dealkylation and 3-hydroxylation of levobupivacaine followed by glucuronidation or sulfation.[95]

ROPIVACAINE

Ropivacaine

The recognized increase in cardiotoxicity of one bupivacaine isomer led to the stereospecific production of ropivacaine as the single "S" (−) enantiomer. Ropivacaine is the propyl analog of mepivacaine (methyl) and bupivacaine (butyl). The pK$_a$ of the tertiary nitrogen is 8.1, and it displays the same degree of protein binding as bupivacaine (~94%). Although ropivacaine has similar properties as bupivacaine, it displays less cardiotoxicity. The shortened alkyl chain gives it approximately one third of the lipid solubility of bupivacaine. Animal studies have shown that ropivacaine dissociates from cardiac sodium channels more rapidly than bupivacaine. This decreases the sodium channel block in the heart and may be responsible for the reduced cardiotoxicity of ropivacaine.[92]

Ropivacaine undergoes extensive metabolism in humans with only 1% of a dose excreted unchanged in the urine.[96] Four metabolites of ropivacaine have been identified from human liver microsome incubations and in vivo studies. The CYP1A2 isoform was found to be responsible for the formation of 3-OH ropivacaine, the primary ropivacaine metabolite. The CYP3A4 isoform was responsible for the formation of 4-OH ropivacaine, 2-OH methyl-ropivacaine, and the *N*-dealkylated metabolite (S)-2′,6′-pipecoloxylidide.[97] Coadministered inhibitors of CYP1A2 may be of clinical importance, CYP3A4 inhibitors seem to be of less clinical relevance.[98]

Ropivacaine is a long-acting amide-type local anesthetic with inherent vasoconstrictor activities, so it does not require the use of additional vasoconstrictors. It is approved for epidural, nerve block, infiltration, and intrathecal anesthesia.

DIBUCAINE

Dibucaine

Dibucaine is a topical amide anesthetic available in over-the-counter creams and ointments used to treat minor conditions such as sunburns and hemorrhoids. Dibucaine has been found to be highly toxic when taken orally, inducing seizures, coma, and death in several children who accidentally ingested it.[99] Metabolites of dibucaine identified in the urine of rats, rabbits, and humans included hydroxylated metabolites of the quinoline ring, monohydroxylated and dihydroxylated metabolites of the *O*-alkyl side chain (2′- and 3′-position), and the *N*-de-ethylated dibucaine metabolite.[100]

ARTICAINE

Articaine

Articaine has a secondary nitrogen with a pK$_a$ of 7.8. It contains an aromatic thiophene ring bioisostere of the phenyl ring found in most other amide anesthetics. The log P of a benzene ring is 2.13 and the thiophene ring log P is 1.81, thus the thiophene ring is more hydrophilic than a phenyl ring. Although the thiophene ring has less lipid solubility than a phenyl ring, articaine is a lipid-soluble compound due to the propylamine, the branched methyl and the substitutions on the thiophene ring. The onset of action of articaine is similar to lidocaine's onset of action. Articaine is available in a 4% solution with epinephrine for use in infiltration and nerve block anesthesia.

Articaine is metabolized rapidly via plasma and tissue carboxyesterase to its primary metabolite, the inactive, water-soluble carboxylic acid. Approximately 40% to 70% of articaine administered epidurally is metabolized to the carboxylic acid, articainic acid. Approximately 4% to 15% of the articainic acid undergoes glucuronide conjugation and only 3% of the dose is recovered unchanged in the urine. The rapid plasma metabolism and reported inactivity of the carboxylic acid metabolite make articaine a potentially safer anesthetic agent when multiple or large doses are necessary.[101,102]

Future Directions of Local Anesthetic Research

One of the issues of local anesthetic use is that they are not specific to sensory nociceptors, the "pain neurons." Local anesthetics also block pressure, touch, and motor axons leading to numbness and loss of muscle control. Recent studies in rats have shown that administering the quaternary lidocaine molecule, QX-314, along with capsaicin allows the permanently charged anesthetic access to pain-sensing neurons only. The quaternary charge on QX-314 prevents it from entering all neurons via simple diffusion through the lipophilic membrane. Capsaicin was found to bind to a protein only found on pain-sensing neurons, TRPV1 channels. When capsaicin binds to TRPV1, the channel opens to allow QX-314 to enter the axoplasm and then access the local anesthetic binding site in the sodium channel from the hydrophilic pathway (Fig. 22.13 hydrophilic pathway C). By specifically blocking the sodium channels of only pain neurons, other nerve function is preserved. This type of pain management would make it possible to have a dental procedure with no pain, yet not leave the entire face numb, or have an epidural during labor and still be able to walk. This is an exciting new opportunity in pain management that is undergoing research presently.[103]

Another area of research is the formulation of local anesthetic liposomes and microspheres. The principle behind this research is that the local anesthetic molecules are amphipathic, with both a hydrophilic and hydrophobic component. The anesthetic molecule can be suspended inside carrier substances made of egg phospholipids and cholesterol liposomes or biodegradable polymers of lactic acid or glycolic acid. The carrier molecule will allow a controlled delivery of the local anesthetic and provide a long duration of action, potentially with less systemic toxicity.[91,104] Carrier molecules are also being designed that combine a local anesthetic with an opioid analgesic that may offer alternative analgesic delivery methods.[105]

◈ R E V I E W   Q U E S T I O N S ◈

1. A nurse anesthetist calls the OR pharmacy to discuss a patient history and get your input on choosing a general anesthetic for an upcoming operation.

   ML is a 32-year-old, 5'4", 460-pound woman who is scheduled for an elective gastroplasty (stomach stapling). She has a history of hypertension (150/98 mm Hg), hyperlipidemia (LDL-cholesterol = 140mg/dL), and a large stage III pressure ulcer on her lower back. The last time that the patient underwent surgery, she could not be roused from the sedation and spent 24 hours in the postanesthetic care unit (PACU). Her prior surgery required 3 hours of general anesthesia maintained with isoflurane. The nurse anesthetist would like to know if one of the other formulary agents offers a shorter recovery time. General anesthetics on the formulary include nitrous oxide, desflurane, sevoflurane, isoflurane, enflurane, and halothane.

2. A medical student was assigned the task of debriding ML's decubitus ulcer and calls the pharmacy to obtain procaine to inject locally before beginning the painful procedure. You review the patient's chart for allergies (no known drug allergies [NKDA]) and notice that the patient is also receiving 1% silver sulfadiazine cream to prevent bacterial colonization of the ulcer. You recommend against using the procaine and suggest a 1% lidocaine with epinephrine instead. Why?

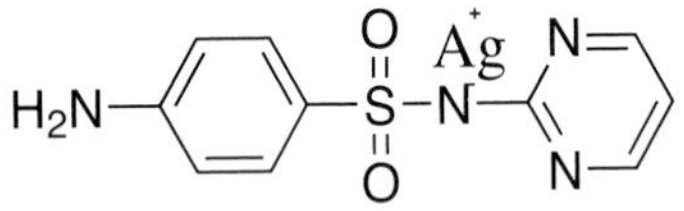

3. An anesthesiologist from the obstetric unit calls to request stat delivery of 20% intralipid to treat an inadvertent intravascular injection of bupivacaine. The patient is in cardiac arrest. Why is the anesthesiologist requesting intralipid?

4. TG, a 45-year-old male woodworker, presents to the ER with an injured index finger. While cleaning a circular saw blade, he accidentally severed the tip (fleshy part, no bone) of his finger. The ER resident calls to request lidocaine 2% with epinephrine 1:200,000 to decrease the pain associated with suturing. You suggest an alternate. Why did you NOT fill the original requested anesthetic?

5. JF, a patient with a severe allergic reaction to 2-chloroprocaine, is having plastic surgery to remove three moles from her face. The physician calls to request your input in choosing a local anesthetic. The plastic surgeon has the five drugs shown at the bottom of this page available in his clinic. Which drug would you recommend that he use?

6. While working as a pharmacy intern at a retail pharmacy, a woman carrying an infant asks you to ring up three tubes of Maximum Strength Vagisil Creme. In conversation with her, you find out that she has been treating her 2-month-old daughter's painful, excoriated diaper rash with the cream for the last week. She claims to have received the advice on a mothers' chat room on the Internet. You observe that her 2-month-old daughter has bluish lips and very pale translucent skin that also has a bluish tint. You immediately advise her to take her daughter to the emergency room. Why?

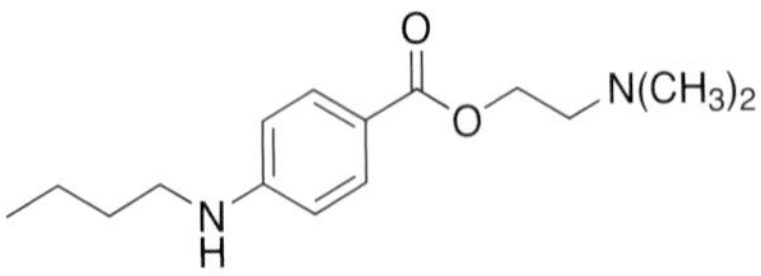

A (Preservative free)

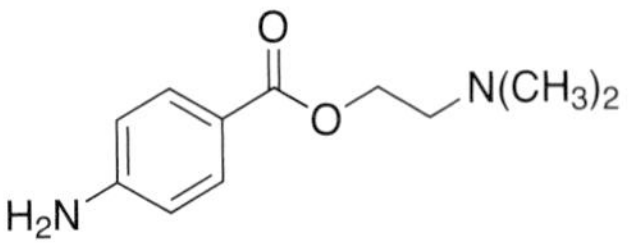

B (Preservative: Methylparaben)

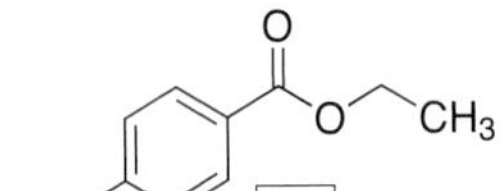

(Preservative: Benzalkonium chloride)

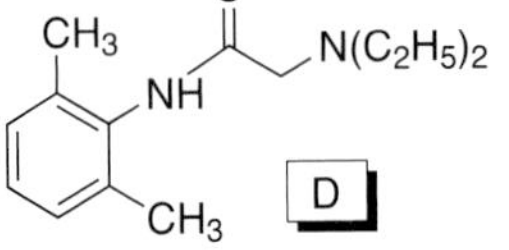

D (Preservative: Benzalkonium chloride)

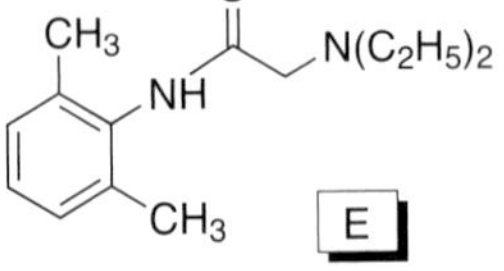

E (Preservative: Methylparaben)

REFERENCES

1. Morton, W. T. G.: Remarks on the Proper Mode of Administering Sulphuric Ether by Inhalation. Boston, MA, Dutton and Wentworth, 1847, pp. 1–44.
2. Antognini, J. F., and Carstens, E.: Br. J. Anaesth. 89:156–166, 2002.
3. Eger, E. I., 2nd.: Am. J. Health. Syst. Pharm. 61 Suppl 4:S3–10, 2004.
4. Castro, B. A., Freedman, L. A., Craig, W. L., et al.: Anesthesiology 101:537–539, 2004.
5. Wu, J., Previte, J. P., Adler, E., et al.: Anesthesiology 101:534–537, 2004.
6. Dunning, M. B., 3rd, Bretscher, L. E., Arain, S. R., et al.: Anesthesiology 106:144–148, 2007.
7. Eger, E. I., 2nd, Halsey, M. J., Harris, R. A., et al.: Anesth. Analg. 88:1395–1400, 1999.
8. Kobin, D. D.: Structure-activity relationships of inhaled anesthetics. In Moody, E., and Skolnick, P. (eds.). Molecular Bases of Anesthesia. New York, CRC Press, 2000, pp. 123–145.
9. Fang, Z., Ionescu, P., Chortkoff, B., et al.: Anesth. Analg. 84:1042–1048, 1997.
10. Targ, A. G., Yasuda, N., Eger, E. I., 2nd, et al.: Anesth. Analg. 68:599–602, 1989.
11. Halsey, M. J.: Br. J. Anaesth. 56 Suppl 1:9S–25S, 1984.
12. Eger, E., II, and Laster, M.: Anesth. Analg. 92:1477–1482, 2001.
13. Eckenhoff, R. G.: Mol. Interv. 1:258–268, 2001.
14. Campagna, J. A., Miller, K. W., and Forman, S. A.: N. Engl. J. Med. 348:2110–2124, 2003.
15. Hemmings, H. C., Akabas, M. H., Goldstein, P. A., et al.: Trends. Pharmacol. Sci. 26:503–510, 2005.
16. Anonymous Inhalants. http://www.drugabuse.gov/PDF/Infofacts/Inhalants06.pdf (accessed October 12, 2007).
17. Stachnik, J.: Am. J. Health. Syst. Pharm. 63:623–634, 2006.
18. Spracklin, D. K., Thummel, K. E., and Kharasch, E. D.: Drug Metab. Dispos. 24:976–983, 1996.
19. Litman, R. S., and Rosenberg, H.: JAMA 293:2918–2924, 2005.
20. Lerman, J., Gregory, G. A., Willis, M. M., et al.: Anesthesiology 61:139–143, 1984.
21. Mazze, R. I.: Anesthesiology 105:843–846, 2006.
22. Evers, A. S., Crowder, C. M., and Balser J. R.: General anesthetics. In Brunton L. L., Lazo, J. L., and Parker, K. L. (eds.). Goodman and Gilman's The Pharmacological Basis of Therapeutics. New York, McGraw-Hill, 2006, pp. 341–368.
23. Goldberg, M. E., Cantillo, J., Larijani, G. E., et al.: Anesth. Analg. 82:1268–1272, 1996.
24. Package Insert Suprane (desflurane, USP). Baxter Healthcare Corporation 2005.
25. Smith, I., Nathanson, M., and White, P. F.: Br. J. Anaesth. 76:435–445, 1996.
26. Iyer, R. A., Baggs, R. B., and Anders, M. W.: J. Pharmacol. Exp. Ther. 283:1544–1551, 1997.
27. Kharasch, E. D., and Jubert, C.: Anesthesiology 91:1267–1278, 1999.
28. Kharasch, E., Schroeder, J., Bammler, T., et al.: Toxicol. Sci. 90:419–431, 2006.
29. Fatheree, R. S., and Leighton, B. L.: Anesthesiology 101:531–533, 2004.
30. Kharasch, E. D., Armstrong, A. S., Gunn, K., et al.: Anesthesiology 82:1379–1388, 1995.
31. Kharasch, E. D., and Thummel, K. E.: Anesthesiology 79:795–807, 1993.
32. Package Insert Ultane (sevoflurane). Abbott Laboratories 2006.
33. Jaaskelainen, S. K., Kaisti, K., Suni, L., et al.: Neurology 61:1073–1078, 2003.
34. Schoenborn, B. P., and Nobbs, C. L.: Mol. Pharmacol. 2:495–498, 1966.
35. Trudell, J., Koblin, D., and Eger, E., 2nd: Anesth. Analg. 87:411–418, 1998.
36. Goto, T., Saito H., Shinkai M., et al.: Anesthesiology 86:1273–1278, 1997.
37. Goto, T.: Can. J. Anaesth. 49:335–338, 2002.
38. Higgins, T. L., Murray, M., Kett, D. H., et al.: Intensive Care Med. 26:S413–421, 2000.
39. Package Insert Diprivan (propofol) Injectable Emulsion. AstraZeneca Rev. 08/2005.
40. McKeage, K., and Perry, C. M.: CNS Drugs 17:235–272, 2003.
41. Fassoulaki, A., Sarantopoulos, C., and Papilas, K.: Can. J. Anaesth. 40:10, 1993.
42. Trapani, G., Altomare, C., Sanna, E., et al.: Curr. Med. Chem. 7:249, 2000.
43. Langley, M. S., and Heel, R. C.: Drugs 35:334–372, 1988.
44. Belelli, D., Lambert, J. J., Peters, J. A., et al.: PNAS 94:11031–11036, 1997.
45. Package Insert Etomidate Injection. Bedford Laboratories 03/2004.
46. Doenicke, A. W., Roizen, M. F., Hoernecke, R., et al.: Br. J. Anaesth. 83:464–466, 1999.
47. Sinha, A. C., and Soliz, J. M.: The Internet J. Anesthesiol. 5, 2002.
48. Lipiner-Friedman, D., Sprung, C. L., Laterre, P. F., et al.: Crit. Care Med. 35:1012–1018, 2007.
49. Giese, J. L., and Stanley, T. H.: Pharmacotherapy 3:251–258, 1983.
50. Hustveit, O., Maurset, A., and Oye, I.: Pharmacol. Toxicol. 77:355–359, 1995.
51. Hirota, K., and Lambert, D. G.: Br. J. Anaesth. 77:441–444, 1996.
52. Hocking, G., and Cousins, M. J.: Anesth. Analg. 97:1730–1739, 2003.
53. Visser, E., and Schug, S. A.: Biomed. Pharmacother. 60:341–348, 2006.
54. Anonymous, Intelligence Bulletin:Ketamine. USDOJ.gov/ndic (accessed June 6, 2007).
55. Hijazi, Y., and Boulieu, R.: Drug Metab. Dispos. 30:853–858, 2002.
56. Williams, M. L., Mager, D. E., Parenteau, H., et al.: Drug Metab. Dispos. 32:786–793, 2004.
57. Catterall, W. A.: Neuron 26:13–25, 2000.
58. Armstrong, C. M., and Hille, B.: Neuron 20:371–380, 1998.
59. Heinemann, S. H., Terlau, H., Stuhmer, W., et al.: Nature 356:441–443, 1992.
60. Elinder, F., Nilsson, J., and Arhem, P.: Physiol. Behav. 92:1–7, 2007.
61. Lipkind, G., and Fozzard, H.: Mol. Pharmacol. 68:1611–1622, 2005.
62. Li, H., Galue, A., Meadows, L., et al.: Mol. Pharmacol. 55:134–141, 1999.
63. Strichartz, G.: J. Gen. Physiol. 62:37–57, 1973.
64. Hille, B.: J. Gen. Physiol. 69:497–515, 1977.
65. Strichartz, G., Sanchez, V., Arthur, G., et al.: Anesth. Analg. 1:158–170, 1990.
66. Chernoff, D. M., and Strichartz, G. R.: Biophys. J. 58:69–81, 1990.
67. Catterall, W. A., and Mackie, K.: Local anesthetics. In Brunton, L. L., Lazo, J. L., and Parker, K. L. (eds.). Goodman and Gilman's The Pharmacological Basis of Therapeutics. New York, The McGraw Hill Companies, 2006, p. 369.
68. Gupta, S. P.: Chem. Rev. 91:1109–1119, 1991.
69. Buchi, J., and Perlia, X.: Design of local anesthetics. In Ariens, E. J. (ed). Drug Design. New York, Academic Press, 1972, Vol. 3, p. 243.
70. Heavner, J. E.: Curr. Opin. Anaesthesiol. 20:336–342, 2007.
71. Tucker, G. T., and Mather, L. E.: Br. J. Anaesth. 47:1029–1030, 1975.
72. Eggleston, S., and Lush, L.: Ann. Pharmacother. 30:851–857, 1996.
73. Tetzlaff, J. E.: Boston, Clinical Pharmacology of Local Anesthetics; Butterworth, 1999, p. 258.
74. Simon, R. A. J.: Allergy Clin. Immunol. 74:623–630, 1984.
75. Karim, A., Ahmed, S., Siddiqui, R., et al.: Am. J. Med. 111:150–153, 2001.
76. Kaendler, L., Dorszewski, A., and Daehnert, I.: Heart 90:e51, 2004.
77. Wilburn-Goo, D., and Lloyd, L.: J. Am. Dent. Assoc. 130:826–831, 1999.
78. Moore, T., Walsh, C., and Cohen, M.: Arch. Intern. Med. 164:1192–1196, 2004.
79. Nunn, D. B.: Adv. Stud. Med. 6:106–108, 2006.
80. Goodell, J., Gilroy, G., and Huntress, J.: Am. J. Health Syst. Pharm. 45:2510–2513, 1988.
81. Lander, J., Weltman, B., and So, S.: Cochrane Database Syst. Rev. 3, 2007.
82. Noorily, A., Noorily, S., and Otto, R.: Anesth. Analg. 81:724–727, 1995.
83. Tush, G., and Kuhn, R.: Ann. Pharmacother. 30:1251–1254, 1996.
84. Dahshan, A., and Donovan, G. K.: Pediatrics 117:e806–809, 2006.
85. Alexson, S. H., Diczfalusy, M., Halldin, M., et al.: Drug Metab. Dispos. 30:643–647, 2002.
86. Wang, J., Backman, J., Taavitsainen, P., et al.: Drug Metab. Dispos. 28:959–965, 2000.
87. Wang, J. S., Backman, J. T., Wen, X., et al.: Pharmacol. Toxicol. 85:201–205, 1999.
88. Hjelm, M., Ragnarsson, B., and Wistrand, P.: Biochem. Pharmacol. 21:2825–2834, 1972.
89. Gaber, K., Harreus, U. A., Matthias, C., et al.: Toxicology 229:157–164, 2007.
90. Paradis, B., and Fournier, L.: Can. J. Anesth. 22:70–75, 1975.
91. Ruetsch, Y. A., Boni, T., and Borgeat, A.: Curr. Top. Med. Chem. 1:175–182, 2001.

92. Whiteside, J. B., and Wildsmith, J. A. W.: Br. J. Anaesth. 87:27–35, 2001.
93. Huang, Y., Pryor, M., Mather, L., et al.: Anesth. Analg. 86:797–804, 1998.
94. Glaser, C., Marhofer, P., Zimpfer, G., et al.: Anesth. Analg. 94:194–198, 2002.
95. Gantenbein, M., Attolini, L., Bruguerolle, B., et al.: Drug Metab. Dispos. 28:383–385, 2000.
96. Halldin, M., Bredberg, E., Angelin, B., et al.: Drug Metab. Dispos. 24:962–968, 1996.
97. Ekstrom, G., and Gunnarsson, U.: Drug Metab. Dispos. 24:955–961, 1996.
98. Arlander, E., Ekström, G., Alm, C., et al.: Clin. Pharmacol. Ther. 64:484–491, 1998.
99. Dayan P. S., Litovitz T. L., Crouch B. I., et al.: Ann. Emerg. Med. 28:442–445, 1996.
100. Igarashi, K., Kasuya, F., and Fukui, M.: J. Pharmacobiodyn. 6:538–550, 1983.
101. Vree, T. B., Simon, M. A. M., Gielen, M. J. M., et al.: Br. J. Clin. Pharmacol. 44:29–34, 1997.
102. van Oss, G. E., Vree, T. B., Baars, A. M., et al.: Eur. J. Anaesthesiol. 6:49–56, 1989.
103. Binshtok, A. M., Bean B. P., and Wu, J.: Nature 449:607–610, 2007.
104. deAraujo, D., Cereda, C. S., Brunetto, G., et al.: Can. J. Anesth. 51:566–572, 2004.
105. Sendil, D., Bonney, I. M., Carr, D. B., et al.: Biomaterials 24:1969–1976, 2003.

$Pka = 10.15$ in $Pg79$

CHAPTER 23

Histamine and Antihistaminic Agents

JACK DERUITER

Histamine or β-imidazolylethylamine is synthesized from L-histidine by histidine decarboxylase, an enzyme that is expressed in many mammalian tissues including gastric-mucosa parietal cells, mast cells, and basophils and the central nervous system (CNS).[1] As a result, histamine plays an important role in human physiology including regulation of the cardiovascular system, smooth muscle, exocrine glands, the immune system, and central nerve function. It is also involved in embryonic development, the proliferation and differentiation of cells, hematopoiesis, inflammation, and wound healing. Histamine exerts its diverse biologic effects through four types of receptors. The involvement of histamine in the mediation of immune and hypersensitivity reactions and the regulation of gastric acid secretion has led to the development of important drug classes useful in the treatment of symptoms associated with allergic and gastric hypersecretory disorders.

HISTAMINE CHEMISTRY

Nomenclature

Histamine, known trivially as 4(5-)(2-aminoethyl)imidazole, structurally is composed of an imidazole heterocycle and ethylamine side chain. The methylene groups of the amino-ethyl side chain are designated α and β. The side chain is attached, via the β-CH_2 group, to the 4-position of an imidazole ring. The imidazole N at position 3 is designated the *pros* (π) N, whereas the N at position 1 is termed the *tele* (τ) N. The side chain N is distinguished as N^α (Fig. 23.1).

Ionization and Tautomerization

Histamine is a basic organic compound (N^π, $pK_{a1} = 5.80$; N $pK_{a2} = 9.40$; N^α, $pK_{a3} = 14.0$) capable of existing as a mixture of different ionic and uncharged tautomeric species (Fig. 23.2).[2,3] Histamine exists almost exclusively (96.6%) as the monocationic conjugate species (αNH_3^+) at physiological pH (7.4). At lower pHs, a higher percentage of the dicationic species exists. In water, the ratio of the concentrations of the tautomers N^τ—H/N^π—H has been calculated to be 4.2, indicating that 80% of the histamine monocation exists as N^τ—H and 20% exists as N^π—H in aqueous solution.[2,3] However, crystalline forms of histamine salts appear to exist primarily as N^τ—H tautomer to facilitate crystal packing. Also, for derivatives of histamine, the ratio of

tautomers is dependent on the presence of imidazole ring substituents as discussed later in this chapter.[4]

Structure–activity relationship studies suggest that the αNH_3^+ monocation is important for agonist activity at histamine receptors and that transient existence of the more lipophilic uncharged histamine species may contribute to diffusion across cell membranes. Other studies support proposal that the N^τ—H tautomer of the histamine monocation is the pharmacophoric species at the H_1-receptor, while a 1,3-tautomeric system is important for selective H_2-agonism.

Stereochemistry

While histamine is an achiral molecule, histamine receptors exert high stereoselectivity toward chiral ligands.[5] Molecular modeling and steric–activity relationship studies of the influence of conformational isomerism suggest the importance of *trans-gauche* rotameric structures in the receptor binding of histamine (Fig. 23.3). Although both conformers exist in solution, studies with conformationally restricted histamine analogs suggest that the *trans*-rotamer of histamine possesses affinity for both H_1- and H_2-receptors, and the *gauche* conformer is preferred for H_3-receptors, but not H_1- or H_2-receptors.[4]

HISTAMINE AS A CHEMICAL MESSENGER

Knowledge of the biodisposition of histamine is important in understanding the involvement of this substance in various pathophysiologies as well as the actions of various ligands that either enhance or block its actions. Each of the steps in the "life cycle" of histamine represents a potential point for pharmacological intervention.

Biosynthesis and Distribution

Histamine is synthesized in Golgi apparatus of its principal storage cells, mast cells, and basophils.[6] Histamine is formed from the naturally occurring amino acid L-hisitidne (S-histidine) via the catalysis of either the pyridoxal phosphate dependent enzyme histidine decarboxylase (HDC, EC 4.1.1.22) or L-aromatic amino acid decarboxylase (L-AAAD) (Fig. 23.4). Substrate specificity is higher for HDC versus L-AAAD. HDC inhibitors (HDCIs) include α-fluoromethylhistidine (FMH), a mechanism-based inhibitor, and certain flavonoids.[7] Although useful as pharmacologic probes, HDCIs have not proved to be useful clinically.

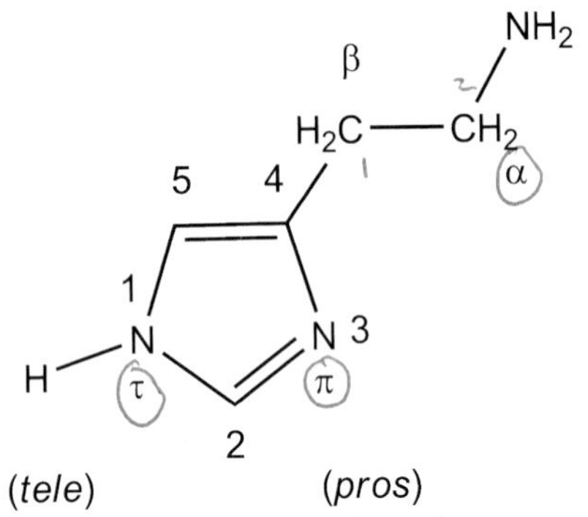

Figure 23.1 ● Histamine.

Histamine is found in almost all mammalian tissues in concentrations ranging from 1 to more than 100 μg/g. Mast cells and histamine are in particularly high concentration in skin and the mucosal cells of the bronchi, intestine, urinary tract, and tissues adjacent to the circulation. It is found in higher concentrations in mammalian cerebrospinal fluid than in plasma and other body fluids.

Storage and Release

Most histamine is biosynthesized and stored as protein complexes in mast cells (complexed with heparin) and basophilic granulocytes (complexed with chondroitin).[8,9] Protein-complexed histamine is stored in secretory granules and released by exocytosis in response to a wide variety of immune (antigen and antibody) and nonimmune (bacterial products, xenobiotics, physical effects, and cholinergic effects) stimuli. The release of histamine as one of the mediators of

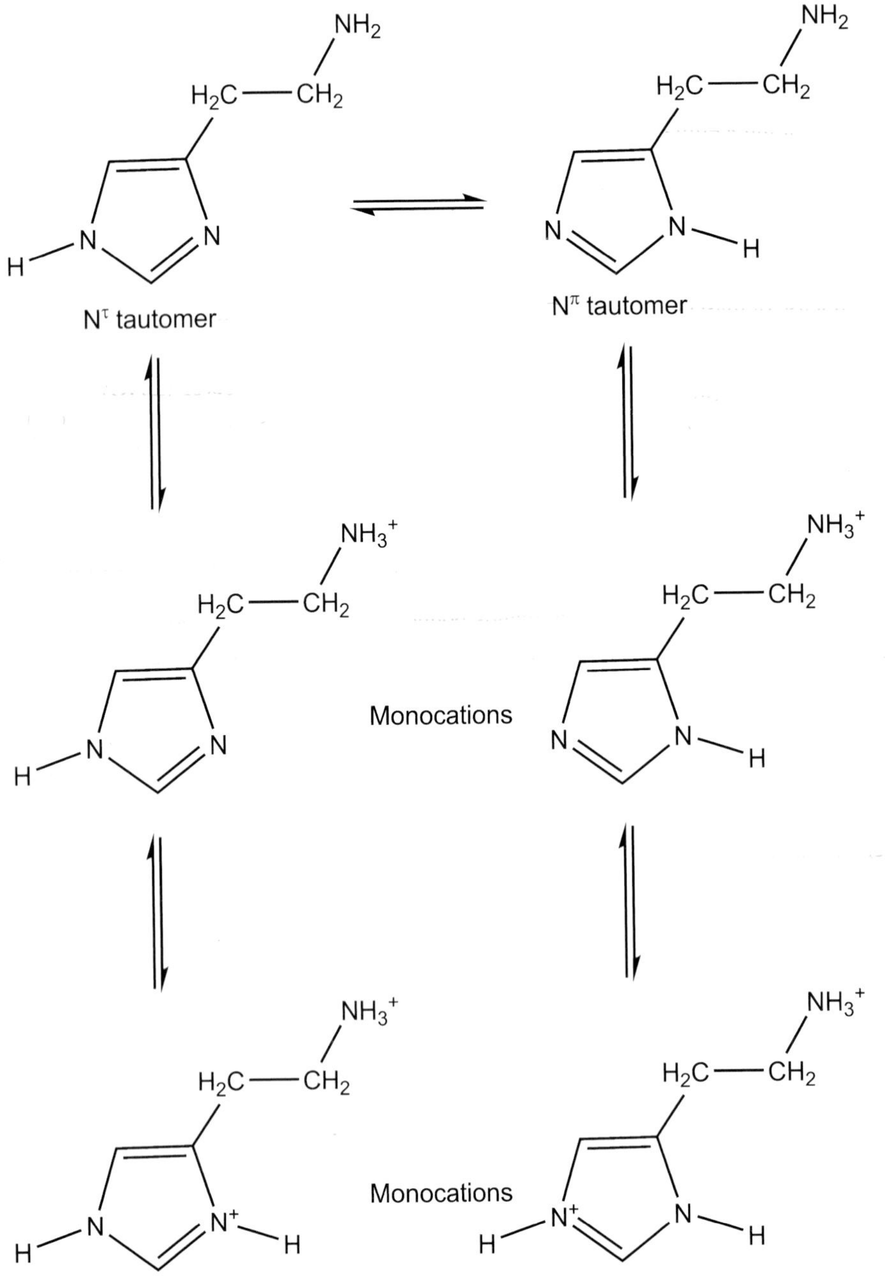

Figure 23.2 ● Histamine tautomers and cations.

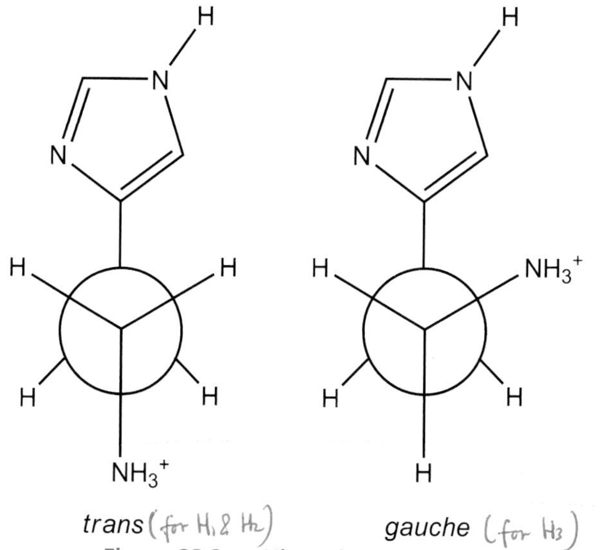

trans (for H₁ & H₂) *gauche* (for H₃)

Figure 23.3 ● Histamine rotamers.

hypersensitivity reactions is initiated by the interaction of an antigen-IgE complex with the membrane of a histamine storage cell. This interaction triggers activation of intracellular phosphokinase C (PKC), leading to accumulation of inositol phosphates, diacylglycerol, and calcium. Exocytotic release of histamine follows the degranulation of histamine storage cells.[10] Degranulation also results in the release of other mediators of inflammation including prostaglandins, leukotrienes, platelet-activating factor, kinins, etc.[10] The release of mast cell mediators can be inhibited by several agents as described in the sections that follow. Histamine is released from mast cells in the gastric mucosa by gastrin and acetylcholine. Neurochemical studies also suggest that histamine is stored in and released from selected neuronal tracts in the CNS.

Histamine Receptors and Histamine-Mediated Physiologic Functions

Once released, the physiological effects of histamine are mediated by specific cell-surface receptors. Extensive pharmacological and molecular biology studies have revealed the presence of at least four different histamine receptor subtypes in mammalian systems designated as H_1, H_2, H_3, and H_4 (Table 23.1).[10] All histamine receptor subtypes are heptahelical transmembrane molecules (TM1-TM7) that transduce extracellular signals via G-proteins to intracellular second-messenger systems. These receptors have constitu-

tive receptor G-protein–signaling activity that is independent of histamine agonist binding.[10,11] Thus, they exist in two conformations that are in equilibrium—an active (constitutive) and inactive state. The four histamine receptor subtypes differ in their expression, location, primary structure, precise signal transduction processes, and physiologic functions as indicated in Table 23.1 and detailed here. In general, H_1- and H_2-receptors appear to be more widely expressed than H_3- and H_4-receptors.[10]

Histamine H_1-receptor expression is widespread including CNS neurons, the smooth muscle of respiratory, gastrointestinal (GI), uterine tissues, epithelial and endothelial cells, neutrophils, eosinophils, monocytes, dendritic cells, T cells, B cells, hepatocytes, and chondrocytes.[10] This receptor is composed of 487 amino acids and has a molecular mass of 56 kd. Its seven transmembrane domains consist of a short intracellular C-terminal tail (17 amino acids), N-terminal glycosylation sites, phosphorylation sites for protein kinases A and C, and a large intracellular loop (212 amino acids, TM3).[12,13] Based on data from site-directed mutagenesis studies, the third (TM3) and fifth (TM5) transmembrane domains are responsible for binding of H_1-receptor ligands. An acidic aspartate residue in TM3 (position 107) appears to be responsible for binding of the protonated amino group of the ethylamine side chain of histamine via ionic interactions. An asparagine (position 207) of the TM5 domain appears to interact with the N^τ-nitrogen atom of the imidazole ring of histamine and lysine (200) interacts with the nucleophilic N^π-nitrogen of the natural ligand.[12,13]

Signal transduction at the H_1-receptor involves the activation of $G_{\alpha q11}$ that stimulates intracellular phospholipase C (PLC) to hydrolyze phosphatidylinositide to inositol-1,4,5-triphosphate (IP_3) and 1,2-diacylglycerol (DAG). IP_3 promotes intracellular calcium release, whereas DAG may stimulate various biochemical pathways including phospholipase A_2 and D, NFκB-mediated gene transcription, as well as cyclic adenosine monophosphate (cAMP) and nitric oxide synthase (NOS) production.[10–13] Human H_1-receptors have approximately 45% homology with muscarinic M_1- and M_2-receptors, perhaps accounting for some of the overlap in ligands bound by each receptor subtype. H_1-receptor polymorphisms have been described, although it is not yet clear how they influence the histamine binding or clinical response to H_1-antihistamine drugs.[14]

As a result of widespread tissue localization and the varied functions of these tissues, H_1-receptors mediate a host of physiologic processes including pruritus, pain, vasodilation, vascular permeability, hypotension, flushing, headache, tachycardia, bronchoconstriction, stimulation of airway vagal

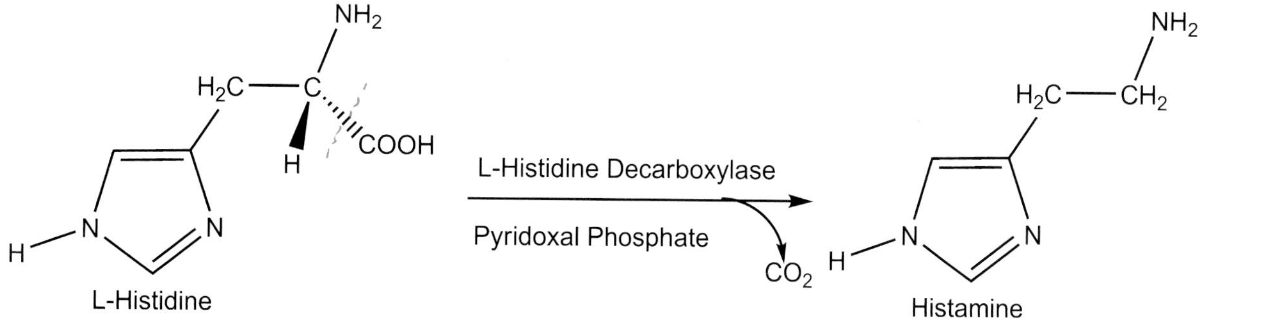

Figure 23.4 ● Histamine biosynthesis.

TABLE 23.1 **Histamine Receptor Subtypes**

Characteristic	H$_1$-Receptor	H$_2$-Receptor	H$_3$-Receptor	H$_4$-Receptor
Receptor proteins in humans	487 amino acids, 56 kd	359 amino acids, 40 kd	445 amino acids, 70 kd; splice variants	390 amino acids
Chromosomal location	3p25, 3p14–21	5q35.3	20q13.33	18q11.2
G-protein coupling	Gαq11	Gαs	Gi/o	Gi/o
Activated intracellular signals	Ca2+, cGMP, phospholipase A2, C, and D, NFκB, cAMP, NOS	cAMP, Ca2+, phospholipase C, protein kinase C, c-fos	Ca2+, MAP kinase; inhibition of cAMP	Ca2+, MAP kinase; inhibition of cAMP
Inverse agonists for clinical use	First- and second-generation antihistamines	H$_2$-blockers	None to date	None to date

Source: Simons, F. E. R.: Advances in H$_1$-antihistamines. N. Engl. J. Med. 351:2203–2217, 2004.

afferent nerves and cough receptors, and decreased atrioventricular-node conduction time. With respect to the cells involved in the immune response, released histamine acting at H$_1$-receptors causes increased cellular adhesion–molecule expression and chemotaxis of eosinophils and neutrophils, increased antigen-presenting–cell capacity, costimulatory activity on B cells, blocking of humoral immunity and IgE production, induction of cellular immunity (Th1), and increased interferon-gamma (IFN-γ) autoimmunity.[9,10,15,16] These processes contribute to the allergic inflammation associated with histamine release and are the basis for antihistamine drug therapy for the treatment of allergy. It should be noted, however, that other mediators released with histamine also contribute to these immunologic and allergenic actions.[15,16] In the CNS H$_1$-receptor activation influences cycles of sleeping and waking, food intake, thermal regulation, emotions and aggressive behavior, locomotion, memory, and learning.[10]

H$_2$-receptors are expressed in various tissues where they mediate gastric acid secretion, vascular permeability, hypotension, flushing, headache, tachycardia, chronotropic and inotropic activity, bronchodilatation and respiratory mucus production. This receptor is composed of 359 amino acids and has a molecular mass of 40 kd. Like the H$_1$-receptor, this receptor has N-terminal glycosylation sites and phosphorylation sites in the C-terminus.[10,12,13] It also has an aspartate residue in TM3 and threonine/aspartate and tyrosine/aspirate residues in TM5, which bind agonists. The most notable difference between structures of cloned H$_1$- and H$_2$-receptors is the much shorter third intracellular loop and longer C-terminal loop of the H$_2$-receptor protein.

In most tissues, signal transduction of the H$_2$-receptor involves the activation of G$_{\alpha s}$, which stimulates adenylate cyclase promoting the synthesis of cAMP. In some tissues, H$_2$-receptors may be linked to G$_q$ proteins that stimulate PLC to form IP$_3$ and DAG, which regulate intracellular calcium levels and other processes including protein kinases.[10,12,13] A more detailed discussion of the role of H$_2$-receptors in gastric acid secretion is included under "Histamine H$_2$-Antagonist" later in this chapter.

In addition to regulation of gastric acid secretion and cardiovascular functions listed previously, H$_2$-receptors modulate immune function by decreasing eosinophil and neutrophil chemotaxis, inducing interleukin-10, suppressing interleukin-12 by dendritic cells, developing Th2 or tolerance-inducing dendritic cells, inducing humoral immunity, suppressing cellular immunity, and suppressing Th2 cells and cytokines.[10] Thus, this receptor also plays an indirect role in allergy, autoimmunity, malignant disease, and graft rejection. It may also have a neuroendocrine role in the CNS.

The highest density of H$_3$-receptors occurs in the CNS, mainly in the striatum, substantia nigra, and the cortex.[10,17] In the CNS, this receptor subtype may be a presynaptic heteroreceptor and regulate histamine, dopamine, serotonin, noradrenaline, and acetylcholine release. H$_3$-receptors also play a lesser role in peripheral nerve and tissues where they appear to prevent excessive bronchoconstriction; mediate pruritus (no mast-cell involvement) and may be involved in the control of neurogenic inflammation through local neuron–mast cell feedback loops. The H$_3$-receptor consists of 445 amino acids and has a mass of 70 kd. It is coupled to a G$_{i/o}$ protein, which inhibits the action of adenylate cyclase and regulates MAP kinase and intracellular calcium levels. There is little sequence homology between H$_3$- and H$_1$- and H$_2$-receptors (only 20% per receptor subtype).[17]

H$_4$-receptors appear to be involved in the differentiation of hematopoietic cells (myeloblasts and promyelocytes) and to modulate immune function by increasing cytosolic calcium in eosinophils, increasing eosinophil chemotaxis and increasing interleukin-16 production.[10] Thus, these receptor subtypes may also be involved in the allergic inflammatory response. A role for this receptor subtype in the CNS remains to be defined. The H$_4$-receptor is composed of 390 amino acids and is coupled to a G$_{i/o}$ protein, which transmits intracellular signals similar to H$_3$-receptors.[10,18]

The role of histamine in the inflammation of allergy merits additional discussion, because so many histamine-based therapeutic products target this process. Inflammation results from a complex set of cellular events that involve redundant mediators and signals. Histamine is released from the granules of mast cells and basophils (also known as FcεRI+ cells) along with tryptase and other preformed mediators, as well as leukotrienes, prostaglandins, and other newly generated mediators. This release in response to cross-linking of surface IgE by allergen or through mechanisms that are independent of IgE. While most of the effects of histamine in allergic disease are mediated via H$_1$-receptors, hypotension, tachycardia, flushing, and headache occur as a result of histamine action at both the H$_1$- and H$_2$-receptors in the vasculature. Also, cutaneous itch and nasal congestion may occur through both the H$_1$- and H$_3$-receptors. In addition to its role in the early allergic response to antigen, histamine acts as a stimulatory signal for the production of cytokines and the expression of cell-adhesion molecules and class II antigens, thereby contributing to the late allergic response.[9–11]

In addition to those actions, histamine exerts other important and variable immunomodulatory effects through its receptor subtypes.[10,19] First, the expression of the receptors changes according to the stage of cell differentiation and local tissue influences. Second, depending on the predominance of the type of receptor, histamine may have proinflammatory or anti-inflammatory effects. Through the H_1-receptor, histamine has proinflammatory activity and is involved in the development of several aspects of antigen-specific immune response, including the maturation of dendritic cells and the modulation of the balance of type 1 helper (Th1) T cells and type 2 helper (Th2) T cells. Histamine may induce an increase in the proliferation of Th1 cells and in the production of interferon and may block humoral immune responses by means of this mechanism. It also induces the release of proinflammatory cytokines and lysosomal enzymes from human macrophages and has the capacity to influence the activity of basophils, eosinophils, and fibroblasts. Finally, histamine may play a role in autoimmunity and malignant disease through the H_1-receptor.

Termination of Histamine Action

Three principal ways exist to terminate the physiological effects of histamine[3,20,21]:

- Cellular uptake: Animal studies have documented the uptake of histamine by many cells. In particular, uptake is a temperature- and partially Na^+-dependent process in rabbit gastric glands and the histamine is metabolized once in the cell.
- Desensitization of cells: Some H_1-receptor–containing tissues exhibit a homogeneous loss of sensitivity to the actions of histamine, perhaps as a result of receptor modification.
- Metabolism: The most common pathway for terminating histamine action involves enzymatic inactivation, as discussed in more detail here.

Released histamine is rapidly inactivated by metabolism via two pathways as shown in Figure 23.5. One pathway involves N^τ-methylation via the enzyme histamine N-methyltransferase (HMT; EC 2.1.1.8). This enzyme is widely distributed in mammalian tissues and catalyzes the transfer of a methyl group from *S*-adenosyl-L-methionine (SAM) to the ring *tele*-nitrogen of histamine, producing N^τ-methylhistamine and *S*-adenosyl-L-homocysteine (Fig. 23.5). The other pathway of catabolism involves oxidative deamination by diamine oxidase (DAO; EC 1.4.3.6), yielding imidazole acetaldehyde, which is further oxidized to imidazole acetic acid by aldehyde dehydrogenases (ALD-DH). Similarly, N^τ-methylhistamine is converted by both DAO and monoamine oxidase (MAO), followed by ALD-DH to N-methyl imidazole acetic acid (Fig. 23.5). All of these metabolites are devoid of histamine receptor agonist activity.

Functions of Histamine as Related to Pharmacological Intervention

Histamine exhibits a wide variety of both physiological and pathological functions in different tissues and cells. The actions of histamine that are of interest from both a pharmacological and therapeutic point of view include (a) its important, but limited, role as a chemical mediator of hypersensitivity and allergic inflammatory reactions, (b) a major role in the regulation of gastric acid secretion, and (c) an emerging role as a neurotransmitter in the CNS.

ANTIHISTAMINES

The term *antihistamine* historically has referred to drugs that block the actions of histamine at H_1-receptors rather than other histamine receptor subtypes. The development of antihistamine drugs began decades ago with the discovery by Fourneau and Bovet[22] that piperoxan could protect animals from the bronchial spasm induced by histamine. This finding was followed by the synthesis of several *N*-phenylethylenediamines with antihistamininic activities superior to those of piperoxan.[23] Further traditional structure–activity studies in this series, based largely on the principles of isosterism and functional group modification, led to the introduction in the 1940s to 1970s of various H_1-antihistamine containing the diarylalkylamine framework.[23,24] These antihistamines, referred to now as the first-generation or classical antihistamines, are related structurally and include several aminoalkyl ethers, ethylenediamines, piperazines, propylamines, phenothiazines, and dibenzocycloheptenes. In addition to H_1-antihistaminic action, these compounds display an array of other pharmacological activities that contribute either toward additional therapeutic applications, or limit use as adverse reactions. More recently, several second-generation or "nonsedating" antihistamines have been developed and introduced.[10,23] The second-generation agents are derivatives of several first-generation agents, but have been modified to be more specific in pharmacologic action and limited in their tissue distribution or accumulation profiles.

Mechanism of Action

It is now known that H_1-antihistamines act as inverse agonists that combine with and stabilize the inactive form of the H_1-receptor, shifting the equilibrium toward the inactive state.[10] Thus, they effectively antagonize the actions of histamine at H_1-receptors. Historically, H_1-antihistamines have been evaluated in vitro in terms of their ability to inhibit histamine-induced spasms in an isolated strip of guinea pig ileum. Antihistamines may be evaluated in vivo in terms of their ability to protect animals against the lethal effects of histamine administered intravenously or by aerosol.

To distinguish antagonism of histamine from other modes of action, the index pA is applied in in vitro assays. The index pA_2 is defined as the inverse of the logarithm of the molar concentration of the antagonist that reduces the response of a double dose of the agonist to that of a single one. The more potent H_1-antihistamines exhibit a pA_2 value significantly higher than 6. Although there are many pitfalls to be avoided in the interpretation of structure–activity relationship (SAR) studies using pA_2 values, the following example illustrates distinguishing competitive antagonism. pA_2 values for pyrilamine (mepyramine) antagonism range from 9.1 to 9.4 with human bronchi and guinea pig ileum.[24,25] By contrast, the pA_2 value in guinea pig (H_2-receptor) is 5.3. Thus, one may conclude that pyrilamine is a weak, noncompetitive inhibitor of histamine at the H_2-receptors and a competitive inhibitor at H_1-receptors. The structural features required for effective interaction of these receptors are discussed next. Some H_1-antihistamines can also block histamine release. The concentrations, however, are considerably higher than those required to produce significant histamine receptor blockade. The H_1-antihistamines do not, however, block antibody production or antigen–antibody interactions.[10,26]

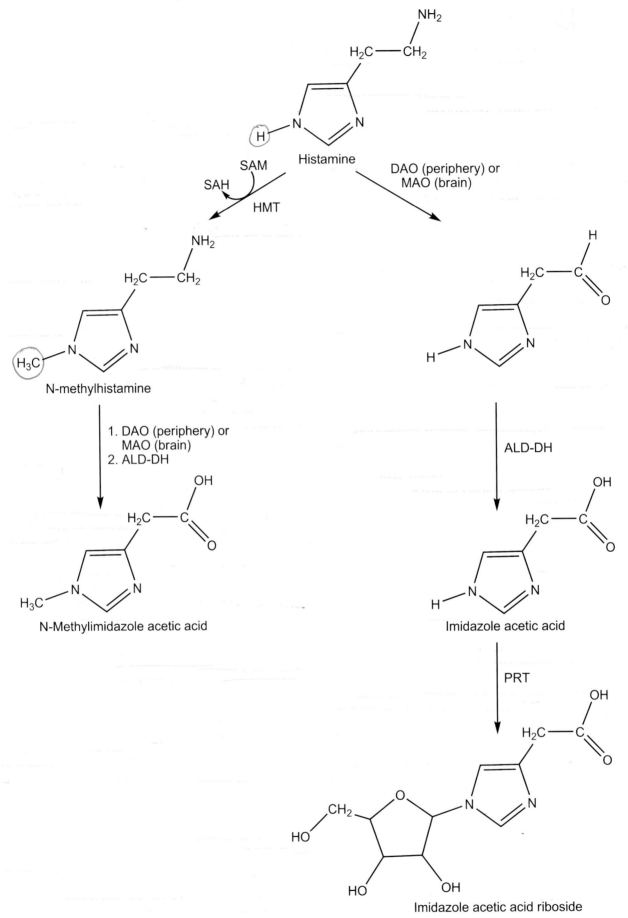

Figure 23.5 ● Metabolism of histamine. (ALD-DH, aldehyde dehydrogenase; PRT, phosphoribosyltransferase.)

Structure–Activity Relationships at H$_1$-Receptors

The H$_1$-antihistamines are now commonly subdivided into two broad groups—the first-generation or classical antihistamines and the second-generation or "nonsedating" antihistamines—based primarily on their general pharmacological profiles.[10,23,27] The differences between these two series are discussed in more detail in the sections that follow. The most detailed published SAR analyses for antihistamines, however, focus on the structural requirements for the first-generation agents.[22–24] From these studies, the structural requirements for H$_1$-antihistaminic action were identified as shown in Figure 23.6. In this structure, Ar is aryl (including phenyl, substituted phenyl, and heteroaryl groups such as 2-pyridyl); Ar' is a second aryl or arylmethyl group; X is a connecting atom of O, C, or N; (CH$_2$)$_n$ represents a carbon chain, usually ethyl; and NRR' represents a basic, terminal amine function. The nature of the connecting atom as well as the diaryl substitution pattern and amine moiety has been used to subclassify the first-generation antihistamines as indicated in the succeeding sections.

This diaryl substitution pattern is present in both the first- and second-generation antihistamines and is essentially a significant H$_1$-receptor affinity.[22–24] Furthermore, several SAR studies suggest that the two aryl moieties must be able to adopt a noncoplanar conformation relative to each other for optimal interaction with the H$_1$-receptor.[28] The two aromatic systems may be linked, as in the tricyclic antihistamines (phenothiazines, dibenzocycloheptanes, and heptenes), but again they must be noncoplanar for effective receptor interaction. Most H$_1$-antihistamines contain substituents in one of the aryl rings (usually benzene), and these influence histamine potency as well as biodisposition, as discussed for the individual classes of compounds in the succeeding sections.

In many of the first-generation, or classical, antihistamines, the terminal nitrogen atom is a simple dimethyl moiety. The amine may also be part of a heteroyclic structure, however, as illustrated by the piperazines, some propylamines (pyrrolidines and piperidines), some phenthiazines, the dibenzocycloheptenes, and the second-generation antihistamines. In all cases, the amino moiety is basic, with pK$_a$s ranging from 8.5 to 10, and thus is presumed to be protonated when bound on the receptor. The amine moiety is also important in the development of stable, solid dosage forms through salt formation.

The carbon chain of typical H$_1$-antihistamines consists of two or three atoms.[22–24] As a result, the distance between the central point of the diaryl ring system and the terminal nitrogen atom in the extended conformation of these compounds ranges from 5 to 6 angstroms (Å). A similar distance between these key moieties is observed for those antihistamines with less conformational freedom. In some structural series, branching of the carbon chain results in reduced antihistaminic activity. There are exceptions, however, as evidenced by promethazine, which has greater activity than its nonbranched counterpart. When the carbon adjacent to the terminal nitrogen atom is branched, the possibility of asymmetry exists. Stereoselective H$_1$-receptor binding is typically not observed, however, when chirality exists at this site.[29] Also, in compounds with an asymmetrically substituted unsaturated carbon chain (pyrrobutamine and triprolidine), one geometric isomer typically displays higher receptor affinity than the other.

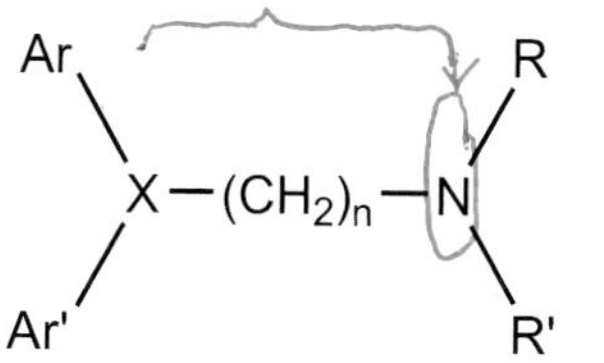

The X connecting moiety of typical H$_1$-antihistamines may be a saturated carbon–oxygen moiety or simply a carbon atom. This group, along with the carbon chain, appears to serve primarily as a spacer group for the key pharmacophoric moieties. Many antihistamines containing a carbon atom in the connecting moiety are chiral and exhibit stereoselective receptor binding. For example, in the pheniramine series and carbinoxamine, this atom is chiral, and in vitro analyses indicate that enantiomers with the S configuration have higher H$_1$-receptor affinity.[30]

Generally, the first- and second-generation antihistamines are substantially more lipophilic than the endogenous agonist, histamine (or the H$_2$-antagonists).[31] This lipophilicity difference results primarily from the presence of the two aryl rings and the substituted amino moieties and thus may simply reflect the different structural requirements for antagonist versus agonist action at H$_1$-receptors.

The nature of the connecting moiety and the structural nature of the aryl moieties have been used to classify the antihistarnines as indicated in the sections that follow. Furthermore, variations in the diaryl groups, X-connecting moieties, and the nature of substitution in the alkyl side chain or terminal nitrogen among the various drugs account for differences observed in antihistaminic potency as well as pharmacological, biodisposition, and adverse reaction profiles. The ability of these drugs to display an array of pharmacological activities is largely because they can interact with H$_1$-receptors throughout the body, and that they contain the basic pharmacophore required for binding to muscarinic as well as adrenergic and serotonergic receptors (Table 23.2). The relationships of antihistamine structure to these overlapping actions (H$_1$-antihistaminic, anticholinergic, and local anesthetic) have been analyzed.

General Pharmacological and Therapeutic Considerations

The classical antihistamines have been used extensively for the symptomatic treatment (sneezing, rhinorrhea, and itching of eyes, nose, and throat) of allergic rhinitis (hay fever, pollinosis), chronic idiopathic urticaria, and several other histamine-related diseases.[10] These uses are clearly attributed to their ability to counter the action of histamine at peripheral H$_1$-receptors, which mediate the immune and inflammatory processes characteristic of these pathologies. These drugs best relieve the symptoms of allergic diseases at the beginning of the season when pollen counts are low. The antihistamines also reduce the number, size, and duration of wheals and itching in chronic urticaria when used promptly. Most clinical evidence suggests that there is no significant difference in therapeutic efficacy for first- and second-generation agents in the treatment of these conditions. The antihistamines have been widely used to relieve the symptoms of

Figure 23.6 ● General antihistamine structure.

TABLE 23.2 General Pharmacologic Properties of Selected "Antihistamines"

Antihistamine	Dose (mg)	Dosing Int. (hrs)	Sedative Effects	Anti-H1 Activity	Anti-M Activity	Antiemetic
First Generation: Propylamines						
Brompheniramine	4	4–6	+	+++	++	—
Chlorpheniramine	4	4–6	±	++	++	—
Dexchlorpheniramine	2	4–6	+	+++	++	—
Triprolidine	2.5	4–6	+	++/+++	++	—
Phenindamine	25	4–6	±	++	++	—
First Generation: Ethanolamines (Aminoalkyl Ethers)						
Clemastine	1	12	++	++	+++	++/+++
Carbinoxamine	4–8	6–8	++	+/++	+++	++/+++
Diphenhydramine	25–50	6–8	+++	+	+++	++/+++
First Generation: Ethylenediamines						
Pyrilamine	25–50	6–8	+	+/++	±	—
Tripelennamine	25–50	4–6	++	+/++	±	—
First Generation: Phenothiazines						
Promethazine	12.5–25	6–24	+++	+++	+++	++++
Trimeprazine	2.5	6	++	++/+++	+++	++++
Methdilazine	8	6–12	+	++/+++	+++	++++
First Generation: Piperazines (Cyclizines)						
Hydroxyzine	25–100	4–8	+++	++/+++	++	+++
First Generation: Dibenzocycloheptenes/Heptanes						
Azatadine	1–2	12	++	++	++	—
Cyproheptadine	4	8	++	++	++	—
First Generation: Phthalazinone						
Azelastine	0.5	12	±	++/+++	±	—
Second Generation (Peripherally Selective): Piperazine						
Cetirizine/Levocetirizine*	5* to 10	24	±	++/+++	±	—
Second Generation (Peripherally Selective): Piperidines						
Astemizole	10	24	±	++/+++	±	—
Fexofenadine	60	12	±	—	±	—
Loratadine /Desloratadine	10	24	±	++/+++	±	—

Source: Facts and Comparisons 4.0, Wolters Kluwer Health, Amsterdam, Netherlands, 2009.
++++, very high; +++, high; ++, moderate; +, low; ±, low to none; — no data.

asthma and upper respiratory infections including the common cold, otitis media, and sinusitis. Most clinical evidence[10] does not support such use unless asthma or infection is accompanied by allergic inflammation. Also, the antihistamines should not be used alone in analphylaxis, but may be used with epinephrine to relieve any H_1-receptor–mediated symptoms.[10]

As the aforementioned general pharmacological profiles suggests, many antihistamines can interact with various neurotransmitter receptors and other biomacromolecular targets.[10] This is most evident among the first-generation agents, many of which function as antagonists at muscarinic receptors and, to a lesser extent, adrenergic, serotonergic, and dopamine receptors. The first-generation agents also tend to achieve and maintain higher levels in the brain than the second-generation agents, resulting in CNS-based pharmacologic actions.[10] Although some of these non–target-receptor interactions may have therapeutic value (as discussed next), more frequently they are manifested as adverse reactions that limit drug use. This is particularly true of the peripheral anticholinergic effects produced by these drugs and of interactions with several neurotransmitter systems in the CNS that result in sedation, fatigue, and dizziness (see Table 23.2).

Several first-generation antihistamines, particularly the phenothiazines and aminoalkyl ethers, have antiemetic actions

and thus may be useful in the treatment of nausea and vomiting and for vertigo and motion sickness.[10,26,27] Several of the phenothiazines have limited use in parkinsonism as a result of their ability to block central muscarinic receptors.[10,26,27] Antihistamines, including promethazine, pyrilamine, tripelennamine, and diphenhydramine, also display local anesthetic activity that may be therapeutically useful.[32]

Many of the first-generation antihistamines readily penetrate the blood-brain barrier (BBB) because of their lipophilicity, and maintain significant CNS concentrations because they are not substrates for P-glycoprotein efflux pump that are expressed on endothelial cells of the CNS vasculature. The lack of affinity by P-glycoprotein efflux pumps appears to be directly related to the relatively low molecular weight and small size of the first-generation antihistamines.[10,33] Blockade of central H_1-receptors results in sedation, an effect that has contributed to the historical use of antihistamines as nonprescription sleep aids, as well as drugs for perioperative sedation.[10] However, the sedative actions of antihistamines are undesired effects in the treatment of allergy-based diseases. Furthermore, the blockade of central H_1-receptors also results in decreased cognitive and psychomotor performance, as well as increased appetite and weight gain, all considered to be therapy-limiting adverse effects.[10,33]

TABLE 23.3 Antihistamine Pharmacokinetic Properties

H_1-Antihistamine (Metabolite)	T_{max} after a Single Dose (hrs)	Terminal Elim. Half-life (hrs)	% Elim. Unchanged in Urine/ Feces	Clinically Relevant DIs?	Onset, Dur. of Action (hrs)	Usual Adult Dose	Dose Adjustment Required for Impairment?
First-Generation Antihistamines							
Chlorpheniramine	2.8±0.8	27.9±8.7	—	Possible	3, 24	4 mg 3–4 times per day 12 mg SRF)/2 times per day	—
Diphenhydramine	1.7±1.0	9.2±2.5	—	Possible	2, 12	25–50 mg 3–4 times per day or at bedtime	Hepatic
Doxepin	2	13	—	Possible	—	25–50 mg 3 times daily or at bedtime	Hepatic
Hydroxyzine	2.1±0.4	20.0±4.1	—	Possible	2, 24	25–50 mg 3 times daily or at bedtime	Hepatic
Second-Generation Antihistamines		↓ metab.					
Acrivastine	1.4±0.4	1.4–3.1	59/0	Unlikely	1, 8	8 mg 3 times per day	—
Cetirizine	1.0±0.5	6.5–10	60/10	Unlikely	1, 24	5–10 mg daily	Renal and hepatic
Desloratadine	1–3	27	0	Unlikely	2, 24	5 mg daily	Renal and hepatic
Fexofenadine	2.6	14.4	12/80	Unlikely	2, 24	60 mg twice per day or 120 or 180 mg per day	Renal
Levocetirizine	0.8±0.5	7±1.5	86/13	Unlikely	1, 24	5 mg daily	Renal and hepatic
Loratadine (Desloratadine)	1.2±0.3 (1.5±0.7)	7.8±4.2 (24±9.8)	Trace —	Unlikely —	2, 24	10 mg daily	Hepatic

Source: Simons, F. E. R.: Advances in H_1-antihistamines. N. Engl. J. Med. 351:2203–2217, 2004.

Cardiac toxic effects induced by H_1-antihistamines occur rarely and are independent of H_1-receptor occupation.[10,33,34] As mentioned previously, first-generation H_1-antihistamines have antimuscarinic and α-adrenergic blockade activity and thus may cause dose-related prolongation of the QT interval. The first two second-generation H_1-antihistamines, astemizole and terfenadine, were found to be even more cardiotoxic than the first-generation agents, especially when used in combination with other drugs. This led to their withdrawal from the market. The cardiac effects of the second-generation antihistamines are discussed in more detail in the next section of this chapter.

The primary objective of antihistamine drug development over the past several decades has centered on developing new drugs with higher selectivity for H_1-receptors and lacking undesirable CNS and cardiovascular actions.[10,33,34] These efforts led to the introduction of the second-generation antihistamines, which are classified as "nonsedating" and have little antagonist activity at other neurotransmitter receptors, including muscarinic receptors, and cardiac ion channels at therapeutic concentrations. The pharmacological properties of these agents will be discussed in more detail.

There are relatively few published studies concerning the pharmacokinetic and biodisposition profiles of the first-generation antihistamines.[10,31] Generally, the compounds are orally active and well absorbed, but oral bioavailability may be limited by first-pass metabolism. The metabolites formed depend on drug structure to a large extent but commonly involve the tertiary amino moiety. This functionality may be subject to successive oxidative *N*-dealkylation, deamination, and amino acid conjugation of the resultant acid. The amine group may also undergo *N*-oxidation (which may be reversible) or direct glucuronide conjugation. First-generation agents with unsubstituted and activated aromatic rings (phenothiazines) may undergo aromatic hydroxylation to yield

phenols, which may be eliminated as conjugates. More detailed pharmacokinetic data are available for the second-generation agents and are included in the monographs that follow and Table 23.3.

The H_1-antihistamines display various significant drug interactions when coadministered with other therapeutic agents. For example, MAO inhibitors prolong and intensify the anticholinergic actions of the antihistamines. Also, the sedative effects of these agents may potentiate the depressant activity of barbiturates, alcohol, narcotic analgesics, and other depressants.[10,23,31]

First-Generation Antihistamine Classes

AMINOALKYL ETHERS (ETHANOLAMINES)

The aminoalkyl ether antihistamines are characterized by the presence of a CHO connecting moiety (X) and a two- or three-carbon atom chain as the linking moiety between the key diaryl and tertiary amino groups (Fig. 23.7). Most compounds in this series are simple *N*, *N*-dimethylethanolamine derivatives and are so classified in several texts. Clemastine and diphenylpyraline differ from this basic structural pattern, in that the basic nitrogen moiety and at least part of the carbon chain are part of a heterocyclic ring system and

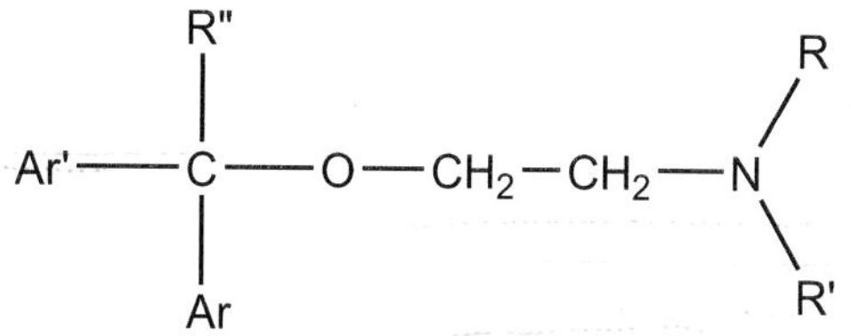

Figure 23.7 ● General structure of the aminoalkyl ethers.

there are three carbon atoms between the oxygen and nitrogen atoms. The basic nitrogen in all of these compounds is not only essential for binding affinity, but also serves as a moiety for the formation of stable, solid salts.

The simple diphenyl derivative diphenhydramine was the first clinically useful member of the ethanolamine series and serves as the prototype. Other therapeutically useful derivatives of diphenhydramine have been obtained by para substitution of methyl (methyldiphenhydramine), methoxy (medrylamine), chloro (chlorodiphenhydramine), or bromo (bromodiphenhydramine) on one of the phenyl rings. These derivatives reportedly have better therapeutic profiles than diphenhydramine because of reduced adverse effects.[10,31] Replacement of one of the phenyl rings of the diphenhydramine with a 2-pyridyl group, as in doxylamine and carbinoxamine, enhances antihistaminic activity as demonstrated by pA_2 values in vitro and therapeutic dosing data (Table 23.2). These compounds display oral antihistaminic activities 40 and 2 greater, respectively, than diphenhydramine in animal test models.[31]

As a result of an asymmetrically substituted benzylic carbon, most of the aminoalkyl ethers are optically active. Most studies indicate indicate that the individual enantiomers differ significantly in antihistaminic activity, with activity residing predominantly in the S-enantiomers.[30,35]

The diaryl tertiary aminoalkyl ether structure that characterizes these compounds also serves as a pharmacophore for muscarinic receptors (Table 23.2). As a result, the drugs in this group possess significant anticholinergic activity, which contributes not only to their therapeutic use as antiemetic, motion sickness, and anti-Parkinson drugs but also to their adverse effect profile (dry mouth, blurred vision, urinary retention, constipation, tachycardia). Drowsiness, as well as other CNS effects, is a common side effect to the tertiary aminoalkyl ethers, presumably as a result of the ability of these compounds to penetrate the BBB and occupy central H_1-receptors. Although this central action is exploited in over-the-counter (OTC) sleeping aids, it may interfere with the performance of tasks requiring mental alertness.[10,26,27] The frequency of GI side effects in this series of antihistamines is relatively low, compared with the ethylenediamine antihistamines.[10,26,27]

In spite of their long and extensive use, pharmacokinetic data on this series of compounds are relatively limited. Most members of this series appear to be extensively metabolized by pathways including *N*-oxidation and successive oxidative *N*-dealkylation followed by aldehyde oxidation and amino acid conjugation.[31] The known kinetic properties of representative members of this class of antihistamines are summarized in Table 23.3.[10]

The structures of the aminoalkyl ether derivatives with physicochemical properties, basic therapeutic activty data, and dosage form information are provided in the monographs that follow.

✶ *Diphenhydramine Hydrochloride, Tannate, and Citrate.* Diphenhydramine hydrochloride, 2-(diphenylmethoxy)-*N*,*N*-dimethylethanamine hydrochloride (Benadryl), is an oily, lipid-soluble free base available as the bitter-tasting hydrochloride salt, which is a stable, white crystalline powder soluble in water (1:1), alcohol (1:2) and chloroform (1:2). The salt has a pK_a value of 9, and a 1% aqueous solution has a pH of about 5. The other salts display comparable properties.

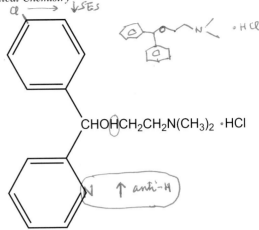

$CHOHCH_2CH_2N(CH_3)_2 \cdot HCl$

Diphenhydramine Hydrochloride

In addition to antihistaminic action, diphenhydramine exhibits antidyskinetic, antiemetic, antitussive and antimuscarinic, and sedative properties. In the usual dose range of 25 to 400 mg, diphenhydramine is not a highly active H_1-antihistamine. Conversion to a quaternary ammonium salt does not alter the antihistaminic action greatly but does increase the anticholinergic action.

As an antihistaminic agent, diphenhydramine is recommended in various allergic conditions and, to a lesser as an antitussive and Parkinsonism drug. It is also used in OTC sleep-aid products. It is administered either orally or parenterally in the treatment of urticaria, seasonal rhinitis (hay fever), and some dermatoses. The most common side effect is drowsiness, and the concurrent use of alcohol and other CNS depressants should be avoided.

Dosage forms: Tablets (12.5, 25, and 50 mg); capsules (25 and 50 mg); oral disintegrating strips (12.5 and 25 mg); solutions, elixirs, and syrups (12.5 mg/5 mL); suspension (25 mg/5 mL); and injection (50 mg/mL).
Usual adult doses:
- Antihistamine: 25 to 50 mg every 4 to 6 hours (maximum of 300 mg/day)
- Antitussive liquid: 25 to 50 mg every 4 hours (liquid) or 25 mg every 4 hours (syrup); do not exceed 300 mg/day
- Motion sickness: 25 to 50 mg every 4 to 6 hours (maximum of 300 mg/day)

Dimenhydrinate. The 8-chlorotheophyllinate (theoclate) salt of diphenhydramine, 8-chlorotheophylline 2-(diphenylmethoxy)-*N*,*N*-dimethylethylamine (Dramamine), is a white crystalline, odorless powder that is highly soluble in water and freely soluble in alcohol and chloroform.

Dimenhydrinate is recommended for nausea of motion sickness and for hyperemesis gravidarum (nausea of pregnancy). For the prevention of motion sickness, the dose should be taken at least 0.5 hour before beginning a trip. The cautions listed for diphenhydramine should be observed.

Dosage forms: Tablets (50 mg), liquid (12.5 mg/5 mL, 15.62 mg/5 mL), injection (50 mg/mL)
Usual dosage (motion sickness):
- Adult/children >12 years of age: 1 to 2 chewable tablets or tablets (50–100 mg) every 4 to 6 hours, not to exceed 8 chewable tablets or tablets (400 mg) in 24 hours

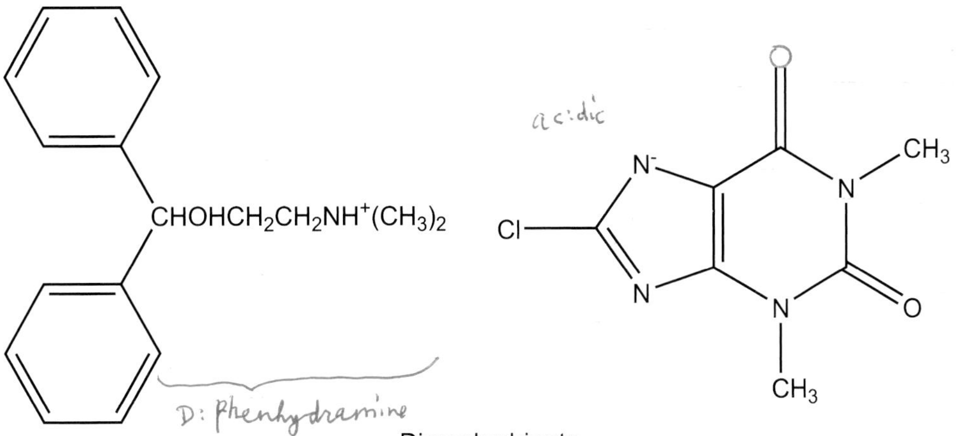

CHOHCH$_2$CH$_2$NH$^+$(CH$_3$)$_2$

D: Phenhydramine

Dimenhydrinate

acidic

CH$_3$

CH$_3$

- Children 6 to younger than 12 years of age: ½ to 1 chewable tablet or tablet (25–50 mg) every 6 to 8 hours, not to exceed 3 tablets in 24 hours
- Children 2 to younger than 6 years of age: ¼ to ½ chewable tablet or tablet (12.5–25 mg) every 6 to 8 hours, not to exceed 1 ½ tablets in 24 hours

Bromodiphenhydramine Hydrochloride. Bromodiphenhydramine hydrochloride, 2-[(4-bromophenyl)-phenylmethoxy]-*N*, *N*-dimethylethanamine hydrochloride (Ambodryl Hydrochloride), is a white to pale buff crystalline powder that is freely soluble in water and in alcohol. Relative to diphenhydramine, bromodiphenhydramine is more lipid soluble and was twice as effective in protecting against the lethal effects of histamine aerosols.

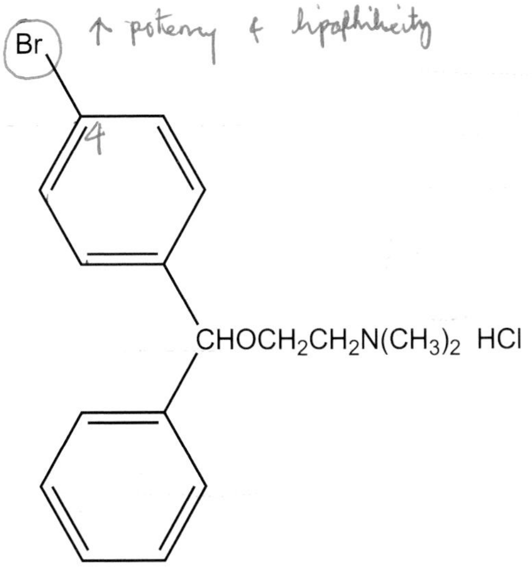

↑ potency & lipophilicity

Br

/4

CHOCH$_2$CH$_2$N(CH$_3$)$_2$ HCl

Bromodiphenhydramine Hydrochloride

Dosage forms: Capsules and elixir
Usual adult dose: Oral, 25 mg/4 to 6 hours

Doxylamine Succinate. The acid succinate salt (bisuccinate) of doxylamine, 2-[α-[2-(dimethylamino)ethoxy]-α-methylbenzyl]pyridine bisuccinate (Decapryn Succinate), is a white to creamy-white powder with a characteristic odor. It is soluble in water (1:1), alcohol (1:2), and chloroform (1:2). A 1% solution has a pH of about 5.

Doxylamine succinate is comparable in potency to diphenhydramine. It is indicated for the relief of seasonal

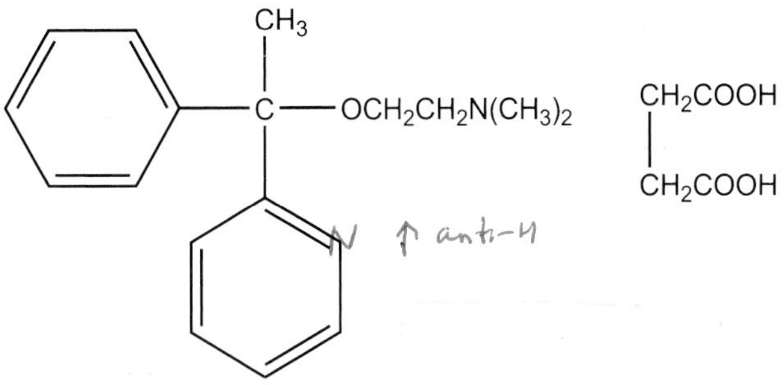

CH$_3$

C—OCH$_2$CH$_2$N(CH$_3$)$_2$

CH$_2$COOH
|
CH$_2$COOH

N ↑ anti-H

Doxylamine Succinate

rhinitis symptoms, but is also used as a nighttime sedative. Concurrent use of alcohol and other CNS depressants should be avoided.

Dosage forms: Tablets (5 mg), oral suspension (1 mg/mL), and oral liquid (2.5 mg/2.5 mL)
Usual adult dose: Oral, 12.5 to 25 mg/4 to 6 hours

Carbinoxamine Maleate. Carbinoxamine is available as a bitter bimaleate salt, (d, l)-2-[*p*-chloro-α-[2-(dimethylamino)ethoxy]benzyl]pyridine bimaleate (Clistin), which is a white crystalline powder that is very soluble in water and freely soluble in alcohol and in chloroform. The pH of a 1% solution is between 4.6 and 5.1.

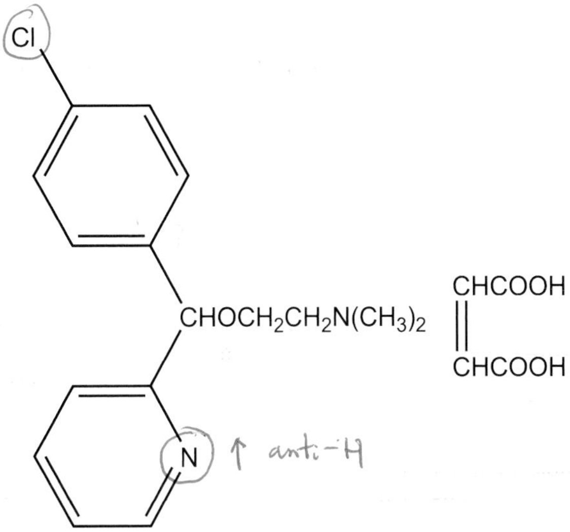

Cl

CHOCH$_2$CH$_2$N(CH$_3$)$_2$

CHCOOH
||
CHCOOH

N *↑ anti-H*

Carbinoxamine Maleate

Carbinoxamine is a potent antihistaminic and is available as the racemic mixture. It differs structurally from chlorpheniramine only in having an oxygen atom separate the asymmetric carbon atom from the aminoethyl side chain. The more active *levo* isomer of carbinoxamine has the (S) absolute configuration[30] and can be superimposed on the more active *dextro* isomer (S configuration) of chlorpheniramine.

Dosage forms: Tablets (4 and 8 mg), capsules (10 mg), liquid (1.67 mg/5 mL), solution (4 mg/5 mL), and suspension (3.2 mg/5 mL)
Usual dose (tablets):
- Adults and children 12 years of age and older: 1 tablet (8 mg) twice daily
- Children 6 to 12 years of age: ½ tablet twice daily (every 12 hours). The tablets are not recommended for children younger than 6 years of age.

Clemastine Fumarate. Dextrorotatory clemastine, R,R-2[2[1-(4-chlorophenyl)-1-phenylethoxy]ethyl]-1-methylpyrrolidine hydrogen furnarate (1:1) (Tavist), has two chiral centers, each of which has the (R) absolute configuration. A comparison of the activities of the enantiomers indicates that the asymmetric center close to the terminal side chain nitrogen is of lesser importance to antihistaminic activity.[36]

This member of the ethanolamine series is characterized by a long duration of action, with an activity that reaches a maximum in 5 to 7 hours and persists for 10 to 12 hours. It is well absorbed when administered orally, and it is excreted primarily in the urine. The side effects are those usually encountered with this series of antihistamines. Clemastine is closely related to chlorphenoxamine, which is used for its central cholinergic-blocking activity. Therefore, it is not surprising that clemastine has significant antimuscarinic activity.

Dosage forms: Tablets (1.34 and 2.68 mg) and syrup (0.67 mg/5 mL)
Usual adult dose:
- Allergic rhinitis: 1.34 mg every 12 hours or twice daily (maximum 8.04 mg/day for the syrup or 2.68 mg in 24 hours for the tablets) for adults; 0.67 mg twice daily (maximum 4.02 mg) for children 6 to 12 years of age (syrup only)
- Urticaria/angioedema: 2.68 mg twice daily, not to exceed 8.04 mg/day for adults; 1.34 mg twice daily, not to exceed 4.02 mg/day for children 6 to 12 years of age (syrup only)

Diphenylpyraline Hydrochloride. Diphenylpyraline hydrochloride, 4-(diphenylmethoxy)-1-methylpiperidine hydrochloride (Hispril, Diafen) is a white or slightly off-white crystalline powder that is soluble in water or alcohol. Diphenylpyraline is structurally related to diphenhydramine with the aminoalkyl side chain incorporated in a piperidine ring. It is a potent antihistaminic, and the usual dose is 2 mg 3 or 4 times daily.

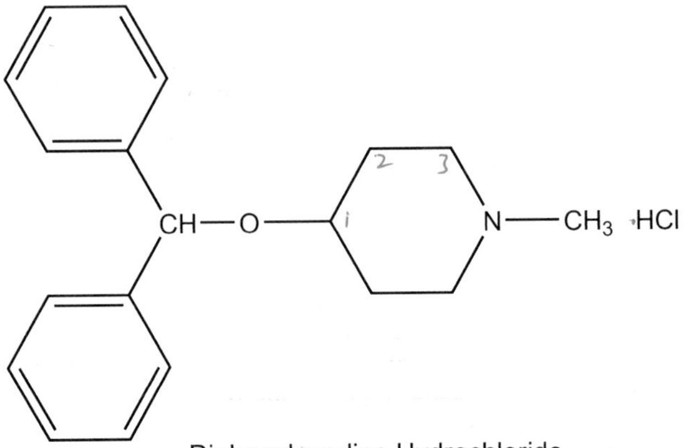

Diphenylpyraline Hydrochloride

Dosage forms: Extended-release capsules (5 mg)
Usual adult dose: Oral, 5 mg/12 hours

ETHYLENEDIAMINES

The ethylenediamine antihistamines are characterized by the presence of a nitrogen-connecting atom (X) and a two-carbon atom chain as the linking moiety between the key diaryl and tertiary amino moieties (Fig. 23.8). All compounds in this series are simple diarylethylenediamines except antazoline, in which the terminal amine and a portion of the carbon chain are included as part of an imidazoline ring system. Because it differs significantly in its pharmacological profile, antazoline is not always classified as an ethylenediamine derivative.

Phenbenzamine was the first clinically useful member of this class and served as the prototype for the development of more effective derivatives. Replacement of the phenyl moiety of phenbenzamine with a 2-pyridyl system yielded

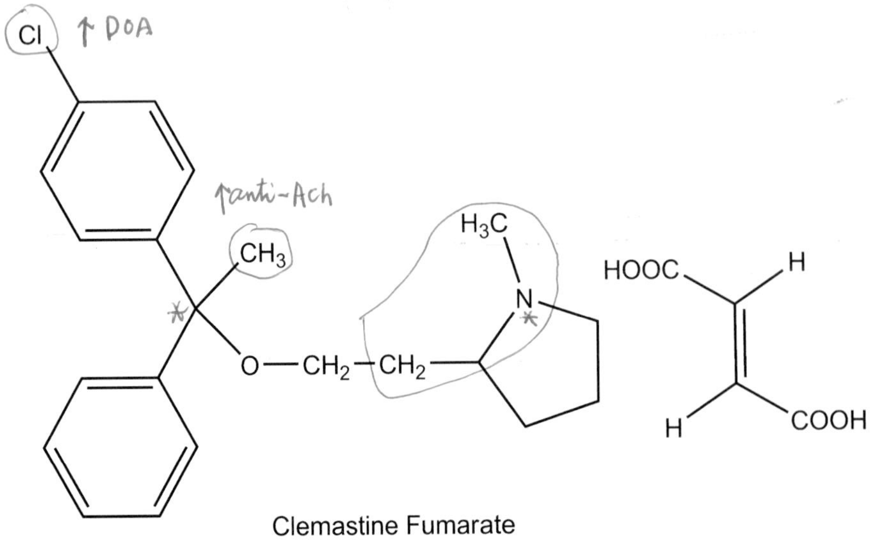

Clemastine Fumarate

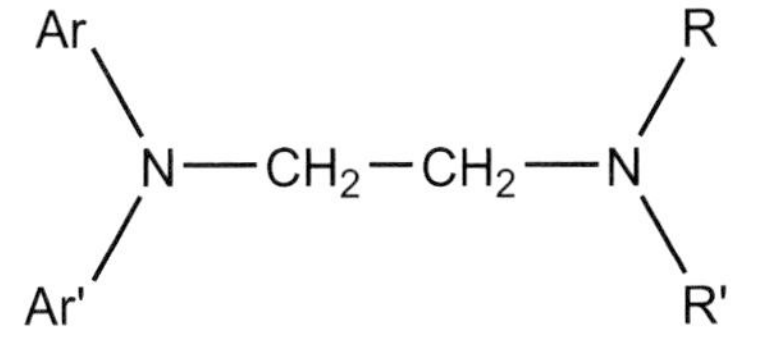

Figure 23.8 ● General structure of the ethylenediamines.

tripelennamine, a significantly more effective histamine receptor blocker as was also observed in the aminoalkyl ether series described previously.[31] Substitution of a *para* methoxy (pyrilamine or mepyramine), chloro (chloropyramine), or bromo (bromtripelennamine) further enhances activity, as observed earlier. Replacement of the benzyl group of tripelennamine with a 2-thienylmethyl group provided methapyrilene, and replacement of tripelennamine's 2-pyridyl group with a pyrimidinyl moiety (along with *p*-methoxy substitution) yielded thonzylamine, both of which function as potent H_1-receptor antagonists.[31]

In all of these compounds, the aliphatic or terminal amino group is required for H_1-blocking activity and is significantly more basic than the nitrogen atom bonded to the diaryl moiety; the nonbonded electrons on the diaryl nitrogen are delocalized by the aromatic ring, and the resultant reduction in electron density on nitrogen decreases basicity. Thus, the aliphatic amino group in the ethylenediamines is sufficiently basic for the formation of pharmaceutically useful salts.

Historically, the ethylenediamines were among the first useful antihistamines. They are moderately effective H_1-antihistamines based on pA_2 values and doses, but they also display a relatively high frequency of CNS depressant and GI side effects.[27,31] The anticholinergic and antiemetic actions of these compounds are relatively low compared with those of most other classical, first-generation antihistamines (Table 23.2). The piperazine- and phenothiazine-type antihistamines also contain the ethylenediamine moiety, but these agents are discussed separately because they exhibit significantly different pharmacological properties.

Relatively little information is available concerning the pharmacokinetics of this series of compounds. Tripelennamine is metabolized in humans by *N*-glucuronidation, *N*-oxidation, and pyridyl oxidation followed by phenol glucuronidation. It is anticipated that other members of this series are similarly metabolized.[31] The known pharmacokinetic properties of representative members of this class of antihistamines are summarized in Table 23.3.

The structures of the salt forms of the marketed ethylenediamine antihistamines, along with physicochemical properties, therapeutic activity profiles, and dosage form information, are provided in the monographs that follow.

Tripelennamine Citrate. Tripelennamine citrate, 2-[benzyl[2-dimethylamino)-ethyl]amino]pyridine citrate (1:1), PBZ (Pyribenzamine Citrate), is available as a monocitrate salt, which is a white crystalline powder freely soluble in water and in alcohol. A 1% solution has a pH of 4.25. For oral administration in liquid dose forms, the citrate salt is less bitter and thus more palatable than the hydrochloride. Because of the difference in molecular weights, the doses of the two salts must be equated −30 mg of the citrate salt is equivalent to 20 mg of the hydrochloride salt.

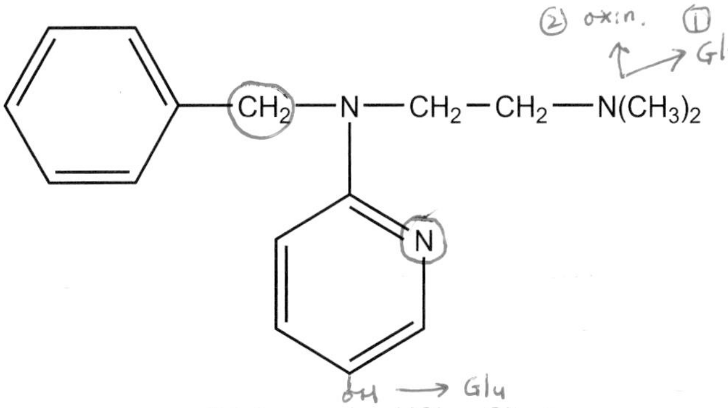

Triplennamine HCl or Citrate

Dosage forms: Elixir
Usual adult dose: Oral, 25 to 50 mg/4 to 6 hours

Tripelennamine Hydrochloride. Tripelennamine hydrochloride is a white crystalline powder that darkens slowly on exposure to light. The salt is soluble in water (1:0.77) and in alcohol (1:6). It has a pK_a of about 9, and a 0.1% solution has a pH of about 5.5.

Tripelennamine, the first ethylenediamine developed in the United States and is well absorbed when given orally. It appears to be as effective as diphenhydramine and may have the advantage of fewer and less severe side reactions. Drowsiness may occur, however, and may impair the ability to perform tasks requiring alertness. The concurrent use of alcoholic beverages should be avoided.

Dosage forms: Tablets, extended-release tablets
Usual adult dose: Oral tablets, 25 to 50 mg/4 to 6 hours; extended-release tablets, 100 mg/8 to 12 hours

Pyrilamine Maleate. Pyrilamine, 2-[4-methoxybenzyl [2-dimethylamino)ethyl]-amino]pyridine, is available as the acid maleate salt (1:1), which is a white crystalline powder with a faint odor and a bitter, saline taste. The salt is soluble in water (1:0.4) and freely soluble in alcohol. A 10% solution has a pH of approximately 5. At a pH of 7.5 or above, the free base begins to precipitate.

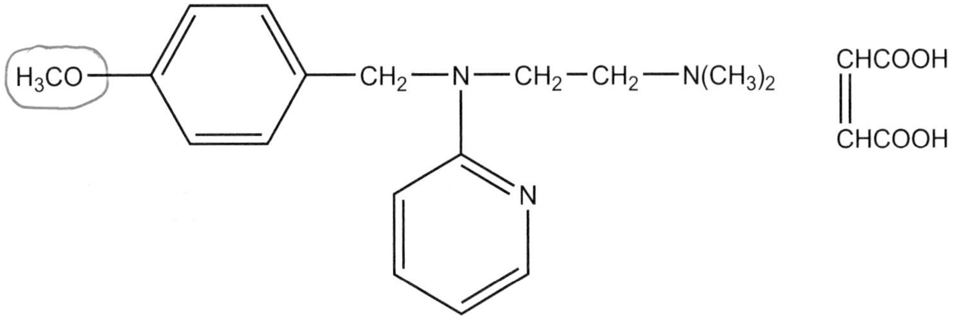

Pyrilamine Maleate

Pyrilamine differs structurally from tripelennamine by having a methoxy group in the *para* position of the benzyl radical. It differs from its more toxic and less potent precursor phenbenzamine (Antergan) by having a 2-pyridyl group on the nitrogen atom in place of a phenyl group.

Clinically, pyrilamine and tripelennamine are considered among the less potent antihistaminics. They are highly potent, however, in antagonizing histamine-induced contractions of guinea pig ileum.[22] Because of the pronounced local anesthetic action, the drug should not be chewed, but taken with food.

Dosage forms: Tablets
Usual adult dose: Oral, 25 to 50 mg/6 to 8 hours

X *Methapyrilene Hydrochloride.* Methapyrilene hydrochloride, 2-[[2-(dimethylamino)-ethyl]-2-thienylarnino] pyridine monohydrochloride (Histadyl) is available as the bitter-tasting, white crystalline powder that is soluble in water (1:0.5), in alcohol (1:5), and in chloroform (1:3). Its solutions have a pH of about 5.5. It differs structurally from tripelennamine in having a 2-thiophene—methylene group in place of the benzyl group. The thiophene ring is considered isosteric with the benzene ring, and the isosteres exhibit similar activity. A study of the solid-state conformation of methapyrilene hydrochloride showed that the *trans*-conformation is preferred for the two ethylenediamine nitrogen atoms. The Food and Drug Administration declared methapyrilene a potential carcinogen in 1979, and all products containing it have been recalled.

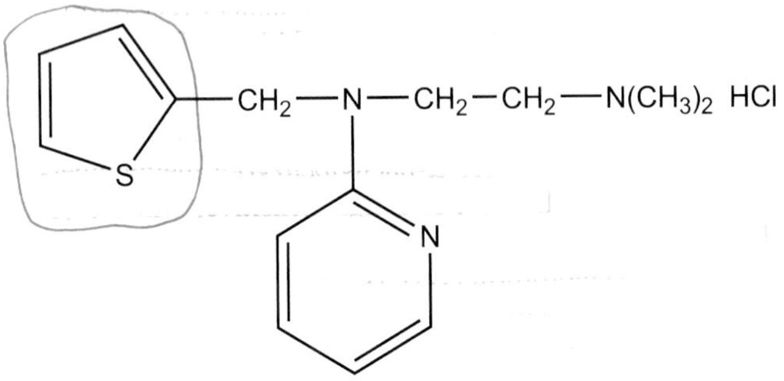

Methapyrilene Hydrochloride

X *Thonzylamine Hydrochloride.* Thonzylamine hydrochloride, 2-[[2-(dimethylamino)-ethyl](p-methoxybenzyl)amino]pyrimidine hydrochloride, is a white crystalline powder soluble in water (1:1), in alcohol (1:6), and in chloroform (1:4). A 2% aqueous solution has a pH of 5.5. It is similar in activity to tripelennamine but is claimed to be less toxic. The usual dose is 50 mg taken up to 4 times daily. It is available in certain combination products.

X *Antazoline Phosphate.* Antazoline phosphate, 2-[(N-benzylanilino)methyl]-2-imidazoline dihydrogen phosphate, is a bitter, white to off-white crystalline powder that is soluble in water. It has a pKa of 10.0, and a 2% solution has a pH of about 4.5. Antazoline, like the ethylenediamines, contains an N-benzylanilino group linked to a basic nitrogen through a two-carbon chain.

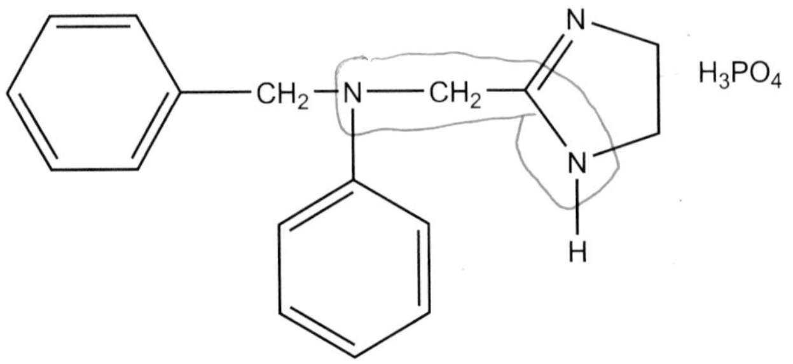

Antazoline Phosphate

Antazoline is less active than most of the other antihistaminic drugs, but it is characterized by the lack of local irritation. The more soluble phosphate salt is applied topically to the eye in a 0.5% solution. The less soluble hydrochloride is given orally. In addition to its use as an antihistamine, antazoline has more than twice the local anesthetic potency of procaine and also exhibits anticholinergic actions.

PIPERAZINES (CYCLIZINES)

The piperazines or cyclizines can also be considered ethylenediamine derivatives or cyclic ethylenediamines (cyclizines); in this series, however, the connecting moiety (X) is a CHN group, and the carbon chain, terminal amine functionality, and the nitrogen atom of the connecting group are all part of a piperazine moiety (Fig. 23.9). Both nitrogen atoms in these compounds are aliphatic and thus display comparable basicities. The primary structural differences within this series involve the nature of the *para* aromatic ring substituent (H or Cl) and, more importantly, the nature of the terminal piperazine nitrogen substituent.

The piperazines are moderately potent antihistaminics with a relatively high potential to cause drowsiness and psychomotor and cognitive dysfunction (Table 23.2).[26,27,31] The activity of the piperazine-type antihistaminics is characterized by a slow onset, but a long duration of action. These

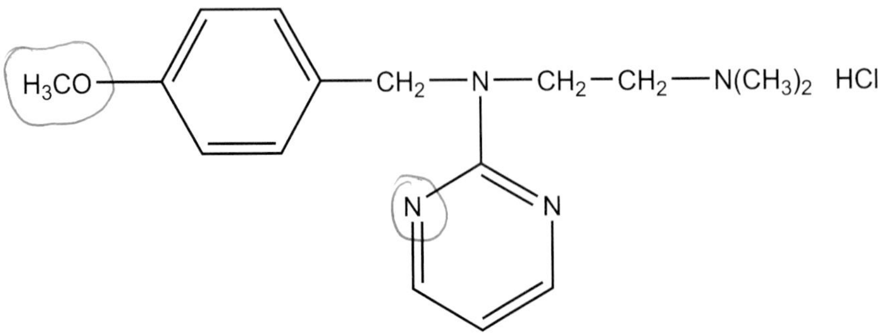

Thonzylamine Hydrochloride

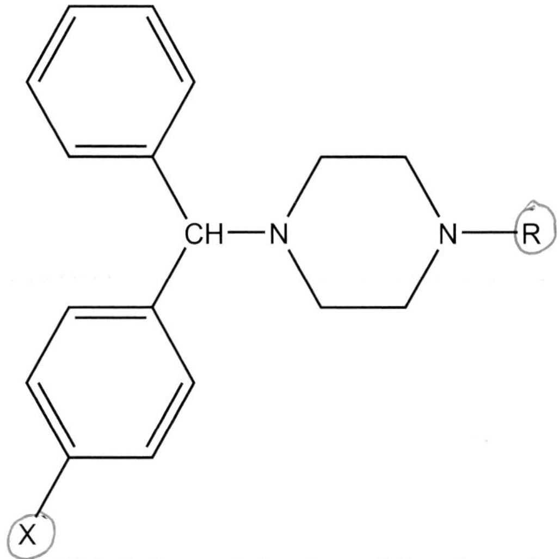

Figure 23.9 ● General structure of the piperazines.

agents exhibit peripheral and central antimuscarinic activity, and thereby diminish vestibular stimulation and act on the medullary chemoreceptor trigger zone.[10,26,27] Thus, as a group, these agents have found significant use as antiemetics and antivertigo agents and in the treatment of motion sickness (Table 23.2).

Some members of this series have exhibited a strong teratogenic potential, inducing several malformations in animal models. The *N*-dealkylayed metabolites, the norchlorcyclizines, have been proposed as responsible for the teratogenic effects of the parent drugs.[37] Although teratogenicity has not been observed in humans, its use during pregnancy is discouraged. Metabolic studies in this series of compounds have focused primarily on cyclizine and chlorcyclizine, and these compounds undergo similar biotransformation. The primary pathways involve *N*-oxidation and *N*-demethylation, and both of these metabolites are devoid of antihistaminic activity.

The structures of the marketed salt forms of the piperazine antihistamines, along with physicochemical properties, basic therapeutic activity profiles, and dosage form information, are provided in the monographs that follow. The known kinetic properties of representative members of this class of antihistamines are summarized in Table 23.3.

Cyclizine Hydrochloride. Cyclizine hydrochloride, 1-(diphenylmethyl)-4-methylpiperazine monohydrochloride

(Marezine), occurs as a light-sensitive, white crystalline powder with a bitter taste. It is slightly soluble in water (1:115), in alcohol (1:115), and in chloroform (1:75). It is used primarily in the prophylaxis and treatment of motion sickness. The lactate salt (Cyclizine Lactate Injection, *United States Pharmacopoeia* [*USP*]) is used for intramuscular (IM) injection because of the limited water solubility of the hydrochloride. The injection should be stored in a cold place, because if it is stored at room temperature for several months, a slight yellow tint may develop. This does not indicate a loss in biologic potency.

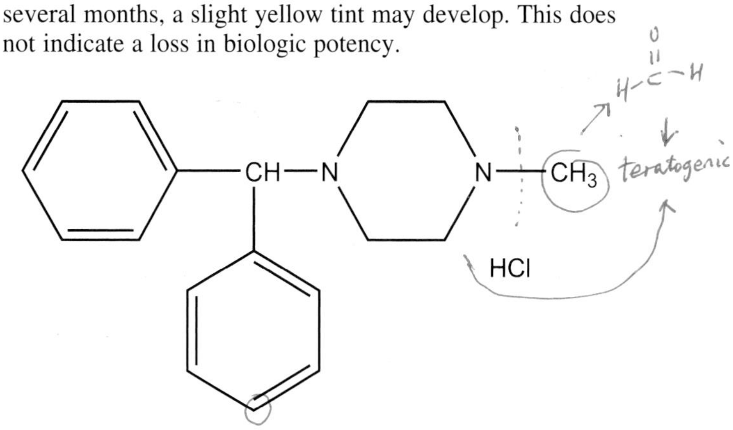

Cyclizine Hydrochloride or Lactate

Dosage forms: Tablets HCl (25 and 50 mgHCl) and injection (lactate)

Usual adult dose: 1 tablet every 4 to 6 hours for adults and children 12 years of age and older; ½ tablet every 6 to 8 hours, not to exceed 1½ tablets in 24 hours for children from 6 to 12 years of age

Chlorcyclizine Hydrochloride. Chlorcyclizine hydrochloride, 1-(*p*-chloro-α-phenylbenzyl)-4-methylpiperazine monohydrochloride, is a light-sensitive, white crystalline powder that is soluble in water (1:2), in alcohol (1:11), and in chloroform (1:4). A 1% solution has a pH between 4.8 and 5.5. Disubstitution or substitution of halogen in the 2- or 3-position of the benzhydryl rings results in a much less potent compound. Chlorcydizine is indicated for the symptomatic relief of urticaria, hay fever, and certain other conditions.

Meclizine Hydrochloride. Meclizine hydrochloride, 1-(*p*-chloro-α-phenylbenzyl)-4-(*m*-methylbenzyl)piperazine dihydrochloride monohydrate (Bonine, Antivert), is a tasteless, white or slightly yellowish crystalline powder that

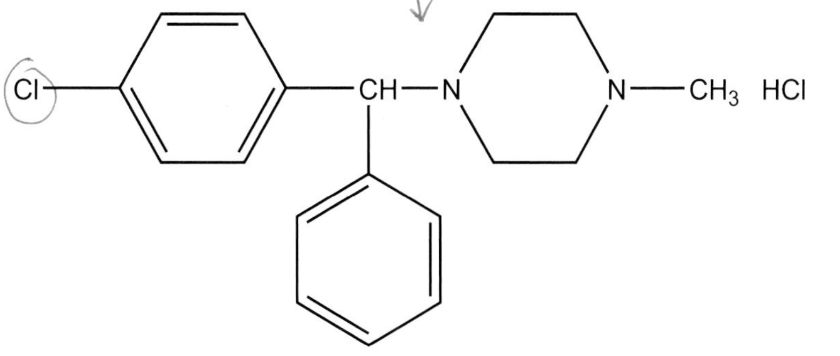

Chlorcyclizine Hydrochloride

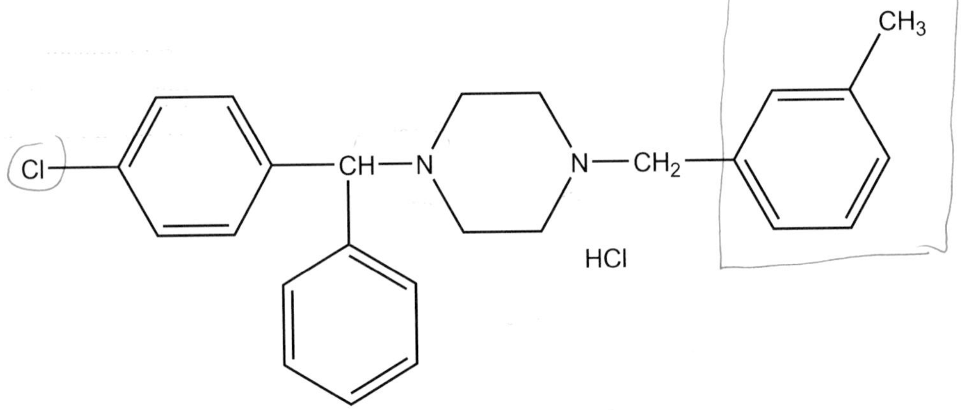

Meclizine Hydrochloride

is practically insoluble in water (1:1,000). It differs from chlorcyclizine in having an *N-m*-methylbenzyl group in place of the *N*-methyl group. Although it is a moderately potent antihistaminic, meclizine is used primarily as an antinauseant in the prevention and treatment of motion sickness and in the treatment of nausea and vomiting associated with vertigo.

Dosage forms: Tablets (12, 5, 25, 50 mg) and capsules (25 mg)
Usual adult dose:
- Motion sickness: 25- to 50-mg meclizine HCl should be taken 1 hour prior
- Vertigo: 25 to 100 mg daily in divided doses

λ *Buclizine Hydrochloride.* Buclizine hydrochloride, 1-(*p*-tertbutylbenzyl)-4-(*p*-chloro-α-phenylbenzyl)piperazine dihydrochloride (Bucladin-S), is a white to slightly yellow crystalline powder that is insoluble in water. The highly lipid-soluble buclizine has CNS depressant, antiemetic, and antihistaminic properties. This drug has been discontinued in the United States.

PROPYLAMINES (MONOAMINOPROPYL OR ALKYLAMINE DERIVATIVES)

The propylamine antihistamines are characterized structurally by an sp^3 or sp^2 carbon-connecting atom with a carbon chain of two additional carbons linking the key tertiary amino and diaryl pharmacophore moieties (Fig. 23.10). Those propylamines with a saturated carbon-connecting moiety are commonly referred to as the pheniramines. All of the pheniramines consist of a phenyl and a 2-pyridyl aryl group and a terminal dimethylamino moiety. These compounds differ only in the phenyl substituent at the *para* position: H (pheniramine), Cl (chlorpheniramine), and Br (brompheniramine). The halogenated pheniramines are significantly more potent (20–50 times) and have a longer duration of action than pheniramine.[31]

All pheniramines are chiral molecules, and the halogen-substituted derivatives have been resolved by crystallization of salts formed with d-tartaric acid. Antihistaminic activity resides almost exclusively in the *S*-stereoisomers (200–1,000 times higher H_1-receptor binding affinities).[30,38] The pheniramines are widely used in OTC products for seasonal allergies.

The propylamines with an unsaturated connecting moiety include the simple open-chain alkene derivatives pyrrobutarnine and triprolidine and the cyclic alkene analogs dirnethindene and phenindamine. In the open-chain propylamines, a coplanar aromatic double-bond system appears to be an important factor for antihistaminic activity. Also, these compounds are asymmetric and the *E*-isomers are significantly more potent than the *Z*-isomers.[4,39] The pyrrolidino group of these compounds is the side chain tertiary amine that imparts greatest antihistaminic activity. The conformational rigidity of the cyclic alkene propylamines has provided a useful model to determine distances between the key diaryl and tertiary pharmacophoric moieties in H_1-antagonists, a distance of 5 to 6 Å.[39]

The antihistamines in this group are among the most active H_1-antagonists in terms of pA_2 values and doses (Table 23.2 and 23.3). They also have greater receptor selectivity and

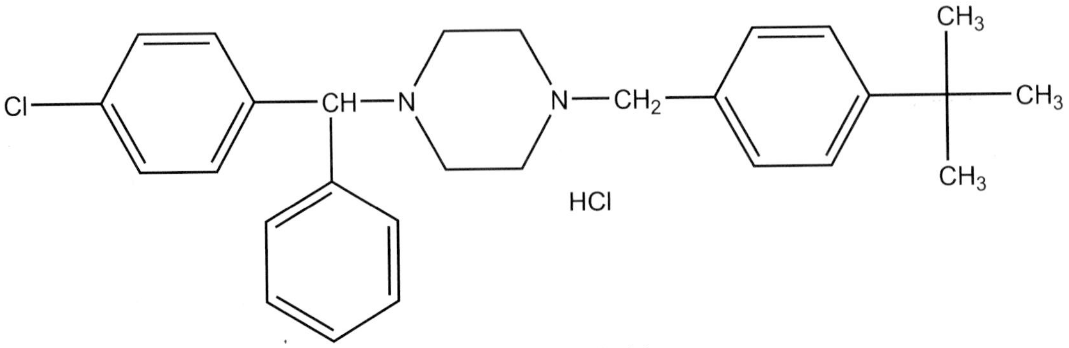

Buclizine Hydrochloride

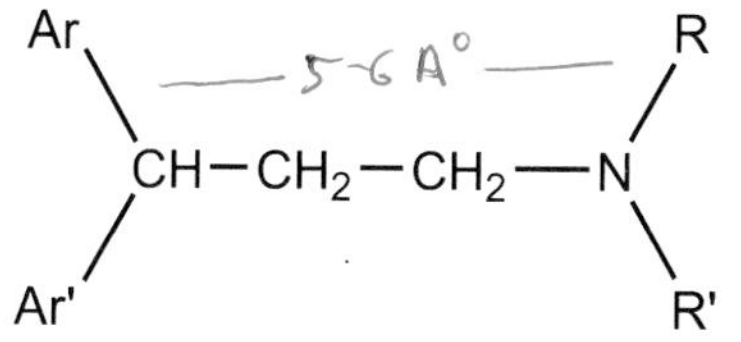

Figure 23.10 ● General structure of the propylamines.

fewer anticholingeric and CNS side effects than other first-generation antihistamines. The propylamines have relatively long half-lives and are in many OTC preparations for once-a-day treatment of mild allergy symptoms. Although they produce less sedation, a significant proportion of patients do experience this effect.

In the propylamine series, the phamacokinetics of chlorpheniramine have been studied most extensively in humans.[10,31] Oral bioavailability is relatively low (30%–50%) and may be limited by first-pass metabolism. The primary metabolites for this compound and other members of this series are the mono- and di-N-dealkylation products. Complete oxidation of the terminal amino moiety followed by glycine conjugation has also been reported for brompheniramine. In general, the members of this group have long half-lives, allowing for once-daily dosing. Chlorpheniramine's plasma half-life ranges from about 12 to 28 hours, depending on the route of administration (Table 23.3). The known kinetic properties of representative members of this class of antihistamines are summarized in Table 23.3.

The structures of the marketed salt forms of the propylamine antihistamines, along with physicochemical properties, basic therapeutic activity profiles, and dosage form information, are provided in the monographs that follow.

Pheniramine Maleate. Pheniramine maleate, 2-[α-[2-dimethylaminoethyl]benzyl]-pyridine bimaleate (Trimeton, Inhiston), is a white crystalline powder, with a faint amine-like odor, which is soluble in water (1:5) and very soluble in alcohol. This drug is the least potent member of the series and is marketed as the racemate. The usual adult dose is 20 to 40 mg 3 times daily. It is available in certain combination products.

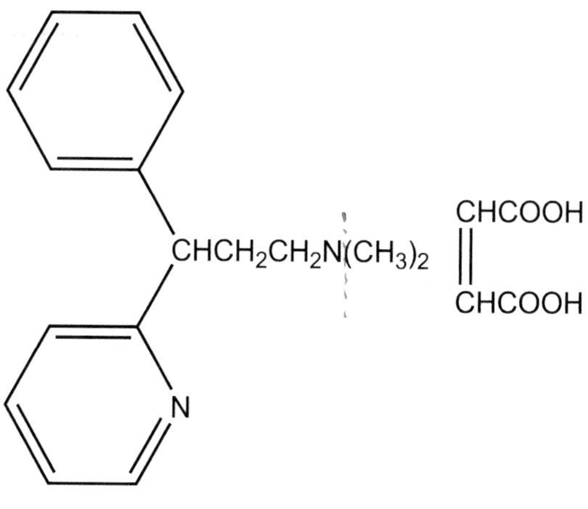

Pheniramine Maleate

Chlorpheniramine Maleate. Chlorpheniramine maleate, (±)2-[p-chloro-α-[2-dimethylamino)ethyl]benzyl]pyridine bimaleate (Chlor-Trimeton), is a white crystalline powder that is soluble in water (1:3.4), in alcohol (1:10), and in chloroform (1:10). It has a pKa of 9.2, and an aqueous solution has a pH between 4 and 5. Chlorination of pheniramine in the *para* position of the phenyl ring increases potency 10-fold with no appreciable change in toxicity. Most of the antihistaminic activity resides with the dextro isomer (see under "Dexchlorpheniramine Maleate"). The usual dose is 2 to 4 mg 3 or 4 times a day. It has a half-life of 12 to 15 hours.

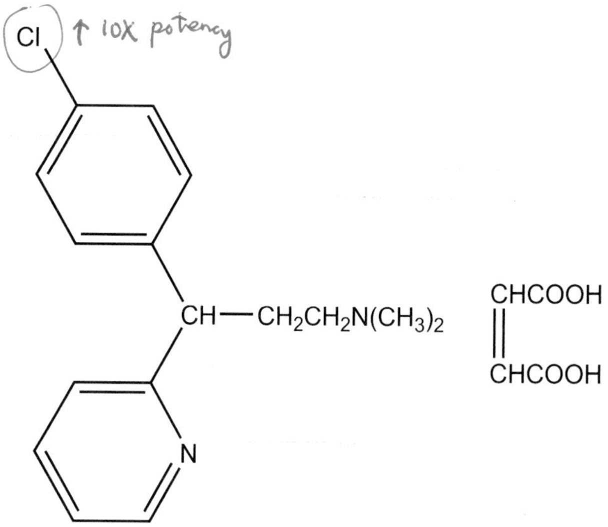

Chlorpheniramine Maleate
Dextrochlorpheniramine Maleate

Dosage forms: Tablets (2, 4, 8, and 12 mg), extended-release capsules (8 and 12 mg), syrup (2 mg/5 mL), and oral suspension (4 and 8 mg/5 mL)
Usual adult dose: Oral, 4 mg/4 to 6 hours; extended release, 8 to 12 mg/8 to 12 hours; IM, intravenous (IV), or subcutaneous, 5 to 40 mg

Dexchlorpheniramine Maleate. Dexchlorpheniramine (Polaramine) is the dextrorotatory enantiomer of chlorpheniramine. In vitro and in vivo studies of the enantiomers of chlorpheniramine showed that the antihistaminic activity exists predominantly in the dextro isomer. As mentioned previously, the dextro isomer has the (S) configuration, which is superimposable on the (S) configuration of the more active levorotatory enantiomer of carbinoxamine.[30]

Dosage forms: Extended-release tablets (4 and 6 mg), syrup (2 mg/5mL)
Usual adult dose: 4 or 6 mg at bedtime or every 8 to 10 hours

Brompheniramine Maleate and Tannate. Brompheniramine maleate, (+)2-[p-bromo-α-[2-(dimethylamino) ethyl]benzyl]pyridine bimaleate (Dimetane), differs from chlorpheniramine by the substitution of a bromine atom for the chlorine atom. Its actions and uses are like those of chlorpheniramine. It has a half-life of 25 hours, which is almost twice that of chlorpheniramine.

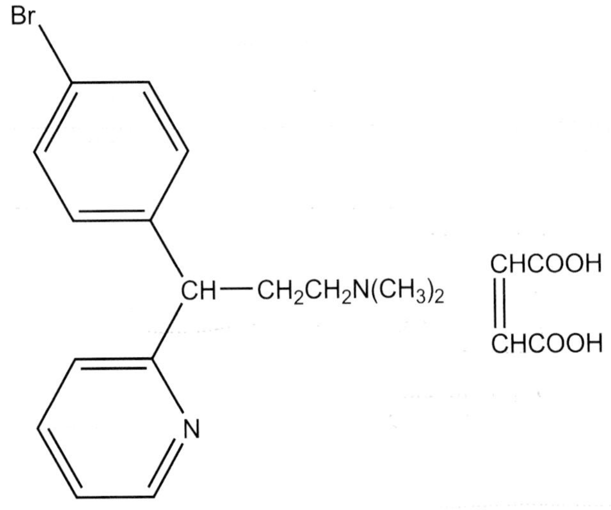

Brompheniramine Maleate

Dosage forms: Tablets (6 and 12 mg), oral drops (1 mg), capsules (12 mg), liquid (2 mg/5mL), oral suspension (4, 8, 10, and 12 mg/5 mL)

Usual adult dose: 1or 2 tablets (6–12 mg) every 12 hours, or 5 to 10 mL of solution or suspension

Dexbrompheniramine Maleate. Like the chlorine derivative, the antihistaminic activity of brompheniramine exists predominantly in the dextro isomer, dexbrompheniramine maleate (D-isomer), and is of comparable potency.

Pyrrobutamine Phosphate. Pyrrobutamine phosphate, (E)-1-[4-(4-chlorophenyl)-3-phenyl-2-butenyl]pyrrolidine diphosphate (Pyronil), is a white crystalline powder that is soluble to the extent of 10% in warm water. Pyrrobutamine was investigated originally as the hydrochloride salt, but the diphosphate was absorbed more readily and completely. Clinical studies indicate that it is long acting, with a comparatively slow onset of action. The weak antihistaminic properties of several analogs point to the importance of having a planar ArC=CH-CH$_2$N unit and a pyrrolidino group as the side chain tertiary amine.[39]

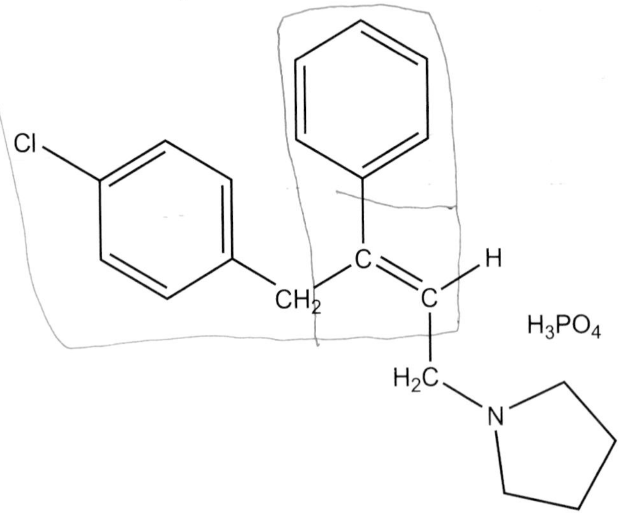

Pyrrobutamine Phosphate

Triprolidine Hydrochloride. Triprolidine hydrochloride, (E)-2-[3-(1-pyrrolidinyl)-1-*p*-tolylpropenyl]pyridine mono-hydrochloride monohydrate (Actidil), is a white crystalline

powder with a slight, but unpleasant, odor. It is soluble in water and in alcohol, and its solutions are alkaline to litmus.

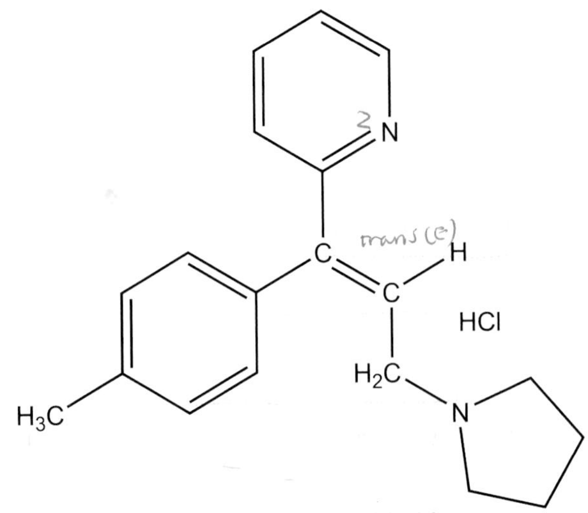

Triprolidine Hydrochloride

The antihistaminic activity is confined mainly to the geometric isomer in which the pyrrolidinomethyl group is *trans* to the 2-pyridyl group. Pharmacological studies confirm the high activity of triprolidine and the superiority of (E) over corresponding (Z) isomers as H$_1$-antihistamines.[39] At guinea pig ileum sites, the affinity of triprolidine for H-receptors was more than 1,000 times the affinity of its (Z) diasteromer.

The relative potency of triprolidine is of the same order as that of dexchlorpheniramine. The peak effect occurs about 3.5 hours after oral administration, and the duration of effect is about 12 hours.

Dosage forms: Oral liquid (1.25 mg/5 mL) and oral suspension (2.5 mg/5 mL)

Usual adult dose: 10 mL every 4 to 6 hours; do not exceed 40 mL in 24 hours

Phenindamine Tartrate. Phenindamine tartrate, 2,3,4,9-tetrahydro-2-methyl-9-phenyl-1H-indeno[2, 1-c]pyridine bitartrate, occurs as a creamy-white powder, usually with a faint odor and sparingly soluble in water (1:40). A 2% aqueous solution has a pH of about 3.5. It is most stable in the pH range of 3.5 to 5.0 and is unstable in solutions of pH 7 or higher. Oxidizing substances or heat may cause isomerization to an inactive form.

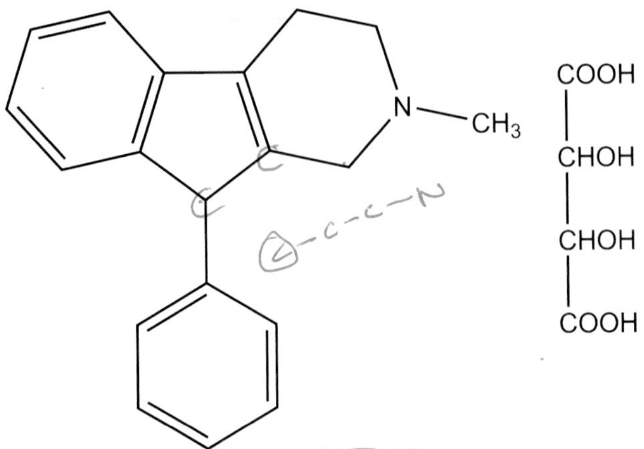

Phenindamine Tartrate

Structurally, phenindamine can be regarded as an unsaturated propylamine derivative, in that the rigid ring system contains a distorted, *trans*-alkene. Like the other commonly used antihistamines, it may produce drowsiness and sleepiness; it may also cause a mildly stimulating action in some patients and insomnia when taken just before bedtime.

Dosage forms: Tablets (25 mg)
Usual adult dose: 1 tablet every 4 to 6 hours, not to exceed 6 tablets in 24 hours

Dimethindene Maleate. Dimethindene maleate, (±)2-[1-[2-[2-dimethylamino)ethyl]-inden-3-yl]ethyl]pyridine bimaleate (1:1) (Forhistal Maleate), is a white to off-white crystalline powder that has a characteristic odor and is sparingly soluble in water. This potent antihistaminic agent may be considered a derivative of the unsaturated propylamines. The principal side effect is some sedation or drowsiness. The antihistaminic activity resides mainly in the levorotatory isomer.

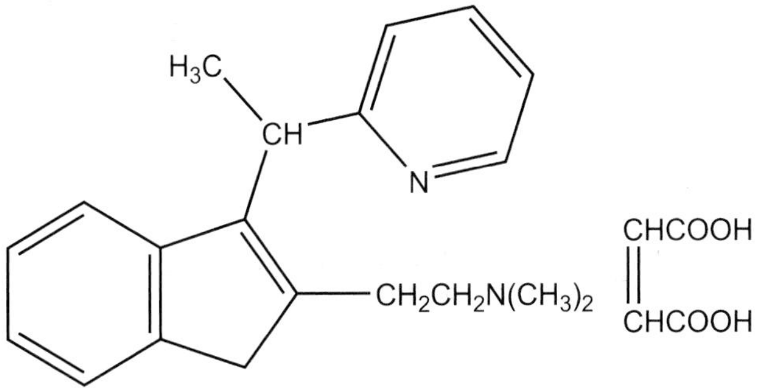

Dimethindene Maleate

PHENOTHIAZINES

Beginning in the mid-1940s, several antihistaminic drugs were been discovered as a result of bridging the aryl units of agents related to the ethylenediamines. The search for effective antimalarials led to the investigation of phenothiazine derivatives in which the bridging entity is sulfur. Subsequent testing found that the phenothiazine class of drugs had not only antihistaminic activity but also a pharmacological profile of its own, considerably different from that of the ethylenediamines (Fig. 23.11). Thus began the era of development of useful psychotherapeutic agents, the phenothiazine antipsychotics.

The phenothiazine derivatives that display therapeutically useful antihistaminic actions contain a two- or three-carbon, branched alkyl chain between the ring system and terminal nitrogen atom. This differs significantly from the phenothiazine antipsychotic series in which an unbranched propyl chain is required. The branched alkyl chain contains a chiral carbon, giving rise to optical isomerism. The enantiomers of the pro-

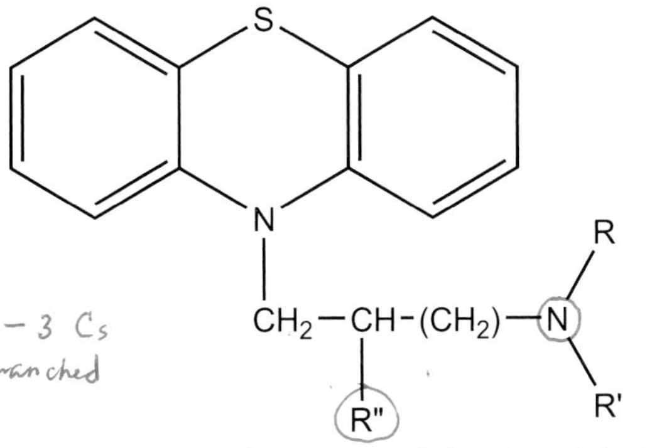

Figure 23.11 ● General structure of the phenothiazines.

totype of this class, promethazine, have been resolved and found to possess similar antihistaminic and other pharmacological properties as described later.[40,41] This is in contrast with results of studies of the pheniramines and carbinoxamine compounds in which the chiral center is closer to the aromatic moieties of the molecule. Thus, asymmetry appears to have less influence on antihistaminic activity when the chiral center lies near the positively charged side-chain nitrogen. In general, the combination of lengthening of the side chain and substitution of lipophilic groups in the 2-position of the aromatic ring results in compounds with decreased antihistaminic activity and increased psychotherapeutic properties. Also, unlike the phenothiazine antipsychotics, the heterocyclic ring of the antihistamines is unsubstituted.

Promethazine, the parent member of this series, is a moderately potent antihistamine based on pA_2 values and doses with pronounced sedative effects (Table 23.2). It is a relatively long-acting antihistamine as a result of slow metabolic inactivation, perhaps because of sterically hindered cytochrome *N*-dealkylation. In addition to its antihistaminic and sedating action, it is a potent antiemetic, anticholinergic, and significantly potentiates the action of analgesic and other sedative drugs.[30] The other members of this series display a similar pharmacological profile and thus may cause drowsiness and impair the ability to perform tasks requiring alertness. Also, concurrent administration of alcoholic beverages and other CNS depressants with the phenothiazines should be avoided.[10]

Although few pharmacokinetic data are available for the phenothiazine antihistamines, the metabolism of a close structural analog promethazine has been studied in detail.[31] This compound undergoes mono- and di-*N*-dealkylation, sulfur oxidation, aromatic oxidation at the 3-position to yield the phenol, and *N*-oxidation. Several of these metabolites, particularly the phenol, may yield glucuronide conjugates. It is expected that the phenothiazine antihistamines would display similar metabolic profiles.

Promethazine Hydrochloride. Promethazine hydrochloride, (±)10-[2-(dimethylamino)-propyl]phenothiazine monohydrochloride (Phenergan), occurs as a white to faint yellow crystalline powder that is very soluble in water, in hot absolute alcohol, and in chloroform. Its aqueous solutions are slightly acid to litmus.

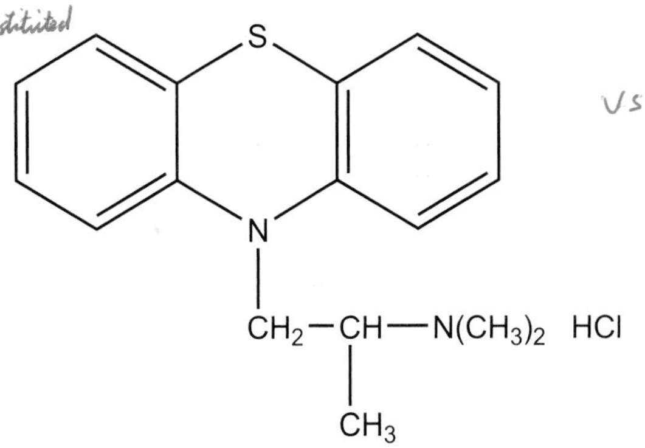

Promethazine Hydrochloride

Dosage forms: Tablets (12.5, 25, and 50 mg), oral syrup (6.25 mg/5 mL), rectal suppositories (12.5, 25, and 50 mg), injection (25 and 50 mg/mL)
Usual adult dose:
• Allergy: 25 mg taken before retiring; however, 12.5 mg may be taken before meals or on retiring, if necessary

- Transfusion reactions: 25-mg doses to control minor transfusion reactions
- Motion sickness: 25 mg taken 30 to 60 minutes before travel and repeated 8 to 12 hours later, if necessary
- Nausea and vomiting: 12.5 to 25 mg every 4 to 6 hours as necessary
- Prophylactic dosage: 25 mg every 4 to 6 hours as necessary for prophylactic dosing (given during surgery and the postoperative period) and 25 to 50 mg with analgesics postoperatively or preoperatively
- Sedation: 25 to 50 mg for nighttime, presurgical, or obstetrical sedation

Trimeprazine Tartrate. Trimeprazine tartrate, (±)10-[3-(dimethylamino)-2-methylpropyl] phenothiazine tartrate (Temaril), occurs as a white to off-white crystalline powder that is freely soluble in water and soluble in alcohol. Its antihistaminic action is reported to be from 1.5 to 5 times that of promethazine. Clinical studies have shown it has a pronounced antipruritic action that may be unrelated to its histamine-antagonizing properties.

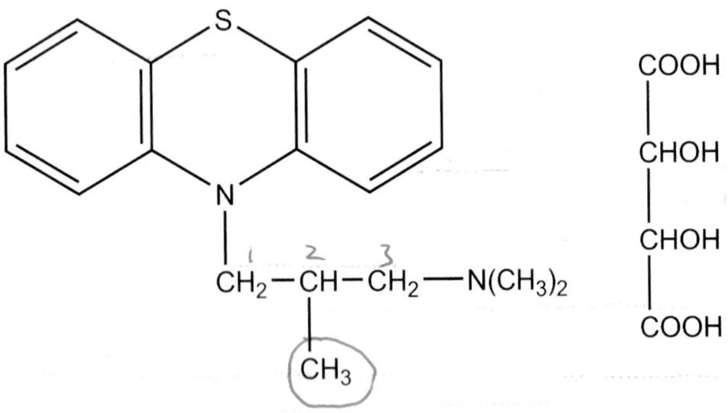

Trimeprazine Tartrate

Dosage forms: Syrup and tablets
Usual adult dose: Oral, 2.5 mg 4 times a day

Methdilazine. Methdilazine, 10-[(1-methyl-3-pyrrolidinyl)methyl]phenothiazine (Tacaryl), is a light-tan crystalline powder that has a characteristic odor and is practically insoluble in water. Methdilazine, as the free base, is used in chewable tablets because its low solubility in water contributes to its tastelessness. Some local anesthesia of the buccal mucosa may be experienced if the tablet is chewed and not swallowed promptly.

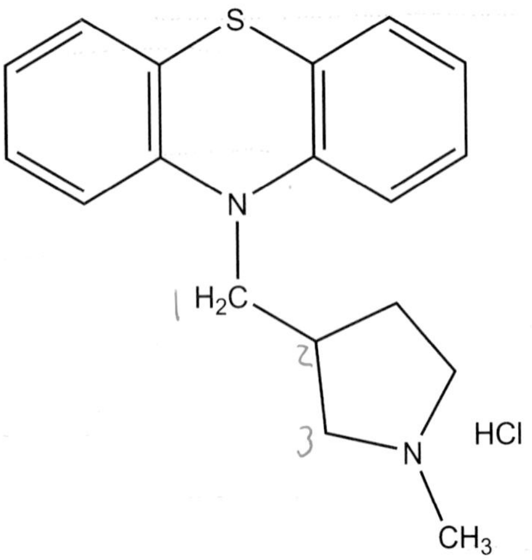

Methdilazine Hydrochloride

Methdilazine Hydrochloride. Methdilazine hydrochloride (Tacaryl Hydrochloride), also occurs as a light-tan crystalline powder with a slight characteristic odor. The salt is freely soluble in water and in alcohol, however. The activity is like that of methdilazine, and it is administered orally for its antipruritic effect.

DIBENZOCYCLOHEPTENES AND DIBENZOCYCLOHEPTANES

The dibenzocycloheptene and dibenzocycloheptane antihistamines may be regarded as phenothiazine analogs in which the sulfur atom has been replaced by an isosteric vinyl group (cyproheptadine) or a saturated ethyl bridge (azatadine), and the ring nitrogen has been replaced by an sp^2 carbon atom (Fig. 23.12). The two members of this series are closely related in structure; azatadine is an aza (pyridyl) isostere of cyproheptadine in which the 10,11-double bond is reduced. These agents are potent antihistamines with moderate sedation and anticholinergic potential, and little antiemetic activity (Table 23.2).

Cyproheptadine Hydrochloride. Cyproheptadine hydrochloride, 4-(5H-dibenzo-[a,d]-cyclohepten-5-ylidine)-1-methylpiperidine hydrochloride sesquihydrate (Periactin), is slightly soluble in water and sparingly soluble in alcohol.

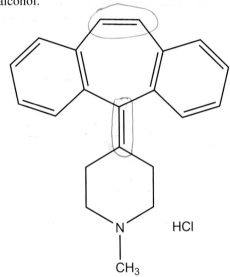

Cyproheptadine Hydrochloride

Cyproheptadine possesses both antihistamine and antiserotonin activity and is used as an antipruritic agent. It is indicated for the treatment of hypersensitivity reactions, perennial, and seasonal allergic rhinitis; vasomotor rhinitis; allergic conjunctivitis, uncomplicated allergic skin manifestations of urticaria and angioedema; amelioration of allergic reactions to blood or plasma; and cold urticaria. It is also used off-label for nightmares associated with posttraumatic stress disorder (PTSD), prevention of migraine, suppression of vascular headaches, and appetite stimulation. Sedation is the most prominent side effect, and this is usually brief, disappearing after 3 or 4 days of treatment.

Dosage forms: Tablets (4 mg) and syrup (2 mg/5 mL)
Usual adult dose: Oral, 4 mg 3 or 4 times a day

Azatadine Maleate. Azatadine maleate, 6,11-dihydro-11-(1-methyl-4-piperidylidene)-5H-benzo-[5,6]cyclo-

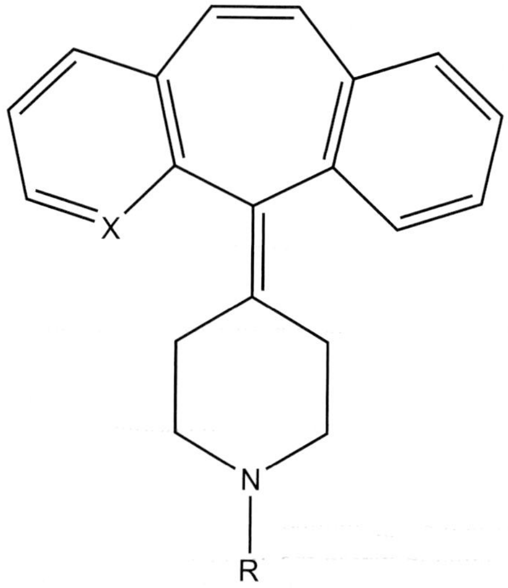

Figure 23.12 ● General structure of the dibenzocyclo-heptenes and dibenzocycloheptanes.

hepta(1,2-b]pyridine maleate (1:2) (Optimine), is a potent, long-acting antihistaminic with antiserotonin activity. In early testing, azatadine exhibited more than three times the potency of chlorpheniramine in the isolated guinea pig ileum screen and more than seven times the oral potency of chlorpheniramine in protection of guinea pigs against a double lethal dose of intravenously administered histamine.[41]

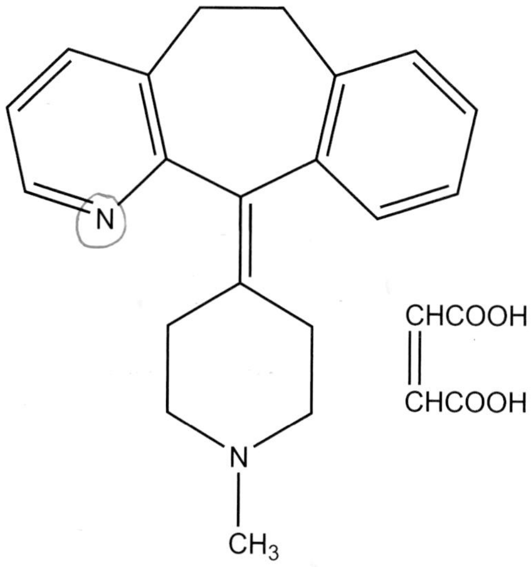

Azatadine Maleate

Dosage forms: Tablets (1 mg)
Usual dosage: 1 to 2 mg twice daily

Second-Generation Antihistamines

Initial design efforts toward new or second-generation antihistamines focused on developing agents with a lower sedation potential and reduced binding affinities for nontarget proteins including muscarinic, adrenergic, and serotonergic receptors. These efforts led to the introduction of astemizole and terfenadine, derivatives of the first-generation agents with substantially larger N-tertiary amine substituents (Fig. 23.13). Astemizole and terfenadine proved to be nonsedating and target-receptor selective, but extensive clinical use uncovered serious cardiovascular toxicities (QT prolongation and

arrhythmias).[10,33,34] These cardiac actions appear to result from the blockade of the rapid component of delayed rectifier potassium current (IKr) by astemizole and terfenadine, even at therapeutic concentrations. Blocking the rectifier current causes prolongation of the monophasic cardiac action potential and QT interval, as well as induction of early after-depolarizations and dispersion (slowing) of repolarization, resulting in torsades de pointes.[10] Furthermore, such cardiac effects were observed more commonly when astemizole and terfenadine were administered with other drugs that inhibit their cytochrome metabolism, such as the imidazole antifungals (ketoconazole, itraconazole) and the macrolides (erythromycin, clarithromycin). Through this drug interaction, astemizole and terfenadine levels would rise and the incidence of untoward cardiac events increases. As a result of these concerns, both astemizole and terfenadine have been withdrawn from the U.S. market. The newer second-generation H₁-antihistamines described later have significantly reduced IKr current-blocking capacity, and have demonstrated significantly lower cardiotoxicity in clinical use.

Further drug design efforts resulted in the discovery of new second-generation agents, which retained the nonsedating and receptor-selectivity properties, but lacked the cardiotoxicity of astemizole and terfenadine. These newer agents are structurally diverse, but are derivatives of first-generation drugs, containing larger, polar functionality connected either to the terminal tertiary amine, or as a substituent of one of the aromatic rings. The new second-generation drugs currently on the market include acrivastine, an alkene-acid derivative of triprolidine; cetirizine and levocetirizine, oxidation metabolites of hydroxyzine; desloratadine, an oxidation–hydrolysis metabolite of loratadine; and fexofenadine, an oxidative metabolite of terfenadine.[10] In addition to their H₁-receptor selectivity, these second-generation agents do not accumulate in the CNS because their hydrophilicity (in some cases) and high affinity for P-glycoprotein efflux pumps of cells associated with the BBB.[10,42,43] The propensity of these drugs to occupy CNS H₁-receptors varies from 0% for fexofenadine to 30% for cetirizine. The properties of these drugs are described in more detail in the monographs that follow.[44]

Fexofenadine Hydrochloride. Fexofenadine hydrochloride, (±)-4-[1-hydroxy-4-[4-(hydroxyldiphenyl-methyl)-1-piperinyl]butyl-α,α-dimethylbenzeneacetic acid (Allegra), occurs as a white to off-white crystalline powder that is freely soluble in methanol and ethanol, slightly soluble in chloroform and water, and insoluble in hexane. This compound is marketed as a racemate and exists as a zwitter-ion in aqueous media at physiological pH.

Fexofenadine is a primary oxidative metabolite of terfenadine.[45] Terfenadine was developed during a search for new butyrophenone antipsychotic drugs as evidenced by the presence of the N-phenylbutanol substituent. It also contains a diphenylmethyl-piperidine moiety analogous to that found in the piperazine antihistamines. Terfenadine is a selective, long-acting (>12 hours) H₁-antihistamine with little affinity for muscarinic, serotonergic, or adrenergic receptors. The histamine receptor affinity of this compound is believed to be related primarily to the presence of the diphenylmethylpiperidine moiety. The prolonged action results from very slow dissociation from these receptors. The lack of anticholinergic, adrenergic, or serotonergic actions appears to be linked to the presence of the N-phenylbutanol substituent (Table 23.2). This substituent contributes to P-glycoprotein efflux pump affinity,

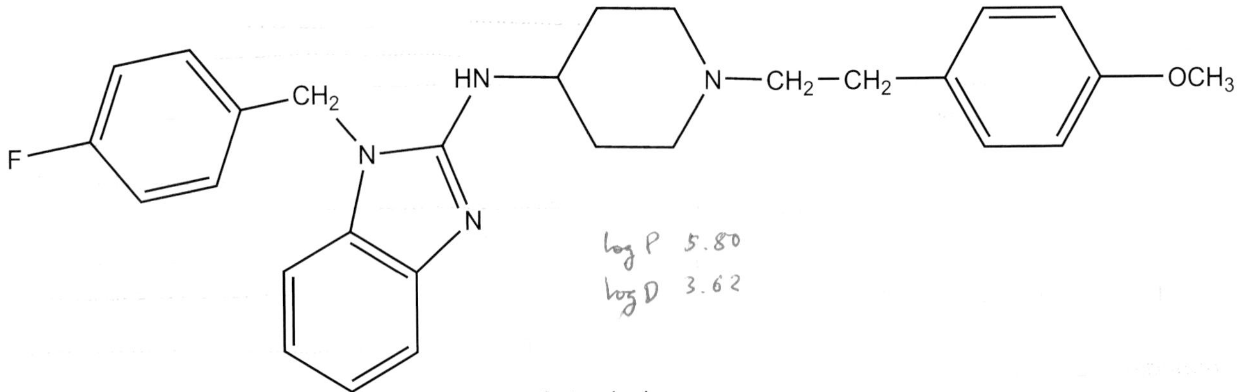

log P 5.80
log D 3.62

Astemizole

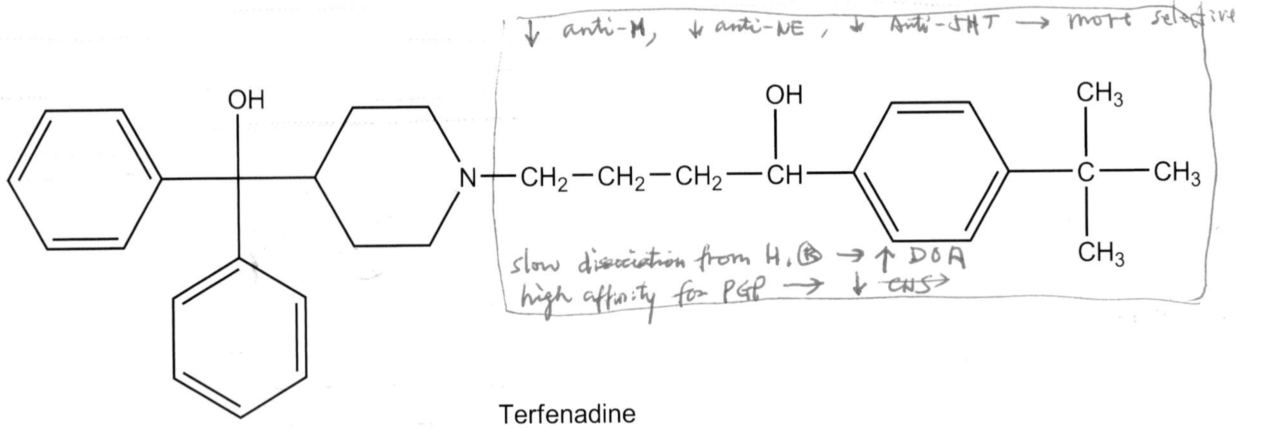

↓ anti-M, ↓ anti-NE, ↓ Anti-5HT → more selective

slow dissociation from H₁Ⓡ → ↑ DOA
high affinity for PGP → ↓ CNS→

Terfenadine

Figure 23.13 ● Structures of terfenadine and astemizole.

which serves to limit accumulation of terfenadine in the CNS. Terfenadine undergoes significant first-pass cytochrome P450 (CYP)-based metabolism, with the predominant metabolite being fexofenadine, an active metabolite resulting from methyl group oxidation. When drugs that inhibit this transformation, such as the imidazole antifungals and macrolides, are used concurrently, terfenadine levels may rise to toxic levels, resulting in potentially fatal heart rhythm problems that were described. The observation that fexofenadine displays antihistaminic activity comparable with that of terfenadine but is less cardiotoxic led to its development as an alternative to terfenadine for the relief of the symptoms of seasonal allergies.

Fexofenadine, like terfenadine, is a selective peripheral H_1-receptor ligand that produces no clinically significant anticholinergic effects or α_1-adrenergic receptor blockade at therapeutic doses (Table 23.2). No sedative or other CNS effects have been reported for this drug, and animal studies indicate that fexofenadine does not cross the BBB. In vitro studies also suggest that unlike terfenadine, fexofenadine does not block potassium channels in cardiocytes. Furthermore, in drug interaction studies, no prolongation of the QTc interval or related heart rhythm abnormalities were detected when fexofenadine was administered concurrently with erythromycin or ketoconazole.[10,46]

Fexofenadine is indicated for the treatment of seasonal allergic rhinitis and chronic idiopathic urticaria. It is rapidly absorbed after oral administration, producing peak serum concentrations in about 2.5 hours. Fexofenadine is 60% to 70% plasma protein bound. Unlike its parent drug, only 5% of the total dose of fexofenadine is metabolized. The re-

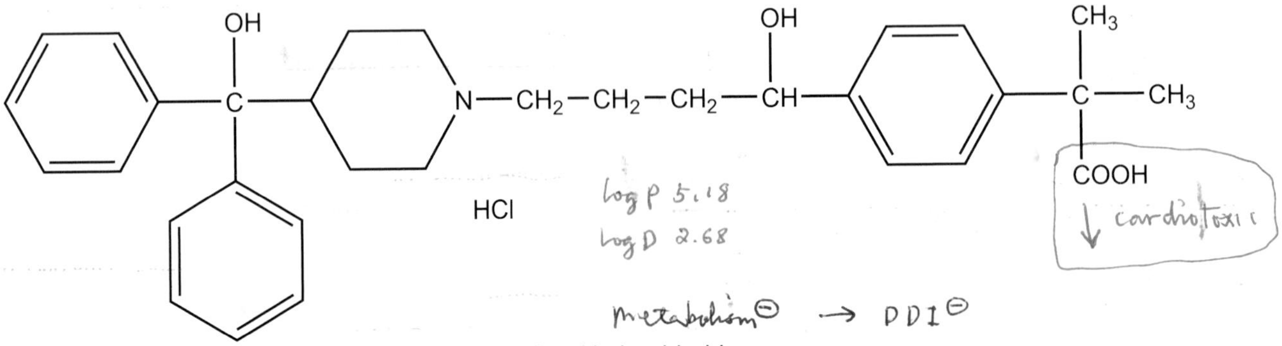

HCl

log P 5.18
log D 2.68

↓ cardiotoxic

metabolism⊖ → PD1⊖

Fexofenadine Hydrochloride

mainder is excreted primarily in the urine; the mean elimination half-life is about 14 hours (Table 23.3).[10]

Dosage form: Tablets (30, 60, and 180 mg), oral disintegrating tablets (30 mg), and an oral suspension (6 mg/mL)
Usual doses:
- Chronic idiopathic urticaria: 60 mg twice daily or 180 mg once daily in adults and children >12; lower doses are recommended in children
- Seasonal allergic rhinitis: 60 mg twice daily or 180 mg once daily in adults and children >12; lower doses are recommended in children

Loratadine. Loratadine, 4-(8-chloro-5, 6-dihydro- 11H-benzo[5,6]-cyclohepta[1,2-b]pyridin-1 1-ylidene-1-carboxylic acid ethyl ester, is a white to off-white powder insoluble in water but very soluble in acetone, alcohols, and chloroform. Loratadine is structurally related to the antihistamines azatadine and cyproheptadine, and to some tricyclic antidepressants. It differs from azatadine, in that a neutral carbamate group has replaced the basic tertiary amino moiety, and a phenyl ring has been substituted with a chlorine atom.

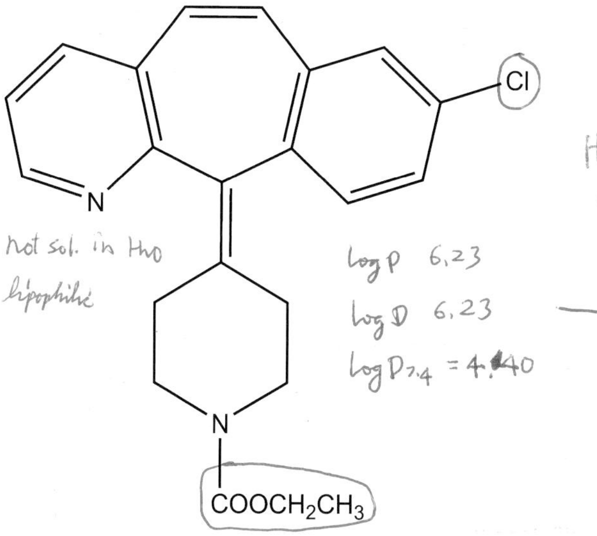

not sol. in H₂O
lipophilic

Log P 6.23
Log D 6.23
Log D₇.₄ = 4.40

Loratadine

Loratadine is a selective peripheral H_1-antihistamine with a receptor-binding profile like that of the other members of this series, except that it has more antiserotonergic activity (Table 23.2). Thus, it produces no substantial CNS or autonomic side effects or cardiac toxicity. Loratadine displays potency comparable with that of astemizole and greater than that of terfenadine.

Loratadine is indicated for the relief of nasal and nonnasal symptoms of seasonal allergic rhinitis. It is rapidly absorbed after oral administration, producing peak plasma levels in about 1.5 hours. This drug is extensively metabolized by oxidation of the carbamate methylene group, a reaction catalyzed by CYP3A4 and, to a lesser extent, CYP2D6 (Table 23.3). This oxidation metabolite readily undergoes *O*-demethylation and decarboxylation to form the descarboethoxy metabolite (desloratadine), which appears to be responsible for antihistaminic activity.[47–49] In the presence of a CYP3A4 inhibitor ketoconazole, loratadine is metabolized to descarboethoxyloratadine predominantly by CYP2D6. Concurrent administration of loratadine with either ketoconazole, erythromycin (both CYP3A4 inhibitors),

or cimetidine (CYP2D6 and CYP3A4 inhibitor) is associated with substantially increased plasma concentrations of loratadine.[10,48] Both parent drug and active metabolite have elimination half-lives ranging from 8 to 15 hours. The metabolite is excreted renally as a conjugate (Table 23.3).[10]

Dosage forms: Tablets (5 and 10 mg), oral disintegrating tablets (5 and 10 mg), syrup (5 mg/5 mL)
Usual adult dose (allergic rhinitis): 10 mg once daily (adults and children 6 years of age and older), 5 mg (chewable tablets, syrup) once daily for children 2 to 5 years of age

Desloratadine. Desloratadine, 8-chloro-6,11-dihydro-11-(4-piperdinylidene)-5*H*-benzo[5,6]cyclohepta[1,2-*b*]pyridine (Clarinex) is a white to off-white powder that is slightly soluble in water, but very soluble in ethanol and propylene glycol. It is the proposed active metabolite loratadine and has a very similar receptor binding and safety profile (Table 23.2). It is indicated for the symptomatic relief of pruritus and reduction in the number and size of hives in chronic idiopathic urticaria patients 6 months of age and older and for the relief of the nasal and nonnasal symptoms of perennial allergic rhinitis (in patients 6 months of age and older) and seasonal allergic rhinitis (in patients 2 years of age and older).

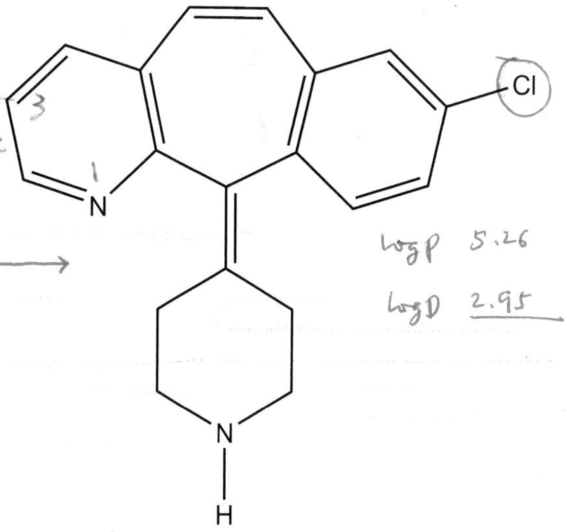

HO — 3 active

Log P 5.26
Log D 2.95

Desloratadine

Desloratadine is extensively metabolized to 3-hydroxydesloratadine, also an active metabolite, which is subsequently glucuronidated (Table 23.3). The cytochrome enzymes responsible for the formation of 3-hydroxydesloratadine have not been reported. Coadministration of desloratadine with CYP3A4 inhibitors results in marginal increases in plasma concentrations of desloratadine and 3-hydroxydesloratadine, but no significant changes in safety or efficacy.[48] The mean elimination half-life of desloratadine is about 6 hours, and the drug and its metabolites are eliminated in the urine and feces (Table 23.3).

Dosage forms: Tablets (5 mg), rapidly disintegrating tablets (2.5 and 5.0 mg), syrup (2.5 mg/5 mL)
Usual doses:
Adults and children 12 years of age and older: 5 mg once daily
Children 6 to 11 years of age: 2.5 mg once daily

Cetirizine. Cetirizine, (±)-[2-[4-[(4-chlorophenyl)phenylmethyl]-1-piperazinyl]ethoxy]acetic acid (Zyrtec), is a racemic compound available as a white crystalline powder that

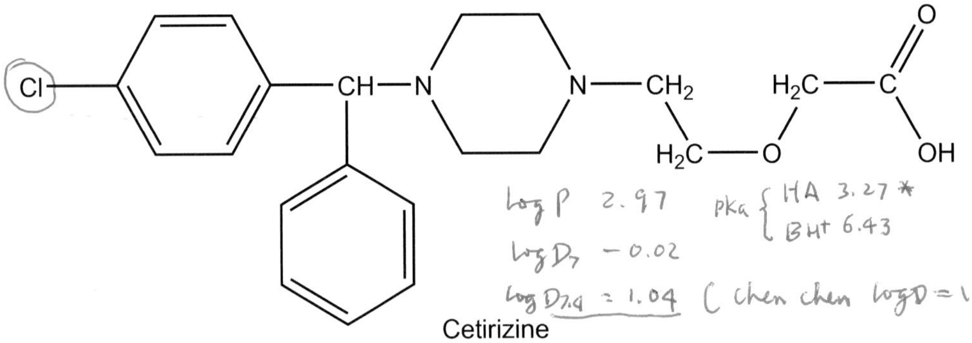

H₂O – Sol.

Cetirizine

Log P 2.97   pka { HA 3.27 *
                    { BH⁺ 6.43
Log D₇ – 0.02
Log D₂.₄ = 1.04 (chen chen logD = 1.5)

is water soluble. Cetirizine is the primary acid metabolite of hydroxyzine, resulting from complete oxidation of the primary alcohol moiety. This compound is zwitterionic and relatively polar and thus does not penetrate or accumulate in the CNS.[10,50,51] Before its introduction in the United States, cetirizine was one of the most widely prescribed H_1-antihistamines in Europe. It is highly selective in its interaction with various neuronal binding sites and highly potent ($\gg$ terfenadine) as well (Table 23.2). The advantages of this compound appear to be its long action (once-daily dosing), rapid onset of activity, minimal CNS effects and a lack of clinically significant effects on cardiac rhythm.[10,50]

Cetirizine produces qualitatively different effects on psychomotor and psychophysical functions from the first-generation antihistamines.[10,50] The drug has been associated with dose-related somnolence, however, so patients should be advised that cetirizine may interfere with the performance of certain jobs or activities. Other effects of this drug include fatigue, dry mouth, pharyngitis, and dizziness. Because the drug is extensively eliminated by a renal route, its adverse reactions may be more pronounced in individuals suffering from renal insufficiency. No cardiotoxic effects, such as QT prolongation, are observed with the new drug when used at its recommended or higher doses or when coadministered with imidazole antifungals and macrolide antibiotics.[10] Other typical drug interactions of H_1-antihistamines, however, apply to cetirizine and concurrent use of this drug with alcohol and other CNS depressants should be avoided.

Cetirizine is indicated for the temporary relief of runny nose, sneezing, itching of the nose or throat, and/or itchy, watery eyes caused by hay fever or other upper respiratory allergies. It also relieves itching caused by hives (urticaria), but it will not prevent hives or an allergic skin reaction from occurring.

Dose-proportional C_{max} values are achieved within 1 hour of oral administration of cetirizine. Food slows the rate of cetirizine absorption but does not affect the overall extent. Consistent with the polar nature of this carboxylic acid drug, less than 10% of peak plasma levels have been measured in the brain. Cetirizine is not extensively metabolized, and more than 60% of a 10-mg oral dose is excreted in the urine (>60% as unchanged drug) and 10% is recovered in the feces (Table 23.3). The drug is highly protein bound (93%) and has a terminal half-life of 8.3 hours. The clearance of cetirizine is reduced in elderly subjects and in renally and hepatically impaired patients.

Dosage forms: Tablets (5 and 10 mg) and oral syrup (1 mg/mL)
Usual adult dose (allergies/hay fever and urticaria): 5 to 10 mg once daily depending on the severity of symptoms, up to maximum of 10 mg/day in adults and chil-

dren 6 or older; 2.5 mg once daily of the oral solution for children younger than the age of 6

Levocetirizine Dihydrochloride. Levocetirizine dihydrochloride, (R)-[2-[4-[(4-chlorophenyl) phenylmethyl]-1-piperazinyl] ethoxy] acetic acid dihydrochloride, (Xyzal) is a white, crystalline powder and is water soluble. This R-enantiomer is has a 30-fold higher affinity than the S-enantiomer, and dissociates more slowly from H_1-receptors.[51] Pharmacologically, it displays the same receptor and CNS selecitivity profile as the racemate, cetirizine (Table 23.2), and thus the same therapeutic advantages. Levocetirizine is indicated for the relief of symptoms associated with allergic rhinitis (seasonal and perennial) in adults and children 6 years of age and older and for the treatment of the uncomplicated skin manifestations of chronic idiopathic urticaria in adults and children 6 years of age and older. Its pharmacokinetics and clearance profile are essentially the same as the racemate, cetirizine (Table 23.3).

Dosage forms: Tablets (5 mg) and solution (2.5 mg/5 mL)
Usual dose: 5 mg (one tablet or 10-mL oral solution) once daily in the evening for adults and children 12 years of age and older; 2.5 mg (half of a tablet or 5-mL oral solution) once daily in the evening for children 6 to 11 years old

Acrivastine. Acrivastine, (E, E)-3-[6-[1-(4-methylphenyl)-3-(1-pyrrolidinyl)-1-propenyl-2-pyridinyl]-2-propenoic acid (Semprex), is a fixed-combination product of the antihistamine acrivastine (8 mg) with the decongestant pseudoephedrine (60 mg). Acrivastine is an odorless, white to pale cream crystalline powder that is soluble in chloroform and alcohol and slightly soluble in water.

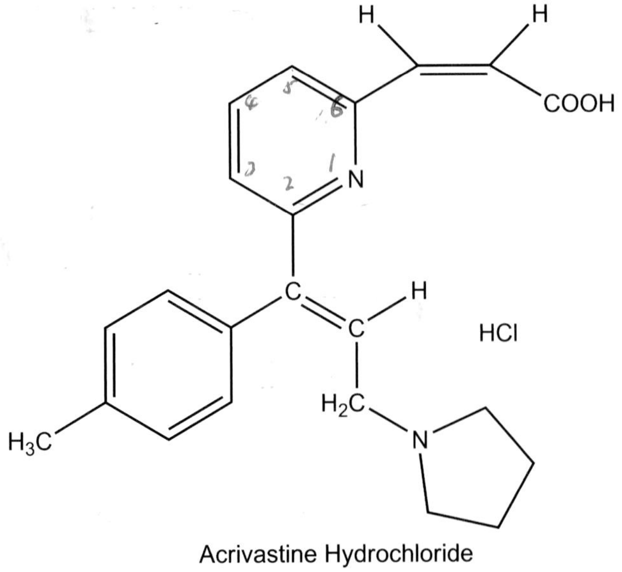

Acrivastine Hydrochloride

Acrivastine is an analog of triprolidine containing a carboxyethenyl moiety at the 6-position of the pyridyl ring. Acrivastine shows antihistaminic potency and duration of action comparable to those of triprolidine (Table 23.2). Unlike triprolidine, acrivastine does not display significant anticholinergic activity at therapeutic concentrations. Also, the enhanced polarity of this compound resulting from carboxyethenyl substitution limits BBB accumulation, and thus, this compound produces less sedation than triprolidine.

Limited pharmacokinetic data are available for this compound. Orally administered drug has a half-life of about 1.7 hours and a total body clearance of 4.4 mL/min per kilogram. The mean peak plasma concentrations are reported to vary widely, and the drug appears to penetrate the CNS poorly. The metabolic fate of acrivastine has not been reported.

Dosage forms: Tablets: various combination products
Usual adult dose: Oral, 8 or 60 mg 3 to 4 times a day

⬡ INHIBITION OF HISTAMINE RELEASE: MAST CELL STABILIZERS

The discovery of the bronchodilating activity of the natural product khellin, obtained from the plant *Ammi visnaga*, led to the development of the bis(chromones) as compounds that stabilize mast cells and inhibit the release of histamine and other mediators of inflammation.[52] The first therapeutically significant member of this class was cromolyn sodium. Further research targeting more effective agents resulted in the introduction of nedocromil, followed more recently by pemirolast and lodoxantide. Generally, the mast cell stabilizers inhibit activation of, and mediator release from, various inflammatory cell types associated with allergy and asthma, including eosinophils, neutrophils, macrophages; mast cells, monocytes, and platelets. In addition to histamine, these drugs inhibit the release of leukotrienes (C4, D4, E4) and prostaglandins.[53,54] In vitro studies suggest that these drugs stimulate the protein kinase C-mediated phosphorylation of moesin. This phosphorylated protein then binds with key proteins on the secretory granule (such as actin) and stabilizes them to prevent exocytosis. Other studies suggest that the bischromones indirectly inhibit calcium ion entry into the mast cell and that this action prevents mediator release.

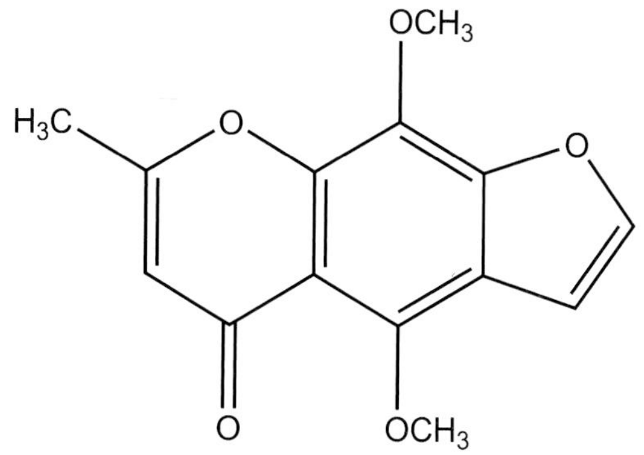

Khellin

In addition to their inhibition of mediator release, some of these drugs also inhibit the chemotaxis of eosinophils at the site of application (i.e., ocular tissue).[54] In lung tissue, pretreatment with the mast cell stabilizers cromolyn and nedocromil blocks the immediate and delayed bronchoconstrictive reactions induced by the inhalation of antigens. These drugs also attenuate the bronchospasm associated with exercise, cold air, environmental pollutants, and certain drugs (aspirin). However, the mast cell stabilizers do not have intrinsic bronchodilator, antihistamine, anticholinergic, vasoconstrictor, or glucocorticoid activity, and, when delivered by inhalation at the recommended dose, have no known therapeutic systemic activity. The structures, chemical properties, pharmacological profiles, and dosage data for these agents are provided in the monographs that follow.

Cromolyn Sodium. Cromolyn sodium, disodium 1,3-bis(2-carboxychromon-5-yloxy)-2-hydroxypropane (Intal), is a hygroscopic, white, hydrated crystalline powder that is soluble in water (1:10). It is tasteless at first but leaves a very slightly bitter aftertaste. The pK of cromolyn is 2. It is available as a solution for a nebulizer, an aerosol spray, a nasal solution, an ophthalmic solution, and an oral concentrate.

Nebulized and aerosol cromolyn has been used for prophylactic management of bronchial asthma and prevention of exercise-induced bronchospasm.[52] Cromolyn nasal solution is used for the prevention and treatment of allergic rhinitis, and oral concentrate is used to treat the histaminic symptoms of mastocytosis (diarrhea, flushing, headaches, vomiting, urticaria, abdominal pain, nausea, and itching). Topical cromolyn (eye drops) is used to treat allergic conjunctivitis and keratitis. In the treatment of asthma, cromolyn efficacy is manifested by decreased severity of clinical symptoms, or need for

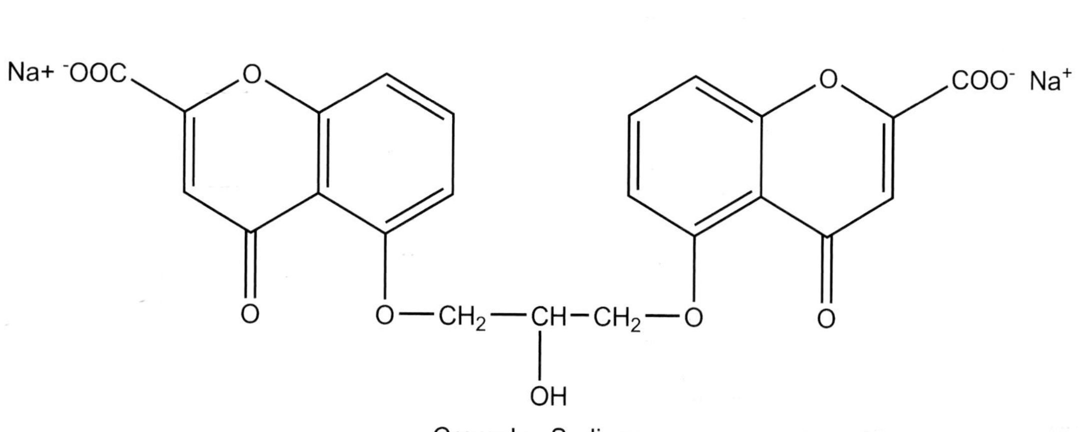

Cromolyn Sodium

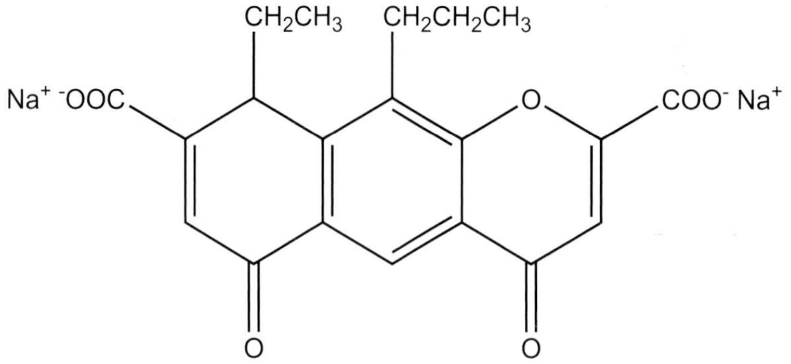

Nedocromil disodium

concomitant therapy, or both. Long-term use is justified if the drug significantly reduces the severity of asthma symptoms; permits a significant reduction in, or elimination of, steroid dosage; or improves management of those who have intolerable side effects to sympathomimetic agents or methylxanthines. For cromolyn to be effective, it must be administered at least 30 minutes prior to antigen challenge and administered at regular intervals (see dosing information that follows). When inhaled, the powder does produce irritation in some patients. Also, overuse of cromolyn can result in tolerance.

Dosage forms: Oral concentrate (100 mg/5 mL), nasal solution (40 mg/mL), solution for inhalation (20 mg/2 mL), aerosol (800 mg), ophthalmic solution (4%)
Usual adult dose:
- Inhalation solution (adults and children at least 2 years of age): 20 mg (one ampule per vial) bynebulization 4 times/day at regular intervals
- Aerosol (asthma in adults and children at least 5 years of age): 2 metered sprays inhaled 4 times per day at regular intervals
- Nasal solution (adults and children): one spray in each nostril 3 to 6 times daily at regular intervals every 4 to 6 hours
- Oral: two ampules 4 times per day 30 minutes before meals and at bedtime
- Ophthalmic: 1 drop of a 2% to 4% solution 4 to 6 times daily; Oral: two ampules 4 times a day 30 minutes before meals and at bedtime

Nedocromil Sodium. Nedocromil sodium, disodium 9-ethyl-6, 9-dihydro-4,6-dioxo-10-propyl-4H-pyrano[3, 2-g]quinoline-2,8-dicarboxylate (Tilade), is structurally related to cromolyn and displays similar, but broader, pharmacological actions.[52] It was available as an aerosol in a metered-dose inhaler for asthma treatment, and currently remains available as ophthalmic solution for the treatment of itching associated with allergic conjunctivitis. The inhalation formulation was marketed for maintenance therapy in the management of patients with mild-to-moderate bronchial asthma, but since has been withdrawn.

Dosage forms: Ophthalmic solution (2% or 20 mg/mL)
Usual adult dose: 1 or 2 drops in each eye twice a day at regular intervals

Lodoxamide Tromethamine. Lodoxamide tromethamine, N, N'-(2-chloro-5-cyano-m-phenylene)dioxamic acid (Alomide), is a white crystalline, water-soluble powder. The only significant structural similarity between lodoxamide and cromolyn and nedocromil is the presence of two acidic groups. Lodoxamide is indicated in the treatment of the ocular disorders including vernal keratoconjunctivitis, vernal conjunctivitis, and vernal keratitis.[55] Lodoxamide is available as a 0.1% solution, with each milliliter containing 1.78 mg of lodoxamide tromethamine equivalent to 1 mg of lodoxamide. The solution contains the preservative benzalkonium chloride (0.007%) as well as mannitol, hydroxypropyl methylcellulose, sodium citrate, citric acid, edetate disodium, tyloxapol, hydrochloric acid and/or sodium hydroxide (to adjust pH), and purified water.

The dose for adults and children older than 2 years of age is 1 to 2 drops in each affected eye 4 times daily for up to 3 months. The most frequently reported ocular adverse experiences were transient burning, stinging, or discomfort on instillation.

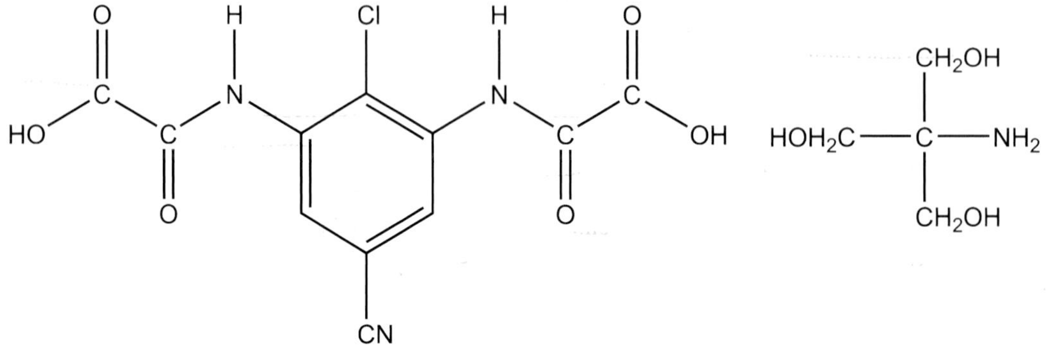

Lodoxamide Tromethamine

Pemirolast Potassium Ophthalmic Solution.
Pemirolast potassium, 9-methyl-3-(1H-tetrazol-5-yl)-4H-pyrido[1, 2-α]pyrimidin-4-one potassium (Alamast), is a yellow, water-soluble powder. It can be considered an analog of one portion of the cromolyn structure in which the carboxyl group has been replaced with an isosteric tetrazole moiety. Pemirolast is indicated for the prevention of itching of the eye caused by allergic conjunctivitis. The commercial preparation is available as a 0.1% sterile ophthalmic solution for topical administration to the eyes. Each milliliter of this solution contains 1 mg of pemirolast potassium, as well as the preservative lauralkonium chloride (0.005%), and glycerin, phosphate buffers, and sodium hydroxide to maintain a solution pH of 8.0. The solution has an osmolality of 240 mOsm/L. The recommended dose is 1 to 2 drops instilled into each affected eye 4 times a day. This drug product is for ocular administration only and not for injection or oral use and should be used with caution during pregnancy or while nursing.[56]

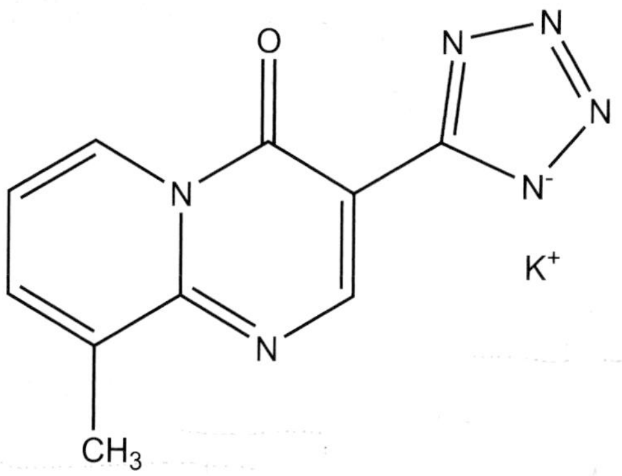

Pemirolast Potassium

RECENT ANTIHISTAMINE DEVELOPMENTS: THE "DUAL-ACTING" ANTIHISTAMINES

Over the several past decades, there has been considerable interest in the development of novel antihistaminic compounds with dual mechanisms of action including H₁-receptor antihistaminic action and mast cell stabilization. Currently available drugs that exhibit such dual antihistaminic actions include azelastine and ketotifen. These compounds contain the basic pharmacophore to produce relatively selective antihistaminic action (diarylalkylamines) as well as inhibition of the release of histamine and other mediators (e.g., leukotrienes and PAP) from mast cells involved in the allergic response. In vitro studies suggest that these compounds also decrease chemotaxis and activation of eosinophils. Azelastine and ketotifen currently are indicated for the treatment of itching of the eye associated with allergic conjunctivitis. Their antiallergy actions occur within minutes after administration and may persist for up to 8 hours. The structures, chemical properties, pharmacological profiles, and dosage data for these agents are provided in the monographs that follow.

Azelastine Hydrochloride Ophthalmic Solution.
Azelastine hydrochloride, (±)-4-[(4-chlorophenyl)methyl]-2-(hexahydro-1-methyl-1H-azepin-4-yl)-1-(2H)-phthalazinone monohydrochloride (Optivar), is a white crystalline powder that is sparingly soluble in water, methanol, and propylene glycol and slightly soluble in ethanol, octanol, and glycerine. The commercial preparation is available as a 0.05% sterile ophthalmic solution for topical administration to the eyes. Each milliliter of azelastine solution contains 0.5-mg azelastine hydrochloride equivalent to 0.457 mg of azelastine base, the preservative benzalkonium chloride (0.125 mg), and inactive ingredients including disodium edetate dihydrate, hydroxypropylmethylcellulose, sorbitol solution, sodium hydroxide, and water for injection. The solution has a pH of approximately 5.0 to 6.5 and an osmolality of approximately 271 to 312 mOsm/L.

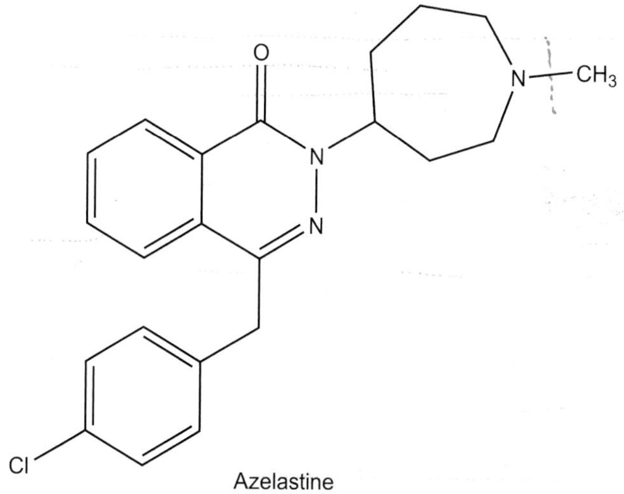

Azelastine

DiPiro, nasal only

The recommended dose of azelastine solution is 1 drop instilled into each affected eye twice a day. This drug product is for ocular administration only and not for injection or oral use. Absorption of azelastine following ocular administration is relatively low (less than 1 ng/rnL). Absorbed drug undergoes extensive oxidative *N*-demethylation by CYP, and the parent drug and metabolite are eliminated primarily in the feces. The most frequently reported adverse reactions are transient eye burning or stinging, headaches, and bitter taste. Azelastine solution should be used with caution during pregnancy or while nursing, because its safety has not been studied under these circumstances.[57]

Ketotifen Fumarate Ophthalmic Solution.
Ketotifen fumarate, 4-(1-methyl-4-piperidylidene)-4H-benzo[4,5]cyclohepta[1,2-b]thiophen-10(9H)-one hydrogen fumarate (Zaditor), is a fine crystalline powder. Ketotifen is a ketothiophene isostere analog of the dibenzocycloheptane antihistamines. The solution contains 0.345 mg of ketotifen fumarate, which is equivalent to 0.25 mg of ketotifen. The solution also contains the preservative benzalkonium chloride (0.01%) as well as glycerol, sodium hydroxide and/or hydrochloric acid (to adjust pH), and purified water. It has a pH of 4.4 to 5.8 and an osmolality of 210 to 300 mOsm/kg.

Ketotifen Fumarate

The recommended dose of ketotifen solution is 1 drop instilled into each affected eye every 8 to 12 hours. The most frequently reported adverse reactions are conjunctival infection, headaches, and rhinitis. This drug product is for ocular administration only and not for injection or oral use. Ketotifen solution should be used with caution during pregnancy or while nursing, because its safety has not been studied under these circumstances.[58]

HISTAMINE H₂-ANTAGONISTS

Drugs whose pharmacological action primarily involves antagonism of the action of histamine at its H₂-receptors find therapeutic application in the treatment of acid-peptic disorders including heartburn, gastroesophageal reflux disease (GERD), erosive esophagitis, gastric and duodenal ulcers, and gastric acid pathologic hypersecretory diseases such as Zollinger-Ellison syndrome. They are also useful in combination with H₁-antihistamines for the treatment of chronic urticaria and for the itching of anaphylaxis and pruritis.[59–62]

Gastric Acid Secretion

A characteristic feature of the mammalian stomach is its ability to secrete acid as part of its processes to digest food for absorption later in the intestine. The presence of acid and proteolytic pepsin enzymes, whose formation is facilitated by the low gastric pH, is generally assumed to be required for the hydrolysis of proteins and other food constiuents. The acid secretory unit of the gastric mucosa is the parietal (oxyntic) cell. Parietal cells contain an H^+, K^+-ATPase or hydrogen ion pump that secretes proton (H^+) in exchange for the uptake of K^+ ion (Fig, 23.14).[61,62] Secretion of acid by gastric parietal cells is stimulated by various mediators at receptors located on the basolateral membrane, including histamine agonism of H₂-receptors (cellular), gastrin activity at G receptors (blood), and acetylcholine (ACh) at M₂ muscarinic receptors (neuronal). Gastric and muscarinic receptors modulate acid secretion through calcium-dependent processes, while the H₂-receptor is coupled to adenylate cy-

clase (Fig. 23.14). The adenylate cyclase pathway, and therefore acid secretion, is inhibited by intracellular prostaglandins of the E series. These prostaglandins also stimulate other GI epithelial cells to secrete mucous and bicarbonate, and enhance blood flow through gastric tissues. All of these prostaglandin-mediated actions have acid-neutralizing and gastric tissue protective properties referred to generally as "cytoprotection." When there is hypersecretion of gastric acid or breakdown of muscosal cell defenses, including bacterial infection, gastric tissues and contiguous structures (esophagus, intestines) may become compromised and ulcerated.[61,62]

Peptic Ulcer Disease

Peptide ulcer disease (PUD) is a group of upper GI tract disorders characterized by mucosal erosions equal to or greater than 0.5 cm that result from the erosive action of acid and pepsin.[63] Duodenal ulcer and gastric ulcer are the most common forms, although PUD may occur in the esophagus or small intestine. Factors involved in the pathogenesis and recurrence of PUD include hypersecretion of acid and pepsin and GI infection by *Helicobacter pylori*, a Gram-negative spiral bacterium. *H. pylori* have been found in virtually all patients with duodenal ulcers and approximately 75% of patients with gastric ulcers. Some risk factors associated with recurrence of PUD include cigarette smoking, chronic use of ulcerogenic drugs (e.g., nonsteroidal anti-inflammatory drugs [NSAIDs]), male gender, age, alcohol consumption, emotional stress, and family history. About 4% of gastric ulcers are caused by a malignancy, whereas duodenal ulcers are generally benign.

The goals of PUD therapy are to promote healing, relieve pain, and prevent ulcer complications and recurrences. Medications used to heal or reduce ulcer recurrence include antacids, histamine H₂-antagonists, protective mucosal barriers, proton pump inhibitors (PPIs), prostaglandins, and bismuth salt and combinations of these drugs with antibiotics to eradicate *H. pylori* infection.

Structural Derivation of the "H₂-Antagonists"

The H₂-antagonists are used to treat acid indigestion (an OTC application), GERD, peptic ulcers, and pathologic hypersecretory disorders, as well as some of the symptoms of urticaria and anaphylaxis. Cimetidine, the original member of this drug class, was developed by a classical structure–activity study beginning with the endogenous agonist, histamine as shown in Table 23.4.[64] Methylation of the 5-position of the imidazole heterocycle of histamine produced a selective agonist at atrial histamine receptors (H₂). The guanidino analog of histamine was then found to possess weak antagonist activity to the acid-secretory actions of histamine. Increasing the length of the side chain from two to four carbons, coupled with replacement of the strongly basic guanidino group by a neutral methyl thiourea function, led to development of burimamide, the first full H₂-receptor antagonist, albeit one of low potency. The low potency of burimamide was postulated to be related to its nonbasic, electron-releasing side chain, which favors the nonpharmacophoric N$^\pi$—H imidazole tautomer over the basic, electron-withdrawing side chain in histamine, which predominantly presents the higher-affinity N$^\tau$—H imidazole tautomer to the

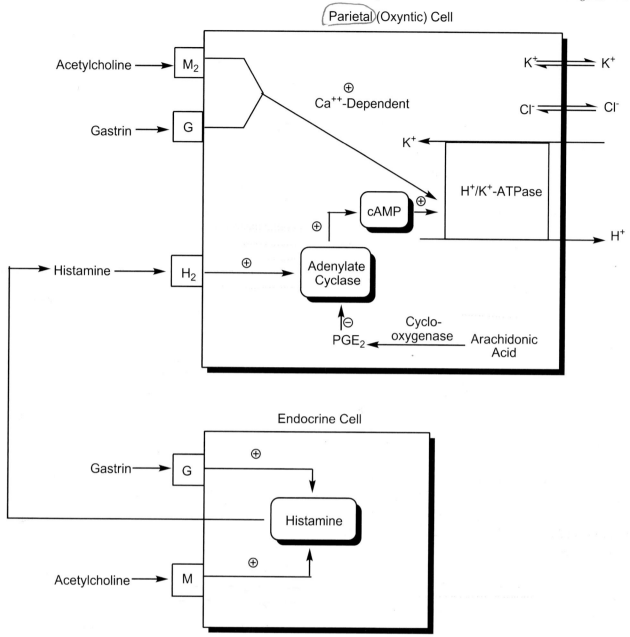

Figure 23.14 ● Hormonal regulation of acid secretion by parietal cells.

receptor. Insertion of an electronegative thioether function in the side chain in place of a methylene group favors the N^7—H tautomer, and introduction of the 5-methyl group favors H_2 selectivity and led to metiamide, an H_2-blocker of higher potency and oral bioavailability than burimamide. Unfortunately, drug-related toxicities including agranulocytosis prevented further development of this compound. However, replacement of the thiourea moiety of metiamide with a cyano-imino function produced cimetidine, the first clinically effective and relatively safe member of this therapeutic class (Table 23.4).[64]

Introduction of cimetidine into medicine revealed an effective gastric antisecretory agent that promotes the healing of duodenal ulcers. Cimetidine is not without several limitations, however. Because it is short acting, it requires a frequent-dosing schedule. Also, cimetidine was found to possess antiandrogenic activity, which can lead to gynecomastia, and to

cause confusional states in some elderly patients and decreased renal function. Also, cimetidine inhibits CYP isozymes and renal tubular secretion, resulting in clinically significant drug interactions.[65] The drug interaction potential and several adverse effects (gynecomastia) of cimetidine appear to be directly related to the presence of the imidazole group. These limitations prompted additional drug design and development efforts, which revealed that the imidazole ring was not required for H_2-antagonist activity (discussed next). In fact, replacement of the imidazole ring with a furan (ranitidine) or a thiazole (famotidine, nizatidine) heterocycle with a basic ring substitutent (guanidine or dimethylaminomethyl) not only enhances both potency and selectivity of H_2-antagonism, but also reduces cytochrome and renal secretory drug interactions.[64]

The pharmacokinetic properties of the H_2-antagonists are summarized in Table 23.5.[66] Cimetidine, ranitidine, and

TABLE 23.4 Development of H$_2$-Antagonists

Structure–Activity Relationship	Structure
Histamine: Nonselective histamine receptor agonist (H$_1$ = H$_2$)	
5-Methylhistamine: Selective H$_2$-agonist (H$_2$ > H$_1$)	
N$^\alpha$-Guanylhistamine: Partial H$_2$-receptor agonist (weak antagonist)	
Burimamide: Full H$_2$-receptor antagonist; but low potency and poor oral bioavailability	
Metiamide: Full H$_2$-receptor antagonist with higher potency and improved oral bioavailability; but toxicity resulting from the thiourea	
Cimetidine: Full H$_2$-receptor antagonist with higher potency and improved oral bioavailability and low systemic toxicity	

TABLE 23.5 Potency and Pharmacokinetics of the H$_2$-Antagonists

H$_2$-Blocker	Relative Potency	Oral Bioaval	Metabolites	% Dose Metab	Elimination
Cimetidine	1	63–78	S-oxide, Hydroxy-methyl	25	Renal
Famotidine	40	37–45	S-oxide	30	Renal
Nizatidine	10	98	N2-desmethyl, N-oxide	37	Renal
Ranitidine	6	52	N-desmethyl, N-oxide, S-oxide	30	Renal, biliary

Source: Facts and Comparisons 4.0, Wolters Kluwer Health, Amsterdam, Netherlands, 2009.

famotidine have lower oral bioavailabilities than nizatidine as a result of greater first-pass metabolism. Based on their common structural features, most of these agents are metabolized by *S*- and *N*-oxidation. The imidazole ring of cimetidine serves as an addition site for oxidative metabolism, as do the *N,N*-dimethyl functionalities of nizatidine and ranitidine. All of these metabolites are presumed to be inactive, or at least less active than the parent drugs. Also, a significant proportion of the dose of each of the H$_2$-antagonists is excreted renally in unmetabolized form. The half-lives of these agents range from 1 to 4 hours, with nizatidine having the shortest half-life.[66] The properties of the individual H$_2$-antagonists that are in clinical use in the United States are described and compared in the monographs that follow.

Cimetidine, USP. Cimetidine, N^{π}-cyano-*N*-methyl-*N'*-[2-[[5-methylimidazol-4-yl)methyl]thio]ethyl]guanidine (Tagamet), is a colorless crystalline solid that is slightly soluble in water (1.14% at 37°C). The solubility is greatly increased by the addition of dilute acid to protonate the imidazole ring (apparent pK_a of 6.8). At pH 7, aqueous solutions are stable for at least 7 days. Cimetidine is a relatively hydrophilic molecule with an octanol/water partition coefficient of 2.5.

Cimetidine inhibits the hepatic metabolism of drugs biotransformed by various CYP isozymes, delaying elimination and increasing serum levels of these drugs. Thus, concomitant therapy with cimetidine and drugs metabolized by hepatic cytochrome isozymes or in patients with renal or hepatic impairment may require dosage adjustment. This is particulary true for drugs with relatively low therapeutic indices including warfarin-type anticoagulants, phenytoin, propranolol, nifedipine, benzodiazepines, certain tricyclic antidepressants, lidocaine, theophylline, and metronidazole.[66] Additionally, cimetidine administration may increase gastric pH and decrease the absorption of drugs such as the azole antifungals (e.g., ketoconazole), which require an acidic environment for dissolution.[66] If concurrent azole therapy is required, it is best to administer it at least 2 hours before cimetidine administration. Cimetidine has a weak antiandrogenic effect, and it may cause gynecomastia in patients treated for 1 month or more.

Cimetidine exhibits relatively good bioavailability (60%–70%) and a plasma half-life of about 2 hours, which is increased in renal and hepatic impairment and in the elderly. Approximately 30% to 40% of a cimetidine dose is metabolized (*S*-oxidation, 5-CH$_3$ hydroxylation), and the parent drug and metabolites are eliminated primarily by renal excretion.[66] Antacids interfer with cimetidine absorption and should be administered at least 1 hour before or after a cimetidine dose.

Dosage forms: Tablet (200, 300, 400, 800 mg), liquid (300 mg/5 mL), injection (150/mL and 6 mg/mL)
Usual adult oral dose:
- Benign gastric ulcer: 800 or 300 mg 4 times a day
- Duodenal ulcer: 800 or 300 mg 4 times a day (with meals and at bedtime); maintenance dose, 400 mg 4 times a day
- Gastroesophageal reflux disease, erosive: 1,600 mg daily in divided doses (800 mg twice daily or 400 mg 4 times per day) for 12 weeks
- Heartburn relief or prevention (OTC): 200 mg with water as symptoms occur or right before or any time up to 30 minutes before eating food or drinking; maximum dosage, 400 mg/day
- Pathological hypersecretory conditions: 300 mg 4 times per day with meals and at bedtime; maximum dosage, 2,400 mg/day
- Usual pediatric dose: Oral, 20 to 40 mg (base) per kilogram of body weight 4 times a day with meals and at bedtime

Famotidine, USP. Famotidine, *N'*-(aminosulfonyl)-3-[[[2[(diamnomethylene)amino]-4-thiazolyl]methyl]thio]propanimidamide (Pepcid), is a white to pale-yellow crystalline compound that is very slightly soluble in water and practically insoluble in ethanol. It is a thiazole bioisotere of cimetidine that contains a guanidine substituent that may mimic the imizadole of cimetidine.

Famotidine is a competitive inhibitor of histamine H$_2$-receptors with a potency significantly greater than cimetidine. It inhibits basal and nocturnal gastric secretion as well as secretion stimulated by food and pentagastrin. Its current labeling indications are for the short-term treatment of duodenal and benign gastric ulcers, GERD, pathological hypersecretory conditions (e.g., Zollinger-Ellison syndrome), and heartburn (OTC only).[66]

No cases of gynecomastia, increased prolactin levels, or impotence have been reported, even at the higher dosage levels used in patients with pathological hypersecretory conditions. Studies with famotidine in humans, in animal models, and in vitro have shown no significant interference with the disposition of compounds metabolized by cytochrome isozymes. No significant interactions have been detected with warfarin, theophylline, phenytoin, diazepam, aminopyrine, and antipyrine.

Famotidine is incompletely absorbed (37%–45% bioavailability).[66] The drug is eliminated by renal (65%–70%) and metabolic (30%–35%) routes. Famotidine sulfoxide is the only metabolite identified in humans. The effects of food or antacid on the bioavailability of famotidine are not clinically significant.

Cimetidine

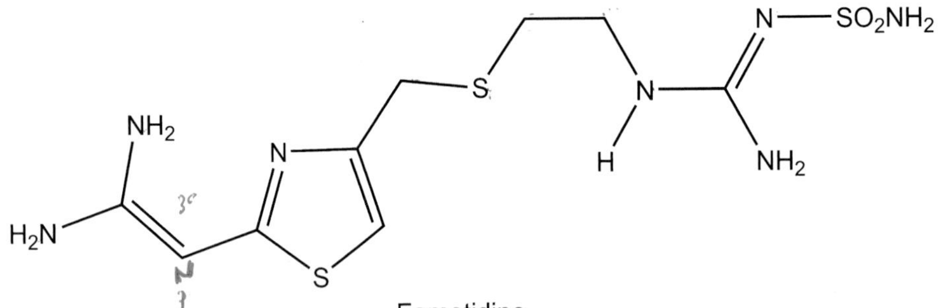

Famotidine

Dosage forms: Tablets (20 and 40 mg), oral disintegrating tablets (20 and 40 mg), gelcaps (10 mg), oral suspension (40 mg/5 mL), injection (10 mg/mL and 20 mg/50 mL)

Usual adult oral dose:
- Benign gastric ulcer: 40 mg once daily (bedtime)
- Duodenal ulcer: Treatment dose, 40 mg once to twice a day at bedtime; maintenance dose, 20 mg once daily at bedtime
- Gastroesophageal reflux disease: 20 mg twice a day
- Heartburn: 10 to 20 mg for relief or 1 hour before a meal for prevention
- Esophagitis, including erosions and ulcerations: 20 or 40 mg twice a day
- Pathological hypersecretory conditions: individualize dosage; typically 20 mg every 6 hours
- Severe Zollinger-Ellison syndrome: up to 160 mg every 6 hours

Ranitidine, USP. Ranitidine, *N*-[2-[[[5-(dimethylamino)methyl]-2-furanyl]methyl]thiol] ethyl]-*N'*-methyl-2-nitro-l,1-ethenediamine (Zantac), is a white solid, which in its hydrochloride salt form is highly soluble in water. It is an aminoalkyl furan derivative with pK_a values of 2.7 (side chain) and 8.2 (dimethylamino). Ranitidine is more potent than cimetidine, but less potent than famotidine. Like other H$_2$-antagonists, it does not appear to bind to other receptors.[66]

Bioavailability of an oral dose of ranitidine is about 50% and is not significantly affected by the presence of food.[66] Some antacids may reduce ranitidine absorption and should not be taken within 1 hour of administration of this drug. The plasma half-life of the drug is 2 to 3 hours, and it is excreted along with its metabolites in the urine. Three metabolites, ranitidine *N*-oxide, ranitidine *S*-oxide, and desmethyl ranitidine,

have been identified. Ranitidine is only a weak inhibitor of the hepatic cytochrome isozymes, and recommended doses of the drug do not appear to inhibit the metabolism of other drugs. However, there have been isolated reports of drug interactions (warfarin, triazolam) that suggest that ranitidine may affect the bioavailability of certain drugs by some unidentified mechanism, perhaps by pH-dependent effect on absorption or a change in volume of distribution.[66]

In addition to being available in various dosage forms as the hydrochloride salt, ranitidine is also available as a bismuth citrate salt for use with the macrolide antibiotic clarithromycin in treating patients with an active duodenal ulcer associated with *H. pylori* infection. Eradication of *H. pylori* reduces the risk of duodenal ulcer recurrence.

Dosage forms: Tablets (75, 150, and 300 mg of HCl salt); effervescent tablets (25 and 150 mg); capsules (150 and 300 mg); syrup (15 mg/mL as HCl salt); injection (1 and 25 mg/mL as HCl salt)

Usual adult oral dose:
- Erosive esophagitis: 150 mg 4 times daily initially and then 150 mg twice daily for maintenance
- Benign gastric ulcer: 150 mg twice a day
- Duodenal ulcer: 150 mg twice a day or 300 mg daily initially and then 150 mg once daily for maintenance
- Heartburn (OTC only): Initial dosage for relief 1 tablet, can be used up to twice daily for maintenance
- Gastroesophageal reflux disease: 150 mg twice a day
- Pathological hypersecretory conditions: 150 mg twice a day

Nizatidine. Nizatidine, *N*-[2-[[[2-(dimethylamino)methyl]-4-thiazolyl]methyl]thio]-ethyl]-*N'*-methyl-2-nitro-1,1-ethenediamine (Axid), is an off-white to buff crystalline solid that is soluble in water, alcohol, and chloroform. It is a thaizole derivative of ranitidine and has pK_as of 2.1 (side

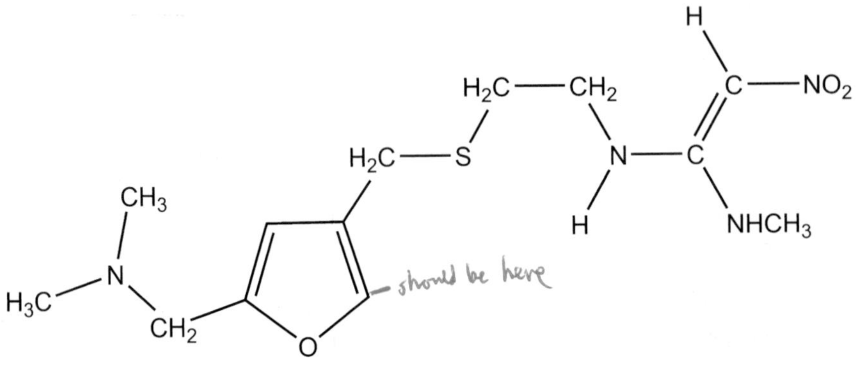

Ranitidine

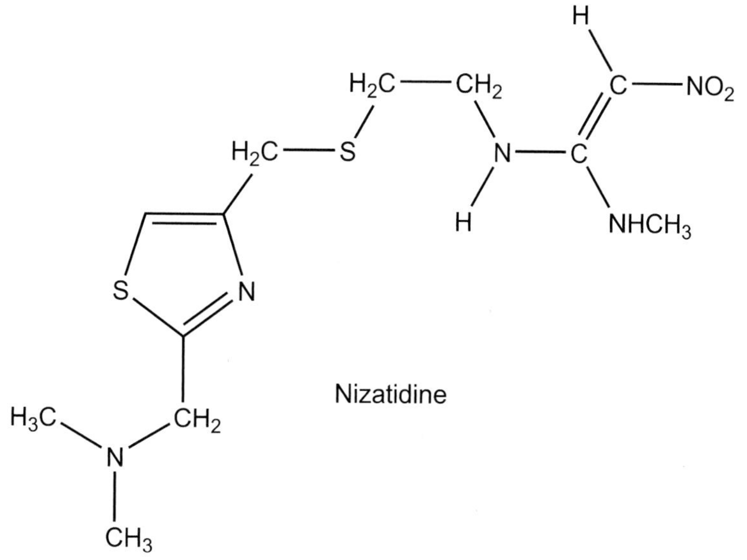

$$H_2C - CH_2$$

Nizatidine

chain) and 6.8 (dimethylamino). Nizatidine's mechanism of action is similar to other H_2-antagonists, as is its receptor selectivity. It is more potent than cimetidine.

Nizatidine has excellent oral bioavailability (>90%). The effects of antacids or food on its bioavailability are not clinically significant.[66] The elimination half-life is 1 to 2 hours. It is excreted primarily in the urine (90%) and mostly as unchanged drug (60%). Metabolites include nizatidine sulfoxide (6%), N-desmethylnizatidine (7%), and nizatidine N-oxide (dimethylaminomethyl function).[66] Nizatidine has no demonstrable antiandrogenic action, effects on other hormones, or inhibitory effects on cytochrome isozymes involved in the metabolism of other drugs.

Dosage forms: Tablets (75 mg), capsules (150 and 300 mg), oral solution (15 mg/mL)
Usual adult oral dose:
- Benign gastric ulcer: 150 mg twice a day or 300 mg once daily at bedtime.
- Duodenal ulcer: Treatment, 300 mg once to twice a day; maintenance, 150 mg once daily
- GERD: 150 mg twice a day
- Heartburn (OTC products only): 1 tablet with a full glass of water, up to 2 tablets in 24 hours.
- Hypersecretory condition: 150 mg twice a day

Other Antiulcer and Gastric Acid Hypersecretory Disease Therapies: Proton Pump Inhibitors

The final step in acid secretion in the parietal cell is the extrusion or "pumping" of protons into the lumen of stomach by the membrane H^+, K^+-ATPase pump as described previously (Fig. 23.14). Thus, inhibition of this proton pump acts beyond the site of action of second messengers (e.g., calcium and cAMP) and is independent of the action of secretogogues histamine, gastrin, and acetylcholine. Thus, acid pump inhibitors block both basal and stimulated acid secretion.

In 1972, a group of Swedish medicinal chemists discovered that certain pyridylmethyl benzimidazole sulfides were capable of functioning as H^+, K^+-ATPase or PPIs.[67,68] These compounds were subsequently converted to sulfoxide

derivatives, which exhibited highly potent, irreversible inhibition of the proton pump. The benzimidazole PPIs are prodrugs that are rapidly converted to a sulfenamide intermedate in the highly acidic environment of gastric parietal cells. The weakly basic benzimidazole PPIs accumulate in these acidic compartments on the luminal side of the tubuvesicular and canalicular structures of the parietal cells. The benzimidazole PPIs are then chemically converted by acid to a sulfenamide intermediate that inhibits the proton pump via covalent interaction with sulfhydryl groups with cysteine residues of the H^+, K^+-ATPase pump (Fig. 23.15).[67,68] All of the PPIs have been shown to react with cysteine 813 of pump, but some bind to additional pump sulfhydryl residues as well.[69] For example, omeprazole and esomeprazole also react with cysteine 892, and pantoprazole with cysteine 822 and lansoprazole to cysteine 321.[69,70] Cysteines 321, 813, and 822 are all in the proton-transport domain of the H^+, K^+-ATPase system, whereas cysteine 892 is on the external luminal surface and does not affect pump transport ability.[69,70] The bioaccumulation and activation of the PPIs within the acidic environment of the parietal cell also ensures specificity of pharmacologic action. The acid lability of the benzimidazole PPIs dictates that these drugs must be formulated as delayed-release, enteric-coated granular dosage forms.

To date, five structually related benzimidazole sulfoxide PPIs have been approved for use in the United States to treat various gastric acid hypersecretory disorders. These include omeprazole, esomeprazole (the active enantiomers of omeprazole), lansoprazole, patoprazole, and rabeprazole. The PPIs differ only in the nature and degree and pyridine and imidazole ring substituents, which has an impact on pK_a values and pharmacokinetic properties. The extent of initial PPI protonation and, thereby, parietal cell accumulation is governed by the pK_a of the pyridine ring nitrogen that ranges from 3.8 for lansoprazole and pantoprazole to 4.5 for rabeprazole (Table 23.6).[71] Thus, all drugs are believed to be concentrated at their physiologic site of action to a similar extent. The rate of conversion of PPIs to their active sulfenamides, however, is determined largely by the pK_a of the benzimidazole group (pK_a2). Omeprazole, lansoprazole, and rabeprazole with higher pK_a2s (0.62–0.79) undergo

Benzimidazole PPI

Covalent complex with PPI and Proton Pump

Sulfenamide

Figure 23.15 ● Mechanism of action of PPIs.

TABLE 23.6 pKₐs of the Proton Pump Inhibitors

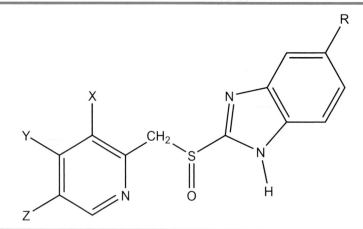

PPI	X	Y	X	R	pKₐ1	pKₐ2
Omeprazole	CH_3	CH_3O	CH_3	CH_3O	4.06	0.79
Lansoprazole	CH_3	CF_3CH_2O	H	H	3.83	0.62
Pantoprazole	CH_3O	CH_3O	H	CHF_2O	3.83	0.11
Rabeprazole	CH_3	$CH_3OCH_2CH_2CH_2O$	H	H	4.53	0.62

Source: Sachs, G., Shin, J. M., and Howden, C. W.: Review article: the clinical pharmacology of proton pumps inhibitors. Aliment. Pharmacol. Ther. 23(Suppl. 2):2–8, 2006.

TABLE 23.7 FDA Indications for Antihypersecretory Agents

Drug	Heartburn	GERD	Erosive Esophagitis	Benign Gastric Ulcer	Duodenal Ulcer	NSAID-Induced Ulcers	Pathological Hypersecretory Conditions*
Cimetidine	X	X		X	X		X
Ranitidine	X	X	X	X	X		
Nizatidine	X	X		X	X		
Famotidine	X	X		X	X		X
Omeprazole	X	X	X	X	X		X
Esomeprazole		X	X		X	X	X
Lansoprazole		X	X	X	X	X	X
Pantoprazole		X	X		X		X
Rabeprazole		X	X		X		X

Source: Facts and Comparisons 4.0, Wolters Kluwer Health, Amsterdam, Netherlands, 2009.
*Including Zollinger-Ellison syndrome.

benzimidazole protonation and sulfenamide formation faster than pantoprazole with a pK_a2 of 0.11.[71]

The duration of PPI antisecretory action is determined by several factors including the extent and nature of cysteine residues inactivated, pump protein turnover, activation of inactive pumps, and reactivation of inhibited pumps by endogenous reducing agents capable of breaking the PPI-pump disulfide bonds.[72–74] PPIs that inactivate cysteine 822 (pantoprazole) tend to have the longest duration of effect, because this cyteine residue is on the pump transport domain, is resistant to reductive reactivation, and therefore, requires replacement by new pump protein. Thus, pantoprazole has an effective half-life of 46 hours, whereas omeprazole is 28 hours, and lansoprazole is less than 15 hours.[72–75] The significance of the differences in rates of PPI activation or duration of action does not appear to have overwhelming clinical significance.

Most clinical data suggests that these PPIs are more effective in the short term than the H₂-blockers in healing duodenal ulcers and erosive esophagitis and can even heal esophagitis resistant to treatment with the H₂-antagonists.[73,74] In addition, the benzimidazole PPIs are reported to have antimicrobial activity against *H. pylori*, and thus, possess efficacy in treating gastric ulcers or with one or more antimicrobials, in eradicating infection by this organism. A host of clinical trials have been performed in an attempt to compare the relative clinical efficacies of the PPIs in various hypersecretory disease states (see Table 23.7 for indications). Often the results of these studies have been difficult to interpret because of many variables in PPI formulation, dosage strength, pharmacokinetic properties, diagnostic criteria, etc. Most studies have concluded, however, that comparable dosage strengths and formulations of all of these agents are therapeutically interchangeable in terms of clinical efficacy.[73,74] The PPIs also share a very similar adverse reaction profile, with the most common adverse effects involving abdominal pain, diarrhea, and headache. Several other, more severe, adverse reactions (serious allergy, blood dyscrasias) have been reported rarely with PPI use, but have not been linked causally with the drugs.[73,74]

The PPIs vary in their oral bioavialability from 30% (omeprazole) to 80% (lansoprazole), and bioavailability generally increases upon repeated dosing. All, except rabeprazole, achieve peak plasma levels by about 2 hours (Table 23.8).[66] All of PPIs are eliminated almost entirely as cytochrome-based metabolites and, with the exception of lansoprazole, predominantly by the renal route. Virtually no unchanged drug is excreted in the urine and feces. The cytochrome isozymes primarily involved in PPI metabolism in-

TABLE 23.8 Pharmacokinetic Properties of the Proton Pump Inhibitors

PPI	Oral Bioavail*	T_{max}	PPB	Plasma $t_{1/2}$			Linear Kinetics?
Omeprazole	30%–40%	0.5–3.5 hr	95%	0.7 hr	Hydroxy acid sulfide and sulfone	77% urine as metabolites	No
Esomeprazole	64%	1.6 hr	97%	0.9 hr	Hydroxy, desmethyl, sulfone	80% urine as metabolites	No
Lansoprazole	80%	1.7 hr	97%	1.2 hr	Hydroxylated sulfinyl and sulfone	33% urine as metabolites; 66% feces as metabolites	Yes
Pantoprazole	77%	2.5 hr	98%	1.2 hr	Demethylation, with subsequent sulfation	71% urine as metabolites; 18% feces as metabolites	Yes
Rabeprazole	52%	2–5 hr	96%	1.0 hr	Thioether carboxylic acid, its glucuronide, sulfone, mercapturic acid	90% urine as metabolites	Yes

Source: Facts and Comparisons 4.0, Wolters Kluwer Health, Amsterdam, Netherlands, 2009.
*Increases with repeated once-daily dosing.

clude CYP2C19 and CYP3A4, and these catalyze pyridine ring methyl oxidation (CYP2C19: omeprazole, esomeprazole), benzimidazole ring *O*-demethylation (CYP2C19: omeprazole and esomeprazole) and sulfoxide oxidation (all PPIs as illustrated in Fig. 23.16) for omeprazole.[75,76] The primary metabolite of omeprazole, a racemate, is 5-hydroxymethylomeprazole, whereas the main metabolite formed from esomeprazole (the *S*-isomer) is the sulfone.[75,76] Lansoprazole, pantoprazole, and rabeprazole lack the pyridyl 5-methyl group and benzimidazole 5-methoxy group, so they do not undergo these oxidative processes (see structures that follow).[75,76]

As a result of their metabolic clearance profiles, the PPIs, and especially omeprazole, can interact with other drugs that are also processed by CYP2C19 and CYP3A4 isozymes (Table 23.9). Inhibition of oxidative metabolism by omeprazole (but not esomeprazole) is responsible for prolonging the clearance of benzodiazepines, phenytoin, and warfarin.[66] Lansoprazole decreases theophylline concentration slightly and may decrease the efficacy of oral contraceptives. Pantoprazole and rabeprazole appear to be free of these interactions. Further, the profound and long-lasting inhibition of gastric acid secretion by the PPIs may interfere with the bioavailability of drugs when gastric pH is an important determinant, such as the azole antifungals (e.g.,

ketoconazole), ampicillin, iron salts, digoxin, and cyanocobalamin (Table 23.9).[66]

Omeprazole. Omeprazole, 5-methoxy-2-(((4-methoxy-3, 5-dimethyl-2-pyridinyl)methyl) sulfinyl)-1H-benzimidazole (Losec), is a white to off-white crystalline powder with very slight solubility in water. Omeprazole is an amphoteric compound (pyridine N, pK$_a$ 4.06; benzimidazole N-H, pK$_a$ 0.79), and consistent with the proposed mechanism of action of the substituted benzimidazoles, is acid labile. Hence, the omeprazole product is formulated as delayed-release capsules containing enteric-coated granules.

The absolute bioavailability of orally administered orneprazole is 30% to 40% related to substantial first-pass biotransformation (Table 23.8).[66] The drug has a plasma half-life of about 1 hour. Most (77%) of an oral dose of omeprazole is excreted in the urine as metabolites with insignificant antisecretory activity. The primary metabolites of omeprazole are 5-hydroxyomeprazole (CYP2C19) and omeprazole sulfone (CYP3A4). The antisecretory actions of omeprazole persist for 24 to 72 hours, long after the drug has disappeared from plasma, which is consistent with its suggested mechanism of action involving irreversible inhibition of the proton pump.

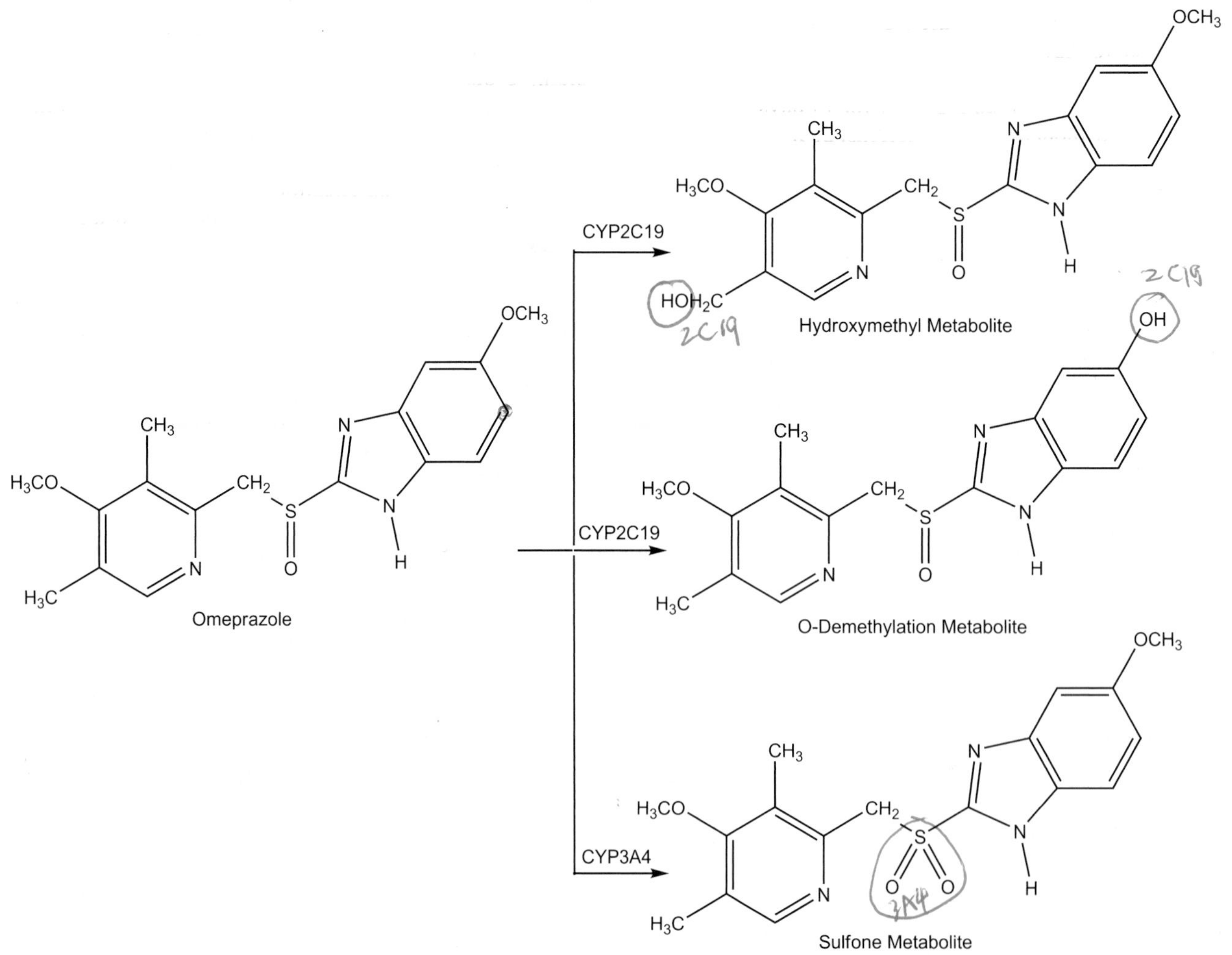

Figure 23.16 • Metabolic transformations of benzimidazole PPIs.

TABLE 23.9 PPI Drug Interactions

PPI Drug Interaction	Mechanism of Drug Interaction
Azole antifungals	Inhibition of PPI (especially omeprazole, esomeprazole) metabolism, resulting in significantly higher drug levels. PPIs may reduce the GI absorption of azoles by elevating gastric pH and reducing azole solubility in the GI tract
Macrolide antibiotics	Inhibition of PPI (especially omeprazole, esomeprazole) metabolism, resulting in significantly higher drug levels.
Herbals (e.g., ginkgo biloba, St. John's wort	Certain herbals may induce the metabolism of PPIs, especially omeprazole, reducing their plasma concentrations and efficacy.
Hydantoins (e.g., phenytoin)	PPIs, especially omeprazole, may increase serum hydantoin levels. Dose adjustment may be required.
Benzodiazepines (e.g., diazepam, triazolam)	PPIs, especially omeprazole and esomeprazole, may decrease the oxidative metabolism of certain benzodiazepines, thereby reducing their clearance, increasing their half-life and serum levels, and increasing the risk of benzodiazepine-associated adverse effects. Benzodiazepine dosage should be decreased (or dosing interval increased).
Cilostazol, digoxin	PPIs, especially omeprazole, may increase the plasma concentrations of these drugs, thereby increasing their therapeutic effect and adverse effect potential. Consider dosage adjustment of cilostazol.
Protease inhibitors (e.g., atazanavir, indinavir)	PPIs may reduce the absorption and plasma levels certain protease inhibitors. Concurrent use of atazanavir and omeprazole is not recommended.
Warfarin	PPIs may increase the hypoprothrombinemic effects of warfarin. The anticoagulant efficacy of warfarin should be monitored when starting or stopping omeprazole.

Source: Facts and Comparisons 4.0, Wolters Kluwer Health, Amsterdam, Netherlands, 2009.

Omeprazole is approved for the treatment of heartburn, GERD, duodenal ulcer, erosive esophagitis, gastric ulcer, and pathological hypersecretory conditions.

Dosage form: Delayed-release tablets (20 mg) and capsules (20 and 40 mg)

Usual adult doses:
- Heartburn (OTC): 20 mg daily for 14 days
- GERD without esophageal lesions: 20 mg/daily for up to 4 weeks
- GERD with erosive esophagitis: 20 mg/daily for 4 to 8 weeks; an additional 4 weeks of treatment may be beneficial
- Duodenal ulcer: 20 mg/day for 4 or more weeks
- Duodenal ulcer associated with *H. pylori*: Triple therapy with omeprazole 20 mg plus clarithromycin 500 mg plus amoxicillin 1,000 mg, each twice daily for 10 days. If an ulcer is present at the initiation of therapy, continue omeprazole 20 mg for an additional 14 days.
- Erosive esophagitis: 20 mg daily for 4 to 8 weeks; not beyond 12 months

- Gastric ulcer: 40 mg once a day for 4 to 8 weeks
- Pathological hypersecretory conditions: 60 mg daily for as long as indicated; dosages up to 120 mg 3 times per day have been administered.

Esomeprazole Magnesium. Esomeprazole magnesium, *S*-bis(5-rnethoxy-2-[(*S*)-[(4-methoxy-3,5-dimethyl-2-pyridinyl)methyl]sulfinyl]-1H-benzimidazole-l-yl) magnesium trihydrate (Nexium), is the *S*-enantiomer of omeprazole. The benzimidazole PPIs contain a chiral sulfur atom that form an enantiomeric pair that is stable and insoluble under standard conditions. The *S*-isomer of omeprazole has slightly greater PPI activity, and its intrinsic clearance is approximately three times lower than that of R-omeprazole (15 vs. 43 μL/min). The lower clearance of S-omeprazole is related to slower metabolic clearance by the CYP2C19 isozyme.[66,76] Although R-omeprazole is primarily transformed to the 5-hydroxy metabolite, the *S*-isomer is metabolized by *O*-demethylation and sulfoxidation, which contribute little to intrinsic clearance (Table 23.7).

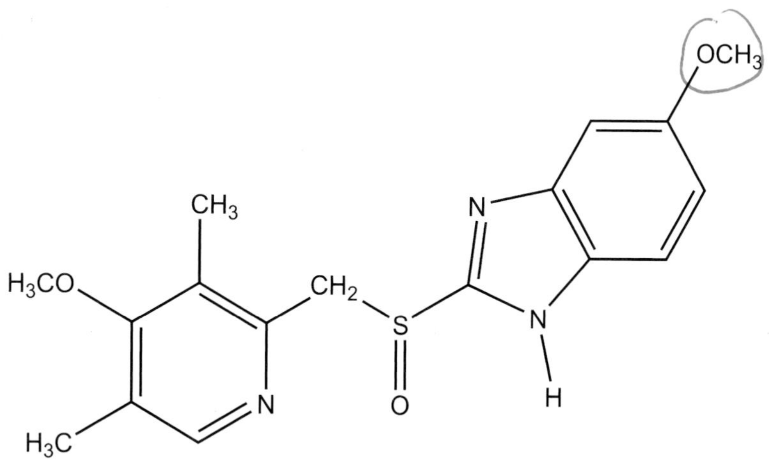

Omeprazole

Dosage forms: Delayed-release capsules (20 or 40 mg), powder for suspension (10, 20, and 40 mg), and powder for injection (20 and 40 mg)

Usual adult doses:

- Symptomatic gastroesophageal reflux disease: 20 mg daily usually for 4 weeks
- Erosive esophagitis: 20 or 40 mg daily usually for 4 to 8 weeks
- Duodenal ulcer associated *H. pylori* eradication: Triple therapy with esomeprazole (40 mg once daily), amoxicillin (1,000 mg twice daily), and clarithromycin (500 mg twice daily), each for 10 days
- Risk reduction of NSAIDs-associated gastric ulcer: 20 or 40 mg daily for up to 6 months
- Pathological hypersecretory conditions, including Zollinger-Ellison syndrome: 40 mg twice daily but doses of up to 240 mg daily have been used

Lansoprazole. Lansoprazole, 2-[[[3-methyl-4-(2,2,2-trifluoroethoxy)-2-pyridyl]methyl]sulfinyl]-1H-benzimidazole (Prevacid), is a white to brownish white, odorless crystalline powder that is practically insoluble in water. Lansoprazole is a weak base (pyridine N, pK$_a$ 3.83.) and a weak acid (benzimidazole N-H, pK 0.62). Like other PPIs, lansoprazole is essentially a prodrug that, in the acidic biophase of the parietal cell, forms an active metabolite that irreversibly interacts with the target ATPase of the pump. Lansoprazole must be formulated as encapsulated enteric-coated granules for oral administration to protect the drug from the acidic environment of the stomach.

In the fasting state, about 80% of a dose of lansoprazole (vs. 50% of omeprazole) reaches the systemic circulation, where it is 97% bound to plasma proteins (Table 23.8).[66] The drug is metabolized in the liver (sulfone and hydroxy metabolites) and excreted in bile and urine, with a plasma half-life of about 1.5 hours.

Dosage form: Delayed-release and orally disintegrating tablets (15 and 30 mg), delayed-release capsules (5 and 30 mg), delayed-release granules for oral suspension (15 and 30 mg), and a powder for injection (30 mg/vial)

Usual adult dose:

- GERD: 15 mg once daily for up to 8 weeks
- Erosive esophagitis: Initially 30 mg once daily for up to 8 weeks. For adults who do not heal within 8 weeks (5%–10%), an additional 8 weeks of treatment may be given. Then, 15 mg once daily to maintain healing of erosive esophagitis.

- Gastric ulcer: 30 mg once daily for up to 8 weeks
- Gastric associated with NSAIDs: 30 mg once daily for up to 8 weeks to promote healing 15 mg once daily for up to 12 weeks to reduce the risk of NSAID-induced ulcer. Controlled studies did not extend beyond indicated duration.
- Duodenal ulcer: Short-term treatment: 15 mg once daily for 4 weeks for short-term treatment and 15 mg once daily to maintain healing of duodenal ulcers
- Duodenal ulcer associated with *H. pylori*: Dual therapy with lansoprazole (30 mg) and amoxicillin (1 g) both taken 3 times/day (every 8 hours) for 14 days for patients intolerant or resistant to clarithromycin
- Duodenal ulcer associated with *H. pylori*: Triple therapy with lansoprazole (30 mg) plus clarithromycin (500 mg) and amoxicillin (1 g), all taken twice daily (every 12 hours) for 10 or 14 days
- Hypersecretory conditions, including Zollinger-Ellison syndrome: Usually an initial dose of 60 mg once daily; dosages up to 90 mg twice daily have been administered

Pantoprazole Sodium. Pantoprazole sodium, racemic-sodium 5-(difluoromethoxy)-2-[[3,4-dimethoxy-2-pyridinyl)methyl]sulfinyl]-1H-benzimidazole sesquihydrate is a white to off-white crystalline powder that is freely soluble in water, very slightly soluble in phosphate buffer at pH 7.4, and practically insoluble in n-hexane. The benzimidazole of this drug has a weakly basic nitrogen (pyridine N, pK$_a$ 3.83) and an benzimidazole proton (pK$_a$ 0.11), facilitating formulation as a sodium salt. The stability of the compound in aqueous solution is pH dependent; the rate of degradation increases with decreasing pH. At ambient temperature, the degradation half-life is approximately 2.8 hours at pH 5.0 and approximately 220 hours at pH 7.8.

The absorption of pantoprazole is rapid (C$_{max}$ of 2.5 μg/mL, T$_{max}$ 2.5 hours) after single or multiple oral 40-mg doses. Pantoprazole is well absorbed (77% bioavailability). Administration with food may delay its absorption but does not alter pantoprazole bioavailability. Pantoprazole is distributed mainly in extracellular fluid. The serum protein binding of pantoprazole is about 98%, primarily to albumin. Pantoprazole is extensively metabolized in the liver through the CYP system, including *O*-demethylation (CYP2C19), with subsequent sulfation. Other metabolic pathways include sulfur oxidation by CYP3A4 (Table 23.8).[66] There is no evidence that any of the pantoprazole metabolites have significant pharmacological activity. Approximately 71% of a dose

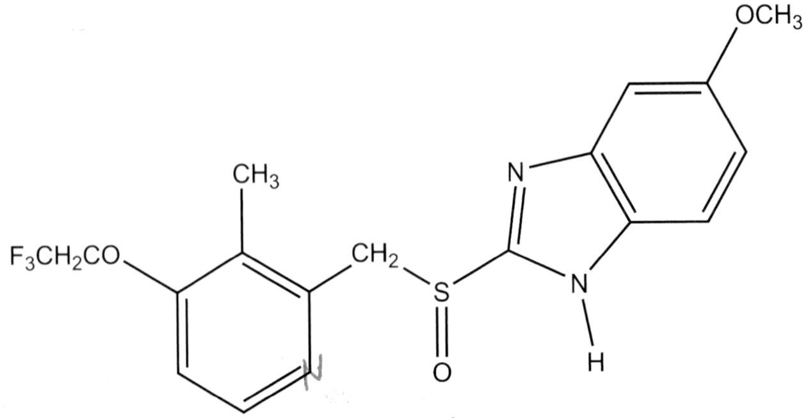

Lansoprazole

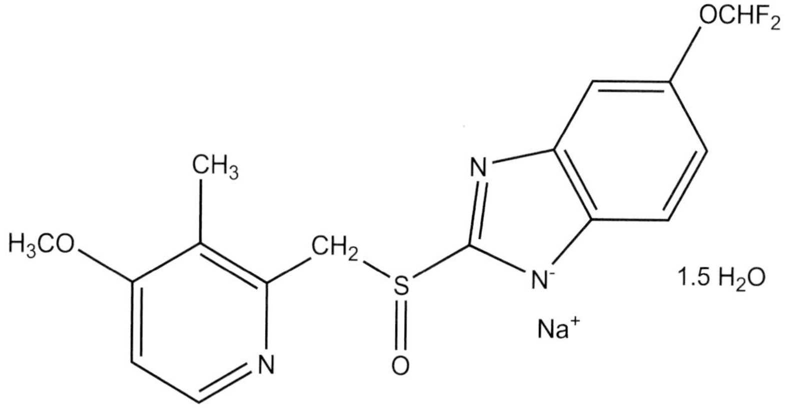

Pantoprazole Sodium

of pantoprazole is excreted in the urine, with 18% excreted in the feces through biliary excretion.

Dosage forms: Delayed-release tablets (20 and 40 mg), delayed-release oral suspension (40 mg), and a powder for injection (40 mg)

Usual adult dose:
- Erosive esophagitis (maintenance): Usually 40 mg once daily for up to 8 weeks. For those patients who have not healed after 8 weeks of treatment, an additional 8-week course of pantoprazole may be considered. The maintenance dose is 40 mg daily.
- Pathological hypersecretory conditions, including Zollinger-Ellison syndrome: The usual starting dosage is 40 mg twice daily. Adjust dosage regimens to individual patient needs and continue for as long as clinically indicated. Doses of up to 240 mg daily have been administered.

Rabeprazole Sodium. Rabeprazole sodium, 2[[[4-(3-methoxypropoxy)-3-methyl-2-pyridinyl]methyl]sulfinyl]-1H-benzimidazole sodium salt (Aciphex), is a white to slightly yellowish white solid. It is very soluble in water and methanol, freely soluble in ethanol, chloroform, and ethyl acetate, and insoluble in ether and hexane. Rabeprazole is a weak base (pyridine N, pK_a 4.53) and a weak acid (benzimidazole N-H, pK_a 0.62), faciliting sodium salt formation.

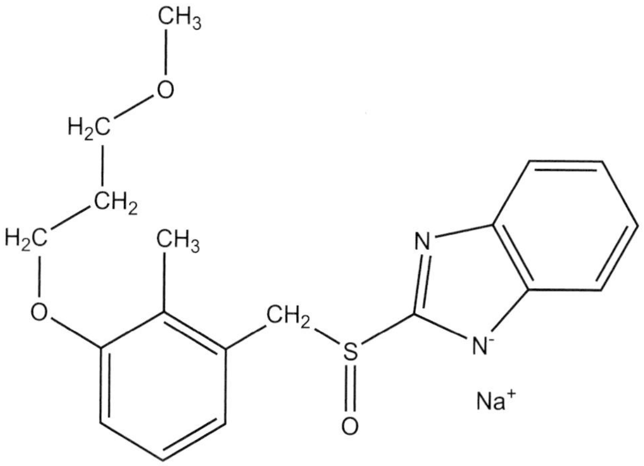

Rabeprazole Sodium

Rabeprazole sodium is formulated as enteric-coated, delayed-release tablets to allow the drug to pass through the stomach relatively intact. After oral administration of 20-mg peak plasma concentrations (C_{max}) occur over a range of 2 to 5 hours (T_{max}). Absolute bioavailability for a 20-mg oral tablet of rabeprazole (vs. IV administration) is approximately 52% (Table 23.8).[66] The plasma half-life of rabeprazole ranges from 1 to 2 hours. The effects of food on the absorption of rabeprazole have not been evaluated. Rabeprazole is 96% bound to human plasma proteins. Rabeprazole is extensively metabolized in the liver. The thioether and sulfone are the primary metabolites measured in human plasma resulting from CYP3A oxidation. Additionally, desmethyl rabeprazole is formed via the action of CYP2C19. Approximately 90% of the drug is eliminated in the urine, primarily as thioether carboxylic acid and its glucuronide and mercapturic acid metabolites. The remainder of the dose is recovered in the feces. No unchanged rabeprazole is excreted in the urine or feces (Table 23.8).[66]

Dosage form: Delayed-release tablets (20 mg)

Usual adult dose:
- Duodenal ulcers (healing): Usually 20 mg once daily after the morning meal for a period of up to 4 weeks
- Erosive or ulcerative GERD: 20 mg once daily for 4 weeks. If symptoms do not resolve completely after 4 weeks, an additional course of treatment may be considered.
- *H. pylori* eradication: Triple therapy with rabeprazole (20 mg), amoxicillin (1 g), and clarithromycin (500 mg)
- Treatment of pathological hypersecretory conditions: Usually 60 mg once daily, but doses should be adjusted to individual patient needs and should continue for as long as clinically indicated. Some patients may require divided doses. Dosages of up to 100 mg daily and 60 mg twice daily have been administered.

CHEMICAL COMPLEXATION

The sulfate esters and sulfonate derivatives of polysaccharides and lignin form chemical complexes with the enzyme pepsin. These complexes have no proteolytic activity. Because polysulfates and polysulfonates are poorly absorbed from the GI tract, specific chemical complexation appears to be a desirable mechanism of pepsin inhibition.[77] Unfortunately, these polymers are also potent anticoagulants.

The properties of chemical complexation and anticoagulant action are separable by structural variation. In a comparison of selected sulfated saccharides of increasing number of monosaccharide units, from disaccharides through starch-derived polysaccharides of differing molecular size, three conclusions are supported by the data: (a) the anticoagulant activity of sulfated saccharide is positively related to molecular size; (b) anticoagulant activity is absent in the disaccharides; and (c) the inhibition of pepsin activity and the protection against experimentally induced ulceration depend on the degree of sulfation and not on molecular size.[77] The readily available disaccharide sucrose has been used to develop a useful antiulcer agent, sucralfate.

Sucralfate. Sucralfate, 3,4,5,6-tetra-(polyhydroxyaluminum)-α-D-glucopyranosyl sulfate-2,3,4,5-tetra-(polyhydroxyaluminum)-β-D-fructofuranoside sulfate (Carafate), is the aluminum hydroxide complex of the octasulfate ester of sucrose. It is practically insoluble in water and soluble in strong acids and bases. It has a pK_a value between 0.43 and 1.19.

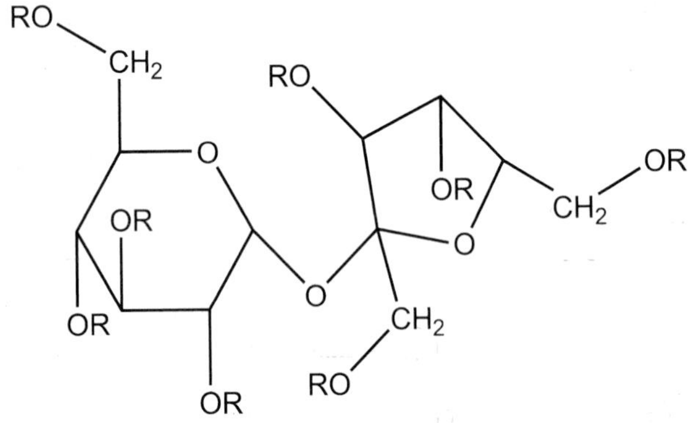

Sucralfate R = SO$_3$[Al$_2$(OH)$_5$]

Sucralfate is minimally absorbed from the GI tract by design, and thus exerts its antiulcer effect through local rather than systemic action. It has negligible acid-neutralizing or buffering capacity in therapeutic doses. Although its mechanism of action has not been established, studies suggest that sucralfate binds preferentially to the ulcer site to form a protective barrier that prevents exposure of the lesion to acid and pepsin. In addition, it adsorbs pepsin and bile salts. Either would be very desirable modes of action.

The simultaneous administration of sucralfate may reduce the bioavailability of certain agents (e.g., tetracycline, phenytoin, digoxin, or cimetidine).[78] It further recommends restoration of bioavailability by separating administration of these agents from that of sucralfate by 2 hours. Presumably, sucralfate binds these agents in the GI tract.[78] The most frequently reported adverse reaction to sucralfate is constipation (2.2%). Antacids may be prescribed as needed but should not be taken within 0.5 hour before or after sucralfate.

Dosage forms: Tablets (1 g) and suspension (1 g/10 mL)
Usual adult dose: 1 g (10 mL or 2 teaspoons of the oral suspension) 4 times a day on an empty stomach. Oral, 1 g 4 times a day on an empty stomach. Treatment should be continued for 4 to 8 weeks.

PROSTAGLANDINS

The prostaglandins are endogenous 20-carbon unsaturated fatty acids biosynthetically derived from arachidonic acid. These bioactive substances and their synthetic derivatives have been of considerable research and development interest as potential therapeutic agents because of their widespread physiological and pharmacological actions on the cardiovascular system, GI smooth muscle, the reproductive system, the nervous system, platelets, kidney, the eye, etc. Prostaglandins of the E, F, and I series are found in significant concentrations throughout the GI tract. The GI actions of the prostaglandins include inhibition of basal and stimulated gastric acid and pepsin secretion in addition to prevention of ulcerogen or irritant-induced gross mucosal lesions of the stomach and intestine (termed cytoprotection). The prostaglandins can both stimulate (PGFs) and inhibit (PGEs and PGIs) intestinal smooth muscle contractility and accumulation of fluid and electrolytes in the gut lumen (PGEs). Therapeutic application of the natural prostaglandins in the treatment of GI disorders is hindered by their lack of pharmacological selectivity coupled with a less-than-optimal biodisposition profile.

Misoprostol. Misoprostol, ($\pm$)-methyl 11α, 16-dihydroxy-16-methyl-9-oxoprost-13E-en-1-oate, is a semisynthetic derivative of PGE$_1$ that derives some pharmacological selectivity as well as enhanced biostability from its 16-methyl, 16-hydroxy substitutions. A mixture of misoprostol diastereomers are present in the commercial product, but most of the activity is associated with the 11r, 16S-isomer.[79] Misoprostol exhibits both antisecretory and cytoprotectant effects characteristic of the natural prostaglandins and has a therapeutically acceptable biodis-

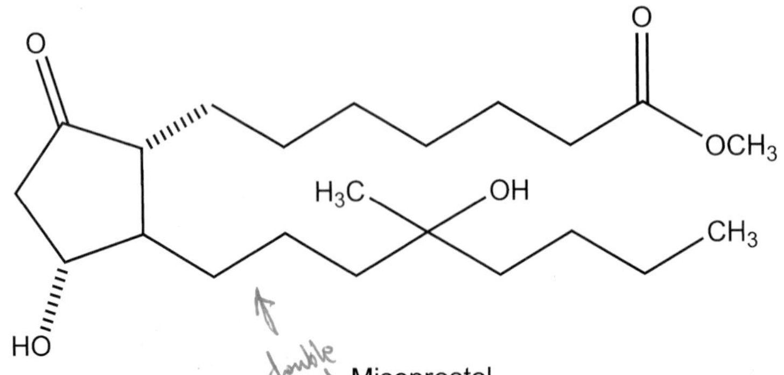

Misoprostol

position profile. Although the antisecretory effects of misoprostol are thought to be related to its agonistic actions at parietal cell prostaglandin receptors, its cytoprotective actions are proposed to be related to increases in GI mucus and bicarbonate secretion, increases in mucosal blood flow, and/or prevention of back diffusion of acid into the gastric mucosa.[80]

Misoprostol is rapidly absorbed following oral administration and undergoes rapid deesterification to the pharmacologically active free acid with a terminal half-life of 20 to 40 minutes. Misoprostol is commonly used to prevent NSAID-induced gastric ulcers in patients at high risk of complications from a gastric ulcer, such as elderly patients and patients with a history of ulcer. Misoprostol has also been used in treating duodenal ulcers unresponsive to histamine H_2-antagonists; the drug does not prevent duodenal ulcers, however, in patients taking NSAIDS. Misoprostol can cause miscarriage, often associated with potentially dangerous bleeding.

Dosage form: 100- and 200-μg tablets
Usual adult dose: Oral, 200 mg 4 times a day with food

◉ HISTAMINE H₃- AND H₄-RECEPTOR LIGANDS

As discussed earlier, H_3-receptors are presynaptic receptors that regulate the release of histamine (autoreceptors) and other neurotransmitters (heteroreceptor).[10,17] The H_3-heteroreceptors have been identified in CNS, stomach, lung and cardiac tissues where they appear to regulate neurotransmitter release from histaminergic, noradrenergic, dopaminergic, cholinergic, serotoninergic, and peptidergic neurons. Histaminergic nerves are located in the hippocampus and project into many brain regions where they regulate sleep, alertness, feeding behavior, and memory. Thus, H_3-receptor antagonists have a potential therapeutic role in learning and memory impairment, attention-deficit hyperactivity disorder, obesity, and even epilepsy. Furthermore, studies of the regulation of inflammatory processes, gastroprotection, and cardiovascular function suggest several therapeutic possibilities for peripherally acting histamine H_3-agonists.[10] To date, no histamine H_3-receptor ligands have been approved for marketing in the United States.

Potent H_3-agonists (Fig. 23.17) are obtained by simple modifications of the histamine molecule.[81,82] The imidazole

ring is a common structural feature in almost all H_3-agonists. Methylation of the aminoethyl side chain of histamine favors H_3 activity. Introduction of one or two methyl groups to give α-methylhistamine and α,α-dimethylhistamine yields potent H_3-agonists that show little selectivity among the histamine receptors. The increased potency of α-methylhistamine is ascribed almost completely to its R-enantiomer (H_3/H_1 ratio = 17). The clinical use of R-α-methylhistamine is compromised by rapid catabolism by histamine-N-methyltransferase. Azomethine derivatives of R-α-methylhistamine have been developed and shown to possess anti-inflammatory and antinociceptive properties. Other H_3-agonists include the isothiourea derivative, imetit, a highly selective, full agonist that is more potent than R-α-methylhistamine. A third type of H_3-agonist is immepip, which may be considered as a histamine analog with an elongated and cyclized side chain. Immepip is both a highly selective and potent H_3-agonist.[81,82]

A large number of H_3-antagonists have been described.[83] In general, antagonist structures conform to the general representation shown in Figure 23.18. The heterocycle component of this general structure is most commonly a 4-monosubstituted imidazole or bioisosteric equivalent. Chains A and B can be of various structures and lengths, and there is also wide latitude in the structural requirements for the polar group. Halogenated phenyl, cycloalkyl, and heteroaryl structures are usually found for the lipophilic moiety.

Thioperamide (Fig. 23.18) was the first potent H_3-antagonist to be described. This agent enhances arousal and/or vigilant patterns in a dose-dependent fashion in animals, suggesting possible use of CNS-acting H_3-antagonists in treating sleep disorders characterized by excessive daytime sleep, such as narcolepsy.[83] Other H_3 structures are shown in Figure 23.18, including the natural product verongamine, isolated from a sea sponge.

As discussed earlier, the H_4-receptor appears to be involved in the differentiation of hematopoietic cells (myeloblasts and promyelocytes) and to modulate immune function by modulating eosinophil calcium levels and chemotaxis. Several H_3-agonists (R-α-methylhistamine, imetit) and antagonists (thioperamide) are also ligands for H_4-receptors.[84] Based on its physiological role in immune and inflammatory processes, H_4-antagonists may have utility in various autoimmune (rheumatoid arthritis, asthma) and allergic disorders (allergic rhinitis, etc.).[10] To date, no histamine H_4-receptor ligands have been approved for marketing in the United States.

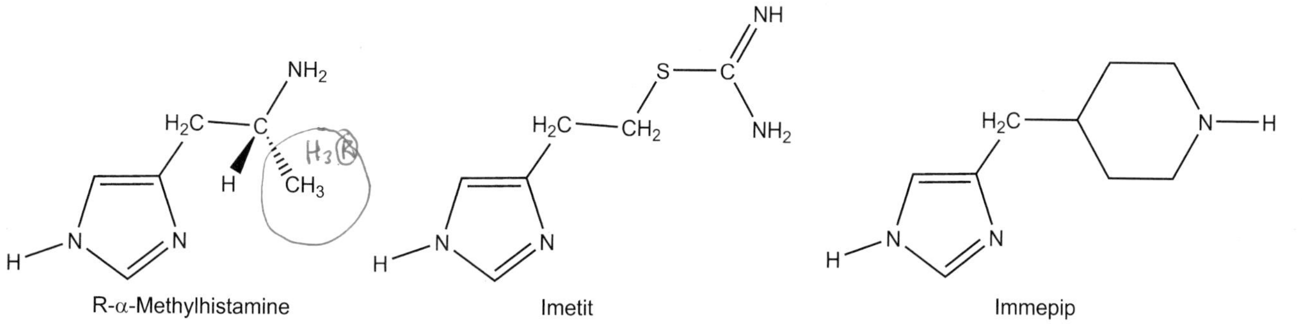

Figure 23.17 ◆ Histamine H_3-receptor agonists.

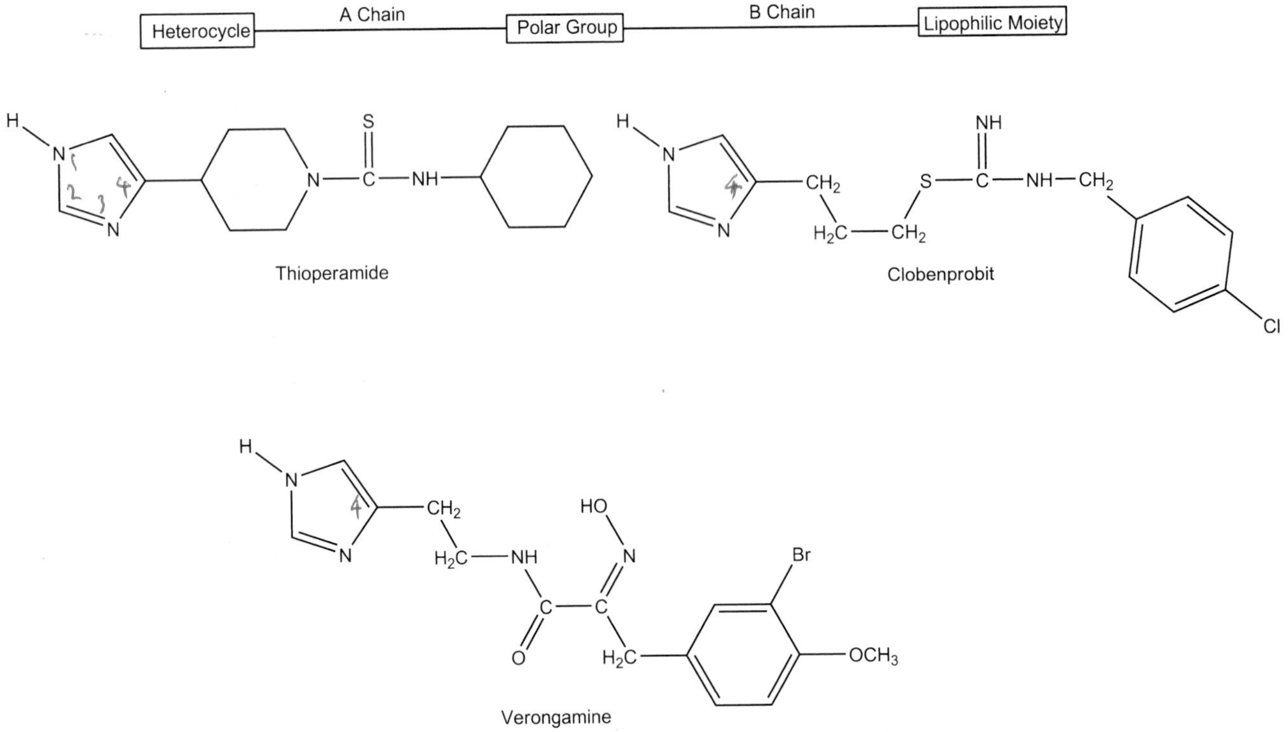

Figure 23.18 ● Histamine H$_3$-receptor antagonists.

REVIEW QUESTIONS

1. Briefly describe how the various histamine receptor subtypes are structurally and functionally similar. In what ways are the histamine receptor subtypes different?

2. What are the primary metabolic pathways of histamine inactivation?

3. Rank (from highest to lowest) diphehydramine, chlorpheniramine, and cetirizine with respect to their relative sedation potential and antimuscarinic activity.

4. Show the mechanism whereby omeprazole is converted to its pharmacologically active form in the presence of acid.

5. What are the primary enzymes involved in the metabolism of most PPIs and what reactions do they catalyze? What is the therapeutic significance of PPI metabolism?

REFERENCES

1. Babe, K. S. J., and Serfin, W. E.: Histamine, bradykinin, and their antagonists. In Hardman, J. G., Limbird, L. E., Mollinoff, P. B., et al. (eds.). Goodman and Gilman's The Pharmacological Basis of Therapeutics, 9th ed. New York, McGraw-Hill, 1995, pp. 581–600.
2. Saxena, A. K., and Saxena, M.: Prog. Drug Res. 39:35, 1992.
3. Durant, G. I., Ganellin, C. R., and Parsons, M. E.: J. Med. Chem. 18: 905–909, 1975.
4. Cooper, D. G., Young, R. C., Durant, G. H., et al.: In Emmett, J. C., (ed.). Comprehensive Medicinal Chemistry. The Rational Design, Mechanistic Study and Therapeutic Application of Chemical Compounds, vol 3. Membranes and Receptors. Oxford: Permagon Press, 1990, pp. 343–421.
5. Casy, A. F.: The Steric Factor in Medicinal Chemistry. Dissymmetric Probes of Pharmacological Receptors. New York, Plenum Press, 1993, Chap. 11.
6. Falus, A.: Histamine and Inflammation. Austin, TX: R. G. Landes, 1994, Chap. 1.1, p. 2.
7. Watanabe, T., Yamatodani, A., Maeyama K., et al.: Trends Pharmacol. Sci. 1009. 11:363–367.
8. Marone, G., Genovese, A., Granata F., et al.: Clin. Exp. Allergy. 32:1682–1689, 2002.
9. Oliver, J. M., Kepley, C. I., Ortega, E., et al.: Immunopharm. 48: 269–281, 2000.
10. Simons, F. E. R.: N. Engl. J. Med. 351:2203–2217, 2004.
11. Leurs, R., Church, M. K., and Taglialatela, M.: Clin. Exp. Allergy. 32:489–498, 2002.
12. Bakker, R. A., Timmerman, H., and Leurs, R.: Histamine receptors: specific ligands, receptor biochemistry, and signal transduction. In Simons, F. E. R., (ed.). Histamine and H$_1$-antihistamines in Allergic Disease, 2nd ed. New York, Marcel Dekker, 2002, pp. 27–64.
13. Leurs, R., Smit, M. J., and Timmerman, H.: Pharmacol. Ther. 66:413–463, 1995.
14. Hall, I. P.: Eur. Respir. J. 15:449–451, 2000.
15. Church, M. K., Shute, J. K., and Jensen, H. M.: Mast cell derived mediators. In Adkinson, N. F., Yunginer, J. W., Busse, W. W., et al. (eds.). Middleton's Allergy: Principles and Practice, 6th ed. Philadelphia, Mosby, 2003, pp. 189–212.
16. Goetzl, E. J.: Lipid mediators of hypersensitivity and inflammation. In Adkinson, N. F., Yunginer, J. W., Busse, W. W., et al. (eds.). Middleton's Allergy: Principles and Practice, 6th ed. Philadelphia, Mosby, 2003, pp. 213–230.
17. Leurs, R., Bakker, R. A., Timmerman, H., et al.: Nature Rev. Drug Discov. 4:107–120, 2005.
18. Leurs, R., Timmerman, H., and Watanabe, T.: Trends Phamacol. Sci. 22:337–339, 2001.
19. Akdis, C. A., and Blaser, K.: J. Allergy Clin. Immunol. 112:15–22, 2003.

20. Maslinski, C., and Fogel, W. A.: Catabolism of histamine. In Uvnas, B. (ed.). Histamine and Histamine Antagonists, Handbook of Experimental Pharmacology, vol. 97. New York, Springer-Verlag, 1991, Chap. 5.
21. Schayer, R. C., and Cooper, J. A. D.: J. Appl. Physiol. 9:481–483, 1956.
22. Fourneau, B., and Bovet, D.: Arch. Int. Pharmacodyn. 46:178–191, 1993.
23. Witiak, D. T.: Antiallergenic agents. In Burger, A. (ed.). Medicinal Chemistry, 3rd ed. New York, Wiley Interscience, 1970, p. 1643.
24. Casy, A. F.: Chemistry of anti-H₁ histamine antagonists. In Rocha e Silva, M. (ed.). Handbook of Experimental Pharmacology, vol. 18/2. New York, Springer-Verlag, 1978, p. 175.
25. Paton, D. M.: Receptors for histamine. In Schachter, M. (ed.). Histamine and Antihistamines. New York, Pergamon Press, 1973, p. 3.
26. Rocha e Silva, M., and Antonio, A.: Bioassay of antihistaminic action. In Rocha e Silva, M. (ed.). Handbook of Experimental Pharmacology, vol. 18/2. New York, Springer-Verlag, 1978, p. 381.
27. Biel, J. H., and Martin, Y. C.: Organic synthesis as a source of new drugs. In Gould, R. F. (ed.). Drug Discovery, Advances in Chemistry Series no. 108. Washington, DC, American Chemical Society, 1971, p. 81.
28. Ahlquist, R. P.: Am. J. Physiol. 153:586, 1948.
29. Lin, T. M., et al.: Ann. N. Y. Acad. Sci. 99:30, 1962.
30. Ash, A. S. F., and Schild, H. O.: Br. J. Pharmacol. Chemother. 27:427, 1966.
31. Black, J. W., et al.: Nature 236:385, 1972.
32. Metzler, D. E., and Ikawa Mand Sneil, E. E. J.: Am. Chem. Soc. 76: 648, 1954.
33. Taglialatela, M., Timmerman, H., and Annunziato, L.: Trends Pharmacol. Sci. 21:52–56, 2000.
34. Woosley, R. L.: Ann. Rev. Pharmacol. Toxicol. 36:233–252, 1996.
35. Casy, A. F., et al.: Chirality. 4:356–366, 1992.
36. Ednoether, A., and Weber, H. P.: Helv. Chim. Acta. 59:2462–2468, 1976.
37. Ganellin, C. R., and Parsons, M. E.: Bristol, UK, Wright, 1982.
38. Shafi'ee, A., and Hite, G.: J. Med Chem. 12:266–270, 1969.
39. Hanna, P. E., and Ahmed, A. E.: J. Med. Chem. 16:963–968, 1973.
40. van den Brink, F. G., and Lien, B. 3.: Competitive and noncompetitive antagonism. In Rocha e Silva, M. (ed.). Handbook of Experimental Pharmacology, vol. 18/2. New York, Springer-Verlag, 1978, p. 333.
41. Nauta, W. T., and Rekker, R. F.: Structure-activity relationships of Hi-receptor antagonists. In Rocha e Silva, M. (ed.). Handbook of Experimental Pharmacology, vol. 18/2. New York, Springer-Verlag, 1978.
42. Chishty, M., et al.: J. Drug Target. 9:223–228, 2001.
43. Chen, C., Hanson, E., Watson, J. W., et al.: Drug Metab. Dispos. 31:312–318, 2003.
44. Tashiro, M., Mochizuki, H., Iwabuchi, K., et al.: Life Sci. 72: 409–414, 2002.
45. Garteiz, D. A., Hook, R. H., Walker, B. J., et al.: Arzneim-Forsch. 32:1185–1190, 1982.
46. Nobles, W. L., and Blanton, C. D.: 3. Pharm. Sci. 53:115, 1964.
47. Toldy, L., et al.: Acta Chim. Acad. Sci. Hung. 19: 273, 1959.
48. Gupta, S., Banfield, C., Kantesaria, B., et al.: Clin. Ther. 23:451–466, 2001.
49. Yumibe, N., Huie, K., Chen, K. J., et al.: Biochem. Pharmacol. 51:165–172, 1996.
50. Curran, M. P., Scott, L. J., and Perry, C. M.: Drugs. 64: 523–561, 2004.
51. Gillard, M., Van Der Perren, C., Moguilevsky, N., et al.: Mol. Pharmacol. 61:391–399, 2002.
52. Holgate, S. T.: The chromones: cromolyn sodium and nedocromil sodium. In Adkinson, N. F., Yunginer, J. W., Busse, W. W., et al. (eds.). Middleton's Allergy: Principles and Practice, 6th ed. Philadelphia, Mosby, 2003, pp. 915–927.
53. Douglas, W. W.: Histamine and 5-hydroxytryptamine (serotonin) and their antagonists. In Gilman, A. G., Goodman, L. S., Rail, T. W., et al. (eds.). Goodman and Gilman's The Pharmacological Basis of Therapeutics, 7th ed. New York, Macmillan, 1985, p. 605.
54. Cook, E. B., Stahl, J. L., Barney N. P., et al.: Med. Chem. Rev. 1:333–347, 2004.
55. Caldwell, D. R., Verin, P., Hartwich-Young, R., et al.: Am. J. Ophthalmol. 113:632–637, 1992.
56. Tanaka, M.: Drugs Today 28:29–31, 1992.
57. McTavish, D., and Sorkin, E. M.: Drugs 38:778–800, 1989.
58. Martin, U., and Romer, D.:Arzneimittelforschung 28:770–782, 1978.
59. Feldman, M., and Burton, M. E.: N. Engl. J. Med. 323:1672–1680, 1990.
60. Feldman, M., and Burton, M. E.: N. Engl. J. Med. 323:1749–1755, 1990.
61. Roberts, S., and McDonald, I. M.: Inhibitors of gasatric acid secretion. In Abraham, D. J., (ed.). Burger's Medicinal Chemistry and Drug Discovery, vol 4. Autocoids, Diagnostics and Drugs from New Biology, 6th ed. Hoboken, NJ, Wiley-Interscience, 2003, pp. 85–127.
62. Sachs, G.: Pharmacotherapy. 23:S68–S73, 2003.
63. Soil, A. H.: N. Engl. J. Med. 322:909–916, 1990.
64. Ganellin, C. R.: Discovery of cimetidine. In Roberts, S. M., Price, B. J., (eds.). Medicinal Chemistry, The role of organic chemistry in drug research. London, Academic Press, 1985, pp. 93–118.
65. Somogyi, A., and Muirhead, M.: Clin. Phrmacokinet. 12:321–366, 1987.
66. Facts and Comparisons 4.0, Wolters Kluwer Health, Amsterdam, Netherlands, 2009.
67. Brandstrom, A., Lindberg, P., and Junggren, U.: Scand. J. Gastroenterol. 20(Suppl. 108):15–22, 1985.
68. Lindberg, P., Brandstrom, A., Wallmark, B., et al.: Med. Res. Rev. 10:1–54, 1990.
69. Munson, K., Garcia, R., and Sachs, G.: Biochemistry 44:5267–5284, 2005.
70. Shin, J. M., and Sachs, G.: Biochem. Pharmacol. 68:2117–2127, 2004.
71. Shin, J. M., Choo, Y. M., and Sachs, G. J.: Am. Chem. Soc. 126:7800–7811, 2004.
72. Shin, J. M., and Sachs, G.: Gastroenterology 123:1588–1597, 2002.
73. Sachs, G., Shin, J. M., and Howden, C. W.: Aliment. Pharmacol. Ther. 23(Suppl. 2):2–8, 2006.
74. Yacyshyn, B. R., and Thomson, A. B. R.: Digestion. 66:67–78, 2002.
75. Andersson, T.: Clin. Pharmacokinet. 31:9–28, 1996.
76. Andersson, T.: Clin. Pharmacokinet. 43:279–285, 2004.
77. Nagashima, R., and Yoshida, N.: Arzneim.-Forsch. 29:1668–1676, 1979.
78. Marks, I. N.: J. Clin. Gastroenterol. 9(Suppl 1):18–22, 1987.
79. Won-Kin, S., Kachur, J. F., and Gaginella, T. S.: Prostaglandins 46:221–231, 1993.
80. Monk, J. P., and Clissold, S. P.: Drugs 33:1–30, 1987.
81. Leurs, R., and Timmerman, H.: Prog. Drug Res. 39:127, 1992.
82. Phillips, J. G., Au, S. M., Yates, S. L., et al.: Annu. Rep. Med. Chem. 33:31–40, 1998.
83. Stark, H., Ligneau, X., Arrang, J. M., et al.: Bioorg. Med. Chem. Lett. 8:2011–2016, 1998.
84. Lim, H. D., van Rijn, R. M., Ling, P., et al.: J. Pharmacol. Exp. Ther. 314:1310–1321, 2005.

Analgesics

CAROLYN J. FRIEL AND MATTHIAS C. LU

The terms *analgesics* and *analgetic drugs* are often used interchangeably to describe a diverse group of pain medications such as opioids, nonsteroidal anti-inflammatory drugs (NSAIDs), and triptans, each with very different mechanisms of action for relieving pains of a wide array of causes.

Analgesics can be broadly categorized, according to their therapeutic use, into several drug classes: (a) the opioids (or narcotic analgesics), which play a major role in the relief of acute pain and in the management of moderate to severe chronic pain; (b) the NSAIDs and acetaminophen, which are the most widely used analgesic drugs for relieving mild to moderate pain and reducing fever; (c) the triptans (the antimigraine medications), which are specifically designed and targeted for acute and abortive treatment of migraine and cluster headaches; and (d) a new emerging class of analgesics known as analgesic adjuvants that include tricyclic antidepressants such as amitriptyline, anticonvulsants such as gabapentin and pregabalin, and topical analgesics such as lidocaine patches that can be used to treat neuropathic pains.

In this chapter, only the first three classes of pain medications are covered. The main objectives of this chapter will be focusing on their mechanism of action, structure–activity relationships (SARs), pharmacokinetic properties, and their clinical applications for pain management. Readers should consult other chapters under anticonvulsants, antidepressants, and local anesthetics for a detailed discussion of drugs used for treating neuropathic and other incidental pains associated with minor cuts, burns, and insect bites.

⬡ PAIN AND PAIN MANAGEMENT

Pain, one of the most common complaints for which patients seek medical attention, is also the hardest to manage despite the availability of many analgesic medications as well as other nonpharmacologic treatment options. Pain management, especially the use of opioids in patients with chronic pains, is one of the most troublesome public health issues for patients, doctors, and other healthcare providers.[1,2] As early as the 1970s, the National Institutes of Health formed a committee, at the request of the president, to investigate therapies for rare diseases, but the initial focus was on pain management. The committee found that the problem associated with the use of the opioid analgesics was a lack of training of physicians in pain management and misinformation among healthcare providers because of fear of psychological dependence (commonly referred to as addiction), disciplinary action, or adverse effects such as tolerance and physical dependence of the pain medications.[2,3] As a result, many patients with moderate to severe pain are often undertreated or untreated.[3–5] Another possible reason for treatment failure is the fact that pain perception may also vary among individuals especially across racial and ethnic origins.[6]

Origin of Pain

Pain differs in its underlying causes, symptoms, and neurobiological mechanisms and has been classified into three major types: physiological (nociceptive), inflammatory, and neuropathic.[7,8] Physiological pain is the most common and is often caused by an injury to body organs or tissues. It is further categorized, according to the source of the pain, into cutaneous pains (skin and surface tissues), somatic pains (ligaments, tendons, bones, blood vessels), and visceral pains (body organs and internal cavities). Inflammatory pain originates from an infection or inflammation as a result of the initial tissue or organ damage. Neuropathic pain is a very complex, chronic pain, resulting from injury of the nervous systems.[9] Neuropathic pain may originate from limb amputation, spinal surgery, viral infections such as shingles, or worsening of disease states associated with diabetes, acquired immunodeficiency syndrome (AIDS), or multiple sclerosis. The pharmacological interventions are very complex and often require the use of other analgesic adjuvants not covered in this chapter. Readers should consult a recent review for a practical guide to the current clinical management of neuropathic pain.[10]

Acute and Chronic Pain

Pain may be acute or chronic.[11] Acute pain is often severe but usually lasts only until the removal of the source that triggered the pain. Acute pain includes nociceptive, somatic, or visceral pain, postoperative and posttraumatic pain, burn pain, acute pain during childbirth, acute headache, etc. Acute and postoperative pains are most often treated with the opioid analgesics.

Chronic pain, on the other hand, is defined as a pain lasting longer than 6 months that persists even when the initial cause has been resolved through appropriate medical intervention. Chronic pain can be further divided into chronic malignant pain (e.g., cancer, human immunodeficiency virus [HIV]/AIDS, amyotrophic lateral sclerosis, multiple sclerosis, end-stage organ failure) and chronic nonmalignant pain (e.g., lower-back pain, chronic degenerative arthritis, osteoarthritis (OA), rheumatoid arthritis (RA), migraine and chronic headache, and bond pain). Pain therapy in patients with chronic pain only provides transient pain relief but does not resolve the underlying pathological process.[7] Chronic pain is also often associated with behavior and psychological components that make effective pain management quite subjective and difficult to resolve.[10,12,13] Chronic pain is also the leading cause of disability among the elderly; the prevalence of pain may be as high as 80%.[3]

Significant advances in understanding the pathophysiology and neurobiology of pain have occurred in the past 10 years.[5,13–17] However, a full discussion of complex pain-signaling mechanisms and the etiology of pain is beyond the scope of this chapter.

Approaches to Pain Management

The World Health Organization (WHO), through its *Access to Controlled Medications Programme*, has brought together an international, multidisciplinary group of experts to discuss and formulate a series of WHO guidelines, including the "three-step analgesic ladder" on pain management.[11,18] The use of the WHO three-step analgesic ladder has allowed physicians to select the most appropriate drug treatment regimen and has resulted in adequate analgesia for their patients, according to a 10-year prospective study published in 1995.[18] This guideline has now been adapted for treating other noncancer pains.[19] According to this analgesic ladder model (see Fig. 24.1), the choice of analgesic therapy is based on assessment of pain intensity. Thus, nonopioid analgesics such as acetaminophen and NSAIDs are the drugs of choice for mild pain. The patients should continue on this regimen for as long as they are receiving adequate pain control, although an analgesic adjuvant may be added to help relieve the side effects associated with pain medications. For moderate pain, a combination of an NSAID (or acetaminophen) and a weak opioid such as codeine should be used. Morphine, fentanyl, and other potent opioids are reserved only for severe pain, especially in patients who are terminally ill, to control pain and to improve their quality of life.[11]

OPIOIDS

Opioid Receptor Discovery and Endogenous Ligands

There was no direct evidence for the existence of specific opioid receptors until the 1970s when Goldstein et al.[20] found that radiolabeled levorphanol bound stereospecifically to certain mouse brain fractions. They hypothesized that this compound bound to an "opiate receptor." This prediction gained credence in 1973 when additional studies showed that opioid agonists and opioid antagonists compete for the same binding site. Building on these studies, Pert[21] was able to show that the pharmacologic potencies of the opioid drugs were proportional to their ability to compete with the antagonist for opioid receptor binding.

As it seemed unlikely that these receptors evolved in response to a plant alkaloid, the search for endogenous ligands was intense. The discovery and identification of endogenous substrates for the opioid receptor by Hughes[22,23] in 1975 further confirmed the existence of an opioid receptor and intensified the SAR studies of the analgesic opioids. The endogenous peptide ligands for the opioid receptors were originally isolated from pig brains but have been found in every mammal studied. The first

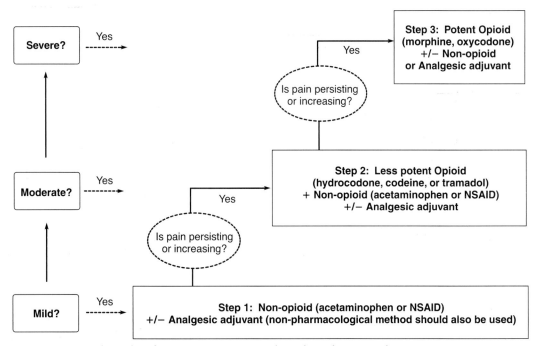

WHO 3-Step Analgesic Ladder - Is the pain...

Figure 24.1 ● Algorithm for pain management based on the WHO three-Step Analgesic Ladder. (Source: http://www.who.int/cancer/palliative/painladder/en/.)

Met-enkephalin = Tyr^1-Gly^2-Gly^3-Phe^4-Met^5(OH)   Leu-enkephalin = Tyr^1-Gly^2-Gly^3-Phe^4-Leu^5(OH)

endogenous peptide was termed *enkephalin*, which was found to be a mixture of the two pentapeptides that only differ in their terminal amino acid.

Both methionine-enkephalin (Met-enkephalin) and leucine-enkephalin (Leu-enkephalin) were shown to inhibit the contraction of electrically stimulated guinea pig ileum (GPI) and mouse vas deferens (MVD). These two tests are still used as screening methods for opioid activity. Naloxone completely reversed the inhibitory effects of enkephalin, which led Hughes to infer that the peptides were acting on an opioid receptor.[22] The central administration of enkephalins in rats produced short analgesic activity. The transient nature of the enkephalins' actions correlated with the rapid degradation of the enkephalin Tyr-Gly bond by aminopeptidases. Much synthetic work has been done in an attempt to increase the duration of action of the opioid peptides and maintain their analgesic effect.

SARs of Enkephalins

TYR^1

The first amino acid of the pentapeptide shows a distinct preference for tyrosine. Most changes to this amino acid, either by substituting with other amino acids or masking the phenolic hydroxyl (OH) or amino function, produce an inactive or weakly active peptide.

GLY^2

Replacing the naturally occurring L-Gly with various D-amino acids produces a peptide that is resistant to peptide cleavage by aminopeptidases. Replacement with D-Ser is the most effective replacement, and all L-amino acid analogs had low activities. Substituting D-amino acids for L-amino acids produces stable peptides, and the stereochemical change may give the peptide access to additional binding sites on the receptors; both of these actions may explain their increased potencies. Replacing the Gly^2 with D-Ala^2 while simultaneously replacing the L-Leu^5 with D-Leu^5 produces the peptide known as D-Ala^2, D-Leu^5 enkephalin (DADLE), which is commonly used as a selective δ-agonist.

GLY^3

Almost all changes to this amino acid result in a drop in potency, unless they are also accompanied by another change such as replacing the Gly^2 with D-Ala^2 as described above.

PHE^4

The aromatic nature of the fourth residue is required for high activity. When combined with the D-Ala^2 replacement, the addition of an electron withdrawing, lipophilic substituent (e.g.,

NO$_2$, Cl, and Br) in the para position of Phe^4 greatly increases activity. Para substitutions with electron donating, hydrophilic functional groups (e.g., NH$_2$ and OH) abolish activity.

MET^5/LEU^5

Position 5 appears to tolerate more residue changes than the other positions. Many amino acid substitutions at this position maintain activity (e.g., Ala, Gly, Phe, Pro). Even the loss of the fifth residue to yield the tetrapeptide Tyr^1-Gly^2-Gly^3-Phe^4 maintains weak activity in both the GPI and MVD assays. The protected peptide, Tyr^1-D-Ala^2-Gly^3-MePhe^4-Gly-ol^5, known as DAMGO is highly selective for the μ-receptor.

The pituitary gland, hypothalamus, and the adrenal medulla all produce various opioid peptides. Many of these materials were found to be fragments of β-lipotropin (β-LPT) a 91 amino acid peptide. β-LPT has no opioid activity itself. The fraction containing amino acids 61–91 is designated β-endorphin (a word derived from combining *end*ogenous and m*orphin*e). It is much more potent than the enkephalins in both in vivo and in vitro tests. The search for opioid peptides continued, and additional precursor proteins were discovered. Many additional precursor proteins synthesized in the pituitary, adrenal glands, and brain terminals were found to contain sequences of amino acids that were enkephalins or other active opioid peptides. It appears that naturally occurring peptides may serve roles as both short-acting analgesics and long-term neuronal or endocrine modulators. Acupuncture, running, or other physical activity may induce the release of neuropeptides although studies exist that both confirm and refute these claims.[24,25] A complete discussion on the neuropeptides is beyond the scope of this chapter. Some examples of opioid peptides are given in Figure 24.2.[26–29]

Opioid Receptors

The discovery of the endogenous opioid peptides paralleled the development of radiolabeling techniques. During the 1970s, researchers were able to label opioid receptors with reversible radioactive ligands that allowed pharmacological actions of specific receptors and their locations to be identified. These techniques allowed for the identification of opioid receptor locations in the brain. Additional pharmacological advances in gene expression studies led to the identification of peripheral opioid receptor locations.[30] Opioid receptors are distributed throughout the brain, spinal cord, and peripheral tissues. The distribution of specific opioid receptor subtypes (μ, δ, and κ) usually overlaps. In rats, high concentrations of all three genes for the μ-, δ-, and κ-receptors were found in the hypothalamus and cerebral

Endogenous Precursor Proteins
Pro-opimelanocortin $\longrightarrow$ ACTH + β LPH $\longrightarrow$ γ-LPH + β endorphin
Pro-enkephalin A^{263} $\longrightarrow$ 4Met-enkephalin + Leu-enkephalin
Pro-enkephalin B^{256} $\longrightarrow$ β neo-endorphin$^{175-183}$ + dynorphin$^{209-225}$ + Leu-enkephalin$^{228-232}$

Endogenous Opioid Peptide sequences
β Endorphin = Tyr-Gly-Gly-Phe-Met^5-Thr-Ser-Glu-Lys-Ser^{10}-Gln-Thr-Pro-Leu-Val^{15}-Thr-Leu-Phe-Lys-Asn^{20}-Ala-Ile-Ile-Lys-Asn^{25}-Ala-Tyr-Lys-Lys-Gly-Glu^{31} = δ and μ opioid receptor ligand
Endomorphin-1 = Tyr-Pro-Trp-Phe-NH$_2$ = μ receptor agonist
Endomorphin-2 = Tyr-Pro-Phe-Phe-NH$_2$ = μ receptor agonist

Dynorphin = Tyr-Gly-Gly-Phe-Leu^5-Arg-Arg-Ile-Arg-Pro^{10}-Lys-Leu-Lys^{13} = κ opioid selectivity
α-Neoendorphin = Tyr-Gly-Gly-Phe-Leu^5-Arg-Lys-Tyr-Pro-Lys^{10}
β-Neoendorphin = Tyr-Gly-Gly-Phe-Leu^5-Arg-Lys-Tyr-Pro^9

Nociceptin = Phe-Gly-Gly-Thr-Gly^5-Ala-Arg-Lys-Ser-Ala^{10}-Lys-Ala-Asn-Gln^{14} = orphanin receptor
Orphanin FQ = Phe-Gly-Gly-Phe-Thr^5-Gly-Ala-Arg-Lys-Ser^{10}-Ala-Arg-Lys-Leu-Ala-Asn-Gln^{17}

Exogenous Opioid Peptide sequences "Exorphins"
DADLE = Tyr-D-Ala-Gly-Phe-D-Leu = δ selective agonist
DPDPE = Tyr-D-Pen-Gly-Phe-D-Pen = δ selective agonist
DSLET = Tyr-D-Ser-Gly-Phe-Leu-Thr = δ selective agonist
Casomorphin (cow's milk μ opioid receptor agonist) = Tyr-Pro-Phe-Pro-Gly-Pro-Ile^7
Dermorphin (South American frog skin μ opioid receptor agonist) = Tyr-D-Ala-Phe-Gly-Tyr-Pro-Ser^7-NH$_2$
Gluten exorphins (multiple peptides from wheat having opioid agonist and antagonist activity)

Figure 24.2 ● Endogenous and exogenous opioid peptides.

cortex. Intermediate concentrations were found in the small intestine, adrenal gland, testes, ovary, and uterus. Low concentrations of all the three gene transcripts were found in the lung and kidney. The gene for the μ-opioid receptor was not found in the stomach, heart, endothelium, or synovium of the rat.[30] Opioid receptors are also found on the peripheral terminals of sensory neurons in inflamed rat paws.[31] Thus, the central and peripheral distribution of opioid receptors is complex. This complicates the interpretation of pharmacological data of individual drugs that may have overlapping binding at multiple opioid receptor subtypes. In addition, opioid receptors form homodimers and heterodimers with opioid receptors and nonopioid receptors such as the α_{2a}-adrenergic receptors resulting in different pharmacologic actions and altered coupling to second messengers.[32]

Genes for the four major opioid receptor subtypes have been cloned; the MOP = μ-receptor (mu for morphine), the KOP = κ-receptor (kappa for ketocyclazocine), the DOP = δ-receptor (delta for deferens because it was originally discovered in the MVD), and the NOP = nociception/orphanin FQ receptor (named as an orphan receptor because the endogenous/exogenous ligand was unknown at its time of discovery).[33] The opioid receptor subtypes share extensive residue homology in their transmembrane (TM) domains with most of the variation found in the extracellular loops (Fig. 24.3).[33] All of the opioid receptors belong to the G-protein–coupled receptor class and as such, they are composed of seven TM domains. When the receptor is activated, a portion of the G protein diffuses within the membrane and causes an inhibition of adenylate cyclase activity. The decreased enzyme activity results in a decrease in cyclic adenosine monophosphate (cAMP) formation, which regulates numerous cellular processes. One process that is inhibited is the opening of voltage-gated calcium influx channels on nociceptive C-fibers. This results in the hyperpolarazation of the nerve cell and decreased firing and release of pain neurotransmitters such as glutamate and substance P.[34]

OPIOID LIGAND BINDING SITE

There are no x-ray crystal structures reported for any opioid receptor, and most modeling work has been based on the crystal structure of rhodopsin. Many groups have attempted to find the specific binding site through homology modeling, molecular dynamics, site-directed mutagenesis, chimeric receptors, truncated receptors, and SAR studies. As of yet, no definitive model of the ligand-binding site is available. The opioid-binding site for all four opioid receptors is believed to be an inner cavity formed by conserved residues on TM helices TM3, TM4, TM5, TM6, and TM7.[33,35] Not all groups agree that the binding pocket is formed via TM domains; some evidence suggest that the amino terminus is an important determinant of ligand binding affinity as well.[36] The ligand specificity that each receptor shows may be a result of differences in the extracellular loops that form lids on the binding cavities or differences in amino acids within the binding cavity. Within the cavity, agonists are thought to bind toward the bottom of the cavity via interactions with a conserved Asp from TM3 and a His from TM6. Molecular modeling calculations show that the phenolic OH of the Tyr^1 opioid peptide, or the ring A OH of nonpeptide opioids, forms a hydrogen bond with the conserved His on TM6. The Tyr^1-charged nitrogen, or the N$^+$ of the nonpeptide agonist, forms an ionic bond with the conserved Asp of TM3. Antagonist ligands are thought to bind deeper in the binding pocket but retain the ionic bond with the Asp of TM3. The bulky substituent on the charged nitrogen of antagonists is believed to insert itself between TM3 and TM6, preventing the shifts required for activation. Thus, antagonists prevent the necessary movement of TM3 and TM6 resulting in functional antagonism.[33,35]

THE μ-RECEPTOR

Mu receptors are found primarily in the brainstem and medial thalamus.[34] Endogenous peptides for the μ-receptor include endomorphin-1, endomorphin-2, and β-endorphin

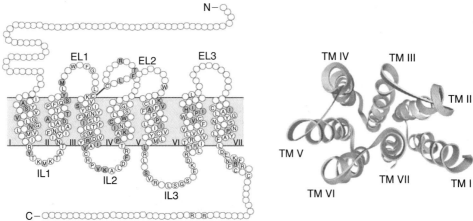

Figure 24.3 ● Structure of opioid receptors. (*Left*) Serpentine model of the opioid receptor. Each transmembrane helix is labeled with a roman number. The white empty circles represent nonconserved amino acids among the MOP, DOP, KOP, and NOP receptors. White circles with a letter represent identical amino acids among all four opioid receptors. Violet circles represent further identity between the MOP-R, DOP-R, and KOP-R. Green circles highlight the highly conserved fingerprint residues of family A receptors, Asn I:18 in TM1, AspII:10 in TM2, CysIII:01 in TM3, TrpIV:10 in TM4, ProV:16 in TM5, ProVI:15 in TM6, and ProVII:17 TM7. Yellow circles depict the two conserved cystines in EL loops 1 and 2, likely forming a disulfide bridge. (IL, intracellular loop, and EL, extracellular loop.) (*Right*) Proposed arrangement of the seven transmembrane helices of opioid receptors as viewed from the top (extracellular side). The seven transmembrane helices are arranged sequentially in a counterclockwise manner. Each transmembrane helix is labeled with a roman number. (Reprinted with permission from the *Annual Review of Biochemistry*, Volume 73 © 2004 by Annual Reviews.)

(Fig. 24.2). Exogenous agonists for the μ-receptor include drugs from the five structural classes discussed later in this chapter (4,5-epoxymorphinan, morphinan, benzomorphan, 4-phenyl/4-anilido piperidines, and the diphenylheptanes) and exogenous peptides such as dermorphin isolated from the skin of South American frogs. Recently, human neuroblastoma cells have been shown to be capable of synthesizing morphine via biosynthesis from radiolabeled tyramine. The synthetic route involves at least 19 steps and is similar, but not exact, to the synthetic route used by the poppy plant.[37] The exact role of endogenous morphine is unknown at this time. In general, agonists at the μ-receptor produce analgesia, respiratory depression, decreased gastrointestinal (GI) motility, euphoria, feeding, and the release of hormones. Agonists are also responsible for the addictive effects of the opioid analgesics. Most clinically used opioid drugs bind to the μ-opioid receptor.

THE δ-RECEPTOR

Opioid peptides for the δ-receptor include the endogenous peptides described previously, Met and Leu enkephalin, as well as some synthetic peptides such as DADLE, DSLET, and DPDPE (see Fig. 24.2 for amino acid sequences). These peptides have high affinity for the receptor but low bioavailability and thus limited clinical usefulness. They are used in animal in vitro studies as probes for δ-receptor location and function.

In an attempt to distinguish the amino acids responsible for δ-receptor ligand specificity, point mutations of the δ-receptor, and μ/δ-receptor chimeras were constructed.[38] The altered receptors had a decreased ability to bind to δ-receptor selective peptide and nonpeptide ligands, when amino acids in the extracellular top of TM6 and TM7 and the extracellular loop (EC loop 3) that connected them were mutated.

Specifically, amino acids Try^{284}, Val^{296}, and Val^{297} were crucial to selective δ-ligand binding. These amino acids may provide recognition sites on the receptor that the ligand would have to pass through to reach the putative binding site deeper in the TM cavity. Befort et al.[39] also used site-directed point mutant receptors along with molecular modeling to identify Tyr^{129} in TM3 as the most crucial amino acid for ligand binding. In addition, they found a role for amino acid Tyr^{308} (TM7) in ligand binding.

Nonpeptide agonists and antagonists have been designed to further study the function of the δ-receptor. The first nonpeptide lead compound selective for the δ-receptor came from screening. Modifications to the lead compound led to the identification of SNC-80 as a potent agonist specific for the δ-receptor (Fig. 24.4). This compound has weak antinociceptive effects in monkeys, an effect that can be reversed with the δ-antagonist naltrindole (NTI) (Fig. 24.4).[40] A series of SNC-80 analog, prepared by multiple groups, found that the amide nitrogen appears to be the most sensitive to modifications and may play an important role in δ-receptor selectivity.[41] Portoghese designed 7-spiroindanyloxymorphone (SIOM) (Fig. 24.4) based on the idea that the indole of NTI is acting as an "address" mimic of the Phe^4 phenyl group of enkephalin. The "address–message" concept proposes that one part of the molecule may act as an "address," essentially directing the chemical to the correct receptor by binding specifically to that receptor, and another part of the molecule acts as the "message," which gives the compound the biological action. The indole of NTI was replaced with a spiroindane functional group equivalent address in SIOM. The N-methyl group of SIOM confers an agonist message as opposed to the antagonist message of the NTI cyclopropyl methyl.[42] Additional agonists for the δ-receptor have been

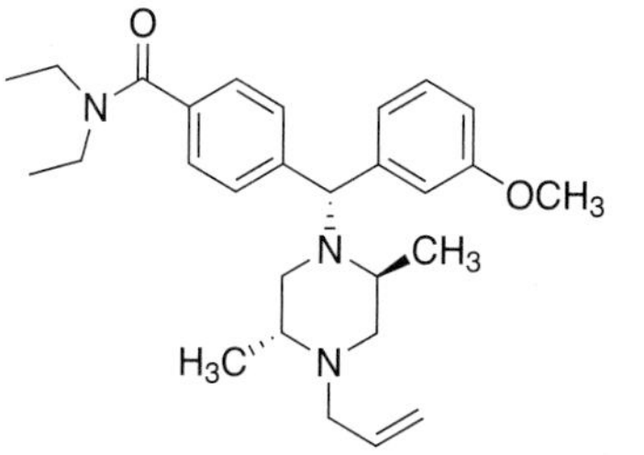

(+) SNC-80
δ receptor agonist

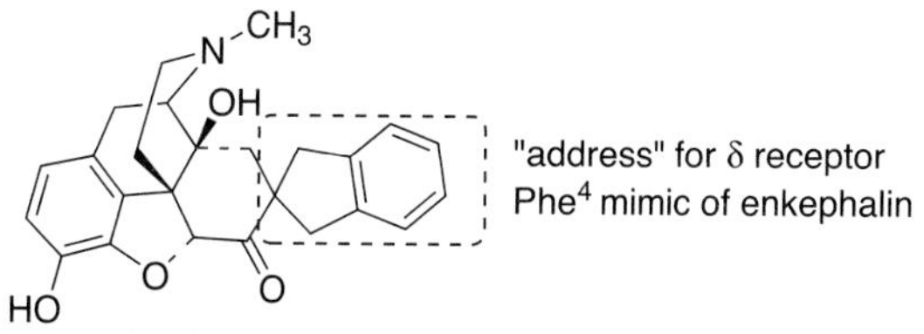

7-spiroindanyloxymorphone (SIOM)
δ receptor agonist

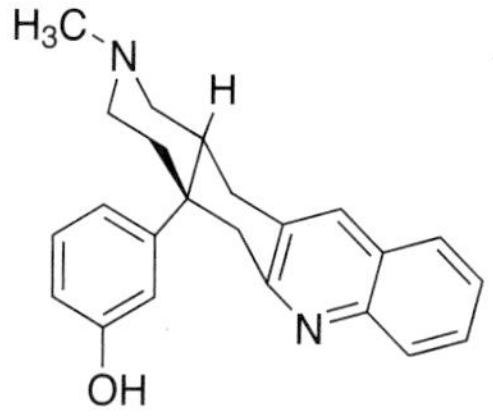

TAN-67
δ receptor agonist

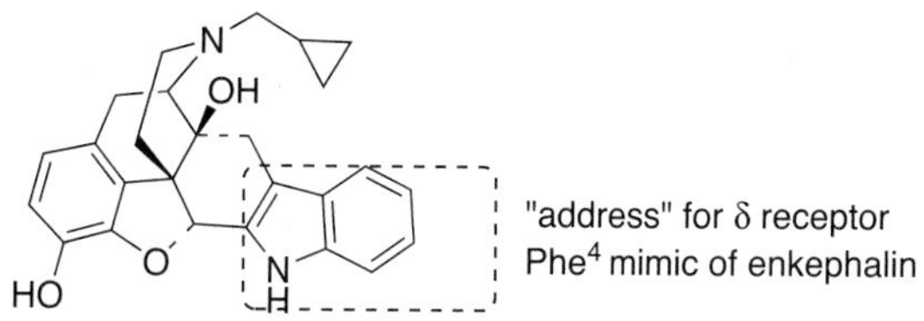

Naltrindole (NTI)
δ receptor antagonist

Figure 24.4 ● Selective δ-receptor ligands.

developed based on the octahydroisoquinoline structure with five-membered ring spacers being δ-receptor antagonists and six-membered ring spacers, agonists. TAN-67 is the most extensively studied in this class (Fig. 24.4).[41] The δ-receptor tolerates multiple chemical structures, and no pharmacophore has been identified that can accommodate all of the diverse structures.[38,43]

Transgenic mice lacking the δ-receptor have been generated and found to display increased levels of anxiety. In addition, δ-receptor agonist show antidepressant activity in rat models.[32,44] These results suggest that ligands targeting this receptor may represent new leads for the treatment of schizophrenia, bipolar disorders, and depression. There are few clinical reports of selective δ-receptor agonist use in humans, although they are reported to have proconvulsive activity that may limit their use.[44]

THE κ-RECEPTOR

Kappa receptors are primarily found in the limbic, brain stem, and spinal cord.[34] The κ-receptor shows less structural homology to the μ-receptor than the δ-receptor does. (Fig. 24.3) Unlike the μ- and δ-receptors that bind the (enkephalin) peptide sequence Tyr-Gly-Gly-Phe-(Leu/Met), the κ-receptor does not. The κ-receptor shows a clear preference for binding peptides with an arginine in position 6 as seen in the dynorphin peptides (Fig. 24.2).[45]

The structure of some κ-agonists and an antagonist can be seen in Figure 24.5.[46,47] TRK-820 is a κ-agonist displaying approximately 15 times selectivity toward κ-receptors versus μ-receptors.[46] The 4,5-epoxymorphinan structure of TRK-820 is proposed to mimic the tyrosine–glycine moiety of endogenous opioid peptides, in effect the agonist message. The additional 6β-substituent constitutes the address directing the compound to the κ-receptor. Spiradoline was one of the earliest compounds to show improved κ-receptor selectivity (125 times over μ-receptors). SARs on this class of compounds revealed that methyl-substituted nitrogen amides, a methylene spacer between the amide and the aromatic ring and the (−) isomer were all required for κ-activity. The dichlorophenyl ring could be replaced with a 4-benzothiophene or a 4-benzofuran for increased potency and κ-receptor selectivity.[41] Salvinorin A (Fig. 24.5) a nonnitrogen-containing natural compound found in the herb sage is a potent agonist at the κ-receptor.[48] The hallucinogenic properties of *salvia divinorum* (sage) have been known for hundreds of years but recently, these properties have been exploited by online groups attempting to sell legal hallucinogenic compounds. The κ-antagonist nor-binaltorphimine (nor-BNI) was made by incorporating a rigid pyrrole spacer linking two κ-pharmacophores. Nor-BNI is used in the laboratory to determine if κ-receptors are involved in an observed activity.[41] The second pharmacophore of nor-BNI is not required for κ-antagonism, and compounds that are missing the second aromatic ring have been found to be even more selective and potent antagonists at the κ-receptor.

In clinical trials, most κ-agonists produce dysphoria and thus may be less psychologically addicting but also less acceptable to patients. Some compounds with κ-agonist activity (e.g., pentazocine, nalbuphine) are available, but the clinical development of pure κ-agonists has been limited by the centrally mediated side effects. Spiradoline was developed under the premise that a selective κ-agonist would be an analgesic without the μ-opioid–mediated problems associated with addiction and respiratory depression. Clinical trials in humans found that spiradoline did not produce analgesic effects within a dose range that did not also cause dysphoria, diuresis, and sedation.[47] The selective κ-agonist TRK-820 shows some promise for the treatment of uremic pruritus, the itch associated with dialysis.[49]

THE ORPHANIN RECEPTOR/FQ/NOP$_1$

The traditional opioid peptides do not elicit any biological effect at the orphanin receptor. An endogenous peptide for the orphanin receptor has been found and termed orphanin FQ or *nociceptin* (Fig. 24.2). This 17 amino acid peptide can reverse the analgesic effects of morphine thus is antiopioid

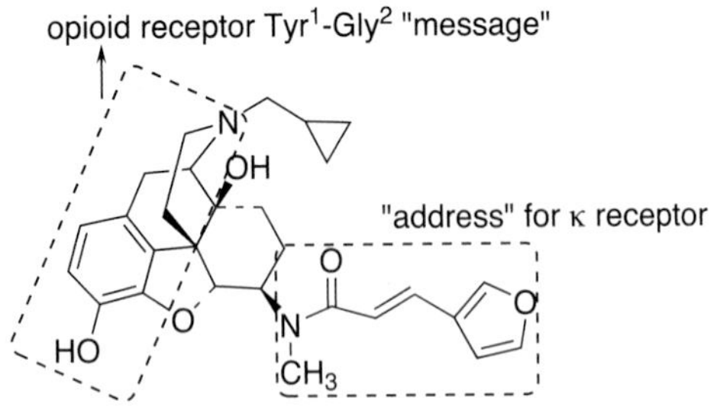

opioid receptor Tyr¹-Gly² "message"

"address" for κ receptor

TRK-820
κ receptor agonist
modest selectivity (15x over μ)

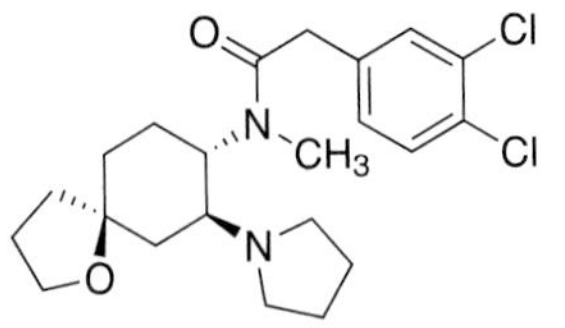

(-) spiradoline
κ receptor agonist (125 x over μ)

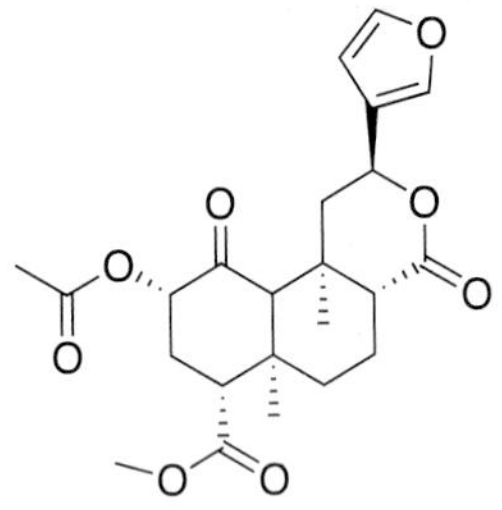

salvinorin A
κ receptor agonist

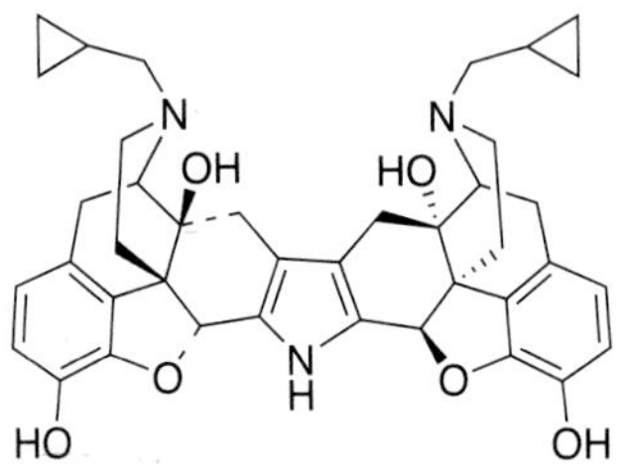

Nor-binaltorphimine (nor-BNI)
κ receptor antagonist

Figure 24.5 ● Selective κ-receptor ligands.

in some situations.[50] The carboxy-terminal half of the receptor may serve as the portion that excludes binding to the μ-, δ-, and κ-opioid ligands. The functional role of the receptor is still being investigated, but selective agonists have been shown to delay gastric emptying and decrease gastric secretory functions in rats.[51] In addition, this receptor is found on airway nerves, and agonists decrease bronchospasms in guinea pigs and cats. This receptor is a target for the design of novel peripherally acting antitussive agents, although no compounds are on the market at present.

STRUCTURE–ACTIVITY RELATIONSHIPS

Relating the structure of the chemical ligand to the physiologic activity it induces can only be accomplished by looking at each receptor type individually. The chemically diverse nature of agonists and antagonists found for the μ-, δ-, and κ-receptors is testimony to the adaptability of the

receptors to multiple chemical backbones and tolerance for divergent functional groups. The reader is referred to reviews of the κ- and δ-receptor for detailed SARs for ligands at those receptors.[41] A summary review of the SARs of the μ-receptor compounds is included in the drug monograph section below. For the purpose of this chapter, the drug classes covered will be 4,5-epoxymorphinans, morphinans, benzomorphans, 4-phenylpiperidines/4-anilidopiperidines, diphenylheptanes, and the miscellaneous category.

⬡ DRUG MONOGRAPHS

4,5-Epoxymorphinans

A summary of the SARs of the 4,5-epoxymorphinan structure can be seen in Figure 24.6, and these are discussed in the succeeding individual drug monographs.

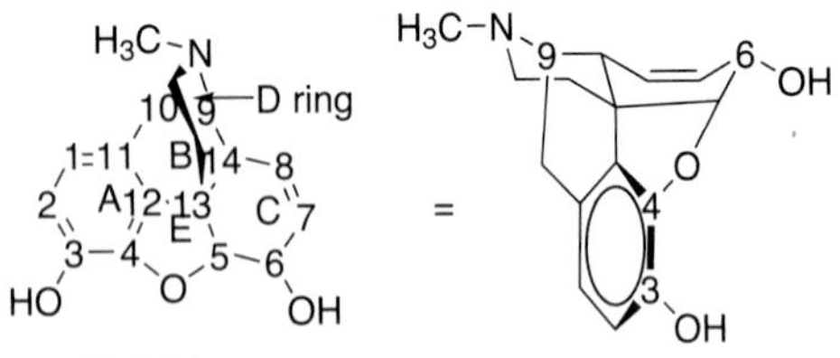

Morphine

Changes on Morphine that increase analgesic activity
C6 - OH to OAc
C3 and C6 - OH to OAc
C6 - OH to O-Sulfate or O-glucuronide
C6 - OH to =O and C7-C8 single bond
C6 - OH to H and C7-C8 single bond
C14 - H to βOH
N - CH₃ to CH₂CH₂Ph
N - CH₃ to CH₂CH₂furan
N - CH₃ to CH₂C=OPh
Removal of C4-C5 ether link

Changes on Morphine that produce antagonists
N - CH₃ to CH₂CH=CH₂
N - CH₃ to CH₂⬤

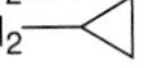

Figure 24.6 ● Summary of functional group changes on morphine structure.

MORPHINE

The prototype ligand for the μ-receptor is morphine. The numbering and ring lettering (A, B, C. . .) can be seen in Figure 24.6. Morphine contains 5 chiral centers and has 16 optical isomers (not 32 because of the restriction of C-9 to C-13 ethanamino bridge). The naturally occurring, active form of morphine is the levorotatory enantiomorph with the stereochemistry 5(R), 6(S), 9(R), 13(S), and 14 (R). The x-ray determined conformation of morphine is a "T" shape with the A, B, and E rings forming the vertical portion, and the C and D ring forming the top (Fig. 24.6).[41]

Morphine was isolated from opium in 1806 by a German pharmacist, Seturner. He named the compound "morphine" after the Greek god of dreams "Morpheus." The first mention of the opium poppy was found in Iraq on clay tablets inscribed in cuneiform script in about 3000 BC.[52] Opium has been used throughout history and is found in ancient Egyptian, Greek, Roman, Arabic, Indian, and Chinese writing. Opium is isolated from the opium poppy, *Papaver somniferum*, by lancing the unripe pod and collecting and drying the latex that seeps from the incision. Opium contains over 40 different alkaloids with most alkaloids represented in the following five structures: morphine (8%–17%), codeine (0.7%–5%), thebaine (0.1%–2.5%), papaverine (0.5%–1.5%), and noscapine (1%–10%).[52]

Although the total synthesis of morphine has been accomplished by various chemical processes, it is still produced from the poppy latex.[53] Thus far, no synthetic pathway is efficient enough to make it competitive with the preparation of morphine from either isolation or semisynthesis from a precursor compound from the poppy plant. The endogenous synthesis of morphine in human neuroblastoma cells has been elegantly described.[37] The function of endogenous morphine is unknown at this time, but the genes and enzymes involved in morphine biosynthesis may become targets for novel drugs used to treat pain.

Morphine is the prototype μ-receptor agonist; it is the drug to which all other μ-agonists are compared. The pharmacological properties of morphine are well documented and include analgesia, its primary use. For equivalent analgesic effect, the oral dose must be 3 times the intravenous (IV) dose to account for the morphine lost to first-pass hepatic metabolism. The equianalgesic dose of morphine congeners can be seen in Figure 24.7.

Morphine is extensively metabolized via phase II conjugation to morphine-3-glucuronide (~60%), morphine-6-glucuronide (~9%), and, to a lesser extent, the *N*-demethylated metabolite (~3%)[54] (Fig. 24.8). Much controversy exists on the contribution of the metabolites of both codeine-6-glucuronide and morphine-6-glucuronide to their analgesic effect. In some studies, the 6-glucuronide metabolite of both drugs contributes significantly to their potency.[55–57] In other studies, the 6-glucuronide metabolites of morphine and codeine produces very little analgesic effect.[58,59]

Morphine, or another potent opioid drug, is introduced in the WHO stepladder when pain is severe and no relief is obtained from NSAIDs or a combination of NSAIDs and a less potent opioid. Morphine is a monoacidic base and readily forms water-soluble salts with most acids. Because morphine itself is poorly soluble in water (1 g/5,000 mL at 25°C), the

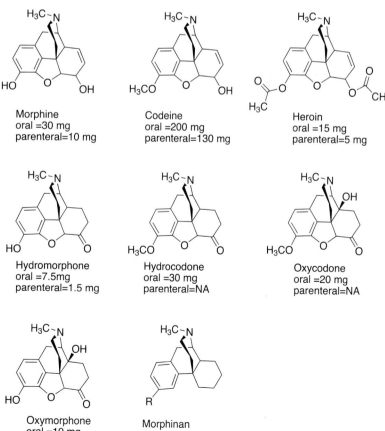

Morphine
oral =30 mg
parenteral=10 mg

Codeine
oral =200 mg
parenteral=130 mg

Heroin
oral =15 mg
parenteral=5 mg

Hydromorphone
oral =7.5mg
parenteral=1.5 mg

Hydrocodone
oral =30 mg
parenteral=NA

Oxycodone
oral =20 mg
parenteral=NA

Oxymorphone
oral =10 mg
parenteral=1 mg

Morphinan
R= OH (-) Levorphanol oral = 2 mg
R= OCH₃ (+) Dextromethorphan

Figure 24.7 ● 4,5-Epoxymorphinans and morphinans.

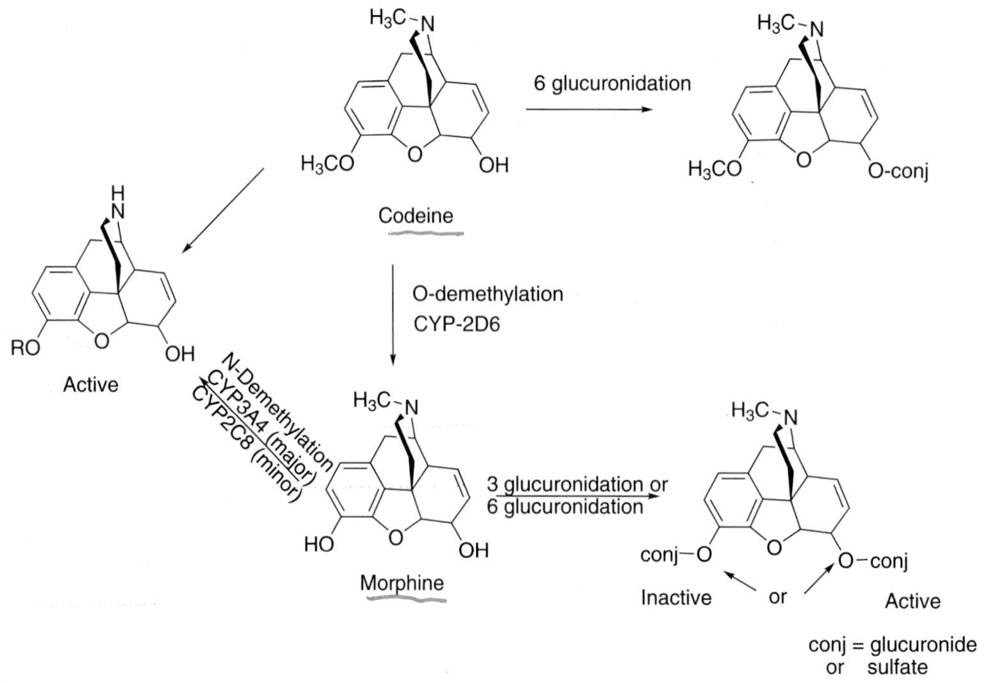

Figure 24.8 ● Metabolism of morphine and codeine.

sulfate salt is formed for both oral, IV, and suppository use. The usual starting parenteral dose of morphine in adults is 2.5 to 5 mg q 4 hours. Morphine is available for oral use both as an immediate release and sustained release formulation. The immediate release preparations are dosed q 4 hours, and the sustained release formulations are dosed q 12 to q 24 hours depending on the formulation.

CODEINE

Codeine is an alkaloid that occurs naturally in opium, but the amount present is usually too small to be of commercial importance. Consequently, most commercial codeine is prepared from morphine by methylating the phenolic OH group. It occurs as levorotatory, colorless, efflorescent crystals, or as a white crystalline powder. It is light sensitive. Codeine is a monoacidic base and readily forms salts with acids, with the most important being the sulfate and the phosphate. The acetate and methylbromide derivatives have been used to a limited extent in cough preparations.

The general pharmacological action of codeine is similar to that of morphine, but it does not possess the same analgesic potency. The equianalgesic dose of parenteral morphine 3 to 5 mg q 4 hours is codeine 30 to 65 mg q 4 hours. The equianalgesic dose of oral morphine 10 mg q 4 hours is codeine 60 mg q 4 hours. The decreased potency also leads to a lower addiction potential compared with morphine. Side effects include respiratory depression, mioisis, constipation, nausea, itching, dry mouth, and drowsiness. Approximately 5% of codeine is metabolized to morphine via *O*-demethylation. (Fig. 24.8) The enzyme responsible for the *O*-demethylation of codeine is cytochrome P450 (CYP) 2D6. This enzyme exhibits genetic polymorphism with an estimated 7% to 10% of Caucasians designated as poor metabolizers, and thus only able to form traces of morphine after codeine is administered.[60] The analgesic component of codeine has long been assumed to

be the *O*-demethylated metabolite, morphine. If codeine has no analgesic potency itself, then patients who lack this enzyme should have no analgesic effect to administered codeine. This has been shown not to be the case, so codeine itself may posses analgesic activity, or codeine-6-glucuronide may be the active analgesic.[56,57]

Codeine's role as an effective antitussive agent has been questioned. A Cochrane evidence-based review of the literature shows that codeine is no more effective than placebo for acute cough in children or adults.[61] Codeine is available in several combination products with either aspirin, ibuprofen, or acetaminophen for the treatment of moderate pain.

HEROIN

Heroin, was first commercially synthesized in 1898 by Bayer company in Germany as an alternate analgesic to morphine. Heroin is the 3,6 diacetylated form of morphine (Fig. 24.7). The laboratory researchers, which also used the acetylation process to convert salicylic acid into acetyl salicylic acid (aspirin), believed that heroin would be an effective analgesic with no addictive properties. This was unfortunately not the case. They named the product "heroin" because it made the test subjects, including some of the chemists, feel "heroic." With both OH groups protected as an ester, heroin can pass through the blood-brain barrier quicker than morphine and lead to the euphoric "rush" that becomes so addictive to addicts, especially after IV injection. Once heroin is in the brain, it is quickly metabolized to 3-acetylmorphine, which has low to zero activity at the μ-receptor and 6-acetylmorphine, which is 2 to 3 times more potent at the μ-receptor than morphine.[62]

Heroin is not available as a prescription product in the United States, although it is available in some countries to treat pain associated with cancer and myocardial infarctions. It remains one of the most widely used narcotics for illicit purposes and places major economic burdens on society.

HYDROMORPHONE

Hydromorphone, (Dilaudid) is a synthetic derivative of morphine prepared by the catalytic hydrogenation and dehydrogenation of morphine under acidic conditions, using a large excess of platinum or palladium.[63] Oxidation of the 6-OH of morphine resulted in a compound with decreased potency. Reducing the 7,8 double bond of morphine increased the flexibility of the molecule and resulted in a compound with slightly enhanced binding. Making both of these structural changes to morphine-produced hydromorphone, a compound approximately 5 times as potent as morphine. Hydromorphone was introduced in 1926 and is available as an immediate release tablet, a liquid, and a suppository. A sustained release form is available in some countries but not in the United States. The sustained release form was removed from the U.S. market in 2005 when studies showed that drinking 8 oz of alcohol (40%) could cause the drug to be released from the capsule immediately and lead to concentrations that were 5.5 times higher than in patients that did not drink alcohol. This potentially lethal combination prompted the Food and Drug Administration (FDA) to remove it from the market.

HYDROCODONE

Hydrocodone is the 3 methoxy version of hydromorphone. The loss of the 3-OH group yields a compound that is approximately 4 to 5 times less potent than hydromorphone, thus about equal to morphine. Unlike codeine, the agonist activity of hydrocodone does not require 3-*O*-demethylation, although it does occur via CYP2D6 representing 4.6% of total clearance.[64] The protected 3-position has better brain penetration, and the 7,8-dihydro-6-keto C ring contributes to the increased binding of the compound to the μ-receptor.

There are no pure hydrocodone products available on the U.S. market. All FDA-approved products containing hydrocodone are combination products. Like codeine, hydrocodone is marketed as an antitussive agent. It is available combined with the anticholinergic agent homatropine as a syrup and a tablet. The addition of the anticholinergic agent is to discourage abuse. It is also available in a delayed release suspension form (Tussionex). This formulation uses a sulfonated styrene divinylbenzene copolymer complexed with hydromorphone and chlorpheniramine that acts as a cation-exchange resin slowly releasing the drugs over a 12-hour period. Hydrocodone is also marketed in combination with acetaminophen (Vicodin, Lortab) or aspirin (Lortab ASA) for the treatment of pain. The dose of acetaminophen consumed by the patient must be closely monitored, and prescriptions that allow for greater than 4 grams of acetaminophen per 24-hour period should not be dispensed.

OXYCODONE

Oxycodone is synthesized from the natural opium alkaloid thebaine. Oxycodone is the 14 beta-hydroxyl version of hydrocodone. This additional functional group gives oxycodone greater potency (1.5 times orally) than hydrocodone presumably by increasing receptor affinity. The oral bioavailability of oxycodone is 65% to 87%.[65] The metabolism of oxycodone follows the similar pattern of opioid metabolism with *N*-demethylation, *O*-demethylation, and their glucuronides all identified. Per the manufacturer, the analgesic effect of oxycodone correlates well with oxycodone plasma concentrations, not the minimal amount of oxymorphone formed, thus

oxycodone is not assumed to be a prodrug. There are no large-scale studies of oxycodone used for analgesia in CYP2D6 poor metabolizers that can confirm this.

Oxycodone is marketed in combination with acetaminophen (Percocet), aspirin (Percodan), and ibuprofen (Combunox). It has been available for over 50 years as an immediate-release tablet, and in 1995 an extended-release tablet was approved by the FDA (OxyContin). OxyContin is manufactured in eight strengths from 10 to 160 mg, and the high-dose preparations quickly became attractive to drug abusers. The extended-release tablets are crushed and then injected or snorted to give an immediate high. The Drug Abuse Warning Network (DAWN) is a public health surveillance system that monitors drug-related emergency room visits and drug-related deaths. In 1995, they estimated that 598,542 emergency room visits involved the nonmedical use of a pharmaceutical (e.g., antidepressant, anxiolytic, stimulant). Of these ER visits, 160,363 visits were attributed to opiates with an estimated 42,810 involving oxycodone or an oxycodone combination. Methadone and hydrocodone/combinations were estimated to be similar to oxycodone.[66]

OXYMORPHONE

Oxymorphone is the 14 beta-hydroxyl version of hydromorphone, analogous to the hydrocodone, oxycodone pair discussed above. Although the addition of the 14 beta-hydroxyl group to hydrocodone (30 mg) yielded oxycodone (20 mg), a more potent drug, the opposite is true for the conversion of hydromorphone (7.5 mg) to oxymorphone (10 mg). The reason for this is that the oral bioavailability of oxymorphone (10%) is lower than that of hydromorphone (35%) because of decreased absorption and increased first-pass metabolism. Presumably, the addition of the OH group does increase its binding affinity at the receptor as the injectable form of oxymorphone (1 mg) is more potent than injectable hydromorphone (1.5 mg).

Oxymorphone is available as a suppository (5 mg), an injection (1 mg/mL), an immediate-release tablet (5 mg, 10 mg), and in 2003 the FDA approved a sustained release formulation (Opana ER 5 mg, 10 mg, 20 mg, and 40 mg). The 12-hour coverage of the extended release tablet provides another option for those patients suffering from chronic pain. The side effect profile of the extended release formulations of morphine, oxycodone, and oxymorphone are similar, and there appears to be no clear advantage of one over the other.

Morphinans

The morphinans were made by removing the E ring of morphine, the 4,5-ether bridge, in an attempt to simplify the structure (Fig. 24.7).

LEVORPHANOL

Levorphanol tartrate is the levorotatory form of methorphan and is approximately 7.5 times more potent than morphine orally. The loss of the 4,5-epoxide and the 7,8-double bond allows levorphanol greater flexibility and presumable leads to the increased binding affinity at all opioid receptor subtypes compared with morphine. The plasma half-life of levorphanol is about 6 to 8 hours but displays great interperson variability and may increase upon repeated dosing. The excretion of levorphanol is dependent on the kidneys, so caution must be used in renally compromised patients.[67]

The analgesic effect of levorphanol may not match the long plasma half-life, and patients must be closely monitored for drug accumulation and respiratory depression. Levorphanol has strong agonist activity at the μ-, κ-, and δ-opioid receptors and has also been shown to be a noncompetitive *N*-methyl-D-aspartate (NMDA)-receptor antagonist.[68] The pharmacodynamic properties of levorphanol are sufficiently different to make it an attractive alternate for patients that receive inadequate pain relief from morphine. Levorphanol is available as a 2-mg oral tablet (Levo-Dromoran), and a 2-mg/mL solution for injection.

DEXTROMETHORPHAN

Dextromethorphan is the dextrorotatory form of levorphanol with a methoxy group on the 3-position (Fig. 24.7). It is available in more than 140 over-the-counter (OTC) cough and cold formulations.[69] Evidence-based reviews have been unable to conclude that it is more effective than placebo in reducing cough.[61,70] Like (+) and (−) levorphanol, (+) dextromethorphan is a potent NMDA antagonist and, in higher than recommended doses, has the potential for causing dissociative anesthetic effects similar to ketamine or phencyclidine (PCP). The OTC status and availability of pure dextromethorphan powder online has contributed greatly to its abuse in recent years. DAWN reports that in 2004, there were approximately 12,500 emergency room visits involving dextromethorphan with 44% of those involving abuse of the drug.[71] The *2006 National Survey on Drug Abuse* report shows that nearly 1 million persons aged 12 to 25 years (1.7%) misused OTC cough and cold medications in the past year.[69]

Dextromethorphan's ability to antagonize the NMDA receptor has led to its use to treat phantom pain, diabetic neuropathy, and postoperative acute pain.[72,73]

Benzomorphans

Structural simplification of the morphine ring system further, by removing the C ring of the morphinan structure, yields the benzomorphans also referred to as the *benzazocines*.

Pentazocine

PENTAZOCINE

The benzomorphans are prepared synthetically and thus result in several stereoisomers. The active benzomorphans are those that have the equivalent bridgehead carbons in the same absolute configuration of morphine (carbons 9, 13, and 14 of morphine). The only benzomorphan in clinical use is pentazocine, which is prepared as the 2(R), 6(R), 11(R) enantiomer (*Chemical Abstracts* numbering).[74] Pentazocine is a mixed agonist/antagonist displaying differing intrinsic activity at the opioid receptor subtypes. At the μ-receptor, pentazocine is a partial agonist and a weak antagonist.

According to the manufacturer, a 50-mg dose of pentazocine has about the same analgesic potency as 60 mg of codeine and about 1/50th the antagonistic activity of nalorphine.[74] Pentazocine is also an agonist at the κ-receptor, and this may be responsible for the higher percentage of patients that experience dysphoria with pentazocine versus morphine.[75] Some evidence also exists that women respond better to κ-agonists than men.[76,77] Pentazocine is available in a 50-mg tablet along with a low dose of the antagonist naloxone 0.5 mg (Talwin NX). Naloxone 0.5 mg orally is expected to have no pharmacological effect but is included to dissuade IV drug abusers from dissolving and injecting Talwin NX.

4-Phenylpiperidines and 4-Anilidopiperidines

Further structural simplification of the benzomorphan ring system, via removal of the B ring of the benzomorphans yields the 4-substituted piperidines. The resultant structures are flexible and, without the B ring locking the A ring in an axial position relative to the piperidine (D) ring, the A ring can exist in either an axial or an equatorial position. Much SAR work has been conducted on theses compounds, and the reader is referred to Casy's book for a detailed review.[62]

MEPERIDINE

Meperidine (Demerol) (Fig. 24.9) was discovered in 1939 during a serendipitous screening of compounds being studied for antispasmodic activity. Mice given meperidine were noted to carry their tails in an erect position (the Straub tail reaction), which was indicative of narcotic analgesia. This led to the study of meperidine and derivatives as analgesic agents. Meperidine was found to have low potency at the receptor compared with morphine (0.2%) but much higher penetration into the brain resulting in a compound with about 10% of the potency of morphine.[41] Meperidine is an agonist at the μ-receptor and a 300-mg oral or 75-mg IV dose is reported to be equianalgesic with morphine 30-mg oral or 10-mg IV dose.

The 4-ethyl ester was found to be the optimal length for analgesic potency. Increasing or decreasing the chain length decreased activity.[41] Structural changes that increase the potency of meperidine include the introduction of an m-hydroxyl on the phenyl ring, substituting the methyl on the N for a phenylethyl or a *p*-aminophenylethyl.[41] Replacing the *N*-methyl with an *N*-allyl or *N*-cyclopropylmethyl group does not generate an antagonist, unlike the similar substitution of the morphine congeners. Meperidine quickly penetrates the blood-brain barrier and thus has a quick onset of activity and a high abuse potential. Meperidine is metabolized to normeperidine (Fig. 24.10) by the liver enzymes CYP3A4 and CYP2C18 and in the brain by CYP2B6. Meperidine and normeperidine are also metabolized by liver carboxylesterases.[78,79] The metabolism to normeperidine has clinical consequences. The duration of analgesia of meperidine may be shorter than the 3- to 4-hour half-life of the drug. This may necessitate frequent dosing to relieve pain, and thus the excessive formation of normeperidine. Normeperidine has been shown to cause central nervous system (CNS) excitation that presents clinically as tremors, twitches, "shaky feelings," and multifocal myoclonus potentially followed by grand mal seizures.[80] Patients at the greatest risk of developing normeperidine toxicity are those that are on high doses, long durations (greater than 3 days), have

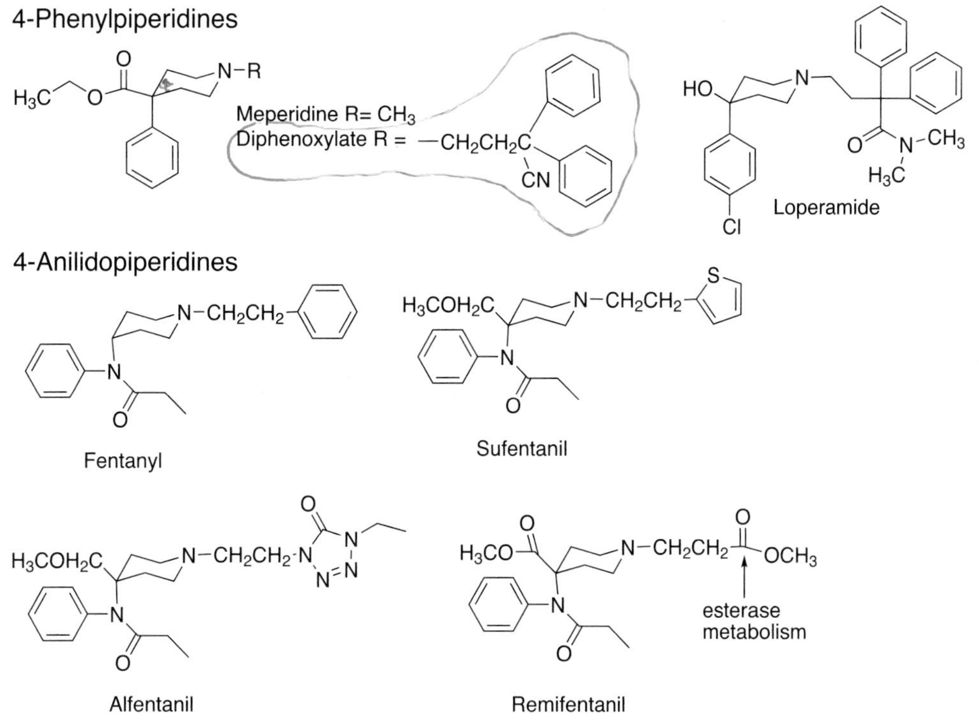

4-Phenylpiperidines

Meperidine R= CH₃
Diphenoxylate R = —CH₂CH₂C(CN)(phenyl)₂

Loperamide

4-Anilidopiperidines

Fentanyl

Sufentanil

Alfentanil

Remifentanil

esterase metabolism

Figure 24.9 ● 4-Phenylpiperidines and 4-anilidopiperidines.

renal dysfunction, thus cannot eliminate the normeperidine, and those on CYP inducers.[81]

In addition to the CNS toxicity of normeperidine, meperidine has also been found to be a weak serotonin reuptake inhibitor and has been involved in serotonin toxicity reactions when used with monoamine oxidase inhibitors or serotonin reuptake inhibitors.[82] Meperidine is available in tablet, liquid, and injectable forms. The use of meperidine should be limited to those patients that have true allergies to the morphine-type opioids, and patients should be monitored for toxicity.

DIPHENOXYLATE

Diphenoxylate (Fig. 24.9) is a weak opioid agonist and is available combined with atropine (Lomotil) for use as an antidiarrheal agent. At low doses, the opioid effect is minimal,

and the atropine is added to dissuade abuse. One study found both codeine and loperamide to be superior to diphenoxylate for treating chronic diarrhea.[83] The manufacturer has strict dosing guidelines for pediatric use because opioid intoxication and deaths from diphenoxylate have been reported.[84]

LOPERAMIDE

Loperamide (Imodium) is a 4-phenylypiperidine with a methadone-like structure attached to the piperidine nitrogen (Fig. 24.9). It acts as an antidiarrheal by directly binding to the opiate receptors in the gut wall. Loperamide inhibits acetylcholine and prostaglandin release, decreasing peristalsis and fluid secretion thus increasing the GI transit time and reducing the volume of fecal matter.[85,86] Loperamide is

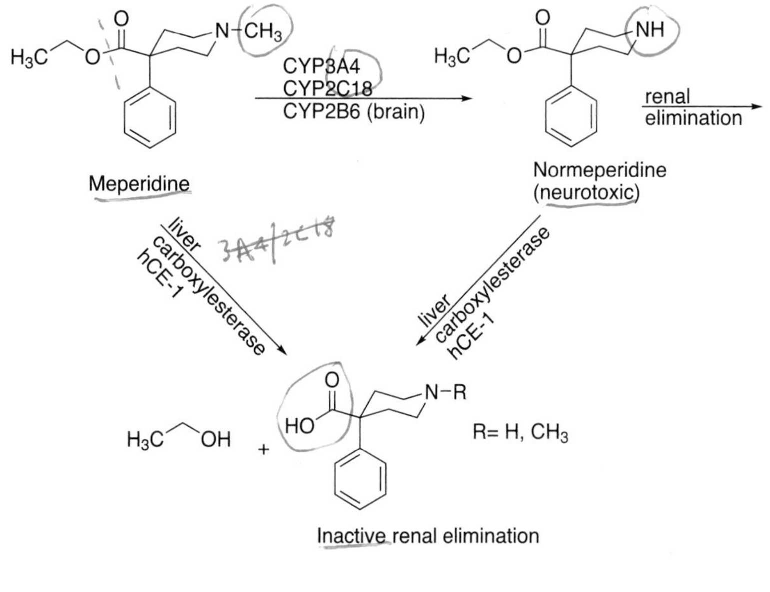

Figure 24.10 ● Metabolism of meperidine.

sufficiently lipophilic to cross the blood-brain barrier, yet it displays no CNS-opioid effects. The reason for this is that it is actively pumped out of the brain via the P-glycoprotein pump (MDR1).[87] Knockout mice with the P-glycoprotein pump genetically removed were given radiolabeled loperamide and sacrificed 4 hours later. The [^{3}H]loperamide concentrations were measured and compared with wild-type mice. A 13.5-fold increase in loperamide concentration was found in the brain of the knockouts. In addition, the mice lacking the P-glycoprotein pump displayed pronounced signs of central opiate agonism.[87] Loperamide is available as 2-mg capsules for treatment of acute and chronic diarrhea. Recommended dosage is 4 mg initially, with 2 mg after each loose stool for a maximum of 16 mg/d.

FENTANYL

When the 4-phenyl substituent of meperidine was replaced with a 4-aniline with a nitrogen connection, the potency increased. This led to the development of the 4-anilidopiperidine series of compounds seen in Figure 24.9. Fentanyl (Sublimaze) was the first compound marketed and was found to be almost 500 times more potent than meperidine. The high lipophilicity of fentanyl gave it a quick onset, and the quick metabolism led to a short duration of action. The combination of potency, quick onset, and quick recovery led to the use of fentanyl as an adjunct anesthetic. In addition to the injectable formulation, fentanyl is available in a unique transdermal system (Duragesic). This formulation is beneficial to many chronic pain sufferers unable to take oral medication. The transdermal system releases fentanyl from the drug reservoir patch into the skin, forming a depot layer. The fentanyl is then absorbed into the systemic circulation. Patches are replaced every 72 hours, and serum concentrations of fentanyl can be maintained relatively constant. A transmucosal lollipop form (Actiq) for breakthrough pain only in opioid tolerant cancer patients is also available.

The SAR studies of the 4-phenylpiperidine analgesics found that the propionamide is the optimal chain length. Adding polar groups to the 4-piperidine carbon (CH$_2$OCH$_3$ in sufentanil and alfentanil, COOCH$_3$ in remifentanil) increases potency. The piperidine nitrogen of fentanyl contains a phenethyl substituent that appears to be the correct chain length for optimal potency. Molecular docking studies speculate that the phenethyl group of fentanyl binds to a crevice between TM2 and TM3 of the μ-opioid receptor. This model also aligns the cationic nitrogen of fentanyl with the conserved Asp but leaves the aromatic pocket of the ring unoccupied.[88] Substituting the *N*-phenethyl group with bioisosteres led to the development of fentanyl congeners alfentanil, sufentanil, and remifentanil.

ALFENTANIL

The addition of a methoxy methyl on the 4-piperidine and the substitution of the phenethyl ring for an ethyl-substituted tetrazole-one yielded a compound with about one fourth to one third the potency of fentanyl (Fig. 24.9). Although less potent, it has a quicker onset of action, a shorter duration of action, and thus a better, safety profile for use as an anesthetic adjunct. The piperidine amine has a pK$_a$ of 6.5 compared with fentanyl's pK$_a$ of 8.4. This results in a higher proportion of unionized drug for alfentanil leading to quicker penetration through the blood-brain barrier and thus onset of action.[41] Alfentanil (Alfenta) is available as an IV injection for use as an analgesic adjunct for induction of general anesthesia and to maintain analgesia during general surgical procedures.

SUFENTANIL

Sufentanil (Sufenta) contains the same 4 methoxy methyl substituent as alfentanil along with an isosteric replacement of the phenyl of the phenethyl group with a thiophene ring (Fig. 24.9). The resulting compound is about 7 times more potent than fentanyl with an immediate onset of action and a similar recovery time compared with fentanyl. Sufentanil is only available in an injectable formulation and is also used as an anesthetic adjunct.

REMIFENTANIL

Remifentanil (Ultiva) was designed as a "soft drug." Soft drugs are designed to undergo metabolism quickly and thus have ultrashort durations of action. In place of the ethyl aromatic ring seen on the other piperidine opioids, remifentanil has an ester group (Fig. 24.9). This ester group is metabolized by esterases in the blood and tissue to a weakly active metabolite (1:300–1:1,000 the potency of remifentanil).[89] The n-octanol/water partition coefficient of remifentanil is 17.9. The pK$_a$ of remifentanil is 7.07, thus it is predominately unionized at physiological pH. Both of these properties account for its rapid distribution across the blood-brain barrier (<1 minute). The ester hydrolysis leads to a quick recovery (5–10 minutes) independent of duration of drug administration, renal, or liver function. The favorable pharmacodynamics of remifentanil have led to its use for induction and maintenance of surgical anesthesia.

Diphenylheptanes

METHADONE

Methadone (Dolophine) (Fig. 24.11) is a synthetic opioid approved for analgesic therapy and for the maintenance and treatment of opioid addiction. Methadone is marketed as the

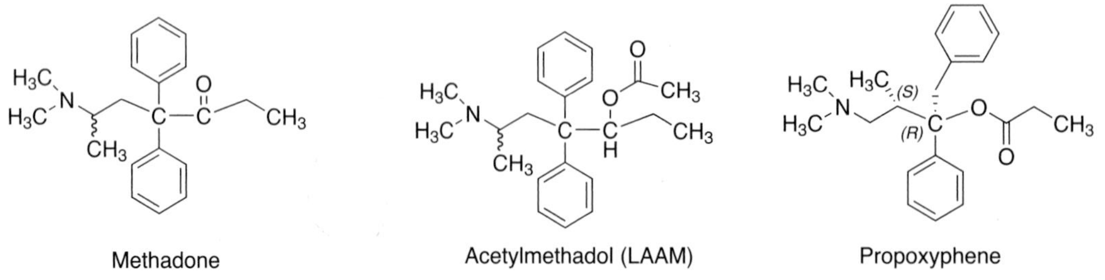

Figure 24.11 ● Diphenylheptanes.

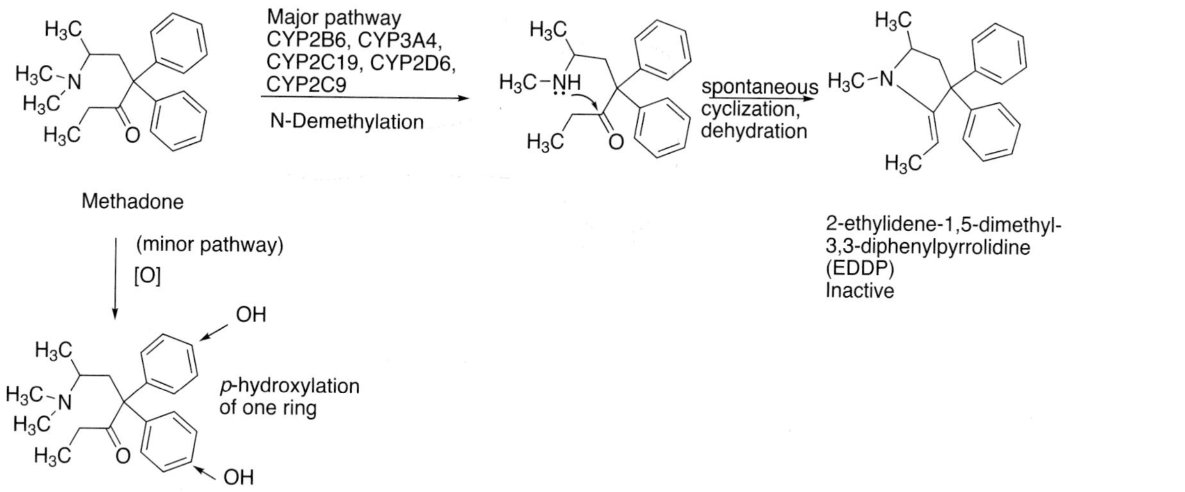

Figure 24.12 ● Metabolism of methadone.

racemate, although the opioid activity resides in the R-enantiomer (7–50 times more potent than the S-enantiomer). Methadone may only be dispensed for the treatment of opioid addiction by a program certified by the Federal Substance Abuse and Mental Health Services Administration. Methadone is a μ-receptor agonist with complex and highly variable pharmacokinetic parameters. Bioavailability following oral administration ranges from 36% to 100%. Steady-state volume of distribution ranges between 1.0 to 8.0 L/kg. Methadone is highly bound to plasma α_1-acid glycoprotein (85%–90%), and $t_{1/2}$ elimination ranged between 8 and 59 hours. The wide range in parameters leads to difficulty when trying to switch from one opioid to methadone for either treatment of pain or substance abuse. Methadone doses and administration schedules need to be individualized and closely monitored. The metabolism and elimination of methadone also lead to much interpatient variability and can be effected by genetic CYP levels, drug–drug interactions, and the pH of the urine (Fig. 24.12).[90] The major metabolic pathway of methadone metabolism is via *N*-demethylation to an unstable product that spontaneously cyclizes to form the inactive 2-ethylidene-1,5-dimethyl-3,3-diphenylpyrrolidine (EDDP). Initial reports concluded that CYP3A4 was the major isoform responsible for this pathway, but more recent reports indicate that CYP2B6 is primarily responsible for the *N*-demethylation.[91–95]

Adverse effects of methadone include all of the standard opioid effects including constricted pupils, respiratory depression, physical dependence, extreme somnolence, coma, cardiac arrest, and death. In addition, QT interval prolongation and torsades de pointes have been reported. The QT interval prolongation reported for methadone was also observed in another diphenylheptane, levomethadyl, or levo-α-acetylmethadol (LAAM) (Orlaam) that was also used to treat opioid addiction. The severe cardiac-related adverse events resulted in the removal of LAAM from the U.S. market in 2003.

PROPOXYPHENE

Most of the structural changes to the methadone skeleton resulted in compounds with decreased opioid potencies, thus most of these compounds, with the exception of LAAM were not developed. Propoxyphene is a derivative of methadone marketed in 1957 as the enantiomerically pure (2S, 3R)-4-(Dimethylamino)-3-methyl-1,2,-diphenyl-2-butanol propionate (ester). It is only about 1/10th as potent as morphine as an analgesic yet retains all the same opioid adverse effects. One propoxyphene 65-mg capsule has the same analgesic effect of 650 mg of aspirin or 1,000 mg of acetaminophen, thus overdoses of propoxyphene can occur if patients do not follow the prescribed dose. Between 1981 and 1999, 2,110 accidental deaths were reported because of propoxyphene. Propoxyphene and all propoxyphene combination products are listed using the Beers criteria as medications to avoid in patients older than 65 years of age.[96] The metabolism of propoxyphene also contributes to the potential dangers of the drug. Propoxyphene is metabolized via *N*-demethylation to form norpropoxyphene. Norpropoxyphene has been shown to build up in cardiac tissues and result in naloxone-insensitive cardiotoxicity.[97] The weak analgesic action and potential risk to the patient have some health practitioners advocating to remove all drugs containing propoxyphene from the market.[98] The hydrochloride salt is marketed as Darvon, the napsylate salt as Darvon-N, both salts are also available combined with acetaminophen (Darvocet, Darvocet-N) and a propoxyphene, aspirin, caffeine product is also available.

Miscellaneous

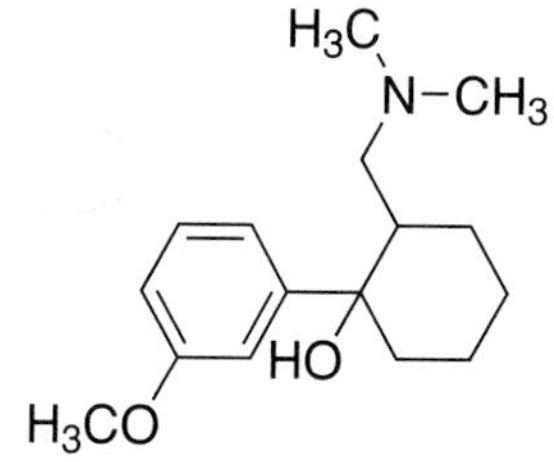

(+/-)Tramadol

TRAMADOL

Tramadol (Ultram) is an analgesic agent with multiple mechanisms of action. It is a weak μ-agonist with approximately 30% of the analgesic effect antagonized by the opioid antagonist naloxone. Used at recommended doses, it has minimal effects on respiratory rate, heart rate, blood pressure, or GI transit times. Structurally, tramadol resembles codeine with the B, D, and E ring removed. The manufacturer states that patients allergic to codeine should not receive tramadol, because they may be at increased risk for anaphylactic reactions.[99] Tramadol is synthesized and marketed as the racemic mixture of two (the [2S, 3S] [-] and the [2R, 3R] [+]) of the four possible enantiomers.[100] The (+) enantiomer is about 30 times more potent than the (−) enantiomer; however, racemic tramadol shows improved tolerability.[101,102] Neurotransmitter reuptake inhibition is also responsible for some of the analgesic activity with the (−) enantiomer primarily responsible for norepinephrine reuptake and the (+) enantiomer responsible for inhibiting serotonin reuptake.[101,103] Like codeine, tramadol is O-demethylated via CYP2D6 to a more potent opioid agonist having 200-fold higher affinity for the opioid receptor than the parent compound. Tramadol was initially marketed as nonaddictive, and a 3-year follow up study showed that the abuse potential is very low, but not zero. Most abusers of tramadol have abused opioid drugs in the past.[104] Both enantiomers of tramadol and the major O-demethylated metabolite are proconvulsive, and tramadol should not be used in patients with a low-seizure threshold including patients with epilepsy.[101]

Mixed Agonist/Antagonist

Nalbuphine

NALBUPHINE

Nalbuphine (Nubain) is structurally a member of the phenanthrene class of compounds and resembles oxymorphone with a cyclobutyl methyl group on the nitrogen, equivalent to naloxone's substitution. It was introduced in 1979 as an agonist/antagonist with the hope of becoming an effective pain reliever with little abuse potential. Although the abuse potential of nalbuphine is low, it is not zero, and increasing reports of diversion and abuse can be found in the literature and the Internet.[105] At low parenteral doses (<0.5 mg), it has an analgesic potency approximately two thirds that of morphine, and it has a similar degree of respiratory depression. However, escalating doses above 30 mg does not produce further respiratory depression.[106] The oral bioavailability of nalbuphine is only 12%, and the drug is only marketed as an injectable.[107] Patents have been filed for an oral extended-release formulation, and it is presently in phase II testing.[108] The pharmacologic profile of nalbuphine in animal studies includes agonist activity at the κ-receptor and antagonist activity at the μ-receptor.[109] Clinical studies have shown that nalbuphine, and κ-agonists in general, may have better analgesic activity in female patients compared with male patients.[77] Used as the sole opioid agent, nalbuphine has been used successfully to treat the pain of labor, cesarean section, dental extraction, hip replacement, and hysterectomy surgery.[110] Nalbuphine also may have a role in

treating opioid-induced pruritus, because it can reverse the pruritus without reversing the analgesic effect when used in low doses. Nalbuphine is marketed as an injectable (10 and 20 mg/mL). The usual dose is 10 mg administered subcutaneously, intramuscularly, or intravenously at 3- to 6-hour intervals, with a maximal daily dose of 160 mg.

Butorphanol

BUTORPHANOL

Structurally, butorphanol is a morphinan and shares the same cyclobutyl methyl group on the nitrogen as nalbuphine. Like nalbuphine, butorphanol is an agonist at the κ-receptor but at the μ-receptor butorphanol is both a partial agonist and an antagonist.[111] The affinity for opioid receptors in vitro is 1:4:25 for the μ-, δ-, and κ-receptors respectively.[111] The high affinity for the κ-receptors is proposed to give butorphanol its analgesic properties and is also responsible for the CNS adverse effects such as hallucinations, psychosis, and paranoid reactions. Butorphanol binds with μ-receptors as a partial agonist, and administration to humans maintained on high-potency μ-agonists such as morphine may precipitate withdrawal. Butorphanol was found to produce convulsions in morphine-deprived, morphine-dependent monkeys.[112]

The parenteral injection is used for moderate to severe pain associated with orthopedic procedures, obstetric surgery, and burns. The recommended dose is 1 mg IV or 2 mg intramuscular (IM) every 3 to 4 hours as needed. Early studies proposed a "ceiling effect" for butorphanol's antinociception and respiratory depressant effect. More recently, the WHO Expert Committee on Drug Dependence performed a critical review of butorphanol and found no ceiling effect to the respiratory depressant effect of parenteral butorphanol in monkeys and humans.[112] The nasal preparation (Stadol NS) is an effective analgesic for the relief of moderate to severe pain such as migraine attacks, dental, or other surgical pain where an opioid is appropriate. The nasal spray is administered 1 mg (1 spray in one nostril) with an additional spray 60 to 90 minutes later if adequate pain relief is not achieved. Respiratory depression is not an issue with normal doses of the nasal preparation, but CNS side effects are the same as parenteral butorphanol. Increased reports of abuse and addiction of the nasal spray led the FDA to change the product to a Schedule IV drug in 1997.

Buprenorphine

BUPRENORPHINE

Buprenorphine is a semisynthetic, highly lipophilic opiate derived from thebaine. Pharmacologically, it is classified as a mixed μ-agonist/antagonist (a partial agonist) and a weak κ-antagonist. It has a high affinity for the μ-receptors (1,000 times greater than morphine) and a slow dissociation rate leading to its long duration of action (6–8 hours).[113] At recommended doses, it acts as an agonist at the μ-receptor with approximately 0.3 mg IV equianalgesic to 10 mg of IV morphine. One study in humans found that buprenorphine displays a ceiling effect to the respiratory depression, but not the analgesic effect over a dose range of 0.05 to 0.6 mg.[114] In practice, this makes buprenorphine a safer opiate (when used alone) than pure μ-agonists. Relatively few deaths from buprenorphine overdose (when used alone) have been reported.[113] The tight binding of the drug to the receptor also has led to mixed reports on the effectiveness of using naloxone to reverse the respiratory depression. In animal studies, normal doses of the pure antagonist naloxone were unable to remove buprenorphine from the receptor site and precipitate withdrawal. In a human study designed to precipitate withdrawal from buprenorphine, a naloxone dose (mean = 35 mg) 100 times the dose usually needed to precipitate withdrawal in methadone-dependent subjects was used. For comparison, approximately 0.3 mg, 4 mg, 4 mg, and 10 mg of naloxone would be required to precipitate withdrawal from heroin, butorphanol, nalbuphine, or pentazocine respectively.[115]

The unique pharmacologic and pharmacokinetic profile of buprenorphine made it a drug of interest for the treatment of opioid dependence. The first study of buprenorphine for this purpose was published in 1978 and confirmed that buprenorphine was an acceptable alternative to methadone for addicts and that it blocked the effects of large single doses of morphine for at least 24 hours.[116] Early clinical studies showed that the oral bioavailability of buprenorphine was low because of intestinal and liver metabolism. Therefore, a sublingual (SL) formulation (Subutex) was developed that would bypass this metabolism. The SL tablet has a bioavailability of 55% but varies widely among individuals.[116] SL buprenorphine is also available combined with naloxone (Suboxone) in sufficient quantity (25% of the buprenorphine dose) to discourage crushing and injecting the SL tablet. SL naloxone is 0% to 10% bioavailable, and it does not change the absorption or action of the SL buprenorphine. Abrupt withdrawal of chronically administered buprenorphine produces mild to moderate opioid withdrawal symptoms peaking between 3 and 5 days following the last buprenorphine dose. These symptoms require no therapeutic intervention. Suboxone and Subutex are the first medications approved for office-based treatment of opioid dependence under the Drug Addiction Treatment Act of 2000. U.S. pharmacists may only dispense these medications when prescribed by physicians that meet special train-

ing criteria and are registered with the Center for Substance Abuse Treatment, a component of the Substance Abuse and Mental Health Services Administration. A transdermal buprenorphine patch is available outside the United States for use in chronic pain.[117] This product is currently undergoing phase III clinical trials in the United States.

Buprenorphine is oxidatively metabolized by *N*-dealkylation by hepatic CYP3A4 and to a lesser extent CYP2C8 to the active metabolite norbuprenorphine. Both the parent and major metabolite undergo glucuronidation at the phenolic-3 position. Minor metabolites include hydroxylation of the aromatic ring of buprenorphine and norbuprenorphine at an unspecified site.[118]

Opioid Antagonists

NALTREXONE

Naltrexone (Fig. 24.13) is a pure opioid antagonist at all opioid receptor subtypes with the highest affinity for the μ-receptor. Naltrexone is orally bioavailable and blocks the effects of opiate agonists for approximately 24 hours after a single dose of 50 mg. It produces no opioid agonist effects and is devoid of any intrinsic actions other than opioid receptor blockade. Theoretically, it should work well to treat opioid dependence but in clinical practice, patients have shown poor compliance and high relapse rates. Naltrexone has also been studied to treat alcohol dependence with mixed results. To address the compliance issues and effectively remove the "choice" of taking the antagonist, naltrexone was developed into an extended-release injectable microsphere formulation for IM injection once a month (Vivitrol). This formulation provides steady-state plasma concentrations of naltrexone threefold to fourfold higher than the 50-mg oral dose 4 times a day.[119] Currently, Vivitrol is only indicated for the treatment of alcohol dependence. A Cochrane review found insufficient evidence from randomized controlled trials to evaluate its effectiveness for treating opioid dependence.[120] Currently, phase II and phase III clinical trials of an implantable pellet form of naltrexone are being conducted for treating opioid dependence.

The CYP450 system is not involved in naltrexone metabolism. Naltrexone is reduced to the active antagonist 6-β-naltrexol by dihydrodiol dehydrogenase, a cytosolic enzyme. Naltrexone has a black box warning, because it has the potential to cause hepatocellular injury when given in excessive doses.[119]

NALOXONE

Naloxone (Narcan) (Fig. 24.13) is a pure antagonist at all opioid receptor subtypes. Structurally, it resembles oxymorphone except that the methyl group on the nitrogen is replaced by an allyl group. This minor structural change

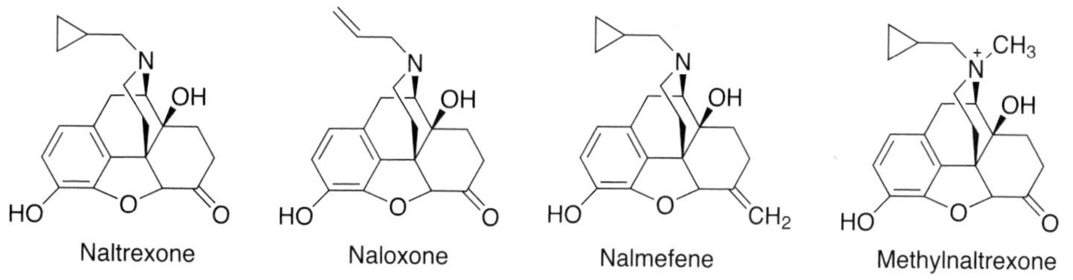

Figure 24.13 ● Opioid antagonists.

Naltrexone   Naloxone   Nalmefene   Methylnaltrexone

retains high binding affinity to the receptor, but no intrinsic activity. It is used to reverse the respiratory depressant effects of opioid overdoses.

Naloxone is administered intravenously with an onset of action within 2 minutes. Because it is competing with the opioid for the receptor sites, the dose and frequency of administration will depend on the amount and type of narcotic being antagonized. Overdoses of long-acting opioids (methadone) may require multiple IV doses of naloxone or continuous infusions. Neonates born to opioid-exposed mothers may be given IV naloxone at birth to reverse the effects of opiates.

Very few metabolism studies on naloxone have been conducted, although the major metabolite found in the urine is naloxone-3-glucuronide.[121,122]

NALMEFENE

Nalmefene (Revex) is a pure opioid antagonist that is the 6-methylene analog of naltrexone. It is available as a solution for IV, IM, or subcutaneous (SC) administration to reverse the effects of opioids after general anesthesia and in the treatment of overdose. It is longer acting than naloxone but otherwise has a similar pharmacodynamic and metabolic (3-glucuronidation) profile. Nalmefene has higher oral bioavailability (approximately 40%)[123] than naloxone or naltrexone and is currently being investigated as an oral treatment for pathological gambling[124] and alcohol abuse.[125]

METHYLNALTREXONE

Methylnaltrexone (Relistor) is the methylated, quaternary form of naltrexone (Fig. 24.13). The permanently charged nitrogen prevents the drug from crossing the blood-brain barrier. Thus, it only acts as an antagonist at peripheral opioid receptors. Relistor was approved in April 2008 to treat opioid-induced constipation in patients receiving palliative care. It is administered as a SC injection once every other day.

● NONSTEROIDAL ANTI-INFLAMMATORY DRUGS

NSAIDs including aspirin and acetaminophen, two of the oldest pain medications, are among the most widely prescribed drugs worldwide for the treatment of rheumatic arthritis and other degenerative inflammatory joint diseases.[126,127] Although NSAIDs are very effective in relieving mild to moderate pains and inflammation, their use is also often associated with many undesirable side effects, including GI irritation and bleeding, platelet dysfunction, kidney damage, and bronchospasm.[126–129]

With the exception of acetaminophen (Tylenol) and the newer "coxibs" drugs, the conventional NSAIDs (also commonly referred to as the *aspirin-like drugs*), share very similar therapeutic and side effect profiles. The conventional NSAIDs exert their therapeutic action by inhibiting two isoforms of cyclooxygenase (COX-1, the constitutive isozyme and COX-2, the inducible isozyme), which is the rate-limiting enzyme responsible for the biosynthesis of the proinflammatory prostaglandins (PGs) such as the PGD_2, PGE_2,

$PGF_{2\alpha}$, and PGI_2 and thereby modulating pain transmission, attenuating inflammation, and reducing fever.[127,128] They also produce their undesirable side effects such as GI bleeding, ulcerations, or renal impairments by blocking the same cyclooxygenases responsible for synthesizing PGs that modulate platelet activity (TXA_2 and PGI_2), gastric acid secretion and cytoprotection (PGE_2 and PGI_2), and renal blood flow (PGE_2).[128–132]

In early 1990, Vane et al.[133,134] hypothesized that the undesirable side effects of the conventional NSAIDs are a result of inhibition of the COX-1 isozyme, whereas the therapeutic effects are related mainly to their inhibitory action on the inducible COX-2 isozyme. This hypothesis has stimulated extensive drug development and hasty market introductions of many selective COX-2 inhibitors, or coxibs drugs.[130,135] However, all of the marketed coxibs drugs except celecoxib (Celebrex), the first FDA-approved COX-2 drug in 1998, have been withdrawn from the market because of the potential risk of a cardiovascular event, including heart attack or stroke, especially in cardiac patients.[136] Recent clinical trials have placed all NSAIDs under surveillance for their potential cardiovascular risk, thus the indiscriminate use of any NSAIDs including naproxen in cardiac patients should be avoided.[135–137]

Mechanism of Action and NSAID-Induced Side Effects

For aspirin and many of the conventional NSAIDs, despite their worldwide use as pain medications for over a century, their mechanism of action was not completely known until 1971 when Vane first identified the cyclooxygenases as their molecular targets.[128] Cyclooxygenase (also known as prostaglandin endoperoxide synthase or PGH synthase) is the rate-limiting enzyme responsible for the biosynthesis of PGs.

PGs are short-lived, lipidlike molecules that play a vital role in modulating many important physiological and pathophysiological functions including pain, inflammation, gastric acid secretion, wound healing, and renal function. They are biosynthesized via a tissue-specific cyclooxygenase pathway (COX-1 or COX-2) either on an as-needed basis (mostly via the COX-1 isozyme) or via the induced and overexpressed COX-2 isozyme because of an injury, inflammation, or infection.[126,129] Some of the salient features of the cyclooxygenase pathway involved in the biosynthesis of these PGs from arachidonic acid (AA) (5,8,11,14-eicosatetraenoic acid), a polyunsaturated fatty acid released from membrane phospholipids by the action of phospholipase A_2, are depicted in Figure 24.14.

As stated earlier, all classes of NSAIDs strongly inhibit prostaglandin synthesis in various tissues, especially at the site of the tissue damage or inflammation. This inhibition occurs at the stage of oxidative cyclization of AA, catalyzed by the rate-limiting enzyme, cyclooxygenase (or PGH synthase), to the hydroperoxy-endoperoxide (prostaglandin G_2, PGG_2) and its subsequent reduction to key intermediate, prostaglandin H_2 (PGH_2) needed for all prostaglandin biosynthesis.[138]

Blockade of PGH_2 production, thus prevents its further conversion, by tissue-specific terminal prostaglandin synthases or isomerases, into different biologically active PGs

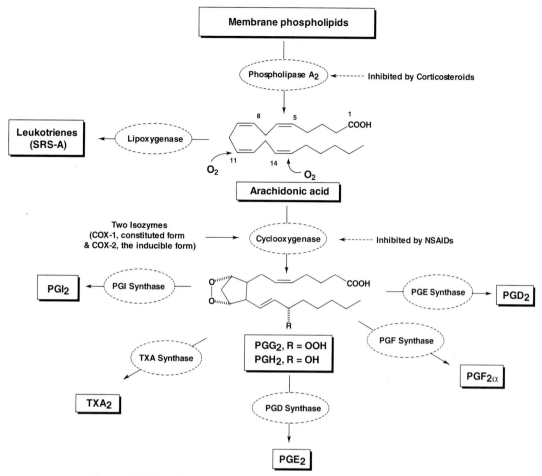

Figure 24.14 ● Conversion of arachidonic acid to prostaglandins.

including PGE$_2$, PGD$_2$, PGF$_{2\alpha}$, PGI$_2$ (prostacyclin), and thromboxane A$_2$ (TXA$_2$) (Fig. 24.14).[138,139]

Among the PGs synthesized by the action of either COX-1 or COX-2 isozymes, PGI$_2$ and PGE$_2$ made at the site of injury (via COX-2 isozyme in the inflammatory cells such as monocytes and macrophages) and also in the brain, are known to play a dominant role in mediating inflammation and inducing hyperanalgesia.[132] However, their synthesis in the GI tract (via COX-1 isozyme) and in the renal tubules (via COX-1 and COX-2 isozymes), is essential to provide cytoprotective action for restoring the integrity of the stomach lining and maintaining renal functions in an otherwise compromised kidney as a result of constant insult.[132,138] Thus, inhibition of PGE$_2$ synthesis by the conventional NSAIDs in the parietal cells removes its ability to modulate histamine-mediated release of gastric acid from the parietal cells, whereas blockade of PGI$_2$ and PGE$_2$ synthesis in the epithelial cells in the stomach linings also prevents their action on the biosynthesis and release of bicarbonate and mucous gel desperately needed to repair damage resulting from erosion caused by gastric acid and other aggressive factors.[127,129,132] Thus, it should not be surprising to note that NSAID-induced gastric ulcers can only be prevented clinically with coadministration of misoprostol, a stable PGE analog, but not with either the histamine H$_2$-antagonists, sucralfate, or any proton pump inhibitors such as omeprazole.[127] Furthermore, maintenance of kidney function,

especially in patients with congestive heart failure, liver cirrhosis, or renal insufficiency, is reliant on the action of PGI$_2$ and PGE$_2$ to restore normal renal blood flow. Thus, NSAID use (both COX-1 and COX-2 inhibitors) will increase the risk of renal ischemia and therefore is contraindicated in these patients.[129]

The readers should consult Chapter 26 of this text on "Prostanglandins, Leukotrienes, and Other Eicosanoids" for a detailed discussion of PGs, their physiological and pathophysiological functions, and their corresponding PG receptors.

Structure–Activity Relationships of NSAIDs

It is well established that the therapeutic potency of the conventional NSAIDs are highly correlated with their ability to induce upper GI toxicity.[127] But, are all NSAIDs other than coxibs really equally effective in the treatment of pain and inflammation? Some insight might be found by exploring how these chemically diverse classes of drugs bind to their molecular targets (i.e., their selectivity for COX-2 relative to COX-1).[140] Thus, the benefit/risk profile of individual NSAIDs, as reflected by their COX selectivity, may be more clinically relevant for predicting the risk of GI complications. Table 24.1 summarizes a few representative drugs from different NSAID classes with their recommended daily

TABLE 24.1 Comparison of Relative Risk of NSAID-Induced Gastrointestinal Complication

Drug	Trade Name	Dosing Range (Total Daily Dose)	Relative Risk for GI complication	COX-2/COX-1 Selectivity Ratio
Not on NSAIDs or Aspirin			1.0	—
Celecoxib	Celebrex	100–200 mg BID[a] (200–400 mg)	—	0.7
Meloxicam	Mobic	7.5–15 mg daily	—	0.37
Ibuprofen	Advil, Motrin	200–600 mg TID[b] (0.6–1.8 g)	2.9 (1.7–5.0)	0.9
Sulindac	Clinoril	150–200 mg BID (300–600 mg)	2.9 (1.5–5.6)	29 (on active sulfide)
Aspirin	—	325–650 mg QID[c] (1.3–2.6 g)	3,1 (2.0–4.8)	>100
Naproxen	Aleve, Naprosyn	125–500 mg BID (0.5–1.0 g)	3.1 (1.7–5.9)	3.0
Diclofenac	Voltaren	25–50 mg TID (75–150 mg)	3.9 (2.3–6.5)	0.5
Ketoprofen	Orudis	50–100 mg TID (150–300 mg)	5.4 (2.6–11.3)	61
Indomethacin	Indocin	25–50 mg TID (75–150 mg)	6.3 (3.3–12.2)	80
Piroxicam	Feldene	10–20 mg daily	18.0 (8.2–39.6)	3.3

[a]BID, bis in die (twice a day).
[b]TID, ter in die (3 times a day).
[c]QID, quater in die (4 times a day).

dosages and their relative risks of bleeding peptic ulcer complications.[130,141,142]

ENZYMATIC STRUCTURE OF CYCLOOXYGENASES

Cyclooxygenases (COX-1 and COX-2) are heme-containing, membrane-bound proteins that share a high degree of sequence identity and also have very similar active site topography.[138,143–145] Note that the homologous residues of the COX-2 isozyme are numbered in parallel with the similar amino acid residues found at the active site of COX-1 isozyme for easier comparison of their structural differences in the following discussion (i.e., the actual Arg-106 of human COX-2 [hCOX-2] is numbered as Arg-120).[143] The actual hCOX-2 assignments for these residues are provided in parentheses.

Thus, despite their similarity, the active site for hCOX-2 is approximately 20% larger than the COX-1 binding site because of the replacement of Ile-523 in COX-1 with a smaller Val-523 in hCOX-2 (Val-509).[138,144,145] There are a total of 24 amino acid residues lining the largely hydrophobic AA binding site with only one difference between the isozymes (i.e., Ile-523 in COX-1 and Val-509 in hCOX-2). The hCOX-2 isozyme has an additional hydrophilic side pocket accessible for drug binding, extended from the main binding pocket.[143] The size and nature of this hydrophilic side pocket for binding in hCOX-2 is a result of further substitutions Ile-434 and His-513 in COX-1 with a smaller Val-434 (Val 420 in hCOX-2) and a more basic Arg-513 (Arg-499 in hCOX-2).[146] Thus, it is not surprising that this basic amino acid residue in hCOX-2 (Arg-499) may provide an additional binding interaction for selective COX-2 inhibitors such as celecoxib.[144] Although there is only a very limited amount of published data showing how the substrate, AA, binds to cyclooxygenases, the relative positioning of the double bonds in AA at the active site, proposed by Gund and Shen based on the conformational analysis of indomethacin and other conventional NSAIDs, is still currently valid.[147]

Interestingly, Arg-120 (Arg-104 in hCOX-2) is the only positively charged amino acid residue in the COX active site, on one end of the active site as depicted by Luong[144,148] and is responsible for binding, via an ionic interaction, with the carboxylate anion of the substrate

(AA) or the conventional NSAIDs. The amino acid residue Tyr-385 (Tyr-371 in hCOX-2) is located on the opposite end of the COX active site and is believed to serve as the catalytic residue for activating molecular oxygen and its initial addition to the Δ^{11}-double bond of the substrate to form PGG$_2$.[143–148] Furthermore, the presence of an amino acid residue, Ser-530 (Ser-516 in hCOX-2) is believed to be involved only in the irreversible inactivation by aspirin and NSAID action but not contributing to any substrate binding.[143]

BINDING OF NSAID TO CYCLOOXYGENASE

Most NSAIDs possess a free carboxylic acid (COOH) for an ionic interaction with the positively charged arginine residue at the active site of the cyclooxygenases (i.e., Arg-120 in COX-1 or Arg-106 in COX-2 isozymes). This acidic moiety is further linked to an aromatic (or heteroaromatic) ring for binding to either the Δ^5-double-bond or Δ^8-double-bond binding regions, and an additional center of lipophilicity in the form of an alkyl chain (e.g., ibuprofen) or an additional aromatic ring (e.g., indomethacin) for binding to the Δ^{11}-double-bond binding region.

A hypothetical binding model for indomethacin and related analogs to the COX-1 isozyme is shown in Figure 24. 15-A, based on the crystallographic and SAR data found in the literature.[146,149] The suggested orientation and placement of the N-p-chlorobenzoyl group to the Δ^{11}-double-bond binding region and the indole ring to the Δ^5- and Δ^8-double-bond binding regions is made from assuming that a preferred, lower-energy conformation of indomethacin is essential for its binding to COX isozymes[147], and the fact that this orientation also allows correct positioning of the amide carbonyl oxygen for possible binding interactions to Ser-530 and the 5-methoxy group to Ser-355 at the active site of the enzymes.[146]

Additional support for this model can be obtained from the observation that the (Z)-isomer of sulindac, an indene isosteric analog of indomethacin, is much more potent than the corresponding (E)-isomer and the fact that replacement of the 5-methoxy group with a fluorine atom on the indole ring further enhances its analgesic action.[145,149] Furthermore, because there is limited space available for binding around either Leu-384 or Ile-523 (i.e., both around the Δ^{11}-double-bond binding region), it is not surprising to see a facile conversion of the indomethacin from a nonselective COX inhibitor into a potent and highly selective COX-2 inhibitor with just a simple substitution of the *p*-chlorine with a larger bromine atom or by addition of two chlorine atoms to the *o,o'* positions of the *N-p*-chlorobenzoyl group reported by Kalgutkar et al.[150] This observation can explain why a lower risk for GI complications was reported with sulindac than indomethacin, because it requires metabolic activation, via reduction of its bulky sulfoxide moiety into a much smaller methyl sulfide for binding into the Leu-384 pocket. The fact that kidneys possess a high level of the flavin-containing monooxygenases for deactivating the active metabolite of sulindac back into its inactive sulfoxide or sulfone, further provided evidence for this binding model.[149,151]

With this binding model, it is also possible to see why the relative therapeutic potency of the conventional NSAIDs and their ability to induce GI complication is in the order: indomethacin >ketoprofen ~diclofenac >naproxen >ibuprofen. Ibuprofen is the least potent because it can only bind to the Δ^5-double-bond region with additional weak van der Waals interactions to the Δ^{11}-double-bond region. Naproxen is slightly more active than ibuprofen, because its naphthalene ring, isosteric to the indole ring, can interact with both the Δ^5- and Δ^8-double-bond regions. Ketoprofen and diclofenac are slightly less potent than indomethacin because of the absence of an additional ring for binding to either the Δ^5- or the Δ^8-double-bond regions.

BINDING OF CELECOXIB TO COX-2 ISOZYME

The hypothetical binding model for binding of celecoxib, the only selective "coxibs" type COX-2 inhibitor shown on Figure 24.15B, is purely speculative, based only on the crystallographic binding data reported for SC-558 (the *p*-bromophenyl analog of celecoxib) with the murine COX-2 isozyme.[146] However, the celecoxib selectivity toward the COX-2 isozyme is most likely a result of the extension of the sulfonamide moiety into the extra hydrophilic-binding pocket, surrounded by His-90 (His-76 in hCOX-2) and Arg-513 (Arg-499 in hCOX-2). The opening of this additional pocket for binding is the result of the replacement of Ile-523

in the COX-1 with a smaller valine residue (Val 509 in hCOX-2). It should be pointed out that a similar hydrophilic pocket does exist in the COX-1 isozyme, but it is inaccessible because of the bulkier Ile-523 residue that guards the entrance to this side pocket of the COX-1 isozyme (see Fig. 24.15-A).

The COX-2/COX-1 selectivity ratios, estimated by different research groups, can be quite different (e.g., the reported selectivity ratio for celecoxib ranges any where from 0.003–0.7; for piroxicam, the range is 3.3–600). Thus, the selectivity ratios included in Table 24.1, obtained from one such study, is only valid for comparing their differences among these NSAIDs. Furthermore, recent reviews comparing the SAR among different structural classes of COX-2 inhibitors have indicated that there is little or no common pharmacophore required for their COX-2 selectivity, but minor changes within the structure type, in terms of molecular shape, lipophilicity, electronic density, flexibility, polarity, and hydrogen-bonding properties, can all have drastic effects in its COX selectivity.[152,153]

PIROXICAM AND MELOXICAM: THE DIFFERENCE IN THEIR COX SELECTIVITY

Piroxicam and meloxicam have nearly identical structural features but also have at least a ninefold difference in selectivity for meloxicam to COX-2 isozyme and an even larger difference in their relative risks for GI complications (i.e., piroxicam has the highest risk among NSAIDs, whereas meloxicam has very little or no such side effects) (Table 24.1). A closer comparison of their structure (Fig. 24.16), however, reveals no apparent reason for these differences, either in size, lipophilicity, or electronic properties, between the 2-pyridyl group (in piroxicam) and the 5-methyl-2-thiazoyl group (meloxicam) that may alter their ability to bind COX isozymes. It is unlikely that these drastic differences in their COX selectivity, especially the drug-induced GI toxicity, could be due solely to the binding of the parent molecules with such minor changes in their structures. Thus, could the observed differences, especially the differences in drug-induced GI side effects, be attributed to the involvement of an active metabolite of piroxicam and/or meloxicam?

The metabolism of piroxicam to its major active metabolite, 5'-hydroxypiroxicam and meloxicam to its

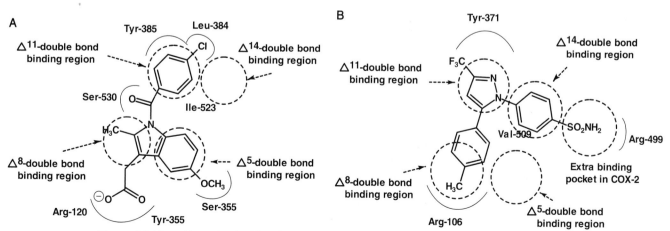

Figure 24.15 ● Hypothetical binding models of indomethacin to COX-1 and Celecoxib to COX-2. **A.** Binding of the conventional NSAID, indomethacin, to the active site of COX-1; **B.** Binding of celecoxib, a selective COX-2 inhibitor to the active site of COX-2 with crystallographic maps suggested by Luong et al. (Flexibility of the NSAID binding site in the structure of human cyclooxygenase-2. Nat. Struct. Biol. 1996;3:927–933)

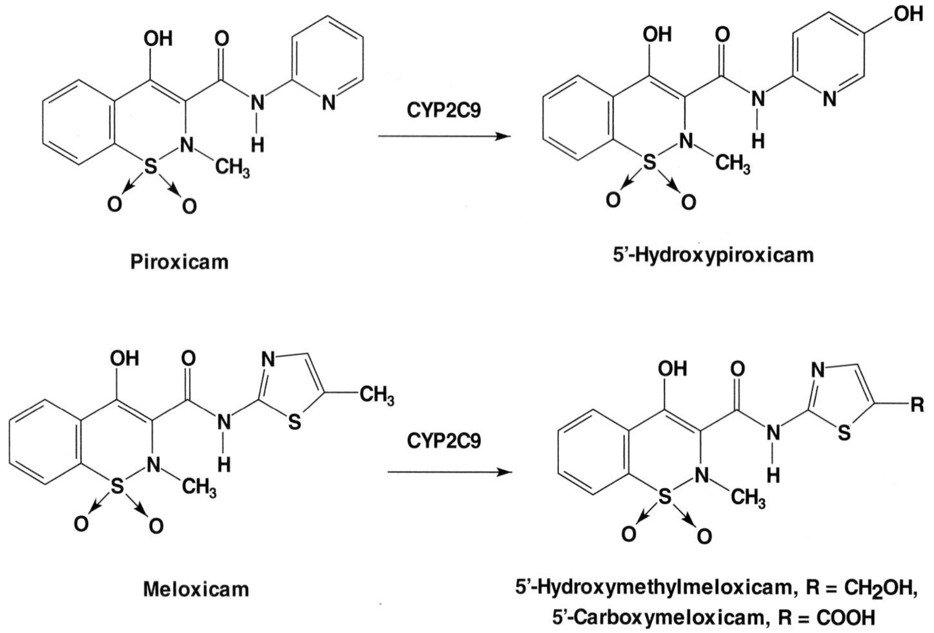

Figure 24.16 ● Metabolism of piroxicam and meloxicam.

5′-hydroxy-methylmeloxicam and 5′-carboxymeloxicam metabolites are shown in Figure 24.16.[154–156] Thus, with the proposed binding interaction of indomethacin described earlier (Fig. 24.15), it is reasonable to assume that the pyridyl group of the piroxicam or the 5′-hydroxypyridyl group of its active metabolite will be directed to bind to the Δ^{11}-double-bond binding region (especially the active metabolite caused by an additional H-bonding to the Tyr-385 residue), in a similar manner as the *N-p*-chlorobenzoyl group of the indomethacin. This would also allow the OH group of the acidic enol carboxamide moiety of the piroxicam or its active metabolite to position itself for binding to the Ser-530 residue of the COX-1 isozyme. However, a similar binding interaction of the active metabolites of meloxicam, especially the 5′carboxy metabolite, to the active site of the COX-1 isozyme may not be possible, because it will reorient itself for a stronger ionic interaction with the Arg-120 of the COX-1 isozyme. Thus, they can fit only into the active site of the COX-2 isozyme because the binding of an acidic moiety to Arg-106 in the active site of the COX-2 isozyme is believed to play a lesser role in the inhibitory action of the COX-2 selective inhibitors like celecoxib[152] (i.e., the most acidic moiety, sulfonamide is extended into the side pocket instead of binding to Arg-106).

ASPIRIN AND ITS COX-1 SELECTIVITY

Aspirin covalently modifies COX-1 and hCOX-2 isozymes by acetylating the OH group of Ser-530 in COX-1 and Ser-516 in hCOX-2 isozymes. This is made possible by an ionic attraction between the carboxylate anion of aspirin and the arginine cation of Arg-120 in COX-1 (or Arg-106 in hCOX-2), thereby positioning the acetyl group of aspirin for acetylating the COX isozymes. Even though both COX isozymes are irreversibly acetylated by aspirin, acetylation of Ser-530 totally blocks the accessibility of substrate AA from entering into the active site, whereas an acetylated hCOX-2 is still able to form a significant amount of PGG_2.[143] Thus, aspirin, among all conventional NSAIDs,

exhibits the highest selectivity toward the COX-1 isozyme, especially the COX-1 isozyme present in the platelets.

Aspirin and Salicylic Acid Derivatives

Aspirin and the salicylates were among the first group of NSAIDs introduced into medicine for their use as analgesics to relieve pain and as antipyretics to reduce fever.[157] As early as 1763, the Reverend Edward Stone of Chipping Norton in Oxfordshire, England reported the use of dried willow bark to parishioners suffering from rheumatic fever.[129,158] The active ingredient of willow bark was isolated by Leroux, in 1827 and named salicin, which is a salicylic acid containing glycoside. After these discoveries, Cahours (1844) obtained salicylic acid from oil of wintergreen (methyl salicylate), and Kolbe and Lautermann (1860) prepared it synthetically from phenol. Sodium salicylate was introduced in 1875 by Buss, followed by the introduction of phenyl salicylate by Nencki in 1886. Aspirin, or acetylsalicylic acid, was first prepared in 1853 by Gerhardt but remained obscure until Felix Hoffmann from Bayer discovered its pharmacological activities in 1899. It was tested and introduced into medicine by Dreser (1899), who named it *aspirin* by taking the *a* from acetyl and *spirin*, an old name for salicylic or spiric acid, derived from its natural source of spirea plants.

Most of the salicylic acid drugs (commonly referred to as the salicylates) are either marketed as salts of salicylic acid (sodium, magnesium, bismuth, choline, or triethanolamine) or as ester or amide derivatives (aspirin, salsalate, salicylamide). (Fig. 24.17) Children, between the ages of 3 and 12, who are recovering from flu or chicken pox, should not be taking aspirin or any salicylates because of the perceived risks of a rare disease known as Reye syndrome.[159]

MECHANISM OF ACTION OF SALICYLATES

Salicylates, in general, exert their antipyretic action in febrile patients by increasing heat elimination of the body via the mobilization of water and consequent dilution of

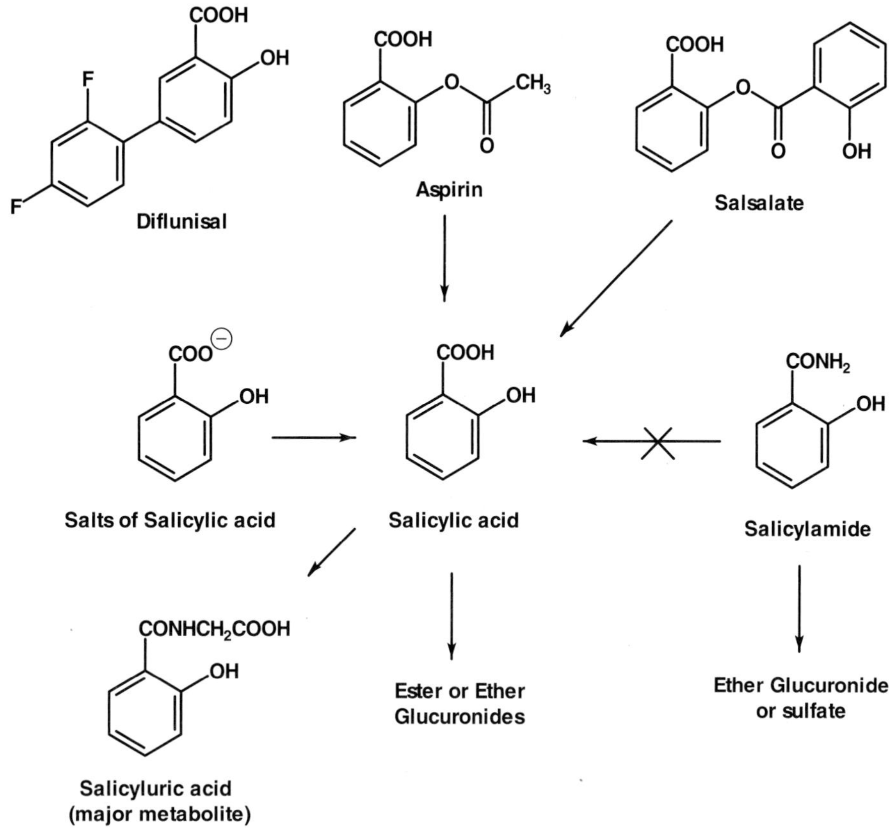

Figure 24.17 ● Salicylates and their metabolism.

the blood. This brings about perspiration, causing cutaneous dilatation. This does not occur with normal temperatures. The antipyretic and analgesic actions are believed to work by inhibiting cyclooxygenase and reducing the levels of PGE_2, a proximal mediator of the febrile response, in the hypothalamic area of the brain that regulates body temperature.[157]

It is well established that a low daily dose of aspirin (75–100 mg or one tablet of baby aspirin) is sufficient to completely block platelet TXA_2 production and its ability to induce platelet aggregation after only 1 week of dosing, thereby preventing the risk of a cardiovascular event, including myocardial infarction and ischemic stroke.[160,161] This antiplatelet action of aspirin is because COX-2 is not expressed in platelets; therefore, aspirin can selectively and irreversibly inhibit platelet TXA_2 production for 8 to 10 days (i.e., until new platelets are formed) at such a low dose (i.e., via the irreversible acetylation of Ser-530 of the COX-1 isozymes discussed earlier). However, the analgesic, antipyretic, and anti-inflammatory action of aspirin is more complex and may involve other mechanisms of action than simply based on its ability to irreversibly inhibit the COX isozymes.[157,162,163] Furthermore, it is worth noting that up to 50% of the oral analgesic dose of aspirin is rapidly deacetylated before it reaches general circulation, and its major active metabolite, salicylic acid, is found to have comparable in vivo antipyretic and anti-inflammatory properties to aspirin but is a very weak inhibitor of cyclooxygenases (i.e., in vitro binding studies).[164] Several possible mechanisms of action have recently been suggested for aspirin and especially the salicylates including blocking the induction of the COX-2 isozyme at the genetic levels,[165] turning off the

nuclear factor-κB-mediated polymorphonuclear leukocyte apoptosis signaling[166,167] or blocking the activation of the mitogen-activated kinase, Erk signaling associated with inflammatory responses.[168]

PHARMACOKINETICS OF SALICYLATES

The salicylates, being acidic in nature, are readily absorbed from the stomach and the small intestine. However, their absorption depends strongly on the pH of the environment, thus coadministration of an antacid or other buffering agents should be avoided because it greatly hinders their absorption and reduces their bioavailability and onset of action. They are also highly bound to plasma proteins, a major source of potential drug interactions with other medications.

Salicylic acid undergoes extensive phase-II metabolism (see Fig. 24.17) and is excreted via the kidneys as the water-soluble glycine conjugate, salicyluric acid, the major metabolite ($>75\%$) or as the corresponding acyl glucuronides (i.e., the ester type, via the COOH) or O-glucuronides (i.e., the ether type, via the phenolic OH) ($\sim 15\%$). Alkalinization of the urine increases the rate of excretion of the free salicylates.

Aspirin

Aspirin, acetylsalicylic acid (Aspro, Empirin), was introduced into medicine by Dreser in 1899.

Aspirin occurs as white crystals or as a white crystalline powder and must be kept under dry conditions. It is not advisable to keep aspirin products in the kitchen or bathroom cabinets, because aspirin is slowly decomposed into acetic and salicylic acids in the presence of heat and moisture. Several proprietaries (e.g., Bufferin) use compounds such as sodium bicarbonate, aluminum glycinate, sodium citrate, aluminum hydroxide, or magnesium trisilicate to counteract aspirin's acidic property. One of the better antacids is dihydroxyaluminum aminoacetate. Aspirin is unusually effective when prescribed with calcium glutamate. The more stable, nonirritant calcium acetylsalicylate is formed, and the glutamate portion (glutamic acid) maintains a pH of 3.5 to 5. Practically all salts of aspirin, except those of aluminum and calcium, are unstable for pharmaceutical use. These salts appear to have fewer undesirable side effects and induce analgesia faster than aspirin. A timed release preparation of aspirin is available. It does not appear to offer any advantages over aspirin, except for bedtime dosage.

Aspirin is used as an analgesic for minor aches and pains and as an antipyretic to reduce fever. Although higher doses of aspirin can also be used to treat inflammation, its use is often associated with many unwanted side effects including ulcers, stomach bleeding, and tinnitus. A low dosage form of aspirin, 81 mg, equivalent to the dose recommended for infants (the "baby aspirin"), is recommended as a daily dose for individuals who are at even a low cardiovascular risk. Several large studies have found that this low dose of aspirin reduces the number of heart attacks and thrombotic strokes.[160,161] Other salicylates and NSAIDs have not shown similar effects. In fact, a recent report indicated using ibuprofen can interfere with aspirin's cardiovascular benefits, and they should not be taken within 12 hours of each other.[169]

Aspirin and other potent NSAIDs (except salicylates) are also known to precipitate asthma attacks and other hypersensitivity reactions in up to 10% of the patients who have any type of respiratory problems.[170] This hypersensitivity reaction is believed to occur as a result of shifting the substrate, AA from the inhibited cyclooxygenase pathway to the lipoxygenase pathway (see Fig. 24.14), therefore resulting in overproduction of anaphylactic leukotrienes because of the blockade of the cyclooxygenase pathway by aspirin and other potent NSAIDs.[171]

Salsalate
Salsalate, salicylsalicylic acid (Amigesic, Disalcid, Salflex), is the ester formed between two salicylic acid molecules. It is rapidly hydrolyzed to salicylic acid following its absorption. It reportedly causes less gastric irritation than aspirin, because it is relatively insoluble in the stomach and is not absorbed until it reaches the small intestine.

Diflunisal
Diflunisal (Dolobid), is a longer acting and more potent drug than aspirin because of its hydrophobic, 2,4-difluorophenyl group attached to the 5-position of the salicyclic acid. In a large-scale comparative study with aspirin, it was also better tolerated with less GI complications than aspirin.[172] It is marketed in tablet form for treating mild to moderate postoperative pain as well as RA and OA.

Diflunisal is highly protein bound. Its metabolism is subject to a dose-dependent, saturable, and capacity-limited glucuronide formation.[173] This unusual pharmacokinetic profile is a result of an enterohepatic circulation and the reabsorption of 65% of the drug and its glucuronides, followed by cleavage of its unstable, acyl glucuronide back to the active drug. Thus, diflunisal usage in patients with renal impairment should be closely monitored.

Sodium Salicylate
Sodium salicylate may be prepared by the reaction, in aqueous solution, by adding equal molar ratio of salicylic acid and sodium bicarbonate; evaporating to dryness yields the white salt. In solution, particularly in the presence of sodium bicarbonate, the salt will darken on standing. This is the salt of choice for salicylate medication and usually is administered with sodium bicarbonate to lessen gastric distress, or it is administered in enteric coated tablets. However, the use of sodium bicarbonate is ill advised, because it decreases the plasma levels of salicylate and increases the excretion of free salicylate in the urine.

Sodium salicylate, even though not as potent as aspirin for pain relief, also has less GI irritation and is useful for patients who are hypersensitive to aspirin.

OTHER SALTS OF SALICYLIC ACID

Sodium thiosalicylate (Rexolate) is the sulfur or thio analog of sodium salicylate. It is more soluble and better absorbed, thus allowing lower dosages. It is recommended for gout, rheumatic fever, and muscular pains, but it is available only for injection.

Magnesium salicylate (Mobidin, Magan) is a sodium-free salicylate preparation for use when sodium intake is restricted. It is claimed to produce less GI irritation.

Choline salicylate (Arthropan) is extremely soluble in water and is available as a flavored liquid. It is claimed to be absorbed more rapidly than aspirin, giving faster peak blood levels. It is used when salicylates are indicated. It is also available in combination with magnesium salicylate (Trilisate, Tricosal, Trisalcid, CMT) for the relief of minor to moderate pains and fever associated with arthritis, bursitis, tendinitis, menstrual cramps, and others.

Salicylamide
Salicylamide, *o*-hydroxybenzamide, is a derivative of salicylic acid that is fairly stable to heat, light, and moisture. It reportedly exerts a moderately quicker and deeper analgesic effect than aspirin because of quicker CNS penetration. Its metabolism differs from aspirin, because it is not metabolized to salicylic acid but rather excreted exclusively as the ether glucuronide or sulfate.[174] Thus, as a result of lack of contribution from salicylic acid, it has a lower analgesic and antipyretic efficacy than that of aspirin. However, it can be used in place of salicylates for patients with a demonstrated sensitivity to salicylates. It is also excreted much more rapidly than other salicylates, which accounts for its lower toxicity. It is available in several nonprescription products, in combination with acetaminophen and phenyltoloxamine (e.g., Rid-A Pain compound, Cetazone T, Dolorex, Ed-Flex, Lobac) or with aspirin, acetaminophen, and caffeine (e.g., Saleto, BC Powder).

The Conventional Nonselective Cyclooxygenase Inhibitors

With the removal of rofecoxib (Vioxx) from the market and the concern of cardiovascular risk associated with celecoxib (Celebrex), the conventional NSAIDs, being more potent than aspirin and related salicylates, once again become the drug of choice for the treatment of RA and other inflammatory diseases.[130] The conventional NSAIDs vary considerably in terms of their selective inhibitory action for COX-2 relative to COX-1 isozymes and also their relative drug-induced toxicities discussed earlier in this text. Although several drugs in this class are available OTC, they are no safer than prescription medications with regard to their drug-induced GI liability.[127] The conventional NSAIDs, as a group, are highly protein bound and exhibit both pharmacokinetic as well as pharmacodynamic interactions with many drugs, especially anticoagulants, diuretics, lithium, and other arthritis medications.

For the purpose of comparing their SAR, toxicity, and metabolic biotransformations, the conventional NSAIDs are further divided into several chemical classes.

ARYL- AND HETEROARYLACETIC ACIDS

This group of NSAIDs has received the most intensive attention for new clinical candidates. As a group, they show high analgesic potency in addition to their potent anti-inflammatory activity, needed for treating inflammatory diseases. Among the members of this class shown in Figure 24.18, ketorolac, indomethacin, and tolmetin have the highest risk of GI complications because of their higher affinity for the COX-1 isozymes, whereas etodolac has the lowest risk because of its COX-2 selective inhibitory action. Both sulindac and nabumetone are prodrugs that require activation, and therefore have lower risk of causing GI irritation than indomethacin.[130]

Indomethacin

From the time of its introduction in 1965, indomethacin (Indocin) has been widely used as an analgesic to relieve inflammatory pain associated with RA, OA and ankylosing spondylitis, and, to a lesser extent, in gout. Although both its analgesic and anti-inflammatory activities are well established, its use is often limited because of frequent GI distress and potential drug interactions, especially with warfarin furosemide, and lithium (i.e., it elevates blood levels of lithium as a result of reducing renal blood flow and therefore increases lithium toxicities).

Following oral administration, indomethacin is rapidly absorbed and is 90% protein bound at therapeutic plasma concentrations.[175] The drug has a biological half-life of about 5 to 10 hours and a plasma clearance of 1 to 2.5 ml/kg per minute. It is metabolized to its inactive, *O*-desmethyl, *N*-deschlorobenzoyl-, and *O*-desmethyl, *N*-deschlorobenzoylindomethacin metabolites.[175]

Sulindac

Sulindac, (*Z*)-5-fluoro-2-methyl-1-([*p*-(methylsulfinyl) phenyl]methylene)-1*H*-indene-3-acetic acid (Clinoril), is an NSAID prodrug that contains a chiral sulfoxide moiety but is marketed as the racemate because it undergoes in vivo reduction by the hepatic enzymes into its achiral, active metabolite, methyl sulfide that exhibits potent and nonselective COX inhibition similar to indomethacin.[151]

The parent sulfoxide has a plasma half-life of 8 hours, and the active methyl sulfide metabolite is 16.4 hours. The more polar and inactive sulfoxide is virtually the only form excreted into the renal tubules, thus sulindac is believed to have minimal nephrotoxicity associated with indomethacin.[176] The long half-life of sulindac is caused by the extensive enterohepatic circulation and reactivation of the inactive sulfoxide excreted. Coadministration of aspirin is contraindicated because it considerably reduces the sulfide blood levels. Careful monitoring of patients with a history of ulcers is recommended. Gastric bleeding, nausea, diarrhea, dizziness, and other adverse effects have been noted with sulindac, but with a lower frequency than with aspirin. Sulindac is recommended for RA, OA, and ankylosing spondylitis.

Tolmetin

Tolmetin sodium (Tolectin), is an arylacetic acid derivative with a pyrrole as the aryl group. This drug is well absorbed

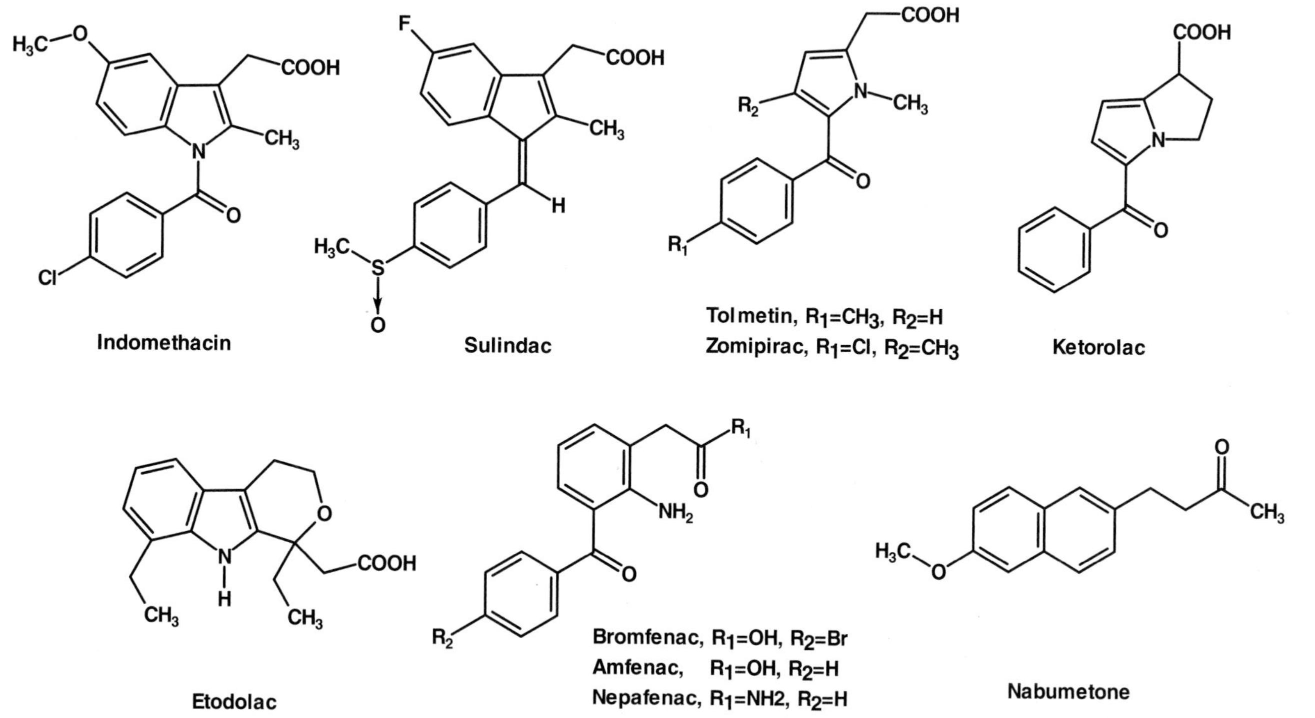

Tolmetin, R₁=CH₃, R₂=H
Zomipirac, R₁=Cl, R₂=CH₃

Bromfenac, R₁=OH, R₂=Br
Amfenac, R₁=OH, R₂=H
Nepafenac, R₁=NH2, R₂=H

Indomethacin **Sulindac** **Ketorolac** **Etodolac** **Nabumetone**

Figure 24.18 ● Aryl- and heteroarylacetic acid derivatives.

and has a relatively short plasma half-life (1 hour). It is recommended for use in the management of acute and chronic RA. Its efficacy is similar to aspirin and indomethacin, but with less frequency of the adverse effects and tinnitus associated with aspirin. It does not potentiate coumarin-like drugs nor alter the blood levels of sulfonylureas or insulin. However, tolmetin, and especially its closely related drug, zomepirac (i.e., with a *p*-chlorobenzoyl group and an additional methyl group on the pyrrole ring), can produce a rare but fatal anaphylactic reaction because of irreversible binding of their unstable acyl glucuronides.[177] Zomepirac was withdrawn from market because it is eliminated only via the ester-type, acyl glucuronide.[178] It is possible that tolmetin is less toxic in this regard because it undergoes additional hepatic benzylic hydroxylation via its *p*-methyl group and is excreted as its stable ether glucuronide.

Ketorolac

Ketorolac tromethamine (Toradol), marketed as a mixture of (R)- and (S)-ketorolac enantiomers, is a potent NSAID analgesic indicated for the treatment of moderately severe, acute pain. It should be noted that the pharmacokinetic disposition of ketorolac in humans is subject to marked enantioselectivity. Thus, it is important to monitor the individual blood levels so an accurate assessment of its therapeutic action can be made correctly.[179] However, it should be noted that, being one of the conventional NSAIDs with highest risk of GI complications, its administration should not exceed 5 days.

Nabumetone

Nabumetone (Relafen), a nonacidic NSAID prodrug, is classified as an arylacetic acid, because it undergoes rapid hepatic metabolism to its active metabolite, 6-methoxy-2-naphthylacetic acid.[180] Similar to the other arylacetic acid drugs, it is used in short- or long-term management of RA and OA. Being nonacidic, it does not produce significant primary insult to the GI mucosa lining and also has no effect on prostaglandin synthesis in gastric mucosa, thus producing minimum secondary GI damage when compared with other conventional NSAIDs.

Etodolac

Etodolac (Lodine, Ultradol), a chiral, COX-2 selective NSAID drug that is marketed as a racemate, possesses an indole ring as the aryl portion of this group of NSAID drugs. It shares many similar properties of this group and is indicated for short- and long-term management of pain and OA.

Similar to ketorolac, etodolac exhibits several unique enantioselective pharmacokinetic properties.[181] For example, the "inactive" (R)-enantiomer has approximately a 10-fold higher plasma concentration than the active (S)-enantiomer. Furthermore, the active (S)-enantiomer is less protein bound than its (R)-enantiomer and therefore has a very large volume of distribution. It is well absorbed with an elimination half-life of 6 to 8 hours. Etodolac is extensively metabolized into three major inactive metabolites, 6-hydroxy etodolac (via aromatic hydroxylation), 7-hydroxy-etodolac (via aromatic hydroxylation), and 8-(1'-hydroxylethyl) etodolac (via benzylic hydroxylation), which are eliminated as the corresponding ether glucuronides.[182] Its unstable, acyl glucuronide, however, is subject to enterohepatic circulation and reactivation to the parent drug, similar to other NSAIDS in this class.

In a recent study comparing its gastric safety profile with those of meloxicam, diclofenac, and indomethacin, etodolac

was found to have the highest safety index among these NSAIDs in arthritic rats.[183] Thus, etodolac is an example of a COX-2 selective drug with a much better safety profile among the first generation of NSAIDs developed through the traditional route of using only animal model studies. Its selective COX-2 inhibitory action, which was not realized until much later, explains its much lower risk of the GI side effects among first-generation NSAIDs.

Amfenac, Bromfenac, and Nepafenac

Amfenac (Fenazox), its amide prodrug, nepafenac (Nevanac), and the related analog, bromofenac, are amphoteric because of the presence of an additional aromatic amine group. They are less likely to be absorbed into the general circulation. They are approved for use as topical ocular anti-inflammatory agents for the treatment of postoperative ocular pain, inflammation, and posterior segment edema.[184] The only observed side effects of these drugs are all related to tissues around the eye including abnormal ocular sensation, eye redness and irritation, burning and stinging, and conjunctival or cornea edema.

ARYL- AND HETEROARYLPROPANOIC ACIDS

These are perhaps the most widely used drugs worldwide because three members of this class, ibuprofen, naproxen, and ketoprofen, are now available without a prescription (Fig. 24.19). Their indiscriminate use, however, by the general public without a doctor's prescription, has resulted in an increased incidence of complications in adolescents, including acute and chronic renal failure.[185]

All of the members of this class (except oxaprozin) contain a chiral carbon in the α-position of the acetic acid side chain. Even though most are marketed as racemates, only the (S)-enantiomer was found to have any inhibitory activity against the COX isozymes. Thus, the (S)-enantiomer is believed to be solely responsible for the observed therapeutic action as well as the drug-induced GI side effects and nephrotoxicity. Furthermore, in most cases, the inactive (R)-enantiomer is epimerized in vivo, via the 2-arylpropionyl coenzyme-A epimerase to its active (S)-enantiomer.[186]

Ibuprofen

Ibuprofen, 2-(4-isobutylphenyl)propionic acid (Motrin, Advil, Nuprin), was introduced into clinical practice following extensive clinical trials. It appears to have comparable efficacy to aspirin in the treatment of RA, but with a lower incidence of side effects. It has also been approved for use in the treatment of primary dysmenorrhea, which is thought to be caused by an excessive concentration of PGs and endoperoxides.[187] However, a recent study indicates that concurrent use of ibuprofen and aspirin may actually interfere with the cardioprotective effects of aspirin, at least in patients with established cardiovascular disease.[169] This is because ibuprofen can reversibly bind to the platelet COX-1 isozymes, thereby blocking aspirin's ability to inhibit TXA_2 synthesis in platelets.

Naproxen

Naproxen (Naprosyn, Anaprox), marketed as the (S)-enantiomer, is well absorbed after oral administration, giving peak plasma levels in 2 to 4 hours and a half-life of 13 hours. Naproxen is highly protein bound and displaces most protein-bound drugs. It is recommended for use in RA, OA,

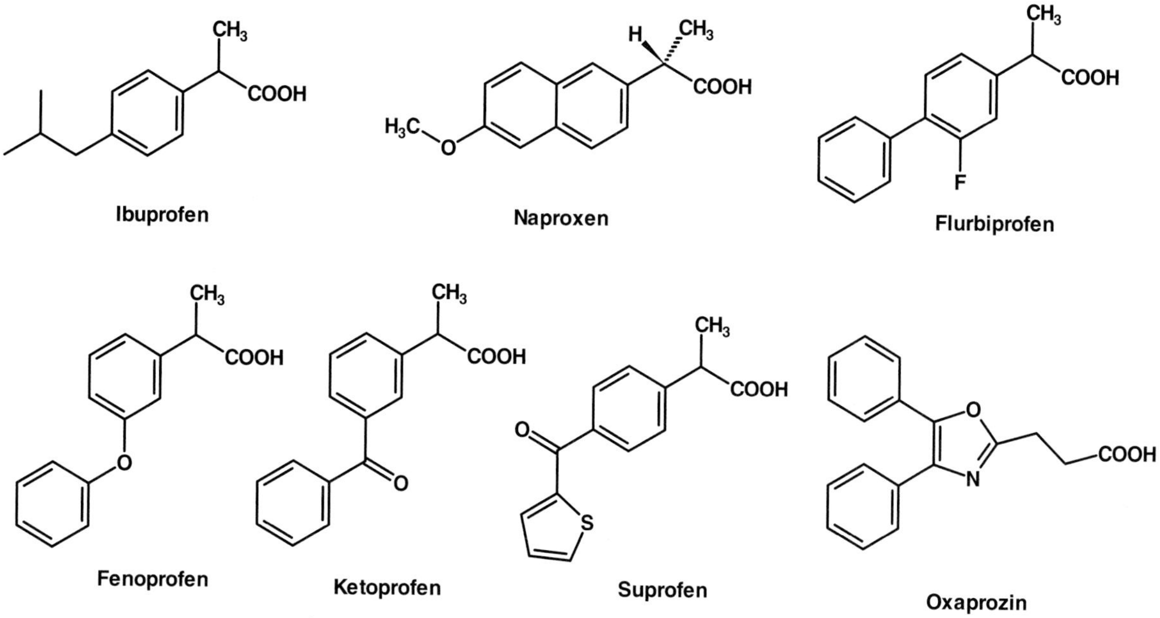

Figure 24.19 ● Aryl- and heteroarylpropionic acids.

acute gouty inflammation, and in primary dysmenorrhea. It shows good analgesic activity (i.e., 400 mg is comparable to 75–150 mg of oral meperidine and superior to 65 mg of propoxyphene and 325 mg of aspirin plus 30 mg of codeine). It is also available OTC as 200-mg tablets (Aleve).

Fenoprofen

Fenoprofen (Nalfon), is rapidly absorbed orally, reaches peak plasma levels within 2 hours, and has a short plasma half-life (3 hours). It is highly protein bound, just like the other NSAIDs, thus caution is needed when it is used concurrently with other medications including hydantoins, sulfonamides, and sulfonylureas. It is recommended for RA and OA, at an oral dose of 300 to 600 mg for 3 or 4 times per day, but not exceeding 3 g/d to avoid any serious side effects. It should be noted that in a comparison study of all NSAIDs, fenoprofen is the one that has been most closely associated with a rare acute interstitial nephritis.[188] For mild to moderate pain relief, the recommended dosage is 200 mg given every 4 to 6 hours, as needed.

Ketoprofen and Suprofen

Ketoprofen (Orudis, Rhodis) and suprofen (Profenal) are closely related to fenoprofen in their structures, properties, and indications. Even though ketoprofen has been approved for OTC use (Orudis KT, Actron), its GI side effects are similar to indomethacin (Table 24.1), and therefore its use should be closely monitored, especially in patients with GI or renal problems.

Flurbiprofen

Flurbiprofen (Ansaid, Ocufen, Froben), is another drug in this class indicated for both acute and long-term management of RA and OA but with a more complex mechanism of action. Unlike the other drugs in this class, it does not undergo chiral inversion (i.e., the conversion of the "inactive" [R]-enantiomer to the active, [S]-enantiomer). Similar to aspirin and other salicylates, both flurbiprofen enantiomers block COX-2 induction as well as inhibiting the nuclear factor-κB-mediated polymorphonuclear leukocyte apoptosis

signaling[189]; therefore, both enantiomers are believed to contribute equally to its overall anti-inflammatory action.

(R)-flurbiprofen is actually a strong clinical candidate for the treatment of Alzheimer disease, because it has been shown to reduce Aβ42 production by human cells.[190]

Oxaprozin

Oxaprozin, 4,5-diphenyl-2-oxazolepropionic acid (Daypro), differs from the other members of this group in being an arylpropionic acid derivative. It shares the same properties and side effects of other members in this group. It is indicated for the short- and long-term management of OA and RA, administered as a once-daily dose of 600- to 1,200-mg dose because of its long duration of action.[191]

N-ARYLANTHRANILIC ACIDS (FENAMATES) AND STRUCTURALLY RELATED ANALOGS

This class of NSAIDs shares one common structural feature that is not present in the other classes discussed earlier. Unlike other classes discussed earlier, the second aromatic ring in this class is connected to the main aromatic carboxylic acid containing ring through a secondary amine linkage (rather than carbonyl group or other nonbasic linker) and at the ortho position rather than at the meta or para position (see their structures in Fig. 24.20). As a result of this structural feature, this class of NSAIDs appears to have a lower risk of causing GI irritation. Recent crystallographic evidence suggests that diclofenac binds to COX isozymes in an inverted conformation with its carboxylate group hydrogen-bonded to Tyr-385 and Ser-530.[192] This finding provides a reason why diclofenac and especially its related analog, lumicoxib, have much greater selectivity toward COX-2 isozymes.

Mefenamic Acid

Mefenamic acid (Ponstel, Ponstan) is one of the oldest NSAIDs, introduced into the market in 1967 for mild to moderate pain and for primary dysmenorrhea. It is rapidly

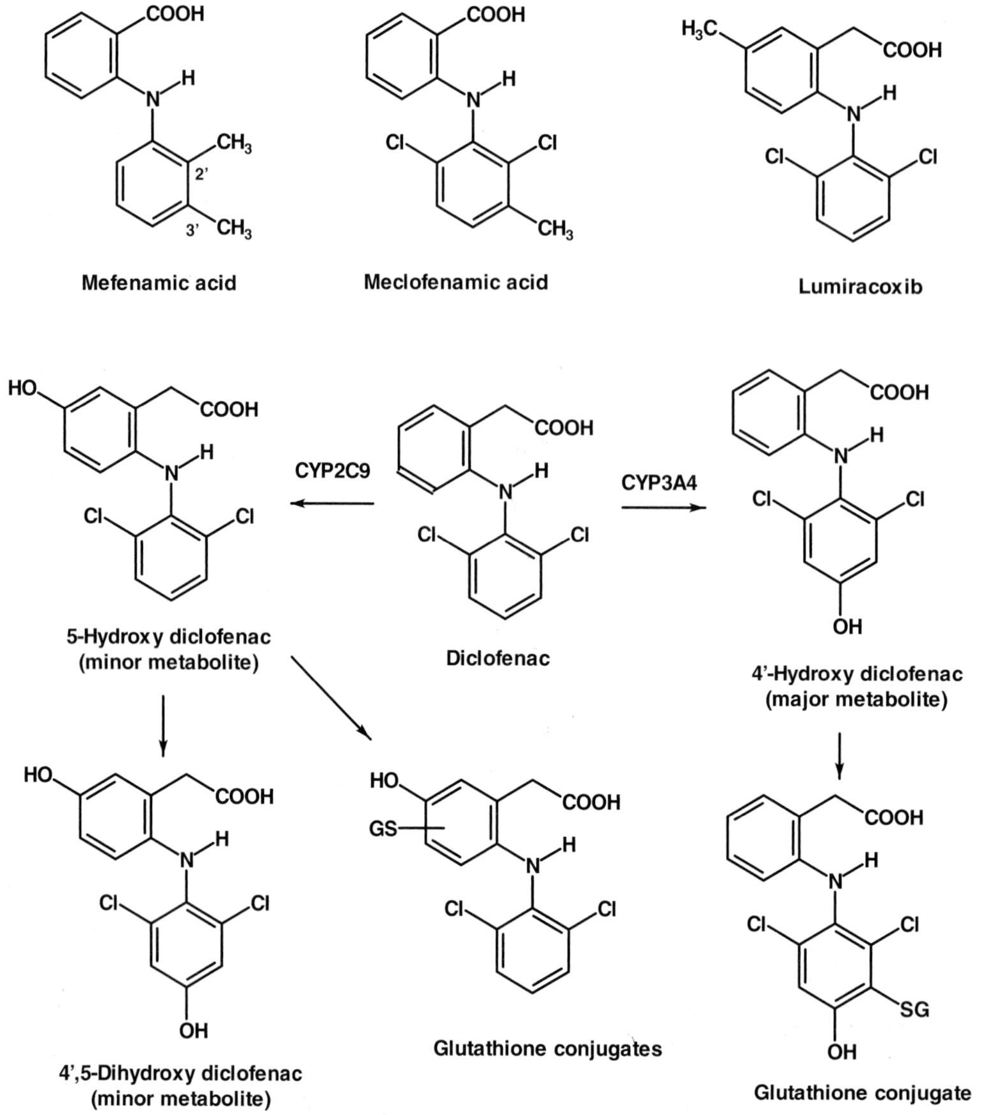

Figure 24.20 • Fenamates and metabolism of diclofenac.

absorbed with peak plasma levels occurring 2 to 4 hours after oral administration. It undergoes hepatic benzylic hydroxylation of its 3′methyl group regioselectively into two inactive metabolites, 3′-hydroxymethylmefenamic acid and the 3′carboxylate metabolite (via further oxidation of the benzylic alcohol group). The parent drugs and these metabolites are conjugated with glucuronic acid and excreted primarily in the urine. Thus, although patients with known liver deficiency may be given lower doses, it is contraindicated in patients with preexisting renal dysfunction.

Common side effects associated with its use include diarrhea, drowsiness, and headache. The possibility of blood disorders has also prompted limitation of its administration to 7 days. It is not recommended for children or during pregnancy.

Meclofenamate
Meclofenamate sodium (Meclomen) is available for use in the treatment of acute and chronic RA, OA, and primary dysmenorrhea. It is metabolized in a similar manner to mefenamic acid discussed above, thus a similar restriction is also applied to meclofenamate. The most significant side effects are GI, including diarrhea.

Diclofenac and Lumiracoxib
Diclofenac sodium (Voltaren), is indicated for short- and long-term treatment of RA, OA, and ankylosing spondylitis. The potassium salt (Cataflam), which is faster acting, is indicated for the management of acute pain and primary dysmenorrhea. Diclofenac was first marketed in Japan in 1974 but was not approved for its use in the United States until 1989, perhaps because of concerns about its hepatotoxicity. Diclofenac is also available in combination with misoprostol (Arthrotec).

Unlike the other NSAIDs, diclofenac appears to be more hepatotoxic and, in rare cases, can cause severe liver damage. This idiosyncratic hepatotoxicity has been attributed to the formation of reactive benzoquinone imines, similar to acetaminophen, which will be discussed later.[193] Diclofenac undergoes hepatic CYP2C9/3A4 catalyzed aromatic hydroxylations to give 4′-Hydroxy-diclofenac as its major inactive metabolite (~30%) and 5-hydroxy- and 4′5-dihydroxy-diclofenac as its minor metabolites (Fig. 24.20). These hydroxylated metabolites are excreted, normally, such as their glucuronides. Similar to that of acetaminophen, both the 4′ and 5-hydroxylated metabolites can be further activated to their reactive quinone imines (not shown in the

Figure), which are normally deactivated by glutathione, the host defensive mechanism, to its inactive glutathione conjugates shown in Figure 24.20. Thus, it is reasonable to assume that patients with low levels of glutathione are more susceptible to diclofenac toxicity, and their use in these patients should be avoided.

Lumiracoxib (Prexige), one of the most COX-2 selective inhibitors marketed in Australia (2004), the United Kingdom (2005), and the United States (2007), was the mainstay of therapy for OA, RA, and acute pain. It differs from diclofenac with an additional methyl substituted onto the 5-position of phenylacetic acid ring. It is extensively metabolized by CYP2C9, just like diclofenac, into three major inactive metabolites, 5-carboxy, 4′-hydroxy, and 4′-hydroxy-5-carboxy derivative, through the oxidation of the 5-methyl group and hydroxylation of the dichloroaromatic ring.[194] Although no evidence of formation of potentially reactive metabolites was reported, the 4′-hydroxy derivatives are the major inactive metabolites eliminated (as the glucuronides), so it is not surprising to learn that lumiracoxib was withdrawn from market in October, 2007 because of several cases of serious adverse liver reactions to the drug, including two deaths and two liver transplants. Thus, patients with low glutathione levels or glucuronyl transferase activity as a result of drug interactions or aging are susceptible for forming reactive metabolites that are not found with healthy individuals, the subjects used in the original metabolic study.[194]

OXICAMS

Oxicams, are first-generation NSAIDs that lack a free carboxylic acid side chain but with an acidic enolic 1,2-benzothiazine carboxamide ring (see Fig. 24.16). Only two members of this class, piroxicam and meloxicam, are available in the United States for the management of inflammatory arthritis. Tenoxicam (Mobiflex), a close isosteric analog of piroxicam (i.e., with a 1,2-thiazole ring replacing the benzene ring fused to the thiazine ring), is available in Canada but with a pharmacodynamic and pharmacokinetic profile similar to piroxicam. As discussed earlier, piroxicam and meloxicam have very different affinities for the COX isozymes, and therefore exhibit very different risks for GI complications.

Piroxicam

Piroxicam (Feldene) is the most widely used oxicam because of its once-daily dosing schedule. It is well absorbed after oral administration and has a plasma half-life of 50 hours, thus requiring a dose of only 20 to 30 mg once daily.[195] It undergoes extensive hepatic metabolism, catalyzed by CYP2C9 to give 5-hydroxypiroxicam as its major metabolite (See Fig. 24.16).[154] Several piroxicam prodrugs have been synthesized via derivatization of the enol alcohol group (amipiroxicam, droxicam, and pivoxicam) to reduce piroxicam-induced GI irritation.[195]

Meloxicam

Meloxicam (Mobic) is a selective COX-2 inhibitor among oxicams indicated for use in RA and OA. It also has a relatively long half-life of 15 to 20 hours and has a much lower rate of serious GI side effects and a lower than average risk of nephropathy when compared with other conventional NSAIDs.[196] The recommended dose is 7.5 mg once daily with a maximum of 15 mg/d. Meloxicam is metabolized in humans mainly by CYP2C9 (with a minor contribution via

CYP3A4) to 5′-hydroxymethylmeloxicam and 5′-carboxymeloxicam (see Fig. 24.16).[156]

In large-scale comparative trials, meloxicam was found to be at least as effective as most conventional NSAIDs in the treatment of rheumatic disease or postoperative pain, but has demonstrated a more favorable GI tolerability profile.[158]

The Selective COX-2 Inhibitors

As stated earlier, the development and hasty market introduction of the first selective coxibs drugs, celecoxib (Celebrex), and rofecoxib (Vioxx) in 1999, was based on Vane's[133,134] hypothesis that blocking an inducible COX-2 isozyme retains all of the therapeutic effects but none of the side effects of the conventional NSAIDs. Shortly after their market introduction, the results of a preliminary Vioxx gastrointestinal outcomes research (VIGOR) trial was reported in 2000 that raised concern and much debate on the cardiovascular safety of all selective COX-2 inhibitors.[135–137,197] Several additional coxibs drugs including valdecoxib (Bextra), etoricoxib (Arcoxia), and parecoxib sodium (Dynastat), were introduced into the worldwide market during 2002. The potential cardiovascular risk was not taken seriously until late 2004 when rofecoxib (Vioxx) was voluntary withdrawn from the worldwide market, based on an additional risk assessment from a 3-year randomized, placebo-controlled, double-blind clinical trial.[197] To date, all but the least potent of COX-2 drugs, celecoxib (Celebrex), have been removed from the worldwide market, therefore depriving an otherwise, rational choice of pain medications, especially for arthritic patients who are at higher risk of serious GI complications.[137]

An overexpression of COX-2 was found in multiple cancer types, especially in colorectal cancer,[198,199] thus future roles of the selective COX-2 inhibitors may be realized in the chemoprevention of cancers and other inflammatory degenerative diseases. The reader should consult several excellent reviews on these latest developments.[200–202]

CELECOXIB

Celecoxib (Celebrex) was the first selective COX-2 inhibitor drug introduced into the market in 1998 for use in the treatment of RA, OA, acute pain, and menstrual pain. The real benefit is that it has caused fewer GI complications when compared with other conventional NSAIDs. It has also been approved for reducing the number of adenomatous colorectal polyps in familial adenomatous polyposis (FAP).

Celecoxib is well absorbed and undergoes rapid oxidative metabolism via CYP2C9 to give its inactive metabolites (Fig. 24.21).[203] Thus, a potential drug interaction exists between celecoxib and warfarin because the active isomer of warfarin is primarily degraded by CYP2C9.

The Analgesic Antipyretics: Acetaminophen (Paracetamol) and Related Analogs

From a historical perspective, acetaminophen (paracetamol) and the related analgesic antipyretic drugs such as acetanilide, antipyrine, and dipyrone were introduced into the market about the same time as aspirin and the other salicylates (i.e., acetanilide, 1886; phenacetin, 1887; and acetaminophen, 1893).[204] They were once the most widely used analgesic

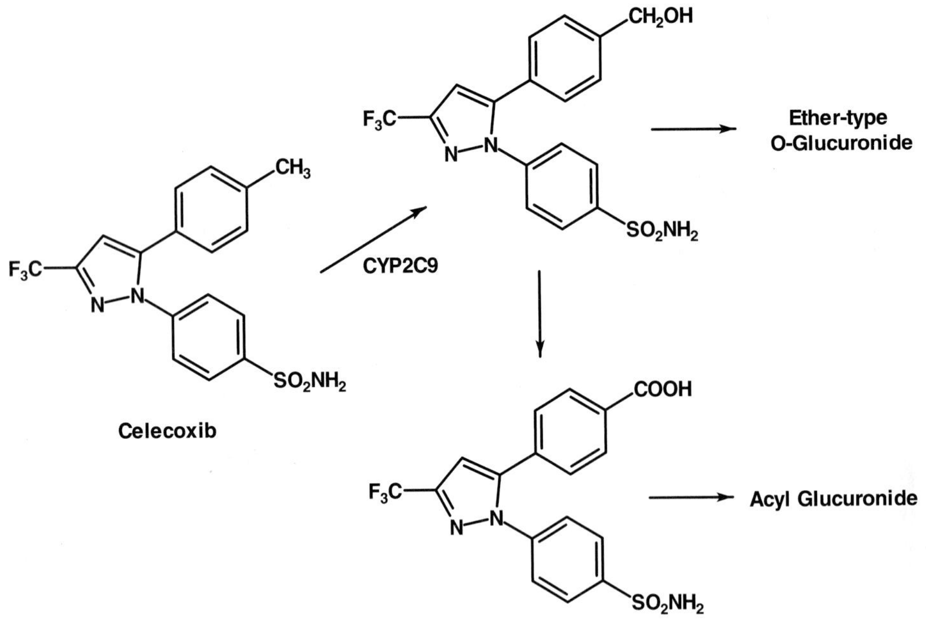

Figure 24.21 • Metabolic biotransformation of celecoxib.

antipyretics for relieving pain and reducing fever because, unlike aspirin and salicylates, they do not cause ulceration or increase bleeding time.[204] Among these agents, phenacetin was once a very popular analgesic antipyretic drug, more so than acetaminophen, because it was perceived to be safer than acetaminophen toward the stomach (i.e., less acidic in nature). Its use was continued until the late 1970s, even though Brodie and Axelrod had already reported in 1949 that acetaminophen was the active metabolite of acetanilide and phenacetin.[205] In their elegant studies, acetanilide was found to undergo hepatic metabolism (i.e., via an aromatic hydroxylation) to acetaminophen, whereas only a small amount of the drug was hydrolyzed to give aniline, which can be further *N*-hydroxylated to phenylhydroxylamine, the compound believed to be responsible for acetanilide toxicity because of methemoglobin formation. Phenacetin, on the other hand, was found to undergo mostly *O*-dealkylation to acetaminophen, whereas a small amount was converted by deacetylation to *p*-phenetidine, also responsible for methemoglobin formation.

Phenacetin only fell out of favor around 1980 when it was found to cause renal and urinary tract tumors in experimental animal models.[206] Because of the toxicity described above, both acetanilide and phenacetin are now no longer available, thus acetaminophen is the only drug in this class that is still widely used worldwide because it is a safer and better tolerated pain medication.

MECHANISM OF ACTION: ACETAMINOPHEN AND THE COX-3 PUZZLE

Acetaminophen and other analgesic antipyretics have similar analgesic and antipyretic efficacies to the conventional NSAIDs such as aspirin, ibuprofen, or diclofenac. However, unlike the conventional NSAIDs, they lack the antiplatelet effects of aspirin or the GI side effects associated with NSAIDs. Acetaminophen also has little or no anti-inflammatory properties.[207–209] Although it has been in use for nearly a century, the mechanism of action of acetaminophen and related analgesic antipyretics remains unknown, but it is generally assumed that they work centrally by blocking a brain-specific enzyme, perhaps a COX-3 isozyme, responsible for the biosynthesis of prostaglandin.[210]

In 2002, Simmons et al.,[211] through cloning studies, identified a distinct variant of the canine COX-1 isozyme found only in the canine brain, which was designated as the COX-3 isozyme and hypothesized this isozyme as the target for acetaminophen and related analgesic-antipyretic drugs because this isozyme was selectively inhibited by acetaminophen, phenacetin, antipyrine, and dipyrone. This hypothesis was further supported by the findings that acetaminophen produces analgesia and induces hypothermia centrally and that both of these actions are accompanied by a dose-dependent reduction of brain PGE_2 levels that is not observed with diclofenac, a conventional NSAID.[209] In addition, the peripheral levels of PGE_2/PGI_2 levels were reduced only by diclofenac but not by acetaminophen.[210] Moreover, acetaminophen-induced hypothermia was reduced in COX-1 but not COX-2 gene-deleted animal studies.[209,212] These observations appear to provide additional support for hypothesis that the analgesia and hypothermia of acetaminophen are indeed mediated by inhibition of a distinct COX isozyme present only in the brain. However, most of the recent studies focusing on finding this elusive human COX-3 isozyme have not been successful.[207,213,214] Moreover, a similar COX-1 variant identified and expressed in humans (this isozyme was designated as COX-1b) was not inhibited by acetaminophen even though it is active in catalyzing PGH_2 synthesis in the brain. Thus, although the COX-3 isozyme may indeed be the molecular target responsible for acetaminophen action in canines, its role in humans is still unproven.[213,214]

In a recent commentary, Aronoff et al.[208] suggested an alternative target (mechanism) by which acetaminophen (APAP) blocks the cyclooxygenase action. Their hypothesis is based on the fact that acetaminophen acts as a reducing cosubstrate, thus actively competing with PGG_2 for its conversion to PGH_2, catalyzed by the peroxidase (POX) action of COX enzymes. Figure 24.22 summarizes some of the key mechanism of COX's action suggested by Aronoff et al.[208] and includes the additional hypothesis suggested by Gram and Scott[215] that acetaminophen acts by depleting the stores

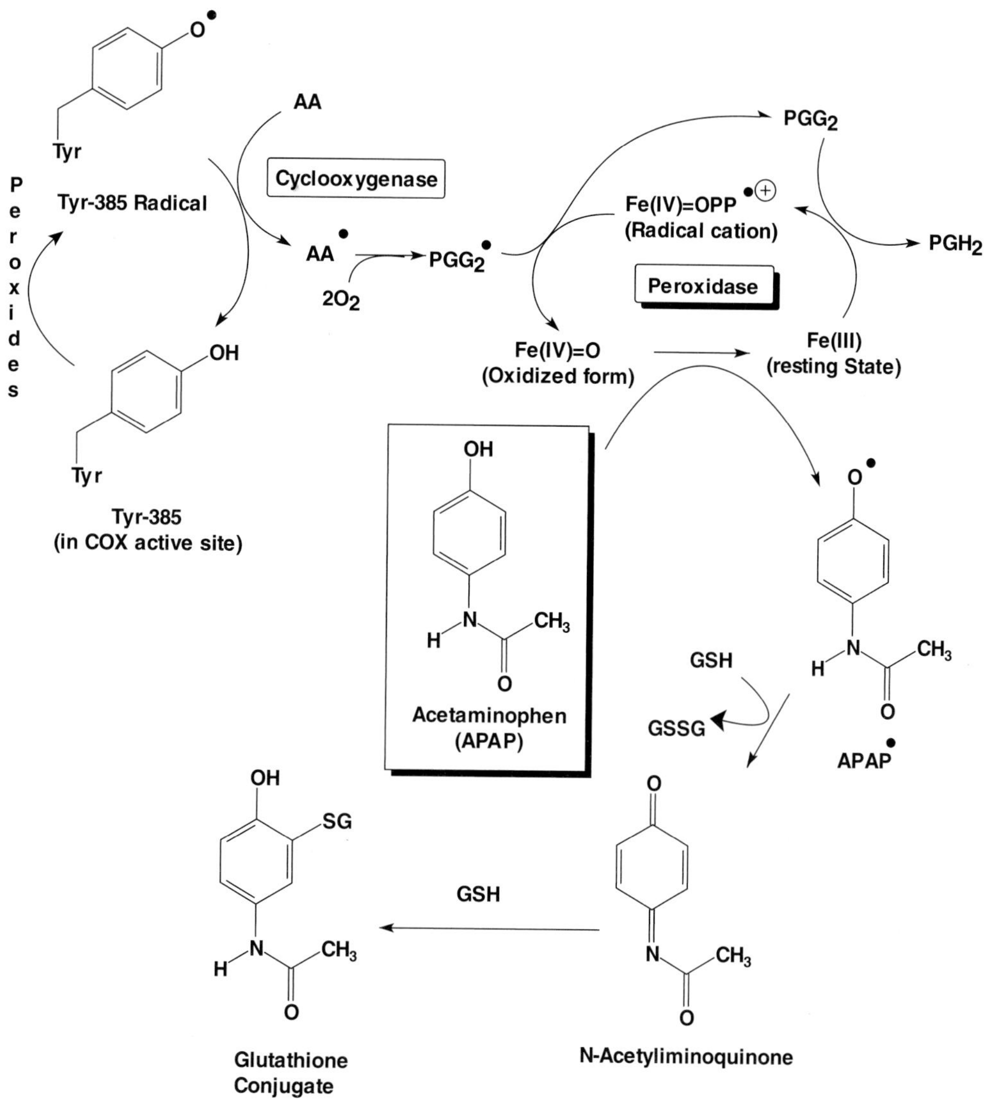

Figure 24.22 ● Mechanism of action of acetaminophen on PGH₂ synthesis.

of glutathione (GSH), which is a known cofactor for PGE synthase. Thus, with this illustration, it is now possible to see why acetaminophen's action depends on the level of peroxide generated in solution (i.e., PGG₂ and other lipid peroxides, generated by the lipoxygenase pathway), and its effectiveness varies with COX activity.[207] At low peroxide concentrations, acetaminophen can compete effectively with the electron transfer mechanism between the Tyr-385 residue and the heme radical, which generates the tyrosine radical in the active site of COX enzymes for the production of PGG₂, it also prevents the regeneration of Fe (IV) (APAP causes the formation of Fe (III), thus ↓ activity of POX), a process that is essential for starting a new POX cycle as shown in Fig. 24.22. However, acetaminophen is ineffective during inflammation because the higher concentration of PGG₂ or other peroxides, produced in the inflamed cells as a consequence of induction of the COX-2 isozyme and lipoxygenase, can overcome the acetaminophen inhibition by degrading acetaminophen in the synovial fluids as depicted in Figure 24.22 (i.e., conversion of APAP to its inactive glutathione conjugate shown).

This mechanism would also explain the recent findings that acetaminophen, unlike NSAIDs, cannot inhibit COX activity in broken cells, and the observation that only the inhibitory effects of acetaminophen, not indomethacin or diclofenac, were abolished by increasing intracellular oxidation conditions with the addition of cell-permeable hydroperoxide, *t*-butyl-OOH.[216] This hypothesis would also provide an additional reason why depletion of glutathione is the main cause of acetaminophen toxicity discussed under the next section. In summary, APAP does not compete with AA for the binding site on the COX enzyme. Its mechanism of action is via inhibiting the peroxidase activity of the COX enzyme.

TOXICITY IN ACETAMINOPHEN AND PHENACETIN

Acetaminophen and phenacetin can be metabolized to reactive hepatotoxic and renal toxic metabolites by various mechanisms.[217] Readers should consult a more detailed discussion in the drug metabolism chapter of this text. Figure 24.23 summarizes only the salient features for the purpose of discussing phenacetin/acetaminophen-induced liver and renal toxicities.

Acetanilide and phenacetin are hydroxylated or *O*-dealkylated, respectively via CYP1A2 to their active metabolite, acetaminophen.[206] In healthy individuals, acetaminophen is primarily eliminated as its *O*-sulfates and *O*-glucuronides, with only a small amount of the

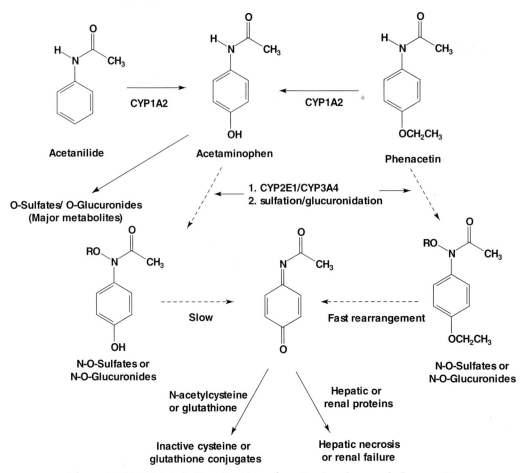

Figure 24.23 • Metabolic activation of acetaminophen and phenacetin.

N-hydroxylated metabolite (via CYP2E1/CYP3A4 isozymes), which can be sulfated or glucuronidated.[217,218] Small amounts of these *O*-sulfates, if accumulated in liver or renal tubules, can slowly rearrange to form the reactive *N*-acetyliminoquinone metabolites, shown in Figure 24.23. However, these reactive metabolites, once formed, are immediately deactivated by glutathione, the body's defense mechanism for detoxifying reactive metabolites.

In contrast, a similar *N*-*O*-sulfate of phenacetin will immediately rearrange to this reactive metabolite, *N*-acetyliminoquinone, whereas the corresponding *N*-*O*-glucuronide can also be slowly converted to this reactive metabolite.[217] Thus, it is not surprising that acetaminophen is a much safer drug than phenacetin with regard to their relative toxicities (i.e., with occasional use, most of acetaminophen is eliminated as its *O*-sulfates and *O*-glucuronides). However, it should be pointed out that acetaminophen-induced toxicity can be greatly increased by concurrent use of alcoholic beverages, especially in alcoholic individuals. This is because both CYP2E1 and CYP3A4 isozymes are induced by alcohol consumption.[218] Moreover, heavy caffeine use, together with alcohol, would further increase the risk of alcohol-mediated acetaminophen hepatotoxicity.[219] *N*-acetylcysteine is typically given as an antidote to treat possible acetaminophen poisoning even before plasma levels of acetaminophen are determined. Similar to glutathione, it deactivates the *N*-acetyliminoquinone metabolite before it changes to covalently bind cellular proteins (Fig. 24.23).

ACETAMINOPHEN

Acetaminophen (also known as paracetamol, APAP), a well established analgesic/antipyretic drug, is frequently used by itself OTC (Panado, Tempra, Tylenol) or in combination with codeine (Tylenol 3), hydrocodone (Vicodin), or oxycodone (Percocet) for the treatment of mild to moderate pain and to reduce fever. It is available in several nonprescription forms and is also marketed in combination with aspirin and caffeine (Excedrin, Vanquish).

Unlike aspirin or ibuprofen, acetaminophen is well tolerated with a low incidence of GI side effects. It also has good oral bioavailability, a fast onset and a plasma half-life of approximately 2 hours after dosing. Although it is a relatively safe pain medication, several precautions should be recognized, including not exceeding the recommended maximum dosage of 4 g/d. A lower daily dose of less than 2 g/d is required in patients who are chronic alcoholics or have renal complications.[220]

DISEASE-MODIFYING ANTIRHEUMATIC DRUGS

RA is one of the most common chronic, inflammatory autoimmune diseases, affecting approximately 1% of the world's adult population.[221] It is characterized by persistent inflammation of the synovial lining of the joints that causes pain, swelling, and stiffness of the upper and lower extremities. RA, if left untreated, can lead to permanent joint cartilage and bone damage that eventually results in disability and a significant impairment of quality of life.[221,222] A typical treatment of RA may involve a combination of physical and drug therapy including aspirin, other NSAIDs, or glucocorticoids initially to provide symptomatic relief of pain and swelling, and one or more of the disease-modifying antirheumatic drugs (DMARDs) to slow down the underlying disease progression and to limit further joint damage.[223,224]

DMARDs, sometime also referred to as the "slow-acting antirheumatic drugs," include a diverse class of synthetic drugs such as methotrexate, hydroxychloroquine, sulfasalazine, leflunomide, azathioprine, organic gold compounds, or immunobiologicals useful for treating the persistent inflammatory conditions associated with RA. DMARDs have very different mechanisms of action that allow physicians to individualize treatment strategies to slow down the clinical and radiographic progression of RA,

even though it takes between 6 weeks to 6 months to fully realize any of their therapeutic effects.[222,224–226]

In this chapter, only a few of the commonly used synthetic DMARDs are covered to exemplify different treatment strategies. Readers interested in more detailed information regarding the structure–activity and mechanism of actions of these DMARDs and related analogs should consult other chapters in antimalarials (chloroquine and hydroxychloroquine), anti-infectives (sulfasalazine), and antineoplastic agents (methotrexate, azathioprine, leflunomide). Recent advances in new disease-modifying anti-tumor necrosis factor agents such as etanercept, adalimumab, and infliximab are covered in a separate chapter entitled "Immunobiologicals" in this text as well as in several recent reviews.[221,222,225–227]

Synthetic Disease-Modifying Antirheumatic Drugs

Figure 24.24 contains the chemical structures of the DMARDs and their metabolites mentioned in this section.

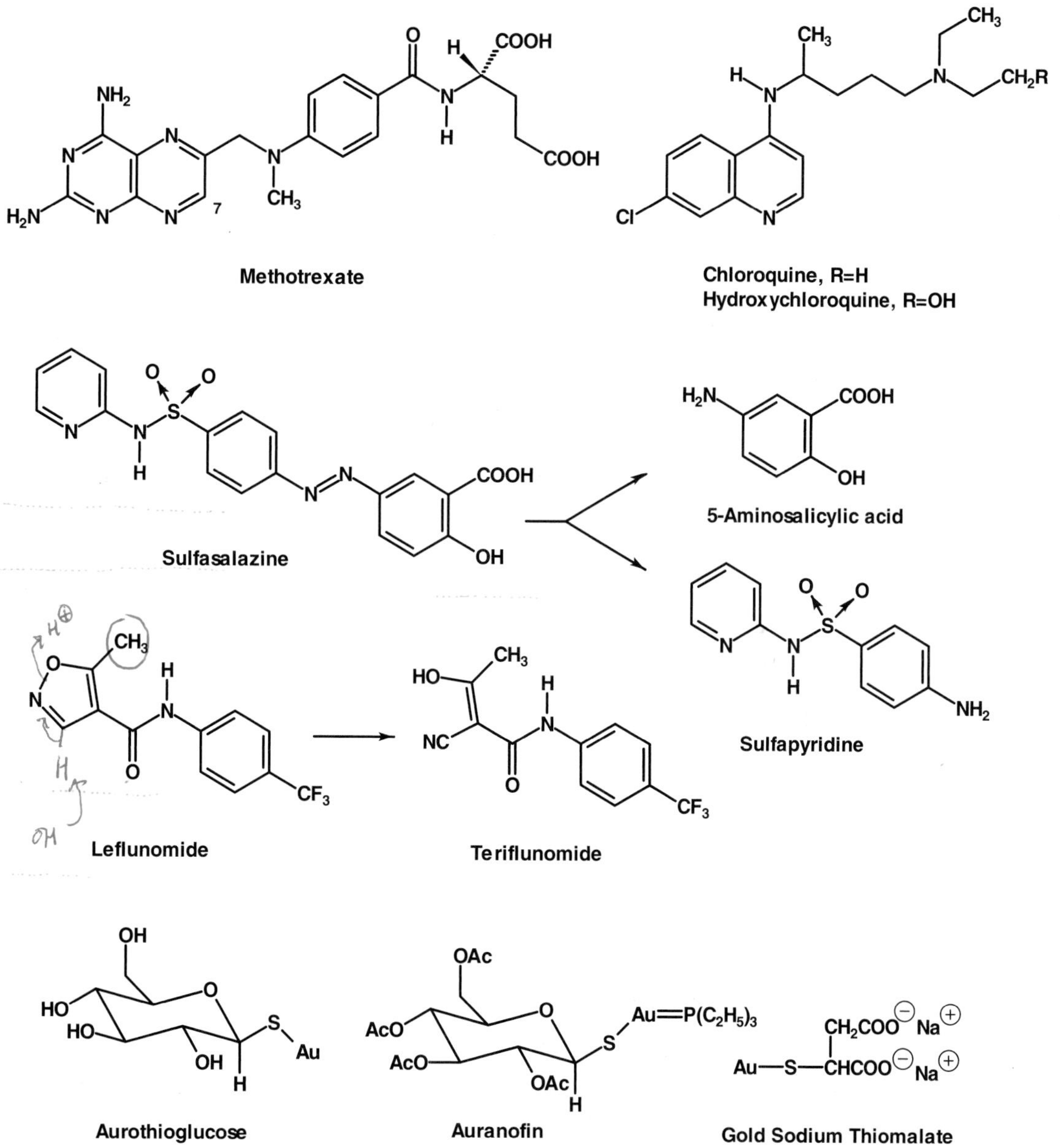

Figure 24.24 ● Disease-modifying antirheumatic drugs.

Readers should consult other chapters in this text for additional information regarding these drugs.

METHOTREXATE

Methotrexate (MTX, Rheumatrex), an antifolate drug used in cancer treatment, has also been used in the disease management of RA since the 1950s. Because of its quicker therapeutic onset among all DMARDs and its demonstrated efficacy, tolerability, and low cost, MTX has been the first-line therapy for RA patients who are not responsive to NSAIDs alone.[224,226,227] Recent findings have indicated that other DMARDs should only be used for patients who are refractory to MTX.[224,226]

At least four anti-inflammatory mechanisms of action have been suggested for MTX's ability to slow down RA disease progression.[222,228] First, MTX, being a folate antagonist, prevents antigen-dependent T-cell proliferation by blocking de novo pyrimidine biosynthesis, via a reversible inhibition of dihydrofolate reductase.[228] It also inhibits folate-mediated production of spermine and spermidine in synovial tissue. These polyamines are believed to be the toxic compounds responsible for causing tissue injury in RA. MTX can also reduce intracellular glutathione concentration, thereby altering the cellular redox state that suppresses the formation of reactive oxygen radicals in synovial tissue. Lastly, MTX, similar to sulfasalazine, infliximab, and IL-4, can also inhibit osteoclastogenesis (i.e., bone erosion) in patients with RA, by modulating the interaction of the receptor activator of nuclear factor κB, its ligand, and osteoprotegrin.[229]

Methotrexate is usually administered in a once-weekly dose in the range of 15 to 17.5 mg. Although it has good oral bioavailability ($\sim$70%), it is more efficacious via IM or SC routes, because its uptake from the GI tract is mediated by a saturable transporter, known as the reduced folate carrier-1.[225,228] Most of the administered dose of methotrexate is eliminated in the urine via its 7-hydroxymethotrexate metabolite.

Common side effects of MTX include nausea, anemia, and GI mucosa ulcerations. The use of folinic acid supplement to reduce MTX-mediated toxicities, however, is not recommended for RA patients, because high dosages of folinic acid will compete with MTX for the same transporter for absorption from the GI tract and for cellular uptake. Thus, it may also reverse MTX's anti-inflammatory effects in RA patients.[228] Moreover, MTX can cause birth defects in unborn children, thus it is contraindicated for women during pregnancy.

HYDROXYCHLOROQUINE AND CHLOROQUINE

Hydroxychloroquine (Plaquenil, Quineprox) is an older drug used to treat malaria that is used more often in the treatment of RA and lupus erythematosus. Although its mechanism of action is not known, its ability to interfere with lipopolysaccharide-induced TNF-α gene expression, thereby preventing TNF-α release from mononuclear phagocytes has been suggested.[230] It is usually taken orally with food or milk to prevent stomach irritation and is preferred over chloroquine because of a lower incidence of ocular toxicity. However, long-term use of this medication requires periodic retinal examinations because of rare but potentially preventable retinopathy associated with its use, especially at a daily dose over 6.5 mg/kg.[231]

SULFASALAZINE

Sulfasalazine (Azufidine) is an azo prodrug that is reduced by the bacterium present in the lower intestine to its active metabolites, sulfapyridine and 5-aminosalicylic acid (5-ASA or mesalamine). It has been used for the treatment of RA or ankylosing spondylitis, and inflammatory bowel diseases (IBDs) such as ulcerative colitis and Crohn disease.

It is generally agreed that the therapeutic effects of sulfasalazine in treating IBDs are due mainly through its active metabolite, 5-ASA. 5-ASA is believed to work, via similar mechanisms of action to the salicylates discussed earlier, by blocking prostaglandin synthesis in the lower intestine.[165–168] On the other hand, because 5-ASA is completely ionized and very little of this metabolite can enter into systemic circulation, the antirheumatic effects of sulfasalazine have been attributed to its other active metabolite, sulfapyridine.[232] In a more recent study, sulfasalazine and sulfapyridine were found to inhibit 5-aminoimidazole-4-carboxamide ribonucleotide transformylase, an enzyme involved in de novo purine biosynthesis.[233] Sulfasalazine also inhibits neutrophil function, reduces immunoglobulin levels, and interferes with T-cell function via suppression of NF-κB activation.[233] Furthermore, like methotrexate, sulfasalazine has also been shown to inhibit osteoclastogenesis, thereby preventing bone erosion in arthritic patients.[229,234]

It should be pointed out that approximately one third of the patients treated long term with sulfasalazine discontinued the drug because of dose-related adverse effects including nausea, dyspepsia, vomiting, headache, rash, gastric distress, especially in patients on a daily dosage of greater than 4 g (or a serum sulfapyridine levels above 50 mg/mL).

LEFLUNOMIDE

Leflunomide (Arava), an isoxazole prodrug, is an orally active DMARD marketed in 1998 for the treatment of RA. It is well absorbed and extensively metabolized in vivo to its active metabolite, 2-cyano-3-hydroxy-2-buteneamide (teriflunomide), resulting from a reductive ring opening of the isoxazole ring (see Fig. 24.24). Unlike MTX, teriflunomide blocks T-cell proliferation by inhibiting dihydroorotate dehydrogenase, the rate-limiting enzyme in the de novo biosynthesis of pyrimidine that is believed to be responsible for the immunosuppressive properties of leflunomide.[235,236] For this reason, it is not surprising that leflunomide has a very comparable therapeutic efficacy to the first-line DMARD, MTX as shown in several extended open clinical trials.[237] However, even though leflunomide is well tolerated like MTX, several cases of toxic neuropathy have been observed during its use, thus careful monitoring of the patient's neurological status during treatment is mandatory.[237] Like MTX, leflunomide is contraindicated in pregnancy or in women considering pregnancy.

THE GOLD COMPOUNDS

The gold salts, gold sodium thiomalate (Aurolate), aurothioglucose (Solganal), and auranofin (Ridaura) have been known to be effective in the treatment of RA for more than 60 years.[225] Recent findings have suggested that, auranofin, an orally active gold salt, inhibits Nuclear factor κB (NF-κB) activation TLR4-mediated activation of the signaling pathway that leads to the blocking of the formation of inflammatory gene product such as cytokines and COX-2.[238] Because zinc is a necessary component of NF-κB, a transcription factor that is critical for its DNA binding, Yang et al.[239] suggested that auranofin works by oxidizing the zinc containing thiolate anions of NF-κB into a disulfide, thus abolishing the DNA binding requirement for gene expression. However, few patients take gold salt therapy for longer than 5 years because of their toxicities including mucocutaneous reactions, proteinuria, and cytopenias.[222]

OTHER DISEASE-MODIFYING ANTIRHEUMATIC DRUGS

Other DMARDs that can be used in the treatment of RA include penicillamine (Cuprimine), a metabolite of penicillin, or the cytotoxic anticancer drugs such as chlorambucil (Leukeran), Azathioprine (Imuran) and cycophosphamide (Cytoxan), or the other immunosuppressants such as cyclosporine (Sandimmune) and mycophenolate mofetil (MMF). However, most of these drugs are less commonly used because of their toxicities.

⬢ DRUGS USED IN THE MANAGEMENT OF GOUT AND HYPERURICEMIA

In contrast to RA discussed earlier, gout is somewhat unique, in that its cause is well known, therefore gouty inflammation can be effectively controlled and treated with medications.[240,241] Gout is one of the most common causes of acute inflammatory arthritis in men older than 40 years old, characterized by the deposition of monosodium urate crystals in the joints and cartilage.[242] Phagocytosis of urate crystals by human neutrophils (and macrophage) induces the synthesis and release of a glycoprotein, the crystal-induced chemotactic factor (CCF), which is believed to be the initial stimulus in the development of acute gouty attacks.[243] Gouty arthritis is also more prevalent in men than in women by a ratio of approximately 6 to 1.

Hyperuricemia

Hyperuricemia is defined as having serum uric acid levels of greater than 7.0 mg/dL in men or more than 6.0 mg/dL in women. Although recurrent attacks of gouty arthritis in a patient are typically associated with hyperuricemia, most people with high serum urate levels are asymptomatic and may never develop gout.[241,244] Uric acid is a normal metabolic end product of purine nucleotide catabolism (i.e., adenine and guanine), but unlike other mammals, humans lack a critical enzyme, urate oxidase (uricase), needed to further break down uric acid into more water-soluble allantoin (Fig. 24.25).[241,245,246]

Risk Factors

In addition to hyperuricemia, other factors that may also increase the risk of development of gout include hypertension, renal insufficiency, obesity, and the use of thiazides or loop

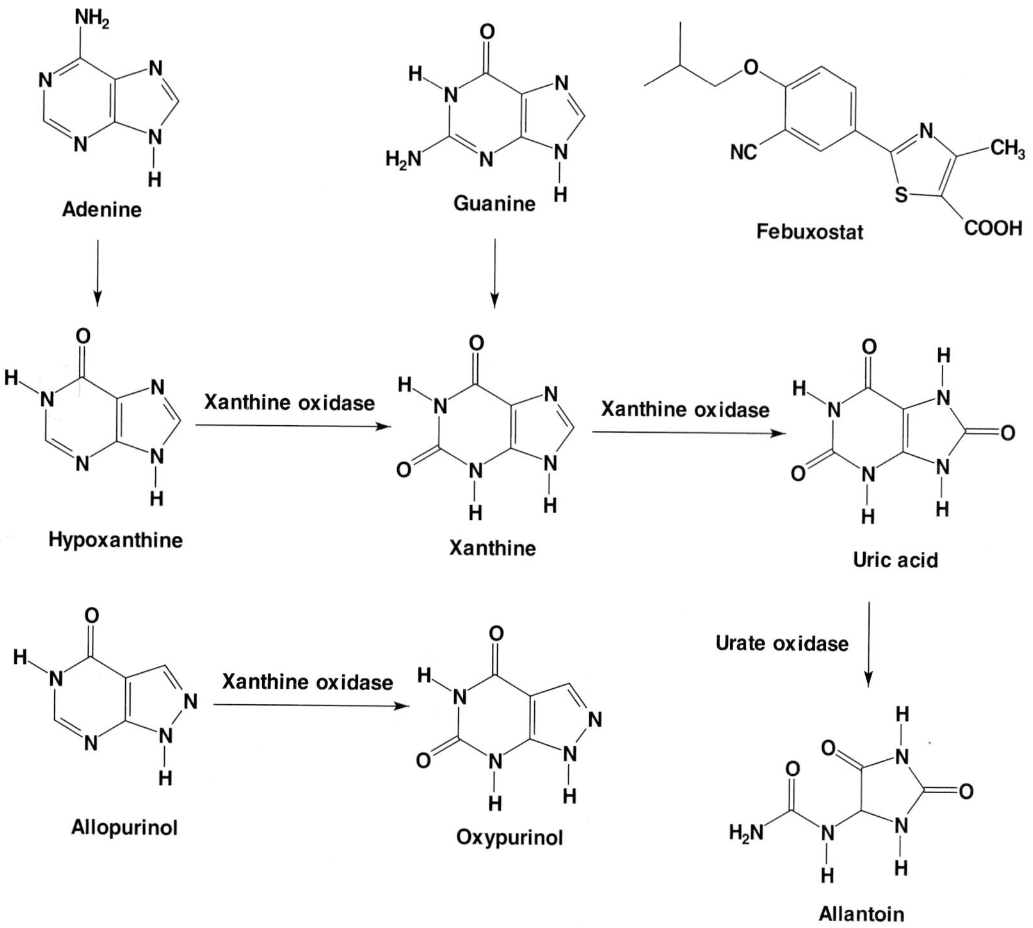

Figure 24.25 ● Catabolism of purine nucleotides and xanthine oxidase inhibitors.

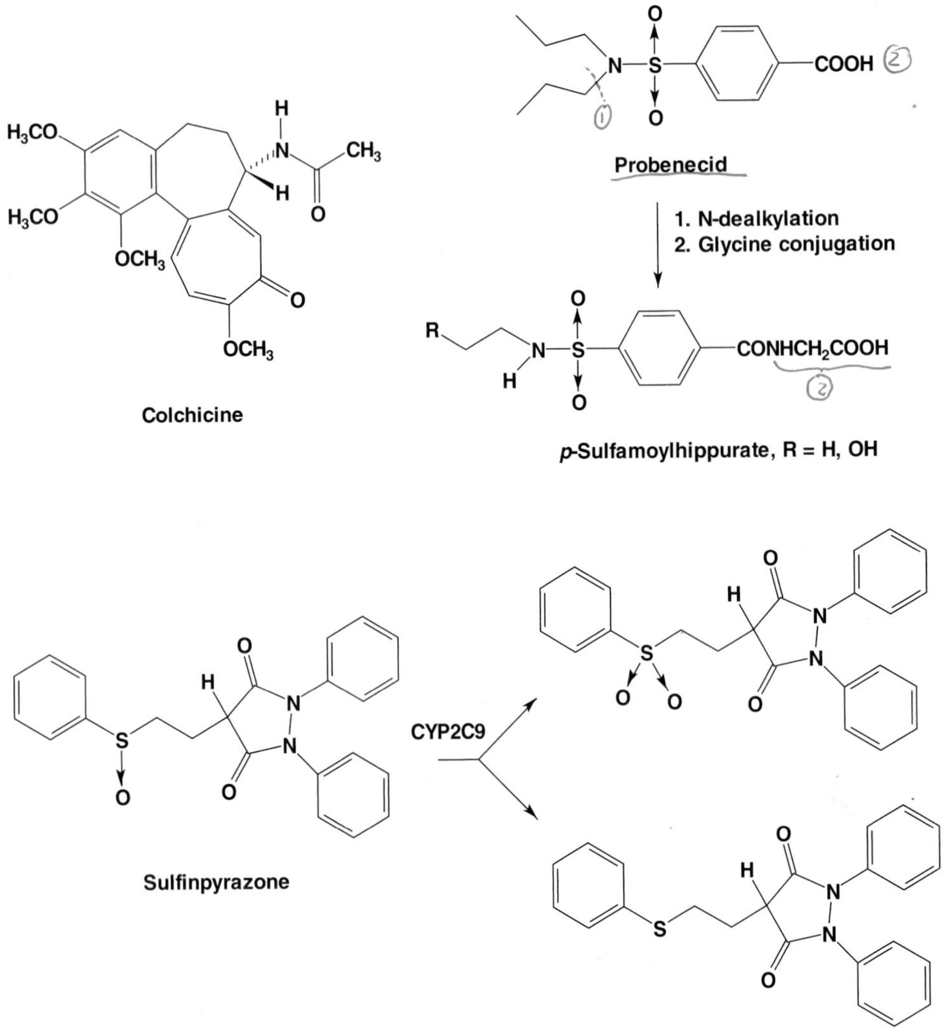

Figure 24.26 ● Colchicine and uricosuric acids.

diuretics, or high intake of alcoholic beverages and purine-rich foods such as meats, liver, bacon, fish, and beans.[241,242] The prevalence of gout also increases in organ-transplant patients who are treated with cyclosporine. Furthermore, early onset of gout (between 20 and 30 years of age) is most likely a result of hereditary disorders of purine metabolism, especially in those who have a hypoxanthine-guanine phosphoribosyltransferase deficiency, thus it should be evaluated before proper treatment is given.[245,247]

Treatment of Acute Gouty Arthritis

The main goal of the pharmacotherapy of acute gouty arthritis is a rapid resolution of pain and debility. The treatment of choice in the United States is the use of NSAIDs for patients with an established diagnosis of uncomplicated gout (i.e., those with heart failure, renal insufficiency, or GI disease).[241,248] For patients who have active peptic ulcers or renal impairment, the choice is either an IM dose of *corticotropin* (ACTH) or an intra-articular injection of glucocorticoids. The chemical aspects of corticosteroids and their therapeutic uses are covered in a separate chapter in this text. Colchicine is generally reserved for prophylaxis of recurrent, acute flare-ups of gouty arthritis or in patients in whom the diagnosis of gout is not yet confirmed.[245,248]

COLCHICINE

Colchicine is an alkaloid isolated from the dried corns and seeds of *Colchicum autumnale L.*, commonly known as autumn crocus or meadow saffron, (see Fig. 24.26 for structure). It is specifically indicated for acute treatment of gouty arthritis because of its ability to block the production and release of the CCF that mediates the inflammatory response because of urate crystals, a mechanism different from colchicine's antimitotic action, which is being investigated for its anticancer properties.[243] It is often quite effective in aborting an acute gouty attack if given within the first 10 to 12 hours after the onset of arthritis.[248,249]

Colchicine can be administered orally or intravenously. A low oral dose of 0.6 mg is taken every 1 to 2 hours, until either the resolution of gouty symptoms or the occurrence of GI toxicities such as increased peristalsis, abdominal discomfort, nausea and vomiting, and diarrhea.[248] Most of the severe systemic toxicity associated with IV administration of colchicine has been linked to an inappropriate use of the drug.[250] Several recent findings comparing the safety and efficacy of colchicine to that of NSAIDs and corticosteroids, have provided strong evidence for eliminating the IV use of colchicine in the treatment of acute gouty arthritis because improper IV dosing can cause severe bone marrow suppression, renal failure, and death.[251,252] Moreover, oral colchicine is also recommended only as a second-line therapy for acute gout treatment when NSAIDs or corticosteroids are contraindicated or ineffective.[252] Concomitant use of oral colchicine with any of the cholesterol-lowering statins including pravastatin (Pravachol) should also be avoided because of increased risk of axonal neuromyopathy that can progress to rhabdomyolysis with renal failure.[253] This is because most of the statins and colchicine are metabolized in liver primarily by the hepatic CYP3A4 isozymes. Colchicine can also induce acute myopathy in patients when used with pravastatin even though it is not metabolized by CYP3A4, because they share the same P-glycoprotein efflux transporter system.[253]

Control of Hyperuricemia

In general, if a patient who has hyperuricemia and the recurrence of gouty arthritis attacks (i.e., less than two attacks/year), their gout can usually be controlled by maintaining serum urate levels below the limit of solubility (i.e., at 6 mg/dL or lower) with drugs that block uric acid synthesis by inhibiting xanthine oxidase or with uricosuric drugs that promote uric acid elimination from the renal tubules.[244,245,248]

XANTHINE OXIDASE INHIBITORS: ALLOPURINOL, OXYPURINOL, FEBUXOSTAT

Allopurinol (Zyloprim, Progout) is the only xanthine oxidase inhibitor available in this class. It is rapidly metabolized to its active isomer oxypurinol (Oxyprim), an experimental drug currently in phase III trials, that has a half-life of approximately 15 hours but was found to exhibit a similar side effect profile to that of allopurinol (i.e., 40% of those allergic to allopurinol have similar cross-reactivity to this drug).[240] Allopurinol and its active metabolite, oxypurinol, works by effectively competing with the substrate hypoxanthine and xanthine, respectively, because of their structural similarity to xanthine, for xanthine oxidase, thus blocking uric acid formation from purine nucleosides, adenine, and guanine as shown in Figure 24.25. Similarly, allopurinol (or oxypurinol) may also exhibit potential drug interactions with other medications such as didanosine (antiviral agent), azathioprine and mercaptopurine (anticancer drugs), and theophylline (asthma drug). For example, if a patient is given a prescription for allopurinol and azathioprine (Imuran), then the dose of azathioprine should be reduced by at least 50% to avoid the risk of myelosuppression by azathioprine.[254]

Febuxostat is a novel and selective, nonpurine inhibitor of xanthine oxidase currently awaiting FDA approval for treatment of chronic gout. It is more effective, at a daily dose of 80 or 120 mg, than allopurinol at the commonly recommended daily dose of 300 mg in lowering serum urate levels.[255,256] Unlike allopurinol, it has minimal effects on other enzymes involved in purine and pyrimidine metabolisms.

URICOSURIC AGENTS: PROBENECID AND SULFINPYRAZONE

Probenecid (Benemid) and sulfinpyrazone (Anturane) are uricosuric agents that work by preventing uric acid reabsorption from the renal proximal tubules (see Fig. 24.26 for structures).[257] They are only effective in patients with normal renal function who are not taking any medications such as the thiazide diuretics that compete for uric acid excretion via the organic anion transporter system (OATS) at the renal proximal tubules. In addition, patients who are using probenecid should also be counseled to avoid using any salicylates at doses greater than 81 mg/d or sulfonamide-containing diuretics such as furosemide, because concomitant use of any salicylates or diuretics can negate its uricosuric activity.[242]

Probenecid

Probenecid (Benemid) is the most widely used uricosuric agent in the United States. It is selectively excreted into the renal tubules by OATS. It is extensively metabolized via *N*-dealkylation or ω-oxidation, followed by phase II conjugation into the active metabolite, *p*-sulfamyl hippurate, which exhibits a high affinity, similar to *p*-aminohippurate, for binding to OATS, thereby preventing uric acid reabsorption from the renal proximal tubules (Fig. 24.26)[257]

Sulfinpyrazone

Sulfinpyrazone (Anturane) produces its uricosuric action in a similar manner to that of probenecid and is indicated for the treatment of chronic and recurrent gouty arthritis. It is well absorbed with approximately 50% of the administered dose excreted as unchanged drug into the renal tubules. The rest of the drug is primarily metabolized via CYP2C9 into the corresponding sulfide and sulfone metabolites, thus it can potentiate the anticoagulant effect of warfarin.[258]

⬡ TRIPTANS

Triptans are safe and effective drugs for abortive, but not for prophylactic, treatment of moderate to severe migraine and cluster headaches.[259] Because of their higher affinity and selectivity for the serotonin 5-HT$_{1B/1D}$ receptors at the trigeminal nerve fibers and dural vasculature, they are able to induce vasoconstrictions at these sites, thereby relieving pain from cranial vasodilatation and reducing neurogenic inflammation associated with these disorders.[259,260] However, triptans are often contraindicated in patients with uncontrolled hypertension, especially those with coronary vascular diseases, even though there are far fewer 5-HT$_{1B}$ receptors found in coronary blood vessels and in the peripheral vasculatures than in the cranial blood vessels.[261] Thus, special attention should also be given to assess the safety and tolerability profile of the triptans when choosing among available drugs because of their pharmacokinetic differences.[261,262]

Pathophysiology of Migraine

Migraine, a recurrent and debilitating headache disorder, affects about 12% of the worldwide population with a higher prevalence in women (~18%) than in men (~6%).[259] In the most recent classification and diagnostic criteria for headache disorders published by the Headache Classification Committee of the International Headache Society, the terms, *common* and *classical* migraines have been replaced with *migraine without aura* and *migraine with aura*, respectively.[263] The patients often describe their migraine attack as having an intense pulsating and throbbing headache lasting from 4 hours to 3 days, if not properly treated.[259,260] In addition to this excruciating pain, migraine patients often have other symptoms like nausea, vomiting, sensitivity to light (photophobia), sound (phonophobia), or movements that can also severely impact their quality of life.

Although the etiology of migraines remains poorly understood, activation of the meningeal nociceptors at the intracranial trigeminovascular system (TGVS, also referred to as the trigeminal pain pathway) is believed to play a key role in promoting headache and other symptoms associated with migraines.[264–266] Several theories have been suggested to explain the underlying causes for the symptoms associated with migraines.[259] Only two of the most prominent theories are briefly discussed under this section.

THE VASCULAR THEORY OF MIGRAINES

According to the vascular theory, the vasodilatation of cranial carotid arteriovenous anastomoses (sites of many 5-$HT_{1B/1D}$ receptors) and meningeal, dural, cerebral, or pial vessels (primary sites of 5-HT_{1B} receptors) plays an important role in the pathogenesis of migraines and is responsible for the pain associated with migraine headaches.[259,261] The fact that sumatriptan-induced cranial vasoconstriction is selectively blocked by a selective 5-HT_{1B} antagonist, and not by a 5-HT_{1D} antagonist, lends further support to this vascular theory of migraines.[267]

THE NEUROGENIC INFLAMMATION THEORY OF MIGRAINES

This theory suggests that migraine headaches occur as a result of an abnormal firing of meningeal nociceptors at the TGVS. Activation of trigeminal neurons releases vasoactive peptides including calcitonin gene-related peptide (CGRP, a vasodilator peptide), substance P, and neurokinin A (both play an important role in pain transmission as well as activation of immune responses and neurogenic inflammation) onto dural tissue where these peptides produce a local response known as neurogenic inflammation.[259] These peptides induce cranial vasodilatation, especially at the dural membranes surrounding the brain (mainly a result of CGRP), thus producing the pain associated with migraine attacks. Further evidence supporting this theory as the underlying cause of migraines can be found from a recent study linking the dural mast cell degranulation to the prolonged activation of the trigeminal pain pathway and neurogenic inflammation.[268]

The discovery of these vasoactive peptides provides new targets for the future design of nonvasoconstrictors, nontriptan drugs such as CGRP antagonists for the acute and preventive treatment of migraine and cluster headaches.[259,269]

Structure–Activity Relationship

All clinically available triptans possess comparable pharmacodynamic properties. They all bind and stimulate serotonin 5-$HT_{1B/1D}$ with affinity in the low nanomolar ranges, thus they are equally effective for the acute treatment of migraine.[262,270] However, they all have different pharmacokinetic properties and side effect profiles that vary in type and severity.[261] Thus, they are not equally efficacious in preventing migraine recurrence because of the differences in their elimination half-lives.[262] They also differ in their potential to induce drug-related CNS side effects, especially somnolence and paresthesia that may lead to a patient's noncompliance of an otherwise effective migraine treatment.[270]

Table 24.2 summarizes the pharmacokinetic properties of clinically available triptans that contributes to their efficacy, safety, and tolerability.[259,262,270–274] A quick glance at their chemical structures (see Fig. 24.27) reveals two general structural types, which might provide insights for assessing some of these differences.

The 3-alkylaminoethyl containing triptans (sumatriptan, zolmitriptan, rizatriptan, and almotriptan) are substrates for the hepatic monoamine oxidase type A (MAO-A) because

TABLE 24.2 Pharmacokinetic Properties of the Triptans[a]

Drug	Trade Name	Bioavailability Oral (%)	Onset Time (min)	Plasma Half-life (h)	Metabolizing Enzyme[a,b]	Drug Interactions	% CNS Side Effects
Sumitriptan	Imitrex Imigrain	14	10–15 (iv) 15–30 (nasal) 30–90 (PO)	2	MAO-A	MAOIs especially MAO-A inhibitors	1.7–6.3
Zolmitriptan	Zomig, Zomig-ZMT	40–48	10–15 (nasal) 45–60 (PO)	3	CYP1A2 MAO-A	MAOIs, SSRIs, Cimethidine	9.9–11.5
Naratriptan	Amerge Naramig	63 (men) 74 (women)	60–180 (PO)	5–6.3	Renal/CYP isozymes		1.9
Rizatriptan	Maxalt Maxalt-MLT	45	30–120 (PO)	2–3	MAO-A	MAOIs especially MAO-A inhibitors, Propranolol	6.1–9.4
Almotriptan	Axert	70–80	60–180 (PO)	3.3	MAO-A CYP3A4		1.5
Frovatriptan	Prova	60	120–180 (PO)	26	CYP1A2	Fluvoxamine, ciprofloxacin, mexiletine	6.0
Eletriptan	Relpax	50	30–60 (PO)	3.6–5.5	CYP3A4	Ketoconazole and other CYP3A4 inhibitors	2.6–14.6

[a]Compiled from data reported in the following references (1, 4, 12, and 13).
[b]Primary mode of metabolism listed first.

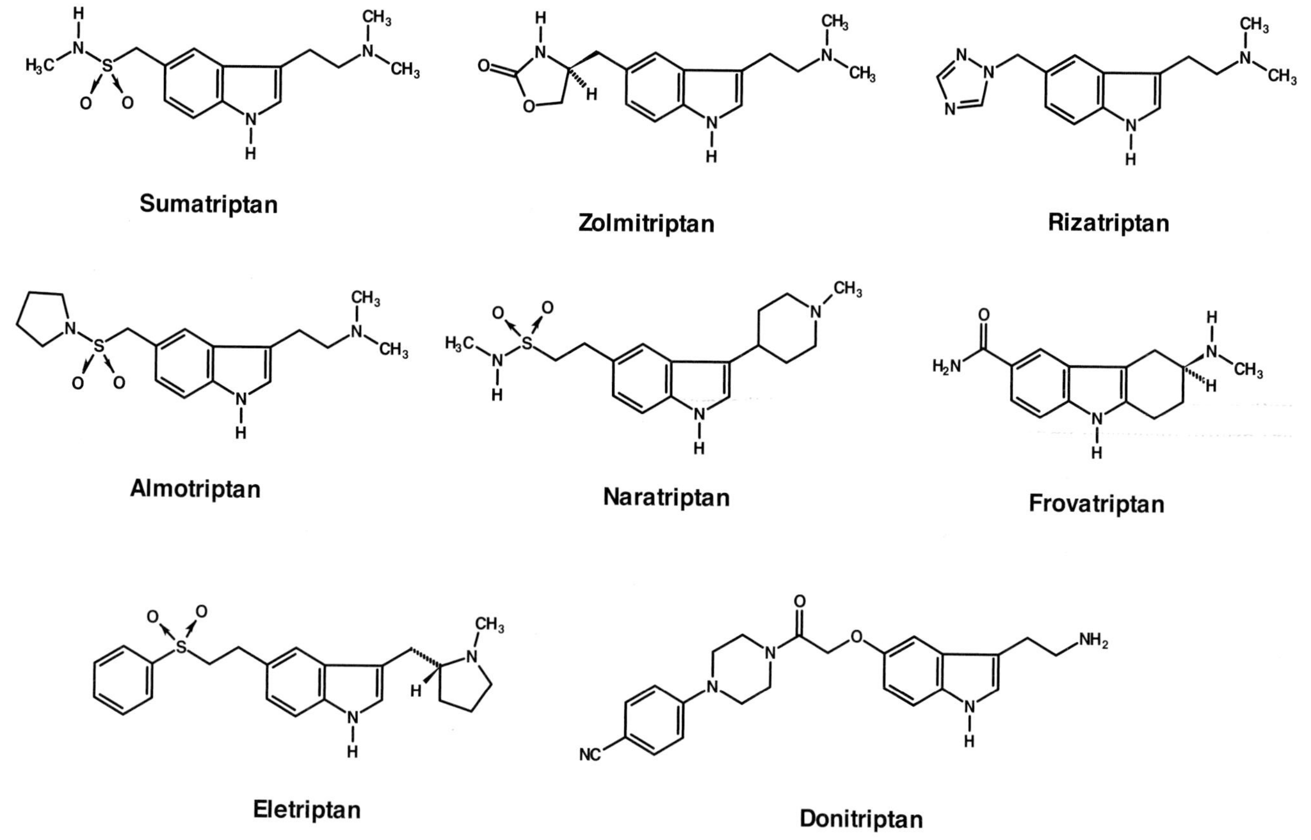

Figure 24.27 ● Triptans.

of their structural resemblance to 5-HT, the preferred substrate for MAO-A. They all have a relatively short duration of action (i.e., 2–3 hours) because of first-pass metabolic inactivation by the MAO-A into an indole acetic acid metabolite that is rapidly eliminated as their corresponding glucuronides. Thus, the use of these triptans requires repeat dosing to prevent the recurrence of migraine attack. They are also contraindicated with concomitant use of any MAO inhibitors, especially inhibitors of MAO-A such as the antidepressant drug, moclobemide (Aurorix, Mauerix).[261,273]

Eletriptan, frovatriptan, and naratriptan, on the other hand, with their 3-alkylamino side chain fused into a carbocyclic ring structure, all have much longer elimination half-lives and lower incidence of headache recurrence reported.[273] This is because they are not a substrate for MAO-A (amphetamine is not a substrate for MAO because it has an additional methyl group α to the terminal amine function). These triptans are mainly degraded by the hepatic CYP isozymes (CYP1A2, 2D6, 3A4), but their bioavailability may be altered with a drug that inhibits or induces these CYP isozymes.[275] For example, eletriptan is primarily metabolized by CYP3A4 isozyme, thus it is not advisable to use eletriptan with a CYP3A4 inhibitor such as ketoconazole, or nefazodone without appropriately adjusting their dosages.[275]

The highest reported incidences of drug-induced CNS toxicities were found with eletriptan (14% at 80-mg dose), zolmitriptan (11.5% at 5-mg dose) and rizatriptan (9.4% at 10-mg dose). They all have N-demethylated, active metabolites that can easily gain entry into the brain because of their high lipophilicity.[270] Thus, the presence of this active metabolite in the brain and the high lipophilicity of the parent triptan have been suggested as a factor for contributing to the observed CNS side effects of the triptans.[270] This hypothesis is further supported by the fact that frovatriptan has a much lower CNS toxicity because of the greater water solubility of its N-demethylated active metabolite that prevents it from entering the brain, whereas sumatriptan, almotriptan, and naratriptan all have a very low reported incidence of CNS side effects because they have no clinically significant active metabolites.[270,276]

Donitriptan, a unique high-efficacy and high-selectivity 5-HT$_{1B/1D}$ agonist (i.e., with high-intrinsic activity approaching that of the endogenous agonist 5-HT) currently in late-stage clinical trials, is a novel arylpiperazole derivative with much better consistency of pain relief and a lower incidence of migraine recurrence.[277] Furthermore, unlike sumatriptan, it can also block capsaicin-sensitive trigeminal sensory nerves from releasing CGRP, resulting in selective cranial vasodilatation and central nociception.[278]

Mechanism of Action

Triptans are specifically designed to bind to the 5-HT$_{1B/1D}$ receptors based on the findings that 5-HT$_{1B}$ receptors are present in the cranial blood vessels[279,280] and 5-HT$_{1B/1D}$ receptors are found in the trigeminal pain pathway.[280,281] Three distinct mechanisms have been suggested to explain the actions of triptans: (a) Triptans abort migraine headache by its agonist action at the 5-HT$_{1B}$ receptors, thereby inducing vasoconstriction of the meningeal, dural, or pial blood vessels.[279] (b) Triptans also inhibit neurogenic inflammation via its presynaptic stimulation of 5-HT$_{1D}$ receptors and/or through its additional action at the 5-HT$_{1B/1D}$ receptors.[281] (c) Triptans relieve migraine pain transmission most likely because of its inhibitory action at the trigeminal pain pathway mediated via 5-HT$_{1B/1D/1F}$ receptors.[259,279,280]

Antimigraine Drugs Acting on 5-HT$_{1B/1D}$ Receptors

SUMATRIPTAN (IMITREX)

Sumatriptan was the first triptan approved (1991) for the acute treatment of migraine headaches. It has the lowest oral bioavailability among all triptans because of its low lipophilicity. The availability of many different dosage forms (i.e., an oral tablet, a SC injection, a nasal spray formulation, and a suppository) allows the flexibility of tailoring therapy to the needs of the individual patients, thus making sumatriptans a very useful drug for an acute treatment of migraine headaches.[262,282] It also has a very fast onset of action via SC injection or nasal spray administration. However, sumatriptan is contraindicated with monoamine oxidase inhibitors because it is primarily degraded by hepatic MAO-A. Thus, it may require frequent dosing as a result of its short duration of action to prevent migraine recurrence.[262,282]

ZOLMITRIPTAN (ZOMIG, ZOMIG-ZMT)

Zolmitriptan, the second triptan marketed (approved in 1997), has a much better bioavailability (40%–48%) than sumatriptan. It is rapidly absorbed after oral or nasal spray administration. It also has an orally disintegrating tablet formulation (Zomig ZMT), which can be taken without water. Zolmitriptan undergoes rapid *N*-demethylation via CYP1A2 to a more potent, active metabolite, *N*-desmethylzolmitriptan, which is 2 to 6 times more potent than the parent drug.[262,283] This active metabolite was detected 5 minutes after dosing and accounts for about two thirds of the plasma concentration of the administered dose of the parent drug.[284] Thus, it is reasonable to assume that the therapeutic effects and especially the CNS side effects of zolmitriptan must be in part attributed to the plasma levels of this active metabolite, at least until it is further degraded by hepatic MAO-A to its inactive indole acetic acid derivatives.[262,283]

NARATRIPTAN (AMERGE, NARAMIG)

Naratriptan, the third triptan approved in 1998, is one of the most lipophilic triptans marketed to date. It has a much improved bioavailability (63% in men and 74% in women), a greater affinity for 5-HT$_{1B/1D}$ receptors (3–6 times), and a lower recurrence rate than sumatriptan because of its much longer elimination half-life.[262,285] Naratritan also has a favorable CNS side effect profile when compared with sumatriptan or zolmitriptan because of its metabolic stability, thereby lacking a *N*-demethylated active metabolite and a significant renal excretion (>70% of naratriptan is excreted unchanged and the rest of the administered dose is degraded via several CYP isozymes).[262,270,286]

RIZATRIPTAN (MAXALT)

Rizatriptan, approved in 1998, is a fast-acting triptan because of its moderate lipophilicity yet has a very short elimination half-life similar to sumatriptan (i.e., like sumatriptan, it is mainly metabolized by MAO-A). The only advantages of this drug when compared with sumatriptan are that it has a slightly faster onset and that it has an orally disintegrating tablet formulation which can be taken without water.[262]

ALMOTRIPTAN (AXERT)

Almotriptan, marketed in 2000, has the highest oral bioavailability among all triptans (see Table 24.2). It is metabolized by both MAO-A and CYP3A4, thus has a more favorable side effects profile when compared with sumatriptan. However, it is only available in a 12.5 mg tablet form.

FROVATRIPTAN (FROVA)

Frovatriptan is a newer triptan introduced into the market in 2001. With the incorporation of a 3-alkylamino side chain into a carbazole ring structure, it is not a substrate for MAO-A or CYP3A4. Thus, unlike the other clinically available triptans, it possesses a much longer duration of action with fewer drug–drug interactions with MAO inhibitors or with drugs metabolized by the CYP3A4 isozymes.[274,276] It is primarily metabolized by CYP1A2 to give its active metabolite, *N*-desmethyl-frovatriptan, which has about one third of the binding affinity for 5-HT$_{1D/1B}$ receptors but with three times longer plasma half-life of the parent drug.[276,287]

Frovatriptan also has the highest affinity for brain 5-HT$_{1B}$ receptors and the longest elimination half-life among all triptans.[273,288] The only disadvantage of this drug is its slower onset of action because of its greater water solubility. However, it is a drug of choice for patients with long-lasting migraines or if recurrence is a problem.[273]

ELETRIPTAN (RELPAX)

Eletriptan, introduced into the market in 2002, is the newest triptan with highest affinity for 5-HT$_{1B}$, 5-HT$_{1D}$, and 5-HT$_{1F}$ receptors. It is one of the most lipophilic triptans marketed to date and is well tolerated and safe across its dosing range of 20 to 80 mg.[275] However, it is metabolized primarily (>90%) by CYP3A4 isozyme to its active metabolite, the *N*-desmethyleletriptan, which accounts for approximately 10% to 20% of the plasma concentration of that observed for parent drug.[289] Thus, coadministration of eletriptan with potent CYP3A4 inhibitors such as ketoconazole, itraconazole, nefazodone, troleandomycin, clarithromycin, ritonavir, and nelfinavir may require dose reduction and closer monitoring for CNS side effects.[262,275] Furthermore, because eletriptan and its active metabolite, *N*-desmethyleletriptan, are also substrates for the P-glycoprotein efflux pumps that are responsible for their removal from the brain, coadministration of eletriptan with a known P-glycoprotein inhibitor and/or inducer such as digoxin, diltiazem, verapamil, or St. John's Worth would result in higher brain levels of its active metabolite, and thus a higher rate of the CNS side effects reported for this drug.[290]

1. A patient is brought to the emergency room via ambulance. He is unresponsive to questions, has a respiratory rate of 4 breaths per minute, and an arterial oxygen saturation (SpO_2) of 82% measured by finger pulse oximetry. On physical exam, multiple injection (track) marks are identified on his forearms, and the patient also displays a cutaneous rash over his trunk. The suspected diagnosis is a heroin overdose. The nurse calls the pharmacy for 50 mg of diphenhydramine to treat the cutaneous rash. You do not dispense it, why?

2. A new mom comes to your pharmacy to refill her codeine prescription, prescribed for episiotomy pain. She is concerned because her 2-week-old breastfed baby is extremely lethargic, sleeps all day, and seems unresponsive to stimulus. You recommend that she bring the baby to the emergency room immediately. What genetic polymorphism do you suspect the mom has? What danger does this pose to her breastfed infant?

3. A patient presents to your pharmacy with a prescription for Vicodin ES; 2 tablets q 6 hours around the clock; #240; refills = zero. You do not dispense it, why?

4. A 72-year-old man who has been taking the antiarrythmic drug quinidine for 4 years self treats his diarrhea with Imodium (loperamide). His son calls your pharmacy to report that his father is very sleepy, his pupils are pinpoints, and he is acting "very strange." You suspect that loperamide is having CNS effects. What is the pharmacological reason behind the quinidine-loperamide drug–drug interaction?

5. Diflunisal is a potent, long acting nonselective COX inhibitor. Explain how this drug binds to the COX-1 enzyme, and how it is eliminated from the body.

6. Provide a biochemical reason why acetaminophen, unlike aspirin and other NSAIDS, is a centrally acting analgesic/antipyretic drug that has no anti-inflammatory activity.

7. Provide a possible rationale for why CYP3A4 inducers can increase the clearance of diclofenac, yet CYP3A4 inhibitors have little or no effect on its pharmacokinetic profile.

8. Sulindac, a potent nonselective COX inhibitor, is said to have a lower risk of stomach bleeding and nephrotoxicity than other aspirin-like NSAIDs such as indomethacin. Explain.

9. Provide a possible chemical/biochemical rationale why frovatriptan has a much lower CNS toxicity than eletriptan.

REFERENCES

1. Anonymous. U.S. Department of Health, Education and Welfare. The Interagency Committee on New Therapies for Pain and Discomfort: Report to the White House, 1979.
2. Katz, N. P., Adams, E. H., Benneyan, J. C., et al.: Clin. J. Pain 23:103–118, 2007.
3. Staats, P. S.: J. Pain Symptom Manage. 24:S4–S9, 2002.
4. Fields, H. L.: Pain 129:233–234, 2007.
5. Hobson, A. R., and Aziz, Q.: News Physiol. Sci. 16:109–114, 2003.
6. Riley, J. L., III, Wade, J. B., Myers, C. D., et al.: Pain 100:291–298, 2002.
7. Loeser, J. D., and Melzack, R.: Lancet 353:1607–1609, 1999.
8. Besson, J. M.: Lancet 353:1610–1615, 1999.
9. Zimmermann, M.: Eur. J. Pharmacol. 429:23–37, 2001.
10. Baliki, M. N., Chialvo, D. R., Geha, P. Y., et al.: J. Neurosci. 26:12165–12173, 2006.
11. Kumar, N.: World Health Organization Normative Guidelines on Pain Management-Report of a Delphi Study. 2007.
12. Koyama, T., McHaffie, J. G., Laurienti, P. J., et al.: Proc. Natl. Acad. Sci. U. S. A. 102:12950–12955, 2005.
13. Price, D. D.: Science 288:1769–1772, 2000.
14. Price, D. D., Greenspan, J. D., and Dubner, R.: Pain 106:215–219, 2003.
15. Seminowicz, D. A., and Davis, K. D.: Pain 130:8–13, 2007.
16. Goffaux, P., Redmond, W. J., Rainville, P., et al.: Pain 130:137–143, 2007.
17. Jensen, T. S., and Baron, R.: Pain 102:1–8, 2003.
18. Zech, D. F. J., Grond, S., Lynch, J., et al.: Pain 63:65–76, 1995.
19. Barakzoy, A. S., and Moss, A. H.: J. Am. Soc. Nephrol. 17:3198–3203, 2006.
20. Goldstein, A., Lowney, L. I., and Pal, B. K.: Proc. Natl. Acad. Sci. U. S. A. 68:1742–1747, 1971.
21. Pert, C. B., and Snyder, S. H.: Proc. Natl. Acad. Sci. U. S. A. 70:2243–2247, 1973.
22. Hughes, J., Smith, T. W., and Kosterlitz, H. W.: Nature 258:577–579, 1975.
23. Morley, J. S.: Annu. Rev. Pharmacol. Toxicol. 20:81–110, 1980.
24. Clement-Jones, V., McLoughlin, L., Tomlin, S., et al.: Lancet 2:946–949, 1980.
25. Kenyon, J. N., Knight, C. J., and Wells, C.: Acupunct. Electrother. Res. 8:17–24, 1983.
26. Tseng, L. F., Narita, M., Suganuma, C., et al.: J. Pharmacol. Exp. Ther. 292:576–583, 2000.
27. New, D. C., and Wong, Y. H.: Neurosignals 11:197–212, 2002.
28. Klavdieva, M. M.: Neuroendocrinol. 17:247–280, 1996.
29. Zioudrou, C., Streaty, R. A., and Klee, W. A.: J. Biol. Chem. 254:2446–2449, 1979.
30. Wittert, G., Hope, P., and Pyle, D.: Biochem. Biophys. Res. Commun. 218:877–881, 1996.
31. Stein, C., Hassan, A., Przewlocki, R., et al.: Proc. Natl. Acad. Sci. U. S. A. 87:5935–5939, 1990.
32. Corbett, A. D., Henderson, G., McKnight, A. T., et al.: Br. J. Pharmacol. 147 Suppl 1:S153–S162, 2006.
33. Waldhoer, M., Bartlett, S. E., and Whistler, J. L.: Annu. Rev. Biochem. 73:953–990, 2004.
34. Trescot, A. M., Datta, S., Lee, M., et al.: Pain Physician 11:S133–S153, 2008.
35. Pogozheva, I. D., Lomize, A. L., and Mosberg, H. I.: Biophys. J. 75:612–634, 1998.
36. Chaturvedi, K., Shahrestanifar, M., and Howells, R. D.: Brain Res. Mol. Brain Res. 76:64–72, 2000.
37. Boettcher, C., Fellermeier, M., Boettcher, C., et al.: Proc. Natl. Acad. Sci. U. S. A. 102:8495–8500, 2005.
38. Valiquette, M., Vu, H. K., Yue, S. Y., et al.: J. Biol. Chem. 271:18789–18796, 1996.
39. Befort, K., Tabbara, L., Kling, D., et al.: J. Biol. Chem. 271:10161–10168, 1996.
40. Negus, S. S., Gatch, M. B., Mello, N. K., et al.: J. Pharmacol. Exp. Ther. 286:362–375, 1998.
41. Aldrich, J. V., and Vigil-Cruz, S. C.: Narcotic analgesics. In Abraham D. J., (ed.). Burger's Medicinal Chemistry and Drug Discovery. New York, John Wiley and Sons, 2003.
42. Portoghese, P. S., Moe, S. T., and Takemori, A. E.: J. Med. Chem. 36:2572–2574, 1993.

43. Portoghese, P. S., Sultana, M., Nagase, H., et al.: J. Med. Chem. 31:281–282, 1988.
44. Broom, D. C., Jutkiewicz, E. M., Rice, K. C., et al.: Jpn. J. Pharmacol. 90:1–6, 2002.
45. Mansour, A., Hoversten, M. T., Taylor, L. P., et al.: Brain Res. 700:89–98, 1995.
46. Nagase, H., Hayakawa, J., Kawamura, K., et al.: Chem. Pharm. Bull. (Tokyo) 46:366–369, 1998.
47. Wadenberg, M. G.: CNS Drug Rev. 9:187–198, 2003.
48. Chavkin, C., Sud, S., Jin, W., et al.: J. Pharmacol. Exp. Ther. 308:1197–1203, 2004.
49. Wang, Y., Tang, K., Inan, S., et al.: J. Pharmacol. Exp. Ther. 312:220–230, 2005.
50. Reinscheid, R. K., Higelin, J., Henningsen, R. A., et al.: J. Biol. Chem. 273:1490–1495, 1998.
51. Broccardo, M., Guerrini, R., Morini, G., et al.: Peptides 28:1974–1981, 2007.
52. Schiff, P. L. J.: Amer. J. Pharm. Educ. 66:186–194, 2002.
53. Novak, B. H., Hudlicky, T., Reed, J. W., et al.: Curr. Org. Chem. 4:343–362, 2000.
54. McQuay, H. J., and Moore, R. A.: Opioid problems, and morphine metabolism and excretion. In Handbook of experimental pharmacology. Springer Verlag KG, 1997, vol. 130, pp. 335–360.
55. Buetler, T., Wilder-Smith, O., Wilder-Smith, C., et al.: Br. J. Anaesth. 84:97–99, 2000.
56. Lotsch, J., Skarke, C., Schmidt, H., et al.: Clin. Pharmacol. Ther. 79:35–48, 2006.
57. Vree, T. B., van Dongen, R. T., and Koopman-Kimenai, P. M.: Int. J. Clin. Pract. 54:395–398, 2000.
58. Skarke, C., Darimont, J., Schmidt, H., et al.: Clin. Pharmacol. Ther. 73:107–121, 2003.
59. Lotsch, J., Kobal, G., and Geisslinger, G.: Clin. Neuropharmacol. 21:351–354, 1998.
60. Eckhardt, K., Li, S., Ammon, S., et al.: Pain 76:27–33, 1998.
61. Schroeder, K., and Fahey, T.: Cochrane Database Syst. Rev. (4):CD001831, 2004.
62. Casy, A. F., and Parfitt, R. T.: Opioid Analgesics Chemistry and Receptors. New York, Plenum Press, 1986, pp. 518.
63. Willette, R. E.: Ch. 22 Analgesic agents. In Block, J. H., and Beale, J. M., Jr., (eds.). Wilson and Gisvold's Textbook of Organic Medicinal and Pharmaceutical Chemistry, 11th ed. New York, Lippincott Williams and Wilkins, 2004, pp. 731–766.
64. Kaplan, H. L., Busto, U. E., Baylon, G. J., et al.: J. Pharmacol. Exp. Ther. 281:103–108, 1997.
65. Poyhia, R., Seppala, T., Olkkola, K. T., et al.: Br. J. Clin. Pharmacol. 33:617–621, 1992.
66. Anonymous. Drug Abuse Warning Network, 2005: National estimates of drug-related emergency department visits Series D-29, DHHS Publication No. (SMA) 07-4256, Rockville, MD, accessed January 28, 2008.
67. Prommer, E. E.: J. Palliat. Med. 10:1228–1230, 2007.
68. Stringer, M., Makin, M. K., Miles, J., et al.: d-morphine, but not l-morphine, has low micromolar affinity for the non-competitive N-methyl-D-aspartate site in rat forebrain. Possible clinical implications for the management of neuropathic pain. Neurosci. Lett. 295:21–24, 2000.
69. Anonymous. Substance Abuse and Mental Health Services Administration, Office of Applied Studies. The NSDUH Report: Misuse of Over-the-Counter Cough and Cold Medications among Persons Aged 12 to 25. Rockville, MD, January 10, 2008.
70. Smith, S. M., Schroeder, K., and Fahey, T.: Cochrane Database Syst. Rev. (1):CD001831, 2008.
71. Ball, J., and Alexson, S. H.: The Dawn Report: Emergency Department Visits Involving Dextromethorphan. Rockville MD, Substance Abuse and Mental Health Services Administration, 2006, 32, 1–4.
72. Abraham, R. B., Marouani, N., and Weinbroum, A. A.: Ann. Surg. Oncol. 10:268–274, 2003.
73. Sindrup, S. H., and Jensen, T. S.: Pain 83:389–400, 1999.
74. Anonymous. Package Insert: Talwin Nx. September 2006, 7.
75. Zacny, J. P., Hill, J. L., Black, M. L., et al.: J. Pharmacol. Exp. Ther. 286:1197–1207, 1998.
76. Gear, R. W., Gordon, N. C., Heller, P. H., et al.: Neurosci. Lett. 205:207–209, 1996.
77. Gear, R. W., Miaskowski, C., Gordon, N. C., et al.: Pain 83:339–345, 1999.
78. Zhang, J., Burnell, J. C., Dumaual, N., et al.: J. Pharmacol. Exp. Ther. 290:314–318, 1999.
79. Latta, K. S., Ginsberg, B., and Barkin, R. L.: Am. J. Ther. 9:53–68, 2002.
80. Simopoulos, T. T., Smith, H. S., Peeters-Asdourian, C., et al.: Arch. Surg. 137:84–88, 2002.
81. Seifert, C. F., and Kennedy, S.: Pharmacotherapy 24:776–783, 2004.
82. Tissot, T. A.: Anesthesiology 98:1511–1512, 2003.
83. Palmer, K. R., Corbett, C. L., and Holdsworth, C. D.: Gastroenterology 79:1272–1275, 1980.
84. McCarron, M. M., Challoner, K. R., and Thompson, G. A.: Pediatrics 87:694–700, 1991.
85. Baker, D. E.: Rev. Gastroenterol. Disord. 7 Suppl 3:S11–S18, 2007.
86. Sandhu, B. K., Tripp, J. H., Candy, D. C., et al.: Gut 22:658–662, 1981.
87. Schinkel, A. H., Wagenaar, E., Mol, C. A., et al.: J. Clin. Invest. 97:2517–2524, 1996.
88. Subramanian, G., Paterlini, M. G., Portoghese, P. S., et al.: J. Med. Chem. 43:381–391, 2000.
89. Westmoreland, C. L., Hoke, J. F., Sebel, P. S., et al.: Anesthesiology 79:893–903, 1993.
90. Anonymous. Dolophine Hydrochloride CII (Methadone Hydrochloride Tablets, USP) Package Insert, Roxane Laboratories, Inc., Revised 10/2006.
91. Gerber, J. G., Rhodes, R. J., and Gal, J.: Chirality 16:36–44, 2004.
92. Foster, D. J., Somogyi, A. A., and Bochner, F.: Br. J. Clin. Pharmacol. 47:403–412, 1999.
93. Iribarne, C., Berthou, F., Baird, S., et al.: Chem. Res. Toxicol. 9:365–373, 1996.
94. Totah, R. A., Sheffels, P., Roberts, T., et al.: Anesthesiology 108:363–374, 2008.
95. Wang, J., and DeVane, C. L.: Drug Metab. Dispos. 31:742–747, 2003.
96. Fick, D. M., Cooper, J. W., Wade, W. E., et al.: Arch. Intern. Med. 163:2716–2724, 2003.
97. Ulens, C., Daenens, P., and Tytgat, J.: Cardiovasc. Res. 44:568–578, 1999.
98. Willens, J. S.: Pain Manag. Nurs. 7:43–43, 2006.
99. Anonymous. Tramadol HCl Tablets, Ultram, Package Insert, Ortho-McNeil, Revised December 1999.
100. Evans, G. R., Henshilwood, J. A., and O'Rourke, J.: Tetrahedron Asymmetry 12:1663–1670, 2001.
101. Potschka, H., Friderichs, E., and Loscher, W.: Br. J. Pharmacol. 131:203–212, 2000.
102. Scott, L. J., and Perry, C. M.: Drugs 60:139–176, 2000.
103. Raffa, R. B., Friderichs, E., Reimann, W., et al.: J. Pharmacol. Exp. Ther. 267:331–340, 1993.
104. Raffa, R. B.: J. Clin. Pharm. Ther. 33:101–108, 2008.
105. Anonymous. DEA Office of Diversion Control, Nalbuphine. (http://www.deadiversion.usdoj.gov/drugs_concern/nalbuphine.htm), 2008.
106. Anonymous. Nubaine (Nalbuphine Hydrochloride), Package Insert, Endo Pharmaceuticals Inc., Updated January, 2005.
107. Aitkenhead, A. R., Lin, E. S., and Achola, K. J.: Br. J. Clin. Pharmacol. 25:264–268, 1988.
108. Anonymous. Press Release: Penwest Begins Dosing Phase IIa Clinical Study of Nalbuphine ER. (http://www.penwest.com/2008).
109. De Souza, E., Schmidt, W., and Kuhar, M.: J. Pharmacol. Exp. Ther. 244:391–402, 1998.
110. Gunion M. W., Marchionne A. M., and Anderson, C. T. M.: Acute Pain 6:29–39, 2004.
111. Commiskey, S., Fan, L. W., Ho, I. K., et al.: J. Pharmacol. Sci. 98:109–116, 2005.
112. Anonymous. Critical Review of Butorphanol; WHO 34th Expert Committee on Drug Dependence (ECDD) 2006. http://www.who.int/medicines/areas/quality_safety/4.1Buthorphanol CritReview.pdf.
113. Megarbane, B., Hreiche, R., Pirnay, S., et al.: Toxicol. Rev. 25:79–85, 2006.
114. Dahan, A., Yassen, A., Romberg, R., et al.: Br. J. Anaesth. 96:627–632, 2006.
115. Kosten, T. R., Morgan, C., and Kleber, H. D.: NIDA Res. Monogr. 121:101–119, 1992.
116. Lewis, J. W., and Walter, D.: NIDA Res. Monogr. 121:5–11, 1992.
117. Griessinger, N., Sittl, R., and Likar, R.: Curr. Med. Res. Opin. 21:1147–1156, 2005.
118. Picard, N., Cresteil, T., Djebli, N., et al.: Drug Metab. Dispos. 33:689–695, 2005.

119. Anonymous. Vivitrol (naltrexone for extended-release injectable suspension) Package Insert Manufactured by Alkermes, Inc. Marketed by Cephalon, Inc. Revised 11/10/05.

120. Lobmaier, P., Kornor, H., Kunoe, N., et al.: Cochrane Database Syst. Rev. (2):CD006140, 2008.

121. Fujimoto, J. M.: Proc. Soc. Exp. Biol. Med. 133:317–319, 1970.

122. Weinstein, S. H., Pfeffer, M., Schor, J. M., et al.: J. Pharm. Sci. 60:1567–1568, 1971.

123. Costantini, L. C., Kleppner, S. R., McDonough, J., et al.: Int. J. Pharm. 283:35–44, 2004.

124. Grant, J. E., Potenza, M. N., Hollander, E., et al.: Am. J. Psychiatry 163:303–312, 2006.

125. Mason, B. J., Salvato, F. R., Williams, L. D., et al.: Arch. Gen. Psychiatry 56:719–724, 1999.

126. Fiorucci, S., Meli, R., Bucci, M., et al.: Biochem. Pharmacol. 2001, 62:1433–1438.

127. Champion, G. D., Feng, P. H., Azuma, T., et al.: Drugs 53:6–19, 1997.

128. Vane, J. R.: Nat. New Biol. 231:232–235, 1971.

129. Vane, J. R., and Botting, R. M.: Inflamm. Res. 47 Suppl 2:S78–S87, 1998.

130. Warner, T. D., Giuliano, F., Vojnovic, I., et al.: Proc. Natl. Acad. Sci. U. S. A. 96:7563–7568, 1999.

131. Meyer-Kirchrath, J., and Schror, K.: Curr. Med. Chem. 7:1121–1129, 2000.

132. Zeilhofer, H. U.: Biochem. Pharmacol. 73:165–174, 2007.

133. Vane, J.: Nature 367:215–216, 1994.

134. Vane, J. R., and Botting, R. M.: Inflamm. Res. 44:1–10, 1995.

135. McGettigan, P., and Henry, D.: JAMA 296:1633–1644, 2006.

136. Howard, P. A., and Delafontaine, P.: J. Am. Coll. Cardiol. 43:519–525, 2004.

137. Graham, D. J.: JAMA 296:1653–1656, 2006.

138. Vane, J. R., Bakhle, Y. S., and Botting, R. M.: Annu. Rev. Pharmacol. Toxicol. 38:97–120, 1998.

139. Charlier, C., and Michaux, C.: Eur. J. Med. Chem. 38:645–659, 2003.

140. Fenner, H.: Semin. Arthritis Rheum. 26:28–33, 1997.

141. Garcia Rodriguez, L. A., and Jick, H.: Lancet 343:769–772, 1994.

142. Langman, M. J., Weil, J., Wainwright, P., et al.: Lancet 343:1075–1078, 1994.

143. Smith, W. L., DeWitt, D. L., and Garavito, R. M.: Annu. Rev. Biochem. 69:145–182, 2000.

144. Marnett, L. J., and Kalgutkar, A. S.: Curr. Opin. Chem. Biol. 2:482–490, 1998.

145. Kiefer, J. R., Pawlitz, J. L., Moreland, K. T., et al.: Nature 405:97–101, 2000.

146. Kurumbail, R. G., Stevens, A. M., Gierse, J. K., et al.: Nature 384:644–648, 1996.

147. Gund, P., and Shen, T. Y.: J. Med. Chem. 20:1146–1152, 1977.

148. Luong, C., Miller, A., Barnett, J., et al.: Nat. Struct. Biol. 3:927–933, 1996.

149. Duggan, D., Hooke, K., Risley, E., et al.: J. Pharmacol. Exp. Ther. 201:8–13, 1977.

150. Kalgutkar, A. S., Crews, B. C., Rowlinson, S. W., et al.: Proc. Natl. Acad. Sci. U. S. A. 97:925–930, 2000.

151. Hamman, M. A., Haehner-Daniels, B. D., Wrighton, S. A., et al.: Biochem. Pharmacol. 60:7–17, 2000.

152. van Ryn, J., Trummlitz, G., and Pairet, M.: Curr. Med. Chem. 7:1145–1161, 2000.

153. Dannhardt, G., and Laufer, S.: Curr. Med. Chem. 7:1101–1112, 2000.

154. McKinney, A. R., Suann, C. J., and Stenhouse, A. M.: Rapid Commun. Mass Spectrom. 18:2338–2342, 2004.

155. Busch, U.: Drug Metab. Dispos. 26:576–584, 1998.

156. Ludwig, E., Schmid, J., Beschke, K., et al.: J. Pharmacol. Exp. Ther. 290:1–8, 1999.

157. Aronoff, D. M., and Neilson, E. G.: Am. J. Med. 111:304–315, 2001.

158. Del Tacca, M., Colucci, R., Fornai, M., et al.: Clin. Drug Investig. 22:799–818, 2002.

159. Orlowski, J. P., Hanhan, U. A., and Fiallos, M. R.: Drug Saf. 25:225–231, 2002.

160. Patrono, C., Garcia Rodriguez, L. A., Landolfi, R., et al.: N. Engl. J. Med. 353:2373–2383, 2005.

161. Patrono, C. N.: Engl. J. Med. 330:1287–1294, 1994.

162. Amann, R., and Peskar, B. A.: Eur. J. Pharmacol. 447:1–9, 2002.

163. Wu, K. K.: Circulation 102:2022–2023, 2002.

164. Riendeau, D., Charleson, S., Cromlish, W., et al.: Can. J. Physiol. Pharmacol. 75:1088–1095, 1997.

165. Xu, X. M., Sansores-Garcia, L., Chen, X. M., et al.: Proc. Natl. Acad. Sci. U. S. A. 96:5292–5297, 1999.

166. Negrotto, S., Malaver, E., Alvarez, M. E., et al.: J. Pharmacol. Exp. Ther. 319:972–979, 2006.

167. Zheng, L., Howell, S. J., Hatala, D. A., et al.: Diabetes 56:337–345, 2007.

168. Pillinger, M. H., Capodici, C., Rosenthal, P., et al.: Proc. Natl. Acad. Sci. U. S. A. 95:14540–14545, 1998.

169. MacDonald, T. M., and Wei, L.: Lancet 361:573–574, 2003.

170. Szczeklik, A., Sanak, M., Nizankowska-Mogilnicka, E., et al.: Curr. Opin. Pulm. Med. 10:51–56, 2004.

171. Gilroy, D. W., Lawrence, T., Perretti, M., et al.: Nat. Rev. Drug Discov. 3:401–416, 2004.

172. Huskisson, E. C., Williams, T. N., Shaw, L. D., et al.: Curr. Med. Res. Opin. 5:589–592, 1978.

173. Loewen, G. R., Herman, R. J., Ross, S. G., et al.: Br. J. Clin. Pharmacol. 26:31–39, 1988.

174. Xu, X., Hirayama, H., and Pang, K. S.: Drug Metab. Dispos. 17:556–563, 1989.

175. Helleberg, L.: Clin. Pharmacokinet. 6:245–258, 1981.

176. Basivireddy, J., Jacob, M., Pulimood, A. B., et al.: Biochem. Pharmacol. 67:587–599, 2004.

177. Ding, A., Ojingwa, J. C., McDonagh, A. F., et al.: Proc. Natl. Acad. Sci. U. S. A. 90:3797–3801, 1993.

178. Smith, P. C., McDonagh, A. F., and Benet, L. Z.: J. Clin. Invest. 77:934–939, 1986.

179. Hayball, P. J., Wrobel, J., Tamblyn, J. G., et al.: Br. J. Clin. Pharmacol. 37:75–78, 1994.

180. Haddock, R. E., Jeffery, D. J., Lloyd, J. A., et al.: Xenobiotica 14:327–337, 1984.

181. Brocks, D. R., and Jamali, F.: Clin. Pharmacokinet. 26:259–274, 1994.

182. Strickmann, D. B., Chankvetadz, B., Blaschke, G., et al.: J. Chromatogr. A 887:393–407, 2000.

183. Tachibana, M., Inoue, N., Yoshida, E., et al.: Pharmacology 68:96–104, 2003.

184. Gamache, D. A., Graff, G., Brady, M. T., et al.: Inflammation 24:357–370, 2000.

185. Nakahura, T., Griswold, W., Lemire, J., et al.: J. Adolesc. Health 23:307–310, 1998.

186. Reichel, C., Brugger, R., Bang, H., et al.: Mol. Pharmacol. 51:576–582, 1997.

187. Mehlisch, D.: J. Clin. Pharmacol. 28:S29–S33, 1988.

188. Porile, J., Bakris, G., and Garella, S.: J. Clin. Pharmacol. 30:468–475, 1990.

189. Tegeder, I., Niederberger, E., Israr, E., et al.: FASEB J. 15:2–4, 2001.

190. Morihara, T., Chu, T., Ubeda, O., et al.: J. Neurochem. 83:1009–1012, 2002.

191. Miller, L. G.: Clin. Pharm. 11:591–603, 1992.

192. Rowlinson, S. W., Kiefer, J. R., Prusakiewicz, J. J., et al.: J. Biol. Chem. 278:45763–45769, 2003.

193. Tang, W., Stearns, R. A., Bandiera, S. M., et al.: Drug Metab. Dispos. 27:365–372, 1999.

194. Mangold, J. B., Gu, H., Rodriguez, L. C., et al.: Drug Metab. Dispos. 32:566–571, 2004.

195. Olkkola, K. T., Brunetto, A. V., and Mattila, M. J.: Clin. Pharmacokinet. 26:107–120, 1994.

196. Engelhardt, G., Homma, D., Schlegel, K., et al.: Inflamm. Res. 44:423–433, 1995.

197. Dogne, J. M., Supuran, C. T., and Pratico, D.: J. Med. Chem. 48:2251–2257, 2005.

198. Sano, H., Kawahito, Y., Wilder, R. L., et al.: Cancer Res. 55:3785–3789, 1995.

199. Kulkarni, S., Rader, J. S., Zhang, F., et al.: Clin. Cancer Res. 7:429–434, 2001.

200. Zha, S., Yegnasubramanian, V., Nelson, W. G., et al.: Cancer Lett. 215:1–20, 2004.

201. FitzGerald, G. A.: Nat. Rev. Drug Discov. 2:879–890, 2003.

202. Pruthi, R. S., Kouba, E., Carson, C. C., 3rd, et al.: Urology 68:917–923, 2006.

203. Tang, C., Shou, M., Mei, Q., et al.: J. Pharmacol. Exp. Ther. 293:453–459, 2000.

204. Brune, K.: Acute Pain 1:33–40, 1997.

205. Brodie, B. B., and Axelrod, J.: J. Pharmacol. Exp. Ther. 97:58–67, 1949.

206. Peters, J. M., Morishima, H., Ward, J. M., et al.: Toxicol. Sci. 50:82–89, 1999.

207. Kis, B., Snipes, J. A., and Busija, D. W.: J. Pharmacol. Exp. Ther. 315:1–7, 2005.

208. Aronoff, D. M., Oates, J. A., and Boutaud, O.: Clin. Pharmacol. Ther. 79:9–19, 2006.

209. Botting, R., and Ayoub, S. S.: Fatty Acids 72:85–87, 2005.

210. Botting, R. M.: Clin. Infect. Dis. 31 Suppl 5:S202–S210, 2000.

211. Chandrasekharan, N. V., Dai, H., Roos, K. L., et al.: Proc. Natl. Acad. Sci. U. S. A. 99:13926–13931, 2002.

212. Ayoub, S. S., Colville-Nash, P. R., Willoughby, D. A., et al.: Eur. J. Pharmacol. 538:57–65, 2006.

213. Censarek, P., Freidel, K., Hohlfeld, T., et al.: Eur. J. Pharmacol. 551:50–53, 2006.

214. Nossaman, B. D., Baber, S. R., Nazim, M. M., et al.: Pharmacology 80:249–260, 2007.

215. Graham, G. G., and Scott, K. F.: Am. J. Ther. 12:46–55, 2005.

216. Lucas, R., Warner, T. D., Vojnovic, I., et al.: FASEB J. 19:635–637, 2005.

217. Hinson, J. A.: Environ. Health Perspect. 49:71–79, 1983.

218. Sinclair, J., Jeffery, E., Wrighton, S., et al.: Biochem. Pharmacol. 55:1557–1565, 1998.

219. DiPetrillo, K., Wood, S., Kostrubsky, V., et al.: Toxicol. Appl. Pharmacol. 185:91–97, 2002.

220. Vale, J. A., and Proudfoot, A. T.: Lancet 346:547–552, 1995.

221. Smith, R. J.: Drug Discov. Today 10:1598–1606, 2005.

222. Gaffo, A., Saag, K. G., and Curtis, J. R.: Am. J. Health. Syst. Pharm. 63:2451–2465, 2006.

223. O'Dell, J. R., Leff, R., Paulsen, G., et al.: Arthritis Rheum. 46:1164–1170, 2002.

224. van der Kooij, S. M., de Vries-Bouwstra, J. K., Goekoop-Ruiterman, Y. P., et al.: Ann. Rheum. Dis. 66:1356–1362, 2007.

225. Gabriel, S. E., Coyle, D., and Moreland, L. W.: Pharmacoeconomics 19:715–728, 2001.

226. Bertele', V., Assisi, A., Di Muzio, V., et al.: Eur. J. Clin. Pharmacol. 63:879–889, 2007.

227. Simmons, D. L.: Drug Discov. Today 11:210–219, 2006.

228. Cronstein, B. N.: Pharmacol. Rev. 57:163–172, 2005.

229. Lee, C. K., Lee, E. Y., Chung, S. M., et al.: Arthritis Rheum. 50:3831–3843, 2004.

230. Weber, S. M., and Levitz, S. M.: J. Immunol. 165:1534–1540, 2000.

231. Mavrikakis, I., Sfikakis, P. P., Mavrikakis, E., et al.: Ophthalmology 110:1321–1326, 2003.

232. Pullar, T., Hunter, J. A., and Capell, H. A.: Br. Med. J. (Clin. Res. Ed) 290:1535–1538, 1985.

233. Cronstein, B. N., Montesinos, M. C., and Weissmann, G.: Proc. Natl. Acad. Sci. U. S. A. 96:6377–6381, 1999.

234. Gadangi, P., Longaker, M., Naime, D., et al.: J. Immunol. 156:1937–1941, 1996.

235. Strand, V., Cohen, S., Schiff, M., et al.: Arch. Intern. Med. 159:2542–2550, 1999.

236. Magne, D., Mezin, F., Palmer, G., et al.: Inflamm. Res. 55:469–475, 2006.

237. Martin, K., Bentaberry, F., Dumoulin, C., et al.: Pharmacoepidemiol. Drug Saf. 16:74–78, 2007.

238. Youn, H. S., Lee, J. Y., Saitoh, S. I., et al.: Biophys. Res. Commun. 350:866–871, 2006.

239. Yang, J. P., Merin, J. P., Nakano, T., et al.: FEBS Lett. 361:89–96, 1995.

240. Wortmann, R. L.: Curr. Opin. Rheumatol. 17:319–324, 2005.

241. Kim, K. Y., Ralph Schumacher, H., Hunsche, E., et al.: Clin. Ther. 25:1593–1617, 2003.

242. Rott, K. T., and Agudelo, C. A.: JAMA 289:2857–2860, 2003.

243. Spilberg, I., Mandell, B., Mehta, J., et al.: J. Clin. Invest. 64:775–780, 1979.

244. Shoji, A., Yamanaka, H., and Kamatani, N.: Arthritis Rheum. 51:321–325, 2004.

245. Terkeltaub, R. A.: N. Engl. J. Med. 349:1647–1655, 2003.

246. Wu, X., et al.: Proc. Natl. Acad. Sci. U. S. A. 91:742–746, 1994.

247. Simmonds, H. A., Duley, J. A., Fairbanks, L. D., et al.: J. Inherit. Metab. Dis. 20:214–226, 1997.

248. Hoskison, T. K., and Wortmann, R. L.: Scand. J. Rheumatol. 35:251–260, 2006.

249. Ahern, M. J., Reid, C., Gordon, T. P., et al.: Aust. N. Z. J. Med. 17:301–304, 1987.

250. Wallace, S. L., and Singer, J. Z.: J. Rheumatol. 15:495–499, 1988.

251. Schlesinger, N.: Expert Opin. Drug Saf. 6:625–629, 2007.

252. Schlesinger, N., Schumacher, R., Catton, M., et al.: Cochrane Database Syst. Rev. (4):CD006190, 2006.

253. Alayli, G., Cengiz, K., Canturk, F., et al.: Ann. Pharmacother. 39:1358–1361, 2005.

254. Mikuls, T. R., MacLean, C. H., Olivieri, J., et al.: Arthritis Rheum. 50:937–943, 2004.

255. Bruce, S. P.: Ann. Pharmacother. 40:2187–2194, 2006.

256. Becker, M. A., Schumacher, H. R., Jr, Wortmann, R. L., et al.: N. Engl. J. Med. 353:2450–2461, 2005.

257. Roch-Ramel, F., and Guisan, B.: News Physiol. Sci. 14:80–84, 1999.

258. He, M., Kunze, K. L., and Trager, W. F.: Drug Metab. Dispos. 23:659–663, 1995.

259. Arulmozhi, D. K., Veeranjaneyulu, A., and Bodhankar, S. L.: Vascul. Pharmacol. 43:176–187, 2005.

260. Striessnig, J.: Drug Discov. Today Dis. Mech. 2:453–462, 2005.

261. Martin, V. T., and Goldstein, J. A.: Am. J. Med. 118(Suppl 1):36S–44S, 2005.

262. Rapoport, A. M., Tepper, S. J., Sheftell, F. D., et al.: Neurol. Sci. 27 Suppl 2:S123–S129, 2006.

263. Anonymous. Cephalalgia 24:1–160, 2004.

264. Strassman, A. M., Raymond, S. A., and Burstein, R.: Nature 384:560–564, 1996.

265. Pietrobon, D., and Striessnig, J.: Nat. Rev. Neurosci. 4:386–398, 2003.

266. Waeber, C., and Moskowitz, M. A.: Neurology 64:S9–S15, 2005.

267. De Vries, P., Sanchez-Lopez, A., Centurion, D., et al.: Eur. J. Pharmacol. 362:69–72, 1998.

268. Levy, D., Burstein, R., Kainz, V., et al.: Pain 130:166–176, 2007.

269. Goadsby, P. J.: Curr. Opin. Neurol. 18:283–288, 2005.

270. Dodick, D. W., and Martin, V.: Cephalalgia 24:417–424, 2004.

271. Armstrong, S. C., and Cozza, K. L.: Psychosomatics 43:502–504, 2002.

272. Rapoport, A. M., and Tepper, S. J.: Arch. Neurol. 58:1479–1480, 2001.

273. Tepper, S. J., and Millson, D.: Expert Opin. Drug Saf. 2:123–132, 2003.

274. Geraud, G., Keywood, C., and Senard, J. M.: Headache 43:376–388, 2003.

275. Mathew, N. T., Hettiarachchi, J., and Alderman, J.: Headache 43:962–974, 2003.

276. Buchan, P., Wade, A., Ward, C., et al.: Headache 42 Suppl 2:S63–S73, 2002.

277. John, G. W., Perez, M., Pauwels, P. J., et al.: CNS Drug Rev. 6:278–289, 2000.

278. Munoz-Islas, E., Gupta, S., Jimenez-Mena, L. R., et al.: Br. J. Pharmacol. 149:82–91, 2006.

279. De Vries, P., Villalon, C. M., and Saxena, P. R.: Eur. J. Pharmacol. 375:61–74, 1999.

280. Ahn, A. H., and Basbaum, A. I.: Pain 115:1–4, 2005.

281. Burstein, R., Jakubowski, M., and Levy, D.: Pain 115:21–28, 2005.

282. Adelman, J. U., and Adelman, R. D.: Clin. Ther. 23:772–788; discussion 771, 2001.

283. Uemura, N., Onishi, T., Mitaniyama, A., et al.: Clin. Drug Investig. 25:199–208, 2005.

284. Kilic, B., Ozden, T., Toptan, S., et al.: Chromatographia Supplement 6:S129–S133, 2007.

285. Lambert, G. A.: CNS Drug Rev. 11:289–316, 2005.

286. Rapoport, A. M., Tepper, S. J., Bigal, M. E., et al.: CNS Drugs 17:431–447, 2003.

287. Buchan, P., Keywood, C., Wade, A., et al.: Headache 42 Suppl 2:S54–S62, 2002.

288. Comer, M. B.: Headache 42 Suppl 2:S47–S53, 2002.

289. Evans, D. C., O'Connor, D., Lake, B. G., et al.: Drug Metab. Dispos. 31:861–869, 2003.

290. Armstrong, S. C., Cozza, K. L., and Sandson, N.: Psychosomatics 44:255–258, 2003.

Steroid Hormones and Therapeutically Related Compounds

PHILIP J. PROTEAU

C H A P T E R   O V E R V I E W

Steroid hormones and related products represent one of the most widely used classes of therapeutic agents. These drugs are used primarily in birth control, hormone-replacement therapy (HRT), inflammatory conditions, and cancer treatment. Most of these agents are chemically based on a common structural backbone, the steroid backbone. Although they share a common structural foundation, the variations in the structures provide specificity for the unique molecular targets. Five general groups of steroid hormones are discussed: estrogens, progestins, androgens, glucocorticoids (GCs), and mineralocorticoids (MCs). The structural bases for the differences in actions and the various therapeutic uses for these compounds are explored. Several review articles and texts provide excellent coverage of the pharmacology and chemistry of steroid hormones.[1–3]

STEROID NOMENCLATURE, STEREOCHEMISTRY, AND NUMBERING

As shown in Figure 25.1, nearly all steroids are named as derivatives of cholestane, androstane, pregnane, or estrane. The standard system of numbering is illustrated with 5α-cholestane (the H8 and H9 protons have been omitted here for clarity).

The absolute stereochemistry of the molecule and any substituents is shown with solid (β) and dashed (α) bonds. Most carbons have one β bond and one α bond, with the β bond lying closer to the "top" or C18 and C19 methyl side of the molecule. Both α- and β-substituents may be axial or equatorial. This system of designating stereochemistry can best be illustrated by the use of 5α-androstane (Fig. 25.2).

The stereochemistry of the H at C5 is always indicated in the name. The stereochemistry of the other H atoms is not indicated, unless it differs from 5α-cholestane. Changing the stereochemistry of any of the ring juncture or backbone carbons (shown in Fig. 25.1 with a heavy line on 5α-cholestane) greatly changes the shape of the steroid, as seen in the examples of 5α, 8α-androstane and 5β-androstane (Fig. 25.2).

Because of the immense effect that "backbone" stereochemistry has on the shape of the molecule, the International Union of Pure and Applied Chemistry (IUPAC) rules[4] strongly recommend that the stereochemistry at all backbone carbons be clearly shown. That is, all hydrogens along the

backbone should be drawn. When the stereochemistry is not known, a wavy line is used in the drawing. Methyls are explicitly indicated as CH_3.

The terms *cis* and *trans* are occasionally used in steroid nomenclature to indicate the backbone stereochemistry among rings. For example, 5α steroids are A/B *trans*, and 5β-steroids are A/B *cis*. The terms *syn* and *anti* are used analogously to *trans* and *cis* for indicating stereochemistry in bonds connecting rings (e.g., the C9:C10 bond that connects rings A and C). The use of these terms is indicated in Figure 25.2.

The position of double bonds can be designated in any of the various ways shown below in Figure 25.3. Double bonds from C8 may go toward C9 or C14, and those from C20 may go toward C21 or C22. In such cases, both carbons are indicated in the name if the double bond is not between sequentially numbered carbons (e.g., 5α-androst-8(14)-ene or 5α-$\Delta8(14)$-androstene; see Fig. 25.3). These principles of modern steroid nomenclature are applied to naming several common steroid drugs shown in Figure 25.1.

Such common names as *testosterone* and *cortisone* are obviously much easier to use than the long systematic names. Substituents must always have their position and stereochemistry clearly indicated, however, when common names are used (e.g.,17α-methyltestosterone, 9α-fluorocortisone).

Steroid drawings sometimes appear with lines drawn instead of methyls (CH_3), and backbone stereochemistry is not indicated unless it differs from that of 5α-androstane (Fig. 25.4). This manner of representation should be used only when there is no ambiguity in the implied stereochemistry.

STEROID BIOSYNTHESIS

Steroid hormones in mammals are biosynthesized from cholesterol, which in turn is made in vivo from acetyl-coenzyme A (acetyl-CoA) via the mevalonate pathway. Although humans do obtain approximately 300 mg of cholesterol per day in their diets, a greater amount (about 1 g) is biosynthesized per day. A schematic outline of these biosynthetic pathways is shown in Figure 25.5.

Conversion of cholesterol to pregnenolone is the rate-limiting step in steroid hormone biosynthesis. It is not the enzymatic transformation itself that is rate limiting; however, the translocation of cholesterol to the inner mitochondrial membrane of steroid-synthesizing cells is rate limiting.[5] A key protein involved in the translocation is the

(text continues on page 822)

Numbering and Primary Steroid Names

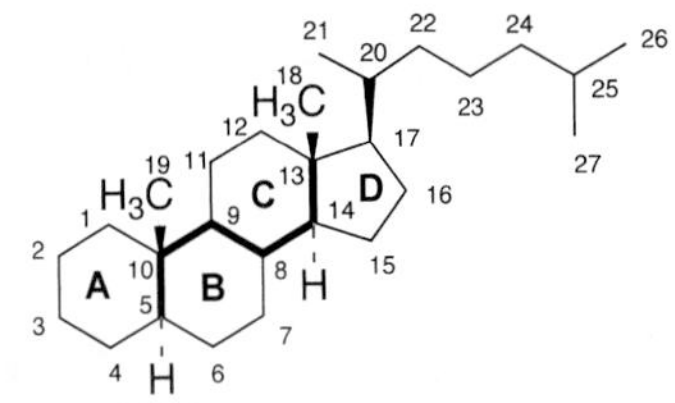

5α-Cholestane

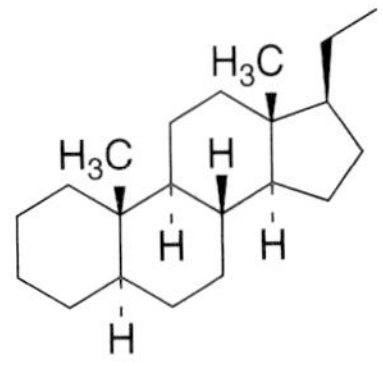

5α-Pregnane

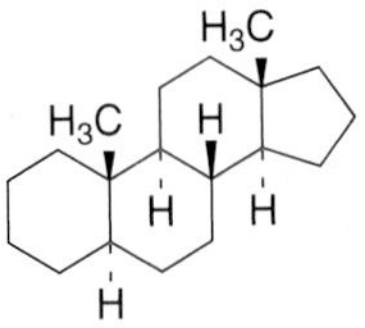

5α-Androstane

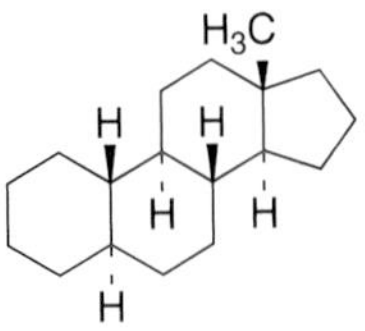

5α-Estrane

Examples of Common and Systematic Names

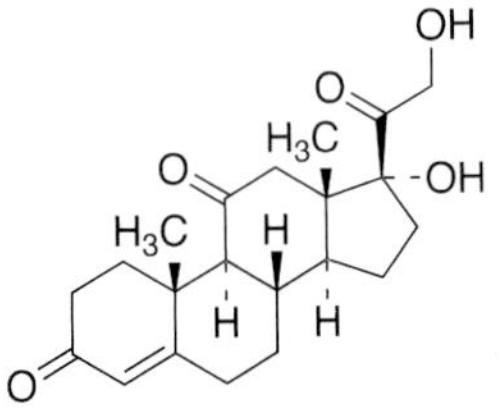

Cortisone
(17,21-Dihydroxypregn-4-ene-
3,11,20-trione)

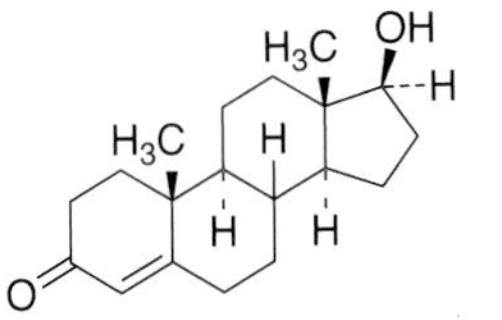

Testosterone
(17β-Hydroxyandrost-4-en-3-one)

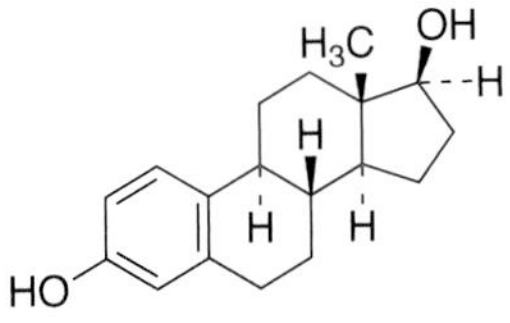

17β-estradiol
(Estra-1,3,5(10)-triene-3,17β-diol)

Figure 25.1 ● Steroid nomenclature and numbering.

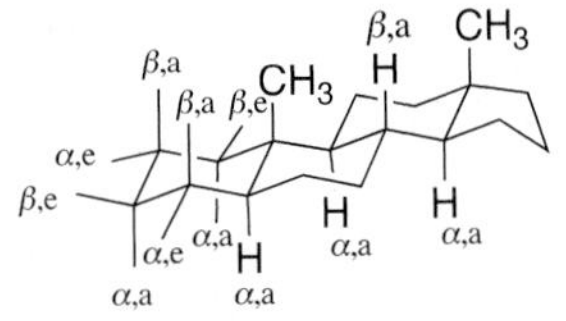

a = axial
e = equatorial
α = alpha bond
β = beta bond

5α-Androstane

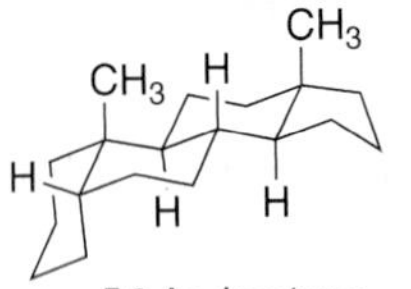

5β-Androstane

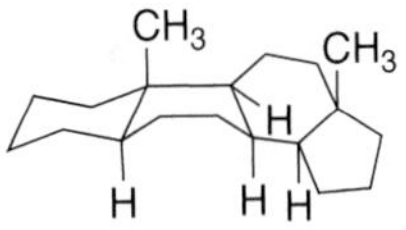

5α,8α-Androstane

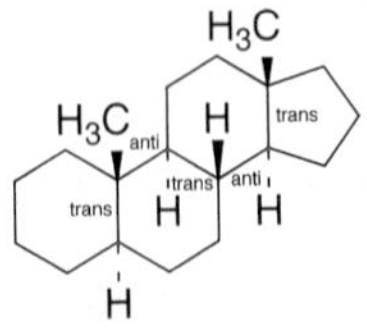

Figure 25.2 ● Steroid nomenclature—stereochemistry.

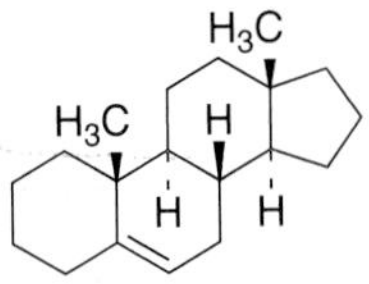

5-Androstene or
Δ⁵-Androstene or
Androst-5-ene

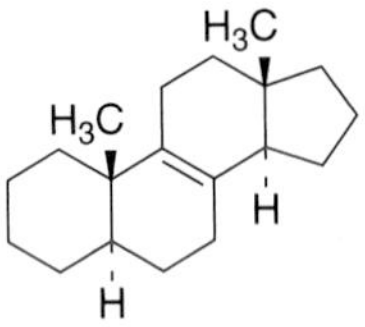

5α-Androst-8-ene or
5α-Δ⁸-Androstene

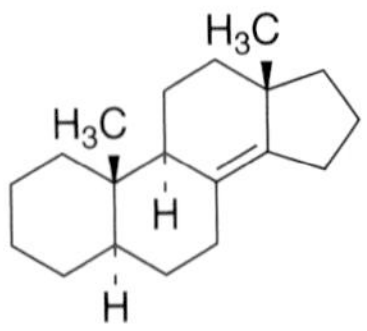

5α-Androst-8(14)-ene or
5α-Δ⁸⁽¹⁴⁾-Androstene

Figure 25.3 ● Steroid nomenclature—double bonds.

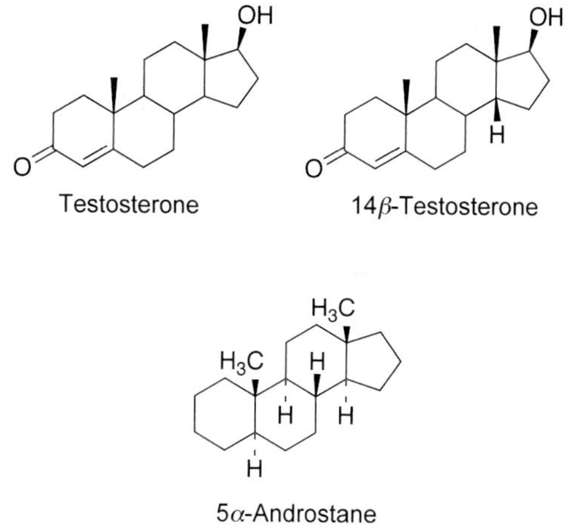

Testosterone

14β-Testosterone

5α-Androstane

Figure 25.4 ● Alternative representations of steroids.

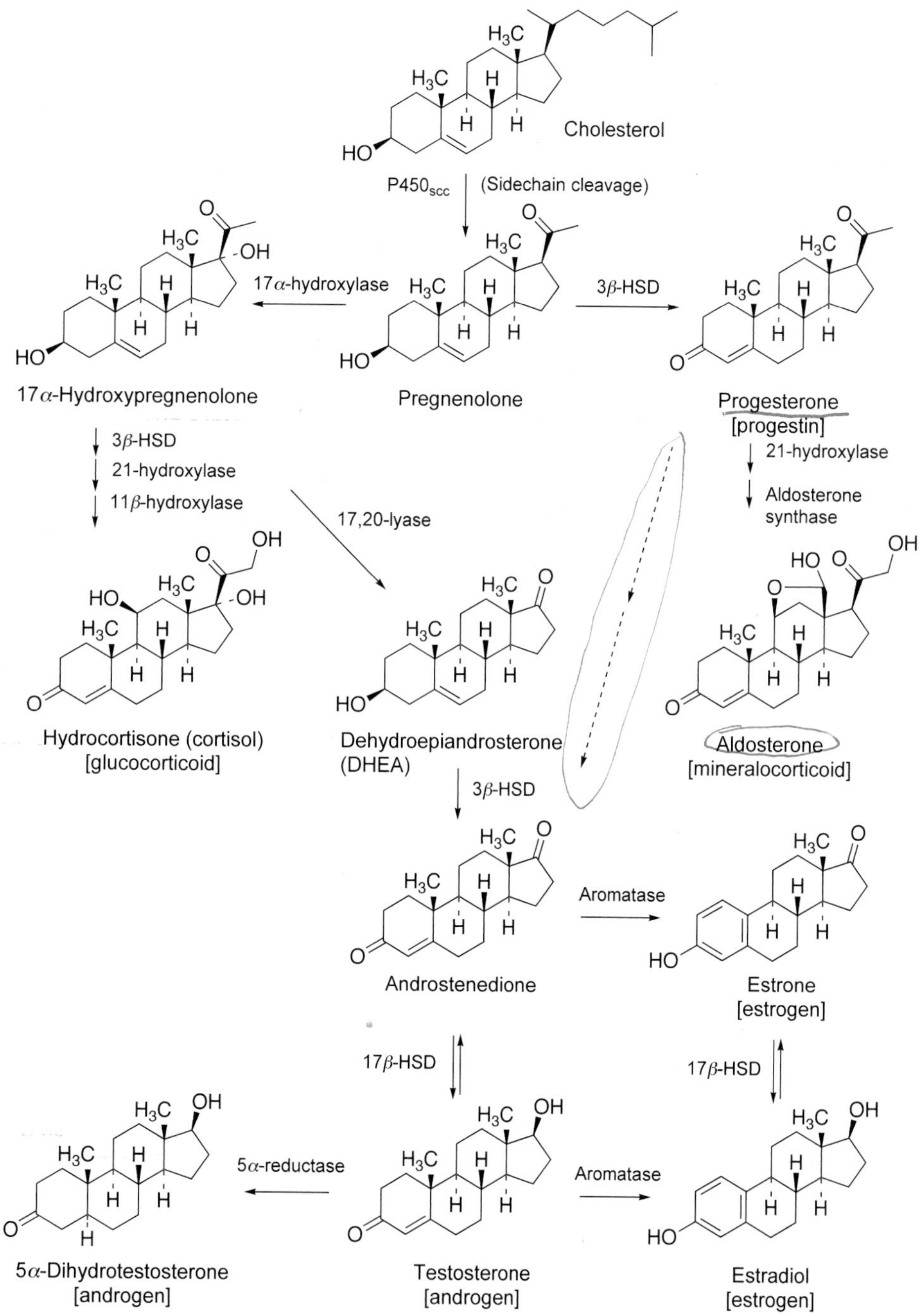

Cholesterol

P450$_{scc}$ (Sidechain cleavage)

17α-Hydroxypregnenolone

Pregnenolone

Progesterone
[progestin]

17α-hydroxylase

3β-HSD

3β-HSD
21-hydroxylase
11β-hydroxylase

17,20-lyase

21-hydroxylase

Aldosterone synthase

Hydrocortisone (cortisol)
[glucocorticoid]

Dehydroepiandrosterone
(DHEA)

Aldosterone
[mineralocorticoid]

3β-HSD

Androstenedione

Aromatase

Estrone
[estrogen]

17β-HSD

17β-HSD

5α-reductase

Aromatase

5α-Dihydrotestosterone
[androgen]

Testosterone
[androgen]

Estradiol
[estrogen]

Figure 25.5 ● Outline of the biosynthesis of steroid hormones. (3β-HSD, 3β-hydroxysteroid dehydrogenase/Δ$^{5-4}$-isomerase; 17β-HSD, 17β-hydroxysteroid dehydrogenase.)

Steroidogenic Acute Regulatory protein (StAR). Defects in the StAR gene lead to congenital lipoid adrenal hyperplasia, a rare condition marked by a deficiency of adrenal and gonadal steroid hormones.[6] The enzymes involved in the transformation of cholesterol to the hormones are mainly cytochromes P450 and dehydrogenases. The main routes of biosynthesis of the hormones are depicted in Figure 25.5. Estradiol, testosterone, progesterone, aldosterone, and hydrocortisone are representatives of the distinct steroid–receptor ligands that are shown. Further metabolic fates of these compounds are presented under the specific structural class.

An enzyme-denoted cytochrome P450$_{scc}$ (SCC stands for side-chain cleavage) mediates the cleavage of the C17 side chain on the D ring of the sterol to provide pregnenolone, the C21 precursor of the steroids. This enzyme mediates a three-step process involved in the oxidative metabolism of the side chain. Successive hydroxylations at C20 and C22 are followed by oxidative cleavage of the C20–C22 bond, providing pregnenolone. Pregnenolone can be either directly converted into progesterone or modified for synthesis of GCs, estrogens, and androgens. Introduction of unsaturation into the A ring leads to the formation of progesterone. Specifically, oxidation of the alcohol at C3 to the ketone provides a substrate in which isomerization of the $\Delta^{5,6}$-double bond to the $\Delta^{4,5}$-double bond is facilitated. This transformation is mediated by a bifunctional enzyme, 3β-hydroxysteroid dehydrogenase/Δ^{5-4} isomerase (3β-HSD). This enzyme can act on several 3-ol-5-ene steroids in addition to pregnenolone. Hydroxylation at C17 provides the precursor for both sex steroid hormones and GCs. Cytochrome P450c17 hydroxylates pregnenolone and progesterone to provide the corresponding 17α-hydroxylated compounds. 17α-Hydroxypregnenolone can be converted to 17α-hydroxyprogesterone by 3β-HSD. Cytochrome P450c17 is also a bifunctional enzyme, with lyase activity in addition to the hydroxylase action. The C17,20-lyase activity is crucial for the formation of sex hormones. The lyase oxidatively removes the two carbons at C17, providing the C17 ketone. In the case of 17α-hydroxypregnenolone, the product is dehydroepiandrosterone (DHEA). If 17α-hydroxyprogesterone is the substrate for the lyase, androstenedione results. The conversion of 17α-hydroxyprogesterone to androstenedione is limited in humans, although in other species this is an important pathway. DHEA is converted to androstenedione by the action of 3β-HSD. Androstenedione can either be converted to testosterone by the action of 17β-hydroxysteroid dehydrogenase (17β-HSD) or be transformed into estrone by aromatase, a unique cytochrome P450 that aromatizes the A ring of certain steroid precursors. Testosterone is aromatized to 17β-estradiol by the same enzyme. 17β-HSD acts on estrone to form 17β-estradiol. If testosterone is acted on by 5α-reductase, 5α-dihydrotestosterone (DHT), an androgen important in the prostate, is produced.

The major route to GCs diverges at 17α-hydroxypregnenolone. Instead of oxidative cleavage at C17, 3β-HSD acts on this substrate to provide 17α-hydroxyprogesterone. Small amounts of 17α-hydroxyprogesterone can be produced directly from progesterone, although this is not a major pathway in humans. Sequential action of 21-hydroxylase (Cyp21) and 11β-hydroxylase (Cyp11B1) provides hydrocortisone, the key GC in humans.

If progesterone is directly acted on by 21-hydroxylase (Cyp21), 11-deoxycorticosterone is produced, a precursor to the MC aldosterone. In tissues where aldosterone is synthesized, aldosterone synthase (Cyp11B2), the multifunctional enzyme, mediates the hydroxylation at C11, as well as the two-step oxidation of C18 to an aldehyde, providing aldosterone, which exists predominantly in the cyclic-hemiacetal form.

CHEMICAL AND PHYSICAL PROPERTIES OF STEROIDS

With few exceptions, the steroids are white crystalline solids. They may be in the form of needles, leaflets, platelets, or amorphous particles, depending on the particular compound, the solvent used in crystallization, and the skill and luck of the chemist. Because the steroids have 17 or more carbon atoms, it is not surprising that they tend to be water insoluble. Addition of hydroxyls or other polar groups (or decreasing carbons) increases water solubility slightly, as expected. Salts are the most water soluble. Examples are shown in Table 25.1. As a class, the 4-en-3-one steroids are light sensitive and should be kept in light-resistant containers.

CHANGES TO MODIFY PHARMACOKINETIC PROPERTIES OF STEROIDS

As with many other compounds described in previous chapters, the steroids can be made more lipid soluble or more water soluble by making suitable ester derivatives of hydroxyl (OH) groups. Derivatives with increased lipid solubility are often made to decrease the release rate of the drug from intramuscular (IM) injection sites (i.e., in depot preparations). More lipid-soluble derivatives also have improved skin absorption properties and thus, are preferred for dermatological preparations. Derivatives with increased water solubility are needed for intravenous preparations. Since hydrolyzing enzymes are found throughout mammalian cells especially in the liver, converting OH groups to esters does not significantly modify the activity of most compounds.

TABLE 25.1 Solubilities of Steroids

	Solubility (g/100 mL)		
	CHCl$_3$	EtOH	H$_2$O
Cholesterol	22	1.2	Insoluble
Testosterone	50	15	Insoluble
Testosterone propionate	45	25	Insoluble
Dehydrocholic acid	90	0.33	0.02
Estradiol	1.0	10	Insoluble
Estradiol benzoate	0.8	8	Insoluble
Betamethasone	0.1	2	Insoluble
Betamethasone acetate	10	3	Insoluble
Betamethasone NaPO$_4$ salt	Insoluble	15	50
Hydrocortisone	0.5	2.5	0.01
Hydrocortisone acetate	1.0	0.4	Insoluble
Hydrocortisone NaPO$_4$ salt	Insoluble	1.0	75
Prednisolone	0.4	3	0.01
Prednisolone acetate	1.0	0.7	Insoluble
Prednisolone NaPO$_4$ salt	0.8	13	25

Some steroids (e.g., estradiol, progesterone, and testosterone) are particularly susceptible to rapid metabolism after absorption or rapid inactivation in the gastrointestinal tract before absorption. These inactivation processes limit the effectiveness of these hormones as orally available drugs, although micronized forms of estradiol and progesterone are available for oral administration. Sometimes, a simple chemical modification can decrease the rate of inactivation and, thereby, increase the drug's half-life or make it possible to be taken orally.

Examples of common chemical modifications are illustrated in Figure 25.6. Drugs such as testosterone *cy*clopentylpro*pionate* (cypionate) and methylprednisolone

sodium succinate are prodrugs that require hydrolysis to release the active hormone in the body.

⬡ STEROID HORMONE RECEPTORS

Steroid hormones regulate tissue-specific gene expression. The individual hormones exhibit remarkable tissue selectivity, even though their structural differences are relatively minor. Estrogens such as estradiol increase uterine cell proliferation, for example, but not prostate cell proliferation. Androgens such as testosterone do the reverse, but neither androgens nor estrogens affect stomach epithelium. The

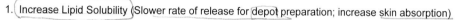

1. Increase Lipid Solubility (Slower rate of release for depot preparation; increase skin absorption)

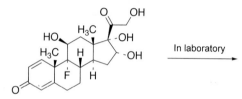

2. Increase Water Solubility (Suitable for IV use)

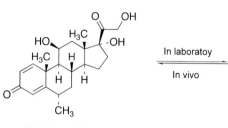

3. Decrease Inactivation

Figure 25.6 ● Common steroid modifications to alter therapeutic utility. (*, prodrug.)

basis for this selectivity is the presence of selective steroid hormone receptors in individual tissues. This section provides an overview of steroid hormone receptors and their mode of action.[1,2]

The steroid receptors themselves are key players in gene expression, but many other proteins are involved in this process. Chaperone proteins, for example, help fold the receptor proteins into the proper three-dimensional shape for binding the steroid ligand. Together, the steroid hormone receptor and associated proteins (Fig. 25.7; details on next page) make up the mature-receptor complex. Transcription (or repression of transcription) occurs when all the necessary associated proteins have been recruited to the DNA–receptor complex. In addition to the major effects on transcription, some effects of steroid hormones are mediated via rapid, nongenomic mech-anisms. Some of these actions appear to involve classical steroid hormone receptors, whereas others rely on novel membrane receptors.[7–9] This is an active area of study and will help explain all the various actions of steroid hormones.

Structure of Steroid Hormone Receptors

The complementary DNAs (cDNAs) of all the major steroid hormone receptors have been cloned, giving the complete amino acid sequence of each. Although the whole three-dimensional structure of a steroid hormone receptor has not been solved (structures of the ligand-binding domains of the steroid hormone receptors have been elucidated; see next page in this section), the functional role of each part is well known (see Fig. 25.8).[10] The organization of the domains for all types of steroid hormone receptors is the same, but the number of amino acids for each receptor varies:

1. *N-terminal (A/B) domain.* Once the steroid–receptor complex has bound to the target gene(s), this domain (also called the *A/B modulator domain*) activates the hormone response elements adjacent to the genes. The hormone response elements are on the DNA adjacent to the target gene. They contain about 12 to 18 base-pair DNA sequences and consist of two "half sites" that are separated by a variable spacer. In the nucleus, steroid hormone–receptor

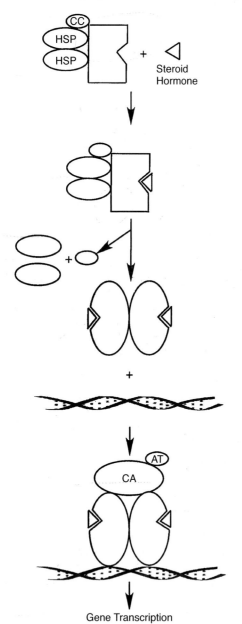

Figure 25.7 ● Generic structural model of a steroid hormone–receptor complex and its activation for gene transcription. (AT, histone acetyltransferase; CA, coactivator; CC, cochaperone; HSP, heat shock protein; SHR, steroid hormone receptor.)

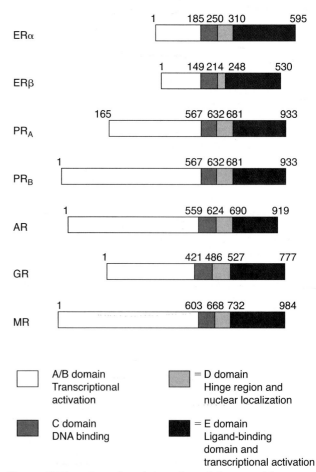

Figure 25.8 ● Functional domains of the steroid hormone receptors. (AR, androgen receptor; ER, estrogen receptor; GR, glucocorticoid receptor; MR, mineralocorticoid receptor; and PR, progesterone receptor.)

complexes exist as dimers; the dimeric structure allows access to both half sites. The nucleotide sequence and spacing between the half sites are essential for the specificity of the various steroid–hormone complexes. After the dimer binds and all accessory proteins have been recruited to the receptor–DNA complex, transcription is initiated.

2. *DNA-binding (C) domain.* This short section is made up of about 65 amino acids, organized into two zinc finger motifs that are important for recognition and binding to the DNA response elements. The zinc fingers are also responsible for dimerization of the receptor.

3. *Hinge (D) domain.* This variable linker region appears to be involved with nuclear localization and transport (translocation) of the steroid–receptor complex into the nucleus.

4. *C-terminal ligand-binding (E) domain (LBD).* The C-terminal domain includes about 250 amino acids. This section has the steroid hormone–binding site and is also involved with ligand-dependent transcriptional activation, receptor dimerization, binding to chaperone proteins (discussed later), and in some cases, repressing ("silencing") particular genes.

ESTROGEN RECEPTORS

There are two distinct estrogen receptors (ERs), estrogen receptor α (ER$_\alpha$) and estrogen receptor β (ER$_\beta$), which are encoded by different genes.[11] The ERs have distinct tissue distributions and can have distinct actions on the target genes. ER$_\alpha$ can be found in high abundance in the uterus, vagina, and ovaries, as well as in the breast, the hypothalamus, endothelial cells, and vascular smooth muscle. ER$_\beta$ is found in greatest abundance in the ovaries and the prostate, with reduced occurrence in the lungs, brain, and vasculature.[12] Although many ligands bind with similar affinities to both receptor subtypes, some ligands are selective for one or the other receptor.[13–15]

PROGESTERONE RECEPTORS

The progesterone receptor (PR) can also be found in two forms, but these are derived from a single gene. PR$_A$ has had 164 amino acids truncated from the N-terminus of PR$_B$, providing a receptor that has different interactions with target genes and associated proteins. PR$_B$ mainly mediates the stimulatory actions of progesterone. PR$_A$ acts as a transcriptional inhibitor of ER, androgen receptor (AR), glucocorticoid receptor (GR), mineralocorticoid receptor (MR), and PR$_B$.[12] These differential actions are believed to be a result of interactions with different coactivators and corepressors. The DNA- and ligand-binding domains for the two receptors are identical.

ANDROGEN, GLUCOCORTICOID, AND MINERALOCORTICOID RECEPTORS

The AR, GR, and MR are present in only a single form. Only one gene and one protein are known for each receptor. Mutant forms of AR[16] and GR[17] are known, and evidence is mounting that some of these mutant receptors are associated with disease states.

X-RAY CRYSTALLOGRAPHY AND STEROID FIT AT THE RECEPTOR

The x-ray structures have now been solved for the ligand-binding domains of all the steroid hormone receptors (ER$_\alpha$

and ER$_\beta$,[18–20] PR,[21] AR,[22] GR,[23,24] and MR[25]). The x-ray crystal structures of the ER, PR, and AR have revealed a key difference that leads to the unique ligand specificity of the ERs.[19,26] In the region of the ligand-binding domain, where the A ring of steroids binds, are key residues that bind to either the phenolic A ring of estrogens or the enone A ring of progesterone or testosterone. In the case of the ER, glutamate and arginine residues are important in a hydrogen-bonding network that involves the phenolic hydroxyl. In contrast to this structural arrangement, the PR and AR have glutamine and arginine residues that hydrogen bond to the A-ring enones of progesterone and testosterone. The change from glutamate, a hydrogen-bond acceptor, to glutamine, a hydrogen-bond donor, is critical for the discrimination between estrogens and other steroid hormones. The structures of the GR and MR LBDs also reveal the features that provide the specificities for these two receptors. In the LBD of the GR, key proline and glutamine residues are replaced by serine and leucine, respectively, in the MR.[25] The proline residue results in a slightly more open-binding pocket, which can accommodate larger residues at the 17α-position, as seen in many GR ligands, and the glutamine side chain can hydrogen bond with the 17α-hydroxyl, which is seen in GRs, but is absent in aldosterone.

The x-ray crystal structures of the steroid hormones themselves have also provided important information. Although the conformations of rigid molecules in crystals and their preferred conformations in solution with receptors can differ, it is now clear from x-ray crystallography studies of steroids, prostaglandins, thyroid compounds, and many other drug classes that this technique can be a powerful tool in understanding drug action and in designing new drugs.[27–29] The relationship is straightforward: steroid drugs usually do not have a charge and, as a result, are held to their receptors by relatively weak forces of attraction. The same is true for steroid molecules as they "pack" into crystals. In both events, the binding energy is too small to hold any but low-energy conformations. In short, the steroid conformation observed in steroid crystals is often the same or very similar to that at the receptor.

Structure of Steroid Hormone–Receptor Complexes

Steroid hormone–receptor complexes include the steroid hormone receptor as well as other proteins, predominantly chaperone (heat shock) proteins, cochaperones, and immunophilins (Fig. 25.7).[30,31] Their role is to "chaperone" the correct conformation and folding of complex proteins, which is otherwise much more difficult as temperatures increase. At normal physiological temperatures, the chaperone proteins assist the proper folding of large proteins such as steroid hormone receptors. The individual components vary depending on the type of steroid hormone receptor. Without the chaperones, the steroid hormone-binding site on the receptor does not have the proper folding and conformation for optimal steroid binding.

Once the steroid hormone binds to the receptor, a conformational change of the receptor occurs, and the mature receptor complex dissociates (Fig. 25.7). The receptor is dimerized, phosphorylated, and transported into the nucleus, if necessary. There, the zinc fingers on the steroid hormone receptor bind to the target gene(s) in the DNA.

Additional proteins are recruited to the receptor–DNA complex prior to initiation or repression of transcription.[32] These additional proteins include coactivators or corepressors and histone acetyltransferases. Typically, the receptor–DNA–coactivator complex displays histone acetyltransferase action, which relaxes the chromatin structure, allowing binding of RNA polymerase II and the subsequent initiation of transcription. If corepressors are recruited to the complex, deacetylation of the histone complex is facilitated, preventing transcription.

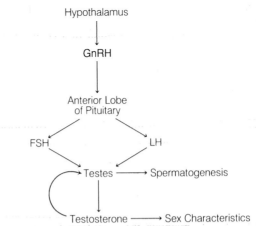

Figure 25.10 ● Regulation of spermatogenesis.

⬡ GONADOTROPIN-RELEASING HORMONE AND GONADOTROPINS

The gonadotropins are peptides that have a close functional relationship to estrogen, progesterone, and testosterone. They are called *gonadotropins* because of their actions on the gonads. As shown in Figures 25.9 to 25.11, they control ovulation, spermatogenesis, and development of sex organs, and they maintain pregnancy. An additional peptide, gonadotropin-releasing hormone (GnRH), regulates release of the gonadotropins. Included in this group are the following:

- GnRH
- Luteinizing hormone (LH)
- Follicle-stimulating hormone (FSH)
- Chorionic gonadotropin (CG; hCG is human chorionic gonadotropin), a glycopeptide produced by the placenta; its pharmacological actions are essentially the same as those of LH

Gonadotropin-Releasing Hormone

The hypothalamus releases GnRH, a peptide that stimulates the anterior pituitary to secrete LH and FSH in males and females. This peptide controls and regulates both male and female reproduction (Figs. 25.9 and 25.10). GnRH is a modified decapeptide (10 amino acids): PyroGlu-His-Trp-Ser-Tyr-Gly-Leu-Arg-Pro-Gly-NH$_2$. The pyroglutamate at the N-terminus and the C-terminal amide distinguish this pep-

tide from unmodified decapeptides. Analogs of GnRH that are used therapeutically are covered in Chapter 20.

Pituitary Gonadotropins: Luteinizing Hormone and Follicle-Stimulating Hormone

The pituitary gonadotropins LH and FSH, their structures, genes, receptors, biological roles, and their regulation (including by negative feedback actions of steroid hormones) have been studied intensively.[33,34] FSH, LH, and CG are all glycopeptide dimers with the same α subunit but different β-subunits.

In females, LH and FSH regulate the menstrual cycle (see Figs. 25.9 and 25.11). At the start of the cycle, plasma concentrations of estradiol and other estrogens (Fig. 25.11) and progesterone are low. FSH and LH stimulate several ovarian follicles to enlarge and begin developing more rapidly than others. After a few days, only one follicle continues developing to the release of a mature ovum. The granulosa cells of the maturing follicles begin secreting estrogens, which then cause the uterine endometrium to thicken. Vaginal and cervical secretions increase. Gonadotropins and estrogen reach their

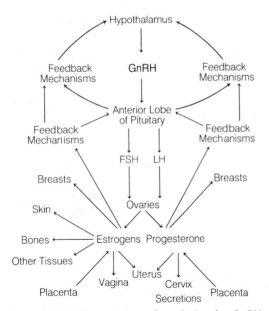

Figure 25.9 ● Regulation of ovulation by GnRH.

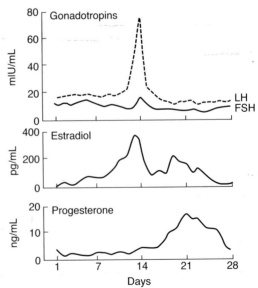

Figure 25.11 ● Hormone changes in the normal menstrual cycle.

maximum plasma concentrations at about day 14 of the cycle. The release in LH causes the follicle to break open, releasing a mature ovum. Under the stimulation of LH, the follicle changes into the corpus luteum, which begins secreting progesterone as well as estrogen.

The increased concentrations of estrogens and progesterone regulate the hypothalamus and the anterior pituitary by a feedback inhibition process that decreases GnRH, LH, and FSH production. The result is that further ovulation is inhibited. As described later in this chapter, this is the primary mechanism by which steroid birth control products inhibit ovulation.

If fertilization does not occur by about day 25, the corpus luteum begins to degenerate, slowing down its production of hormones. The concentrations of estrogens and progesterone become too low to maintain the vascularization of the endometrium, and menstruation results.

The pharmacological actions of hCG are essentially the same as those of LH. In females during pregnancy, the hCG secreted by the placenta maintains the corpus luteum to continue secretion of estrogen and progesterone, thus inhibiting ovulation and menstruation.

In males (Fig. 25.10), LH stimulates testosterone synthesis by the testes, and together, testosterone and LH promote spermatogenesis (sperm production) and development of the testes. Testosterone is also essential for the development of secondary sex characteristics in males. FSH stimulates production of proteins and nutrients required for sperm maturation.

SEX HORMONES

Although estrogens and progesterone are usually called female sex hormones and testosterone is called a male sex hormone, all of these steroids are biosynthesized in both males and females. For example, examination of the biosynthetic pathway in Figure 25.5 reveals that progesterone serves as a biosynthetic precursor to hydrocortisone and aldosterone and, to a lesser extent, to testosterone and estrogens. Testosterone is one of the precursors of estrogens. Estrogens and progesterone are produced in much larger amounts in females, however, as is testosterone in males. These hormones play profound roles in reproduction, in the menstrual cycle, and in giving women and men their characteristic physical differences.

Several modified steroidal compounds, as well as some nonsteroidal compounds, have estrogenic activity. A large number of synthetic or semisynthetic steroids with biological activities similar to those of progesterone have been made, and these are commonly called *progestins.* Although the estrogens and progestins have had their most extensive use as chemical contraceptive agents for women and in HRT, their wide spectrum of activity has given them a diversity of therapeutic uses in women, as well as a few uses in men.

Testosterone has two primary kinds of activities: androgenic (promoting male physical characteristics) and anabolic (muscle building). Many synthetic and semisynthetic androgenic and anabolic steroids have been prepared. Despite efforts to prepare selective anabolic agents (e.g., for use in aiding recovery from debilitating illness or surgery), all "anabolic" steroids have androgenic effects. The androgenic

agents are mainly used in males, but they do have some therapeutic usefulness in women (e.g., in the palliation of certain sex organ cancers).

In summary, although many sex hormone products have their greatest therapeutic uses in either women or men, nearly all have some uses in both sexes. Nevertheless, the higher concentrations of estrogens and progesterone in women and of testosterone in men cause the development of the complementary reproductive systems and characteristic physical differences of women and men.

Estrogens[35]

ENDOGENOUS ESTROGENS

The active endogenous estrogens are estradiol, estrone, and estriol. Estradiol provides the greatest estrogenic activity, with less activity for estrone, and the least activity with estriol. This range of activity parallels the affinity of these estrogens for the ER,[36] but the in vivo activities of these compounds are also affected by interconversions between active and inactive metabolites.

BIOSYNTHESIS

The estrogens are synthesized by the action of the enzyme aromatase on androstenedione or testosterone (Fig. 25.5). They are normally produced in relatively large quantities in the ovaries and the placenta, in lower amounts in the adrenal glands, and in trace quantities in the testes. In postmenopausal women, most estrogens are synthesized in adipose tissue and other nonovarian sites. About 50 to 350 μg/d of estradiol are produced by the ovaries (especially the corpus luteum) during the menstrual cycle. During the first months of pregnancy, the corpus luteum produces larger amounts of estradiol and other estrogens; the placenta produces most of the circulating hormone in late pregnancy. During pregnancy, the estrogen blood levels are up to 1,000 times higher than during the menstrual cycle.

METABOLISM OF ESTROGENS

The metabolism of natural estrogens has been reviewed in detail.[37] The three primary estrogens in women are 17β-estradiol, estrone, and estriol (16α,17β-estriol). Although 17β-estradiol is produced in the greatest amounts, it is quickly oxidized (see Fig. 25.12) to estrone, the estrogen found in highest concentration in the plasma. Estrone, in turn, is converted to estriol, the major estrogen found in human urine, by hydroxylation at C16 (to provide the 16α-hydroxyl) and reduction of the C17 ketone (17β-hydroxyl). Estradiol can also be directly converted to estriol. In the human placenta, the most abundant estrogen synthesized is estriol. In both pregnant and nonpregnant women, however, the three primary estrogens are also metabolized to small amounts of other derivatives (e.g., 2-hydroxyestrone, 2-methoxyestrone, 4-hydroxyestrone, and 16β-hydroxy-17β-estradiol). Only about 50% of therapeutically administered estrogens (and their various metabolites) are excreted in the urine during the first 24 hours. The remainder are excreted into the bile and reabsorbed; consequently, several days are required for complete excretion of a given dose.

Conjugation appears to be very important in estrogen transport and metabolism. Although the estrogens are unconjugated in the ovaries, significant amounts of conju-

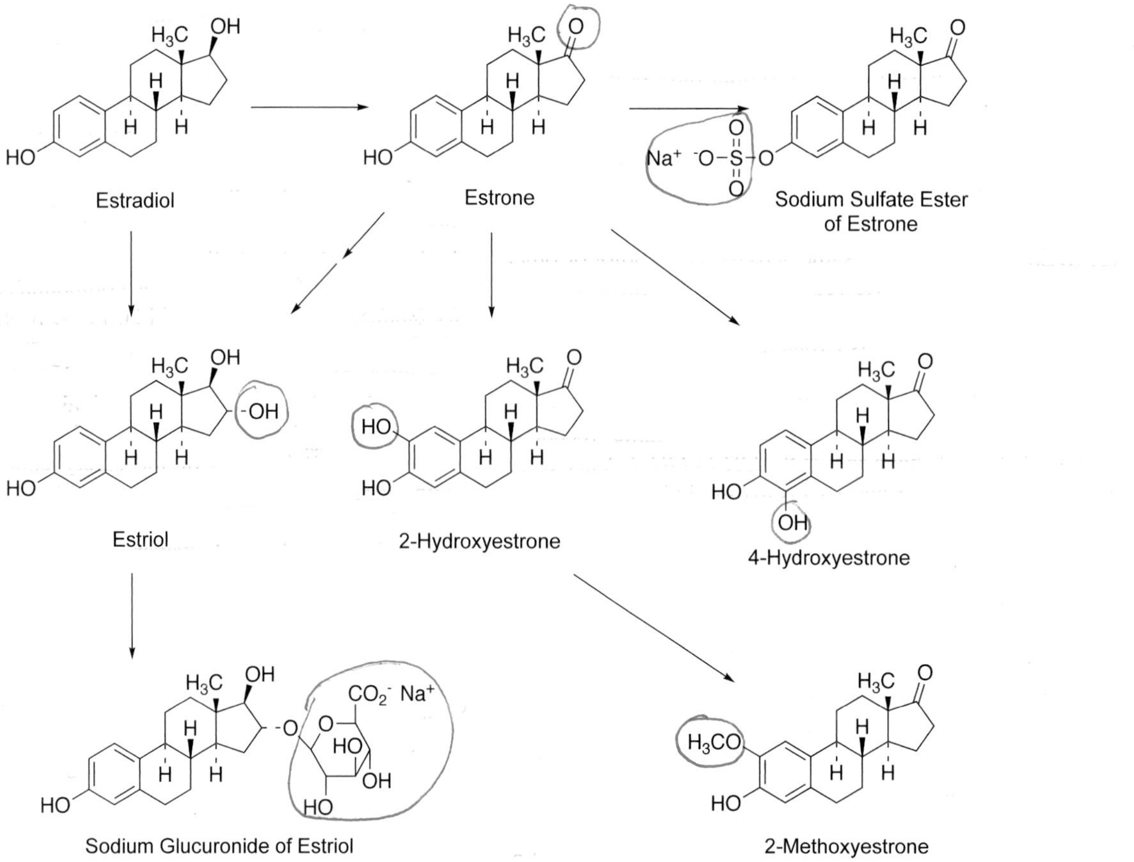

7 metabolites

Figure 25.12 ● Metabolites of 17β-estradiol and estrone.

gated estrogens may predominate in the plasma and other tissues. Most of the conjugation takes place in the liver. The primary estrogen conjugates found in plasma and urine are glucuronides and sulfates. As sodium salts, they are quite water soluble. The sodium glucuronide of estriol and the sodium sulfate ester of estrone are shown in Figure 25.12.

BIOLOGICAL ACTIVITIES OF ESTROGENS[12]

In addition to having important roles in the menstrual cycle (described previously), the estrogens and, to a lesser extent, progesterone are largely responsible for the development of secondary sex characteristics in women at puberty. The estrogens cause a proliferation of the breast ductile system, and progesterone stimulates development of the alveolar system. The estrogens also stimulate the development of lipid and other tissues that contribute to breast shape and function. Pituitary hormones and other hormones are also involved. Fluid retention in the breasts during the later stages of the menstrual cycle is a common effect of the estrogens.

The estrogens directly stimulate the growth and development of the vagina, uterus, and fallopian tubes and, in combination with other hormones, play a primary role in sexual arousal and in producing the body contours of the mature woman. Pigmentation of the nipples and genital tissues and growth stimulation of pubic and underarm hair (possibly with the help of small amounts of testosterone) are other results of estrogen action.

The physiological changes at menopause emphasize the important roles of estrogens in a young woman. Breast and reproductive tissues atrophy, the skin loses some of its

suppleness, coronary atherosclerosis and gout become potential health problems for the first time, and the bones begin to lose density because of decreased mineral content.

STRUCTURAL CLASSES: ESTROGENS

As shown in Figure 25.13, there are three structural classes of estrogens: steroidal estrogens, diethylstilbestrol and other synthetic compounds, and phytoestrogens (Each class is summarized in the sections that follow). The steroidal estrogens include the naturally occurring estrogens found in humans and other mammals, as well as semisynthetic derivatives of these compounds. Because of rapid metabolism, estradiol itself has poor oral bioavailability. The addition of a 17α-alkyl group to the estradiol structure blocks oxidation to estrone. Ethinyl estradiol is therefore very effective orally, whereas estradiol itself is not. Most of the therapeutically useful steroidal estrogens are produced semisynthetically from natural precursors such as diosgenin, a plant sterol.

Steroidal Estrogens—Conjugated Estrogens, Esterified Estrogens. Conjugated estrogens (sometimes called equine estrogens) are estradiol-related metabolites originally obtained from the urine of horses, especially pregnant mares. Premarin, the major conjugated estrogen product on the market, is a mixture of numerous components that is obtained from mare urine. Equine estrogens are largely mixtures of estrone sulfate and equilin sodium sulfate. Little or no equilin and equilenin are produced in humans. The sulfate groups must be removed metabolically to release the active estrogens. Conjugated estrogens that derive exclusively from plant precursors are also on the market. Esterified estrogens are also mainly a combination of estrone sodium sulfate and equilin sodium sulfate, but in a different ratio to that in conjugated estrogens. The esterified estrogens are now prepared exclusively from plant sterols.

Diethylstilbestrol. At first glance, it might be surprising that synthetic nonsteroidal molecules such as diethylstilbestrol (DES) could have the same activity as estradiol or other estrogens. DES can be viewed, however, as a form of estradiol with rings B and C open and a six-carbon ring D. The activity of DES analogs was explained in 1946.[38] It was proposed that the distance between the two DES phenol OH groups was the same as the 3-OH to 17-OH distance of estradiol; therefore, they could both fit the same receptor. Medicinal chemists have shown the OH-to-OH distance to be actually 12.1 Å in DES and 10.9 Å in estradiol. In aqueous solution, however, estradiol has two water molecules that are hydrogen bonded to the 17-OH. If one of the two water mol-

ecules is included in the distance measurement, there is a perfect fit with the two OH groups of DES (Fig. 25.14). This suggests that water may have an important role for estradiol in its receptor site. It is now generally accepted that the estrogens must have a phenolic moiety for binding, but some investigators propose that the receptor may be flexible enough to accommodate varying distances between the two key hydroxyls. This point about estrogens needing a phenolic ring for high-affinity binding to the ER is critical. Steroids with a phenolic A ring and related phenolic compounds lack high-affinity binding to the other steroid hormone receptors. Although DES was used for many years, it was discovered that the daughters of women who had taken DES during pregnancy (DES babies) had a high risk of vaginal, cervical, and uterine abnormalities, along with a low risk of vaginal clear cell adenocarcinoma.[39] Because of the safety concerns associated with DES, it was completely removed from the U.S. market in the late 1990s. DES is still available as an estrogen for use in veterinary medicine, however.

1. Steroidal Estrogens and Derivatives

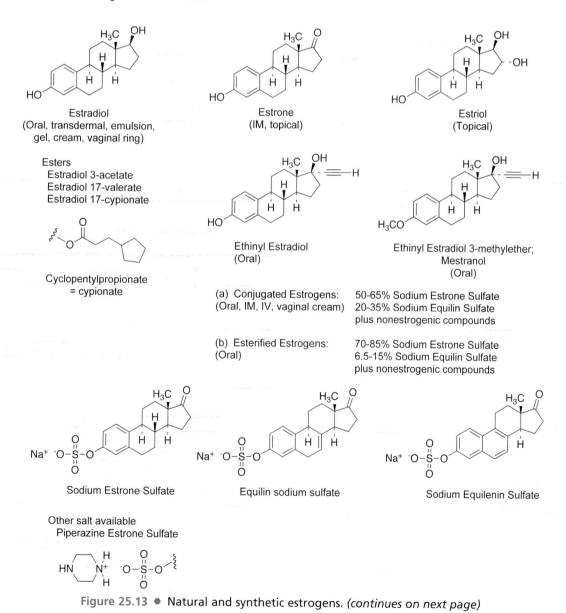

Figure 25.13 ● Natural and synthetic estrogens. *(continues on next page)*

1. Steroidal Estrogens and Derivatives (cont.)

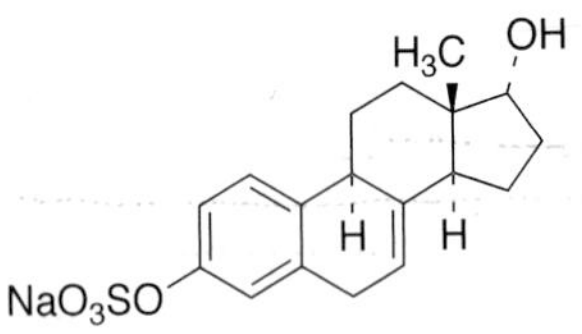

Sodium 17α-Dihydroequilin Sulfate

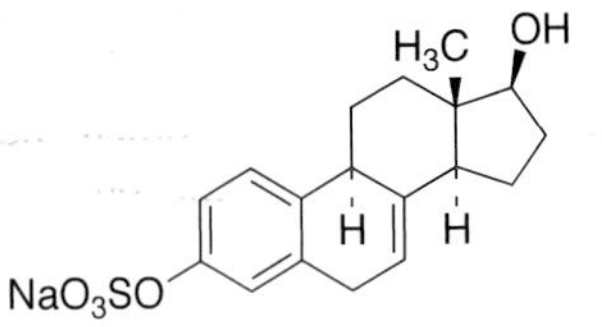

Sodium 17β-Dihydroequilin Sulfate

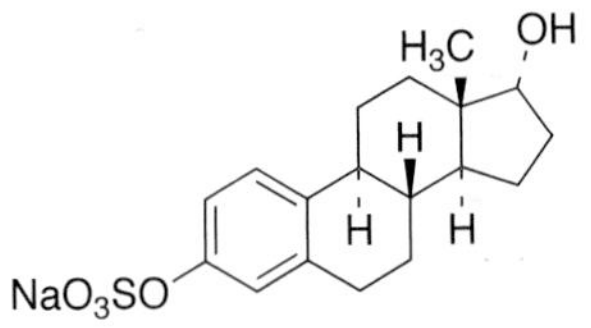

Sodium 17α-Estradiol Sulfate

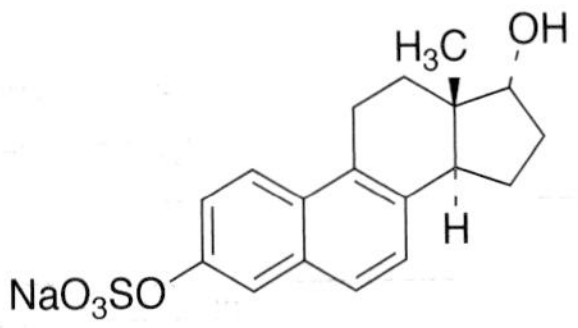

Sodium 17α-Dihydroequilenin Sulfate

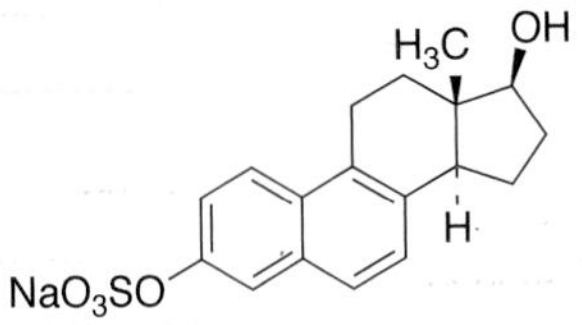

Sodium 17β-Dihydroequilenin Sulfate

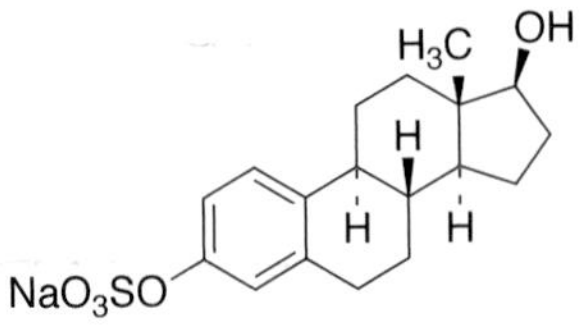

Sodium 17β-Estradiol Sulfate

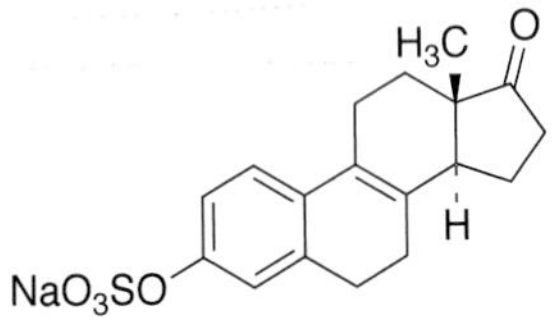

Sodium Δ^{8,9}-Dehydroestrone Sulfate

2. Diethylstilbestrol and Other Synthetic Compounds

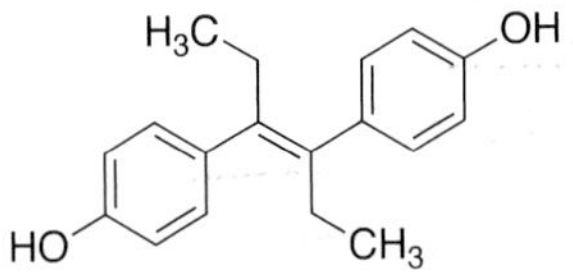

Diethylstilbestrol

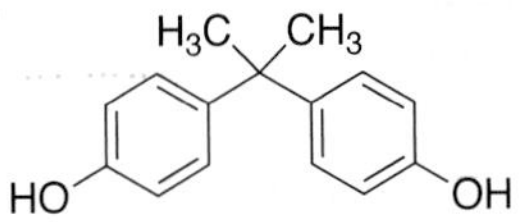

Bisphenol A

3. Estrogens from Plants (Phytoestrogens)

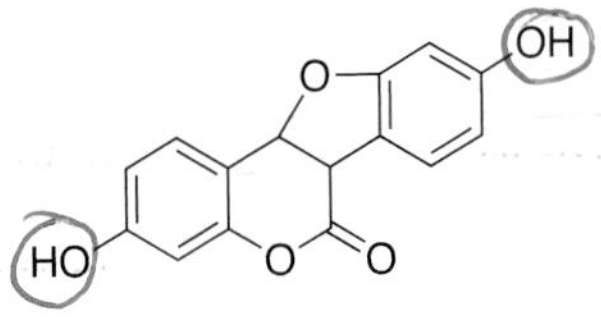

Coumestrol

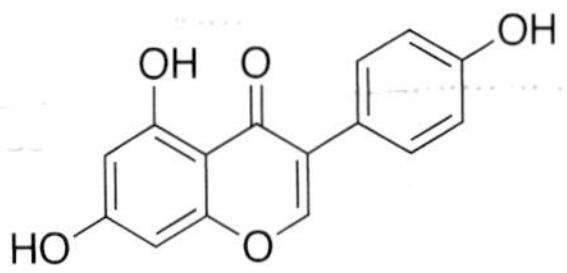

Genistein

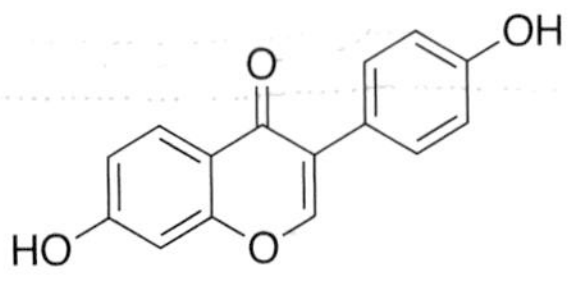

Daidzein

Figure 25.13 • *(Continued)*

Another synthetic compound, bisphenol A, shares some structural features of DES, in that it has two phenolic groups, but in this case only a single dimethylated carbon separates the two rings, rather than the substituted double bond in DES. As might be expected, the reduced distance between the phenolic hydroxyls and the greater flexibility in the structure lead to an affinity for the ERs several orders of magnitude less than estradiol or DES.[40] Although bisphenol A is only weakly estrogenic, it is still considered to be an "environmental estrogen" and is present in small quantities in a wide range of plastic products. The low-level exposure of humans to bisphenol A, although currently considered to have minimal health risks, continues to be the focus of numerous studies.[41]

Phytoestrogens. Several natural plant substances that have general structural features similar to those of DES and estradiol also have estrogenic effects and have been termed *phytoestrogens*.[42] These include genistein, from soybeans and a species of clover; daidzein, from soybeans; and coumestrol, found in certain legumes. Genistein and daidzein are examples of isoflavones. These and others have antifertility activity in animals.[43] Many claims have been made about the beneficial effects of consuming products containing these phytoestrogens, including preventing and treating cardiovascular disease, reducing postmenopausal symptoms, and preventing osteoporosis. Because of the numerous other components present in many of the commercial products as well as a lack of well-

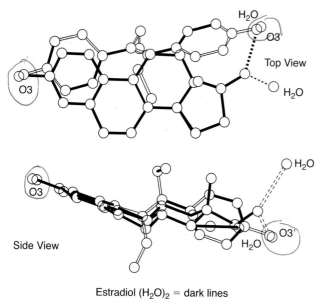

Estradiol $(H_2O)_2$ = dark lines
DES = light lines

Figure 25.14 ◆ Computer graphics. Superposition of estradiol $(H_2O)_2$ *(dark lines)* with DES *(light lines)*. (Courtesy of Medical Foundation of Buffalo, Inc.)

designed studies to test the effects of the phytoestrogens themselves, however, positive health effects specifically because of direct hormonal action of the phytoestrogens are uncertain. Questions have also been raised about a possible contribution of phytoestrogens to an increased incidence of breast cancer. These concerns, however, are contradicted by studies that suggest a chemoprotective role for soy products containing phytoestrogens (this could well be due to other components of the mixture).[44] The long history of use of soy products in the world and no global correlations with increased breast cancer risks suggest that any connection between phytoestrogens in general and breast cancer is quite small.[45]

Recent studies have demonstrated that genistein and other phytoestrogens binds preferentially to ER_β over ER_α.[46,47] The clinical relevance of this difference in binding is unclear, but further research is being vigorously pursued to understand the distinctions between the phytoestrogens and classical estrogens.[44]

THERAPEUTIC USES OF ESTROGENS

Birth Control. A major use of estrogens is for inhibition of ovulation, in combination with progestins. Steroidal birth control agents containing estrogens are discussed in the section on chemical contraception later in this chapter.

Hormone Replacement Therapy. Another major use of estrogens is in HRT for postmenopausal women. For this use, a progestin is often included to oppose the effects of estrogens on endometrial tissue. HRT is covered in more depth later in the chapter.

Treatment of Estrogen Deficiency from Ovarian Failure or after Oophorectomy. Estrogen therapy, usually with a progestin, is common in cases of ovarian failure and after an oophorectomy.

Treatment of Advanced, Inoperable Breast Cancer in Men and Postmenopausal Women and of Advanced, Inoperable Prostate Cancer in Men. Estrogens are used to treat inoperable breast cancer in men and in postmenopausal women, but estrogen therapy can actually stimulate existing breast cancers in premenopausal women. The selective ER modulator tamoxifen is reported to have fewer side effects; hence, it is usually preferred. Estrogens have also been used to treat inoperable prostate cancer, but GnRH analogs are now generally preferred because of fewer unwanted side effects.

Estrogens and Cancer. Many years of study have firmly established an association between estrogen use and increased risk of breast cancer. The risk is associated, however, with the timing of estrogen exposure, the estrogen dose, the length of use, and the type of estrogen used.[48] A patient should discuss the potential risks of breast cancer with her doctor carefully before starting estrogen therapy. Unopposed estrogens in HRT for postmenopausal women are also linked to an increased risk of endometrial carcinoma, which is the basis for inclusion of a progestin in many forms of HRT.[49]

ESTROGEN PRODUCTS

Estrogens are commercially available in a wide variety of dosage forms: oral tablets, vaginal creams and foams, transdermal patches, and IM dosage preparations.

Estradiol, United States Pharmacopeia (USP). Estradiol, estra-1,3,5(10)-triene-3,17β-diol, is the most active of the natural steroid estrogens. Although its 17β-OH group is vulnerable to bacterial and enzymatic oxidation to estrone (Fig. 25.12), it can be temporarily protected as an ester at C3 or C17, or permanently protected by adding a 17α-alkyl group (e.g., 17α-ethinyl estradiol, the most commonly used estrogen in oral contraceptives). The increased oil solubility of the 17β-esters (relative to estradiol) permits the esters to remain in oil at the IM injection site for extended periods. These derivatives illustrate the principles of steroid modification shown in Figure 25.6. Transdermal estradiol products avoid first-pass metabolism, allowing estradiol to be as effective as oral estrogens for treating menopausal symptoms. A new transdermal spray, Evamist, was approved in 2007. Estradiol itself is typically not very effective orally because of rapid metabolism, but an oral formulation of micronized estradiol that allows more rapid absorption of the drug is available (Estrace). In addition to the oral and transdermal products, estradiol is also available in gel, cream, and vaginal ring formulations. The commercially available estradiol esters are the following:

Estradiol 3-acetate, *USP* (oral; vaginal ring)
Estradiol 17-valerate, *USP* (IM injection)
Estradiol 17-cypionate, *USP* (IM injection)

Estrone, USP. Estrone, 3-hydroxyestra-1,3,5(10)-trien-17-one, is less active than estradiol but more active than its metabolite, estriol. As the salt of its 3-sulfate ester, estrone is the primary ingredient in conjugated estrogens, *USP*, and esterified estrogens, *USP*. Although originally obtained from the urine of pregnant mares (about 10 mg/L), estrone is now prepared synthetically. Estrone itself is not available in commercial oral formulations, but can be obtained at compounding pharmacies as a topical formulation. Oleoyl-estrone, the C3 ester of estrone with oleic acid, is in phase II clinical trials for the treatment of obesity. This acyl estrone derivative reduces fat stores by a mechanism not involving the ER,[50] although some of the oleoyl-estrone is hydrolyzed to estrone in vivo.

Piperazine Estrone Sulfate (3-Sulfoxy-Estra-1,3,5(10)-Trien-17-One Piperazine Salt), USP

All the estrone 3-sulfate salts have the obvious pharmaceutical advantage of increased water solubility and better oral availability. Acids convert the salts to the free 3-sulfate esters and cause some hydrolysis of the ester. This does not seem to affect absorption adversely, but precipitation of the free sulfate esters in acidic pharmaceutical preparations should be avoided. The dibasic piperazine molecule acts as a buffer, giving it somewhat greater stability.

Conjugated Estrogens, USP

The term *conjugated estrogens* refers to the mix of sulfate conjugates of estrogenic components isolated from pregnant mare urine (Premarin). These compounds are also referred to as CEE (conjugated equine estrogens). Conjugated estrogens contain 50% to 65% sodium estrone sulfate and 20% to 35% sodium equilin sulfate (based on the total estrogen content of the product). Premarin also contains the sulfate esters of 17α-estradiol, 17α-dihydroequilin, and 17β-dihydroequilin, in addition to other minor components. Although most commonly used in HRT to treat postmenopausal symptoms, the conjugated estrogens are used for the entire range of indications described previously, except birth control.

Synthetic Conjugated Estrogens

Cenestin, referred to as "synthetic conjugated estrogens, A" is a mixture of nine estrogenic substances (Fig. 25.13): sodium estrone sulfate, sodium equilin sulfate, sodium equilenin sulfate, sodium 17α-estradiol sulfate, sodium 17β-estradiol sulfate, sodium 17α-dihydroequilin sulfate, sodium 17β-dihydroequilin sulfate, sodium 17α-dihydroequilenin sulfate, and sodium 17β-dihydroequilenin sulfate. These estrogenic substances are synthesized from soy sterols. The term *synthetic* has been added before conjugated estrogens to indicate that this product is distinct from (not equivalent to) the conjugated estrogens derived from mare urine. The "A" following the name indicates that this is the first approved mixture of synthetic conjugated estrogens. Enjuvia is "synthetic conjugated estrogens, B." Subsequent synthetic conjugated estrogen products will be named in order, with the final descriptors "C, D, E," etc. Enjuvia contains $\Delta^{8,9}$-dehydroestrone sulfate, in addition to the nine estrogenic substances listed previously. Cenestin and Enjuvia are both approved for the treatment of moderate-to-severe vasomotor symptoms and vulvar and vaginal atrophy associated with menopause.

Esterified Estrogens, USP

Esterified estrogens (Menest) contain some of the same sulfate conjugates of estrogens present in conjugated estrogens, but the ratios of these components and the composition of minor components of the products differ. These products contain 75% to 85% sodium estrone sulfate and 6% to 15% sodium equilin sulfate, in such proportion that the total of these two components is 90% of the total esterified estrogens content. The esterified estrogens find the same uses as the conjugated estrogens.

Estriol, USP. Estriol, estra-1,3,5(10)-triene-3,16α,17β-triol, is available for compounding into several different formulations for use in HRT. It can be used alone or in combinations with estradiol (Bi-Est) or with estradiol and estrone (Tri-Est).

Ethinyl Estradiol, USP. 17α-Ethinyl estradiol has the greatest advantage over other estradiol products of being orally active. It is equal to estradiol in potency by injection but is 15 to 20 times more orally active. The primary metabolic path for ethinyl estradiol is 2-hydroxylation by cytochrome P450 isozyme 3A4 (CYP3A4), followed by conversion to the 2- and 3-methyl ethers by catechol-*O*-methyltransferase. The 3-methyl ether of ethinyl estradiol is mestranol, *USP*, used in oral contraceptives. Mestranol is a prodrug that is 3-*O*-demethylated to the active ethinyl estradiol. An oral dose of about 50 μg of mestranol has an estrogenic action approximately equivalent to 35 μg of oral ethinyl estradiol. The demethylation is mainly mediated by CYP2C9.[51]

SELECTIVE ESTROGEN RECEPTOR MODULATORS AND ANTIESTROGENS

Whereas estrogens have been very important in chemical contraception and HRT, compounds that can antagonize the ER have been of great interest for the treatment of estrogen-dependent breast cancers. Tumor biopsies have shown ER to be present in about 60% of primary breast cancers, and most are responsive to estrogen blockade. Unfortunately, most of these ER-related breast cancers also develop resistance to antiestrogen therapy within 5 years. In contrast, only about 6% of nonmalignant breast tissues have significant ER present. Three compounds that are used clinically for estrogen antagonist action in the treatment of breast cancer are tamoxifen, toremifene, and fulvestrant (Fig. 25.15). Two additional agents that can antagonize ERs are clomiphene, which is used as an ovulation stimulant, and raloxifene, which is used for the prevention and treatment of osteoporosis.

Tamoxifen and clomiphene were traditionally called *ER antagonists* or *antiestrogens.* Referring to these compounds as ER antagonists, however, does not accurately portray how these compounds work in vivo. Although tamoxifen is an ER antagonist in breast tissue, it has agonist actions on endometrium, liver, bone, and cardiovascular system. Because of the differential agonist and antagonist effects of these types of compounds on the ER, depending on the specific tissue, a new term was coined: *selective estrogen receptor modulators* (SERMs). A SERM is a drug that has tissue-specific estrogenic activity. Although many compounds exhibit SERM activity, a few agents are antagonists in all tissues. These compounds are termed *antiestrogens,* and fulvestrant is one example (Fig. 25.15). Tamoxifen and clomiphene are often referred to in older literature as *antiestrogens.*

Tamoxifen has seen extensive use in treating primary breast cancers that are ER dependent.[52,53] For premenopausal women with metastatic disease, tamoxifen is an alternative and adjuvant with oophorectomy, ovarian irradiation, and mastectomy. Tamoxifen use, however, is not problem free. Tamoxifen increases the incidence of endometrial polyps, hyperplasia and carcinoma, and uterine sarcomas. The risk of endometrial cancer resulting from tamoxifen is, however, much lower than the "modest but highly significant reductions in morbidity and mortality of breast cancer."[54] Because

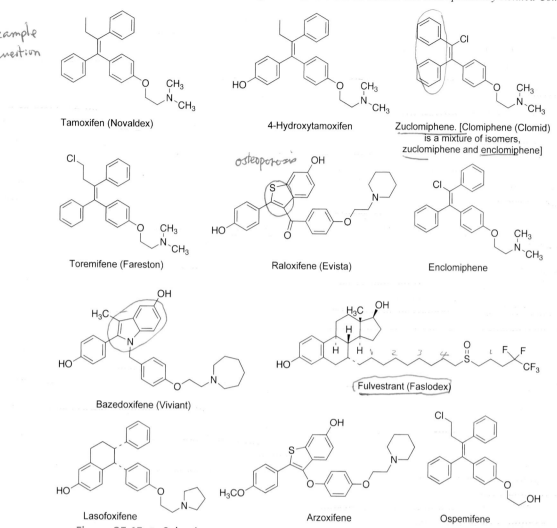

Example Question

Tamoxifen (Novaldex)

4-Hydroxytamoxifen

Zuclomiphene. [Clomiphene (Clomid) is a mixture of isomers, zuclomiphene and enclomiphene]

Toremifene (Fareston)

osteoporosis

Raloxifene (Evista)

Enclomiphene

Bazedoxifene (Viviant)

Fulvestrant (Faslodex)

Lasofoxifene

Arzoxifene

Ospemifene

Figure 25.15 ● Selective estrogen receptor modulators (SERMs) and antiestrogens.

of the increased risk of endometrial cancer with tamoxifen therapy, tamoxifen should be used to prevent breast cancer only in women at high risk. Women without a family history of breast cancer or other risks should not use tamoxifen in this manner.

Raloxifene is another SERM, but its profile of activity differs from that of tamoxifen. Raloxifene is an ER antagonist in both breast and endometrial tissue, but has agonist action on bone and acts as an estrogen agonist in lowering total cholesterol and low-density lipoprotein (LDL). The subtle structural differences between the two drugs underlie the distinct activity profiles.[55] The agonist action on bone tissue is the basis for the use of this drug for treating osteoporosis.

A key question is why do compounds like tamoxifen and raloxifene exhibit antagonist action in some tissues, but agonist action in other tissues? Major developments in the past few years are beginning to provide the answer to this question.[15,56–58] Tamoxifen,[59] raloxifene, and estradiol[18] all bind to the ER at the same site, but their binding modes are different. In addition, each induces a distinct conformation in the transactivation region of the ligand-binding domain.[18] These unique conformations dictate how the receptor–ligand complex will interact with coregulator proteins (coactivators or corepressors).[56] In all tissues, the estradiol–ER complex recruits coactivators, so gene transcription is stimulated.

In breast tissue, both raloxifene- and tamoxifen-bound receptors prevent the association with coactivators, but rather recruit corepressors, so antagonist action is observed. In uterine tissue, however, the raloxifene–ER complex recruits corepressors, whereas the tamoxifen–ER complex recruits a coactivator, SRC-1, which leads to agonist action.[57] An additional factor involved in this agonist action of tamoxifen is the context in which the liganded receptor interacts with the target gene. The liganded ER can interact directly with DNA or can interact indirectly by being tethered to other transcription factors. When the tamoxifen-bound receptor interacts in a tethered manner with the target genes in uterine tissue, the SRC-1 coactivator is recruited, and gene transcription is promoted.[56,57] A deeper understanding of how the liganded receptors interact with target genes and the mechanisms for recruitment of coregulators may help explain the phenomenon of tamoxifen resistance, which results from increased tamoxifen agonism in breast tissue.[56]

Bazedoxifene is a new SERM that should soon be marketed for the treatment of osteoporosis. Bazedoxifene incorporates an indole ring system in place of the benzothiophene of raloxifene. Bazedoxifene was the result of a screening program that selected for compounds that did not stimulate breast or uterine tissue.[60] Lasofoxifene, arzoxifene, and ospemifene are the other newer SERMs that are in the late stage of development (Fig. 25.15).[61] Lasofoxifene can be viewed as a constrained, saturated analog of 4-hydroxytamoxifen. A new drug application (NDA) was filed with the Food and Drug Administration (FDA) in late 2007 and the review is still in progress. Structurally, arzoxifene is most similar to raloxifene, with an ether bridge, rather than a carbonyl bridge, attached to the benzothiophene core. Arzoxifene is being investigated (phase III) for treating osteoporosis and for preventing breast cancer. Ospemifene is an analog of toremifene, which has an OH in place of the *N,N*-dimethyl amino substituent. It is in phase III clinical trials for the treatment of vaginal atrophy in postmenopausal women.

Clomiphene is another drug that exhibits antiestrogen actions, but it is not used for treating breast cancer or osteoporosis; rather, it is used for increasing the odds of a successful pregnancy. Clomiphene's therapeutic application as an ovulation stimulant results from its ability to increase GnRH production by the hypothalamus. The mechanism is presumably a blocking of feedback inhibition of ovary-produced estrogens (via ER antagonism). The hypothalamus and pituitary interpret the false signal that estrogen levels are low and respond by increasing the production of GnRH. The increased GnRH, in turn, leads to increased secretion of LH and FSH, maturation of the ovarian follicle, and ovulation (as described previously in this chapter; see Fig. 25.9). Support for the feedback inhibition mechanism is provided by tests with experimental animals in which clomiphene has no effect in the absence of a functioning pituitary gland.

Multiple births occur about 10% of the time with patients taking clomiphene, and birth defects in 2% to 3% of live newborns. Vasomotor "hot flashes" occur about 10% of the time, and abnormal enlargement of the ovaries about 14%. Abdominal discomfort should be discussed immediately with the physician.

SERM AND ANTIESTROGEN PRODUCTS

Tamoxifen Citrate, USP. Tamoxifen, 2-[4-(1,2-diphenyl-1-butenyl)phenoxy]-*N,N*-dimethylethanamine (Nolvadex), is a triphenylethylene SERM used to treat early and advanced breast carcinoma in postmenopausal women. Tamoxifen is used as adjuvant treatment for breast cancer in women following mastectomy and breast irradiation. It reduces the occurrence of contralateral breast cancer in patients receiving adjuvant tamoxifen therapy. It is also effective in the treatment of metastatic breast cancer in both women and men. In premenopausal women with metastatic breast cancer, tamoxifen is an alternative to oophorectomy or ovarian irradiation. Tamoxifen can be used preventatively to reduce the incidence of breast cancer in women at high risk. Antiestrogenic and estrogenic side effects can include hot flashes, nausea, vomiting, platelet reduction, and (in patients with bone metastases) hypercalcemia. Like all triphenylethylene derivatives, it should be protected from light.

The major metabolite of tamoxifen is *N*-desmethyltamoxifen, which reaches steady-state levels higher than tamoxifen itself. It is believed that *N*-desmethyltamoxifen contributes significantly to the overall antiestrogenic effect. Another metabolite, 4-hydroxytamoxifen, is a more potent antiestrogen than tamoxifen, but because it is only a minor metabolite of tamoxifen, it probably does not contribute significantly to the therapeutic effects. 4-Hydroxytamoxifen, with its greater affinity for the ERs, however, has been used extensively in pharmacological studies of these receptors. Tamoxifen concentrations are reduced if coadministered with rifampin, a cytochrome P450 inducer.

Toremifene Citrate, USP. Toremifene, 2-[4-[(1Z)-4-chloro-1,2-diphenyl-1-butenyl]phenoxy]-*N,N*-dimethylethanamine (Fareston), differs structurally from tamoxifen only by having a chloroethyl group (rather than an ethyl group) attached to the triphenylethylene structure. As might be expected, the pharmacological actions of toremifene and tamoxifen are quite similar. Toremifene is also a SERM, with estrogen antagonist action in breast tissue but agonist action in the endometrium, on bone tissue, and on serum lipid profiles. Recent clinical data indicate that the incidence of endometrial cancer is lower with toremifene use than with tamoxifen.[62] Toremifene is used in the treatment of metastatic breast cancer in postmenopausal women.

Raloxifene, USP. Raloxifene, [6-hydroxy-2-(4-hydroxyphenyl)benzo[*b*]thien-3-yl][4-[2-(1-piperidinyl)ethoxy]phenyl]methanone (Evista), is a benzothiophene derivative that differs slightly from the triphenylethylene SERMs. A key structural difference is the carbonyl "hinge" that connects the modified phenolic side chain to the benzothiophene ring system. This hinge is the key structural element that leads to the differing actions at the ERs.[55] Raloxifene, unlike tamoxifen and toremifene, has antagonist properties on the endometrium and breast tissue and agonist properties on bone and the cardiovascular system. The lack of agonist action on endometrial tissue has been suggested as a reason for the lack of endometrial cancer associated with raloxifene use. Raloxifene is approved for the prevention and treatment of osteoporosis in postmenopausal women. It has also been investigated for preventing breast cancer in comparison with tamoxifen. Recent studies indicates that it has similar effectiveness to tamoxifen, but has a preferable side effect profile.[63]

Bazedoxifene, USP. Bazedoxifene, 1-[[4-[2-(azepan-1-yl)ethoxy]phenyl]methyl]-2-(4-hydroxyphenyl)-3-methyl-indol-5-ol (Viviant), was declared to be "approvable" by the FDA in 2007 for the prevention of postmenopausal osteoporosis. As of mid-2009, final approval in the United States is still pending. Bazedoxifene was approved in Europe in 2009 for the treatment of post–menopausal osteoporosis.

Fulvestrant, USP. Fulvestrant, 7α-[9-[(4,4,5,5,5-pentafluoropentyl)sulfinyl]nonyl]estra-1,3,5(10)-triene-3,17β-diol (Faslodex), is an antagonist structurally based on the estradiol structure, with a long, substituted alkyl chain attached at the 7α-position of the steroid skeleton. When bound to the ERs, this alkyl chain induces a conformation of the receptor distinctive from that formed upon estradiol or tamoxifen binding, preventing agonist action. Fulvestrant is a pure antagonist at both ER_α and ER_β and an ER downregulator (stimulates degradation of the ER), completely lacking the agonist activity that is seen with tamoxifen or raloxifene. The different pharmacological profile of fulvestrant allows the use of this agent in women who have had disease progression after prior antiestrogen therapy (typically tamoxifen), providing an alternative to aromatase inhibitors.[64]

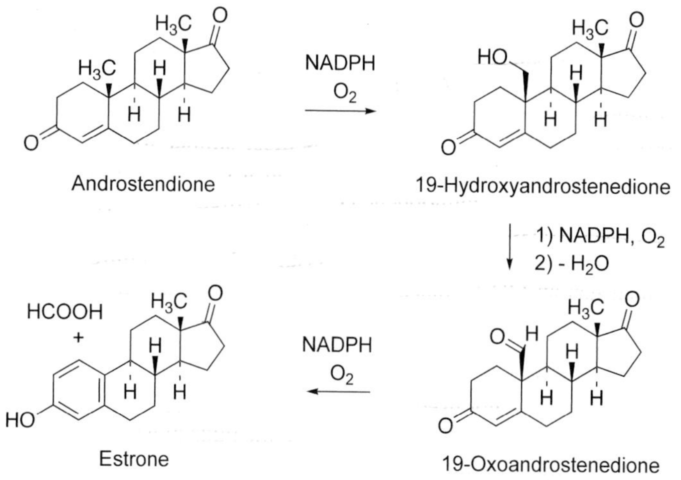

Figure 25.16 ● Conversion of androstenedione to estrone by aromatase.

Clomiphene Citrate, USP. Clomiphene citrate, 2-[4(2-chloro-1,2-diphenylethenyl)phenoxy]-*N,N*-diethyl-ethanamine (Clomid), is used as an ovulation stimulant in women desiring pregnancy. Although early literature refers to clomiphene as an estrogen antagonist, it is more accurately a SERM.[65] Clomiphene is chemically a mixture of two geometric isomers, zuclomiphene, the *cis*-isomer, and enclomiphene, the *trans*-isomer. In animal studies, these isomers have different estrogenic actions in different tissues. Zuclomiphene appears to have weak agonist actions on all tissues studied, whereas enclomiphene has antagonist actions on uterine tissue, but agonist action on bone tissue.[66] The actions of clomiphene in humans are likely a composite of the actions of the two isomers.

AROMATASE INHIBITORS

Aromatase is a cytochrome P450 enzyme complex that catalyzes the conversion of androstenedione to estrone and testosterone to estradiol (Figs. 25.5 and 25.16).[67–69] The complex is made up of reduced nicotinamide adenine dinucleotide phosphate (NADPH)-cytochrome P450 reductase, and cytochrome P450 hemoprotein. In the first two steps, the C19 methyl is hydroxylated to CH_2OH, and then to an alde-

hyde hydrate form that dehydrates to provide the C19 aldehyde. In the final aromatization step, the C19 carbon is oxidatively cleaved to formate. A hydride shift, proton transfer, and free radical pathways have been proposed, with *cis*-elimination of the 1β and 2β hydrogens.[70] In premenopausal women, aromatase is primarily found in ovaries, but in postmenopausal women, aromatase is largely in muscle and adipose tissue.

As discussed previously with SERMs, some types of breast cancer are estrogen dependent. Because the aromatase reaction is unique in steroid biosynthetic pathways, it would be anticipated that aromatase inhibitors would be very specific in their estrogen biosynthesis blockade. This has proved to be true, and aromatase inhibitors offer a useful approach to decreasing estrogen levels in the treatment of estrogen-dependent breast cancer. Initially, aromatase inhibitors were used as second-line therapy in postmenopausal women who failed on tamoxifen therapy. Recent studies have indicated, however, that the newer aromatase inhibitors can be used as first-line therapy and possibly for cancer prevention in patients at high risk.[71]

Aromatase inhibitors include both steroidal and nonsteroidal compounds. Examples of aromatase inhibitors are shown in Fig. 25.17. The first-generation aromatase inhibitors

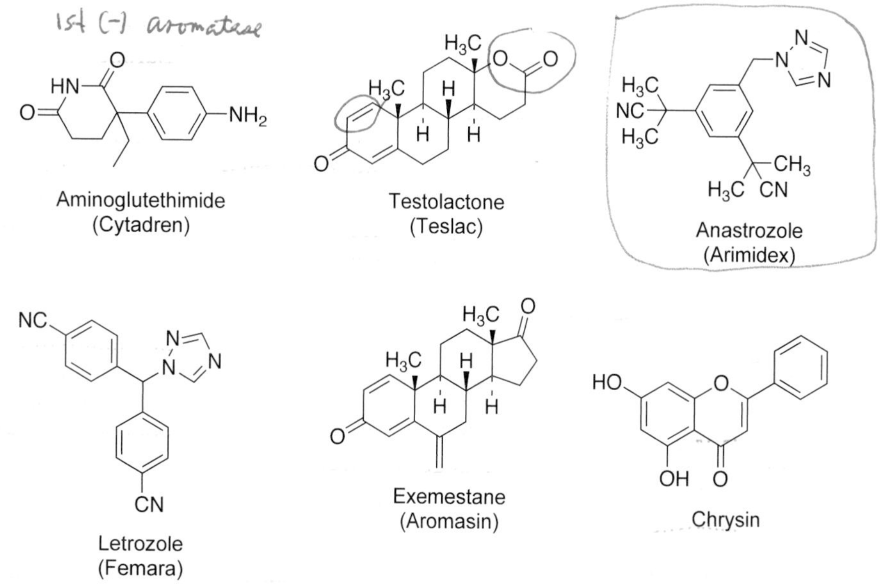

Figure 25.17 ● Aromatase inhibitors.

were aminoglutethimide, a nonsteroidal compound, and the steroid-based testolactone, two compounds that were developed before it was recognized that their effectiveness in breast cancer treatment was caused by aromatase inhibition.[72] Aminoglutethimide also inhibits other P450s involved in steroid hormone biosynthesis, which limits its use in breast cancer treatment. The newer drugs are more potent and more specific inhibitors of aromatase than the earlier compounds.

Exemestane is a newer steroidal aromatase inhibitor. It is an enzyme activated irreversible ("suicide") inhibitor of aromatase. It is orally available and highly selective for aromatase. Its structure reflects only minor structural modifications to the natural substrate, androstenedione.

The nonsteroidal aromatase inhibitors are competitive inhibitors that bind to the enzyme active site by coordinating the iron atom present in the heme group of the P450 protein. Aside from aminoglutethimide, the first selective aromatase inhibitor to be marketed in the United States was anastrozole (Arimidex). Anastrozole incorporates a triazole ring into its structure that can coordinate to the heme iron. Letrozole is another triazole-containing inhibitor that is also effective in the treatment of breast cancer.

Currently available inhibitors suppress plasma estrogen levels (estradiol, estrone, and estrone sulfate) by 80% to 95%. Earlier aromatase inhibitors, such as aminoglutethimide and testolactone, suppressed plasma estrogens to a lesser extent. The side effects often seen with aminoglutethimide because of additional inhibition of other biosynthetic enzymes are avoided with the newest agents. The selectivity of these drugs for aromatase is quite high.

As with the SERMs, these drugs are only effective when the breast cancer cells are "ER positive," meaning that they respond and proliferate in the presence of estrogen. Aromatase inhibitors can cause fetal harm in pregnant women and are therefore contraindicated.

Additional nonsteroidal inhibitors are based on the flavone structure. Chrysin is a flavonoid natural product that has aromatase inhibitory action in vitro similar to that of aminoglutethimide.[73] It is isolated from *Passiflora coerulea* and other plants. While this compound is not used therapeutically as an aromatase inhibitor, it has found questionable use as a nutritional supplement either alone or in combination with anabolic steroids to enhance muscle building and athletic performance. The theory for use is that an aromatase inhibitor allows the estrogenic side effects of androgenic compounds to be reduced. Although various nutritional supplement products containing chrysin are available, it is unclear whether or not significant aromatase inhibition is being achieved in vivo. The oral bioavailability of chrysin is very low, mainly as a result of efficient conversion to the corresponding glucuronide and sulfate conjugates, so the plasma concentration of free chrysin is minimal.[74]

AROMATASE INHIBITOR PRODUCTS

Anastrozole, USP. Anastrozole, $\alpha,\alpha,\alpha',\alpha'$-tetramethyl5-(1*H*-1,2,4-triazol-1-ylmethyl)-1,3-benzenediacetonitrile, was the first specific aromatase inhibitor approved in the United States. It is indicated for first-line treatment of postmenopausal women with advanced or metastatic breast cancer, for second-line treatment of postmenopausal patients with advanced breast cancer who have had disease progression following tamoxifen therapy, and for adjuvant treatment of women with early breast cancer. Patients who did not respond to tamoxifen therapy rarely respond to anastrozole.

Anastrozole reduces serum estradiol approximately 80% after 14 days of daily dosing. Because of an elimination half-life of 50 hours, anastrozole is effective with once-daily dosing (1 mg). Metabolism of anastrozole includes hydroxylation and glucuronidation, as well as *N*-dealkylation to produce triazole. The metabolites of anastrozole are inactive. Although anastrozole can inhibit CYPs 1A2, 2C9, and 3A4 with K_i values in the low micromolar range, the concentrations of anastrozole reached under standard therapeutic dosing are much lower, so anastrozole should lack significant P450 interactions.[75]

Letrozole, USP. Letrozole, 4,4′-(1*H*-1,2,4-triazol-1-ylmethylene)dibenzonitrile (Femara), is used for most of the same indications as anastrozole. It reduces concentrations of estrogens by 75% to 95%, with maximal suppression achieved within 2 to 3 days. Letrozole is specific for aromatase inhibition, with no additional effects on adrenal corticoid biosynthesis. CYPs 3A4 and 2A6 are involved in the metabolism of letrozole to the major carbinol metabolite, which is inactive. The loss of the triazole ring, which is involved in coordination of the heme iron, would explain the loss of activity. Letrozole strongly inhibits CYP2A6 in vitro, with moderate inhibition of CYP2C19. The effect of this in vitro inhibition on the pharmacokinetics of coadministered drugs is unknown. Tamoxifen reduces the levels of letrozole significantly if they are used together, so combination treatment with these agents is not recommended.[76]

Exemestane, USP. Exemestane, 6-methylenandrosta-1,4-diene-3,17-dione (Aromasin), is the first steroid-based aromatase inhibitor approved for the treatment of breast cancer in the United States. It is a mechanism-based inactivator that irreversibly inhibits the enzyme. Plasma estrogen levels are reduced by 85% to 95% within 2 to 3 days, and effects last 4 to 5 days. Exemestane does not inhibit any of the major cytochromes P450 and has essentially no interaction with steroid receptors, with only a very weak affinity for the AR. The 17β-hydroxyexemestane reduction product, however, has much higher affinity for the AR than the parent (still several fold less than DHT, 0.28% for parent vs. 30% for metabolite). The clinical significance of the affinity is likely minimal because of the low levels of the metabolite produced.

Aminoglutethimide, USP. Aminoglutethimide, 3-(4-aminophenyl)-3-ethyl-2,6-piperidinedione, is mainly used to treat Cushing syndrome, a condition of adrenal steroid excess, a use in which the $P450_{scc}$ inhibition of this compound is exploited rather than its aromatase inhibition. Aminoglutethimide is a weak inhibitor of aromatase and has been used successfully in the treatment of estrogen-dependent breast cancer. Because of the development of more selective aromatase inhibitors, the use of aminoglutethimide for its ability to inhibit aromatase is not supported.

Testolactone, USP. Testolactone, 13-hydroxy-3-oxo-13,17-secoandrosta-1,4-dien-17-oic acid Δ-lactone (Teslac), was originally synthesized as a possible anabolic steroid, considering its structural similarity to testosterone. The key structural difference from anabolic steroids is the D-ring lactone instead of the typical cyclopentyl ring. Although considered in many texts an androgen or anabolic steroid (it is a Schedule III drug because of its classification as an anabolic steroid), testolactone lacks androgenic effects in vivo. Its action is believed to be caused by irreversible inhibition of aromatase. It is a relatively weak inhibitor of aromatase, but the irreversible nature of the inhibition can lead to prolonged effects. Its relatively weak inhibition of aromatase and its undesirable dosage schedule (5 × 50-mg tablets q.i.d.) give this older agent only limited use in breast cancer treatment because of better available options.

Progestins

ENDOGENOUS PROGESTINS

The key endogenous steroid hormone that acts at the PRs is progesterone. All other endogenous steroids lack significant progestational action.

BIOSYNTHESIS

Progesterone is produced in the ovaries, testes, and adrenal glands. Much of the progesterone that is synthesized from pregnenolone is immediately converted to other hormonal intermediates and is not secreted. See the biosynthetic pathway (Fig. 25.5). The corpus luteum secretes the most progesterone, 20 to 30 mg/d during the last or "luteal" stage of the menstrual cycle. Normal men secrete about 1 to 5 mg of progesterone daily.

METABOLISM OF PROGESTERONE

Progesterone has a half-life of only about 5 minutes when taken orally, because of rapid metabolism. Progesterone can be transformed to many other steroid hormones (Fig. 25.5) and, in that sense, has numerous metabolic products. The principal excretory product of progesterone metabolism, however, is 5β-pregnane-3α,20α-diol and its conjugates (Fig. 25.18). The steps that are involved in the formation of

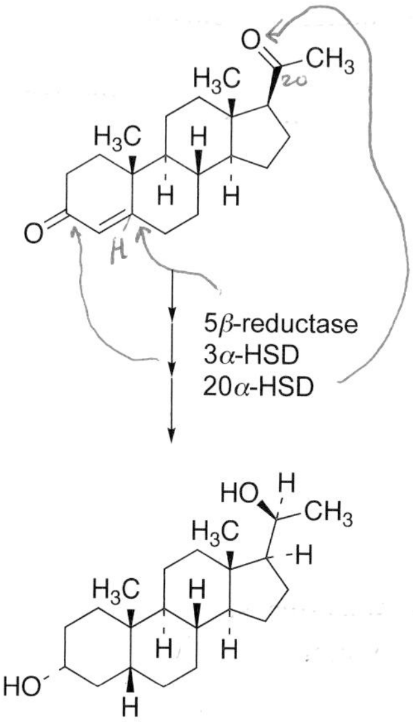

5β-Pregnane-3α,20S-diol
(5β-Pregnane-3α,20α-diol)

Figure 25.18 ● Progesterone metabolism (timing of the reduction steps can vary). (HSD, hydroxysteroid dehydrogenase.)

this metabolite are reduction of the C4-5 double bond, reduction of the C3 ketone providing the 3α-ol, and reduction of the C20 ketone. The reduction at C5 must precede the reduction of the C3 ketone, but the timing of the C20 can vary, depending on the tissue.[77,78] Structural features that can block reduction at C5 or C20 have greatly increased the half-lives of progesterone derivatives.

BIOLOGICAL ACTIVITIES OF THE PROGESTINS[12]

Like the estrogens, progesterone has various pharmacological actions, with the main target tissues being the uterus, the breast, and the brain. Progesterone decreases the frequency of the hypothalamic pulse generator and increases the amplitude of LH pulses released from the pituitary. The actions of progesterone in the uterus include development of the secretory endometrium. When release of progesterone from the corpus luteum at the end of the menstrual cycle declines, menstruation begins. Progesterone also acts to thicken cervical secretions, decreasing cervical penetration by sperm. Progesterone is critical for the maintenance of pregnancy by suppressing menstruation and decreasing uterine contractility. Progesterone has important actions in the breasts during pregnancy, acting in conjunction with estrogens to prepare for lactation.

A thermogenic action is also associated with progesterone. During the menstrual cycle, progesterone mediates a slight temperature increase near midcycle and maintains the increased temperature until the onset of menstruation. The exact mechanism for this temperature increase is not known. Progesterone and its metabolites have additional central effects, which are being actively explored (see "Neurosteroids" section at the end of the chapter).[79]

STRUCTURAL CLASSES—PROGESTINS

Progestins are compounds with biological activities similar to those of progesterone. They include three structural classes: (a) progesterone and derivatives, (b) testosterone and 19-nortestosterone derivatives, and (c) miscellaneous synthetic progestins (Fig. 25.19). Progesterone itself has low oral bioavailability because of poor absorption and almost complete metabolism in one passage through the liver. A recently available oral formulation is micronized progesterone in gelatin capsules. The micronized drug is much more readily absorbed, allowing oral delivery of progesterone, even though the dose must be much higher than a parenteral dose to compensate for extensive liver metabolism. Adding 17α-acyl groups slows metabolism of the 20-one, whereas a 6-methyl group enhances activity and reduces metabolism. Medroxyprogesterone acetate (MPA) is a particularly potent example (Table 25.2).

The structural requirements of the PR have been studied in detail.[27,28] The progesterone 4-en-3-one ring A is a key to binding but only when it is in a conformation quite different from that of testosterone or the GCs. Reviews of this work contain stereo drawings that show the required conformations in three dimensions.[27,28] Structural features modifying the steroid D ring are also important for optimal interactions with the PR.

Two important discoveries led to the development of the nortestosterone derivatives. One was the discovery that 19-norprogesterone still maintained significant progestational activity. The second was that 17α-alkynyl testosterone

Data from Salhanick, H. A., et al.: Metabolic Effects of Gonadal Hormones and Contraceptive Steroids. New York, Plenum Press, 1969.

TABLE 25.2 Comparative Progestational Activity of Selected Progestins

	Relative Oral Activity	Activity SC
Progesterone	(nil)	1
17 α-Ethinyltestosterone (ethisterone)	1	0.1
17 α-Ethinyl-19-nortestosterone (norethindrone)	5–10	0.5–1
Norethynodrel	0.5–1	0.05–1
17 α-Hydroxyprogesterone caproate	2–10	4–10
Medroxyprogesterone acetate	12–25	50
19-Norprogesterone		5–10
Norgestrel		3
Dimethisterone	12	

(ethisterone) had greater progestational than androgenic activity. Although the 19-nortestosterones do have androgenic side effects, their primary activity, nevertheless, is progestational. In addition to causing a marked increase in progestational activity, the 17α-alkynyl group also blocks metabolic or bacterial oxidation to the corresponding 17-ones. Thus, by adding a 17α-ethinyl group to testosterone, one can simultaneously decrease androgenic activity, promote good progestational activity, and have an orally active compound as well. Table 25.2 illustrates the relative progestational activity of several progestins. A further modification to the nortestosterones yields progestins with minimal androgenic activities. Changing the alkyl group at C13 from a methyl to an ethyl group, as in levonorgestrel, reduces the androgenic effects, while maintaining the progestational effects.

The most exciting new research area relating to progestins is the development of nonsteroidal PR agonists. Tanoproget is the most successful example to date (phase II trials).[80] As can be seen in Figure 25.19, tanaproget is completely unrelated to progesterone, but it still has high affinity and selectivity for the PR. The nonsteroidal nature of tanaproget offers

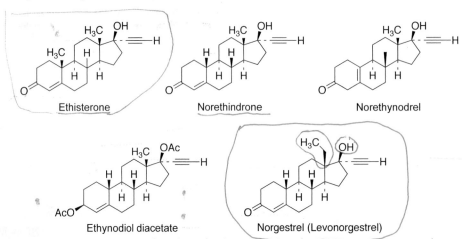

Figure 25.19 • Natural and synthetic progestins. *(continues on next page)*

2. Synthetic Progestins – (continued)

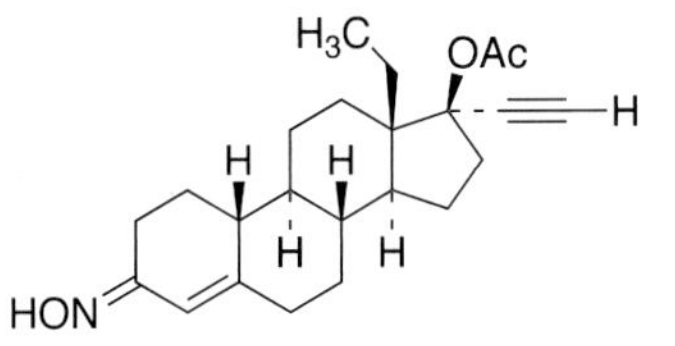

Norgestimate

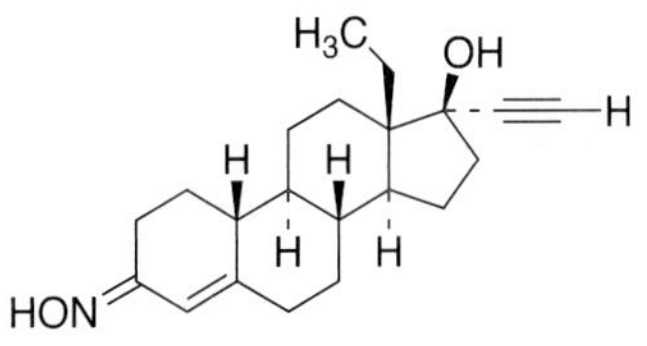

Norelgestromin

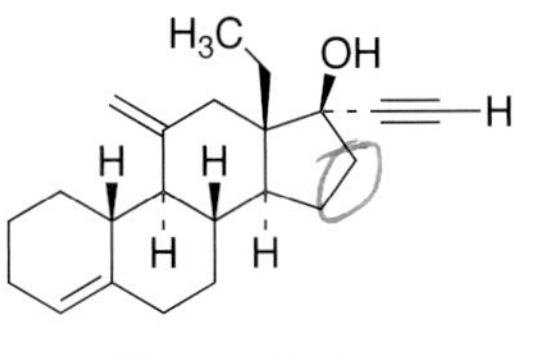

Desogestrel

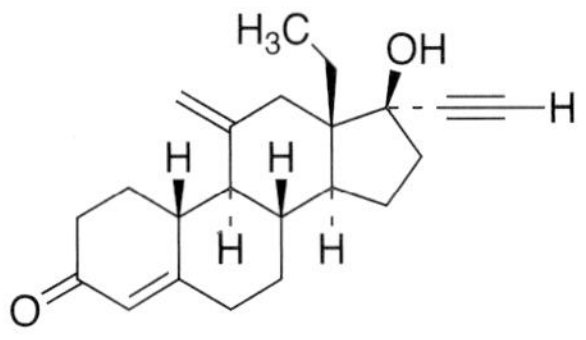

Etonogestrel

3. Miscellaneous Synthetic Progestins

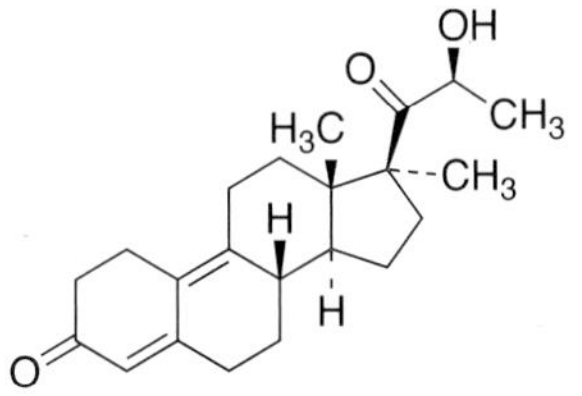

Trimegestone

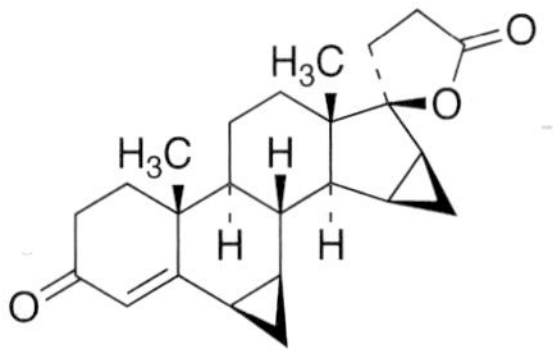

Drospirenone

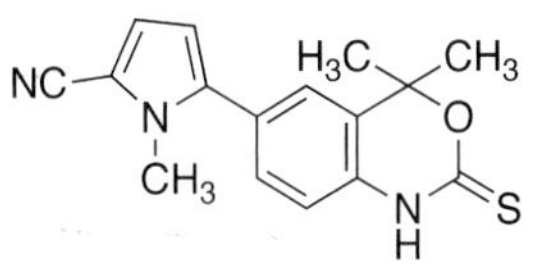

Tanaproget PR agonist (phase II)

Figure 25.19 ● *(Continued)*

the potential for a different side effect profile compared with the other progestins. While there is still a long road before approval of nonsteroidal progestins like tanaproget, there is great enthusiasm that a new class of progestins can be developed.

THERAPEUTIC USES OF PROGESTINS

Progestin therapy may cause menstrual irregularities, such as spotting or amenorrhea. Weight gain and acne have been associated with testosterone and 19-nortestosterone analog, in part because of their slight androgenic effects.

Birth Control. A significant use of the progestins, as of the estrogens, is inhibition of ovulation. Steroidal birth control agents are discussed in the following section on chemical contraception.

Reduction of the Risk of Endometrial Cancer from Postmenopausal Estrogens. As discussed in the section on therapeutic uses of estrogens, several studies have suggested that the combination of a progestin with an estrogen may significantly reduce the risk of endometrial cancer in women taking postmenopausal estrogens. Because of this, a progestin is often included in HRT.

Primary and Secondary Amenorrhea and Functional Uterine Bleeding Caused by Insufficient Progesterone Production or Estrogen–Progesterone Imbalance. Progestins have been used very effectively to treat primary and secondary amenorrhea, functional uterine bleeding, and related menstrual disorders caused by hormonal deficiency or imbalance.

Breast or Endometrial Carcinoma. Progestins can be used for palliative treatment of advanced carcinoma of the breast or endometrium. These agents should not be used in place of surgery, radiation, or chemotherapy.

PROGESTIN PRODUCTS

The progestins are primarily used in oral contraceptive products and in hormone replacement regimens for women. They are also used to treat several gynecological disorders: dysmenorrhea, endometriosis, amenorrhea, and dysfunctional uterine bleeding. Estrogens are given simultaneously in most of these situations.

Progesterone, USP. Progesterone, pregn-4-en-3,20-dione, is so rapidly metabolized that it is not particularly effective orally, being only one twelfth as active as intramuscularly. An oral formulation of micronized progesterone (Prometrium) is available. Progesterone given intramuscularly can be very irritating. A vaginal gel containing 4% or 8% progesterone offers an alternative dosage form. Progesterone was originally obtained from animal ovaries but is now prepared synthetically from plant sterol precursors. The discovery of 19-nortestosterones with progesterone activity made synthetically modified progestins of tremendous therapeutic importance.

Progesterone (and all other steroid 4-ene-3-ones) is light sensitive and should be protected from light.

Hydroxyprogesterone Caproate, USP. Hydroxyprogesterone caproate, 17-hydroxypregn-4-ene-3,20-dione hexanoate, is much more active and longer acting than progesterone (see Table 25.2), probably because the 17α ester hinders reduction to the 20-ol. In contrast, hydroxyprogesterone itself lacks progestational activity. The caproate ester is given only intramuscularly. The ester greatly increases oil solubility, allowing it to be slowly released from depot preparations, as one would predict from Figure 25.6. Although only currently available through compounding pharmacies, a new formulation (Gestiva) was deemed approvable by the FDA in late 2006 for the prevention of preterm labor, pending further studies.

Medroxyprogesterone Acetate, USP. MPA, 17-acetyloxy-6α-methylpregn-4-ene-3,20-dione (Provera), adds a 6α-methyl group to the basic 17α-hydroxyprogesterone structure to greatly decrease the rate of reduction of the 4-ene-3-one system. The 17α-acetate group also decreases reduction of the 20-one, similar to the 17α-caproate. MPA is very active orally (see Table 25.2) and has such a long duration of action intramuscularly that it cannot be routinely used intramuscularly for treating many menstrual disorders. The IM formulation is useful in the palliative treatment of advanced endometrial, breast, and renal carcinomas. MPA also has an important role in several birth control products (Depo-Provera, Depo-SubQ Provera 104).

Megestrol Acetate, USP. Megestrol acetate, 17-hydroxy-6-methylpregna-4,6-diene-3,20-dione acetate (Megace), is a progestin used primarily for the palliative management of recurrent, inoperable, or metastatic endometrial or breast carcinoma. Megestrol acetate has also been indicated for appetite enhancement in patients with AIDS. The biochemical basis for this use of megestrol is unclear.

Nomegestrol Acetate, USP. Nomegestrol acetate, 17-hydroxy-6-methyl-19-norpregna-4,6-diene-3,20-dione acetate, is being investigated as the progestin component of a new oral contraceptive, in combination with the estrogen estradiol. This new combination, NOMAC/E2, is in phase III trials and would be the first oral contraceptive to utilize estradiol itself as the estrogenic component. Structurally, NOMAC is considered a nor-progesterone derivative that lacks the C19 methyl group in megestrol acetate.

Norethindrone, USP, and Norethynodrel, USP. Norethindrone, 17α-ethinyl-19-nortestosterone, and its $\Delta^{5(10)}$-isomer, norethynodrel, might appear at first glance to be subtle copies of each other. One would predict that the $\Delta^{5(10)}$-double bond would isomerize in the stomach's acid to the Δ^4-position. However, the two drugs were actually developed simultaneously and independently; hence, neither can be considered a copy of the other. Furthermore, norethindrone is about 10 times more active than norethynodrel (see Table 25.2), indicating that isomerization is not as facile in vivo as one might predict. Although they are less active than progesterone when given subcutaneously, they have the important advantage of being orally active. The discovery of the potent progestin activity of 17α-ethinyltestosterone (ethisterone) and 19-norprogesterone preceded the development of these potent progestins. Both are orally active, with the 17α-ethinyl group blocking oxidation to the less active 17-one. The rich electron density of the ethinyl group and the absence of the 19-methyl group greatly enhance progestin activity. Both compounds were of great importance as progestin components of oral contraceptives, although currently, use of norethynodrel is minimal. Norethindrone, *USP*, and norethindrone acetate,

USP, are widely used for all the usual indications of the progestins, as well as being components of oral contraceptives. Because these compounds retain key features of the testosterone structure, including the 17β-OH, it is not surprising that they possess some androgenic side effects.

Ethynodiol Diacetate, USP. Ethynodiol diacetate, 19-norpregn-4-en-20-yne-$3\beta,17\alpha$-diol diacetate, is a prodrug of norethindrone. A combination of hydrolysis of both esters and oxidation of the C3 alcohol to the ketone is necessary to provide the fully active progestin.[81]

Norgestrel, USP, and Levonorgestrel, USP. Norgestrel, (17α)-$(\pm)$-13-ethyl-17-hydroxy-18,19-dinorpregn-4-en-20-yn-3-one, and levonorgestrel, (17α)-$(-)$-13-ethyl-17-hydroxy-18,19-dinorpregn-4-en-20-yn-3-one, have a C13 ethyl group instead of the C13 methyl but have progestational properties similar to those of norethindrone, with decreased androgenic effects. The ethyl group apparently provides unfavorable steric interactions with the AR that reduce the affinity compared with that with the PRs. Norgestrel is a racemic mixture, while levonorgestrel is the single active levorotatory enantiomer. Norgestrel is used only in oral contraceptives. Levonorgestrel is used in both oral combination birth control products and polymeric implants that provide contraception for up to 5 years.

Desogestrel, USP. Desogestrel, (17α)-13-ethyl-11-methylene-18,19-dinorpregn-4-en-20-yn-17-ol, is a 19-nortestosterone analog with good progestin activity. Like the other progestins, it is orally active and used in combination with an estrogen in oral contraceptives. Desogestrel is a prodrug that must be oxidized to the 3-one in vivo to have progestational action. CYPs 2C9 and 2C19 have been implicated in the initial hydroxylation of desogestrel at C3.[82]

Norgestimate, USP. Norgestimate, (17α)-17-acetyloxy-13-ethyl-18,19-dinor-pregn-4-en-20yn-3-one oxime, is a 19-nortestosterone, 3-oxime prodrug that is orally active and used with an estrogen in oral contraceptive products. It has minimal androgenic action. Norgestimate is metabolized to 17-deacetylnorgestimate (norelgestromin) and norgestrel, which provide the progestational action.[83]

Norelgestromin, USP. Norelgestromin, (17α)-13ethyl-17-hydroxy-18,19-dinor-pregn-4-en-20-yn-3-one, oxime, is the progestin component in the contraceptive patch (Ortho-Evra). First-pass metabolism in the liver is avoided by the transdermal application. Hepatic metabolism does occur, however, and norgestrel, an active metabolite, and other hydroxylated and conjugated metabolites are formed.

Etonogestrel, USP. Etonogestrel, 17α-13-ethyl-17hydroxy-11-methylene-18,19-dinorpregn-4-en-20-yn-3-one,3-ketodesogestrel, is the active metabolite of desogestrel. It is the progestin component in a newer implantable contraceptive (Implanon) and in the vaginal contraceptive ring (NuvaRing).

Drospirenone, USP. Drospirenone, 3-oxo-$6\beta,7\beta:15\beta$, 16β-dimethylene-17α-pregn-4-en-21,17-carbolactone, differs structurally from all the other commercially available progestins. Its structure is similar to that of spironolactone, an MR antagonist, and it does have antimineralocorticoid activity as well as progestational activity. It is also reported to have some antiandrogenic effects. The spirolactone at C17 and the two cyclopropyl groups at C6-

C7 and C15-C16 contribute to these unique actions. Drospirenone is the progestin component in the newer oral contraceptives, Yasmin and Yaz, and in the HRT product, Angeliq.

Trimegestone. Trimegestone, 17β-(S)-lactoyl-17-methyl-estra-4,9-dien-3-one, is a highly modified norprogesterone derivative. The key structural differences are a 17β-lactoyl group in place of the typical acetyl group, a 17α-methyl, and a C9-C10 double bond. Trimegestone lacks androgenic action and has little to no affinity for the ER and GR.[84] Although already approved for treating HRT in Sweden in combination with estradiol, it is still in development in the United States for its use in HRT and as a component of oral contraceptives.

Progesterone Receptor Antagonists and Selective Progesterone Receptor Modulators

Mifepristone (Mifeprex), a PR antagonist, is approved by the FDA to induce abortion in the first 49 days of pregnancy (Fig. 25.20). Mifepristone acts directly by antagonizing the effects of progesterone at PRs, as well as indirectly by causing a decrease in progesterone secretion from the corpus luteum. These combined effects lead to an increase in the level of prostaglandins, which stimulates uterine contractions.

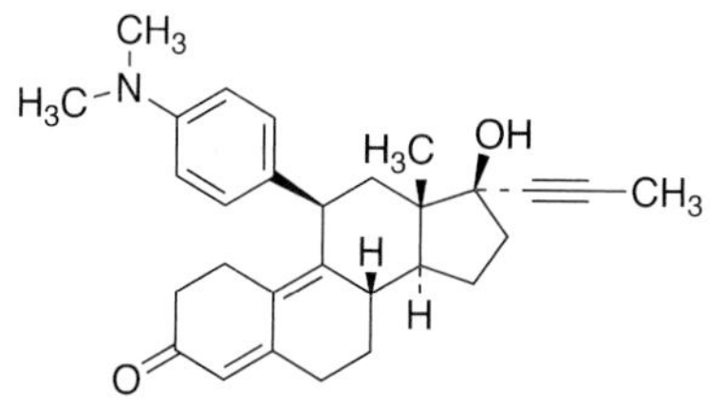

Mifepristone (Mifeprex; RU 486)

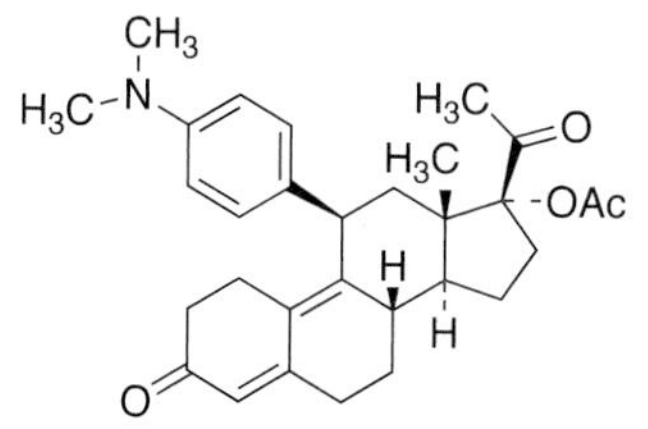

CDB-2914

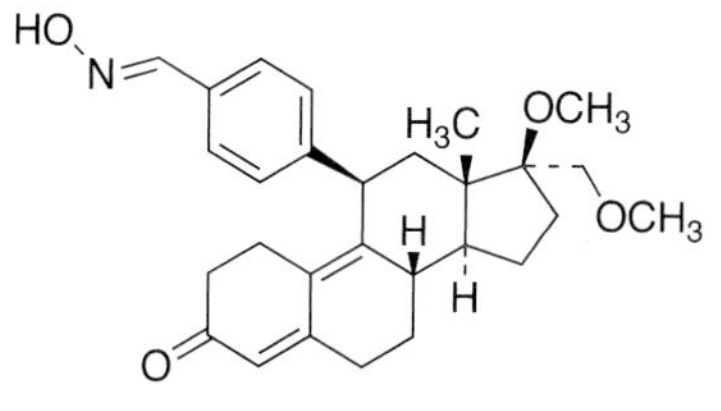

Asoprisnil

Figure 25.20 ● Progesterone receptor antagonists and SPRM.

Mifepristone also causes a softening of the cervix, which aids in expulsion of the fertilized ovum. Mifepristone treatment is followed by the use of misoprostol, a prostaglandin E₂ analog, to ensure a complete abortion. Mifepristone also has antagonist action at GR.

Another PR antagonist that is in development is CDB-2914. It is a norprogesterone derivative that has the same 11β-aryl substituent as seen in mifepristone, although it has less GR antagonism than mifepristone.[85] CDB-2914 is in phase III trials as an emergency contraceptive.

Compounds that have both agonist and antagonist properties at PRs, depending on the target tissue, have been called selective progesterone receptor modulators (SPRMs), which are analogous to the SERMs. Several are currently in development for various conditions, with asoprisnil being one that has been examined in phase III clinical trials for the treatment of uterine fibroids.[86] Asoprisnil has antagonist properties in breasts and partial agonist actions in the uterus and vagina.[87] Structurally, asoprisnil is a nortestosterone derivative with an 11β-aryl group bearing an oxime in the 4' position. O-Demethylation at C-17β produces a metabolite that also acts an SPRM.

CHEMICAL CONTRACEPTIVE AGENTS

The most notable achievement in chemical contraception came in the late 1950s and early 1960s with the development of oral contraceptive agents—"the pill." Since then, various contraceptive products have been introduced, including hormone-releasing intrauterine devices, polymer implants, injectable formulations, and a transdermal patch. In addition, postcoital contraceptives and abortifacients have been developed. Despite the advances in chemical contraceptive agents for women, no hormonal male contraceptives are currently available, although limited research in this area has been conducted. In the following pages, each of these approaches to chemical contraception is discussed. Individual compounds are discussed previously with the estrogens and progestins.

Ovulation Inhibitors and Related Hormonal Contraceptives

HISTORY[88–91]

In the 1930s, several research groups found that injections of progesterone inhibited ovulation in rats, rabbits, and guinea pigs.[92–94] In the early 1940s, it was discovered that estrogens, progesterone, or both could be used to prevent ovulation in women.[95,96] In 1965, it was reported that progesterone given from day 5 to day 25 of the menstrual cycle would inhibit ovulation in women.[97] During this time, Djerassi et al.[98] of Syntex and Colton[99] of G. D. Searle and Co. reported the synthesis of norethindrone and norethynodrel. These progestins possessed very high progestational and ovulation-inhibiting activity.

Extensive animal and clinical trials confirmed in 1956 that Searle's norethynodrel and Syntex's norethindrone were effective ovulation inhibitors in women. In 1960, Searle marketed Enovid (a mixture of norethynodrel and mestranol), and in 1962, Ortho marketed Ortho-Novum (a mixture of norethindrone and mestranol) under contract with Syntex. Norethindrone has remained the most extensively used progestin in oral contraceptives, but several other useful agents have been developed.

THERAPEUTIC CLASSES AND MECHANISMOF ACTION

The modern hormonal contraceptives fall into several major categories (Table 25.3), each with its own mechanism of contraceptive action. Individual compounds are discussed with the estrogens and progestins in the previous section.

Combination Tablets: Mechanism of Action. Although recognized in the early 1940s that either estrogens or progestins could inhibit ovulation, it was subsequently found that combinations were highly effective. Some problems, such as

TABLE 25.3 Comparison of Steroid Contraceptive Regimens

1. Combination—Monophasic

Products are available in 21- or 28-day dispensers and refills. The 28-day dispensers contain several inert (or Fe21-containing) tablets of a different color, taken daily after the 21 days of active tablets. Doses of active tablets are shown.

Brand	Progestin	Estrogen
Necon 1/50	Norethindrone, 1 mg	Mestranol, 50 μg
Norinyl 1 + 50	Norethindrone, 1 mg	Mestranol, 50 μg
Ortho-Novum 1/50	Norethindrone, 1 mg	Mestranol, 50 μg
Ovcon 50	Norethindrone, 1 mg	Ethinyl estradiol, 50 μg
Demulen 1/50	Ethynodiol diacetate, 1 mg	Ethinyl estradiol, 50 μg
Zovia 1/50E	Ethynodiol diacetate, 1 mg	Ethinyl estradiol, 50 μg
Ovral-28	Norgestrel, 0.5 mg	Ethinyl estradiol, 50 μg
Ogestrel	Norgestrel, 0.5 mg	Ethinyl estradiol, 50 μg
Necon 1/35	Norethindrone, 1 mg	Ethinyl estradiol, 35 μg
Norinyl 1 + 35	Norethindrone, 1 mg	Ethinyl estradiol, 35 μg
Nortrel 1/35	Norethindrone, 1 mg	Ethinyl estradiol, 35 μg
Ortho-Novum 1/35	Norethindrone, 1 mg	Ethinyl estradiol, 35 μg
Modicon	Norethindrone, 0.5 mg	Ethinyl estradiol, 35 μg
Necon 0.5/35	Norethindrone, 0.5 mg	Ethinyl estradiol, 35 μg
Nortrel 0.5/35	Norethindrone, 0.5 mg	Ethinyl estradiol, 35 μg
Ovcon-35	Norethindrone, 0.4 mg	Ethinyl estradiol, 35 μg
Ortho-Cyclen	Norgestimate, 0.25 mg	Ethinyl estradiol, 35 μg
Demulen 1/35	Ethynodiol diacetate, 1 mg	Ethinyl estradiol, 35 μg
Zovia 1/35E	Ethynodiol diacetate, 1 mg	Ethinyl estradiol, 35 μg
Yasmin	Drospirenone, 3 mg	Ethinyl estradiol, 30 μg
Loestrin 21 1.5/30	Norethindrone acetate, 1.5 mg	Ethinyl estradiol, 30 μg
Loestrin Fe 1.5/30	Norethindrone acetate, 1.5 mg	Ethinyl estradiol, 30 μg
Microgestin Fe 1.5/30	Norethindrone acetate, 1.5 mg	Ethinyl estradiol, 30 μg
Lo/Ovral	Norgestrel, 0.3 mg	Ethinyl estradiol, 30 μg
Low-Ogestrel	Norgestrel, 0.3 mg	Ethinyl estradiol, 30 μg
Desogen	Desogestrel, 0.15 mg	Ethinyl estradiol, 30 μg
Ortho-Cept	Desogestrel, 0.15 mg	Ethinyl estradiol, 30 μg
Apri	Desogestrel, 0.15 mg	Ethinyl estradiol, 30 μg
Levlen	Levonorgestrel, 0.15 mg	Ethinyl estradiol, 30 μg
Levora	Levonorgestrel, 0.15 mg	Ethinyl estradiol, 30 μg
Nordette	Levonorgestrel, 0.15 mg	Ethinyl estradiol, 30 μg
Alesse	Levonorgestrel, 0.1 mg	Ethinyl estradiol, 20 μg
Aviane	Levonorgestrel, 0.1 mg	Ethinyl estradiol, 20 μg
Levlite	Levonorgestrel, 0.1 mg	Ethinyl estradiol, 20 μg
Loestrin 21 1/20	Norethindrone acetate, 1 mg	Ethinyl estradiol, 20 μg
Loestrin Fe 1/20	Norethindrone acetate, 1 mg	Ethinyl estradiol, 20 μg
Microgestin Fe 1/20	Norethindrone acetate, 1 mg	Ethinyl estradiol, 20 μg

2. Combination—Biphasic

Products are available in 21- or 28-day dispensers and refills. They are taken on the same schedule of 21 days plus 7 days of no (or inert) tablets as the monophasics above, except Mircette. Doses of active tablets are shown.

Brand	Progestin and Estrogen
Jenest-28	7 days: Norethindrone, 0.5 mg, and ethinyl estradiol, 35 μg 14 days: Norethindrone, 1 mg, and ethinyl estradiol, 35 μg
Necon 10/11	10 days: Norethindrone, 0.5 mg, and ethinyl estradiol, 35 μg 11 days: Norethindrone, 1 mg, and ethinyl estradiol, 35 μg
Ortho-Novum 10/11 21	10 days: Norethindrone, 0.5 mg, and ethinyl estradiol, 35 μg 11 days: Norethindrone, 1 mg, and ethinyl estradiol, 35 μg
Mircette	21 days: Desogestrel, 0.15 mg, and ethinyl estradiol, 20 μg 5 days: Ethinyl estradiol, 10 μg 2 days: Inert

3. Combination—Triphasic

Products are available in 21- or 28-day dispensers and refills. They are taken on the same schedule of 21 days plus 7 days of no (or inert) tablets as the monophasics. Doses of active tablets are shown.

Brand	Progestin and Estrogen
Ortho-Novum 7/7/7	7 days: Norethindrone, 0.5 mg, and ethinyl estradiol, 35 μg
	7 days: Norethindrone, 0.75 mg, and ethinyl estradiol, 35 μg
	7 days: Norethindrone, 1 mg, and ethinyl estradiol, 35 μg
Ortho-Tri-Cyclen	7 days: Norgestimate, 0.18 mg, and ethinyl estradiol, 35 μg
	7 days: Norgestimate, 0.215 mg, and ethinyl estradiol, 35 μg
	7 days: Norgestimate, 0.25 mg, and ethinyl estradiol, 35 μg
Trinorinyl	7 days: Norethindrone, 0.5 mg, and ethinyl estradiol, 35 μg
	9 days: Norethindrone, 1 mg, and ethinyl estradiol, 35 μg
Tri-Levlen	5 days: Norethindrone, 0.5 mg, and ethinyl estradiol, 35 μg
	6 days: Levonorgestrel, 0.05 mg, and ethinyl estradiol, 30 μg
	5 days: Levonorgestrel, 0.075 mg, and ethinyl estradiol, 40 μg
Tri-Phasil	10 days: Levonorgestrel, 0.125 mg, and ethinyl estradiol, 30 μg
	6 days: Levonorgestrel, 0.05 mg, and ethinyl estradiol, 30 μg
	5 days: Levonorgestrel, 0.075 mg, and ethinyl estradiol, 40 μg
Trivora	10 days: Levonorgestrel, 0.125 mg, and ethinyl estradiol, 30 μg
	6 days: Levonorgestrel, 0.05 mg, and ethinyl estradiol, 30 μg
	5 days: Levonorgestrel, 0.075 mg, and ethinyl estradiol, 40 μg
	10 days: Levonorgestrel, 0.125 mg, and ethinyl estradiol, 30 μg
Estrostep	5 days: Norethindrone acetate, 1 mg, and ethinyl estradiol, 20 μg
	7 days: Norethindrone acetate, 1 mg, and ethinyl estradiol, 30 μg
	9 days: Norethindrone acetate, 1 mg, and ethinyl estradiol, 35 μg

4. Progestin Only

An active tablet is taken each day of the year.

Brand	Progestin	Dose
Micronor	Norethindrone	0.35 mg
Nor-Q.D.	Norethindrone	0.35 mg
Ovrette	Norgestrel	0.075 mg

5. Injectable Depot Hormonal Contraceptives

Brand	Drug	Dosage Cycle
Depo-Provera	Medroxyprogesterone acetate alone	150 mg/month
		150 mg every 3 months
Lunelle	Medroxyprogesterone acetate (MPA), 25 mg, and estradiol cypionate (E2C), 5 mg/0.5 mL	0.5-mL IM injection once in deltoid, gluteus maximus, or anterior thigh every 28–30 days

6. Transdermal Contraceptive Patch

Brand	Release Rate	Total Hormone Content	Dosage Cycle
Ortho-Evra	0.15-mg norelgestromin, 0.02 mg, ethinyl estradiol/24 hours	6-mg norelgestromin, 0.075 mg, ethinyl estradiol	One patch each week for 3 weeks, 1 week no patch.

7. Hormone-Releasing Implants, IUDs, and Vaginal Rings

Brand	Drug	Dosage Cycle
Progestasert	Progesterone-releasing IUD	38-mg dose in IUD lasts 1 year
Mirena	Levonorgestrel-releasing intrauterine system (LRIS)	52-mg dose in LRIS provides contraception for up to 5 years
Norplant	6 Silastic capsules with 36-mg levonorgestrel; all 6 capsules are inserted subdermally in the middle upper arm	Contraceptive efficacy lasts for 5 years if the implants are not removed

(table continues on page 844)

TABLE 25.3 **Comparison of Steroid Contraceptive Regimens** *(continued)*

Brand	Drug	Dosage Cycle
Implanon	One polymeric rod with 68-mg etonorgestrel, released at a rate of ~40 μg/day.	Contraceptive efficacy lasts up to 3 years if the implant is not removed
NuvaRing	11.7 mg etonogestrel, 2.7-mg ethinyl estradiol in a flexible, polymeric vaginal ring	Vaginal ring is inserted for 3 weeks duration, then 1 week off before insertion of a new ring

8. Emergency Contraceptives

Brand	Drug	Dosage
Plan B	0.75-mg levonorgestrel	The first dose (1 tablet) should be taken as soon as possible within 72 hours of intercourse; the second dose (1 tablet) must be taken 12 hours later
Preven	0.25-mg levonorgestrel, 0.05-mg ethinyl estradiol	The first dose (2 tablets) should be taken as soon as possible within 72 hours of intercourse; the second dose (2 tablets) must be taken 12 hours later

breakthrough (midcycle) bleeding, were also reduced by the use of a combination of progestin and estrogen.

It is now believed that the combination tablets suppress the production of LH, FSH, or both by a feedback-inhibition process (see Fig. 25.9). Without FSH or LH, ovulation is prevented. The process is similar to the natural inhibition of ovulation during pregnancy, caused by the release of estrogens and progesterone from the placenta and ovaries. An additional effect comes from the progestin causing the cervical mucus to become very thick, providing a barrier for the passage of sperm through the cervix. Because pregnancy is impossible without ovulation, however, the contraceptive effects of thick cervical mucus or alterations in the lining of the uterus (to decrease the probability of implantation of a fertilized ovum) would appear to be quite secondary. Nevertheless, occasional ovulation may occur, and thus the alterations of the cervical mucus and the endometrium may actually serve an important contraceptive function (especially, perhaps, when the patient forgets to take one of the tablets). During combination drug treatment, the endometrial lining develops enough for withdrawal bleeding to occur about 4 or 5 days after taking the last active tablet of the series (see Table 25.3).

Monophasic (Fixed) Combinations
The monophasic combinations of a progestin and estrogen contain the same amount of drug in each active tablet (see Table 25.3). As discussed later in this chapter, the trend in prescribing has been toward lower doses of estrogen. As estrogen levels are reduced, however, breakthrough bleeding (or spotting) becomes an annoying side effect for some patients at early to midcycle. Spotting after midcycle or amenorrhea appears to be related to too little progestin relative to the estrogen. The biphasic and triphasic combinations were developed to solve these breakthrough-bleeding problems in some patients.

Biphasic and Triphasic (Variable) Combinations
In the natural menstrual cycle, progesterone plasma concentrations peak late in the cycle. The higher estrogen/progesterone ratio early in the cycle is believed to assist in development of the endometrium. The higher progesterone concentration later contributes to proliferation of the endometrium and a resultant "normal" volume of menstrual flow. The biphasic and triphasic combinations attempt to mimic this variation in estrogen/progestin levels, and thereby reduce the incidence of spotting associated with low-dose monophasic combinations. With proper selection of patients, the goal has been achieved; but in other patients, the incidence of spotting has not decreased appreciably.

Extended Oral Contraceptive Therapy
Several oral contraceptive products that offer women the option to reduce the number of menstrual cycles are now available. Three of these use a 91-day cycle as opposed to the current 28-day cycles typically used for oral contraceptives. The key difference with this approach is that the number of menstrual cycles during the year would be reduced from 12 to 4. The monophasic products, Seasonale and Quasense, have levonorgestrel (0.15 mg) and ethinyl estradiol (30 μg) as the progestin and estrogen, respectively. The dosing regimen has 84 days of hormones, followed by a week of inert tablets. Seasonique is a biphasic contraceptive using the same progestin and estrogen, but with 7 days of 10-μg ethinyl estradiol tablets, instead of inert tablets. The latest addition to extended oral contraceptive therapy is Lybrel, a low-dose product that is dosed continuously, completely eliminating monthly periods. Lybrel uses 90-μg levonorgestrel and 20-μg ethinyl estradiol in each tablet. Although regular menstrual periods will be eliminated, many women in the clinical trials experienced unscheduled breakthrough bleeding.

HOW SAFE?

The safety of the pill has been investigated extensively because of the widespread use of these drugs in healthy young women. Overall, oral contraceptives have an excellent safety profile in healthy, nonsmoking women of child-bearing age.[100] Early studies, based largely on the earlier products that contained high doses of estrogen, showed an alarming incidence of thromboembolic disease (blood clots). More recent studies have shown a greatly reduced risk of cardiovascular effects with lower estrogen doses. Another concern has been an association between estrogens and increased cancer risk. Recent reanalysis of clinical data supports a slightly increased risk of breast cancer in women taking oral contraceptives, but the risk subsides within 10 years of discontinuation of use.[101] This small increase in incidence of breast cancer is not greatly affected by duration of use, dose, age at first use, or progestin component. In addition, use of oral contraceptives has shown a decreased risk for endometrial and ovarian cancers.[101]

The overall results of these studies have been that (a) the sequential contraceptive products with their high doses of estrogen have been removed from American markets; (b) most combination contraceptives now marketed contain less than 50 μg of estrogen per dose (see Table 25.3); (c) progestin-only or minipill products are available (see Table 25.3); and (d) a few groups of women who should definitely not take oral contraceptives (e.g., women with a history of thromboembolic disease or other cardiovascular disease, women who are heavy smokers over the age of 35, and women with a history of breast cancer in their immediate family) have been identified. The actual incidence of "pill-induced" cardiovascular death for nonsmoking young women is quite small, and there is not a widespread link between oral contraceptive use and cancer. Cigarette smoking increases the risk of thromboembolic disorders associated with oral contraceptive use, so women should be counseled to abstain from smoking while using oral contraceptives.

Progestin Only (Minipill). The estrogen component of sequential and combination oral contraceptive agents has been related to some side effects, with thromboembolism being a concern. One solution to this problem has been to develop new products with decreased estrogen content. The minipill contains no estrogen at all.

Although higher doses of progestin are known to suppress ovulation, minipill doses of progestin do not suffice to suppress ovulation in all women. Some studies have indicated that increased viscosity of the cervical mucus (or sperm barrier) could account for much of the contraceptive effect. Low doses of progestin have also been found to increase the rate of ovum transport and to disrupt implantation. There is a good probability that most, or all, of these factors contribute to the overall contraceptive effect of the minipill. The incidence of pregnancy with the minipill is slightly higher than with combination products, although still very low when the minipill is used as directed.

Depo-Provera. MPA IM injection (Depo-Provera) provides contraception for 3 months after a single 150-mg IM dose. Most women experience some irregular bleeding or spotting and often experience small weight gain. Fertility returns for most women within the first 12 months after discontinuance of Depo-Provera. Contraception typically continues for a few weeks beyond the 3-month term, giving patients a short grace period if the subsequent IM dose is delayed. A related product is Depo-SubQ Provera 104. This is a formulation designed for subcutaneous injection and uses 104 mg of MPA for the same 3-month period of effectiveness.

Transdermal Contraceptives. One transdermal contraceptive patch, Ortho-Evra, is available. The product contains norelgestromin and ethinyl estradiol. A patch is applied once a week for 3 weeks, followed by a week with no patch. The pregnancy rate for this product is 1 in 100, a rate similar to that often observed with oral contraceptives. Reports of increased risk of blood clots relative to the use of the pill appeared several years after the introduction of Ortho-Evra, which led the FDA to strengthen the warning associated with the use of this product.

Progesterone IUD. The low progestin doses of the minipill seem to have a direct effect on the uterus and associated reproductive tract. Therefore, it would seem possible to lower the progestin dose even more if the drug was released in the reproductive tract itself.

The Progestasert IUD (Progesterone Intrauterine Contraceptive System, *USP*) has 38 mg of microcrystalline progesterone dispersed in silicone oil. The dispersion is contained in a flexible polymer in the approximate shape of a T. The polymer acts as a membrane to permit 65 μg of progesterone to be released slowly into the uterus each day for 1 year. The progesterone-containing IUD has had some of the therapeutic problems of other IUDs, including a relatively low patient continuation rate, some septic abortions, and some perforations of uterus and cervix.

Levonorgestrel-Releasing Intrauterine System (LRIS). Because the Progestasert system provided evidence that a progestin-releasing intrauterine device was an effective contraceptive, another intrauterine system has been developed with use of a different progestin. Mirena is a plastic T-shaped frame, with the stem of the "T" containing 52 mg of levonorgestrel. The levonorgestrel is released slowly, at a dose lower than in a pill (approximately one-seventh strength), directly to the lining of the uterus. This local release and absorption of the hormone helps to reduce systemic progesterone-type side effects. The contraceptive effectiveness of this device lasts up to 5 years.

Mirena acts as a contraceptive in two ways: it thickens the mucus at the cervix, preventing sperm from getting through, and it also thins the lining of the uterus, preventing implantation. In some women it also prevents ovulation. An additional feature of the LRIS is that menstrual periods are typically lighter than usual. The LRIS may be useful to alleviate the difficulties associated with heavy periods, even in patients who do not need contraception.

There is a small chance that the device may dislodge in the early months of use. Although the LRIS releases a reduced amount of progestin, it does slightly increase progesterone levels in the bloodstream. This increased progesterone can cause side effects including headache, water retention, breast tenderness, or acne, although these are typically mild. Bleeding problems are the most common side effect, but this effect usually ceases after 3 to 6 months of use.

Intrauterine Ring. Another contraceptive option is a flexible polymeric ring, approximately 2.1 inches in diameter, that contains etonogestrel and ethinyl estradiol (NuvaRing). The ring is inserted into the vagina by the woman herself and remains inserted for 3 weeks. The spent ring is removed for 1 week to allow menstrual period. A new ring is inserted 1 week after the removal of the prior ring. The ring contains 11.7 mg of etonogestrel and 2.7 mg of ethinyl estradiol, with a release rate of 0.12-mg etonogestrel per day and 0.015 mg of ethinyl estradiol per day. Unlike a diaphragm, the placement of the vaginal ring contraceptive device is not critical. Clinical trials suggest a 1% to 2% pregnancy rate for women using the ring as indicated. Like other hormone-based contraceptives, the ring should not be used by women who have cardiovascular disease, blood clots, or hormone-dependent breast cancer. Women should also abstain from smoking while using the ring.

CONTRACEPTIVE IMPLANTS

Norplant. The first implantable contraceptive was Norplant, a set of six flexible Silastic (dimethylsiloxane/methylvinylsiloxane copolymer) capsules that contain levonorgestrel. The capsules implanted in the midportion of the upper arm provided contraception for up to 5 years. Contraceptive efficacy was very high, but the insertion and removal procedures required extra training of physicians, a feature that reduced the desirability of this product. Although Norplant was extremely effective as a contraceptive, various legal issues, public concerns, and production issues led the manufacturers to discontinue production of Norplant. Norplant II, a two-rod implantable system that had reduced problems with insertion and removal, was approved by the FDA but was never marketed in the United States. This system, however, is available as the product Jadelle in various other countries.

The implantable system that has replaced Norplant in the United States is Implanon, a single-rod system (40×2 mm) that releases etonogestrel (3-ketodesogestrel) rather than the levonorgestrel. The contraceptive efficacy is up to 3 years. With a single polymer rod and a specially designed applicator system, the insertion/removal difficulties with Norplant should be avoided.

POSTCOITAL CONTRACEPTIVES

Two products specifically designated for postcoital or emergency contraception have been approved. Plan B uses a high-dose, progestin-only approach, whereas Preven combines a progestin and an estrogen (Table 25.3). Both must be taken within 72 hours of unprotected intercourse, followed by another dose 12 hours later. Plan B had its status changed in 2006 to over-the-counter for women 18 years of age or older. Women younger than 18 years old must still obtain a prescription. These treatments are intended only for use in short-term emergency situations.

Combined Estrogen/Progestin Hormone Replacement Therapy

Similar to the combined estrogen and progestin oral contraceptives, combination estrogen/progestin products are available for use in HRT in women. In contrast to the oral contraceptives, in which the estrogen component is almost always ethinyl estradiol, the estrogen component of HRT products is typically conjugated estrogens or estradiol. The progestin component for HRT is often MPA or norethindrone acetate. Table 25.4 lists the currently available combination products. Both oral tablets and a transdermal patch are used.

TREATMENT OF VASOMOTOR SYMPTOMS OF MENOPAUSE AND ATROPHIC VAGINITIS

Estrogens have been very useful in treating the hot flashes associated with early menopause, as well as atrophic vaginitis and other vaginal symptoms of inadequate estrogen production. The evidence that they result in enhanced mood and improved cognitive function in postmenopausal women is less clear, however, and more studies are needed to sort out the competing claims in these areas.[102,103] Based on the results of the Women's Health Initiative (WHI) studies of HRT, however, the lowest effective doses should be used for as short of a duration as necessary for the management of postmenopausal symptoms (see below).

OSTEOPOROSIS PREVENTION AND TREATMENT[104–106]

Osteoporosis is an enormous public health problem, responsible for approximately 1.5 million fractures in the United States each year. Because of the prevalence of osteoporosis, especially in older women, the prevention and treatment of this condition have received much attention. Prior to menopause, a good diet and exercise are essential for young women, to decrease the risk of osteoporosis later in life. After menopause, supplemental estrogens can have a positive effect relative to osteoporosis. Estrogens mainly act by decreasing bone resorption, so estrogens are better at preventing bone loss than restoring bone mass. Estrogens taken after menopause (often with a supplemental progestin) have been unequivocally shown to greatly decrease the incidence and severity of osteoporosis, especially when combined with good nutrition and exercise. The long-term use of estrogens plus a progestin for preventing osteoporosis, however, should be carefully evaluated in light of the WHI studies examining HRT for lowering the risk of heart disease (see next page). Alternatives to estrogens for the prevention of osteoporosis, such as raloxifene and bisphosphonates, should also be considered.

TABLE 25.4 Combined Progestin/Estrogen Hormone Replacement Therapy Products (Available in Tablets or a Transdermal Patch)

Brand	Progestin	Estrogen
Prempro	Medroxyprogesterone acetate, 2.5 or 5 mg	Conjugated estrogens, 0.625 mg
Premphase[a]	Medroxyprogesterone acetate, 5 mg	Conjugated estrogens, 0.625 mg
Femhrt	Norethindrone acetate, 1 mg	Ethinyl estradiol, 5 μg
Activella	Norethindrone acetate, 0.5 mg	Estradiol, 1 mg
Ortho-Prefest[b]	Norgestimate, 0.09 mg	Estradiol, 1 mg
CombiPatch	Norethindrone acetate, 0.14 or 0.25 mg	Estradiol, 50 μg

[a]Premphase is dosed 14 days of estrogen-only tablets (0.625-mg conjugated estrogens), followed by 14 days of combined progestin/estrogen.
[b]Ortho-Prefest is dosed 15 days of estradiol (1 mg) alone, then 15 days of the combined progestin/estrogen.

After years of general recommendations for the beneficial use of estrogens after menopause for lowering the risk of heart disease, the results of a long-term study with conjugated estrogens supplemented with a progestin have indicated that the risks of this approach outweigh the benefits. The WHI trial, which enrolled over 16,000 postmenopausal women between 1993 and 1998, was terminated early in 2002 because of an unacceptably high level of adverse effects relative to the benefits gained. With long-term use (average follow-up of 5.2 years), there was a slight increase in the incidence of coronary heart disease, as well as an increase in breast cancer risk. Although there was a slight decrease in the risk of colorectal cancer and fewer hip fractures, the effects on the heart and breast argue against the use of estrogens plus a progestin for the prevention of coronary heart disease in postmenopausal women. A second WHI trial with estrogen alone in postmenopausal women without a uterus was halted in 2004. In this study, with an average of 7 years of follow-up, no effect was seen on heart disease, but there was an increase in stroke risk as well as a decrease in hip fractures. In both studies, a single drug regimen was used (0.625 mg of conjugated equine estrogens alone or with 2.5 mg of MPA), so care should be taken in extending these results to other regimens and products. Several years after the studies were stopped, the medical profession is still analyzing and debating the results of the WHI trials.[108,109] It is fair to say that there are many important health issues associated with HRT and each patient should discuss the costs and benefits of HRT with their physicians and pharmacists. In addition to the WHI studies indicating an increase in breast cancer risk, the Million Women Study conducted in the United Kingdom indicated an additional risk of ovarian cancer for women using HRT, with an increase in risk correlating with the duration of use.[110]

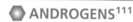 ANDROGENS[111]

Endogenous Androgens

Testosterone and its more potent reduction product 5α-DHT are produced in significantly greater amounts in males than in females, but females also produce low amounts of these "male" sex hormones. These endogenous compounds have two important activities: androgenic activity (promoting male sex characteristics) and anabolic activity (muscle building).

DHEA and androstenedione are referred to as *adrenal androgens*, although this nomenclature is somewhat misleading. DHEA and androstenedione are biosynthetic precursors to the androgens but have only low affinity for the AR themselves.[112,113] Therefore, DHEA or androstenedione can have androgenic actions, but only after in vivo conversion to testosterone and DHT. DHEA and androstenedione are, however, also precursors to the estrogens, so estrogenic actions may also occur.

Biosynthesis

As shown in Figure 25.5, testosterone can be synthesized through pregnenolone, DHEA, and androstenedione. About 7 mg/d is synthesized by young human adult males. Labeling experiments have also shown that it can be biosynthesized from androst-5-ene-3β,17β-diol, a reduction product of DHEA.

Testosterone is primarily produced by the interstitial cells of the testes, synthesized largely from cholesterol made in Sertoli cells. DHT is also secreted by the testes, as well as being produced in other tissues. The ovaries and adrenal cortex synthesize androstenedione and DHEA, which can be rapidly converted to testosterone in many tissues. Testosterone levels in the plasma of men are 5 to 100 times higher than those in the plasma of women.

Testosterone is produced in the testes in response to LH release by the anterior pituitary, as shown in Figure 25.10. Testosterone and DHT inhibit the production of LH and FSH by a feedback-inhibition process. This is quite similar to the feedback inhibition by estrogens and progestins in FSH and LH production.

Metabolism of Androgens

Testosterone is rapidly converted to 5α-DHT in many tissues by the action of 5α-reductase. Depending on the tissue, this is either to activate testosterone to the more potent androgen, DHT (e.g., in the prostate), or a step in the metabolic inactivation of this androgen. The primary route for metabolic inactivation of testosterone and DHT is oxidation to the 17-one. The 3-one group is also reduced to the 3α- (major) and 3β-ols (minor). The metabolites are shown in Figure 25.21. Androsterone is the major urinary metabolite and was the first "androgenic" steroid isolated. These metabolites are excreted mainly as the corresponding glucuronides. Other minor metabolites have also been detected.[111]

Biological Activities of Androgens[114]

Testosterone and DHT cause pronounced masculinizing effects, even in the male fetus. They induce the development of the prostate, penis, and related sexual tissues. At puberty, the secretion of testosterone by the testes increases greatly, leading to an increase in facial and body hair, deepening of the voice, increased protein anabolic activity and muscle mass, rapid growth of long bones, and loss of some subcutaneous fat. Spermatogenesis begins, and the prostate and seminal vesicles increase in activity. Sexual organs increase in size. The skin becomes thicker, and sebaceous glands increase in number, leading to acne in many young people. The androgens also play important roles in male psychology and behavior. In women, testosterone plays a role in libido, mood, muscle mass and strength, as well as bone density.[115,116]

Structural Classes: Anabolic Androgenic Steroids

The androgens, also known as anabolic androgenic steroids (AAS), include all of the therapeutic agents whose main actions are mediated by the AR. The inclusion of both *anabolic* and *androgenic* in referring to these compounds reflects the fact that no products are currently available in which the anabolic properties of androgens can be separated from the androgenic properties. The commonly used AAS are shown in Figure 25.22. Several recent reviews on AAS have been published.[111,117]

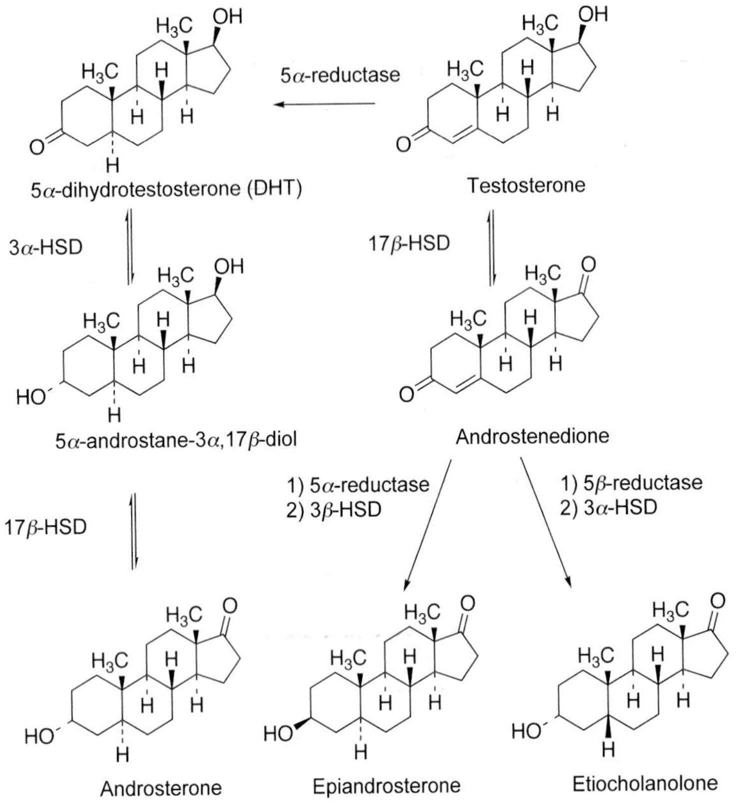

Figure 25.21 ● Metabolism of testosterone and 5α-DHT (conjugates of the metabolites are also formed). (HSD, hydroxysteroid dehydrogenase.)

SEMISYNTHETIC ANALOGS

Because bacterial and hepatic oxidation of the 17β-hydroxyl to the 17-one is a key component of metabolic inactivation, 17α-alkyl groups have been added to prevent oxidation of the alcohol. Even though 17α-methyltestosterone is only about half as active as testosterone, it can be taken orally because its half-life is longer than that of testosterone. 17α-ethyltestosterone has greatly reduced activity, as shown in Table 25.5.[98] As mentioned previously, addition of an α-alkynyl group provides more progestogenic action than androgenic

action, although some activities at AR are retained. A disadvantage of the 17α-methyl testosterones is hepatotoxicity. Hepatic disturbances, jaundice (occasionally), and death (in rare cases) may occur, particularly in the high doses often used by athletes (see next section).

Table 25.5 illustrates some structure–activity effects of the androgens, such as the greatly decreased activity of the 17α-ol isomer of testosterone (epitestosterone). A carbonyl group at C3 and a 17β-OH on a steroid backbone are key structural features required for high affinity at the AR. Hundreds of different AAS have been synthesized and studied. The goal of many synthetic programs was to make a compound that possessed the anabolic properties of testosterone but lacked its androgenic actions. Although numerous compounds were prepared that did display improved anabolic/androgenic ratios in vitro, no compounds completely lacked androgenic action.[117] Also, the high anabolic/androgenic ratios did not appear to be maintained when these drugs were used in humans. Despite the inability to prepare a strictly anabolic steroid, several trends were noticed in the structure–activity relationships for the hundreds of AAS that have been prepared.[111] Removal of the C19 methyl, 5α-reduction, and replacement of C2 with an oxygen are all structural changes that tend to increase anabolic activity. Although most of the androgens have a carbonyl at C3, stanozolol (Fig. 25.22) represents an "anabolic" steroid that lacks the C3 carbonyl, but still is active. As with other compounds that have been discussed, OH groups in the testosterones are often converted to the corresponding esters to prolong activity or to provide some protection from oxidation.

Therapeutic Uses of Anabolic Androgenic Steroids

The primary use of AAS is in androgen replacement therapy in men, either at maturity or in adolescence. The cause of

TABLE 25.5 Androgenic Activities of Some Androgens

Compound	μg Equivalent to an International Unit
Testosterone (17 β-ol)	15
Epitestosterone (17 α-ol)	400
17 α-Methyltestosterone	25–30
17 α-Ethyltestosterone	70–100
17 α-Methylandrostane-3α, 17 β-diol	35
17 α-Methylandrostane-3-one-17 β-ol	15
Androsterone	100
Epiandrosterone	700
Androstane-3α, 17 β-diol	20–25
Androstane-3α, 17 α-diol	350
Androstane-3β, 17 β-diol	500
Androstane-17β-ol-3-one	20
Androstane-17α-ol-3-one	300
Δ5-Androstene-3α, 17β-diol	35
Δ5-Androstene-3β, 17β-diol	500
Androstanedione-3, 17	120–130
Δ4-Androstenedione	120

Data are from Djerassi, C., Miramontes, L., Rosenkranz, G., et al.: Steroids. LIV. Synthesis of 19-Nor-17α-ethynyltestosterone and 19-Nor-17α-methyltestosterone. J. Am. Chem. Soc. 76:4092–4094, 1954.

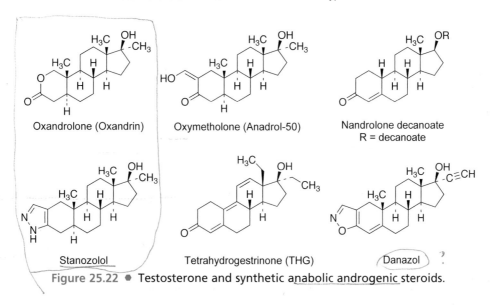

Figure 25.22 ● Testosterone and synthetic anabolic androgenic steroids.

testosterone deficiency may be either hypogonadism or hypopituitarism.

The use of the AAS for their anabolic activity or for uses other than androgen replacement has been limited because of their masculinizing actions. This has greatly limited their use in women and children. Although anabolic activity is often needed clinically, especially in patients with AIDS, none of the products presently available is free of significant androgenic side effects.

The masculinizing (androgenic) side effects in females include hirsutism, acne, deepening of the voice, clitoral enlargement, and depression of the menstrual cycle. Furthermore, AAS generally alter serum lipid levels and increase the probability of atherosclerosis, characteristically a disease of men and postmenopausal women.

The masculinizing effects of the AAS preclude their use in most circumstances in women. Secondary treatment of advanced or metastatic breast carcinoma in selected patients is generally considered to be the only indication for large-dose, long-term androgen therapy in women. In lower doses, androgen replacement therapy is more often being considered for use in menopausal and post-menopausal women for the positive effects on libido, mood, vasomotor symptoms, and muscle mass, all areas negatively affected by decreased testosterone levels in aging women.[118]

Androgens are also used to relieve bone pain associated with osteoporosis and to treat certain anemias, although this use has greatly decreased because of the availability of erythropoietin. In all cases, use of these agents requires caution.

Androgens and Sports

The use of androgens for their anabolic effects (hence the term *anabolic steroids*) by athletes began in the late 1940s and has, at times, been widespread.[119] Prior to urine testing requirements, it was estimated that up to 80% of competitive weight lifters and about 75% of professional football players used these drugs, along with various other athletes. Despite the growing awareness of the dangers of anabolic steroid use over the past 20 years, abuse of steroids is still a problem in many competitive sports. The recent Bay Area Laboratory Co-Operative (BALCO) scandal involving professional athletes in baseball, football, and track, and the continuing steroid problems seen in cycling illustrate this phenomenon all too well.

Some of the specific risks associated with the use/abuse of AAS are[120]:

In both sexes
Increased risk of coronary heart disease, stroke, or obstructed blood vessels

Increased aggression and antisocial behavior (known as "steroid rage")

Liver tumors, peliosis hepatis (blood-filled cysts), and jaundice (for 17α-alkylated androgens only)

In men

Testicular atrophy with consequent sterility or decreased sperm count and abnormal motility and morphology

Impotence

Enlarged prostate

Breast enlargement (for androgens that can be converted to estrogens)

In women

Clitoral enlargement

Facial and body hair growth

Baldness

Deepened voice

Breast diminution

Because of these risks, the International Olympic Committee, numerous professional sports organizations, and the National Collegiate Athletic Association (NCAA) banned all anabolic drugs. Testing of elite athletes for performance-enhancing drugs of all types, as mentioned previously, is now commonplace.

Although numerous anabolic steroids have been synthesized and used/abused by athletes, most likely all of the androgens have been used by athletes in an attempt to improve strength and increase muscle mass. In the early years, the 17α-alkylated steroids with high anabolic/androgenic ratios in vitro were used with the belief that the anabolic properties of these drugs were greater than those of other androgens such as testosterone. With the ban on the use of steroids in most sports and the prevalence of drug testing, however, the 17α-alkylated steroids have fallen out of favor because of the ease of detecting these compounds by mass spectrometry. This has led to a greater use of testosterone and its esters, as well as the androgen precursors androstenedione ("andro"), androstenediol, androstanediol, and DHEA. The belief is that because these steroids all occur naturally, detecting them will be much more difficult. Although it is true that assays for the endogenous steroids must now discriminate deviations from normal ratios, it is possible to detect the abuse of these compounds. Pharmaceutical testosterone, for example, can be detected by a urine test examining the ratio of testosterone glucuronide to epitestosterone glucuronide and by determining the carbon isotope ratio that can distinguish between synthetic and natural testosterone.[121] Another approach to avoid detection is the synthesis and use of designer steroids, chemicals that have not been previously described and therefore are not actively pursued in drug screens. Tetrahydrogestrinone (THG) (see Figure 25.22) is a designer steroid associated with the BALCO scandal. THG is a derivative of the progestin, gestrinone, that was unknown prior to 2003.[122] In 2004, THG and the testosterone precursors (except DHEA) were reclassified as Schedule III controlled substances.

Many studies have attempted to determine if taking anabolic steroids improves athletic performance.[123,124] Some failed to use controls (athletes who trained in an identical manner but did not take anabolic steroids). Others failed to use placebos in at least a single-blind research design (neither the treated nor control groups knowing that they were taking).

An additional problem with many of the studies has been that typical therapeutic doses have been tested for their anabolic properties in clinical settings, whereas athletes typically use much higher doses.[117] Although short-term enhancements in strength and increases in muscle mass have been observed, many negative side effects can be expected with long-term steroid use. It would be fair to say, therefore, that the benefit of anabolic steroids to athletic performance is uncertain. The risks of using these drugs appear to outweigh their benefits.

Anabolic Androgenic Steroid Products

Therapeutic uses of the androgens are discussed previously. 17β-Esters and 17α-alkyl products are available for a complete range of therapeutic uses. These drugs are contraindicated in men with prostate cancer; in men or women with heart, kidney, or liver disease; and in pregnancy. Diabetics using the androgens should be carefully monitored. Androgens potentiate the action of oral anticoagulants, causing bleeding in some patients, and they may also interfere with some laboratory tests. Female patients may develop virilization side effects, and doctors should be warned that some of these effects may be irreversible (e.g., voice changes). All the anabolic agents currently commercially available (oxymetholone, oxandrolone, nandrolone decanoate) have significant androgenic activity; hence, virilization is a potential problem for all women patients. Many of the anabolic agents are orally active, as one would predict by noting a 17α-alkyl group in many of them (see Fig. 25.22). Those without the 17α-alkyl (nandrolone decanoate) are active only intramuscularly. The 17α-alkyl products may induce liver toxicity in some patients.

***Testosterone*, USP.** Testosterone, 17β-hydroxyandrost-4-en-3-one, is a naturally occurring androgen in men. In women, it mainly serves as a biosynthetic precursor to estradiol but also has other hormonal effects. It is rapidly metabolized to relatively inactive 17-ones (see Fig. 25.21), however, preventing significant oral activity. Testosterone is available in a transdermal delivery system (patch), a gel formulation, a buccal system, and as implantable pellets. Testosterone 17β-esters are available in long-acting IM depot preparations illustrated in Figure 25.22, including the following:

- Testosterone cypionate, *USP*: Testosterone 17β-cyclopentylpropionate
- Testosterone enanthate, *USP*: Testosterone 17β-heptanoate
- Testosterone propionate, *USP*: Testosterone 17β-propionate

In addition, a NDA for testosterone undecanoate (Nebido) was filed in 2007 for approval as a long-acting preparation for the treatment of male hypogonadism. It is already approved for this use in Europe.

***Methyltestosterone*, USP.** Methyltestosterone, 17β-hydroxy-17-methylandrost-4-en-3-one, is only about half as active as testosterone (intramuscularly), but it has the great advantage of being orally active.

***Fluoxymesterone*, USP.** Fluoxymesterone, 9α-fluoro-11β,17β-dihydroxy-17-methylandrost-4-en-3-one, is a highly potent, orally active androgen, about 5 to 10 times more potent than testosterone. It can be used for all the indications discussed previously, but its great androgenic activity has made it useful primarily for treatment of the androgen-deficient male.

Oxymetholone, **USP.** Oxymetholone, 17β-hydroxy-2-(hydroxymethylene)-17-methylandrostan-3-one, is approved for the treatment of various anemias.

Oxandrolone, **USP.** Oxandrolone, 17β-hydroxy-17-methyl-2-oxaandrostan-3-one, is approved to aid in the promotion of weight gain after weight loss following surgery, chronic infections, or severe trauma and to offset protein catabolism associated with long-term corticosteroid use. Oxandrolone is also used to relieve bone pain accompanying osteoporosis. It has been used to treat alcoholic hepatitis and HIV wasting syndrome.

Nandrolone Decanoate, **USP.** Nandrolone decanoate, 17β-hydroxyestr-4-en-3-one 17-decanoate, has been used in the management of certain anemias, but the availability of erythropoietin has greatly reduced this use.

Danazol and Endometriosis

✱*Danazol,* **USP.** Danazol, 17α-pregna-2,4-dien-20-yno-[2,3-*d*]isoxazol-17-ol, is a weak androgen that, in spite of the 17α-ethinyl group, has little estrogenic or progestogenic activity. Danazol has been called a synthetic steroid with diverse biological effects.[125] Danazol binds to sex hormone–binding globulin (SHBG) and decreases the hepatic synthesis of this estradiol and testosterone carrier. Free testosterone thus increases. Danazol inhibits FSH and LH production by the hypothalamus and pituitary. It binds to PRs, GRs, ARs, and ERs. Although the exact mechanism of action is unclear, danazol alters endometrial tissue so that it becomes inactive and atrophic, which allows danazol to be an effective treatment for endometriosis. Danazol is also used to treat hereditary angioedema and fibrocystic breast disease.

Antiandrogens

Various compounds (Fig. 25.23) have been intensively studied as AR antagonists, or antiandrogens.[126,127] Antiandrogens are of therapeutic use in treating conditions of hyperandrogenism (e.g., hirsutism, acute acne, and premature baldness) or androgen-stimulated cancers (e.g., prostatic carcinoma). The ideal antiandrogen would be nontoxic, highly active, and devoid of any hormonal activity. Both steroidal and nonsteroidal antiandrogens have been investigated, but only nonsteroidal antiandrogens have been approved for use

in the United States. Cyproterone acetate, a steroidal antiandrogen, is used in Europe. The steroidal antiandrogens typically have actions at other steroid receptors that limit their use. The nonsteroidal antiandrogens, while lacking hormonal activity, bind with lower affinity to the AR than the endogenous hormones.

FLUTAMIDE, BICALUTAMIDE, AND NILUTAMIDE

Three nonsteroidal antiandrogens are in clinical use in the United States—flutamide, bicalutamide, and nilutamide (Fig. 25.23). They are mainly used in the management of prostate cancer. Flutamide was the first of these compounds approved for use by the FDA, but liver toxicity and thrice-daily dosing offered room for improvement. It was also determined that a metabolite of flutamide, hydroxyflutamide, had greater antiandrogen action than the parent. Bicalutamide, which has greater potency than flutamide, incorporates an OH into its structure at the same relative position as in hydroxyflutamide. Bicalutamide is dosed once a day and has less toxicity than flutamide and nilutamide, making it a preferred choice when initiating therapy.

Prostate cancer is strongly androgen sensitive, so by blocking AR, the cancer can be inhibited or slowed. Studies have shown that these drugs completely inhibit the action of testosterone and other androgens by binding to AR. In clinical trials when given as a single agent for prostate cancer, serum testosterone and estradiol increase. But when given in combination with a GnRH agonist, such as goserelin or leuprolide, bicalutamide and flutamide do not affect testosterone suppression, which is the result of GnRH. GnRH agonists greatly decrease gonadal function—the medical equivalent of castration in men. Thus, the combination of GnRH with bicalutamide or flutamide blocks the production of testosterone in the testes and AR in the prostate.

Antiandrogen Products

Flutamide, **USP.** Flutamide, 2-methyl-*N*-[4-nitro-3-(trifluoromethyl)phenyl]propanamide, is dosed 3 times daily (250-mg dose; 750-mg total daily dose). A major metabolite of flutamide, hydroxyflutamide, is a more potent AR antagonist than the parent compound. This metabolite, which is present at a much higher steady-state concentration than is flutamide, contributes a significant amount of the

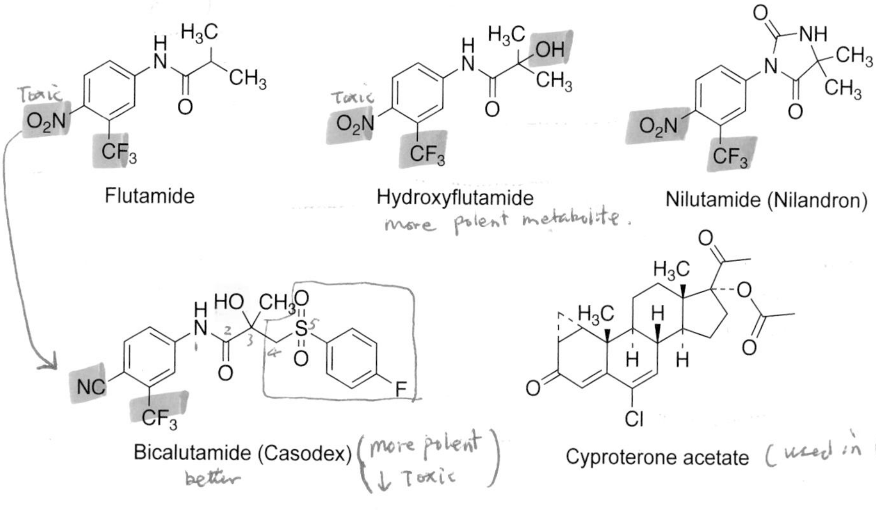

Figure 25.23 ● Antiandrogens.

Flutamide

Hydroxyflutamide

Nilutamide (Nilandron)

Bicalutamide (Casodex)

Cyproterone acetate

antiandrogen action of this drug. A limiting factor in the use of flutamide is hepatotoxicity in from 1% to 5% of patients. Although the hepatotoxicity usually is reversible following cessation of treatment, rare cases of death associated with hepatic failure have been reported to be associated with flutamide therapy. Diarrhea is also a limiting side effect with flutamide therapy for some patients.

Bicalutamide, USP. Bicalutamide, *N*-4-cyano-3-(trifluoromethyl)phenyl-3-[(4-fluorophenyl)sulfonyl]-2-hydroxy-2-methyl-propanamide (Casodex), is more potent than flutamide and has a much longer half-life (5.9 days vs. 6 hours for hydroxyflutamide). Because of the longer half-life, bicalutamide is used for once-a-day (50 mg) treatment of advanced prostate cancer. Bicalutamide is available as a racemic mixture, but both animal and human studies with the AR show that the R-enantiomer has higher affinity for the AR than the S-enantiomer.[128]

Nilutamide, USP. Nilutamide, 5,5-dimethyl-3-[4-nitro-3-(trifluoromethyl)phenyl]-2,4-imidazolidinedione, is used in combination with surgical castration for the treatment of metastatic prostate cancer. Nilutamide, which has an elimination half-life of approximately 40 hours, can also be used in once-daily dosing, but it has side effects that limit its use—visual disturbances, alcohol intolerance, and allergic pneumonitis.

Inhibition of 5α-Reductase

5α-DHT is important for maintaining prostate function in men. The formation of DHT is mediated by 5α-reductase, an enzyme that has two distinct forms, type I and type II.[129,130] The type I enzyme is located in the liver and some peripheral tissues and is involved mainly in the metabolism of testosterone and other A-ring enones. The type II enzyme is located in the prostate gland and testes and is responsible for the conversion of testosterone to DHT for androgenic action. Blocking this enzyme is one approach for controlling androgen action. The review by Harris and Kozarich provides an excellent background and details the development of finasteride, the first 5α-reductase inhibitor approved for use in the United States (Fig. 25.24).[131]

DHT also plays a major role in the pathogenesis of benign prostatic hyperplasia (BPH). Finasteride, (5α,17β)-*N*-(1,1-dimethylethyl)-3-oxo-4-azaandrost-1-ene-17-carboxamide (Proscar, Propecia), is a potent, slow, tight-binding inhibitor of 5α-reductase that functions by a unique mechanism. Finasteride is activated by the enzyme and irreversibly binds to the NADP cofactor, yielding a finasteride–NADP complex that is only slowly released from the enzyme active site, producing essentially irreversible inhibition of the enzyme (Fig. 25.25).[132] The turnover from the finasteride–5α-reductase complex is very slow ($t_{1/2}$~30 days).

Finasteride is a relatively selective inhibitor of type II 5α-reductase. This enzyme is present in high levels in the prostate and at lower levels in other tissues. Because of the strong connection to the formation of DHT in the prostate, it was theorized that specific inhibition of this isoform would yield the greatest therapeutic effect. Other studies suggest, however, that the type I isoform may also play a role in the progression of hormone-dependent prostate cancer.[133] Because of this, dual 5α-reductase inhibitors have been developed. Dutasteride, (5α,17β)-*N*-{2,5

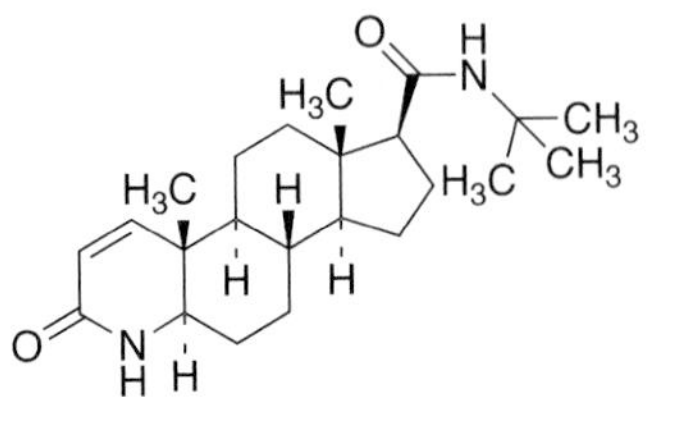

Finasteride
(Proscar, Propecia)

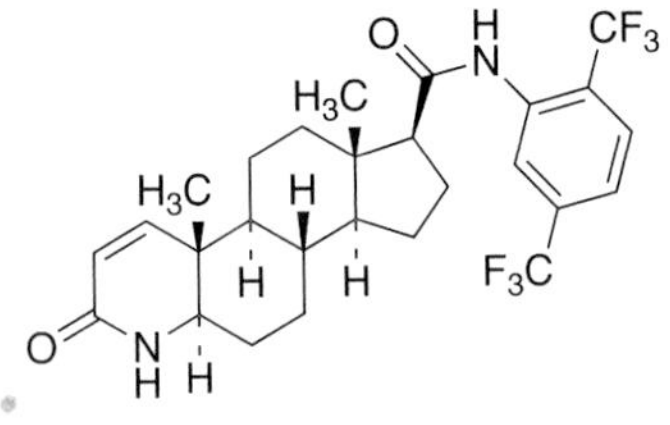

Dutasteride
(Avodart)

Figure 25.24 ● Steroid 5α-reductase inhibitors.

bis(trifluoromethyl)phenyl}-3-oxo-4-azaandrost-1-ene-17-carboxamide (Avodart) a newer drug for treating BPH, inhibits both isoforms of the enzyme (Fig. 25.24). Dutasteride bears an aromatic amide at C17, rather than the *t*-butyl amide seen in finasteride. Both drugs are effective at treating BPH, but a recent retrospective study suggests that rates of acute urinary retention are lower with dutasteride.[134] It is not yet known, however, if this reduced urinary retention is a result of the dual inhibition nature of dutasteride. Dutasteride inhibits 5α-reductase by the same mechanism as finasteride and has a long terminal elimination half-life, which is approximately 5 weeks at steady state. In addition to the treatment of BPH, dutasteride is being investigated for its ability to delay the progression of prostate cancer.[135]

A second use of finasteride is in the treatment of male pattern baldness. The conversion of testosterone to DHT in advancing years leads to thinning of hair in men. Inhibition of this conversion was envisioned as a possible baldness treatment. After finasteride was shown to be safe and effective in the treatment of BPH, a lower dose formulation was studied for treating male pattern baldness. The trials were a success, and Propecia (1 mg/d) was the result. Although finasteride preferentially inhibits the type II enzyme, it is believed to be the peripheral type I 5α-reductase that is being targeted for the baldness treatment. Dutasteride is also being investigated for use as a baldness treatment.

An important warning for the use of both finasteride and dutasteride is that pregnant women should not handle or in any way be exposed to the active ingredients of these drugs. Exposure to either of these 5α-reductase inhibitors could cause abnormalities of a male baby's external genitalia.

Saw palmetto (*Serenoa repens*) extract is an herbal product used to treat BPH, and it has been suggested that the effects may be attributed to a constituent of the extract with 5α-reductase inhibition, but other mechanisms have also been proposed.[136] Further studies and identification of a specific component that inhibits 5α-reductase are necessary.

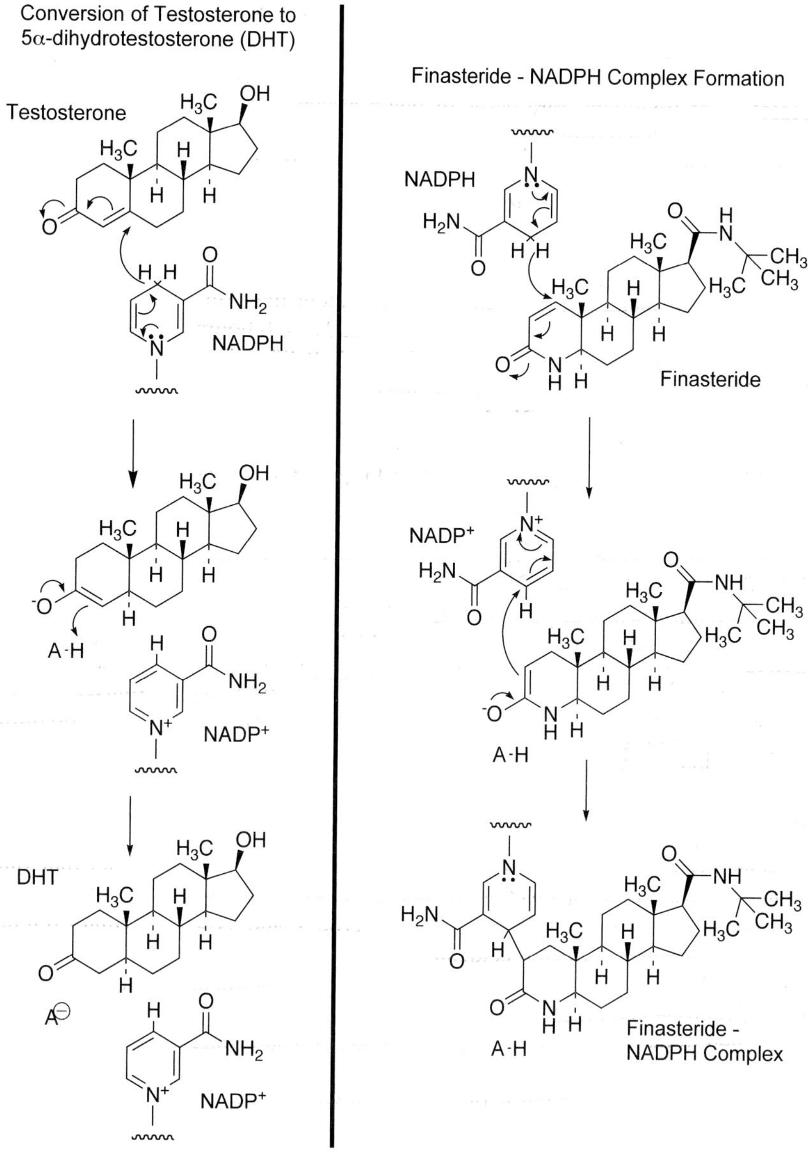

Conversion of Testosterone to
5α-dihydrotestosterone (DHT)

Finasteride - NADPH Complex Formation

Figure 25.25 ● Comparison of 5α-reductase action on testosterone and finasteride. This scheme is an oversimplification of the exact mechanisms, but it indicates that when finasteride is bound at the active site of 5α-reductase, NADPH is positioned closer to C1 of finasteride than to the normal C5 of testosterone, leading to essentially irreversible inhibition.

Future Directions: SARMs[137,138]

Selective androgen receptor modulators or SARMs are the newest developments among the potential androgen drugs. A parallel to the SERMs and SPRMs, SARMs are molecules that have differential actions at ARs in distinct tissues. The lead compounds furthest along in development are non-steroidal AR ligands that have anabolic properties in muscle and bone, with only partial agonist action in the prostate. Two of these lead compounds, LGD2226 and S4 (Fig. 25.26) are in phase I/II trials, with potential to treat age-related muscle wasting and osteoporosis, in both men and women. As can be seen from Figure 25.26, S4 shares structural similarities with the antiandrogen bicalutamide.

◆ ADRENAL CORTEX HORMONES

Endogenous Corticosteroids

The adrenal glands (which lie just above the kidneys) secrete over 50 different steroids, including precursors for other steroid hormones. The most important hormonal

steroids produced by the adrenal cortex, however, are aldosterone and hydrocortisone. Aldosterone is the primary *MC* in humans (i.e., it causes significant salt retention). Hydrocortisone is the primary *GC* in humans (i.e., it has its primary effects on intermediary metabolism). The GCs have

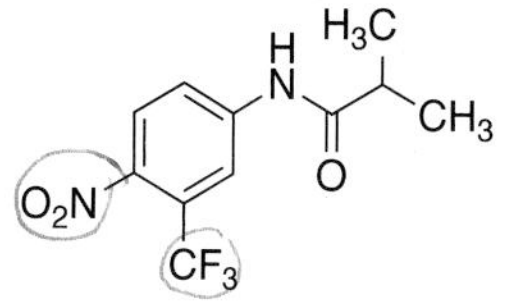

LGD2226

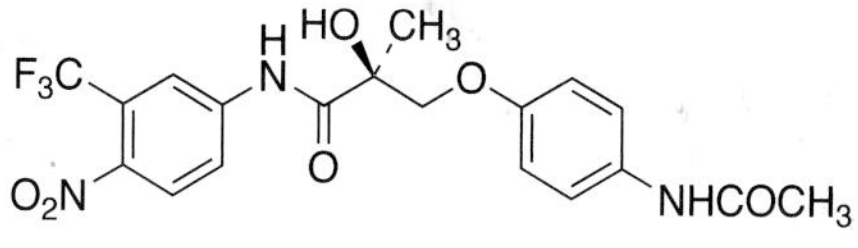

S4

Figure 25.26 ● SARMs.

become very important in modern medicine, especially for their anti-inflammatory effects.

Aldosterone and, to a lesser extent, other MCs maintain a constant electrolyte balance and blood volume. The GCs have key roles in controlling carbohydrate, protein, and lipid metabolism.

Biosynthesis

As shown in the scheme in Figure 25.27, aldosterone and hydrocortisone are biosynthesized from pregnenolone through a series of steps involving hydroxylations at C17, C11, and C21 that convert pregnenolone to hydrocortisone. Deficiencies in any of the enzymes cause congenital adrenal hyperplasia. Defects in the gene regulation, as well as the enzymes that catalyze the hydroxylation, have been studied intensively.[139–141] Investigators have linked defects in particular genes or steroid-binding sites to the pathophysiology of patients with the corresponding metabolic diseases.[141]

These disorders are usually caused by an inability of the adrenal glands to carry out 11β-, 17α-, or 21-hydroxylations. The most common is a lack of 21-hydroxylase activity, which will result in decreased production of hydrocortisone and a compensatory increase in adrenocorticotropic hormone (ACTH) production. Furthermore, the resultant buildup of 17α-hydroxyprogesterone will lead to an increase of testosterone. The 21-hydroxylase is important for the synthesis of both MCs and GCs. When 11β-hydroxylase activity is low,

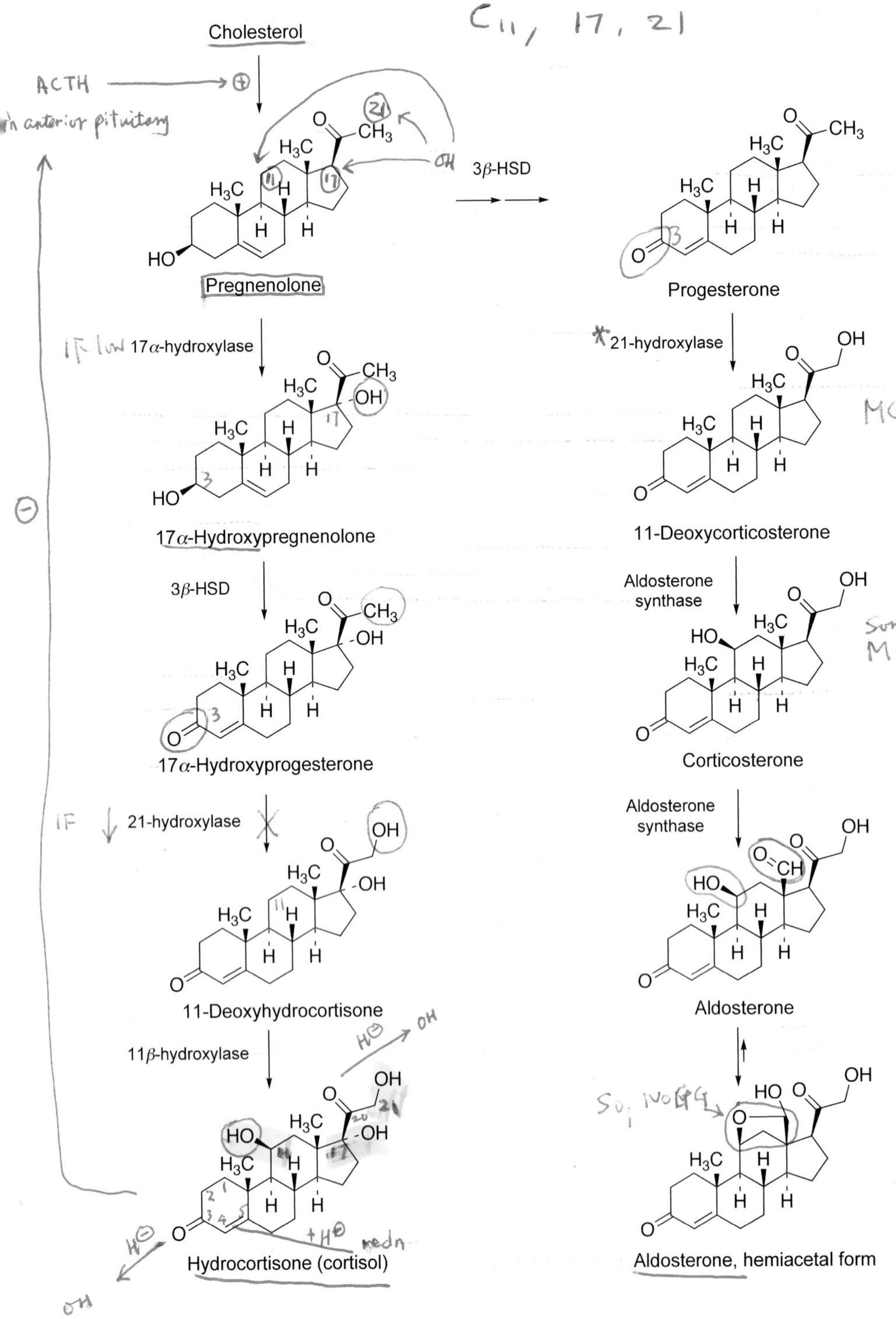

Figure 25.27 ● Biosynthesis of hydrocortisone and aldosterone.

large amounts of 11-deoxycorticosterone will be produced. Because 11-deoxycorticosterone is a potent MC, there will be symptoms of MC excess, including hypertension. When 17α-hydroxylase activity is low, there will be decreased production of testosterone and estrogens as well as hydrocortisone.

Although the details are not completely known, the 39-amino acid peptide ACTH (corticotropin) produced by the anterior pituitary is necessary for the conversion of cholesterol to pregnenolone. ACTH acts at the ACTH receptor, a G-protein–coupled receptor that activates adenylyl cyclase, leading to increased cyclic adenosine monophosphate (cAMP) levels. Activation of the ACTH receptors has short- and long-term effects on steroidogenesis. The short-term phase involves an increase in the supply of cholesterol for use by cytochrome P450$_{scc}$ in the formation of pregnenolone. The long-term effects are caused by an increased transcription of steroidogenic enzymes.[142] An overall result of ACTH action is increased synthesis and release of hydrocortisone. Hydrocortisone then acts by feedback inhibition to suppress the formation of additional ACTH (ACTH is discussed in more detail in Chapter 27).

The release of the primary MC aldosterone depends only slightly on ACTH. Aldosterone is an active part of the angiotensin–renin–blood pressure cycle that controls blood volume. A decrease in blood volume stimulates the kidneys to secrete the enzyme renin. Renin, in turn, converts angiotensinogen to angiotensin, which stimulates the adrenal cortex to release aldosterone. Aldosterone then causes the kidneys to retain sodium, and blood volume increases. When the blood volume has increased sufficiently, renin production decreases, until blood volume drops again.

Metabolism of Hydrocortisone

Hydrocortisone and cortisone are enzymatically interconvertible, and thus one finds metabolites with both the 11-keto and the 11β-hydroxy functionality. Most of the metabolic processes occur in the liver, with the metabolites excreted primarily in the urine. Although many metabolites have been isolated, the primary routes of catabolism are (a) reduction of the C4,5 double bond to yield 5β-pregnanes, (b) reduction of the 3-one to give 3α-ols, and (c) reduction of the 20-one to the corresponding 20α- and 20β-ols. These are the same steps that are involved in progesterone metabolism. The two primary metabolites are tetrahydrocortisol and tetrahydrocortisone and their conjugates. The cortols (20α and 20β), cortolones (20α and 20β), and 11β-hydroxyetiocholanolone are some of the minor metabolites of hydrocortisone (Fig. 25.28).

Biological Activities of Mineralocorticoids and Glucocorticoids[142]

The adrenocortical steroids permit the body to adjust to environmental changes, to stress, and to changes in the diet. Aldosterone and, to a lesser extent, other MCs maintain a constant electrolyte balance and blood volume, and the GCs have key roles in controlling carbohydrate, protein, and lipid metabolism.

Aldosterone increases sodium reabsorption in the kidneys. An increase in plasma sodium concentration, in turn, will lead to increased blood volume, because blood volume and urinary excretion of water are directly related to the plasma sodium

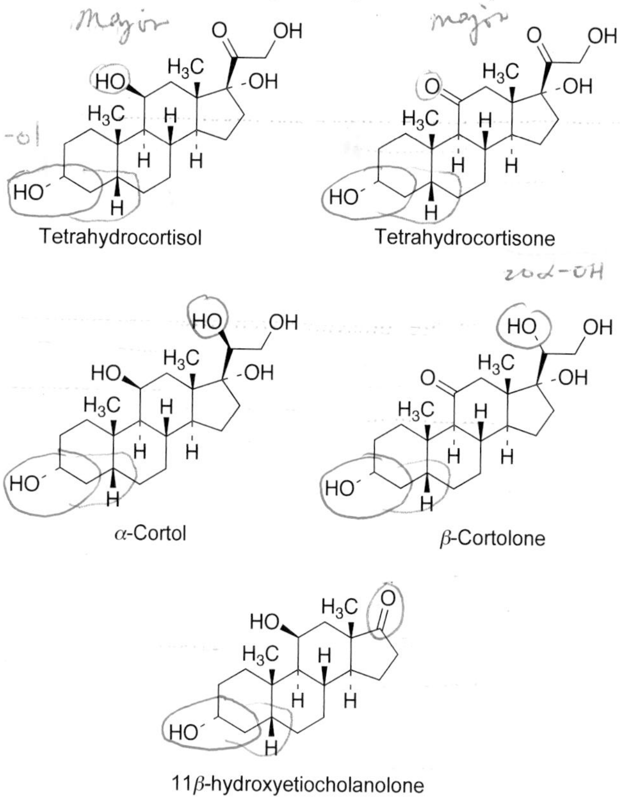

Figure 25.28 ● Metabolites of cortisone and hydrocortisone.

concentration. Simultaneously, aldosterone increases potassium ion excretion. 11-Deoxycorticosterone is also quite active as a MC. Similar actions are exhibited with hydrocortisone and corticosterone, but to a much smaller degree.

Aldosterone controls the movement of sodium ions in most epithelial structures involved in active sodium transport. Although aldosterone acts primarily on the distal convoluted tubules of the kidneys, it also acts on the proximal convoluted tubules and collecting ducts. Aldosterone controls the transport of sodium in sweat glands, small intestine, salivary glands, and the colon. In all of these tissues, aldosterone enhances the inward flow of sodium ions and promotes the outward flow of potassium ions.

The GCs have many physiological and pharmacological actions. They control or influence carbohydrate, protein, lipid, and purine metabolism. They also affect the cardiovascular and nervous systems and skeletal muscle. They regulate growth hormone gene expression. In addition, GCs have anti-inflammatory and immunosuppressive actions that arise through complex mechanisms.

GCs stimulate glycogen storage synthesis by inducing the synthesis of glycogen synthase and stimulate gluconeogenesis in the liver. They have a catabolic effect on muscle tissue, stimulating the formation and transamination of amino acids into glucose precursors in the liver. The catabolic actions in Cushing syndrome are demonstrated by wasting of the tissues, osteoporosis, and reduced muscle mass. Lipid metabolism and synthesis increase significantly in the presence of GCs, but the actions usually seem to depend on the presence of other hormones or cofactors. A lack of adrenal cortex steroids also causes depression, irritability, and even psychoses, reflecting significant effects on the central nervous system.

ANTI-INFLAMMATORY/IMMUNOSUPPRESSIVE MOA ACTIONS OF GLUCOCORTICOIDS[143–147]

GR complexes may activate or repress the genes to which they associate. Repression in particular may have an important role in GC anti-inflammatory actions. GCs inhibit the transcription of genes encoding cytokines such as interferon-γ, tumor necrosis factor-α (TNF-α), the interleukins, and granulocyte/monocyte colony-stimulating factor, all factors involved in the immune system and inflammatory responses.[142] GCs inhibit the production and release of other mediators of inflammation, including prostaglandins, leukotrienes, and histamine. In addition, GCs inhibit the expression of the gene encoding collagenase, an important enzyme involved with inflammation.

RESISTANCE TO GLUCOCORTICOIDS[148–150]

A few patients with chronic inflammatory illnesses such as asthma, rheumatoid arthritis, and lupus develop resistance to the anti-inflammatory effects of the GCs. The mechanism is not fully understood but appears to be a decrease in the binding or activation ability of GR complexes and their target or "activator" genes. Disruption of the translocation of the GR to the nucleus has also been implicated in GC resistance.[151]

Structural Classes: Mineralocorticoids and Glucocorticoids[152]

Medically important adrenal cortex hormones and synthetic MCs and GCs are shown in Figure 25.29. Because salt re-

1. Mineralocorticoids (High Salt Retention)

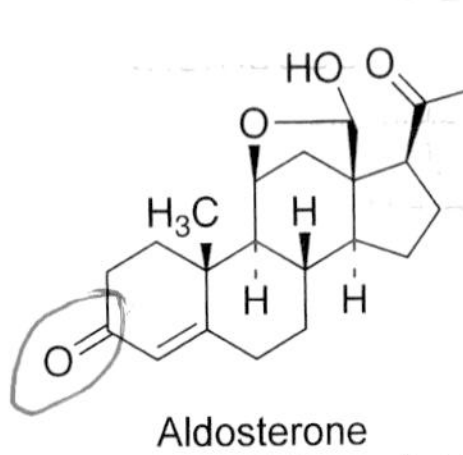

Aldosterone
(not commercially available)

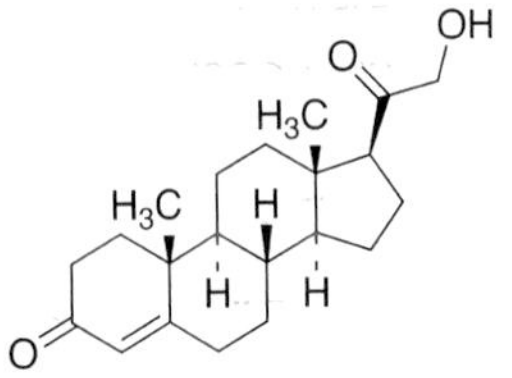

11-Deoxycorticosterone
(not commercially available)

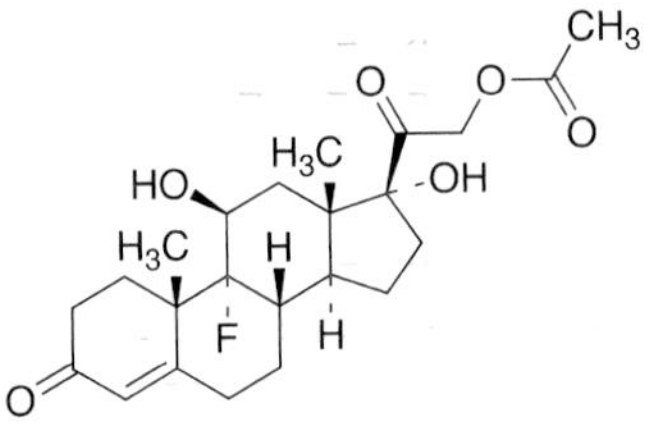

Fludrocortisone Acetate

2. Glucocorticoids with Moderate to Low Salt Retention

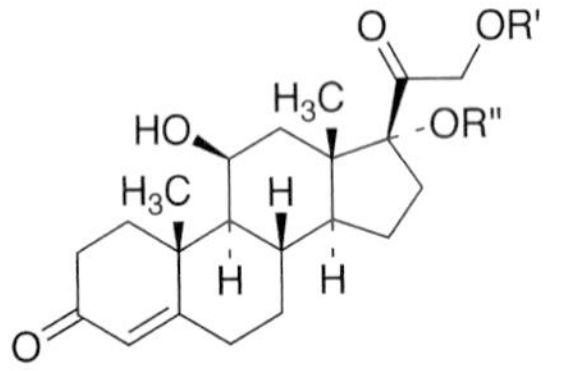

Hydrocortisone (R' = R" = H)
(or cortisol)

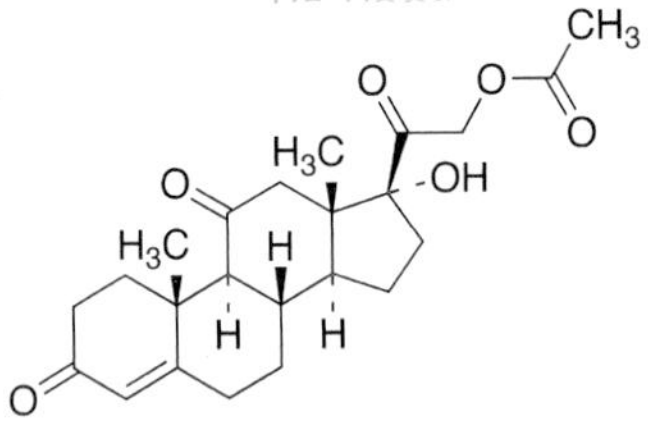

Cortisone acetate

Esters available
  Hydrocortisone acetate: R'= COCH$_3$, R" = H
  Hydrocortisone buteprate: R' = COCH$_2$CH$_3$
                          R" = COCH$_2$CH$_2$CH$_3$
  Hydrocortisone butyrate: R' = H, R" = COCH$_2$CH$_2$CH$_3$
  Hydrocortisone cypionate: R' =

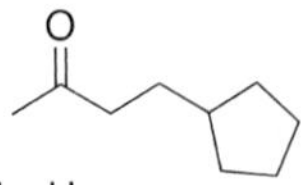

  R" = H
  Hydrocortisone valerate: R'= H, R" = COCH$_2$CH$_2$CH$_2$CH$_3$

21-Salts available (R" = H)
  Hydrocortisone Sodium Phosphate: R' = PO$_3^{2-}$ (Na$^+$)$_2$
  Hydrocortisone Sodium Succinate:
                R' = COCH$_2$CH$_2$CO$_2^-$ Na$^+$

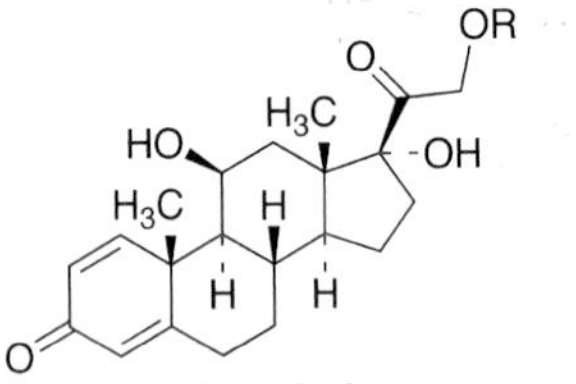

Prednisolone

Esters available
  Prednisolone acetate: R = COCH$_3$

Salts available
  Prednisolone Sodium Phosphate:
                R = PO$_3^{2-}$ (Na$^+$)$_2$
  Prednisolone Sodium Succinate:
                R = COCH$_2$CH$_2$CO$_2^-$ Na$^+$

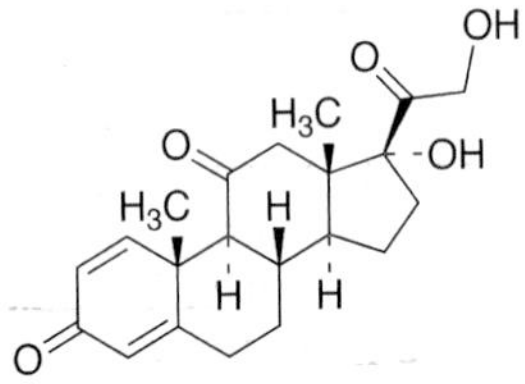

Prednisone

Figure 25.29 ● Natural and synthetic corticosteroids. *(continues on next page)*

3. Glucocorticoids with Very Little or No Salt Retention

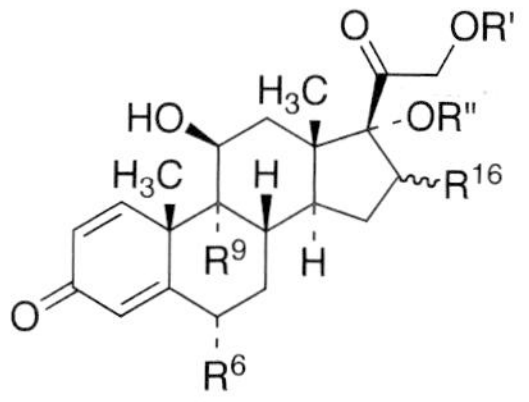

Betamethasone
R^6 = H
R^9 = F
R^{16} = ▬CH$_3$
R' = R" = H

Dexamethasone
R^6 = H
R^9 = F
R^{16} = --CH$_3$
R' = R" = H

Diflorasone diacetate
R^6 = R^9 = F
R^{16} = ▬CH$_3$
R' = R" = COCH$_3$

Methylprednisolone
R^6 = CH$_3$
R^9 = R^{16} = H
R' = R" = H

Prednicarbate
R^6 = R^9 = R^{16} = H
R' = R" = COCH$_2$CH$_3$

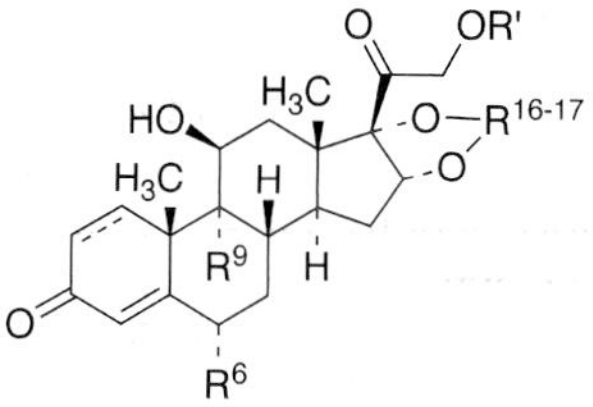

R^{16-17} = I =

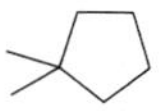

= II =   CH$_3$
           CH$_3$

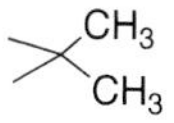

Amcinonide
1-ene
R^6 = H
R^9 = F
R^{16-17} = I
R' = COCCH$_3$

Desonide
1-ene
R^6 = R^9 = H
R^{16-17} = II
R' = H

Fluocinolone acetonide
1-ene
R^6 = R^9 = F
R^{16-17} = II
R' = H (fluocinonide is
the C21 acetate)

Flurandrenolide
R^6 = F
R^9 = H
R^{16-17} = II
R' = H

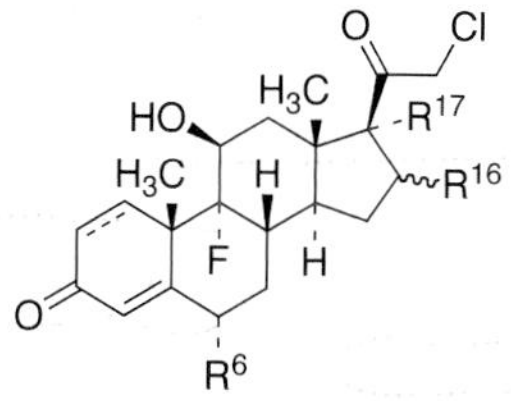

Clobetasol propionate
1-ene
R^6 = H
R^{16} = ▬CH$_3$
R^{17} = OCOCH$_2$CH$_3$

Halobetasol propionate
1-ene
R^6 = F
R^{16} = ▬CH$_3$
R^{17} = OCOCH$_2$CH$_3$

Halcinonide
R^6 = H
$R^{16,17}$ = acetonide

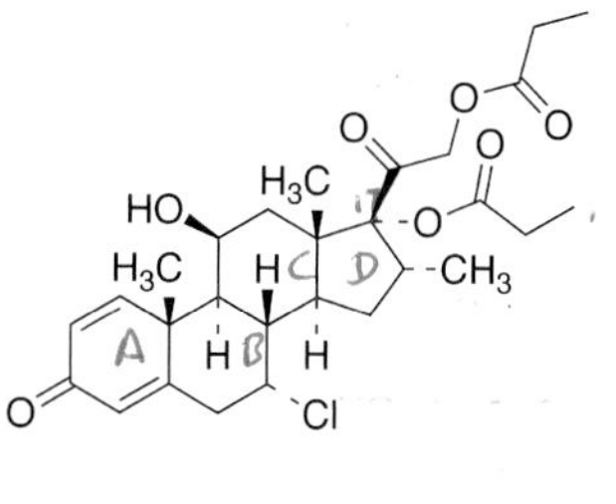

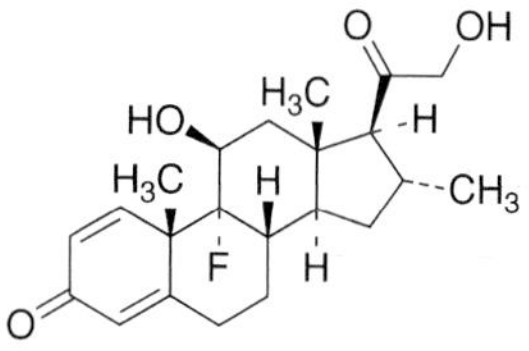

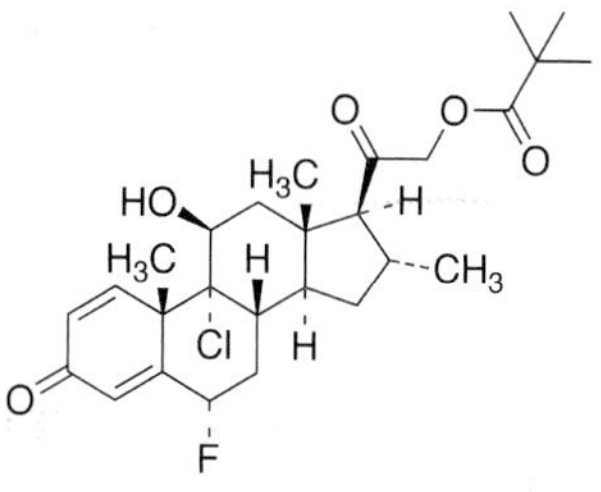

Alclometasone dipropionate

Desoximetasone

Clocortolone pivalate

Figure 25.29 ● *(Continued)*

tention activity is usually underesirable, the drugs are classified by their salt retention activities. As illustrated in Figure 25.29, the adrenal cortex hormones are classified by their biological activities into three major groups.

MINERALOCORTICOIDS

The MCs are adrenal cortex steroids and analogs with high salt-retaining activity. They are used mainly for treatment of Addison disease, or primary adrenal insufficiency. The naturally occurring hormone aldosterone has an 11β-OH and an 18-CHO that naturally bridge to form a hemiacetal (as drawn in Fig. 25.27). Aldosterone is too expensive to produce commercially; therefore, other semisynthetic analogs

have taken its place for treatment of Addison disease. Adding a 9α-fluoro group to hydrocortisone greatly increases both salt retention and anti-inflammatory activity. Deoxycorticosterone (11-deoxy), an intermediate in the biosynthesis of aldosterone, has lower MC activity than aldosterone (20-fold) but may play a role if the 11β-hydroxylase is deficient. Deoxycorticosterone is not available for therapeutic uses.

Extensive modifications have been made to the basic hydrocortisone structure to alter the properties of GCs. Modifications at all sites of the steroid backbone have been tried. Aside from addition of a double bond at C1–C2, the most beneficial changes are made to rings B and D of the steroid skeleton and modification of the C17 side chain.

TABLE 25.6 Effects of Substituents on Glucocorticoid/Mineralocorticoid Activity

Functional Group	Glycogen Deposition	Anti-inflammatory Activity	Effects on Urinary Sodium[a]
9α-Fluoro	10	7–10	+++
9α-Chloro	3–5	3–4	++
1-Dehydro	3–4	3–4	–
6α-Methyl	2–3	1–2	---
16α-Hydroxy	0.4–0.5	0.1–0.2	----
17α-Hydroxy	1–2	4	
21-Hydroxy	4–7	25	++

Adapted from Rodig, O.R.: In Burger, A. (ed.). Medicinal Chemistry, Part 2, 3rd ed. New York, Wiley-Interscience, 1970. Used with permission.
[a]+, retention; −, excretion.

Table 25.6 summarizes the relative effects of various substituents seen in commercially available products on salt retention and GC activity. The salt-retaining actions are approximately additive. For example, the 3+ increase in salt retention of a 9α-fluoro group can be eliminated by the 3– decrease of a 6α-methyl.

GLUCOCORTICOIDS WITH MODERATE-TO-LOW SALT RETENTION

The GCs with moderate-to-low salt retention include cortisone, hydrocortisone, and their 1-enes prednisolone and prednisone. As shown in Table 25.7, an 11β-OH maintains good topical anti-inflammatory activity, but 11-ones have little or none. The 11β-hydroxysteroid dehydrogenase in the skin oxidizes an 11β-hydroxyl to an 11-ketone.[153] For activation of an 11-one GC for topical action, reduction at C11 would be necessary. The 1-ene of prednisolone and prednisone increases anti-inflammatory activity about fourfold and somewhat decreases salt retention. This increase in activity may be a result of a change in shape of ring A.[28] Specifically, analogs more active than hydrocortisone appear to have their ring A bent underneath the molecule to a much greater extent than hydrocortisone.

The 11β-OH of hydrocortisone is of major importance in binding to the receptors. Cortisone is reduced in vivo to yield hydrocortisone as the active agent. The increased activity of 9α-halo derivatives may be a result the electron-withdrawing inductive effect on the 11β-OH, making it more acidic and, therefore, better able to form hydrogen bonds with the receptor. A 9α-halo substituent also reduces oxidation of the 11β-OH to the inactive 11-one.

GLUCOCORTICOIDS WITH VERY LITTLE OR NO SALT RETENTION

Cortisone and hydrocortisone, and even prednisone and prednisolone, have too much salt-retaining activity in the doses needed for some therapeutic purposes. Over the past several decades, several substituents have been discovered that greatly decrease salt retention. They include 16α-hydroxy, 16α,17α-ketal, 6α-methyl, and 16α- and 16β-methyl. Other substituents have been found to increase both GC and MC activities: 9α-fluoro, 9α-chloro, and 21-hydroxy.

As a result of the great economic benefit of having a potent anti-inflammatory product on the market, pharmaceutical manufacturers have made numerous combinations of these various substituents. In almost every case, a 16-

TABLE 25.7 Approximate Relative Activities of Corticosteroids[a]

	Anti-inflammatory Activity	Topical Activity	Salt-Retaining Activity	Equivalent Dose (mg)
Mineralocorticoids				
Aldosterone	0.2	0.2	800	
Deoxycorticosterone	0	0	40	
Fludrocortisone	10	5–40	800	2
Glucocorticoids				
Hydrocortisone	1	1	1	20
Cortisone	0.8	0	0.8	25
Prednisolone	4	4	0.6	5
Prednisone	3.5	0	0.6	5
Methylprednisolone	5	5	0	4
Triamcinolone acetonide	5	5–100	0	4
Triamcinolone		1–5		
Fluocinolone acetonide		Over 40		
Flurandrenolide		Over 20		
Fluocinolone		Over 40		
Fluocinonide		40–100		
Betamethasone	35	5–100	0	0.6
Dexamethasone	30	10–35	0	0.75

[a]The data in this table are only approximate. Blanks indicate that comparative data are not available to the author or that the product has only one use (e.g., topical). Data were taken from several sources, and there is an inherent risk in comparing such data. The table should, however, serve as a guide to relative activities.

methyl or a modified 16-hydroxy (to eliminate salt retention) has been combined with another substituent to increase GC or anti-inflammatory activity. The number of permutations and combinations has resulted in a redundant array of analogs with very low salt retention and high anti-inflammatory activity.

A primary goal of these highly anti-inflammatory drugs has been to increase topical potency. As shown in Table 25.7, some are as much as 100 times more active topically than hydrocortisone. Relative potency is as follows:

Very high potency
  Augmented betamethasone dipropionate ointment, 0.05% *hyp* 4.23
  Clobetasol propionate, 0.05% 4.18
  Diflorasone diacetate ointment, 0.05% 2.91
High potency
  Amcinonide, 0.1% 3.80
  Betamethasone dipropionate ointment, 0.05% 4.23
  Desoximetasone, 0.25% 2.40
  Diflorasone diacetate cream, 0.05%
  Fluocinonide, 0.05% 2.91
  Halcinonide, 0.1% 3.32
  Halobetasol propionate, 0.05%
  Triamcinolone acetonide, 0.5%
Medium potency
  Betamethasone valerate, 0.1%
  Clocortolone pivalate, 0.1%
  Desoximetasone, 0.05%
  Fluocinolone acetonide, 0.025%
  Fluticasone propionate, 0.005%
  Hydrocortisone butyrate, 0.1%
  Hydrocortisone valerate, 0.2%
  Mometasone furoate, 0.1%
  Prednicarbate, 0.1%
  Triamcinolone acetonide, 0.1%
Low potency *↑GC*
  Alclometasone dipropionate, 0.05%
  Desonide, 0.05%
  Fluocinolone acetonide, 0.01%
  Triamcinolone acetonide cream, 0.1%
Lowest potency
  Hydrocortisone, 1.0% 1.43
  Hydrocortisone, 2.5% 1.43
  which 2 are not active topically?

Although, as shown in Table 25.7, cortisone and prednisone are not active topically, most other GCs are active. Some compounds, such as clobetasol and betamethasone dipropionate, have striking activity topically. Skin absorption is favored by increased lipid solubility of the drug.

Absorption of topical GCs can also be greatly affected by the extent of skin damage, concentration of the GC, cream or ointment base used, and similar factors. One must not assume, therefore, from a study of Table 25.7 that, for example, a 0.25% cream of prednisolone is necessarily exactly equivalent in anti-inflammatory potency to 1% hydrocortisone. Nevertheless, the table can serve as a preliminary guide. Furthermore, particular patients may seem to respond better to one topical anti-inflammatory GC than to another, irrespective of the relative potencies shown in Table 25.7.

RISK OF SYSTEMIC ABSORPTION

The topical corticosteroids do not typically cause significant absorption effects when used on small areas of intact skin.

When these compounds are used on large areas of the body, however, systemic absorption may occur, especially if the skin is damaged or if occlusive dressings are used. Up to 20% to 40% of hydrocortisone given rectally may also be absorbed.

which for Addison disease?

Therapeutic Uses of Adrenal Cortex Hormones

The adrenocortical steroids are used primarily for their GC effects, including immunosuppression, anti-inflammatory activity, and antiallergic activity. The MCs are used only for treatment of Addison disease. Addison disease is caused by chronic adrenocortical insufficiency and may be due to either adrenal or anterior pituitary failure. The GCs are also used in the treatment of congenital adrenal hyperplasias.

The symptoms of Addison disease illustrate the great importance of the adrenocortical steroids in the body and, especially, the importance of aldosterone. These symptoms include increased loss of body sodium, decreased loss of potassium, hypoglycemia, weight loss, hypotension, weakness, increased sensitivity to insulin, and decreased lipolysis.

Hydrocortisone is also used during postoperative recovery after surgery for Cushing syndrome—excessive adrenal secretion of GCs. Cushing syndrome can be caused by bilateral adrenal hyperplasia or adrenal tumors and is treated by surgical removal of the tumors or resection of hyperplastic adrenal gland(s).

The use of GCs during recovery from surgery for Cushing syndrome illustrates a most important principle of GC therapy: abrupt withdrawal of GCs may result in adrenal insufficiency, showing clinical symptoms similar to those of Addison disease. For that reason, patients who have been on long-term GC therapy must have the dose reduced gradually. Furthermore, prolonged treatment with GCs can cause adrenal suppression, especially during times of stress. The symptoms are similar to those of Cushing syndrome, such as rounding of the face, hypertension, edema, hypokalemia, thinning of the skin, osteoporosis, diabetes, and even subcapsular cataracts.

The GCs are used in the treatment of collagen vascular diseases, including rheumatoid arthritis and disseminated lupus erythematosus. Although there is usually prompt remission of redness, swelling, and tenderness by the GCs in rheumatoid arthritis, continued long-term use may lead to serious systemic forms of collagen disease. As a result, the GCs should be used infrequently in rheumatoid arthritis.

The GCs are used extensively topically, orally, and parenterally to treat inflammatory conditions. They also usually relieve the discomforting symptoms of many allergic conditions—intractable hay fever, exfoliative dermatitis, generalized eczema, and others. The GCs are also used to treat asthmatic symptoms unresponsive to bronchodilators. They are especially useful in inhaled formulations (see section on page 863). The GCs' lymphocytopenic actions make them particularly useful for treatment of chronic lymphocytic leukemia in combination with other antineoplastic drugs.

The adrenocortical steroids are contraindicated or should be used with great caution in patients who have (a) peptic ulcer (in which the steroids may cause hemorrhage), (b) heart disease, (c) infections (the GCs suppress the body's normal infection-fighting processes), (d) psychoses (since behavioral disturbances may occur during steroid therapy),

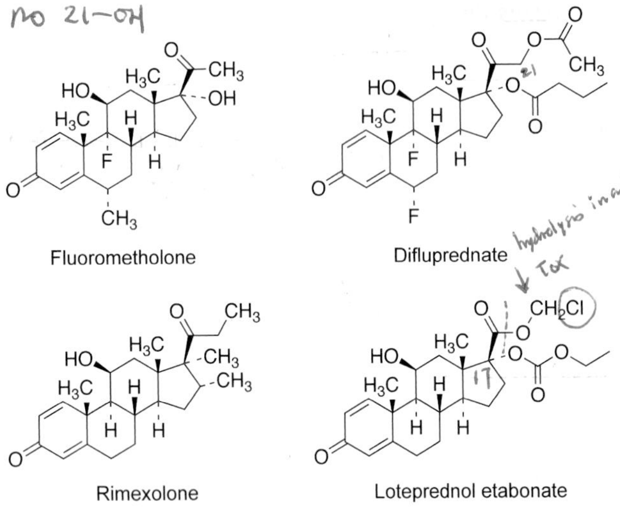

Fluorometholone

Difluprednate

Rimexolone

Loteprednol etabonate

Figure 25.30 ● Ophthalmic glucocorticoids.

(e) diabetes (the GCs increase glucose production, so more insulin may be needed), (f) glaucoma, (g) osteoporosis, or (h) herpes simplex involving the cornea.

When administered topically, the GCs present relatively infrequent therapeutic problems, but their anti-inflammatory action can mask symptoms of infection. Many physicians prefer not giving a topical anti-inflammatory steroid until after an infection is controlled with topical antibiotics. The immunosuppressive activity of the topical GCs can also prevent natural processes from curing the infection. Topical steroids actually may also cause dermatoses in some patients.

Finally, as discussed previously with the oral contraceptives, steroid hormones should not be used during pregnancy. If it is absolutely necessary to use GCs topically during pregnancy, they should be limited to small areas of intact skin and used for a limited time.

Mineralocorticoid and Glucocorticoid Products

The corticosteroids used in commercial products are shown in Figures 25.29, 25.30, and 25.31. The structures illustrate the usual changes (see Fig. 25.6) made to modify solubility of the products and, therefore, their therapeutic uses. In particular, the 21-hydroxyl can be converted to an ester to make it less water soluble to modify absorption or to a phosphate ester salt or hemisuccinate ester salt to make it more water soluble and appropriate for intravenous use. The products also reflect the structure–activity relationship changes discussed previously to increase anti-inflammatory activity or potency or decrease salt retention.

Again, patients who have been on long-term GC therapy must have the dose reduced gradually. This "critical rule" and indications are discussed previously under the heading, "Therapeutic Uses of Adrenal Cortex Hormones." Dosage schedules and gradual dosage reduction can be quite complex and specific for each indication.

Many of the GCs are available in topical dosage forms, including creams, ointments, aerosols, lotions, and solutions. They are usually applied 3 to 4 times a day to well-cleaned areas of affected skin. Ointments are usually prescribed for dry, scaly dermatoses. Lotions are well suited for weeping dermatoses. Creams are of general use for many other

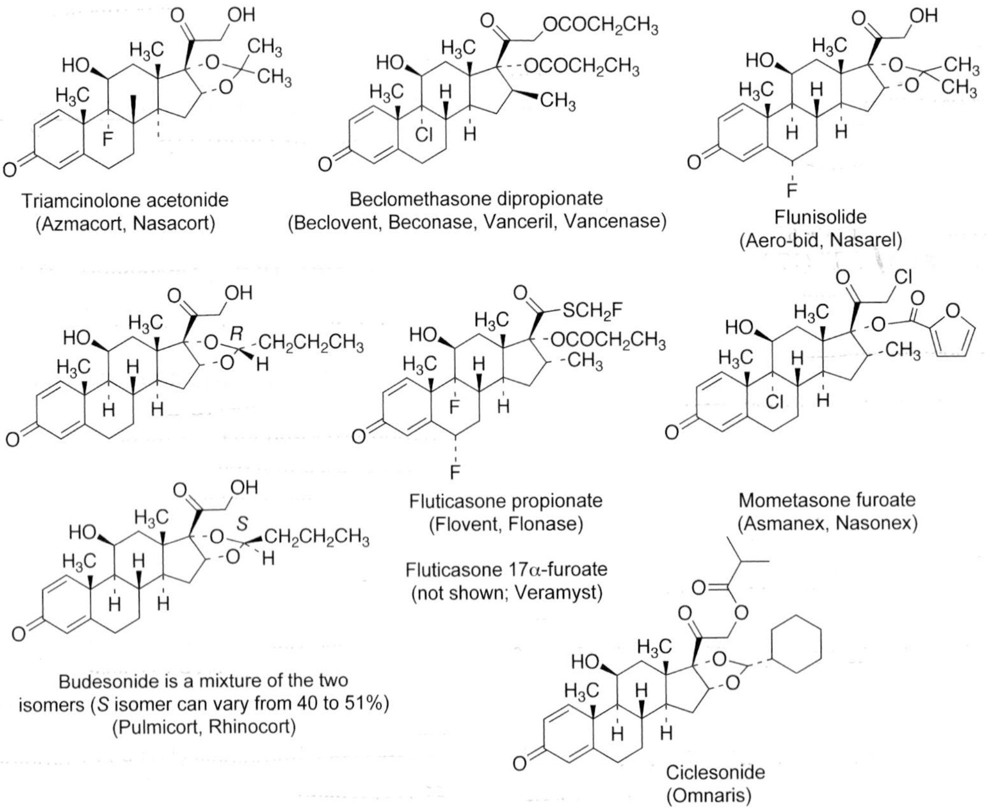

Triamcinolone acetonide
(Azmacort, Nasacort)

Beclomethasone dipropionate
(Beclovent, Beconase, Vanceril, Vancenase)

Flunisolide
(Aero-bid, Nasarel)

Fluticasone propionate
(Flovent, Flonase)

Mometasone furoate
(Asmanex, Nasonex)

Fluticasone 17α-furoate
(not shown; Veramyst)

Budesonide is a mixture of the two
isomers (S isomer can vary from 40 to 51%)
(Pulmicort, Rhinocort)

Ciclesonide
(Omnaris)

Figure 25.31 ● Glucocorticoids used to treat asthma and allergic rhinitis (some are also used topically).

dermatoses. When applied to very large areas of skin or to damaged areas of skin, significant systemic absorption can occur. The use of an occlusive dressing can also greatly increase systemic absorption.

The GCs that are mainly used for inflammation of the eye are shown in Figure 25.30. These compounds differ structurally from other GRs, in that the 21-hydroxyl is missing from medrysone, fluorometholone, and rimexolone, while loteprednol etabonate has a modified ester at C17 that leads to rapid degradation upon systemic absorption.

MINERALOCORTICOIDS

Fludrocortisone Acetate, USP. Fludrocortisone acetate, 21-acetyloxy-9-fluoro-11β,17-dihydroxypregn-4-ene-3,20-dione, 9α-fluorohydrocortisone (Florinef Acetate), is used only for the treatment of Addison disease and for inhibition of endogenous adrenocortical secretions. As shown in Table 25.7, it has up to about 800 times the MC activity of hydrocortisone and about 11 times the GC activity. Its potent activity stimulated the synthesis and study of the many fluorinated steroids shown in Figure 25.29. Although its great salt-retaining activity limits its use to Addison disease, it has sufficient GC activity that in some cases of the disease, additional GCs need not be prescribed.

GLUCOCORTICOIDS WITH MODERATE-TO-LOW SALT RETENTION

Hydrocortisone, USP. Hydrocortisone, 11β,17,21-trihydroxypregn-4-ene-3,20-dione, is the primary natural GC in humans. Despite the large number of synthetic GCs, hydrocortisone, its esters, and its salts remain a mainstay of modern adrenocortical steroid therapy and the standard for comparison of all other GCs and MCs (see Table 25.7). It is used for all the indications mentioned previously. Its esters and salts illustrate the principles of chemical modification to modify pharmacokinetic use shown in Figure 25.6. The commercially available salts and esters (see Fig. 25.29) include:

1 Hydrocortisone acetate, *USP* (21-acetate)
2 Hydrocortisone buteprate = hydrocortisone probutate, *USP* (17-butyrate, 21-propionate)
3 Hydrocortisone butyrate, *USP* (17-butyrate)
4 Hydrocortisone sodium phosphate, *USP* (21-sodium phosphate)
5 Hydrocortisone sodium succinate, *USP* (21-sodium succinate)
6 Hydrocortisone valerate, *USP* (17-valerate)

Cortisone Acetate, USP. Cortisone acetate, 21-(acetyloxy)-17-hydroxypregn-4-ene-3,11,20-trione, is the 21-acetate of naturally occurring cortisone with good systemic anti-inflammatory activity and low-to-moderate salt-retention activity after its in vivo conversion to hydrocortisone acetate. This conversion is mediated by 11β-hydroxysteroid dehydrogenase. It is used for the entire spectrum of uses discussed previously under the heading, "Therapeutic Uses of Adrenal Cortex Hormones"—collagen diseases, Addison disease, severe shock, allergic conditions, chronic lymphocytic leukemia, and many other indications. Cortisone acetate is relatively ineffective topically, mainly because it must be reduced in vivo to hydrocortisone. Its plasma half-life is only about 30 minutes, compared with 90 minutes to 3 hours for hydrocortisone.

Prednisolone, USP. Prednisolone, Δ¹-hydrocortisone, 11β,17,21-trihydroxypregna-1,4-diene-3,20-dione, has less salt-retention activity than hydrocortisone (see Table 25.7), but some patients have more frequently experienced complications such as gastric irritation and peptic ulcers. Because of low MC activity, it cannot be used alone for adrenal insufficiency. Prednisolone is available in various salts and esters to maximize its therapeutic utility (see Fig. 25.29):

Prednisolone acetate, *USP* (21-acetate)
Prednisolone sodium phosphate, *USP* (21-sodium phosphate)
Prednisolone sodium succinate, *USP* (21-sodium succinate)
Prednisolone tebutate, *USP* (21-tebutate)

Prednisone, USP. Prednisone, Δ¹-cortisone, 17,21-dihydroxypregna-1,4-diene-3,11,20-trione, has systemic activity very similar to that of prednisolone, and because of its lower salt-retention activity, it is often preferred over cortisone or hydrocortisone. Prednisone must be reduced in vivo to prednisolone to provide the active GC.

GLUCOCORTICOIDS WITH VERY LITTLE OR NO SALT RETENTION

Most of the key differences between the many GCs with minimal salt retention (see Fig. 25.29) have been summarized in Tables 25.6 and 25.7. The tremendous therapeutic and, therefore, commercial importance of these drugs has stimulated the proliferation of new compounds and their products. Many compounds also are available as salts or esters to give the complete range of therapeutic flexibility illustrated in Figure 25.29. When additional pertinent information is available, it is given below the drug name. The systemic name for each drug is provided after the common name.

Alclometasone Dipropionate, USP. Alclometasone dipropionate, 7α-chloro-11β-hydroxy-16α-methyl-17,21-bis(1-oxopropoxy)-pregna-1,4-diene-3,20-dione (Aclovate), is one of the few commercially used GRs that bears a halogen substituent in the 7α-position.

Amcinonide, USP. Amcinonide, 21-(acetyloxy)-16α,17-[cyclopentylidenebis(oxy)]-9-fluoro-11β-hydroxy-pregna-1,4-diene-3,20-dione (Cyclocort).

Beclomethasone Dipropionate, USP. Beclomethasone dipropionate, 9-chloro-11β-hydroxy-16β-methyl-17,21-bis-(1-oxopropoxy)-pregna-1,4-diene-3,20-dione (Beconase, QVAR), is used in nasal sprays and aerosol formulations to treat allergic rhinitis and asthma (see section on page 863).

Betamethasone, USP. Betamethasone, 9-fluoro-11β,17,21-trihydroxy-16β-methylpregna-1,4-diene-3,20-dione, is available as a variety of ester derivatives.

Betamethasone valerate, *USP* (17-valerate)
Betamethasone acetate, *USP* (21-acetate)
Betamethasone sodium phosphate, *USP* (21-sodium phosphate)
Betamethasone dipropionate, *USP* (17-propionate, 21-propionate)

Budesonide, USP. Budesonide, 16α,17-[butylidenebis-(oxy)]-11β,21-dihydroxypregna-1,4-diene-3, 20-dione

(Entocort), in oral capsules is used to treat Crohn disease. The affinity for the GC is approximately 200-fold greater than that of hydrocortisone and 15-fold greater than that of prednisolone. Budesonide is a mixture of epimers, with the 22R form having twice the affinity for the GR of the S epimer. This GC is metabolized by CYP3A4, and its levels can be increased in the presence of potent CYP3A4 inhibitors. Budesonide is also used in an inhaled formulation for the treatment of asthma (see next page).

Clobetasol Propionate, USP. Clobetasol propionate, 21-chloro-9-fluoro-11β-hydroxy-16β-methyl-17-(1-oxopropoxy)-pregna-1,4-diene-3,20-dione (Temovate).

Clocortolone Pivalate, USP. Clocortolone pivalate, 9-chloro-21-(2,2-dimethyl-1-oxopropoxy)-6α-fluoro-11β-hydroxy-16α-methylpregna-1,4-diene-3,20-dione (Cloderm), along with desoximetasone, lacks the C17α oxygen functionality that is present in other GCs but still retains good GC activity.

Desonide, USP. Desonide, 11β,21-dihydroxy-16α,17-[(1-methylethylidene)bis(oxy)]pregna-1,4-diene-3,20-dione (DesOwen, Tridesiol).

Desoximetasone, USP. Desoximetasone, 9-fluoro-11β, 21-dihydroxy-16α-methylpregna-1,4-diene-3,20-dione, like clocortolone pivalate, lacks a C17α OH group in its structure.

Dexamethasone, USP. Dexamethasone, 9-fluoro-11β, 17,21-trihydroxy-16α-methylpregna-1,4-diene-3,20-dione, is the 16α-isomer of betamethasone.

Dexamethasone acetate, *USP* (21-acetate)
Dexamethasone sodium phosphate, *USP* (21-sodium phosphate)

Diflorasone Diacetate, USP. Diflorasone diacetate, 17, 21-bis(acetyloxy)-6α,9-difluoro-11β-hydroxy-16α-methylpregna-1,4-diene-3,20-dione.

Difluprednate. *Difluprednate*, 21-(acetyloxy)-6α,9-difluoro-11β-hydroxy-17-(1-oxobutoxy)pregna-1,4-diene-3,20-dione is being developed (phase III) as a topical ophthalmic emulsion to treat inflammatory eye diseases.

Flunisolide, USP. Flunisolide, 6α-fluoro-11β,21-dihydroxy-16α,17-[(1-methylethylidene)bis(oxy)]pregna-1,4-diene-3,20-dione. (See following section for use of flunisolide in the treatment of asthma.)

Fluocinolone Acetonide, USP. Fluocinolone acetonide, 6α,9-difluoro-11β,21-dihydroxy-16α,17-[(1-methylethylidene)bis(oxy)]pregna-1,4-diene-3,20-dione, also known as 6α-fluorotriamcinolone acetonide, is the 21-acetate derivative of fluocinolone acetonide and is about 5 times more potent than fluocinolone acetonide in at least one topical activity assay.

Fluorometholone, USP. Fluorometholone, 9-fluoro-11β,17-dihydroxy-6α-methylpregn-4-ene-3,20-dione (Fluor-Op, FML), lacks the typical C21 OH group of GCs and is used exclusively in ophthalmic products. The 17-acetate of fluorometholone is also used as an ophthalmic suspension (Flarex).

Flurandrenolide, USP. Flurandrenolide, 6α-fluoro-11β,21-dihydroxy-16 α,17-[(1-methylethylidene)bis(oxy)]

pregn-4-ene-3,20-dione, although available as a tape product, can stick to and remove damaged skin, so it should be avoided with vesicular or weeping dermatoses.

Fluticasone Propionate, USP. Fluticasone propionate, S-(fluoromethyl) 6α,9-difluoro-11β-hydroxy-16α-methyl-3-oxo-17α-(1-oxopropoxy)androsta-1,4-diene-17-carbothio-ate (Cutivate), is threefold to fivefold more potent than dexamethasone in receptor binding assays (see also the following section on inhaled corticosteroids).

Halcinonide. Halcinonide, 21-chloro-9-fluoro-11β-hydroxy-16α,17-[(1-methylethylidene)bis(oxy)]pregn-4-ene-3,20-dione, was the first chloroGC marketed. Like many other potent GCs, it is used only topically.

Halobetasol Propionate, USP. Halobetasol propionate, 21-chloro-6α,9-difluoro-11β-hydroxy-16β-methyl-17-(1-oxopropoxy)pregna-1,4-diene-3,20-dione.

Loteprednol Etabonate, USP. Loteprednol etabonate, chloromethyl 17α-[(ethoxycarbonyl)oxy]-11β-hydroxy-3-oxoandrosta-1,4-diene-17-carboxylate (Alrex, Lotemax), has a modified carboxylate at the C17 position rather than the typical ketone functionality. This modification maintains affinity for the GR but allows facile metabolism to inactive metabolites. This limits the systemic action of the drug. Loteprednol etabonate is used as an ophthalmic suspension that has greatly reduced systemic action because of rapid metabolism to the inactive carboxylate (Fig. 25.30).

Methylprednisolone, USP. Methylprednisolone, 11β, 17,21-trihydroxy-6α-methyl-1,4-pregnadiene-3,20-dione, is available unmodified or as ester derivatives.

Methylprednisolone acetate, *USP*
Methylprednisolone sodium succinate, *USP*

Mometasone Furoate, USP. Mometasone furoate, 9,21-dichloro-17α-[(2-furanylcarbonyl)oxy]-11β-hydroxy-16α-methylpregna-1,4-diene-3,20-dione (Elocon), is a high-potency GC available in cream, lotion, or ointment formulations for topical use. In addition, mometasone furoate monohydrate is formulated for treating allergic rhinitis and asthma (see following section).

Prednicarbate, USP. Prednicarbate, 17-[(ethoxycarbonyl)oxy]-11β-hydroxy-21-(1-oxopropoxy)pregna-1,4-diene-3,20-dione, is a prednisolone derivative with a C21 propionate ester and a C17 ethyl carbonate group. It is available for use only in a 0.1% topical cream. Prednicarbate is a medium-potency GC.

Rimexolone, USP. Rimexolone, 11β-hydroxy-16α, 17α-dimethyl-17-(1-oxopropyl)androsta-1,4-diene-3-one, like medrysone and fluorometholone, lacks the C21 OH group. In addition, rimexolone has an additional methyl group in the 17α-position, a site where an OH group is typically found. Rimexolone is available as a suspension for ophthalmic use (Fig. 25.30).

Triamcinolone, USP. Triamcinolone, 9-fluoro-11β,16α, 17,21-tetrahydroxypregna-1,4-diene-3,20-dione.

Triamcinolone acetonide, *USP*: Triamcinolone-16α, 17-acetonide
Triamcinolone hexacetonide, *USP*: Triamcinolone acetonide 21-[3-(3,3-dimethyl)butyrate]
Triamcinolone diacetate, *USP*: 16,21-Diacetate

Triamcinolone acetonide is approximately 8 times more potent than prednisone in animal inflammation models. Topically applied triamcinolone acetonide is a potent anti-inflammatory agent (see Table 25.7), about 10 times more so than triamcinolone. The plasma half-life is approximately 90 minutes, although the plasma half-life and biological half-lives for GCs do not correlate well. The hexacetonide is slowly converted to the acetonide in vivo and is given only by intra-articular injection. Only triamcinolone and the diacetate are given orally. The acetonide and diacetate may be given by intra-articular or intrasynovial injection. In addition, the acetonide may be given by intrabursal or, sometimes, IM or subcutaneous injection. A single IM dose of the diacetate or acetonide may last up to 3 or 4 weeks. Plasma levels with IM doses of the acetonide are significantly higher than with triamcinolone itself. The acetonide is also used to treat asthma and allergic rhinitis (see following section).

INHALED CORTICOSTEROIDS FOR ASTHMA AND ALLERGIC RHINITIS

The National Asthma Education and Prevention Program has provided recent recommendations on the treatment of asthma, including a strong recommendation for the first-line use of inhaled corticosteroids for severe and moderate persistent asthma in all age groups. The corticosteroids currently used in inhaled formulations are all relatively potent topical corticosteroids that have the advantage of rapid deactivation/inactivation for the portion of the dose that is swallowed. The development of GCs that are efficiently inactivated metabolically when swallowed has greatly reduced the systemic side effects associated with the use of steroids in asthma treatment. The older corticosteroids that are used orally (e.g., methylprednisolone, prednisolone, and prednisone) have much greater systemic side effects, and their use should be limited, if possible. Although systemic side effects are reduced, they are not completely eliminated. The side effects can vary with the steroid used and the frequency of administration.

The six GCs that are currently approved for use in the United States for asthma as inhaled formulations are beclomethasone dipropionate, budesonide, flunisolide, fluticasone propionate, mometasone furoate, and triamcinolone acetonide (Fig. 25.31). Ciclesonide (Alvesco) is the newest GC being pursued for use in the treatment of asthma. Ciclesonide is in phase III clinical trials and may be available in the United States within a few years. It is already approved to treat asthma in Europe and Canada. Clinical trials suggest that it may have better tolerability than some of the currently available inhaled steroids.

The following agents are also available in nasal inhalers for the treatment of allergic rhinitis. Details are provided below for the mode of metabolic inactivation involved for each of these products. Although all of these agents have much lower systemic effects than the oral steroids, some systemic effects, as measured by suppression of the hypothalamic–pituitary–adrenal (HPA) axis, have been observed for these products. Ciclesonide (2006) and fluticasone furoate (Veramyst, 2007), with a 17-furoate in place of the 17-propionate, were both also recently approved for treating allergic rhinitis.

GLUCOCORTICOIDS FOR ASTHMA AND ALLERGIC RHINITIS

Beclomethasone Dipropionate.
Beclomethasone dipropionate (Beclovent, Beconase, Vanceril, Vancenase) (BDP) is rapidly converted in the lungs to beclomethasone 17-monopropionate (17-BMP), the metabolite that provides the bulk of the anti-inflammatory activity. The monopropionate also has higher affinity for the GR than either the dipropionate or beclomethasone. The portion of BDP that is swallowed is rapidly hydrolyzed to 17-BMP, 21-BMP (which arises by a transesterification reaction from 17-BMP), and beclomethasone itself.[154] Beclomethasone has much less GC activity than the monopropionate.[155]

Budesonide.
Budesonide (Pulmicort Turbohaler, Rhinocort) is extensively metabolized in the liver, with 85% to 95% of the orally absorbed drug metabolized by the first-pass effect. The major metabolites are 6β-hydroxybudesonide and 16α-hydroxyprednisolone, both with less than 1% of the activity of the parent compound. Metabolism involves the CYP3A4 enzyme, so coadministration of budesonide with a known CYP3A4 inhibitor should be monitored carefully.

Ciclesonide.
Ciclesonide (Omnaris) is a prodrug that requires hydrolysis of the isobutyrate ester at C21 to form the active corticosteroid (des-ciclesonide). It has minimal oral bioavailability due to extensive metabolism, mainly by CYP3A4. The metabolites of ciclesonide have not been fully characterized.

Flunisolide.
The portion of a flunisolide (AeroBid, Nasarel) dose that is swallowed is rapidly converted to the 6β-hydroxy metabolite after first-pass metabolism in the liver. The 6β-hydroxy metabolite is approximately as active as hydrocortisone itself, but the small amount produced usually has limited systemic effects. Water-soluble conjugates are inactive.

Fluticasone Propionate.
The main metabolite of fluticasone propionate (Flovent, Flonase) found in circulation in humans is the 17β-carboxylate derivative. As expected, a charged carboxylate in place of the normal acetol functionality at C17 greatly reduces affinity for the GR (2,000-fold less than the parent), and this metabolite is essentially inactive. The metabolite is formed via the CYP3A4 system, so care should be taken if fluticasone propionate is coadministered with a CYP3A4 inhibitor such as ketoconazole or ritonavir. Clinically induced Cushing syndrome has been observed when inhaled fluticasone propionate was administered concurrently with ritonavir.[156] Fluticasone is also available in an inhaled formulation in combination with the long-acting β2-agonist salmeterol (Advair Diskus).

Mometasone Furoate.
Mometasone furoate (Asmanex, Nasonex) undergoes extensive metabolism to multiple metabolites. No major metabolites are detectable in human plasma after oral administration, but the 6β-hydroxy metabolite is detectable by use of human liver microsomes. This metabolite is formed via the CYP3A4 pathway.

Triamcinolone Acetonide.
The three main metabolites of triamcinolone acetonide (Azmacort, Nasacort) are 6β-hydroxytriamcinolone acetonide, 21-carboxytriamcinolone acetonide, and 6β-hydroxy-21-carboxytriamcinolone acetonide. All are much less active than the parent compound. The 6β-hydroxyl group and the 21-carboxy group are both structural features that greatly reduce GC action. The increased water solubility of these metabolites also facilitates more rapid excretion.

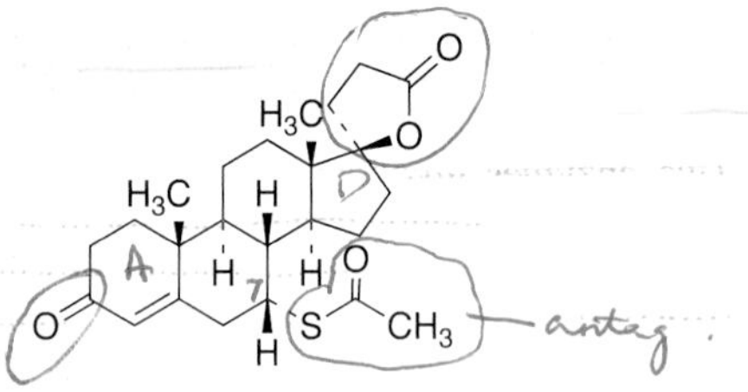

Spironolactone (Aldolactone)

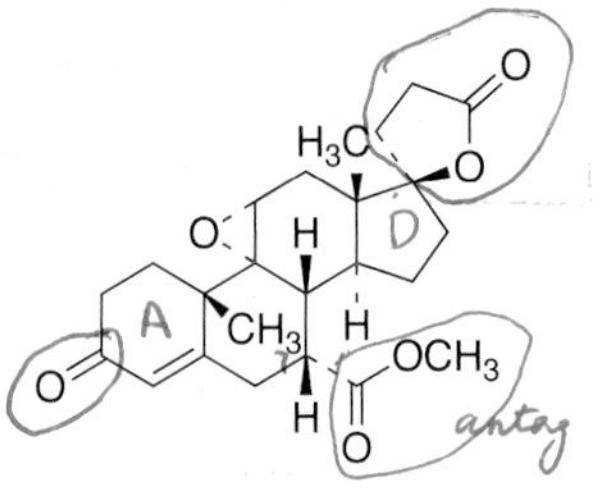

Eplerenone (Inspra)

Figure 25.32 • Aldosterone receptor antagonists.

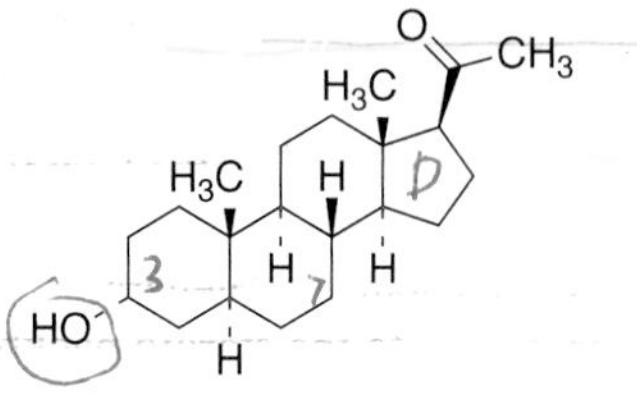

Allopreganolone
(3α-Hydroxy-5α-pregnan-20-one)
(3α, 5α-Tetrahydroprogesterone)

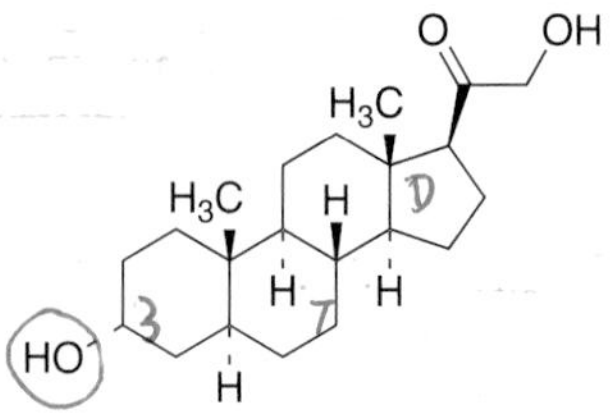

Allotetrahydrodeoxycorticosterone
(3α,21-Dihydroxy-5α-pregnan-20-one)

Figure 25.33 • Neurosteroid examples.

Mineralocorticoid Receptor Antagonists (Aldosterone Antagonists)

Antagonism of the MR can have profound effects on the renin–angiotensin system, thus having significant cardiac effects. Structurally, these compounds have an A-ring enone, essential for recognition by the receptor, but the 7α-substituent and the D-ring spirolactone provide structural elements that lead to antagonism (Fig. 25.32).

Spironolactone, USP. Spironolactone, 7α-(acetylthio)-17α-hydroxy-3-oxopregn-4-ene-3-one-21-carboxylic acid γ-lactone (Aldactone) is an aldosterone antagonist of great medical importance because of its diuretic activity. Spironolactone is discussed in Chapter 18.

Eplerenone, USP. Eplerenone, 9,11α-epoxy-17α-hydroxy-3-oxopregn-4-ene-7α,21-dicarboxylic acid, γ-lactone, methyl ester (Inspra), is a newer aldosterone antagonist that is used for the treatment of hypertension.

NEUROSTEROIDS[79,157,158]

Although the main effects of the steroid hormones described in this chapter have been focused on sexual development, maintenance of sexual organ function, and inflammatory processes, steroids also play important roles in the brain. Two terms have been developed to describe the specific steroids that act on the nervous system, neurosteroids and neuroactive steroids. Neurosteroids are synthesized in the brain, either from cholesterol or from other steroid hormones, and have their specific actions in the nervous system. Neuroactive steroids are synthesized in other steroidogenic tissues, but have their actions in the brain after transport from the site of synthesis. Many of the neurosteroids are the same as steroid hormones acting peripherally, but some have unique roles in the brain. Neurosteroids include pregnenolone, progesterone, and DHEA, as well as their sulfate esters. Metabolites of progesterone and 11-deoxycorticosterone, allopregnanolone and allotetrahydrodeoxycorticosterone (allotetrahydroDOC; Fig. 25.33), respectively, represent neurosteroids with specific central actions.

In addition to the action of neurosteroids/neuroactive steroids via traditional steroid receptors (progesterone, estradiol), many neurosteroids act at different sites, especially the neurosteroids with a 3α-hydroxyl (Fig. 25.33). Allopregnanolone and allotetrahydroDOC are positive modulators of GABA$_A$ receptors, while pregnenolone sulfate and DHEA sulfate are negative modulators of the GABA$_A$ receptors. DHEA sulfate and pregnenolone sulfate also have actions at NMDA receptors and sigma type 1 receptors, while progesterone interacts with kainite, glycine, 5HT$_3$, and nicotinic acetylcholine receptors. Although much of the neurosteroid research has been conducted in animal models, the clinical significance of neurosteroids is an area of growing interest.[79] Neurosteroids have been hypothesized to have neuroprotective effects, anxiolytic effects, and may play roles in modulating seizures. The actions of steroids in the brain will undoubtedly be the focus of much more research in the years to come.

ACKNOWLEDGMENT

I would like to thank Debra Peters for assistance with the illustration of several figures. I would also like to express my appreciation to the authors of various review articles on the steroids and the authors of previous versions of this text. Without the dedication and hard work of these individuals, the assembly of this chapter would have been a much more challenging task.

● R E V I E W   Q U E S T I O N S ●

1. What is the natural precursor in the human body to all the steroid hormones (estrogens, progestins, androgens, and corticosteroids)? Explain the general steps necessary to convert this precursor to the steroid backbones necessary for the specific steroid hormones. Also indicate the enzyme involved in the key steps. *Steroid syn*

2. Tamoxifen and raloxifene both mediate their main pharmacological actions via the the ERs. Tamoxifen is an antagonist in breast tissue and an agonist in the endometrium and bone. Raloxifene, in contrast, is an antagonist in the breast and the endometrium and an agonist in bone tissue. Explain how these two drugs can have these varied effects in separate tissues, despite both binding at the same site on the ER. *ER antagonists*

3. Levonorgestrel has several structural differences relative to progesterone, yet still is a drug with useful progestational activity. Describe these structural differences and indicate how they affect the therapeutic properties of this drug. *ER*

4. The three structures depicted all illustrate a common structural modification seen in steroid hormone drugs, even though each structure represents a different class of steroid hormone. What is the common structural modification and how does it affect the action of each of these drugs? For each of the structures, provide the specific class of steroid hormone that is represented.

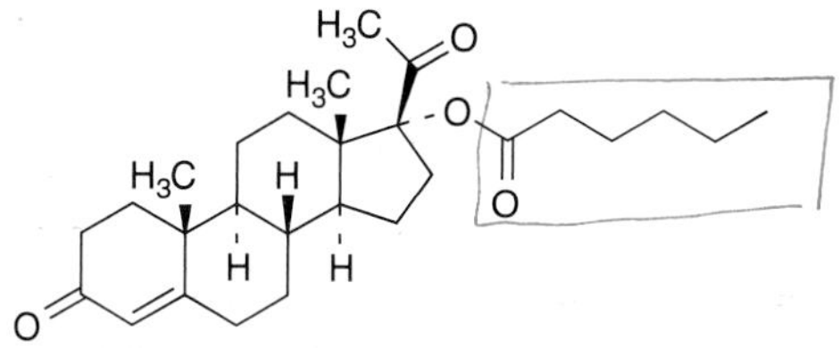

A

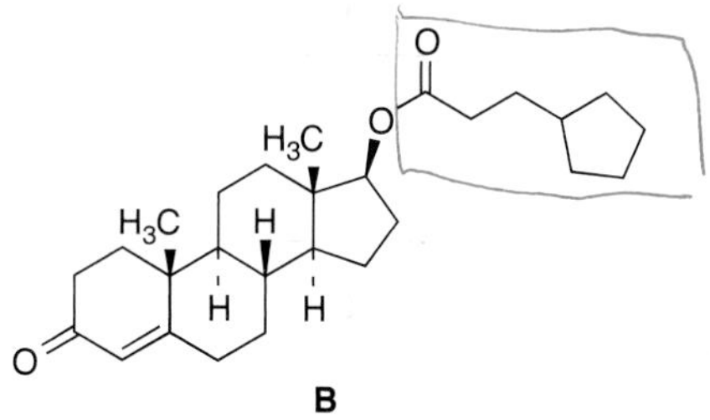

B

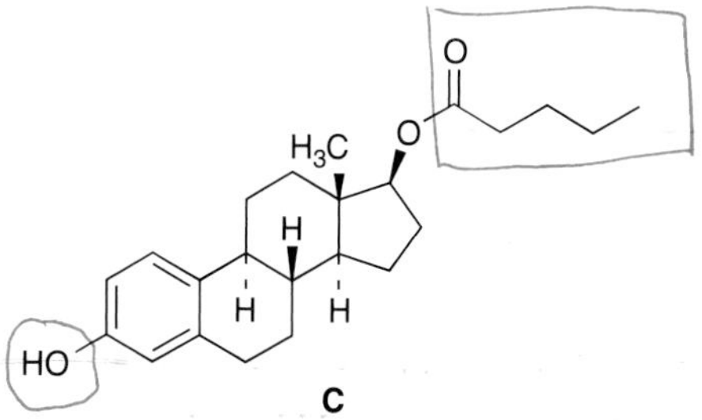

C

5. Two enzymes involved in steroid hormone biosynthesis are useful therapeutic targets, one for treating breast cancer and the other for treating benign prostatic hypertrophy (BPH). What are these two enzymes and what biosynthetic conversions do they mediate? Provide the name of an inhibitor of each enzyme that is used as a drug. *sex Hormone*

6. Based on structural features, which of the following represents a corticosteroid that would have strong anti-inflammatory properties, but would have minimal MC (water-retention) action? Explain your choice, specifically identifying key structural features. *GC*

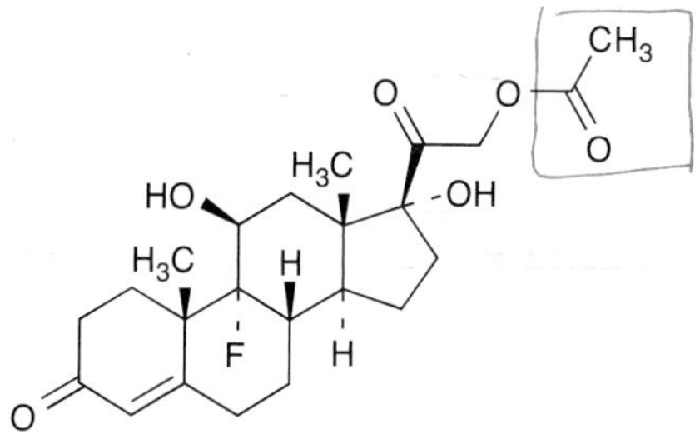

A

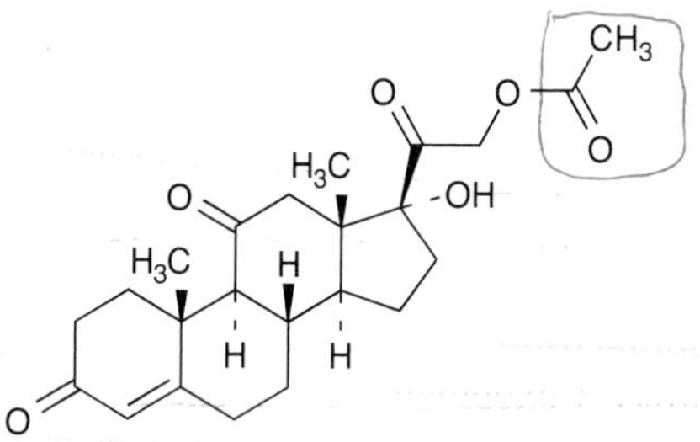

B

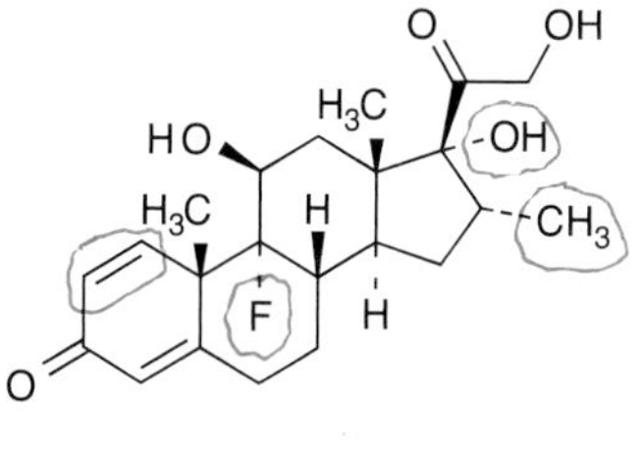

C

REFERENCES

1. Brunton, L. L., Lazo, J. S., and Parker, K. L.: Goodman & Gilman's The Pharmacological Basis of Therapeutics. New York, McGraw-Hill, 2006.
2. Norman, A. W., and Litwack, G.: Hormones, 2nd ed. San Diego, Academic Press, 1997.
3. Brueggemeier, R., and Li, P.-K.: Fundamentals of steroid chemistry and biochemistry. In Abraham, D. J. (ed.). Burger's Medicinal Chemistry and Drug Discovery, 6th ed. Hoboken, Interscience, 2003, pp. 593–627.
4. Moss, G. P.: Eur. J. Biochem. 186:429–458, 1989.
5. Stocco, D. M.: Annu. Rev. Physiol. 63:193–213, 2001.
6. Lin, D., Sugawara, T., and Strauss, J. F., et al.: Science 267:1828–1831, 1995.
7. Wehling, M., and Losel, R.: J. Steroid Biochem. Mol. Biol. 102:180–183, 2006.
8. Vasudevan, N., and Pfaff, D. W.: Endocr. Rev. 28:1–19, 2007.
9. Tasker, J. G., Di, S., and Malcher-Lopes, R.: Endocrinology 147:5549–5556, 2006.
10. Aranda, A., and Pascual, A.: Physiol. Rev. 81:1269–1304, 2001.
11. Mosselman, S., Polman, J., and Dijkema, R.: FEBS Lett. 392:49–53, 1996.
12. Loose-Mitchell, D. S., and Stancel, G. M.: Estrogens and progestins. In Brunton, L. L., Lazo, J. S., and Parker, K. L. (eds.). Goodman and Gilman's The Pharmacological Basis of Therapeutics, 11th ed. New York, McGraw-Hill, 2006, pp. 1541–1571.
13. Harris, H. A., Katzenellenbogen, J. A., and Katzenellenbogen, B. S.: Endocrinology 143:4172–4177, 2002.
14. Harris, H. A., Bapat, A. R., Gonder, D. S., et al.: Steroids 67:379–384, 2002.
15. Katzenellenbogen, B. S., Sun, J., Harrington, W. R., et al.: Ann. N. Y. Acad. Sci. 949:6–15, 2001.
16. Gelmann, E. P.: J. Clin. Oncol. 20:3001–3015, 2002.
17. DeRijk, R. H., Schaaf, M., and de Kloet, E. R.: J. Steroid Biochem. Mol. Biol. 81:103–122, 2002.
18. Brzozowski, A. M., Pike, A. C., Dauter, Z., et al.: Nature 389:753–758, 1997.
19. Tanenbaum, D. M., Wang, Y., Williams, S. P., et al.: Proc. Natl. Acad. Sci. U. S. A. 95:5998–6003, 1998.
20. Pike, A. C., Brzozowski, A. M., Hubbard, R. E., et al.: EMBO J. 18:4608–4618, 1999.
21. Williams, S. P., and Sigler, P. B.: Nature 393:392–396, 1998.
22. Sack, J. S., Kish, K. F., Wang, C., et al.: Proc. Natl. Acad. Sci. U. S. A. 98:4904–4909, 2001.
23. Bledsoe, R. K., Montana, V. G., Stanley, T. B., et al.: Cell 110:93–105, 2002.
24. Kauppi, B., Jakob, C., Farnegardh, M., et al.: J. Biol. Chem. 278:22748–22754, 2003.
25. Li, Y., Suino, K., Daugherty, J., et al.: Mol. Cell. 19:367–380, 2005.
26. Ekena, K., Katzenellenbogen, J. A., and Katzenellenbogen, B. S.: J. Biol. Chem. 273:693–699, 1998.
27. Duax, W. L.: Biochemical Actions of Hormones, vol 11. New York, Academic Press, 1984.
28. Duax, W. L., Griffin, J. F., Weeks, C. M., et al.: J. Steroid Biochem. 31:481–492, 1988.
29. Hanson, J. R.: Nat. Prod. Rep. 19:381–389, 2002.
30. Cheung, J., and Smith, D. F.: Mol. Endocrinol. 14:939–946, 2000.
31. Pratt, W. B., and Toft, D. O.: Endocr. Rev. 18:306–360, 1997.
32. DeFranco, D. B.: Mol. Endocrinol. 16:1449–1455, 2002.
33. Burns, K. H., and Matzuk, M. M.: Endocrinology 143:2823–2835, 2002.
34. Themmen, A. P. N., and Huhtaniemi, I. T.: Endocr. Rev. 21:551–583, 2000.
35. Ruenitz, P. C.: Chapter 13. Female sex hormones, contraceptives, and fertility drugs. In Abraham, D. J. (ed.). Burger's Medicinal Chemistry and Drug Discovery, 6th ed., vol 3. Hoboken, Wiley-Interscience, 2003.
36. Rich, R. L., Hoth, L. R., Geoghegan, K. F., et al.: Proc. Natl. Acad. Sci. U. S. A. 99:8562–8567, 2002.
37. Martin, C. R.: Endocrine Physiology. New York, Oxford University Press, 1985.
38. Schuler, F. S.: Science 103:221, 1946.
39. Mittendorf, R.: Teratology 51:435–445, 1995.
40. Kuiper, G. G., Lemmen, J. G., Carlsson, B., et al.: Endocrinology 139:4252–4263, 1998.
41. Kaiser, J.: Science 317: 884–885, 2007.
42. Jordan, V. C., Mittal, S., Gosden, B., et al.: Environ. Health Perspect. 61:97–110, 1985.
43. Adams, N. R.: J. Anim. Sci. 73:1509–1515, 1995.
44. Rice, S., and Whitehead, S. A.: Endocr. Relat. Cancer 13:995–1015, 2006.
45. Setchell, K. D.: J. Am. Coll. Nutr. 20:354S–362S, discussion: 381S-383S, 2001.
46. An, J., Tzagarakis-Foster, C., Scharschmidt, T. C., et al.: J. Biol. Chem. 276:17808–17814, 2001.
47. Zhao, L., and Brinton, R. D.: J. Med. Chem. 48:3463–3466, 2005.
48. Hilakivi-Clarke, Cabanes, A., Olivo, S., et al.: J. Steroid Biochem. Mol. Biol. 80:163–174, 2002.
49. Shapiro, S., Kelly, J. P., Rosenberg, L., et al.: N. Engl. J. Med. 313:969–972, 1985.
50. Ferrer-Lorente, R., Garcia-Pelaez, B., Fernandez-Lopez, J. A., et al.: Steroids 69:661–665, 2004.
51. Schmider, J., Greenblatt, D. J., von Moltke, L. L., et al.: J. Clin. Pharmacol. 37:193–200, 1997.
52. Cummings, F. J.: Clin. Ther. 24 (Suppl C):C3–25, 2002.
53. Carlson, R. W.: Breast Cancer Res. Treat. 75 (Suppl 1):S27–32, discussion: S33–S35, 2002.
54. Ross, D., and Whitehead, M.: Curr. Opin. Obstet. Gynecol. 7:63–68, 1995.
55. Grese, T. A., Sluka, J. P., Bryant, H. U., et al.: Proc. Natl. Acad. Sci. U. S. A. 94:14105–14110, 1997.
56. Katzenellenbogen, B. S., and Katzenellenbogen, J. A.: Science 295:2380–2381, 2002.
57. Shang, Y., and Brown, M.: Science 295:2465–2468, 2002.
58. Musa, M. A., Khan, M. O., and Cooperwood, J. S.: Curr. Med. Chem. 14:1249–1261, 2007.
59. Shiau, A. K., Barstad, D., Loria, P. M., et al.: Cell 95:927–937, 1998.
60. Komm, B. S., and Lyttle, C. R.: Ann. N. Y. Acad. Sci. 949:317–326, 2001.
61. Gennari, L., Merlotti, D., Valleggi, F., et al.: Drugs Aging 24:361–379, 2007.
62. Harvey, H. A., Kimura, M., and Hajba, A.: Breast 15:142–157, 2006.
63. Vogel, V. G., Costantino, J. P., Wickerham, D. L., et al.: JAMA 295:2727–2741, 2006.
64. Wardley, A. M.: Int. J. Clin. Pract. 56:305–309, 2002.
65. Goldstein, S. R., Siddhanti, S., Ciaccia, A. V., et al.: Hum. Reprod. Update 6:212–224, 2000.
66. Turner, R. T., Evans, G. L., Sluka, J. P., et al.: Endocrinology 139:3712–3720, 1998.
67. Brueggemeier, R. W.: Am. J. Ther. 8:333–344, 2001.
68. Recanatini, M., Cavalli, A., and Valenti, P.: Med. Res. Rev. 22:282–304, 2002.
69. Simpson, E. R., Clyne, C., Rubin, G., et al.: Annu. Rev. Physiol. 64:93–127, 2002.
70. Osawa, Y., Higashiyama, T., Fronckowiak, M., et al.: J. Steroid Biochem. 27:781–789, 1987.
71. Simpson, E. R., and Dowsett, M.: Recent Prog. Horm. Res. 57:317–338, 2002.
72. Cocconi, G.: Breast Cancer Res. Treat. 30:57–80, 1994.
73. Campbell, D. R., and Kurzer, M. S.: J. Steroid Biochem. Mol. Biol. 46:381–388, 1993.
74. Walle, T., Otake, Y., Brubaker, J. A., et al.: Br. J. Clin. Pharmacol. 51:143–146, 2001.
75. Grimm, S. W., and Dyroff, M. C.: Drug Metab. Dispos. 25:598–602, 1997.
76. Dowsett, M., Pfister, C., Johnston, S. R., et al.: Clin. Cancer Res. 5:2338–2343, 1999.
77. Charbonneau, A.: Biochim. Biophys. Acta. 1517:228–235, 2001.
78. Blom, T., Ojanotko-Harri, A., Laine, M., et al.: J. Steroid Biochem. Mol. Biol. 44:69–76, 1993.
79. Mellon, S. H., and Griffin, L. D.: Trends Endocrinol. Metab. 13:35–43, 2002.
80. Fensome, A., Bender, R., Chopra, R., et al.: J. Med. Chem. 48:5092–5095, 2005.
81. Briggs, M. H.: Curr. Med. Res. Opin. 3:95–98, 1975.
82. Gentile, D. M., Verhoeven, C. H., Shimada, T., et al.: J. Pharmacol. Exp. Ther. 287:975–982, 1998.
83. Kuhnz, W., Fritzemeier, K. H., Hegele-Hartung, C., et al.: Contraception 51:131–139, 1995.
84. Zhang, Z., Lundeen, S. G., Zhu, Y., et al.: Steroids 65:637–643, 2002.
85. Attardi, B. J., Burgenson, J., Hild, S. A., et al.: J. Steroid Biochem. Mol. Biol. 88:277–288, 2004.

86. Chabbert-Buffet, N., Meduri, G., Bouchard, P., et al.: Hum. Reprod. Update 11:293–307, 2005.
87. DeManno, D., Elger, W., Garg, R., et al.: Steroids 68:1019–1032, 2003.
88. Djerassi, C.: The Politics of Contraception. New York, W.W. Norton, 1979.
89. Lednicer, D. (ed.): Contraception, The Chemical Control of Fertility. New York, Marcel Dekker, 1969.
90. Chester, E.: Woman of Valor, Margaret Sanger. New York, Simon and Schuster, 1992.
91. Asbell, B.: The Pill. New York, Random House, 1995.
92. Makepeace, A. W., et al.: Am. J. Physiol. 119:512, 1937.
93. Selye, H., Tache, Y., and Szabo, S.: Fertil. Steril. 22:735–740, 1971.
94. Dempsey, E. W.: Am. J. Physiol. 120:926, 1937.
95. Kurzrok, R.: J. Contraception 2:27, 1937.
96. Sturgis, S. H., and Albright, F.: Endocrinology 26:68, 1940.
97. Pincus, G.: The Control of Fertility. New York, Academic Press, 1965.
98. Djerassi, C., Miramontes, L., Rosenkranz, G., et al.: J. Am. Chem. Soc. 76:4092–4094, 1954.
99. Colton, F. B.: U.S. Patent 2,691,028. 1954.
100. Borgelt-Hansen, L.: J. Am. Pharm. Assoc. (Wash.) 41:875–886, 2001.
101. La Vecchia, C., Altieri, A., Franceschi, S., et al.: Drug Saf. 24:741–754, 2001.
102. Sherwin, B. B.: J. Neuroendocrinol. 19:77–81, 2007.
103. Genazzani, A. R., Pluchino, N., Luisi, S., et al.: Hum. Reprod. Update 13:175–187, 2007.
104. Gennari, L., Becherini, L., Falchetti, A., et al.: J. Steroid Biochem. Mol. Biol. 81:1–24, 2002.
105. Riggs, B. L., Khosla, S., and Melton, L. J.: Endocr. Rev. 23:279–302.
106. Notelovitz, M.: J. Reprod. Med. 47:71–81, 2002.
107. Rossouw, J. E., et al.: JAMA 288:321–33, 2002.
108. Harman, S. M., Naftolin, F., Brinton, E. A., et al.: Ann. N. Y. Acad. Sci. 1052:43–56, 2005.
109. Mastorakos, G., Sakkas, E. G., Xydakis, A. M., et al.: Ann. N. Y. Acad. Sci. 1092:331–340, 2006.
110. Beral, V., Bull, D., Green, J., et al.: Lancet 369:1703–1710, 2007.
111. Brueggemeier, R.: Chapter 14. Male sex hormones, analogs, and antagonists. In Abraham, D. J. (ed.). Burger's Medicinal Chemistry and Drug Discovery, 6th ed., vol 3. Hoboken, Wiley, 2003.
112. George, F. W.: Endocrinology 138:871–877, 1997.
113. Williams, M. R., Ling, S., Dawood, T., et al.: J. Clin. Endocrinol. Metab. 87:176–181.
114. Snyder, P. J.: Androgens. In Brunton, L. L., Lazo, J. S., and Parker, K. L. (eds.). Goodman and Gilman's The Pharmacological Basis of Therapeutics, 11th ed. New York, McGraw-Hill, 2006.
115. Davis, S. R., and Tran, J.: Trends Endocrinol. Metab. 12:33–37, 2001.
116. Padero, M. C., Bhasin, S., and Friedman, T. C.: J. Am. Geriatr. Soc. 50:1131–1140, 2002.
117. Kuhn, C. M.: Recent Prog. Horm. Res. 57:411–434, 2002.
118. Burd, I. D., and Bachmann, G. A.: Curr. Womens Health Rep. 1:202–205, 2001.
119. Hoberman, J. M., and Yesalis, C. E.: Sci. Am. 272:76–81, 1995.
120. Bahrke, M. S., and Yesalis, C. E.: Curr. Opin. Pharmacol. 4:614–620, 2004.
121. Saudan, C., Baume, N., Robinson, N., et al.: Br. J. Sports Med. 40(Suppl 1):i21–4, 2006.
122. Death, A. K., McGrath, K. C., Kazlauskas, R., et al.: J. Clin. Endocrinol. Metab. 89:2498–2500, 2004.
123. Hartgens, F., and Kuipers, H.: Sports Med. 34:513–554, 2004.
124. Foster, Z. J., and Housner, J. A.: Curr. Sports Med. Rep. 3:234–241, 2004.
125. Dmowski, W. P.: J. Reprod. Med. 35: 69–74, 1990.
126. Reid, P., Kantoff, P., and Oh, W.: Invest. New Drugs 17:271–284, 1999.
127. Singh, S. M., Gauthier, S., and Labrie, F.: Curr. Med. Chem. 7:211–247.
128. Mukherjee, A., Kirkovsky, L., Yao, X. T., et al.: Xenobiotica 26:117–122, 1996.
129. Li, X., Chen, C., Singh, S. M., et al.: Steroids 60:430–441, 1995.
130. Jin, Y., and Penning, T. M.: Best Pract. Res. Clin. Endocrinol. Metab. 15:79–94, 2001.
131. Harris, G. S., and Kozarich, J. W.: Curr. Opin. Chem. Biol. 1:254–259, 1997.
132. Bull, H. G., Garcia-Calvo, M., Andersson, S., et al.: J. Am. Chem. Soc. 118:2359–2365, 1996.
133. Thomas, L. N., Douglas, R. C., Vessey, J. P., et al.: J. Urol. 170:2019–2025, 2003.
134. Issa, M. M., Runken, M. C., Grogg, A. L., et al.: Am. J. Manag. Care 13(Suppl 1):S10–S16, 2007.
135. Fleshner, N., Gomella, L. G., Cookson, M. S., et al.: Contemp. Clin. Trials, 2007.
136. Buck, A. C.: J. Urol. 172:1792–1799, 2004.
137. Gao, W., and Dalton, J. T.: Drug Discov. Today 12:241–248, 2007.
138. Omwancha, J., and Brown, T. R.: Curr. Opin. Investig. Drugs 7:873–881, 2006.
139. Stowasser, M., and Gordon, R. D.: J. Steroid Biochem. Mol. Biol. 78:215–229, 2001.
140. Peter, M., Dubuis, J. M., and Sippell, W. G.: Horm. Res. 51:211–222, 1999.
141. Dacou-Voutetakis, C., Maniati-Christidi, M., and Dracopoulou-Vabouli, M.: J. Pediatr. Endocrinol. Metab. 14(Suppl 5):1303–1308, 2001.
142. Schimmer, B. P., and Parker, K. L.: Adrenocorticotropic hormone; adrenocortical steroids and their synthetic analogs; inhibitors of the synthesis and actions of adrenocortical hormones. In Brunton, L. L., Lazo, J. S., and Parker, K. L. (eds.). Goodman and Gilman's The Pharmacological Basis of Therapeutics, 11th ed. New York, McGraw-Hill, 2006.
143. Amsterdam, A., Tajima, K., and Sasson, R.: Biochem. Pharmacol. 64:843–850, 2002.
144. Van Laethem, F., Baus, E., Andris, F., et al.: Cell Mol. Life Sci. 58:599–1606, 2001.
145. Karin, M., and Chang, L.: J. Endocrinol. 169:447–451, 2001.
146. Sternberg, E. M.: J. Endocrinol. 169:429–435, 2001.
147. De Bosscher, K., Vanden Berghe, W., and Haegeman, G.: J. Neuroimmunol. 109:16–22, 2000.
148. Chikanza, I. C.: Ann. N. Y. Acad. Sci. 966: 39–48, 2002.
149. Loke, T. K., Sousa, A. R., Corrigan, C. J., et al.: Curr. Allergy Asthma Rep. 2:144–150, 2002.
150. Kino, T., and Chrousos, G. P.: J. Endocrinol. 169:437–445, 2001.
151. Goleva, E., Kisich, K. O., and Leung, D. Y.: J. Immunol. 169:5934–5940.
152. Avery, M. A., and Woolfrey, J. R.: Anti-inflammatory steroids. In Abraham, D. J. (ed.). Burger's Medicinal Chemistry and Drug Discovery, 6th ed., vol 3. Hoboken, Wiley-Interscience, 2003.
153. Hennebold, J. D., and Daynes, R. A.: Arch. Dermatol. Res. 290:413–419, 1998.
154. Foe, K., Cheung, H. T., Tattam, B. N., et al.: Drug Metab. Dispos. 26:132–137, 1998.
155. Daley-Yates, P. T., Price, A. C., Sisson, J. R., et al.: Br. J. Clin. Pharmacol. 51:400–409, 2001.
156. Clevenbergh, P., Corcostegui, M., Gerard, D., et al.: J. Infect. 44:94–195, 2002.
157. Baulieu, E. E.: Recent Prog. Horm. Res. 52:1–32, 1997.
158. Tsutsui, K.: J. Steroid Biochem. Mol. Biol. 102:187–194, 2006.

Prostaglandins, Leukotrienes, and Essential Fatty Acids

THOMAS J. HOLMES, JR.

CHAPTER OVERVIEW

Lipidomics, which is the quantitative measurement of specifically identified, highly fat-soluble materials found naturally in the human body, is a subset of metabolomics, whose goal is to establish patterns of occurrence or change of intermediary metabolites that might help characterize conditions of health or disease. Prostaglandins, leukotrienes, and essential fatty acids are just three of the many fat-soluble, naturally occurring "targets" or "markers" for such investigations. Other lipids of high interest include cholesterol, steroid hormones, triglycerides, sphingolipids, phospholipids, glycolipids, the fat-soluble vitamins (A, D, E, K, Q), and the myriad derivatives of these compounds. Essential fatty acids are those polyunsaturated fatty acids (PUFA) that must be included in the human diet to maintain health. Various omega-3 and omega-6 fatty acids are included in this group. The prostaglandins (PGA through PGJ) are one group of naturally occurring 20-carbon fatty acid derivatives produced by the oxidative metabolism of 5,8,11,14-eicosatetraenoic acid, an omega-6 fatty acid, which is also called *arachidonic acid*. Other so-called eicosanoids produced in the complex biologic oxidation scheme called the *arachidonic acid cascade* are thromboxane A_2 (TXA_2), the leukotrienes (LKT A–F), and the highly potent antithrombotic agent prostacyclin (PGI_2). Although eicosanoid-derived agents in current human clinical therapy are few, the promise of future contributions from this area is presumed to be very great. This promise stems from the fact that intermediates of arachidonic acid metabolism play an essential modulatory role in many normal and disease-related cellular processes. In fact, much of the pain, fever, swelling, nausea, and vomiting associated with "illness," in general is probably a result of excessive prostaglandin production in damaged tissues.

ESSENTIAL FATTY ACIDS

The fatty acids that are absolutely necessary to maintain the health of humans are generally polyunsaturated, even-numbered organic acids derived from plants or marine animals. For example, the essential fatty acids linoleic acid (18:2) and alpha-linolenic acid (ALA,18:3) are respectively omega-6 and omega-3 18-carbon fatty acids, which occur naturally in olive oil as well as other oil-rich plants and seeds. Other PUFA, such as eicosapentaenoic acid (EPA; 20:5) and docasahexaenoic acid (DHA; 22:6) are omega-3 fatty acids that occur in the oils of cold-water ocean fish and have been found to be beneficial to the cardiovascular health of humans. The nomenclature for these PUFA is presented in Table 26.1.

In general, the designation (18:2) indicates that the fatty acid contains 18 carbon atoms and two double bonds, and the omega designation indicates the position of the double bond relative to the last carbon in the fatty acid. Thus, an 18:2 omega-3 fatty acid would have its last double bond terminating at the third carbon from the 18th carbon of the fatty acid (likewise omega-6 indicating the last double bond terminating at the sixth carbon from the end). Omega-9 fatty acids, such as oleic acid (18:1), are not considered essential to the diet but often occur in natural mixtures of unsaturated fatty acids. The omega designation has been transformed to an "n" designation (i.e., n-3, n-6, n-9) in some publications. A delta superscript designation indicates the position of each double bond relative to the carboxylic acid terminus. All double bonds occurring in natural fatty acids are of the *cis*-configuration. The production of harmful *trans*-unsaturated fatty acids (and their triglyceride ester derivatives) occurs as a result of commercial "partial" hydrogenation methods designed to raise the boiling point (cooking temperature) for vegetable oils used in deep-frying popular foods. Partial hydrogenation of vegetable oils was initially considered beneficial in that completely saturated fats (no double bonds) derived from animal fats (i.e., lard) could be replaced in the cooking process.

HISTORY OF EICOSANOID DISCOVERY

Early in the past century (1931), it was noted by Kurzrok and Lieb[1] that human seminal fluid could increase or decrease spontaneous muscle contractions of uterine tissue under controlled conditions. This observed effect on uterine musculature was believed to be induced by an acidic vasoactive substance formed in the prostate gland, which was later (1936) termed *prostaglandin* by von Euler.[2] Much later (1950s), it was found that the acidic extract contained not one but several structurally related prostaglandin substances.[3] These materials subsequently were separated, purified, and characterized as the prostaglandins (PGA through PGJ), varying somewhat in degree of oxygenation and dehydrogenation and markedly in biologic activity (see Table 26.2). Specific stereochemical syntheses of the prostaglandins provided access to sufficient quantities of purified materials for wide-scale biologic evaluation and confirmed the structural characterization of these complex substances.[4]

TABLE 26.1 Nomenclature of Unsaturated Fatty Acids

Oleic acid	HOOC—CH_2—CH_2—CH_2—CH_2—CH_2—CH_2—CH_2— CH=CH—CH_2—CH_2—CH_2—CH_2—CH_2—CH_2— CH_2—CH_3	18:1 omega-9 n-9 delta-9
Linoleic acid	HOOC—CH_2—CH_2—CH_2—CH_2—CH_2—CH_2—CH_2— CH=CH—CH_2—CH=CH—CH_2—CH_2—CH_2— CH_2—CH_3	18:2 omega-6 n-6 delta-9, -12
Alpha-linolenic acid (ALA)	HOOC—CH_2—CH_2—CH_2—CH_2—CH_2—CH_2—CH_2— CH=CH—CH_2—CH=CH—CH_2—CH=CH—CH_2—CH_3	18:3 omega-3 n-3 delta-9, -12, -15
Arachidonic acid	HOOC—CH_2—CH_2—CH_2—CH_2—CH=CH—CH_2—CH= CH—CH_2—CH=CH—CH_2—CH=CH—CH_2—CH_2— CH_2—CH_2—CH_3	20:4 omega-6 n-6 delta-5, -8, -11, -14
Eicosapentaenoic acid (EPA)	HOOC—CH_2—CH_2—CH_2—CH=CH—CH_2—CH= CH—CH_2—CH=CH—CH_2—CH=CH—CH_2—CH= CH—CH_2—CH_3	20:5 omega-3 n-3 delta-5, -8, -11, -14, -17
Docosahexaenoic acid (DHA)	HOOC—CH_2—CH_2—CH=CH—CH_2—CH=CH—CH_2— CH=CH—CH_2—CH=CH—CH_2—CH=CH—CH_2—CH= CH—CH_2—CH_3	22:6 omega-3 n-3 delta-4, -7, -10, -13, -16, -19

TABLE 26.2 Biological Activities Observed with the Eicosanoids

Substance	Observed Biological Activity
PGD_2	Weak inhibitor of platelet aggregation Mast cell allergic response
PGE_1	Vasodilation Inhibitor of lipolysis Inhibitor of platelet aggregation Bronchodilatation Stimulates contraction of gastrointestinal smooth muscle
PGE_2	Stimulates hyperalgesic response Renal vasodilatation Stimulates uterine smooth muscle contraction Protects gastrointestinal epithelia from acid degradation Reduces secretion of stomach acid
PGF_2	Elevates thermoregulatory set point in anterior hypothalamus Stimulates breakdown of corpus luteum (luteolysis) in animals Stimulates uterine smooth muscle contraction
PGI_2	Potent inhibitor of platelet aggregation Potent vasodilator Increases cAMP levels in platelets
PGJ_2	Stimulates osteogenesis Inhibits cell proliferation
TXA_2	Potent inducer of platelet aggregation Potent vasoconstrictor Decreases cAMP levels in platelets Stimulates release of ADP and serotonin from platelets
LTB_4	Increases leukocyte chemotaxis and aggregation
LTC/D_4	Slow-reacting substances of anaphylaxis Potent and prolonged contraction of guinea pig ileum smooth muscle Contracts guinea pig lung parenchymal strips Bronchoconstrictive in humans Increased vascular permeability in guinea pig skin (augmented by PGEs)
5- or 12-HPETE	Vasodilatation of rat and rabbit gastric circulation Inhibits induced platelet aggregation
5- or 12-HETE	Aggregates human leukocytes Promotes leukocyte chemotaxis

Although many scientists have contributed to a refined characterization of the eicosanoid biosynthetic pathways and the biologic consequences of this cascade (currently dubbed "eicosanomics"), the discerning and persistent pioneering efforts of Sune Bergström, Bengt Samuellson, and John R. Vane were recognized by the award of a shared Nobel Prize in Medicine in 1982. These scientists not only dedicated themselves to the chemical and biologic characterization of the eicosanoid substances, but also were the first to realize the profound significance of the arachidonic acid cascade in disease processes, particularly inflammation. These individuals first proved that the mechanism of the anti-inflammatory action of aspirin and related nonsteroidal anti-inflammatory drugs (NSAIDs) was a direct result of their inhibitory effect on prostaglandin formation. It was shown subsequently that the analgesic and antipyretic effects of these NSAIDs, as well as their proulcerative and anticoagulant side effects, also result from their effect on eicosanoid metabolism (e.g., inhibition of cyclooxygenases 1 and 2 [COX-1 and COX-2]) (see the "Selected Reading" listed at the end of this chapter for comprehensive reviews of the diverse biological roles of the eicosanoids).

EICOSANOID BIOSYNTHESIS

Prostaglandins and other eicosanoids are produced by the oxidative metabolism of free arachidonic acid. Under normal circumstances, arachidonic acid is not available for metabolism as it is present as a conjugated component of the phospholipid matrix of most cellular membranes. Release of free arachidonic acid, which subsequently may be oxidatively metabolized, occurs by stimulation of phospholipase (PLA_2) enzyme activity in response to some traumatic event (e.g., tissue damage, toxin exposure, or hormonal stimulation). It is believed that the clinical anti-inflammatory effect of glucocortical steroids (i.e., hydrocortisone) is a result of their ability to suppress PLA_2 activity via lipocortins and thus prevent the release of free arachidonic acid.[5] Modulation of PLA_2 activity by alkali metal ions, toxins, and various therapeutic agents has become a major focus of biologic research because of the changes in eicosanoid production and the dramatic biological effects accompanying PLA_2 stimulation or suppression. Although it was initially believed that the inflammatory response (swelling, redness, pain) was principally a result of PGE_2, recent interest has focused on the interrelationships of PGE-type eicosanoids with the cytokines, such as interleukins-1 and -2, in the modulation of inflammatory reactions.[6]

Two different routes for oxygenation of arachidonic acid have been identified: the cyclooxygenase pathway (Fig. 26.1) and the lipoxygenase pathway (Fig. 26.2). The relative significance of each of these pathways may vary in a particular tissue or disease state. The cyclooxygenase pathway, so named because of the unusual bicyclic endoperoxide (PGG_2) produced in the first step of the sequence, involves the highly stereospecific addition of two molecules of oxygen to the arachidonic acid substrate, followed by subsequent enzyme-controlled rearrangements to produce an array of oxygenated eicosanoids with diverse biologic activities (see Table 26.2). The first enzyme in this pathway, PGH-synthase, is a hemoprotein that catalyzes both the addition of oxygen (to form PGG_2) and the subsequent reduction (peroxidase activity) of the 15-position hydroperoxide to the 15-(S)-configuration alcohol (PGH_2).[7] PGH-synthase (also called *cyclooxygenase-1[COX-1]* or *-2 [COX-2]*, and formerly *PG-synthetase*) has been the focus of intense investigation because of its key role as the first enzyme in the arachidonic acid cascade.[8] It is this enzyme in constitutive (COX-1) or inducible form (COX-2) that is susceptible to inhibition by NSAIDs, leading to relief of pain, fever, and inflammation.[6,9] This enzyme is also inhibited by the ω-3 (omega-3) fatty acids (EPA and docosahexaenoic acid [DHA]) found in certain cold-water fish, which are provided commercially as nutritional supplements, leading to beneficial cardiovascular effects.[10] Cyclooxygenase will

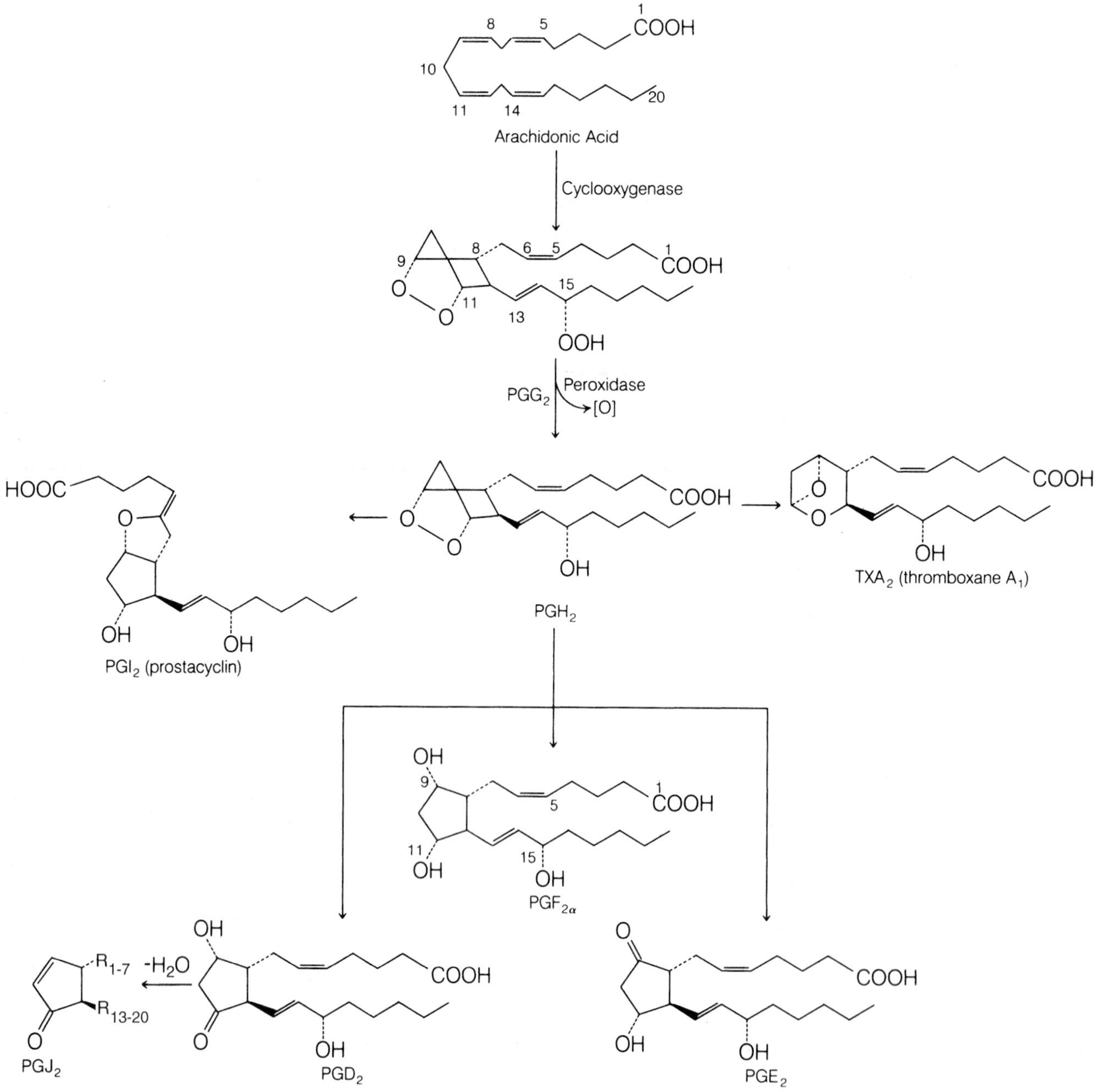

Figure 26.1 ● Cyclooxygenase pathway.

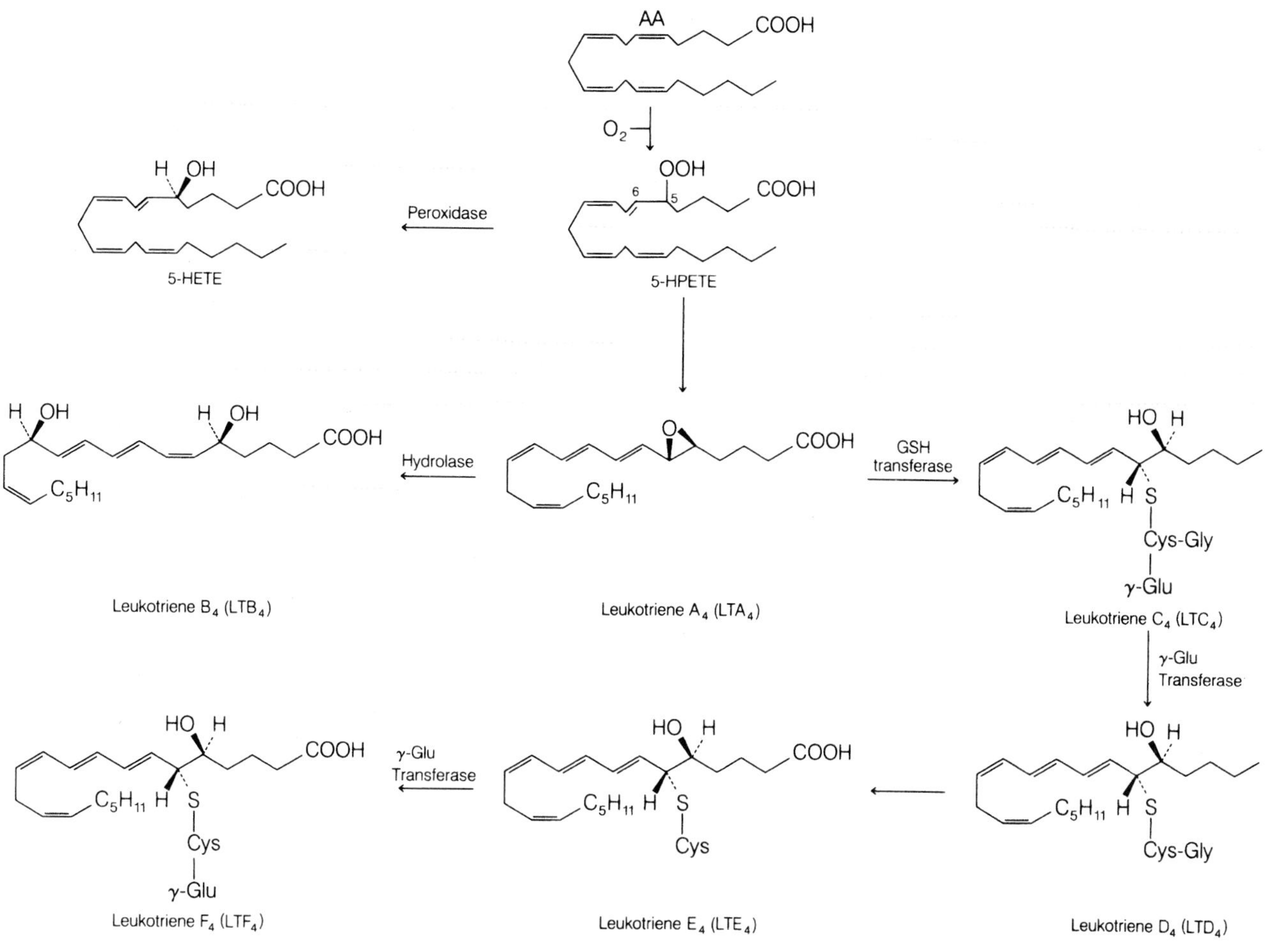

Figure 26.2 ● Lipoxygenase pathway.

metabolize 20-carbon fatty acids with one more or one less double bond than arachidonic acid, leading to prostaglandins of varied degrees of unsaturation (e.g., PGE_1 or PGE_3, for which the subscript number indicates the number of double bonds in the molecule).

Prostaglandin H_2 serves as a branch-point substrate for specific enzymes, leading to the production of the various prostaglandins, TXA_2, and PGI_2. Even though most tissues can produce PGH_2, the relative production of each of these derived eicosanoids is highly tissue specific and may be subject to secondary modulation by various cofactors. The complete characterization of enzymes involved in branches of the cyclooxygenase pathway and their genetic origins is currently under way.[11]

Specific cellular or tissue responses to the eicosanoids are apparently a function of available surface receptor recognition sites.[12] The various tissue responses observed on eicosanoid exposure is outlined in Table 26.2. Nontissue-selective inhibitors of the cyclooxygenase pathway, such as aspirin, thus may exert a diversity of therapeutic effects or side effects (e.g., decreased uterine muscle contraction and platelet aggregation, gastric ulceration, lowering of elevated body temperature, central and peripheral pain relief, and decreased vascular perfusion) based on the inhibitor's tissue distribution profile.

The lipoxygenase pathway of arachidonic acid metabolism (Fig. 26.2) produces various acyclic lipid peroxides

(hydroperoxyeicosatetraenoic acids [HPETEs]) and derived alcohols (hydroxyeicosatetraenoic acids [HETEs]).[13] Although the specific biologic function of each of these lipoxygenase-derived products is not completely known, they are believed to play a major role as chemotactic factors that promote cellular mobilization toward sites of tissue injury. In addition, the glutathione (GSH) conjugates LKT-C_4 and LKT-D_4 are potent, long-acting bronchoconstrictors that are released in the lungs during severe hypersensitivity episodes (leading to their initial designation as the "slow-reacting substances of anaphylaxis" [SRSAs]). Because of the presumed benefit of preventing formation of LKTs in asthmatic patients, much research effort is being dedicated to the design and discovery of drugs that might selectively inhibit the lipoxygenase pathway of arachidonic acid metabolism, without affecting the cyclooxygenase pathway.[14] Zileuton (Zyflo by Abbott Laboratories) specifically inhibits the 5-lipoxygenase (5-LO) pathway. It has been proposed that aspirin hypersensitivity in susceptible individuals may result from effectively "shutting down" the cyclooxygenase metabolic route, allowing only the biosynthesis of lipoxygenase pathway intermediates, including the bronchoconstrictive LKTs.[14] Other drugs (i.e., Singulair) have been developed, which block the receptors for certain leukotrienes. Considerable effort has also been directed toward discovering inhibitors of 5-LO activating protein (FLAP), which affects this pathway.[15]

DRUG ACTION MEDIATED BY EICOSANOIDS

The ubiquitous nature of the eicosanoid-producing enzymes implies their significance in various essential cellular processes. In addition, the sensitivity of these enzymes to structurally varied hydrophobic materials, particularly carboxylic acids and phenolic antioxidants, implies their susceptibility to influence by various exogenously administered agents.

The only group of drugs that has been thoroughly characterized for its effect on arachidonic acid metabolism is the NSAIDs. This large group of acidic, aromatic molecules exerts a diverse spectrum of activities (mentioned previously in this chapter) by inhibition of the first enzyme in the arachidonic acid cascade, PGH-synthase. Such agents as salicylic acid, phenylbutazone, naproxen, sulindac, and ibuprofen presumably act by a competitive, reversible inhibition of arachidonic acid oxygenation.[16] Aspirin and certain halogenated aromatics (including indomethacin, flurbiprofen, and meclomen) appear to inhibit PGH-synthase in a time-dependent, irreversible manner.[17] Since this irreversible inhibition appears critical for aspirin's significant effect on platelet aggregation and, therefore, prolongation of bleeding time,[18] this discovery has led clinicians to recommend the daily consumption of low doses of aspirin (81 mg) in patients at risk for myocardial infarction (MI; heart attack), particularly a second MI.

Interestingly, aspirin's primary competitor in the commercial analgesic marketplace, acetaminophen, is a rather weak inhibitor of arachidonic acid oxygenation in vitro.[19] This, in fact, is a characteristic of reversible, noncompetitive, phenolic antioxidant inhibitors in general.[20] This determination, in concert with its lack of in vitro anti-inflammatory activity (while maintaining analgesic and antipyretic activity equivalent to that of the salicylates), has led to the proposal that acetaminophen is more active as an inhibitor of cyclooxygenases in the brain, where peroxide levels (which stimulate cyclooxygenase activity) are lower, than in inflamed peripheral joints, where lipid peroxide levels are high.[16] In fact, when in vitro experimental conditions are modified to reduce the so-called peroxide tone, acetaminophen becomes as effective an inhibitor as aspirin in reducing arachidonic acid metabolism.[19]

COX-2 INHIBITORS

The newer anti-inflammatory COX-2 inhibitors were claimed to show greater inhibitory selectivity for the inducible form of cyclooxygenase.[21] Although not absolute, this selectivity provides a potential therapeutic advantage by reducing side effects, particularly gastric irritation and ulceration.[22] Unfortunately, this altered profile of activity is not totally risk free. The manufacturer of rofecoxib (Vioxx) issued a warning (April 2002) regarding the use of this product in patients with a medical history of ischemic heart disease, and this product was removed from the market in 2004. COX-2 inhibitors do not share the same beneficial effects as aspirin in preventing cardiovascular thrombotic events.

DESIGN OF EICOSANOID DRUGS

The ability to capitalize successfully on the highly potent biologic effects of the various eicosanoids to develop new therapeutic agents currently seems an unfulfilled promise to medicinal chemists. Although these natural substances are highly potent effectors of various biologic functions, their use as drugs has been hampered by the following factors: (a) their chemical complexity and relative instability, which have limited, to some extent, their large-scale production and formulation for clinical testing; (b) their susceptibility to rapid degradation in vivo (Fig. 26.3), which limits their effective bioactive half-life; and (c) their propensity to affect diverse tissues (particularly the gastrointestinal tract, which may lead to severe nausea and vomiting) if they enter the systemic circulation, even in small amounts. Caution is always recommended with the use of prostaglandin analogs in women of childbearing age because of their potential for inducing dramatic contraction of uterine muscles, possibly leading to miscarriage.

Several approaches have been used to overcome these difficulties. First, structural analogs of particular eicosanoids have been synthesized that are more resistant to chemical and metabolic degradation but maintain, to a large extent, a desirable biologic activity. Although commercial production and formulation may be facilitated by this approach, biological potency of these analogs is usually reduced by several orders of magnitude. Also, systemic side effects may become troublesome because of broader tissue distribution as a result of the increased biological half-life.

Structural alterations of the eicosanoids have been aimed primarily at reducing or eliminating the very rapid metabolism of these potent substances to relatively inactive metabolites (see Fig. 26.3). Several analogs are presented in Table 26.3 to illustrate approaches that have led to potentially useful eicosanoid drugs. Methylation at the 15- or 16-position will eliminate or reduce oxidation of the essential 15-(S)-alcohol moiety. Esterification of the carboxylic acid function may affect formulation or absorption characteristics of the eicosanoid, whereas esterase enzymes in the bloodstream or tissues would be expected to quickly regenerate the active therapeutic agent. Somewhat surprisingly, considering the restrictive configurational requirements at the naturally asymmetric centers, various hydrophobic substituents (including phenyl rings) may replace the saturated alkyl chains, with retention of bioactivity.

A second major approach has been aimed at delivering the desired agent, either a natural eicosanoid or a modified analog, to a localized site of action by a controlled delivery method. The exact method of delivery may vary according to the desired site of action (e.g., uterus, stomach, lung) but has included aerosols and locally applied suppository, gel formulations, or cyclodextrin complexes. The recent commercial development of prostaglandin PGF-type derivatives for use in the eye to lower intraocular pressure (IOP) in glaucoma (discussed under "Prostaglandins for Ophthalmic Use") relies on their potent therapeutic effects coupled with their limited distribution from this site of administration.[23]

Prostaglandins

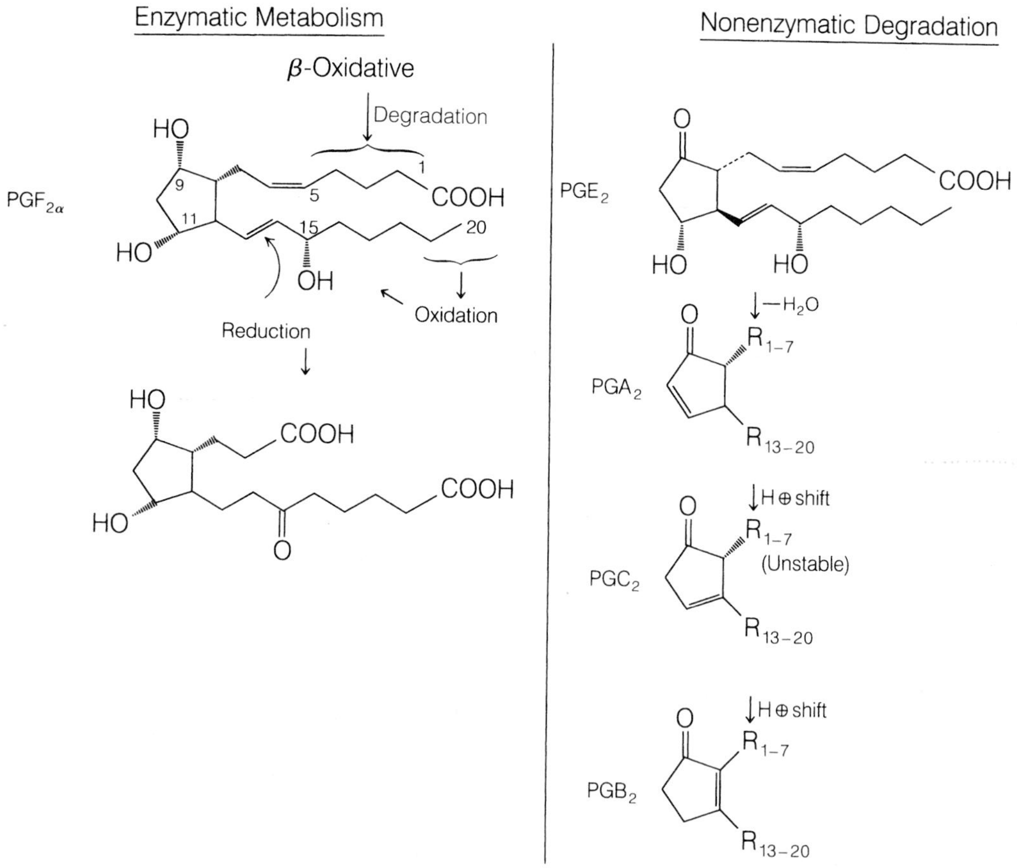

Enzymatic Metabolism

Nonenzymatic Degradation

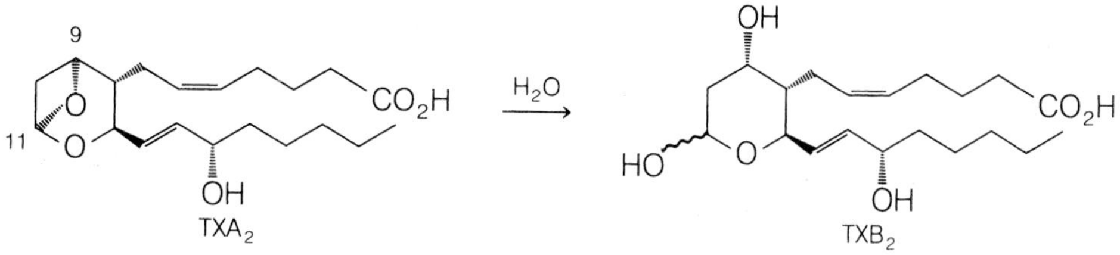

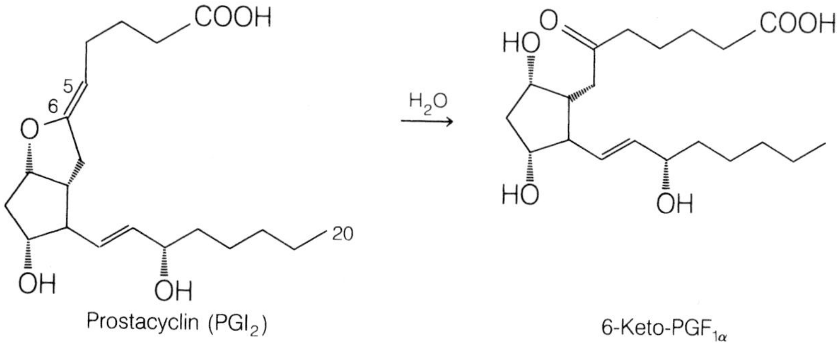

Figure 26.3 ● Eicosanoid degradation.

TABLE 26.3   Prostaglandin Analogs under Investigation as Receptor Ligands and Future Drug Candidates

Structure	Name	Activity
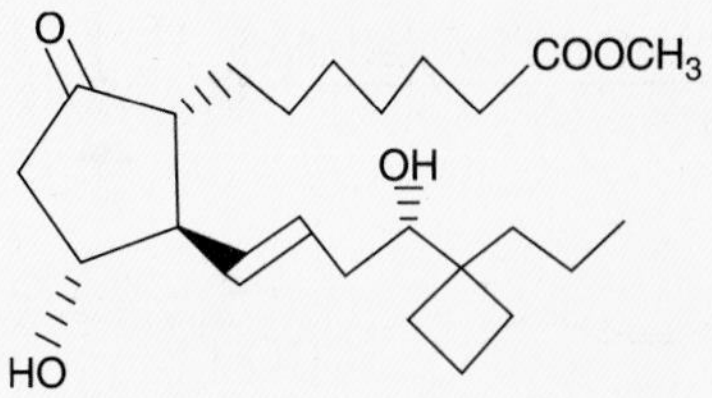	Butaprost	EP$_2$-receptor ligand
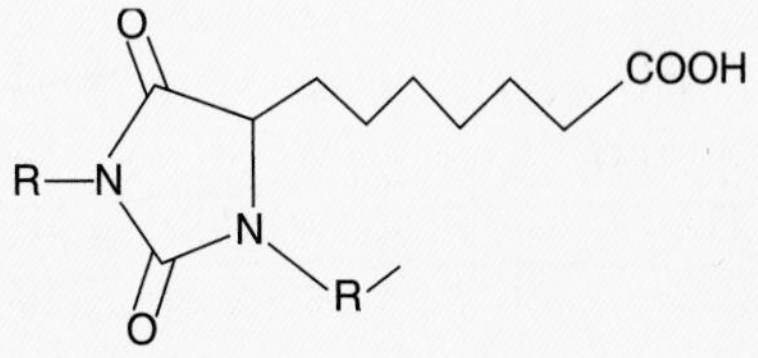	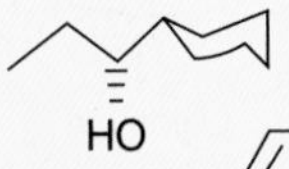 BW245C: R = H BWA 868C: R = CH$_2$ 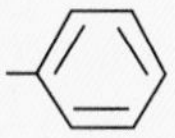 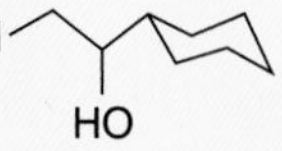	DP-receptor ligands
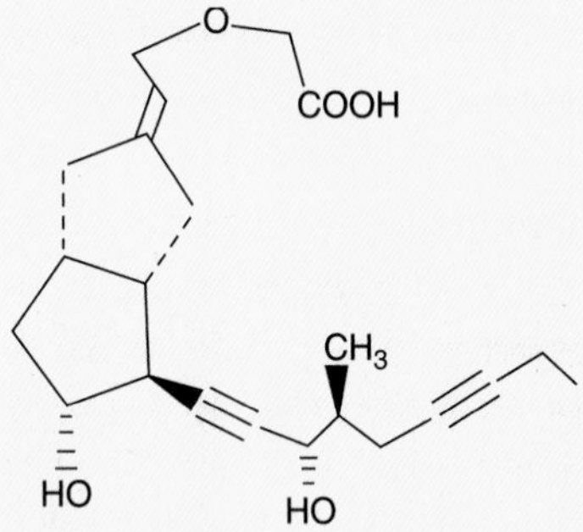	Cicaprost	IP-receptor ligand
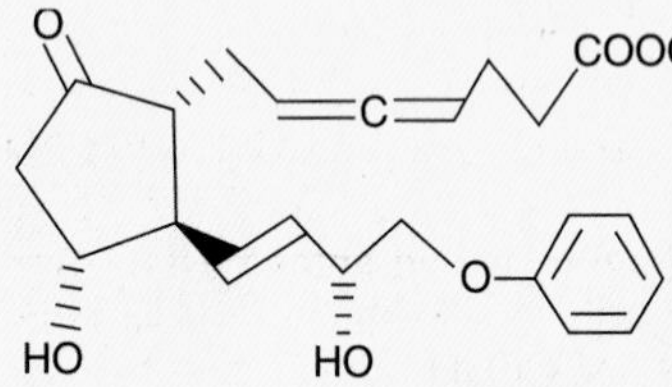	Enprostil (Roche)	EP$_3$-receptor ligand antiulcer therapy
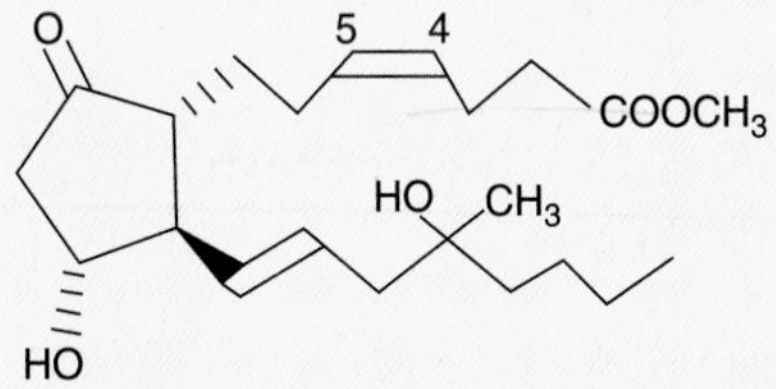	Enisoprost (Searle)	Orphan status: cyclosporine toxicity
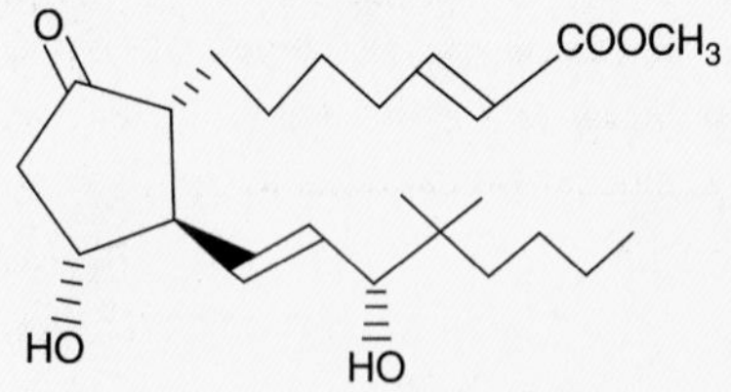	Gemeprost (Cervagem by Ono Pharmaceuticals)	Abortifacient
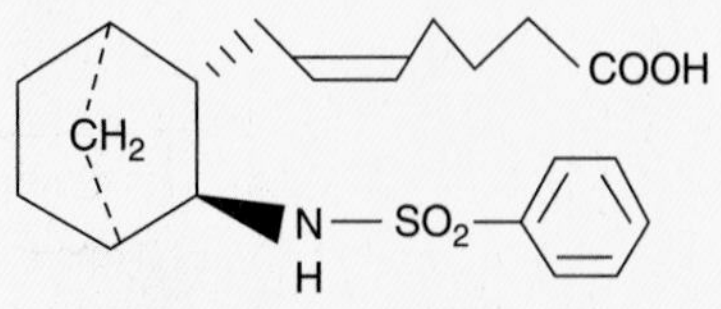	S-145	TP-receptor ligand

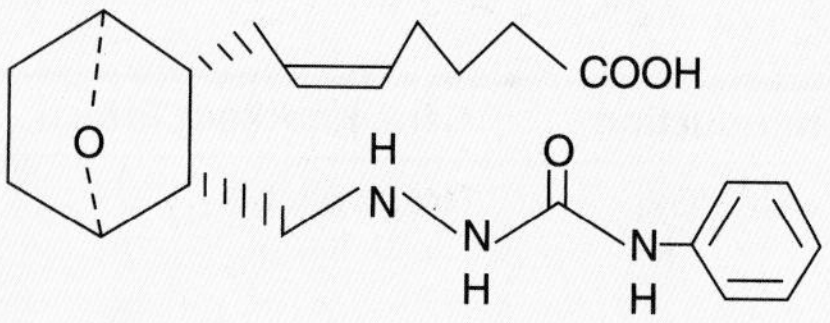	SQ-29548	TP-receptor ligand
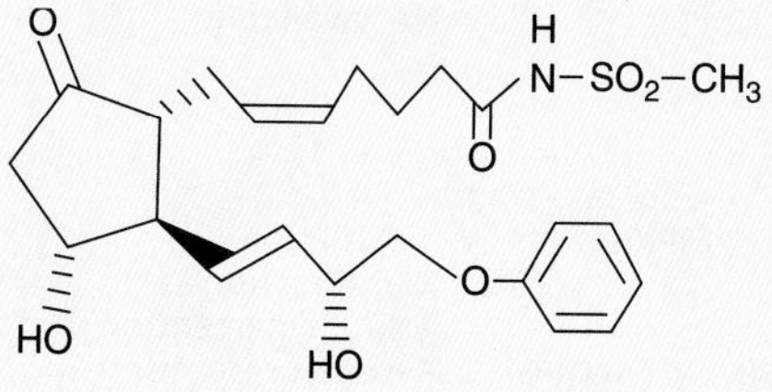	Sulprostone (Glofil Banca Dati Sanitaria Farmaceutical)	EP-receptor ligand Oxytoxic
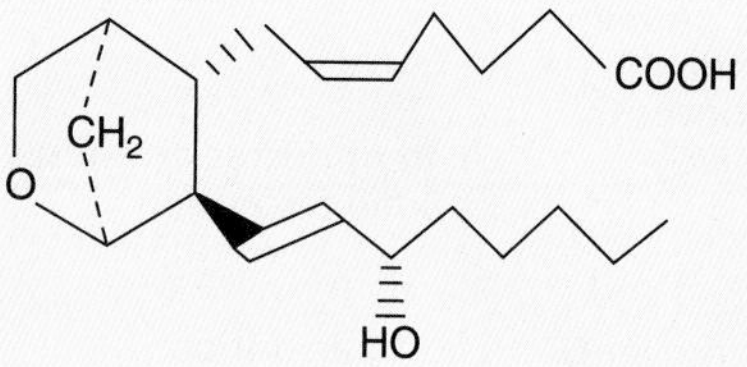	U-46619	TP-receptor ligand

EICOSANOID RECEPTORS

Another approach to developing new therapies based on the known biological activities of the prostaglandins and leukotrienes requires characterization of the naturally occurring tissue receptors for these agents. A thorough knowledge of the tissue distribution (localization) of such receptors and their binding characteristics would allow the design of receptor-specific agonists or antagonists, which might not possess the same limitations as the natural eicosanoids, but could affect tissue function nonetheless.[24]

An excellent historical description of prostanoid receptor isolation and characterization has been published[25]; and, a review of developments in this field is available.[12] Basically, prostanoid receptors are identified by their primary eicosanoid agonist (e.g., DP, EP, IP, and TP), although subclassification of PGE receptors has been necessary (e.g., EP_1, EP_2, EP_3, and EP_4), and separate DP_1 and DP_2 have also recently been proposed. In fact, subtypes of the EP_3 receptor (EP_{3A}, EP_{3B}, EP_{3C}, EP_{3D}) and TP receptor (TP_α, TP_β) have also been proposed. Complete characterization of receptors (and subtypes) includes tissue localization, biological effect produced, cellular signal transduction mechanism, inhibitor sensitivity, protein structure, and genetic origin. Not all receptors, or subtypes, have been completely characterized in this way, but significant progress toward this goal has occurred recently. Table 26.4 indicates characteristics of the prostanoid receptors identified thus far.

Although receptor studies have required the use of non-human species (principally, the mouse, but also rat, cow, sheep, and rabbit), a high correlation of structural homology of receptor subtypes between species (approximately 80%–90%) has been observed, whereas structural homology among receptor subtypes is relatively low (30%–50%). All prostanoid receptors, however, are believed to belong to a "rhodopsin-type" superfamily of receptors that function via G-protein–coupled transduction mechanisms. Three general classes of prostanoid receptors are proposed[12]: (a) *relaxant*, including DP, EP_2, EP_4, and IP, which promote smooth muscle relaxation by raising intracellular cyclic adenosine monophosphate (cAMP) levels; (b) *contractile*, including EP_1, FP, and TP, which promote smooth muscle contraction via calcium ion mobilization; and (c) *inhibitory*, such as EP_3, which prevents smooth muscle contraction by lowering intracellular cAMP levels. Although structural and functional characterization of prostanoid receptors has permitted the identification and differentiation of selective receptor ligands (Table 26.3) (both agonists and antagonists), overlapping tissue distributions and common signal transduction mechanisms present formidable obstacles to the development of specific pharmacological therapies.

COMMERCIALLY AVAILABLE ESSENTIAL FATTY ACID SUPPLEMENTS

Lovaza (omega-3-acid ethyl esters) is available from Reliant Pharmaceuticals by prescription only. Formerly known as Omacar, this mixture of omega-3 fatty acid ethyl esters is recommended to reduce very high (500 mg/dL or above) triglyceride blood levels in adults. This product is administered orally and has similar precautions to usage as the available over-the-counter (OTC) products discussed below.

OTC fatty acid supplements ("fish oil" capsules) are widely available as mixtures of omega-3 PUFA containing predominantly DHA and EPA. The primary therapeutic claim for these products is improved cardiovascular health, however, other health claims for these products are broad and may be unsubstantiated. A comprehensive listing of claims and references to supportive evidence has been published.[26] The recommended minimum oral daily dose for these products is 500 mg of combined DHA and EPA. Suggested dosages for specific indications may be 2 to 3 times this level. The natural antioxidant vitamin E may be included in these

TABLE 26.4 **Prostanoid Receptor Characteristics**

Receptor	Principle Ligands	Tissue/Action	Transduction	Gene Knockout Effect
DP_1	PGD_2 BW245C BWA868C	Ileum/muscle relaxation Brain (leptomeninges)/ sleep induction	↑cAMP/Gs	Not available
DP_2	BAY μ3405	Eosinophil chemoattractant (CRTH2)	↑Ca^{2+}	↓Asthmatic response
EP_1	PGE_2 17-phenyl-PGE_2 Sulprostone Iloprost Bimatoprost	Kidney/papillary ducts Lung/bronchoconstriction Stomach/smooth muscle contraction	↑Ca^{2+}	Not available
EP_2 (inducible)	PGE_2; PGE_1 Butaprost (misoprostol)	Lung/bronchodilation Uterus/implantation	↑cAMP/G_s	↓Ovulation ↓Fertilization ↑Na^+ hypertension Pyrogen response
EP_3	PGE_2; PGE_1 Sulprostone Misoprostol Enprostil Gemeprost	Gastric/antisecretory Gastric/cytoprotective Uterus/inhibits contraction Brain/fever response	EP_{3A} ↓ cAMP/G_i EP_{3B} ↑ cAMP/G_s EP_{3C} ↑ cAMP/G_s EP_{3D} ↑PI turnover/G_q	
EP_4	PGE_2; PGE_1 Misoprostol	Ductus arteriosus/relaxant Kidney/glomerulus Gastric antrum/mucous secretion Uterus/endometrium	↑cAMP/G_s	Patent ductus arteriosus ↓Bone resorption
FP	$PGF_{2\alpha}$ Fluprostenol Carboprost Latanoprost Unoprostone Travoprost Bimatoprost	Eye/decreases intraocular pressure Corpus luteum/luteolysis Lung/bronchoconstriction	↑PI turnover/G_q	Lost parturition
IP	PGI_2 Iloprost Cicaprost Beraprost	Platelets/aggregation Arteries/dilation DRG neurons/pain Kidney/afferent arterioles (↑GFR)	↑cAMP/Gs	↑Thrombosis ↓Inflammatory edema
TP	TXA_2 S-145 SQ-29548 U-46619	Lung/bronchoconstriction Kidney/↓ GFR Arteries/constriction Thymus/↓ immature thymocytes	TP_α ↓ cAMP TP_β ↑ cAMP	↑Bleeding

Source: Narumiya, S., Sugimoto, Y., and Ushikubi, F.: Physiol. Rev. 79:1193–1226, 1999.

products as a "preservative" or cobeneficial nutritional supplement. At lower recommended dosages, side effects are generally minimal (i.e., fishy aftertaste or burping; potential diarrhea), however, caution is recommended for patients on anticoagulant therapy who might experience an exaggerated "blood-thinning" effect caused by displacement of protein-bound anticoagulant in the bloodstream.

EICOSANOIDS APPROVED FOR HUMAN CLINICAL USE

Prostaglandin E₂. PGE₂ Dinoprostone (Prostin E2; Cervidil) is a naturally occurring prostaglandin that is administered in a single dose of 10 mg by controlled-release (0.3 mg/hr) vaginal insert to induce cervical ripening. Use of this agent will potentiate the effects of oxytocin.

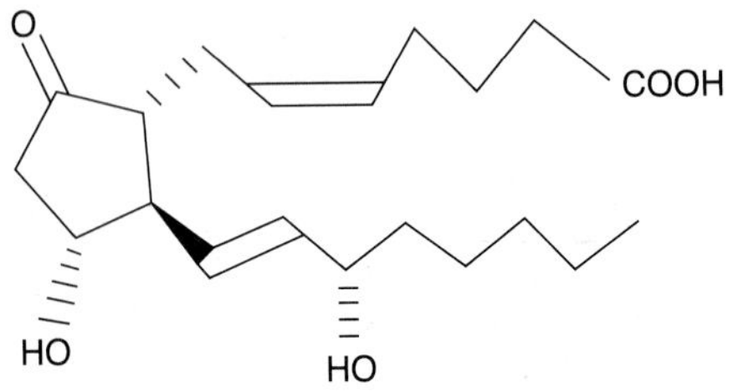

Carboprost Tromethamine. Carboprost tromethamine, 15-(S)-methyl-PGF₂α (Hemabate), is a prostaglandin derivative that has been modified to prevent metabolic oxidation of the 15-position alcohol function. This derivative may be administered in a hospital setting only in a dose of 250 μg by deep intramuscular injection to induce abortion or to ameliorate severe postpartum hemorrhage.

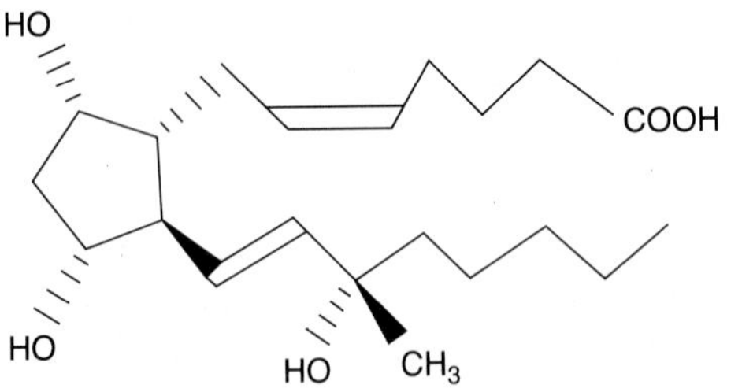

Prostaglandin E₁, United States Pharmacopeia (USP). PGE₁, Alprostadil (Prostin VR Pediatric), is a naturally occurring prostaglandin that has found particular use in maintaining a patent (opened) ductus arteriosus in infants with congenital defects that restrict pulmonary or systemic blood flow.

Alprostadil must be administered intravenously continually at a rate of approximately 0.1 μg/kg/min to temporarily maintain the patency of the ductus arteriosus until corrective surgery can be performed. Up to 80% of circulating alprostadil may be metabolized in a single pass through the lungs. Because apnea has been observed in 10% to 12% of neonates with congenital heart defects, this product should be administered *only* when ventilatory assistance is immediately available. Other commonly observed side effects include decreased arterial blood pressure, which should be monitored during infusion; inhibited platelet aggregation, which might aggravate bleeding tendencies; and diarrhea. Prostin VR Pediatric is provided as a sterile solution in absolute alcohol (0.5 mg/mL) that must be diluted in saline or dextrose solution before intravenous administration. A liposomal preparation is available (Liposome Company) to extend the biological half-life of the active prostaglandin.

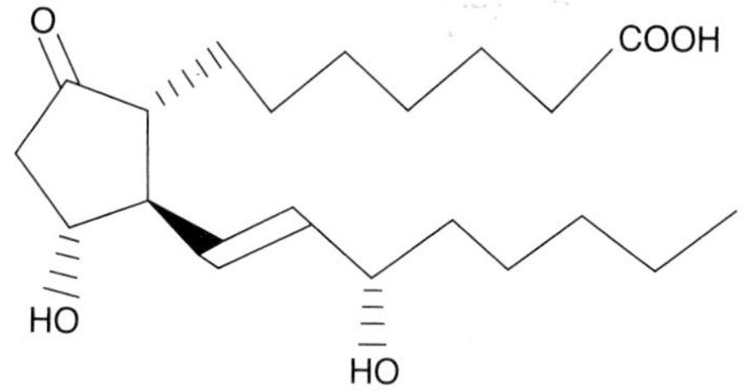

Alprostadil (Caverject) is also available in glass vials for reconstitution to provide 1 mL of solution containing either 10 or 20 μg/mL for intercavernosal penile injection to diagnose or correct erectile dysfunction in certain cases of impotence. The availability of orally administered drugs to treat erectile dysfunction has reduced the therapeutic use of this agent.

Prostaglandin E₁ Cyclodextrin. This cyclic polysaccharide complex of PGE_1 (Vasoprost) is available as an orphan drug for the treatment of severe peripheral arterial occlusive disease when grafts or angioplasty are not indicated. Cyclodextrin complexation is used to enhance water solubility and reduce rapid metabolic inactivation.

Misoprostol. Misoprostol, (16-(R,S)-methyl-16-hydroxy)-PGE_1, methyl ester (Cytotec), is a modified prostaglandin analog that shows potent gastric antisecretory and gastroprotective effects when administered orally. Misoprostol is administered orally in tablet form in a dose of 100 to 200 μg 4 times a day to prevent gastric ulceration in susceptible individuals who are taking NSAIDs. Misoprostol is combined with the NSAID diclofenac (Voltaren) in an analgesic product (Arthrotec by Pharmacia), which is potentially safe for long-term antiarthritic therapy. This prostaglandin derivative absolutely should be avoided by pregnant women because of its potential to induce abortion. In fact, the combined use of intramuscular methotrexate and intravaginal misoprostol has been claimed to be a safe and effective, noninvasive method for the termination of early pregnancy.[27]

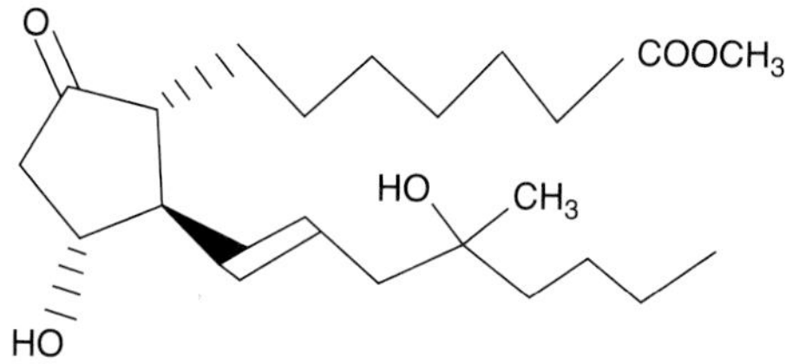

Lubiprostone. This product is marketed as Amitiza by Sucampo Pharmaceuticals, Inc. and Takeda Pharmaceuticals America, Inc. to relieve chronic idiopathic constipation in adults. The recommended oral dosage is 24 μg 2 times a day with food. Precautions and side effects are similar to those for other prostaglandin-derived products.

Prostacyclin (PGI₂). Marketed as the sodium salt (epoprostenol; Flolan by GlaxoSmithKline), this product is administered by continuous infusion of a recently prepared solution (within 48 hours) for the treatment of primary pulmonary hypertension (PPH). The chemical stability of this compound in aqueous solution is limited, and the biological half-life is less than 6 minutes. The potent vasodilatory, platelet antiaggregatory effect, and vascular smooth muscle antiproliferatory effect of this naturally occurring eicosanoid produce a dramatic but short-lived therapeutic effect in PPH patients. Because continuous uninterrupted administration of the drug by portable infusion pump is necessary to prevent symptoms of rebound pulmonary hypertension, distribution of this product is restricted.[28]

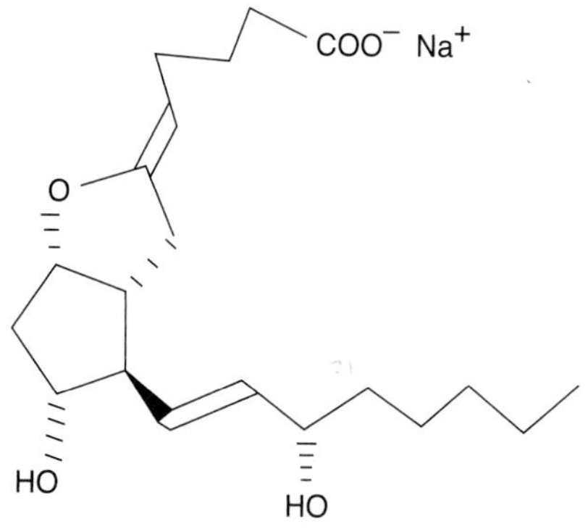

Iloprost. This more chemically and biologically stable derivative of prostacyclin is available as a solution (10 μg/mL) for nasal inhalation (Ventavis by Actelion) via a precisely calibrated inhalation device for the treatment of pulmonary arterial hypertension (PAH). Patients inhale 6 to 8 puffs of aerosolized iloprost every 2 to 3 hours to produce a direct vasodilatory effect on pulmonary blood vessels, thereby decreasing vascular resistance. Side effects of coughing, flushing, headaches, and jaw pain have been most commonly reported.

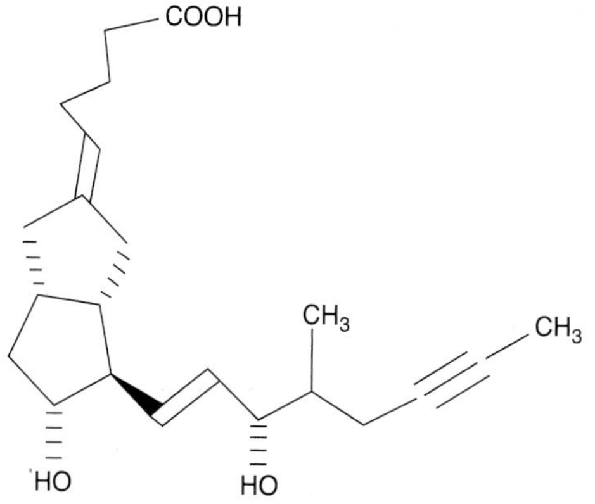

⬡ PROSTAGLANDINS FOR OPHTHALMIC USE

Several prostaglandin analogs have recently come to market for the treatment of open-angle glaucoma or ocular hypertension in patients who have not benefited from other available therapies. These products are marketed as sterile solutions for use in the eye (as indicated). Each of these agents is presumed to lower IOP by stimulation of FP receptors to open the uveoscleral pathway, thus increasing aqueous humor outflow. Commonly occurring side effects reported for this product group include conjunctival hyperemia, increased pigmentation and growth of eyelashes, ocular pruritus, and increased pigmentation of the iris and eyelid. Contact lenses should be removed during and after (15 minutes) administration of these products.

Bimatoprost (Lumigan) is supplied as a sterile 0.03% ophthalmic solution in 2.5- and 5.0-mL sizes. The recommended dosage of bimatoprost is limited to one drop into the affected eye once daily in the evening. Increased usage may decrease its beneficial effect. If used concurrently with other IOP-lowering drugs, a waiting period of 5 minutes should separate administrations.

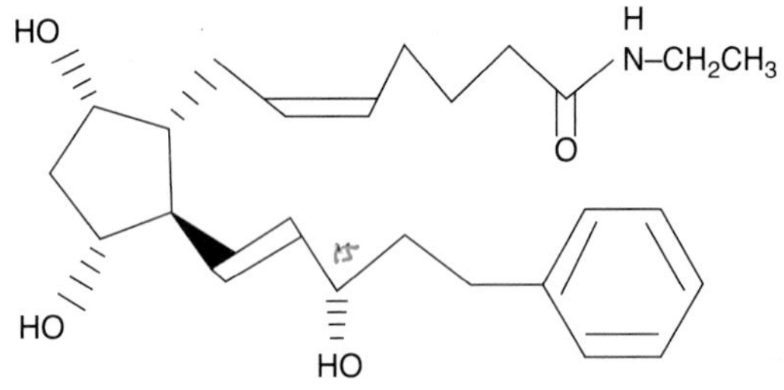

Latanoprost (Xalatan) is available as a 0.005% sterile ophthalmic solution in a 2.5-mL dispenser bottle. Latanoprost is also marketed as a combination ophthalmic product with the β-adrenergic blocking agent, timolol, which apparently enhances IOP-lowering by decreasing the production of aqueous humor. Cautions and side effects are similar to those for other ophthalmic prostanoids.

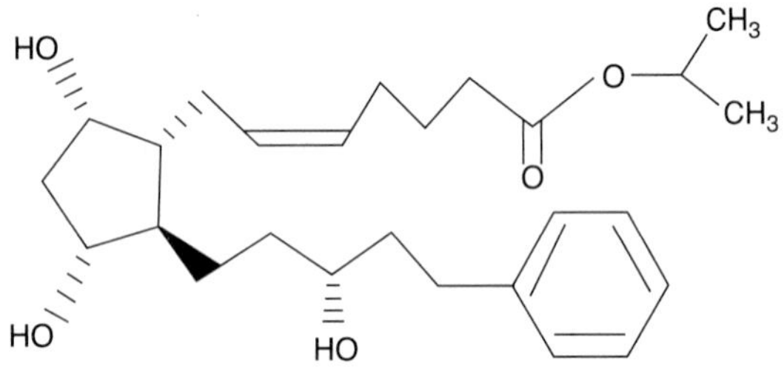

Travoprost (Travatan and Travatan-Z) is supplied as a 2.5- or 5.0-mL sterile 0.004% ophthalmic solution in a 4.0- or 7.5-mL size container. Travoprost is claimed to be the most potent and FP-specific analog in this product category.[29] Cautions and side effects are similar to those given previously.

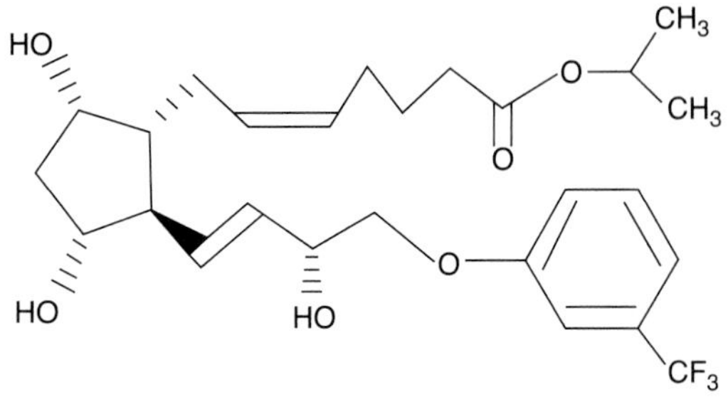

Unoprostone (Rescula) is supplied as a 0.15% sterile ophthalmic solution. Unoprostone is somewhat unusual in that it is a docosanoid (22-carbon atom) $PGF_{2\alpha}$ analog marketed as the isopropyl ester. The natural 15-position alcohol is oxidized to the ketone as would be expected to occur in vivo. Cautions and side effects are similar to those given previously.

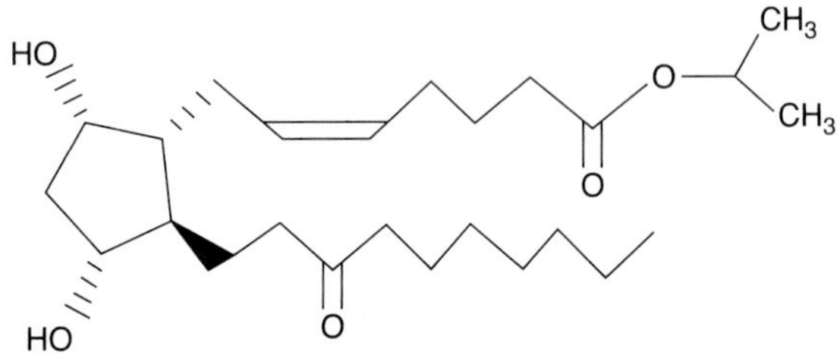

⬡ VETERINARY USES OF PROSTANOIDS

Since McCracken and coworkers[30] demonstrated that $PGF_{2\alpha}$ acts as a hormone in sheep to induce disintegration of the corpus luteum (luteolysis), salts of this prostaglandin and various analogs have been marketed to induce or synchronize estrus in breed animals. This procedure allows artificial insemination of many animals during one insemination period. The following two products are currently available for this purpose.

Cloprostenol Sodium. Cloprostenol sodium (Estrumate) is available as the sodium salt from Bayer Agricultural Division or Bayvet Division of Miles Laboratory as an aqueous solution containing 250 mg/mL.

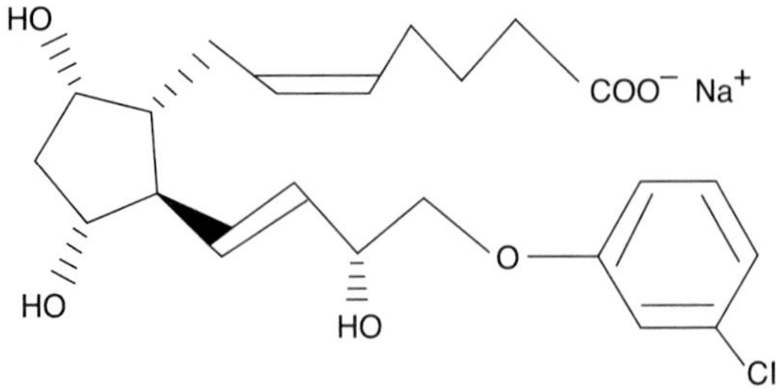

Dinoprost Trimethamine. Dinoprost trimetamine (Lutalyse) marketed by Upjohn Veterinary is a pH-balanced aqueous solution of the trimethylammonium salt of $PGF_{2\alpha}$ (5 mg/mL).

⬡ EICOSANOIDS IN CLINICAL DEVELOPMENT FOR HUMAN TREATMENT

Numerous prostaglandin analogs are under investigation for the treatment of human diseases (see Table 26.3). Efforts are being focused in the areas of gastroprotection as antiulcer therapy, fertility control, the development of thrombolytics (e.g., prostacyclin or thromboxane synthetase inhibitors) to treat cerebrovascular or coronary artery diseases, and the development of antiasthmatics through modulation of the lipoxygenase pathway. However, future application of eicosanoids to the treatment of cancer, hypertension, or immune system disorders cannot be ruled out. Thus, although progress in this area has been slow, the expanded use of eicosanoids or eiconsanoid analogs as therapeutic agents in the future is almost ensured.

◆ R E V I E W   Q U E S T I O N S ◆

1. Why is the initial enzyme in the arachidonic acid cascade called cyclooxygenase?

2. Name three major categories of highly potent chemical mediators of biological processes produced by the arachidonic acid cascade.

3. What chemical and biological properties of natural prostaglandins cause difficulties in the development of successful commercial drug products derived from this group?

4. Name several classes of therapeutic drug products, which provide their beneficial effects through interference with the arachidonic acid cascade.

5. Why are all prostanoid drug products strictly contraindicated in the treatment of women of childbearing age?

6. What particular birth defect may be successfully treated using PGE$_1$?

7. Name the two omega-3 fatty acids, which are usually present in the highest concentrations in over-the-counter nutritional supplement formulations?

8. Which eye disease may be successfully treated by local administration of a dilute solution of PGF$_2$ analogs?

9. Lubiprostone (Amitiza) is recommended for treatment of what condition based on the natural effect of prostaglandins to strongly stimulate contraction of smooth muscles in the GI tract?

10. Why does increased unsaturation (more double bonds) increase the ease of oxidation for long chain fatty acids?

REFERENCES
1. Kurzrok, R., and Lieb, C.: Proc. Soc. Exp. Biol. 28:268, 1931.
2. von Euler, U. S.: J. Physiol. (Lond.) 88:213, 1937.
3. Bergstrom, S., et al.: Acta Chem. Scand. 16:501, 1962.
4. Nicolaou, K. C., and Petasis, N. A.: In Willis, A. L. (ed.). Handbook of Eicosanoids, Prostaglandins and Related Lipids, vol. I, part B. Boca Raton, FL, CRC Press, 1987, pp. 1–18.
5. Flower, R. J., Blackwell, G. J., and Smith, D. L.: In Willis, A. L. (ed.). Handbook of Eicosanoids, Prostaglandins and Related Lipids, vol. II. Boca Raton, FL, CRC Press, 1989, pp. 35–46.
6. Parnham, M. J., Day, R. O., and Van den Berg, W. B.: Agents Actions 41:C145–C149, 1994.
7. Van der Donk, W. A., Tsai, A. L., and Kulmacz, R. J.: Biochemistry 41:15451–15458, 2002.
8. Smith, W. L., Dewitt, D. L., and Garavito, R. M.: Annu. Rev. Biochem. 69:145–182, 2000.
9. Vane, J. R., Bakhle, Y. S., and Botting, R. M.: Annu. Rev. Pharmacol. Toxicol. 38:97–120, 1998
10. Smith, W. L.: Curr. Opin. Cell Biol. 17:174–182, 2005.
11. Kang, Y. J., Mbonye, U. R., DeLong, C. J., et al.: Prog. Lipid Res. 46:108–125, 2007.
12. Narumiya, S., Sugimoto, Y., and Ushikubi, F.: Physiol. Rev. 79:1193–1226, 1999.
13. Kuhn, H.: Prostaglandins Other Lipid Mediat. 62:255–270, 2000.
14. Szczeklik, A.: Adv. Prostaglandin Thromboxane Leukot. Res. 22:185–198, 1994.
15. Friesen, R. W., and Riendeau, D.: In Doherty, A. M. (ed.). Annu. Rep. Med. Chem. 40:199–214, 2005.
16. Lands, W. E. M., Jr.: Trends Pharmacol. Sci. 1:78, 1981.
17. Rome, L. H., and Lands, W. E. M.: Proc. Natl. Acad. Sci. U. S. A. 72:4863, 1975.
18. Higgs, G. A., et al.: Proc. Natl. Acad. Sci. U. S. A. 84:1417, 1987.
19. Hanel, A. M., and Lands, W. E.: Biochem. Pharmacol. 31:3307, 1982.
20. Kuehl, F. A., et al.: In Ramwell, P. (ed.). Prostaglandin Synthetase Inhibitors: New Clinical Applications. New York, Alan R. Liss, 1980, pp. 73–86.
21. Cryer, B., and Feldman, M.: Am. J. Med. 104:413–421, 1998.
22. Warner, T. D., Giuliano, F., Vojnovic, I., et al.: Proc. Natl. Acad. Sci. U. S. A. 96:7563–7568, 1999.
23. Susanna, R., Jr., Giampani, J., Borges, A. S., et al.: Opthalmology 108:259–263, 2001.
24. Medina, J. C., and Liu, J.: In Wood, A. (ed.). Annu. Rep. Med. Chem. 41:221–235, 2006.
25. Coleman, R. A., Smith, W. L., and Narumiya, S.: Pharmacol. Rev. 46:205–229, 1994.
26. Ulbricht, C. E., and Basch, E. M. (eds.): Natural Standards Herb and Supplement Reference: Evidence-Based Clinical Reviews. St. Louis, MO, Elsevier Mosby, 2005, pp. 267–301.
27. Hausknecht, R. V.: N. Engl. J. Med. 333:537–540, 1995.
28. Am. J. Health Syst. Pharm. 53:976, 982, 1996.
29. Sharif, N. A., Davis, T. L., and Williams, G. W.: J. Pharm. Pharmacol. 51:685–694, 1999.
30. McCracken, J. A., et al.: Nature 238:129, 1972.

SELECTED READING
Batt, D. G.: 5-Lipoxygenase inhibitors and their anti-inflammatory activities. Prog. Med. Chem. 29:1–63, 1992.
Chandra, R. K. (ed.): Health Effects of Fish and Fish Oils. St. John's, Newfoundland, ARTS Biomedical Publishers and Distributors, 1989.
Edqvist, L. E., and Kindahl, H. (eds.): Prostaglandins in Animal Reproduction. New York, Elsevier, 1984.
Fukushima, M.: Biological activities and mechanisms of action of PGJ$_2$ and related compounds: an update. Prostaglandins Leukot. Essent. Fatty Acids 47:1–12, 1992.
Gryglewski, R. J., and Stock, G. (eds.): Prostacyclin and Its Stable Analogue Iloprost. New York, Springer-Verlag, 1987.
Pace-Asciak, C. R.: Mass spectra of prostaglandins and related products. Adv. Prostaglandin Thromboxane Leukot. Res. 18:1–565, 1989.
Rainsford, K. D.: Anti-Inflammatory and Anti-Rheumatic Drugs, vols. 1–3. Boca Raton, FL, CRC Press, 1985.
Robinson, H. J., and Vane, J. R. (eds.): Prostaglandin Synthetase Inhibitors. New York, Raven Press, 1974.
Thaler-Dao, H., dePaulet, A. C., and Paoletti, R.: Icosanoids and Cancer. New York, Raven Press, 1984.
Vane, J. R., and O'Grady, J. (eds.): Therapeutic Applications of Prostaglandins. Boston, Edward Arnold, 1993.

Proteins, Enzymes, and Peptide Hormones

STEPHEN J. CUTLER AND HORACE G. CUTLER

CHAPTER OVERVIEW

This chapter describes the role human proteins, enzymes, and peptides play in regulating the mammalian system. It supports the fact that proteins play a critical role in the mechanisms of molecular biology and the role cellular components play in human physiology. This, in turn, not only serves in the development of natural proteins as therapeutic agents, but also in the development of novel synthetic congeners and genetic derivatives. For pharmacists to be good practitioners, it is necessary that they understand how proteins influence normal physiological function as well as to how they can be used in manipulating diseases.

Proteins are essential to all living matter and perform numerous functions as cellular components. Fundamental cellular events are catalyzed by proteins called *enzymes*, while other proteins serve as architectural constituents of protoplasm and cell membranes. Most important are the classes of hormones that are characterized as proteins or proteinlike compounds because of their polypeptidic structure.

Protein chemistry, essential in understanding the mechanisms of molecular biology and how cellular components participate in physiology, is also key to certain aspects of medicinal chemistry. An examination of the chemical nature of proteins explains the action of those medicinal agents that are proteins, or proteinlike compounds, and elucidates their physicochemical and biochemical properties. This, in turn, relates to their mechanisms of action. Furthermore, in medicinal chemistry, drug–receptor interactions are directly related to structure–activity relationships (SARs) and aid in the process of rational drug design. Drug receptors are considered to be macromolecules, some of which appear to be proteins or proteinlike.

Recombinant DNA (rDNA) technology[1] has had a dramatic impact on our ability to produce complex proteins and polypeptides structurally identical with those found in vivo. Many of the endogenous proteins or polypeptides have exhibited neurotransmitter and hormonal properties that regulate various important physiological processes. rDNA-derived technology products currently being used are discussed in this chapter.

Although this chapter reviews the medicinal chemistry of proteins, it includes some enzymology, not only because many drugs affect enzyme systems and vice versa, but also because basic discoveries in enzymology have been practically applied to the study of drug–receptor interactions. Hence, a basic introduction to enzymes is included.

PROTEIN HYDROLYSATES

In therapeutics, agents affecting volume and composition of body fluids include various classes of parenteral products. Ideally, it would be desirable to have available parenteral fluids that provide adequate calories and important proteins and lipids to mimic, as closely as possible, an appropriate diet. Unfortunately, this is not the case. Usually, sufficient carbohydrate is administered intravenously to prevent ketosis, and in some cases, it is necessary to give further sources of carbohydrate by vein to reduce protein waste. Sources of protein are made available in the form of protein hydrolysates, and these can be administered to induce a favorable balance.

Protein deficiencies in human nutrition are sometimes treated with protein hydrolysates. The lack of adequate protein may result from several conditions, but the problem is not always easy to diagnose. The deficiency may be caused by insufficient dietary intake, temporarily increased demands (as in pregnancy), impaired digestion or absorption, liver malfunction, increased catabolism, or loss of proteins and amino acids (e.g., in fevers, leukemia, hemorrhage, surgery, burns, fractures, or shock).

Protein Hydrolysate. Protein hydrolysate is a solution of amino acids and short-chain oligopeptides that represent the approximate nutritive equivalent of the casein, lactalbumin, plasma, fibrin, or other suitable protein from which it is derived by acid, enzymatic, or other hydrolytic methods. It may be modified by partial removal, and restoration or addition of one, or more, amino acids. It may contain dextrose, or another carbohydrate suitable for intravenous infusion. Not less than 50% of the total nitrogen present is in the form of α-amino nitrogen. It is a yellowish to red-amber transparent liquid with a pH of 4 to 7.

Parenteral preparations are used to maintain a positive nitrogen balance in patients who exhibit interference with ingestion, digestion, or absorption of food. For such patients, the material to be injected must be nonantigenic and must not contain pyrogens or peptides of high–molecular weight. Injection may result in untoward effects such as nausea, vomiting, fever, vasodilatation, abdominal pain, twitching and convulsions, edema at the site of injection, phlebitis, and thrombosis. Sometimes, these reactions are caused by inadequate cleanliness or too-rapid administration.

⬡ AMINO ACID SOLUTIONS

Amino acid solutions contain a mixture of essential and nonessential crystalline amino acids, with or without electrolytes (e.g., Aminosyn, ProcalAmine, Travasol, Novamine). Although oral studies have shown a comparison between protein hydrolysates and free amino acid diets,[2] protein hydrolysates are being replaced by crystalline amino acid solutions for parenteral administration because the free amino acids are used more efficiently than the peptides produced by the enzymatic cleavage of protein hydrolysates.[3]

⬡ PROTEINS AND PROTEINLIKE COMPOUNDS

The chemistry of proteins is complex, with many facets not completely understood. Protein structure is usually studied in basic organic chemistry and, to a greater extent, in biochemistry, but for the purposes of this chapter, some of the more important topics are summarized, with emphasis on relationships to medicinal chemistry. Much progress has been made in understanding the more sophisticated features of protein structure[4] and its correlation with physicochemical and biological properties. With the total synthesis of ribonuclease in 1969, new approaches to the study of SARs among proteins have involved the synthesis of modified proteins.

Many types of compounds important in medicinal chemistry are classified structurally as proteins, including enzymes, antigens, and antibodies. Numerous hormones are low–relative-molecular-mass proteins and so are called *simple proteins*. Fundamentally, all proteins are composed of one or more polypeptide chains; that is, the primary organizational level of protein structure is the polypeptide (polyamide) chain composed of naturally occurring amino acids bonded to one another by amide linkages (Fig. 27.1). The specific physicochemical and biological properties of proteins depend not only on the nature of the specific amino acids and their sequence within the polypeptide chain but also on conformational characteristics.

Conformational Features of Protein Structure

As stated, the polypeptide chain is considered to be the primary level of protein structure, and the folding of the polypeptide chains into a specific coiled structure is maintained through hydrogen-bonding interactions (intramolecular) (Fig. 27.2). The folding pattern is the secondary level of protein structure. The intramolecular hydrogen bonds involve the partially negative oxygens of amide carbonyl groups and the partially positive hydrogens of the amide —NH. Additional factors, such as ionic bonding between positively and negatively charged groups and disulfide bonds, help stabilize such folded structures.

The arrangement and interfolding of the coiled chains into layers determine the tertiary and higher levels of protein structure. Such final conformational character is determined by various types of interaction, primarily hydrophobic forces and, to some extent, hydrogen bonding and ion pairing.[4,5] Hydrophobic forces are implicated in many biological phenomena associated with protein structure and interactions.[6] The side chains (R groups) of

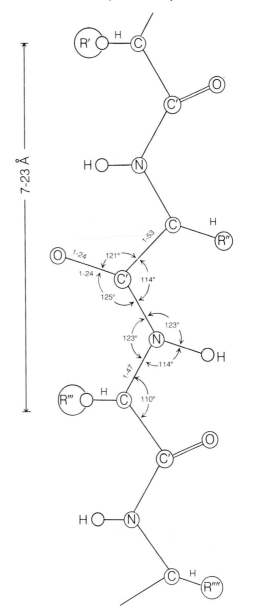

Figure 27.1 ● Diagrammatic representation of a fully extended polypeptide chain with the bond lengths and the bond angles derived from crystal structures and other experimental evidence. (From Corey, R. B., and Pauling, L.: Proc. R. Soc. Lond. Ser. B 141:10, 1953.)

various amino acids have hydrocarbon moieties that are hydrophobic, and they have minimal tendency to associate with water molecules, whereas water molecules are strongly associated through hydrogen bonding. Such hydrophobic R groups tend to get close to one another, with exclusion of water molecules, to form "bonds" between different segments of the chain or between different chains. These are often termed *hydrophobic bonds, hydrophobic forces,* or *hydrophobic interactions.*

The study of protein structure has required several physicochemical methods of analysis.[4] Ultraviolet spectrophotometry has been applied to the assessment of conformational changes that proteins undergo. Conformational changes can be investigated by the direct plotting of the difference in absorption of the protein under various sets of conditions.

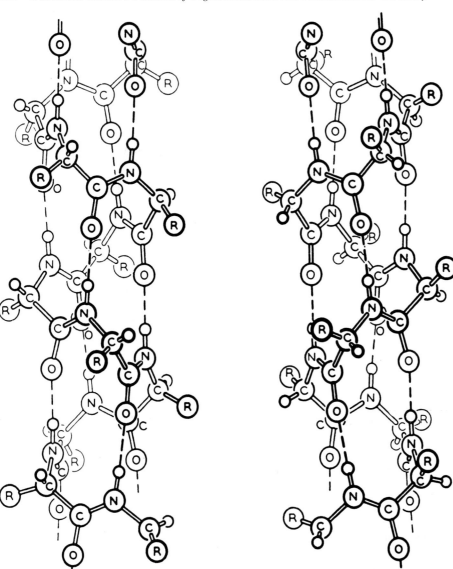

Figure 27.2 ● Left-handed and right-handed α-helices. The R and H groups on the α-carbon atom are in the correct position corresponding to the known configuration of the L-amino acids in proteins. (From Pauling, L., and Corey, R. B.: unpublished drawings.)

X-ray analysis has been most useful in the elucidation of the structures of several proteins (e.g., myoglobulin and lysozyme). Absolute determinations of conformation and helical content can be made by x-ray diffraction analysis. Optical rotation of proteins has also been studied fruitfully. The specific rotations of proteins are always negative, and extreme changes in pH (when the protein is in solution) and conditions that promote denaturation (urea solutions, increased temperatures) tend to augment the negative optical rotation. Accordingly, it is thought that the changes in rotation are caused by conformational changes (i.e., changes in protein structure at the secondary and higher levels of organization). Optical rotatory dispersion has also been used to study conformational alterations and differences among globular proteins. Additionally, circular dichroism methodology has been involved in structural studies. The shape and the magnitude of rotatory dispersion curves and circular dichroism spectra are very sensitive to conformational alterations; thus, the effects of enzyme inhibitors on conformation can be analyzed. Structural studies have included the investigation of the tertiary structures of proteins in high-frequency nuclear magnetic resonance (NMR).[7,8]

NMR spectroscopy has been of some use in the study of interactions between drug molecules and proteins such as enzymes, proteolipids, and others. NMR has been applied to the study of binding of atropine analogs to acetylcholinesterase[9] and interactions involving cholinergic ligands and housefly brain and torpedo electroplax.[10] NMR was also used in the determination of the tertiary structure of the capsid protein of the human immunodeficiency virus (HIV).[11]

Factors Affecting Protein Structure

Conditions that promote the hydrolysis of amide linkages affect protein structure (see under "Protein Hydrolysates" previously in this chapter). The highly ordered conformation of a protein can be disorganized (without hydrolysis of the amide linkages), and in the process, the protein's biological activity is lost. This process, customarily called *denaturation*, involves unfolding of the polypeptide chains, loss of the native conformation of the protein, and disorganization of the uniquely ordered structure, without the cleavage of covalent bonds (e.g., cooked egg albumin). The rupture of native disulfide bonds is usually considered a more extensive and drastic change than denaturation. Criteria for the detection of denaturation involve detection of previously masked —SH, imidazole, and —NH$_2$ groups; decreased solubility; increased susceptibility to the action of proteolytic enzymes; decreased diffusion constant and increased viscosity of protein solution; loss of enzymatic activity if the protein is an enzyme; and modification of antigenic properties.

Purification and Classification

It might be said that it is old-fashioned to classify proteins according to the following system, since so much progress has been made in understanding protein structure. Nevertheless, an outline of this system of classification is given because the terms used are still found in the pharmaceutical and medical literature. Table 27.1 includes the classification and characterization of simple proteins. Before classification, the protein material must be purified as much as possible, which is a very challenging task. Several criteria are used to determine homomolecularity, including crystallinity, constant solubility at a given temperature, osmotic pressure in different solvents, diffusion rate, electrophoretic mobility, dielectric constant, chemical assay, spectrophotometry, and quantification of antigenicity. The methodology of purification is complex; procedures can involve various techniques of chromatography (column), electrophoresis, ultracentrifugation, and others. High-performance liquid chromatography (HPLC) has been applied to the separation of peptides (e.g., the purification of some hypothalamic peptides by a combination of chromatographic methods including HPLC).[12,13]

Conjugated proteins contain a nonprotein structural component in addition to the protein moiety, whereas simple proteins contain only the polypeptide chain of amino acid units. Nucleoproteins are conjugated proteins containing nucleic acids as structural components. Glycoproteins are carbohydrate-containing conjugated proteins (e.g., thyroglobulin). Phosphoproteins contain phosphate moieties (e.g., casein). Lipoproteins are lipid bearing. Metalloproteins have some bound metal. Chromoproteins, such as hemoglobin or cytochrome, have some chromophoric moiety.

Properties of Proteins

The classification in Table 27.1 is based on solubility properties. Fibrous proteins are water insoluble and highly resistant to hydrolysis by proteolytic enzymes; the collagens, elastins, and keratins are in this class. Globular proteins (albumins, globulins, histones, and protamines) are relatively water soluble; they are also soluble in aqueous solutions containing salts, acids, bases, or ethanol. Enzymes, oxygen-carrying proteins, and protein hormones are globular proteins.

Another important characteristic of proteins is their amphoteric behavior. In solution, proteins migrate in an electric field, and the direction and rate of migration are a function of the net electrical charge of the protein molecule, which in turn depends on the pH of the solution. The isoelectric point is the pH value at which a given protein does not migrate in an electric field; it is a constant for any given protein and can be used as an index of characterization. Proteins differ in rate of migration and in their isoelectric points. Electrophoretic analysis is used to determine purity and for quantitative estimation because proteins differ in electrophoretic mobility at any given pH.[4]

Because they are ionic in solution, proteins bind with cations and anions depending on the pH of the environment. Sometimes, complex salts are formed, and precipitation takes place (e.g., trichloroacetic acid is a precipitating agent for proteins and is used for deproteinizing solutions).

Proteins possess chemical properties characteristic of their component functional groups, but in the native state, some of these groups are "buried" within the tertiary protein structure and may not react readily. Certain denaturation procedures can expose these functions and allow them to respond to the usual chemical reagents (e.g., an exposed —NH$_2$ group can be acetylated by ketene; —CO$_2$H can be esterified with diazomethane).

Color Tests and Miscellaneous Separation and Identification Methods

Proteins respond to the following color tests: (a) biuret, pink to purple with an excess of alkali and a small amount of copper sulfate; (b) ninhydrin, a blue color when boiled with ninhydrin (triketohydrindene hydrate), which is intensified by the presence of pyridine; (c) Millon test for tyrosine, a brick-red color or precipitate when boiled with mercuric nitrate in an excess of nitric acid; (d) Hopkins-Cole test for tryptophan, a violet zone with a salt of glyoxylic acid and stratified over sulfuric acid; and (e) xanthoproteic test, a brilliant

TABLE 27.1 Simple (True) Proteins

Class	Characteristics	Occurrence
Albumins	Soluble in water, coagulable by heat and reagents	Egg albumin, lactalbumin, serum albumin, leucosin of wheat, legumelin of legumes
Globulins	Insoluble in water, soluble in dilute salt solution, coagulable	Edestin of plants, vitelline of egg, serum globulin, lactoglobulin, amandin of almonds, myosin of muscles
Prolamines	Insoluble in water or alcohol, soluble in 60%–80% alcohol, not coagulable	Found only in plants (e.g., gliadin of wheat, hordein of barley, zein of corn, and secalin of rye)
Glutelins	Soluble only in dilute acids or bases, coagulable	Found only in plants (e.g., glutenin of wheat and oryzenin of rice)
Protamines	Soluble in water or ammonia, strongly alkaline, not coagulable	Found only in the sperm of fish (e.g., salmine from salmon)
Histones	Soluble in water, but not in ammonia, predominantly basic, not coagulable	Globin of hemoglobin, nucleohistone from nucleoprotein
Albuminoids	Insoluble in all solvents	In keratin of hair, nails, and feathers; collagen of connective tissue; chondrin of cartilage; fibroin of silk; and spongin of sponges

orange zone when a solution in concentrated nitric acid is stratified under ammonia. Almost all so-called alkaloidal reagents will precipitate proteins in slightly acid solution.

The qualitative identification of the amino acids found in proteins and other substances has been simplified greatly by the application of paper chromatographic techniques to the proper hydrolysate of proteins and related substances. End-member degradation techniques for the detection of the sequential arrangements of the amino acid residues in polypeptides (proteins, hormones, enzymes, etc.) have been developed to such a high degree with the aid of paper chromatography that very small samples of the polypeptides can be used. These techniques, together with statistical methods, have led to the elucidation of the amino acid sequences in oxytocin, vasopressin, insulin, hypertensin, glucagon, corticotropins, and others.

Ion exchange chromatography has been applied to protein analysis and to the separation of amino acids. The principles of ion exchange chromatography can be applied to the design of automatic amino acid analyzers with appropriate recording instrumentation.[4] One- or two-dimensional thin-layer chromatography has been used to accomplish separations not possible with paper chromatography. Another method for separating amino acids and proteins involves a two-dimensional analytical procedure that uses electrophoresis in one dimension and partition chromatography in the other. The applicability of HPLC was noted previously.[12,13]

Products

Gelatin, NF. Gelatin, NF, is a protein obtained by the partial hydrolysis of collagen, an albuminoid found in bones, skin, tendons, cartilage, hoofs, and other animal tissues. The products seem to be of great variety, and from a technical standpoint, the raw material must be selected according to the purpose intended (Table 27.2). This is because collagen is usually accompanied in nature by elastin and, especially, mucoids such as chondromucoid, which enter into the product in a small amount. The raw materials for official gelatin, and that used generally for food, are skins of calf or swine and bones. The bones are first treated with hydrochloric acid to remove the calcium compounds and then are digested with lime for a prolonged period, which solubilizes most other impurities. The fairly pure collagen is extracted with hot water at a pH of about 5.5, and the aqueous solution of gelatin is concentrated, filtered, and cooled to a stiff gel. Calf skins are treated in about the same way, but those from hogs are not given any lime treatment. The product derived from an acid-treated precursor is known as type A and exhibits an isoelectric point between

pH 7 and 9; that for which alkali is used is known as type B and exhibits an isoelectric point between pH 4.7 and 5. The minimum gel strength officially is that a 1% solution kept at 0°C for 6 hours must show no perceptible flow when the container is inverted.

Gelatin occurs in sheets, shreds, flakes, or coarse powder. It is white or yellowish, has a slight but characteristic odor and taste, and is stable in dry air but subject to microbial decomposition when moist or in solution. It is insoluble in cold water but swells and softens when immersed and gradually absorbs 5 to 10 times its own weight of water. It dissolves in hot water to form a colloidal solution; it also dissolves in acetic acid and in hot dilute glycerin. Gelatin commonly is bleached with sulfur dioxide, but the medicinal product must not have more than 40 parts per million of sulfur dioxide. A proviso is made, however, for the manufacture of capsules or pills, which may have certified colors added, may contain as much as 0.15% sulfur dioxide, and may have a lower gel strength.

Gelatin is used in the preparation of capsules, in the coating of tablets, and, with glycerin, as a vehicle for suppositories. It has also been used as a vehicle when slow absorption is desired for drugs. When dissolved in water, the solution becomes somewhat viscous, and in cases of shock, these solutions may be used to replace the loss in blood volume. Presently, this replacement is accomplished more efficiently with blood plasma, which is safer to use. In hemorrhagic conditions, it is sometimes administered intravenously to increase the clotting of blood or is applied locally for the treatment of wounds.

The most important value in therapy is as an easily digested and adjuvant food. Notably, it fails to provide any tryptophan and is lacking in adequate amounts of other essential amino acids; approximately 60% of the total amino acids consist of glycine and the prolines. Nevertheless, when supplemented, it is very useful in various forms of malnutrition, gastric hyperacidity or ulcer, convalescence, and general diets of the sick. It is especially useful in the preparation of modified milk formulas for feeding infants.

Gelatin Film, Absorbable, United States Pharmacopoeia (USP). Gelatin film, absorbable (Gelfilm), is a sterile, nonantigenic, absorbable, water-insoluble gelatin film. The gelatin films are prepared from a solution of specially prepared gelatin–formaldehyde combination, by spreading on plates and drying under controlled humidity and temperature. The film is available as light yellow, transparent, brittle sheets 0.076 to 0.228 mm thick. Although insoluble in water, they become rubbery after being in water for a few minutes.

Gelatin Sponge, Absorbable, USP. Gelatin sponge absorbable (Gelfoam, Surgifoam) is a sterile, absorbable, water-insoluble, gelatin-based sponge that is a light, nearly white, nonelastic, tough, porous matrix. It is stable to dry heat at 150°C for 4 hours. It absorbs 50 times its own weight of water or 45 times oxalated whole blood.

It is absorbed in 4 to 6 weeks when used as a surgical sponge. When applied topically to control capillary bleeding, it should be moistened with sterile isotonic sodium chloride solution or thrombin solution.

Venoms. Cobra (Naja) venom solution, from which the hemotoxic and proteolytic principles have been removed,

TABLE 27.2 **Pharmaceutically Important Protein Products**

Name *Proprietary Name*	Category
Gelatin, NF	Pharmaceutical acid (encapsulating agent; suspending agent; tablet binder and coating agent)
Gelatin film, absorbable, USP Gelfilm	Local hemostatic
Gelatin sponge, absorbable, USP Gelfoam, Surgiform	Local hemostatic

has been credited with virtues because of its toxins and has been injected intramuscularly as a nonnarcotic analgesic in doses of 1 mL/day. Snake venom solution of the water moccasin is used subcutaneously in doses of 0.4 to 1.0 mL as a hemostatic in recurrent epistaxis and thrombocytopenic purpura and as a prophylactic before tooth extraction and minor surgical procedures. Stypven, from the Russell viper, is used topically as a hemostatic and as a thromboplastic agent in Quick's modified clotting-time test. Ven-Apis, the purified and standardized venom from bees, is furnished in graduated strengths of 32, 50, and 100 bee-sting units. It is administered topically in acute and chronic arthritis, myositis, and neuritis.

The frog venom, caerulein, isolated from the red-eyed tree frog *Agalychnis callidryas* mimics the effects of cholecystokinin and has been used in radiography procedures to contract the gallbladder. In addition, sauvagine, an anxiolytic, has been isolated from *A. callidryas*. Finally, bombesin, a 14-amino acid peptide that also possesses anxiolytic properties, has been isolated from the European fire-bellied frog. Although not a complete list of the peptides isolated from frogs, these provide an insight into the ancient defense mechanisms these reptiles possess and the possibility of exploitation for such uses as analgetics, antimicrobials (especially against resistant organisms), and cardiovascular agents.

Nucleoproteins. The aforementioned nucleoproteins are found in the nuclei and cytoplasm of all cells. They can be deproteinized by several methods. The compounds that occur in yeast are usually treated by grinding with a very dilute solution of potassium hydroxide, adding picric acid in excess, and precipitating the nucleic acids with hydrochloric acid, leaving the protein in solution. The nucleic acids are purified by dissolving in dilute potassium hydroxide, filtering, acidifying with acetic acid, and finally precipitating with a large excess of ethanol.

The nucleoproteins found in the nucleus of eukaryotic cells include various enzymes, such as DNA and RNA polymerases (involved in nucleic acid synthesis), nucleases (involved in the hydrolytic cleavage of nucleotide bonds), isomerases, and others. The nucleus of eukaryotic cells also contains specialized proteins, such as tubulin (involved in the formation of mitotic spindle before mitosis) and histones. Histones are proteins rich in the basic amino acids arginine and lysine, which together make up one fourth of the amino acid residues. Histones combine with negatively charged double-helical DNA to form complexes that are held together by electrostatic interactions. Histones package and order the DNA into structural units called *nucleosomes*. Because of the enormous amount of research on histones, the reader is encouraged to evaluate the "Selected Reading" list provided at the end of this chapter.

⬡ ENZYMES

Proteins that have catalytic properties are called *enzymes* (i.e., enzymes are biological catalysts of protein nature). Some enzymes have full catalytic reactivity per se; these are considered simple proteins because they do not have a nonprotein moiety. Other enzymes are conjugated proteins, and the nonprotein structural components are necessary for reactivity. Occasionally, enzymes require metallic ions. Because enzymes are proteins or conjugated proteins, the general review of protein structural studies presented previously in this chapter (e.g., protein conformation and denaturation) is fundamental to the following topics. Conditions that affect denaturation of proteins usually have an adverse effect on the activity of the enzyme.

General enzymology is discussed effectively in numerous standard treatises, and one of the most concise discussions appears in the classic work by Ferdinand,[14] who includes reviews of enzyme structure and function, bioenergetics, and kinetics and appropriate illustrations with a total of 37 enzymes selected from the six major classes. For additional basic studies of enzymology, the reader should refer to this classic monograph and to a comprehensive review of this topic.[15]

Relation of Structure and Function

Koshland[16] has reviewed concepts concerning correlations of protein conformation and conformational flexibility of enzymes with enzyme catalysis. Enzymes do not exist initially in a conformation complementary to that of the substrate. The substrate induces the enzyme to assume a complementary conformation. This is the so-called induced-fit theory. There is proof that proteins do possess conformational flexibility and undergo conformational changes under the influence of small molecules. This does not mean that all proteins must be flexible; nor does it mean that conformationally flexible enzymes must undergo conformational changes when interacting with all compounds. Furthermore, a regulatory compound that is not directly involved in the reaction can exert control on the reactivity of the enzyme by inducing conformational changes (i.e., by inducing the enzyme to assume the specific conformation complementary to the substrate). (Conceivably, hormones as regulators function according to the foregoing mechanism of affecting protein structure.) So-called flexible enzymes can be distorted conformationally by molecules classically called *inhibitors*. Such inhibitors can induce the protein to undergo conformational changes, disrupting the catalytic functions or the binding function of the enzyme. In this connection, it is noteworthy how the work of Belleau[17] and the molecular perturbation theory of drug action relate to Koshland's studies presented previously in this textbook.

Evidence continues to support the explanation of enzyme catalysis based on the active site (reactive center) of amino acid residues, which is considered to be that relatively small region of the enzyme's macromolecular surface involved in catalysis. Within this site, the enzyme has strategically positioned functional groups (from the side chains of amino acid units) that participate cooperatively in the catalytic action.[18]

Some enzymes have absolute specificity for a single substrate; others catalyze a particular type of reaction that various compounds undergo. In the latter, the enzyme is said to have *relative specificity*. Nevertheless, compared with other catalysts, enzymes are outstanding in their specificity for certain substrates.[19] The physical, chemical, conformational, and configurational properties of the substrate determine its complementarity to the enzyme's reactive center. These factors, therefore, determine whether a given compound satisfies the specificity of a particular enzyme. Enzyme specificity must be a function of the nature, including conformational and chemical reactivity, of the reactive center, but when the enzyme is a conjugated protein with a coenzyme moiety, the nature of the coenzyme also contributes to specificity characteristics.

In some instances, the active center of the enzyme is apparently complementary to the substrate molecule in a strained configuration, corresponding to the "activated" complex for the reaction catalyzed by the enzyme. The substrate molecule is attracted to the enzyme, and the forces of attraction cause it to assume the strained state, with conformational changes that favor the chemical reaction; that is, the enzyme decreases the activation energy requirement of the reaction to such an extent that the reaction proceeds appreciably faster than it would in the absence of the enzyme. If enzymes were always completely complementary in structure to the substrates, then no other molecule would be expected to compete successfully with the substrate in combination with the enzyme, which, in this respect, would be similar in behavior to antibodies. Occasionally, however, an enzyme complementary to a strained substrate molecule attracts a molecule resembling the strained substrate molecule more strongly; for example, the hydrolysis of benzoyl-L-tyrosylglycineamide is practically inhibited by an equal amount of benzoyl-D-tyrosylglycineamide. This example illustrates a type of antimetabolite activity.

Several types of interaction contribute to the formation of enzyme–substrate complexes: attractions between charged (ionic) groups on the protein and the substrate, hydrogen bonding, hydrophobic forces (the tendency of hydrocarbon moieties of side chains of amino acid residues to associate with the nonpolar groups of the substrate in a water environment), and London forces (induced dipole interactions).

Many studies of enzyme specificity have involved proteolytic enzymes (proteases). Configurational specificity can be exemplified by the aminopeptidase that cleaves L-leucylglycylglycine but does not affect D-leucylglycylglycine. D-Alanylglycylglycine is cleaved slowly by this enzyme. These phenomena illustrate the significance of steric factors; at the active center of aminopeptidase, the closeness of approach affects the kinetics of the reaction.

One can easily imagine how difficult it is to study the reactivity of enzymes on a functional group basis because the mechanism of enzyme action is so complex.[16] Nevertheless, the —SH group probably is found in more enzymes as a functional group than are the other polar groups. In some enzymes (e.g., urease), the less readily available SH groups are necessary for biological activity and cannot be detected by the nitroprusside test, which is used to detect freely reactive SH groups.

A free —OH group of the tyrosyl residue is necessary for the activity of pepsin. Both the —OH of serine and the imidazole portion of histidine appear to be necessary parts of the active center of certain hydrolytic enzymes, such as trypsin and chymotrypsin, and furnish the electrostatic forces involved in a proposed mechanism (Fig. 27.3), in which E denotes enzyme and the other symbols are self-evident. (Alternative mechanisms have been proposed[15]; esterification and hydrolysis were studied extensively by M. L. Bender.[19a–d] D. M. Blow reviewed studies concerning the structure and mechanism of chymotrypsin.[19e])

These two groups (i.e., —OH and =NH) could be located on separate peptide chains in the enzyme as long as the specific three-dimensional structure formed during activation of the zymogen brought them near enough to form a hydrogen bond. The polarization of the resulting structure would cause the serine oxygen to be the nucleophilic agent that attacks the carbonyl function of the substrate. The complex is stabilized by the simultaneous "exchange" of the hydrogen bond from the serine oxygen to the carbonyl oxygen of the substrate.

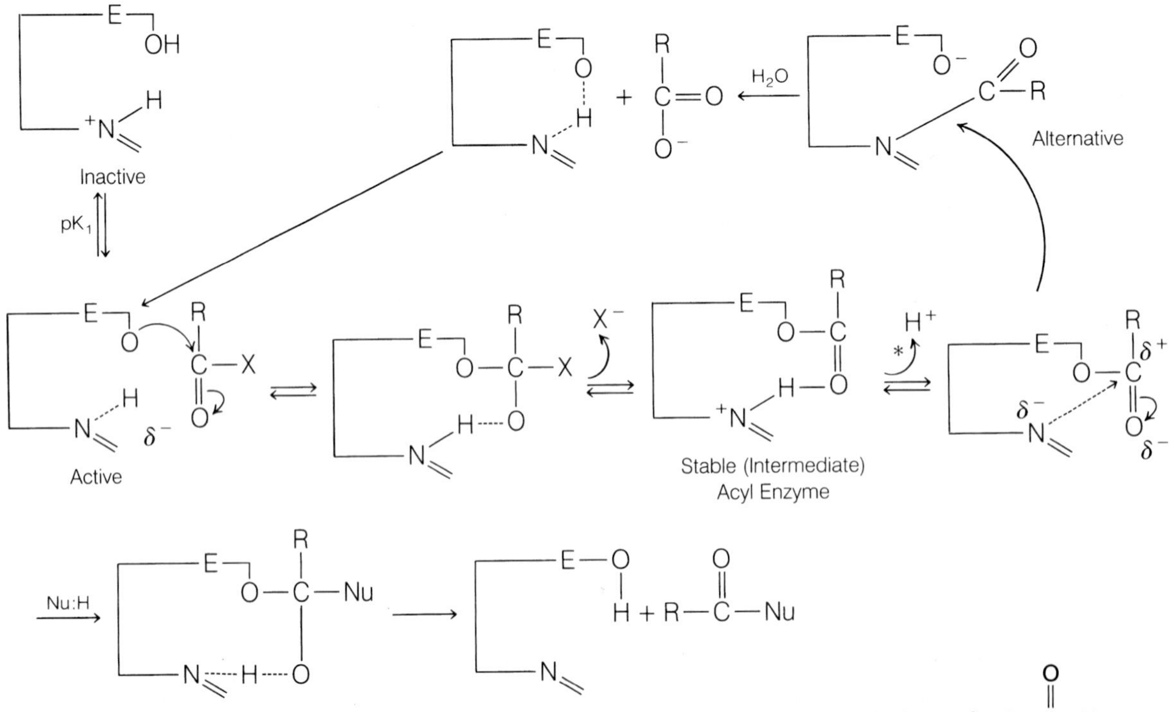

Figure 27.3 • Proposed generalized mechanism for enzyme-catalyzed hydrolysis of R—C(=O)—X.

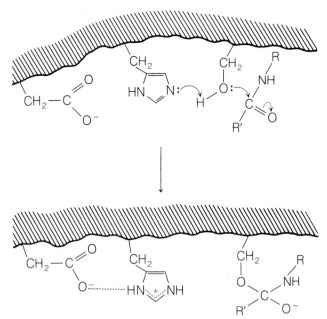

Figure 27.4 ● Generalized mechanism of protease catalysis. (Roberts, J. D.: Chem. Eng. News 57:23, 1979.)

The intermediate acylated enzyme is written with the proton on the imidazole nitrogen. The deacylation reaction involves the loss of this positive charge simultaneously with the attack of the nucleophilic reagent (abbreviated Nu:H).

Roberts[20] used nitrogen-15 (^{15}N) NMR to study the mechanism of protease catalysis. A schematic summary of the generalized mechanism is represented in Figure 27.4. It is concluded that the tertiary N-1 nitrogen of the histidine unit within the reactive center of the enzyme deprotonates the hydroxyl of the neighboring serine unit and simultaneously the hydroxyl oxygen exerts a nucleophilic attack on the carbonyl carbon of the amide substrate, as depicted in the scheme. A tetrahedral intermediate is implicated, and the carboxylate group of the aspartate unit (the third functional group within the reactive center) stabilizes the developing imidazolium ion by hydrogen bonding to the N-3 hydrogen. Finally, decomposition of the anionic tetrahedral intermediate toward product formation (amine and acylated serine) is promoted by prior protonation of the amide nitrogen by the imidazolium group.

A possible alternative route to deacylation would involve the nucleophilic attack of the imidazole nitrogen on the newly formed ester linkage of the postulated acyl intermediate, leading to the formation of the acyl imidazole. The latter is unstable in water, hydrolyzing rapidly to give the product and regenerated active enzyme.

The reaction of an alkyl phosphate in such a scheme may be written in an entirely analogous fashion, except that the resulting phosphorylated enzyme would be less susceptible to deacylation through nucleophilic attack. The diagrammatic scheme in Figure 27.5 has been proposed to explain the function of the active thiol ester site of papain. This ester site is formed and maintained by the folding energy of the enzyme (protein) molecule.

Zymogens (Proenzymes)

Zymogens, also called *proenzymes*, are enzyme precursors. These proenzymes are said to be activated when they are transformed to the enzyme. Activation usually involves catalytic action by some proteolytic enzyme. Occasionally, the activators merely effect a reorganization of the tertiary structure (conformation) of the protein so that the groups involved within the reactive center become functional (i.e., unmasked).

Synthesis and Secretion of Enzymes

Exportable proteins (enzymes), such as amylase, ribonuclease, chymotrypsin(ogen), trypsin(ogen), and insulin, are synthesized on the ribosomes. They pass across the membrane of the endoplasmic reticulum into the cisternae and directly into a smooth vesicular structure, which effects further transportation. They are finally stored in highly concentrated form within membrane-bound granules called *zymogen granules*. The exportable protein content of zymogen granules may reach a value of 40% of the total protein of the gland cell. In these enzyme sequences, the newly synthesized exportable protein (enzyme) is not free in the cell sap. The stored exportable digestive enzymes are released into the extracellular milieu and the hormones into adjacent capillaries. Release of these proteins is initiated by specific inducers. For example, cholinergic agents (but not epinephrine) and Ca^{2+} effect a discharge of amylase, lipase, or others into the medium, increased glucose levels stimulate the secretion of insulin, and so on. This release of the reserve enzymes and hormones is completely independent of the synthetic process, as long as the stores in the granules are not depleted. Energy oxidative phosphorylation does not play an important role in these releases. Electron microscope studies indicate a fusion of the zymogen granule membrane with the cell membrane so that the granule opens directly into the extracellular lumen of the gland.

Classification

There are various systems for the classification of enzymes. The International Union of Biochemistry system includes some of the terminology used in the literature of

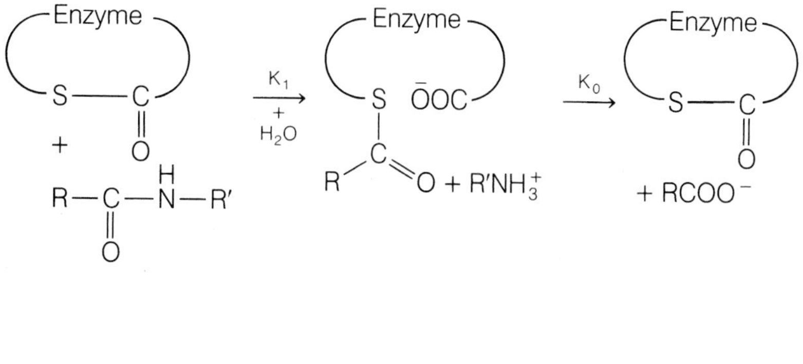

Figure 27.5 ● Proposed scheme for the action of papain.

medicinal chemistry, and in many instances the terms are self-explanatory. For example, transferases catalyze transfer of a group (e.g., methyltransferase); hydrolases catalyze hydrolysis reactions (e.g., esterases and amidases); and lyases catalyze nonhydrolytic removal of groups, leaving double bonds. There are also oxidoreductases, isomerases, and ligases. Other systems are sometimes used to classify and characterize enzymes, and the following terms are frequently encountered: *lipase, peptidase, protease, phosphatase, kinase, synthetase, dehydrogenase, oxidase,* and *reductase.*

Products

Pharmaceutically important enzyme products are listed in Table 27.3.

Pancreatin, USP.   Pancreatin (Panteric) is a substance obtained from the fresh pancreas of the hog or the ox and contains a mixture of enzymes, principally pancreatic amylase (amylopsin), protease, and pancreatic lipase (steapsin). It converts not less than 25 times its weight of *USP* Potato Starch Reference Standard into soluble carbohydrates and not less than 25 times its weight of casein into proteoses. Pancreatin of higher digestive power may be brought to this

standard by admixture with lactose, sucrose containing not more than 3.25% of starch, or pancreatin of lower digestive power. Pancreatin is a cream-colored amorphous powder with a faint, characteristic, but not offensive, odor. It dissolves slowly but incompletely in water and is insoluble in alcohol. It acts best in neutral or faintly alkaline media, and excessive acid or alkali renders it inert. Pancreatin can be prepared by extracting the fresh gland with 25% alcohol or with water and subsequently precipitating with alcohol. Besides the enzymes mentioned, it contains some trypsinogen, which can be activated by intestinal enterokinase; chymotrypsinogen, which is converted by trypsin to chymotrypsin; and carboxypeptidase.

Pancreatin is used largely for predigestion of food and for the preparation of hydrolysates. The value of its enzymes orally must be very small because they are digested by pepsin and acid in the stomach, although some of them may escape into the intestines without change. Even if they are protected by enteric coatings, it is doubtful they could be of great assistance in digestion.

Trypsin Crystallized, USP.   Trypsin crystallized is a proteolytic enzyme crystallized from an extract of the pancreas gland of the ox, *Bos taurus.* It occurs as a white to yellowish

TABLE 27.3 **Pharmaceutically Important Enzyme Products**

Name Proprietary Name	Preparations	Category	Application	Usual Adult Dose[a]	Usual Dose Range[a]
Pancreatin, *USP* *Panteric*	Pancreatin capsules, *USP* Pancreatin tablets, *USP*	Digestive aid		325 mg–1 g	
Trypsin crystallized, *USP*	Trypsin crystallized for aerosol, *USP*	Proteolytic enzyme		Aerosol, 125,000 *USP* units in 3 mL of saline daily	
Pancrelipase, *USP* *Cotazym*	Pancrelipase capsules, *USP* Pancrelipase tablets, *USP*	Digestive aid			An amount of pancrelipase equivalent to 8,000–24,000 *USP* units of lipolytic activity before each meal or snack, or to be determined by the practitioner according to the needs of the patient
Chymotrypsin, *USP* *Chymar*	Chymotrypsin for ophthalmic solution, *USP*	Proteolytic enzyme (for zonule lysis)	1–2 mL by irrigation to the posterior chamber of the eye, under the iris, as a solution containing 75–150 U/mL		
Dornase Alfa *Pulmozyme*	Aerosol	Proteolytic enzyme	Nebulizer		
Hyaluronidase for injection, *USP* *Alidase, Wydase*	Hyaluronidase injection, *USP*	Spreading agent		Hypodermoclysis, 150 *USP* hyaluronidase units	
Imiglucerase *Cerezyme*	Injection	Proteolytic enzyme			Dose based on body weight; range is 15–60 U/kg IV over 1–2 hours
Sutilains, *USP* *Travase*	Sutilains ointment, *USP*	Proteolytic enzyme	Topical, ointment, b.i.d. to q.i.d.		

[a]See *USP* DI for complete dosage information.

white, odorless, crystalline or amorphous powder, and 500,000 *USP* trypsin units are soluble in 10 mL of water or saline TS.

Trypsin has been used for several conditions in which its proteolytic activities relieve certain inflammatory states, liquefy tenacious sputum, and so forth. Many side reactions are encountered, however, particularly when it is used parenterally, which mitigate against its use.

Pancrelipase, USP. Pancrelipase (Cotazym) has a greater lipolytic action than other pancreatic enzyme preparations. Hence, it is used to help control steatorrhea and in other conditions in which pancreatic insufficiency impairs the digestion of fats in the diet.

Chymotrypsin, USP. Chymotrypsin (Chymar) is extracted from mammalian pancreas and is used in cataract surgery. A dilute solution is used to irrigate the posterior chamber of the eye to dissolve the fine filaments that hold the lens.

Dornase Alpha, USP. Dornase alpha (Pulmozyme) is a highly purified solution of recombinant human deoxyribonuclease I (rhDNAse). It is indicated for use in cystic fibrosis because of its ability to liquefy secretions from the lung effectively. It accomplishes this by cleaving the extracellular DNA in purulent sputum and reducing the viscosity and elasticity of the secretion.

Hyaluronidase for Injection, USP. Hyaluronidase for injection (Alidase, Wydase) is a sterile, dry, soluble enzyme product prepared from mammalian testes and capable of hydrolyzing the mucopolysaccharide hyaluronic acid. It contains not more than 0.25 μg of tyrosine for each *USP* hyaluronidase unit. Hyaluronidase in solution must be stored in a refrigerator. Hyaluronic acid, an essential component of tissues, limits the spread of fluids and other extracellular material, and because the enzyme destroys this acid, injected fluids and other substances tend to spread farther and faster than normal when administered with this enzyme. Hyaluronidase may be used to increase the spread and consequent absorption of hypodermoclytic solutions; to diffuse local anesthetics, especially in nerve blocking; and to increase diffusion and absorption of other injected materials, such as penicillin. It also enhances local anesthesia in surgery of the eye and is useful in glaucoma because it causes a temporary drop in intraocular pressure.

Hyaluronidase is practically nontoxic, but caution must be exercised in the presence of infection because the enzyme may cause a local infection to spread, through the same mechanism. It should never be injected in an infected area. Sensitivity to the drug is rare.

The activity of hyaluronidase is determined by measuring the reduction in turbidity of a substrate of native hyaluronidate and certain proteins, or by measuring the reduction in viscosity of a buffered solution of sodium, or potassium hyaluronidate. Each manufacturer defines its product in turbidity or viscosity units, but values are not the same because they measure different properties of the enzyme.

Imiglucerase Injection. Imiglucerase injection (Cerezyme) is a form of human placental glucocerebrosidase from which the terminal mannose residues have been removed. This product is produced through recombinant tech-nology and is used to treat type 1 Gaucher disease because its ability to hydrolyze glucocerebroside prevents the accumulation of this lipid in organs and tissues.

Sutilains, USP. Sutilains (Travase) is a proteolytic enzyme obtained from cultures of *Bacillus subtilis* and used to dissolve necrotic tissue occurring in second- and third-degree burns as well as bed sores and ulcerated wounds.

Many substances are contraindicated during the topical use of sutilains. These include detergents and anti-infectives that denature the enzyme preparation. The antibiotics penicillin, streptomycin, and neomycin do not inactivate sutilains. Mafenide acetate is also compatible with the enzyme.

Streptokinase. Streptokinase (Kabikinase, Streptase) is a catabolic 47,000-d protein secreted by group C β-hemolytic streptococci. It is a protein with no intrinsic enzymatic activity. Streptokinase activates plasminogen to plasmin, a proteolytic enzyme that hydrolyzes fibrin and promotes the dissolution of thrombi. Plasminogen is activated when streptokinase forms a 1:1 stoichiometric complex with it. Allergic reactions to streptokinase occur commonly because of antibody formation in individuals treated with it. Furthermore, the antibodies inactivate streptokinase and reduce its ability to prolong thrombin time. Streptokinase is indicated for acute myocardial infarction, for local perfusion of an occluded vessel, and before angiography, by intravenous, intra-arterial, and intracoronary administration, respectively.

Urokinase. Urokinase (Abbokinase) is a glycosylated serine protease consisting of 411 amino acid residues, which exists as two polypeptide chains connected by a single disulfide bond. It is isolated from human urine or tissue culture of human kidneys. The only known substrate of urokinase is plasminogen, which is activated to plasmin, a fibrinolytic enzyme. Unlike streptokinase, urokinase is a direct activator of plasminogen. Urokinase is nonantigenic because it is an endogenous enzyme and, therefore, may be used when streptokinase use is impossible because of antibody formation. It is administered intravenously or by the intracoronary route. Its indications are similar to those of streptokinase.

Alteplase. Alteplase (Activase) is a tissue plasminogen activator (t-PA) produced by rDNA technology. It is a single-chain glycoprotein protease consisting of 527 amino acid residues. Native t-PA is isolated from a melanoma cell line. The single-chain molecule is susceptible to enzymatic digestion to a two-chain molecule, in which the two chains remain linked with a disulfide bond. Both forms of the native t-PA are equipotent in fibrinolytic (and plasminogen-activating) properties. It is an extrinsic plasminogen activator associated with vascular endothelial tissue, which preferentially activates plasminogen bound to fibrin. The fibrinolytic action of alteplase (t-PA) is confined to thrombi, with minimal systemic activation of plasminogen. It is produced commercially by rDNA methods by inserting the alteplase gene (acquired from human melanoma cells) into ovarian cells of the Chinese hamster, serving as host cells. The melanoma-derived alteplase is immunologically and chemically identical with the uterine form. Alteplase is indicated for the intravenous management of acute myocardial infarction.

Papain, USP. Papain (Papase), the dried and purified latex of the fruit of *Carica papaya* L. (Caricaceae), can digest protein in either acidic or alkaline media; it is best at a pH between 4 and 7 and at 65°C to 90°C. It occurs as light brownish gray to weakly reddish brown granules, or as a yellowish gray to weakly yellow powder. It has a characteristic odor and taste and is incompletely soluble in water to form an opalescent solution. The commercial material is prepared by evaporating the juice, but the pure enzyme has also been prepared and crystallized. In medicine, it has been used locally in various conditions similar to those for which pepsin is used. It has the advantage of activity over a wider range of conditions, but it is often much less reliable. Intraperitoneal instillation of a weak solution has been recommended to counteract a tendency to develop adhesions after abdominal surgery, and several enthusiastic reports have been made about its value under these conditions. Papain has been reported to cause allergies in persons who handle it, especially those who are exposed to inhalation of the powder.

Bromelains. Bromelains (Ananase) is a mixture of proteolytic enzymes obtained from the pineapple plant. It is proposed for use in the treatment of soft-tissue inflammation and edema associated with traumatic injury, localized inflammation, and postoperative tissue reactions. The swelling that accompanies inflammation may be caused by occlusion of the tissue spaces with fibrin. If this is true, enough Ananase would have to be absorbed and reach the target area after oral administration to act selectively on the fibrin. This is yet to be established, and its efficacy as an anti-inflammatory agent is inconclusive. An apparent inhibition of inflammation, however, has been demonstrated with irritants such as turpentine and croton oil (granuloma pouch technique). Ananase is available in 50,000-U tablets for oral use.

Diastase. Diastase (Taka-Diastase) is derived from the action of a fungus, *Aspergillus oryzae* Cohn (Ahlburg), on rice hulls or wheat bran. It is a yellow, hygroscopic, almost tasteless powder that is freely soluble in water and can solubilize 300 times its weight of starch in 10 minutes. It is used in doses of 0.3 to 1.0 g in the same conditions as malt diastase. Taka-Diastase is combined with alkalies as an antacid in Takazyme, with vitamins in Taka-Combex, and in other preparations.

⬡ HORMONES

The hormones discussed in this chapter may be classified structurally as polypeptides, proteins, or glycoproteins. These hormones include metabolites elaborated by the hypothalamus, pituitary gland, pancreas, gastrointestinal tract, parathyroid gland, liver, and kidneys. A comprehensive review of the biochemistry of these polypeptides and other related hormones is beyond the scope of this chapter. For a detailed discussion, the reader should refer to the review by Wallis et al.[21] and other literature cited throughout this chapter.

Hormones from the Hypothalamus

Spatola provides an excellent, although somewhat dated, review on the physiological and clinical aspects of hypothalamic-releasing hormones.[22] Through use of these hormones, the central nervous system regulates other essential endocrine systems, including the pituitary, which in turn controls still other systems (e.g., the thyroid).

Thyroliberin (thyrotropin-releasing hormone [TRH]) is the hypothalamic hormone responsible for the release of the pituitary's thyrotropin. Thyrotropin stimulates the production of thyroxine and liothyronine by the thyroid. The latter thyroid hormones, by feedback regulation, inhibit the action of TRH on the pituitary. TRH is a relatively simple tripeptide that has been characterized as pyroglutamyl-histidyl-prolinamide. TRH possesses interesting biological properties. In addition to stimulating the release of thyrotropin, it promotes the release of prolactin. It has also some central nervous system effects that have been evaluated for antidepressant therapeutic potential, but the results of clinical studies are not yet considered conclusive.

Gonadoliberin, as the name implies, is the gonadotropin-releasing hormone (Gn-RH), also known as *luteinizing hormone–releasing hormone* (LH-RH). This hypothalamic decapeptide stimulates the release of luteinizing hormone (LH) and follicle-stimulating hormone (FSH) by the pituitary. LH-RH is considered to be of potential therapeutic importance in the treatment of hypogonadotropic infertility in both males and females.[23]

$$(\text{pyro})^1\text{Glu} \quad \overset{10}{\text{Gly-NH}_2}$$

Luteinizing Hormone-Releasing Hormone
(LH-RH)

A hypothalamic growth-releasing factor (GRF), also called somatoliberin, continues to be under intensive investigation. Its identification and biological characterization remain to be completed, but physiological and clinical data support the existence of hypothalamic control of pituitary release of somatotropin.

Somatostatin is another very interesting hypothalamic hormone.[22] It is a tetradecapeptide possessing a disulfide bond linking two cysteine residues, 3 and 14, in the form of a 38-member ring. Somatostatin suppresses several endocrine systems. It inhibits the release of somatotropin and thyrotropin by the pituitary. It also inhibits the secretion of insulin and glucagon by the pancreas. Gastrin, pepsin, and secretin are intestinal hormones that are likewise affected by somatostatin. The therapeutic potential of somatostatin is discussed later in relation to the role of glucagon in the pathology of human diabetes.

Other hypothalamic hormones include the luteinizing hormone release-inhibiting factor (LHRIF), prolactin-releasing factor (PRF), corticotropin-releasing factor (CRF), melanocyte-stimulating hormone-releasing factor (MRF), and melanocyte-stimulating hormone release-inhibiting factor (MIF).

As the foregoing discussion illustrates, the hypothalamic endocrine system performs many essential functions affecting other endocrine systems. In turn, the thalamus and cortex exert control on the secretion of these (hypothalamic) factors. A complete review of this field is beyond the scope of this chapter; the interested reader should refer to the literature cited.[21-23]

Pituitary Hormones

The pituitary gland, or the hypophysis, is located at the base of the skull and is attached to the hypothalamus by a stalk. The pituitary gland plays a major role[21] in regulating activity of the endocrine organs, including the adrenal cortex, the gonads, and the thyroid. The neurohypophysis (posterior pituitary), which originates from the brain, and the adenohypophysis (anterior pituitary), which is derived from epithelial tissue, are the two embryologically and functionally different parts of the pituitary gland. The adenohypophysis is under the control of hypothalamic regulatory hormones, and it secretes adrenocorticotropic hormone (ACTH), growth hormone (GH), LH, FSH, prolactin, and others. The neurohypophysis is responsible for the storage and secretion of the hormones vasopressin and oxytocin, controlled by nerve impulses traveling from the hypothalamus.

ADRENOCORTICOTROPIC HORMONE

ACTH (adrenocorticotropin, corticotropin) is a medicinal agent that has been the center of much research. In the late 1950s, its structure was elucidated, and the total synthesis was accomplished in the 1960s. Related peptides also have been synthesized, and some of these possess similar physiological action. Human ACTH has 39 amino acid units within the polypeptide chain.

SAR studies of ACTH[24] showed that the COOH-terminal sequence is not particularly important for biological activity. Removal of the NH$_2$-terminal amino acid results in complete loss of steroidogenic activity. Full activity has been reported for synthetic peptides containing the first 20 amino acids. A peptide containing 24 amino acids has full steroidogenic activity, without allergenic reactions. This is of practical importance because natural ACTH preparations sometimes produce clinically dangerous allergic reactions.

Corticotropin exerts its major action on the adrenal cortex, promoting steroid synthesis by stimulating the formation of pregnenolone from cholesterol.[25] An interaction between ACTH and specific receptors is implicated in the mechanism leading to stimulation of adenylate cyclase and acceleration of steroid production. The rate-limiting step in the biosynthesis of steroids from cholesterol is the oxidative cleavage of the side chain of cholesterol, which results in the formation of pregnenolone. This rate-limiting step is regulated by cyclic adenosine monophosphate (cAMP). Corticotropin, through cAMP, stimulates the biosynthesis of steroids from cholesterol by increasing the availability of free cholesterol. This involves activation of cholesterol esterase by phosphorylation. Corticotropin also stimulates the uptake of cholesterol from plasma lipoproteins. Other biochemical effects exerted by ACTH include stimulation of phosphorylase and hydroxylase activities. Glycolysis also is increased by this hormone. Enzyme systems that catalyze processes involving the production of reduced nicotinamide adenine dinucleotide phosphate (NADPH) are also stimulated. (NADPH is required by the steroid hydroxylations that take place in the overall transformation of cholesterol to hydrocortisone, the major glucocorticoid hormone.) Pharmaceutically important ACTH products are listed in Table 27.4.

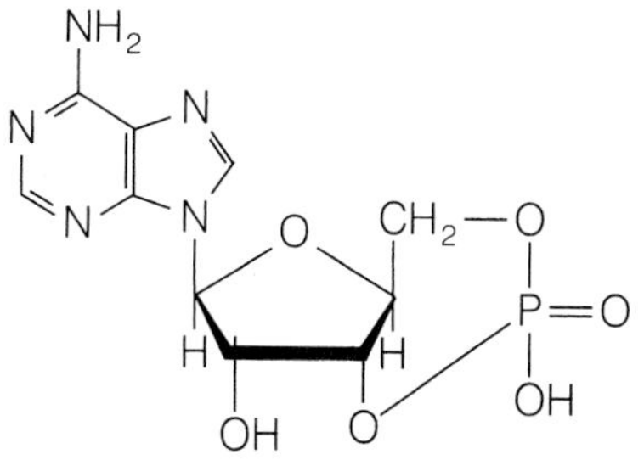

cAMP

Corticotropin Injection, USP. Adrenocorticotropin injection (ACTH injection, Acthar) is a sterile preparation of the principle, or principles derived from the anterior lobe of the pituitary of mammals used for food by humans. It occurs as a colorless or light straw-colored liquid, or a soluble, amorphous solid by drying such liquid from the frozen state. It exerts a tropic influence on the adrenal cortex. The solution has a pH range of 3 to 7 and is used for its adrenocorticotropic activity.

Repository Corticotropin Injection, USP. ACTH purified (ACTH-80, corticotropin gel, purified corticotropin) is corticotropin in a solution of partially hydrolyzed gelatin to be used intramuscularly for a more uniform and prolonged maintenance of activity.

Sterile Corticotropin Zinc Hydroxide Suspension, USP. Sterile corticotropin zinc hydroxide suspension is a sterile suspension of corticotropin, adsorbed on zinc hydroxide, which contains no less than 45 and no more than 55 μg of zinc for each 20 *USP* corticotropin units. Because of its prolonged activity caused by slow release of corticotropin, an initial dose of 40 *USP* units can be administered intramuscularly, followed by a maintenance dose of 20 U 2 or 3 times a week.

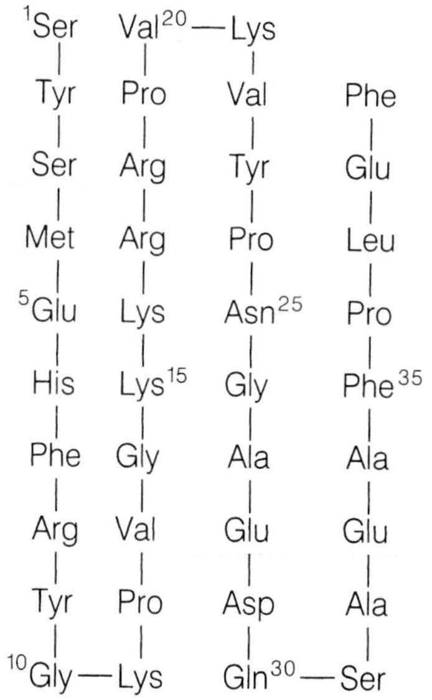

Corticotropin

Cosyntropin. Cosyntropin (Cortrosyn) is a synthetic peptide containing the first 24 amino acids of natural corticotropin. Cosyntropin is used as a diagnostic agent to test for adrenal cortical deficiency. Plasma hydrocortisone concentration is determined before and 30 minutes after the administration of 250 μg of cosyntropin. Most normal re-

TABLE 27.4 Pharmaceutically Important Adrenocorticotropic Hormone Products

Preparation *Proprietary Name*	Category	Usual Adult Dose[a]	Usual Dose Range[a]	Usual Pediatric Dose[a]
Corticotropin injection, *USP* Corticotropin for injection, *USP* *Acthar*	Adrenocorticotropic hormone; adrenocortical steroid (anti-inflammatory): diagnostic aid (adrenocortical insufficiency)	Adrenocorticotropic hormone: parenteral, 20 *USP* units, q.i.d. Adrenocortical steroid (anti-inflammatory): parenteral, 20 *USP* units q.i.d. Diagnostic aid (adrenocortical insufficiency): rapid test—IM or IV, 25 *USP* units, with blood sampling in 1 hour; adrenocortical steroid output— IV infusion, 25 U in 500–1,000 mL of 5% dextrose injection over a period of 8 hours on each of 2 successive days, with 24-hour urine collection each day	Adrenocorticotropic hormone: 40–80 U/day; adrenocortical steroid (anti-inflammatory): 40–80 U/day	Parenteral, 0.4 U/kg of body weight or 12.5 U/m^2 of body surface, q.i.d.
Repository corticotropin injection, *USP* *Acthar Gel, Cortrophin Gel*	Adrenocorticotropic hormone; adrenocortical steroid (anti-inflammatory); diagnostic aid (adrenocortical insufficiency)	Adrenocorticotropic hormone: IM or SC, 40–80 U every 24–72 hours; IV infusion, 40–80 U in 500 mL of 5% dextrose injection given over an 8-hour period, q.d. Adrenocortical steroid (anti-inflammatory): IM or SC, 40–80 U every 24–72 hours; IV infusion, 40–80 U in 500 mL of 5% dextrose injection given over an 8-hour period, q.d. Diagnostic aid (adrenocortical insufficiency): IM, 40 U b.i.d. on each of 2 successive days, with 24-hour urine collection each day		Adrenocorticotropic hormone: parenteral, 0.8 U/kg of body weight or 25 U/m^2 of body surface per dose
Sterile corticotropin zinc hydroxide suspension, *USP* *Cortrophin-Zinc*	Adrenocorticotropic hormone; adrenocortical steroid (anti-inflammatory); diagnostic aid (adrenocortical insufficiency)	Adrenocorticotropic hormone: IM, initial, 40–60 U/day, increasing interval to 48, then 72 hours: reduce dose per injection thereafter; maintenance, 20 U/day to twice weekly Adrenocortical steroid (anti-inflammatory): IM, initial, 40–60 U/day, increasing interval to 48, then 72 hours; reduce dose per injection thereafter; maintenance, 20 U/day to twice weekly Diagnostic aid (adrenocortical insufficiency): IM, 40 U on each of 2 successive 24-hour periods		
Cosyntropin *Cortrosyn*	Diagnostic aid (adrenocortical insufficiency)	IM or IV, 250 μg		Children 2 years of age or less, 0.125 mg

[a]See *USP* DI for complete dosage information.

sponses result in an approximate doubling of the basal hydrocortisone concentration in 30 to 60 minutes. If the response is not normal, adrenal insufficiency is indicated. Such adrenal insufficiency could be a result of either adrenal or pituitary malfunction, and further testing is required to distinguish between the two. Cosyntropin (250 μg infused within 4–8 hours) or corticotropin (80–120 U/day for 3–4 days) is administered. Patients with functional adrenal tissue should respond to this dosage. Patients who respond accordingly are suspected of hypopituitarism, and the diagnosis can be confirmed by other tests for pituitary function. Patients who have Addison disease, however, show little or no response.

Corticorelin. Corticorelin (Acthrel) is a synthetic peptide that may be used as an injectable in the determination of pituitary responsiveness. It possesses the amino acid sequence found in corticotropin-releasing hormone that is responsible for stimulating the release of ACTH.

MELANOTROPINS (MELANOCYTE-STIMULATING HORMONE)

Melanocyte-stimulating hormone (MSH) is elaborated by the intermediate lobe of the pituitary gland and regulates pigmentation of skin in fish, amphibians, and, to a lesser extent, humans. Altered secretion of MSH has been implicated in causing changes in skin pigmentation during the menstrual cycle and pregnancy. The two major types of melanotropin, α-MSH and β-MSH, are derived from ACTH and β-lipotropin, respectively. α-MSH contains the same amino acid sequence as the first 13 amino acids of ACTH; β-MSH has 18 amino acid residues. A third melanotropin, γ-melanotropin, is derived from a larger peptide precursor, proopiomelanocortin (POMC). Some important endocrinological correlations include inhibitory actions of hydrocortisone on the secretion of MSH and the inhibitory effects of epinephrine and norepinephrine on MSH action.

LIPOTROPINS (ENKEPHALINS AND ENDORPHINS)

Opiates, such as opium and morphine, have been known for centuries as substances that relieve pain and suffering. Neuropharmacologists have theorized that opiates interact with receptors in the brain that are affected by endogenous substances that function as regulators of pain perception. The important breakthrough came in 1975, with the isolation of two peptides with opiatelike activity[26] from pig brains. These related pentapeptides, called methionine-enkephalin (metenkephalin) and leucine-enkephalin (leuenkephalin), are abundant in certain nerve terminals and have been found in the pituitary gland.

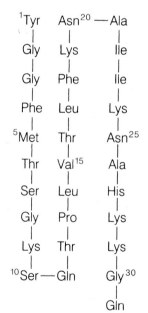

β-Endorphin (sheep)

An examination of the structures of enkephalins revealed that the amino acid sequence of metenkephalin was identical with the sequence of residues 61 to 65 of β-lipotropin (β-LPH), a larger peptide found in the pituitary gland. This discovery suggested that β-LPH might be a precursor for other larger peptides containing the metenkephalin sequence. Soon after the structural relationship between β-LPH and metenkephalin was established, longer peptides, called *endorphins*, were isolated from the intermediate lobe of the pituitary gland. The endorphins (α, β, and γ) contained the metenkephalin amino acid sequence and possessed morphinelike activity.[27] The longest of these peptides, β-endorphin, a 31-residue peptide (residues 61–91 of β-LPH), is about 20 to 50 times more potent than morphine as an analgesic and has a considerably longer duration of action than enkephalins. Numerous enkephalin analogs and derivatives have been prepared, and their biological activity has been evaluated. Like morphine, β-endorphin and the enkephalins can induce tolerance and dependence.

In addition to the enkephalins and endorphins, several other opioid peptides have been extracted from pituitary, adrenal, and nervous tissue, including dynorphins and neoendorphins. The peptides β-LPH, ACTH, and γ-MSH are derived from the same precursor, POMC.

The endorphins and enkephalins have a wide range of biological effects, and most of their actions are in the central nervous system. Their actions include inhibition of release of dopamine in brain tissue and inhibition of release of acetylcholine from neuromuscular junctions. The role of endorphins and enkephalins as inhibitory neurotransmitters agrees well with the observed biological effects of these peptides in lowering response to pain and other stimuli. The role of endorphins and enkephalins as neurotransmitters and neuromodulators, with emphasis on receptor interactions, has been reviewed.[28] Also, see Chapter 24 in this textbook.

GROWTH HORMONE (SOMATOTROPIN)

GH is a 191-residue polypeptide elaborated by the anterior pituitary. The amino acid sequence of GH has been determined, and comparison with growth hormones of different species has revealed considerable structural variation.[29] In addition, the structure and properties of human GH have been reviewed.[30]

The major biological action of GH is to promote overall somatic growth. Deficiency in the secretion of this hormone can cause dwarfism, and an overproduction of this hormone can cause acromegaly and giantism. Secretion of this hormone is stimulated by growth hormone–releasing hormone (GH-RH), a 44-residue polypeptide secreted by the hypothalamus. Secretion of GH is inhibited by somatostatin.

GH stimulates protein synthesis, both in the skeletal muscles and in the liver. In the liver, GH stimulates uptake of amino acids and promotes the synthesis of all forms of RNA. It stimulates glucagon secretion by the pancreas, increases synthesis of glycogen in muscles, augments the release of fatty acids from adipose tissue, and increases osteogenesis. It also causes acute hypoglycemia followed by elevated blood glucose concentration and, perhaps, glycosuria.

GH has been recognized as an effective replacement therapy for GH-deficient children. The supply of GH, however, was very limited because its source was the pituitary glands of human cadavers, and several reports of deaths in children with Creutzfeldt-Jakob disease (caused by viral contamination of GH) halted the distribution of GH in 1977. Both of these problems were solved with the application of rDNA technology in the commercial production of somatrem and somatropin.

Somatrem (Systemic). Somatrem (Protropin) is a biosynthetic form of human GH that differs from the pituitary-derived GH and recombinant somatotropin by addition of an extra amino acid, methionine. Because of its structural difference from the natural GH, patients receiving somatrem may develop antibodies, which may result in a decreased response to it. Somatrem is administered intramuscularly or subcutaneously, and the therapy is continued as long as the patient responds, until the patient reaches mature adult height, or until the epiphyses close. The dosage range is 0.05 to 0.1 IU.

Somatropin (rDNA Origin). Somatropin for injection (Humatrope) is a natural-sequence human GH of rDNA origin. Its composition and sequence of amino acids are identical with those of human GH of pituitary origin. It is administered intramuscularly or subcutaneously. The dosage range is 0.05 to 0.1 IU.

PROLACTIN

Prolactin (PRL), a hormone secreted by the anterior pituitary, was discovered in 1928. It is a 198-residue polypeptide with general structural features similar to those of GH. PRL stimulates lactation of parturition.

Gonadotropic Hormones

The two principal gonadotropins elaborated by the adenohypophysis are FSH and LH. LH is also known as *interstitial cell–stimulating hormone*. The gonadotropins along with thyrotropin form the incomplete glycoprotein group of hormones. FSH and LH may be produced by a single cell, the gonadotroph. The secretion of FSH and LH is controlled by the hypothalamus, which produces LH-RH. LH-RH stimulates the secretion of both FSH and LH, although its effects on the secretion of LH are more pronounced.

FOLLICLE-STIMULATING HORMONE

FSH promotes the development of ovarian follicles to maturity as well as spermatogenesis in testicular tissue. It is a glycoprotein, and the carbohydrate component is considered to be associated with its activity. Urofollitropin (Bravelle) is a highly purified, human-derived FSH that is indicated for ovulation induction.

LUTEINIZING HORMONE

LH is another glycoprotein. It acts after the maturing action of FSH on ovarian follicles, stimulates production of estrogens, and transforms the follicles into *corpora lutea*. LH also acts in the male to stimulate the Leydig cells that produce testosterone.

MENOTROPINS

Pituitary hormones prepared from the urine of postmenopausal women whose ovarian tissue does not respond to gonadotropin are available for medicinal use as the product menotropins (Pergonal). The latter has FSH and LH gonadotropin activity in a 1:1 ratio. Menotropins are useful in the treatment of anovular women whose ovaries respond to pituitary gonadotropins but who have a gonadotropin deficiency caused by either pituitary or hypothalamus malfunction. Usually, menotropins are administered intramuscularly in an initial dose of 75 IU of FSH and 75 IU of LH daily for 9 to 12 days, followed by 10,000 IU of chorionic gonadotropin 1 day after the last dose of menotropins.

Thyrotropin

The thyrotropic hormone, also called *thyrotropin* and *thyroid-stimulating hormone* (TSH), is a glycoprotein consisting of two polypeptide chains. This hormone promotes production of thyroid hormones by affecting the kinetics of the mechanism by which the thyroid concentrates iodide ions from the bloodstream, thereby promoting incorporation of the halogen into the thyroid hormones and release of hormones by the thyroid.

TSH (Thyropar) appears to be a glycoprotein (relative molecular mass [M_r] 26,000–30,000) containing glucosamine, galactosamine, mannose, and fucose, whose homogeneity is yet to be established. It is produced by the basophil cells of the anterior lobe of the pituitary gland. TSH enters the circulation from the pituitary, presumably traversing cell membranes in the process. After exogenous administration, it is widely distributed and disappears very rapidly from circulation. Some evidence suggests that the thyroid may directly inactivate some of the TSH by an oxidation mechanism that may involve iodine. TSH thus inactivated can be reactivated by certain reducing agents. TSH regulates the production by the thyroid gland of thyroxine, which stimulates the metabolic rate. Thyroxine feedback mechanisms regulate the production of TSH by the pituitary gland.

The decreased secretion of TSH from the pituitary is a part of a generalized hypopituitarism that leads to hypothyroidism. This type of hypothyroidism can be distinguished from primary hypothyroidism by the administration of TSH in doses sufficient to increase the uptake of radioiodine, or to elevate the blood or plasma protein-bound iodine (PBI) as a consequence of enhanced secretion of hormonal iodine (thyroxine). Interestingly, massive doses of vitamin A inhibit the secretion of TSH. Thyrotropin is used as a diagnostic agent to differentiate between primary and secondary hypothyroidism. Its use in hypothyroidism caused by pituitary deficiency has limited application; other forms of treatment are preferable.

Somatostatin

Somatostatin was discovered in the hypothalamus. It is elaborated by the δ-cells of the pancreas and elsewhere in the body. Somatostatin is an oligopeptide (14 amino acid residues) and is referred to as *somatotropin release–inhibiting factor* (SRIF).

Its primary action is inhibiting the release of GH from the pituitary gland. Somatostatin also suppresses the release of both insulin and glucagon. It causes a decrease in both cAMP levels and adenylate cyclase activity. It also inhibits calcium ion influx into the pituitary cells and suppresses glucose-induced pancreatic insulin secretion by activating and deactivating potassium ion and calcium ion permeability, respectively. The chemistry, SARs, and potential clinical applications have been reviewed.[22,31]

```
           ¹Ala
            |
           Gly
            |
        Cys-S-S-Cys
         |        |
        Lys      Ser
         |        |
       ⁵Asn      Thr
         |        |
        Phe      Phe
         |        |
        Phe      Thr¹⁰
         |        |
        Trp ———— Lys
```
Somatostatin

A powerful new synthetic peptide that mimics the action of somatostatin, octreotide acetate (Sandostatin), is approved by the Food and Drug Administration (FDA) for the treatment of certain rare forms of intestinal endocrine cancers, such as malignant carcinoid tumors and vasoactive intestinal peptide-secreting tumors (VIPomas). Octreotide acetate is indicated for long-term treatment of severe diarrhea associated with these carcinomas.

An octaoeotide somatostatin analog, lanreotide acetate (Somatuline Depot), was introduced in 2007 for the long-term treatment of acromegaly. Lanreotide is an inhibitor of various endocrine functions, but its main effects are associated with inhibiting insulin-like growth factor-1 (IGF-1).

Although not an analog of somatostatin but having inhibitory effects on IGF-1 is mecasermin (Increlex). It is designed to replace natural IGF-1 in patients who are deficient in the hormone.

Placental Hormones

HUMAN CHORIONIC GONADOTROPIN

Human chorionic gonadotropin (hCG) is a glycoprotein synthesized by the placenta. Estrogens stimulate the anterior pituitary to produce placentotropin, which in turn stimulates hCG synthesis and secretion. hCG is produced primarily during the first trimester of pregnancy. It exerts effects that are similar to those of pituitary LH.

hCG is used therapeutically in the management of cryptorchidism in prepubertal boys. It also is used in women in conjunction with menotropins to induce ovulation when the endogenous availability of gonadotropin is not normal.

HUMAN PLACENTAL LACTOGEN

Human placental lactogen (hPL) also is called *human choriomammotropin* and *chorionic growth-hormone prolactin*. This hormone exerts numerous actions. In addition to mammotropic and lactotropic effects, it exerts somatotropic and luteotropic actions. It is a protein composed of 191 amino acid units in a single-peptide chain with two disulfide bridges.[23] hPL resembles human somatotropin.

Neurohypophyseal Hormones (Oxytocin, Vasopressin)

The posterior pituitary (neurohypophysis) is the source of vasopressin, oxytocin, α- and β-MSH, and coherin. The

synthesis, transport, and release of these hormones have been reviewed by Brownstein.[32] Vasopressin and oxytocin are synthesized and released by neurons of the hypothalamic–neurohypophyseal system. These peptide hormones, and their respective neurophysin carrier proteins, are synthesized as structural components of separate precursor proteins, and these proteins appear to be partially degraded into smaller bioactive peptides in the course of transport along the axon.

```
        Gly(NH₂)                      Gly(NH₂)
           |                             |
          Leu                           Arg
           |                             |
  NH₂     Pro                   NH₂     Pro
   |       |                     |       |
 ¹Cys-S-S-Cys                  ¹Cys-S-S-Cys
   |       |                     |       |
  Tyr     Asn⁵                  Tyr     Asn⁵
   |       |                     |       |
  Ile ——— Gln                   Phe ——— Gln
```
   Oxytocin   Vasopressin

The structures of vasopressin and oxytocin have been elucidated, and these peptides have been synthesized. Actually, three closely related nonapeptides have been isolated from mammalian posterior pituitary: oxytocin and arginine vasopressin from most mammals and lysine vasopressin from pigs. The vasopressins differ from one another in the nature of the eighth amino acid residue: arginine and lysine, respectively. Oxytocin has leucine at position 8, and its third amino acid is isoleucine instead of phenylalanine. Several analog of vasopressin have been synthesized and their antidiuretic activity evaluated. Desmopressin, 1-desamino-8-arginine-vasopressin, is a synthetic derivative of vasopressin. It is a longer-acting and more potent antidiuretic than vasopressin, with much less pressor activity. Desmopressin is much more resistant to the actions of peptidases because of the deamination at position 1, which accounts for its longer duration of action. The substitution of D- for L-arginine in position 8 accounts for its sharply lower vasoconstrictive effects.

Vasopressin also is known as the *pituitary antidiuretic hormone* (ADH). This hormone can effect graded changes in the permeability of the distal portion of the mammalian nephron to water, resulting in either conservation or excretion of water; thus, it modulates the renal tubular reabsorption of water. ADH has been shown to increase cAMP production in several tissues. Theophylline, which promotes cAMP by inhibiting the enzyme (phosphodiesterase) that catalyzes its hydrolysis, causes permeability changes similar to those caused by ADH. Cyclic AMP also effects similar permeability changes; hence, it is suggested that cAMP is involved in the mechanism of action of ADH.

The nonrenal actions of vasopressin include its vasoconstrictor effects and neurotransmitter actions in the central nervous system, such as regulation of ACTH secretion, circulation, and body temperature.

ADH is therapeutically useful in the treatment of diabetes insipidus of pituitary origin. It also has been used to relieve intestinal paresis and distention.

Oxytocin is appropriately named because of its oxytocic action. Oxytocin exerts stimulant effects on the smooth muscle of the uterus and mammary gland and has a relaxing effect on vascular smooth muscle when administered in high doses. It is considered the drug of choice to induce labor, particularly in cases of intrapartum hypotonic inertia. Oxytocin also is used in inevitable or incomplete abortion after the 20th week of gestation. It also may be used to prevent or control hemorrhage and to correct uterine hypotonicity. In some cases, oxytocin is used to promote milk ejection; it acts by contracting the myoepithelium of the mammary glands. Oxytocin is usually administered parenterally by intravenous infusion, intravenous injection, or intramuscular injection. Oxytocin citrate buccal tablets are also available, but the rate of absorption is unpredictable, and buccal administration is less precise. Topical administration (nasal spray) 2 or 3 minutes before nursing to promote milk ejection is sometimes recommended.[33] See Table 27.5 for product listing.

Oxytocin Injection, USP. Oxytocin injection is a sterile solution in water for injection of oxytocic principle prepared by synthesis, or obtained from the posterior lobe of the pituitary of healthy, domestic animals used for food by humans. The pH is 2.5 to 4.5; expiration date, 3 years.

Oxytocin preparations are widely used with or without amniotomy to induce and stimulate labor. Although injection is the usual route of administration, the sublingual route is extremely effective. Sublingual and intranasal spray (Oxytocin Nasal Solution, *USP*) routes of administration also will stimulate milk letdown.

Vasopressin Injection, USP. Vasopressin injection (Pitressin) is a sterile solution of the water-soluble pressor principle of the posterior lobe of the pituitary of healthy, domestic animals used for food by humans; it also may be prepared by synthesis. Each milliliter possesses a pressor activity equal to 20 *USP* posterior pituitary units; expiration date, 3 years.

Vasopressin Tannate. Vasopressin tannate (Pitressin Tannate) is a water-insoluble tannate of vasopressin administered intramuscularly (1.5–5.0 pressor units daily) for its prolonged duration of action by the slow release of vasopressin. It is particularly useful for patients who have diabetes insipidus, but it should never be used intravenously.

Felypressin. Felypressin, 2-L-phenylalanine-8-L-lysine vasopressin, has relatively low antidiuretic activity and little oxytocic activity. It has considerable pressor (i.e., vasoconstrictor) activity, which differs from that of epinephrine (i.e., following capillary constriction in the intestine it lowers the pressure in the vena portae, whereas epinephrine raises the portal pressure). Felypressin also causes increased renal blood flow in the cat, whereas epinephrine brings about a fall in renal blood flow. Felypressin is five times more effective as a vasopressor than is lysine vasopressin and is recommended in surgery to minimize blood flow, especially in obstetrics and gynecology.

Lypressin. Lypressin is synthetic 8-L-lysine vasopressin, a polypeptide similar to ADH. The lysine analog is considered more stable, and it is absorbed rapidly from the nasal mucosa. Lypressin (Diapid) is pharmaceutically available as a topical solution, spray, 50 pressor units (185 μg)/mL in 5-mL containers. Usual dosage, topical (intranasal), one or more sprays applied to one or both nostrils one or more times daily.

Desmopressin Acetate. Desmopressin acetate (DDAVP, Stimate) is synthetic 1-desamino-8-D-arginine vasopressin. Its efficacy, ease of administration (intranasal), long duration of action, and lack of side effects make it the drug of choice for the treatment of central diabetes insipidus. It may also be administered intramuscularly or intravenously. It is preferred to vasopressin injection and oral antidiuretics for use in children. It is indicated in the management of temporary polydipsia and polyuria associated with trauma to, or surgery in, the pituitary region.

TABLE 27.5 Neurohypophyseal Hormones: Pharmaceutical Products

Preparation *Proprietary Name*	Category	Usual Adult Dose[a]	Usual Pediatric Dose[a]
Oxytocin injection, *USP* *Pitocin, Syntocinon*	Oxytocic	IM, 3–10 U after delivery of placenta; IV, initially no more than 1–2 mU/minute, increased every 15–30 minutes in increments of 1–2 mU	
Oxytocin nasal solution, *USP* *Syntocinon*	Oxytocic	1 spray or 3 drops in one or both nostrils 2–3 minutes before nursing or pumping of breasts	
Vasopressin injection, *USP* *Pitressin*	Antidiuretic posterior pituitary hormone	IM or SC, 2.5–10 U t.i.d. or q.i.d. as necessary	IM or SC, 2.5–10 U t.i.d. or q.i.d. as necessary
Sterile vasopressin tannate oil suspension *Pitressin*	Antidiuretic posterior pituitary hormone	IM, 1.5–5 U every 1–3 days	IM, 1.25–2.5 U every 1–3 days
Desmopressin acetate nasal solution *DDAVP*	Antidiuretic posterior pituitary hormone	Maintenance: intranasal, 2–4 μg/day, as a single dose or in 2–3 divided doses	Maintenance: intranasal, 2–4 μg/kg of body weight per day or 5–30 mg/day or in 2–3 divided doses
Desmopressin acetate injection *DDAVP, Stimate*	Antidiuretic posterior pituitary hormone	IV or SC, 2–4 μg/day usually in 2 divided doses in the morning or evening	IV, 3 μg/kg of body weight diluted in 0.9% sodium chloride injection *USP*

[a]See *USP* DI for complete dosage information.

Pancreatic Hormones

Relationships between lipid and glucose levels in the blood and the general disorders of lipid metabolism found in diabetic subjects have received the attention of many chemists and clinicians. To understand diabetes mellitus, its complications, and its treatment, one has to begin with the basic biochemistry of the pancreas and the way carbohydrates are correlated with lipid and protein metabolism. The pancreas produces insulin, as well as glucagon; β-cells secrete insulin, and α-cells secrete glucagon. Insulin is considered first.

INSULIN

One of the major triumphs of the 20th century occurred in 1922, when Banting and Best[34] extracted insulin from dog pancreas. Advances in the biochemistry of insulin have been reviewed with emphasis on proinsulin biosynthesis, conversion of proinsulin to insulin, insulin secretion, insulin receptors, metabolism, effects by sulfonylureas, and so on.[35–38]

Insulin is synthesized by the islet β-cells from a single-chain, 86-amino-acid polypeptide precursor, proinsulin.[39] Proinsulin itself is synthesized in the polyribosomes of the rough endoplasmic reticulum of the β-cells from an even larger polypeptide precursor, preproinsulin. The B chain of preproinsulin is extended at the NH$_2$-terminus by at least 23 amino acids. Proinsulin then traverses the Golgi apparatus and enters the storage granules, where the conversion to insulin occurs.

The subsequent proteolytic conversion of proinsulin to insulin is accomplished by the removal of the Arg–Arg residue at positions 31 and 32 and the Arg-Lys residue at positions 64 and 65 by an endopeptidase that resembles trypsin in its specificity and a thiol-activated carboxypeptidase B-like enzyme.[40]

The actions of these proteolytic enzymes on proinsulin result in the formation of equimolar quantities of insulin and the connecting C-peptide. The resulting insulin molecule consists of chains A and B, with 21 and 31 amino acid residues, respectively. The chains are connected by two disulfide linkages, with an additional disulfide linkage within chain A (Fig. 27.6).

The three-dimensional structure of insulin was determined by x-ray analysis of single crystals. These studies demonstrated that the high bioactivity of insulin depends on the integrity of the overall conformation. The biologically active form of the hormone is thought to be the monomer. The receptor-binding region consists of A-1 Gly, A-4 Glu, A-5 Gln, A-19 Tyr, A-21 Asn, B-12 Val, B-16 Tyr, B-24 Phe, and B-26 Tyr. The three-dimensional crystal structure appears to be conserved in solution and during its receptor interaction.

The amino acid sequence of insulins from various animal species has been examined.[35] Details of these are shown in

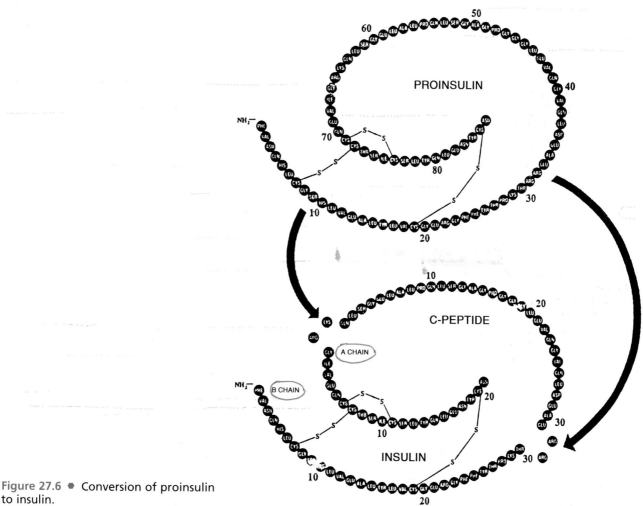

Figure 27.6 ● Conversion of proinsulin to insulin.

TABLE 27.6 Some Sequence Differences in Insulins of Various Species

Species	A Chain				B Chain			
	1	8	9	10	-1	1	29	30
Human	Gly.	Thr.	Ser.	Ile.		Phe.	Lys.	Thr.
Pork	Gly.	Thr.	Ser.	Ile.		Phe.	Lys.	Ala.
Beef	Gly.	Ala.	Ser.	Val.		Phe.	Lys.	Ala.
Sheep	Gly.	Ala.	Gly.	Val.		Phe.	Lys.	Ala.
Horse	Gly.	Thr.	Gly.	Ile.		Phe.	Lys.	Ala.
Rabbit	Gly.	Thr.	Ser.	Ile.		Phe.	Lys.	Ser.
Chicken	Gly.	His.	Asn.	Thr.		Ala.	Lys.	Ala.
Cod	Gly.	His.	Arg.	Pro.	Met.	Ala.	Lys.	—
Rat I[a]	Gly.	Thr.	Ser.	Ile.		Phe.	Lys.	Ser.
Rat II[a]	Gly.	Thr.	Ser.	Ile.		Phe.	Met.	Ser.

See Reference 55 for details.
[a]Asp substitution for Glu at position 4 on A chain.

Table 27.6. It is apparent from the analysis that frequent changes in sequence occur within the interchain disulfide ring (positions 8, 9, and 10). The hormonal sequence for porcine insulin is the closest to that of humans, differing only by the substitution of an alanine residue at the COOH-terminus of the B chain. Porcine insulin, therefore, is a good starting material for the synthesis of human insulin.

Insulin composes 1% of pancreatic tissue, and secretory protein granules contain about 10% insulin. These granules fuse with the cell membrane with simultaneous liberation of equimolar amounts of insulin and the C-peptide. Insulin enters the portal vein, and about 50% is removed in its first passage through the liver. The plasma half-life of insulin is approximately 4 minutes, compared with 30 minutes for the C-peptide.

Usually, exogenous insulin is weakly antigenic. Insulin antibodies have been observed to neutralize the hypoglycemic effect of injected insulin. The antibody-binding sites on insulin are quite different from the sites involved in binding of insulin with its receptors.[41]

Regulation of insulin secretion is affected by numerous factors, such as food, hormonal and neuronal stimuli, and ionic mechanisms.[42] In humans, the principal substrate that stimulates the release of insulin from the islet β-cells is glucose. In addition to glucose, other substrates (e.g., amino acids, free fatty acids, and ketone bodies) also can stimulate insulin secretion directly. Secretin and ACTH can directly stimulate insulin secretion. Glucagon and other related peptides can increase the secretion of insulin, whereas somatostatin inhibits its secretion.

Autonomic neuronal mechanisms also play an important role in regulating insulin release. In the sympathetic nervous system, α-adrenergic agonists inhibit insulin release, whereas β-adrenergic agonists stimulate the release of insulin. In the parasympathetic nervous system, cholinomimetic drugs stimulate insulin release.

"Clinical" insulin that has been crystallized five times and then subjected to countercurrent distribution (2-butanol:1% dichloroacetic acid in water) yields about 90% insulin A, with varying amounts of insulin B together with other minor components. A and B differ by an amide group and have the same activity. End-member analysis, sedimentation, and diffusion studies indicate an M_r of about 6,000. The value of 12,000 M_r for insulin containing trace amounts of zinc (obtained by physical methods) is probably a bimolecular

association product through the aid of zinc. Insulin was the first protein for which a complete amino acid sequence was determined. The extensive studies of Sanger[43] and others elucidated the amino acid sequence and structure of insulin. Katsoyannis[44] and others followed with the synthesis of A and B chains of human, bovine, and sheep insulin. The A and B chains were combined to form insulin in 60% to 80% yields, with a specific activity comparable to that of the natural hormone.

The total synthesis of human insulin was reported by Rittel et al.[45] These workers selectively synthesized the final molecule appropriately cross-linked by disulfide (-S-S-) groups in yields ranging between 40% and 50%, whereas earlier synthetic methods involved random combination of separately prepared A and B chains of the molecule.

rDNA technology has been applied successfully in the production of human insulin on a commercial scale. Human insulin is produced in genetically engineered *Escherichia coli*.[46] Eli Lilly and Co., in cooperation with Genentech, began marketing rDNA-derived human insulin (Humulin) in 1982. There are two available methods of applying rDNA technology in the production of human insulin. The earlier method involved insertion of genes, for production of either the A or the B chain of the insulin molecule, into a special strain of *E. coli* (KI2) and subsequently combining the two chains chemically to produce an insulin that is structurally and chemically identical with pancreatic human insulin. The second, and more recent, method involves the insertion of genes for the entire proinsulin molecule into special *E. coli* cells that are then grown via fermentation. The connecting C-peptide is then enzymatically cleaved from proinsulin to produce human insulin.[47] Human insulin produced by rDNA technology is less antigenic than that from animal sources.

Although insulin is readily available from natural sources (e.g., porcine and bovine pancreatic tissue), partial syntheses and molecular modifications have been developed as the basis for SAR studies. Such studies have shown that amino acid units cannot be removed from the insulin peptide chain A without significant loss of hormonal activity. Several amino acids of chain B, however, are not considered essential for activity. Up to the first six and the last three amino acid units can be removed without significant decrease in activity.[23]

Two insulin analogs, which differ from the parent hormone in that the NH2-terminus of chain A (A[1]) glycine has been replaced by L- and D-alanine, respectively, have been synthesized by Cosmatos et al.[48] for SAR studies. The relative potencies of the L and D analogs reveal interesting SARs. The L- and D-alanine analogs are 9.4% and 95%, respectively, as potent as insulin in glucose oxidation. The relative binding affinity to isolated fat cells is reported to be approximately 10% for the L and 100% for the D analog. Apparently, substitution on the α carbon of A^1 glycine of insulin, with a methyl in a particular configuration, interferes with the binding; hence, the resulting analog (that of L-alanine) is much less active. Methyl substitution in the opposite configuration affects neither the binding nor the bioactivity.

Molecular modifications of insulin on the amino groups appear to reduce bioactivity, but modifications of the ε-amino group of lysine number 29 on chain B (B-29) may yield active analogs. Accordingly, May et al.[49] synthesized N-ε-(+)-biotinyl insulin, which was equipotent with natural insulin. Complexes of this biotinyl-insulin derivative with avidin also were prepared and evaluated biologically; these complexes showed a potency decrease to 5% of that of insulin. Such complexes conjugated with ferritin are expected to be useful in the development of electron microscope stains of insulin receptors.

Alteration in the tertiary structure of insulin appears to drastically reduce biological activity as well as receptor binding. The three-dimensional structure provided by x-ray crystallography of the insulin monomer has revealed an exposed hydrophobic face that is thought to be involved directly in interacting with the receptor.[50] Thus, loss of biological activity in insulin derivatives, produced by chemical modification, can be interpreted in terms of adversely affecting this hydrophobic region. Also, species variation in this hydrophobic region is very unusual.

Insulin is inactivated in vivo by (a) an immunochemical system in the blood of insulin-treated patients, (b) reduction of disulfide bonds (probably by glutathione), and (c) insulinase (a proteolytic enzyme) that occurs in liver. Pepsin and chymotrypsin hydrolyze some peptide bonds that lead to inactivation. Insulin is inactivated by reducing agents such as sodium bisulfite, sulfurous acid, and hydrogen.

Advances in the area of insulin's molecular mechanisms have been reviewed[36–38,51] with emphasis on receptor interactions, effect on membrane structure and functions, effects on enzymes, and the role of second messengers. The insulin receptor is believed to be a glycoprotein complex with a high M_r. The receptor is thought to consist of four subunits: two identical α units with an M_r of about 130,000 d and two identical β units with an M_r of 95,000 d, joined together by disulfide bonds. The α subunits are primarily responsible for binding insulin to its receptor, and the β subunits are thought to possess intrinsic protein kinase activity that is stimulated by insulin. The primary effect of insulin may be a kinase stimulation leading to phosphorylation of the receptor as well as other intracellular proteins.[52,53] Additionally, insulin binding to its receptors may result in the generation of a soluble intracellular second messenger (possibly a peptide) that may mediate some insulin activity relating to activation of enzymes such as pyruvate dehydrogenase and glycogen synthetase. The insulin–receptor complex becomes internalized and may serve as a vehicle for translocating insulin to the lysosomes, in which it may be broken down and recycled back to the plasma membrane. The half-life of insulin is about 10 hours.

The binding of insulin to its target tissue is determined by several factors. The number of receptors in the target tissue and their affinity for insulin are two important determinants. These factors vary substantially from tissue to tissue. Another important consideration is the concentration of insulin itself. Elevated levels of circulating insulin decrease the number of insulin receptors on target cell surfaces and vice versa. Other factors that affect insulin binding to its receptors include pH, temperature, membrane lipid composition, and ionic strength.[53] It is conceivable, therefore, that conditions associated with insulin resistance, such as obesity and type 1 and type 2 diabetes mellitus, could be caused by altered receptor kinase activity, or impaired generation of second messengers (low-M_r peptides), increased degradation of the messenger, or fewer substrates (enzymes involved in metabolic activity) for the messenger or receptor kinase.[54]

Metabolic Effects of Insulin. Insulin has pronounced effects on the metabolism of carbohydrates, lipids, and proteins.[55] The major tissues affected by insulin are muscle (cardiac and skeletal), adipose tissue, and liver. The kidney is much less responsive, and others (e.g., brain tissue and red blood cells) do not respond at all. The actions of insulin are highly complex and diverse. Because many of the actions of insulin are mediated by second messengers, it is difficult to distinguish between its primary and secondary actions.

In muscle and adipose tissue, insulin promotes transport of glucose and other monosaccharides across cell membranes; it also facilitates transport of amino acids, potassium ions, nucleosides, and ionic phosphate. Insulin also activates certain enzymes—kinases and glycogen synthetase in muscle and adipose tissue. In adipose tissue, insulin decreases the release of fatty acids induced by epinephrine or glucagon. cAMP promotes fatty acid release from adipose tissue; therefore, it is possible that insulin decreases fatty acid release by reducing tissue levels of cAMP. Insulin also facilitates the incorporation of intracellular amino acids into protein.

Insulin is believed to influence protein synthesis at the ribosomal level in various tissues.[56] In skeletal muscles, insulin predominantly stimulates translation by increasing the rate of initiation of protein synthesis and the number of ribosomes. In the liver, the predominant effect is on transcription. In cardiac muscles, insulin is believed to decrease the rate of protein degradation.

In the liver, there is no barrier to the transport of glucose into cells; nevertheless, insulin influences liver metabolism, decreasing glucose output, decreasing urea production, lowering cAMP levels, and increasing potassium and phosphate uptake. The lower cAMP levels result in decreased activity of glycogen phosphorylase, leading to diminished glycogen breakdown and increased activity of glycogen synthetase. It appears that insulin induces specific hepatic enzymes involved in glycolysis while inhibiting gluconeogenic enzymes. Thus, insulin promotes glucose use through glycolysis by increasing the synthesis of glucokinase, phosphofructokinase, and pyruvate kinase. Insulin decreases the availability of glucose from gluconeogenesis by suppressing pyruvate carboxylase, phosphoenolpyruvate carboxykinase, fructose-1,6-diphosphatase, and glucose-6-phosphatase.

Insulin's effects on lipid metabolism also are important. In adipose tissue, it has an antilipolytic action (i.e., an effect opposing the breakdown of fatty acid triglycerides). It also decreases the supply of glycerol to the liver. Thus, at these two sites, insulin decreases the availability of precursors for the formation of triglycerides. Insulin is necessary for the activation and synthesis of lipoprotein lipases, enzymes responsible for lowering very low-density lipoprotein (VLDL) and chylomicrons in peripheral tissue. Other effects include stimulation of the synthesis of fatty acids (lipogenesis) in the liver.

Diabetes mellitus is a systemic disease caused by a decrease in the secretion of insulin or reduced sensitivity or responsiveness to insulin by target tissue (insulin receptor activity). The disease is characterized by hyperglycemia, hyperlipidemia, and hyperaminoacidemia. Diabetes mellitus frequently is associated with the development of microvascular and macrovascular diseases, neuropathy, and atherosclerosis. Various types of diabetes have been recognized and classified and their pathophysiology discussed.[57]

The two major types of diabetes are type 1, insulin-dependent diabetes mellitus (IDDM), and type 2, non–insulin-dependent diabetes mellitus (NIDDM). Type 1 diabetes (also known as juvenile-onset diabetes) is characterized by a destruction of pancreatic β-cells, resulting in a deficiency of insulin secretion. Autoimmune complexes and viruses have been mentioned as two possible causes of β-cell destruction. Generally, in type 1 diabetes, receptor sensitivity to insulin is not decreased. Type 2 diabetes, also known as adult-onset diabetes, is characterized primarily by insulin receptor defects or postinsulin receptor defects. There is no destruction of β-cells, and insulin secretion is relatively normal. In reality, however, the two types of diabetes show a considerable overlap of clinical features.[57]

Diabetes mellitus is associated with both microangiopathy (damage to smaller vessels, e.g., the eyes and kidney) and macroangiopathy (damage to larger vessels, e.g., atherosclerosis). Hyperlipidemia (characterized by an increase in the concentration of lipoproteins such as VLDL, intermediate density lipoprotein [IDL], and LDL) has been implicated in the development of atherosclerosis and is known to occur in diabetes. Severe hyperlipidemia may lead to life-threatening attacks of acute pancreatitis. It also seems that severe hyperlipidemia causes xanthoma. Considering the effects of insulin on lipid metabolism, as summarized previously, one can rationalize that in type 2 diabetes, in which the patient may actually have an absolute excess of insulin, in spite of the evidence of glucose tolerance tests, the effect of the excessive insulin on lipogenesis in the liver may suffice to increase the levels of circulating triglycerides and VLDL. In type 1 diabetes, with a deficiency of insulin, the circulating level of lipids may rise because too much precursor is available, with fatty acids and carbohydrates going to the liver.

The relationship between the carbohydrate metabolic manifestations of diabetes and the development of microvascular and macrovascular diseases has been studied extensively.[58,59] It is becoming increasingly clear that hyperglycemia plays a major role in the development of vascular complications of diabetes, including intercapillary glomerulosclerosis, premature atherosclerosis, retinopathy with its specific microaneurysms and retinitis proliferans, leg ulcers, and limb gangrene. First, hyperglycemia causes an increase in the activity of lysine hydroxylase and galactosyl transferase, two important enzymes involved in glycoprotein synthesis. Increased glycoprotein synthesis in the collagen of kidney basement membrane may lead to the de-

velopment of diabetic glomerulosclerosis. Second, increased uptake of glucose by noninsulin-sensitive tissues (e.g., nerve Schwann cells and ocular lens cells) occurs during hyperglycemia. Intracellular glucose is converted enzymatically first to sorbitol and then to fructose. The buildup of these sugars inside the cells increases the osmotic pressure in ocular lens cells and Schwann cells, resulting in increased water uptake and impairing cell functions. Some forms of diabetic cataracts and diabetic neuropathy are believed to be caused by this pathway. Third, hyperglycemia may precipitate nonenzymatic glycosylation of various proteins in the body, including hemoglobin, serum albumin, lipoprotein, fibrinogen, and basement membrane protein. Glycosylation is believed to alter the tertiary structures of proteins and possibly their rate of metabolism. The rate of glycosylation is a function of plasma glucose concentration and the duration of hyperglycemia. Needless to say, this mechanism might play an important role in both macrovascular and microvascular lesions. Finally, hyperglycemia increases the rate of aggregation and agglutinization of circulating platelets. Platelets play an important role in promoting atherogenesis. The increase in the rate of platelet aggregation and agglutinization leads to the development of microemboli, which can cause transient cerebral ischemic attacks, strokes, and heart attacks.[57]

Concepts of the therapeutics of diabetes mellitus have been reviewed by Maurer.[60] This review emphasizes that insulin therapy does not always prevent serious complications. Even diabetic patients considered under insulin therapeutic control experience wide fluctuations in blood glucose concentration, and it is hypothesized that these fluctuations eventually cause the serious complications of diabetes (e.g., kidney damage, retinal degeneration, premature atherosclerosis, cataracts, neurological dysfunction, and a predisposition to gangrene).

Insulin Preparations. The various commercially available insulin preparations are listed in Table 27.7. Amorphous insulin was the first form made available for clinical use. Further purification afforded crystalline insulin, which is now commonly called "regular insulin." Insulin injection, *USP*, is made from zinc insulin crystals. For some time, regular insulin solutions have been prepared at a pH of 2.8 to 3.5; if the pH were increased above the acidic range, particles would be formed. More highly purified insulin, however, can be maintained in solution over a wider pH range, even when unbuffered. Neutral insulin solutions have greater stability than acidic solutions; neutral insulin solutions maintain nearly full potency when stored up to 18 months at 5°C and 25°C. As noted in Table 27.7, the various preparations differ in onset and duration of action. A major disadvantage of regular insulin is its short duration of action (5–7 hours), which necessitates its administration several times daily.

Many attempts have been made to prolong the duration of action of insulin, for example, development of insulin forms less water soluble than the highly soluble (in body fluids) regular insulin. Protamine insulin preparations proved to be less soluble and less readily absorbed from body tissue. Protamine zinc insulin (PZI) suspensions were even longer acting (36 hours) than protamine insulin; these are prepared by mixing insulin, protamine, and zinc chloride with a buffered solution. The regular insulin/PZI ratios in clinically useful preparations range from 2:1 to 4:1.

TABLE 27.7 Insulin Preparations

Name	Particle Size (μm)	Action	Composition	pH	Duration (hours)
Insulin injection,[a] *USP*		Prompt	Insulin + $ZnCl_2$	2.5–3.5	5–7
Prompt insulin zinc suspension,[a] *USP*	2[b]	Rapid	Insulin + $ZnCl_2$ + buffer	7.2–7.5	12
Insulin zinc suspension,[a] *USP*	10–40 (70%) 2 (30%)[b]	Intermediate	Insulin + $ZnCl_2$ + buffer	7.2–7.5	18–24
Extended insulin zinc suspension,[a] *USP*	10–40	Long acting	Insulin + $ZnCl_2$ + buffer	7.2–7.5	24–36
Globin zinc insulin injection[a] *USP*		Intermediate	Globin[c] + $ZnCl_2$ + insulin	3.4–3.8	12–18
Protamine zinc insulin suspension,[d] *USP*		Long acting	Protamine[e] + insulin + Zn	7.1–7.4	24–36
Isophane insulin suspension,[a] *USP*	30	Intermediate	Protamine[f] $ZnCl_2$ insulin buffer	7.1–7.4	18–24

[a]Clear or almost clear.
[b]Amorphous.
[c]Globin (3.6–4.0 mg/100 *USP* units of insulin) prepared from beef blood.
[d]Turbid.
[e]Protamine (1.0–1.5 mg/100 *USP* units of insulin) from the sperm or the mature testes of fish belonging to the genus *Oncorhynchus* or *Salmo*.
[f]Protamine (0.3–0.6 mg/100 *USP* units of insulin).

Isophane insulin suspension incorporates some of the qualities of regular insulin injection and is usually long acting enough (although not as much as PZI) to protect the patient from first day to the next (the term *isophane* is derived from the Greek *iso* and *phane*, meaning equal and appearance, respectively). Isophane insulin is prepared by careful control of the protamine/insulin ratio and the formation of a crystalline entity containing stoichiometric amounts of insulin and protamine. (Isophane insulin also is known as *NPH;* the *N* indicates neutral pH, the *P* stands for protamine, and the *H* for Hegedorn, the developer of the product.) NPH insulin has a quicker onset and a shorter duration of action (28 hours) than PZI. NPH is given in single morning doses and normally exhibits greater activity during the day than at night. NPH and regular insulin can be combined conveniently and effectively for many patients with diabetes.

The posology of various insulin preparations is summarized in Table 27.7.

A major concern with PZI and NPH insulins is the potential antigenicity of protamine (obtained from fish). This concern led to the development of lente insulins. By varying the amounts of excess zinc, by using an acetate buffer (instead of phosphate), and by adjusting the pH, two types of lente insulin were prepared. At high concentrations of zinc, a microcrystalline form precipitates and is called *ultralente*. Ultralente insulin is relatively insoluble and has a slower onset and a longer duration of action than PZI. At a relatively low zinc concentration, an amorphous form precipitates and is called *semilente insulin*. The latter is more soluble and has a quicker onset and a shorter duration of action than regular insulins. A third type of insulin suspension, lente insulin, is a 70:30 mixture of ultralente and semilente insulins. Lente insulin has a rapid onset and an intermediate duration of action (comparable to that of NPH insulin). Lente insulins are chemically incompatible with the PZI and NPH insulins because of the different buffer system used in the preparation of these insulins (an acetate buffer is used in lente insulins and a phosphate buffer is used in PZI and NPH insulins). Dosage and sources are summarized in Table 27.8.

Additionally, regular insulin will remain fast acting when combined with NPH but not when added to lente. The rapid action of regular insulin is neutralized by the excess zinc present in lente insulin.[54] Similar products[61] containing rDNA-derived human insulin (instead of the bovine- and porcine-derived insulin) are available.

Progress in alternative routes of delivery of insulin has been prompted by problems associated with conventional insulin therapy, mentioned previously. First, various types of electromechanical devices (infusion pumps) have been developed with the aim of reducing fluctuations in blood glucose levels associated with conventional insulin therapy (subcutaneous injections). These continuous-infusion pumps are either close-loop or open-loop systems. The ultimate goal of research in this area is to develop a reliable implantable (miniature) device for long-term use that would eliminate the need for daily administration and monitoring of blood glucose levels. The second area of research studies alternative routes of administration such as oral, nasal, and rectal. Preliminary results indicate that absorption of insulin at these sites is not uniform and is unpredictable. The third approach to correcting the problems of conventional insulin therapy is to supplement the defective pancreas by transplantation with a normally functioning pancreas from an appropriate donor. The major problem with this approach is rejection of the donor pancreas by the recipient, as well as problems associated with the draining of exocrine enzymes. A modified procedure transplants only viable pancreatic islet cells or fetal or neonatal pancreas. The possibility remains, however, that in type 1 diabetes, the newly transplanted pancreatic β-cells could be destroyed by the same autoimmune process that caused the disease in the first place.

GLUCAGON

Glucagon, **USP.** The hyperglycemic–glycogenolytic hormone elaborated by the α-cells of the pancreas is known as glucagon. It contains 29 amino acid residues in the sequence shown. Glucagon has been isolated from the amorphous fraction of a commercial insulin sample (4% glucagon).

TABLE 27.8 Dosage and Source of Insulin Preparations

USP Insulin Type	Strengths and Sources	Usual Adult Dose[a]
Insulin injection (regular insulin, crystalline zinc insulin, Cispro)	U-40 mixed, U-100 mixed: purified beef, pork; purified pork; biosynthetic human; semisynthetic human U-500: purified pork	Diabetic hyperglycemia: SC, as directed by physician 15–30 minutes before meals up to t.i.d. or q.i.d.
Isophane insulin suspension (NPH insulin)	U-40 mixed, U-400 mixed: beef; purified beef, pork; purified pork; biosynthetic human; semisynthetic human	SC, as directed by physician, q.d. 30–60 minutes before breakfast; an additional dose before breakfast may be necessary for some patients about 30 minutes before a meal or at bedtime
Isophane insulin suspension (70%) and insulin injection (30%)	U-100: purified pork; semisynthetic human	SC, as directed by physician, q.d. 15–30 minutes before breakfast, or as directed
Insulin zinc suspension (Lente insulin)	U-40 mixed, U-100 mixed: beef; purified beef; purified pork; biosynthetic human; semisynthetic human	SC, as directed by physician, q.d. 30–60 minutes before breakfast; an additional dose may be necessary for some patients about 30 minutes before a meal or at bedtime
Extended insulin zinc suspension (Ultralente insulin)	U-40 mixed, U-100 mixed: beef; purified beef	SC, as directed by physician, q.d. 30–60 minutes before breakfast
Prompt insulin zinc suspension (Semilente insulin)	U-40 mixed, U-100 mixed: beef; purified pork	SC, as directed by physician, q.d. 30–60 minutes before breakfast; an additional dose may be necessary for some patients about 30 minutes before a meal or at bedtime
Protamine zinc insulin suspension (PZI Insulin)	U-40 mixed, U-100 mixed: purified pork	SC, as directed by physician, q.d. 30–60 minutes before breakfast

[a]See *USP* DI for complete dosage information.
SC, subcutaneously.

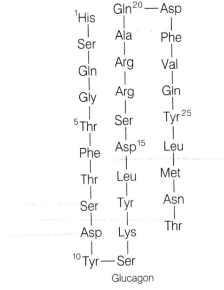

Glucagon

Attention has been focused on glucagon as a factor in the pathology of human diabetes. According to Unger et al.,[62] the following observations support this implication of glucagon: elevated glucagon blood levels (hyperglucagonemia) have been observed in association with every type of hyperglycemia; when secretion of both glucagon and insulin is suppressed, hyperglycemia is not observed unless the glucagon levels are restored to normal by the administration of glucagon; the somatostatin-induced suppression of glucagon release in diabetic animals and humans restores blood sugar levels to normal and alleviates certain other symptoms of diabetes.

Unger et al.[62] propose that although the major role of insulin is regulation of the transfer of glucose from the blood to storage in insulin-responsive tissues (e.g., liver, fat, and muscle), the role of glucagon is regulation of the liver-mediated mobilization of stored glucose. The principal consequence of high concentrations of glucagon is liver-mediated release into the blood of abnormally high concen-trations of glucose, thereby causing persistent hyperglycemia. This indicates that a relative excess of glucagon is an essential factor in the development of diabetes.

Glucagon's solubility is 50 μg/mL in most buffers between pH 3.5 and 8.5. It is soluble, 1 to 10 mg/mL, in the pH ranges 2.5 to 3.0 and 9.0 to 9.5. Solutions of 200 μg/mL at pH 2.5 to 3.0 are stable for at least several months at 4°C if sterile. Loss of activity by fibril formation occurs readily at high concentrations of glucagon at room temperature, or above, at pH 2.5. The isoelectric point appears to be at pH 7.5 to 8.5. Because it has been isolated from commercial insulin, its stability properties should be comparable to those of insulin.

As with insulin and some of the other polypeptide hormones, glucagon-sensitive receptor sites in target cells bind glucagon. This hormone–receptor interaction leads to activation of membrane adenylate cyclase, which catalyzes cAMP formation. Thus, intracellular cAMP levels are elevated. The mode of action of glucagon in glycogenolysis is basically the same as the mechanism of epinephrine (i.e., stimulation of adenylate cyclase). Subsequently, the increase in cAMP activates the protein kinase that catalyzes phosphorylation of phosphorylase kinase to phosphophosphorylase kinase. The latter is necessary for the activation of phosphorylase to form phosphorylase *a*. Finally, phosphorylase *a* catalyzes glycogenolysis, which is the basis for the hyperglycemic action of glucagon. Although both glucagon and epinephrine exert hyperglycemic action through cAMP, glucagon affects liver cells and epinephrine affects both muscle and liver cells.

Fain[63] reviewed the many phenomena associated with hormones, membranes, and cyclic nucleotides, including several factors that activate glycogen phosphorylase in rat liver. These factors involve not only glucagon but also vasopressin and the catecholamines. Glucagon and β-catecholamines mediate their effects on glycogen phosphorylase through cAMP, but may involve other factors as well.

Glucagon exerts other biochemical effects. Gluconeogenesis in the liver is stimulated by glucagon, and this is accompanied by enhanced urea formation. Glucagon inhibits the incorporation of amino acids into liver proteins. Fatty acid synthesis is decreased by glucagon. Cholesterol formation is also reduced. Glucagon activates liver lipases, however, and stimulates ketogenesis. Ultimately, the availability of fatty acids from liver triglycerides is elevated, fatty acid oxidation increases acetyl-CoA and other acyl-CoAs, and ketogenesis is promoted. As glucagon effects elevation of cAMP levels, release of glycerol and free fatty acids from adipose tissue also is increased.

Glucagon, whose regulatory effect on carbohydrate and fatty acid metabolism is well understood, is therapeutically important. It is recommended for the treatment of severe hypoglycemic reactions caused by the administration of insulin to diabetic or psychiatric patients. Of course, this treatment is effective only when hepatic glycogen is available. Nausea and vomiting are the most frequently encountered reactions to glucagon.

Usual dose: parenteral, adults, 500 μg to 1 mg (0.5–1.0 U), repeated in 20 minutes if necessary; pediatric, 25 μg/kg of body weight, repeated in 20 minutes if necessary.

Gastrointestinal Hormones

There is a formidable array of polypeptide hormones of the gastrointestinal tract that includes secretin, pancreozymin–cholecystokinin, gastrin, motilin, neurotensin, vasoactive intestinal peptide, somatostatin, and others. The biosynthesis, chemistry, secretion, and actions of these hormones have been reviewed.[64]

GASTRIN

Gastrin is a 17-residue polypeptide isolated from the antral mucosa. It was isolated originally in two different forms. In one of the forms, the tyrosine residue in position 12 is sulfated. Both forms are biologically active. Cholinergic response to the presence of food in the gastrointestinal tract provides the stimulus for gastrin secretion. The lowering of pH in the stomach inhibits the secretion of gastrin. The effects of structural modification of gastrin on gastric acid secretion have been reviewed.[65] These studies revealed that the four residues at the COOH terminus retain significant biological activity and that the aspartate residue is the most critical for activity. The most important action of gastrin is to stimulate the secretion of gastric acid and pepsin. Other actions of gastrin include increased secretion of pancreatic enzymes; contraction of smooth muscles; water and electrolyte secretion by the stomach and pancreas; water and electrolyte absorption by the small intestine; and secretion of insulin, glucagon, and somatostatin. A synthetic pentapeptide derivative, pentagastrin, is currently used as a gastric acid secretagogue.

Pentagastrin. Pentagastrin (Peptavlon), a physiological gastric acid secretagogue, is the synthetic pentapeptide derivative: N-*t*-butyloxycarbonyl-β-alanyl-L-tryptophyl-L-methionyl-L-aspartyl-L-phenylalanyl amide. It contains the COOH-terminal tetrapeptide amide (H · Try · Met · Asp · Phe · NH$_2$), which is considered to be the active center of the natural gastrins. Accordingly, pentagastrin appears to have the physiological and pharmacological properties of the gastrins, including stimulation of gastric secretion, pepsin secretion, gastric motility, pancreatic secretion of water and bicarbonate, pancreatic enzyme secretion, biliary flow and bicarbonate output, intrinsic factor secretion, and contraction of the gallbladder.

Pentagastrin is indicated as a diagnostic agent to evaluate gastric acid secretory function, and it is useful in testing for anacidity in patients with suspected pernicious anemia, atrophic gastritis or gastric carcinoma, hypersecretion in suspected duodenal ulcer or postoperative stomal ulcers, and Zollinger-Ellison tumor.

Pentagastrin is usually administered subcutaneously; the optimal dose is 6 μg/kg. Gastric acid secretion begins approximately 10 minutes after administration, and peak responses usually occur within 20 to 30 minutes. The usual duration of action is from 60 to 80 minutes. Pentagastrin has a relatively short plasma half-life, perhaps less than 10 minutes. The available data from metabolic studies indicate that pentagastrin is inactivated by the liver, kidney, and tissues of the upper intestine.

Contraindications include hypersensitivity or idiosyncrasy to pentagastrin. It should be used with caution in patients with pancreatic, hepatic, or biliary disease.

SECRETIN

Secretin is a 27-amino-acid polypeptide that is structurally similar to glucagon. The presence of acid in the small intestine is the most important physiological stimulus for the secretion of secretin. The primary action of secretin is on pancreatic acinar cells that regulate the secretion of water and bicarbonate. Secretin also promotes the secretion of pancreatic enzymes, to a lesser extent. Secretin inhibits the release of gastrin and, therefore, gastric acid. It also increases stomach-emptying time by reducing the contraction of the pyloric sphincter.[64]

$$
\begin{array}{ccc}
 & \text{Ala} - \text{Tyr-SO}_3\text{H} & \\
 & | & | \\
\text{(pyro)}^1\text{Glu} & \text{Glu}^{10} & \text{Gly} \\
| & | & | \\
\text{Gly} & \text{Glu} & \text{Trp} \\
| & | & | \\
\text{Pro} & \text{Glu} & \text{Met}^{15} \\
| & | & | \\
\text{Trp} & \text{Glu} & \text{Asp} \\
| & | & | \\
^5\text{Met} - \text{Glu} & \text{Phe-NH}_2
\end{array}
$$

Gastrin

$$
\begin{array}{ccc}
^1\text{His} & \text{Gln}^{20} - \text{Arg} \\
| & | & | \\
\text{Ser} & \text{Leu} & \text{Leu} \\
| & | & | \\
\text{Asp} & \text{Arg} & \text{Leu} \\
| & | & | \\
\text{Gly} & \text{Ala} & \text{Gln} \\
| & | & | \\
^5\text{Thr} & \text{Ser} & \text{Gly}^{25} \\
| & | & | \\
\text{Phe} & \text{Asp}^{15} & \text{Leu} \\
| & | & | \\
\text{Thr} & \text{Arg} & \text{Val-NH}_2 \\
| & | & \\
\text{Ser} & \text{Leu} & \\
| & | & \\
\text{Gly} & \text{Arg} & \\
| & | & \\
^{10}\text{Leu} - \text{Ser} &
\end{array}
$$

Secretin

CHOLECYSTOKININ–PANCREOZYMIN

It was thought originally that cholecystokinin and pancreozymin were two different hormones. Cholecystokinin was thought to be responsible for contraction of the gallbladder, whereas pancreozymin was believed to induce secretion of pancreatic enzymes. It is now clear that both actions are caused by a single 33-residue polypeptide, referred to as *cholecystokinin–pancreozymin* (CCK-PZ). CCK-PZ is secreted in the blood in response to the presence of food in the duodenum, especially long-chain fatty acids. The five COOH-terminal amino acid residues are identical with those in gastrin. The COOH-terminal octapeptide retains full activity of the parent hormone.

^{1}Lys His^{20} — Arg
| | |
Ala Ser Ile
| | |
Pro Pro Ser
| | |
Ser Asp Asp
| | |
^{5}Gly Leu Arg^{25}
| | |
Arg Ser^{15} Asp
| | |
Val Gln Tyr-SO$_3$H
| | |
Ser Leu Met Phe-NH$_2$
| | | |
Met Asn Gly Asp
| | | |
^{10}Ile — Lys Trp^{30} — Met

Cholecystokinin

The octapeptide is found in the gut as well as the central nervous system. SARs of cholecystokinin have been reviewed.[64] The COOH-terminal octapeptide is present in significant concentrations in the central nervous system. Its possible actions here, the therapeutic implications in the treatment of Parkinson disease and schizophrenia, and its SAR have been reviewed.[65]

VASOACTIVE INTESTINAL PEPTIDE

Vasoactive intestinal peptide (VIP) is widely distributed in the body and is believed to occur throughout the gastrointestinal tract. It is a 28-residue polypeptide with structural similarities to secretin and glucagon. It causes vasodilatation and increases cardiac contractibility. VIP stimulates bicarbonate secretion, relaxes gastrointestinal and other smooth muscles, stimulates glycogenesis, inhibits gastric acid secretion, and stimulates insulin secretion. Its hormonal and neurotransmitter role has been investigated.[66]

GASTRIC INHIBITORY PEPTIDE

Gastric inhibitory peptide (GIP) is a 43-amino-acid polypeptide isolated from the duodenum. Secretion of GIP into the blood is stimulated by food. The primary action of GIP is inhibition of gastric acid secretion. Other actions include stimulation of insulin and glucagon secretion and stimulation of intestinal secretion.[64]

MOTILIN

Motilin is a 22-residue polypeptide isolated from the duodenum. Its secretion is stimulated by the presence of acid in the duodenum. Motilin inhibits gastric motor activity and delays gastric emptying.

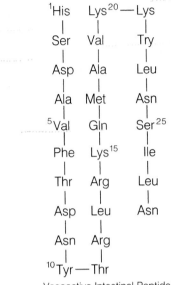

Vasoactive Intestinal Peptide

NEUROTENSIN

Neurotensin is a 13-amino-acid peptide, first isolated from bovine hypothalamus. It has now been identified in the intestinal tract. The ileal mucosa contains 90% of the total neurotensin of the body. It is implicated as a releasing factor for several adenohypophyseal hormones. It causes vasodilatation, increases vascular permeability, and increases gastrin secretion. It decreases secretion of gastric acid and secretin.

Parathyroid Hormone

This hormone is a linear polypeptide containing 84 amino acid residues. SAR studies[67] of bovine parathyroid hormone revealed that the biological activity is retained by an NH$_2$-terminal fragment consisting of eight amino acid residues. It regulates the concentration of calcium ion in the plasma within the normal range, in spite of variations in calcium intake, excretion, and anabolism into bone. In addition, for this hormone, cAMP is implicated as a second messenger. Parathyroid hormone activates adenylate cyclase in renal and skeletal cells, and this effect promotes formation of cAMP from ATP. The cAMP increases the synthesis and release of the lysosomal enzymes necessary for the mobilization of calcium from bone.

Parathyroid Injection, USP. Parathyroid injection has been used therapeutically as an antihypocalcemic agent for the temporary control of tetany in acute hypoparathyroidism.

Teriparatide (Forteo). Teriparatide is a recombinant form of parathyroid hormone, which is used for the treatment of osteoporosis in men and postmenopausal women. The N-terminal region possesses 34 amino acids, which are identical to the biologically active region of the 84-amino acid sequence of human parathyroid hormone. It has been shown to act on osteoblasts to stimulate new bone growth and improve bone density.

CALCITONIN

Calcitonin (thyrocalcitonin) is a 32-amino-acid polypeptide hormone secreted by parafollicular cells of the thyroid glands in response to hypocalcemia. The entire 32-residue peptide appears to be required for activity, because smaller fragments are totally inactive. Common structural features of calcitonin isolated from different species are a COOH-terminal prolinamide, a disulfide bond between residues 1 and 7 at the NH_2 terminus, and a chain length of 32 residues. Calcitonin inhibits calcium resorption from bone, causing hypocalcemia, with parallel changes in plasma phosphate concentration. In general, calcitonin negates the osteolytic effects of parathyroid hormone.

The potential therapeutic uses of calcitonin are in the treatment of hyperparathyroidism, osteoporosis and other bone disorders, hypercalcemia of malignancy, and idiopathic hypercalcemia.

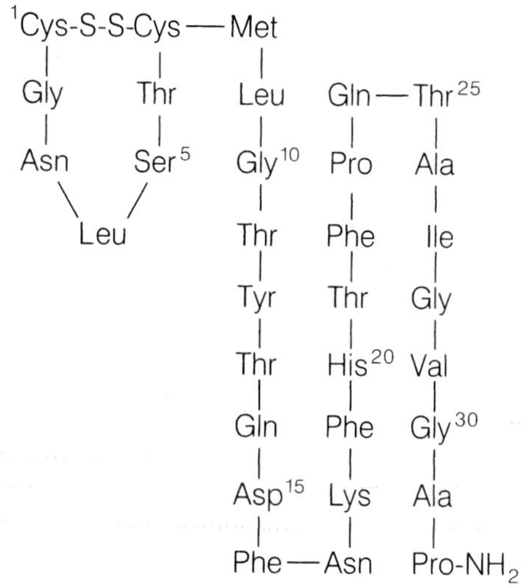

Calcitonin

Angiotensins

The synthesis of angiotensins in the plasma is initiated by the catalytic action of renin (a peptidase elaborated by the kidneys) on angiotensinogen, an α-globulin produced by the liver and found in the plasma. The hydrolytic action of renin on angiotensinogen yields angiotensin I, a decapeptide consisting of the first 10 residues of the NH_2-terminal segment of angiotensinogen. Angiotensin I has weak pharmacological activity. It is converted to angiotensin II, an octapeptide, by the catalytic actions of angiotensin-converting enzyme (ACE). Angiotensin II is a highly active peptide and is hydrolyzed to angiotensin III, a heptapeptide, by an aminopeptidase. Angiotensin III retains most of the pharmacological activity of its precursor. Further degradation of angiotensin III leads to pharmacologically inactive peptide fragments.

Angiotensin II is the most active form; hence, it is the most investigated angiotensin for pharmacological action and SARs. The two primary actions of angiotensin II are vasoconstriction and stimulation of synthesis and secretion of aldosterone by the adrenal cortex. Both of these actions lead to hypertension.

Mechanisms and sites of action of angiotensin agonists and antagonists in terms of biological activity and receptor interactions have been reviewed.[68] Additionally, com-

pounds that inhibit ACE have found therapeutic use as antihypertensive agents (e.g., captopril). The synthesis and the biological activity of several ACE inhibitors have been reviewed.[69] Further, the agents used to target this enzyme are discussed in the cardiovascular section of this textbook.

Angiotensin Amide. Angiotensin amide (Hypertensin) is a synthetic polypeptide (1-L-aspariginyl-5-L-valine angiotensin octapeptide) and has twice the pressor activity of angiotensin II. It is pharmaceutically available as a lyophilized powder for injection (0.5–2.5 mg diluted in 500 mL of sodium chloride injection or 5% dextrose for injection) to be administered by continuous infusion. The pressor effect of angiotensin is due to an increase in peripheral resistance; it constricts resistance vessels but has little or no stimulating action on the heart and little effect on the capacitance vessels. Angiotensin has been used as an adjunct in various hypotensive states. It is mainly useful in controlling acute hypotension during administration of general anesthetics that sensitize the heart to the effects of catecholamines.

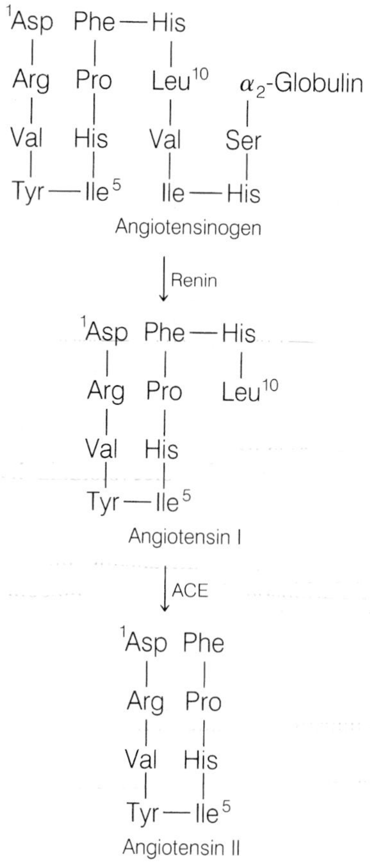

Plasmakinins

Bradykinin and kallidin are potent vasodilators and hypotensive agents that have different peptide structures: bradykinin is a nonapeptide, whereas kallidin is a decapeptide. Kallidin is lysyl-bradykinin; that is, it has an additional lysine at the NH_2 terminus of the chain. These two compounds are made available from kininogen, a blood globulin, on hydrolysis. Trypsin, plasmin, or the proteases of certain snake venoms can catalyze the hydrolysis of kininogen.

```
            Arg      ¹Lys    Arg¹⁰
             |         |       |
    ¹Arg    Phe       Arg     Phe
      |      |         |       |
    Pro     Pro       Pro     Pro
      |      |         |       |
    Pro     Ser       Pro     Ser
      |      |         |       |
    Gly —— Phe⁵      ⁵Gly —— Phe
      Bradykinin       Kallidin
```

Bradykinin is one of the most powerful vasodilators known; 0.05 to 0.5 $\mu g/kg$ intravenously can decrease blood pressure in all mammals investigated so far.

Although the kinins per se are not used as medicinals, kallikrein enzyme preparations that release bradykinin from the inactive precursor have been used in the treatment of Raynaud disease, claudication, and circulatory diseases of the eyegrounds. (*Kallikreins* is the term used to designate the group of proteolytic enzymes that catalyze the hydrolysis of kininogen, forming bradykinin.)

SUBSTANCE P

Substance P is a polypeptide consisting of 11 amino acid residues. It has been implicated in the transmission of "painful" sensory information through the spinal cord to higher centers in the central nervous system.[70–72] Substance P is localized in the primary afferent sensory fibers. Other pharmacological effects are vasodilatation, stimulation of smooth muscles, stimulation of salivary secretion, and diuresis. In addition, this neuropeptide contributes to some inflammatory responses. Approximately 50% of the known neuropeptides are synthesized as biologically inactive glycine extended precursors that require a carboxy-terminal posttranslational amidation for biological activity. Amidation enzymes are responsible for the conversion of the carboxyl group of the neuropeptide to the corresponding amide group and include the two amidating enzymes peptidylglycine α-monooxygenase (PAM) and peptidylamidoglycolate lyase (PGL), which work sequentially to produce the inflammatory neuropeptide Substance P from an inactive precursor peptide. Much research is being performed to exploit this mechanism of inflammation.

```
           Met-NH₂
             |
    ¹Arg    Leu¹⁰
      |      |
    Pro     Gly
      |      |
    Lys     Phe
      |      |
    Pro     Phe
      |      |
    ⁵Gln —— Gln
        Substance P
```

Thyroglobulin

Thyroglobulin, a glycoprotein, is composed of several peptide chains; it also contains 0.5% to 1% iodine and 8% to 10% carbohydrate in the form of two types of polysaccharide. The formation of thyroglobulin is regulated by TSH. Thyroglobulin has no hormonal properties. It must be hydrolyzed to release the hormonal iodothyronines thyroxine and liothyronine (see "Thyroid Hormones" in Chapter 19).

⬡ BLOOD PROTEINS

The blood is the transport system of the organism and thus performs important distributive functions. Considering the multitude of materials transported by the blood (e.g., nutrients, oxygen, carbon dioxide, waste products of metabolism, buffer systems, antibodies, enzymes, and hormones), its chemistry is very complex. Grossly, approximately 45% consists of the formed elements that can be separated by centrifugation, and of these, only 0.2% is other than erythrocytes. The 55% of removed plasma contains approximately 8% solids, of which a small portion (less than 1%) can be removed by clotting to produce defibrinated plasma, called *serum*. Serum contains inorganic and organic compounds, but the total solids are chiefly protein, mostly albumin, and the rest nearly all globulin. The plasma contains the protein fibrinogen, which is converted by coagulation to insoluble fibrin. The separated serum has an excess of the clotting agent thrombin.

Serum globulins can be separated by electrophoresis into α-, β-, and γ-globulins, which contain most of the antibodies. The immunological importance of globulins is well-known. Many classes and groups of immunoglobulins are produced in response to antigens or even to a single antigen. The specificity of antibodies has been studied from various points of view, and Richards et al.[73] have suggested that even though immune sera appear to be highly specific for antigen binding, individual immunoglobulins may not only interact with several structurally diverse determinants, but may bind such diverse determinants to different sites within the combining region.

The importance of the blood coagulation process has been obvious for a long time. Coagulation mechanisms are covered in several biochemistry texts (see under "Selected Reading"), so a brief summary suffices here. The required time for blood clotting is normally 5 minutes, and any prolongation beyond 10 minutes is considered abnormal. Thrombin, the enzyme responsible for the catalysis of fibrin formation, originates from the inactive zymogen prothrombin; the prothrombin–thrombin transformation depends on calcium ions and thromboplastin. The fibrinogen–fibrin reaction catalyzed by thrombin involves proteolytic cleavage (partial hydrolysis), polymerization of the fibrin monomers from the preceding step, and actual clotting (hard clot formation). The final process forming the hard clot occurs in the presence of calcium ions and the enzyme fibrinase.

Thrombin, USP. Thrombin is a sterile protein substance prepared from prothrombin of bovine origin. It is used as a topical hemostatic because it can clot blood, plasma, or a solution of fibrinogen without addition of other substances. Thrombin also may initiate clotting when combined with gelatin sponge or fibrin foam.

For external use it is applied topically to the wound, as a solution containing 100 to 2,000 National Institutes of Health (NIH) units/mL in sodium chloride irrigation or sterile water for injection or as a dry powder.

Hemoglobin

Erythrocytes contain 32% to 55% hemoglobin, about 60% water, and the rest as stroma. Stroma can be obtained, after hemolysis of the corpuscles by dilution, through the process of centrifuging and consists of lecithin, cholesterol, inorganic salts, and a protein, stromatin. Hemolysis of the corpuscles, or "laking" as it is sometimes called, may be brought about by hypotonic solution, by fat solvents, by bile salts that dissolve the lecithin, by soaps or alkalies, by saponins, by immune hemolysins, and by hemolytic sera, such as those from snake venom and numerous bacterial products.

Hemoglobin (Hb) is a conjugated protein; the prosthetic group heme (hematin) and the protein (globin), which is composed of four polypeptide chains, are usually in identical pairs. The total M_r is about 66,000, including four heme molecules. The molecule has an axis of symmetry and, therefore, is composed of identical halves with an overall ellipsoid shape of the dimensions $55 \times 55 \times 70$ Å.

Iron in the heme of hemoglobin (ferrohemoglobin), is in the ferrous state and can combine reversibly with oxygen to function as a transporter of oxygen.

$$Hb + O_2 \leftrightarrow Oxyhemoglobin\ (HbO_2)$$

In this process, the formation of a stable oxygen complex, the iron remains in the ferrous form because the heme moiety lies within a cover of hydrophobic groups of the globin. Both Hb and O_2 are magnetic, whereas HbO_2 is diamagnetic because the unpaired electrons in both molecules have become paired. When oxidized to the ferric state (methemoglobin or ferrihemoglobin), this function is lost. Carbon monoxide combines with hemoglobin to form carboxyhemoglobin (carbonmonoxyhemoglobin) to inactivate it.

The stereochemistry of the oxygenation of hemoglobin is very complex, and it has been investigated to some extent. Some evidence from x-ray crystallographic studies reveals that the conformations of the α and β chains are altered when their heme moieties complex with oxygen, thus promoting complexation with oxygen. It is assumed that hemoglobin can exist in two forms, the relative position of the subunits in each form being different. In the deoxy form, α and β subunits are bound to each other by ionic bonds in a compact structure that is less reactive toward oxygen than is the oxy form. Some ionic bonds are cleaved in the oxy form, relaxing the conformation. The latter conformation is more reactive to oxygen.

⬡ IMPACT OF BIOTECHNOLOGY ON THE DEVELOPMENT AND COMMERCIAL PRODUCTION OF PROTEINS AND PEPTIDES AS PHARMACEUTICAL PRODUCTS

Over the past decade and a half, far-reaching and revolutionary breakthroughs in molecular biology, especially research involving gene manipulations (i.e., genetic engineering), have led the way in the development of new biotechnology-derived products for the treatment of diseases. The term *biotherapy* has been coined to describe the clinical and diagnostic use of biotechnology-derived products. Generally, these products are proteins, peptides, or nucleic acids that are structurally and/or functionally similar to naturally occurring biomolecules. The large-scale production of these complex biomolecules was beyond the capabilities of traditional pharmaceutical technologies. According to the 1995 survey[74] conducted by the Pharmaceutical Research and Manufacturers of America, there are currently more than 230 biotechnology-derived products in various stages of development and 24 approved biotechnology-derived products available in the market. The currently approved biotechnology products are listed

in Table 27.9. There are 14 approval applications pending at the FDA and 49 in the third and final stage of clinical testing. A detailed discussion of the various processes and methodologies involved in biotechnology and the wide array of biotechnology-derived pharmaceutical products is beyond the scope of this chapter and is covered in Chapter 4. There are several reference sources[72,75–77] available.

Since the emphasis in this chapter is on proteins, peptides, and enzymes, the discussion of biotechnology processes and products is limited to these topics. The various biotechnology-derived products[74] include enzymes, receptors, hormones and growth factors, cytokines, vaccines, monoclonal antibodies, and nucleic acids (genes and antisense RNA).

Biotechnology techniques are constantly changing and expanding; however, the two primary techniques responsible for the development of most of the products are rDNA technology and monoclonal antibody technology. The emphasis in this chapter is on rDNA technology and products derived from this technology. The monoclonal antibody technology and resulting products are discussed elsewhere in this book. Excellent references[78,79] are available for review. The following discussion of rDNA technology assumes that the reader has thorough comprehension of the normal process of genetic expression in human cells (i.e., replication, transcription, and translation). Several biochemistry textbooks are available for review.

rDNA Technology

rDNA technology frequently has been referred to as *genetic engineering* or *gene cloning*. A comprehensive discussion of the process and application of rDNA technology is available in several good reviews.[72,75–77] The concept of genetic engineering is based on the fact that the genetic material (DNA) in all living organisms is made of the same four building blocks, that is, four different deoxymononucleotides. Therefore, genetic material from one organism or cell may be combined with the genetic material of another organism or cell. Because every single protein, regardless of its source, is produced as a result of expression of a specific gene coding for it, the application of this technology in the mass production of desired human proteins is obvious. A number of human diseases are caused by deficiencies of desired proteins or peptides. For example, insulin deficiency is a major cause of diabetes, and human growth hormone deficiency causes dwarfism. If a human gene coding for a deficient protein is identified and isolated, then it may be combined with fast-replicating, nonchromosomal bacterial DNA (i.e., plasmids). The recombined DNA is placed back into the bacteria, which then are grown in ideal media. The plasmids replicate and the genes within the plasmid are expressed, including the human gene, resulting in large quantities of the desired human protein.

The major steps in a typical rDNA process used in commercial-scale synthesis of human proteins are summarized in Figure 27.7 and discussed in the following:

1. Identification and isolation of the desired gene: The possible nucleotide sequence of a desired gene can be ascertained by (a) isolating and determining the amino acid sequence of the protein expressed by the gene and then determining the possible nucleotide sequences for the corresponding mRNA and the DNA (gene), (b) isolating

TABLE 27.9 Approved Biotechnology of Drugs and Vaccines

Product Name	Company	Indication (Date of U.S. Approval)
Actimmune Interferon gamma-1b	Genentech[a] (San Francisco, CA)	Management of chronic granulomatous disease (December 1990)
Activase Alteplase, recombinant	Genentech[a] (San Francisco, CA)	Acute myocardial infarction (November 1987); acute massive pulmonary embolism (June 1990)
Aldurazyme Laronidase	Genzyme	Mucopolysaccharidosis I (May 2003)
Alferon N Interferon alfa-n3 (injection)	Interferon Sciences (New Brunswick, NJ)	Genital warts (October 1989)
Betaseron Interferon beta-1b, recombinant	Berlex Laboratories[a] (Wayne, NJ) Chiron[a] (Emeryville, CA)	Relapsing, remitting multiple sclerosis (July 1993)
Cerezyme Imiglucerase for injection (recombinant glucocerebrosidase)	Genzyme (Cambridge, MA)	Treatment of Gaucher disease (May 1994)
Engerix-B Hepatitis B vaccine (recombinant)	SmithKline Beecham[a] (Philadelphia, PA)	Hepatitis B (September 1989)
Epogen Epoetin alfa (rEPO)	Amgen[a] (Thousand Oaks, CA)	Treatment of anemia associated with chronic renal failure, including patients on dialysis and not on dialysis, and anemia in Retrovir-treated, HIV-infected patients (June 1989); treatment of anemia caused by chemotherapy in patients with nonmyeloid malignancies (April 1993)
Fabrazyme Agalsidase beta	Genzyme	Fabry disease (April 2003)
Procrit[c] Epoetin alfa (rEPO)	Ortho Biotech[a] (Raritan, NJ)	Treatment of anemia associated with chronic renal failure, including patients on dialysis and not on dialysis, and anemia in Retrovir-treated, HIV-infected patients (December 1990); treatment of anemia caused by chemotherapy in patients with nonmyeloid malignancies (April 1993)
Humatrope Somatropin (rDNA origin) for injection	Eli Lilly[a] (Indianapolis, IN)	Human growth hormone deficiency in children (March 1987)
Humulin Human insulin (rDNA origin)	Eli Lilly[a] (Indianapolis, IN)	Diabetes (October 1982)
Intron A Interferon alfa-2b (recombinant)	Schering-Plough[a] (Madison, NJ)	Hairy cell leukemia (June 1986); genital warts (June 1988); AIDS-related Kaposi sarcoma (November 1988); hepatitis C (February 1991); hepatitis B (July 1992)
KoGENate Antihemophiliac factor (recombinant)	Miles[a] (West Haven, CT)	Treatment of hemophilia A (February 1993)
Leukine Sargramostim (yeast-derived GM-CSF)	Immunex[a] (Seattle, WA)	Autologous bone marrow transplantation (March 1991)
Myozyme Alglucosidase alfa	Genzyme	Treatment of Pompe disease (April 2006)
Naglazyme Galsulfase	BioMarin	Mucopolysaccharidosis VI (May 2005)
Neupogen Filgrastim (rG-CSF)	Amgen[a] (Thousand Oaks, CA)	Chemotherapy-induced neutropenia (February 1991); autologous or allogeneic bone marrow transplantation (June 1994); chronic severe neutropenia (December 1994)
Nutropin Somatropin for injection	Genentech[a] (San Francisco, CA)	Growth failure in children due to chronic renal insufficiency, growth hormone inadequacy in children (March 1994)
OncoScint CR/OV Satumomab pendetide	CYTOGEN[a] (Princeton, NJ)	Detection, staging, and follow-up of colorectal and ovarian cancers (December 1992)
Orencia Abatacept	Bristol-Myers	Treatment of rheumatoid arthritis (December 2005)
ORTHOCLONE OKT 3 Muromonab-CD3	Ortho Biotech[a] (Raritan, NJ)	Reversal of acute kidney transplant rejection (June 1986); reversal of heart and liver transplant rejection (June 1993)

Product Name	Company	Indication (Date of U.S. Approval)
Proleukin Aldesleukin (interleukin-2)	Chiron[a] (Emeryville, CA)	Renal cell carcinoma (May 1992)
Protropin Somatrem for injection	Genentech[a] (San Francisco, CA)	Human growth hormone deficiency in children (October 1985)
Pulmozyme DNAse (dornase alpha)	Genentech[a] (San Francisco, CA)	Cystic fibrosis (December 1993)
Rebif Interferon beta-1a	Serono Labs	Treatment of multiple sclerosis (March 2002)
RECOMBINATE Antihemophilic factor recombinant (rAHF)	Baxter Healthcare/Hyland Division (Glendale, CA) Genetics Institute[b] (Cambridge, MA)	Hemophilia A (December 1992)
RECOMBIVAX HB Hepatitis B vaccine (recombinant), MSD	Merck[a] (Whitehouse Station, NJ)	Hepatitis B prevention (July 1986)
ReoPro Abciximab	Centocor (Malvern, PA) Eli Lilly[a] (Indianapolis, IN)	Antiplatelet prevention of blood clots (December 1994)
Roferon-A Interferon alfa-2a, recombinant	Hoffmann-La Roche[a] (Nutley, NJ)	Hairy cell leukemia (June 1986); AIDS-related Kaposi sarcoma (November 1988)

Adapted from Biotechnology Medicines in Development: Approved Biotechnology Drugs and Vaccines [survey]. Pharmaceutical Research and Manufacturers of America, 1995, p. 20.
[a]PhRMA member company.
[b]PhRMA research affiliate.
[c]Procrit was approved for marketing under Amgen's epoetin alfa PLA. Amgen manufactures the product for Ortho Biotech. Under an agreement between the two companies, Amgen licensed to Ortho Pharmaceuticals the U.S. rights to epoetin for indications in human use excluding dialysis and diagnostics.

the mRNA and determining its nucleotide sequence, and (c) using DNA probes to "fish out" the desired gene from the genomic library (cellular DNA chopped up into segments 10,000–20,000 nucleotides long).

2. Constructing rDNA: Once the desired human gene is identified and isolated, it is recombined with genes of microbial cells that are known to have rapid rates of cell division. To accomplish this task, bacterial enzymes known as *restriction endonucleases* are used. More than 100 different variations of these hydrolytic enzymes, which act like scissors in hydrolyzing the phosphodiester bonds of DNA at specific sites (i.e., nucleotide sequences), are available. The use of a specific restriction endonuclease both to obtain the human gene and to open a site on the microbial gene allows easy formation of the hybrid (recombined) DNA molecule because of the "sticky" ends on both genes. The ends of the human gene and the microbial DNA vector are "glued" together by enzymes known as *DNA ligases*. The human genes are placed in specific locations on the microbial DNA vectors to ensure expression of the human gene when the microbial cells divide. Plasmids are the most commonly used microbial DNA. These extrachromosomal circular DNAs replicate independently of the chromosomes and are much smaller than chromosomal DNA. Plasmids are easy to manipulate and are considered excellent vectors to carry human genes. Other microbial cells used as hosts are yeast cells. Mammalian cells, such as Chinese hamster ovary cells, are used when glycosylation of the rDNA-derived protein is essential for biological activity (e.g., erythropoietin). Nonmammalian cells cannot glycosylate proteins.

3. Cloning: The cells carrying the recombined human gene are then allowed to grow in appropriate media. As the cells divide, the rDNA replicates and expresses its products, including the desired human protein as well as the normal bacterial proteins.

4. Isolation and purification of rDNA-derived protein: From this complex mixture containing bacterial proteins, cell components, chemicals used in preparing the media, etc., isolating and purifying the desired human protein is a daunting task indeed. This requires sophisticated isolation techniques, such as complex filtrations, precipitations, and HPLC. The primary goal of the purification process is to ensure that the protein isolated will retain the biological activity of the native protein in the body. The rDNA-derived protein is then formulated into a pharmaceutical product that is stable during transportation, storage, and administration to a patient.

BIOTECHNOLOGY-DERIVED PHARMACEUTICAL PRODUCTS

More than 2 dozen FDA-approved biotechnology-derived pharmaceutical products are listed in Table 27.9. There are more than 200 other products in various stages of development.[74] The FDA-approved products fall loosely into five major categories: enzymes, hormones, lymphokines, hematopoietic factors, and biologicals. A detailed discussion of all of these products is beyond the scope of this chapter. Because most of these products are proteins or peptides, a cursory evaluation of them and their uses[80] follows.

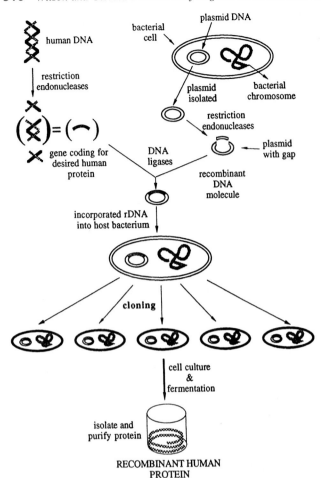

Figure 27.7 • Summary of a typical rDNA process used in the commercial-scale production of human proteins.

rDNA-DERIVED ENZYMES

Alteplase, Recombinant. Alteplase (Activase) was discussed previously.

Dornase Alpha. Dornase alpha, rhDNAse (Pulmozyme), is a mucolytic enzyme identical with the natural human DNAse and is used in the treatment of cystic fibrosis. Patients with cystic fibrosis suffer from decreased pulmonary function and infections caused by the secretion of thick mucus. Proteins contained in the mucus are bound to extracellular DNA, produced as a result of disintegration of bacteria in the lungs. This enzyme is involved in cleaving extracellular DNA and separates DNA from proteins, allowing proteolytic enzymes to break down proteins and thus decrease the viscosity of mucus in the lungs.[81] Proteins bound to extracellular DNA are not susceptible to proteolytic enzymes.[82] Dornase alpha is a glycoprotein containing 260 amino acids that is commercially produced in genetically engineered Chinese hamster ovary cells.

Dornase alpha is indicated for the treatment of cystic fibrosis in conjunction with other available therapies, such as antibiotics, bronchodilators, and corticosteroids. Adult dosage is 2.5 mg inhaled once daily, administered via a recommended nebulizer. Dornase alpha should not be mixed or diluted with other agents in the nebulizer because of the possibility of adverse physicochemical changes that may affect

activity. Common adverse effects include sore throat, hoarseness, and facial edema.

Imiglucerase. Imiglucerase (Cerezyme)[80] is a glycoprotein containing 497 amino acid residues and is *N*-glycosylated at four different positions. It is an analog of the natural human enzyme β-glucocerebrosidase and contains arginine at position 495 instead of the histidine in the natural enzyme. It is commercially produced in genetically engineered Chinese hamster ovary cells.

Like the natural enzyme, imiglucerase catalyzes the hydrolysis of glucocerebroside, a glycolipid, to glucose and ceramide within the lysosomes of phagocytic cells. Gaucher disease is caused by a deficiency of this enzyme, which results in the accumulation of glucocerebroside within tissue macrophages. The glycolipid-engorged macrophages are known as *Gaucher cells* and are responsible for the numerous clinical manifestations of Gaucher disease. The common clinical manifestations of Gaucher disease are severe anemia, thrombocytopenia, and skeletal complications that include osteonecrosis and osteopenia.

Imiglucerase is indicated for the long-term replacement therapy of Gaucher disease. It is administered intravenously at an initial dose of 2.5 to 60 U/kg, infused over 1 to 2 hours. This dose is usually repeated every 2 weeks. Both the dose and the frequency of administration may be varied, however, depending on the response.[83] Common adverse effects include dizziness, headache, abdominal discomfort, nausea, and rash.

rDNA-DERIVED HORMONES

The rDNA-derived hormones include insulin human injection *USP* (Humulin R, Novolin R, Velosulin Human), growth hormone (somatotropin; Humatrope), and somatrem (Protropin). All of these products, as well as other products containing human insulin, have been discussed in this chapter.

rDNA-DERIVED CYTOKINES

Interferons. [80] Interferons are natural glycoproteins produced by virtually all eukaryotic cells; they possess immunomodulating, antiviral, and cytotoxic activities. This family of glycoproteins is produced by cells in response to a wide range of stimuli.[84] In humans, interferons bind to cellular receptors, which leads to the synthesis of more than a dozen proteins that contribute to viral resistance. The antiviral effects of interferons may be caused by inhibition of the synthesis of viral mRNA or proteins or prevention of viral penetration or uncoating.[85,86] Based on their antigenic subtypes, the interferons are classified into three major groups: α, β, and γ. α-Interferon and β-interferon are produced by virtually all cells in response to a viral infection and various other stimuli. γ-Interferon is produced specifically by the T lymphocytes and the natural killer (NK) cells. γ-Interferons have greater immunoregulatory, but lower antiviral, effects than α- or β-interferons.[86] More than 12 subspecies of α-interferons, 1 β-interferon, and 2 γ-interferons are known to exist. In general, the interferons are glycoproteins consisting of 165 to 166 amino acid residues. There are four rDNA-derived α-interferons available for clinical use around the world and three available in the United States (described next). All α-interferons exhibit antiviral and antiproliferative activity, enhance phagocytic activity, and augment specific cytoxicity of lymphocytes for certain target cells.[87] The most common adverse effects of α- and β-interferons include flulike symptoms, bone marrow suppression, neurotoxic effects, hypocalcemia, anorexia and other gastrointestinal symptoms, and weight loss.

Interferon Alfa-2a, Recombinant. Interferon alfa-2a, recombinant (Roferon), is produced from genetically engineered *E. coli* and contains 165 amino acid residues. At position 23, interferon alfa-2a has a lysine residue. The pharmaceutical product contains a single α-interferon subtype. A murine monoclonal antibody is used during purification by affinity chromatography. Interferon alfa-2a is used in the treatment of hairy cell leukemia and acquired immunodeficiency syndrome (AIDS)-related Kaposi sarcoma. It is absorbed well after intramuscular or intravenous administration and has a half-life of 5 to 7 hours when administered by the intramuscular route. The solution should be stored in the refrigerator at 36°F to 46°F and should not be frozen or shaken.

Peginterferon Alfa-2a, Recombinant. Interferon alfa-2a, recombinant (Roferon), is produced from genetically engineered *E. coli*. It is interferon, alfa-2a utilizing a 40 kd polyethylene glycol (PEG) strand to allow for stable therapeutic serum levels of alpa-2a for up to 168 hours on a single dose. This process is known as PEGylation and involves the process of attaching strands of the polymer PEG to molecules in an attempt to make them safer and more effective as therapeutic agents. The physiochemical changes in the drug increase systemic retention as well as influence the binding affinity to the cell receptors. The therapeutic usefulness of peginterferon alpfa-2a is in the treatment of hepatitis C.

Interferon Alfa-2b, Recombinant. Interferon alfa-2b, recombinant (Intron A), also contains a single subtype of α-interferon. It is a glycoprotein containing 165 amino acid residues and is commercially produced from genetically engineered *E. coli*. It differs from interferon alfa-2b in possessing an arginine residue at position 23. It is used in the treatment of hairy cell leukemia, condyloma acuminata (genital warts), AIDS-related Kaposi sarcoma, hepatitis C, and hepatitis B. It is administered intramuscularly or subcutaneously with a half-life of 2 to 3 hours and via intravenous infusion with a half-life of 8 hours. The reconstituted solution is stable for 1 month when stored at a temperature of 36°F to 46°F.

Interferon Alfa-n3 (Injection). Interferon alfa-n3 (Alferon N) is a polyclonal mixture of up to 14 natural α-interferon subtypes and contains 166 amino acid residues. Its commercial production involves induction of pooled units of human leukocytes with an avian virus (Sendai virus). The purification process involves immunoaffinity and filtration chromatography. It is indicated primarily by intralesional injection for the treatment of genital warts. The solution should be stored at a temperature of 36°F to 46°F and should not be shaken.

Interferon Beta-1a. Interferon beta-1a (Rebif, Avonex), has biological effects similar to those of natural β-interferon and α-interferons. Unlike beta-1b, which is produced in modified *E. coli*, beta-1a is produced in mammalian cells. It has been shown to slow the progression of multiple sclerosis as well as reduce the rate of relapse of this disease.

Interferon Beta-1b, Recombinant. Interferon beta-1b, recombinant (Betaseron), has biological effects similar to those of natural β-interferon and α-interferons. The natural β-interferon is a glycoprotein containing 166 amino acid residues. The rDNA product differs from the natural form, in that it is not glycosylated, it lacks the amino-terminal methionine, and it has serine in the place of methionine at position 17.[88] It is used for a wide variety of indications via intravenous, intramuscular, subcutaneous, intrathecal, and intralesional routes. Its primary indication is for the prevention of exacerbations in patients suffering from relapsing/remitting multiple sclerosis. Recommended dosage is 8 million units, administered subcutaneously, every other day. It also is indicated in the treatment of malignant glioma and malignant melanoma. Recommended temperature for storage is 36°F to 46 °F, and unused reconstituted solution should be discarded.

Aldesleukin. Aldesleukin, interleukin-2 (Proleukin),[80] is an rDNA-derived lymphokine that differs structurally from native interleukin-2 (IL-2) but has biological activity similar to that of the natural lymphokine.[89] Natural IL-2 is produced primarily by the peripheral blood lymphocytes and contains 133 amino acid residues. The immunoregulatory effects of aldesleukin include enhancing mitogenesis of lymphocytes, stimulating the growth of IL-2–dependent cell lines, enhancing cytotoxicity of lymphocytes, inducing lymphokine-activated killer (LAK) cells and NK cells, and inducing interferon-γ production. The exact mechanism of the antitumor activity of aldesleukin in humans is unknown.

The rDNA process involves genetically engineered *E. coli* (pBR 322 plasmids). The gene for IL-2 was synthesized after first isolating and identifying the mRNA from the human Jurkat cell line and then preparing the complementary DNA (cDNA). The IL-2 gene was genetically engineered before it was hybridized into pBR 322 plasmid. Further manipulation of the hybridized plasmid resulted in the production of a modified IL-2, aldesleukin.[90] Aldesleukin differs structurally from the native IL-2 in that the former is not glycosylated, it lacks the N-terminal alanine residue, and it has serine in the place of cysteine at position 125. Noncovalent, molecular aggregation of aldesleukin is different from IL-2, and the former exists as a microaggregate of 27 molecules.

The primary indication for aldesleukin is in the treatment of adult metastatic renal carcinoma. It is administered via intravenous infusion in doses of 10,000 to 50,000 U/kg every 8 hours for 12 days. It is primarily metabolized by the kidneys, with no active form found in the urine. Aldesleukin causes serious adverse effects in patients, including fever, hypotension, pulmonary congestion and dyspnea, coma, gastrointestinal bleeding, respiratory failure, renal failure, arrhythmias, seizures, and death.

rDNA-DERIVED HEMATOPOIETIC FACTORS

Hematopoietic growth factors are glycoproteins produced by a number of peripheral and marrow cells. More than 200 billion blood cells are produced each day; and the hematopoietic factors, along with other lymphopoietic factors such as the stem cell factor and the interleukins, are involved in the proliferation, differentiation, and maturation of various types of blood cells derived from the pluripotent stem cells.

Erythropoietin.[80] Erythropoietin is a heavily glycosylated protein containing 166 amino acid residues. It is produced primarily by the peritubular cells in the cortex of the kidney, and up to 15% is produced in the liver. It is the principal hormone responsible for stimulating the production of red blood cells from erythroid progenitor cells, erythrocyte burst-forming units, and erythrocyte colony-forming units.[91] Small amounts of erythropoietin are detectable in the plasma; however, most of the hormone is secreted by the kidneys in response to hypoxia or anemia, when levels of the hormone can rise more than 100-fold.

Decreased erythropoietin production is one of several potential causes of anemia of chronic renal disease. Other causes of anemia of chronic renal disease include infection or inflammatory condition in the kidneys, iron deficiency, marrow damage, and vitamin or mineral deficiency. Regardless of the underlying disease causing renal failure, erythropoietin levels decrease in patients with renal failure. Until rDNA technology was used to produce commercial quantities of erythropoietin, it was obtained from the urine of patients suffering from severe aplastic anemia. This process of obtaining natural hormone was costly and time-consuming and produced only small quantities of the hormone.

Epoetin Alfa.   Epoetin alfa, rEPO (Epogen, Procrit), is the recombinant human erythropoietin produced in Chinese hamster ovary cells into which the human erythropoietin gene has been inserted. These mammalian cells glycosylate the protein in a manner similar to that observed in human cells.[92]

Epoetin alfa is indicated in anemic patients with chronic renal failure, including both those who require regular dialysis and those who do not. Epoetin alfa is also indicated in anemia associated with AIDS, treatment of AIDS with zidovudine, frequent blood donations, and neoplastic diseases. It is indicated to prevent anemia in patients who donate blood prior to surgery for future autologous transfusions and to reduce the need for repeated maintenance transfusions.[93] The hormone is available as an isotonic buffered solution, which is administered by the intravenous route. The solution should not be frozen or shaken and is stored at 36°F to 46°F.

Colony-Stimulating Factors.[80]   Colony-stimulating factors are natural glycoproteins produced in lymphocytes and monocytes. These factors bind to cell-surface receptors of hematopoietic progenitor cells and stimulate proliferation, differentiation, and maturation of these cells into recognizable mature blood cells.[93] Colony-stimulating factors produced by rDNA technology have the same biological activity as the natural hormones. Currently, there are two colony-stimulating factors commercially produced by rDNA technology. These products are discussed next.

Filgrastim.   Filgrastim, rG-CSF (Neupogen), is a 175-amino acid polypeptide produced in genetically engineered *E. coli* cells containing the human granulocyte colony-stimulating factor (G-CSF) gene. Filgrastim differs from the natural hormone in that the former is not glycosylated and contains an additional methionine group at the N-terminus, which is deemed necessary for expression of the gene in *E. coli.*

Filgrastim specifically stimulates the proliferation and maturation of neutrophil granulocytes and, hence, is considered lineage specific. Accepted indications for filgrastim include the following: (a) to decrease the incidence of febrile neutropenia in patients with nonmyeloid malignancies who receive myelosuppressive chemotherapeutic agents, thus

lowering the incidence of infections in these patients; (b) to accelerate myeloid recovery in patients undergoing autologous bone marrow transplantation; and (c) in AIDS patients, to decrease the incidence of neutropenia caused by the disease itself, or by drugs used to treat the disease. The usual starting dose for filgrastim is 5 μg/kg per day in patients with nonmyeloid cancer who receive myelosuppressive chemotherapy.

Filgrastim solution should be stored at 36°F to 46°F and used within 24 hours of preparation. The solution should not be shaken or allowed to freeze. Any solution left at room temperature for more than 6 hours should be discarded. The most frequent adverse effects of filgrastim are medullary bone pain, arthralgia, and myalgia.

Sargramostim.   Sargramostim, rGM-CSF (Leukine), is a glycoprotein commercially produced in genetically engineered yeast cells. Its polypeptide chain contains 127 amino acids. It differs from the natural hormone by substitution of leucine at position 23 and variations in the glycosylation.[94] Sargramostim is a lineage-nonspecific hematopoietic factor, because it promotes the proliferation and maturation of granulocytes (neutrophils and eosinophils) and monocytes (macrophages and megakaryocytes).

The primary indication for sargramostim is in myeloid engraftment following autologous bone marrow transplantation and hematopoietic stem cell transplantation. Handling, storage precautions, and adverse effects are similar to those for filgrastim.

RDNA-DERIVED MISCELLANEOUS PRODUCTS

Antihemophilic Factor.   Antihemophilic factor (factor VIII) (Humate-P, Hemophil M, Koate HP, Monoclate-P) is a glycoprotein found in human plasma and a necessary cofactor in the blood-clotting mechanism. This high–molecular-weight glycoprotein has a complex structure with several components (subcofactors).[95] The commercially available concentrates derived from blood collected from volunteer donors by the American Red Cross Blood Services are used primarily for the treatment of patients with hemophilia A. Because the commercially available products are purified concentrates derived from blood pooled from millions of donors, the major precautions in using the products relate to transmission of viruses, such as hepatitis virus, herpesvirus, and HIV. This major problem has been alleviated, mostly because of the development and marketing of rDNA-derived antihemophilic factors.

Antihemophilic Factor (Recombinant).   Antihemophilic factor (recombinant), rAHF (KoGENate, Helixate), is an rDNA-derived factor VIII expressed in genetically engineered baby hamster kidney cells.[96] KoGENate has the same biological activity as the human plasma-derived antihemophilic factor (pdAHF). The purification process for rAHF includes monoclonal antibody immunoaffinity chromatography to remove any protein contaminants.

rAHF is indicated for the treatment of hemophilia A and is administered by the intravenous route. Patients suffering from hemophilia A exhibit a decrease in the activity of plasma clotting factor VIII. This product temporarily prevents bleeding episodes in hemophiliacs and may be used to prevent excessive bleeding during surgical procedures in these patients. A major advantage of the rAHF over the natural factor VIII is the lack of virus in the product. rAHF does not contain von Willebrand factor; therefore, it is not indicated in the treatment of von Willebrand disease. Patients receiving rAHF should be monitored carefully for the development of antibodies.

Bioclate is an rDNA-derived factor VIII expressed in genetically engineered Chinese hamster ovary cells. It has the same biological activity as pdAHF and is structurally similar. Its indications and adverse effects are similar to those for KoGENate.

● R E V I E W   Q U E S T I O N S ●

1. The rennin–angiotensin system plays an important role in regulation of blood pressure. As such, this pathway encompasses the conversion of an approximately 400-amino acid sequence to a decapeptide, then to the biologically active octapeptide and is an excellent target for drug therapy to manage hypertension. Describe the starting protein and its conversion to the biologically active metabolite. Be sure to include the enzymes involved in the conversion of the protein and peptides.

2. In the digestion and absorption of dietary protein:
   a. pepsinogen is converted to pepsin by gastrin via a proteolysis reaction.
   b. chymotrypsinogen is activated by trypsin.
   c. carboxypeptidase activates pepsinogen in the stomach.
   d. hydrochloric acid activates aminopeptidase.

3. Clinically, which of the following is used to dissolve necrotic tissue of second- and third-degree burn patients?
   a. streptokinase
   b. sutilains
   c. trypsin
   d. dornase
   e. lypressin

4. While working in your basement you discover a method of producing proteins and peptides that has never been described in the literature. What is the significance of being able to produce cytokines such as interferons?

5. You have discovered a protein that is capable of blocking the progression of Alzheimer disease. The sources of this protein are very limited, and you need additional material to complete a phase II clinical trial. Describe how you would use rDNA technology to produce more of this wonder drug.

REFERENCES

1. Ahmad, F., et al. (eds.): From Gene to Protein: Translation into Biotechnology, vol. 19. New York, Academic Press, 1982.
2. Boza, J. J., et al.: Eur. J. Nutr. 39(6):237, 2000.
3. American Medical Association Department of Drugs: Drug Evaluations, 6th ed. New York, John Wiley & Sons, 1986, pp. 867–870.
4. Stryer, L.: Biochemistry, 5th ed. New York, W. H. Freeman & Co., 2002, Chap. 3.
5. Corey, R. B., and Pauling, L.: Proc. R. Soc. Lond. Ser. B 141:10, 1953. (See also Adv. Protein Chem. 8:147, 1957)
6. Tanford, C.: The Hydrophobic Effect: Formation of Micelles and Biological Membranes, 2nd ed. New York, John Wiley & Sons, 1979.
7. McDonald, C. C., and Phillips, W. D.: J. Am. Chem. Soc. 89:6332, 1967.
8. Rienstra, C. M., et al.: Proc. Natl. Acad. Sci. U. S. A. 99(16):10260, 2002.
9. Kato, G., and Yung, J.: Mol. Pharmacol. 7:33, 1971.
10. Elefrawi, M. E., et al.: Mol. Pharmacol. 7:104, 1971.
11. Tang, C., Ndassa, Y., and Summers, M. F.: Nat. Strict. Biol. 9(7):537, 2002.
12. Kodak, A., et al.: Endocrinology 143(2):411, 2002.
13. Catrina, S. B., Cocilescu, M., and Andersson, M.: J. Cell Mol. Med. 5(2):195, 2001.
14. Ferdinand, W.: The Enzyme Molecule. New York, John Wiley & Sons, 1976.
15. Stryer, L.: Biochemistry, 5th ed. New York, W. H. Freeman & Co., 2002, Chap. 4.
16. Koshland, D. E.: Sci. Am. 229:52, 1973 (see also Annu. Rev. Biochem. 37:359, 1968).
17. Belleau, B.: J. Med. Chem. 7:776, 1964.
18. Lowe, J. N., and Ingraham, L. L.: An Introduction to Biochemical Reaction Mechanisms. Englewood Cliffs, NJ, Prentice-Hall, 1974.
19. Hanson, K. R., and Rose, I. A.: Acc. Chem. Res. 8:1, 1975 (see also Science 193:121, 1976).
19a. Bender, M. L.: J. Am. Chem. Soc. 79:1258, 1957.
19b. Bender, M. L.: J. Am. Chem. Soc. 80:5338, 1958.
19c. Bender, M. L.: J. Am. Chem. Soc. 82:1900, 1960.
19d. Bender, M. L.: J. Am. Chem. Soc. 86:3704, 5330, 1964.
19e. Blow, D. M.: Acc. Chem. Res. 9:145, 1976.
20. Roberts, J. D.: Chem. Eng. News, 57:23, 1979.
21. Wallis, M., Howell, S. L., and Taylor, K. W.: The Biochemistry of the Peptide Hormone. Chichester, U. K., John Wiley & Sons, 1986.
22. Spatola, A. F.: Annu. Rep. Med. Chem. 16:199, 1981.
23. Brueggemeier, R. W.: Peptide and protein hormones. In Wolff, M. E. (ed.): Burger's Medicinal Chemistry, vol. 3, 5th ed. New York, John Wiley & Sons, 1996, pp. 464–465.
24. Otsuka, H., and Inouye, L. K.: Pharmacol. Ther. [B] 1:501, 1975.
25. Schimmer, B. P., and Parker, K. L.: In Hardman, J. G., and Limbird, L. E. (eds.). Goodman and Gilman's The Pharmacological Basis of Therapeutics, 10th ed. New York, Macmillan, 2001, pp. 1650–1655.
26. Hughes, J., et al.: Nature 258:577, 1975.
27. Gutstein, H. B., and Akil, H.: In Hardman, J. G., and Limbird, L. E. (eds.). Goodman and Gilman's The Pharmacological Basis of Therapeutics, 10th ed. New York, Macmillan, 2001, pp. 569–579.
28. Snyder, S. H.: Science 224:22, 1984.
29. Wallis, M.: J. Mol. Evol. 17:10, 1981.
30. Lewis, U. J., Sinha, Y. N., and Lewis, G. P.: Endocr. J. 47(Suppl.):S1–8, 2000.
31. Janecka, A., Zubrzycka, M., and Janecki, T.: J. Pept. Res. 58(2):91, 2001.
32. Brownstein, M. J.: Science 207:373, 1980.
33. Drug Information for the Health Care Professional, vol. 1, 22nd ed. Rockville, MD, U. S. Pharmacopeial Convention, 2002, p. 2275.
34. Banting, F. G., and Best, C. H.: J. Lab. Clin. Med. 7:251, 1922.
35. Wallis, M., Howell, S. L., and Taylor, K. W.: The Biochemistry of Peptide Hormones. Chichester, U. K., John Wiley & Sons, 1985, pp. 257–297.
36. Alrefai, H., Allababidi, H., Levy, S., et al.: Endocrine 18(2):105, 2002.
37. Newgard, C. B.: Diabetes 51(11):3141, 2002.
38. De Meyts, P., and Whittaker, J.: Nat. Rev. Drug Discov. 1(10):769, 2002.
39. Steiner, D. F., et al.: Recent Prog. Horm. Res. 25:207–282, 1969.
40. Docherty, K., et al.: Proc. Natl. Acad. Sci. U. S. A. 79:4613, 1982.
41. Arquilla, E. R., et al.: In Steiner, D. F., and Freinkel, N. (eds.). Handbook of Physiology, Sect. 7: Endocrinology, vol. 1. Washington, DC, American Physiological Society, 1972, pp. 159–173.
42. Gerich, J., et al.: Annu. Rev. Physiol. 38:353, 1976.

43. Sanger, F.: Annu. Rev. Biochem. 27:58, 1958.
44. Katsoyannis, P. G.: Science 154:1509, 1966.
45. Rittel, W., et al.: Helv. Chim. Acta 67:2617, 1974.
46. Chance, R. E., et al.: Diabetes Care 4:147, 1981.
47. Johnson, I. S.: Diabetes Care 5(Suppl. 2):4, 1982.
48. Cosmatos, A., et al.: J. Biol. Chem. 253:6586, 1978.
49. May, J. M., et al.: J. Biol. Chem. 253:686, 1978.
50. Blundell, T. L., et al.: Crit. Rev. Biochem. 13:141, 1982.
51. Larner, J.: Diabetes 37:262, 1988.
52. Kasuga, M., et al.: Science 215:185, 1982.
53. Gerich, J. E.: In Diabetes Mellitus, 9th ed. Indianapolis, Eli Lilly & Co., 1988, p. 53.
54. Galloway, J. A.: In Diabetes Mellitus, 9th ed. Indianapolis, Eli Lilly & Co., 1988, pp. 109–122.
55. Wallis, M., et al.: The Biochemistry of the Polypeptide Hormones. Chichester, U. K., John Wiley & Sons, 1985, p. 280.
56. Jefferson, L. S.: Diabetes 29:487, 1980.
57. Feldman, J. M.: In Diabetes Mellitus, 9th ed. Indianapolis, Eli Lilly & Co., 1988, pp. 28–42.
58. Pirat, J.: Diabetes Care 1(part 1):168–188, (part 2):252–263, 1978.
59. Raskin, P., and Rosenstock, J.: Ann. Intern. Med. 105:254, 1986.
60. Maurer, A. C.: Am. Sci. 67:422, 1979.
61. USP DI: Drug Information for the Health Care Professional, vol. I, 22nd ed. Rockville, MD, U. S. Pharmacopeial Convention, 2002, pp. 1701–1730.
62. Unger, R. J., et al.: Science 188:923, 1975.
63. Fain, J. N.: Recept. Recogn. Ser. A 6:3, 1978.
64. Wallis, M., Howell, S. L., and Taylor, K. W.: The Biochemistry of the Polypeptide Hormones. Chichester, U. K., John Wiley & Sons, 1985, pp. 318–335.
65. Emson, P. C., and Sandberg, B. E.: Annu. Rep. Med. Chem. 18:31, 1983.
66. Miller, R. J.: J. Med. Chem. 27:1239, 1984.
67. Adams, A. E., et al.: Mol. Endocrinol. 12(11):1673, 1998.
68. Bumpus, F. M.: Fed. Proc. 36:2128, 1977.
69. Ondetti, M. A., and Cushman, J.: J. Med. Chem. 24:355, 1981.
70. Ogonowski, A. A., et al.: J. Pharm. Exp. Ther. 280:846–853, 1997.
71. May, S. W., and Pollock, S. H.: U. S. Patent #6,495,514. Issued December 2002.
72. Pezzuto, J. M., Johnson, M. E., and Manasse, H. R. (eds.): Biotechnology and Pharmacy. New York, Chapman & Hall, 1993.
73. Richards, F. F., et al.: Science 187:130, 1975.
74. Biotechnology Medicines in Development [survey], Pharmaceutical Research and Manufacturers of America, Washington, DC, 1995.
75. Zito, S. W. (ed.): Pharmaceutical Biotechnology: A Programmed Text. Lancaster, PA, Technomic Publishing, 1992.
76. Hudson, R. A., and Black, C. D.: Biotechnology—The New Dimension in Pharmacy Practice: A Working Pharmacists' Guide. Columbus, OH, Council of Ohio Colleges of Pharmacy, 1992, p. 1.
77. Primrose, S. B.: Modern Biotechnology. Boston, Blackwell Scientific Publications, 1987.
78. Hudson, R. A., and Black, C. D.: Biotechnology—The New Dimension in Pharmacy Practice: A Working Pharmacists' Guide, Council of Ohio Colleges of Pharmacy, 1992, p. 2.
79. Birch, J. R., and Lennox, E. S. (eds.): Monoclonal Antibodies: Principles and Applications. New York, John Wiley & Sons, 1995.
80. Gelman, C. R., Rumack, B. H., and Hess, A. J. (eds.): DRUGDEX (R) System. Englewood, CO, MICROMEDEX, Inc. (expired 11/30/95).
81. Shak, S., et al.: Recombinant human DNAse I reduces viscosity of cystic fibrosis sputum. Proc. Natl. Acad. Sci. U. S. A. 87:9188, 1990.
82. Lieberman, J., and Kurnick, N. B.: Nature 196:988, 1962.
83. Brady, R. O., et al.: Prog. Clin. Biol. Res. 95:669, 1982.
84. Kirkwood, J. M., and Ernstoff, M. S.: J. Clin. Oncol. 2:336, 1984.
85. Houglum, J. E.: Clin. Pharm. 2:202, 1983.
86. Hayden, F. G.: Antiviral agents. In Hardman, J. G., and Limbird, L. E. (eds.). Goodman and Gilman's The Pharmacological Basis of Therapeutics, 10th ed. New York, Macmillan, 2001, pp. 1332–1335.

87. USP DI: Drug Information for the Health Care Professional, vol. I, 22nd ed. Rockville, MD, U. S. Pharmacopeial Convention, 2002, pp. 1730–1733.
88. Von Hoff, D. D., and Huong, A. M.: J. Interferon Res. 8:813, 1988.
89. Doyle, M. V., Lee, M. T., and Fong, S.: J. Biol. Response Mod. 4:96, 1985.
90. Kato, K., et al.: Biochem. Biophys. Res. Commun. 130:692, 1985.
91. Erslev, A. J.: Erythropoietin coming of age. N. Engl. J. Med. 316:101, 1981.
92. Lin, F. K., et al.: Proc. Natl. Acad. Sci. U. S. A. 82:7580, 1985.
93. USP DI: Drug Information for the Health Care Professional, vol. I, 22nd ed. Rockville, MD, U. S. Pharmacopeial Convention, 2002, pp. 941–947.
94. Lee, F., et al.: Proc. Natl. Acad. Sci. U. S. A. 82:4360, 1985.
95. Fulcher, C., and Zimmerman, T.: Proc. Natl. Acad. Sci. U. S. A. 79:1648, 1982.
96. Lawn, R. M., and Vehar, G. A.: Sci. Am. 254:48, 1986.

SELECTED READING

Birch, J. R., and Lennox, E. S. (eds.): Monoclonal Antibodies: Principles and Applications. New York, John Wiley & Sons, 1995.

Boyer, P. D. (ed.): The Enzymes, 3rd ed. New York, Academic Press, 1970.

Brockerhoff, H., and Jensen, R. G.: Lipolytic Enzymes. New York, Academic Press, 1974.

Ferdinand, W.: The Enzyme Molecule. New York, John Wiley & Sons, 1976.

Galloway, J. A., Potvin, J. H., and Shuman, C. R. (eds.): Diabetes Mellitus, 9th ed. Indianapolis, Eli Lilly & Co., 1988.

Grollman, A. P.: Inhibition of protein biosynthesis. In Brockerhoff, H., and Jensen, R. G. (eds.). Lipolytic Enzymes. New York, Academic Press, 1974, pp. 231–247.

Hardman, J. G., and Limbird, L. E. (eds.). Goodman and Gilman's The Pharmacological Basis of Therapeutics, 10th ed. New York, Macmillan, 2001.

Haschemeyer, R. H., and de Harven, E.: Electron microscopy of enzymes. Annu. Rev. Biochem. 43:279, 1974.

Hruby, V. J., de Chavez, C. G., and Kavarana, M.: Peptide and protein hormones, peptide neurotransmitters, and therapeutic agents. In Abraham, D. J. (ed.) Burger's Medicinal Chemistry and Drug Discovery, vol. 4, 6th ed. New York, John Wiley & Sons, 2003.

Jenks, W. P.: Catalysis in Chemistry and Enzymology. New York, McGraw-Hill, 1969.

Lowe, J. N., and Ingraham, L. L.: An Introduction to Biochemical Reaction Mechanisms. Englewood Cliffs, NJ, Prentice-Hall, 1974. (This book includes elementary enzymology including mechanisms of coenzyme function.)

Mildvan, A. S.: Mechanism of enzyme action. Annu. Rev. Biochem. 43:357, 1974.

Pezzuto, J. M., Johnson, M. E., and Manasse, H. R. (eds.): Biotechnology and Pharmacy. New York, Chapman & Hall, 1993.

Pikes, S. J., and Parks, C. R.: The mode of action of insulin. Annu. Rev. Pharmacol. 14:365, 1974.

Schaeffer, H. J.: Factors in the design of reversible and irreversible enzyme inhibitors. In Ariens, E. J. (ed.). Drug Design, vol. 2. New York, Academic Press, 1971, pp. 129–159.

Stryer, L. S.: Biochemistry, 5th ed. New York, W. H. Freeman & Co., 2002.

Tager, H. S., and Steiner, D. F.: Peptide hormones. Annu. Rev. Biochem. 43:509, 1974.

Waife, S. O. (ed.): Diabetes Mellitus, 8th ed. Indianapolis, Eli Lilly & Co., 1980.

Wallis, M., Howell, S. L., and Taylor, K. W.: The Biochemistry of the Peptide Hormones. Chichester, U. K., John Wiley & Sons, 1985.

Wilson, C. A.: Hypothalamic amines and the release of gonadotrophins and other anterior pituitary hormones. Adv. Drug Res. 8:119–204, 1974.

CHAPTER 28

Vitamins

MICHAEL J. DEIMLING, M. O. FARUK KHAN, AND GUSTAVO R. ORTEGA

CHAPTER OVERVIEW

The medicinal chemistry of vitamins is fundamental not only to the therapeutics of nutritional problems but also to the understanding of the biochemical actions of other medicinal agents that directly or indirectly affect the metabolic functions of vitamins and coenzymes. Notable in this regard is the interrelationship between folic acid and vitamin B_{12} in the development of megaloblastic anemia, as well as the efficacy of warfarin in relation to vitamin K status. In addition, vitamins may rarely be used in treatments unrelated to their role as a vitamin. The use of retinoic acid in acne, niacin in hyperlipidemias, and hydroxocobalamin in the treatment of cyanide poisoning are a few that are discussed within this chapter. Accordingly, this chapter includes a brief summary of the history, chemistry, kinetics, biochemistry, therapeutic use, adverse effects (hypervitaminosis), and available vitamin products that can assist the clinician in a better understanding of the role vitamins play in both health and disease.

The use of vitamins, especially as multivitamins, has increased significantly as a result of a move toward the practice of healthier lifestyles. There are two approaches to the use of vitamins that are not always clearly distinct. The first is in the treatment of known or suspected deficiencies, or to prevent deficiencies as bodily needs change as seen during pregnancy, disease, or aging. In this approach, health consequences are caused by vitamin deficiency, and the vitamins restore health by resolving the deficiency. There are numerous studies that prove the efficacy of using vitamins to treat their known deficiency syndromes or to prevent deficiencies. However, there is evidence that vitamin deficiencies may cause more health problems than are currently known. The role of vitamin deficiencies in cancer, cardiovascular disease, bone health, and immune disorders, among others, continue to be examined although the results are often conflicting. Certainly, the maintenance of adequate vitamin intake, either through diet or a multivitamin supplement, is to be encouraged.

The second approach is the use of a vitamin or group of vitamins in doses above that required for prevention of deficiency, to provide an overall health benefit, or to prevent or treat disease. Study results are even more controversial in this area because of conflicting results and, more importantly, the gathered evidence that excessive use of certain vitamins, under some circumstances, may actually be harmful. It remains controversial whether there is clear and convincing evidence to suggest that the use of vitamins in doses above their recommended dietary allowance (RDA), singly or in combination, provides any health benefit or can prevent or treat disease.

One difficulty in assessing the role of vitamins, and other nutrients, in health and disease is the finding that often more than one is involved in a physiological or disease process. This is seen in studies on bone mineralization where administering calcium in the presence of vitamin D deficiency, or vitamin D in the presence of a calcium-deficient diet, may miss the importance of calcium and/or vitamin D supplementation. We now realize that vitamin K is also involved in bone formation and this third factor, among others, must be considered. However, studies examining multiple factors are complex and not easily performed. Another complicating factor comes from the continually expanding use of fortification. Total vitamin intake is often unknown, even in the absence of supplementation, as a result of intake from multiple sources unnaturally high in vitamin content. For a summary, refer to the National Institutes of Health (NIH) State-of-the-Science Conference on Multivitamin/Mineral Supplements and Chronic Disease Prevention.[1]

INTRODUCTION

A complete history of the vitamins would have to begin with the earliest written historical records. For millennia, different cultures have recorded the use of dietary substances to successfully treat disease; some of which we now know are a result of vitamin deficiency. Patients afflicted with one of these deficiencies were successfully treated as a result of the empirical or fortuitous selection of dietary substances rich in the deficient vitamin(s). However, the basis for these deficiency diseases and why these treatments were successful was not systematically examined until the late 1800s to early 1900s.

The search for vitamins began in earnest in the early 1900s when researchers first began to realize that synthetic diets consisting of sufficient amounts of purified carbohydrates, proteins, fats, minerals, water, and calories failed to sustain growth in animals. Although there were many important contributors to the eventual discovery of the concept of vitamins and the individual chemicals that comprise them, only a few key papers are presented here. These help explain the terminology of vitamins in general; more detail is included with the individual vitamins. In 1911, Funk[2] described a substance that could cure polyneuritis in birds that was found in the aqueous phase of an extract of rice polishings. Later in 1912, Funk[3] published an excellent summary of the state of vitamin discovery, and for the first time proposed the use of the word *vitamine*, which has been often stated to be derived from a combination of the latin, *vita* (life) or alternatively from *vital*, and *amine*, which comes from the chemical term *am* (from ammonia) for nitrogen and the suffix *-ine*, which means basic in the chemical sense. Early work of Funk indicated that the curative substance for bird polyneuritis found in rice polishings was necessary for life, contained nitrogen, and was basic, hence the name.

Also in 1912, Sir Frederick Gowland Hopkins[4] clearly demonstrated that growth retardation found in rats fed purified diets could be reversed by the addition of small amounts of milk. The amount added was not sufficient to be quantitatively important with respect to its caloric value or nutritive value as a source of protein, carbohydrate, fat, or minerals. Therefore, Hopkins suggested that there must be some, yet unidentified, factors in the milk that are required for growth, but only in very small amounts. He referred to these substances as *accessory factors*. McCollum and Davis[5–8] in a series of papers showed that rats fed a diet of purified milk sugar, protein, minerals, and lard or olive oil, which provided sufficient calories, also failed to grow. Furthermore, they found that addition of small amounts of butterfat, egg yolk, or lipid extracts of either of these two substances would quickly restore growth. In 1916, McCollum and Kennedy[9] suggested that the term *vitamine* be dropped for two reasons. First, the use of the prefix *vita* implied that these were the only substances vital for life; however, other dietary substances were known to be required for life, such as essential amino acids. Second, the ending *amine* implied they contained basic nitrogen, proof of which was lacking. Because the substance they were examining was fat soluble and the accessory factor described by Funk was water soluble, the suggestion was made to refer to these as *fat-soluble A* and *water-soluble B*. Deficiency of an *antiscorbutic substance* in the diet was thought to result in scurvy, and Drummond[10] proposed the term *water-soluble C* in 1919.

In 1920, Drummond[11] proposed an alternative. He noted that the ending *-ine* was used in chemical nomenclature to denote a basic substance, and there was no evidence that any of the dietary factors was basic, much less amines. Nor was there an expectation that future discoveries would be basic. He therefore suggested dropping the final "-e" and using the term *vitamin*, which would be acceptable under the rules of chemical nomenclature. He further suggested using the terms vitamin A and vitamin B for the fat-soluble A and water-soluble B, which had been suggested by McCollum and Kennedy, and continuing with subsequent letters, such as C, as new vitamins were discovered. Other names were also proposed, but none as historically important as these.

This terminology continued for the most part, through the discovery of many of the remaining vitamins. The only alteration is that, except for vitamin C, the water-soluble vitamins were grouped into the *vitamin B complex*, instead of, or in addition to, using alphabetic letters as originally suggested, and they were then numbered as vitamin B[1], vitamin B[2], etc. This terminology was a result of the early crude extracts of water-soluble B vitamin actually containing several vitamins, not just one as originally thought, and as the extracts were resolved into individual vitamins, the series B[1], B[2], etc. developed. Jansen[12] noted in 1935 that there were no similarities in the structure or action of the B vitamins and that assigning letters was prone to error. He suggested using their proper names, for example *ascorbic acid* instead of *vitamin C*, and this practice has, for the most part, been adopted by the major

chemistry standards organization, the International Union of Pure and Applied Chemistry (IUPAC).

It continues to be traditional to classify these compounds as either lipid-soluble or water-soluble vitamins. This classification is convenient because members of each category possess important properties in common although they are much more diverse than this simple division suggests. Some designations were later proved to be duplicates, or shown not to be vitamins; hence, we are left with A, B, C, D, E, and K as the only letters to commonly designate the vitamins. Currently, there are 13 substances recognized as vitamins.

The vitamins are arranged in this chapter in the traditional groupings of the fat-soluble vitamins, vitamin A, D, E, and K, followed by the water-soluble vitamins, using their historical B-complex vitamin number such as vitamin B[1], vitamin B[2], etc., with vitamin C at the end. Because the preferred names of many of the water-soluble vitamins no longer follow this convention, Table 28.1 lists the designation and order used in this chapter, followed by the preferred name(s) and other known names.

Two organizations provide guidelines for daily vitamin intake in the United States. The first, the Food and Drug Administration (FDA), regulates the labeling of foods and dietary supplements with respect to their nutritional content, including vitamins. The current labeling requirements for vitamins, established following the Dietary Supplement Health and Education Act (DSHEA) of 1994 and published in the Code of Federal Regulations[13] (CFR) under Title 21, Section 101.9, requires that the vitamin content of food and dietary supplements be listed as a percentage of the daily value (DV). The DV for nutrients is determined by using the daily reference value (DRV) if the nutrient is a source of energy, such as protein, carbohydrates, and fats, or by using the reference daily intake (RDI) for vitamins and minerals. The RDI replaces the previously used term, USRDA (United States Recommended Daily Allowance), to prevent confusion with the RDAs (see later) published by the National Academy of Sciences. The RDI for each of the vitamins as published in 21CFR101.9 is listed in Table 28.2, and the percent DV that is placed on the food or dietary supplement label is determined by dividing the content of one serving of the food by the RDI and multiplying by 100.

The second organization that provides nutritional guidelines is the Nutrition Board of the National Academy of

TABLE 28.1 Nomenclature of Water-Soluble Vitamins

Historical Name	Preferred Name(s)	Other Names
Vitamin B[1]	Thiamine	Thiamin, aneurine, aneurin
Vitamin B[2]	Riboflavin	Vitamin G, riboflavine, lactoflavin
Vitamin B[3]	Niacin, niacinamide	Nicotinic acid, nicotinamide, vitamin PP
Vitamin B[5]	Pantothenic acid	
Vitamin B[6]	Vitamin B[6]	Pyridoxine, pyridoxin
Vitamin B[7]	Biotin	Vitamin H
Vitamin B[9]	Folate, folic acid	Vitamin M, vitamin B[c], folacin
Vitamin B[12]	Cobalamins	Cyanocobalamin, extrinsic factor (EF)
Vitamin C	Ascorbic acid	Antiscorbutic substance

TABLE 28.2 Reference Daily Intakes for Vitamins Used in Food Labeling

Vitamin	Reference Daily Intake
Vitamin A	5,000 IU[a]
Vitamin C	60 mg
Vitamin D	400 IU
Vitamin E	30 IU
Vitamin K	80 μg
Thiamin	1.5 mg
Riboflavin	1.7 mg
Niacin	20 mg
Vitamin B$_6$	2 mg
Folate	400 μg
Vitamin B$_{12}$	6 μg
Biotin	300 μg
Pantothenic acid	10 mg

[a]International Units.

Sciences, Institute of Medicine.[14] Its guidelines are published in the form of dietary reference intakes (DRIs), which include several ways of evaluating the proper intake of vitamins and minerals. The estimated average requirement (EAR) is defined as the "average daily nutrient intake level that is estimated to meet the nutrient needs of half of the healthy individuals in a life stage or gender group." If an EAR can be determined for a vitamin, then the RDA is calculated using statistical methods and is defined as an "estimate of the daily average dietary intake that meets the needs of nearly all (97%–98%) healthy members of a particular life stage and gender group." Generally, the RDA is the most specific guide for daily vitamin intake available. However, when there is not enough data to support determination of an EAR, and thus an RDA, the nutrition board sets a level known as the adequate intake (AI), which is defined as the "recommended average daily nutrient intake level based on observed or experimentally determined approximations of estimates of nutrient intake by a group (or groups) of apparently healthy people who are assumed to be maintaining an adequate nutritional state." Finally, the tolerable upper intake level (UL) is defined as the "highest average nutrient intake level likely to pose no risk of adverse health effects for nearly all people in a particular group." Table 28.3 contains the current DRIs, in terms of the RDA (when available) or the AI (when the RDA is not available) for the vitamins covered in this chapter.

Finally, the World Health Organization[15] (WHO) is in the process of *harmonizing* (WHO term for standardizing) nutrient values so that they can be useful internationally. This is necessary because of the wide variety of terms and corresponding approaches to defining dietary standards seen across the globe. WHO recommends using the term *nutrient intake value* (NIV) to encompass all nutrient-based dietary standards, not just vitamins. In order to simplify terminology, WHO recommends only two NIVs. First, the average nutrient requirement (ANR) represents the mean requirement in a healthy population required to achieve a specific outcome. Second, the upper nutrient level (UNL) is defined as "the highest level of habitual nutrient intake that is likely to pose no risk of adverse health effects in almost all individuals in the general population."

Another important distinction is the difference between the natural vitamin content of foods and the vitamin content following enrichment or fortification. A good example would be vitamins in whole grain products. These naturally serve as an excellent source of certain vitamins; however, when they are processed as is the case with the production of white flour, much of the vitamin content is lost. To effectively prevent vitamin deficiencies, many developed countries, including the United States, require that the lost vitamins be added to approximate the natural levels. This process is called *enrichment*. *Fortification* is the addition of vitamins above the levels found naturally in the food. For example, many ready-to-eat cereals are fortified with vitamins, which can then become an excellent source of a vitamin, although the grain used in the cereal is not a natural source of the vitamin. We try to distinguish between foods that are good natural sources and those that have become significant sources through fortification.

FAT-SOLUBLE VITAMINS

The fat-soluble vitamins include vitamins A, D, E, and K. These compounds possess other characteristics in common besides solubility. They are usually associated with the lipids in foods and are absorbed from the intestine with these dietary lipids. Other than vitamin K, the fat-soluble vitamins are stored in the liver and, thus, conserved by the organism; whereas storage of the water-soluble vitamins is usually not significant. This leads to a greater potential for toxicity associated with long-term accumulation of the fat-soluble vitamins following ingestion of large doses that is not generally seen with the water-soluble vitamins.

Vitamin A

The discovery of vitamin A is often attributed to the original paper by McCollum and Davis[5] in 1912 demonstrating that dietary fats contained substances, other than the fats themselves, necessary for proper growth. In 1931, vitamin A was isolated from fish oil[16] and the structure was confirmed the next year.[17] Vitamin A was first synthesized in 1947,[18] but studies of the molecular mechanism of action in the visual process were not significantly productive until the 1960s. One of the major contributors in elucidating the visual function of vitamin A was George Wald,[19] a corecipient of the Nobel Prize for Physiology or Medicine in 1967 for his work that is summarized in a 1968 paper. Since the original isolation of the substance referred to as vitamin A, several compounds have been found naturally or synthesized to have biological activity similar to vitamin A. Of particular dietary importance in this regard are the provitamin A cartenoids which are converted into active forms of vitamin A in vivo.

Dietary vitamin A is obtained naturally from foods of animal origin, either as free vitamin A or combined as the biologically active esters, chiefly of palmitic and some myristic and dodecanoic acids. The highest sources of natural vitamin A are livers of animals, especially herbivorous, poultry, and fish. Vitamin A is also found in egg yolk; however, the whites are not a good source. Vitamin A can also be obtained from foods fortified with this vitamin such as ready-to-eat breakfast cereals, milk, butter, and margarine.

The provitamin A carotenoids are obtained from plant sources and comprise some of the best sources of this vitamin. The provitamin As are found in deep green, yellow,

TABLE 28.3 Dietary Reference Intakes for Vitamins

Life Stage Group	Vitamin A (μg/d)[a]	Vitamin D (μg/d)[b,c]	Vitamin E (mg/d)[d]	Vitamin K (μg/d)	Thiamine (mg/d)	Riboflavin (mg/d)	Niacin (mg/d)[e]	Pantothenic Acid (mg/d)	Vitamin B6 (mg/d)	Biotin (μg/d)	Folate (μg/d)[f]	Vitamin B12 (μg/d)	Vitamin C (mg/d)
Infants													
0–6 mo	400*	5*	4*	2*	0.2*	0.3*	2*	1.7*	0.1*	5*	65*	0.4*	40*
7–12 mo	500*	5*	5*	2.5*	0.3*	0.4*	4*	1.8*	0.3*	6*	80*	0.5*	50*
Children													
1–3 y	300	5*	6	30*	0.5	0.5	6	2*	0.5	8*	150	0.9	15
4–8 y	400	5*	7	55*	0.6	0.6	8	3*	0.6	12*	200	1.2	25
Males													
9–13 y	600	5*	11	60*	0.9	0.9	12	4*	1.0	20*	300	1.8	45
14–18 y	900	5*	15	75*	1.2	1.3	16	5*	1.3	25*	400	2.4	75
19–30 y	900	5*	15	120*	1.2	1.3	16	5*	1.3	30*	400	2.4	90
31–50 y	900	5*	15	120*	1.2	1.3	16	5*	1.3	30*	400	2.4	90
51–70 y	900	10*	15	120*	1.2	1.3	16	5*	1.7	30*	400	2.4	90
>70 y	900	15*	15	120*	1.2	1.3	16	5*	1.7	30*	400	2.4	90
Females													
9–13 y	600	5*	11	60*	0.9	0.9	12	4*	1.0	20*	300	1.8	45
14–18 y	700	5*	15	75*	1.0	1.0	14	5*	1.2	25*	400[i]	2.4	65
19–30 y	700	5*	15	90*	1.1	1.1	14	5*	1.3	30*	400[i]	2.4	75
31–50 y	700	5*	15	90*	1.1	1.1	14	5*	1.3	30*	400[i]	2.4	75
51–70 y	700	10*	15	90*	1.1	1.1	14	5*	1.5	30*	400	2.4	75
>70 y	700	15*	15	90*	1.1	1.1	14	5*	1.5	30*	400	2.4	75
Pregnancy													
14–18 y	750	5*	15	75*	1.4	1.4	18	6*	1.9	30*	600[i]	2.6	80
19–30 y	770	5*	15	90*	1.4	1.4	18	6*	1.9	30*	600[i]	2.6	85
31–50 y	770	5*	15	90*	1.4	1.4	18	6*	1.9	30*	600[i]	2.6	85
Lactation													
14–18 y	1,200	5*	19	75*	1.4	1.6	17	7*	2.0	35*	500	2.8	115
19–30 y	1,300	5*	19	90*	1.4	1.6	17	7*	2.0	35*	500	2.8	120
31–50 y	1,300	5*	19	90*	1.4	1.6	17	7*	2.0	35*	500	2.8	120

Adapted with permission from Otten, J. J., Hellwig, J. P., and Meyers, L. D. (eds.): Dietary Reference Intakes: The Essential Guide to Nutrient Requirements. Washington D.C., The National Academies Press, 2006, pp. 532–533.

Numbers represent the Recommended Dietary Allowances (RDA) unless marked with an asterisk (*), in which case they represent the Adequate Intake (AI). See source for more detailed information.

aAs retinol activity equivalents (RAEs).
bAs cholecalciferol.
cIn the absence of adequate exposure to sunlight.
dAs α-tocopherol.
eAs niacin equivalents (NE).
fAs dietary folate equivalents (DFE).

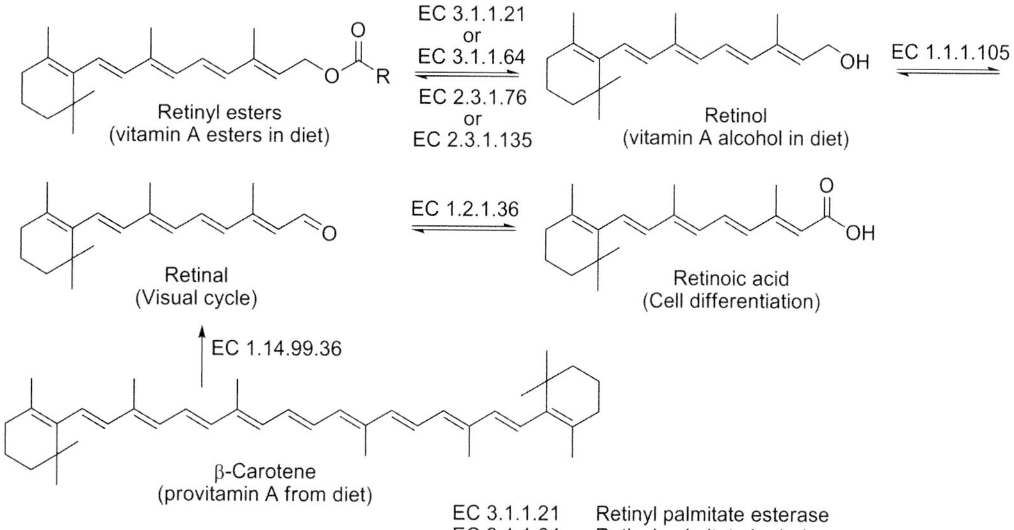

EC 3.1.1.21
or
EC 3.1.1.64

EC 2.3.1.76
or
EC 2.3.1.135

Retinyl esters
(vitamin A esters in diet)

EC 1.1.1.105

Retinol
(vitamin A alcohol in diet)

EC 1.2.1.36

Retinal
(Visual cycle)

Retinoic acid
(Cell differentiation)

EC 1.14.99.36

β-Carotene
(provitamin A from diet)

EC 3.1.1.21	Retinyl palmitate esterase
EC 3.1.1.64	Retinyl palmitate hydrolase
EC 2.3.1.76	Acyl CoA:retinol acyltransferase (ARAT)
EC 2.3.1.135	Lecithin:retinol acyltransferase (LRAT)
EC 1.1.1.105	Retinol dehydrogenase
EC 1.2.1.36	Retinal dehydrogenase
EC 1.14.99.36	β-Carotene 15,15'-monooxygenase

Figure 28.1 ● Interconversions of β-carotene and preformed dietary retinoids.

and orange fruits and vegetables, such as carrots, spinach, broccoli, kale, collard and turnip greens, mangoes, apricots, nectarines, pumpkins, and sweet potatoes.

CHEMISTRY

Vitamin A belongs to a class of compounds referred to as the *retinoids*, which consist of four isoprenoid units joined in a head-to-tail manner.[20] All double bonds in the isoprenoid units are implied to be in the *E* (*trans*) configuration unless stated otherwise. Currently, the term *retinoid* is applied to retinol and its naturally occurring derivatives plus synthetic analogs, which need not have vitamin A activity. *Vitamin A* is currently used as a generic descriptor for all retinoids that exhibit the biological activity of retinol, the original substance identified as vitamin A. The term *vitamin A₁* and all-*trans* retinol have been used to refer to retinol whereas *vitamin A₂*

was used to refer to 3,4-dehydroretinol. *Retinoate analogs* are used to refer to "compounds that control epithelial differentiation and prevent metaplasia, without possessing the full range of activities of vitamin A."[21] Retinal (formerly all-*trans* retinal), the form of vitamin A that takes part in the visual cycle, and retinoic acid (formerly all-*trans* retinoic acid), the form that takes part in cell differentiation, are the two active forms of vitamin A (Fig. 28.1). About 60 β-carotenes, out of 700 carotenoids that have been identified, exhibit vitamin A activity in the body and are termed the provitamin As or provitamin A carotenoids. The important carotenoids regarded as the provitamin As are α-, β-, and γ-carotenes and cryptoxanthin (Fig. 28.2). β-Carotene is the most important provitamin A carotenoid. The transformations of preformed vitamin As and β-carotene are shown in Figure 28.1.

Vitamin A activity has been historically expressed as *United States Pharmacopeia* (*USP*) units, international units (IU), retinol equivalents (RE), or β-carotene equivalents. The *USP* units and IU are equivalent. Each unit expresses the activity of 0.3 μg of retinol. Thus, 1 mg of retinol has the activity of 3,333 units. Other equivalents are listed in Table 28.4. This system does not take into account the incomplete absorption and rate-limited bioconversion of the provitamin A carotenoids into the active form, retinal. One RE represents the biological activity of 1 μg of retinol, 6 μg of β-carotene, or 12 μg of α-carotene or β-cryptoxanthin. The RE was used

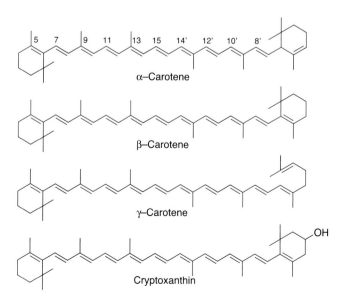

α–Carotene

β–Carotene

γ–Carotene

Cryptoxanthin

Figure 28.2 ● Provitamin A carotenoids.

TABLE 28.4 Weight of Various Vitamin A Sources Equivalent to 1 International Unit

Retinoid	μg
Retinol	0.3
Retinol acetate	0.334
Retinol propionate	0.359
Retinol palmitate	0.55
β-Carotene	0.6

TABLE 28.5 Weight of Various Vitamin A Sources Equivalent to 1 Retinol Equivalent or 1 Retinol Activity Equivalent

Vitamin A Source	REs[1] (μg)	RAEs[2] (μg)
Retinol	1	1
β-Carotene	6	12
α-Carotene	12	24
β-Cryptoxanthin	12	24

[1]Retinol Equivalents.
[2]Retinol Activity Equivalents.

to convert all dietary sources of vitamin A into a single unit for easy comparison and accounts for inefficiencies in absorption and rate-limited bioconversion of the provitamin A carotenoids.[22] The current unit used to express vitamin A activity is the retinol activity equivalents (RAE). This came about from the finding that the absorption of the provitamin A carotenoids is 50% less than originally thought. The only difference in this system is that the provitamin A carotenoids are one half the activity assumed when using REs (see Table 28.5).

The stereochemistry of vitamin A and related compounds is complex, and the study of the structural relationships among vitamin A and its stereoisomers has been complicated by the common use of several numbering systems (Fig. 28.3). The first numbering system (A) is the one currently recommended by IUPAC and is used throughout this text. The second system (B) places emphasis on the conjugated π system, whereas the third (C) is used by the *USP Dictionary of USAN and International Drug Names*.

The conjugated double-bond systems found in vitamin A and β-carotene, as well as the attached ring in the form of β-ionone or dehydro-β-ionone found in 3,4-dehydroretinol, are essential for activity. When any of these is saturated, activity is lost. The ester and methyl ethers of vitamin A have a biological activity on a molar basis equal to that of vitamin A. Retinoic acid (vitamin A acid) is biologically active but is not stored in the liver.

For steric reasons, the number of isomers of vitamin A most likely to occur is limited. These are all-*trans*, 9-*cis*, 13-*cis*, and the 9,13-di-*cis*. A *cis* linkage at double bond 7 or 11 encounters steric hindrance. The 11-*cis* isomer is twisted as well as bent at this linkage; nevertheless, this is the only isomer that is active in vision and is synthesized in retinyl pigmented epithelial cells from all-*trans*-retinyl esters by the action of isomerase followed by hydrolysis.

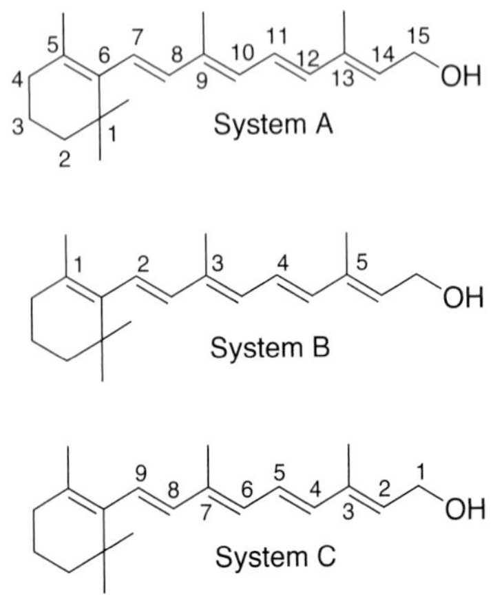

KINETICS

Vitamin A is absorbed in the intestine via the same pathway used for dietary lipids, requiring bile salts, dietary fat, and pancreatic juice. Retinyl esters are hydrolyzed in the intestinal lumen to retinol by pancreatic triacylglycerol lipase (EC 3.1.1.3) and the brush border enzyme lysophospholipase (EC 3.1.1.5). The retinol is absorbed into the enterocytes by facilitated diffusion at normal concentrations. At pharmacological doses, however, retinol can be absorbed by passive diffusion.[23,24] Bioavailability for most forms of preformed vitamin A is 70% to 90%. Upon cellular entry, retinol associates with a retinol binding protein (RBP), most likely RBP2. RBPs represent a group of proteins involved in intracellular and intercellular binding and transport of vitamin A. These intracellular proteins function in the transport and metabolism of retinol and retinoic acid by solubilizing them in aqueous media and presenting them to the appropriate enzymes while protecting them from catabolizing enzymes.[25] These proteins also limit the concentration of free retinoids within the cell.

Provitamin A carotenoids are absorbed by passive diffusion and also depend on absorbable fats and bile. It is currently assumed that one twelfth of normal dietary β-carotene but only one twenty-fourth of the other provitamin A carotenoids is absorbed and bioconverted. This explains the low activity of the provitamin A carotenoids in relation to retinol as shown in Table 28.5. The enterocytes are the main site of β-carotene transformation to retinal,[26] but the enzymes that catalyze the transformation also occur in hepatic and other tissue. Up to 20% to 30% of provitamin A carotenoids are absorbed unchanged. Following absorption by the enterocytes, β-carotene is symmetrically cleaved into retinal by β-carotene 15,15'-monooxygenase (EC 1.14.99.36), which requires molecular oxygen.[27] β-Carotene can give rise to two molecules of retinal; whereas with the other three carotenoids, only one molecule is possible by this transformation. This is a result of the composition of β-carotene, which has a structure identical to retinal in both halves of the molecule, whereas the other provitamin As have a structure identical to retinal in one half of the molecule (see Fig. 28.2). Asymmetric cleavage of the carotenoids by β-carotene-9,10-monooxygenase has also been reported,[26,28,29] but its role in humans is not fully resolved. The retinal formed from the provitamin As is then reduced to retinol by retinol dehydrogenase (EC 1.1.1.105) or alcohol dehydrogenase (EC 1.1.1.1).

Within the enterocytes, the retinol is esterified by three enzymes, diacylglycerol *O*-acyltransferase (DGAT, EC 2.3.1.20), retinol *O*-fatty-acyltransferase (EC 2.3.1.76), also known as acyl-coenzyme A (CoA):retinol acyltransferase (ARAT), and phosphatidylcholine-retinol *O*-acyltransferase (EC 2.3.1.135), also known as lecithin:retinal acyltransferase (LRAT). LRAT esterifies retinol bound to RBP2, whereas ARAT can esterify unbound retinol. It has been proposed that LRAT esterifies retinol at normal doses, while ARAT esterifies excess retinol.[30] It has also been suggested that high doses of retinol may increase retinoic acid formation in the enterocytes through a retinoic acid responsive element (RARE) that promotes RBP2 expression.[31]

The retinyl esters are incorporated into chylomicrons, which in turn enter the lymph. Once in the general circula-

Figure 28.3 • Vitamin A numbering systems.

tion, chylomicrons are converted into chylomicron remnants, which are cleared primarily by the liver but possibly other tissues.[30] As the esters enter the hepatocytes, they are hydrolyzed to retinol which is then bound to RBP1 or RBP4. These are released into the blood or transferred to liver stellate cells for storage. Within the stellate cells, the retinol bound to RBP is esterified for storage by LRAT and ARAT. Stellate cells contain up to 80% of the bodies vitamin A stores.[32] The RBP–retinol complex released into the general circulation from hepatocytes or stellate cells is extensively bound to transthyretin (TTR), which protects RBP-retinol from glomerular filtration and subsequent renal excretion.[33] Retinol alone is taken up by target cells, probably by passive diffusion, from circulating RBP-retinol and once inside, is bound to RBP1 and possibly RBP2. Other retinoids may also circulate in plasma in low amounts, such as free retinol and 13-*cis* retinoic acid, but these are most likely bound to albumin.

Elimination of vitamin A generally involves the glucuronidation of retinol or retinoic acid followed by renal or biliary excretion that may result in enterohepatic cycling. Other pathways for oxidizing retinoids to more polar substances also exist. Normally, no unchanged retinol is excreted. Retinal, retinoic acid, and other metabolites are, however, found in the urine and feces.

BIOCHEMISTRY

Vitamin A is involved in numerous biochemical functions. The best-known action of vitamin A is in its function in the chemistry of vision. The requirement for vitamin A for proper visual response to light in the retina has been well characterized. However, its role in cellular growth and differentiation continues to expand.

The molecular mechanism of action of vitamin A, in the form of 11-*cis* retinal, in the visual process has been under investigation for many years.[34,35] Figure 28.4 represents the

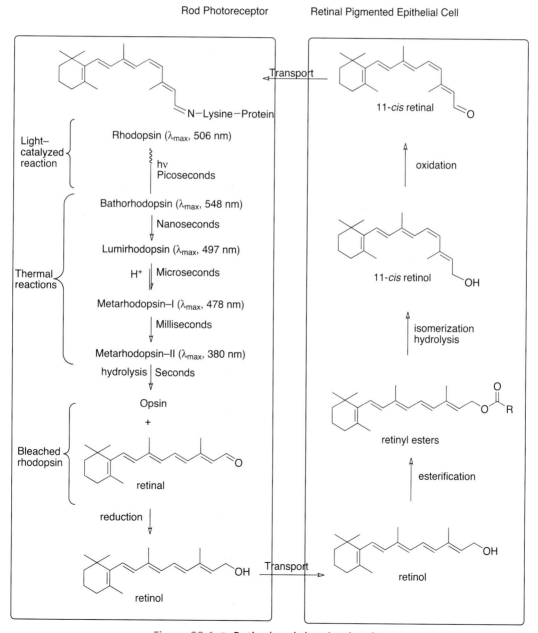

Figure 28.4 ● Retinol and the visual cycle.

chemical changes that take place in the visual cycle involving the rhodopsin system in the rod cells of the retina. Uptake of retinol from blood by the epithelial cells of the retina is followed by re-esterification and conversion to the 11-*cis* retinol form. This is converted to the aldehyde, 11-*cis* retinal, which is the form used in the visual pathway. In contrast to the cone cells of the retina, which are responsible for color vision and only function well in the presence of ample light, the vitamin A–dependent rods are essential for vision over a wide range of light intensity, especially low levels. This system is responsible for vision in the dark, which explains the night blindness seen in vitamin A–deficient individuals.

Vitamin A is also intimately involved in cellular differentiation during embryonic development and the maintenance of cellular differentiation in various tissues in the adult. The molecular mechanism of vitamin A, in the form of retinoic acid, in this area is more complex.[36,37] This form of vitamin A acts through retinoic acid receptors (RARs) which are a member of the steroid/thyroid hormone superfamily of receptors. These act as ligand-dependent transcription factors that regulate gene expression. Several RARs have been identified: RARα (RARA), RARβ (RARB), and RARγ (RARG). These differ in their tissue distribution and the level of expression during cell development and differentiation. Following cytoplasmic RAR-retinoic acid binding, the complex forms a heterodimer with the retinoid X receptor (RXR). The heterodimer translocates to the nucleus and binds to a RARE or retinoid X response element (RXRE) on DNA associated with the promoter region of target genes and, together with coactivators, regulates target gene transcription. Several RXR receptors have also been identified including RXRα (RXRA), RXRβ (RXRB), and RXRγ (RXRG), and they have been shown to be also involved in the intracellular action of vitamin D. They have a different tissue distribution from the RARs. A specific ligand for RXR has been identified as 9-*cis*-retinoic acid, which can also bind to RARs; however, the physiological role of this retinoid is not known. Retinoic acid can bind only to RARs. 9-*cis* retinoic acid may, therefore, represent a third active form of vitamin A.[38,39] Several synthetic retinoids have been synthesized that bind selectively to RXR receptors, and these are referred to as *rexinoids*.

The biological effects of retinoic acid are mediated through various proteins, numbering in the hundreds, which are controlled at the nuclear level by this form of the vitamin. Ultimately, effects are seen in cell differentiation, both during embryonic development and in the adult. Effects on reproduction, growth, immune function, hematopoiesis, epithelium, central nervous system (CNS) function, and cancer have also been observed, among others. This widespread involvement in biological function explains the myriad of effects seen in deficiency and overdoses of this vitamin.

Deficiency of this vitamin leads to several disorders collectively referred to as vitamin A deficiency disorders (VADD). Preschool-age children are especially susceptible to and develop more serious forms of VADD leading to increased mortality which may approach 50% in poor societies.[40] A deficiency of vitamin A is manifested chiefly by keratinization of the mucous membranes throughout the body. This degeneration is more pronounced in the eye than in any other part of the body and gives rise to a condition known as xerophthalmia which results in drying and thickening of the conjunctiva tand cornea. This may ultimately lead to corneal destruction and permanent blindness.

Vitamin A deficiency also results in poor dark adaptation of the eyes referred to as night blindness (*nyctalopia*). Immune insufficiency develops resulting in a tendency to infection. Anemia results from hematopoietic failure in the marrow. In children, growth failure and wasting also occurs. Deficiency of vitamin A can also give rise to dryness and scaliness of the skin in adults.

THERAPEUTIC USES

Vitamin A is used in the treatment of known or suspected vitamin A deficiency. Vitamin A deficiency in developed countries such as the United States is not likely of dietary origin but is more likely caused by malabsorption as is seen in sprue, hepatic cirrhosis, biliary, or pancreatic diseases. Interestingly, vitamin A levels decrease during infection with the measles virus (rubeola) resulting in increased morbidity and mortality, especially in children with preexisting vitamin A deficiency. Vitamin A supplementation has been shown to decrease mortality by 50% and prevent blindness in children developing measles if given at the time of diagnosis. Of course, vaccination is of prime importance; however, in underdeveloped countries where the rate of vaccination is low, vitamin A supplementation is a beneficial alternative.[41] Retinoate analogs have been developed for use in the treatment of dermatological conditions such as psoriasis and acne. Some therapies for cancer by retinoate analogs have also been established, and newer therapies against various cancers are under investigation.[37]

Both natural and synthetic carotenoids decrease acute photosensitivity in porphyria in a manner unrelated to its vitamin activity.[42] Most β-carotene is converted to retinol during absorption, but the fraction that is absorbed unchanged is distributed widely and accumulates in the skin. This can provide protection against sun exposure in patients with erythropoietic protoporphyria. It does not provide total protection against the sun, but patients who respond to its treatment can remain in the sun the same as normal individuals. Discontinuance of the drug results in a return of hypersensitivity. β-Carotene does not function as a sunscreen in normal patients and should not be used as such. Carotenodermia, a result of accumulation in the skin, is the major side effect. Tanning capsules containing β-carotene and/or the carotenoid and canthaxanthin, uses this effect.

β-Carotene has also been investigated for possible protective effects in cancer. Early studies suggested a protective effect in lung cancer, but recent studies of lung, prostate, colon, breast, or nonmelanoma skin cancer did not show a protective effect.[43] Surprisingly, the results of several later studies suggest that increased intake of β-carotene might increase the risk of lung cancer in smokers.[1,44] Studies also do not show any protective effects in cardiovascular disease.[1,43]

HYPERVITAMINOSIS

The toxicities of vitamin A have been known since before the vitamin was discovered,[45] and can lead to both short- and long-term effects.[46–48] Short-term doses of 0.5 to 4 million IU can lead, within hours to several days, to CNS effects including increased intracranial pressure, headache, irritability, and seizures; gastrointestinal effects including nausea, vomiting, and pain; dermatological effects such as desquamation; ophthalmic effects such as papilledema, scotoma, and photophobia; and liver damage. Most of these reactions have been reported in infants following treatment with large doses of vitamin A, but some have resulted from ingestion of food rich in vitamin A, such as liver, especially from polar bears.

Long-term intake of doses of vitamin A lower than the intake required for short-term toxicity but still above that required by the body can lead to long-term effects, including effects on the skin, liver, CNS, and bone. Although the amount required varies, doses as low as 15,000 IU/day have led to some adverse effects. Higher doses, generally above 100,000 IU/day, are required to see all the reported adverse effects. In patients with low body weight, malnutrition, or liver or renal disease, the doses required for long-term adverse effects may be still lower.

Dermatological adverse effects include drying of the skin and mucosa, dermatitis, pruritus, swelling and fissuring of the lips, and rarely loss of body hair. Hepatic effects include hypertrophy and hyperplasia of the hepatic stellate cells, hepatomegaly, fibrosis, and cirrhosis, which can lead to portal hypertension, ascites, and jaundice. Splenomegaly is also seen. CNS effects include increased intracranial pressure (pseudotumor cerebri) leading to headache, visual disturbances (e.g., diplopia), drowsiness, vomiting, seizures, and a bulging fontanel in infants. Finally, pain in the bone and joints, with accompanying tenderness and reduced bone mineralization[49] have also been reported.

The teratogenic effects of vitamin A are also well-known.[50] Intake of as little as 10,000 IU/day during pregnancy may increase the risk of birth defects, and the risk increases with increasing intake of vitamin A.[51,52] Birth defects include cardiovascular, craniofacial, neural tube, and urogenital and musculoskeletal abnormalities.

β-Carotene, in contrast, is relatively nontoxic as are the other provitamin A carotenoids.[47,53] After long-term exposure to high levels of β-carotene (30–180 mg/day for 15 years), patients have not developed any problems other than skin discoloration and asymptomatic hypercarotonemia. Furthermore, β-carotene is not teratogenic. The most likely mechanism is the incomplete absorption and slow rate of conversion of β-carotene to retinol in the intestinal cells.[54] However, a recent systematic review and meta-analysis found an increase in overall mortality in studies using β-carotene.[43,55] This, coupled with the finding that β-carotene may increase the risk of lung cancer in smokers, as discussed previously, suggests that it may not be as nontoxic as originally thought when used chronically.

PRODUCTS

Vitamin A contains retinol (vitamin A alcohol) or its esters from edible fatty acids (chiefly acetic and palmitic acids). It is available from various manufacturers under many names. Dosage forms vary from oral tablets, capsules, and solutions to topical ointments and creams. It is also available as an injectable in the form of vitamin A palmitate (Aquasol A) that is intended for intramuscular (IM) injection. Vitamin A is also available as a component of multivitamins from many different sources.

The provitamin A carotenoids are also widely available, primarily β-carotene, from various sources under many names. Oral liquids, tablets, and capsules are available, containing β-carotene, either singly or in combination as multivitamin preparations.

Retinoate analogs are also available for the treatment of dermatological conditions and cancer. Table 28.6 lists the current products on the market and their approved uses, whereas Figure 28.5 shows their corresponding structure.

Vitamin D

The recognition in 1919 that rickets was the result of a nutritional deficiency led to the isolation of antirachitic compounds from food products.[56] The role of sunlight in the prevention of rickets was noted at the same time.[57] Early studies showed that vitamin A preparations available at the time, in addition to their growth-promoting properties, could also cure xerophthalmia and rickets. Thus, the early assumption was that all of these were because of the deficiency of vitamin A. A preliminary report by Funk and Dubin[58] in 1921 was the first to suggest the presence of a vitamin in yeast extracts that was distinctly different from vitamin A and vitamin B, which the authors named vitamin D. It is interesting that the authors believed the new vitamin D was another of the B vitamins, which at that point in history was known to consist of at least two different vitamins. McCollum et al.[59] clearly showed in 1922 that vitamin A and the antirachitic factor were, in fact, two separate vitamins. The synthesis of both major forms of vitamin D, ergocalciferol and cholecalciferol, was accomplished in 1977.[60]

The highest natural source of vitamin D is fatty fish such as herring, catfish, salmon, mackerel, and tuna or oils derived from fish such as cod liver oil. Eggs, from hens fed vitamin D, and butter also contain small amounts of vitamin D. The most common source of vitamin D in developed countries, such as the United States, is fortified foods such as milk, ready-to-eat cereals, and some fruit juices. Cholecalciferol or ergocalciferol is usually used in fortification or supplementation.

CHEMISTRY

Chemically, the various forms of vitamin D are broken-open steroids referred to as *secosteroids*. The term vitamin D is currently applied to all steroids possessing biological activity like that of cholecalciferol.[61] Irradiation of yeast ergosterol yields a 1:1 mixture of ergocalciferol and lumisterol known as vitamin D_1. Because all the activities reside in the ergocalciferol, the term vitamin D_1 is no longer used. The photoconversion of ergocalciferol (ercalciol, previously calciferol, vitamin D_2) from ergosterol is shown in Figure 28.6. Cholecalciferol (calciol, previously vitamin D_3) is the form produced in vivo from the action of sunlight on 7-dehydrocholesterol (Fig. 28.7) in the skin. 22,23-Dihydroergocalciferol was known as Vitamin D_4. (24S)-Ethylcalciol (formerly sitocalciferol), made from 7-dehydrositosterol, was known as vitamin D_5. Note the structural differences between ergocalciferol and cholecalciferol shown in Figure 28.6 and Figure 28.7. The ergocalciferol side chain contains a double bond between C^{22} and C^{23} and a methyl group on C^{24}.

KINETICS

The gastrointestinal absorption of the vitamin Ds requires bile, pancreatic juice, and dietary fat. Following formation

Generic Name	Trade Name	Dosage Form	Use
Acitretin	Soriatane	Capsule	Psoriasis
Adapalene	Differin	Cream or gel	Acne vulgaris
Alitretinoin	Panretin	Gel	Kaposi sarcoma
Bexarotene	Targretin	Capsule	T-cell lymphomas
Isotretinoin	Accutane, Isotrex	Capsule Topical preparation	Acne vulgaris
Tazarotene	Tazorac, Avage	Cream or gel	Psoriasis
Tretinoin	Retin-A, Renova, Avita, Altinac, Atralin,	Cream or gel	Acne vulgaris
	Vesanoid	Capsule	Leukemia

oxygen and reduced NADPH. The enzyme is found on the inner mitochondrial membrane,[63] and the rate correlates with substrate concentration. Following secretion into the blood, calcidiol and other forms of vitamin D are associated with group-specific component (vitamin D–binding protein [GC]) formerly referred to as vitamin D–binding protein (VDBP). The calcidiol bound to GC is the major circulating form of the vitamin and may be stored in fats and muscle for prolonged periods. GC binding helps in the transport of vitamin Ds in blood and also prolongs the circulatory half-lives by making them less susceptible to hepatic metabolism and biliary excretion.[64] Albumin and lipoproteins also bind vitamin Ds but with lower affinity than GC. The circulating levels of calcidiol are proportional to vitamin D intake and synthesis; thus, plasma levels of calcidiol have been used to indicate vitamin D status.[65]

The epithelial cells of the proximal convoluted tubules in the kidneys convert calcidiol to calcitriol [previously $1\alpha,25$-dihydroxyvitamin D_3, $1\alpha,25(OH)_2D_3$] by the enzyme calcidiol 1-monooxygenase (EC 1.14.13.13) also known previously as $25(OH)D_3$ 1α-hydroxylase. The activity of this mitochondrial, cytochrome P450 enzyme is increased by parathyroid hormone and hypophosphatemia and decreased by calcitriol and Ca^{2+}.[66] Understanding this final step is crucial because renal disease can lead to deficiency of the active calcitriol and subsequent derangements in calcium and bone metabolism. Treatment is only effective if a vitamin D preparation that already has the 1α-hydroxy is used. Similar to cholecalciferol, ergocalciferol also requires hydroxylation in the liver and kidney to become fully active as shown in Figure 28.9.

In a classical sense, cholecalciferol, the form produced in animals, is not a true vitamin because it is produced in the

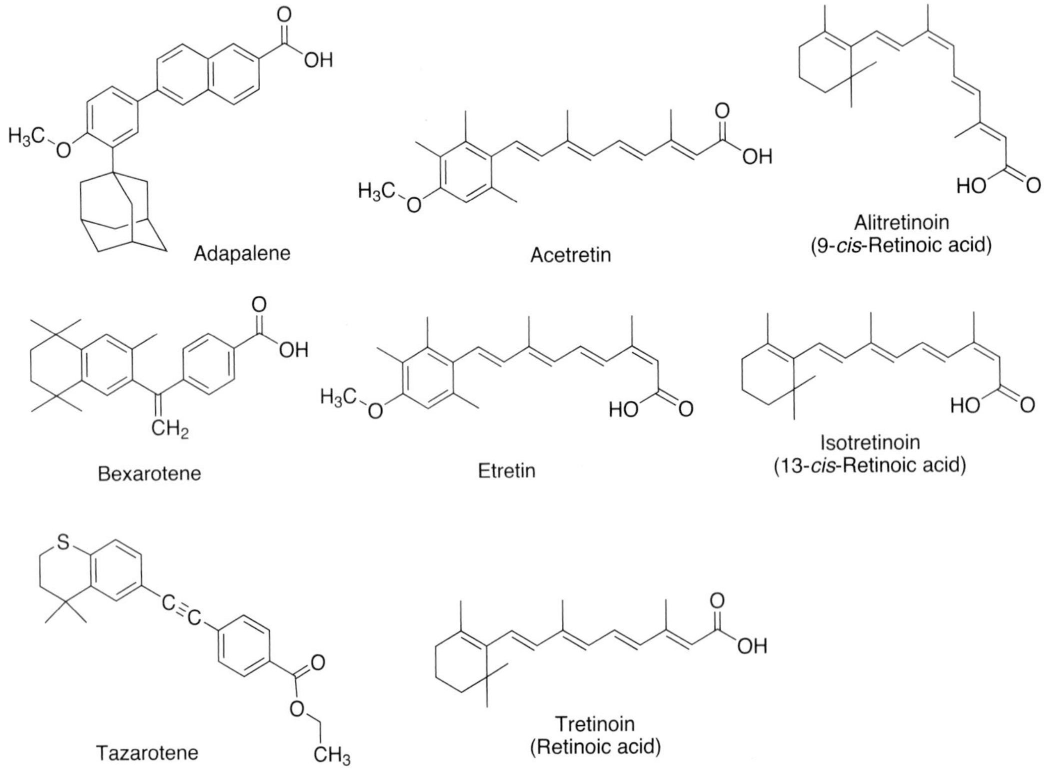

of micelles in the intestinal lumen, vitamin D esters are hydrolyzed, and free vitamin D, usually as cholecalciferol or ergocalciferol, is absorbed by passive diffusion into the enterocytes. There, it is incorporated into chylomicrons and secreted into the lymph where it enters the circulation.[62] Cholecalciferol and ergocalciferol were once thought to be the active forms of vitamin D; however, they have now been identified as provitamins because they require hydroxylation by the liver and the kidney to be fully active.

As shown in Figure 28.8, the first step occurs in the liver, following uptake from chylomicron remnants, by the enzyme vitamin D_3 25-hydroxylase (EC 1.14.15.-). This enzyme converts the provitamin to calcidiol (previously 25-hydroxyvitamin D_3, $25(OH)D_3$) and requires both molecular

Figure 28.5 ● Structures of clinically used retinoate analogs.

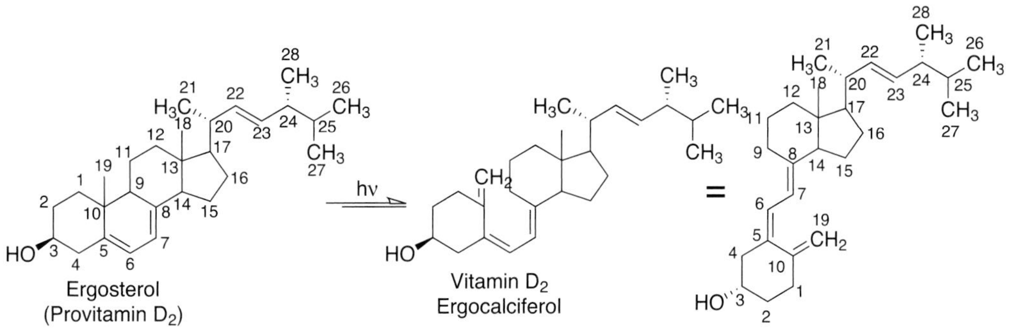

Figure 28.6 ● Photoactivation of ergosterol to ergocalciferol.

skin from 7-dehydrocholesterol by UV radiation (Fig. 28.7) in the range of 290 to 300 nm.[66] 7-Dehydrocholesterol is produced from cholesterol by the enzyme 7-dehydrocholesterol reductase (EC 1.3.1.21). Only when exposure to sunlight is inadequate does cholecalciferol become a vitamin in the historical sense. As shown in Figure 28.7, upon exposure to UV irradiation, 7-dehydrocholesterol is converted rapidly to previtamin D₃. Previtamin D₃ undergoes slow thermal conversion to cholecalciferol and the biologically inactive lumisterol and tacalciol (formerly tachysterol₃). Excess exposure increases production of the inactive compounds. The slow conversion of previtamin D₃ to cholecalciferol ensures adequate supplies when the exposure is brief. Further, lumisterol and tacalciol can be converted back to previtamin D₃ and thus serve as a reservoir.[66] It has been estimated that a 10-minute exposure of just the uncovered hands and face will produce sufficient cholecalciferol.[67] Inadequate photo conversion to cholecalciferol is most likely to occur in northern latitudes during the winter months, in people with dark-colored skin or in people who routinely use clothing or sunscreens to reduce their sun exposure, such as the elderly.

The mechanism responsible for the movement of cholecalciferol from the skin to the blood is not known. In the blood, cholecalciferol is bound primarily to GC. This protein selectively removes cholecalciferol from the skin

because it has low affinity for 7-dehydrocholesterol, previtamin D₃, lumisterol, and tacalciol.

Catabolism of vitamin D is initiated by the enzyme 1,25-dihydroxyvitamin D₃ 24-hydroxylase (EC 1.14.13.-), whose expression is stimulated by calcitriol, itself. 24-Hydroxylation is followed by oxidation to the ketone. Subsequent hydroxylation at C²³ leads to cleavage of the side chain, resulting in the biologically inactive product calcitronic acid.[68,69] The 24-hydroxy metabolites are excreted primarily in the bile.

BIOCHEMISTRY

Similar to retinoic acid, the vitamin D receptor (VDR) is a member of the steroid/thyroid hormone superfamily of receptors. These act as ligand-dependent transcription factors that regulate gene expression. In intestine, bone, kidney, and other tissues, calcitriol binds to VDR localized in the cytoplasm, and the complex forms a heterodimer with a retinoid RXR. RXRs are also involved in vitamin A action and the reader is referred to that section for more information. This complex translocates to the nucleus and binds to vitamin D response elements (VDREs) associated with the promoter region of target genes and, together with coactivators, regulates target gene transcription. Over 50 genes have been identified that are controlled by calcitriol.

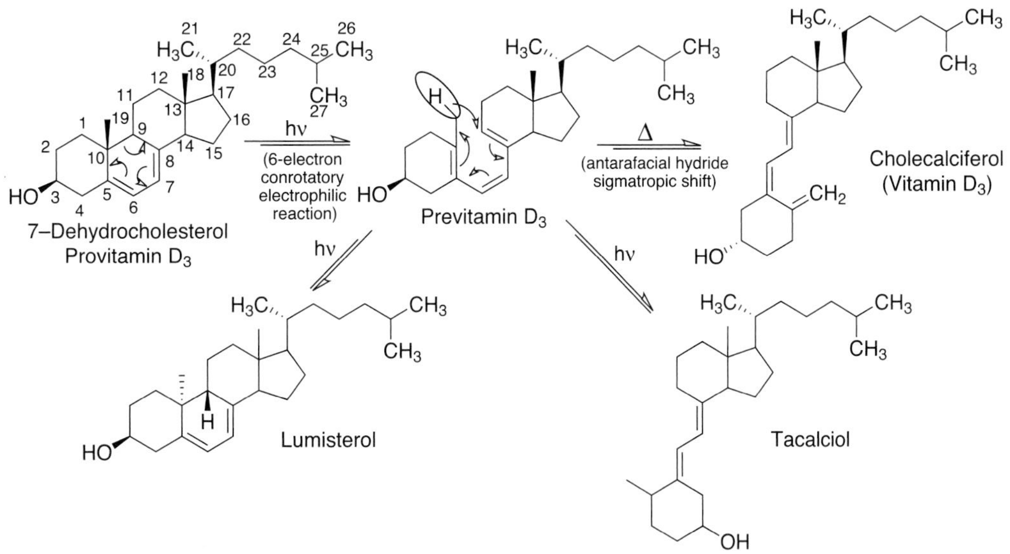

Figure 28.7 ● Photoactivation of 7-dehydrocholesterol to cholecalciferol.

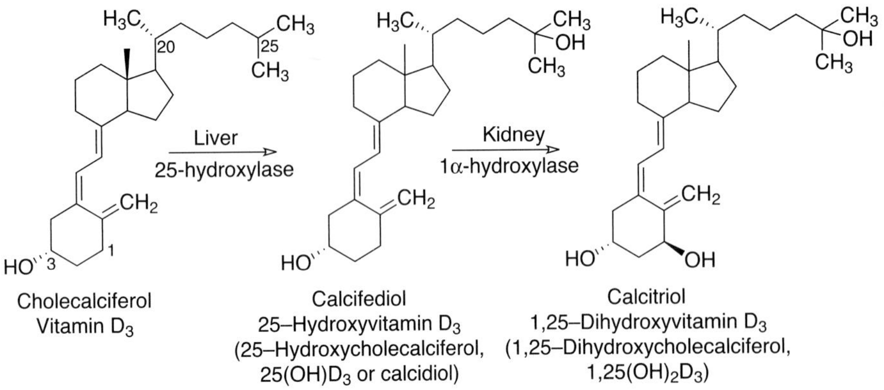

Figure 28.8 ● Cholecalciferol bioactivation.

One of the most well-known effects of calcitriol is to maintain calcium homeostasis. Phosphate metabolism is also affected. The mechanism of action promoting Ca^{2+} transport in the intestine involves calcitriol-mediated formation of a calcium-binding protein, calbindin, which is known to exist in at least two forms in humans, calbindin 1, 28kDa (CALB1) and S100 calcium binding protein G (S100G), also known as calbindin-D9k. A calcium-dependent ATPase, Na^+, and calbindin are necessary for intestinal Ca^{2+} transport and act to enhance the transcellular movement resulting in increased absorption of dietary Ca^{2+}. Transient receptor potential cation channel, subfamily V, member 6 (TRPV6), which controls the rate of cellular entry of Ca^{2+}, is also found to be increased in intestinal cells under the control of calcitriol. Calcitriol also promotes intestinal phosphate absorption, mobilization of Ca^{2+} and phosphate from bone, and renal reabsorption of Ca^{2+} and phosphate. Also involved are parathyroid hormone and calcitonin.

VDRs have also been identified in tissues not normally associated with bone mineral homeostasis. Besides the intestines, kidneys, and osteoblasts, vitamin D receptors have been located in the parathyroid gland, the pancreatic islet cells, the mammary epithelium, the skin keratinocytes, muscle, and the immune cells. Activation in the latter has potent antiproliferative and immunomodulatory functions. Thus, calcitriol and its analogous VDR ligands have therapeutic potential in the treatment of inflammatory diseases (rheumatoid and psoriatic arthritis), dermatological conditions (psoriasis, keratosis), osteoporosis, suppression of parathyroid hormone, cancers (including colon, prostate, and breast), and autoimmune diseases.[70] It has been suggested that vitamin D exerts its anticancer effects through its role as a nuclear transcription factor that regulates cell growth, dif-ferentiation, apoptosis, and other cancer-developing cellular mechanisms.[71]

The classic form of vitamin D deficiency universally recognized is rickets. In young infants, the entire skull is soft (craniotabes), and problems in bone development lead to delays in sitting, crawling, and walking. Osteomalacia (evident on x-rays) and deformities of the bones eventually lead to deformities in the rib cage, bowlegs or knock-knees, bone pain, and a predisposition to fractures. Bone deformities may become permanent if not treated with vitamin D at an early stage. Vitamin D deficiency in children and adults also leads to myopathies, which can lead to weakness, and hypocalcemia, which can lead to paresthesia, muscle spasms, and tetany. Recent studies conclude that an increased rate of overall mortality in the general population is associated with low levels of vitamin D.[72] The same study also demonstrated that vitamin D deficiency increases the risk of cancer, diabetes, and hypertension.

THERAPEUTIC USES

Cholecalciferol and ergocalciferol are used in the treatment of known or suspected vitamin D deficiency or the prevention of vitamin D deficiency when bodily needs are increased as seen in pregnancy. Calcitriol can also be used, especially when an immediate effect is desired as in severe deficiencies because it is the active form of vitamin D found in the body. This would involve treatment of rickets, osteomalacia, muscle pain, and hypocalcemia that can result from vitamin D deficiency. Vitamin D is also useful, particularly when used with calcium supplementation, to treat osteoporosis.[44,73] Vitamin D can also be used to treat hypophosphatemia or hypocalcemia because of other causes, such as hypoparathyroidism.

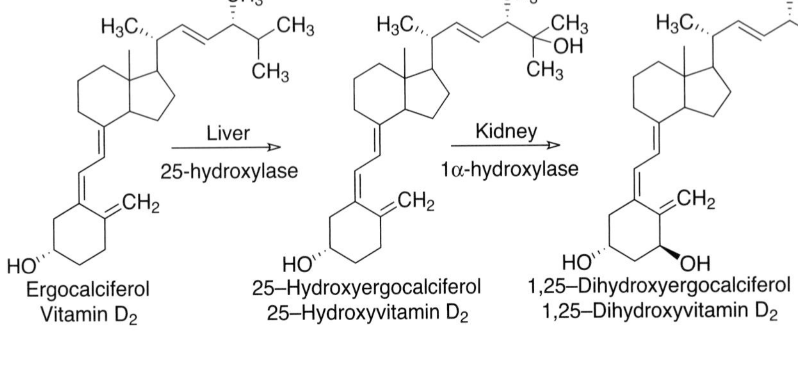

Figure 28.9 ● Ergocalciferol bioactivation.

TABLE 28.7 **Vitamin D Products**

Generic Name	Trade Name	Dosage Form	Use
Calcifediol	Calderol	Capsule	Vitamin D therapy
Calcipotriene	Dovonex	Ointment, cream, or scalp solution	Plaque psoriasis
Calcitriol	Rocaltrol, Calcijex	Capsule, oral solution, injection	Vitamin D therapy, renal osteodystrophy, hypocalcemia, hypoparathyroidism
Cholecalciferol	Delta-D, various	Capsules, tablet, injection, cream, ointment	Vitamin D therapy, hypoparathyroidism, hypophosphatamia
Dihydrotachysterol	DHT	Capsule, oral solution, tablet	Hypoparathyroidism
Doxercalciferol	Hectorol	Capsule	Renal osteodystrophy
Ergocalciferol	Drisdol, various	Oral softgel, capsule, oral solution, tablet	Vitamin D therapy, hypoparathyroidism, hypophosphatamia
Paricalcitol	Zemplar	Injection, capsule	Renal osteodystrophy

Uremia associated with renal failure can result in hypocalcemia and secondary hyperparathyroidism as a result of insufficient conversion of calcidiol to calcitriol by the diseased kidneys. This results in renal osteodystrophy, a metabolic bone disease involving abnormal mineralization. Patients are often on dialysis by the time these problems occur. Treatment with calcitriol, or other active analogs of vitamin D with a 1α-hydroxy group (see Table 28.7) helps to increase Ca^{2+} levels, as well as decrease parathyroid hormone levels essentially controlling these effects. Doses used do not result in extraskeletal calcification or increase the rate of decline in renal function as can be seen with excessive doses of vitamin D.

Beneficial effects have been shown for high levels of calcitriol in patients with advanced prostate cancer[74] and colorectal cancer[75] although this is not a proven therapy. These investigational treatments require high doses of vitamin D and the resultant hypercalcemia limits the usefulness. Vitamin D analogs with a decreased tendency to cause hypercalcemia and hypercalciuria are being developed and investigated. Although the issue of vitamin D in heart health is not resolved yet, an inverse correlation was found between cardiovascular events and serum vitamin D (as calcidiol or calcitriol) levels—low vitamin D levels are associated with hypertension, elevated very low-density lipoprotein (VLDL) triglycerides, and impaired insulin metabolism.[76,77] Calcipotriene represents a vitamin D analog used for its antiproliferative effects and the ability to promote cellular differentiation in the epidermis and is effective in the treatment of psoriasis.[78]

HYPERVITAMINOSIS

Hypervitaminosis D apparently cannot arise from excessive exposure to sunlight[79] but only occurs following ingestion of large quantities of synthetic vitamin D. The precise amount to produce toxicity would depend on the dose and duration of exposure, however, doses of 100,000 IU daily for 4 days have not resulted in toxicity.[80] Toxicity involves derangements of calcium metabolism, resulting in hypercalcemia and metastatic calcification of soft tissue. Most problems result from the hypercalcemia, which typically causes muscular weakness, anorexia, nausea, vomiting, and depression of the CNS (which can result in coma and death). In addition, deposition of calcium salts in the kidneys (nephrocalcinosis) and the tubules (nephrolithiasis) can lead to potentially irreversible renal damage. Early signs are polyuria and nocturia because of damage to the renal concentrating mechanism.

PRODUCTS

Table 28.7 is a list of the currently available products, and Figure 28.10 shows their structures. Most vitamin supplements containing vitamin D singly, or in combination with other vitamins as multivitamin preparations, contain cholecalciferol. However, ergocalciferol can also be used These are available in various preparations under many different names as oral capsules, tablets, solutions, and powders. Table 28.7 also shows the vitamin D analogs used in the treatment of renal osteodystrophy that occurs as a result of secondary hyperparathyroidism in patients unable to convert calcidiol to the active calcitriol. This is most often seen in severe renal failure, especially in patients on dialysis. Each of these products already has the 1α-hydroxy, so the need for bioactivation by the kidney is circumvented. Finally, calcipotriene is available for the treatment of psoriasis.

Vitamin E

Since the early 1920s, it was known that rats fed only cow's milk cannot produce offspring. In 1922, Evans and Bishop[81] discovered an unrecognized dietary factor essential for reproduction. In 1924, Sure[82] named the principle that could rectify this deficiency vitamin E. When the compound known as vitamin E was isolated from wheat germ oil in 1936 by Evans et al.,[83] it was named α-tocopherol, from the Greek words *tokos* meaning "childbirth," *phero* meaning "to bear," and "-ol" indicating an alcohol. The structure[84] and synthesis[85] of α-tocopherol were reported in 1938. Since then, several other closely related compounds have been discovered from natural sources, and this family of natural products took the generic name tocopherols.

The tocopherols are especially abundant in wheat germ, rice germ, corn germ, other seed germs, lettuce, soya, and cottonseed oil. All green plants contain some tocopherols, and there is evidence that some green leafy vegetables and rose hips contain more than wheat germ. It is probably synthesized by leaves and translocated to the seeds. All four tocopherols have been found in wheat germ oil; α-, β-, and γ-tocopherols have been found in cottonseed oil. Corn oil contains predominantly γ-tocopherol and thus furnishes a convenient source for the isolation of this difficult member of the tocopherols. δ-Tocopherol is 30% of the mixed tocopherols of soya bean oil. Palm oil contains about 30% of tocopherols and 70% of tocotrienols. Cereals like oat, rye, and barley contain small amounts of tocotrienols.

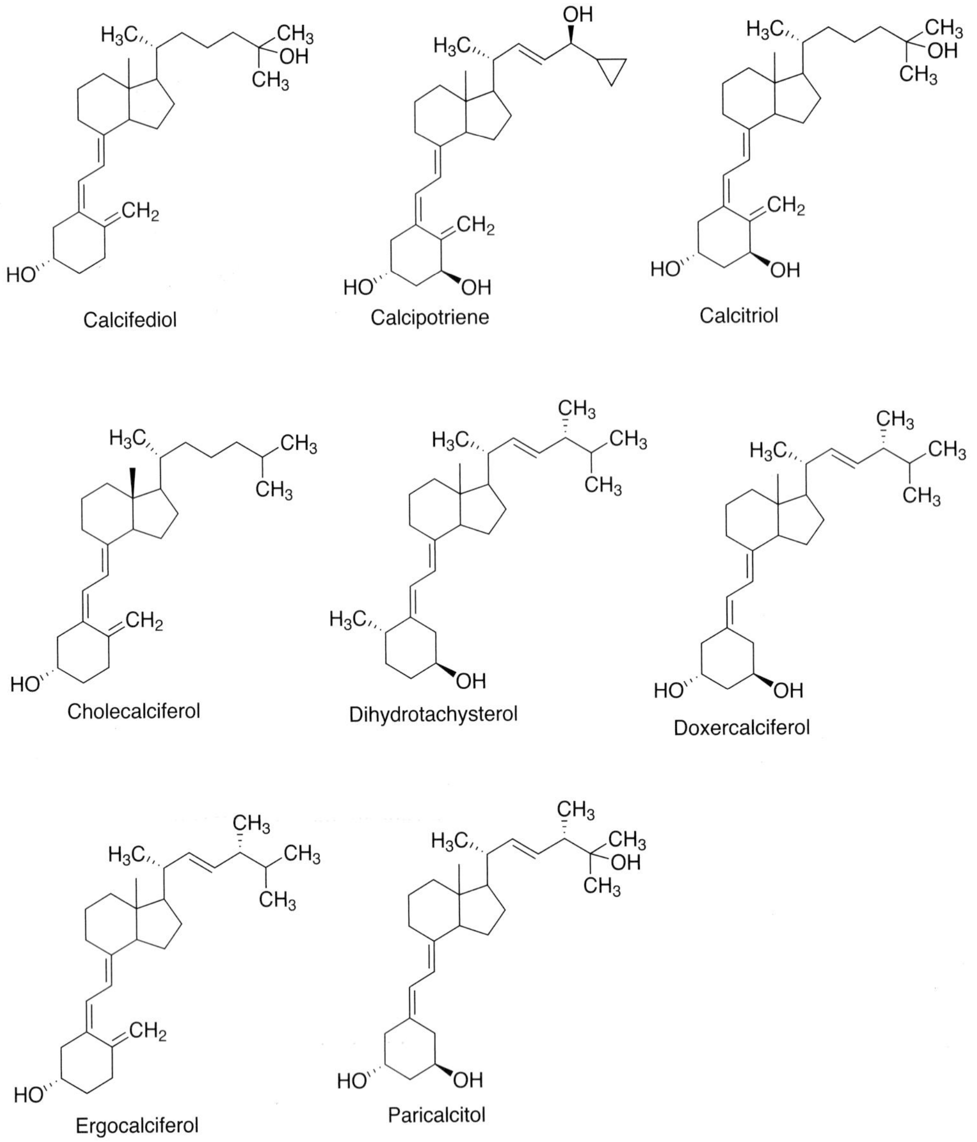

Calcifediol

Calcipotriene

Calcitriol

Cholecalciferol

Dihydrotachysterol

Doxercalciferol

Ergocalciferol

Paricalcitol

Figure 28.10 • Structures of vitamin D products.

CHEMISTRY

Several tocopherols have been isolated. Some have the 4′,8′,12′-trimethyltridecyl-saturated side chain; others have unsaturation in the side chain. It has been suggested that these polyunsaturated tocols be named tocotrienols. The best-known tocopherol is α-tocopherol, which has the greatest biological activity. The base structure, represented in Figure 28.11, shows that the tocopherols are methyl-substituted tocol derivatives: α-tocopherol is 5,7,8-trimethyltocol; β-tocopherol is 5,8-dimethyltocol; the γ-compound is 7,8-dimethyltocol; and δ-tocopherol is 8-methyltocol. The tocotrienols have similar substituents. Vitamin E is a generic descriptor for all tocol and tocotrienol derivatives that have biological activity similar to α-tocopherol.[86] Currently, eight of these tocols, four tocopherols and four tocotrienols, are considered the vitamin E family. These tocols possess two important structural components, the chromanol ring and the side chain, and differ by the methylation patterns of the chromanol ring (α-, β-, γ-, and δ-) and presence or absence of double bonds in the side chain (no double bond in tocopherols whereas three double bonds in tocotrienols).

Natural (+)-α-tocopherol has the configuration 2R,4′R,8′R. The natural tocotrienol has a 2R,3′E,7′E configuration. The tocopherols are diterpenoid natural products biosynthesized from a combination of four isoprenoid units; geranylgeranyl pyrophosphate is the key intermediate that leads to these compounds.

(+)-α-Tocopherol is about 1.36 times as effective as (±)-α-tocopherol in rat antisterility bioassays. As mentioned previously, (+)-α-tocopherol is the naturally occurring form of α-tocopherol with 2R,4′R,8′R configuration. (±)-α-Tocopherol is synthetic, and is called all-*rac*-α-tocopherol. The configuration at C[2] is critical and the Nutrition Board of the National Academy of Sciences, Institute of Medicine recognized in 2000 that 2R-forms of α-tocopherol meet the human requirements. β-Tocopherol is about half as active as α-tocopherol, and the γ- and δ-tocopherols are only 0.01 times as active as α-tocopherol.

The esters of tocopherol (e.g., acetate, propionate, and butyrate) are more active than the parent compound because of better bioavailability.[87] This is also true of the phosphoric acid ester of (±)-δ-tocopherol when it is administered

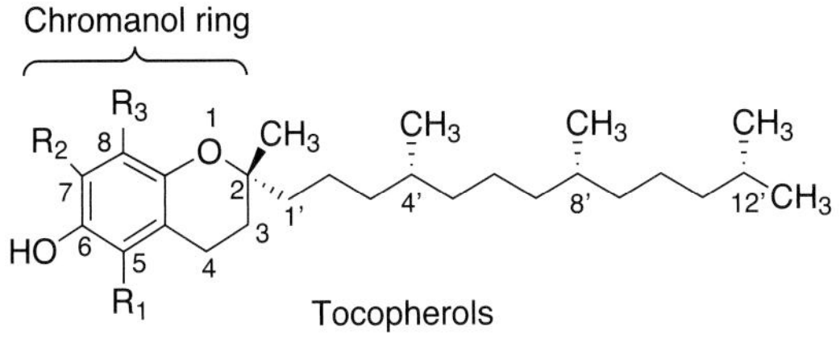

Tocopherols

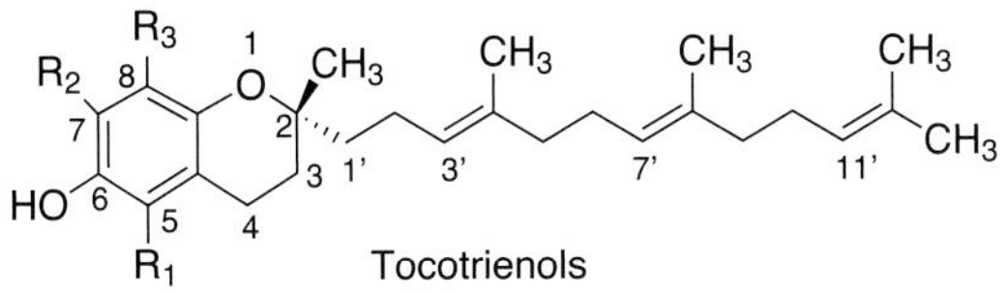

Tocotrienols

α	$R_1 = R_2 = R_3 = CH_3$
β	$R_1 = R_3 = CH_3$; $R_2 = H$
γ	$R_2 = R_3 = CH_3$; $R_1 = H$
δ	$R_1 = R_2 = H$; $R_3 = CH_3$

Figure 28.11 ● Tocopherols and tocotrienols.

parenterally.[88] The ethers of the tocopherols are inactive, because unlike esters that are readily hydrolyzed to the active antioxidant chromanol form by esterases, ethers are relatively metabolically more stable and as such do not possess antioxidant property.

Oxidation of the tocopherols to their corresponding quinones also leads to inactive compounds. Replacement of the methyl groups on the chromanol ring by ethyl groups decreases activity. The introduction of a double bond in the 3,4-position of α-tocopherol reduces its activity by about two thirds. Reduction of the size of the long alkyl side chain or the introduction of double bonds in this side chain markedly reduces activity.

KINETICS

Bile salts and dietary lipids play critical roles in the absorption of vitamin E and their esters into intestinal epithelial cells through micellization. Pancreatic lipases facilitate the micellization of vitamin E as a consequence of hydrolysis of non–vitamin E lipids by forming mixed micells. The vitamin E esters (e.g., α-tocopherol acetate), on the other hand, require hydrolysis by the pancreatic lipases prior to micellization and uptake into the enterocytes. The uptake of vitamin E from the mixed micells is thought to be a passive diffusion process; however, the role of a scavenger receptor class B type I (SR-BI) has also been suggested.

The intracellular trafficking of vitamin E may involve its incorporation into chylomicrons. Both α- and γ-tocopherols are equally incorporated into chylomicrons, which are then secreted into the lymphatic system. An ATP-binding cassette, subfamily A, member 1 (ABCA1) transport protein-directed efflux of vitamin E from epithelial cells into HDL followed by direct transport into the portal vein has also been suggested as an important alternative pathway for vitamin E absorption. Dietary fats increase chylomicron-mediated absorption while a low-fat diet increases HDL-mediated absorption of vitamin E.[89] The absence of dietary fat results in little absorption of vitamin E.[90] Despite a low-fat diet, high bioavailability was reported when vitamin E was added with emulsifier onto fortified breakfast cereal, suggestive of micellization as a critical factor for its absorption.[91] No apparent differences in intestinal absorption of various forms of vitamin E (e.g., α- and γ-tocopherols or *RRR*- and *SRR*-α-tocopherols) have been observed.[92] Overall, 20% to 80% of vitamin E is absorbed from the intestinal lumen into the bloodstream. The liver is an important storage site. γ-Tocopherol is secreted primarily into the bile while α-tocopherol enters the circulation, where it is found in much higher levels than γ-tocopherol, even though the latter predominates in the diet. This difference is attributed to a liver cytosolic binding protein, α-tocopherol transfer protein (α-TTP) that is selective for α-tocopherol.

The tocopherols in lymph are associated with chylomicrons and VLDLs. Circulating tocopherols are also carried by α-TTP, which preferentially incorporates them into blood low-density lipoproteins (LDLs). The tocopherols are readily and reversibly bound to most tissues, including adipose tissue, and the vitamin is thus stored. The vitamin is concentrated in membrane structures, such as mitochondria, endoplasmic reticulum, and nuclear and plasma membranes.

Although “Simon metabolites” (tocopheronic acid and its γ-lactone) were first identified as the primary vitamin E metabolites by in vitro sample oxidation, the biologically relevant are the 2-carboxyethyl-6-hydroxychroman (CEHC) products (Fig. 28.12). Thus α-, β-, γ-, and δ-CEHCs are identified as metabolites of the respective tocopherols. The terminal methyl group is oxidized to a carboxylic acid and shortened by several steps of β-oxidation to produce CEHC. The CEHC metabolites undergo glucuronide and sulfate conjugations, and most of the CEHC metabolites are found in urine as these conjugates. These metabolites are also excreted in the bile and vitamin E may undergo some enterohepatic circulation.[92]

BIOCHEMISTRY

For decades, there has been significant interest in investigating the biochemical functions of vitamin E, but it is still difficult to explain many of the biochemical derangements caused by vitamin E deficiency in animals. There seems to be general agreement that one of the primary metabolic

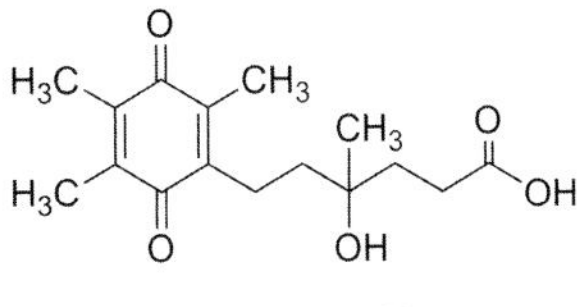

Tocopheronic acid

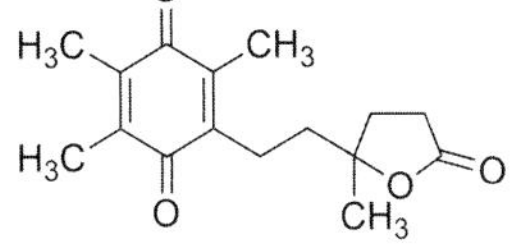

Tocopheronolactone

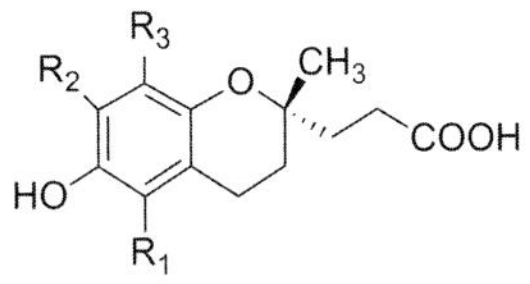

Carboxylethyl hydroxychroman (CEHC)

α	$R_1 = R_2 = R_3 = CH_3$
β	$R_1 = R_3 = CH_3$; $R_2 = H$
γ	$R_2 = R_3 = CH_3$; $R_1 = H$
δ	$R_1 = R_2 = H$; $R_3 = CH_3$

Figure 28.12 ● Vitamin E metabolites.

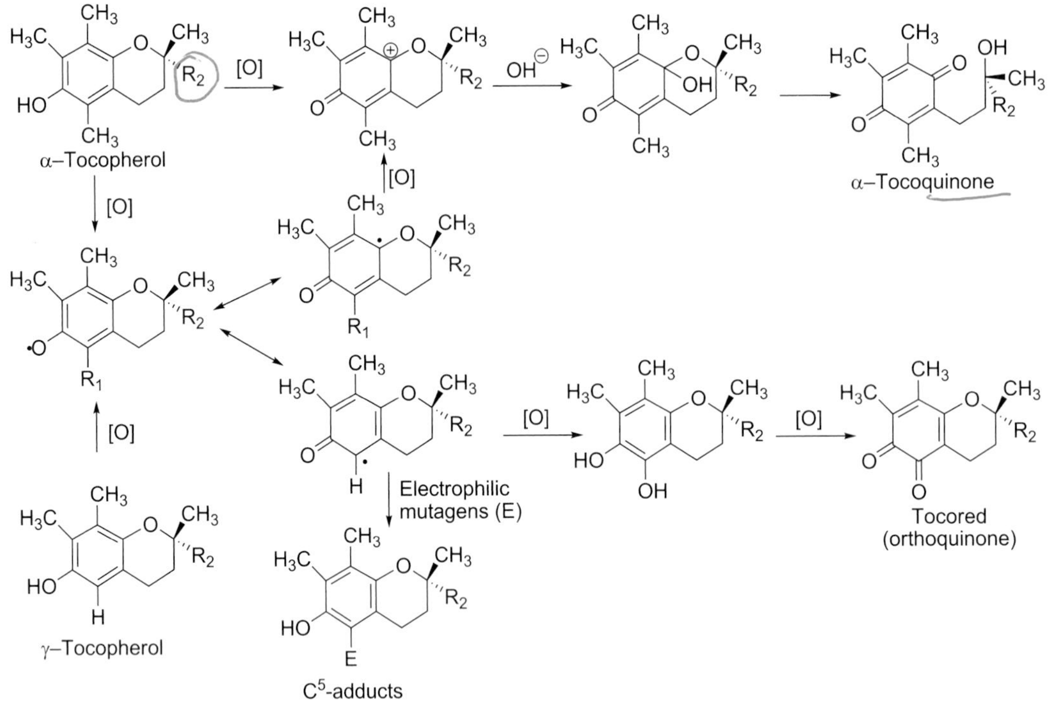

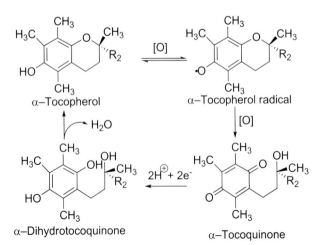

Figure 28.13 ● Antioxidant mechanisms of α- and γ-tocopherols. (R$_1$, H, or CH$_3$; R$_2$, Phytyl.)

functions of the vitamin is preventing the oxidation of lipids, particularly unsaturated fatty acids. Through this antioxidant effect, α-tocopherol plays an important role in protecting cell membranes made of lipids and LDLs. The α-tocopherol donates its electrons to the free radicals to neutralize them, thus protecting the cellular lipids from oxidative damage. In this process, α-tocopherol loses its antioxidant capacity by forming the α-tocoquinone (Fig. 28.13). It is generally accepted that other antioxidants like vitamin C or glutathione can restore vitamin E from its single electron oxidation state, tocopherol radical. Although several reports suggested that once it is fully oxidized to the tocoquinone form, it will not be regenerated back to vitamin E, reports are also available showing that it can be regenerated back in presence of glutathione according to the mechanism shown in Figure 28.14.[93,94]

Because of the methylation level, which enhances the nucleophilicity and reactivity of the 6-OH group, the α-isoforms of both tocopherol and tocotrienol are the most potent antioxidants among all the vitamin E family. Although α-tocotrienol is believed to be a more potent antioxidant than the α-tocopherol for many factors (e.g., higher recycling efficiency, more uniform distribution within the microsomal membrane bilayer and more efficient interaction with lipid free radicals) misleading results have been demonstrated because of the high affinity of α-TTP for α-tocopherol. α-Tocopherol is biologically the most important isoform because of its high affinity for α-TTP, which results in high bioavailability and bioactivity.[95]

Biochemical functions of the vitamin E family are diverse and may include actions other than their well-documented antioxidant activities. α-Tocopherol not only strongly inhibits platelet and other cell adhesion but also inhibits cell proliferation, protein kinase C, 5-lipooxygenase, and phospholipase A$_2$ and activates protein phosphatase 2A and diacylglycerol kinase, which are unrelated to its antioxidant activity. These actions reflect the specific interactions of α-tocopherol with enzymes, structural proteins, lipids, and transcription factors. γ-Tocopherol and CEHC metabolic products of vitamin E exhibit many other functions including anti-inflammatory, antineoplastic, natriuretic, and also cardioprotective functions.[96]

During the last 5 years, interest in the action of tocotrienols has increased with the inclusion of a substantial amount of vitamin E research directed toward that of α-tocotrienol. Numerous unique biochemical functions of α-tocotrienol have been discovered that include prevention of inducible neurodegeneration by regulating specific mediators of cell death, hypocholesterolemic effects by suppressing 3-hydroxy-3-methyl-glutaryl-CoA (HCG-CoA) reductase activity, and protection against stroke. It has also been reported that tocotrienols, but not tocopherols, suppress the growth of breast cancer cells.[96]

Figure 28.14 ● Interconversion of α-tocopherol and α-tocoquinone.

The diseases caused by vitamin E deficiency in animals are not well correlated with that in human. The sterility in rats and nutritional muscular dystrophies in other lower animal including monkeys, rabbits, lambs, and chicks are well documented. Reversible neurological disorders in humans and hemolytic anemia in premature infants because of vitamin E deficiency have been seen.

The antioxidant function does not explain all the biochemical abnormalities caused by vitamin E deficiency. Moreover, vitamin E is not the only in vivo antioxidant. Two enzyme systems, glutathione reductase and *o*-phenylenediamine peroxidase, also function in this capacity.[97] It has been postulated that vitamin E has a role in the regulation of protein synthesis. Other actions of this vitamin have also been investigated, for example, effects on muscle creatine kinase and liver xanthine oxidase. Vitamin E deficiency leads to an increase in the turnover of creatine kinase. Vitamin E–deficient animals also exhibit increased liver xanthine oxidase activity, which is because of increased de novo synthesis.[97]

Although it has been difficult to establish clinical correlates of vitamin E deficiency in humans, Bieri and Farrell[97] have summarized some useful generalizations and conclusions. These workers noted that the infant, especially the premature infant, is susceptible to tocopherol deficiency because of ineffective transfer of the vitamin from placenta to fetus and that growth in infants requires greater availability of the vitamin. In adults, the tocopherol storage depots provide adequate availability that is not readily depleted, but intestinal malabsorption syndromes, when persistent, can lead to depletion of the storage depots. Children with cystic fibrosis suffer from severe vitamin E deficiency caused by malabsorption. Tropical sprue, celiac disease, gastrointestinal resections, hepatic cirrhosis, biliary obstruction, and excessive ingestion of mineral oil may also cause long-term malabsorption.

THERAPEUTIC USES

Vitamin E is used in the treatment of known or suspected vitamin E deficiency. The use of vitamin E to prevent or treat a wide variety of diseases has been examined quite extensively and in some cases has been found to be of some benefit, although the effect is frequently minimal. Vitamin E may help in Alzheimer disease, dysmenorrhea, nonalcoholic fatty liver, and tardive dyskinesias, to name a few. However, in most cases, and especially for common diseases, there is often no proven benefit or the studies are contradictory.

Vitamin E has been extensively studied for the prevention of cardiovascular disease, but evidence against any benefit continues to accumulate.[44,98] Indeed, some studies show that vitamin E supplementation may actually increase stroke risk[98] or all cause mortality.[55] It has also been suggested that megadoses of tocopherol be used in the treatment of peripheral vascular disease. Although some studies support this proposal, experts in the field state that further clinical studies are necessary to make a definitive recommendation. Nevertheless, it continues to be popular and controversial to consider the beneficial effects, and investigations of megavitamin E therapy for cardiovascular disease continue to appear in the literature.[97]

The failure to demonstrate the protective effects against heart diseases by vitamin E supplements may be because they contain only α-tocopherol. To effectively remove the

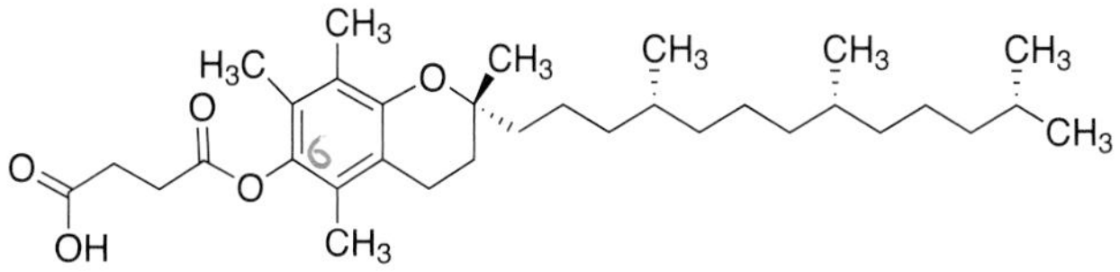

Figure 28.15 ◆ α-Tocopheryl succinate.

peroxide damage in these cells by electrophilic peroxynitrites or other mutagens, γ-tocopherol is also needed that, in addition to forming the orthoquinone, acts in vivo as a trap for these membrane-soluble electrophilic mutagens forming stable adducts through the nucleophilic C^5, which is blocked in α-tocopherol (Fig. 28.13). It has been suggested that because α-tocopherol supplementation suppresses γ-tocopherol levels, a combination of the two tocopherols in the ratios found in the diet may be more useful than α-tocopherol, alone.[99]

The well-documented antioxidant property of the tocopherols led to their examination for anticancer activity without any consistent success;[43,100] although some studies have shown a reduction in prostate cancer in smokers.[44] It is interesting that the ethers (RO-), esters (RCOO-), and amides (RCONH-) at C^6 of the chromanol ring (α-tocopheryl succinate ester is the prototype, Fig. 28.15) have shown to be potent antineoplastic agents. The antineoplastic potency of the tocopherol analogs is not related to their antioxidant property, which was proven by synthesizing a series of "redox-silent" analogs and testing them against various neoplastic cell lines. The detailed molecular biology studies revealed that these are mainly mitocans (mitochondrially targeted anticancer drugs) that selectively destabilize the mitochondria in malignant cells and suppressed cancer in preclinical models. Although they are fully recognized as potent anticancer agents, detailed clinical studies for their therapeutic application are yet to be completed.[101]

HYPERVITAMINOSIS

Vitamin E used in high doses, as high as 3,200 mg/day, has a proven record of safety.[47] Various reports, many single case reports, or uncontrolled studies have suggested adverse effects such as interference with clotting, weakness, decreased thyroid hormone levels, and gastrointestinal upset. The importance of these is unknown. The only notable adverse effects have occurred in premature infants given large doses of this vitamin. Hepatotoxicities have been seen in premature infants of less than 1,500 g birth weight given vitamin E intravenously, and the incidence of necrotizing enterocolitis and sepsis increased under similar conditions following oral or intravenous (IV) dosing.

PRODUCTS

Vitamin E is available from numerous sources as oral capsules, liquids, and tablets under various names. Vitamin E is also available as a component of numerous multivitamin preparations. The forms of vitamin E used in these products are shown in Table 28.8. Vitamin E activity is currently expressed in terms of the (+)-α-tocopherol equivalents based on the former *USP* units and mass. One former *USP* unit is equal to one former IU.

TABLE 28.8 Relative Potencies of Various Commercial Forms of Vitamin E

Form of Vitamin E	Potency
Potency (in former *USP* units) of 1 mg	
($\pm$)-α-Tocopherol	1.1
($\pm$)-α-Tocopherol acetate	1
($\pm$)-α-Tocopherol acid succinate	0.89
(+)-α-Tocopherol	1.49
(+)-α-Tocopherol acetate	1.36
(+)-α-Tocopherol acid succinate	1.21

Vitamin K

Lipid-free diet research by Henrik Dam[102] starting in 1929 and culminating in 1935[103] resulted in the discovery of an antihemorrhagic factor that Dam named *vitamin K* (from the German word *Koagulation*). Along with the work of Edward A. Doisy, the structure of vitamin K was determined in 1939[104] and synthesis accomplished in 1965.[105] For their work, Dam and Doisy shared the 1943 Nobel Prize in Medicine. Originally, the term vitamin K was applied to the vitamin isolated from alfalfa, and a similar principle from putrified fish meal was named *vitamin K₂*. The original vitamin K was thereafter referred to as vitamin K_1. In 1960, IUPAC recommended the terms phylloquinone for vitamin K_1 with the official abbreviation of "K" and farnoquinone for the originally isolated vitamin K_2.[106] Several compounds chemically related to vitamin K_2, differing only in the number of 5-carbon prenyl (isoprenoid) units attached, were subsequently discovered, and in 1973, IUPAC adopted the term *menaquininones* (MK) to refer to this group of substances.[107] The menaquinones differ in the number of prenyl units attached and specific compounds are designated menaquinone-n (MK-n) where *n* represents the number of prenyl side chains. The original vitamin K_2 is now known as MK-6. For this discussion, the term vitamin K will be used to denote both phylloquinone and menaquinones when appropriate. Also of note, the *USP* generic name for phylloquinone in pharmaceutical preparations is phytonadione, and this is the preferred term among medical practitioners. Throughout this text, these two terms will be used in their best context.

Naturally occurring vitamin K is found in two forms depending on whether the source is plants or bacteria. Plants produce phylloquinone whereas bacteria produce menaquinones. Dietary sources from plants include leafy green vegetables; such as collard greens, spinach, and salad greens; soy and canola oils; and margarine. Broccoli, brussels sprouts, cabbage, and olive oil also contain appreciable quantities. The major bacterial source is the intestinal flora, especially Gram-positive organisms; however, their contribution to overall vitamin K intake is unknown.

CHEMISTRY

Chemically, all vitamin Ks are 2-methyl 1,4-naphthoquinone derivatives containing variable aliphatic side chains at C^3. Phylloquinone (Fig. 28.16) invariably contains a phytyl side chain. Menaquinones (Fig. 28.17) are a series of compounds that have a longer side chain with more unsaturation. This side chain may be composed of 1 to 13 prenyl (isoprenyl) units.

Many other closely related compounds possess vitamin K activity. Of particular historical note are the water-soluble menadione (2-methyl-1,4-naphthoquinone; vitamin K_3), which is no longer marketed because of toxicities, and menadiol (2-methylnaphthalene-1,4-diol; vitamin K_4). Menadione contains the naphthoquinone ring without any attached prenyls and can be thought of as MK-0 (see Fig. 28.17). Menadiol is menadione with the two keto groups reduced to hydroxyls. Both compounds are bioactivated to the active form through alkylation. Phylloquinone naturally occurs as a *trans*-isomer and has an *R,R,E* configuration. The synthetic, commercially available form is a mixture of *cis*- and *trans*-isomers, with no more than 20% *cis*.

KINETICS

Phylloquinone is absorbed in the proximal intestine[108] via the same pathway used for dietary lipids, requiring bile salts, dietary fat, and pancreatic juice. The extent of absorption depends on the dietary source. Pharmaceutical preparations of purified phylloquinone may have bioavailabilities as high as 80%, whereas the bioavailability from plant sources, although rich in phylloquinone, may be lower than 10%.[109] This is thought to be because of the inefficiency in extracting the vitamin K from the plant cells during the digestive process. Still, these plant sources are likely the most important natural source of vitamin K in the diet. An additional source of vitamin K is the menaquinones, which are synthesized by the gut flora. These are likely absorbed from the ileum similar to phylloquinone. The contribution to

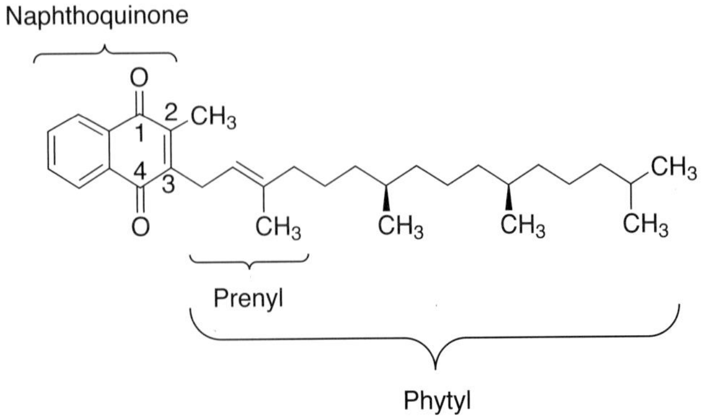

Figure 28.16 ● Phylloquinone (2–Methyl–3–phytyl–1, 4–naphthoquinone).

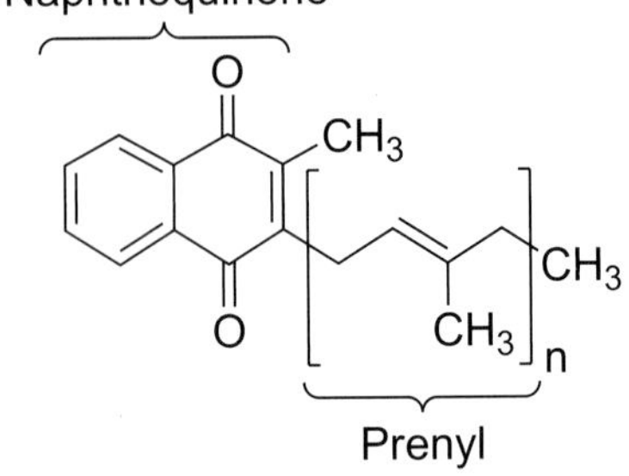

Figure 28.17 ● Menaquinone general structure. Menaquinone-4 (n = 4) and menaquinone-6 (n = 6) are the most common forms.

overall dietary intake is unresolved[110] but these help explain the high level of vitamin K activity in feces.

Following absorption by the enterocytes, and similar to other dietary fats, phylloquinone and menaquinones are found in the newly formed chylomicrons, which are released into the lymph and bloodstream. The primary form of circulating vitamin K activity is phylloquinone. Conversion of the chylomicrons into chylomicron remnants and their subsequent association with apolipoprotein E result in receptor-mediated uptake by cells through pinocytosis. Historically, phylloquinone uptake by hepatic cells was thought to be the predominant process; however, it is now recognized that uptake by osteoblast precursor cells also occurs and explains the ultimate delivery to osteoblasts inside bone tissue.[111] Approximately 90% of the vitamin K found in the liver is in the form of menaquinones and the remainder is phylloquinone.[110] In contrast to other fat-soluble vitamins, no significant storage occurs. The major urinary metabolites are glucuronide conjugates of carboxylic acids derived from shortening of the side chain.

BIOCHEMISTRY

The accepted mechanism for vitamin K is to function as a cofactor in the posttranslational synthesis of γ-carboxyglutamic acid (Gla) from glutamic acid (Glu) residues.[112] The discovery of Gla in 1974[113,114] clarified the mechanism of vitamin K and led to the identification of additional vitamin K–dependent proteins. All vitamin K–dependent proteins contain propeptide possessing Glu residues. Vitamin K participates in the carboxylation of several specific Glu residues to form Gla residues, which function as Ca^{+2}-binding sites on the vitamin K–dependent proteins (see Fig. 28.18). Further, the Gla residues are found in essentially the same region, near the amino terminus, and this region is called the *Gla domain*.[115] Of the 14 known vitamin K–dependent proteins, four function as procoagulants, three function as anticoagulants, two are involved in bone and extracellular matrix homeostasis, one in cell proliferation, and four represent transmembrane proteins whose function has not been identified. All of these proteins have considerable structural homology. All contain 10 to 12 Gla residues, which are important for their proper activity.[116] For example, prothrombin has 10 Gla residues; loss of just two residues decreases its coagulation activity by 80%.

This synthesis of Gla residues from Glu residues requires reduced vitamin K (a hydroquinone, KH_2), carbon dioxide, and molecular oxygen. Although the reaction does not require ATP, it uses the energy from the oxidation of KH_2 to execute the carboxylation of glutamic acid.[117] The enzyme, γ-glutamyl carboxylase (GGCX; EC 6.4.-.-), must create a carbanion by extracting a proton from the glutamate γ-carbon. This requires a base with a pK_a of 26 to 28. The anion of the hydroquinone, however, has a pK_a of only about 9.

A proposed mechanism (Fig. 28.19) for this carboxylation creates such a base from vitamin K.[118,119] Vitamin K is reduced to its hydroquinone form (vitamin KH_2). Molecular oxygen is incorporated into the conjugate acid form of vitamin KH_2 to form a peroxy anion, which subsequently forms a dioxetane intermediate. The peroxy bond is cleaved by the adjacent enolate anion to produce an intermediate sufficiently basic to deprotonate the α-carbon. Extraction of the proton allows the carboxylase to carboxylate the Glu residue. The vitamin K intermediate is converted to vitamin K oxide, which must be reduced back to vitamin K. Vitamin K oxide is recycled back to vitamin K by vitamin K–epoxide reductase (VKOR; EC 1.1.4.1) and NAD(P)H dehydrogenase (quinone) (EC 1.6.5.2), also known as vitamin K reductase. Both of these enzymes are dithiol dependent and are inhibited by the 4-hydroxycoumarin anticoagulants such as warfarin.

Historically, the most well-known function of vitamin K is in the formation of four of the procoagulation factors, specifically factors VII, IX, X, and prothrombin. The Gla residues function as Ca^{2+} ion bridges linking the blood-clotting protein to phospholipids on endothelial cells and platelets. Binding to membrane surfaces is critical in the activation of these proteins.[120] Prothrombin and factors VII, IX, and X participate in the cascade of reactions leading to fibrin clot formation.

Vitamin K in mammals also maintains adequate levels of the vitamin K–dependent proteins C (PROC), S (PROS1), and Z (PROZ), which have anticoagulant activity. PROC exerts its anticoagulant effect by inactivating activated factors V_a and VIII_a.[121] PROC is first activated by prothrombin. This activation requires a cell surface receptor, thrombomodulin (THBD), and also Ca^{2+} and PROS1. PROC also increases fibrinolysis by inactivating the major inhibitor of tissue plasminogen activator.[122] PROS1 is found in the plasma and is bound to complement component 4 binding protein, alpha (C4BPA) and functions as a cofactor in the PROC inactivation of activated factor V_a. PROS1 also acts as a cofactor in the downregulation of factor X activation.[123] PROZ binds to serpin peptidase inhibitor, clade A (alpha-1 antiproteinase, antitrypsin), member 10 (SERPINA10) and downregulates coagulation by inhibiting activated factor X_a.[124]

There are two vitamin K–dependent proteins involved in bone structure, bone Gla protein (BGLAP, osteocalcin) and matrix Gla protein (MGP). BGLAP is present in the highest amounts in bone, dentin, and other mineralized tissue and contains three Gla residues. MGP is found in bone

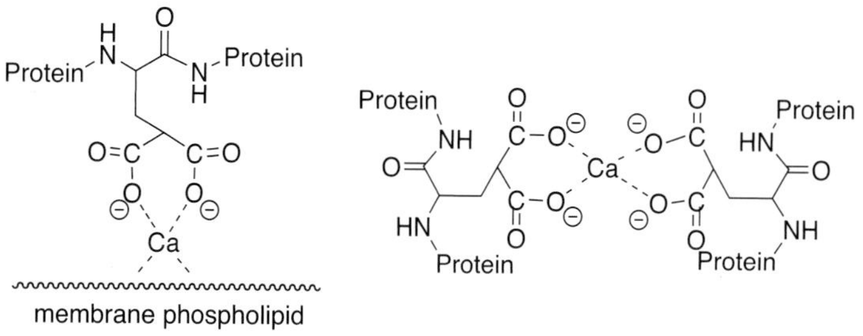

Figure 28.18 ● Calcium binding to Gla residues on vitamin K–dependent proteins.

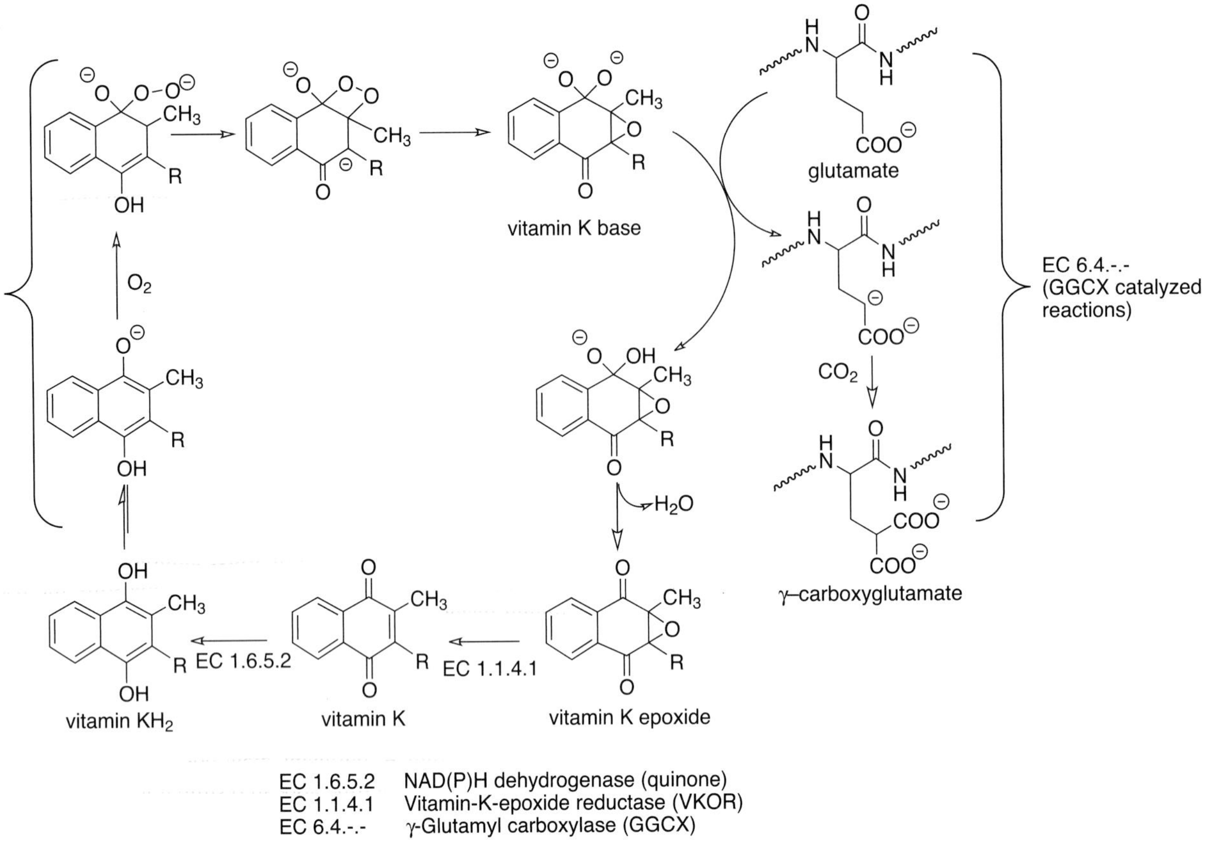

EC 1.6.5.2   NAD(P)H dehydrogenase (quinone)
EC 1.1.4.1   Vitamin-K-epoxide reductase (VKOR)
EC 6.4.-.-   γ-Glutamyl carboxylase (GGCX)

Figure 28.19 ● The vitamin K cycle showing its role in γ-carboxylation of glutamate by GGCX. (R, phytyl side chain.)

and cartilage, but is probably widely distributed in the body, and contains five Gla residues.[125] Both of these are important in regulating bone mineralization, in conjunction with vitamin D, calcium and other hormones. Specifically, vitamin D increases the synthesis of BGLAP propeptide whereas vitamin K is required for its activation through formation of Gla residues. Deficiency of vitamin K or the use of vitamin K antagonists, such as warfarin, can result in mineral loss and bone malformation. Although maintenance of adequate vitamin K intake is important for bone maintenance, high doses of vitamin K may not lead to remineralization. It is important to note that proper maintenance of bone structure is multifaceted with at least two key vitamins, K and D, involved and several other factors. Studies of individual vitamins and their role in bone health may be misleading because increasing intake of a single vitamin may not be sufficient to offset deficiencies in other biomolecules involved in overall bone homeostasis. The promotion of bone formation by vitamin K_2 is not solely mediated through its action on Gla proteins; however, it can also directly stimulate messenger ribonucleic acid (mRNA) production of osteoblast mRNA markers and regulate transcription of bone-specific genes.[126]

Another vitamin K–dependent Gla protein, growth arrest-specific 6 (GAS6), was the most recently discovered which contains 10 to 11 Gla residues.[127] GAS6 is a protein initially found to increase approximately 30-fold during the G_0 phase of the cell cycle suggesting a role in cell proliferation. Several biological roles related to this function have been elucidated since then, including effects on apoptosis,

immune function, inflammation, and cell differentiation, among others.[128] Of particular interest is the possible role in diabetic nephropathy.[129] Current studies are underway to define the function of this protein, with particular interest in the possible role in cancer. Early evidence indicates a possibility of the menaquinones in decreasing the occurrence of hepatocellular carcinoma.[130] The menaquinone analog, menatetrenone, has also been shown to reduce the recurrence rate of hepatocellular carcinoma.[131] This work may ultimately lead to an understanding of any value that vitamin K may have in the prevention or treatment of other cancers.

The latest Gla-containing proteins with unknown functions have wide tissue distribution and are rich in proline residues; thus they have been named proline rich Gla 1 (PRRG1) and proline rich Gla 2 (PRRG2)[132] and transmembrane Gla proteins 3 and 4 (TGP3 and TGP4).[133]

Vitamin K deficiency typically results in an increased clotting time and hemorrhagic disorders. This can manifest as easy bruising, continual bleeding from puncture wounds, mucosal hemorrhage such as gastrointestinal or urinary tract bleeding and intracranial hemorrhaging can occur in infants. Dietary deficiency of vitamin K is rare; most cases are caused by decreased absorption (e.g., intestinal polyposis, chronic ulcerative colitis, intestinal fistula, intestinal obstruction, and sprue), liver disease (e.g., atrophy, cirrhosis, or chronic hepatitis), or biliary disease (e.g., obstructive jaundice, biliary fistulas, insufficient or abnormal bile). Vitamin K deficiency can also lead to decreased bone mineralization.

THERAPEUTIC USES

Phytonadione is indicated in the treatment of known or suspected vitamin K deficiency that may result from dietary deficiency, malabsorption, hepatic, or biliary disease. Phytonadione is also used in the prophylactic treatment of vitamin K deficiency bleeding (VKDB) of the newborn, previously known as hemorrhagic disease of the newborn. In the average infant, the birth values of prothrombin content are adequate, but during the first few days of life, they appear to fall rapidly, even dangerously low, and then slowly recover spontaneously. This transition period was and is critical because of the numerous sites of hemorrhagic manifestations, traumatic or spontaneous, that may prove serious, if not fatal. Several controversial studies linked IM phytonadione administration to newborns with an increased risk of the development of childhood cancer. However, the current position of the American Academy of Pediatrics (AAP) is that these studies were flawed and later large-scale studies showed no association. Therefore, the 2003 policy statement of the AAP recommended 0.5 mg to 1 mg of vitamin K_1 (phytonadione) intramuscularly at birth as a prophylactic measure.[134] This was reaffirmed in 2006.[135]

Phytonadione, or other vitamin K products, should not be administered to patients receiving coumarin anticoagulants, such as warfarin, during routine therapy as these can antagonize their effects. However, phytonadione is indicated in the treatment of overdoses of vitamin K–epoxide reductase inhibitors, such as warfarin, or other drugs that can interfere with vitamin K utilization in the clotting process. Of particular note is the requirement in this one use for an active form of vitamin K. Specifically, the only marketed product is phytonadione. Inactive forms, such as menadiol, are not bioactivated with sufficient rapidity to be used as antidotes in this situation. Finally, vitamin K may also have some utility in preventing bone loss as is seen in osteoporosis.[125]

HYPERVITAMINOSIS

Phytonadione is considered relatively nontoxic even at high doses. Rare cases of hemolytic anemia have been reported, and the manufacturer has reported anaphylactic reactions following use of the injectable product. Menadiol is also considered relatively nontoxic. Menadione, in contrast, can produce hemolytic anemia, hyperbilirubinemia, and kernicterus in newborns, especially premature infants. In addition, menadione can cause hemolytic anemia in patients with glucose-6-phosphate dehydrogenase deficiency.[45] For these reasons, it is no longer marketed in the United States.

PRODUCTS

Phytonadione is available as oral tablets and capsules from numerous sources under various names. A popular prescription product for oral tablets is Mephyton. Phytonadione is also available as an injectable for IM use. It is also available in numerous multivitamin preparations under various names. Menadiol is also available in some markets.

◉ WATER-SOLUBLE VITAMINS

Although the water-soluble vitamins are structurally diverse, they are put in a general class to distinguish them from the lipid-soluble vitamins. This class includes the B-complex vitamins and ascorbic acid (vitamin C). The term *B-complex* refers to combinations including all eight B vitamins: thiamine (B_1), riboflavin (B_2), niacin (B_3), pantothenic acid (B_5), pyridoxine (B_6), biotin (B_7), folic acid (B_9), and cyanocobalamin (B_{12}). Dietary deficiencies of any of the B vitamins commonly are complicated by deficiencies of other members of the group, so treatment with B-complex preparations is usually indicated.

Vitamin B₁

Thiamine, the preferred name for vitamin B_1, holds a prominent place in the history of vitamin discovery because beriberi, the disease resulting from insufficient thiamine intake, was one of the earliest recognized deficiency diseases. Its relationship to polyneuritis in birds was noted in the early work of Funk,[3] and his work with pigeons led to the discovery that a water-soluble substance in rice polishings was curative. The early designation of water-soluble B was replaced with vitamin B by Drummond[11] when suggesting the use of *vitamin* instead of *vitamine*. Complicating early animal studies was the inconsistency in the deficiency syndromes observed by the various investigators. Early work on vitamin B using crude extracts showed that this vitamin also had growth-promoting properties in rats fed vitamin B–deficient diets. In addition, vitamin B–deficient diets could also result in dermatitis, which at that time appeared similar to human pellagra. Oftentimes, the source used for vitamin B and the animal model studied determined the experimental results observed.

The antineuritic water-soluble B vitamin that cured polyneuritis in birds and the growth-promoting water-soluble B vitamin were proposed to be two different vitamins by Emmett and Luros[136] in 1920. This was later confirmed by other investigators.[137] In 1927, the British Accessory Food Factors Committee recommended vitamin B_1 for the antineuritic water-soluble B and vitamin B_2 for the growth-promoting, also called the antipellagra, water-soluble B. The American Society of Biological Chemists recommended the name vitamin B for the antineuritic factor and vitamin G for the growth-promoting factor. Eventually, the British system became the standard. In 1960, the IUPAC Commission on the Nomenclature of Biological Chemistry[106] adopted the name *thiamine*. In 1966, IUPAC[138] proposed the name *thiamin,* and in 2004, reverted once again to *thiamine* although *thiamin* is still in common use. Thiamine has also been referred to as aneurine.[12] The isolation of thiamine was elusive; however, it was finally isolated and crystallized from rice polishings by Jansen and Donath[139] in 1926. The structure and synthesis was published 10 years later in 1936.[140]

One of the richest natural sources of thiamine is pork. Whole grain and whole-grain products, such as yeast, beans, and peas, are also excellent sources. Beef and chicken as well as some fish are also good sources. In developed countries, including the United States, fortified products, especially ready-to-eat cereals, are a significant dietary source of thiamine.

CHEMISTRY

The chemical structures of thiamine and its coenzyme form, thiamine diphosphate (ThDP), are shown in Figure 28.20. ThDP is composed of a diphosphate terminated side chain, a five-membered thiazolium ring, and a six-membered aminopyrimidine ring. Thiamine hydrochloride (Fig. 28.21),

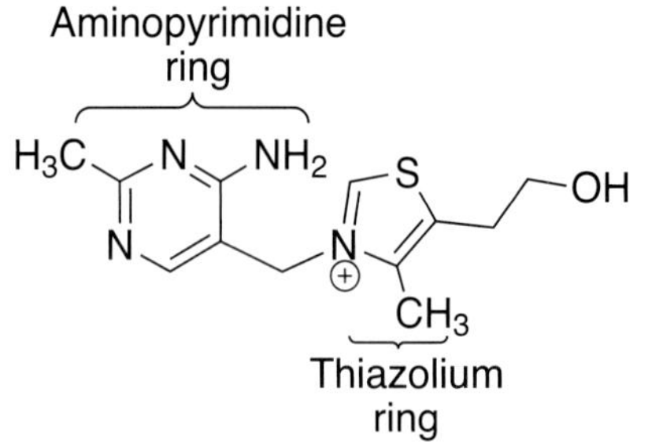

Thiamine

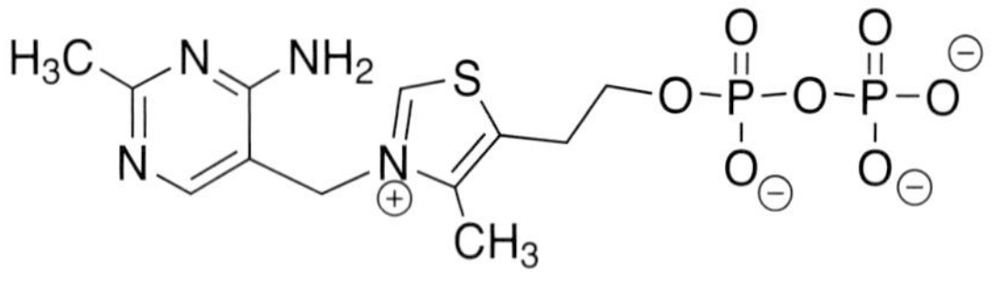

Thiamine diphosphate

Figure 28.20 ● Thiamine and thiamine diphosphate.

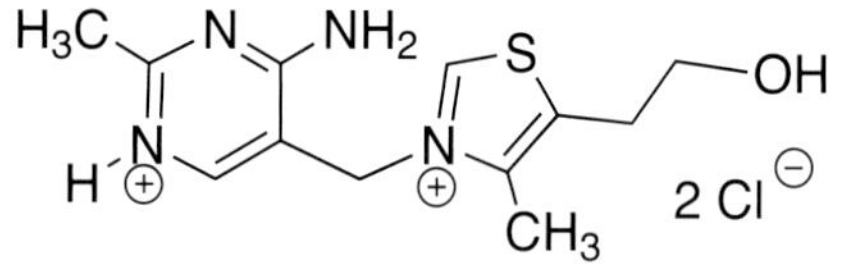

Figure 28.21 ● Thiamine hydrochloride.

a common form available for vitamin supplementation, is stable in acid but unstable in aqueous solutions with a pH above 5. Under these conditions, it undergoes decomposition of the thiazolium ring forming an inactive product (Fig. 28.22). Exposure of thiamine to air or to oxidizing agents such as hydrogen peroxide, permanganate, or alkaline potassium ferricyanide oxidizes it readily to thiochrome (Fig. 28.23). Thiochrome exhibits a vivid blue fluorescence; hence, this reaction is the basis for the quantitative fluorometric assay of thiamine in the *USP*.

KINETICS

ThDP, either from the diet or from production by the intestinal microflora of the colon, is hydrolyzed in the intestinal lumen to free thiamine. Movement of thiamine into and through cells is primarily through transport carriers because it has a quaternary nitrogen, which limits diffusion. Thiamine is transported into the intestinal enterocytes via the human thiamine transporters, (hTHTR)-1 and hTHTR-2.[141] These transporters are now known as solute carrier family 19, member 2 (SLC19A2) and member 3 (SLC19A3), respectively, and are related to the reduced folate carrier (RFC) for folates, which is member 1 (SLC19A1). This carrier-mediated process is saturable at relatively low micromolar concentrations, and higher concentrations can be absorbed through passive diffusion.[142] Once inside the cell, some thiamine is phosphorylated to form ThDP, and the rest is transported across the basolateral membrane into the blood where it freely distributes to other tissues. Phosphorylation of thi-

amine in the cell is thought to be the driving force behind the transport mechanism. Tissues requiring thiamine use SLC19A2 and SLC19A3 to transport thiamine into the cell where it is then phosphorylated. These same transporters also explain entry of thiamine into the CNS. Excess thiamine is readily excreted by the kidneys.

BIOCHEMISTRY

Thiamine is converted to the active ThDP by direct pyrophosphate transfer from ATP using thiamine diphosphokinase (EC 2.7.6.2), which is regulated through a riboswitch; a conformational transition in the RNA transcripts encoding the synthetic enzyme that is induced by the binding of the ThDP itself.[143] ThDP performs important metabolic functions by assisting in making or breaking bonds between carbon and sulfur, oxygen, hydrogen, nitrogen, and carbon. Thus, it plays the central role in several important anabolic and catabolic intermediary pathways (see Table 28.9), such as glycololysis, the citric acid cycle, and amino acid metabolism. Broadly all these enzymes are categorized as decarboxylase- or transferase-type enzymes based on their mechanism of action; all share certain mechanistic similarities as shown in Figure 28.24.[143]

The whole catalytic cycle can be divided into three steps: activation, first half-reaction, and the second half-reaction. The C^2 carbon of ThDP is first activated by deprotonation forming a nucleophilic ylide. ThDP first tautomerizes into an unusual imino form, and the nitrogen atom of the imine then abstracts the proton. Overall, the conformation of ThDP is maintained by the enzymes so as to favor activation by positioning $N^{4'}$ of the amino pyrimidine group in close proximity to the C^2 of the thiazolium ring. The first half-reaction involves nucleophilic attack on a substrate carbonyl cleaving the substrate (e.g., pyruvate for decarboxylase and a ketose sugar for transketolase) to release the first product—CO_2 for decarboxylases, and an aldose with two less carbons for transketolase—leaving behind an enamine complex. This is common to all types of ThDP-dependent enzymatic reactions. The second half-reaction is specialized for each category of ThDP-dependent enzyme, which involves the nucleophilic attack of the enamine intermediate on the incoming second substrate to release the final product. In case of pyruvate or paralogous decarboxylases, this second substrate is a proton producing an aldehyde and releasing the ThDP, whereas in the case of transketolase, this second substrate is an aldose sugar producing a ketose sugar with two more carbon atoms and releasing the ThDP.[143]

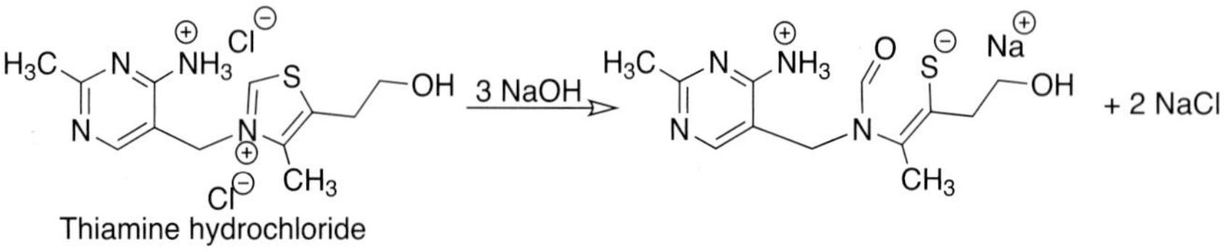

Thiamine hydrochloride

Figure 28.22 ● Alkaline decomposition of thiamine.

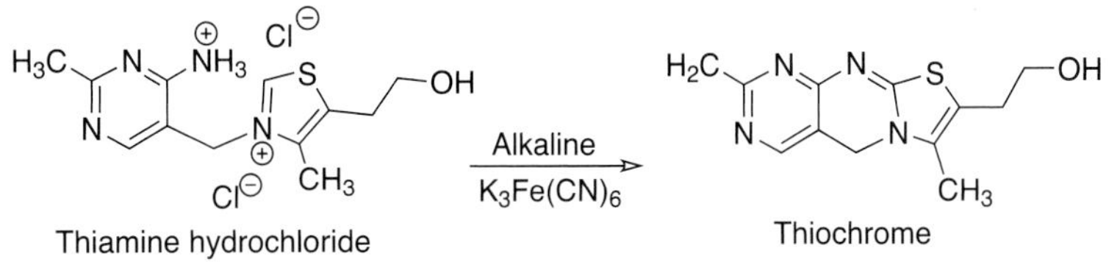

Figure 28.23 ● Oxidation of thiamine to thiochrome.

Thiamine hydrochloride

Alkaline
$K_3Fe(CN)_6$

Thiochrome

TABLE 28.9 Thiamine Diphosphate–Dependent Enzymes

Enzyme	EC Number	Function
Pyruvate dehydrogenase (acetyl-transferring)	1.2.4.1	Glycolysis, gluconeogenesis, amino acid synthesis
Oxoglutarate dehydrogenase (succinyl-transferring)	1.2.4.2	Citric acid cycle (TCA cycle)
3-Methyl-2-oxobutanoate dehydrogenase (2-methylpropanoyl-transferring)	1.2.4.4	Valine, leucine, and isoleucine degradation
Transketolase	2.2.1.1	Pentose phosphate pathway
Branched-chain-2-oxoacid decarboxylase	4.1.1.72	Decarboxylation of α-keto acids

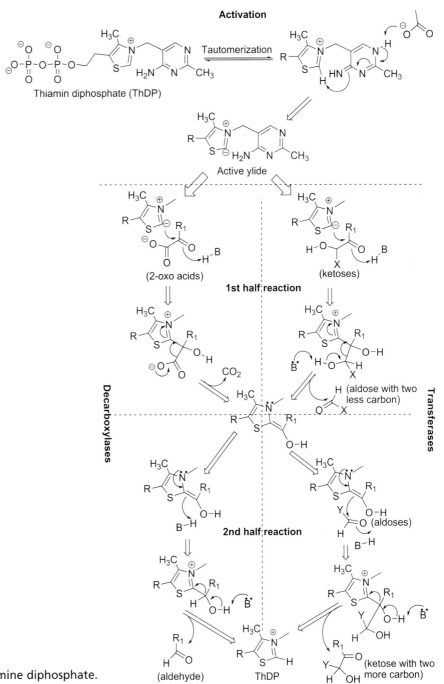

Figure 28.24 ● Catalytic cycle of thiamine diphosphate.

All ThDP-dependent enzymes need a proton donor to initiate the first half-reaction and a proton acceptor to complete the second half-reaction. In most cases, the aminopyrimidine $N^{4'}$ in concert with an invariant glutamate is the proton donor-acceptor in the first half-reaction, although there are no universally conserved residues for the second half-reaction, and differ according to the enzyme class.[143]

In the decarboxylation of pyruvate, the coenzyme interacts with pyruvic acid to form the so-called active aldehyde. This active aldehyde intermediates then interacts with thioctic acid to form acetyl-thioctate, which is responsible for acetylating CoA-SH to form acetyl-CoA. In deficiency states, the oxidation of α-keto acids is decreased, resulting in increased pyruvate levels in the blood.

THERAPEUTIC USES

Thiamine, as the base or as the hydrochloride salt, is indicated in the treatment or prophylaxis of known or suspected thiamine deficiencies. Severe thiamine deficiency is called *beriberi*, which is very rare in developed countries. The most likely cause of thiamine deficiency in the United States is the result of chronic alcoholism, which leads to multiple vitamin deficiencies as a result of poor dietary intake. The major organs affected are the nervous system (dry beriberi), which manifests as neurological damage, the cardiovascular system (wet beriberi), which manifests as heart failure and edema, and the gastrointestinal tract. Thiamine administration reverses the gastrointestinal, cardiovascular, and neurological symptoms; however, if the deficiency has been severe or of prolonged duration, the neurological damage may be permanent. A severe form of neurological damage seen in alcoholics, Wernicke encephalopathy or Wernicke-Korsakoff syndrome, has a high fatality rate and requires immediate therapy with thiamine.

Very high doses of thiamine (30–90 mg/day) are required in the treatment of thiamine-responsive megaloblastic anemia (TRMA),which is a rare genetic disorder resulting from a single point mutation in the thiamine transporter gene.[144] Thiamine antagonists have been examined for their antineoplastic activity; however, there are no current treatments based on this strategy.

HYPERVITAMINOSIS

Thiamine doses of 5 mg/day for 4 to 5 weeks has resulted in headache, insomnia, irritability, increased heart rate, and weakness. In addition, thiamine can cause anaphylactic reactions following parenteral use.

PRODUCTS

Thiamine, as thiamine hydrochloride or thiamine mononitrate, is available from numerous sources as oral capsules, liquids, and tablets under various names. Thiamine hydrochloride is also available in injectable form. Thiamine is also available as a component of numerous multivitamin preparations. Thiamine mononitrate is more stable than the hydrochloride in the dry state and is less hygroscopic.

Vitamin B₂

The discovery of the vitamin we now call riboflavin developed from an early work with vitamin B before the knowledge that it was more than one vitamin. The reader is referred to the history of vitamin B_1 because the histories are identical until the discovery that vitamin B was actually two vitamins leading to the designation of vitamin B_1 and vitamin B_2. The discovery of vitamin B_2 was also complicated by the inconsistent experimental results seen among researchers as they focused on the dermatological effects of vitamin B_2–deficient diets. The conflicting results were eventually found to be due, in part, to deficiencies in study animals not just of vitamin B_2, but also vitamin B_3 (niacin), the cause of human forms of pellagra, and/or vitamin B_6 (pyridoxine), another cause of dermatitis. Likewise, treatments with vitamin B_2 were inconsistent because the early sources of this vitamin contained other B vitamins. Vitamin B_2 was eventually isolated from egg whites in 1933[146] and produced synthetically in 1935.[147] The name *riboflavine* was officially accepted in 1960[106]; although the term was in common use before then. In 1966, IUPAC[138] changed it to *riboflavin*, which is in common use today.

Riboflavin is synthesized by all green plants and by most bacteria and fungi. Therefore, riboflavin is found, at least in small amounts, in most foods. Foods that are naturally high in riboflavin include milk and other dairy products, meat, eggs, fatty fish, and dark green vegetables. Fortified cereals have become an important source of riboflavin in the western diet including the United States.

CHEMISTRY

Chemically, riboflavin is an *N*-glycoside of flavin, also known as lumichrome, and the sugar, ribitol (Fig. 28.25). Flavin is derived from the Latin word *flavus* for "yellow" because of the yellow color of its crystals and yellow fluorescence under UV light. Riboflavin is heat stable but easily degraded by light. Its systematic names are 7,8-dimethyl-10-ribitylisoalloxazine and 7,8-dimethyl-10-(D-ribo-2,3,4,5-tetrahydroxypentyl)isoalloxazine.

KINETICS

Dietary riboflavin must be liberated as free riboflavin prior to absorption; therefore, covalently bound forms are unavailable for absorption. Most dietary riboflavin is in the form of noncovalently bound coenzymes, primarily flavin mononucleotide (FMN) and flavin adenine dinucleotide (FAD), and free riboflavin is liberated following the action of the digestive enzymes. Riboflavin is absorbed in the upper ileum by an active, saturable carrier; although passive diffusion may also occur at high concentrations. The number of carriers appears to be regulated in direct proportion to the need for riboflavin. Following absorption, riboflavin is phosphorylated in the mucosal cell, which aids active transport through a trapping mechanism, followed by release of free riboflavin into the bloodstream.[148,149]

Riboflavin is also synthesized by the microflora of the large intestine, and small amounts are absorbed by an active carrier present in the colonic cells. Excess riboflavin is excreted by the kidney, primarily unchanged, although small amounts may appear as metabolites. Fecal levels are usually high because of synthesis by the microflora of the colon and are not an indicator of increased excretion or decreased absorption.

BIOCHEMISTRY

Riboflavin is the precursor in the biosynthesis of the prosthetic groups of the coenzymes FMN and FAD as shown in

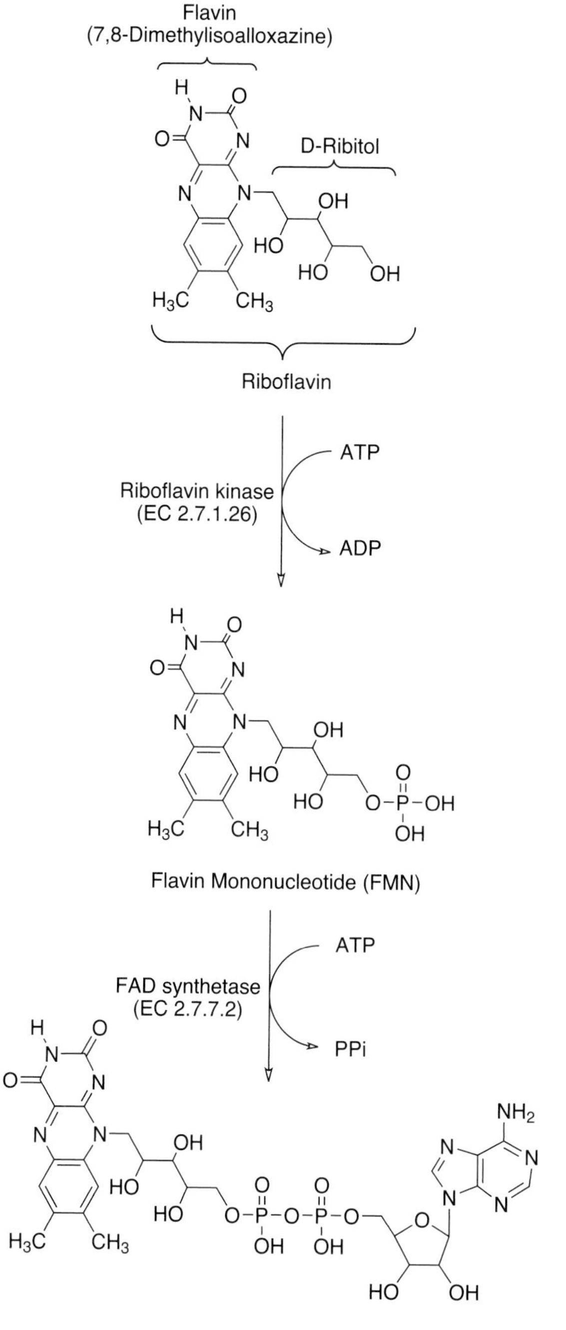

Figure 28.25 ● **Bioactivation of riboflavin to FMN and FAD.**

by riboflavin kinase (EC 2.7.1.26). Amitriptyline, imipramine, and chlorpromazine can inhibit riboflavin kinase resulting in a functional riboflavin deficiency. FAD originates from an FMN and ATP reaction that involves reversible dinucleotide formation catalyzed by FAD synthetase (EC 2.7.7.2). FMN and FAD function in combination with many enzymes, often characterized as flavoproteins, as the prosthetic groups of their coenzymes and rarely as the actual coenzyme. In some instances, the FAD or FMN is found covalently bound to the enzyme.

Flavoproteins function under aerobic or anaerobic conditions as oxidases and dehydrogenases. Examples include glucose oxidase, xanthine oxidase, cytochrome reductase, and acyl-CoA dehydrogenase. The riboflavin moiety of the complex is considered a hydrogen-transporting agent functioning as a hydrogen acceptor. The hydrogen donors may be NADH, NADPH, or other suitable substrate. The isoalloxazine rings accept two hydrides stepwise to form the dihydroriboflavin derivative (Fig. 28.26).

THERAPEUTIC USES

Severe riboflavin deficiency is known as *ariboflavinosis*, and treatment or prevention of this condition is the only proven use of riboflavin. Ariboflavinosis is most commonly associated with multiple vitamin deficiency as a result of alcoholism in developed countries. Because of the large number of enzymes requiring riboflavin as a coenzyme, deficiencies can lead to a wide range of abnormalities. In adults seborrheic dermatitis, photophobia, peripheral neuropathy, anemia, and oropharyngeal changes including angular stomatitis, glossitis, and cheilosis, are often the first signs of riboflavin deficiency. In children, cessation of growth can also occur. As the deficiency progresses, more severe pathologies develop until death ensues. Riboflavin deficiency may also produce teratogenic effects and alter iron handling leading to anemia.[150]

HYPERVITAMINOSIS

There are no known toxicities associated with large doses of riboflavin. This is most likely because of the capacity-limited uptake that, in the presence of high doses, down regulates, thereby limiting absorption from the intestines. Renal filtration and excretion of riboflavin can also increase significantly in the presence of high plasma levels.[149]

PRODUCTS

Riboflavin or riboflavin 5′-monophosphate is available from numerous sources as oral capsules, liquids, and tablets under various names. Riboflavin is also available as a component of numerous multivitamin preparations.

Vitamin B₃

Vitamin B₃ was formerly called nicotinic acid; however, the term niacin is now preferred to avoid any confusion with the

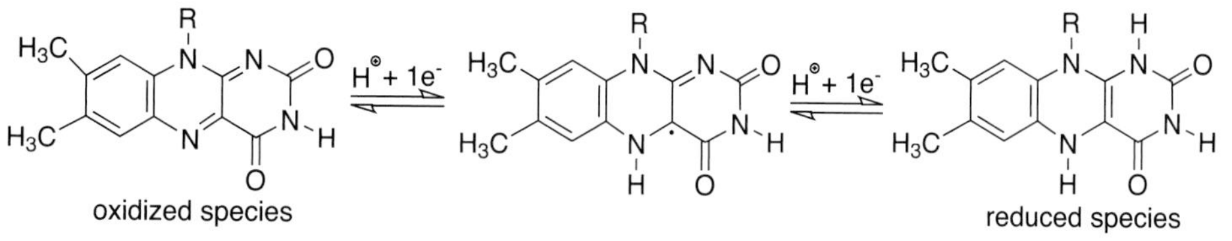

Figure 28.25. FMN is actually named incorrectly because it is not a nucleotide. The metabolic functions of this vitamin involve these two enzyme cofactors, which participate in numerous, vital oxidation–reduction processes. FMN (riboflavin 5′-phosphate) is produced from the vitamin and ATP

Figure 28.26 ● **Oxidation and reduction of the isoalloxazine rings.**

alkaloid, nicotine. Niacinamide, also known as nicotinamide, refers to the amide derivative of niacin that is equivalent in vitamin activity. Some texts use niacin to refer to nicotinic acid, niacinamide, and any derivatives with vitamin activity comparable to niacin. Furthermore, research and chemistry-based resources use the terms nicotinic acid and nicotinamide; whereas pharmacy resources use niacin and niacinamide. For example, enzyme nomenclature uses the former, whereas facts and comparisons uses the latter. This section uses each term in its best context.

The synthesis and structural identification of niacin actually predated its discovery as a vitamin. Niacin had been prepared from nicotine since at least 1898. Niacin had also been purified and identified in 1913 as a component of yeast and rice polishings by Funk[151] in his quest to discover the vitamin later called thiamine. The discovery of niacin as a vitamin was complicated, as discussed under vitamin B_2, by the early misconception that animal forms of pellagra and the human form were caused by the same vitamin deficiency. Ultimately, it was the study of human pellagra and black tongue disease in dogs, also caused by niacin deficiency,[152] that led to the discovery of niacin as a vitamin. In September of 1937, Elvehjem et al.[153] were the first to prove the link between niacin and black tongue disease in dogs. Clinical studies using niacin in human pellagra patients followed, and the first published report of success was in November of 1937.[154]

Niacin can be synthesized by humans into its active forms, nicotinamide adenine dinucleotide (NAD+) and nicotinamide adenine dinucleotide phosphate (NADP+), from the amino acid, tryptophan. Consequently, and analogous to vitamin D, niacin is not a true vitamin by the classic definition of the term. However, because of inherent inefficiencies in the conversion, the use of dietary tryptophan as a replacement for niacin can result in tryptophan deficiency for protein synthesis. This results in a requirement for niacin in the diet as a vitamin or a diet abnormally high in tryptophan. To compensate for this conversion, the DRIs for niacin are expressed in niacin equivalents (NE) that allows for 60 mg of dietary tryptophan to equal 1-mg niacin. Niacin or niacin derived nucleotides can also be synthesized using aspartic acid in plants and microorganisms

Natural sources of niacin include meat (beef, pork, chicken, lamb), fish, and whole grains. As with other B vitamins, fortified ready-to-eat cereals are an important source in developed countries such as the United States.

CHEMISTRY

Niacin is chemically pyridine-3-carboxylic acid (Fig. 28.27). Its coenzyme forms are NADH/NAD+ or NADPH/NADP+ as shown in Figure 28.28.

KINETICS

Niacin appears in the diet in various forms.[155] Some niacin is relatively unavailable for absorption unless the

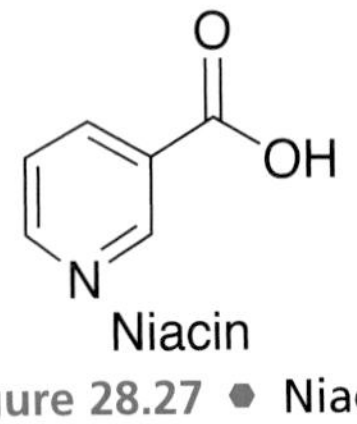

Oxidized form (NAD+, NADP+)

Reduced form (NADH, NADPH)

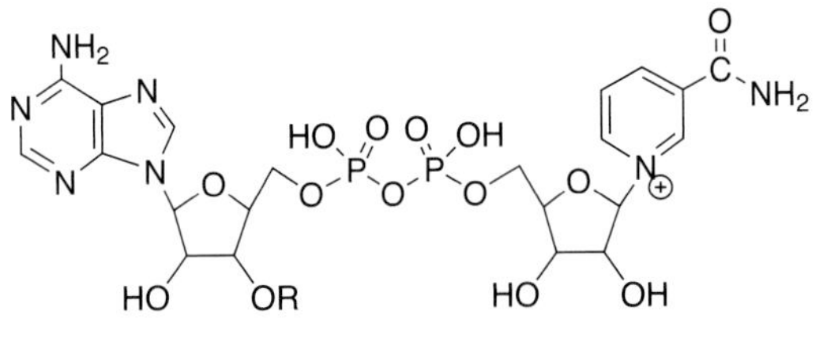

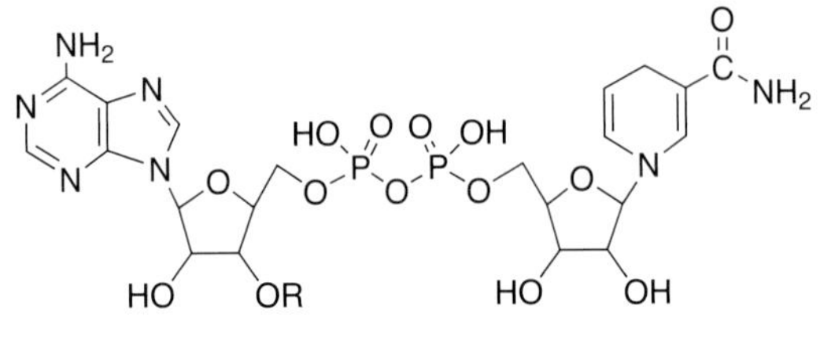

R = H   Nicotinamide adenine dinucleotide

R = PO_3^{2-} Nicotinamide adenine dinucleotide phosphate

Figure 28.28 ● Structures of niacin-derived cofactors.

food is treated in a manner that releases the niacin. For example, some grains (i.e., corn) may contain predominantly niacin esterified to polysaccharides or peptides, referred to as niacytin. This form has a relatively low bioavailability unless treated with alkali in cooking or processing. Coffee beans have a high niacin content in the form of trigonellin (1-methyl nicotinic acid) that is converted to niacin upon roasting. Most dietary niacin from natural sources is in the form of the nucleotide derivatives, NAD+ and NADP+, which are digested by NAD+ diphosphatase (EC 3.6.1.22), followed by hydrolases in the intestine to release nicotinamide. Free nicotinamide and niacin are absorbed through a facilitated diffusion process in the intestine.[156] At physiological doses, little niacin is excreted unchanged. Most is excreted as *N*-methylniacin or the glycine conjugate (nicotinuric acid). After administration of large doses, niacin can be found in the urine unchanged.

BIOCHEMISTRY

Niacin synthesis into the active cofactors, NAD+ and NADP+, is shown in Figure 28.29. Both niacin and niacinamide react with 5-phosphoribosyl-1-pyrophosphate (PRPP) to form the respective mononucleotide derivative, which then reacts with ATP to produce the corresponding dinucleotide product. For niacinamide, this is NAD+; however, for niacin this product is converted to NAD+ by transformation of the carboxyl of the nicotinic acid moiety to the amide using free ammonia. An alternative pathway is to use glutamine through NAD+ synthase (glutamine-hydrolysing) (EC 6.3.5.1); however, this pathway is slower and is most likely not as important. NADP+ is produced from NAD+ by ATP through kinase catalysis.

Figure 28.27 ● Niacin.

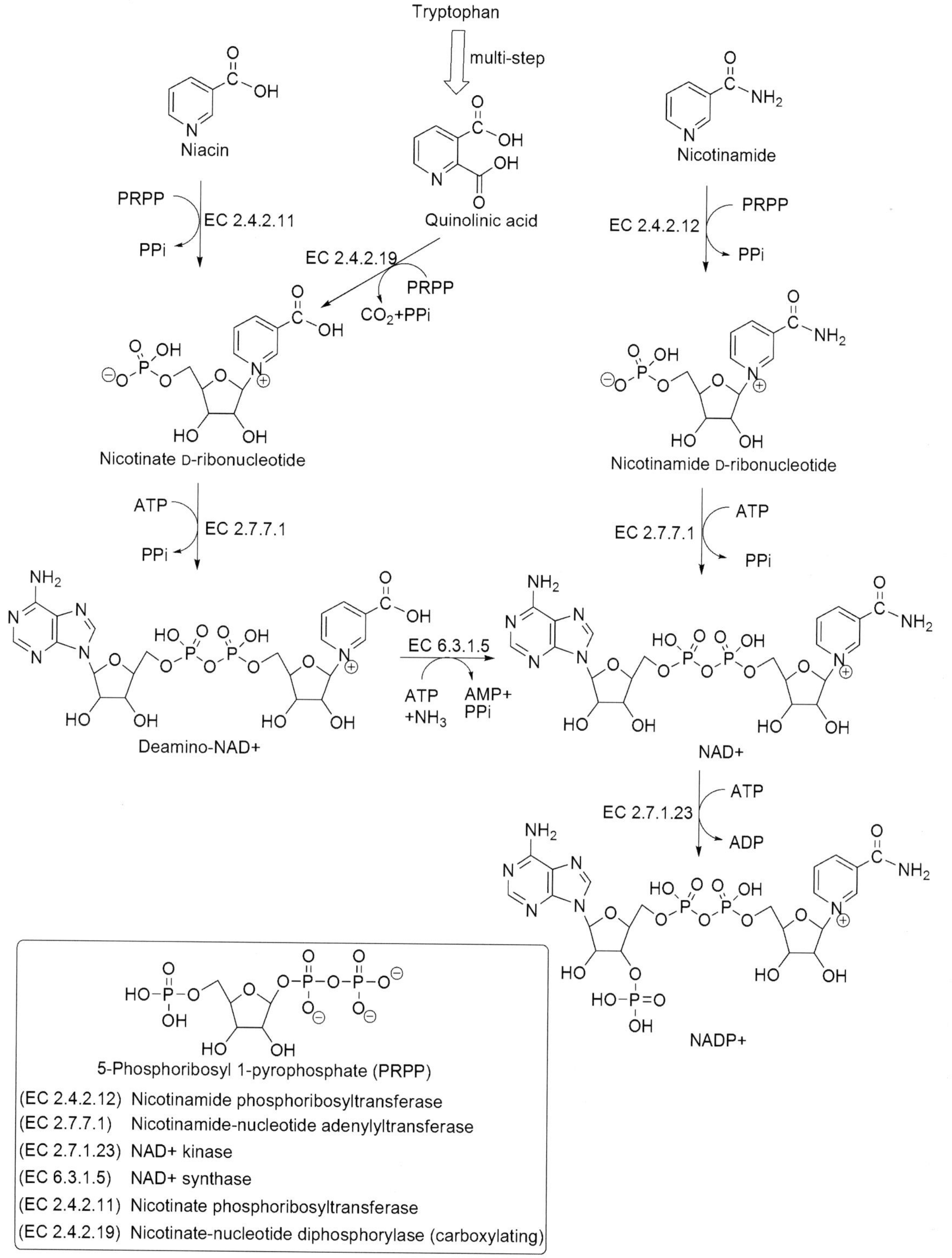

Figure 28.29 ● Biosynthesis of NAD+ and NADP+ from niacin, nicotinamide, or tryptophan.

NAD+ and NADP+ are oxidizing coenzymes for many (>200) dehydrogenases. Some dehydrogenases require NAD+, others require NADP+, and some function with either. The generalized representation in Figure 28.30 illustrates the function of these coenzymes in metabolic oxidations and reductions. The abbreviation NAD+ emphasizes the electrophilicity of the pyridine C^4 moiety (which is the center of reactivity), and the substrate designated could be a

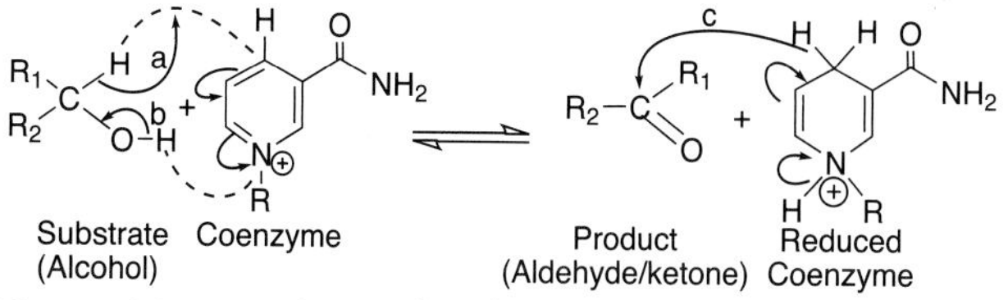

Figure 28.30 ● Generalized representation of the hydride transfer reaction.

primary or secondary alcohol. *Arrow a* in Figure 28.30 symbolizes the function of NAD+ as oxidant in the hydride transfer from the substrate to the coenzyme, forming NADH, reduced coenzyme. The hydroxyl of the substrate is visualized as undergoing deprotonation concertedly by either water or the pyridine nitrogen of NADH. *Arrow b* shows concerted formation of the carbonyl π-bond of the oxidation product. *Arrow c* symbolizes the reverse hydride transfer from reduced coenzyme, NADH, to the carbonyl carbon, and concertedly, as the carbonyl oxygen undergoes protonation, the reduction of the carbonyl group forms the corresponding alcohol. Thus, NAD+ and NADP+ are hydride acceptors, and NADH and NADPH are hydride donors. Although this is a simplistic representation, it shows the dynamism of the oxidation–reduction reactions effected by these coenzymes under appropriate dehydrogenase catalysis. Alternatively, the reduced coenzymes may be used in ATP production through the electron-transport system.

THERAPEUTIC USES

Niacin is used in the treatment of niacin deficiency, which is referred to as pellagra (from the Italian, *pelle* for "skin" and *agra* for "dry"). The major systems affected are the gastrointestinal tract (diarrhea, enteritis and stomatitis), the skin (dermatitis), and the CNS (generalized neurological deficits including dementia). Pellagra has become a rare condition in the United States and other countries that require or encourage enrichment of wheat flour or fortification of cereals with niacin. Because the nucleotide form can be synthesized in vivo from tryptophan, pellagra is most often seen in areas where the diet is deficient in both niacin and tryptophan. Typically, maize (corn)-based diets meet this criteria. Niacin deficiency can also result from diarrhea, cirrhosis, alcoholism, or Hartnup disease. It is interesting that niacin deficiency can also, rarely, result from vitamin B$_6$ deficiency (see Vitamin B$_6$ section).

Niacin, but not niacinamide, is also one of the few vitamins that are useful in the treatment of diseases unrelated to deficiencies. In 1955, Altschul et al.[157] reported that niacin doses of 1 to 4 g/day could lower serum cholesterol levels in humans. Currently, niacin doses of 2 to 4.5 g/day are used in the treatment of hypercholesterolemia and hypertriglyceridemia. Triglycerides, VLDL, and LDL are reduced; HDL is increased. The mechanisms underlying these effects have recently been reviewed.[158,159]

HYPERVITAMINOSIS

Niacin, in doses that range above the DRI but below that required for dyslipidemias, is unlikely to produce adverse effects. However, adverse effects of niacin are seen when this vitamin is used at pharmacological doses above 1 g/day in the treatment of dyslipidemia. Notable adverse effects include flushing because of vasodilation; dermatological effects including dry skin, pruritus and hyperkeratosis; gastrointestinal effects including peptic ulcer, stomach pain, nausea, and diarrhea; elevations in serum uric acid and glucose (in Type 2 diabetics); and rare hepatotoxicity.[159–161] Traditionally, hepatotoxicity has been more associated with the sustained release as compared to the immediate release formulations; however, recent analysis of niacin-ER adverse events suggests the opposite may be true for this formulation.[162]

Of particular note is that niacinamide, even in high doses, is not effective in hyperlipdemias and only rarely produces the vascular, dermatological and hepatotoxicity associated with high doses of niacin. Even gastrointestinal upset is less common with niacinamide. For this reason, niacinamide would be the preferred form for vitamin supplementation, especially if taken in high doses.

PRODUCTS

Niacin is available, in immediate-release form, from numerous sources as oral capsules, liquids, and tablets under various names. Timed-release products of niacin are also available primarily for the treatment of hyperlipidemias. Niacin is also available as a fixed-dose combination with one of the HMG-CoA reductase inhibitors or *statin* antihyperlipidemics (Advicor, Simcor). Niacin is also available as a component of numerous multivitamin preparations. Niacinamide is available from numerous sources as oral capsules, liquids, and tablets under various names. Niacinamide is also available as a component of numerous multivitamin preparations

Vitamin B₅

The first suggestion for the existance of vitamin B$_5$ came from Carter et al.[163] in 1930; although it was never characterized or isolated. In 1933, R. J. Williams[164] and his collaborators found a "growth determinant of universal occurrence" and named it, according to the authors, "*pantothenic acid*, the name being derived from the Greek, meaning *from everywhere*" (probably from the Greek *pantothen*). Pantothenic acid, the preferred term, later became associated with the name *vitamin B$_5$*. The synthesis and structure were reported in 1940.[165] This vitamin is synthesized by most green plants and microorganisms. Excellent sources of the vitamin are liver, egg yolk, whole grains, and fortified ready-to-eat cereals. However, as the original name implies, many foods contain sufficient pantothenic acid to supply dietary needs.

CHEMISTRY

Chemically, pantothenic acid is considered to be a β-alanine derivative of the asymmetric pantoic acid and thus shows asymmetry (Fig. 28.31). Only the naturally occurring D(+)-stereoisomer (with *R* configuration) is biologically active and the L(−)-stereoisomer (with *S* configuration) is inactive. When its carboxylate functional group is attached through an amide linkage with β-mercaptoethylamine, it is known as pantetheine (also spelled *pantotheine*). The biologically active form of pantothenic acid, CoA, is formed when the terminal alcoholic function of pantetheine is attached to ADP 3′-phosphate as shown in Figure 28.32.

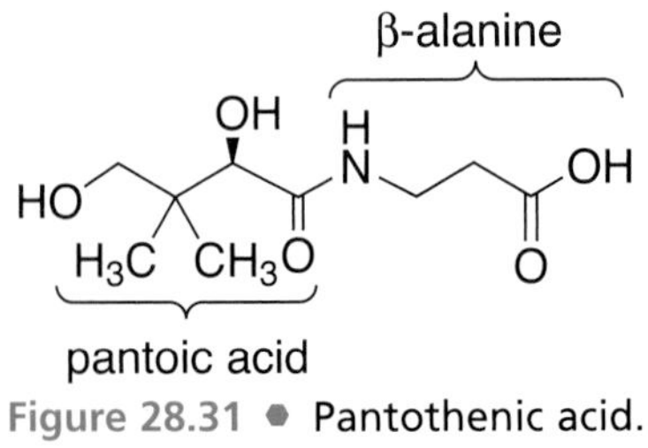

Figure 28.31 ● Pantothenic acid.

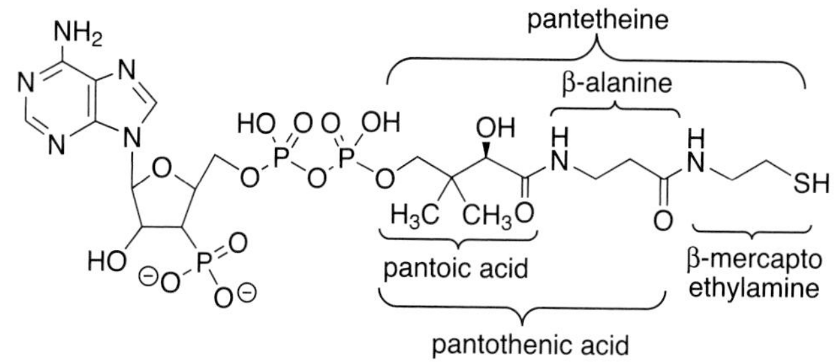

Figure 28.32 ● Coenzyme A structure.

KINETICS

Dietary pantothenic acid occurs primarily in the form of acyl proteins, CoA or pantotheine 4'-phosphate, which are converted into pantetheine in the intestinal lumen. Pantetheine is converted to pantothenic acid by pantetheine hydrolase (EC 3.5.1.92) also found in the intestinal lumen.[166] Enteric bacteria can also provide a source of CoA and pantetheine 4'-phosphate; however, the importance of this source is not known. Pantothenic acid is absorbed from the intestine, more in the jejunum than the ileum, through the sodium-dependent multivitamin transporter (SMVT), which also transports biotin and lipoic acid.[141,148] This explains the ability of these three substances to competitively inhibit absorption of each other. The transporter is driven by the Na$^+$ gradient that exists from the extracellular fluid to the intracellular fluid, transporting 2 Na$^+$ for each monovalent anion of pantothenate, biotin, or lipoate.[167] In addition,

the inside-negative membrane potential may also act as a driving force because a net charge of +1 enters the cell. This same carrier is ubiquitous throughout bodily tissues and probably also accounts for cellular uptake from the blood. Conversion to the active form, acetyl-CoA, most likely occurs inside the cell.

BIOCHEMISTRY

The metabolic functions of pantothenic acid in human biochemistry are mediated through the synthesis of CoA (Fig. 28.33). Pantothenic acid is a structural component of CoA, which is necessary for many important metabolic processes. Pantothenic acid is incorporated into CoA by a series of five enzyme-catalyzed reactions. CoA is involved in the activation of fatty acids before β-oxidation, which requires ATP to form the respective fatty acyl-CoA derivatives. Pantothenic acid also participates in fatty acid β-oxidation in the final step, forming acetyl-CoA. Acetyl-CoA is also formed from pyruvate decarboxylation, in which CoA participates with thiamine diphosphate and lipoic acid, two other important coenzymes. Thiamine diphosphate is the actual decarboxylating coenzyme that functions with lipoic acid to form acetyldihydrolipoic acid from pyruvate decarboxylation. CoA then accepts the acetyl group from acetyldihydrolipoic acid to form acetyl-CoA. Acetyl-CoA is an acetyl donor in many processes and is the precursor in important biosyntheses (e.g., those of fatty acids, steroids, acyl proteins, porphyrins, and acetylcholine). CoA is also intimately involved in the growth of microorganisms, including those pathogenic to humans. This has led to the novel strategy of developing pantothenic acid analogs that selectively inhibit pantothenic acid utilization and/or

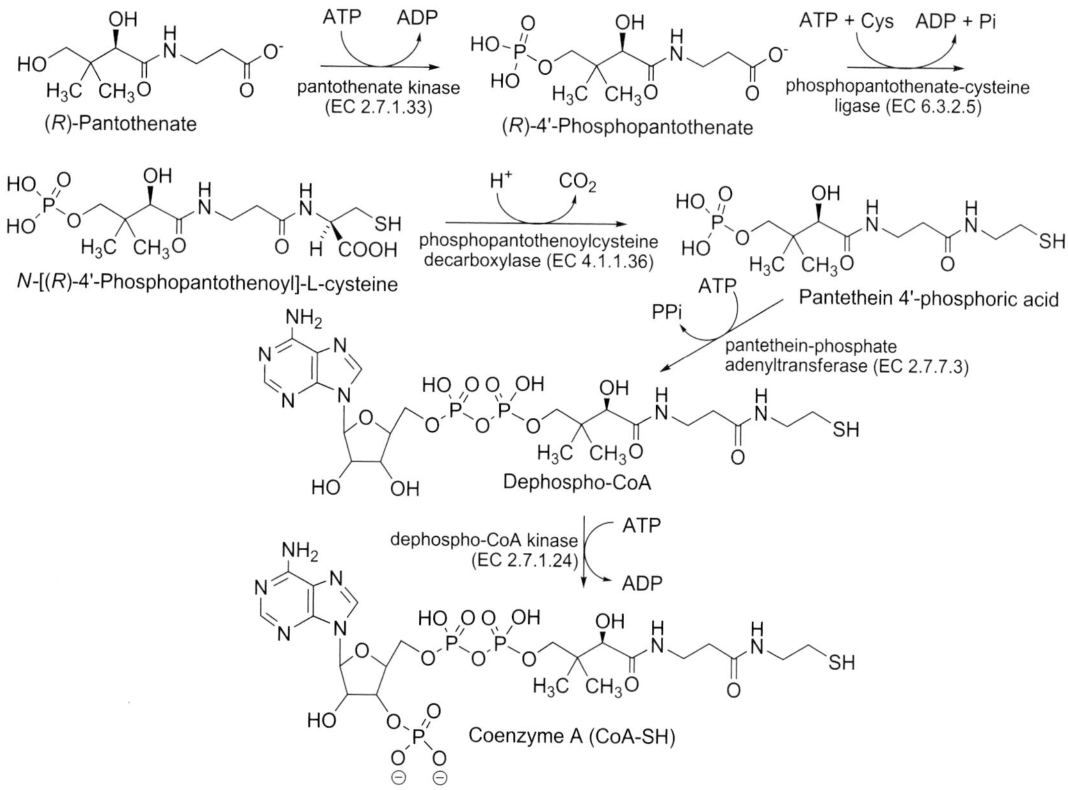

Figure 28.33 ● Biosynthesis of coenzyme A.

biosynthesis in these organisms leading to antibacterial, antifungal, or antimalarial effects.[168]

THERAPEUTIC USES

The only therapeutic indication for pantothenic acid is in treatment of a known or suspected deficiency of this vitamin. Because of the ubiquitous nature of pantothenic acid, deficiency states of this vitamin are only seen experimentally by use of synthetic diets devoid of the vitamin,[169] by use of the vitamin antagonist, ω-methylpantothenic, or both. In a 1991 review, Tahiliani and Beinlich[170] described that the most common symptoms associated with pantothenic acid deficiency were headache, fatigue, and a sensation of weakness. Sleep disturbances and gastrointestinal disturbances, among others, were also noted. The most likely setting for pantothenic acid deficiency is in the setting of alcoholism where a multiple vitamin deficiency exists confounding the exact role of the pantothenic acid deficiency as compared to the other vitamins. Because a deficiency of a single B vitamin is rare, pantothenic acid is commonly formulated in multivitamin or B-complex preparations.

HYPERVITAMINOSIS

Pantothenic acid is considered to be relatively safe. Doses of 10 to 20 g/day have caused diarrhea and water retention.[161]

PRODUCTS

Pantothenic acid is available from numerous sources as oral capsules, liquids, and tablets under various names. The calcium salt of pantothenic acid or the alcohol derivative pantothenol is commonly used in pharmaceutical preparations because it is more stable than the parent compound. Pantothenic acid, or one of its derivative or salt forms, is also available as a component of numerous multivitamin preparations.

Vitamin B₆

The discovery of vitamin B_6 is generally ascribed to Paul György[171] who first realized there was a vitamin that was distinctly different from vitamin B_2 in 1934. Four years later (1938), Lepkovsky[172] was the first to report the isolation of vitamin B_6 in crystalline form although others, including György, followed by just a few months.[173,174] The structure[175,176] and synthesis[177] were published simultaneously in 1939. György[178] proposed the term *pyridoxin*, derived from two of the chemical constituents, *pyrid* of pyridine and *oxo* of methoxy, as a name for the new vitamin in 1939, but *pyridoxine* came into general use thereafter. Other active forms of vitamin B_6 were found,[179] and in 1960, IUPAC[106] used the descriptor *pyridoxine* to refer to all "naturally occurring pyridine derivatives with vitamin B_6 activity." IUPAC[180] terminology was again revised in 1973, and the term *vitamin B_6*, instead of pyridoxine, is the approved generic descriptor for all active forms of the vitamin. *Pyridoxine* is used specifically to refer to 4,5-bis(hydroxymethyl)-2-methylpyridin-3-ol. The term *pyridoxol* is no longer recommended. All active forms of vitamin B_6 and their recommended names are shown in Figure 28.34, along with their interconversions.

Pyridoxine is naturally found in whole grains, meat, poultry, cereals, peanuts, corn, and fish. However, up to 40% of the vitamin may be destroyed during cooking. Food sources contain all three forms, either in their free form or phosphorylated. Plants contain primarily pyridoxine and pyridoxamine, whereas animal sources provide chiefly pyridoxal.

CHEMISTRY

Pyridoxine (PN) is the C^4 hydroxymethyl derivative, pyridoxal (PL) is the C^4 formyl derivative and pyridoxamine (PM) is the C^4 aminomethyl derivative of 5-(hydroxymethyl)-2-methylpyridin-3-ol. Each of these are also converted to their corresponding 5′-phosphate derivatives referred to as pyridoxine 5′-phosphate (PNP), pyridoxal 5′-phosphate (PLP), and pyridoxamine 5′-phosphate (PMP), respectively (see Fig. 28.34). Because of their ability to interconvert, all are considered active forms of vitamin B_6 in vivo. Although PLP is the major coenzyme form, PMP can also function as a coenzyme primarily in aminotransferases. The major metabolite is 4-pyridoxic acid, which is excreted in the urine.

KINETICS

PNP, PLP, and PMP are enzymatically hydrolyzed in the small intestine to PN, PL, and PM prior to absorption. The intestinal absorption of dietary vitamin B_6, in the form of PN, PL, and PM, has historically been ascribed to passive diffusion.[181] Recent evidence suggests that a carrier-mediated process may also be involved.[182] One additional form of vitamin B_6, pyridoxine-5′-β-D-glucoside (Fig. 28.35), is the predominate form in some plants (grains, fruits, and vegetables), and this form has a significantly lower bioavailability than other forms because of incomplete hydrolysis of the glycosidic bond in the intestines.

In the liver, all three forms are interconverted; however, the major form of vitamin B_6 in the liver is PLP.[181] PLP (60%), PN (15%), and PL (14%) circulate in the blood bound to albumin. Vitamin B_6 traverses cell membranes, upon entry or exit, only in the dephosphorylated form. Plasma alkaline phosphatase (EC 3.1.3.1) is responsible for the removal of the phosphate group prior to cellular uptake from the blood.[183] Upon cellular entry via facilitated transport, phosphorylation acts to trap the vitamin and drive the overall process of cellular uptake.[184] Total body stores of vitamin B_6 approximate 170 mg with 75% to 80% found in muscle, primarily as phosphorylase (EC 2.4.1.1), and 5% to 10% in the liver[185] with the remaining portion distributed among the remaining tissues. The muscle pool is thought to be very stable, relatively unavailable to other tissues and highly conserved during deficient intake. Therefore, deficiency of this vitamin is more likely to affect tissues other than muscle, especially newly formed tissues.[185] Excess vitamin B_6 is eventually converted to PL, which is oxidized to 4-pyridoxic acid. This acid is the primary form found in the urine, accounting for essentially all excess dietary vitamin B_6.

BIOCHEMISTRY

PLP functions as a coenzyme[186] that performs many vital functions in human metabolism. More than 140 distinct PLP-dependent enzymes have been cataloged by the Enzyme Commission (EC).[187] It functions in the transaminations and decarboxylations that amino acids generally undergo, and about half of all the PLP-dependent enzymes function as aminotransferases. For example, it functions as

Pyridoxine

EC 2.7.1.35
+ATP

EC 3.1.3.74

Pyridoxine 5'-phosphate

EC 1.4.3.5
+FMN

EC 1.4.3.5
+ FMN

Pyridoxal

EC 2.7.1.35
+ ATP

EC 3.1.3.74

Pyridoxal 5'-phosphate (PLP)

EC 1.4.3.5
+FMN

EC 1.4.3.5
+FMN

EC 1.2.3.1
+ FAD

Pyridoxamine

EC 2.7.1.35
+ ATP

EC 3.1.3.74

Pyridoxamine 5'-phosphate (PMP)

EC 1.4.3.5   pyridoxal 5'-phosphate synthase
EC 2.7.1.35   pyridoxal kinase
EC 3.1.3.74   pyridoxal phosphatase
EC 1.2.3.1   aldehyde oxidase

Pyridoxic acid

Figure 28.34 ● Active forms of vitamin B_6 and the major metabolite pyridoxic acid.

a cotransaminase in the transamination of alanine to form pyruvic acid and as a codecarboxylase in the decarboxylation of dihydroxyphenylalanine (DOPA) to form dopamine. Other biological transformations of amino acids in which pyridoxal can function are racemization, elimination of the α-hydrogen together with a β-substituent (i.e., OH or SH) or a γ-substituent, and probably the reversible cleavage of β-hydroxyamino acids to glycine and carbonyl compounds.

An electromeric displacement of electrons from bonds with the α-carbon (see Fig. 28.36) results in the release of a cation (H, R', or COOH) and, subsequently, leads to various reactions observed with pyridoxal. The extent to which one of these displacements predominates over others depends on the structure of the amino acid and the environment (pH, solvent, catalysts, enzymes, etc.). When this mechanism applies in vivo, the pyridoxal component is linked to the enzyme through the phosphate of the hydroxymethyl group by hydrogen bond networks and/or ionic interactions.

Figure 28.37 shows the role of PLP in the transamination reaction. The first half-reaction involves the initial

proton abstraction from the external aldimine at C_α by the active site lysine, yielding a quinonoid intermediate. Lysin ammonium, thus formed, protonates the $C^{4'}$ of the quinonoid intermediate to generate a ketimine, which is subsequently hydrolyzed to release α-ketogluterate and enzyme-PMP complex (E-PMP).

Diacylglycine decarboxylase (DGD) is an unusual PLP-dependent enzyme that performs both decarboxylation, in the first half-reaction, and transamination, in the second half-reaction (Fig. 28.38). In the first half-reaction, a dialkylamino acid is decarboxylated producing a ketone and releasing the E-PMP form, which in the second half-reaction catalyzes transamination to convert an α-keto acid (e.g., pyruvic acid) into an amino acid (e.g., alanine), regenerating the DGD-PLP form.

Figure 28.35 ● Pyridoxine-5'-β-D-glucoside.

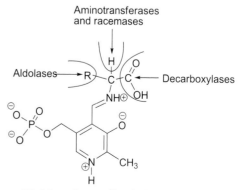

Aminotransferases
and racemases

Aldolases

Decarboxylases

Figure 28.36 ● Generalized vitamin B_6 reactions.

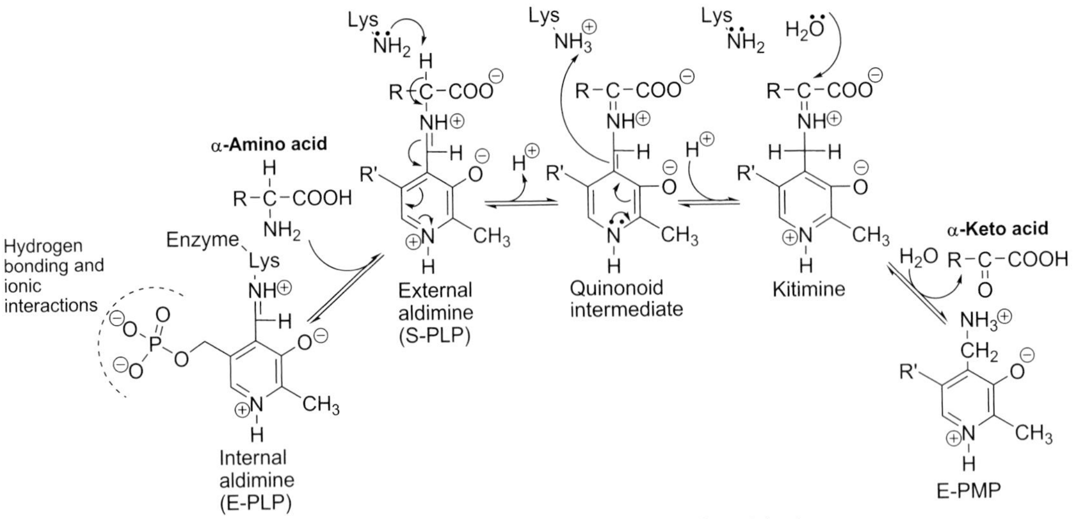

Figure 28.37 • Transamination reactions of pyridoxine.

THERAPEUTIC USES

Pyridoxine is indicated in the treatment and prevention of known or suspected vitamin B_6 deficiency, which is most likely to occur in the setting of alcoholism in developed countries. Vitamin B_6 deficiency-related conditions have been reviewed by Spinneker et al.[184] A hypochromic, microcytic, iron-refractory anemia, a form of sideroblastic anemia, develops because of decreased hemoglobin synthesis. Cognitive defects also develop with impairment in memory function, especially in the elderly. Convulsive seizures occur, and these are particularly problematic in vitamin B_6–deficient infants. Peripheral neuropathy with paresthesia, and burning and thermal sensations is also common. The conversion of tryptophan to niacin is also PLP-dependent and vitamin B_6 deficiency may, rarely, lead to pellagra.[183] All of these conditions respond to increased dietary intake or administration of vitamin B_6.

At least seven genetic disorders that result in a vitamin B_6 deficiency syndrome in the presence of an adequate dietary intake have been identified. These result from defects in enzymes that are responsible for the bioactivation or utilization of vitamin B_6. Chronic use of estrogen-containing oral contraceptives may lead to derangements in tryptophan metabolism, a phenomenon also seen during pregnancy that is thought to result from inhibition of kinureninase (EC 3.7.1.3) by metabolites of estrogenic agents.[188] Vitamin B_6 levels may also be lower in these same groups. All of these conditions respond, at least partially, to treatment with large doses of pyridoxine; although the use of high doses of pyridoxine in pregnancy may not be warranted and its use with contraceptives may lead to failure.[183]

Certain hydrazine derivatives, when administered therapeutically (e.g., isoniazid and hydralazine), can induce a deficiency of the coenzyme PLP by direct inactivation through the mechanism of hydrazone formation with the aldehyde functional group. Cycloserine and penicillamine may act through a similar mechanism.[184] Concurrent administration of pyridoxine can avoid or resolve the relative vitamin B_6 deficiency seen in each of these conditions. Administration of high doses of vitamin B_6 with levodopa, alone, is not recommended because of enhanced conversion of levodopa to dopamine in the periphery resulting in decreased levodopa

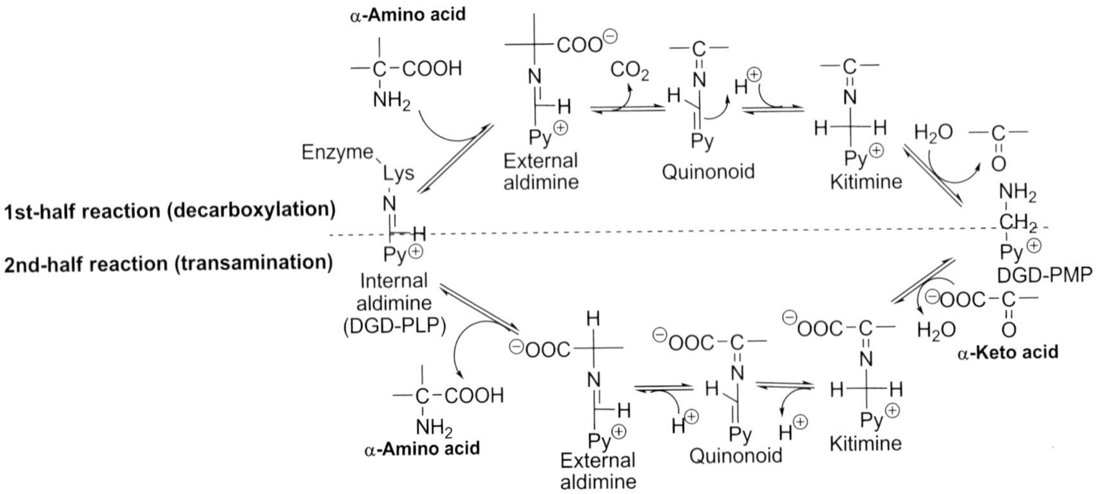

Figure 28.38 • Vitamin B_6–catalyzed decarboxylation and transamination by diacylglycine decarboxylase.

availability to the CNS. The concurrent use of a DOPA decarboxylase inhibitor mitigates this interaction and high doses of vitamin B_6 are without effect on peripheral levodopa conversion. RDA amounts of vitamin B_6 have not been shown to be problematic in either case.

HYPERVITAMINOSIS

Interestingly, peripheral neuropathy, a symptom of vitamin B_6 deficiency, can also occur following ingestion of high doses of pyridoxine. Doses of 2 g/day can produce paresthesia and alter proprioception.[189] Some studies suggest the dose required may be as low as 50 to 500 mg/day. Symptoms may actually increase for several weeks after discontinuing pyridoxine, a phenomenon called *coasting*.[190]

PRODUCTS

Pyridoxine is available from numerous sources under various names as oral formulations in tablet, capsule, powder, lozenge, and solution form. Pyridoxine HCl is avalable for IM or IV injection. Pyrodoxine is also available as a component of numerous multivitamin preparations.

Vitamin B₇

Vitamin B_7 is now referred to as *biotin*. Biotin was first isolated in 1936[191] and identified structurally in 1942.[192] Although this vitamin is known to perform essential metabolic functions in the human, the biotin content of foods, and thus the necessary dietary intake, has not been well established. Good dietary sources of biotin include liver (beef and chicken), meat (beef, pork, chicken), fish, eggs, nuts, and some fruits and vegetables.[193] Enteric microorganisms synthesize biotin from pimeloyl-CoA[194] in the diet and thereby become an additional source of biotin.

CHEMISTRY

Biotin is composed of a tetrahydroimidazolidone (ureido) ring fused with a tetrahydrothiophene ring. A pentanoic acid substituent (at C^5 of pentanoic acid) is attached to the tetrahydrothiophene ring at C^4. The D-isomer (all *cis*) possesses all the activity and the N^1 position is the attachment point for the carboxyl group involved in carboxylation reactions (see Fig. 28.39).

KINETICS

Dietary biotin occurs primarily in the form of protein-bound biotin, which is converted into biotin in the intestinal lumen. Enteric bacteria can also provide a source of protein-bound biotin; however, the importance of this source is not known. Biotin is absorbed from the intestine, more in the jejunum than the ileum, through the SMVT, which also transports

pantothenic acid and lipoic acid.[141,148] This explains the ability of these three substances to competitively inhibit absorption of each other and the ability of some drugs, such as carbamazepine and primidone, to produce biotin deficiency through competitive inhibition of absorption. The transporter is driven by the Na^+ gradient that exists from the extracellular fluid to the intracellular fluid, transporting 2 Na^+ for each monovalent anion of pantothenate, biotin, or lipoate.[167] In addition, the inside-negative membrane potential may also act as a driving force because a net charge of $+1$ enters the cell. This same carrier is ubiquitous throughout bodily tissues and probably also accounts for cellular uptake from the blood. Converson to the active form most likely occurs inside the cell. Greater than 50% of a dose is excreted in the urine as intact biotin. The body appears unable to break the fused imidazolidone and tetrahydrothiophene ring system. The metabolites bisnorbiotin, biotin-*d*, *l*-sulfoxide, bisnorbiotin methyl ketone, and biotin sulfone have been identified in the urine.[141,195]

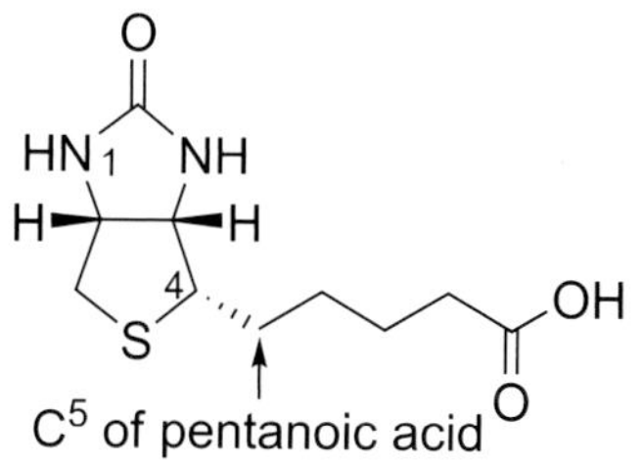

BIOCHEMISTRY

Biotin is required for enzymatic activity of several important carboxylases (Table 28.10). Biotin is first attached to a lysine residue of biotin carboxyl carrier protein (BCCP) by biotin-[propionyl-CoA-carboxylase (ATP-hydrolysing)] ligase (holocarboxylase [HCS], EC 6.3.4.10), which forms the biotinyl domain of the enzyme or separate subunit. The N^1 position is subsequently carboxylated to form carboxybiotin (Fig. 28.40), which is then able to transfer the carboxyl group to other substrates. The source of the carboxyl is either bicarbonate or decarboxylation of another substrate as is seen in transcarboxylation reactions.[196] A typical carboxylation reaction mediated by biotin-BCCP is shown in Figure 28.41. The source of the carboxyl is bicarbonate with ATP supplying energy for the reaction. This is followed by the subsequent transfer of the carboxyl to the substrate with regeneration of the biotin-BCCP complex.

An interesting recent development is the finding that biotin is also attached to histones in the nucleus by the same enzyme involved in attachment to BCCP.[197] The suggestion is that biotin may be involved in genetic regulation; although the exact role remains unknown at this time.

Deficiency states may rarely develop as a result of a biotin-deficient diet, as was observed in early, biotin-deficient TPN solutions,[198] or as a result of prolonged feeding of large quantities of raw egg white.[199] Raw egg white contains avidin, a protein that complexes biotin and interferes with its absorption from the gastrointestinal tract. A relative biotin deficiency has also been shown to occur in

Figure 28.39 ● Biotin.

TABLE 28.10 Biotin-Dependent Enzymes

Enzyme	EC Number	Function
Pyruvate carboxylase	6.4.1.1	Citric acid cycle (TCA cycle)
Acetyl-CoA carboxylase	6.4.1.2	Fatty acid synthesis
Propionyl-CoA carboxylase	6.4.1.3	Conversion of propionyl-CoA to methylmalonyl-CoA
Methylcrotonyl-CoA carboxylase	6.4.1.4	Valine, leucine, and isoleucine degradation

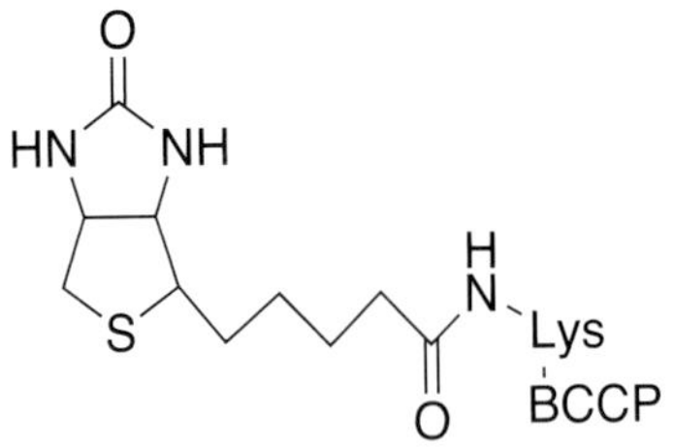

Figure 28.40 • Coenzyme form of biotin.

the case of two identified genetic disorders. Holocarboxylase deficiency is a genetic disorder of biotin-(propionyl-CoA-carboxylase [ATP-hydrolysing]) ligase, the enzyme responsible for the terminal step incorporating biotin into the apoenzyme. Biotinidase (EC 3.5.1.12) deficiency is a genetic disorder of the amidase that releases biotin from the apoenzyme and allows it to be recycled. Both of these lead to multiple carboxylase deficiency (MCD), a condition marked by decreased activity of all biotin-dependent carboxylases and both respond, at least partially, to large doses of biotin.[197] The symptoms of biotin deficiency include dermatitis, conjunctivitis, alopecia, and CNS abnormalities including behavioral, developmental, and psychological effects.[198]

HYPERVITAMINOSIS

There are no known documented cases of toxicity resulting from excessive intake of biotin.

PRODUCTS

Biotin is available as oral tablets, capsules, and lozenges from numerous sources under various names. Biotin content ranges from approximately 300 to 1,000 μg, some-times higher. Biotin is also found in a host of mutlivitamin preparations.

Vitamin B$_9$

Vitamin B$_9$ is now known officially as *folic acid* or *folate*, which is preferred because it is shorter.[200] The term *folic acid* is derived from the Latin word *folium* meaning "leaf" and was coined by Mitchell et al.[201] in 1941 to refer to a substance isolated from spinach leaves that was an essential growth factor in *Streptococcus lactis* R (now classified as *Enterococcus hirae*). Folate crystals were isolated in 1943[202] and the structure reported in 1946.[203]

Natural sources of dietary folate are fruits, vegetables, beans, and peas as well as beef and chicken liver. However, since January 1998, the Federal Government[204] has required folic acid fortification of all enriched cereal-grain products (flour, rice, bread, rolls, buns, pasta, corn, grits, corn meal, farina, macaroni, and noodle products), and these have now become important dietary sources of folate in the United States.[205,206]

CHEMISTRY

The chemical structure of folic acid (Fig. 28.42) was found to be composed of a pteridine heterocyclic system (rings A and B), *p*-aminobenzoic acid (PABA) and Glu; hence the name pteroylglutamate (PteGlu). In plants and bacteria, folic acid is synthesized by converting guanosine triphosphate (GTP) through a multistep sequence into the pteridine heterocycle. This is followed by dihydropteroate synthase (EC 2.5.1.15), which adds the PABA moiety and finally the glutamate residue is added by dihydrofolate synthase (EC 6.3.2.12). It is of note that the antibacterial sulfonamides compete with PABA for the bacterial form of dihydropteroate synthase and, thereby, interfere with bacterial folic acid synthesis. This

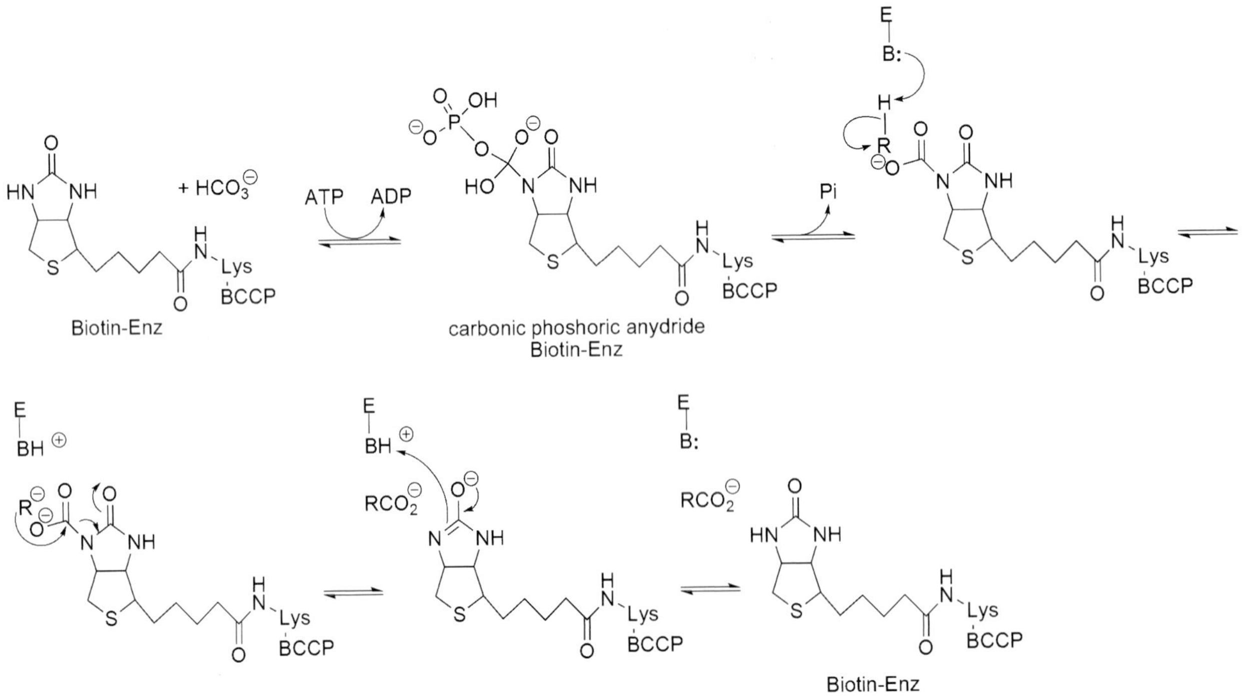

Figure 28.41 • Biotin-mediated carboxylation reaction.

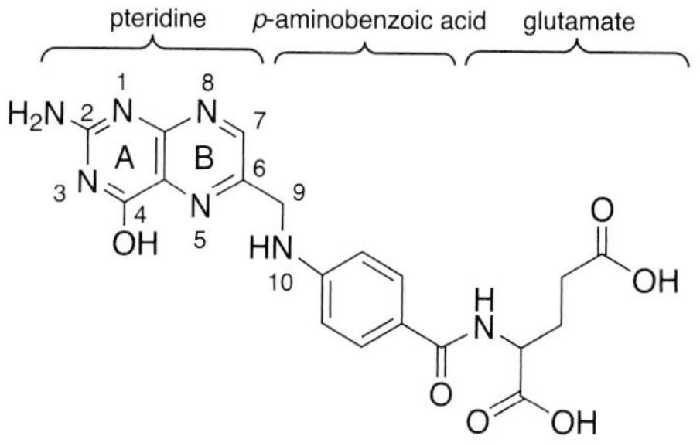

Figure 28.42 ● Folic acid.

results in a selective antibacterial effect because susceptible bacteria cannot utilize preformed folate from the environment.

It was soon noted that PteGlu and naturally occurring folates differed in that the natural forms had a reduced ring B of the pteridine moiety; more than one Glu attached, which is referred to as *pteroylpolyglutamates* (PteGlu$_n$); and a single carbon unit attached to the nitrogen at position 5 or 10. As a result, it was first recommended that folic acid be used to denote the fully oxidized, monoglutamate form without the single carbon unit and folate was used to denote all forms that possess biological activity as the vitamin. Currently, folate (the preferred term) specifically refers to pteroylglutamate and folic acid refers to pteroylglutamic acid.[200] Folate can also be used generically to refer to any of the members of the group of pteroylglutamates, their mixtures, differing one-carbon substituents, level of reduction, or number of glutamate residues. Because of this dual use of the term folate, the authors have chosen to use the term folate only in its generic sense throughout this chapter. This will avoid confusion with the fully oxidized form, folic acid, which is the major form available for vitamin supplementation.

KINETICS

Folates occur in the diet as PteGlu$_n$ that must be hydrolyzed to the monoglutamate form (PteGlu) before absorption. The hydrolysis is catalyzed by gamma-glutamyl hydrolase (EC 3.4.19.9) found in the brush border of the intestinal mucosa. The PteGlu is primarily absorbed by active transport by reduced folate carrier (RFC) in the jejunum and upper duodenum.[141,148] RFC is now known as solute carrier family 19, member 1 (SLC19A1) and is related to the thiamine transporters SLC10A2 and SLC19A3 that were discussed previously. This absorption is saturable and facilitated by the slightly acidic conditions found in these regions. Although the mucosa in these regions possesses dihydrofolate reductase (DHFR, EC 1.5.1.3), most reduction to dihydrofolate (H$_2$PteGlu, formerly called dihydrofolic acid or DHFA) and then to tetrahydrofolate (H$_4$PteGlu, formerly called tetrahydrofolic acid or THFA) and methylation occur in the liver. H$_4$PteGlu is distributed to all tissues, where it is stored as polyglutamates, primarily pentaglutamates or heptaglutamates (H$_4$PteGlu$_5$ or H$_4$PteGlu$_7$). The 5-methyl derivative (5-methyl-PteGlu$_n$) is the main transport and storage form in the body. The body stores 5 to 10 mg with approximately 50% in the liver. The major elimination pathway for the vitamin is biliary excretion as the 5-methyl derivative. Extensive enterohepatic cycling occurs. Only trace amounts are found in the urine. Large doses that exceed the tubular reabsorption limit, however, result in substantial amounts in the urine.

BIOCHEMISTRY

Folic acid, and dietary forms of folate that are not in the reduced state, must undergo reduction of ring B for biological activity. Folic acid is first reduced to H$_2$PteGlu by dihydrofolate reductase (DHFR; EC 1.5.1.3) using NADPH as a cofactor and then to H$_4$PteGlu by the same enzyme. These key steps are important in the understanding of the folate antagonists, such as methotrexate, that inhibit DHFR and, thereby, interfere with the utilization of all folates that are not in the reduced (H$_4$PteGlu) state. Upon cellular uptake, several glutamate residues are attached via tetrahydrofolate synthase (EC 6.3.2.17) to form H$_4$PteGlu$_n$, effectively trapping the folate in the cell (Fig. 28.43).

In its reduced, polyglutamate form (H$_4$PteGlu$_n$), folic acid functions in the transfer of single carbon groups (see Fig. 28.44). H$_4$PteGlu$_n$ is required for several important methylation reactions (Table 28.11) including the biosynthesis of methionine, serine, purine bases, transfer RNA (tRNA), and deoxythymidine triphosphate (dTTP), which is required for DNA synthesis. The most notable methylation reaction involves 5,10-methylene-H$_4$PteGlu$_n$ in the conversion of deoxyuridine monophosphate (dUMP) to deoxythymidine monophosphate (dTMP), the first step in dTTP synthesis, by the enzyme thymidylate synthase (EC 2.1.1.45). Inhibition of DHFR and the resulting depletion of 5,10-methylene-H$_4$PteGlu$_n$ by H$_4$PteGlu analogs, such as methotrexate, is thought to produce an antineoplastic effect by depleting the cellular dTTP, which is required for DNA replication.[207] Likewise, trimethoprim and related drugs produce their antimicrobial effect through high specificity for the bacterial form of the same enzyme.

There is a fundamental relationship between folate and cobalamin in the regulation of active forms of H$_4$PteGlu$_n$. Most of the active forms of H$_4$PteGlu$_n$ are interconvertible through reversible reactions (Fig. 28.44); however, the reduction of 5,10-methylene-H$_4$PteGlu$_n$ to form 5-methyl-H$_4$PteGlu$_n$ is not reversible. The only pathway for conversion of 5-methyl-H$_4$PteGlu$_n$ back to H$_4$PteGlu$_n$ for further utilization is through methionine synthase (EC 2.1.1.13), which converts homocysteine to methionine utilizing methylcobalamin as a cofactor (also see Vitamin B$_{12}$). A deficiency of cobalamin can result in abnormal accumulation of 5-methyl-H$_4$PteGlu$_n$ with a subsequent relative depletion of all other active forms of H$_4$PteGlu$_n$. Depletion of available 5,10-methylene-H$_4$PteGlu$_n$, either through folate deficiency or through cobalamin deficiency, leads to impaired DNA synthesis resulting in the characteristic megaloblastic anemia commonly seen in a deficiency of either of these vitamins. Of great importance for the clinician to remember, administering folic acid to a cobalamin-deficient patient will correct the megaloblastic anemia because it provides a renewed source of reduced H$_4$PteGlu$_n$; however, the neurological damage from the cobalamin deficiency continues unabated.

THERAPEUTIC USES

Folic acid is used in the treatment of known or suspected folate deficiency or increased need as occurs during

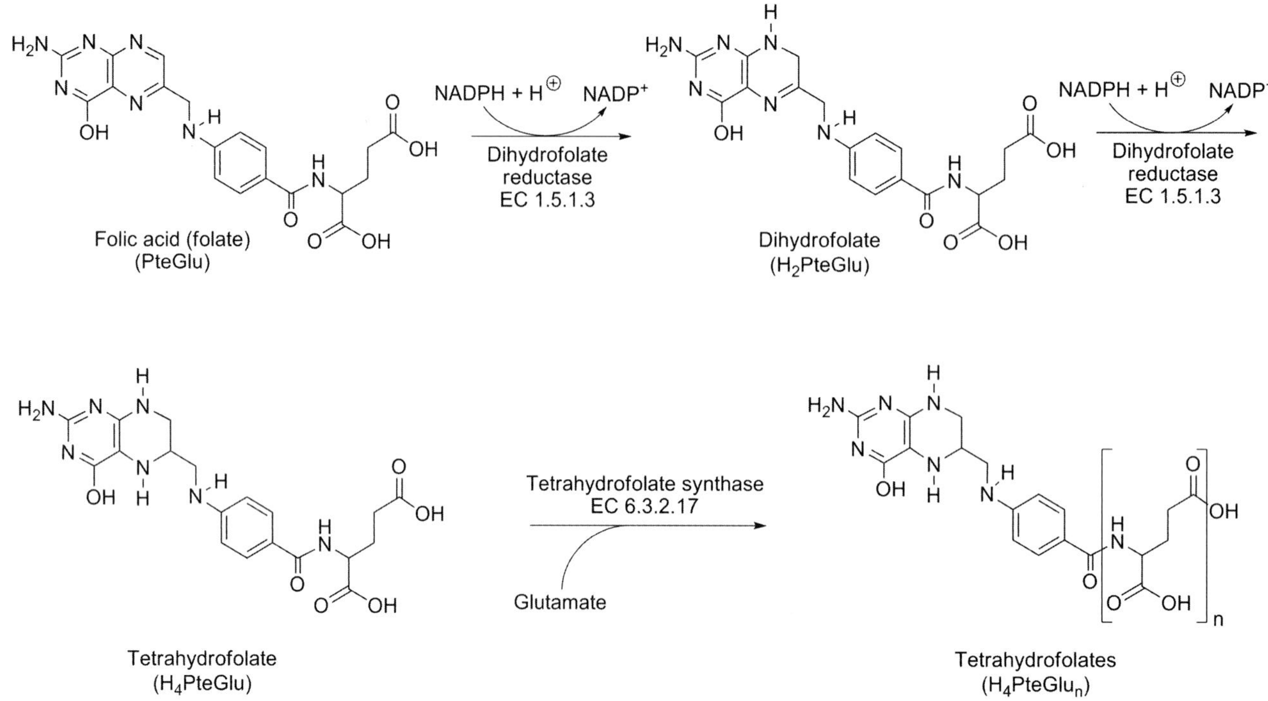

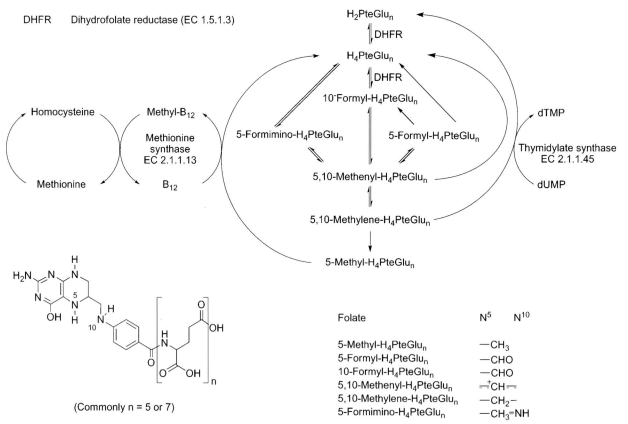

Figure 28.43 ● Bioactivation of folic acid to tetrahydrofolate polyglutamates.

DHFR Dihydrofolate reductase (EC 1.5.1.3)

Folate

Folate	N^5	N^{10}
5-Methyl-H_4PteGlu$_n$	—CH_3	
5-Formyl-H_4PteGlu$_n$	—CHO	
10-Formyl-H_4PteGlu$_n$		—CHO
5,10-Methenyl-H_4PteGlu$_n$	=$^+$CH=	
5,10-Methylene-H_4PteGlu$_n$	—CH_2—	
5-Formimino-H_4PteGlu$_n$	—CH_3=NH	

(Commonly n = 5 or 7)

Figure 28.44 ● Interconversion of active folates.

TABLE 28.11 **Folic Acid–Dependent Enzymes**

Enzyme	EC Number	Function
Methionine synthase	2.1.1.13	Conversion of L-homocysteine to L-methionine
Glycine hydroxymethyltransferase	2.1.2.1	Interconversion of serine and glycine
Phosphoribosylglycinamide formyltransferase	2.1.2.2	Purine synthesis
Phosphoribosylaminoimidazolecarboxamide formyltransferase	2.1.2.3	Purine synthesis
Glutamate formimidoyltransferase	2.1.2.5	Histidine metabolism
Methionyl-tRNA formyltransferase	2.1.2.9	tRNA synthesis
Thymidylate synthase	2.1.1.45	Conversion of dUMP to dTMP in DNA synthesis

pregnancy. The most likely cause of folate deficiency in developed countries is alcoholism. The resulting megaloblastic anemia, thought to result from a deficiency in DNA synthesis, as noted previously, is indistinguishable from that caused by vitamin B_{12} because both vitamins are involved in the same critical biochemical step. Unlike vitamin B_{12}, no neurological abnormalities are associated with folate deficiency. Because folate requirements increase during pregnancy, and maternal folate deficiency has been associated with a risk of neural tube defects in the fetus, folic acid supplementation is recommended, at a minimum, periconceptually.[208,209] Because of the potentially beneficial effects in reducing these birth defects, the FDA has mandated fortification of all enriched cereal-grain products in the United States with folic acid since 1998.[204]

Folic acid has also been shown to reduce homocysteine levels, which is a risk factor for cardiovascular disease independent of other risk factors. However, although there is some evidence that folic acid supplementation may reduce the risk of stroke,[210] the risk of other cardiovascular disease has not been proven to be affected.[211] Some studies suggest that multivitamin preparations with folic acid taken prior to, and during pregnancy, may protect against congenital heart defects. Folate may also decrease the risk of colorectal cancer; however, once colorectal cancer develops it may act as a promoting agent.[212]

One of the biologically active forms of folic acid, leucovorin (5-formyl-H_4PteGlu), is used in the treatment of accidental overdoses of DHFR inhibitors, such as methotrexate, because it does not require bioactivation by DHFR as does folic acid. Leucovorin is also used concomitantly with, or shortly following, methotrexate, trimetrexate, pyrimethamine, trimethoprim, and related drug therapy to decrease the toxicity in sensitive cells. Finally, although leucovorin can be used in place of folic acid in all other uses, there is no therapeutic advantage.

HYPERVITAMINOSIS

High doses of folic acid are rather nontoxic; however, at least one study has shown that 15 mg/day for 1 month can result in gastrointestinal disturbances (including anorexia, nausea, and pain) and CNS effects (including sleep disturbances, vivid dreams, malaise, irritability, and increased excitability).[213] The primary danger of excessive folate intake is the masking of vitamin B_{12} deficiency. Folic acid can correct the anemia caused by vitamin B_{12} deficiency, but it has no effect on the neurological damage. The potential for high doses of folic acid to mask B_{12} deficiency explains why large daily doses of folic acid are best avoided in the general population.

PRODUCTS

Folic acid is available alone in tablet and injectable form, or in combination with other vitamins, in various multivitamin preparations. Leucovorin is a racemic mixture of 6S and 6R 5-formyl-H_4PteGlu and is available as the calcium salt for use in treatment of accidental overdoses of DHFR inhibitors, such as methotrexate, or to decrease their toxicity in sensitive cells. The active 6S-isomer of leucovorin is also available as levoleucovorin calcium (Fusilev) and is dosed at one-half the rate of leucovorin with the same uses. L-Methylfolate (Deplin) is the 6S-isomer of 5-methyl-H_4PteGlu. This is the biologically active isomer of 5-methyl-H_4PteGlu, which is the main transport and storage form (as 5-methyl-H_4PteGlu$_n$) of folates in the body. It is used in tablet form as a *medical food* for the treatment of methylenetetrahydrofolate reductase [NAD(P)H] (EC 1.5.1.20) deficiency (MTHFR deficiency). Medical foods are substances that are regulated by the FDA and are administered enterally under the supervision of a physician intended for the dietary management of a disease that has distinctive nutritional needs.

Vitamin B₁₂

Vitamin B_{12} specifically refers to cyanocobalamin, the form typically found in dietary supplements because of its high stability.[214] However, the immediate precursor to the vitamin B_{12}-derived coenzymes is hydroxocobalamin (vitamin B_{12b}), which is formed in vivo from cyanocobalamin. Cobalamin is used to refer to any of the related cobalt-containing compounds that serve as coenzymes or their biologically active precursors as shown in Figure 28.45.

The discovery of vitamin B_{12} began with the unwitting description by Dr. Thomas Addison in 1855 of patients suffering from an anemia that was later identified as *pernicious anemia*.[215] Following the rapid developments in vitamin discovery in the early 1900s, it was soon determined that a diet high in liver could reverse the effects of pernicious anemia as was clearly shown in 1926 by Minot and Murphy.[216] However, concentration and identification of the vitamin was slow because the only known assay for vitamin B_{12} activity was the reversal of pernicious anemia in human patients. Almost 30 years had passed before Shorb[217] reported in 1947 that liver extract was required for the growth of *Lactobacillus lactis* in similar proportions to that found to treat pernicious anemia. With an inexpensive, rapid assay for vitamin B_{12} activity, the crystalline form was isolated and reported simultaneously just 1 year later by Smith[218] and Ricks et al.[219] who suggested the name vitamin B_{12}. Interestingly, the conversion to cyanocobalamin occurs during the purification process and is not the natural form of

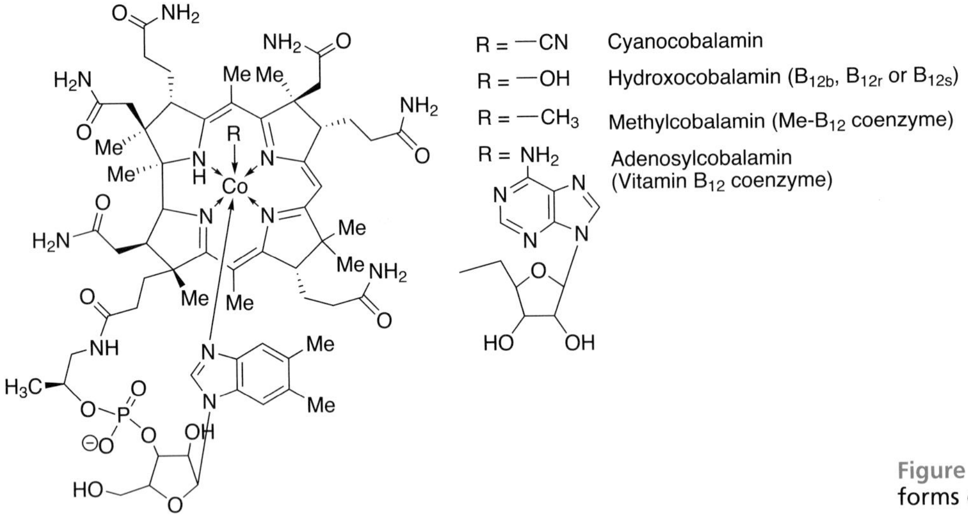

R = —CN   Cyanocobalamin

R = —OH   Hydroxocobalamin (B_{12b}, B_{12r} or B_{12s})

R = —CH_3 Methylcobalamin (Me-B_{12} coenzyme)

R = NH_2 Adenosylcobalamin
                 (Vitamin B_{12} coenzyme)

Figure 28.45 • Biologically active forms of cobalamin.

the vitamin. The structure of cyanocobalamin was announced simultaneously by Hodgkin et al.[220] and Bonnett et al.[221] in 1955 and the complete synthesis completed in 1972.[222]

De novo synthesis of cobalamin is only found in microorganisms. Therefore, cobalmin is found naturally in commercial fermentation processes of antibiotics, such as those of *Streptomyces griseus, Streptomyces olivaceus, and Streptomyces aureofaciens* as well as sewage, Milorganite and others. Some of these fermentations furnish a commercial source of vitamin B_{12}. Animals depend on synthesis by the intestinal flora or, as in humans, foods from animals that have already consumed cobalamin. Excellent dietary sources are meats, eggs, dairy, fish, and shellfish. The only dietary plant products containing the vitamin are legumes, because of their symbiosis with microorganisms, or those that have been fortified with the vitamin.

CHEMISTRY

These are the most complex group of vitamins consisting of a corrin core with a central cobalt atom with +1, +2, or +3 oxidation state. The corrin core has four pyrrol units, two of which are attached directly whereas the others are joined by methylene bridges. Out of six coordination bonds of cobalt, four are bonded to pyrrole nitrogens and the fifth is bound to one of the nitrogen atoms of the dimethylbenzimidazole derivative containing ribose 3-phosphate and aminoisopropanol linked through an amide bond to the side chain of the corrin core. The sixth substituent of the cobalt atom can be —CN, —OH, —CH_3, or a 5'-deoxyadenosyl unit (Fig. 28.45). In hydroxocobalamin, the cobalt atom is in the +3 oxidation state and called vitamin B_{12b} (Co^{3+}), which is reduced by flavoprotein reductase to the vitamin B_{12r} (Co^{2+}) form and then to the vitamin B_{12s} (Co^+) form, which is converted to the methyl coenzyme form. Vitamin B_{12r} (Co^{2+}) is believed to be converted to the adenosylcoenzyme form by cob(I)yrinic acid a, c-diamide adenosyltransferase (EC 2.5.1.17) using ATP.

KINETICS

Dietary cobalamin is protein bound but is released in the stomach through the action of acid and gastric proteases. The primary natural forms are methylcobalamin, deoxyadenosylcobalamin, and hydroxocobalamin with only trace amounts of cyanocobalamin, which is processed similarly except for the initial liberation from protein. Free cobalamin then binds to transcobalamin (TC) I, also called *haptocorrin*, which is a high-affinity cobalamin-binding protein found in all bodily fluids including saliva. As the bound cobalamin enters the small intestine, pancreatic proteases digest TC I releasing free cobalamin, which then binds to intrinsic factor (IF), secreted primarily by parietal cells of the gastric mucosa, forming an intrinsic factor-cobalamin (IF-CBL) complex. In the distal ileum, IF-CBL binds to cubilin, also known as the intrinsic factor cobalamin receptor (IFCR), on the luminal surface and undergoes receptor-mediated endocytosis. Intracellularly, IF is cleaved by the lysozymal enzyme, cathepsin L (EC 3.4.22.15), and the free cobalamin binds to TC II to form TC II-CBL, which is then released into the bloodstream completing the process of transcytosis.[223–225] Dietary supplements that contain cyanocobalamin undergo an additional conversion in the plasma by cyanocobalamin reductase (cyanide-eliminating) (EC 1.16.1.6) to hydroxocobalamin, which serves as the immediate precursor to the cobalamin derived coenzymes.

The average dietary intake of cobalamin is 5 to 30 μg; however, only 1 to 2 μg/meal is absorbed most likely because of saturation of the IF-dependent transport. Small amounts of cobalamin can also be absorbed through passive diffusion; however, this is normally insufficient to prevent deficiency unless the diet consists of abnormally large quantities of foods rich in cobalamin, such as liver. Only 1% of an oral dose of cobalamin is absorbed in patients that lack gastric acid and IF, which explains the large doses, 1,000 to 2,000 μg (1–2 mg) per day, of vitamin B_{12} required in the oral treatment of pernicious anemia.

In the bloodstream, cobalamin is bound not only to TC II but also to plasma haptocorrin, which may function primarily as a storage form of cobalamin. Uptake into cells that need cobalamin is receptor mediated through TC II-CBL receptors (TC II-R). Half of the body stores of cobalamin are in the liver primarily as adenosylcobalamin. Cobalamin is excreted into the bile and undergoes enterohepatic cycling utilizing IF for reabsorption. This explains why deficiency will occur more rapidly in patients with malabsorption of cobalamin than inadequate dietary intake. Excess cobalamin is eliminated unchanged in the feces and urine.

BIOCHEMISTRY

In the biosynthesis of the coenzymes derived from cobalamin, cobalt is reduced from a trivalent to a monovalent state before the organic anionic ligands are attached to the structure. The two types of cobalamins that participate as coenzymes in human metabolism are adenosylcobalamin and methylcobalamin. These coenzymes perform vital functions in methylmalonate–succinate isomerization and in methylation of homocysteine to methionine (Fig. 28.46).

Two enzymes have been shown to be cobalamin dependent in humans. Methylmalonyl-CoA mutase (EC 5.4.99.2) requires 5′-deoxyadenosylcobalamin; this enzyme system catalyzes the methylmalonyl-CoA transformation to succinyl-CoA, which is the major pathway of propionyl-CoA metabolism (Fig. 28.46). This is a free radical mediated rearrangement reaction where cobalamin's role is to serve as the source of free radicals, through homolytic cleavage of the weak Co-C bond, for the abstraction of hydrogen atoms. Propionyl-CoA from odd-chain fatty acid metabolism must be processed through this pathway to succinyl-CoA to enter the Krebs (citric acid) cycle to be either converted to γ-oxaloacetate, leading to gluconeogenesis, or oxidized aerobically to CO_2, with production of ATP. The methylation of homocysteine to form methionine requires methylcobalamin and is catalyzed by methionine synthase (EC 2.1.1.13), a transmethylase that also requires 5-methyl-PteGlu$_n$ and reduced FAD. This lat-

ter reaction forms the basis for the megaloblastic anemia that results from either folic acid or cobalamin deficiency and the masking of cobalamin deficiency by folic acid. The reader is referred to the section on vitamin B$_9$ for a related discussion.

THERAPEUTIC USES

The most common form of cobalamin deficiency, known as pernicious anemia, is now known to be an autoimmune disorder that results from parietal cell destruction. This results in insufficient production of gastric acid and IF and the ensuing malabsorption of cobalamin. Other less common causes of insufficient absorption are hypochlorhydria, gastrectomy, ileocecal resection, celiac disease, and chemical incompatibilities with drugs in the gastric milieu. A deficiency of cobalamin can also result from nutritional deficiencies, increased requirements as is seen in pregnancy, as well as a strict vegetarian diet without adequate supplementation. The symptoms of cobalamin deficiency primarily result from potentially irreversible nerve damage, involving sensory, motor, and cognitive functioning, and the megaloblastic anemia that can be confused with that seen in folate deficiency. The ability of folic acid to reverse megaloblastic anemia seen in cobalamin deficiency, without affecting nerve damage, is discussed in the Vitamin B$_9$ section.

Cyanocobalamin is the form most commonly used in the treatment of cobalamin deficiency; however, hydroxo-

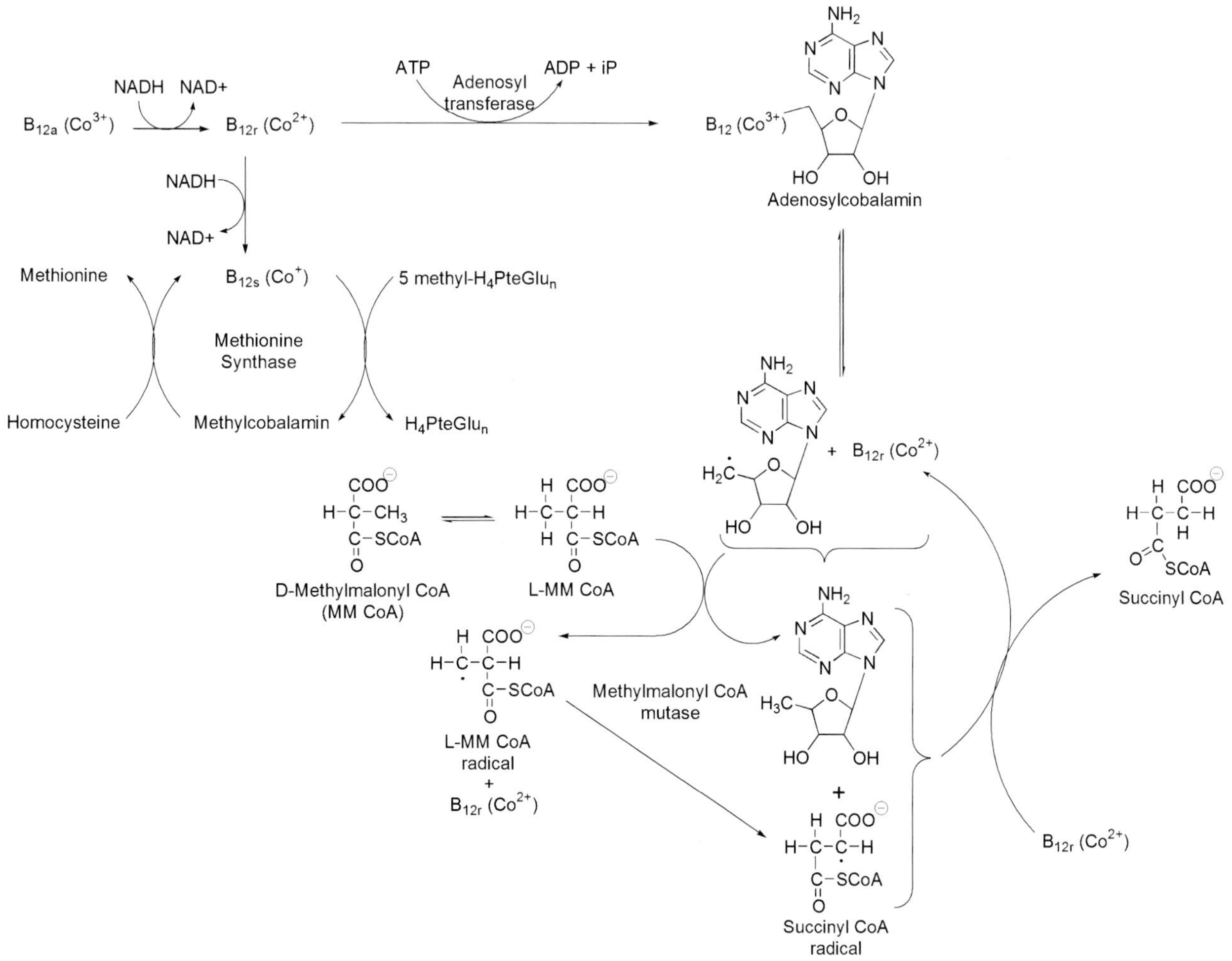

Figure 28.46 ● Coenzymes of vitamin B$_{12}$.

cobalamin is equally efficacious. A rare genetic disorder that results in an inability to convert cyanocobalamin to hydroxocobalamin is the only known instance where hydroxocobalamin would be the preferred treatment.[226] Hydroxocobalamin, but not cycanocobalamin, is also used in the treatment of cyanide toxicity. Administration of large doses results in the conversion of hydroxocobalamin to the nontoxic cyanocobalamin effectively reducing plasma levels of cyanide. In this case, 5 to 10 g of IV hydroxocobalamin may be needed as compared to 1 mg/day in severe pernicious anemia.

HYPERVITAMINOSIS

Milligram doses of cyanocobalamin are generally not associated with toxicity although rare allergic[227] and anaphylactic reactions[228,229] and mild diarrhea have occurred. As further evidence of the safety of vitamin B_{12}, the adverse effects following the use of hydroxocobalmin in the treatment of cyanide poisoning, where the typical dose is 5 to 10 g, have been relatively mild.[230]

PRODUCTS

Cyanocobalamin, the most common form used, is available as oral and sublingual tablets as well as oral lozenges from numerous sources under various names. These products contain anywhere from approximately 50 to 1,000 μg of cyanocobalamin. Cyanocobalamin is also available as a nasal spray for daily use (CaloMist 25 μg/actuation) or weekly use (Nascobal 500 μg/actuation) and as an injectable for intramascular (IM) or deep subcutaneous (SQ) administration. Hydroxocobalamin is available as two, 2.5-g vials (Cyanokit) for the treatment of cyanide poisoning. Hydroxocobalamin is also available in oral and injectable dosage forms from numerous sources under various names. The only advantage for hydroxocobalamin in the treatment of pernicious anemia would be in patients unable to convert cyanocobalamin to hydroxocobalamin as the result of a rare genetic disorder as discussed previously. Cyanocobalamin and hydroxocobalamin are also available in a host of multivitamin preparations.

Vitamin C

Scurvy (from the French word *scorbutus*) has been recognized as a disease afflicting mankind for thousands of years.[231] However, it was not until the early 1500s that natives of North America used teas brewed from pine needles to treat or prevent the symptoms of scurvy without understanding the basis for their curative properties. Citrus fruits such as oranges, lemons, and limes were later identified as equally effective treatments. Only within the last 100 years has a deficiency in vitamin C been definitively identified as the cause of scurvy. In 1932, Waugh and King[232,233] isolated crystalline vitamin C from lemon juice and showed it to be the antiscorbutic factor present in each of these treatments. Interestingly, in a series of papers published at approximately the same time,[234,235] Svirbely and Szent-Györgyi[236] showed that the substance the latter had crystallized from peppers and reported 4 years earlier was the same as vitamin C and not a hexuronic acid as originally proposed. The structure and chemical formula of vitamin C was identified in 1933 by Hirst et al.[237] as one of a series of possible

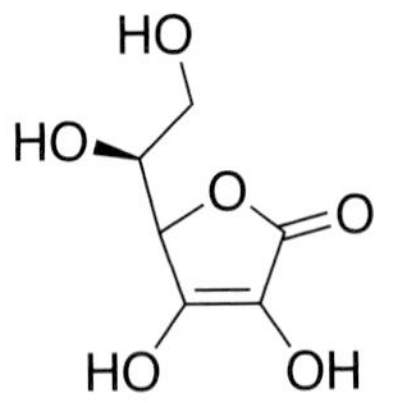

Figure 28.47 • L-Ascorbic acid.

tautomeric isomers. The first synthesis of vitamin C was announced almost simultaneously by Ault et al.[238] and Reichstein[239] in 1933. Since that time, it has been synthesized in several different ways.

Vitamin C can be synthesized by nearly all living organisms, plants, and animals; but primates, guinea pigs, bats, and a few other species cannot produce this vitamin. The consensus is that organisms that cannot synthesize vitamin C lack the liver microsomal enzyme L-gulonolactone oxidase (1.1.3.8), which catalyzes the terminal step of the biosynthetic process. Sato and Udenfriend[240] summarized studies of the biosynthesis of vitamin C in mammals and the biochemical and genetic basis for the incapability of some species to synthesize the vitamin. Because humans are one of the few animal species that cannot synthesize vitamin C, it has to be available as a dietary component.

Dietary sources of ascorbic acid include fruits (especially citrus fruits), vegetables (especially peppers), and potatoes. Although the sources of some commercial products are rose hips and citrus fruits, most ascorbic acid is prepared synthetically.

CHEMISTRY

Vitamin C is now commonly referred to as *ascorbic acid* because of its acidic character and its effectiveness in the treatment and prevention of scorbutus (scurvy). The acidic character is because of the two enolic hydroxyls; the C^3 hydroxyl has a pK_a value of 4.1, and the C^2 hydroxyl has a pK_a of 11.6. All biological activities reside in L-ascorbic acid (Fig. 28.47); therefore, all references to vitamin C, ascorbic acid, ascorbate, and their derivatives refer to this form. The monobasic sodium salt (Fig. 28.48) is the usual salt form.

KINETICS

Dietary ascorbic acid is readily absorbed as ascorbate and dehydroascorbate by facilitated diffusion while ascorbate can also be absorbed by active transport. Large doses can saturate these systems, limiting the amounts absorbed. Once absorbed, it is distributed to all tissues and transported into cells via the same mechanisms.[241,242] Excess ascorbate is metabolized to oxalic acid and excreted by the kidneys (Fig. 28.49), which

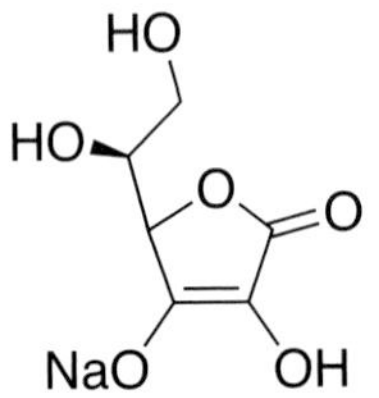

Figure 28.48 • Ascorbate sodium.

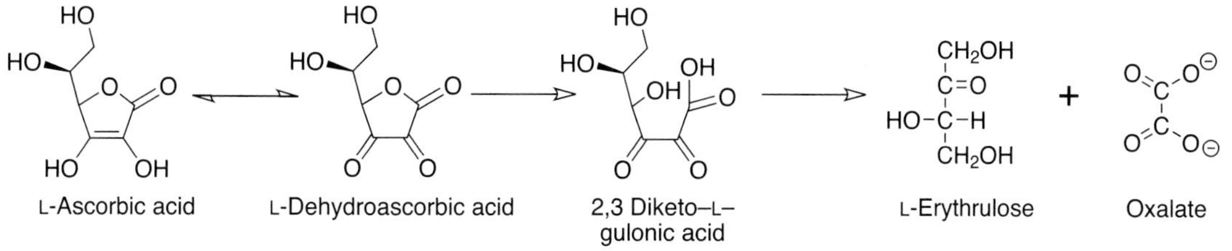

Figure 28.49 ● Oxidation of ascorbic acid.

may form the basis for the formation of kidney stones following ingestion of large doses. Although oxalate is the major urinary metabolite (44%), unchanged ascorbate (20%) and the intermediate metabolite 2,3 diketo-L-gulonic acid (20%) are also found in appreciable quantities.[242]

BIOCHEMISTRY

Ascorbic acid is a required cofactor for several important dioxygenases, functioning as an electron donor in each of these reactions (Table 28.12). These dioxygenases are involved in the hydroxylation of many important biomolecules during their synthetic sequence including collagen, peptide hormones, steroids, and norepinephrine. The resulting oxidized product, semidehydroascorbate (Fig. 28.50), can be reduced back to ascorbic acid through cytochrome-b_5 reductase (EC 1.6.2.2) or thioredoxin-disulfide reductase (EC 1.8.1.9). Alternatively, two molecules of semidehydroascorbate can undergo a disproportionation reaction yielding one molecule of ascorbic acid and one molecule of dehydroascorbate. The latter can also be converted to ascorbic acid by thioredoxin-disulfide reductase (EC 1.8.1.9) or reduction by glutathione that may be enzymatically or nonenzymatically mediated.[242]

THERAPEUTIC USES

Vitamin C is indicated for the treatment and prevention of known or suspect deficiency. Although scurvy occurs infrequently, it is seen in the elderly, infants, alcoholics, and drug users. The array of symptoms associated with scurvy is thought to result from inadequate formation of the products of the key enzymatic reactions for which ascorbate is a cofactor. Especially notable are the derangements in connective tissue formation as a result of the effects on collagen synthesis leading to hemorrhaging, poor wound healing, and defects in bone and dentin. Ascorbate can also be used to enhance absorption of dietary nonheme iron or iron supplements. Ascorbic acid (but not the sodium salt) was historically used to acidify the urine as a result of excretion of unchanged ascorbic acid, although this use has fallen into disfavor. Ascorbate also increases iron chelation by deferoxamine, explaining its use in the treatment of iron toxicity. However, use of ascorbate can also enhance iron absorption, which could aggravate the original iron toxicity and so caution is advised. It is also a useful adjunct in the treatment of methemoglobinemia.

Ascorbic acid is an effective reducing agent and antioxidant; although the daily doses required to produce significant in vivo activity (>1 g) are much higher than the RDA (<100 mg). Because oxidative stress is thought to underlie many disease processes, there has been intense interest in utilizing high doses of the antioxidant vitamins to prevent or treat diseases unrelated to their role as vitamins. There are numerous studies that have examined the effects of vitamin C supplementation alone, or in combination with other vitamins and minerals, yet the only conclusion to be drawn is that there is no clear and convincing evidence that vitamin C is useful in the treatment or prevention of most major disease states. Systematic reviews have not found evidence for general use in the comon cold, cardiovascular disease in general, hypertension, atherosclerosis, cancer, preeclampsia, or overall mortality.[43,55,243,244]

HYPERVITAMINOSIS

High doses of vitamin C can lead to renal, bone, hematological, and gastrointestinal effects.[46] Renal calculi because of oxalate or urate result from enhanced renal excretion of these compounds in the presence of high doses of vitamin C. Increased release of calcium and phosphorus from bone have been observed. Hematological effects include increased absorption of nonheme iron without significant increases in total body iron stores. Diarrhea, likely resulting from an osmotic effect, has been reported following large doses, and ascorbic acid tablets that lodge in the esophagus can cause local erosion. Finally, ascorbic acid has been shown to interfere with several colorimetric redox assays because of its ability to act as a reducing agent.

PRODUCTS

Ascorbic acid is available as oral tablets, capsules, lozenges, crystals, and solutions from various manufacturers. It is also available as an injectable solution and as part

TABLE 28.12 **Ascorbate-Dependent Enzymes**

Enzyme	EC Number	Function
Gamma-butyrobetaine dioxygenase	1.14.11.1	Lysine degradation
Procollagen-proline dioxygenase	1.14.11.2	Collagen synthesis synthesis
Procollagen-lysine 5-dioxygenase	1.14.11.4	Collagen synthesis
Procollagen-proline 3-dioxygenase	1.14.11.7	Collagen synthesis
Trimethyllysine dioxygenase	1.14.11.8	Lysine degradation
Phytanoyl-CoA dioxygenase	1.14.11.18	Fatty acid metabolism
Dopamine beta-monooxygenase	1.14.17.1	Norepinephrine synthesis
Peptidylglycine monooxygenase	1.14.17.3	Peptide hormone synthesis

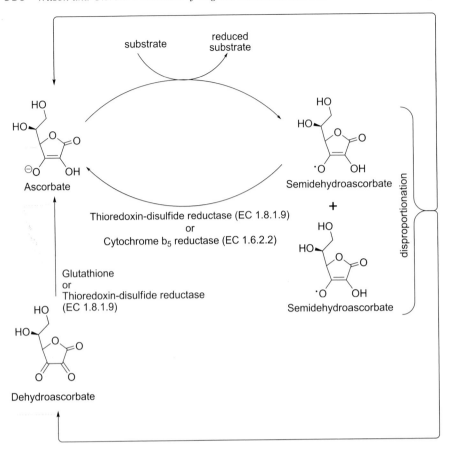

substrate

reduced substrate

Ascorbate

Semidehydroascorbate

Thioredoxin-disulfide reductase (EC 1.8.1.9)
or
Cytochrome b$_5$ reductase (EC 1.6.2.2)

+

Semidehydroascorbate

Glutathione
or
Thioredoxin-disulfide reductase
(EC 1.8.1.9)

disproportionation

Dehydroascorbate

Figure 28.50 ● Ascorbic acid cycle.

of innummerable multivitamin combinations under various names. Ascorbic acid is also available as the sodium salt in an injectable solution and as calcium ascorbate in oral tablets, granules, and powder. These two salts are also formulated into an assortment of multivitamin combinations sold under various names. Several other micronutrient salts of ascorbic acid, such as the potassium salt, are available. Ascorbyl palmitate (ascorbic acid 6 palmitate) is the C^6 palmitic acid ester of ascorbic acid (see Fig. 28.51). This ester of ascorbic acid is a fat-soluble form that releases ascorbic acid in the digestive tract following hydrolysis of the ester bond. Ascorbyl palmitate has also been used in topical preparations designed to protect the skin from UV radiation under the premise that the antioxidant properties,

in a manner similar to the oral use of ascorbic acid, would add to the protectant effects. However, there is evidence that its use in these preparations may actually lead to enhanced skin damage.[245]

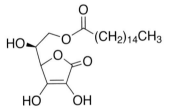

Figure 28.51 ● Ascorbyl palmitate.

● R E V I E W   Q U E S T I O N S ●

1. List the fat-soluble vitamins, the water-soluble vitamins, and the B-complex vitamins.

2. Explain the difference between enrichment and fortification.

3. How do most of the vitamins function? How else might some vitamins function?

4. Which vitamin is involved in proper function of the eye and how is it involved? Would you recommend retinoic acid (Tretinoin) for treatment of a defiency of this vitamin? Explain your reasoning.

5. Vitamin A is very toxic in high doses but the provitamin A carotenoids are not. Explain this difference.

6. Which vitamins can be made in humans and how are they synthesized?

7. Explain the sunlight-mediated production of vitamin D in the skin using structures when appropriate. Does excessive sunlight produce toxic levels of vitamin D?

8. What are tocols? Researchers have shown that all forms of tocols are absorbed from the intestine equally, yet

α-tocopherol is found in the circulation in the highest amounts. Why?

9. Which two vitamins are absorbed via the SMVT and can competitively inhibit each other?

10. What is a severe form of central neurological damage, with a high fatality rate, seen in alcoholics because of a severe vitamin deficiency? Name the vitamin.

11. Controversial results have been found with vitamin E use in cardiovascular diseases. Explain at least one possible chemical reason for this controversy.

12. Vitamin C is an antioxidant vitamin. Explain how the indiscriminate use of large doses may lead to renal, bone, hematological, and gastrointestinal effects.

13. Explain the role of vitamin K in the formation of Gla proteins. List the known biochemical roles of the Gla proteins.

14. Which vitamins have a role in bone mineralization?

15. Explain how leucovorin can treat overdoses of methotrexate, and other DHFR inhibitors, while folic acid is ineffective.

16. What is the danger of treating megaloblastic anemia empirically with folic acid?

17. What is the purpose of fortification of food with folic acid and what foods require fortification?

18. Niacin is used unrelated to its vitamin activity for what cardiovascular disorder? Would you recommend niacinamide instead of niacin for this use because it causes less side effects?

19. What is the major form of vitamin B_6 that takes part in enzymatic reactions? Which form is excreted in the urine? Which other forms of vitamin B_6 are known as active forms because they can be interconverted to the major form used in enzymatic reactions? List the types of reactions cocatalyzed by vitamin B_6.

20. What is pernicious anemia and what is the cause? What chemical form of the deficiency vitamin is most commonly given to treat pernicious anemia? When is this the form to use?

REFERENCES

1. NIH State-of-the-Science Panel: Ann. Intern. Med. 145:64–371, 2006.
2. Funk, C. J.: Physiol. 43:395–400, 1911.
3. Funk, C. J.: State Med. 20:341–368, 1912.
4. Hopkins, F. G.: J. Physiol. 44:425–460, 1912.
5. McCollum, E. V., and Davis, M. J.: Biol. Chem. 15:167–175, 1913.
6. McCollum, E. V., and Davis, M. J.: Biol. Chem. 19:245–250, 1914.
7. McCollum, E. V., and Davis, M. J.: Biol. Chem. 20:641–658, 1915.
8. McCollum, E. V., and Davis, M. J.: Biol. Chem. 21:179–182, 1915.
9. McCollum, E. V., and Kennedy, C. J.: Biol. Chem. 24:491–502, 1916.
10. Drummond, J. C.: Biochem. J. 13:77–80, 1919.
11. Drummond, J. C.: Biochem. J. 14:660, 1920.
12. Jansen, B. C.: Nature 135:267, 1935.
13. Title 21 Code of Federal Regulations, pt.101.9 2007.
14. Otten, J. J., Hellwig, J. P., and Meyers, L. D. (eds.): Dietary Reference Intakes: The Essential Guide to Nutrient Requirements. Washington D.C.: The National Academies Press, 2006, pp. 10–12.
15. King, J. C., and Garza, C.: Food Nutr. Bull. 28:S3–S12, 2007.
16. Karrer, P., Morf, R., and Schöpp, K.: Helv. Chim. Acta 14:1036–1040, 1931.
17. Heilbron, I. M., and Morton, R. A.: Biochem. J. 26:1194–1196, 1932.
18. Isler, O., Huber, W., Ronco, A., et al.: Helv. Chim. Acta 30:1911–1927, 1947.
19. Wald, G.: Science 162:230–239, 1968.
20. IUPAC-IUB Commission on Biochemical Nomenclature: Pure Appl. Chem. 55:721–726, 1983.
21. Liébecg, C.: Eur. J. Biochem. 247:733–739, 1997.
22. Blomhoff, R.: Nutr. Rev. 52(2 Pt 2):S13–S23, 1994.
23. Blomhoff, R., Green, M. H., Green, J. B., et al.: Physiol. Rev. 71:951–990, 1991.
24. Harrison, E. H.: Annu. Rev. Nutr. 25:87–103, 2005.
25. Wolf, G.: Nutr. Rev. 49:1–12, 1991.
26. Kloer, D. P., and Schulz, G. E.: Cell. Mol. Life Sci. 63:2291–2303, 2007.
27. Lindqvist, A., and Andersson, S. J.: Biol. Chem. 277:23942–23948, 2002.
28. Biesalski, H. K., Chichili, G. R., Frank, J., et al.: Vitam. Horm. 75:117–130, 2007.
29. Kiefer, C., Hessel, S., Lampert, J. M., et al.: J. Biol. Chem. 276:14110–14116, 2001.
30. Blomhoff, R., Green M. H., Berg T., et al.: Science 250:399–404, 1990.
31. Norum, K. R., and Blomhoff, R.: Am. J. Clin. Nutr. 56:734–744, 1992.
32. Senoo, H., Kojima, N., and Sato, M.: Vitam. Horm. 75:131–159, 2007.
33. Wolf, G.: Physiol. Rev. 64:873–937, 1984.
34. Lamb, T. D., and Pugh, E. N.: Prog. Retinal Eye Res. 23:307–380, 2004.
35. Imanishi, Y., Lodowski, K. H., and Koutalos, Y.: Biochemistry 46:9674–9684, 2007.
36. Blomhoff, R., and Blomhoff, H. K.: Neurobiol. 66:606–630, 2006.
37. Brtko, J., and Thalhamer, J.: Curr. Pharm. Des. 9:2067–2077, 2003.
38. Desvergne, B.: Vitam. Horm. 75:1–32, 2007.
39. Murphy, K. A., Quadro, L., and White, L. A.: Vitam. Horm. 75:33–67, 2007.
40. West, K. P., Jr.: Food Nutr. Bull. 24:S78–S90, 2003.
41. World Health Organization: Measles. Fact Sheet No. 286. January 2007.
42. Kanofsky, J. R., and Sima, P. D.: J. Photocem. Photobiol. B 87:124–129, 2007.
43. U.S. Preventive Services Task Force: Ann. Intern. Med. 139:51–55, 2003.
44. Fairfield, K. M., and Fletcher, R. H.: JAMA 287:3116–3126, 2002.
45. DiPalma, J. R., and Ritchie, D. M.: Annu. Rev. Pharmacol. Toxicol. 17:133–148, 1977.
46. Penniston, K. L., and Tanumihardjo, S. A.: Am. J. Clin. Nutr. 83:191–201, 2006.
47. Meyers, D. G., Maloley, P. A., and Weeks, D.: Arch. Intern. Med. 156:925–935, 1996.
48. Bendich, A., and Langseth, L.: Am. J. Clin. Nutr. 49:358–371, 1989.
49. Melhus, H., Michaëlsson, K., Kindmark, A., et al.: Ann. Intern. Med. 129:770–778, 1998.
50. Lammer, E. J., Chen, D. T., Hoar, R. M., et al.: N. Engl. J. Med. 313:837–841, 1985.
51. Rothman, K. J., Moore, L. L., Singer, M. R., et al.: N. Engl. J. Med. 21:1369–1373, 1995.
52. Jenkins, K. J., Correa, A., Feinstein, J. A., et al.: Circulation 115:2995–3014, 2007.

53. Diplock, A. T.: Am. J. Clin. Nutr. 62:1510S–1516S, 1995.
54. Micozzi, M. S., Brown, E. D., Taylor, P. R., et al.: Am. J. Clin. Nutr. 48:1061–1064, 1988.
55. Bjelakovic, G., Nikolova, D., Gluud, L. L., et al.: JAMA 297:842–857, 2007.
56. Mellanby, E., and Cantag, M. D.: Lancet 196:407–412, 1919.
57. Huldschinsky, K.: Dtsch. Med. Wochenschr. 45:712–713, 1919.
58. Funk, C., and Dubin, H. E.: Proc. Soc. Exp. Biol. Med. 19:15–16, 1921.
59. McCollum, E. V., Simmonds, N., and Becker, J. E.: J. Biol. Chem. 53:293–312, 1922.
60. Lythgoe, B., Nambudiry, M. E., and Tideswell, J.: Tetrahedron Lett. 18:3685–3688, 1977.
61. IUPAC-IUB Commission on Biochemical Nomenclature: Pure Appl. Chem. 54:1511–1516, 1982.
62. van den Berg, H.: Eur. J. Clin. Nutr. 51:S76–S79, 1997.
63. Saarem, K., Bergseth, S., Oftebro, H., et al.: J. Biol. Chem. 259:10936–10940, 1984.
64. Yagci, A., Werner, A., Murer, H., et al.: Pflugers Arch. 422:211–216, 1992.
65. Holick, M. F.: J. Invest. Dermatol. 77:51–58, 1981.
66. Bikle, D. D.: Sci. Med. 2:58–67, 1995.
67. DeLuca, H. F.: Nutr. Today 28:6–11, 1993.
68. Makin, G., Lohnes, D., Byford, V., et al.: Biochem. J. 262:173–180, 1989.
69. Reddy, G. S., and Tserng, K. Y.: Biochemistry 28:1763–1769, 1989.
70. Nagpal, S., Na, S., and Rathnachalam, R.: Endocrin. Rev. 26:662–687, 2005.
71. Ingraham, B. A., Bragdon, B., and Nohe, A.: Curr. Med. Res. Opin. 24:139–149, 2008.
72. Melamed, M. L., Michos, E. D., Post, W., et al.: Arch. Intern. Med. 168:1629–1637, 2008.
73. Dawson-Hughes, B., Heaney, R. P., Holick, M. F., et al.: Osteoporosis Int. 16:713–716, 2005.
74. Beer, T., and Myrthue, A.: Anticancer Res. 26:2647–2651, 2006.
75. Freedman, D. M., Looker, A. C., Chang, S. C., et al.: J. Natl. Cancer Inst. 99:1594–1602, 2007.
76. Wang, T. J., Pencina, M. J., Booth, S. L., et al.: Circulation 117:503–511, 2008.
77. Lind, L., Hänni, A., Lithell, H., et al.: Am. J. Hypertens. 8:894–901, 1995.
78. van de Kerkhof, P. C.: Skin Pharmacol. Appl. Skin Physiol. 11:2–10, 1998.
79. Fraser, D. R.: Lancet 345:104–107, 1995.
80. Hathcock, J. N., Shao, A., Vieth, R., et al.: Am. J. Clin. Nutr. 85:6–18, 2007.
81. Evans, H. M., and Bishop, K. S.: Science 56:650–651, 1922.
82. Sure, B.: J. Biol. Chem. 58:693–709, 1924.
83. Evans, H. M., Emerson, O. H., and Emerson, G. A.: J. Biol. Chem. 113:319–332, 1936.
84. Fernholz, E.: J. Am. Chem. Soc. 60:700–705, 1938.
85. Karrer, P., Fritzsche, H., and Ringier, B. H.: Helv. Chim. Acta 21:820–825, 1938.
86. IUPAC-IUB Joint Commission on Biochemical Nomenclature: Pure Appl. Chem. 54:1507–1510, 1982.
87. Demole, V., Isler, O., Ringier, B. H., et al.: Helv. Chim. Acta 22:65–68, 1939.
88. Karrer, P., and Bussmann, G.: Helv. Chim. Acta 23:1137–1138, 1940.
89. Rigotti, A.: Mol. Aspects Med. 28:423–436, 2007.
90. Borel, P., Pasquier, B., Armand, M., et al.: Am. J. Physiol. Gastrointest. Liver Physiol. 280:G95–G103, 2001.
91. Leonard, S. W., Good, C. K., Gugger, E. T., et al.: Am. J. Clin. Nutr. 79:86–92, 2004.
92. Mustacich, D. J., Bruno, R. S., and Traber, M. G.: Vitam. Horm. 76:1–21, 2007.
93. van Haaften, R. I., Evelo, C. T., Haenen, G. R., et al.: Biochem. Pharmacol. 61:715–719, 2001.
94. Moore, A. N., and Ingold, K. U.: Free Rad. Biol. Med. 22:931–934, 1997.
95. Sylvester, P. W.: Vitam. Horm. 76:329–355, 2007.
96. Sen, C. K., Khanna, S., Rink, C., et al.: Vitam. Horm. 76:203–261, 2007.
97. Bieri, J. G., and Farrell, P. M.: Vitam. Horm. 34:31–75, 1976.
98. Sesso, H. D., Buring, J. E., Christen, W. G., et al.: JAMA 300:2123–2133, 2008.
99. Christen, S., Woodall, A. A., Shigenaga, M. K., et al.: Proc. Natl. Acad. Sci. U. S. A. 94:3217–3222, 1997.
100. Slatore, C. G., Littman, A. J., Au, D. H., et al.: Am. J. Respir. Crit. Care Med. 177:524–530, 2008.
101. Neuzil, J., Tomasetti, M., Zhao, Y., et al.: Mol. Pharmacol. 71:1185–1199, 2007.
102. Dam, H.: Biochem. Z. 215:475–492, 1929.
103. Dam, H.: Biochem. J. 29:1273–1285, 1935.
104. MacCorquodale, D. W., Cheney, L. C., Binkley, S. B., et al.: J. Biol. Chem. 31:357–370, 1939.
105. Jackman, L. M., Rüegg, R., Ryser, G., et al.: Helv. Chim. Acta 48:1332–1349, 1965.
106. IUPAC Commission on the Nomenclature of Biological Chemistry: J. Am. Chem. Soc. 82:5575–5584, 1960.
107. IUPAC-IUB Commission on Biochemical Nomenclature: Pure Appl. Chem. 38:439–447, 1974.
108. Shearer, M. J., Barkhan, P., and Webster, G. R.: Br. J. Haematol. 18:297–308, 1970.
109. Gijsbers, B. L., Jie, K. G., and Vermeer, C.: Br. J. Nutr. 76:223–229, 1996.
110. Shearer, M. J., Bach, A., and Kohlmeier, M.: J. Nutr. 126:1181S–1186S, 1996.
111. Kohlmeier, M., Salomon, A., Saupe, J., et al.: J. Nutr. 126:1192S–1196S, 1996.
112. Esmon, C. T., Sadowski, J. A., and Suttie, J. W.: J. Biol. Chem. 250:4744–4748, 1975.
113. Stenflo, J., Fernlund, P., Egan, W., et al.: Proc. Natl. Acad. Sci. U. S. A. 71:2730–2733, 1974.
114. Nelsestuen, G. L., Zytkovicz, T. H., and Howard, J. B.: J. Biol. Chem. 249:6347–6350, 1974.
115. Sokoll, L. J., and Sadowski, J. A.: Am. J. Clin. Nutr. 63:566–573, 1996.
116. Suttie, J. W.: FASEB J. 7:445–452, 1993.
117. Olson, R. E., and Suttie, J. W.: Vitam. Horm. 35:59–108, 1977.
118. Dowd, P., Ham, S. W., and Geib, S. J.: J. Am. Chem. Soc. 113:7734–7743, 1991.
119. Dowd, P., Ham, S. W., and Hershline, R.: J. Am. Chem. Soc. 114:7613–7617, 1992.
120. Dowd, P., Hershline, R., Ham, S. W., et al.: Science 269:1684–1691, 1995.
121. Stenflo, J.: Semin. Thromb. Hemost. 10:109–121, 1984.
122. van Hinsbergh, V. W., Bertina, R. M., van Wijngaarden, A., et al.: Blood 65:444–451, 1985.
123. Castoldi, E., and Hackeng, T. M.: Curr. Opin. Hematol. 15:529–36, 2008.
124. Vasse, M.: J. Thromb. Haemost. 100:548–556, 2008.
125. Bügel, S.: Vitam. Horm. 78:393–416, 2008.
126. Stafford, D. W.: J. Thromb. Haemost. 3:1873–1878, 2005.
127. Nakano, T., Higashino, K., Kikuchi, N., et al.: J. Biol. Chem. 270:5702–5705, 1995.
128. Bellido-Martin, L., and de Frutos, P. G.: Vitam. Horm. 78:185–209, 2008.
129. Arai, H., Nagai, K., and Doi, T.: Vitam. Horm. 78:375–392, 2008.
130. Mizuta, T., and Ozaki, I.: Vitam. Horm. 78:435–442, 2008.
131. Mizuta, T., Ozaki, I., Eguchi, Y., et al.: Cancer 106:867–872, 2006.
132. Kulman, J. D., Harris, J. E., Haldeman, B. A., et al.: Proc. Natl. Acad. Sci. U. S. A. 94:9058–9062, 1997.
133. Kulman, J. D., Harris, J. E., Xie, L., et al.: Proc. Natl. Acad. Sci. U. S. A. 98:1370–1375, 2001.
134. Committee on Fetus and Newborn: Pediatrics 112:191–192, 2003.
135. Policy statement AAP publications reaffirmed, May 2006: Pediatrics 118:1266, 2006.
136. Emmett, A. D., and Luros, G. O.: J. Biol. Chem. 43:265–286, 1920.
137. Goldberger, J., and Lillie, R. D.: Public Health Rep. 41:1025–1029, 1926.
138. IUPAC-IUB Commission on Biochemical Nomenclature: J. Biol. Chem. 241:2987–2994, 1966.
139. Jansen, B. C., and Donath, W. F.: Proc. K. Ned. Akad. Wet. 29:1389–1400, 1926.
140. Williams, R. R., and Cline, J. K.: J. Am. Chem. Soc. 58:1504–1505, 1936.
141. Said, H. M., and Mohammed, Z. M.: Curr. Opin. Gastroenterol. 22:140–146, 2006.
142. Gregory, J. F.: Eur. J. Clin. Nutr. 53(Suppl 1):S34–S37, 1997.

143. Frank, R. A., Leeper, F. J., and Luisi, B. F.: Cell. Mol. Life Sci. 64:892–905, 2007.
144. Neufeld, E. J., Fleming, J. C., and Tartaglini, E.: Blood Cells Mol. Dis. 27:135–138, 2001.
145. Singleton, C. K., and Martin, P. R.: Curr. Mol. Med. 1:197–207, 2001.
146. Kuhn, R., György, P., and Wagner-Jauregg, T.: Naturwiss. 21:560–561, 1933.
147. Karrer, P., Schöpp, K., and Benz, F.: Helv. Chim. Acta 18:426–429, 1935.
148. Said, H. M.: Annu. Rev. Physiol. 66:419–446, 2004.
149. Bates, C. J.: Eur. J. Clin. Nutr. 51(Suppl 1):S38–S42, 1997.
150. Powers, H. J.: Am. J. Clin. Nutr. 77:1352–1360, 2003.
151. Funk, C.: J. Physiol. 46:173–179, 1913.
152. Goldberger, J., and Wheeler, G. A.: Public Health Rep. 43:172–217, 1928.
153. Elvehjem, C. A., Madden, R. J., Strong, F. M., et al.: J. Am. Chem. Soc. 59:1767–1768, 1937.
154. Fouts, P. J., Helmer, O. M., Lepkovsky, S., et al.: Proc. Soc. Exp. Biol. Med. 37:405–406, 1937.
155. van den Berg, H.: Eur. J. Clin. Nutr. 51(Suppl 1):S64–S65, 1997.
156. Nabokina, S. M., Kashyap, M. L., and Said, H. M.: Am. J. Physiol. Cell Physiol. 289:C97–C103, 2005.
157. Altschul, R., Hoffer, A., and Stephen, J. D.: Arch. Biochem. Biophys. 54:558–559, 1955.
158. Kamanna, V. S., and Kashyap, M. L.: Am. J. Cardiol. 101:20B–26B, 2008.
159. Gille, A., Bodor, E. T., Ahmed, K., et al.: Annu. Rev. Pharmacol. Toxicol. 48:79–106, 2008.
160. McKenney, J. M., Proctor, J. D., Harris, S., et al.: JAMA 271:672–677, 1994.
161. Alhadeff, L., Gualtieri, C. T., and Lipton, M.: Nutr. Rev. 42:33–40, 1984.
162. Alsheikh-Ali, A. A., and Karas, R. H.: Am. J. Cardiol. 101 (Suppl):9B–13B, 2008.
163. Carter, C. W., Kinnersley, H. W., and Peters, R. A.: Biochem. J. 24:1844–1851, 1930.
164. Williams, R. J., Lyman, C. M., Goodyear, G. H., et al.: J. Am. Chem. Soc. 55:2912–2927, 1933.
165. Williams, R. J., and Major, R. T.: Science 91:246, 1940.
166. van den Berg, H.: Eur. J. Clin. Nutr. 51:S62–S63, 1997.
167. Prasad, P. D., and Ganapathy, V.: Curr. Opin. Clin. Nutr. Metab. Care 3:263–266, 2000.
168. Spry, C., Kirk, K., and Saliba, K. J.: FEMS Microbiol. Rev. 32:56–106, 2008.
169. Fry, P. C., Fox, H. M., and Tao, H. G.: J. Nutr. Sci. Vitaminol. 22:339–346, 1976.
170. Tahiliani, A. G., and Beinlich, C. J.: Vitam. Horm. 46:165–228, 1991.
171. György, P.: Nature 133:498–499, 1934.
172. Lepkovsky, S.: Science 87:169–170, 1938.
173. György, P.: J. Am. Chem. Soc. 60:983–984, 1938.
174. Keresztesy, J. C., and Stevens, J. R.: J. Am. Chem. Soc. 60:1267–1268, 1938.
175. Stiller, E. T., Keresztesy, J. C., and Stevens, J. R.: J. Am. Chem. Soc. 61:1237–1242, 1939.
176. Stiller, E. T., Keresztesy, J. C., and Stevens, J. R.: J. Am. Chem. Soc. 61:1242–1244, 1939.
177. Harris, S. A., and Folkers, K.: J. Am. Chem. Soc. 61:1245–1247, 1939.
178. György, P., and Eckhardt, R. E.: Nature 144:512, 1939.
179. Snell, E. E., Guirard, B. M., and Williams, R. J.: J. Biol. Chem. 143:519–530, 1942.
180. IUPAC-IUB Commission on Biochemical Nomenclature: Pure Appl. Chem. 33:445–452, 1973.
181. Gregory, J. F.: Eur. J. Clin. Nutr. 51(Suppl 1):S43–S48, 1997.
182. Said, H. M., Ortiz, A., and Ma, T. Y.: Am. J. Physiol. Cell Physiol. 285:C1219–C1225, 2003.
183. Bender, D. A.: Eur. J. Clin. Nutr. 43:289–309, 1989.
184. Spinneker, A., Sola, R., Lemmen, V., et al.: Nutr. Hosp. 22:7–24, 2007.
185. Coburn, S. P.: Ann. N. Y. Acad. Sci. 585:76–85, 1990.
186. Snell, E.: Vitam. Horm. 16:77–125, 1958.
187. Percudani, R., and Peracchi, A.: EMBO Rep. 4:850–854, 2003.
188. Ink, S. L., and Henderson, L. M.: Ann. Rev. Nutr. 4:455–470, 1984.
189. Schaumburg, H., Kaplan, J., Windebank, A., et al.: N. Engl. J. Med. 309:445–448, 1983.
190. Parry, G. J., and Bredesen, D. E.: Neurology 35:1466–1468, 1985.
191. Kögl, F., and Tönnis, B.: Z. Physiol. Chem. 242:43–73, 1936.
192. du Vigneaud, V., Melville, D. B., Folkers, K., et al.: J. Biol. Chem. 146:475–485, 1942.
193. Staggs, C. G., Sealey, W. M., McCabe, B. J., et al.: J. Food Compost. Anal. 17(6):767–776, 2004.
194. Marquet, A., and Bui, B. T.: Vitam. Horm. 61:51– 101, 2001.
195. Zempleni, J., and Mock, D.: J. Nutr. 129:494S–497S, 1999.
196. Attwood, P. V., and Wallace, J. C.: Acc. Chem. Res. 35:113–120, 2002.
197. Gravel, R. A., and Narang, M. A.: J. Nutr. Biochem. 16:428–431, 2005.
198. Mock, D. M., Baswell, D. L., Baker, H., et al.: Ann. N. Y. Acad. Sci. 447:314–334, 1985.
199. Scott, D.: Acta Med. Scand. 162:69–70, 1958.
200. IUPAC-IUB Joint Commission on Biochemical Nomenclature: Pure Appl. Chem. 59:833–836, 1987.
201. Mitchell, H. K., Snell, E. E., and Williams, R. J.: J. Am. Chem. Soc. 63:2284, 1941.
202. Pfiffner, J. J., Binkley, S. B., Bloom, E. S., et al.: Science 97:404–405, 1943.
203. Angier, R. B., Booth, J. H., Hutchings, B. L., et al.: Science 103:667–669, 1946.
204. Title 21 Code of Federal Regulations, pt. 136, 137, 139, 2007.
205. Choumenkovitch, S. F., Selhub, J., Wilson, P. W., et al.: J. Nutr. 132:2792–2798, 2002.
206. Dietrich, M., Brown, C., and Block, G.: J. Am. Coll. Nutr. 24:266–274, 2005.
207. Gangjee, A., Jain, H. D., and Kurup, S.: Anticancer Agents Med. Chem. 7:524–542, 2007.
208. ACOG Committee on Practice Bulletins: Obstet. Gynecol. 102:203–213, 2003.
209. Pitkin, R. M.: Am. J. Clin. Nutr. 85:285S–288S, 2007.
210. Wang, X., Qin, X., Demirtas, H., et al.: Lancet 1876–1882, 2007.
211. Bazzano, L. A., Reynolds, K., Holder, K. N., et al.: JAMA 296:2720–2726, 2006.
212. Kim, Y.: Mol. Nutr. Food Res. 51:267–292, 2007.
213. Hunter, R., Barnes, J., Oakeley, H. F., et al.: Lancet 1(7637):61–63, 1970.
214. IUPAC-IUB Commission on Biochemical Nomenclature: Pure Appl. Chem. 48:495–502, 1976.
215. Addison, T.: On the Constitutional and Local Effects of Disease of the Suprarenal Capsules. London, Samuel Highley, 1955.
216. Minot, G. R., and Murphy, W. P.: JAMA 87:470–476, 1926.
217. Shorb, M. S.: J. Biol. Chem. 169:455–456, 1947.
218. Smith, E. L.: Nature 161:638–639, 1948.
219. Rickes, E. L., Brink, N. G., Koniuszy, F. R., et al.: Science 107:396–397, 1948.
220. Hodgkin, D. C., Pickworth, J., Robertson, J. H., et al.: Nature 176:325–328, 1955.
221. Bonnett, R., Cannon, J. R., Johnson, A. W., et al.: Nature 176:328–330, 1955.
222. Woodward, R. B.: Pure Appl. Chem. 33:145–178, 1973.
223. Seetharam, B.: Annu. Rev. Nutr. 19:173–195, 1999.
224. Okuda, K.: J. Gastroenterol. Hepatol. 14:301–308, 1999.
225. Scott, J. M.: Eur. J. Clin. Nutr. 51(Suppl 1):S49–S53, 1997.
226. Cooper, B. A., and Rosenblatt, D. S.: Ann. Rev. Nutr. 7:291–320, 1987.
227. Bigby, M., Jick, S., Jick, H., et al.: JAMA 256:3358–3363, 1986.
228. Ugwu, C.: Age Ageing 10:196–197, 1981.
229. Hovding, G.: Br. Med. J. 3:102, 1968.
230. Shepherd, G.: Ann. Pharmacother. 42:661–669.
231. Carpenter, K. J.: The history of scurvy and vitamin C, New Rochelle, NY, Cambridge University Press, 1986.
232. King, C. G., and Waugh, W. A.: Science 75:357–358, 1932.
233. Waugh, W. A., and King, C. G.: J. Biol. Chem. 97:325–331, 1932.
234. Svirbely, J. L., and Szent-Györgyi, A.: Biochem. J. 26:865–870, 1932.
235. Svirbely, J. L., and Szent-Györgyi, A.: Biochem. J. 27:279–285, 1933.
236. Szent-Györgyi, A.: Biochem. J. 22:1387–1409, 1928.
237. Hirst, E. L.: J. Soc. Chem. Ind. 2:221–222, 1933.
238. Ault, R. G., Baird, D. K., Carrington, H. C., et al.: J. Chem. Soc. 1419–1423, 1933.
239. Reichstein, T., Grüssner, A., and Oppenauer, R.: Helv. Chim. Acta 16:1019–1033, 1933.

240. Sato, P., and Udenfriend, S.: Vitam. Horm. 36:33–52, 1978.
241. Wilson, J. X.: Annu. Rev. Nutr. 25:105–25, 2005.
242. Linster, C. L., and Schaftingen, E. V.: FEBS J. 274:1–22, 2007.
243. Douglas, R. M., Hemilä, H., Chalker, E., et al.: Vitamin C for preventing and treating the common cold (Cochrane Review). In The Cochrane Library, Issue 3, 2007.
244. Rodrigo, R., Guichard, C., and Charles, R.: Fundam. Clin. Pharmacol. 21:111–127, 2007.
245. Meves, A., Stock, S. N., Beyerle, A., et al.: J. Invest. Dermatol. 119:1103–1108, 2002.

SELECTED READING

Otten, J. J., Hellwig, J. P., and Meyers, L. D. (eds.): Dietary Reference Intakes: The Essential Guide to Nutrient Requirements. Washington D.C., The National Academies Press, 2006.
Block, J. H.: Vitamins. In Abraham, D. J. (ed.). Burger's Medicinal Chemistry & Drug Discovery, 6th ed. Hoboken, John Wiley and Sons, Inc. 2003, pp. 359–420.
Leid, M.: Retinoids. In Abraham, D. J. (ed.). Burger's Medicinal Chemistry & Drug Discovery, 6th ed. Hoboken, John Wiley and Sons, Inc. 2003, pp. 317–358.

An Introduction to the Medicinal Chemistry of Herbs

JOHN M. BEALE, JR.

CHAPTER OVERVIEW

According to the World Health Organization, approximately 80% of the world's population uses herbal drugs as part of their normal healthcare routine.[1] The United States is no exception. In the United States, herbal medicines represent the fastest-growing segment of pharmacy trade.[2] Self-medication with herbs cuts across all educational and affluence levels. Senior citizens as well as young, health-conscious persons are using herbs at an incredible rate. The reasons for herbal use are many and certainly cannot be fully enumerated here. Possibly, herbal users desire to assume control over their own healthcare needs. Perhaps the large, "impersonal" healthcare system is unpalatable to many, and they turn to herbal medicines as an alternative. Patients may feel alienated by increasingly busy physicians who have less time to spend with them, and they may turn to herbal drugs because they feel that they can gain some control.

Obviously, if people are going to use herbals as part of their healthcare routine, they must find out about the herbs and what they do. There is no doubt that a definite major factor affecting herbal use is advertising targeted very successfully to specific populations, such as the young professional or the senior citizen. Such advertising is mere pseudoscience, but its flamboyance is a big drawing factor. Herbal ads often convey an attitude that self-medication is safe and effective, and this makes people feel good and as if they do not need the physician who just saw them for 5 minutes. People also tend to believe that natural products are inherently better than synthetic drugs. The natural drugs somehow contain the "vital force" that is going to improve their health. This is actually a belief in the vitalism principle, which Wöhler disproved in 1828.[3] Tyler puts this issue into clear terms: "If it comes in a shrinkwrap, safety-sealed box, or a bottle with a childproof lid, it is not harvested freshly from the earth. It is a manufactured industrial product, no matter how many flowers adorn the wrapper, no matter how many times the label invokes the word 'nature.'"[4]

Certainly, the cost of medical care cannot be overlooked when considering the reasons for interest in alternative forms of medicine. Most herbal medicines are far less expensive than prescription drugs. There is danger, however, in self-medicating with herbal drugs. The old adage that "he who tries to diagnose himself has a fool for a physician" becomes very apropos with herbal medicine. When prescription drugs are dispensed, a patient has access to the information that is available from the physician or pharmacist. This is often not the case with herbal medicinals. In the United States, training of healthcare professionals in the use of herbal drugs has been nearly nonexistent for years. Hence, herbal users are left to their own devices regarding choice, safety, and quality of the herb chosen.

HISTORICAL ASPECTS

Until 1882,[5] several drugs were monographed and described in the *United States Pharmacopoeia* (*USP*). Ginseng, for example, was clearly characterized as a drug and could be labeled and described to patients as such. Today, the Food and Drug Administration (FDA) calls ginseng, legally, a "food for beverage use." Outside the United States, it is common to find ginseng recommended for many different medical conditions.[6] At the time of the 1882 *USP* and into the early 1900s, pharmacists were well trained in the use, preparation, and dispensing of herbals and could advise patients on their herbal selection. This is not always the case today.

The convoluted regulatory efforts that began in 1906 and continue today are well described by Tyler.[7] A group of herbs had been grandfathered against the Federal Food, Drug, and Cosmetic Act of 1938 and the Kefauver-Harris Amendments of 1962. Most purveyors of herbs assumed that these herbs would continue to be salable with the indications on the label—in other words, marketed as drugs. The FDA declared that all of these grandfathered drugs would be considered misbranded and subject to confiscation if any claims of efficacy were not in accordance with the evaluations of 1 of 17 over-the-counter (OTC) drug evaluation panels that had operated between 1972 and 1990. The net result was that it became possible to sell herbal drugs only if no statements regarding prevention or treatment of a disease state were on the label. The FDA assigned three categories into which herbs were placed. Category I[8] (effective) contains only a select few herbal drugs. These are mostly laxatives such as cascara bark and senna leaf (although as Tyler points out, prune juice is excluded). Category II (unsafe or ineffective) contained 142 herbs, and category III (insufficient evidence to judge) contains 116. As applied to herbs and, in fact, the entire OTC classification, the judgments of the FDA have been harmful and nonscientific.

For the most part, herbal manufacturers decided not to fight the FDA and merely removed the disease- or condition-specific information from the labels and continued to sell the herbs as foods or nutritional supplements. With regard to using herbs as food additives, the FDA has maintained a list of substances "generally recognized as safe" (the GRAS list).[9] The list contains about 250 herbs, primarily relating to their use in beverages and cooking and as food additives. The list, of course, contains no references to herbs as drugs.

In 1990, the Nutrition Labeling and Education Act required consistent, scientifically based labeling on all processed foods. Herbal medicines were still left in limbo. Finally, in 1994, the Dietary Safety Health and Education Act included herbal medicines in the definition of dietary supplements. The act ensures consumers' access to supplements on the market as long as they are safe, and it allows structure and function claims on the label. Despite all of these legislative efforts, herbal drugs have been relegated to the grocery shelf as dietary supplements. They are sold with little or no instruction, and the public has no way of ascertaining purity, standardization, or legitimacy of the use for which the product is sold. Indeed, there is more information on the label of a tube of toothpaste than on a bottle of an herbal drug. Herbal manufacturing companies are making efforts to improve products along these lines, but there is a long way to go. Until testing can be done to prove that herbs are safe and effective, they will probably remain in their present circumstances.

For many years, medicinal chemistry was paired with a science called *pharmacognosy*,[10] a course of study of plants with medicinal uses and analytical techniques for detecting active ingredients. Pharmacognosy was an important science, because many of the pharmaceuticals used in the treatment of disease are discovered through the study of ethnobotanical leads and laboratory research. This course of study gave pharmacists the training required to understand, recommend, and counsel on herbs. Today, pharmacognosy is no longer required in most schools, and most practicing pharmacists and physicians have little understanding of herbs.

Medicinal herbs are unlike anything else that appears in the chapters of this book. Although they are unquestionably drugs (a fact that many sellers of herbs will dispute), they are not pure substances. Indeed, most herbal preparations contain many different constituents. Ephedra complex, or *ma huang*, is a sympathomimetic that contains five or six different β-phenethylamine derivatives. At least one of these, (+)-norpseudoephedrine, is a Schedule IV compound. The alkaloid content[11–13] varies widely in commercial ephedra-containing preparations. In one study, for one single product, lot-to-lot variations in the content of (−)-ephedrine, (+)-pseudoephedrine, and (−)-methylephedrine exceeded 180%, 250%, and 1,000%, respectively.[11] Total alkaloid content among 20 products ranged from 0.0 to 18.5 mg/dosage unit, and discrepancies were exhibited between the labeled contents and actual measurements.[12] Another study assayed nine products and found that total alkaloid levels ranged from 0.3 to 56 mg/g of ephedra.[13]

Unlike the situation with ephedra, in many cases, we simply have no idea what the components do. The constituents of some herbal drugs seem to work synergistically and cannot be separated without loss of activity of the preparation. Herbal preparations are most often used as crude mixtures and are not standardized or analyzed for the content of the active principle(s). Hence, the chemistry of medicinal herbs cannot be treated in the same way as that of, say, a pure antibiotic or a calcium channel blocker. The medicinal chemistry of the actions, interactions, and side effects of herbal products is complex and difficult to assess clinically and chemically. Frequently, some of the compounds present in a given herb can be identified, but there may be no obvious way to correlate chemical structure with function. Often, assessment of structure–function relationships with herbal products involves a lot of guessing.

WHAT IS AN HERB?

An herb is a substance of plant origin that, according to one's desires, can be used for culinary or medicinal purposes.[14] Obviously, some are more suited to culinary than medicinal uses, but most herbal substances have some identifiable medicinal use. As mentioned in the previous section, a typical herb may contain dozens of different compounds, so it has rarely been advantageous to separate an herb into its component parts. In fact, doing so may completely inactivate the drug. In an herbal mixture, some compounds can reinforce others and vice versa. It is impossible to predict what will happen. In relatively few cases has the active ingredient of an herb been isolated, characterized thoroughly, and tested for activity. We are left with a situation in which herbs are used in crude form as powders, fluidextracts, and teas. This should not be misconstrued to mean that analysis of herb components is useless. On the contrary, it is essential but just is not done often enough.

HERBAL PURITY AND STANDARDIZATION

In the United States, the issues of herbal purity and adulteration have been neglected for years. Because herbs are not regulated in the United States the same way they are in other countries, the pressure to ensure lot-to-lot standardization and to screen out plant adulterants has been less than optimal. Instances have been reported in the literature[11] in which several bottles of an herb purchased in the same location possessed different concentrations of active ingredient. Ephedra and ginseng are notable examples. Another example is echinacea. This herb is occasionally adulterated with a plant that looks very similar to *Echinacea angustifolia* but has none of the activity of echinacea. Plant parts, insect parts, soil, etc. can all be adulterants. Fortunately, pressure on the herb-producing industry has caused a markedly increased effort to screen and standardize herbs for trade. Possibly, simple high-performance liquid chromatography (HPLC) methods could be used to verify the herb's quality if the time were taken to obtain them. A chromatogram could be supplied to the purchaser to show the purity of the herb. Nevertheless, remember that an herb is a crude material containing multiple pharmacologically active compounds.

AN HERB IS A DRUG

Despite the regulations, an herbal preparation possesses the properties of a drug, albeit a mild one in many cases, and should be treated as such. It is pharmacologically active. It interacts with prescription drugs. It affects the health of the person taking it. Advertisers often tout herbs as "nondrugs" in an attempt to lure consumers. Pharmacists should be cognizant of the truth that herbs are real drugs and that their patients may be self-medicating with them. This practice may affect the outcome of therapy with prescription drugs. For example, suppose a patient is stabilized on Coumadin and starts to take ginkgo. Ginkgo affects platelet-activating factor (PAF)[15] and can effectively cause an overdose effect with Coumadin, and the patient can bleed. Or, suppose a patient taking a monoamine oxidase inhibitor (MAOI) decides to take St. John's wort; the patient may have a toxic reaction.[16] Because pharmacists often do not see what their patients are buying, this is a complex problem.

The herbal drugs available to consumers are far too numerous to discuss in this chapter. This section presents a few of the more commonly used herbs along with their chemistry. Information on other herbs can easily be found in the literature.

⬡ TYPES OF HERBS

Echinacea

The medicinal herb that we call *echinacea*, or the purple coneflower, is indigenous to the Great Plains of the United States and, indeed, can be found in much of the Western Hemisphere. The plant gets its name (coneflower) from the narrow florets, which project downward in a conical array from a prominent center toward a substantial stem that bears one flower. Today, the herb is used as an immunostimulant,[17] as a means of lessening the symptoms and duration of a cold or the flu, and sometimes as a wound healer. Recent reports show that echinacea is the best-selling herb in the United States.[3] Folklore[18] tells us that Native Americans used *E. angustifolia* to treat superficial wounds, snakebite, and the common cold. In the latter part of the 19th century, settlers exchanged information about medicines with the Indians and added echinacea to their own "pharmacopoeia." Echinacea even became one of the first patent medicines, sold by a huckster in Missouri at midcentury. In the early 1900s, echinacea was introduced to the European continent, where it occupies a special place in medical therapy. One estimate stated that, in Germany alone, there are 800 echinacea-containing drugs, including several homeopathic preparations.[19]

Three species are identified as echinacea[20]: *E. angustifolia*, *Echinacea pallida*, and *Echinacea purpurea*. All are used for medicinal purposes, and they have similar properties. There are slight differences among the species with regard to the anatomical distribution of active constituents.

CHEMISTRY

There is no doubt that echinacea has immunomodulating properties. The chemistry of the constituents of the plant has been studied extensively, but it is difficult to correlate a major activity with any plant fraction. Indeed, no single component appears to be responsible for the activity of echinacea. Standardization of echinacea preparations has also proved to be a problem. The consumer is presented with three potential preparations sold under the name "echinacea": *E. purpurea*, *E. angustifolia*, and *E. pallida*. Some medicinal preparations are from the roots (all three species), some from the aerial parts (*E. purpurea*), and some from the whole plant (homeopathic mother tinctures of *E. angustifolia* and *E. pallida*).[20] Another factor that affects the compo-

sition of echinacea preparations is the way in which they are extracted. Expressed juices, teas, hydroalcoholic extracts, and tinctures in alcohol are used, as well as solids. It is rarely possible to obtain reproducibility in these preparations.

In 1916, the National Formulary of the United States listed the roots of both *E. angustifolia* and *E. pallida* as official, and the distinction between the two began to be forgotten. In about 1950, *E. purpurea* was introduced as the primary medicinal plant in Europe. Of the three species, *E. pallida* is the most widely cultivated, the tallest, and has the largest flowers. This is considered the official preparation in the United States. *E. purpurea* root preparations are sometimes adulterated with a similar-looking plant called *Parthenium integrifolium*. HPLC analysis can easily detect the adulteration.[21] This shows how difficult it is to standardize echinacea preparations. Additionally, opinions differ about which plant component is the best for analytical standardization of the drug. Echinacea contains a series of phenylpropanoid glycosides, echinacoside, verbascoside, and 6-*O*-caffeoyl echinacoside (Fig. 29.1).[22,23] These compounds possess no immunostimulating activity. Some argue that the caffeoyl glycoside echinacoside should be the standard, because it is easy to detect and quantitate; others feel that it makes little sense to standardize the echinacea preparation to a compound that has no medicinal activity.

Several fractions of echinacea have been isolated according to polarity and studied for pharmacological activity. The most polar components, the polysaccharides, yielded two immunostimulatory polysaccharides, PS1 and PS2.[24] These stimulate phagocytosis in vivo and in vitro and cause a burst of production of oxygen radicals by macrophages in a dose-dependent way. PS1 is a 4-*O*-methylglucuronoarabinxylan with a molecular weight (MW) of 35,000. PS2 is an acidic arabinorhamnogalactan with an average MW of 45,000. Luettig et al.[25] have shown that different concentrations of polysaccharides from *E. purpurea* could stimulate macrophages to release tumor necrosis factor-α (TNF-α). These constituents also activate B cells and stimulate the production of interleukin-1. Three glycoproteins have also been isolated that exhibit B-cell–stimulating activity and induce the release of interleukin-1, TNF-α, and interferon (IFN) from macrophages, both in vitro and in vivo.[22]

Alcoholic tinctures of the aerial parts and roots of echinacea contain caffeic acid derivatives (Fig. 29.2) and

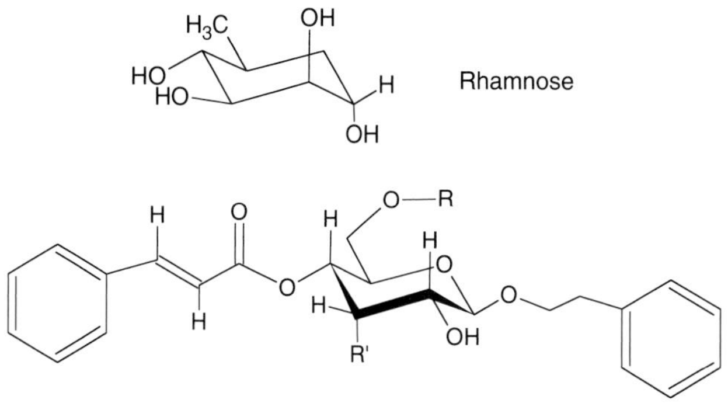

Echinacoside	R=Glucose (1,6-)	R'=Rhamnose (1,3)-
Verbascoside	R=H	R'=Rhamnose (1,3)-
6-*O*-Caffeoylglycoside	R=6-*O*-caffeoylglucose	R'=Rhamnose (1,3)-

Figure 29.1 ● Chemical constituents of *Echinacea*.

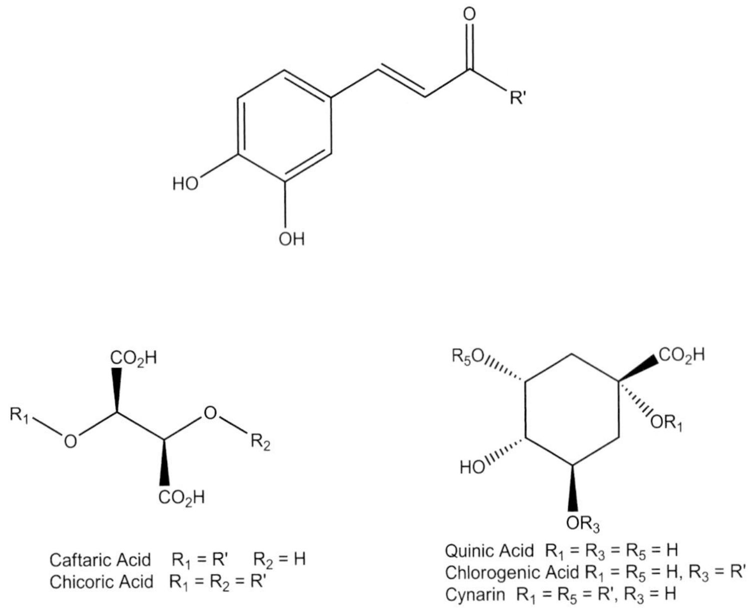

Caftaric Acid $R_1 = R'$ $R_2 = H$
Chicoric Acid $R_1 = R_2 = R'$

Quinic Acid $R_1 = R_3 = R_5 = H$
Chlorogenic Acid $R_1 = R_5 = H$, $R_3 = R'$
Cynarin $R_1 = R_5 = R'$, $R_3 = H$

Figure 29.2 • Caffeic acid derivatives in *Echinacea*.

lipophilic, polyacetylenic compounds (Fig. 29.3). The roots of *E. angustifolia* and *E. pallida* contain 0.3% to 1.7% echinacoside[26] as the principal conjugate in the plant. *E. angustifolia* contains 1,5-*O*-dicaffeoyl quinic acids (quinic, chlorogenic, and cynarin)[27] in the root tissue, allowing distinction by HPLC. Echinacoside has low bacterial and viral activity but does not stimulate the immune system. The most important set of compounds that seem to be found throughout the tissues of all of the echinacea species are the 2,3-*O*-dicaffeoyl tartaric acids, caftaric acid, and chicoric acid.[28] Chicoric acid possesses phagocytic stimulatory activity in vitro and in vivo, whereas echinacoside lacks this activity. Chicoric acid also inhibits hyaluronidase and protects collagen type III from free-radical degradation.

The alkamides[29] (Fig. 29.3) from the roots and flowers of *E. angustifolia* and *E. purpurea* stimulate phagocytosis in model animal systems. There are a host of these compounds distributed throughout the aerial parts of some *Echinacea* species and the roots of most. One such compound, echinacein,[28] displays sialogogue and insect repellent properties and is believed to be the main immunostimulant in echinacea. The alkamides and ketoalkynes[29,30] may very well possess activity. One notable effect is the anti-inflammatory effect of a high–molecular-weight arabinogalactan that is about as potent as indomethacin.[25] The lipophilic fractions, the alkamides, stimulate phagocytosis and inhibit 5-lipoxygenase and cyclooxygenase (COX), blocking the inflammatory process.

It is clear that echinacea can stimulate components of the innate immune system, but no single component seems to be responsible for the effect. Echinacea, if taken at the onset of symptoms of a cold or flu, will lessen the severity of the disease. It is not recommended that one use echinacea longer than 10 to 14 days, however, and persons younger than the age of 12 and those who are immunocompromised should never use this herb.

Feverfew

Feverfew, *Tanacetum parthenium* (L.) Schultz Bip,[31] is an herb that was used in antiquity to reduce fever and pain. The

literature is replete with anecdotal evidence of the usefulness of the herb, and recent clinical studies have added more support. Feverfew is a member of the aster/daisy family. The plant tissues have a pungent smell and very bitter taste. The medicinal principle of feverfew is concentrated in hairy trichomes on the chrysanthemum-like leaves.[32] The plant displays clusters of daisylike flowers with yellow centers and radiating white florets. Recent uses of feverfew are for migraine and arthritis, although the indication for arthritis is disputable. The anecdotal evidence that an herb could successfully treat a condition such as migraine headache, naturally begged for some scientific proof.

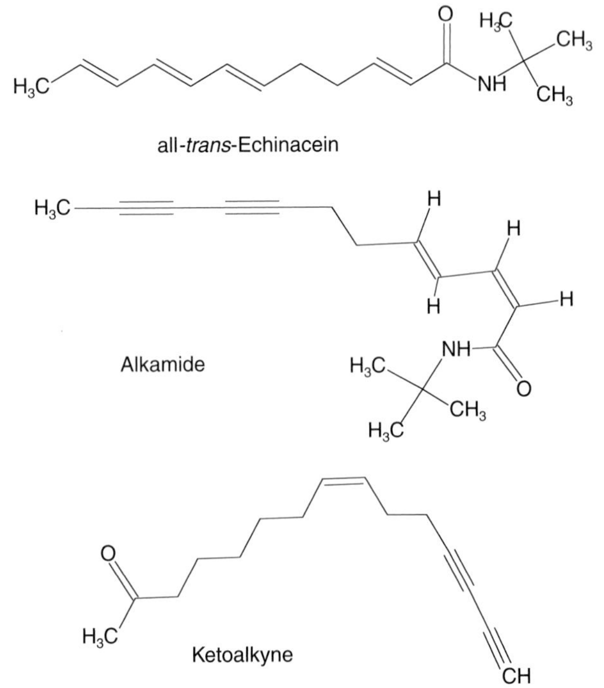

all-*trans*-Echinacein

Alkamide

Ketoalkyne

Figure 29.3 • Lipophilic, polyacetylenic constituents of *Echinacea*.

Two prospective clinical studies using dried whole feverfew leaf have been performed[33,34] to assess the value of the herb in migraine. The two leaf studies on migraine provided good supportive evidence for activity of the herb against migraine. Both studies were double-blinded, placebo-controlled, and standardized on 0.54-mg parthenolide per capsule. In both studies, the feverfew group demonstrated significant decreases in frequency, severity of attacks, and nausea and vomiting. No adverse effects were observed of the nonsteroidal anti-inflammatory drug (NSAID) type.

MECHANISM OF ACTION

Feverfew inhibits prostaglandin synthesis, but not through an effect on COX.[35] The herb also inhibits the synthesis of thromboxane, again by a COX-independent mechanism. Additionally, feverfew inhibits the synthesis of phospholipase A_2 in platelets,[36,37] preventing the liberation of arachidonic acid from membrane phospholipids for subsequent conversion to prostaglandins and thromboxane. Feverfew also inhibits the adenosine diphosphate (ADP)-, collagen-, and thrombin-induced aggregation of platelets, suggesting that the herb has a greater thrombotic effect. In another similar study, dried leaves of feverfew inhibited prostaglandin and thromboxane synthesis in platelets and inhibited platelet aggregation initiated by ADP and collagen.[38] Surprisingly, this study showed that feverfew inhibited the platelet-release reaction by which intracellular storage granules are released.[39] These storage granules contain serotonin, a positive effector in migraine headache. Some of the more surprising findings for feverfew are that it appears to be a selective inhibitor of inducible COX-2,[40] and it has clear effects on vascular tone in animal models.

The pharmacologically active constituent in feverfew has typically been considered to be parthenolide,[41] an amphiphilic sesquiterpene lactone that is biosynthesized from the germacranolide cation. Parthenolide is present in much

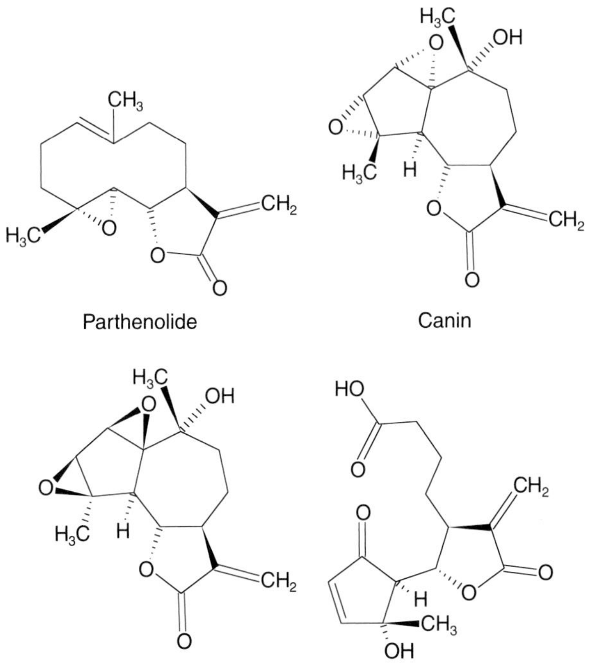

3-β-Hydroxyparthenolide

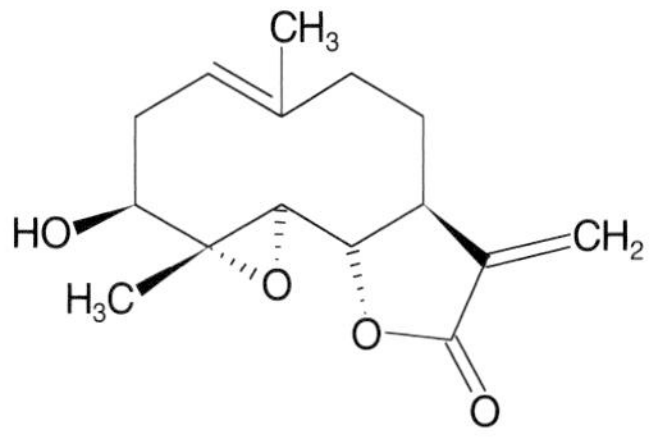

Figure 29.5 ● Chemical constituents of feverfew.

greater quantities than any of the other constituents, and its presence does seem to correlate with activity, at least in dried leaves. Parthenolide is an α-methylene lactone,[42] an α,β-unsaturated molecule that can serve as an acceptor in the Michael reaction. In the Michael reaction, a donor nucleophile such as a thiol can attack the acceptor to form a covalent adduct. If parthenolide functions this way, a biological nucleophile such as a thiol on an enzyme could be bound, inactivating that enzyme. The likelihood of this mechanism has been shown by successfully forming adducts with parthenolide itself in vivo.[43,44] The other components—canin, artecanin, secotanaparthenolide, and 3-β-hydroxyparthenolide (Figs. 29.4 and 29.5) are present in lower concentrations.[45] Their effects may be important to the activity of feverfew, but this is impossible to judge at present. One study that used an extract of the leaf with known parthenolide content failed to show activity, so questions still remain.

Saint John's Wort

Saint John's wort (*Hypericum perforatum*) is a medicinal herb that has been used since the time of Paracelsus (1493–1541) to treat various psychiatric disorders. Today, the herb remains one of the most important psychotropic drugs in Germany and Western Europe for the treatment of depression, anxiety, and nervousness.[46] The drug has recently become popular among consumers in the United States. The demand for the drug in the United States has been fueled by German studies that reported that St. John's wort was equieffective with fluoxetine in the treatment of depression.

Some interesting circumstances give the herb its name. The plant is a low-growing shrub that grows wild in Europe and Western Asia with yellow flowers that bloom around June 24, the traditional birthdate of St. John. If the flowers are rubbed, a red pigment is released. This red substance has traditionally been associated with the blood of St. John released at his beheading.

The medicinal components of St. John's wort are derived from the flowering tops. A 2001 study in *Journal of the American Medical Association*, however, negates about 30 previously published trials and showed that St. John's wort failed to improve major depressive disorder in the first large-scale, multicenter, randomized, placebo-controlled trial in patients diagnosed with major depressive disorder. The herb has a definite mild sedative effect, and in 10 years of controlled clinical trials, it has proved effective in the treatment of *mild* depression.

CHEMISTRY[47]

The red components of Saint John's wort are the anthracene derivatives hypericin, present in about 0.15%,

Parthenolide

Canin

Artecanin

Secotanaparthenolide

Figure 29.4 ● Chemical constituents of feverfew.

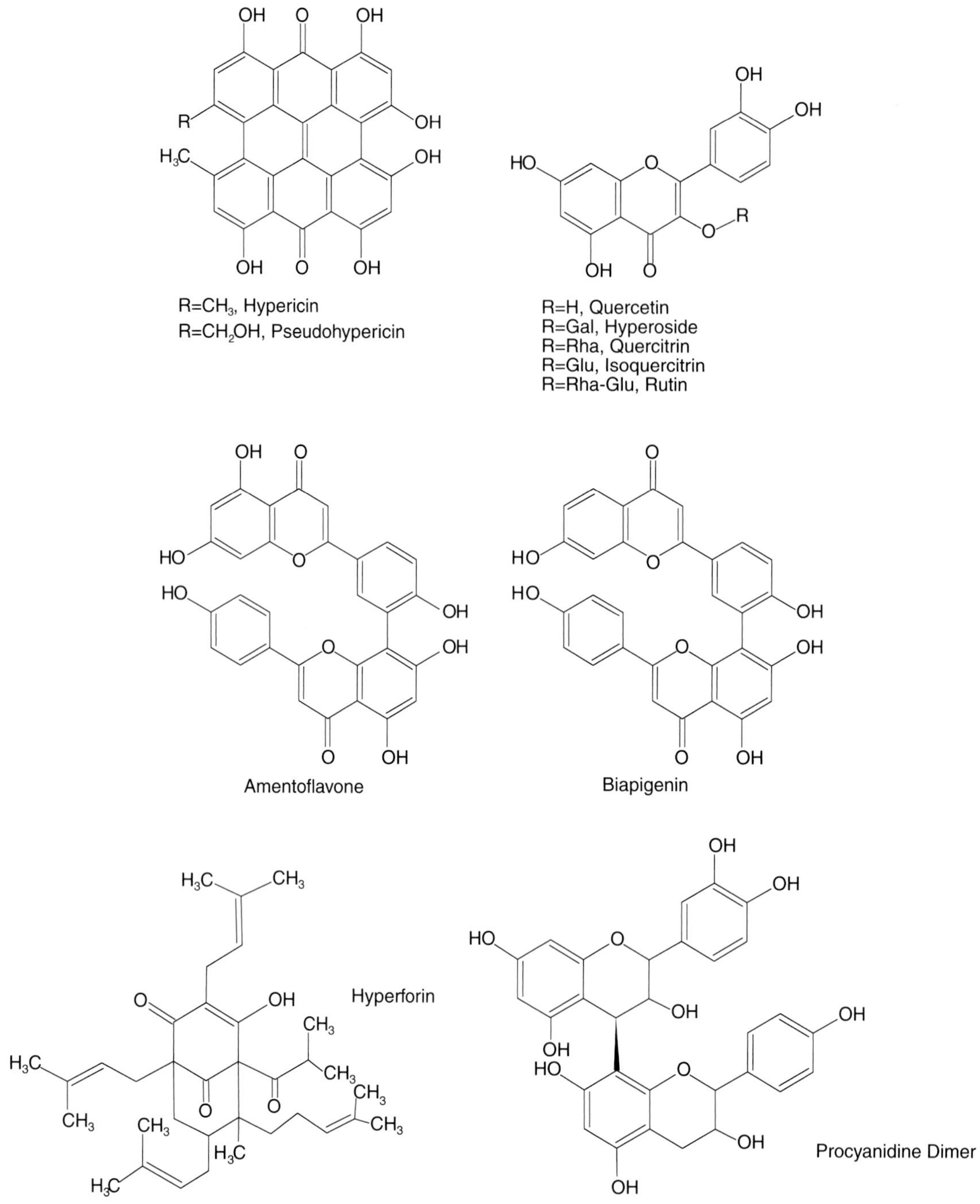

R=CH₃, Hypericin
R=CH₂OH, Pseudohypericin

R=H, Quercetin
R=Gal, Hyperoside
R=Rha, Quercitrin
R=Glu, Isoquercitrin
R=Rha-Glu, Rutin

Amentoflavone

Biapigenin

Hyperforin

Procyanidine Dimer

Figure 29.6 ● Chemical components of St. John's wort.

and pseudohypericin. (Fig. 29.6) Flavonoids present are quercetin, hyperoside, quercitrin, isoquercitrin, and rutin. (Fig. 29.6) Two C–C-linked biflavins, amentoflavone and biapigenin, are present, as is the acylphloroglucinol derivative hyperforin. Procyanidin, a chiral flavone dimer, adds to the list of flavones. Some terpenes and *n*-alkanes are present as minor components. The primary active ingredients have traditionally been held to be the hypericins and the flavone/flavonols, especially the hypericins. In fact, the German Commission E Monograph specifies that the herb should be standardized to hypericin content.

Despite the evidence of efficacy, the mechanism of action of St. John's wort remains unclear. Several possibilities have been put forth. Probably, the most popular one is the MAOI/COMT hypothesis. According to this hypothesis, St. John's wort increases the levels of catecholamines at the brain synapses by inhibiting their inactivation by oxidative deamination (MAOI) and by catechol functionalization (catechol-*O*-methyltransferase [COMT]).[47] Recent studies have shown that hypericins possess such activities only at pharmacologically excessive concentrations. If true, these effects at normal doses are small and do nothing to alleviate depression. Other hypotheses suggest hormonal effects or effects on the dopaminergic system. Hyperforin has become a candidate for the major antidepressant constituent of St. John's wort, supposedly inhibiting serotonin reuptake by elevating free intracellular sodium.

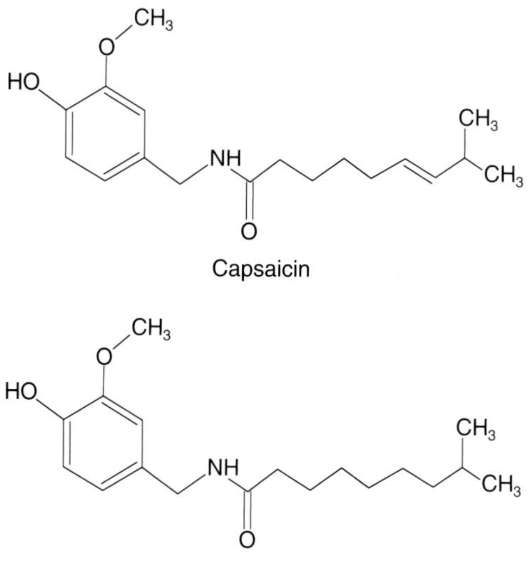

Capsaicin

6,7-Dihydrocapsaicin

Figure 29.7 ● Capsaicin derivatives of *Capsicum*.

St. John's wort also exhibits anti-inflammatory and anti-bacterial activity. Reports of antiviral activity are unsubstantiated. The main adverse effect with St. John's wort is severe phototoxicity. A sunburnlike condition may occur at normal dosages. St. John's wort should never be taken with MAOIs because of the risk of potentiation of the effects. Selective serotonin reuptake inhibitors (SSRIs) likewise should not be taken with St. John's wort because of the risk of serotonergic syndrome.

Dose (capsules standardized to 0.3% hypericin): 300 mg of standardized extract 3 times daily.

The FDA considers St. John's wort to be unsafe.

Capsicum (Capsaicin, Chili Pepper, Hot Pepper)

Pepper plants have been used for years as herbal remedies for pain.[48] The therapeutically useful pepper plants are members of the Solanaceae family. There are two primary species whose dried fruit is commonly used: *Capsicum frutescens* and *Capsicum annum*. The actual active ingredient, capsaicin, is extracted from an oleoresin that represents up to 1.5% of the plant. Two major components in the oleoresin (among several) are capsaicin and 6,7-dihydrocapsaicin. (Fig. 29.7) Volatile oils and vitamins A and C occur in large quantities. The amount of ascorbic acid in the capsaicin oleoresin is reportedly 4 to 6 times that in an orange.[49]

Capsaicin is supplied pharmaceutically as a cream, gel, or lotion. The first application of the preparation produces intense pain and irritation at the site of application, but usually no skin reaction occurs. Repeated applications cause desensitization, and eventually analgesic and anti-inflammatory effects occur. Stimulation of afferent nerve tracts causes a heat sensation.

There are several potential explanations for the alleviation of pain by capsaicin. There is believed to be a compound called *substance P* that mediates pain stimuli from the periphery to the spinal cord. One theory is that capsaicin depletes the neuronal supply of substance P so that pain stimuli cannot reach the brain.[50] Additionally, the methoxyphenol portion of the capsaicin molecule may fit

the COX receptor site and inhibit the lipoxygenase and COX pathways.[49]

Capsaicin is extremely potent, so topical preparations are compounded in percentage strengths of 0.025% to 0.25%. The preparations deplete substance P most effectively if used 3 to 4 times a day. Capsaicin has been suggested as a remedy for postsurgical pain (postamputation and postmastectomy), postherpetic neuralgia, and a variety of other complex pain situations. Relief of pain may occur as quickly as 3 days or may require up to 28 days.

Patients should be instructed to wash their hands well after applying capsaicin. Contact with mucous membranes and the eyes should be avoided. If contact occurs, one should wash with cool running water.

Capsaicin as the oleoresin is used as a "pepper spray" for self-defense. Spraying into the eyes causes immediate blepharospasm, blindness, and incapacitation for up to 30 minutes.

Garlic

Garlic (*Allium sativum*)[51] is an herbal drug with references to medicinal properties that date back thousands of years. Of all the herbal remedies available to consumers, garlic is probably the most extensively researched.[52] Publications about the effects and benefits of garlic occur with great frequency. Garlic is a bulb. It may be used as such, but it is typically dried, powdered, and compressed into a tablet. Usually, the tablets are enteric coated.

CHEMISTRY

Garlic[53] contains a key component, alliin or *S*-methyl-l-cysteine sulfoxide. Additionally, methiin (methylcysteine sulfoxide), cycloalliin, several γ-L-glutamyl-*S*-alkyl-L-cysteines, and alkyl alkanethiosulfinates are present (Fig. 29.8). The tissues also contain enzymes (alliinase, peroxidase, myrosinase), as well as additional sulfur-containing compounds, ajoene, and other minor components. Garlic itself has the highest sulfur content of all of the *Allium* species. When the garlic clove is crushed, the enzyme

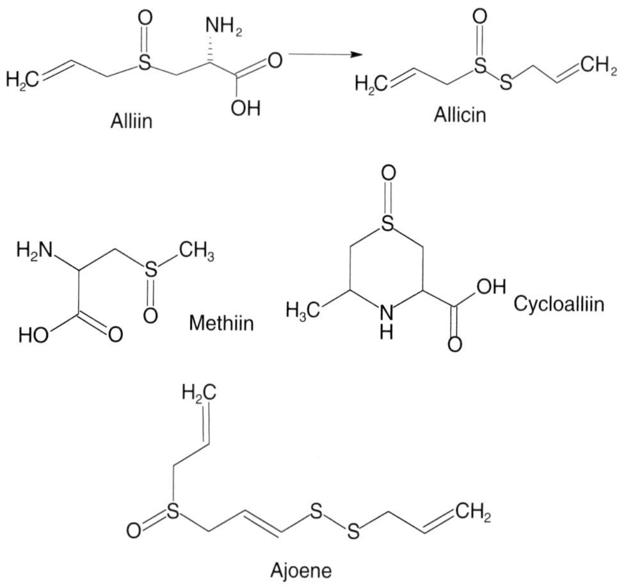

Figure 29.8 ● Chemical components of garlic.

alliinase is released, and alliin is converted to allicin. Allicin gives garlic its characteristic odor and is believed to be the pharmacologically active ingredient from the herb. Alliinase will not survive the acidic environment of the stomach, so enteric-coated tablets are used.

Garlic is most often studied for its lipid-lowering and antithrombotic[54] effects. A cholesterol-lowering effect is well documented in both animals and humans. Garlic lowers serum cholesterol, triglycerides, and low-density lipoprotein (LDL) while increasing high-density lipoprotein (HDL). Jain reported mean reductions of 6% in total serum cholesterol and 11% in LDL. Methylallyltrisulfide in garlic oil potentially inhibits ADP-induced platelet aggregation, and ajoene inhibits platelet aggregation for short periods.

Compared with the statin drugs, there is a paucity of human research data for garlic. There have been no morbidity and mortality studies for garlic, for instance. All that we can really gather from the literature is that there *may* be an effect on patient lipid profiles, but for every positive response, a negative one can be found. Garlic is certainly not harmful and can be used safely as part of a lipid-reduction program, but this should be done under a physician's supervision.

Chamomile

The herb known as chamomile[55] is derived from the plants *Matricaria chamomilla* (German, Hungarian, or genuine chamomile) and *Anthemis nobilis* (English, Roman, or common chamomile). Plants from the two genera have similar activities. The medicinal components are obtained from the flowering tops. The flowers are dried and used for chamomile teas and extracts. Chamomile has been used medicinally for at least 2,000 years. The Romans used the herb for its medicinal properties, which they knew were antispasmodic and sedative. The herb also has a long history in the treatment of digestive and rheumatic disorders.

The activity of chamomile is found in a light blue essential oil that composes only 0.5% of the flower. The blue color is caused by chamazulene, 7-ethyl-1,4-dimethylazulene (Fig. 29.9). This compound is actually a byproduct of processing the herb. The major component of the oil is the sesquiterpene (−)-α-bisabolol. Also present are apigenin, angelic acid, tiglic acid, the terpene precursors (farnesol, nerolidol, and germacranolide) coumarin, scopoletin-7-glucoside, umbelliferone, and herniarin. Much of the effect of chamomile is caused by bisabolol (Fig. 29.9). Bisabolol is a highly active anti-inflammatory agent in various rodent inflammation and arthritis tests. In addition, bisabolol shortens the healing time of burns and ulcers in animal models.

The gastrointestinal (GI) antispasmodic properties of bisabolol and its oxides are well-known. In fact, bisabolol is said to be as potent as papaverine in tests of muscle spasticity. Besides bisabolol, the flavone and coumarin components

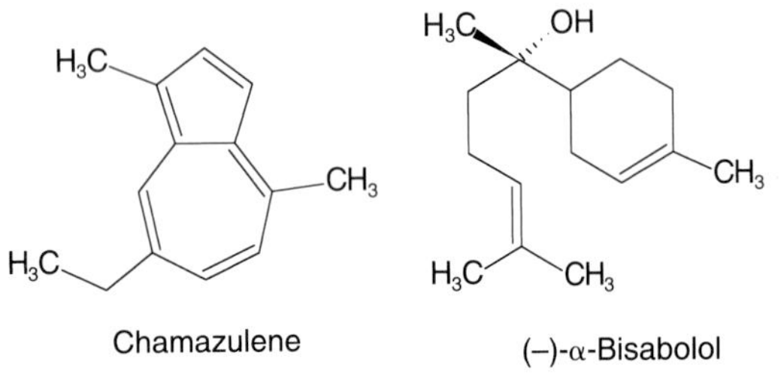

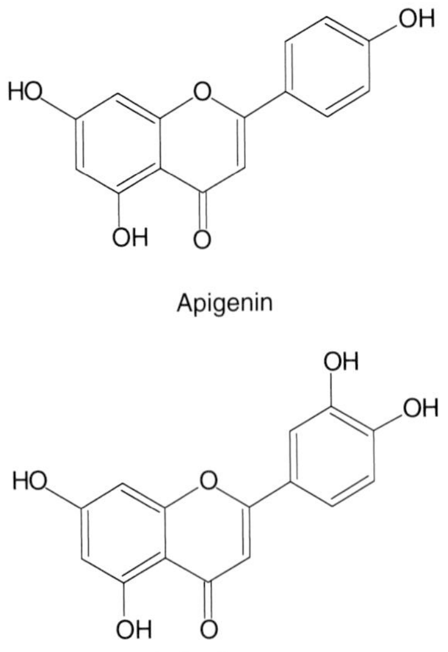

Figure 29.10 ● Anti-inflammatory components of chamomile.

have antispasmodic activities. The blue compound chamazulene possesses both anti-inflammatory and antiallergenic activities, as do the water-soluble components (the flavonoids). Apigenin and luteolin (Fig. 29.10) possess anti-inflammatory potencies similar to that of indomethacin. These flavonoids possess acidic phenolic groups, a spacer, and an aromatic moiety that could fit into the COX receptor. None of these effects has been unequivocally documented in humans. The essential oil possesses low-water solubility, but teas used over a long period of time provide a cumulative medicinal effect. Typically, 1 teaspoon (3 g) of flower head is boiled in hot water for 15 minutes, 4 times a day.

DRUG INTERACTIONS

Chamomile contains coumarins and may enhance the effect of prescription anticoagulants. The herb is an antispasmodic and slows the motility of the GI tract. This action might decrease the absorption of drugs. Chamomile preparations may be adulterated with chamomile pollen. This may cause allergy, anaphylaxis, and atopic dermatitis.

Ephedra

The varieties of ephedra (*Ephedra sinica*, *Ephedra nevadensis*, *Ephedra trifurca*, *ma huang*, natural ecstasy, ephedrine, *Herba Ephedrae*) that possess medicinal activity grow in Mongolia or along the Mongolian border region with China. The plant itself, an evergreen with a pine odor, consists of green canelike structures with small, reddish brown basal leaves. In the fall, the canes, root, and rhizome are harvested and dried in the sun. The dried material furnishes the active ingredients.

ACTIVITY

Ma huang is a sympathomimetic agent. The active principles are β-phenethylamines (Fig. 29.11).[11–13] These agents can stimulate the release of epinephrine and norepinephrine from nerve endings. Ma huang is a sympathomimetic stimulant in the periphery as well as in the central nervous system (CNS). It has positive inotropic and positive chronotropic effects on

Chamazulene   (−)-α-Bisabolol

Figure 29.9 ● Bisabolol, a key component of chamomile.

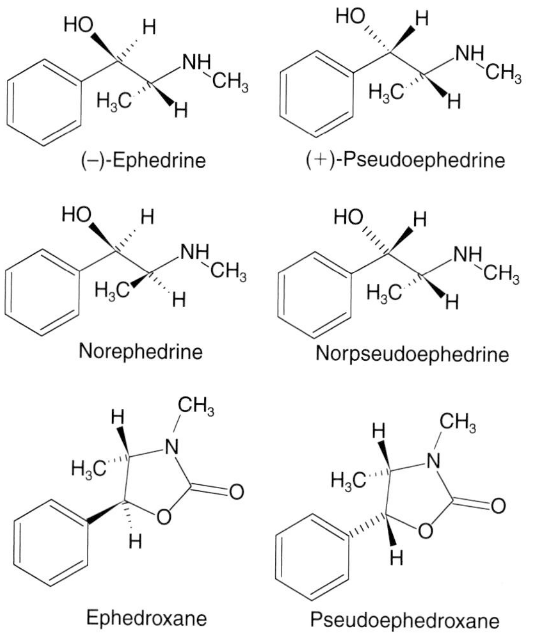

Figure 29.11 ● Beta-phenethylamines in ma huang.

the heart; hence, the herb may be dangerous to people with cardiac disease. The amounts of ephedra-type compounds and the relative composition differ so widely that it is difficult to be certain what one is getting in any given preparation. Ma huang's main active ingredient is the β-phenethylamine compound (−)-ephedrine. Plants grown in China may contain 0.5% to 2.5% of this compound. Many ephedrine congeners are represented in the plant,[11] and many of these possess considerable pharmacological activity. Some are as follows: (−)-ephedrine, (+)-pseudoephedrine, norephedrine, norpseudoephedrine, ephedroxane, and pseudoephedroxane (Fig. 29.11).

Ma huang's principal active ingredient is (−)-ephedrine. This compound is the *erythro*-D(−)-isomer with the 2(S),3(R) configuration. The less potent (+)-pseudoephedrine has the *threo* 2(S),3(S) structure. Ephedrine acts as a mixed agonist on both α- and β-receptors.

PHARMACOLOGICAL EFFECTS

Ephedrine's actions occur through mixed stimulation of the α- and β-adrenergic receptors. The drug is a CNS stimulant that increases the strength and rate of cardiac contraction. Additionally, ephedrine decreases gastric motility, causes bronchodilation, and stimulates peripheral vasoconstriction with the predicted increase in blood pressure. The *threo* isomer (+)-pseudoephedrine causes similar effects but is much less potent than (−)-ephedrine. The claims that ephedra causes increased metabolism and "fat burning" are certainly false, and ephedra lacks anorectic effects. Any reports of successful use of ephedra preparations in weight loss probably reflect the stimulant or "energizing" effect and increased physical activity. In the United States, ephedra has been used as a recreational CNS stimulant (natural ecstasy).

E. nevadensis and *E. trifurca* are typically used in teas. The FDA prohibits preparations with more than 8 mg/dose and advises that one should not take an ephedra product more often than every 6 hours and no more than 24 mg/day. Ephedra should not be used for more than 7 days. Dosages

over the recommended amount may cause stroke, myocardial infarction, seizures, and death.

Ephedra has been closely linked to methamphetamine production. There are movements in many localities to outlaw the herb. There are many drug interactions with ma huang. β-Blockers may enhance the sympathetic effect and cause hypertension. MAOIs may interact with ephedra to cause hypertensive crisis. Phenothiazines might block the α-effects of ephedra, causing hypotension and tachycardia. Simultaneous use of theophylline may cause GI and CNS effects. In pregnancy, ephedra is absolutely contraindicated (uterine stimulation). Persons with heart disease, hypertension, and diabetes should not take ephedra.

Cranberry

The cranberry plant (*Vaccinium macrocarpon, Vaccinium oxycoccus*, and *Vaccinium erythrocarpum*) is a trailing evergreen that grows primarily in acidic swamp areas. The whole berries are divested of seeds and skins, and the rest of the fruit is used as a drink or in capsule form. Cranberry juice has been used, for many years, as a urinary tract disinfectant. In 1923,[56] a report said that the urine of persons who consumed cranberry juice became more acidic. Because an acidic medium hinders the growth of bacteria, it was thought that acidification of the urine inhibited bacterial growth.

An analysis of cranberry juice shows that it contains many different compounds. Citric, malic, benzoic, and quinic acids are present as carboxylic acid components. With pK$_a$'s of 3.5 to 5, these compounds should exist in the ionized form in the urine at pH 5.5, thus lowering the pH. We now know that acidification of the urine is not the entire story. In fact, drinking the cocktail does not appreciably acidify the urine. Two other constituents exist in the juice: mannose and a high–molecular-weight polysaccharide.[57–59] With bacteria that use fimbrial adhesins in infecting the urinary tract, mannose binds and inhibits adhesion of the type 1 mannose-sensitive fimbriae, whereas the high–molecular-weight polysaccharide inhibits binding of the P-type fimbriae. Hence, adhesion of many *Escherichia coli* strains, which cause over half of all urinary tract infections, is inhibited. This inhibition has the effect of blocking infection.

Dosage: Drink between 10 and 16 oz of juice daily.

Ginkgo Biloba

Ginkgo biloba (L.), also known as the maidenhair or Kew tree, has survived essentially unchanged in China for 200 million years.[60] There is a Chinese monograph, describing the use of ginkgo leaves, dating from 2800 BC. Today, ginkgo is extracted by an extremely complex multistep process that concentrates the active constituents and removes the toxic ginkgolic acid.[61]

The ginkgo extract is a complex mixture of both polar and nonpolar components (Fig. 29.12). The more polar fractions contain flavonol and flavone glycosides. The more nonpolar fractions contain some diterpene lactones, known as ginkgetin, ginkgolic acid, and isoginkgetin, and some interesting caged diterpenes known as ginkgolide A, B, C, J, and M.[62] There is also a 15-carbon sesquiterpene (bilobalide) and other minor components. *G. biloba* extract is prepared by picking the leaves, drying them, and constituting them into an acetone-water extract that is standardized to contain 24% flavone glycosides and 6% terpenes.[60]

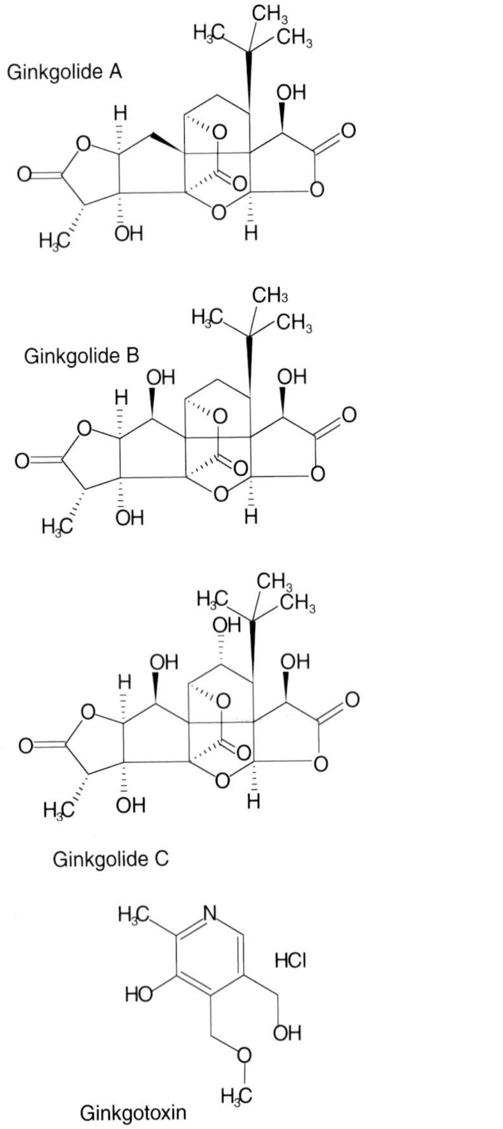

Ginkgolide A

Ginkgolide B

Ginkgolide C

Ginkgotoxin

Figure 29.12 • Chemical components of ginkgo extract.

G. biloba produces vasodilating effects on both the arterial and venous circulation.[60,61] The result is increased tissue perfusion (i.e., in the peripheral circulation) and cerebral blood flow. The extract produces arterial vasodilatation (rodent models), dampens arterial spasticity, and decreases capillary permeability, capillary fragility,[60] erythrocyte aggregation, and blood viscosity. There are several possible explanations for these effects. One possibility is that the compounds in *G. biloba* extract inhibit prostaglandin and thromboxane biosynthesis. It has also been speculated that *G. biloba* extract has an indirect regulatory effect on catecholamines. Ginkgolide B is reportedly a potent inhibitor of PAF.[15] In any case, the effects are caused by a mixture of the constituents, not a single one.

G. biloba has become popular because of its putative abilities to increase peripheral and cerebral circulation. The herb is called an *adaptogen*,[63] a drug that helps persons handle stress. In the periphery, the herb has been compared to pentoxifylline. If the properties are true, the herb could be used for intermittent claudication. If cerebral blood flow can be increased with *G. biloba*, the herb might be useful for disorders of memory that occur with age and Alzheimer disease. The popular use for the herb is to help people think better under stress and to increase the length of time that someone (e.g., a student) can handle mental stress.

Ginseng

Ginseng is the root of the species *Panax quinquefolius*. This form is commonly known as American, or Western, ginseng. The shape of the root is important to many and may make it highly prized. *Panax* means "all" or "man." Sometimes, the root is shaped like the figure of a human. The doctrine of signatures would say that this root would benefit the whole person. Another species of ginseng, *Panax ginseng*, is commonly called Asian, or Korean, ginseng. Chemically, the two species are very similar. Major components are named the *ginsenosides* (Figs. 29.13, 29.14).[64]

The chemical constituents of ginseng are called ginsenosides or *panaxosides*. A total of 12 of these have been isolated but are present in such small quantities that purification is difficult. Sterols, flavonoids, proteins, and vitamins (B_1, B_2, B_{12}, pantothenic acid, niacin, and biotin) are also components with pharmacological activity. The chemistry of ginseng gives a good example of how different compounds in

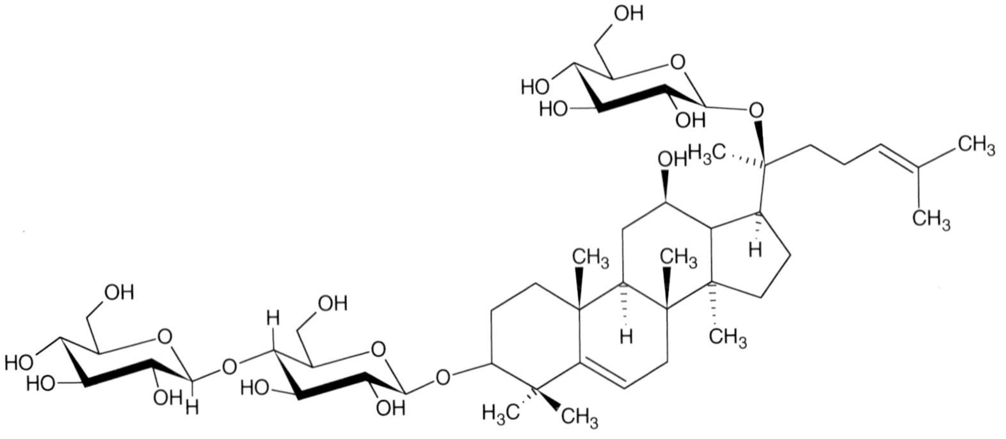

Ginsenoside R$_d$

Figure 29.13 • Structures of ginsenosides.

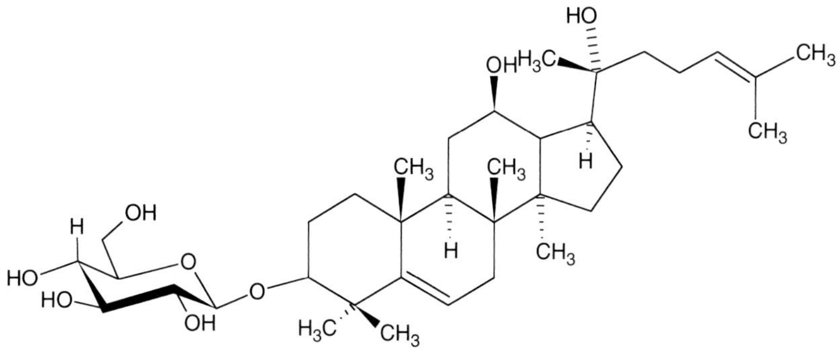

Figure 29.14 ● Structures of ginsenosides.

20 (*R*) Ginsenoside

one herb can have opposing pharmacological effects.[65] Ginsenoside Rb-1 acts as a CNS depressant, anticonvulsant, analgesic, and antipsychotic, prevents stress ulcers, and accelerates glycolysis and nuclear RNA synthesis. Ginsenoside Rg-1 stimulates the CNS, combats fatigue, is hypertensive, and aggravates stress ulcers. Additionally, ginsenosides Rg and Rg-1 enhance cardiac performance, whereas Rb depresses that function. Some of the other ginsenosides display antiarrhythmic activity similar to that of the calcium channel blocker verapamil and amiodarone.

Ginseng is popularly believed to enhance concentration, stamina, alertness, and the ability to do work. Longer-term use in elderly patients is claimed to enhance "well-being." There are few data from human studies. Clinical studies comparing ginseng with placebo on cognitive function tests showed statistically insignificant improvement. Nevertheless, ginseng is a popular herbal product recommended by the German Commission E.

Milk Thistle

Milk thistle (*Silybum marianum*) is a member of the Asteraceae, a family that includes daisies, asters, and thistles. The plant has a wide range around the world and is found in the Mediterranean, Europe, North America, South America, and Australia. The seeds of the milk thistle plant have been used for 2,000 years as a hepatoprotectant.[66,67] This usage can be traced to the writings of Pliny the Elder (AD 23–79) in Rome, who reported that the juice of the plant could be used for "carrying off bile." Culpepper in England reported that milk thistle was useful in "removing obstructions of the liver and spleen and against jaundice."

CHEMISTRY

Milk thistle contains as an active constituent silymarin (Fig. 29.15),[66] which is actually a mixture of three isomeric flavanolignans: silybin (silibinin), silychristin, and silydianin. Silybin is the most active hepatoprotectant and antioxidant compound of the mixture. Also present in the plant are the flavanolignans dehydrosilybin, silandrin, silybinome, and silyhermin. Other lipid-soluble components are apigenin, silybonol, and linoleic, oleic, myristic, stearic, and palmitic acids.

MECHANISM OF ACTION

The silymarin complex is aptly suited for its hepatoprotective actions.[68] Silymarin undergoes enterohepatic cycling, moving from intestine to liver and concentrating in liver cells. Protein synthesis is induced in the liver by silybin, whose steroid structure stimulates both DNA and RNA synthesis. Through these activities, the regenerative capacity of the liver is activated. Silymarin is reported to alter the outer cell membrane structure of liver cells, blocking entrance of toxic substances into the cell. This blockage is so pronounced that it can reduce the death rate from *Amanita phalloides* poisoning. Silymarin's effect can be explained by its antioxidant properties; it scavenges free radicals. By this effect, the level of intracellular glutathione rises, becoming available for other detoxification reactions. Silybin inhibits enzymes such as lipoxygenase,[66] blocking peroxidation of fatty acids and membrane lipid damage. Studies also show that silymarin protects the liver from amitriptyline, nortriptyline, carbon tetrachloride, and cisplatin. When treated, patients with alcoholic cirrhosis showed increased liver function as measured by enzymes. In patients with acute viral hepatitis, silymarin shortened treatment time and improved aspartate aminotransferase (AST) and alanine aminotransferase (ALT) levels.

In liver disease, silymarin appears to have an immunomodulatory effect. The activities of superoxide dismutase (SOD) and glutathione peroxidase are increased, which probably accounts for the effect on free radicals. Silymarin, however, has an anti-inflammatory effect on human platelets. Silybin retards release of histamine from human mast cells and inhibits activation of T lymphocytes. The chemical appears capable of reducing the levels of all immunoglobulin classes and enhances the motility of lymphocytes. Milk thistle extract and its components have shown efficacy in treating hepatotoxin poisoning, cirrhosis, and hepatitis. It also plays a role in blood and

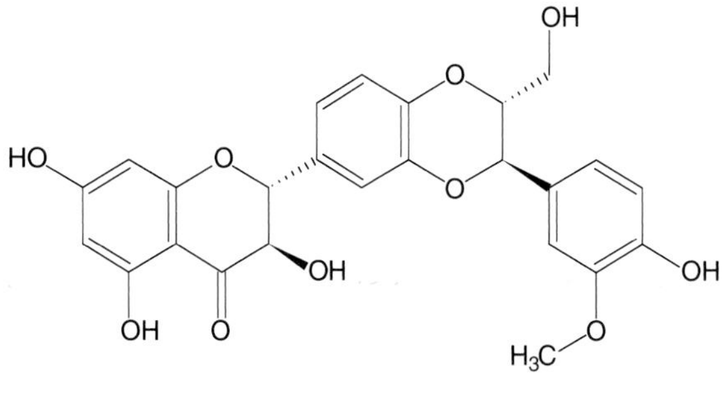

Silymarin

Figure 29.15 ● Silymarin from milk thistle.

immunomodulation and in lipids and biliary function. The overall effect is caused by the electron-scavenging properties of flavanolignans, the enhanced regenerative capacity of the liver, and the alteration of liver cell membranes that blocks toxin entry.

Valerian

Valerian (*Valeriana officinalis*) is found in temperate regions of North America, Europe, and Asia. The dried rhizome of valerian contains an unpleasant-smelling volatile oil that is attributed to isovaleric acid. Despite the odor, valerian is a safe and effective sleep aid.

CHEMISTRY

Three classes of compounds have been linked to the sedative properties of valerian. The rhizome contains monoterpenes and sesquiterpenes (valerenic acid and its acetoxy derivative), iridoids (valepotrioates), and pyridine alkaloids (Fig. 29.16).[69,70] At present, it is not possible to state which class of compound is responsible for the sedative activity. Most researchers believe that the valepotriate is the active component, but some studies have shown that valerenic acid is more potent.

Aqueous and hydroalcoholic extracts of valerian induce the release of [^{3}H]γ-aminobutyric acid (GABA) from synaptosome preparations. The extracts appear to have much the same effects as benzodiazepines, except that valerian does not act on the Na$^+$/K$^+$-ATPase. Valerenic acid inhibits the GABA transaminase. This effect would increase the inhibitory effect of GABA in the CNS.

There is no doubt that valerian is safe and effective as a sleep aid. Used properly, it is one of the more recommendable herbs.

Dose: 400 to 900 mg standardized extract 0.5 to 1 hour before bedtime.

Pennyroyal

Pennyroyal (*Hedeoma pulegeoides*, *Mentha pulegium*) is an example of an extremely toxic herb. The plant is a member

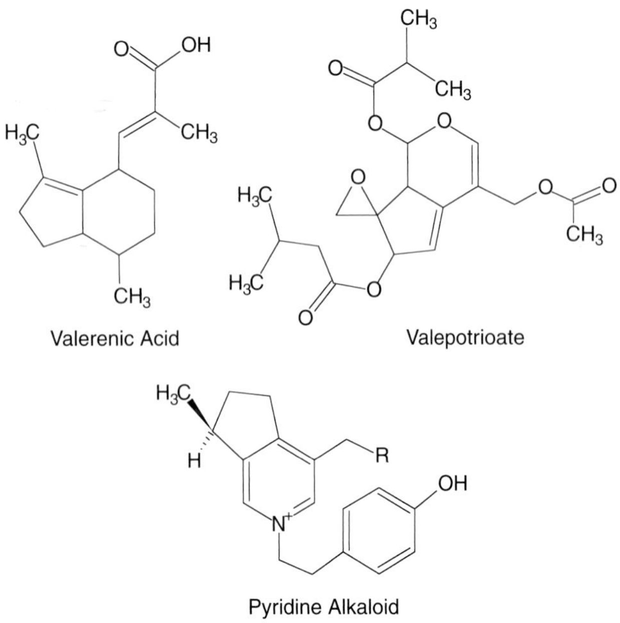

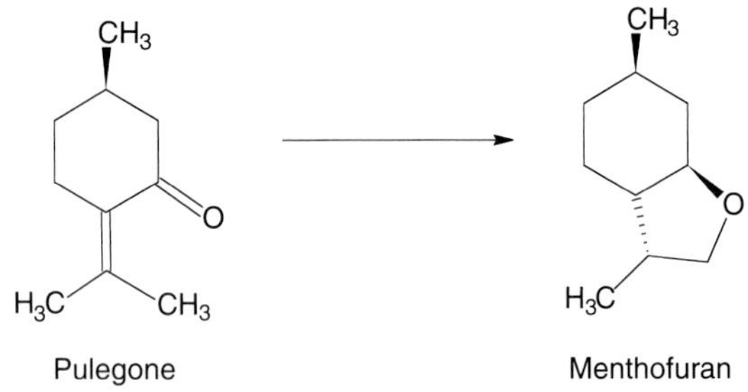

Figure 29.17 ● Pulegone in pennyroyal.

of the mint family, Labiatae. The dried leaves and flowering tops of the plant contain from 16% to 30% oil, consisting of the monoterpene pulegone (Fig. 29.17).[71] The oil also contains tannins, α- and β-pinenes, other terpenes, long-chain alcohols, piperitenones, and paraffin.

The toxicity of pennyroyal is believed to be a result of the pulegone[71] in the oil. Cytochrome P450 catalyzes the metabolism of pulegone to yield the toxic metabolite menthofuran (Fig. 29.17). Possibly, some of the other terpenes undergo oxidation to active metabolites as well. Menthofuran, metabolites of other terpenes, and pulegone itself deplete hepatic glutathione, resulting in liver failure. This mechanistic hypothesis is supported by the fact that administration of acetylcysteine reverses the toxicity.

Pennyroyal has been used as an abortifacient since the time of Pliny the Elder,[72] an insect repellent (the terpenes in the oil have citronellal-like properties), an aid to induce menstruation, and a treatment for the symptoms of premenstrual syndrome. It has also been used as a flea repellent on dogs and cats.

When used as an abortifacient, the drug often causes liver failure and hemorrhage, leading to death. Pennyroyal is sometimes used with black cohosh to accelerate the abortifacient effect. Coma and death have been reported. Pennyroyal is an example of an herb that has no safe uses. It should not be sold.

Herbal Drugs Used in the Treatment of Cancer

Anticancer drugs derived from biological sources are fairly common and are among the most important in the therapeutic armamentarium. Drugs such as doxorubicin, mitomycin C, mithramycin, and bleomycin have been around for a long time and have shed much light on the treatment of cancer. Three plant-derived drugs that have found their way through clinical trials deserve mention here. Two of the most famous are vincristine and vinblastine (Fig. 29.18). These are compounds isolated from the periwinkle plant *Catharanthus roseus*. The Vinca alkaloids bind tightly to tubulin in cells and interfere with its normal function in spindle formation. The Vinca alkaloids make the tubulin less stable. The net result is metaphase arrest of cell division. Paclitaxel (Taxol, Fig. 29.18) was originally isolated from the needles or bark of the Pacific yew. Because it occurs in vanishingly small concentration in the plant, a semisynthetic method for its production was developed. Taxol binds to tubulin like the Vinca alkaloids, but it makes the tubulin structure hyperstable so that it cannot function. Again, the net result is metaphase arrest.

Figure 29.16 ● Chemical constituents of valerian.

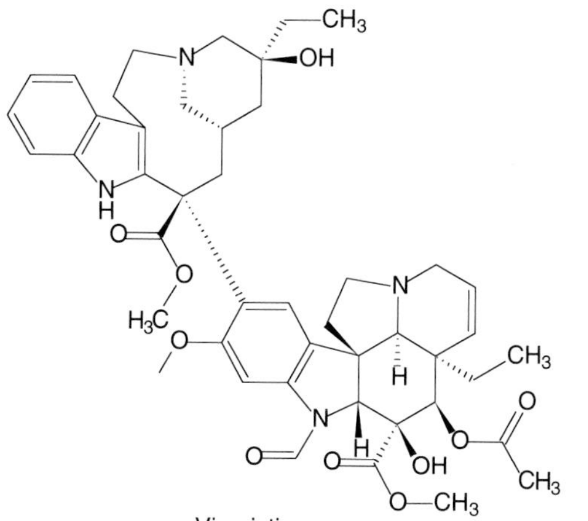

Vincristine

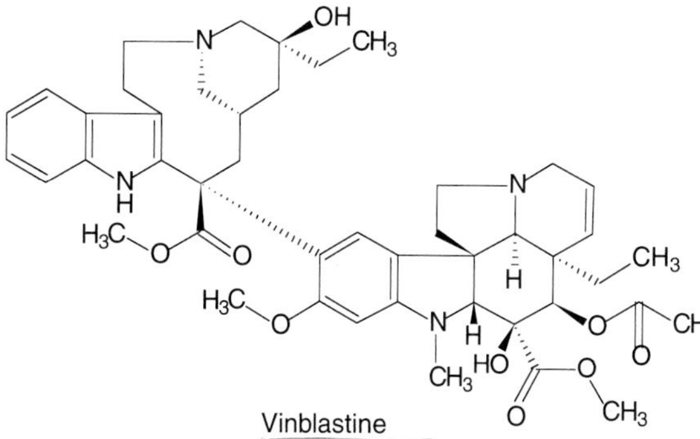

Vinblastine

(57)

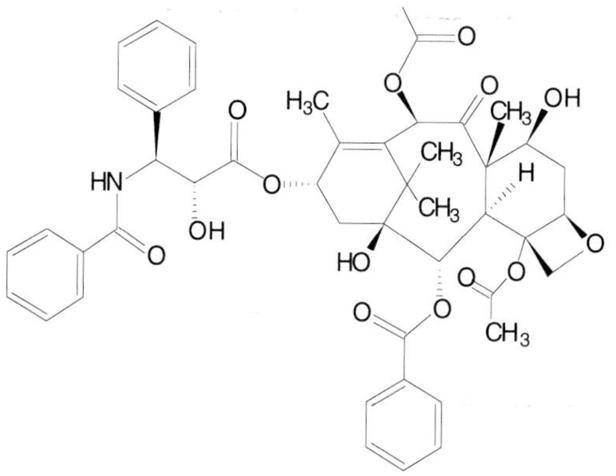

Figure 29.18 ● Vincristine and vinblastine.

Paclitaxel

Licorice

When we think of licorice, we typically think of the popular candy. Licorice, however, has an important history in herbal medicine. Licorice is a perennial shrub that is indigenous to the Mediterranean and is cultivated in the Middle East, Spain, northern Asia, and the United States. The most common variety used for medicinal purposes is *Glycyrrhiza glabra* var. *typica*. Licorice has been used since Roman times and was described in early Chinese writings.

CHEMISTRY

The root and rhizomes of the licorice plant contain ~5% to 9% of a steroidal glycoside called *glycyrrhizin* (Fig. 29.19). In the glycoside form, glycyrrhizin is 150 times sweeter than sugar. Also present are triterpenoids, glucose, mannose, and sucrose. Concentrated aqueous extracts may contain 10% to 20% glycyrrhizin. When the herb is ingested, the intestinal flora catalyze the conversion of glycyrrhizin into glycyrrhetic acid (Fig. 29.19), the pharmacologically active

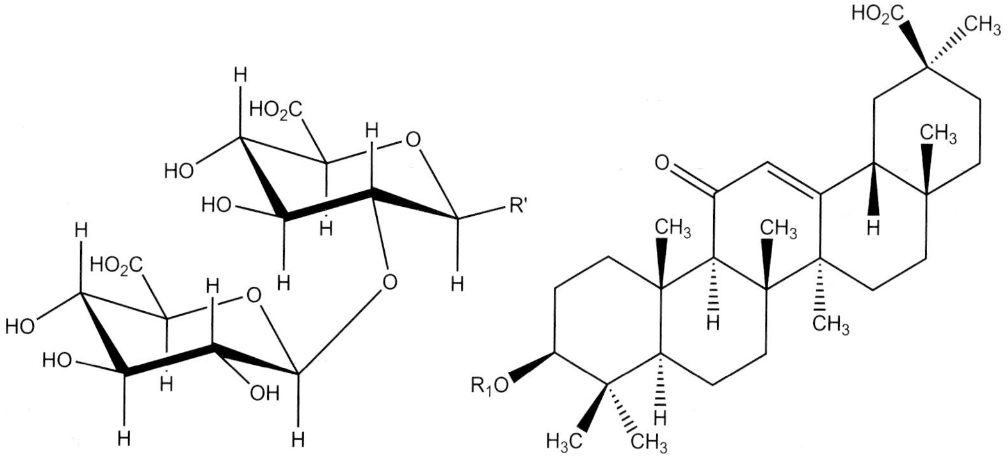

Glycyrrhetic Acid R_1 = H
Glycyrrhizin R_1 = R'

Figure 29.19 ● Chemical components of licorice.

compound. Glycyrrhizin and glycyrrhetic acid possess mild anti-inflammatory properties. Glycyrrhizin appears to stimulate gastric mucus secretion. This may be the origin of the antiulcer properties of licorice. Glycyrrhizin and glycyrrhetic acid do not act directly as steroids. Instead, they potentiate, rather than mimic, endogenous compounds.

There is some interesting folklore relating to the use of licorice. During World War II, a Dutch physician[73] noticed that patients with peptic ulcer disease improved dramatically when treated with a paste containing 40% licorice extract. The physician treated many patients in this way, but during the course of his work, he noticed that there was a serious side effect from the herbal drug. About 20% of his ulcer patients developed a reversible edema of the face and extremities. Since these original observations, many studies have been conducted with licorice root. The findings have remained the same; licorice is useful for peptic ulcer disease, but potentially serious mineralocorticoid side effects are possible (lethargy, edema, headache, sodium and water retention, excess excretion of potassium, and increased blood pressure).

Licorice exerts its protective effects on the gastric mucosa by inhibiting two enzymes, 15-hydroxyprostaglandin dehydrogenase and Δ^{13}-prostaglandin reductase. Inhibition of these enzymes causes their substrates to increase in concentration, increasing the levels of prostaglandins in the gastric mucosa and causing a cytoprotective effect. The acid also inhibits 11-β-hydroxysteroid dehydrogenase,[74] thus increasing the glucocorticoid concentration in mineralocorticoid-responsive tissues, causing increased sodium retention, potassium excretion, and blood pressure.

In the 1960s, a semisynthetic compound based on glycyrrhetic acid, 4-*O*-succinylglycyrrhetic acid (carbenoxolone), was introduced in Europe. It proved effective against peptic ulcer disease, but it was later shown to be inferior to the H₂-receptor antagonists.

Licorice is also an effective demulcent, soothing a sore throat, and is an expectorant and cough suppressant.

Licorice can cause serious adverse reactions. These are mineralocorticoid effects (pseudoprimary aldosteronism), muscle weakness, rhabdomyolysis, and heart failure. Poisoning by licorice is insidious. Long-term high doses are extremely toxic. Licorice can potentiate the digitalis glycosides and cause toxicity. With cardiovascular agents that prolong the QT interval, the effects may be additive.

● R E V I E W   Q U E S T I O N S ●

1. What did the Durham-Humphrey Amendment do to drug commerce?

2. What enzyme is induced by St. John's wort and is responsible for prescription drug interactions with this herb?

3. What drug interaction is commonly observed with *G. biloba* use?

4. What is the most problematic aspect of herbal manufacture in the United States?

5. What is the constituent of St. John's wort that is now believed to be responsible for the antidepressant effect of the herb?

6. What herbal drug has been shown to be an effective hepatoprotectant?

7. What herbal drug is an effective treatment for peptic ulcers, albeit with unfortunate side effects?

8. What is a rhizome?

REFERENCES

1. Strohecker, J.: Alternative Medicine: The Definitive Guide. Puyallup, WA, Future Medicine Publishing, 1994, p. 257.
2. Brevort, P.: HerbalGram 44:33–46, 1998.
3. Solomons, G., and Fryhle, C.: Organic Chemistry, 7th ed. New York, John Wiley & Sons, 2002, pp. 3–4.
4. Tyler, L.: Understanding Alternative Medicine. New York, Haworth Herbal Press, 2000, p. 57.
5. Tyler, V. E.: Herbs of Choice. New York, Pharmaceutical Products Press, 1994, p. 17.
6. Duke, J. A., and Avensu, E. S.: Medicinal Plants of China, vol. 1. Algonac, MI, Reference Publications, 1985, p. 122.
7. Tyler, V. E.: Herbs of Choice. New York, Pharmaceutical Products Press, 1994, pp. 17–31.
8. Blumenthal, M.: HerbalGram 23(49):32–33, 1990.
9. Winter, R.: A Consumer's Dictionary of Food Additives. New York, Crown Publishers, 1984.
10. Tyler, V. E., Brady, L. R., and Robbers, J. E.: Pharmacognosy, 7th ed. Philadelphia, Lea & Febiger, 1976.
11. Gurley, B. J., Gardner, S. F., and Hubbard, M. M.: Am. J. Health Syst. Pharm. 57(10):963–969, 2000.
12. Gurley, B. J., Wang, P., and Gardner, S. F.: J. Pharm. Sci. 87(12):1547–1553, 1988.
13. Betz, J. M., et al.: J. Assoc. Anal. Chem. Int. 80(2):303–315, 1997.
14. Tyler, V. E.: Herbs of Choice. New York, Pharmaceutical Products Press, 1994, p. 1.
15. Koltai, M., et. al.: Drugs 42:9–29, 1991.
16. Suzuki, O., et al.: Planta Med. 50:272–274, 1984.
17. Haas, H.: Arzneipflanzenkunde. Mannheim, B. I. Wissenschafts, Verlag, 1991, pp. 134–135.
18. Moerman, D. E.: Medicinal Plants of Native America. Research Report on Ethnobotany, Contrib. 2, Tech. Rep. no. 19. Ann Arbor, University of Michigan Museum of Anthropology, 1998.
19. Bauer, R.: Echinacea: Biological effects and active principles. In Lawson, L. D., and Bauer, R. (eds.). Phytomedicines of Europe: Chemistry and Biological Activity. American Chemical Society Symposium Series. New York, Oxford University Press, 1998, p. 140.
20. Bauer, R.: Echinacea: Biological effects and active principles. In Lawson, L. D., and Bauer, R. (eds.). Phytomedicines of Europe: Chemistry and Biological Activity. American Chemical Society Symposium Series. New York, Oxford University Press, 1998, p. 141.
21. Bauer, R., Khan, I. A., Lotter, H., et al.: Helv. Chim. Acta 68:2355–2358, 1985.
22. Egert, D., and Beuscher, N.: Planta Med. 58:426–430, 1988.
23. Bauer, R., Khan, I. A., and Wagner, H.: Planta Med. 54:426–430, 1988.

24. Stimpel, M., Proksch, A., Wagner, H., et al.: Infect. Immun. 46:845–849, 1984.
25. Luettig, B., Steinmüller, C., Gifford, G. E., et al.: J. Natl. Cancer Inst. 81:669–675, 1989.
26. Bauer, R., Remiger, P., and Wagner, H.: Dtsch. Apoth. Ztg. 128:174–180, 1988.
27. Egert, D., and Beuscher, N.: Planta Med. 58:163–165, 1992.
28. Jacobson, M.: J. Org. Chem. 32:1646–1647, 1967.
29. Bauer, R., Remiger, P., and Wagner, H.: Phytochemistry 28:505–508, 1989.
30. Bauer, R.: Echinacea: Biological effects and active principles. In Lawson, L. D., and Bauer, R. (eds.). Phytomedicines of Europe: Chemistry and Biological Activity. American Chemical Society Symposium Series. New York, Oxford University Press, 1998, p. 150.
31. Bauer, R.: Echinacea: Biological effects and active principles. In Lawson, L. D., and Bauer, R. (eds.). Phytomedicines of Europe: Chemistry and Biological Activity. American Chemical Society Symposium Series. New York, Oxford University Press, 1998, pp. 158–159.
32. Blakeman, J. P., and Atkinson, P.: Physiol. Plant Pathol. 15:183–192, 1979.
33. Johnson, E. S., Kadam, N. P., Hylands, D. M., et al.: Br. Med. J. 291:569–573, 1985.
34. Murphy, J. J., Heptinstall, S., and Mitchell, J. R. A.: Lancet ii:189–192, 1988.
35. Collier, H. O. J., Butt, N. M., McDonald-Gibson, W. J., et al.: Lancet ii:922–923, 1980.
36. Makheja, A. M., and Bailey, J. M.: Lancet ii:1054, 1981.
37. Makheja, A. M., and Bailey, J. M.: Prostaglandins Leukotrienes Med. 8:653–660, 1982.
38. Thakkar, J. K., Sperelaki, N., Pang, D., et al.: Biochim. Biophys. Acta 750:134–140, 1983.
39. Heptinstall, S., Groenewegen, W. A., Knight, D. W., et al.: In Rose, C. (ed.). Current Problems in Neurology: 4. Advances in Headache Research. Proceedings of the 6th International Migraine Symposium 1987. London, John Libbey & Co. Ltd., 1987, pp. 129–134.
40. Bork, P. M., et al.: FEBS Lett. 402:85–90, 1997.
41. Bohlmann, F., and Zdero, C.: Phytochemistry 21:2543–2549, 1982.
42. Kupchan, S. M., Fessler, D. C., Eakin, M. A., et al.: Science 168:376–377, 1970.
43. Heptinstall, S., Groenewegen, W. A., Spangenberg, P., et al.: Folia Haematol. 115:447–449, 1988.
44. Heptinstall, S., Groenewegen, W. A., Spangenberg, P., et al.: J. Pharm. Pharmacol. 39:459–465, 1987.
45. Heptinstall, S., Awang, D. V. C., Dawson, B. A., et al.: J. Pharm. Pharmacol. 44:391–395, 1992.
46. German Commission E Monograph, 1999.
47. Reuter, H. D.: Chemistry and biology of *Hypericum perforatum* (St. John's Wort). In Lawson, L. D., and Bauer, R. (eds.). Phytomedicines of Europe: Chemistry and Biological Activity. American Chemical Society Symposium Series. New York, Oxford University Press, 1998, pp. 287–298.
48. Tyler, V. E., Brady, L. R., and Robbers, J. E.: Pharmacognosy, 9th ed. Philadelphia, Lea & Febiger, 1988, pp. 148–150.
49. Fetrow, C. W., and Avila, J. R.: Professional's Handbook of Complementary and Alternative Medicines. Springhouse, PA, Springhouse Corporation, 1999, p. 123.
50. Tyler, V. E.: Herbs of Choice. New York, Pharmaceutical Products Press, 1994, p. 125.
51. Gruenwald, J.: HerbalGram 34:60–65, 1995.
52. Koch, H. P., and Lawson, L. D.: Garlic: The Science and Therapeutic Application of *Allium sativum* and Related Species. Baltimore, Williams & Wilkins, 1996, pp. 25–36.
53. Lawson, L. D.: Garlic: A review of its medicinal effects and indicated active compounds. In Lawson, L. D., and Bauer, R. (eds.). Phytomedicines of Europe: Chemistry and Biological Activity. American Chemical Society Symposium Series. New York, Oxford University Press, 1998, pp. 180–186.
54. Koch, H. P., and Lawson, L. D.: Garlic: The Science and Therapeutic Application of *Allium sativum* and Related Species. Baltimore, Williams & Wilkins, 1996, pp. 135–212.
55. Tyler, V. E.: Herbs of Choice. New York, Pharmaceutical Products Press, 1994, pp. 57–58.
56. Blatherwick, N. R., and Long, M. L.: J. Biol. Chem. 57:815–818, 1923.
57. Sabota, A. E.: J. Urol. 131:1013–1016, 1984.
58. Soloway, M. S., and Smith, R. A.: JAMA 260:1465, 1988.
59. Ofek, I., et al.: N. Engl. J. Med. 324:1599, 1991.
60. Tyler, V. E.: Herbs of Choice. New York, Pharmaceutical Products Press, 1994, p. 109.
61. Fetrow, C. W., and Avila, J. R.: Professional's Handbook of Complementary and Alternative Medicines. Springhouse, PA, Springhouse Corporation, 1999, p. 278.
62. Hänsel, R.: Phytopharmaka, 2nd ed. Berlin, Springer-Verlag, 1991, pp. 59–72.
63. Fetrow, C. W., and Avila, J. R.: Professional's Handbook of Complementary and Alternative Medicines. Springhouse, PA, Springhouse Corporation, 1999, p. 279.
64. Fetrow, C. W., and Avila, J. R.: Professional's Handbook of Complementary and Alternative Medicines. Springhouse, PA, Springhouse Corporation, 1999, p. 282.
65. Tyler, V. E.: Herbs of Choice. New York, Pharmaceutical Products Press, 1994, p. 172.
66. Flora, K.: Am. J. Gastroenterol. 93:139–143, 1998.
67. Salmi, A., and Sarna, S.: Scand. J. Gastroenterol. 174:517–521, 1982.
68. Fetrow, C. W., and Avila, J. R.: Professional's Handbook of Complementary and Alternative Medicines. Springhouse, PA, Springhouse Corporation, 1999, p. 430.
69. Hänsel, R.: Phytopharmaka, 2nd ed. Berlin, Springer-Verlag, 1991, pp. 252–259.
70. Krieglstein, J., and Grusla, D.: Dtsch. Apoth. Ztg. 128:2041–2046, 1988.
71. Anderson, I. B.: Ann. Intern. Med. 124:726–734, 1996.
72. Fetrow, C. W., and Avila, J. R.: Professional's Handbook of Complementary and Alternative Medicines. Springhouse, PA, Springhouse Corporation, 1999, p. 499.
73. Nieman, C.: Chem. Drug. 177:741–745, 1962.
74. Baker, M. E., and Fanestil, D. D.: Lancet 337:428–429, 1991.

APPENDIX

Calculated Log P, Log D, and pKₐ

The log P, log D at pH 7, and pK$_a$ values are from Chemical Abstracts Service, American Chemical Society, Columbus, OH, 2009, and were calculated using Advanced Chemistry Development (ACD/Labs) Software V8.14 for Solaris (©1994–2009 ACD/Labs). The pK$_a$ values are for the most acidic HA acid and most weakly acidic BH$^+$ groups. The latter represent the most basic nitrogen. Keep in mind that pK$_a$ values for HA acids that exceed 10 to 11 mean that there will be little, if any, anionic contribution in the pH ranges used in pharmaceutical formulations and in physiological pH ranges. Similarly, for BH$^+$ acids, there will be little, if any, cationic contribution for pK$_a$ values below 2 to 3. Because *Chemical Abstracts* does not report calculated physicochemical values for ionized compounds, including salts and quaternary ammonium compounds, the log P values in this appendix are for the un-ionized form.

Name of Compound	Log P	Log D at pH 7	pKₐ HA	pKₐ BH⁺
Abacavir	0.72	0.72		5.08
Abarelix	5.18	2.08	9.82	10.66
Acarbose	−3.03		12.39	5.90
Acebutolol	2.59	0.52	13.78	9.11
Acetaminophen	0.34	0.34	9.86	
Acetazolamide	−0.26	−0.40	7.44	
Acetic acid	−0.29	−2.49	4.79	
Acetohexamide	2.24	0.03		
Acetohydroxamic acid	−1.59	−1.59	9.26	
Acetylcysteine	−0.15	−3.74	3.25	
Acitretin	5.73	3.52	4.79	
Acyclovir	−1.76	−1.76	9.18	1.89
Adapalene	8.04	5.29	4.23	
Adefovir	2.06	−5.78	1.63	4.07
Adefovir dipivoxil	2.38	2.38		4.63
Adenine	−2.12	−2.12		2.95
Adenosine	−1.46	−1.46	13.11	3.25
Alanine	−0.68	−3.18	9.62	2.31
Alatrofloxacin	0.31	−2.22	0.64	8.12
Albendazole	3.01	2.99	10.46	5.62
Albuterol	0.02	−2.15	9.83	9.22
Alclometasone dipropionate	4.26	4.26	13.73	
Alendronic acid	−3.52	−7.80	0.47	10.56
Alfentanil	2.03			7.59
Alfuzosin	−1.00	−2.69		8.60
Aliskiren	2.74	0.13	12.54	9.78
Alitretinoin	6.83	4.62	4.79	
Allopurinol	−0.48	−0.50	9.20	2.40
Almotriptan	1.89	−0.51		9.48
Alosetron	0.96	0.65		6.71
Alprazolam	2.50	2.50		2.39
Alprostadil (prostaglandin E1)	2.25	0.02	4.77	
Altretamine	2.42	1.90		7.37
Alvimopan	3.38	0.87	3.64	
Amantadine	2.22	−0.79		10.75
Ambrisentan	6.24	2.55	0.93	2.98
Amcinonide	3.80	3.80	13.15	
Amifostine	−1.69	−4.72	1.29	10.16
Amikacin	−3.84		12.94	9.52

Name of Compound	Log P	Log D at pH 7	pKₐ HA	pKₐ BH⁺
Amiloride	1.90	1.88	8.58	1.58
p-Aminobenzoic acid	0.01	−2.12	4.90	2.48
Aminoglutethimide	1.41	1.41	11.60	4.41
Aminolevulinic acid	−0.93	−3.38	4.00	7.37
4-Aminosalicylic acid	0.32	−3.02	3.58	2.21
Amiodarone	8.59	6.29		9.37
Amitriptyline	6.14	3.96		9.24
Amlexanox	4.67	1.65	3.95	
Amlodipine	3.72	2.00		8.73
Amobarbital	2.10	2.05	7.94	
Amoxapine	2.59	1.52		8.03
Amoxicillin	0.61	−2.21	2.61	6.93
Amphetamine	1.81	−0.91		9.94
Amphotericin B	0.18		3.96	8.13
Ampicillin	1.35	−1.54	2.61	6.79
Amprenavir	4.20	4.20	11.54	1.76
Amyl nitrite	2.45	2.45		
Anagrelide	1.13	1.13	11.79	1.48
Anastrozole	0.77	0.77		4.78
Anidulafungin	−3.86	−3.86	9.86	
Anthralin	4.16	3.91	7.16	
Apomorphine	2.47	2.34	9.41	6.50
Apraclonidine	0.30	−1.91		9.11
Aprepitant	4.23	4.17	8.06	4.02
Arginine	−1.78	−5.26	2.51	13.64
Aripiprazole	5.68	5.55		6.50
Aripiprazole	5.60	5.41		6.71
Armodafinil	1.17	1.17		
Articaine	2.44	1.41	13.46	7.99
Ascorbic acid	−2.12	−4.96	4.13	
Asparagine	−1.51	−4.02	2.30	8.34
Aspartic acid	−0.67	−4.17	2.28	9.95
Aspirin	1.19	−2.23	3.48	
Astemizole	5.80	3.62		9.03
Atazanavir	5.51		11.11	4.81
Atenolol	0.10	−2.03	13.88	9.17
Atomoxetine	3.84	1.03		10.12
Atorvastatin	4.22	1.54	4.30	
Atovaquone	6.18	4.14	4.97	
Atropine	1.53	−1.21		9.98
Azacitidine	−1.99	−1.99		3.28
Azathioprine	−0.54	−0.54		0.25

Name of Compound	Log P	Log D at pH 7	pK$_a$ HA	pK$_a$ BH$^+$
Azelaic acid	1.33	−3.01	4.47	
Azelastine	3.71	1.60		9.16
Azithromycin	3.33	0.58	13.30	8.59
Aztreonam	−2.07	7.11		2.36
Baclofen	1.56	−0.94	4.00	10.32
Balsalazide	2.70	−2.29	2.97	
Beclomethasone dipropionate	4.59	4.59	13.08	
Benazepril	5.50	2.31	3.73	5.02
Bendamustine	2.69	0.36	4.50	6.36
Bendroflumethiazide	2.02	2.01	8.63	
Benzocaine	2.49	2.49		2.51
Benzoic acid	1.90	−0.88	4.20	
Benzonatate	0.32	0.32		2.20
Benzoyl peroxide	3.47	3.47		
Benzphetamine	4.43	2.57		8.88
Benzthiazide	2.68	2.67	9.15	
Benztropine	4.96	2.00		10.54
Bepridil	6.43	4.27	9.21	
Besifloxacin	2.57	0.05	6.02	10.22
Betamethasone	2.06	2.06	12.14	
Betamethasone acetate	2.61	2.61	12.05	
Betamethasone dipropionate	4.23	4.23	12.93	
Betamethasone valerate	3.98	3.97	12.67	
Betaxolol	2.69	0.56	13.89	9.17
Bexarotene	8.75	6.07	4.30	
Bicalutamide	4.54	4.54	11.49	
Bimatoprost	1.98	1.98		
Biperiden	4.52	1.89		9.80
Bisoprolol	2.22	0.11	13.86	9.16
Bitolterol	5.25	3.30	13.68	8.97
Bortezomib	2.45	2.44	9.66	
Bosentan	1.15	0.01	5.89	
Brimonidine	0.97	−1.34		9.63
Brinzolamide	0.25	−1.06	9.62	8.29
Bromocriptine	4.63	4.52	9.61	6.45
Brompheniramine	3.57	1.30		9.33
Buclizine	6.24	6.10		6.59
Budesonide	3.24	3.24	12.85	
Bumetanide	2.78	−0.27	3.18	4.48
Bupivacaine	3.64	2.45		8.17
Buprenorphine	3.61	2.40	9.67	8.18
Bupropion	3.47	3.08		7.16
Buspirone	3.43	3.33		6.43
Busulfan	−0.52	−0.52		
Butabarbital	1.56	1.52	7.95	
Butenafine	6.77	5.84		7.87
Butoconazole	6.88	6.69		6.72
Butorphanol	3.94	2.93	10.26	7.97
Cabergoline	2.39	−0.92	13.06	9.41
Caffeine	−0.08	−0.08		1.39
Calcifediol (25-OH-D3)	7.53	7.53		
Calcipotriene	5.43	5.43	13.98	
Calcitriol (1,25-di(OH)-D3)	6.12	6.12		13.98
Candesartan Cilexetil	7.43	4.81	4.22	4.24
Capecitabine	0.97	−0.38	5.67	
Capsaicin	3.31	3.31	9.91	
Captopril	0.27	−2.86	3.82	
Carbamazepine	2.67	2.67	13.94	
Carbenicillin	1.01	−3.99	2.62	
Carbidopa	−0.19	−2.71	3.40	7.91
Carbinoxamine	2.76	1.12	8.65	
Carboprost	2.49	0.27	4.77	
Carisoprodol	2.15	2.15	12.49	

Name of Compound	Log P	Log D at pH 7	pK$_a$ HA	pK$_a$ BH$^+$
Carmustine	1.30	1.30	10.19	
β-Carotene	15.51	15.51		
Carteolol	1.67	−0.42	13.84	9.13
Carvedilol	4.23	3.16	13.90	8.03
Cefaclor	0.19	−2.71	1.95	6.80
Cefadroxil	−0.09	−2.89	3.12	6.93
Cefamandole	1.52	−2.39	2.62	
Cefdinir	−0.73	−5.13	2.80	3.27
Cefditoren pivoxil	1.23	1.13	7.57	2.89
Cefixime	−0.51	−5.53	2.10	2.86
Cefonicid	0.54	−4.46		
Cefoperazone	1.43		2.62	
Cefotaxime	−0.31	−4.24	2.66	2.90
Cefoxitin	0.72	−3.19	2.63	
Cefpodoxime proxetil	0.66	0.57	7.61	2.90
Cefprozil	0.15	−2.67	2.92	6.93
Ceftibuten	−1.06	−5.08	3.00	5.44
Ceftizoxime	−0.92	−4.70	2.99	2.90
Ceftriaxone	−1.76	−5.86	2.57	2.90
Cefuroxime	−0.54	−4.47	2.59	
Celecoxib	3.01	3.01	9.68	
Cephalexin	0.65	−2.22	3.12	6.80
Cephapirin	0.79	−3.05	2.67	4.49
Cephradine	0.98	−1.79	3.12	6.99
Cetirizine	2.97	−0.02	3.27	6.43
Cevimeline	1.12	−1.29		9.51
Chloral hydrate	1.68	1.68	10.54	
Chlorambucil	3.70	1.52	4.86	3.66
Chloramphenicol	1.02	1.02	11.03	
Chlordiazepoxide	2.49	2.49		4.45
Chlorhexidine	4.54	−0.46		11.73
Chloroprocaine	3.38	1.28		9.13
Chloroquine	4.69	1.15		10.48
Chlorothiazide	−0.18	−0.18	9.17	
Chloroxine	3.75	1.51	2.07	7.20
Chlorphenesin carbamate	1.41	1.41	12.99	
Chlorpheniramine	3.39	1.13		9.33
Chlorpromazine	5.36	3.01		9.43
Chlorpropamide	2.21	0.28		
Chlorthalidone	−0.74	−0.74	9.57	
Chlorzoxazone	2.44	2.43	8.92	
Cholecalciferol	9.72	9.72		
Ciclesonide	6.13	6.13		
Ciclopirox	2.59	1.76	6.25	
Cidofovir	−3.38	−7.64	1.61	4.54
Cilastatin	2.42	−1.09	2.09	8.83
Cilostazol	3.04	3.04		
Cimetidine	0.20	−0.11		6.73
Cinacalcet	5.74	3.59		9.19
Cinoxacin	−0.53	−4.58		4.31
Ciprofloxacin	1.31	−1.20	2.74	8.76
Citalopram	2.89	0.41		9.59
Citric acid	−1.72	−7.67	2.93	
Cladribine	0.24	0.24	13.75	1.44
Clarithromycin	3.16	2.00	13.07	8.14
Clavulanic acid	1.98	−5.84	2.78	
Clemastine	5.69	2.83		10.23
Clevidipine	5.46	5.46		2.45
Clindamycin	2.14	0.41	12.87	8.74
Clioquinol	4.32	2.35	2.10	7.24
Clobetasol propionate	4.18	4.18	12.94	
Clocortolone pivalate	4.41	4.41	13.10	
Clodronic acid	−2.38	−7.90	−0.75	
Clofarabine	0.24	0.24		12.56
Clofazimine	7.50	7.43		6.24
Clomiphene	8.01	5.58		9.53
Clomipramine	5.19	2.80		9.49

(table continues on page 978)

Clopidogrel (Plavix) logP = 3.84

non-polar

Name of Compound	Log P	Log D at pH 7	pKa HA	pKa BH+
Clonazepam	3.02	3.02	11.19	1.55
Clonidine	1.41	−0.67		9.16
Clotrimazole	5.76	5.71		6.12
Clozapine	3.48	3.40		6.33
Cocaine	3.08	1.14		8.97
Codeine	2.04	0.83	13.42	8.29
Colchicine	1.03	1.03		
Conivaptan	4.40	4.26		7.32
Cortisone	1.24	1.24	12.29	
Cromolyn	0.20	−4.80	1.85	
Crotamiton	3.10	3.10		
Cyclizine	2.42	1.83		7.46
Cyclobenzaprine	6.22	4.06		9.21
Cyclophosphamide	0.63	0.63		4.09
Cyclopropane	1.69	1.69		
Cycloserine	−1.84	−1.87		5.93
Cyproheptadine	6.62	4.93		8.70
Cystamine	0.62	−2.53		8.97
Cysteamine	0.03	−1.45	7.93	10.47
Cysteine	0.24	−2.31	2.07	11.05
Cytarabine	−2.30	−2.30	13.48	4.47
Dacarbazine	−0.26	−0.26	12.32	4.09
Dalfopristin	−0.94	−2.87	13.32	8.95
Danazol	4.70	4.70	13.10	
Dantrolene	0.95	0.87	7.69	
Dapiprazole	2.44	2.28		6.39
Dapsone	0.94	0.94		1.24
Daptomycin	−4.07	−9.56	4.00	10.06
Darifenacin	4.50	2.30		9.32
Darunavir	3.94	3.94		1.75
Daunorubicin	2.39	0.47	7.15	8.64
Decitabine	−1.93	−1.93		3.49
Deferasirox	6.43	3.42	3.54	
Degarelix	4.45	1.45		10.66
Dehydrocholic acid	1.77	−0.48	4.74	
Delavirdine	−1.23	−3.23	10.10	8.87
Demeclocycline	−0.58	−4.34	4.50	9.68
Desflurane	−1.87	1.87		
Desipramine	3.97	1.05		10.40
Desloratadine	5.26	2.95		9.38
Desonide	2.72	2.72	12.85	
Desoximetasone	2.40	2.40	12.80	
Desvenlafaxine	2.26	0.00	10.04	9.33
Dexamethasone	2.06	2.06	12.14	
Dexamethasone acetate	2.61	2.61	12.05	
Dexlansoprazole	2.76	2.76	8.91	3.64
Dexmedetomidine	3.18	2.85		6.75
Dexrazoxane	−0.37	−0.37	10.74	2.62
Dextromethorphan	4.28	2.22		9.10
Diazepam	3.86	3.86		3.40
Diazoxide	1.07	1.07		
Dibucaine	4.40	1.95	12.90	9.56
Dichloroacetic acid	0.54	−3.54	1.37	
Dichlorphenamide	0.93	0.92	8.95	
Diclofenac	3.28	0.48	4.18	
Dicloxacillin	3.02	−0.90	2.60	
Dicyclomine	6.05	3.87		9.23
Didanosine	−0.92	−0.93	8.67	1.98
Diethylcarbamazine	1.14	1.00		6.57
Diethylpropion	2.95	1.46		8.48
Difenoxin	5.73	3.23	3.57	8.91
Diflorasone diacetate	2.91	2.91	12.69	
Diflunisal	4.32	0.54	2.94	
Difluprednate	3.67	3.67		
Digoxin	1.14	1.14	13.50	
Dihydroergotamine	3.02	1.17	9.64	8.87
Dihydrotachysterol	9.86	9.86		
Dihydroxyacetone	−0.78	−0.78	12.44	
Diltiazem	4.53	2.64		8.91
Dimercaprol	0.84	0.83	8.88	
Dinoprostone (prostaglandin E2)	1.88	−0.36	4.76	
Diphenhydramine	3.66	1.92		8.76
Diphenoxylate	6.57	5.85		7.63
Dipivefrin	1.49	−0.49	13.76	9.01
Dipyridamole	−1.22		13.54	6.37
Disopyramide	2.86	0.07		10.10
Disulfiram	3.88	3.88		0.86
Dobutamine	2.49	−0.31	9.65	10.37
Dofetilide	1.56	0.27	9.68	8.28
Dolasetron	2.40	2.10		7.00
Donepezil	4.70	2.89		8.82
DOPA (dihydroxyphenylalanine)	−0.23	−2.73	2.24	9.30
Dopamine	0.12	−2.36	9.41	9.99
Doripenem	−3.65	−6.15	4.37	9.39
Dorzolamide	−0.21	−2.02	9.48	8.82
Doxapram	3.23	2.67		7.41
Doxazosin	0.65	0.54		6.47
Doxepin	5.08	2.93		9.19
Doxercalciferol	8.15	8.14	13.82	
Doxorubicin	2.29	0.36	7.12	8.64
Doxycycline	−0.26	−3.83	4.50	9.32
Dronabinol	7.64	7.64	9.81	
Droperidol	4.10	2.85		8.23
Duloxetine	3.73	0.97		10.02
Dutasteride	6.85	6.85	13.34	
Dyclonine	4.67	2.83		8.86
Dyphylline	−1.12	−1.12	13.66	0.76
Econazole	5.81	5.64		6.69
Efavirenz	4.90	4.85	7.92	
Eflornithine	0.56	−2.14	1.22	10.45
Eletriptan	3.27	0.36		10.35
Eltrombopag	3.71	0.95	−1.65	
Emedastine	2.06	−0.98		8.91
Emtricitabine	−0.41	−0.41		1.93
Enalapril	2.98	−0.12	3.75	5.50
Enflurane	2.10	2.10		
Entacapone	2.63	1.66	6.07	
Entecavir	−0.96	−0.96	9.48	2.67
Ephedrine	1.05	−1.25	13.96	9.38
Epinastine	3.44	1.44		12.02
Epinephrine	−0.63	−2.75	9.60	9.16
Epirubicin	2.29	0.36	7.12	8.64
Eplerenone	1.05	1.05		
Epoprostenol	2.21	−0.07	4.71	
Eprosartan	4.96	1.46	3.31	8.73
Ergocalciferol	9.56	9.56		
Ergonovine	0.57	0.09		7.30
Ergotamine	3.06	2.65	9.62	7.20
Erlotinib	2.39	2.38		5.06
Ertapenem	−1.28	−4.81	4.03	7.94
Erythromycin	2.83	1.66	13.08	8.14
Escitalopram oxalate	2.89	0.41		9.59
Esmolol	1.91	−0.22	13.88	9.17
Esomeprazole	1.80	1.80	9.08	4.61
Estazolam	3.25	3.25		1.67
Estradiol	4.13	4.13	10.37	
Estradiol cypionate	7.59	7.59	10.35	
Estradiol valerate	6.62	6.62	10.35	
Estramustine	5.75	5.75		
Eszopiclone	0.74	0.53		6.79
Ethacrynic acid	3.38	−0.47	2.80	
Ethambutol	−0.05	−2.56		9.60
Ethanolamine oleate	7.59	6.82		7.68
Ethaverine	5.55	5.43		6.47
Ethinyl estradiol	4.52	4.52	10.34	
Ethionamide	7.22	7.22	12.14	4.34
Ethosuximide	1.14	1.14		9.70
Ethotoin	0.86	0.82	8.00	

Name of Compound	Log P	Log D at pH 7	pKa HA	pKa BH+
Ethylene	1.32	1.32		
Etidronic acid	-3.54	-9.21	0.68	
Etodolac	3.31	0.64	4.31	
Etomidate	3.36	3.36		4.23
Etonogestrel	4.23	4.22		13.02
Etoposide	1.97	1.96	9.95	
Etravirine	4.19	4.19		1.89
Exemestane	3.30	3.30		
Ezetimibe	4.39	4.29	9.66	
Famciclovir	-0.09	-0.09		4.24
Famotidine	2.18	-3.02	7.61	7.75
Febuxostat	4.87	1.73	3.37	
Felbamate	1.20	1.19	12.99	
Felodipine	4.92	4.92		3.96
Fenofibrate	4.80	4.80		
Fenoldopam	1.72	-0.56	8.51	9.53
Fenoprofen	3.84	1.06	4.20	
Fentanyl	3.93	1.90		9.06
Fesoterodine	5.08	2.09		10.60
Fexofenadine	5.18	2.68	4.43	9.56
Finasteride	3.24	3.24		
Flavoxate	5.46	4.18		8.27
Flecainide	3.47	0.55	13.63	10.39
Floxuridine	-1.20	-1.21	8.66	
Fluconazole	0.31	0.30	11.93	5.23
Flucytosine	-2.36	-2.38	8.36	3.68
Fludarabine	-2.32	-2.32	13.05	1.73
Fludrocortisone acetate	1.78	1.78	12.04	
Flumazenil	0.87	0.87		1.42
Flunisolide	2.26	2.26	12.84	
Fluocinolone	0.77	0.77	11.43	
Fluocinolone acetonide	2.34	2.34	12.55	
Fluorescein	3.61	3.60	8.56	
Fluorexon	2.19	-3.86	1.79	9.24
Fluorometholone	2.22	2.21	12.42	
Fluorouracil	-0.78	-2.29	7.88	
Fluoxetine	4.35	1.57		10.05
Fluoxymesterone	2.17	2.17	13.43	
Fluphenazine	4.84	4.29		7.21
Flurandrenolide	1.95	1.95	12.84	
Flurazepam	4.71	2.12		9.76
Flurbiprofen	4.11	1.28	4.14	
Flutamide	4.06	4.06	13.12	
Fluticasone propionate	3.92	3.92	12.59	
Fluvastatin	3.72	1.01	4.28	
Fluvoxamine	3.17	0.86		9.39
Folic acid	-2.63	-7.52	3.55	2.11
Fomepizole	0.78	0.78		3.21
Formaldehyde	0.35	0.35		
Formoterol	1.57	-0.17	8.65	9.09
Foscarnet	-2.53	-7.64	0.66	
Fosfomycin	-2.98	-7.25	1.70	
Fosinopril	5.81	2.65	3.78	
Fosphenytoin	0.47	-4.61	1.72	
Fospropofol	2.70	-1.59	1.67	
Frovatriptan	0.84	-2.06		10.34
Fulvestrant	7.92	7.92	10.27	
Fumaric acid	-0.01	-4.95	3.15	
Furazolidone	-0.04	-0.04		3.12
Furosemide	2.92	-0.80	3.04	
Gabapentin	1.19	-1.31	4.72	10.27
Galantamine	2.12	1.13	13.98	7.94
Ganciclovir	-2.07	-2.07	9.15	3.05
Gatifloxacin	1.59	-0.92		8.82
Gefitinib	4.11	3.61		7.34
Gemcitabine	-0.68	-0.68	11.65	4.47
Gemfibrozil	4.39	2.14	4.75	

Name of Compound	Log P	Log D at pH 7	pKa HA	pKa BH+
Gemifloxacin	1.04	-1.40	6.02	9.15
Glimepiride	2.94	1.27	5.34	
Glipizide	2.19	0.52	5.34	
Glutamic acid	-1.44	-4.92	2.17	9.76
Glutamine	-1.60	-4.10	2.27	9.52
Glutaraldehyde	-0.34	-0.33		
Glutethimide	2.70	2.70	11.36	
Glyburide	3.93	2.28		
Glycerin	-2.32	-2.32	13.52	
Glycine	-1.03	-3.53	2.43	9.64
Granisetron	1.95	-1.00	12.39	10.50
Griseofulvin	2.36	2.36		
Guaifenesin	0.57	0.57	13.38	
Guanadrel	-0.08	-3.18		12.76
Guanethidine	1.07	-3.58		13.43
Guanfacine	1.12	1.12	11.81	3.75
Guanidine	2.57	0.15		9.66
Halcinonide	3.32	3.32	13.25	
Halobetasol propionate	3.92	3.92	12.61	
Halofantrine	8.86	6.50	13.56	9.43
Haloperidol	4.06	2.80	13.90	8.25
Halothane	2.30	2.30		
Heroin	1.52	0.52		7.95
Hexachlorophene	7.20	7.20	6.58	
Histamine	-0.84	-3.68		10.15
Homatropine	1.57	-1.17	12.10	9.98
Hydrochlorothiazide	-0.07	-0.08	8.95	
Hydrocortisone	1.43	1.43	12.48	
Hydrocortisone acetate	1.98	1.98	12.42	
Hydrocortisone buteprate	4.12	4.12		
Hydrocortisone butyrate	2.81	2.80	12.95	
Hydrocortisone cypionate	4.53	4.53	12.33	
Hydrocortisone valerate	3.34	3.34	12.95	
Hydroflumethiazide	0.54	0.54	8.63	
Hydromorphone	-1.23	-0.21	9.61	8.36
Hydroquinone	0.64	0.64	10.33	
Hydroxyamphetamine	1.07	-1.84	9.82	10.71
Hydroxychloroquine	3.54	1.08		8.87
Hydroxyprogesterone caproate	5.74	5.74		
Hydroxyurea	-1.80	-1.80	10.56	
Hydroxyzine	2.31	2.21		6.34
Hyoscyamine sulfate	1.53	-1.21		9.98
Ibandronate	-0.65	-4.89		9.50
Ibandronic acid	-0.65	-4.89	0.43	9.50
Ibuprofen	3.72	1.15	4.41	
Ibutilide fumarate	4.17	1.47	9.57	9.47
Idarubicin	2.16	0.43	7.79	8.64
Ifosfamide	0.63	0.63		4.03
Iloperidone	3.81	2.41		8.39
Iloprost	2.94	0.72	4.77	
Imatinib	1.86	1.18	13.28	7.53
Imipenem	-2.78	-5.28	4.47	10.37
Imipramine	4.46	2.07		9.49
Imiquimod	2.61	0.57		9.04
Indapamide	2.10	2.09	9.35	
Indinavir	2.29	2.26		5.73
Indomethacin	3.11	0.30	4.17	
Inositol	-2.11	-2.11	12.63	
Iodoquinol	4.34	2.14	2.21	7.37
Irinotecan	3.81	1.54	11.00	9.33
Isocarboxazid	1.03	1.03	11.26	1.23
Isoetharine	1.13	-1.03	9.26	9.55
Isoflurane	2.79	2.79		

(table continues on page 980)

Name of Compound	Log P	Log D at pH 7	pKa HA	pKa BH+
Isoniazid	−0.89	−0.89	11.27	3.79
Isoproterenol	0.25	−1.87	9.60	9.16
Isosorbide	−1.75	−1.75		
Isosorbide dinitrate	0.90	0.90		
Isosorbide mononitrate	−0.51	−0.51	13.09	
Isotretinoin	6.83	4.62	4.79	
Isoxsuprine	2.58	1.33	9.47	8.24
Isradipine	3.68	3.67		3.81
Itraconazole	3.29	3.15		6.39
Ixabepilone	1.77	1.77	3.24	
Kanamycin	−2.60		12.94	9.52
Ketamine	2.15	2.01		6.59
Ketoconazole	2.88	2.73		6.54
Ketoprofen	2.81	0.07	4.23	
Ketorolac	2.08	−0.44	4.47	
Ketotifen	4.99	3.25		8.75
Labetalol	2.87	0.99	7.91	9.20
Lacosamide	0.90	0.90		
Lactulose	−2.41	−2.41	11.67	
Lamivudine	−1.02	−1.02	13.83	4.41
Lamotrigine	−0.19	−0.19		3.31
Lanoxin	1.14	1.14	13.50	
Lansoprazole	2.39	2.38	8.48	3.53
Lapatinib	5.14	4.99		6.61
Latanoprost	3.65	3.65		
Leflunomide	1.95	1.95	11.74	
Lenalidomide	−1.09	−1.08	10.75	
Letrozole	1.52	1.52		3.63
Leucovorin	−8.12	−7.91	3.55	5.01
Levalbuterol	0.02	−2.15	9.83	9.22
Levamisole	0.54	−1.26		8.81
Levarterenol	−0.88	−2.19	9.57	8.30
Levetiracetam	−0.67	−0.67		
Levobetaxolol	2.69	0.56	13.89	9.17
Levobunolol	2.86	0.77	13.84	9.13
Levobupivacaine	3.64	2.45		8.17
Levocabastine	4.86	2.36	3.56	9.38
Levocetirizine	2.17	−0.83	3.46	6.22
Levodopa	−0.23	−2.73	2.24	9.30
Levofloxacin	1.49	−1.35	2.27	6.81
Levomethadyl acetate	5.45	3.13		9.40
Levonorgestrel	3.92	3.92	13.10	
Levorphanol	3.63	1.61	10.41	9.01
Levothyroxine (T4; L-thyroxine)	5.96	3.16	2.12	8.94
Lidocaine	2.36	0.83		8.53
Lincomycin	0.86	−0.91	12.91	8.78
Lindane	3.94	3.94		
Linezolid	−0.92	−0.92		3.94
Liothyronine (T3; triiodothyronine)	5.12	2.59	2.13	8.96
Lisdexamfetamine	0.72	−2.88		10.48
Lisinopril	1.75	−1.32	2.18	10.51
Lodoxamide	0.54	−4.46	2.07	
Lomefloxacin	2.33	−0.17	2.40	8.82
Lomustine	2.76	2.76	10.88	
Loperamide	4.95	3.87	13.89	8.05
Lopinavir	5.65	5.64	13.89	
Loracarbef	−0.95	−3.79	3.24	6.84
Loratadine	6.23	6.23		3.80
Lorazepam	2.48	2.48	10.78	0.03
Losartan	3.50	0.89	4.24	3.10
Loteprednol	3.69	3.69		
Lovastatin	4.07	4.07	13.49	
Loxapine	2.99	2.91		6.28
Lubiprostone	2.85	0.63	4.77	
Lysine	−1.04	−4.52	2.48	10.64
Mafenide	−0.80	−2.38	10.16	8.58
Malathion	2.93	2.93		

Name of Compound	Log P	Log D at pH 7	pKa HA	pKa BH+
Mannitol	−4.67	−4.67	13.14	
Maprotiline	4.51	1.52		10.63
Maraviroc	3.60	0.74		10.24
Mebendazole	2.43	2.42	10.29	5.02
Mecamylamine	3.06	−0.02		11.35
Mechlorethamine	1.66	1.33		7.06
Meclizine	5.02	4.83		6.73
Meclofenamate	5.90	2.57	3.59	
Medroxyprogesterone acetate	4.11	4.11		
Medrysone	2.87	2.87		
Mefenamic acid	5.33	2.09	3.69	
Mefloquine	2.87	0.05	13.13	10.13
Megestrol acetate	3.82	3.82		
Meloxicam	2.71	0.22	4.50	3.05
Melphalan	2.40	−0.11	2.12	9.54
Memantine	3.18	0.16		10.79
Meperidine	2.81	1.23		8.55
Mephentermine	2.29	−0.62		10.38
Mephobarbital	1.85	1.81	7.97	
Mepivacaine	2.04	0.93		8.09
Meprobamate	0.70	0.70	13.09	
Mercaptopurine	0.39	0.37	8.46	2.40
Meropenem	−3.13	−5.63	4.47	8.00
Mesalamine	0.46	−2.19	1.90	5.43
Mesoridazine	3.98	1.45		9.66
Metaproterenol	0.13	−2.02	9.12	9.33
Metaraminol	0.07	−1.40	9.75	8.47
Metaxalone	2.42	2.42	12.24	
Metformin	−2.31	−5.41		13.10
Methadone	4.20	2.18		9.05
Methamphetamine	1.94	−0.97		10.38
Methazolamide	0.13	0.13	0.33	
Methenamine	2.17	2.16		5.28
Methimazole	−0.02	−0.02	11.64	1.10
Methionine	0.37	−2.13	2.23	9.26
Methocarbamol	0.55	0.54	13.00	
Methohexital	2.41	2.36	7.92	
Methotrexate	−0.28		3.54	5.09
Methoxsalen	1.31	1.31		
Methoxyflurane	1.66	1.66		
Methsuximide	2.22	2.22		
Methyclothiazide	1.76	1.76	9.36	
Methyldopa	0.13	−2.38	2.28	9.30
Methylergonovine	1.10	0.62		7.30
Methylphenidate	2.55	−0.42		10.55
Methylprednisolone	2.18	2.18	12.48	
Methylprednisolone acetate	2.73	2.73	12.42	
Methyltestosterone	4.02	4.02		
Metipranolol	2.67	0.53	13.91	9.19
Metoclopramide	2.35	−0.15	13.28	9.62
Metolazone	3.16	3.16	10.00	
Metoprolol	1.79	−0.34	13.89	9.17
Metronidazole	−0.02	−0.02		2.58
Metyrosine	0.73	−1.77	2.29	9.35
Mexiletine	2.16	0.58		8.58
Micafungin	−7.49	11.00		
Miconazole	6.42	6.25		6.67
Midazolam	3.67	3.68		5.65
Midodrine	−0.32	−1.14	13.53	7.75
Mifepristone	4.91	4.90	12.94	5.19
Miglitol	−1.40	−1.42	13.71	5.78
Miglustat	0.46	0.22		6.73
Milnacipran	1.23	−1.68		10.36
Milrinone	0.41	0.40	8.83	3.36
Minocycline	−0.27	−3.81	4.50	9.74
Minoxidil	0.69	0.69		4.35
Mirtazapine	2.52	1.38		8.10
Misoprostol	2.91	2.91	13.92	
Mitomycin	0.44	0.44	13.27	4.89

Name of Compound	Log P	Log D at pH 7	pK$_a$ HA	pK$_a$ BH$^+$
Mitotane	5.39	5.39		
Mitoxantrone	2.62	−0.90	7.08	9.22
Modafinil	1.40	1.40		
Moexipril	4.47	1.22	3.57	5.38
Molindone	1.96	1.73		6.83
Mometasone furoate	4.73	4.72	13.08	
Monobenzone	2.96	2.96	10.28	
Monochloroacetic acid	−0.05	−3.95	2.65	
Monoctanoin	2.12	2.12	13.12	
Montelukast	7.85		4.76	
Moricizine	2.67	2.47	10.27	6.77
Morphine	1.27	0.11	9.72	8.14
Moxifloxacin	1.97	−0.53	2.17	10.77
Mupirocin	3.44	1.22	4.78	
Mycophenolate mofetil	4.10	4.00	9.98	6.39
Nabumetone	2.82	2.82		
Nadolol	1.29	−0.84	13.91	9.17
Nafcillin	3.52	−0.40	2.61	
Naftifine	5.67	4.64		7.98
Nalbuphine	1.96	1.53	9.62	7.22
Nalidixic acid	0.18	−3.27	1.20	5.95
Nalmefene	2.82	2.16	9.61	7.56
Naloxone	1.92	1.77	9.38	6.61
Naltrexone	1.97	1.42	9.39	7.40
Nandrolone decanoate	8.14	8.14		
Naphazoline	3.53	0.65		10.27
Naproxen	3.00	0.41	4.40	
Naratriptan	1.81	−0.71	11.52	9.66
Natamycin	0.93	−1.59	3.72	8.13
Nateglinide	4.57	1.26	3.61	
Nebivolol	3.67	2.03		8.65
Nedocromil	2.63	−2.37	2.00	
Nefazodone	3.50	3.19		6.75
Nelarabine	−0.58	−0.58	13.07	4.42
Nelfinavir	6.55	5.91	9.58	7.53
Nepafenac	1.17	1.17		
Neridronic acid	−3.36	−7.48	0.63	10.65
Nevirapine	−0.31	−0.31	10.93	4.74
Niacin	0.82	−2.58	2.17	4.82
Niacinamide	−0.11	−0.11		3.54
Nicardipine	5.22	4.86		7.11
Nicotine	0.72	−0.32		8.00
Nifedipine	3.05	3.05		3.93
Nilotinib	5.15	5.13		5.68
Nilutamide	3.15	3.08	7.73	
Nimodipine	3.94	3.94		4.01
Nisoldipine	4.46	4.46		3.91
Nitazoxanide	0.83	0.83	10.16	
Nitisinone	1.37	−2.30		
Nitrofurantoin	−0.55	−0.63	7.69	1.20
Nitrofurazone	0.09	0.09	11.15	3.87
Nitroglycerin	2.22	2.22		
Nitrous oxide	−1.28	−1.28		
Nizatidine	1.23	0.75		7.31
Norelgestromin	4.40	4.40	12.47	
Norethindrone acetate	3.99	3.99	2.75	8.76
Norfloxacin	1.47	−1.03		
Nortriptyline	5.65	2.86		10.08
Ofloxacin	1.49	−1.35	2.27	6.81
Olanzapine	3.30	3.20		6.37
Olmesartan medoxomil	4.87	2.26	4.23	4.24
Olopatadine	4.37	1.86	4.29	9.19
Olpadronic acid	−2.77	−7.21	−0.09	
Olsalazine	3.94	−1.06	2.70	
Omeprazole	1.80	1.80	9.08	4.61

Name of Compound	Log P	Log D at pH 7	pK$_a$ HA	pK$_a$ BH$^+$
Ondansetron	2.49	1.84		7.54
Orlistat	8.95	8.94		
Orphenadrine	4.12	2.41		8.72
Oseltamivir	1.50	−0.30		8.81
Oxacillin	2.05	−1.87	2.61	
Oxandrolone	3.33	3.33		
Oxaprozin	4.19	1.40	4.19	0.36
Oxazepam	2.31	2.31	10.94	1.68
Oxcarbazepine	1.25	1.25	13.73	
Oxiconazole	5.89	5.82		6.19
Oxybutynin	5.19	3.93	11.94	8.24
Oxycodone	1.84	1.19	13.45	7.53
Oxymetazoline	4.17	1.20	11.96	10.53
Oxymetholone	4.22	1.72	4.50	
Oxymorphone	1.07	0.46	9.40	7.48
Oxytetracycline	−1.22	−4.83	4.50	9.26
Paliperidone	1.52	0.60	13.00	7.86
Palonosetron	2.61	0.45		9.77
Pamidronic acid	−3.40	−7.80	0.18	8.93
Pantoprazole sodium	1.32	1.16	7.36	3.45
Papaverine	3.42	3.33		6.38
Paraldehyde	0.31	0.31		
Paricalcitol	5.83	5.83		
Paromomycin	−3.31		12.93	9.52
Paroxetine	3.89	1.00		10.32
Pemetrexed	−0.70	−5.28	3.46	
Pemirolast	−0.02	−3.12	2.91	
Pemoline	0.52	0.52		1.80
Penbutolol	4.17	2.05	13.90	9.17
Penciclovir	−2.03	−2.03	9.50	3.55
Penicillamine	0.93	−1.60	2.13	11.54
Penicillin G	1.67	−2.25	2.62	
Penicillin V	1.88	−2.04	2.62	
Pentamidine	2.47	−0.65		11.67
Pentazocine	5.00	3.08	10.36	8.90
Pentobarbital	2.10	2.04	7.88	
Pentostatin	−2.82	−3.15	12.88	7.62
Pentoxifylline	0.37	0.37		1.36
Pergolide	3.97	1.44		9.66
Perindopril	3.36	0.27	3.72	5.74
Permethrin	6.74	6.74		
Perphenazine	4.49	3.94		7.22
Phenazopyridine	2.55	2.55		4.16
Phendimetrazine	1.62	1.31		7.02
Phenelzine	1.14	−0.22		8.34
Phenindamine	4.41	3.21		8.07
Phenobarbital	1.71	1.62	7.63	
Phenoxybenzamine	5.18	5.04		6.58
Phentermine	2.16	−0.56		9.94
Phentolamine	3.60	0.70	9.65	10.31
Phenylacetic acid	1.51	−1.18	4.30	
Phenylephrine	−0.30	−2.20	9.76	9.22
Phenytoin	2.52	2.52	8.33	
Physostigmine	1.16	−0.29	12.23	8.44
Phytonadione	12.25	12.25		
Pilocarpine	−0.10	−0.54		7.25
Pimecrolimus	5.21	5.21	9.96	
Pimozide	6.08	3.74	12.11	9.42
Pindolol	1.97	−0.19	13.94	9.21
Pioglitazone	3.16	2.40	6.35	5.56
Piperacillin	1.88	−2.04	2.62	
Pirbuterol	−1.63	−3.17	7.81	8.82
Piroxicam	1.71	−0.78	4.50	3.60
Plerixafor	0.20	−5.89		10.60
Plicamycin	1.39		4.54	
Podofilox	1.29	1.29	13.42	
Polythiazide	1.55	1.54	9.37	
Posaconazole	2.25	2.04		6.50
Pramipexole	1.62	−0.77		9.46

(table continues on page 982)

Name of Compound	Log P	Log D at pH 7	pKa HA	pKa BH+	Name of Compound	Log P	Log D at pH 7	pKa HA	pKa BH+
Pramoxine	3.51	2.95		7.42	Rofecoxib	1.63	1.63		
Pravastatin	1.44	−1.24	4.31		Ropinirole	3.19	0.81		9.47
Praziquantel	2.44	2.44			Ropivacaine	3.11	1.92		8.17
Prazosin	−1.14	−1.25		6.47	Rosiglitazone	2.56	1.71	6.34	6.48
Prednicarbate	3.82	3.82			Rosuvastatin	0.42	−2.29		4.25
Prednisolone	1.69	1.69	12.47		Rotigotine	4.96	3.15	10.50	8.82
Prednisolone acetate	2.24	2.24	12.41		Rufinamide	0.05	0.05		
					Salicylic acid	2.06	−1.68	3.01	
Prednisolone tebutate	4.00	4.00	12.32		Salmeterol	3.16	0.97	9.82	9.23
					Sapropterin	−4.22	−6.01		9.20
Pregabalin	1.12	−1.38	4.23	11.31	Scopolamine	1.34	0.29		8.01
Prilocaine	1.74	0.75		7.95	Secobarbital	2.33	2.27	7.81	
Primaquine	2.67	−0.25		10.38	Selegiline	2.92	2.28		7.53
Primidone	−0.84	−0.84	12.26		Sertaconazole	7.49	7.31		6.69
Probenecid	3.30	0.06	3.69		Sertraline	4.77	2.39		9.47
Procainamide	1.23	−1.43		9.86	Sevoflurane	2.48	2.48		
Procaine	2.91	0.72		9.24	Sibutramine	5.43	2.88		9.68
Procarbazine	0.77	0.11		7.46	Sildenafil	2.28	1.47	9.35	7.74
Prochlorperazine	4.76	3.69		7.82	Silodosin	2.33	0.48		8.86
Procyclidine	4.50	1.55		10.48	Simvastatin	4.41	4.41	13.49	
Progesterone	4.04	4.04			Sirolimus	3.58	3.58	10.40	
Proguanil	2.46	−0.59		11.30	Sitagliptin	1.30	0.88		7.21
Promethazine	4.69	2.73		8.98	Solifenacin	3.70	1.70		9.03
Propafenone	4.63	2.39	13.82	9.31	Sorafenib	5.16	5.16		
Proparacaine HCl	3.55	1.40		9.20	Sorbitol	−4.67	−4.67	13.14	
Propofol	4.16	4.16	11.00		Sotalol	0.32	−1.82	9.55	9.19
Propoxyphene	5.44	3.29		9.19	Sparfloxacin	2.87	0.36	2.27	8.88
Propranolol	3.10	0.99	13.84	9.14	Spectinomycin	1.17	−1.00	9.25	8.56
Propylthiouracil	1.37	1.24	7.63	0.54	Spironolactone	3.12	3.12		
Protriptyline	5.06	2.08		10.61	Stanozolol	5.53	5.53		4.08
Pseudoephedrine	1.05	−1.25	13.96	9.38	Stavudine	−0.91	−0.91	9.57	
Pyrantel	1.37	−1.67		10.97	Streptozocin	−1.55	−1.55	9.36	
Pyrazinamide	−0.37	−0.37		13.91	Succinic acid	−0.59	−4.75	4.24	
Pyridoxine	−1.90	−2.12	8.37	5.06	Sufentanil	3.42	2.16		8.24
Pyrimethamine	2.87	2.67		6.77	Sulconazole	6.03	5.90		6.56
Pyrithione	−0.05	−2.35	4.70		Sulfacetamide	−0.90	−2.14	5.78	0.93
Quazepam	3.87	3.87		0.85	Sulfadiazine	−0.12	−0.74	6.50	1.57
Quetiapine	1.83	1.82		5.34	Sulfadoxine	0.34	−0.56	6.16	3.15
Quinapril	4.73	1.30	3.29	5.38	Sulfasalazine	3.18	−0.63	2.88	1.86
Quinidine	−1.55	1.35	13.05	9.13	Sulfinpyrazone	2.32	−1.01	3.60	
Quinine	3.44	1.35	13.05	9.13	Sulfisoxazole	1.01	−1.12	4.83	1.52
Rabeprazole	1.46	1.44	8.50	4.42	Sulindac	3.56	0.80	4.22	
Raloxifene	6.80	5.12	8.98	8.67	Sumatriptan	0.67	−1.73	11.31	9.49
Raltegravir	−0.68	−3.14	4.50		Sunitinib	3.16	0.54	11.70	9.78
Ramelteon	2.57	2.57			Suprofen	2.42	−0.49	4.07	
Ramipril	3.97	0.85	3.72	5.51	Tacrine	3.32	0.69		9.64
Ranitidine	1.28	−0.13		8.40	Tacrolimus	3.96	3.96	9.96	
Ranolazine	3.47	3.42		6.03	Tadalafil	1.43	1.43		
Rasagiline	2.27	1.66		7.49	Tamoxifen	7.88	6.20		8.69
Regadenoson	−3.09	−3.09			Tamsulosin	2.24	0.51	10.08	8.74
Remifentanil	2.00	1.87		6.55	Tapentadol	3.22	0.85	10.08	9.32
Repaglinide	4.86	2.10	4.19	5.78	Tazarotene	6.22	6.21		0.04
Reserpine	4.37	3.93		7.25	Tazobactam	−1.68	−5.68	2.33	0.88
Retapamulin	5.45	2.47		10.61	Tegaserod	2.19	−0.17		11.21
Retinol	6.84	6.84			Telbivudine	−1.11	−1.11	9.23	
Ribavirin	−2.63	−2.63	12.95	1.00	Telithromycin	4.52	3.36	10.85	8.13
Riboflavin	−2.02	−4.68	4.32		Telmisartan	7.80	4.79	3.83	5.83
Rifabutin	−3.07				Temazepam	3.10	3.10	11.84	1.58
Rifampin	0.49	−1.75	4.92	6.57	Temozolomide	−1.32			
Rifapentine	1.98				Temsirolimus	3.00	3.00	10.40	
Rifaximin	3.22	0.40	8.06	4.42	Teniposide	3.10	3.10		
Riluzole	2.84	2.75		6.38	Tenofovir disoproxil	1.97	1.97		4.67
Rimantadine	3.10	0.03		11.17	Terazosin	−0.96	−1.08		6.47
Rimexolone	4.21	4.21			Terbinafine	6.49	6.15		7.07
Risedronic acid	−2.94	−8.56	0.32	5.09	Terbutaline	0.48	−1.67	9.12	9.33
Risperidone	2.85	1.88		7.91	Terconazole	3.98	3.36		7.46
Ritodrine	1.61	−0.48	9.13		Testolactone	2.72	2.72		
Ritonavir	5.08	5.08	11.47	3.48	Testosterone	3.47	3.47		
Rivastigmine	2.14	0.52		8.62	Testosterone cypionate	6.93	6.93		
Rizatriptan	0.76	−1.64		9.49					

Foye's P789

Name of Compound	Log P	Log D at pH 7	pK$_a$ HA	pK$_a$ BH$^+$	Name of Compound	Log P	Log D at pH 7	pK$_a$ HA	pK$_a$ BH$^+$
Testosterone enanthate	7.03	7.03			Triamcinolone hexacetonide	5.08	5.08	13.15	
Tetrabenazine	3.48	3.37		6.45	Triamterene	1.30	1.22		6.30
Tetracaine	3.49	2.23		8.24	Triazolam	2.67	2.67		2.32
Tetrahydrozoline	3.31	0.38		10.42	Trichlormethiazide	0.57	0.32	7.12	
Theophylline	0.05	0.04	8.60	1.05	Trichloroacetic acid	1.67	−2.42	1.10	
Thiabendazole	2.87	2.86	9.38	3.58	Triclosan	5.82	5.75	7.80	
Thiethylperazine	5.05	3.98		7.82	Trifluoperazine	5.11	4.04		7.82
Thioguanine	−0.26	−0.40	7.44	3.09	Trifluridine	0.01	−0.69	6.40	
Thiopental	3.00	2.93	7.76		Trihexyphenidyl	5.06	2.42		9.83
Thioridazine	6.13	3.60		9.66	Trimethadione	0.31	0.31		
Thiotepa	0.52				Trimethobenzamide	2.91	1.25		
Thiothixene	3.89	2.96		7.74	Trimethoprim	0.79	0.28		7.34
Threonine	−1.23	−3.73	2.19	9.64	Trimetrexate	1.23	−2.03		10.35
Tiagabine	5.65	3.15	3.88	9.44	Trimipramine	4.81	2.51		9.37
Tiaprofenic acid	2.42	−0.47	4.05		Trioxsalen	3.80	3.80		
Ticarcillin	0.69	−4.31	2.62		Triprolidine	4.44	2.36		9.12
Ticlopidine	3.53	3.21		7.05	Troleandomycin	3.36	2.46		7.84
Tigecycline	−0.85	−3.59	4.50	11.05	Tropicamide	1.16	1.14		5.49
Tiludronic acid	−0.51	−6.30	0.45		Trovafloxacin	1.57	−0.95	0.64	8.43
Timolol	−4.30	−1.99	13.38	8.86	Undecylenic acid	3.99	1.77	4.78	
Tinidazole	−0.27	−0.27		2.30	Unoprostone isopropyl ester	4.63	4.63		
Tioconazole	5.79	5.61		6.71	Urea	−2.11	−2.11		0.10
Tiopronin	−0.33	−3.64	3.62		Ursodiol	4.66	2.42	4.76	
Tipranavir	7.21	3.73	4.50		Valacyclovir	0.40	−0.78	9.17	7.75
Tirofiban	4.14	1.64	3.37	11.23	Valdecoxib	1.44	1.44	9.83	
Tizanidine	0.65	−1.47		9.18	Valganciclovir	−0.36	−1.16	9.13	7.73
Tobramycin	−3.44	10.01	13.07	9.52	Valproic acid	2.72	0.54	4.82	
Tocainide	0.76	−0.37		8.10	Valrubicin	5.25	4.89	7.11	
α-Tocopherol	11.86	11.86	11.40		Valsartan	4.38	−0.57	3.69	
Tolazamide	1.71	0.47			Vardenafil	3.03	2.97	9.11	6.11
Tolbutamide	2.34	0.80			Varenicline	0.74	−1.74		9.60
Tolcapone	4.15	1.98	4.78		Venlafaxine HCl	2.91	0.70		9.26
Tolmetin	1.55	−0.98	4.46		Verapamil	4.91	2.91		9.03
Tolnaftate	5.48	5.48			Vidarabine	−1.46	−1.46	13.11	3.25
Tolterodine	5.77	2.80	10.00	10.78	Vinblastine	4.22	3.45	11.36	7.64
Tolvaptan	4.33	4.33			Vincristine	2.84	2.10	11.07	7.64
Topotecan	0.79	0.55	7.20	2.28	Vinorelbine	5.42	5.03	11.34	7.09
Toremifene	7.96	6.32		8.63	Voriconazole	0.72	0.72	12.00	4.98
Torsemide	3.17	0.53	3.08	4.80	Vorinostat	0.86	0.86	9.48	
Tramadol	2.51	0.40		9.16	Warfarin	3.47	0.98	4.50	
Trandolapril	4.53	1.41	3.72	5.51	Xylometazoline	4.91	1.92		10.62
Tranexamic acid	0.32	−2.19	4.77	10.39	Yohimbine	1.91	0.47		8.44
Tranylcypromine	1.21	−0.56		8.78	Zafirlukast	6.15	2.65	3.37	
Travoprost	4.06	4.06	13.50		Zalcitabine	−1.51	−1.51		4.47
Trazodone	1.66	1.52		6.59	Zaleplon	1.00	1.00		
Treprostinil	4.09	0.47	3.19		Zanamivir	−3.75	−6.25	3.92	11.65
Tretinoin	6.83	4.62	4.79		Zileuton	3.74	3.74	9.99	
Triacetin	−0.24	−0.24			Ziprasidone	4.02	2.75	13.34	8.24
Triamcinolone	1.03	1.03	11.58		Zoledronic acid	−2.28	−7.04	0.32	6.78
Triamcinolone acetonide	2.60	2.60	12.69		Zolmitriptan	1.64	−0.78	12.57	9.52
Triamcinolone diacetate	1.82	1.82	11.21		Zolpidem	2.61	2.35		6.91
					Zonisamide	−0.10	−0.10	9.56	

Handwritten annotations:

Log D ICV −1.76

Log D$_{7.4}$ — implication for Drug Development — intestinal and CNS permeability

< 0

0 – 1 — may show a good balance between permeability and solubility at lower values, CNS permeability may suffer

1 – 3 — Good CNS penetration; low metabolic liabilities

3 – 5 — solubility tends to decrease; metabolic liabilities tends to increase

>5 — low solubility; poor bioavailability, erratic absorption; high metabolic liabilities

IOS press. Editors: B. Testa & L. Turski — Virtual ADMET Assessment in Target Selection and Maturation P54, (LogP of 18 β-blockers)

INDEX

Note: Page numbers followed by "*f*" indicate figures; those followed by "*t*" indicate tables. Drugs are listed under the generic name.

$\uparrow$ Log P $\longrightarrow$ {
- $\uparrow$ protein binding
- $\uparrow$ storage in tissue
- more rapid metabolism & elimination

The ideal log P of neutral compd for passive penetration in to the brain is ≈ 2.

Polar surface area (<u>PSA</u>) = the surface area occupied by oxygen and nitrogen AND hydrogen atoms bound to these heteroatoms

① drugs that completely (> 90%) absorbed should have PSAd < 60 $\overset{\circ}{A}^2$.

PSAd $\overset{\circ}{A}^2$	oral absorbed (%)
< 60	> 90
> 140 $\overset{\circ}{A}^2$	< 10%
60-70 (CNS)	

(> 120 $\overset{\circ}{A}^2$ bad)